Pediatric Clinical Practice Guidelines & Policies

• •

A Compendium of Evidence-based Research for Pediatric Practice

17th Edition

American Academy of Pediatrics
141 Northwest Point Blvd
Elk Grove Village, IL 60007-1019
www.aap.org

AMERICAN ACADEMY OF PEDIATRICS
PUBLISHING STAFF

Mark Grimes
Director, Department of Publishing

Jennifer McDonald
Manager, Online Content

Leesa Levin-Doroba
Production Manager, Practice Management

Amanda Helmholz
Editorial Specialist

Peg Mulcahy
Manager, Art Direction and Production

Sean Rogers
Digital Content Specialist

Mary Lou White
Sr. Vice President, Member Engagement and Marketing and Sales

Linda Smessaert
Brand Manager, Clinical and Professional Publications

Mary Louise Carr
Marketing Manager, Clinical Publications

The recommendations in this publication do not indicate an exclusive course of treatment or serve as a standard of medical care. Variations, taking into account individual circumstances, may be appropriate.

Products are mentioned for identification and informational purposes only and do not imply endorsement by the American Academy of Pediatrics.

Every effort has been made to ensure that the drug selection and dosage set forth in this text are in accordance with the current recommendations and practice at the time of publication. It is the responsibility of the health care professional to check the package insert of each drug for any change in indications and dosage and for added warnings and precautions.

This publication has been developed by the American Academy of Pediatrics. The authors, editors, and contributors are expert authorities in the field of pediatrics. No commercial involvement of any kind has been solicited or accepted in the development of the content of this publication.

Printed in the United States of America

9-5/0516

MA0822

ISBN: 978-1-61002-085-5
eBook: 978-61002-086-2
ISSN: 1942-2024

INTRODUCTION TO
PEDIATRIC CLINICAL PRACTICE GUIDELINES & POLICIES: A COMPENDIUM OF EVIDENCE-BASED RESEARCH FOR PEDIATRIC PRACTICE

Clinical practice guidelines have long provided physicians with evidence-based decision-making tools for managing common pediatric conditions. Policy statements issued and endorsed by the American Academy of Pediatrics (AAP) are developed to provide physicians with a quick reference guide to the AAP position on child health care issues. We have combined these two authoritative resources into one comprehensive manual/eBook resource to provide easy access to important clinical and policy information.

This manual contains
- Clinical practice guidelines from the AAP, plus related recommendation summaries, *ICD-10-CM* coding information, and AAP patient education handouts
- Technical report summaries
- Clinical practice guidelines endorsed by the AAP, including abstracts where applicable
- Policy statements, clinical reports, and technical reports issued or endorsed through December 2016, including abstracts where applicable
- Full text of all 2016 AAP policy statements, clinical reports, and technical reports

The eBook, which is available via the code on the inside cover of this manual, builds on content of the manual and points to the full text of all AAP
- Clinical practice guidelines
- Policy statements
- Clinical reports
- Technical reports
- Endorsed clinical practice guidelines and policies

For easy reference within this publication, dates when AAP clinical practice guidelines, policy statements, clinical reports, and technical reports first appeared in the AAP journal *Pediatrics* are provided. In 2009, the online version of *Pediatrics* at http://pediatrics.aappublications.org became the official journal of record; therefore, date of online publication is given for policies from 2010 to present.

Additional information about AAP policy can be found in a variety of professional publications such as

Guidelines for Air and Ground Transport of Neonatal and Pediatric Patients, 4th Edition

Pediatric Nutrition, 7th Edition

Guidelines for Perinatal Care, 7th Edition

Pediatric Environmental Health, 3rd Edition

Care of the Young Athlete, 2nd Edition

Red Book®, 30th Edition, and *Red Book® Online* (http://redbook.solutions.aap.org)

To order these and other pediatric resources, please call 888/227-1770 or visit http://shop.aap.org/books.

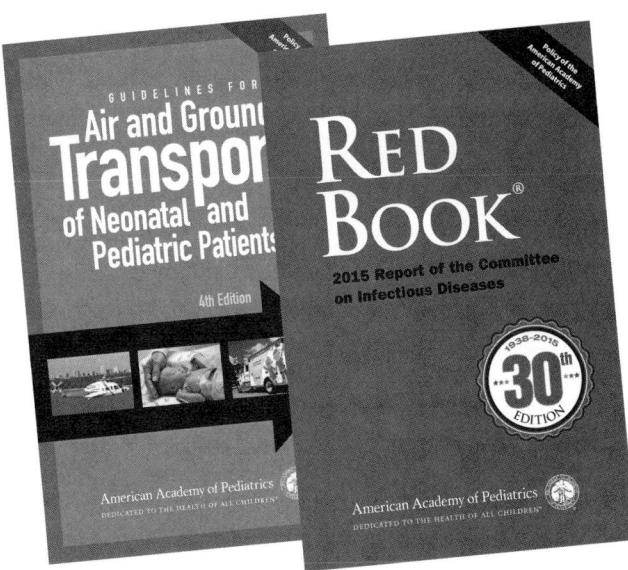

AMERICAN ACADEMY OF PEDIATRICS

The American Academy of Pediatrics (AAP) and its member pediatricians dedicate their efforts and resources to the health, safety, and well-being of infants, children, adolescents, and young adults. The AAP has approximately 66,000 members in the United States, Canada, and Latin America. Members include pediatricians, pediatric medical subspecialists, and pediatric surgical specialists.

Core Values. *We believe*
- In the inherent worth of all children; they are our most enduring and vulnerable legacy.
- Children deserve optimal health and the highest quality health care.
- Pediatricians and subspecialists are the best qualified to provide child health care.
- Multidisciplinary teams including patients and families are integral to delivering the highest quality health care.

The American Academy of Pediatrics is the organization to advance child health and well-being and the profession of pediatrics.

Vision. Children have optimal health and well-being and are valued by society. Academy members practice the highest quality health care and experience professional satisfaction and personal well-being.

Mission. The mission of the American Academy of Pediatrics is to attain optimal physical, mental, and social health and well-being for all infants, children, adolescents, and young adults. To accomplish this mission, the Academy shall support the professional needs of its members.

Table of Contents

SECTION 5

CURRENT POLICIES FROM THE AMERICAN ACADEMY OF PEDIATRICS

SECTION 6

ENDORSED POLICIES

APPENDIX 2

**PPI: AAP PARTNERSHIP FOR
POLICY IMPLEMENTATION** 1555

APPENDIX 3

**AMERICAN ACADEMY OF
PEDIATRICS ACRONYMS** 1559

Section 1

Clinical Practice Guidelines
From the American Academy of Pediatrics
• • • • • • • • • • • • • • • • • • • •

- *Clinical Practice Guidelines*
  EVIDENCE-BASED DECISION-MAKING TOOLS FOR MANAGING COMMON PEDIATRIC CONDITIONS

- *Technical Reports and Summaries*
  BACKGROUND INFORMATION TO SUPPORT AMERICAN ACADEMY OF PEDIATRICS POLICY

- *Quick Reference Tools*
  TOOLS FOR IMPLEMENTING AMERICAN ACADEMY OF PEDIATRICS GUIDELINES IN YOUR
  PRACTICE AND AT THE POINT OF CARE

FOREWORD

To promote the practice of evidence-based medicine, the American Academy of Pediatrics (AAP) provides physicians with evidence-based guidelines for managing common pediatric conditions. The AAP has an established organizational process and methodology for the development of these clinical practice guidelines.

The evidence-based approach to developing clinical practice guidelines requires systematically defining the problem and identifying interventions and health outcomes. Extensive literature reviews and data syntheses provide the basis for guideline recommendations. Clinical practice guidelines also undergo a thorough peer-review process prior to publication and are periodically reviewed to ensure that they are based on the most current data available.

American Academy of Pediatrics clinical practice guidelines are designed to provide physicians with an analytic framework for evaluating and treating common pediatric conditions and are not intended as an exclusive course of treatment or standard of care. When using AAP clinical practice guidelines, physicians should continue to consider other sources of information as well as variations in individual circumstances. The AAP recognizes circumstances in which there is a lack of definitive data and relies on expert consensus in cases in which data do not exist. American Academy of Pediatrics clinical practice guidelines allow for flexibility and adaptability at the local level and should not replace sound clinical judgment.

This manual contains clinical practice guidelines, technical reports, and technical report summaries developed and published by the AAP. Each one contains a summary of data reviewed, results of data analysis, complete evidence tables, and a bibliography of articles included in the review. This manual also contains abstracts and introductions for evidence-based clinical practice guidelines from other organizations that the AAP has endorsed. The AAP is committed to systematically evaluating these documents and disseminating appropriate documents to its membership. Clinical practice guidelines will continually be added to this compendium as they are released or updated. We encourage you to look forward to these future guidelines. Additionally, this edition includes the full text of all policy statements, clinical reports, and technical reports published in 2016 by the AAP as well as abstracts of all active AAP and endorsed policy statements and reports. Policy statements, where possible, should include the quality of evidence and strength of recommendations using a generally acceptable grading system. Both intellectual and financial transparency is essential and should appear in all clinical practice guidelines, as well as policy statements, clinical reports, and technical reports. The companion eBook points to all active AAP and endorsed policy statements and reports published prior to 2016.

If you have any questions about current or future clinical practice guidelines, please contact Kymika Okechukwu, manager of evidence-based practice initiatives at the AAP, at 800/433-9016, extension 4317, or via e-mail at kokechukwu@aap.org.

To order copies of patient education resources that accompany each guideline, please call the AAP at 888/227-1770 or visit http://shop.aap.org/books.

Wayne H. Franklin, MD, MPH, MMM, FAAP
Chairperson, Council on Quality Improvement and Patient Safety

ADHD: Clinical Practice Guideline for the Diagnosis, Evaluation, and Treatment of Attention-Deficit/Hyperactivity Disorder in Children and Adolescents

- *Clinical Practice Guideline*

  - *PPI: AAP Partnership for Policy Implementation*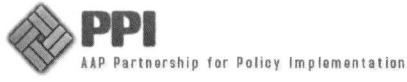
    See Appendix 2 for more information.

CLINICAL PRACTICE GUIDELINE

ADHD: Clinical Practice Guideline for the Diagnosis, Evaluation, and Treatment of Attention-Deficit/Hyperactivity Disorder in Children and Adolescents

SUBCOMMITTEE ON ATTENTION-DEFICIT/HYPERACTIVITY DISORDER, STEERING COMMITTEE ON QUALITY IMPROVEMENT AND MANAGEMENT

KEY WORDS
attention-deficit/hyperactivity disorder, children, adolescents, preschool, behavioral therapy, medication

ABBREVIATIONS
AAP—American Academy of Pediatrics
ADHD—attention-deficit/hyperactivity disorder
DSM-PC—*Diagnostic and Statistical Manual for Primary Care*
CDC—Centers for Disease Control and Prevention
FDA—Food and Drug Administration
DSM-IV—*Diagnostic and Statistical Manual of Mental Disorders, Fourth Edition*
MTA—Multimodal Therapy of ADHD

www.pediatrics.org/cgi/doi/10.1542/peds.2011-2654

doi:10.1542/peds.2011-2654

All clinical practice guidelines from the American Academy of Pediatrics automatically expire 5 years after publication unless reaffirmed, revised, or retired at or before that time.

PEDIATRICS (ISSN Numbers: Print, 0031-4005; Online, 1098-4275).

abstract

Attention-deficit/hyperactivity disorder (ADHD) is the most common neurobehavioral disorder of childhood and can profoundly affect the academic achievement, well-being, and social interactions of children; the American Academy of Pediatrics first published clinical recommendations for the diagnosis and evaluation of ADHD in children in 2000; recommendations for treatment followed in 2001. *Pediatrics* 2011;128: 1007–1022

Summary of key action statements:

1. The primary care clinician should initiate an evaluation for ADHD for any child 4 through 18 years of age who presents with academic or behavioral problems and symptoms of inattention, hyperactivity, or impulsivity (quality of evidence B/strong recommendation).

2. To make a diagnosis of ADHD, the primary care clinician should determine that *Diagnostic and Statistical Manual of Mental Disorders, Fourth Edition* criteria have been met (including documentation of impairment in more than 1 major setting); information should be obtained primarily from reports from parents or guardians, teachers, and other school and mental health clinicians involved in the child's care. The primary care clinician should also rule out any alternative cause (quality of evidence B/strong recommendation).

3. In the evaluation of a child for ADHD, the primary care clinician should include assessment for other conditions that might coexist with ADHD, including emotional or behavioral (eg, anxiety, depressive, oppositional defiant, and conduct disorders), developmental (eg, learning and language disorders or other neurodevelopmental disorders), and physical (eg, tics, sleep apnea) conditions (quality of evidence B/strong recommendation).

4. The primary care clinician should recognize ADHD as a chronic condition and, therefore, consider children and adolescents with ADHD as children and youth with special health care needs. Management of children and youth with special health care needs should follow the principles of the chronic care model and the medical home (quality of evidence B/strong recommendation).

5. Recommendations for treatment of children and youth with ADHD vary depending on the patient's age:

a. For *preschool-aged children (4–5 years of age)*, the primary care clinician should prescribe evidence-based parent- and/or teacher-administered behavior therapy as the first line of treatment (quality of evidence A/strong recommendation) and may prescribe methylphenidate if the behavior interventions do not provide significant improvement and there is moderate-to-severe continuing disturbance in the child's function. In areas where evidence-based behavioral treatments are not available, the clinician needs to weigh the risks of starting medication at an early age against the harm of delaying diagnosis and treatment (quality of evidence B/recommendation).

b. For *elementary school–aged children (6–11 years of age)*, the primary care clinician should prescribe US Food and Drug Administration–approved medications for ADHD (quality of evidence A/strong recommendation) and/or evidence-based parent- and/or teacher-administered behavior therapy as treatment for ADHD, preferably both (quality of evidence B/strong recommendation). The evidence is particularly strong for stimulant medications and sufficient but less strong for atomoxetine, extended-release guanfacine, and extended-release clonidine (in that order) (quality of evidence A/strong recommendation). The school environment, program, or placement is a part of any treatment plan.

c. For *adolescents (12–18 years of age)*, the primary care clinician should prescribe Food and Drug Administration–approved medications for ADHD with the assent of the adolescent (quality of evidence A/strong recommendation) and may prescribe behavior therapy as treatment for ADHD (quality of evidence C/recommendation), preferably both.

6. The primary care clinician should titrate doses of medication for ADHD to achieve maximum benefit with minimum adverse effects (quality of evidence B/strong recommendation).

INTRODUCTION

This document updates and replaces 2 previously published clinical guidelines from the American Academy of Pediatrics (AAP) on the diagnosis and treatment of attention-deficit/hyperactivity disorder (ADHD) in children: "Clinical Practice Guideline: Diagnosis and Evaluation of the Child With Attention-Deficit/Hyperactivity Disorder" (2000)[1] and "Clinical Practice Guideline: Treatment of the School-aged Child With Attention-Deficit/Hyperactivity Disorder" (2001).[2] Since these guidelines were published, new information and evidence regarding the diagnosis and treatment of ADHD has become available. Surveys conducted before and after the publication of the previous guidelines have also provided insight into pediatricians' attitudes and practices regarding ADHD. On the basis of an increased understanding regarding ADHD and the challenges it raises for children and families and as a source for clinicians seeking to diagnose and treat children, this guideline pays particular attention to a number of areas.

Expanded Age Range

The previous guidelines addressed diagnosis and treatment of ADHD in chil- dren 6 through 12 years of age. There is now emerging evidence to expand the age range of the recommendations to include preschool-aged children and adolescents. This guideline addresses the diagnosis and treatment of ADHD in children 4 through 18 years of age, and attention is brought to special circumstances or concerns in particular age groups when appropriate.

Expanded Scope

Behavioral interventions might help families of children with hyperactive/ impulsive behaviors that do not meet full diagnostic criteria for ADHD. Guidance regarding the diagnosis of problem-level concerns in children based on the *Diagnostic and Statistical Manual for Primary Care* (DSM-PC), *Child and Adolescent Version*,[3] as well as suggestions for treatment and care of children and families with problem-level concerns, are provided here. The current DSM-PC was published in 1996 and, therefore, is not consistent with intervening changes to *International Classification of Diseases, Ninth Revision, Clinical Modification* (ICD-9-CM). Although this version of the DSM-PC should not be used as a definitive source for diagnostic codes related to ADHD and comorbid conditions, it certainly may continue to be used as a resource for enriching the understanding of ADHD manifestations. The DSM-PC will be revised when both the DSM-V and ICD-10 are available for use.

A Process of Care for Diagnosis and Treatment

This guideline and process-of-care algorithm (see Supplemental Fig 2 and Supplemental Appendix) recognizes evaluation, diagnosis, and treatment as a continuous process and provides recommendations for both the guideline and the algorithm in this single publication. In addition to the formal recommendations for assessment, diagnosis, and treatment, this guideline provides a single algorithm to guide the clinical process.

Integration With the Task Force on Mental Health

This guideline fits into the broader mission of the AAP Task Force on Mental Health and its efforts to provide a base from which primary care providers can develop alliances with families, work to prevent mental health conditions and identify them early, and collaborate with mental health clinicians.

The diagnosis and management of ADHD in children and youth has been particularly challenging for primary care clinicians because of the limited payment provided for what requires more time than most of the other conditions they typically address. The procedures recommended in this guideline necessitate spending more time with patients and families, developing a system of contacts with school and other personnel, and providing continuous, coordinated care, all of which is time demanding. In addition, relegating mental health conditions exclusively to mental health clinicians also is not a viable solution for many clinicians, because in many areas access to mental health clinicians to whom they can refer patients is limited. Access in many areas is also limited to psychologists when further assessment of cognitive issues is required and not available through the education system because of restrictions from third-party payers in paying for the evaluations on the basis of them being educational and not health related.

Cultural differences in the diagnosis and treatment of ADHD are an important issue, as they are for all pediatric conditions. Because the diagnosis and treatment of ADHD depends to a great extent on family and teacher perceptions, these issues might be even more prominent an issue for ADHD. Specific cultural issues

are beyond the scope of this guideline but are important to consider.

METHODOLOGY

As with the 2 previously published clinical guidelines, the AAP collaborated with several organizations to develop a working subcommittee that represented a wide range of primary care and subspecialty groups. The subcommittee included primary care pediatricians, developmental-behavioral pediatricians, and representatives from the American Academy of Child and Adolescent Psychiatry, the Child Neurology Society, the Society for Pediatric Psychology, the National Association of School Psychologists, the Society for Developmental and Behavioral Pediatrics, the American Academy of Family Physicians, and Children and Adults With Attention-Deficit/Hyperactivity Disorder (CHADD), as well as an epidemiologist from the Centers for Disease Control and Prevention (CDC).

This group met over a 2-year period, during which it reviewed the changes in practice that have occurred and issues that have been identified since the previous guidelines were published. Delay in completing the process led to further conference calls and extended the years of literature reviewed in order to remain as current as possible. The AAP funded the development of this guideline; potential financial conflicts of the participants were identified and taken into consideration in the deliberations. The guideline will be reviewed and/or revised in 5 years unless new evidence emerges that warrants revision sooner.

The subcommittee developed a series of research questions to direct an extensive evidence-based review in partnership with the CDC and the University of Oklahoma Health Sciences Center. The diagnostic review was conducted by the CDC, and the evidence was evaluated in a combined effort of

the AAP, CDC, and University of Oklahoma Health Sciences Center staff. The treatment-related evidence relied on a recent evidence review by the Agency for Healthcare Research and Quality and was supplemented by evidence identified through the CDC review.

The diagnostic issues were focused on 5 areas:

1. ADHD prevalence—specifically: (*a*) What percentage of the general US population aged 21 years or younger has ADHD? (*b*) What percentage of patients presenting at pediatricians' or family physicians' offices in the United States meet diagnostic criteria for ADHD?

2. Co-occurring mental disorders—of people with ADHD, what percentage has 1 or more of the following co-occurring conditions: sleep disorders, learning disabilities, depression, anxiety, conduct disorder, and oppositional defiant disorder?

3. What are the functional impairments of children and youth diagnosed with ADHD? Specifically, in what domains and to what degree do youth with ADHD demonstrate impairments in functional domains, including peer relations, academic performance, adaptive skills, and family functioning?

4. Do behavior rating scales remain the standard of care in assessing the diagnostic criteria for ADHD?

5. What is the prevalence of abnormal findings on selected medical screening tests commonly recommended as standard components of an evaluation of a child with suspected ADHD? How accurate are these tests in the diagnosis of ADHD compared with a reference standard (ie, what are the psychometric properties of these tests)?

The treatment issues were focused on 3 areas:

1. What new information is available

regarding the long-term efficacy and safety of medications approved by the US Food and Drug Administration (FDA) for the treatment of ADHD (stimulants and nonstimulants), and specifically, what information is available about the efficacy and safety of these medications in preschool-aged and adolescent patients?

2. What evidence is available about the long-term efficacy and safety of psychosocial interventions (behavioral modification) for the treatment of ADHD for children, and specifically, what information is available about the efficacy and safety of these interventions in preschool-aged and adolescent patients?

3. Are there any additional therapies that reach the level of consideration as evidence based?

Evidence-Review Process for Diagnosis

A multilevel, systematic approach was taken to identify the literature that built the evidence base for both diagnosis and treatment. To increase the likelihood that relevant articles were included in the final evidence base, the reviewers first conducted a scoping review of the literature by systematically searching literature using relevant key words and then summarized the primary findings of articles that met standard inclusion criteria. The reviewers then created evidence tables that were reviewed by content-area experts who were best able to identify articles that might have been missed through the scoping review. Articles that were missed were reviewed carefully to determine where the abstraction methodology failed, and adjustments to the search strategy were made as required (see technical report to be published). Finally, although published literature reviews did not contribute directly to the evidence

base, the articles included in review articles were cross-referenced with the final evidence tables to ensure that all relevant articles were included in the final evidence tables.

For the scoping review, articles were abstracted in a stratified fashion from 3 article-retrieval systems that provided access to articles in the domains of medicine, psychology, and education: PubMed (www.ncbi.nlm.nih.gov/sites/entrez), PsycINFO (www.apa.org/pubs/databases/psycinfo/index.aspx), and ERIC (www.eric.ed.gov). English-language, peer-reviewed articles published between 1998 and 2009 were queried in the 3 search engines. Key words were selected with the intent of including all possible articles that might have been relevant to 1 or more of the questions of interest (see the technical report to be published). The primary abstraction included the following terms: "attention deficit hyperactivity disorder" or "attention deficit disorder" or "hyperkinesis" and "child." A second, independent abstraction was conducted to identify articles related to medical screening tests for ADHD. For this abstraction, the same search terms were used as in the previous procedure along with the additional condition term "behavioral problems" to allow for the inclusion of studies of youth that sought to diagnose ADHD by using medical screening tests. Abstractions were conducted in parallel fashion across each of the 3 databases; the results from each abstraction (complete reference, abstract, and key words) were exported and compiled into a common reference database using EndNote 10.0.[4] References were subsequently and systematically deduplicated by using the software's deduplication procedure. References for books, chapters, and theses were also deleted from the library. Once a deduplicated library was developed, the semifinal

database of 8267 references was reviewed for inclusion on the basis of inclusion criteria listed in the technical report. Included articles were then pulled in their entirety, the inclusion criteria were reconfirmed, and then the study findings were summarized in evidence tables. The articles included in relevant review articles were revisited to ensure their inclusion in the final evidence base. The evidence tables were then presented to the committee for expert review.

Evidence-Review Process for Treatment

In addition to this systematic review, for treatment we used the review from the Agency for Healthcare Research and Quality (AHRQ) Effective Healthcare Program "Attention Deficit Hyperactivity Disorder: Effectiveness of Treatment in At-Risk Preschoolers; Long-term Effectiveness in All Ages; and Variability in Prevalence, Diagnosis, and Treatment."[5] This review addressed a number of key questions for the committee, including the efficacy of medications and behavioral interventions for preschoolers, children, and adolescents. Evidence identified through the systematic evidence review for diagnosis was also used as a secondary data source to supplement the evidence presented in the AHRQ report. The draft practice guidelines were developed by consensus of the committee regarding the evidence. It was decided to create 2 separate components. The guideline recommendations were based on clear characterization of the evidence. The second component is a practice-of-care algorithm (see Supplemental Fig 2) that provides considerably more detail about how to implement the guidelines but is, necessarily, based less on available evidence and more on consensus of the committee members. When data were lacking, particularly in the

Evidence Quality	Preponderance of Benefit or Harm	Balance of Benefit and Harm
A. Well-designed RCTs or diagnostic studies on relevant population	Strong recommendation	
B. RCTs or diagnostic studies with minor limitations; overwhelmingly consistent evidence from observational studies		Option
C. Observational studies (case-control and cohort design)	Recommendation	
D. Expert opinion, case reports, reasoning from first principles	Option	No Rec
X. Exceptional situations in which validating studies cannot be performed and there is a clear preponderance of benefit or harm	Strong recommendation / Recommendation	

FIGURE 1

Integrating evidence-quality appraisal with an assessment of the anticipated balance between benefits and harms if a policy is conducted leads to designation of a policy as a strong recommendation, recommendation, option, or no recommendation. The evidence is discussed in more detail in a technical report that will follow in a later publication. RCT indicates randomized controlled trial; Rec, recommendation.

process-of-care algorithmic portion of the guidelines, a combination of evidence and expert consensus was used. Action statements labeled "strong recommendation" or "recommendation" were based on high- to moderate-quality scientific evidence and a preponderance of benefit over harm.[6] Option-level action statements were based on lesser-quality or limited data and expert consensus or high-quality evidence with a balance between benefits and harms. These clinical options are interventions that a reasonable health care provider might or might not wish to implement in his or her practice. The quality of evidence supporting each recommendation and the strength of each recommendation were assessed by the committee member most experienced in epidemiology and graded according to AAP policy (Fig 1).[6]

The guidelines and process-of-care algorithm underwent extensive peer review by committees, sections, councils, and task forces within the AAP; numerous outside organizations; and other individuals identified by the subcommittee. Liaisons to the subcommittee also were invited to distribute the draft to entities within their organizations. The re-

sulting comments were compiled and reviewed by the chairperson, and relevant changes were incorporated into the draft, which was then reviewed by the full committee.

ABOUT THIS GUIDELINE

Key Action Statements

In light of the concerns highlighted previously and informed by the available evidence, the AAP has developed 6 action statements for the evaluation, diagnosis, and treatment of ADHD in children. These action statements provide for consistent and quality care for children and families with concerns about or symptoms that suggest attention disorders or problems.

Context

This guideline is intended to be integrated with the broader algorithms developed as part of the mission of the AAP Task Force on Mental Health.[7]

Implementation: A Process-of-Care Algorithm

The AAP recognizes the challenge of instituting practice changes and adopting new recommendations for care. To address the need, a process-of-care algorithm has been devel-

oped and has been used in the revision of the AAP ADHD toolkit.

Implementation: Preparing the Practice

Full implementation of the action statements described in this guideline and the process-of-care algorithm might require changes in office procedures and/or preparatory efforts to identify community resources. The section titled "Preparing the Practice" in the process-of-care algorithm and further information can be found in the supplement to the Task Force on Mental Health report.[7] It is important to document all aspects of the diagnostic and treatment procedures in the patients' records. Use of rating scales for the diagnosis of ADHD and assessment for comorbid conditions and as a method for monitoring treatment as described in the process algorithm (see Supplemental Fig 2), as well as information provided to parents such as management plans, can help facilitate a clinician's accurate documentation of his or her process.

Note

The AAP acknowledges that some primary care clinicians might not be confident of their ability to successfully diagnose and treat ADHD in a child because of the child's age, co-existing conditions, or other concerns. At any point at which a clinician feels that he or she is not adequately trained or is uncertain about making a diagnosis or continuing with treatment, a referral to a pediatric or mental health subspecialist should be made. If a diagnosis of ADHD or other condition is made by a subspecialist, the primary care clinician should develop a management strategy with the subspecialist that ensures that the child will continue to receive appropriate care consistent with a medical home model wherein the pediatrician partners with parents so that both health and mental health needs are integrated.

KEY ACTION STATEMENTS FOR THE EVALUATION, DIAGNOSIS, TREATMENT, AND MONITORING OF ADHD IN CHILDREN AND ADOLESCENTS

Action statement 1: The primary care clinician should initiate an evaluation for ADHD for any child 4 through 18 years of age who presents with academic or behavioral problems and symptoms of inattention, hyperactivity, or impulsivity (quality of evidence B/strong recommendation).

Evidence Profile

- **Aggregate evidence quality:** B.

- **Benefits:** In a considerable number of children, ADHD goes undiagnosed. Primary care clinicians' systematic identification of children with these problems will likely decrease the rate of undiagnosed and untreated ADHD in children.

- **Harms/risks/costs:** Children in whom ADHD is inappropriately diagnosed might be labeled inappropriately, or another condition might be missed, and they might receive treatments that will not benefit them.

- **Benefits-harms assessment:** The high prevalence of ADHD and limited mental health resources require primary care pediatricians to play a significant role in the care of their patients with ADHD so that children with this condition receive the appropriate diagnosis and treatment. Treatments available have shown good evidence of efficacy, and lack of treatment results in a risk for impaired outcomes.

- **Value judgments:** The committee considered the requirements for establishing the diagnosis, the prevalence of ADHD, and the efficacy and adverse effects of treatment as well as the long-term outcomes.

- **Role of patient preferences:** Success with treatment depends on patient and family preference, which has to be taken into account.

- **Exclusions:** None.

- **Intentional vagueness:** The limits between what can be handled by a primary care clinician and what should be referred to a subspecialist because of the varying degrees of skills among primary care clinicians.

- **Strength: strong recommendation.**

The basis for this recommendation is essentially unchanged from that in the previous guideline. ADHD is the most common neurobehavioral disorder in children and occurs in approximately 8% of children and youth[8–10]; the number of children with this condition is far greater than can be managed by the mental health system. There is now increased evidence that appropriate diagnosis can be provided for preschool-aged children[11] (4–5 years of age) and for adolescents.[12]

Action statement 2: To make a diagnosis of ADHD, the primary care clinician should determine that *Diagnostic and Statistical Manual of Mental Disorders, Fourth Edition* (DSM-IV-TR) criteria have been met (including documentation of impairment in more than 1 major setting), and information should be obtained primarily from reports from parents or guardians, teachers, and other school and mental health clinicians involved in the child's care. The primary care clinician should also rule out any alternative cause (quality of evidence B/strong recommendation).

Evidence Profile

- **Aggregate evidence quality:** B.

- **Benefits:** The use of DSM-IV criteria has lead to more uniform categorization of the condition across professional disciplines.

- **Harms/risks/costs:** The DSM-IV system does not specifically provide for developmental-level differences and might lead to some misdiagnoses.

- **Benefits-harms assessment:** The benefits far outweigh the harm.

- **Value judgments:** The committee took into consideration the importance of coordination between pediatric and mental health services.

- **Role of patient preferences:** Although there is some stigma associated with mental disorder diagnoses resulting in some families preferring other diagnoses, the need for better clarity in diagnoses was felt to outweigh this preference.

- **Exclusions:** None.

- **Intentional vagueness:** None.

- **Strength: strong recommendation.**

As with the findings in the previous guideline, the DSM-IV criteria continue to be the criteria best supported by evidence and consensus. Developed through several iterations by the American Psychiatric Association, the DSM-IV criteria were created through use of consensus and an expanding research foundation.[13] The DSM-IV system is used by professionals in psychiatry, psychology, health care systems, and primary care. Use of DSM-IV criteria, in addition to having the best evidence to date for criteria for ADHD, also affords the best method for communication across clinicians and is established with third-party payers. The criteria are under review for the development of the DSM-V, but these changes will not be available until at least 1 year after the publication of this current guideline. The diagnostic criteria have not changed since the previous guideline and are presented in Supplemental Table 2. An anticipated change in the DSM-V is increasing the age limit for when ADHD needs to have first presented from 7 to 12 years.[14]

Special Circumstances: Preschool-aged Children (4–5 Years Old)

There is evidence that the diagnostic criteria for ADHD can be applied to preschool-aged children; however, the subtypes detailed in the DSM-IV might not be valid for this population.[15–21] A review of the literature, including the multisite study of the efficacy of methylphenidate in preschool-aged children, revealed that the criteria could appropriately identify children with the condition.[11] However, there are added challenges in determining the presence of key symptoms. Preschool-aged children are not likely to have a separate observer if they do not attend a preschool or child care program, and even if they do attend, staff in those programs might be less qualified than certified teachers to provide accurate observations. Here, too, focused checklists can help physicians in the diagnostic evaluation, although only the Conners Comprehensive Behavior Rating Scales and the ADHD Rating Scale IV are DSM-IV—based scales that have been validated in preschool-aged children.[22]

When there are concerns about the availability or quality of nonparent observations of a child's behavior, physicians may recommend that parents complete a parent-training program before confirming an ADHD diagnosis for preschool-aged children and consider placement in a qualified preschool program if they have not done so already. Information can be obtained from parents and teachers through the use of validated DSM-IV—based ADHD rating scales. The parent-training program must include helping parents develop age-appropriate developmental expectations and specific management skills for problem behaviors. The clinician may obtain reports from the parenting class instructor about the parents' ability to manage their children, and if the children are

in programs in which they are directly observed, instructors can report information about the core symptoms and function of the child directly. Qualified preschool programs include programs such as Head Start or other public prekindergarten programs. Preschool-aged children who display significant emotional or behavioral concerns might also qualify for Early Childhood Special Education services through their local school districts, and the evaluators for these programs and/or Early Childhood Special Education teachers might be excellent reporters of core symptoms.

Special Circumstances: Adolescents

Obtaining teacher reports for adolescents might be more challenging, because many adolescents will have multiple teachers. Likewise, parents might have less opportunity to observe their adolescent's behaviors than they had when their children were younger. Adolescents' reports of their own behaviors often differ from those of other observers, because they tend to minimize their own problematic behaviors.[23–25] Adolescents are less likely to exhibit overt hyperactive behavior. Despite the difficulties, clinicians need to try to obtain (with agreement from the adolescent) information from at least 2 teachers as well as information from other sources such as coaches, school guidance counselors, or leaders of community activities in which the adolescent participates. In addition, it is unusual for adolescents with behavioral/attention problems not to have been previously given a diagnosis of ADHD. Therefore, it is important to establish the younger manifestations of the condition that were missed and to strongly consider substance use, depression, and anxiety as alternative or co-occurring diagnoses. Adolescents with ADHD, especially when untreated, are at greater risk of substance abuse.[26] In addition, the risks of

mood and anxiety disorders and risky sexual behaviors increase during adolescence.[12]

Special Circumstances: Inattention or Hyperactivity/Impulsivity (Problem Level)

Teachers, parents, and child health professionals typically encounter children with behaviors relating to activity level, impulsivity, and inattention who might not fully meet DSM-IV criteria. The DSM-PC[3] provides a guide to the more common behaviors seen in pediatrics. The manual describes common variations in behavior as well as more problematic behaviors at levels of less impairment than those specified in the DSM-IV.

The behavioral descriptions of the DSM-PC have not yet been tested in community studies to determine the prevalence or severity of developmental variations and problems in the areas of inattention, hyperactivity, or impulsivity. They do, however, provide guidance to clinicians regarding elements of treatment for children with problems with mild-to-moderate inattention, hyperactivity, or impulsivity. The DSM-PC also considers environmental influences on a child's behavior and provides information on differential diagnosis with a developmental perspective.

Action statement 3: In the evaluation of a child for ADHD, the primary care clinician should include assessment for other conditions that might coexist with ADHD, including emotional or behavioral (eg, anxiety, depressive, oppositional defiant, and conduct disorders), developmental (eg, learning and language disorders or other neurodevelopmental disorders), and physical (eg, tics, sleep apnea) conditions (quality of evidence B/strong recommendation).

Evidence Profile

- **Aggregate evidence quality:** B.
- **Benefits:** Identifying coexisting conditions is important for developing the most appropriate treatment plan.
- **Harms/risks/costs:** The major risk is misdiagnosing the conditions and providing inappropriate care.
- **Benefits-harms assessment:** There is a preponderance of benefit over harm.
- **Value judgments:** The committee members took into consideration the common occurrence of coexisting conditions and the importance of addressing them in making this recommendation.
- **Role of patient preferences:** None.
- **Exclusions:** None.
- **Intentional vagueness:** None.
- **Strength: strong recommendation.**

A variety of other behavioral, developmental, and physical conditions can coexist in children who are evaluated for ADHD. These conditions include, but are not limited to, learning problems, language disorder, disruptive behavior, anxiety, mood disorders, tic disorders, seizures, developmental coordination disorder, or sleep disorders.[23,24,27–38] In some cases, the presence of a coexisting condition will alter the treatment of ADHD. The primary care clinician might benefit from additional support and guidance or might need to refer a child with ADHD and coexisting conditions, such as severe mood or anxiety disorders, to subspecialists for assessment and management. The subspecialists could include child psychiatrists, developmental-behavioral pediatricians, neurodevelopmental disability physicians, child neurologists, or child or school psychologists.

Given the likelihood that another condition exists, primary care clinicians should conduct assessments that determine or at least identify the risk of coexisting conditions. Through its Task Force on Mental Health, the AAP has developed algorithms and a toolkit[39] for assessing and treating (or comanaging) the most common developmental disorders and mental health concerns in children. These resources might be useful in assessing children who are being evaluated for ADHD. Payment for evaluation and treatment must cover the fixed and variable costs of providing the services, as noted in the AAP policy statement "Scope of Health Care Benefits for Children From Birth Through Age 26.[40]

Special Circumstances: Adolescents
Clinicians should assess adolescent patients with newly diagnosed ADHD for symptoms and signs of substance abuse; when these signs and symptoms are found, evaluation and treatment for addiction should precede treatment for ADHD, if possible, or careful treatment for ADHD can begin if necessary.[25]

Action statement 4: The primary care clinician should recognize ADHD as a chronic condition and, therefore, consider children and adolescents with ADHD as children and youth with special health care needs. Management of children and youth with special health care needs should follow the principles of the chronic care model and the medical home (quality of evidence B/strong recommendation).

Evidence Profile

- **Aggregate evidence quality:** B.
- **Benefits:** The recommendation describes the coordinated services most appropriate for managing the condition.
- **Harms/risks/costs:** Providing the services might be more costly.
- **Benefits-harms assessment:** There is a preponderance of benefit over harm.
- **Value judgments:** The committee members considered the value of medical home services when deciding to make this recommendation.
- **Role of patient preferences:** Family preference in how these services are provided is an important consideration.
- **Exclusions:** None.
- **Intentional vagueness:** None.
- **Strength: strong recommendation.**

As in the previous guideline, this recommendation is based on the evidence that ADHD continues to cause symptoms and dysfunction in many children who have the condition over long periods of time, even into adulthood, and that the treatments available address symptoms and function but are usually not curative. Although the chronic illness model has not been specifically studied in children and youth with ADHD, it has been effective for other chronic conditions such as asthma,[23] and the medical home model has been accepted as the preferred standard of care.[41] The management process is also helped by encouraging strong family-school partnerships.[42]

Longitudinal studies have found that, frequently, treatments are not sustained despite the fact that long-term outcomes for children with ADHD indicate that they are at greater risk of significant problems if they discontinue treatment.[43] Because a number of parents of children with ADHD also have ADHD, extra support might be necessary to help those parents provide medication on a consistent basis and institute a consistent behavioral program. The medical home and chronic illness approach is provided in the process algorithm (Supplemental Fig 2). An important process in ongoing care is bidirectional communication with teachers and other school and mental health clinicians involved in the child's care as well as with parents and patients.

Special Circumstances: Inattention or Hyperactivity/Impulsivity (Problem Level)

Children with inattention or hyperactivity/impulsivity at the problem level (DSM-PC) and their families might also benefit from the same chronic illness and medical home principles.

Action statement 5: Recommendations for treatment of children and youth with ADHD vary depending on the patient's age.

Action statement 5a: For *preschool-aged children (4–5 years of age)*, the primary care clinician should prescribe evidence-based parent- and/or teacher-administered behavior therapy as the first line of treatment (quality of evidence A/strong recommendation) and may prescribe methylphenidate if the behavior interventions do not provide significant improvement and there is moderate-to-severe continuing disturbance in the child's function. In areas in which evidence-based behavioral treatments are not available, the clinician needs to weigh the risks of starting medication at an early age against the harm of delaying diagnosis and treatment (quality of evidence B/recommendation).

Evidence Profile

- **Aggregate evidence quality:** A for behavior; B for methylphenidate.
- **Benefits:** Both behavior therapy and methylphenidate have been demonstrated to reduce behaviors associated with ADHD and improve function.
- **Harms/risks/costs:** Both therapies increase the cost of care, and behavior therapy requires a higher level of family involvement, whereas methylphenidate has some potential adverse effects.
- **Benefits-harms assessment:** Given the risks of untreated ADHD, the benefits outweigh the risks.
- **Value judgments:** The committee mem-

bers included the effects of untreated ADHD when deciding to make this recommendation.

- **Role of patient preferences:** Family preference is essential in determining the treatment plan.
- **Exclusions:** None.
- **Intentional vagueness:** None.
- **Strength: strong recommendation.**

Action statement 5b: For *elementary school-aged children (6–11 years of age)*, the primary care clinician should prescribe FDA-approved medications for ADHD (quality of evidence A/strong recommendation) and/or evidence-based parent- and/or teacher-administered behavior therapy as treatment for ADHD, preferably both (quality of evidence B/strong recommendation). The evidence is particularly strong for stimulant medications and sufficient but less strong for atomoxetine, extended-release guanfacine, and extended-release clonidine (in that order) (quality of evidence A/strong recommendation). The school environment, program, or placement is a part of any treatment plan.

Evidence Profile

- **Aggregate evidence quality:** A for treatment with FDA-approved medications; B for behavior therapy.
- **Benefits:** Both behavior therapy and FDA-approved medications have been demonstrated to reduce behaviors associated with ADHD and improve function.
- **Harms/risks/costs:** Both therapies increase the cost of care, and behavior therapy requires a higher level of family involvement, whereas FDA-approved medications have some potential adverse effects.
- **Benefits-harms assessment:** Given the risks of untreated ADHD, the benefits outweigh the risks.
- **Value judgments:** The committee members included the effects of untreated

ADHD when deciding to make this recommendation.

- **Role of patient preferences:** Family preference, including patient preference, is essential in determining the treatment plan.
- **Exclusions:** None.
- **Intentional vagueness:** None.
- **Strength: strong recommendation.**

Action statement 5c: For *adolescents (12–18 years of age)*, the primary care clinician should prescribe FDA-approved medications for ADHD with the assent of the adolescent (quality of evidence A/strong recommendation) and may prescribe behavior therapy as treatment for ADHD (quality of evidence C/recommendation), preferably both.

Evidence Profile

- **Aggregate evidence quality:** A for medications; C for behavior therapy.
- **Benefits:** Both behavior therapy and FDA-approved medications have been demonstrated to reduce behaviors associated with ADHD and improve function.
- **Harms/risks/costs:** Both therapies increase the cost of care, and behavior therapy requires a higher level of family involvement, whereas FDA-approved medications have some potential adverse effects.
- **Benefits-harms assessment:** Given the risks of untreated ADHD, the benefits outweigh the risks.
- **Value judgments:** The committee members included the effects of untreated ADHD when deciding to make this recommendation.
- **Role of patient preferences:** Family preference, including patient preference, is essential in determining the treatment plan.
- **Exclusions:** None.
- **Intentional vagueness:** None.
- **Strength: strong recommendation/ recommendation.**

Medication

Similar to the recommendations from the previous guideline, stimulant medications are highly effective for most children in reducing core symptoms of ADHD.[44] One selective norepinephrine-reuptake inhibitor (atomoxetine[45,46]) and 2 selective α_2-adrenergic agonists (extended-release guanfacine[47,48] and extended-release clonidine[49]) have also demonstrated efficacy in reducing core symptoms. Because norepinephrine-reuptake inhibitors and α_2-adrenergic agonists are newer, the evidence base that supports them—although adequate for FDA approval—is considerably smaller than that for stimulants. None of them have been approved for use in preschool-aged children. Compared with stimulant medications that have an effect size [effect size = (treatment mean − control mean)/control SD] of approximately 1.0,[50] the effects of the nonstimulants are slightly weaker; atomoxetine has an effect size of approximately 0.7, and extended-release guanfacine and extended-release clonidine also have effect sizes of approximately 0.7.

The accompanying process-of-care algorithm provides a list of the currently available FDA-approved medications for ADHD (Supplemental Table 3). Characteristics of each medication are provided to help guide the clinician's choice in prescribing medication.

As was identified in the previous guideline, the most common stimulant adverse effects are appetite loss, abdominal pain, headaches, and sleep disturbance. The results of the Multimodal Therapy of ADHD (MTA) study revealed a more persistent effect of stimulants on decreasing growth velocity than have most previous studies, particularly when children were on higher and more consistently administered doses. The effects diminished by the third year of treatment, but no compensatory rebound effects were found.[51] However, diminished growth was in the range of 1 to 2 cm. An uncommon additional significant adverse effect of stimulants is the occurrence of hallucinations and other psychotic symptoms.[52] Although concerns have been raised about the rare occurrence of sudden cardiac death among children using stimulant medications,[53] sudden death in children on stimulant medication is extremely rare, and evidence is conflicting as to whether stimulant medications increase the risk of sudden death.[54–56] It is important to expand the history to include specific cardiac symptoms, Wolf-Parkinson-White syndrome, sudden death in the family, hypertrophic cardiomyopathy, and long QT syndrome. Preschool-aged children might experience increased mood lability and dysphoria.[57] For the nonstimulant atomoxetine, the adverse effects include initial somnolence and gastrointestinal tract symptoms, particularly if the dosage is increased too rapidly; decrease in appetite; increase in suicidal thoughts (less common); and hepatitis (rare). For the nonstimulant α_2-adrenergic agonists extended-release guanfacine and extended-release clonidine, adverse effects include somnolence and dry mouth.

Only 2 medications have evidence to support their use as adjunctive therapy with stimulant medications sufficient to achieve FDA approval: extended-release guanfacine[26] and extended-release clonidine. Other medications have been used in combination off-label, but there is currently only anecdotal evidence for their safety or efficacy, so their use cannot be recommended at this time.

Special Circumstances: Preschool-aged Children

A number of special circumstances support the recommendation to initiate ADHD treatment in preschool-aged children (ages 4–5 years) with behavioral therapy alone first.[57] These circumstances include:

- The multisite study of methylphenidate[57] was limited to preschool-aged children who had moderate-to-severe dysfunction.

- The study also found that many children (ages 4–5 years) experience improvements in symptoms with behavior therapy alone, and the overall evidence for behavior therapy in preschool-aged children is strong.

- Behavioral programs for children 4 to 5 years of age typically run in the form of group parent-training programs and, although not always compensated by health insurance, have a lower cost. The process algorithm (see Supplemental pages s15-16) contains criteria for the clinician to use in assessing the quality of the behavioral therapy. In addition, programs such as Head Start and Children and Adults With Attention Deficit Hyperactivity Disorder (CHADD) (www.chadd.org) might provide some behavioral supports.

Many young children with ADHD might still require medication to achieve maximum improvement, and medication is not contraindicated for children 4 through 5 years of age. However, only 1 multisite study has carefully assessed medication use in preschool-aged children. Other considerations in the recommendation about treating children 4 to 5 years of age with stimulant medications include:

- The study was limited to preschool-aged children who had moderate-to-severe dysfunction.

- Research has found that a number of young children (4–5 years of age) experience improvements in symptoms with behavior therapy alone.

- There are concerns about the possible effects on growth during this rapid growth period of preschool-aged children.

- There has been limited information about and experience with the effects of stimulant medication in children between the ages of 4 and 5 years.

Here, the criteria for enrollment (and, therefore, medication use) included measures of severity that distinguished treated children from the larger group of preschool-aged children with ADHD. Thus, before initiating medications, the physician should assess the severity of the child's ADHD. Given current data, only those preschool-aged children with ADHD who have moderate-to-severe dysfunction should be considered for medication. Criteria for this level of severity, based on the multisite-study results,[57] are (1) symptoms that have persisted for at least 9 months, (2) dysfunction that is manifested in both the home and other settings such as preschool or child care, and (3) dysfunction that has not responded adequately to behavior therapy. The decision to consider initiating medication at this age depends in part on the clinician's assessment of the estimated developmental impairment, safety risks, or consequences for school or social participation that could ensue if medications are not initiated. It is often helpful to consult with a mental health specialist who has had specific experience with preschool-aged children if possible.

Dextroamphetamine is the only medication approved by the FDA for use in children younger than 6 years of age. This approval, however, was based on less stringent criteria in force when the medication was approved rather than on empirical evidence of its safety and efficacy in this age group. Most of the evidence for the safety and efficacy of treating preschool-aged children with stimulant medications has been

from methylphenidate.[57] Methylphenidate evidence consists of 1 multisite study of 165 children and 10 other smaller single-site studies that included from 11 to 59 children (total of 269 children); 7 of the 10 single-site studies found significant efficacy. It must be noted that although there is moderate evidence that methylphenidate is safe and efficacious in preschool-aged children, its use in this age group remains off-label. Although the use of dextroamphetamine is on-label, the insufficient evidence for its safety and efficacy in this age group does not make it possible to recommend at this time.

If children do not experience adequate symptom improvement with behavior therapy, medication can be prescribed, as described previously. Evidence suggests that the rate of metabolizing stimulant medication is slower in children 4 through 5 years of age, so they should be given a lower dose to start, and the dose can be increased in smaller increments. Maximum doses have not been adequately studied.[57]

Special Circumstances: Adolescents

As noted previously, before beginning medication treatment for adolescents with newly diagnosed ADHD, clinicians should assess these patients for symptoms of substance abuse. When substance use is identified, assessment when off the abusive substances should precede treatment for ADHD (see the Task Force on Mental Health report[7]). Diversion of ADHD medication (use for other than its intended medical purposes) is also a special concern among adolescents[58]; clinicians should monitor symptoms and prescription-refill requests for signs of misuse or diversion of ADHD medication and consider prescribing medications with no abuse potential, such as atomoxetine (Strattera [Ely Lilly Co, Indianapolis, IN]) and

extended-release guanfacine (Intuniv [Shire US Inc, Wayne, PA]) or extended-release clonidine (Kapvay [Shionogi Inc, Florham Park, NJ]) (which are not stimulants) or stimulant medications with less abuse potential, such as lisdexamfetamine (Vyvanse [Shire US Inc]), dermal methylphenidate (Daytrana [Noven Therapeutics, LLC, Miami, FL]), or OROS methylphenidate (Concerta [Janssen Pharmaceuticals, Inc, Titusville, NJ]). Because lisdexamfetamine is dextroamphetamine, which contains an additional lysine molecule, it is only activated after ingestion, when it is metabolized by erythrocyte cells to dexamphetamine. The other preparations make extraction of the stimulant medication more difficult.

Given the inherent risks of driving by adolescents with ADHD, special concern should be taken to provide medication coverage for symptom control while driving. Longer-acting or late-afternoon, short-acting medications might be helpful in this regard.[59]

Special Circumstances: Inattention or Hyperactivity/Impulsivity (Problem Level)

Medication is not appropriate for children whose symptoms do not meet DSM-IV criteria for diagnosis of ADHD, although behavior therapy does not require a specific diagnosis, and many of the efficacy studies have included children without specific mental behavioral disorders.

Behavior Therapy

Behavior therapy represents a broad set of specific interventions that have a common goal of modifying the physical and social environment to alter or change behavior. Behavior therapy usually is implemented by training parents in specific techniques that improve their abilities to modify and

TABLE 1 Evidence-Based Behavioral Treatments for ADHD

Intervention Type	Description	Typical Outcome(s)	Median Effect Size[a]
Behavioral parent training (BPT)	Behavior-modification principles provided to parents for implementation in home settings	Improved compliance with parental commands; improved parental understanding of behavioral principles; high levels of parental satisfaction with treatment	0.55
Behavioral classroom management	Behavior-modification principles provided to teachers for implementation in classroom settings	Improved attention to instruction; improved compliance with classroom rules; decreased disruptive behavior; improved work productivity	0.61
Behavioral peer interventions (BPI)[b]	Interventions focused on peer interactions/relationships; these are often group-based interventions provided weekly and include clinic-based social-skills training used either alone or concurrently with behavioral parent training and/or medication	Office-based interventions have produced minimal effects; interventions have been of questionable social validity; some studies of BPI combined with clinic-based BPT found positive effects on parent ratings of ADHD symptoms; no differences on social functioning or parent ratings of social behavior have been revealed	

[a] Effect size = (treatment median − control median)/control SD.
[b] The effect size for behavioral peer interventions is not reported, because the effect sizes for these studies represent outcomes associated with combined interventions. A lower effect size means that they have less of an effect. The effect sizes found are considered moderate.
Adapted from Pelham W, Fabiano GA. *J Clin Child Adolesc Psychol.* 2008;37(1):184–214.

shape their child's behavior and to improve the child's ability to regulate his or her own behavior. The training involves techniques to more effectively provide rewards when their child demonstrates the desired behavior (eg, positive reinforcement), learn what behaviors can be reduced or eliminated by using planned ignoring as an active strategy (or using praising and ignoring in combination), or provide appropriate consequences or punishments when their child fails to meet the goals (eg, punishment). There is a need to consistently apply rewards and consequences as tasks are achieved and then to gradually increase the expectations for each task as they are mastered to shape behaviors. Although behavior therapy shares a set of principles, individual programs introduce different techniques and strategies to achieve the same ends.

Table 1 lists the major behavioral intervention approaches that have been demonstrated to be evidence based for the management of ADHD in 3 different types of settings. The table is based on 22 studies, each completed between 1997 and 2006.

Evidence for the effectiveness of behavior therapy in children with ADHD is derived from a variety of studies[60–62] and an Agency for Healthcare Research and Quality review.[5] The diversity of interventions and outcome measures makes meta-analysis of the effects of behavior therapy alone or in association with medications challenging. The long-term positive effects of behavior therapy have yet to be determined. Ongoing adherence to a behavior program might be important; therefore, implementing a chronic care model for child health might contribute to the long-term effects.[63]

Study results have indicated positive effects of behavior therapy when combined with medications. Most studies that compared behavior therapy to stimulants found a much stronger effect on ADHD core symptoms from stimulants than from behavior therapy. The MTA study found that combined treatment (behavior therapy and stimulant medication) was not significantly more efficacious than treatment with medication alone for the core symptoms of ADHD after correction for multiple tests in the primary analysis.[64] However, a secondary analysis of a combined measure of parent and teacher ratings of ADHD symptoms revealed a significant advantage for the combination with a small effect size of $d = 0.26$.[65] However, the same study also found that the combined treatment compared with medication alone did offer greater improvements on academic and conduct measures when ADHD coexisted with anxiety and when children lived in low socioeconomic environments. In addition, parents and teachers of children who were receiving combined therapy were significantly more satisfied with the treatment plan. Finally, the combination of medication management and behavior therapy allowed for the use of lower dosages of stimulants, which possibly reduced the risk of adverse effects.[66]

School Programming and Supports

Behavior therapy programs coordinating efforts at school as well as home might enhance the effects. School programs can provide classroom adaptations, such as preferred seating, modified work assignments, and test modifications (to the location at which it is administered and time allotted for taking the test), as well as behavior plans as part of a 504 Rehabilitation Act Plan or special education Individualized Education Program (IEP) under the "other health impairment" designation as part of the Individuals With

Disability Education Act (IDEA).[67] It is helpful for clinicians to be aware of the eligibility criteria in their state and school district to advise families of their options. Youths documented to have ADHD can also get permission to take college-readiness tests in an untimed manner by following appropriate documentation guidelines.[68]

The effect of coexisting conditions on ADHD treatment is variable. In some cases, treatment of the ADHD resolves the coexisting condition. For example, treatment of ADHD might resolve oppositional defiant disorder or anxiety.[68] However, sometimes the co-occurring condition might require treatment that is in addition to the treatment for ADHD. Some coexisting conditions can be treated in the primary care setting, but others will require referral and co-management with a subspecialist.

Action statement 6: Primary care clinicians should titrate doses of medication for ADHD to achieve maximum benefit with minimum adverse effects (quality of evidence B/strong recommendation).

Evidence Profile

- **Aggregate evidence quality:** B.
- **Benefits:** The optimal dose of medication is required to reduce core symptoms to or as close to the levels of children without ADHD.
- **Harms/risks/costs:** Higher levels of medication increase the chances of adverse effects.
- **Benefits-harms assessment:** The importance of adequately treating ADHD outweighs the risk of adverse effects.
- **Value judgments:** The committee members included the effects of untreated ADHD when deciding to make this recommendation.
- **Role of patient preferences:** The families' preferences and comfort need to be taken into consideration in developing a titration plan.
- **Exclusions:** None.

- **Intentional vagueness:** None.
- **Strength: strong recommendation.**

The findings from the MTA study suggested that more than 70% of children and youth with ADHD respond to one of the stimulant medications at an optimal dose when a systematic trial is used.[65] Children in the MTA who were treated in the community with care as usual from whomever they chose or to whom they had access received lower doses of stimulants with less frequent monitoring and had less optimal results.[65] Because stimulants might produce positive but suboptimal effects at a low dose in some children and youth, titration to maximum doses that control symptoms without adverse effects is recommended instead of titration strictly on a milligram-per-kilogram basis.

Education of parents is an important component in the chronic illness model to ensure their cooperation in efforts to reach appropriate titration (remembering that the parents themselves might be challenged significantly by ADHD).[69,70] The primary care clinician should alert parents and children that changing medication dose and occasionally changing a medication might be necessary for optimal medication management, that the process might require a few months to achieve optimal success, and that medication efficacy should be systematically monitored at regular intervals.

Because stimulant medication effects are seen immediately, trials of different doses of stimulants can be accomplished in a relatively short time period. Stimulant medications can be effectively titrated on a 3- to 7-day basis.[65]

It is important to note that by the 3-year follow-up of 14-month MTA interventions (optimal medications management, optimal behavioral management, the combination of the 2, or community treatment), all differences among the initial 4

groups were no longer present. After the initial 14-month intervention, the children no longer received the careful monthly monitoring provided by the study and went back to receiving care from their community providers. Their medications and doses varied, and a number of them were no longer taking medication. In children still on medication, the growth deceleration was only seen for the first 2 years and was in the range of 1 to 2 cm.

CONCLUSION

Evidence continues to be fairly clear with regard to the legitimacy of the diagnosis of ADHD and the appropriate diagnostic criteria and procedures required to establish a diagnosis, identify co-occurring conditions, and treat effectively with both behavioral and pharmacologic interventions. However, the steps required to sustain appropriate treatments and achieve successful long-term outcomes still remain a challenge. To provide more detailed information about how the recommendations of this guideline can be accomplished, a more detailed but less strongly evidence-based algorithm is provided as a companion article.

AREAS FOR FUTURE RESEARCH

Some specific research topics pertinent to the diagnosis and treatment of ADHD or developmental variations or problems in children and adolescents in primary care to be explored include:

- identification or development of reliable instruments suitable to use in primary care to assess the nature or degree of functional impairment in children/adolescents with ADHD and monitor improvement over time;
- study of medications and other therapies used clinically but not approved by the FDA for ADHD, such as

electroencephalographic biofeedback;

- determination of the optimal schedule for monitoring children/adolescents with ADHD, including factors for adjusting that schedule according to age, symptom severity, and progress reports;
- evaluation of the effectiveness of various school-based interventions;
- comparisons of medication use and effectiveness in different ages, including both harms and benefits;
- development of methods to involve parents and children/adolescents in their own care and improve adherence to both behavior and medication treatments;
- standardized and documented tools that will help primary care providers in identifying coexisting conditions;
- development and determination of effective electronic and Web-based systems to help gather information to diagnose and monitor children with ADHD;
- improved systems of communication with schools and mental health professionals, as well as other community agencies, to provide effective collaborative care;
- evidence for optimal monitoring by

some aspects of severity, disability, or impairment; and

- long-term outcomes of children first identified with ADHD as preschool-aged children.

SUBCOMMITTEE ON ATTENTION DEFICIT HYPERACTIVITY DISORDER (OVERSIGHT BY THE STEERING COMMITTEE ON QUALITY IMPROVEMENT AND MANAGEMENT, 2005–2011)

WRITING COMMITTEE

Mark Wolraich, MD, Chair – *(periodic consultant to Shire, Eli Lilly, Shinogi, and Next Wave Pharmaceuticals)*

Lawrence Brown, MD – *(neurologist; AAP Section on Neurology; Child Neurology Society) (Safety Monitoring Board for Best Pharmaceuticals for Children Act for National Institutes of Health)*

Ronald T. Brown, PhD – *(child psychologist; Society for Pediatric Psychology) (no conflicts)*

George DuPaul, PhD – *(school psychologist; National Association of School Psychologists) (participated in clinical trial on Vyvanse effects on college students with ADHD, funded by Shire; published 2 books on ADHD and receives royalties)*

Marian Earls, MD – *(general pediatrician with QI expertise, developmental and behavioral pediatrician) (no conflicts)*

Heidi M. Feldman, MD, PhD – *(developmental and behavioral pediatrician; Society for Developmental and Behavioral Pediatricians) (no conflicts)*

Theodore G. Ganiats, MD – *(family physician; American Academy of Family Physicians) (no conflicts)*

Beth Kaplanek, RN, BSN – *(parent advocate, Children and Adults With Attention Deficit Hyperactivity Disorder [CHADD]) (no conflicts)*

Bruce Meyer, MD – *(general pediatrician) (no conflicts)*

James Perrin, MD – *(general pediatrician; AAP Mental Health Task Force, AAP Council on Children With Disabilities) (consultant to Pfizer not related to ADHD)*

Karen Pierce, MD – *(child psychiatrist; American Academy of Child and Adolescent Psychiatry) (no conflicts)*

Michael Reiff, MD – *(developmental and behavioral pediatrician; AAP Section on Developmental and Behavioral Pediatrics) (no conflicts)*

Martin T. Stein, MD – *(developmental and behavioral pediatrician; AAP Section on Developmental and Behavioral Pediatrics) (no conflicts)*

Susanna Visser, MS – *(epidemiologist) (no conflicts)*

CONSULTANT
Melissa Capers, MA, MFA – *(medical writer) (no conflicts)*

STAFF
Caryn Davidson, MA

ACKNOWLEDGMENTS

This guideline was developed with support from the Partnership for Policy Implementation (PPI) initiative. Physicians trained in medical informatics were involved with formatting the algorithm and helping to keep the key action statements actionable, decidable, and executable.

REFERENCES

1. American Academy of Pediatrics, Committee on Quality Improvement and Subcommittee on Attention-Deficit/Hyperactivity Disorder. Clinical practice guideline: diagnosis and evaluation of the child with attention-deficit/hyperactivity disorder. *Pediatrics.* 2000;105(5):1158–1170

2. American Academy of Pediatrics, Subcommittee on Attention-Deficit/Hyperactivity Disorder, Committee on Quality Improvement. Clinical practice guideline: treatment of the school-aged child with attention-deficit/hyperactivity disorder. *Pediatrics.* 2001;108(4):1033–1044

3. Wolraich ML, Felice ME, Drotar DD. *The Classification of Child and Adolescent Mental Conditions in Primary Care: Diagnostic and Statistical Manual for Primary Care (DSM-PC), Child and Adolescent Version.* Elk Grove, IL: American Academy of Pediatrics; 1996

4. *EndNote* [computer program]. 10th ed. Carlsbad, CA: Thompson Reuters; 2009

5. Charach A, Dashti B, Carson P, Booker L, Lim CG, Lillie E, Yeung E, Ma J, Raina P, Schachar R. *Attention Deficit Hyperactivity Disorder: Effectiveness of Treatment in At-Risk Preschoolers; Long-term Effectiveness in All Ages; and Variability in Prevalence, Diagnosis, and Treatment.* Comparative Effectiveness Review No. 44. (Prepared by the McMaster University Evidence-based Practice Center under Contract No. MME2202 290-02-0020.)

AHRQ Publication No. 12-EHC003-EF. Rockville, MD: Agency for Healthcare Research and Quality. October 2011.

6. American Academy of Pediatrics, Steering Committee on Quality Improvement. Classifying recommendations for clinical practice guidelines. *Pediatrics.* 2004;114(3):874–877

7. Foy JM; American Academy of Pediatrics Task Force on Mental Health. Enhancing pediatric mental health care: report from the American Academy of Pediatrics Task Force on Mental Health. Introduction. *Pediatrics.* 2010;125(suppl 3)S69–S174

8. Visser SN, Lesesne CA, Perou R. National estimates and factors associated with medication treatment for childhood

attention-deficit/hyperactivity disorder. *Pediatrics.* 2007;119(suppl 1):S99–S106

9. Centers for Disease Control and Prevention. Mental health in the United States: prevalence of diagnosis and medication treatment for attention-deficit/hyperactivity disorder—United States, 2003. *MMWR Morb Mortal Wkly Rep.* 2005; 54(34):842–847

10. Centers for Disease Control and Prevention. Increasing prevalence of parent-reported attention deficit/hyperactivity disorder among children: United States, 2003–2007. *MMWR Morb Mortal Wkly Rep.* 2010;59(44): 1439–1443

11. Egger HL, Kondo D, Angold A. The epidemiology and diagnostic issues in preschool attention-deficit/hyperactivity disorder. *Infant Young Child.* 2006;19(2):109–122

12. Wolraich ML, Wibbelsman CJ, Brown TE, et al. Attention-deficit/hyperactivity disorder among adolescents: a review of the diagnosis, treatment, and clinical implications. *Pediatrics.* 2005;115(6):1734–1746

13. American Psychiatric Association. *Diagnostic and Statistical Manual of Mental Disorders, 4th ed, Text Revision (DSM-IV-TR).* Washington, DC: American Psychiatric Association; 2000

14. American Psychiatric Association. Diagnostic criteria for attention deficit/hyperactivity disorder. Available at: www.dsm5.org/ProposedRevision/Pages/proposedrevision.aspx?rid=383. Accessed September 30, 2011

15. Lahey BB, Pelham WE, Stein MA, et al. Validity of DSM-IV attention-deficit/hyperactivity disorder for younger children [published correction appears in *J Am Acad Child Adolesc Psychiatry.* 1999;38(2):222]. *J Am Acad Child Adolesc Psychiatry.* 1998;37(7):695–702

16. Pavuluri MN, Luk SL, McGee R. Parent reported preschool attention deficit hyperactivity: measurement and validity. *Eur Child Adolesc Psychiatry.* 1999;8(2): 126–133

17. Harvey EA, Youngwirth SD, Thakar DA, Errazuriz PA. Predicting attention-deficit/hyperactivity disorder and oppositional defiant disorder from preschool diagnostic assessments. *J Consult Clin Psychol.* 2009; 77(2):349–354

18. Keenan K, Wakschlag LS. More than the terrible twos: the nature and severity of behavior problems in clinic-referred preschool children. *J Abnorm Child Psychol.* 2000; 28(1):33–46

19. Gadow KD, Nolan EE, Litcher L, et al. Comparison of attention-deficit/hyperactivity disorder symptoms subtypes in Ukrainian schoolchildren. *J Am Acad Child Adolesc Psychiatry.* 2000;39(12):1520–1527

20. Sprafkin J, Volpe RJ, Gadow KD, Nolan EE, Kelly K. A DSM-IV-referenced screening instrument for preschool children: the Early Childhood Inventory-4. *J Am Acad Child Adolesc Psychiatry.* 2002;41(5): 604–612

21. Poblano A, Romero E. ECI-4 screening of attention deficit-hyperactivity disorder and co-morbidity in Mexican preschool children: preliminary results. *Arq Neuropsiquiatr.* 2006;64(4):932–936

22. McGoey KE, DuPaul GJ, Haley E, Shelton TL. Parent and teacher ratings of attention-deficit/hyperactivity disorder in preschool: the ADHD Rating Scale-IV Preschool Version. *J Psychopathol Behav Assess.* 2007;29(4): 269–276

23. Young J. Common comorbidities seen in adolescents with attention-deficit/hyperactivity disorder. *Adolesc Med State Art Rev.* 2008;19(2): 216–228, vii

24. Freeman R; Tourette Syndrome International Database Consortium. Tic disorders and ADHD: answers from a worldwide clinical dataset on Tourette syndrome [published correction appears in *Eur Child Adolesc Psychiatry.* 2007; 16(8):536]. *Eur Child Adolesc Psychiatry.* 2007;16(1 suppl):15–23

25. Riggs P. Clinical approach to treatment of ADHD in adolescents with substance use disorders and conduct disorder. *J Am Acad Child Adolesc Psychiatry.* 1998;37(3): 331–332

26. Kratochvil CJ, Vaughan BS, Stoner JA, et al. A double-blind, placebo-controlled study of atomoxetine in young children with ADHD. *Pediatrics.* 2011;127(4). Available at: www.pediatrics.org/cgi/content/full/127/4/e862

27. Rowland AS, Lesesne CA, Abramowitz AJ. The epidemiology of attention-deficit/hyperactivity disorder (ADHD): a public health view. *Ment Retard Dev Disabil Res Rev.* 2002;8(3):162–170

28. Cuffe SP, Moore CG, McKeown RE. Prevalence and correlates of ADHD symptoms in the national health interview survey. *J Atten Disord.* 2005;9(2):392–401

29. Pastor PN, Reuben CA. Diagnosed attention deficit hyperactivity disorder and learning disability: United States, 2004–2006. *Vital Health Stat 10.* 2008;(237):1–14

30. Biederman J, Faraone SV, Wozniak J, Mick E, Kwon A, Aleardi M. Further evidence of unique developmental phenotypic correlates of pediatric bipolar disorder: findings from a large sample of clinically referred preadolescent children assessed over the last 7 years. *J Affect Disord.* 2004;82(suppl 1):S45–S58

31. Biederman J, Kwon A, Aleardi M. Absence of gender effects on attention deficit hyperactivity disorder: findings in nonreferred subjects. *Am J Psychiatry.* 2005;162(6): 1083–1089

32. Biederman J, Ball SW, Monuteaux MC, et al. New insights into the comorbidity between ADHD and major depression in adolescent and young adult females. *J Am Acad Child Adolesc Psychiatry.* 2008; 47(4):426–434

33. Biederman J, Melmed RD, Patel A, McBurnett K, Donahue J, Lyne A. Long-term, open-label extension study of guanfacine extended release in children and adolescents with ADHD. *CNS Spectr.* 2008;13(12): 1047–1055

34. Crabtree VM, Ivanenko A, Gozal D. Clinical and parental assessment of sleep in children with attention-deficit/hyperactivity disorder referred to a pediatric sleep medicine center. *Clin Pediatr (Phila).* 2003;42(9): 807–813

35. LeBourgeois MK, Avis K, Mixon M, Olmi J, Harsh J. Snoring, sleep quality, and sleepiness across attention-deficit/hyperactivity disorder subtypes. *Sleep.* 2004;27(3): 520–525

36. Chan E, Zhan C, Homer CJ. Health care use and costs for children with attention-deficit/hyperactivity disorder: national estimates from the medical expenditure panel survey. *Arch Pediatr Adolesc Med.* 2002; 156(5):504–511

37. Newcorn JH, Miller SR, Ivanova I, et al. Adolescent outcome of ADHD: impact of childhood conduct and anxiety disorders. *CNS Spectr.* 2004;9(9):668–678

38. Sung V, Hiscock H, Sciberras E, Efron D. Sleep problems in children with attention-deficit/hyperactivity disorder: prevalence and the effect on the child and family. *Arch Pediatr Adolesc Med.* 2008; 162(4):336–342

39. American Academy of Pediatrics, Task Force on Mental Health. *Addressing Mental Health Concerns in Primary Care: A Clinician's Toolkit* [CD-ROM]. Elk Grove Village, IL: American Academy of Pediatrics; 2010

40. American Academy of Pediatrics, Committee on Child Health Financing. Scope of health care benefits for children from birth through age 26. *Pediatrics.* 2012; In press

41. Brito A, Grant R, Overholt S, et al. The enhanced medical home: the pediatric standard of care for medically underserved children. *Adv Pediatr.* 2008;55:9–28

42. Homer C, Klatka K, Romm D, et al. A review of the evidence for the medical home for children with special health care needs. *Pediatrics*. 2008;122(4). Available at: www.pediatrics.org/cgi/content/full/122/4/e922

43. Ingram S, Hechtman L, Morgenstern G. Outcome issues in ADHD: adolescent and adult long-term outcome. *Ment Retard Dev Disabil Res Rev*. 1999;5(3):243–250

44. Barbaresi WJ, Katusic SK, Colligan RC, Weaver AL, Jacobsen SJ. Modifiers of long-term school outcomes for children with attention-deficit/hyperactivity disorder: does treatment with stimulant medication make a difference? Results from a population-based study. *J Dev Behav Pediatr*. 2007;28(4):274–287

45. Cheng JY, Cheng RY, Ko JS, Ng EM. Efficacy and safety of atomoxetine for attention-deficit/hyperactivity disorder in children and adolescents-meta-analysis and meta-regression analysis. *Psychopharmacology*. 2007;194(2):197–209

46. Michelson D, Allen AJ, Busner J, Casat C, Dunn D, Kratochvil CJ. Once daily atomoxetine treatment for children and adolescents with ADHD: a randomized, placebo-controlled study. *Am J Psychiatry*. 2002; 159(11):1896–1901

47. Biederman J, Melmed RD, Patel A, et al; SPD503 Study Group. A randomized, double-blind, placebo-controlled study of guanfacine extended release in children and adolescents with attention-deficit/hyperactivity disorder. *Pediatrics*. 2008;121(1). Available at: www.pediatrics.org/cgi/content/full/121/1/e73

48. Sallee FR, Lyne A, Wigal T, McGough JJ. Long-term safety and efficacy of guanfacine extended release in children and adolescents with attention-deficit/hyperactivity disorder. *J Child Adolesc Psychopharmacol*. 2009;19(3):215–226

49. Jain R, Segal S, Kollins SH, Khayrallah M. Clonidine extended-release tablets for pediatric patients with attention-deficit/hyperactivity disorder. *J Am Acad Child Adolesc Psychiatry*. 2011;50(2):171–179

50. Newcorn J, Kratochvil CJ, Allen AJ, et al. Atomoxetine and osmotically released methylphenidate for the treatment of attention deficit hyperactivity disorder: acute comparison and differential response. *Am J Psychiatry*. 2008;165(6):721–730

51. Swanson J, Elliott GR, Greenhill LL, et al. Effects of stimulant medication on growth rates across 3 years in the MTA follow-up. *J Am Acad Child Adolesc Psychiatry*. 2007; 46(8):1015–1027

52. Mosholder AD, Gelperin K, Hammad TA, Phelan K, Johann-Liang R. Hallucinations and other psychotic symptoms associated with the use of attention-deficit/hyperactivity disorder drugs in children. *Pediatrics*. 2009;123(2):611–616

53. Avigan M. *Review of AERS Data From Marketed Safety Experience During Stimulant Therapy: Death, Sudden Death, Cardiovascular SAEs (Including Stroke)*. Silver Spring, MD: Food and Drug Administration, Center for Drug Evaluation and Research; 2004. Report No. D030403

54. Perrin JM, Friedman RA, Knilans TK, et al; American Academy of Pediatrics, Black Box Working Group, Section on Cardiology and Cardiac Surgery. Cardiovascular monitoring and stimulant drugs for attention-deficit/hyperactivity disorder. *Pediatrics*. 2008;122(2):451–453

55. McCarthy S, Cranswick N, Potts L, Taylor E, Wong IC. Mortality associated with attention-deficit hyperactivity disorder (ADHD) drug treatment: a retrospective cohort study of children, adolescents and young adults using the general practice research database. *Drug Saf*. 2009;32(11): 1089–1110

56. Gould MS, Walsh BT, Munfakh JL, et al. Sudden death and use of stimulant medications in youths. *Am J Psychiatry*. 2009;166(9):992–1001

57. Greenhill L, Kollins S, Abikoff H, McCracken J, Riddle M, Swanson J. Efficacy and safety of immediate-release methylphenidate treatment for preschoolers with ADHD. *J Am Acad Child Adolesc Psychiatry*. 2006;45(11): 1284–1293

58. Low K, Gendaszek AE. Illicit use of psychostimulants among college students: a preliminary study. *Psychol Health Med*. 2002; 7(3):283–287

59. Cox D, Merkel RL, Moore M, Thorndike F, Muller C, Kovatchev B. Relative benefits of stimulant therapy with OROS methylphenidate versus mixed amphetamine salts extended release in improving the driving performance of adolescent drivers with attention-deficit/hyperactivity disorder. *Pediatrics*. 2006;118(3). Available at: www.pediatrics.org/cgi/content/full/118/3/e704

60. Pelham W, Wheeler T, Chronis A. Empirically supported psychological treatments for attention deficit hyperactivity disorder. *J Clin Child Psychol*. 1998;27(2):190–205

61. Sonuga-Barke E, Daley D, Thompson M, Laver-Bradbury C, Weeks A. Parent-based therapies for preschool attention-deficit/hyperactivity disorder: a randomized, controlled trial with a community sample. *J Am Acad Child Adolesc Psychiatry*. 2001;40(4):402–408

62. Pelham W, Fabiano GA. Evidence-based psychosocial treatments for attention-deficit/hyperactivity disorder. *J Clin Child Adolesc Psychol*. 2008;37(1):184–214

63. Van Cleave J, Leslie LK. Approaching ADHD as a chronic condition: implications for long-term adherence. *J Psychosoc Nurs Ment Health Serv*. 2008;46(8):28–36

64. A 14-month randomized clinical trial of treatment strategies for attention-deficit/hyperactivity disorder. The MTA Cooperative Group. Multimodal Treatment Study of Children With ADHD. *Arch Gen Psychiatry*. 1999;56(12):1073–1086

65. Jensen P, Hinshaw SP, Swanson JM, et al. Findings from the NIMH multimodal treatment study of ADHD (MTA): implications and applications for primary care providers. *J Dev Behav Pediatr*. 2001;22(1):60–73

66. Pelham WE, Gnagy EM. Psychosocial and combined treatments for ADHD. *Ment Retard Dev Disabil Res Rev*. 1999;5(3):225–236

67. Davila RR, Williams ML, MacDonald JT. Memorandum on clarification of policy to address the needs of children with attention deficit disorders within general and/or special education. In: Parker HC*The ADD Hyperactivity Handbook for Schools*. Plantation, FL: Impact Publications Inc; 1991:261–268

68. The College Board. Services for Students With Disabilities (SSD). Available at: www.collegeboard.com/ssd/student. Accessed July 8, 2011

69. Bodenheimer T, Wagner EH, Grumbach K. Improving primary care for patients with chronic illness. *JAMA* 2002;288:1775–1779

70. Bodenheimer T, Wagner EH, Grumbach K. Improving primary care for patients with chronic illness: the chronic care model, Part 2. *JAMA* 2002;288:1909–1914

Attention-Deficit/Hyperactivity Disorder Clinical Practice Guideline Quick Reference Tools

• •

- Action Statement Summary
  — ADHD: Clinical Practice Guideline for the Diagnosis, Evaluation, and Treatment
    of Attention-Deficit/Hyperactivity Disorder in Children and Adolescents
- *ICD-10-CM* Coding Quick Reference for ADHD
- Bonus Features
  — ADHD Coding Fact Sheet for Primary Care Physicians
  — Continuum Model for ADHD
- AAP Patient Education Handouts
  — *Understanding ADHD: Information for Parents About Attention-Deficit/Hyperactivity Disorder*
  — *Medicines for ADHD: Questions From Teens Who Have ADHD*
  — *What Is ADHD? Questions From Teens*

Action Statement Summary

ADHD: Clinical Practice Guideline for the Diagnosis, Evaluation, and Treatment of Attention-Deficit/ Hyperactivity Disorder in Children and Adolescents

Key Action Statement 1

The primary care clinician should initiate an evaluation for ADHD for any child 4 through 18 years of age who presents with academic or behavioral problems and symptoms of inattention, hyperactivity, or impulsivity (quality of evidence B/strong recommendation).

Key Action Statement 2

To make a diagnosis of ADHD, the primary care clinician should determine that *Diagnostic and Statistical Manual of Mental Disorders, Fourth Edition* (DSM-IV-TR) criteria have been met (including documentation of impairment in more than 1 major setting), and information should be obtained primarily from reports from parents or guardians, teachers, and other school and mental health clinicians involved in the child's care. The primary care clinician should also rule out any alternative cause (quality of evidence B/strong recommendation).

Key Action Statement 3

In the evaluation of a child for ADHD, the primary care clinician should include assessment for other conditions that might coexist with ADHD, including emotional or behavioral (eg, anxiety, depressive, oppositional defiant, and conduct disorders), developmental (eg, learning and language disorders or other neurodevelopmental disorders), and physical (eg, tics, sleep apnea) conditions (quality of evidence B/strong recommendation).

Key Action Statement 4

The primary care clinician should recognize ADHD as a chronic condition and, therefore, consider children and adolescents with ADHD as children and youth with special health care needs. Management of children and youth with special health care needs should follow the principles of the chronic care model and the medical home (quality of evidence B/strong recommendation).

Key Action Statement 5

Recommendations for treatment of children and youth with ADHD vary depending on the patient's age.

Key Action Statement 5a

For *preschool-aged children (4–5 years of age)*, the primary care clinician should prescribe evidence-based parent and/or teacher-administered behavior therapy as the first line of treatment (quality of evidence A/strong recommendation) and may prescribe methylphenidate if the behavior interventions do not provide significant improvement and there is moderate-to-severe continuing disturbance in the child's function. In areas in which evidence-based behavioral treatments are not available, the clinician needs to weigh the risks of starting medication at an early age against the harm of delaying diagnosis and treatment (quality of evidence B/recommendation).

Key Action Statement 5b

For *elementary school-aged children (6–11 years of age)*, the primary care clinician should prescribe FDA-approved medications for ADHD (quality of evidence A/strong recommendation) and/or evidence based parent- and/or teacher-administered behavior therapy as treatment for ADHD, preferably both (quality of evidence B/strong recommendation). The evidence is particularly strong for stimulant medications and sufficient but less strong for atomoxetine, extended-release guanfacine, and extended-release clonidine (in that order) (quality of evidence A/strong recommendation). The school environment, program, or placement is a part of any treatment plan.

Key Action Statement 5c

For *adolescents (12–18 years of age)*, the primary care clinician should prescribe FDA-approved medications for ADHD with the assent of the adolescent (quality of evidence A/strong recommendation) and may prescribe behavior therapy as treatment for ADHD (quality of evidence C/recommendation), preferably both.

Key Action Statement 6

Primary care clinicians should titrate doses of medication for ADHD to achieve maximum benefit with minimum adverse effects (quality of evidence B/strong recommendation).

Coding Quick Reference for ADHD
ICD-10-CM
F90.0 Attention-deficit hyperactivity disorder, predominantly inattentive type
F90.1 Attention-deficit hyperactivity disorder, predominantly hyperactive type

ADHD Coding Fact Sheet for Primary Care Physicians

Current Procedural Terminology (Procedure) Codes

Initial assessment usually involves a lot of time determining differential diagnosis, a diagnostic plan, and potential treatment options. Therefore, most pediatricians will report either an office or outpatient evaluation and management (E/M) code using time as the key factor or a consultation code for the initial assessment.

Physician Evaluation and Management Services

*99201	Office or other outpatient visit, *new*[a] patient; self-limited or minor problem, 10 min.
*99202	low to moderate severity problem, 20 min.
*99203	moderate severity problem, 30 min.
*99204	moderate to high severity problem, 45 min.
*99205	high severity problem, 60 min.
*99211	Office or other outpatient visit, *established* patient; minimal problem, 5 min.
*99212	self-limited or minor problem, 10 min.
*99213	low to moderate severity problem, 15 min.
*99214	moderate severity problem, 25 min.
*99215	moderate to high severity problem, 40 min.
*99241	Office or other outpatient *consultation*,[b-d] new or established patient; self-limited or minor problem, 15 min.
*99242	low severity problem, 30 min.
*99243	moderate severity problem, 45 min.
*99244	moderate to high severity problem, 60 min.
*99245	moderate to high severity problem, 80 min.
*+99354	Prolonged physician services in office or other outpatient setting, with direct patient contact; first hour (*use in conjunction with time-based codes* **99201–99215, 99241–99245, 99301–99350, 90837**)
*+99355	each additional 30 min. (*use in conjunction with* **99354**)

- Used when a physician provides prolonged services beyond the usual service (ie, beyond the typical time).
- Time spent does not have to be continuous.
- Prolonged service of less than 15 minutes beyond the first hour or less than 15 minutes beyond the final 30 minutes is not reported separately.
- If reporting E/M service based on time and not key factors (history, examination, medical decision-making), the physician must reach the typical time in the highest code in the code set being reported (eg, **99205, 99215, 99245**) before face-to-face prolonged services can be reported.
- Refer to *Current Procedural Terminology* (*CPT*®) for clinical staff prolonged services.

[a] A new patient is one who has not received any professional services (face-to-face services) rendered by physicians and other qualified health care professionals who may report E/M services using one or more specific *CPT* codes from the physician/qualified health care professional, or another physician/qualified health care professional of the exact same specialty and subspecialty who belongs to the same group practice, within the past 3 years.

[b] Use of these codes (**99241–99245**) requires the following actions:
1. Written or verbal request for consultation is documented in the patient chart.
2. Consultant's opinion, as well as any services ordered or performed, is documented in the patient chart.
3. Consultant's opinion and any services that are performed are prepared in a written report, which is sent to the requesting physician or other appropriate source.

[c] Patients/parents may not initiate a consultation.

[d] For more information on consultation code changes for 2010, see https://www.aap.org/en-us/professional-resources/practice-transformation/getting-paid/Coding-at-the-AAP/Pages/ADHD-Coding-Fact-Sheet.aspx.

+ Codes are *add-on codes*, meaning they are reported separately in addition to the appropriate code for the service provided.

* Indicates a *Current Procedural Terminology*–approved telemedicine service.

Reporting E/M Services Using "Time"

- When counseling or coordination of care dominates (more than 50%) the physician/patient or family encounter (face-to-face time in the office or other outpatient setting or floor/unit time in the hospital or nursing facility), time shall be considered the key or controlling factor to qualify for a particular level of evaluation and management (E/M) services.
- This includes time spent with parties who have assumed responsibility for care of the patient or decision-making, whether or not they are family members (eg, foster parents, person acting in loco parentis, legal guardian). The extent of counseling or coordination of care must be documented in the medical record.
- For coding purposes, face-to-face time for these services is defined as only that time that the physician spends face-to-face with the patient or family. This includes time in which the physician performs such tasks as obtaining a history, performing an examination, and counseling the patient.
- When codes are ranked in sequential typical times (eg, office-based E/M services, consultation codes) and the actual time is between 2 typical times, the code with the typical time closest to the actual time is used.
  — **Example:** A physician sees an established patient in the office to discuss current attention-deficit/hyperactivity disorder (ADHD) medication the patient was placed on. Total face-to-face time was 22 minutes, 15 of which were spent in counseling the mom and patient. Because more than 50% of the total time was spent in counseling, the physician would report the E/M service on the basis of time. The physician would report **99214** instead of **99213** because the total face-to-face time was closer to **99214** (25 minutes) than **99213** (15 minutes).

ADHD Follow-up During a Routine Preventive Medicine Service

- A good time to follow up with a patient regarding his or her attention-deficit/hyperactivity disorder (ADHD) could be during a preventive medicine service.
- If follow-up requires little additional work on behalf of the physician, it should be reported under the preventive medicine service rather than as a separate service.
- If follow-up work requires an additional evaluation and management (E/M) service in addition to the preventive medicine service, it should be reported as a separate service.
- Chronic conditions should be reported only if they are separately addressed.
- When reporting a preventive medicine service in addition to an office-based E/M service and the services are significant and separately identifiable, modifier **25** will be required on the office-based E/M service.
  — **Example:** A 12-year-old established patient presents for his routine preventive medicine service and while he and Mom are there, Mom asks about changing his ADHD medication because of some adverse effects he is experiencing. The physician completes the routine preventive medicine check and then addresses the mom's concerns in a separate service. The additional E/M service takes 15 minutes, about 10 of which the physician spends in counseling and coordinating care; therefore, the E/M service is reported on the basis of time.
    ~ Code **99394** and **99213-25** account for both E/M services and link each to the appropriate *International Classification of Diseases, 10th Revision, Clinical Modification* code.
    ~ Modifier **25** is required on the problem-oriented office visit code (eg, **99213**) when it is significant and separately identifiable from another service.

Physician Non–face-to-face Services

99339   Care Plan Oversight—Individual physician supervision of a patient (patient not present) in home, domiciliary or rest home (e.g., assisted living facility) requiring complex and multidisciplinary care modalities involving regular physician development and/or revision of care plans, review of subsequent reports of patient status, review of related laboratory and other studies, communication (including telephone calls) for purposes of assessment or care decisions with health care professional(s), family member(s), surrogate decision maker(s) (e.g., legal guardian) and/or key caregiver(s) involved in patient's care, integration of new information into the medical treatment plan and/or adjustment of medical therapy, within a calendar month; 15–29 minutes

99340   30 minutes or more

99358   Prolonged physician services without direct patient contact; first hour

+99359   each additional 30 min. (+ *use in conjunction* with **99358**)

99367   Medical team conference by physician with interdisciplinary team of health care professionals, patient and/or family not present, 30 minutes or more

99441   Telephone evaluation and management to patient, parent or guardian not originating from a related E/M service within the previous 7 days nor leading to an E/M service or procedure within the next 24 hours or soonest available appointment; 5–10 minutes of medical discussion

99442   11–20 minutes of medical discussion

99443   21–30 minutes of medical discussion

99444   Online E/M service provided by a physician or other qualified health care professional to an established patient, guardian or health care provider not originating from a related E/M service provided within the previous 7 days, using the internet or similar electronic communications network

Care Management Services

Codes are selected on the basis of the amount of time spent by clinical staff providing care coordination activities. *Current Procedural Terminology* clearly defines care coordination activities. To report chronic care management codes, you must

1. Provide 24/7 access to physicians or other qualified health care professionals or clinical staff.
2. Use a standardized methodology to identify patients who require chronic complex care coordination services.
3. Have an internal care coordination process/function whereby a patient identified as meeting requirements for these services starts receiving them in a timely manner.
4. Use a form and format in the medical record that is standardized within the practice.
5. Be able to engage and educate patients and caregivers as well as coordinate care among all service professionals, as appropriate for each patient.

99490   Chronic care management services, at least 20 minutes of clinical staff time directed by a physician or other qualified health care professional, per calendar month, with the following required elements:
- multiple (two or more) chronic conditions expected to last at least 12 months, or until the death of the patient;
- chronic conditions place the patient at significant risk of death, acute exacerbation/decompensation, or functional decline;
- comprehensive care plan established, implemented, revised, or monitored.

Chronic care management services are provided when medical or psychosocial needs of the patient require establishing, implementing, revising, or monitoring the care plan. If 20 minutes are not met within a calendar month, you do not report chronic care management. Refer to *CPT* for more information.

Psychiatry

+90785   Interactive complexity (Use in conjunction with codes for diagnostic psychiatric evaluation [**90791**, **90792**], psychotherapy [**90832**, **90834**, **90837**], psychotherapy when performed with an evaluation and management service [**90833**, **90836**, **90838**, **99201–99255**, **99304–99337**, **99341–99350**], and group psychotherapy [**90853**])

Psychiatric Diagnostic or Evaluative Interview Procedures

90791   Psychiatric diagnostic interview examination evaluation

90792   Psychiatric diagnostic evaluation with medical services

Psychotherapy

*90832   Psychotherapy, 30 min with patient;

*+90833   with medical E/M (Use in conjunction with **99201–99255**, **99304–99337**, **99341–99350**)

*90834   Psychotherapy, 45 min with patient;

*+90836   with medical E/M services (Use in conjunction with **99201–99255**, **99304–99337**, **99341–99350**)

*90837   Psychotherapy, 60 min with patient;

*+90838   with medical E/M services (Use in conjunction with **99201–99255**, **99304–99337**, **99341–99350**)

+90785   Interactive complexity (Use in conjunction with codes for diagnostic psychiatric evaluation [**90791**, **90792**], psychotherapy [**90832**, **90834**, **90837**], psychotherapy when performed with an evaluation and management service [**90833**, **90836**, **90838**, **99201–99255**, **99304–99337**, **99341–99350**], and group psychotherapy [**90853**])

Refers to specific communication factors that complicate the delivery of a psychiatric procedure. Common factors include more difficult communication with discordant or emotional family members and engagement of young and verbally undeveloped or impaired patients. Typical encounters include
- Patients who have other individuals legally responsible for their care
- Patients who request others to be present or involved in their care such as translators, interpreters, or additional family members

---

+ Codes are *add-on codes,* meaning they are reported separately in addition to the appropriate code for the service provided.

* Indicates a *Current Procedural Terminology*–approved telemedicine service.

- Patients who require the involvement of other third parties such as child welfare agencies, schools, or probation officers

*90846 Family psychotherapy (without patient present), 50 min

*90847 Family psychotherapy (conjoint psychotherapy) (with patient present), 50 min

Other Psychiatric Services/Procedures

90863 Pharmacologic management, including prescription and review of medication, when performed with psychotherapy services (Use in conjunction with **90832**, **90834**, **90837**)
- For pharmacologic management with psychotherapy services performed by a physician or other qualified health care professional who may report E/M codes, use the appropriate E/M codes (**99201–99255**, **99281–99285**, **99304–99337**, **99341–99350**) and the appropriate psychotherapy with E/M service (**90833**, **90836**, **90838**).
- Note code **90862** was deleted.

90887 Interpretation or explanation of results of psychiatric, other medical exams, or other accumulated data to family or other responsible persons, or advising them how to assist patient

90889 Preparation of reports on patient's psychiatric status, history, treatment, or progress (other than for legal or consultative purposes) for other physicians, agencies, or insurance carriers

Psychological Testing

96101 Psychological testing (includes psychodiagnostic assessment of emotionality, intellectual abilities, personality and psychopathology, e.g., MMPI, Rorschach, WAIS), per hour of the *psychologist's or physician's time*, both face-to-face time administering tests to the patient and time interpreting these test results and preparing the report

96102 Psychological testing (includes psychodiagnostic assessment of emotionality, intellectual abilities, personality and psychopathology, e.g., MMPI, Rorschach, WAIS), with *qualified health care professional* interpretation and report, administered by technician, per hour of technician time, face-to-face

96103 Psychological testing (includes psychodiagnostic assessment of emotionality, intellectual abilities, personality and psychopathology, e.g., MMPI, Rorschach, WAIS), administered by a computer, with *qualified health care professional* interpretation and report

96110 Developmental screening, with scoring and documentation, per standardized instrument (Do not use for ADHD screens or assessments)

96111 Developmental testing (includes assessment of motor, language, social, adaptive and/or cognitive functioning by standardized instruments) with interpretation and report

*96116 Neurobehavioral status exam (clinical assessment of thinking, reasoning and judgment, eg, acquired knowledge, attention, language, memory, planning and problem solving, and visual spatial abilities), per

hour of the psychologist's or physician's time, both face-to-face time with the patient and time interpreting test results and preparing the report

96127 Brief emotional/behavioral assessment (eg, depression inventory, attention-deficit/hyperactivity disorder [ADHD] scale), with scoring and documentation, per standardized instrument

Nonphysician Provider Services

99366 Medical team conference with interdisciplinary team of health care professionals, face-to-face with patient and/or family, 30 minutes or more, participation by a nonphysician qualified health care professional

99368 Medical team conference with interdisciplinary team of health care professionals, patient and/or family not present, 30 minutes or more, participation by a nonphysician qualified health care professional

96120 Neuropsychological testing (eg, Wisconsin Card Sorting Test), administered by a computer, with qualified health care professional interpretation and report

*96150 Health and behavior assessment performed by nonphysician provider (health-focused clinical interviews, behavior observations) to identify psychological, behavioral, emotional, cognitive or social factors important to management of physical health problems, 15 min., initial assessment

*96151 re-assessment

*96152 Health and behavior intervention performed by nonphysician provider to improve patient's health and well-being using cognitive, behavioral, social, and/or psychophysiological procedures designed to ameliorate specific disease-related problems, individual, 15 min.

*96153 group (2 or more patients)

*96154 family (with the patient present)

96155 family (without the patient present)

Non–face-to-face Services: Nonphysician

98966 Telephone assessment and management service provided by a qualified nonphysician health care professional to an established patient, parent or guardian not originating from a related assessment and management service provided within the previous seven days nor leading to an assessment and management service or procedure within the next 24 hours or soonest available appointment; 5–10 minutes of medical discussion

98967 11–20 minutes of medical discussion

98968 21–30 minutes of medical discussion

98969 Online assessment and management service provided by a qualified nonphysician health care professional to an established patient or guardian not originating from a related assessment and management service provided within the previous seven days nor using the internet or similar electronic communications network

Miscellaneous Services

99071 Educational supplies, such as books, tapes, or pamphlets, provided by the physician for the patient's education at cost to the physician

---

+ Codes are *add-on codes,* meaning they are reported separately in addition to the appropriate code for the service provided.

* Indicates a *Current Procedural Terminology*–approved telemedicine service.

International Classification of Diseases, 10th Revision, Clinical Modification Codes

- Use as many diagnosis codes that apply to document the patient's complexity and report the patient's symptoms or adverse environmental circumstances.
- Once a definitive diagnosis is established, report the appropriate definitive diagnosis code(s) as the primary code, plus any other symptoms the patient is exhibiting as secondary diagnoses that are not part of the usual disease course or are considered incidental.
- *International Classification of Diseases, 10th Revision, Clinical Modification* codes are only valid on or after October 1, 2015.

Depressive Disorders

F34.1	Dysthymic disorder (depressive personality disorder, dysthymia neurotic depression)
F39	Mood (affective) disorder, unspecified
F30.8	Other manic episode

Anxiety Disorders

F06.4	Anxiety disorder due to known physiological conditions
F40.10	Social phobia, unspecified
F40.11	Social phobia, generalized
F40.8	Phobic anxiety disorders, other (phobic anxiety disorder of childhood)
F40.9	Phobic anxiety disorder, unspecified
F41.1	Generalized anxiety disorder
F41.9	Anxiety disorder, unspecified

Feeding and Eating Disorders/Elimination Disorders

F50.89	Eating disorders, other
F50.9	Eating disorder, unspecified
F98.0	Enuresis not due to a substance or known physiological condition
F98.1	Encopresis not due to a substance or known physiological condition
F98.3	Pica (infancy or childhood)

Impulse Disorders

F63.9	Impulse disorder, unspecified

Trauma- and Stressor-Related Disorders

F43.20	Adjustment disorder, unspecified
F43.21	Adjustment disorder with depressed mood
F43.22	Adjustment disorder with anxiety
F43.23	Adjustment disorder with mixed anxiety and depressed mood
F43.24	Adjustment disorder with disturbance of conduct

Neurodevelopmental/Other Developmental Disorders

F70	Mild intellectual disabilities
F71	Moderate intellectual disabilities
F72	Severe intellectual disabilities
F73	Profound intellectual disabilities
F79	Unspecified intellectual disabilities
F80.0	Phonological (speech) disorder (speech-sound disorder)
F80.1	Expressive language disorder
F80.2	Mixed receptive-expressive language disorder
F80.4	Speech and language developmental delay due to hearing loss (code also hearing loss)
F80.81	Stuttering
F80.82	Social pragmatic communication disorder
F80.89	Other developmental disorders of speech and language
F80.9	Developmental disorder of speech and language, unspecified
F81.0	Specific reading disorder
F81.2	Mathematics disorder
F81.89	Other developmental disorders of scholastic skills
F82	Developmental coordination disorder
F84.0	Autistic disorder (autism spectrum disorder)
F88	Specified delays in development; other
F89	Unspecified delay in development
F81.9	Developmental disorder of scholastic skills, unspecified

Behavioral/Emotional Disorders

F90.0	Attention-deficit hyperactivity disorder, predominantly inattentive type
F90.1	Attention-deficit hyperactivity disorder, predominantly hyperactive type
F90.8	Attention-deficit hyperactivity disorder, other type
F90.9	Attention-deficit hyperactivity disorder, unspecified type
F91.1	Conduct disorder, childhood-onset type
F91.2	Conduct disorder, adolescent-onset type
F91.3	Oppositional defiant disorder
F91.9	Conduct disorder, unspecified
F93.0	Separation anxiety disorder
F93.8	Other childhood emotional disorders (relationship problems)
F93.9	Childhood emotional disorder, unspecified
F94.9	Childhood disorder of social functioning, unspecified
F95.0	Transient tic disorder
F95.1	Chronic motor or vocal tic disorder
F95.2	Tourette's disorder
F95.9	Tic disorder, unspecified
F98.8	Other specified behavioral and emotional disorders with onset usually occurring in childhood and adolescence (nail-biting, nose-picking, thumb-sucking)

Other

F07.81	Postconcussional syndrome
F07.89	Personality and behavioral disorders due to known physiological condition, other
F07.9	Personality and behavioral disorder due to known physiological condition, unspecified
F45.41	Pain disorder exclusively related to psychological factors
F48.8	Nonpsychotic mental disorders, other (neurasthenia)
F48.9	Nonpsychotic mental disorders, unspecified
F51.01	Primary insomnia
F51.02	Adjustment insomnia
F51.03	Paradoxical insomnia
F51.04	Psychophysiologic insomnia
F51.05	Insomnia due to other mental disorder (Code also associated mental disorder)
F51.09	Insomnia, other (not due to a substance or known physiological condition)
F51.3	Sleepwalking (somnambulism)
F51.4	Sleep terrors (night terrors)
F51.8	Other sleep disorders

+ Codes are *add-on codes,* meaning they are reported separately in addition to the appropriate code for the service provided.

* Indicates a *Current Procedural Terminology*–approved telemedicine service.

F93.8 Childhood emotional disorders, other
R46.89 Other symptoms and signs involving appearance and behavior

Substance-Related and Addictive Disorders

If a provider documents multiple patterns of use, only one should be reported. Use the following hierarchy: use–abuse–dependence (eg, if use and dependence are documented, only code for dependence).

When a minus symbol (-) is included in codes **F10–F17**, a last character is required. Be sure to include the last character from the following list:

0 anxiety disorder
2 sleep disorder
8 other disorder
9 unspecified disorder

Alcohol

F10.10 Alcohol abuse, uncomplicated (alcohol use disorder, mild)
F10.14 Alcohol abuse with alcohol-induced mood disorder
F10.159 Alcohol abuse with alcohol-induced psychotic disorder, unspecified
F10.18- Alcohol abuse with alcohol-induced
F10.19 Alcohol abuse with unspecified alcohol-induced disorder
F10.20 Alcohol dependence, uncomplicated
F10.21 Alcohol dependence, in remission
F10.24 Alcohol dependence with alcohol-induced mood disorder
F10.259 Alcohol dependence with alcohol-induced psychotic disorder, unspecified
F10.28- Alcohol dependence with alcohol-induced
F10.29 Alcohol dependence with unspecified alcohol-induced disorder
F10.94 Alcohol use, unspecified with alcohol-induced mood disorder
F10.959 Alcohol use, unspecified with alcohol-induced psychotic disorder, unspecified
F10.98- Alcohol use, unspecified with alcohol-induced
F10.99 Alcohol use, unspecified with unspecified alcohol-induced disorder

Cannabis

F12.10 Cannabis abuse, uncomplicated (cannabis use disorder, mild)
F12.18- Cannabis abuse with cannabis-induced
F12.19 Cannabis abuse with unspecified cannabis-induced disorder
F12.20 Cannabis dependence, uncomplicated
F12.21 Cannabis dependence, in remission
F12.28- Cannabis dependence with cannabis-induced
F12.29 Cannabis dependence with unspecified cannabis-induced disorder
F12.90 Cannabis use, unspecified, uncomplicated
F12.98- Cannabis use, unspecified with
F12.99 Cannabis use, unspecified with unspecified cannabis-induced disorder

Sedatives

F13.10 Sedative, hypnotic or anxiolytic abuse, uncomplicated (sedative, hypnotic, or anxiolytic use disorder, mild)
F13.129 Sedative, hypnotic or anxiolytic abuse with intoxication, unspecified
F13.14 Sedative, hypnotic or anxiolytic abuse with sedative, hypnotic or anxiolytic-induced mood disorder
F13.18- Sedative, hypnotic or anxiolytic abuse with sedative, hypnotic or anxiolytic-induced
F13.21 Sedative, hypnotic or anxiolytic dependence, in remission
F13.90 Sedative, hypnotic or anxiolytic use, unspecified, uncomplicated
F13.94 Sedative, hypnotic or anxiolytic use, unspecified with sedative, hypnotic or anxiolytic-induced mood disorder
F13.98- Sedative, hypnotic or anxiolytic use, unspecified with sedative, hypnotic or anxiolytic-induced
F13.99 Sedative, hypnotic or anxiolytic use, unspecified with unspecified sedative, hypnotic or anxiolytic-induced disorder

Stimulants (eg, caffeine, amphetamines)

F15.10 Other stimulant (amphetamine-related disorders or caffeine) abuse, uncomplicated (amphetamine, other or unspecified stimulant type substance use disorder, mild)
F15.14 Other stimulant (amphetamine-related disorders or caffeine) abuse with stimulant-induced mood disorder
F15.18- Other stimulant (amphetamine-related disorders or caffeine) abuse with stimulant-induced
F15.19 Other stimulant (amphetamine-related disorders or caffeine) abuse with unspecified stimulant-induced disorder
F15.20 Other stimulant (amphetamine-related disorders or caffeine) dependence, uncomplicated
F15.21 Other stimulant (amphetamine-related disorders or caffeine) dependence, in remission
F15.24 Other stimulant (amphetamine-related disorders or caffeine) dependence with stimulant-induced mood disorder
F15.28- Other stimulant (amphetamine-related disorders or caffeine) dependence with stimulant-induced
F15.29 Other stimulant (amphetamine-related disorders or caffeine) dependence with unspecified stimulant-induced disorder
F15.90 Other stimulant (amphetamine-related disorders or caffeine) use, unspecified, uncomplicated
F15.94 Other stimulant (amphetamine-related disorders or caffeine) use, unspecified with stimulant-induced mood disorder
F15.98- Other stimulant (amphetamine-related disorders or caffeine) use, unspecified with stimulant-induced
F15.99 Other stimulant (amphetamine-related disorders or caffeine) use, unspecified with unspecified stimulant-induced disorder

Nicotine (eg, cigarettes)

F17.200 Nicotine dependence, unspecified, uncomplicated (tobacco use disorder, mild, moderate, or severe)
F17.201 Nicotine dependence, unspecified, in remission
F17.203 Nicotine dependence unspecified, with withdrawal
F17.20- Nicotine dependence, unspecified, with
F17.210 Nicotine dependence, cigarettes, uncomplicated

F17.211 Nicotine dependence, cigarettes, in remission
F17.213 Nicotine dependence, cigarettes, with withdrawal
F17.218- Nicotine dependence, cigarettes, with

Symptoms, Signs, and Ill-Defined Conditions

Use these codes in absence of a definitive mental diagnosis or when the sign or symptom is not part of the disease course or considered incidental.

G47.9 Sleep disorder, unspecified
H90.0 Conductive hearing loss, bilateral
H90.11 Conductive hearing loss, unilateral, right ear, with unrestricted hearing on the contralateral side
H90.12 Conductive hearing loss, unilateral, left ear, with unrestricted hearing on the contralateral side
H90.A1 Conductive hearing loss, unilateral, with restricted hearing on the contralateral side
H90.A2 Sensorineural hearing loss, unilateral, with restricted hearing on the contralateral side
H90.A3 Mixed conductive and sensorineural hearing loss, unilateral, with restricted hearing on the contralateral side
(Codes under category **H90** require a 6th digit: 1–right ear, 2–left ear)
K11.7 Disturbance of salivary secretions
K59.00 Constipation, unspecified
N39.44 Nocturnal enuresis
R10.0 Acute abdomen pain
R11.11 Vomiting without nausea
R11.2 Nausea with vomiting, unspecified
R19.7 Diarrhea, unspecified
R21 Rash, NOS
R25.0 Abnormal head movements
R25.1 Tremor, unspecified
R25.3 Twitching, NOS
R25.8 Other abnormal involuntary movements
R25.9 Unspecified abnormal involuntary movements
R27.8 Other lack of coordination (excludes ataxia)
R27.9 Unspecified lack of coordination
R41.83 Borderline intellectual functioning
R42 Dizziness
R48.0 Alexia/dyslexia, NOS
R51 Headache
R62.0 Delayed milestone in childhood
R62.52 Short stature (child)
R63.3 Feeding difficulties
R63.4 Abnormal weight loss
R63.5 Abnormal weight gain
R68.2 Dry mouth, unspecified
T56.0X1A Toxic effect of lead and its compounds, accidental (unintentional), initial encounter

Z Codes

Z codes represent reasons for encounters. Categories **Z00–Z99** are provided for occasions when circumstances other than a disease, injury, or external cause classifiable to categories **A00–Y89** are recorded as *diagnoses* or *problems*. This can arise in 2 main ways.

1. When a person who may or may not be sick encounters health services for some specific purpose, such as to receive limited care or service for a current condition, donate an organ or tissue, receive prophylactic vaccination (immunization), or discuss a problem that is in itself not a disease or an injury

2. When some present circumstance or problem influences the person's health status but is not in itself a current illness or injury

Z13.89 Encounter for screening for other disorder
Z55.0 Illiteracy and low-level literacy
Z55.2 Failed school examinations
Z55.3 Underachievement in school
Z55.4 Educational maladjustment and discord with teachers and classmates
Z55.8 Other problems related to education and literacy
Z55.9 Problems related to education and literacy, unspecified (**Z55** codes exclude those conditions reported with **F80–F89**)
Z60.4 Social exclusion and rejection
Z60.8 Other problems related to social environment
Z60.9 Problem related to social environment, unspecified
Z62.0 Inadequate parental supervision and control
Z62.21 Foster care status (child welfare)
Z62.6 Inappropriate (excessive) parental pressure
Z62.810 Personal history of physical and sexual abuse in childhood
Z62.811 Personal history of psychological abuse in childhood
Z62.820 Parent-biological child conflict
Z62.821 Parent-adopted child conflict
Z62.822 Parent-foster child conflict
Z63.72 Alcoholism and drug addiction in family
Z63.8 Other specified problems related to primary support group
Z65.3 Problems related to legal circumstances
Z71.89 Counseling, other specified
Z71.9 Counseling, unspecified
Z72.0 Tobacco use
Z77.011 Contact with and (suspected) exposure to lead
Z79.899 Other long term (current) drug therapy
Z81.0 Family history of intellectual disabilities (conditions classifiable to **F70–F79**)
Z81.8 Family history of other mental and behavioral disorders
Z83.2 Family history of diseases of the blood and blood-forming organs (anemia) (conditions classifiable to **D50–D89**)
Z86.2 Personal history of diseases of the blood and blood-forming organs
Z86.39 Personal history of other endocrine, nutritional, and metabolic disease
Z86.59 Personal history of other mental and behavioral disorders
Z86.69 Personal history of other diseases of the nervous system and sense organs
Z87.09 Personal history of other diseases of the respiratory system
Z87.19 Personal history of other diseases of the digestive system
Z87.798 Personal history of other (corrected) congenital malformations
Z87.820 Personal history of traumatic brain injury
Z91.128 Patient's intentional underdosing of medication regimen for other reason (report drug code)
Z91.138 Patient's unintentional underdosing of medication regimen for other reason (report drug code)
Z91.14 Patient's other noncompliance with medication regimen
Z91.19 Patient's noncompliance with other medical treatment and regimen
Z91.411 Personal history of adult psychological abuse

+ Codes are *add-on codes,* meaning they are reported separately in addition to the appropriate code for the service provided.
* Indicates a *Current Procedural Terminology*–approved telemedicine service.
CPT® copyright 2015 American Medical Association (AMA). All rights reserved.

Continuum Model for ADHD

The following continuum model from *Coding for Pediatrics 2017* has been devised to express the various levels of service for ADHD. This model demonstrates the cumulative effect of the key criteria for each level of service using a single diagnosis as the common denominator. It also shows the importance of other variables, such as patient age, duration and severity of illness, social contexts, and comorbid conditions, that often have key roles in pediatric cases.

Quick Reference for Codes Used in Continuum for ADHD—Established Patients[a]				
E/M Code Level	**History**	**Examination**	**MDM**	**Time**
99211[b]	NA	NA	NA	5 minutes[b]
99212	Problem-focused	Problem-focused	Straightforward	10 minutes
99213	Expanded problem-focused	Expanded problem-focused	Low	15 minutes
99214	Detailed	Detailed	Moderate	25 minutes
99215	Comprehensive	Comprehensive	High	40 minutes

Abbreviations: ADHD, attention-deficit/hyperactivity disorder; E/M, evaluation and management; MDM, medical decision-making; NA, not applicable.
[a] Use of a code level requires that you meet or exceed 2 of the 3 key components based on medical necessity.
[b] Low level E/M service that may not require the presence of a physician.

Adapted from American Academy of Pediatrics. *Coding for Pediatrics 2017: A Manual for Pediatric Documentation and Payment.* 22nd ed. Elk Grove Village, IL: American Academy of Pediatrics; 2017.

Continuum Model for Attention-Deficit/Hyperactivity Disorder

CPT® Code Vignette	History	Physical Examination	Medical Decision-making
99211[a] Nurse visit to follow up growth or blood pressure prior to renewing prescription for psychoactive drugs	1. Chief complaint 2. Brief HPI, existing medications, and desired/undesired effects	1. Weight, blood pressure 2. Overall appearance	1. Refill existing prescription.
99212 Follow-up visit to recheck prior weight loss in patient with established ADHD otherwise stable on stimulant medication	**Problem focused** 1. Chief complaint 2. Brief HPI, existing medications, and desired/undesired effects	**Problem focused** 1. Weight, blood pressure 2. Overall appearance	**Straightforward** 1. Refill existing prescription.
99213 (Typical time: 15 min) 3- to 6-month follow-up of child with ADHD who is presently doing well using medication and without other problems OR May be reported based on time if more than 50% of the face-to-face encounter is spent in counseling and/or coordination of care	**Expanded problem focused** 1. Reason for the visit 2. Review of medications 3. Effect of medication on appetite, mood, sleep 4. Quality of schoolwork (eg, review report cards) 5. Absence of tics 6. Problem-pertinent ROS	**Expanded problem focused** 1. General multisystem examination or single organ system examination with special reference to neurologic examination	**Low complexity** 1. Review rating scale results and feedback materials from teacher. 2. Discuss 6-month treatment plan with adjustment of medication. 3. Plan for further monitoring.

99214 (Typical time: 25 min)
Follow-up evaluation of an established patient with ADHD with failure to improve on medication and/or weight loss
OR
May be reported based on time if more than 50% of the face-to-face encounter is spent in counseling and/or coordination of care
	Detailed
	All data implicit in **99213** expanded plus pertinent review of PFSH and extended ROS, including gastrointestinal and psychiatric
		Detailed
		1. General multisystem examination or detailed single organ system examination of neurologic system
			Moderate complexity
			1. Review rating scale results and feedback materials from teacher.
			2. Discussion of possible interventions, including, but not limited to,
			  a. Educational intervention
			  b. Alteration in medications
			  c. Obtaining drug levels
			  d. Psychiatric intervention
			  e. Behavioral modification program

Continuum Model for Attention-Deficit/Hyperactivity Disorder (continued)

CPT® Code Vignette	History	Physical Examination	Medical Decision-making
99215 (Typical time: 40 min) Initial evaluation of an established patient experiencing difficulty in classroom, home, or social situation and suspected of having ADHD This could be billed as a consultation if the established patient is referred by school for opinion or advice (not transfer of care) and the criteria for reporting a consultation are met. May be reported based on time if more than 50% of the face-to-face encounter is spent in counseling and/or coordination of care	**Comprehensive** 1. Chief complaint 2. History of the problem, extended 3. Complete PFSH 4. Complete ROS	**Comprehensive** 1. General multisystem examination with special attention to neurologic examination and mental health status	**High complexity** Review of Vanderbilt scales, school record, any other formal evaluations completed to date; discussion of differential diagnoses; possible interventions including, but not limited to, 1. Educational interventions 2. Initiation of medications 3. Obtaining drug levels or ruling out substance abuse, if appropriate 4. Laboratory tests as indicated (eg, complete blood cell count and iron studies, serum lead levels) 5. Psychological and/or psychiatric interventions 6. Behavioral modification program 7. Consideration of neurology consultation 8. Coordination of care services with school, family, and other providers

Abbreviations: ADHD, attention-deficit/hyperactivity disorder; CPT, Current Procedural Terminology; HPI, history of present illness; PFSH, past, family, and social history; ROS, review of systems.

ᵃ There are no required key components for code 99211; however, the nurse must document his or her history, physical examination, and assessment to support medical necessity.

Understanding ADHD:
Information for Parents About
Attention-Deficit/Hyperactivity Disorder

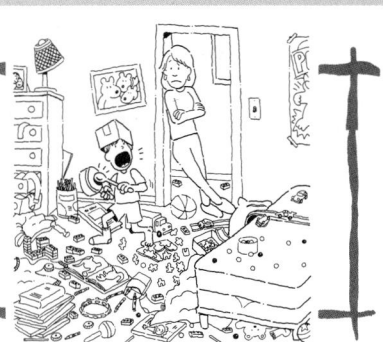

Almost all children have times when their behavior veers out of control. They may speed about in constant motion, make noise nonstop, refuse to wait their turn, and crash into everything around them. At other times they may drift as if in a daydream, unable to pay attention or finish what they start.

However, for some children, these kinds of behaviors are more than an occasional problem. Children with attention-deficit/hyperactivity disorder (ADHD) have behavior problems that are so frequent and severe that they interfere with their ability to live normal lives.

These children often have trouble getting along with siblings and other children at school, at home, and in other settings. Those who have trouble paying attention usually have trouble learning. An impulsive nature may put them in actual physical danger. Because children with ADHD have difficulty controlling this behavior, they may be labeled "bad kids" or "space cadets."

Left untreated, ADHD in some children will continue to cause serious, lifelong problems, such as poor grades in school, run-ins with the law, failed relationships, and the inability to keep a job.

Effective treatment is available. If your child has ADHD, your pediatrician can offer a long-term treatment plan to help your child lead a happy and healthy life. As a parent, you have a very important role in this treatment.

What is ADHD?

ADHD is a condition of the brain that makes it difficult for children to control their behavior. It is one of the most common chronic conditions of childhood. It affects 4% to 12% of school-aged children. ADHD is diagnosed in about 3 times more boys than girls.

The condition affects behavior in specific ways.

What are the symptoms of ADHD?

ADHD includes 3 groups of behavior symptoms: inattention, hyperactivity, and impulsivity. Table 1 explains these symptoms.

Are there different types of ADHD?

Not all children with ADHD have all the symptoms. They may have one or more of the symptom groups listed in Table 1. The symptoms usually are classified as the following types of ADHD:

- **Inattentive only** (formerly known as attention-deficit disorder [ADD])—Children with this form of ADHD are not overly active. Because they do not disrupt the classroom or other activities, their symptoms may not be noticed. Among girls with ADHD, this form is more common.
- **Hyperactive/impulsive**—Children with this type of ADHD show both hyperactive and impulsive behavior, but they can pay attention. They are the least common group and are frequently younger.
- **Combined inattentive/hyperactive/impulsive**—Children with this type of ADHD show a number of symptoms in all 3 dimensions. It is the type that most people think of when they think of ADHD.

How can I tell if my child has ADHD?

Remember, it is normal for all children to show some of these symptoms from time to time. Your child may be reacting to stress at school or home. She may be bored or going through a difficult stage of life. It does not mean she has ADHD.

Sometimes a teacher is the first to notice inattention, hyperactivity, and/or impulsivity and bring these symptoms to the parents' attention.

Perhaps questions from your pediatrician raised the issue. At routine visits, pediatricians often ask questions such as

- How is your child doing in school?
- Are there any problems with learning that you or your child's teachers have seen?
- Is your child happy in school?
- Is your child having problems completing class work or homework?
- Are you concerned with any behavior problems in school, at home, or when your child is playing with friends?

Your answers to these questions may lead to further evaluation for ADHD.

If your child has shown symptoms of ADHD on a regular basis for more than 6 months, discuss this with your pediatrician.

Diagnosis

Your pediatrician will determine whether your child has ADHD using standard guidelines developed by the American Academy of Pediatrics. These diagnosis guidelines are specifically for children 4 to 18 years of age.

It is difficult to diagnose ADHD in children younger than 4 years. This is because younger children change very rapidly. It is also more difficult to diagnose ADHD once a child becomes a teenager.

There is no single test for ADHD. The process requires several steps and involves gathering a lot of information from multiple sources. You, your child, your child's school, and other caregivers should be involved in assessing your child's behavior.

Children with ADHD show signs of inattention, hyperactivity, and/or impulsivity in specific ways. (See the behaviors listed in Table 1.) Your pediatrician will look at how your child's behavior compares to that of other children her own age, based on the information reported about your child by you, her teacher, and any other caregivers who spend time with your child, such as coaches or child care workers.

The following guidelines are used to confirm a diagnosis of ADHD:

- Symptoms occur in 2 or more settings, such as home, school, and social situations, and cause some impairment.
- In a child 4 to 17 years of age, 6 or more symptoms must be identified.
- In a child 17 years and older, 5 or more symptoms must be identified.
- Symptoms significantly impair your child's ability to function in some of the activities of daily life, such as schoolwork, relationships with you and siblings, relationships with friends, or the ability to function in groups such as sports teams.

TABLE 1. Symptoms of ADHD

Symptom	How a child with this symptom may behave
Inattention	Often has a hard time paying attention, daydreams
	Often does not seem to listen
	Is easily distracted from work or play
	Often does not seem to care about details, makes careless mistakes
	Frequently does not follow through on instructions or finish tasks
	Is disorganized
	Frequently loses a lot of important things
	Often forgets things
	Frequently avoids doing things that require ongoing mental effort
Hyperactivity	Is in constant motion, as if "driven by a motor"
	Cannot stay seated
	Frequently squirms and fidgets
	Talks too much
	Often runs, jumps, and climbs when this is not permitted
	Cannot play quietly
Impulsivity	Frequently acts and speaks without thinking
	May run into the street without looking for traffic first
	Frequently has trouble taking turns
	Cannot wait for things
	Often calls out answers before the question is complete
	Frequently interrupts others

- Symptoms start before the child reaches 12 years of age. However, these may not be recognized as ADHD symptoms until a child is older.
- Symptoms have continued for more than 6 months.

In addition to looking at your child's behavior, your pediatrician will do a physical and neurologic examination. A full medical history will be needed to put your child's behavior in context and screen for other conditions that may affect her behavior. Your pediatrician also will talk with your child about how your child acts and feels.

Your pediatrician may refer your child to a pediatric subspecialist or mental health clinician if there are concerns in one of the following areas:
- Intellectual disability (mental retardation)
- Developmental disorder such as speech problems, motor problems, or a learning disability
- Chronic illness being treated with a medication that may interfere with learning
- Trouble seeing and/or hearing
- History of abuse
- Major anxiety or major depression
- Severe aggression
- Possible seizure disorder
- Possible sleep disorder

How can parents help with the diagnosis?

As a parent, you will provide crucial information about your child's behavior and how it affects her life at home, in school, and in other social settings. Your pediatrician will want to know what symptoms your child is showing, how long the symptoms have occurred, and how the behavior affects your

---

Keep safety in mind

If your child shows any symptoms of ADHD, it is very important that you pay close attention to safety. A child with ADHD may not always be aware of dangers and can get hurt easily. Be especially careful around
- Traffic
- Firearms
- Swimming pools
- Tools such as lawn mowers
- Poisonous chemicals, cleaning supplies, or medicines

---

child and your family. You may need to fill in checklists or rating scales about your child's behavior.

In addition, sharing your family history can offer important clues about your child's condition.

How will my child's school be involved?

For an accurate diagnosis, your pediatrician will need to get information about your child directly from your child's classroom teacher or another school professional. Children at least 4 years and older spend many of their waking hours at preschool or school. Teachers provide valuable insights. Your child's teacher may write a report or discuss the following topics with your pediatrician:
- Your child's behavior in the classroom
- Your child's learning patterns
- How long the symptoms have been a problem
- How the symptoms are affecting your child's progress at school
- Ways the classroom program is being adapted to help your child
- Whether other conditions may be affecting the symptoms

In addition, your pediatrician may want to see report cards, standardized tests, and samples of your child's schoolwork.

How will others who care for my child be involved?

Other caregivers may also provide important information about your child's behavior. Former teachers, religious and scout leaders, or coaches may have valuable input. If your child is homeschooled, it is especially important to assess his behavior in settings outside of the home.

Your child may not behave the same way at home as he does in other settings. Direct information about the way your child acts in more than one setting is required. It is important to consider other possible causes of your child's symptoms in these settings.

In some cases, other mental health care professionals may also need to be involved in gathering information for the diagnosis.

Coexisting conditions

As part of the diagnosis, your pediatrician will look for other conditions that show the same types of symptoms as ADHD. Your child may simply have a different condition or ADHD and another condition. Most children with a diagnosis of ADHD have at least one coexisting condition.

Common coexisting conditions include
- **Learning disabilities**—Learning disabilities are conditions that make it difficult for a child to master specific skills such as reading or math. ADHD is not a learning disability. However, ADHD can make it hard for

a child to do well in school. Diagnosing learning disabilities requires evaluations, such as IQ and academic achievement tests, and it requires educational interventions.

- **Oppositional defiant disorder or conduct disorder**—Up to 35% of children with ADHD also have oppositional defiant disorder or conduct disorder. Children with oppositional defiant disorder tend to lose their temper easily and annoy people on purpose, and they are defiant and hostile toward authority figures. Children with conduct disorder break rules, destroy property, get suspended or expelled from school, and violate the rights of other people. Children with coexisting conduct disorder are at much higher risk for getting into trouble with the law or having substance abuse problems than children who have only ADHD. Studies show that this type of coexisting condition is more common among children with the primarily hyperactive/impulsive and combination types of ADHD. Your pediatrician may recommend behavioral therapy for your child if she has this condition.
- **Mood disorders/depression**—About 18% of children with ADHD also have mood disorders such as depression or bipolar disorder (formerly called manic depression). There is frequently a family history of these types of disorders. Coexisting mood disorders may put children at higher risk for suicide, especially during the teenage years. These disorders are more common among children with inattentive and combined types of ADHD. Children with mood disorders or depression often require additional interventions or a different type of medication than those normally used to treat ADHD.
- **Anxiety disorders**—These affect about 25% of children with ADHD. Children with anxiety disorders have extreme feelings of fear, worry, or panic that make it difficult to function. These disorders can produce physical symptoms such as racing pulse, sweating, diarrhea, and nausea. Counseling and/or different medication may be needed to treat these coexisting conditions.
- **Language disorders**—Children with ADHD may have difficulty with how they use language. It is referred to as a pragmatic language disorder. It may not show up with standard tests of language. A speech and language clinician can detect it by observing how a child uses language in her day-to-day activities.

Are there other tests for ADHD?

You may have heard theories about other tests for ADHD. There are no other proven tests for ADHD at this time.

Many theories have been presented, but studies have shown that the following tests have little value in diagnosing an individual child:

- Screening for high lead levels in the blood
- Screening for thyroid problems
- Computerized continuous performance tests
- Brain imaging studies such as CAT scans and MRIs
- Electroencephalogram (EEG) or brain-wave test

While these tests are not helpful in diagnosing ADHD, your pediatrician may see other signs or symptoms in your child that warrant blood tests, brain imaging studies, or an EEG.

What causes ADHD?

ADHD is one of the most studied conditions of childhood, but ADHD may be caused by a number of things.

Research to date has shown

- ADHD is a neurobiologic condition whose symptoms are also dependent on the child's environment.
- A lower level of activity in the parts of the brain that control attention and activity level may be associated with ADHD.
- ADHD frequently runs in families. Sometimes ADHD is diagnosed in a parent at the same time it is diagnosed in the child.
- In very rare cases, toxins in the environment may lead to ADHD. For instance, lead in the body can affect child development and behavior. Lead may be found in many places, including homes built before 1978 when lead was added to paint.
- Significant head injuries may cause ADHD in some cases.
- Prematurity increases the risk of developing ADHD.
- Prenatal exposures, such as alcohol or nicotine from smoking, increase the risk of developing ADHD.

There is little evidence that ADHD is caused by

- Eating too much sugar
- Food additives
- Allergies
- Immunizations

Treatment

Once the diagnosis is confirmed, the outlook for most children who receive treatment for ADHD is encouraging. There is no specific cure for ADHD, but there are many treatment options available.

Each child's treatment must be tailored to meet his individual needs. In most cases, treatment for ADHD should include

- A long-term management plan with
  - Target outcomes for behavior
  - Follow-up activities
  - Monitoring
- Education about ADHD
- Teamwork among doctors, parents, teachers, caregivers, other health care professionals, and the child
- Medication
- Behavior therapy including parent training
- Individual and family counseling

Treatment for ADHD uses the same principles that are used to treat other chronic conditions like asthma or diabetes. Long-term planning is needed because these conditions are not cured. Families must manage them on an ongoing basis. In the case of ADHD, schools and other caregivers must also be involved in managing the condition.

Educating the people involved about ADHD is a key part of treating your child. As a parent, you will need to learn about ADHD. Read about the condition and talk with people who understand it. This will help you manage the ways ADHD affects your child and your family on a day-to-day basis. It will also help your child learn to help himself.

Setting target outcomes

At the beginning of treatment, your pediatrician should help you set around 3 target outcomes (goals) for your child's behavior. These target outcomes will guide the treatment plan. Your child's target outcomes should focus on helping her function as well as possible at home, at school, and in your

Table 2. Common medications

Type of medication	Brand name	Generic name	Duration
Short-acting amphetamine stimulants	Adderall	Mixed amphetamine salts	4 to 6 hours
	Dexedrine	Dextroamphetamine	4 to 6 hours
Short-acting methylphenidate stimulants	Focalin	Dexmethylphenidate	3 to 5 hours
	Methylin	Methylphenidate (tablet, liquid, and chewable tablets)	3 to 5 hours
	Ritalin	Methylphenidate	3 to 5 hours
Mildly extended-release methylphenidate stimulants	Metadate ER	Methylphenidate	4 to 6 hours
	Methylin ER	Methylphenidate	4 to 6 hours
Intermediate-acting extended-release methylphenidate stimulants	Focalin XR	Dexmethylphenidate	6 to 8 hours
	Metadate CD	Methylphenidate	6 to 8 hours
	Ritalin LA	Methylphenidate	6 to 8 hours
Long-acting extended-release amphetamine stimulants	Adderall XR	Mixed amphetamine salts	8 to 12 hours
	Adzeny XR-ODT	Amphetamine	8 to 12 hours
	Dyanavel XR	Amphetamine	8 to 12 hours
	Vyvanse	Lisdexamfetamine	8 to 12 hours
Long-acting extended-release methylphenidate stimulants	Concerta	Methylphenidate	10 to 12 hours
	Daytrana	Methylphenidate (skin patch)	11 to 12 hours
	Quillivant XR	Methylphenidate (liquid)	10 to 12 hours
α-Adrenergic agents (non-stimulant)	Intuniv	Guanfacine	24 hours
	Kapvay	Clonidine	12 hours
Selective norepinephrine reuptake inhibitors (non-stimulant)	Strattera	Atomoxetine	24 hours

Products are mentioned for informational purposes only and do not imply an endorsement by the American Academy of Pediatrics.

Your doctor or pharmacist can provide you with important safety information for the products listed.

community. You need to identify what behaviors are most preventing your child from success.

Here are examples of target outcomes.

- Improved relationships with parents, siblings, teachers, and friends (eg, fewer arguments with brothers or sisters or being invited more frequently to friends' houses or parties)
- Better schoolwork (eg, completing class work or homework assignments)
- More independence in self-care or homework (eg, getting ready for school in the morning without supervision)
- Improved self-esteem (eg, increase in feeling that she can get her work done)

- Fewer disruptive behaviors (eg, decrease in the number of times she refuses to obey rules)
- Safer behavior in the community (eg, when crossing streets)

The target outcomes should be
- Realistic
- Something your child will be able to do
- Behaviors that you can observe and count (eg, with rating scales)

Your child's treatment plan will be set up to help her achieve these goals.

Medication

For most children, stimulant medications are a safe and effective way to relieve ADHD symptoms. As glasses help people focus their eyes to see, these medications help children with ADHD focus their thoughts better and ignore distractions. This makes them more able to pay attention and control their behavior.

Stimulants may be used alone or combined with behavior therapy. Studies show that about 80% of children with ADHD who are treated with stimulants improve a great deal once the right medication and dose are determined.

Two forms of stimulants are available: immediate-release (short-acting) and extended-release (intermediate-acting and long-acting). (See Table 2.) Immediate-release medications usually are taken every 4 hours, when needed. They are the cheapest of the medications. Extended-release medications usually are taken once in the morning.

Children who use extended-release forms of stimulants can avoid taking medication at school or after school. It is important not to chew or crush extended-release capsules or tablets. However, extended-release capsules that are made up of beads can be opened and sprinkled onto food for children who have difficulties swallowing tablets or capsules.

Non-stimulants can be tried when stimulant medications don't work or cause bothersome side effects.

Which medication is best for my child?

It may take some time to find the best medication, dosage, and schedule for your child.

Your child may need to try different types of stimulants or other medication. Some children respond to one type of stimulant but not another.

The amount of medication (dosage) that your child needs also may need to be adjusted. The dosage is not based solely on his weight. Your pediatrician will vary the dosage over time to get the best results and control possible side effects.

The medication schedule also may be adjusted depending on the target outcome. For example, if the goal is to get relief from symptoms mostly at school, your child may take the medication only on school days.

It is important for your child to have regular medical checkups to monitor how well the medication is working and check for possible side effects.

What side effects can stimulants cause?

Side effects occur sometimes. These tend to happen early in treatment and are usually mild and short-lived, but in rare cases they can be prolonged or more severe.

The most common side effects include
- Decreased appetite/weight loss
- Sleep problems
- Social withdrawal

Principles for behavior therapy

Behavior therapy has 3 basic principles.

1. **Set specific doable goals.** Set clear and reasonable goals for your child, such as staying focused on homework for a certain amount of time or sharing toys with friends.
2. **Provide rewards and consequences.** Give your child a specified reward (positive reinforcement) every time she shows the desired behavior. Give your child a consequence (unwanted result or punishment) consistently when she has inappropriate behaviors.
3. **Keep using the rewards and consequences.** Using the rewards and consequences consistently for a long time will shape your child's behavior in a positive way.

Some less common side effects include
- Rebound effect (increased activity or a bad mood as the medication wears off)
- Transient muscle movements or sounds called tics
- Minor growth delay

Very rare side effects include
- Significant increase in blood pressure or heart rate
- Bizarre behaviors

The same sleep problems do not exist for atomoxetine, but initially it may make your child sleepy or upset her stomach. There have been very rare cases of atomoxetine needing to be stopped because it was causing liver damage. Rarely atomoxetine increased thoughts of suicide. Guanfacine can cause drowsiness, fatigue, or a decrease in blood pressure.

More than half of children who have tic disorders, such as Tourette syndrome, also have ADHD. Tourette syndrome is an inherited condition associated with frequent tics and unusual vocal sounds. The effect of stimulants on tics is not predictable, although most studies indicate that stimulants are safe for children with ADHD and tic disorders in most cases. It is also possible to use atomoxetine or guanfacine for children with ADHD and Tourette syndrome. Most side effects can be relieved by
- Changing the medication dosage
- Adjusting the schedule of medication
- Using a different stimulant or trying a non-stimulant (See Table 2.)

Close contact with your pediatrician is required until you find the best medication and dose for your child. After that, periodic monitoring by your doctor is important to maintain the best effects. To monitor the effects of the medication, your pediatrician will probably have you and your child's teacher(s) fill out behavior rating scales, observe changes in your child's target goals, notice any side effects, and monitor your child's height, weight, pulse, and blood pressure.

Stimulants, atomoxetine, and guanfacine may not be an option for children who are taking certain other medications or who have some medical conditions, such as congenital heart disease.

Behavior therapy

Most experts recommend using both medication and behavior therapy to treat ADHD. This is known as a multimodal treatment approach.

There are many forms of behavior therapy, but all have a common goal—to change the child's physical and social environments to help the child improve his behavior.

Table 3. Behavior therapy techniques

Technique	Description	Example
Positive reinforcement	Complimenting and providing rewards or privileges in response to desired behavior.	Child completes an assignment and is permitted to play on the computer.
Time-out	Removing access to desired activity because of unwanted behavior.	Child hits sibling and, as a result, must sit for 5 minutes in the corner of the room.
Response cost	Withdrawing rewards or privileges because of unwanted behavior.	Child loses free-time privileges for not completing homework.
Token economy	Combining reward and consequence. Child earns rewards and privileges when performing desired behaviors. She loses rewards and privileges as a result of unwanted behavior.	Child earns stars or points for completing assignments and loses stars for getting out of seat. Child cashes in the sum of her stars at the end of the week for a prize.

Under this approach, parents, teachers, and other caregivers learn better ways to work with and relate to the child with ADHD. You will learn how to set and enforce rules, help your child understand what he needs to do, use discipline effectively, and encourage good behavior. Your child will learn better ways to control his behavior as a result. You will learn how to be more consistent.

Table 3 shows specific behavior therapy techniques that can be effective with children with ADHD.

Behavior therapy recognizes the limits that having ADHD puts on a child. It focuses on how the important people and places in the child's life can adapt to encourage good behavior and discourage unwanted behavior. It is different from play therapy or other therapies that focus mainly on the child and his emotions.

How can I help my child control her behavior?

As the child's primary caregivers, parents play a major role in behavior therapy. Parent training is available to help you learn more about ADHD and specific, positive ways to respond to ADHD-type behaviors. This will help your child improve. In many cases parenting classes with other parents will be sufficient, but with more challenging children, individual work with a counselor/coach may be needed.

Taking care of yourself also will help your child. Being the parent of a child with ADHD can be tiring and trying. It can test the limits of even the best parents. Parent training and support groups made up of other families who are dealing with ADHD can be a great source of help. Learn stress-management techniques to help you respond calmly to your child. Seek counseling if you feel overwhelmed or hopeless.

Ask your pediatrician to help you find parent training, counseling, and support groups in your community. Additional resources are listed at the end of this publication.

How can my child's school help?

Your child's school is a key partner in providing effective behavior therapy for your child. In fact, these principles work well in the classroom for most students.

Tips for helping your child control his behavior

- **Keep your child on a daily schedule.** Try to keep the time that your child wakes up, eats, bathes, leaves for school, and goes to sleep the same each day.
- **Cut down on distractions.** Loud music, computer games, and TV can be overstimulating to your child. Make it a rule to keep the TV or music off during mealtime and while your child is doing homework. Don't place a TV in your child's bedroom. Whenever possible, avoid taking your child to places that may be too stimulating, such as busy shopping malls.
- **Organize your house.** If your child has specific and logical places to keep his schoolwork, toys, and clothes, he is less likely to lose them. Save a spot near the front door for his school backpack so he can grab it on the way out the door.
- **Reward positive behavior.** Offer kind words, hugs, or small prizes for reaching goals in a timely manner or good behavior. Praise and reward your child's efforts to pay attention.
- **Set small, reachable goals.** Aim for slow progress rather than instant results. Be sure that your child understands that he can take small steps toward learning to control himself.
- **Help your child stay "on task."** Use charts and checklists to track progress with homework or chores. Keep instructions brief. Offer frequent, friendly reminders.
- **Limit choices.** Help your child learn to make good decisions by giving him only 2 or 3 options at a time.
- **Find activities at which your child can succeed.** All children need to experience success to feel good about themselves.
- **Use calm discipline.** Use consequences such as time-out, removing the child from the situation, or distraction. Sometimes it is best to simply ignore the behavior. Physical punishment, such as spanking or slapping, is *not* helpful. Discuss your child's behavior with him when both of you are calm.
- **Develop a good communication system with your child's teacher** so that you can coordinate your efforts and monitor your child's progress.

Classroom management techniques may include
- Keeping a set routine and schedule for activities
- Using a system of clear rewards and consequences, such as a point system or token economy (See Table 3.)
- Sending daily or weekly report cards or behavior charts to parents to inform them about the child's progress
- Seating the child near the teacher
- Using small groups for activities
- Encouraging students to pause a moment before answering questions
- Keeping assignments short or breaking them into sections
- Close supervision with frequent, positive cues to stay on task
- Changes to where and how tests are given so students can succeed (eg, allowing students to take tests in a less distracting environment or allowing more time to complete tests)

Your child's school should work with you and your pediatrician to develop strategies to assist your child in the classroom. When a child has ADHD that is severe enough to interfere with her ability to learn, 2 federal laws offer help. These laws require public schools to cover costs of evaluating the educational needs of the affected child and providing the needed services.

1. The Individuals with Disabilities Education Act, Part B (IDEA) requires public schools to cover costs of evaluating the educational needs of the affected child and providing the needed special education services if your child qualifies because her learning is impaired by her ADHD.
2. Section 504 of the Rehabilitation Act of 1973 does not have strict qualification criteria but is limited to changes in the classroom, modifications in homework assignments, and taking tests in a less distracting environment or allowing more time to complete tests.

If your child has ADHD and a coexisting condition, she may need additional special services such as a classroom aide, private tutoring, special classroom settings, or, in rare cases, a special school.

It is important to remember that once ADHD is diagnosed and treated, children with it are more likely to achieve their goals in school.

Keeping the treatment plan on track

Ongoing monitoring of your child's behavior and medications is required to find out if the treatment plan is working. Office visits, phone conversations, behavior checklists, written reports from teachers, and behavior report cards are common tools for following the child's progress.

Treatment plans for ADHD usually require long-term efforts on the part of families and schools. Medication schedules may be complex. Behavior therapies require education and patience. Sometimes it can be hard for everyone to stick with it. Your efforts play an important part in building a healthy future for your child.

Ask your pediatrician to help you find ways to keep your child's treatment plan on track.

What if my child does not reach his target outcomes?

Most school-aged children with ADHD respond well when their treatment plan includes both medication and behavior therapy. If your child is not achieving his goals, your pediatrician will assess the following factors:
- Were the target outcomes realistic?
- Is more information needed about the child's behavior?
- Is the diagnosis correct?
- Is another condition hindering treatment?
- Is the treatment plan being followed?
- Has the treatment failed?

While treatment for ADHD should improve your child's behavior, **it may not completely eliminate the symptoms** of inattention, hyperactivity, and impulsivity. Children who are being treated successfully may still have trouble with their friends or schoolwork.

However, if your child clearly is not meeting his specific target outcomes, your pediatrician will need to reassess the treatment plan.

Unproven treatments

You may have heard media reports or seen advertisements for "miracle cures" for ADHD. Carefully research any such claims. Consider whether the source of the information is valid. At this time, there is no scientifically proven cure for this condition.

The following methods **need more scientific evidence to prove that they work**:
- Megavitamins and mineral supplements
- Anti–motion-sickness medication (to treat the inner ear)

Teenagers with ADHD

The teenage years can be a special challenge. Academic and social demands increase. In some cases, symptoms may be better controlled as the child grows older; however, frequently the demands for performance also increase so that in most cases, ADHD symptoms persist and continue to interfere with the child's ability to function adequately. According to the National Institute of Mental Health, about 80% of those who required medication for ADHD as children still need it as teenagers.

Parents play an important role in helping teenagers become independent. Encourage your teenager to help herself with strategies such as

- Using a daily planner for assignments and appointments
- Making lists
- Keeping a routine
- Setting aside a quiet time and place to do homework
- Organizing storage for items such as school supplies, clothes, CDs, and sports equipment
- Being safety conscious (eg, always wearing seat belts, using protective gear for sports)
- Talking about problems with someone she trusts
- Getting enough sleep
- Understanding her increased risk of abusing substances such as tobacco and alcohol

Activities such as sports, drama, and debate teams can be good places to channel excess energy and develop friendships. Find what your teenager does well and support her efforts to "go for it."

Milestones such as learning to drive and dating offer new freedom and risks. Parents must stay involved and set limits for safety. Your child's ADHD increases her risk of incurring traffic violations and accidents.

It remains important for parents of teenagers to keep in touch with teachers and make sure that their teenager's schoolwork is going well.

Talk with your pediatrician if your teenager shows signs of severe problems such as depression, drug abuse, or gang-related activities.

- Treatment for candida yeast infection
- EEG biofeedback (training to increase brain-wave activity)
- Applied kinesiology (realigning bones in the skull)
- Reducing sugar consumption
- Optometric vision training (asserts that faulty eye movement and sensitivities cause the behavior problems)

Always tell your pediatrician about any alternative therapies, supplements, or medications that your child is using. These may interact with prescribed medications and harm your child.

Will there be a cure for ADHD soon?

While there are no signs of a cure at this time, research is ongoing to learn more about the role of the brain in ADHD and the best ways to treat the disorder. Additional research is looking at the long-term outcomes for people with ADHD.

Frequently asked questions
Will my child outgrow ADHD?

ADHD continues into adulthood in most cases. However, by developing their strengths, structuring their environments, and using medication when needed, adults with ADHD can lead very productive lives. In some careers, having a high-energy behavior pattern can be an asset.

Why do so many children have ADHD?

The number of children getting treatment for ADHD has risen. It is not clear whether more children have ADHD or more children are receiving a diagnosis of ADHD. Also, more children with ADHD are getting treatment for a longer period. ADHD is now one of the most common and most studied conditions of childhood. Because of more awareness and better ways of diagnosing and treating this disorder, more children are being helped. It may also be the case that school performance has become more important because of the higher technical demand of many jobs, and ADHD frequently interferes with school functioning.

Are schools putting children on ADHD medication?

Teachers are often the first to notice behavior signs of possible ADHD. However, only physicians can prescribe medications to treat ADHD. The diagnosis of ADHD should follow a careful process.

Are children getting high on stimulant medications?

When taken as directed by a doctor, there is no evidence that children are getting high on stimulant drugs such as methylphenidate and amphetamine. At therapeutic doses, these drugs also do not sedate or tranquilize children and do not increase the risk of addiction.

Stimulants are classified as Schedule II drugs by the US Drug Enforcement Administration because there is abuse potential of this class of medication. If your child is on medication, it is always best to supervise the use of the medication closely. Atomoxetine and guanfacine are not Schedule II drugs because they don't have abuse potential, even in adults.

Are stimulant medications gateway drugs leading to illegal drug or alcohol abuse?

People with ADHD are naturally impulsive and tend to take risks. But patients with ADHD who are taking stimulants are not at a greater risk and actually may be at a lower risk of using other drugs. Children and teenagers who have ADHD and also have coexisting conditions may be at higher risk for drug and alcohol abuse, regardless of the medication used.

Resources

Here is a list of support groups and additional resources for more information about ADHD. Check with your pediatrician for resources in your community.

National Resource Center on ADHD
www.help4adhd.org/NRC.aspx

Children and Adults with Attention-Deficit/Hyperactivity Disorder (CHADD)
800/233-4050
www.chadd.org

Attention Deficit Disorder Association

800/939-1019

www.add.org

Center for Parent Information and Resources

www.parentcenterhub.org

National Institute of Mental Health

866/615-6464

www.nimh.nih.gov

Tourette Association of America

888/4-TOURET (486-8738)

www.tourette.org

Listing of resources does not imply an endorsement by the American Academy of Pediatrics (AAP). The AAP is not responsible for the content of external resources. Information was current at the time of publication.

Products are mentioned for informational purposes only and do not imply an endorsement by the American Academy of Pediatrics.

The information contained in this publication should not be used as a substitute for the medical care and advice of your pediatrician. There may be variations in treatment that your pediatrician may recommend based on individual facts and circumstances.

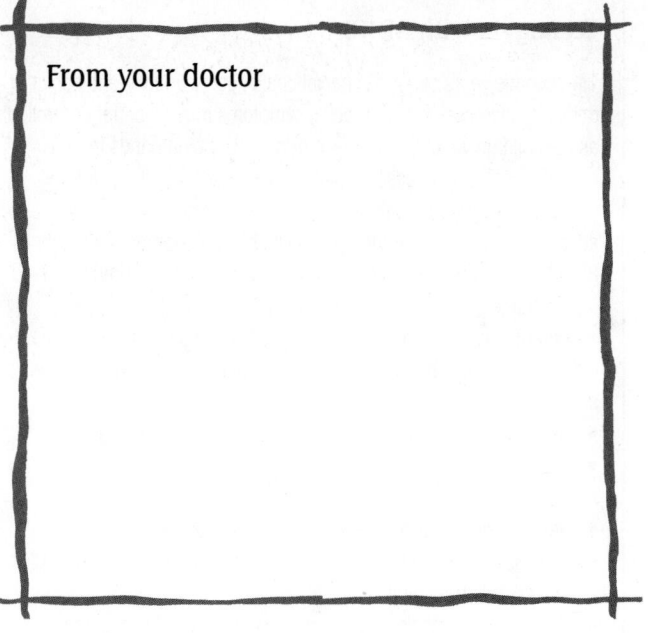

From your doctor

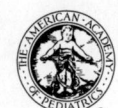

American Academy of Pediatrics

DEDICATED TO THE HEALTH OF ALL CHILDREN™

The American Academy of Pediatrics (AAP) is an organization of 66,000 primary care pediatricians, pediatric medical subspecialists, and pediatric surgical specialists dedicated to the health, safety, and well-being of all infants, children, adolescents, and young adults.

American Academy of Pediatrics
Web site — www.HealthyChildren.org

medicines for ADHD
questions from teens
who have ADHD

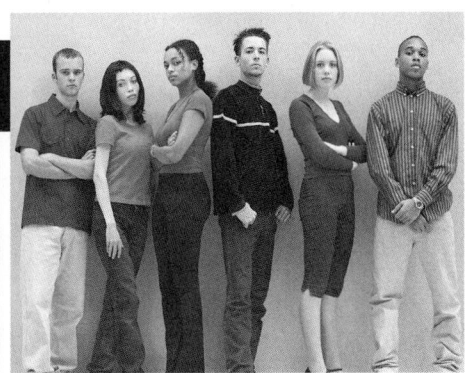

Q: What can I do besides taking medicines?

A: Medicines and behavior therapies are the only treatments that have been shown by scientific studies to work consistently for ADHD symptoms. Medicines are prescribed by a doctor, while behavior therapies usually are done with a trained counselor in behavior treatment. These 2 treatments are probably best used together, but you might be able to do well with one or the other. You can't rely on other treatments such as biofeedback, allergy treatments, special diets, vision training, or chiropractic because there isn't enough evidence that shows they work.

Counseling may help you learn how to cope with some issues you may face. And there are things you can do to help yourself. For example, things that may help you stay focused include using a daily planner for schoolwork and other activities, making to-do lists, and even getting enough sleep. Counseling can help you find an organization system or a checklist.

Q: How can medicines help me?

A: There are several different ADHD medicines. They work by causing the brain to have more *neurotransmitters* in the right places. Neurotransmitters are chemicals in the brain that help us focus our attention, control our impulses, organize and plan, and stick to routines. Medicines for ADHD can help you focus your thoughts and ignore distractions so that you can reach your full potential. They also can help you control your emotions and behavior. Check with your doctor to learn more about this.

Q: Are medicines safe?

A: For most teens with ADHD, stimulant medicines are safe and effective if taken as recommended. However, like most medicines, there could be side effects. Luckily, the side effects tend to happen early on, are usually mild, and don't last too long. If you have any side effects, tell your doctor. Changes may need to be made in your medicines or their dosages.

- **Most common side effects** include decreased appetite or weight loss, problems falling asleep, headaches, jitteriness, and stomachaches.
- **Less common side effects** include a bad mood as medicines wear off (called the rebound effect) and facial twitches or tics.

Q: Will medicines change my personality?

A: Medicines won't change who you are and should not change your personality. If you notice changes in your mood or personality, tell your doctor. Occasionally when medicines wear off, some teens become more irritable for a short time. An adjustment of the medicines by your doctor may be helpful.

Q: Will medicines affect my growth?

A: Medicines will not keep you from growing. Significant growth delay is a very rare side effect of some medicines prescribed for ADHD. Most scientific studies show that taking these medicines has little to no long-term effect on growth in most cases.

Q: Do I need to take medicines at school?

A: There are 3 types of medicines used for teens with ADHD: *short acting* (immediate release), *intermediate acting,* and *long acting.* You can avoid taking medicines at school if you take the intermediate- or long-acting kind. Long-acting medicines usually are taken once in the morning or evening. Short-acting medicines usually are taken every 4 hours.

Q: Does taking medicines make me a drug user?

A: No! Although you may need medicines to help you stay in control of your behavior, medicines used to treat ADHD do not lead to drug abuse. In fact, taking medicines as prescribed by your doctor and doing better in school may help you avoid drug use and abuse. (But never give or share your medicines with anyone else.)

Q: Will I have to take medicines forever?

A: In most cases, ADHD continues later in life. Whether you need to keep taking medicines as an adult depends on your own needs. The need for medicines may change over time. Many adults with ADHD have learned how to succeed in life without medicines by using behavior therapies or finding jobs that suit their strengths and weaknesses.

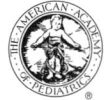

American Academy of Pediatrics

DEDICATED TO THE HEALTH OF ALL CHILDREN™

The American Academy of Pediatrics is an organization of 60,000 primary care pediatricians, pediatric medical subspecialists, and pediatric surgical specialists dedicated to the health, safety, and well-being of infants, children, adolescents, and young adults.

American Academy of Pediatrics
Web site—www.HealthyChildren.org

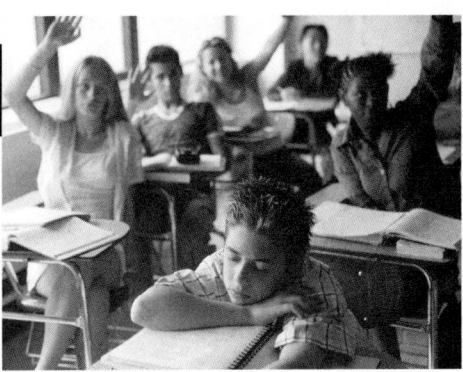

what is ADHD?
questions from teens

Attention-deficit/hyperactivity disorder (ADHD) is a condition of the brain that makes it difficult for people to concentrate or pay attention in certain areas where it is easy for others, like school or homework. The following are quick answers to some common questions:

Q: What causes ADHD?

A: **There isn't just one cause.** Research shows that

- ADHD is a medical condition caused by small changes in how the brain works. It seems to be related to 2 chemicals in your brain called *dopamine* and *norepinephrine.* These chemicals help send messages between nerve cells in the brain—especially those areas of the brain that control attention and activity level.

- ADHD most often runs in families.

- In a few people with ADHD, being born prematurely or being exposed to alcohol during the pregnancy can contribute to ADHD.

- Immunizations and eating too much sugar do NOT cause ADHD. And there isn't enough evidence that shows allergies and food additives cause ADHD.

Q: How can you tell if someone has ADHD?

A: You can't tell if someone has ADHD just by looks. People with ADHD don't look any different, but how they act may make them stand out from the crowd. Some people with ADHD are very hyperactive (they move around a lot and are not able to sit still) and have behavior problems that are obvious to everyone. Other people with ADHD are quiet and more laid back on the outside, but on the inside struggle with attention to schoolwork and other tasks. They are distracted by people and things around them when they try to study; they may have trouble organizing schoolwork or forget to turn in assignments.

Q: Can ADHD cause someone to act up or get in trouble?

A: Having ADHD can cause you to struggle in school or have problems controlling your behavior. Some people may say or think that your struggles and problems are because you are bad, lazy, or not smart. But they're wrong. It's important that you get help so your impulses don't get you into serious trouble.

Q: Don't little kids who have ADHD outgrow it by the time they are teens?

A: Often kids with the hyperactive kind of ADHD get less hyperactive as they get into their teens, but usually they still have a lot of difficulty paying attention, remembering what they have read, and getting their work done. They may or may not have other behavior problems. Some kids with ADHD have never been hyperactive at all, but usually their attention problems also continue into their teens.

Q: If I have trouble with homework or tests, do I have ADHD?

A: There could be many reasons why a student struggles with schoolwork and tests. ADHD could be one reason. It may or may not be, but your doctor is the best person to say for sure. Kids with ADHD often say it's hard to concentrate, focus on a task (for example, schoolwork, chores, or a job), manage their time, and finish tasks. This could explain why they may have trouble with schoolwork and tests. Whatever the problem, there are many people willing to help you. You need to find the approach that works best for you.

Q: Does having ADHD mean a person is not very smart?

A: Absolutely not! People who have trouble paying attention may have problems in school, but that doesn't mean they're not smart. In fact, some people with ADHD are very smart, but may not be able to reach their potential in school until they get treatment.

ADHD is a common problem. Teens with ADHD have the potential to do well in school and live a normal life with the right treatment.

Q: Is ADHD more common in boys?

A: More boys than girls are diagnosed with ADHD—about 2 or 3 boys to every 1 girl. However, these numbers do not include the number of girls with the inattentive type of ADHD who are not diagnosed. Girls with the inattentive type of ADHD tend to be overlooked entirely or do not attract attention until they are older.

Q: What do I do if I think I have ADHD?

A: Don't be afraid to talk with your parents or other adults that you trust. Together you can meet with your doctor and find out if you really have ADHD. If you do, your doctor will help you learn how to live with ADHD and find ways to deal with your condition.

The persons whose photographs are depicted in this publication are professional models. They have no relation to the issues discussed. Any characters they are portraying are fictional.

The information contained in this publication should not be used as a substitute for the medical care and advice of your pediatrician. There may be variations in treatment that your pediatrician may recommend based on individual facts and circumstances.

From your doctor

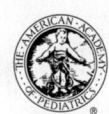

American Academy of Pediatrics

DEDICATED TO THE HEALTH OF ALL CHILDREN™

The American Academy of Pediatrics is an organization of 60,000 primary care pediatricians, pediatric medical subspecialists, and pediatric surgical specialists dedicated to the health, safety, and well-being of infants, children, adolescents, and young adults.

American Academy of Pediatrics
Web site—www.HealthyChildren.org

Brief Resolved Unexplained Events (Formerly Apparent Life-Threatening Events) and Evaluation of Lower-Risk Infants

- *Clinical Practice Guideline*

  - *PPI: AAP Partnership for Policy Implementation*
    See Appendix 2 for more information.

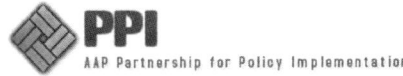

- *Executive Summary*

  - *PPI: AAP Partnership for Policy Implementation*
    See Appendix 2 for more information.

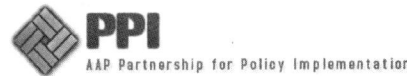

CLINICAL PRACTICE GUIDELINE   Guidance for the Clinician in Rendering Pediatric Care

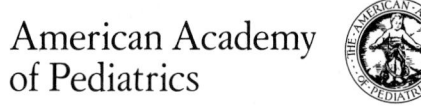

Brief Resolved Unexplained Events (Formerly Apparent Life-Threatening Events) and Evaluation of Lower-Risk Infants

Joel S. Tieder, MD, MPH, FAAP, Joshua L. Bonkowsky, MD, PhD, FAAP, Ruth A. Etzel, MD, PhD, FAAP, Wayne H. Franklin, MD, MPH, MMM, FAAP, David A. Gremse, MD, FAAP, Bruce Herman, MD, FAAP, Eliot S. Katz, MD, FAAP, Leonard R. Krilov, MD, FAAP, J. Lawrence Merritt II, MD, FAAP, Chuck Norlin, MD, FAAP, Jack Percelay, MD, MPH, FAAP, Robert E. Sapién, MD, MMM, FAAP, Richard N. Shiffman, MD, MCIS, FAAP, Michael B.H. Smith, MB, FRCPCH, FAAP, for the SUBCOMMITTEE ON APPARENT LIFE THREATENING EVENTS

abstract

This is the first clinical practice guideline from the American Academy of Pediatrics that specifically applies to patients who have experienced an apparent life-threatening event (ALTE). This clinical practice guideline has 3 objectives. First, it recommends the replacement of the term ALTE with a new term, brief resolved unexplained event (BRUE). Second, it provides an approach to patient evaluation that is based on the risk that the infant will have a repeat event or has a serious underlying disorder. Finally, it provides management recommendations, or key action statements, for lower-risk infants. The term BRUE is defined as an event occurring in an infant younger than 1 year when the observer reports a sudden, brief, and now resolved episode of ≥1 of the following: (1) cyanosis or pallor; (2) absent, decreased, or irregular breathing; (3) marked change in tone (hyper- or hypotonia); and (4) altered level of responsiveness. A BRUE is diagnosed only when there is no explanation for a qualifying event after conducting an appropriate history and physical examination. By using this definition and framework, infants younger than 1 year who present with a BRUE are categorized either as (1) a lower-risk patient on the basis of history and physical examination for whom evidence-based recommendations for evaluation and management are offered or (2) a higher-risk patient whose history and physical examination suggest the need for further investigation and treatment but for whom recommendations are not offered. This clinical practice guideline is intended to foster a patient- and family-centered approach to care, reduce unnecessary and costly medical interventions, improve patient outcomes, support implementation, and provide direction for future research. Each key action statement indicates a level of evidence, the benefit-harm relationship, and the strength of recommendation.

DOI: 10.1542/peds.2016-0590

PEDIATRICS (ISSN Numbers: Print, 0031-4005; Online, 1098-4275).

To cite: Tieder JS, Bonkowsky JL, Etzel RA, et al. Brief Resolved Unexplained Events (Formerly Apparent Life-Threatening Events) and Evaluation of Lower-Risk Infants. *Pediatrics.* 2016;137(5):e20160590

INTRODUCTION

This clinical practice guideline applies to infants younger than 1 year and is intended for pediatric clinicians. This guideline has 3 primary objectives. First, it recommends the replacement of the term apparent life-threatening event (ALTE) with a new term, brief resolved unexplained event (BRUE). Second, it provides an approach to patient evaluation that is based on the risk that the infant will have a recurring event or has a serious underlying disorder. Third, it provides evidence-based management recommendations, or key action statements, for lower-risk patients whose history and physical examination are normal. It does not offer recommendations for higher-risk patients whose history and physical examination suggest the need for further investigation and treatment (because of insufficient evidence or the availability of clinical practice guidelines specific to their presentation). This clinical practice guideline also provides implementation support and suggests directions for future research.

The term ALTE originated from a 1986 National Institutes of Health Consensus Conference on Infantile Apnea and was intended to replace the term "near-miss sudden infant death syndrome" (SIDS).[1] An ALTE was defined as "an episode that is frightening to the observer and that is characterized by some combination of apnea (central or occasionally obstructive), color change (usually cyanotic or pallid but occasionally erythematous or plethoric), marked change in muscle tone (usually marked limpness), choking, or gagging. In some cases, the observer fears that the infant has died."[2] Although the definition of ALTE eventually enabled researchers to establish that these events are separate entities from SIDS, the clinical application of this classification, which describes a constellation of observed, subjective, and nonspecific symptoms, has raised significant challenges for clinicians and parents in the evaluation and care of these infants.[3] Although a broad range of disorders can present as an ALTE (eg, child abuse, congenital abnormalities, epilepsy, inborn errors of metabolism, and infections), for a majority of infants who appear well after the event, the risk of a serious underlying disorder or a recurrent event is extremely low.[2]

CHANGE IN TERMINOLOGY AND DIAGNOSIS

The imprecise nature of the original ALTE definition is difficult to apply to clinical care and research.[3] As a result, the clinician is often faced with several dilemmas. First, under the ALTE definition, the infant is often, but not necessarily, asymptomatic on presentation. The evaluation and management of symptomatic infants (eg, those with fever or respiratory distress) need to be distinguished from that of asymptomatic infants. Second, the reported symptoms under the ALTE definition, although often concerning to the caregiver, are not intrinsically life-threatening and frequently are a benign manifestation of normal infant physiology or a self-limited condition. A definition needs enough precision to allow the clinician to base clinical decisions on events that are characterized as abnormal after conducting a thorough history and physical examination. For example, a constellation of symptoms suggesting hemodynamic instability or central apnea needs to be distinguished from more common and less concerning events readily characterized as periodic breathing of the newborn, breath-holding spells, dysphagia, or gastroesophageal reflux (GER). Furthermore, events defined as ALTEs are rarely a manifestation of a more serious illness that, if left undiagnosed, could lead to morbidity or death. Yet, the perceived potential for recurring events or a serious underlying disorder often provokes concern in caregivers and clinicians.[2,4,5] This concern can compel testing or admission to the hospital for observation, which can increase parental anxiety and subject the patient to further risk and does not necessarily lead to a treatable diagnosis or prevention of future events. A more precise definition could prevent the overuse of medical interventions by helping clinicians distinguish infants with lower risk. Finally, the use of ALTE as a diagnosis may reinforce the caregivers' perceptions that the event was indeed "life-threatening," even when it most often was not. For these reasons, a replacement of the term ALTE with a more specific term could improve clinical care and management.

In this clinical practice guideline, a more precise definition is introduced for this group of clinical events: brief resolved unexplained event (BRUE). The term BRUE is intended to better reflect the transient nature and lack of clear cause and removes the "life-threatening" label. The authors of this guideline recommend that the term ALTE no longer be used by clinicians to describe an event or as a diagnosis. Rather, the term BRUE should be used to describe events occurring in infants younger than 1 year of age that are characterized by the observer as "brief" (lasting <1 minute but typically <20–30 seconds) and "resolved" (meaning the patient returned to baseline state of health after the event) and with a reassuring history, physical examination, and vital signs at the time of clinical evaluation by trained medical providers (Table 1). For example, the presence of respiratory symptoms or fever would preclude classification of an event as a BRUE. BRUEs are also "unexplained," meaning that a clinician is unable to explain the cause of the event after an appropriate history and physical examination. Similarly, an event characterized as choking or gagging associated with spitting up is not included in the BRUE definition, because clinicians will want to pursue the cause of vomiting, which may be related to GER, infection, or central nervous system (CNS) disease. However, until BRUE-specific codes are available, for billing and coding purposes, it is reasonable to apply the ALTE International Classification of Diseases, 9th Revision, and International Classification of Diseases, 10th revision, codes to patients determined to have experienced a BRUE (see section entitled "Dissemination and Implementation").

BRUE DEFINITION

Clinicians should use the term BRUE to describe an event occurring in an infant <1 year of age when the observer reports a sudden, brief, and now resolved episode of ≥1 of the following:

- **cyanosis or pallor**
- **absent, decreased, or irregular breathing**
- **marked change in tone (hyper- or hypotonia)**
- **altered level of responsiveness**

Moreover, clinicians should diagnose a BRUE only when there is no explanation for a qualifying event after conducting an appropriate history and physical examination (Tables 2 and 3).

Differences between the terms ALTE and BRUE should be noted. First, the BRUE definition has a strict age limit. Second, an event is only a BRUE if there is no other likely explanation. Clinical symptoms such as fever, nasal congestion, and increased work of breathing may indicate temporary airway obstruction from viral infection. Events characterized as choking after vomiting may indicate

TABLE 1 BRUE Definition and Factors for Inclusion and Exclusion

	Includes	Excludes
Brief	Duration <1 min; typically 20–30 s	Duration ≥1 min
Resolved	Patient returned to his or her baseline state of health after the event	At the time of medical evaluation:
	Normal vital signs	Fever or recent fever
	Normal appearance	Tachypnea, bradypnea, apnea
		Tachycardia or bradycardia
		Hypotension, hypertension, or hemodynamic instability
		Mental status changes, somnolence, lethargy
		Hypotonia or hypertonia
		Vomiting
		Bruising, petechiae, or other signs of injury/trauma
		Abnormal weight, growth, or head circumference
		Noisy breathing (stridor, sturgor, wheezing)
		Repeat event(s)
Unexplained	Not explained by an identifiable medical condition	Event consistent with GER, swallow dysfunction, nasal congestion, etc
		History or physical examination concerning for child abuse, congenital airway abnormality, etc
Event Characterization		
Cyanosis or pallor	Central cyanosis: blue or purple coloration of face, gums, trunk	Acrocyanosis or perioral cyanosis
	Central pallor: pale coloration of face or trunk	Rubor
Absent, decreased, or irregular breathing	Central apnea	Periodic breathing of the newborn
	Obstructive apnea	Breath-holding spell
	Mixed obstructive apnea	
Marked change in tone (hyper- or hypotonia)	Hypertonia	Hypertonia associated with crying, choking, or gagging due to GER or feeding problems
	Hypotonia	Tone changes associated with breath-holding spell
		Tonic eye deviation or nystagmus
		Tonic-clonic seizure activity
		Infantile spasms
Altered responsiveness	Loss of consciousness	Loss of consciousness associated with breath-holding spell
	Mental status change	
	Lethargy	
	Somnolence	
	Postictal phase	

a gastrointestinal cause, such as GER. Third, a BRUE diagnosis is based on the clinician's characterization of features of the event and not on a caregiver's perception that the event was life-threatening. Although such perceptions are understandable and important to address, such risk can only be assessed after the event has been objectively characterized by a clinician. Fourth, the clinician should determine whether the infant had episodic cyanosis or pallor, rather than just determining whether "color change" occurred. Episodes of rubor or redness are not consistent with BRUE, because they are common in healthy infants. Fifth, BRUE expands the respiratory criteria beyond "apnea" to include absent breathing, diminished breathing, and other breathing irregularities. Sixth, instead of the less specific criterion of "change in muscle tone," the clinician should determine whether there was marked change in tone, including hypertonia or hypotonia. Seventh, because choking and gagging usually indicate common diagnoses such as GER or respiratory infection, their presence suggests an event was not a BRUE. Finally, the use of "altered level of responsiveness" is a new criterion, because it can be an important component of an episodic but serious cardiac, respiratory, metabolic, or neurologic event.

For infants who have experienced a BRUE, a careful history and physical examination are necessary to characterize the event, assess the risk of recurrence, and determine the presence of an underlying disorder (Tables 2 and 3). The recommendations provided in this guideline focus on infants with a lower risk of a subsequent event or serious underlying disorder (see section entitled "Risk Assessment: Lower- Versus Higher-Risk BRUE"). In the absence of identifiable risk factors, infants are at lower risk and laboratory studies, imaging studies, and other diagnostic procedures are unlikely to be useful or necessary. However, if the clinical history or physical examination reveals abnormalities, the patient may be at higher risk and further evaluation should focus on the specific areas of concern. For example,

- possible child abuse may be considered when the event history is reported inconsistently or is incompatible with the child's developmental age, or when, on physical examination, there is unexplained bruising or a torn labial or lingual frenulum;

- a cardiac arrhythmia may be considered if there is a family history of sudden, unexplained death in first-degree relatives; and

- infection may be considered if there is fever or persistent respiratory symptoms.

TABLE 2 Historical Features To Be Considered in the Evaluation of a Potential BRUE

Features To Be Considered

Considerations for possible child abuse:
  Multiple or changing versions of the history/circumstances
  History/circumstances inconsistent with child's developmental stage
  History of unexplained bruising
  Incongruence between caregiver expectations and child's developmental stage, including assigning negative attributes to the child

History of the event
  General description
  Who reported the event?
  Witness of the event? Parent(s), other children, other adults? Reliability of historian(s)?
  State immediately before the event
    Where did it occur (home/elsewhere, room, crib/floor, etc)?
    Awake or asleep?
    Position: supine, prone, upright, sitting, moving?
    Feeding? Anything in the mouth? Availability of item to choke on? Vomiting or spitting up?
    Objects nearby that could smother or choke?
  State during the event
    Choking or gagging noise?
    Active/moving or quiet/flaccid?
    Conscious? Able to see you or respond to voice?
    Muscle tone increased or decreased?
    Repetitive movements?
    Appeared distressed or alarmed?
    Breathing: yes/no, struggling to breathe?
    Skin color: normal, pale, red, or blue?
    Bleeding from nose or mouth?
    Color of lips: normal, pale, or blue?
  End of event
    Approximate duration of the event?
    How did it stop: with no intervention, picking up, positioning, rubbing or clapping back, mouth-to-mouth, chest compressions, etc?
    End abruptly or gradually?
    Treatment provided by parent/caregiver (eg, glucose-containing drink or food)?
    911 called by caregiver?
  State after event
    Back to normal immediately/gradually/still not there?
    Before back to normal, was quiet, dazed, fussy, irritable, crying?

Recent history
  Illness in preceding day(s)?
    If yes, detail signs/symptoms (fussiness, decreased activity, fever, congestion, rhinorrhea, cough, vomiting, diarrhea, decreased intake, poor sleep)
  Injuries, falls, previous unexplained bruising?

Past medical history
  Pre-/perinatal history
  Gestational age
  Newborn screen normal (for IEMs, congenital heart disease)?
  Previous episodes/BRUE?
  Reflux? If yes, obtain details, including management
  Breathing problems? Noisy ever? Snoring?
  Growth patterns normal?
  Development normal? Assess a few major milestones across categories, any concerns about development or behavior?
  Illnesses, injuries, emergencies?
  Previous hospitalization, surgery?
  Recent immunization?
  Use of over-the-counter medications?

Family history
  Sudden unexplained death (including unexplained car accident or drowning) in first- or second-degree family members before age 35, and particularly as an infant?
  Apparent life-threatening event in sibling?
  Long QT syndrome?
  Arrhythmia?

TABLE 2 Continued

Features To Be Considered
Inborn error of metabolism or genetic disease?
Developmental delay?
Environmental history
Housing: general, water damage, or mold problems?
Exposure to tobacco smoke, toxic substances, drugs?
Social history
Family structure, individuals living in home?
Housing: general, mold?
Recent changes, stressors, or strife?
Exposure to smoke, toxic substances, drugs?
Recent exposure to infectious illness, particularly upper respiratory illness, paroxysmal cough, pertussis?
Support system(s)/access to needed resources?
Current level of concern/anxiety; how family manages adverse situations?
Potential impact of event/admission on work/family?
Previous child protective services or law enforcement involvement (eg, domestic violence, animal abuse), alerts/reports for this child or others in the family (when available)?
Exposure of child to adults with history of mental illness or substance abuse?

The key action statements in this clinical practice guideline do not apply to higher-risk patients but rather apply only to infants who meet the lower-risk criteria by having an otherwise normal history and physical examination.

RISK ASSESSMENT: LOWER- VERSUS HIGHER-RISK BRUE

Patients who have experienced a BRUE may have a recurrent event or an undiagnosed serious condition (eg, child abuse, pertussis, etc) that confers a risk of adverse outcomes. Although this risk has been difficult to quantify historically and no studies have fully evaluated patient-centered outcomes (eg, family experience survey), the systematic review of the ALTE literature identified a subset of BRUE patients who are unlikely to have a recurrent event or undiagnosed serious conditions, are at lower risk of adverse outcomes, and can likely be managed safely without extensive diagnostic evaluation or hospitalization.[3] In the systematic review of ALTE studies in which it was possible to identify BRUE patients, the following characteristics most consistently conferred higher risk: infants <2 months of age, those with a history of prematurity, and those with more

than 1 event. There was generally an increased risk from prematurity in infants born at <32 weeks' gestation, and the risk attenuated once infants born at <32 weeks' gestation reached 45 weeks' postconceptional age. Two ALTE studies evaluated the duration of the event.[6,7] Although duration did not appear to be predictive of hospital admission, it was difficult to discern a BRUE population from the heterogeneous ALTE populations. Nonetheless, most events were less than one minute. By consensus, the subcommittee established <1 minute as the upper limit of a "brief event," understanding that objective, verifiable measurements were rarely, if ever, available. Cariopulmonary resuscitation (CPR) was identified as a risk factor in the older ALTE studies and confirmed in a recent study,[6] but it was unclear how the need for CPR was determined. Therefore, the committee agreed by consensus that the need for CPR should be determined by trained medical providers.

PATIENT FACTORS THAT DETERMINE A LOWER RISK

To be designated lower risk, the following criteria should be met (see Fig 1):

- Age >60 days

- Prematurity: gestational age ≥32 weeks and postconceptional age ≥45 weeks

- First BRUE (no previous BRUE ever and not occurring in clusters)

- Duration of event <1 minute

- No CPR required by trained medical provider

- No concerning historical features (see Table 2)

- No concerning physical examination findings (see Table 3)

Infants who have experienced a BRUE who do not qualify as lower-risk patients are, by definition, at higher risk. Unfortunately, the outcomes data from ALTE studies in the heterogeneous higher-risk population are unclear and preclude the derivation of evidence-based recommendations regarding management. Thus, pending further research, this guideline does not provide recommendations for the management of the higher-risk infant. Nonetheless, it is important for clinicians and researchers to recognize that some studies suggest that higher-risk BRUE patients may be more likely to have a serious underlying cause, recurrent event, or an adverse outcome. For example, infants younger than 2 months who experience a BRUE may be more likely to have a congenital or infectious cause and be at higher risk of an adverse outcome. Infants who have experienced multiple events or a concerning social assessment for child abuse may warrant increased observation to better document the events or contextual factors. A list of differential diagnoses for BRUE patients is provided in Supplemental Table 6.

METHODS

In July 2013, the American Academy of Pediatrics (AAP) convened a multidisciplinary subcommittee composed of primary care clinicians

TABLE 3 Physical Examination Features To Be Considered in the Evaluation of a Potential BRUE

Physical Examination
General appearance
Craniofacial abnormalities (mandible, maxilla, nasal)
Age-appropriate responsiveness to environment
Growth variables
Length, weight, occipitofrontal circumference
Vital signs
Temperature, pulse, respiratory rate, blood pressure, oxygen saturation
Skin
Color, perfusion, evidence of injury (eg, bruising or erythema)
Head
Shape, fontanelles, bruising or other injury
Eyes
General, extraocular movement, pupillary response
Conjunctival hemorrhage
Retinal examination, if indicated by other findings
Ears
Tympanic membranes
Nose and mouth
Congestion/coryza
Blood in nares or oropharynx
Evidence of trauma or obstruction
Torn frenulum
Neck
Mobility
Chest
Auscultation, palpation for rib tenderness, crepitus, irregularities
Heart
Rhythm, rate, auscultation
Abdomen
Organomegaly, masses, distention
Tenderness
Genitalia
Any abnormalities
Extremities
Muscle tone, injuries, limb deformities consistent with fracture
Neurologic
Alertness, responsiveness
Response to sound and visual stimuli
General tone
Pupillary constriction in response to light
Presence of symmetrical reflexes
Symmetry of movement/tone/strength

and experts in the fields of general pediatrics, hospital medicine, emergency medicine, infectious diseases, child abuse, sleep medicine, pulmonary medicine, cardiology, neurology, biochemical genetics, gastroenterology, environmental health, and quality improvement. The subcommittee also included a parent representative, a guideline methodologist/informatician, and an epidemiologist skilled in systematic reviews. All panel members declared potential conflicts on the basis of the AAP policy on Conflict of Interest and Voluntary Disclosure. Subcommittee

members repeated this process annually and upon publication of the guideline. All potential conflicts of interest are listed at the end of this document. The project was funded by the AAP.

The subcommittee performed a comprehensive review of the literature related to ALTEs from 1970 through 2014. Articles from 1970 through 2011 were identified and evaluated by using "Management of Apparent Life Threatening Events in Infants: A Systematic Review," authored by

the Society of Hospital Medicine's ALTE Expert Panel (which included 4 members of the subcommittee).[3] The subcommittee partnered with the Society of Hospital Medicine Expert Panel and a librarian to update the original systematic review with articles published through December 31, 2014, with the use of the same methodology as the original systematic review. PubMed, Cumulative Index to Nursing and Allied Health Literature, and Cochrane Library databases were searched for studies involving children younger than 24 months by using the stepwise approach specified in the Preferred Reporting Items for Systematic Reviews and Meta-Analyses (PRISMA) statement.[8] Search terms included "ALTE(s)," "apparent life threatening event(s)," "life threatening event(s)," "near miss SIDS" or "near miss sudden infant death syndrome," "aborted crib death" or "aborted sudden infant death syndrome," and "aborted SIDS" or "aborted cot death" or "infant death, sudden." The Medical Subject Heading "infantile apparent life-threatening event," introduced in 2011, was also searched but did not identify additional articles.

In updating the systematic review published in 2012, pairs of 2 subcommittee members used validated methodology to independently score the newly identified abstracts from English-language articles (*n* = 120) for relevance to the clinical questions (Supplemental Fig 3).[9,10] Two independent reviewers then critically appraised the full text of the identified articles (*n* = 23) using a structured data collection form based on published guidelines for evaluating medical literature.[11,12] They recorded each study's relevance to the clinical question, research design, setting, time period covered, sample size, patient eligibility criteria, data source, variables collected, key results, study

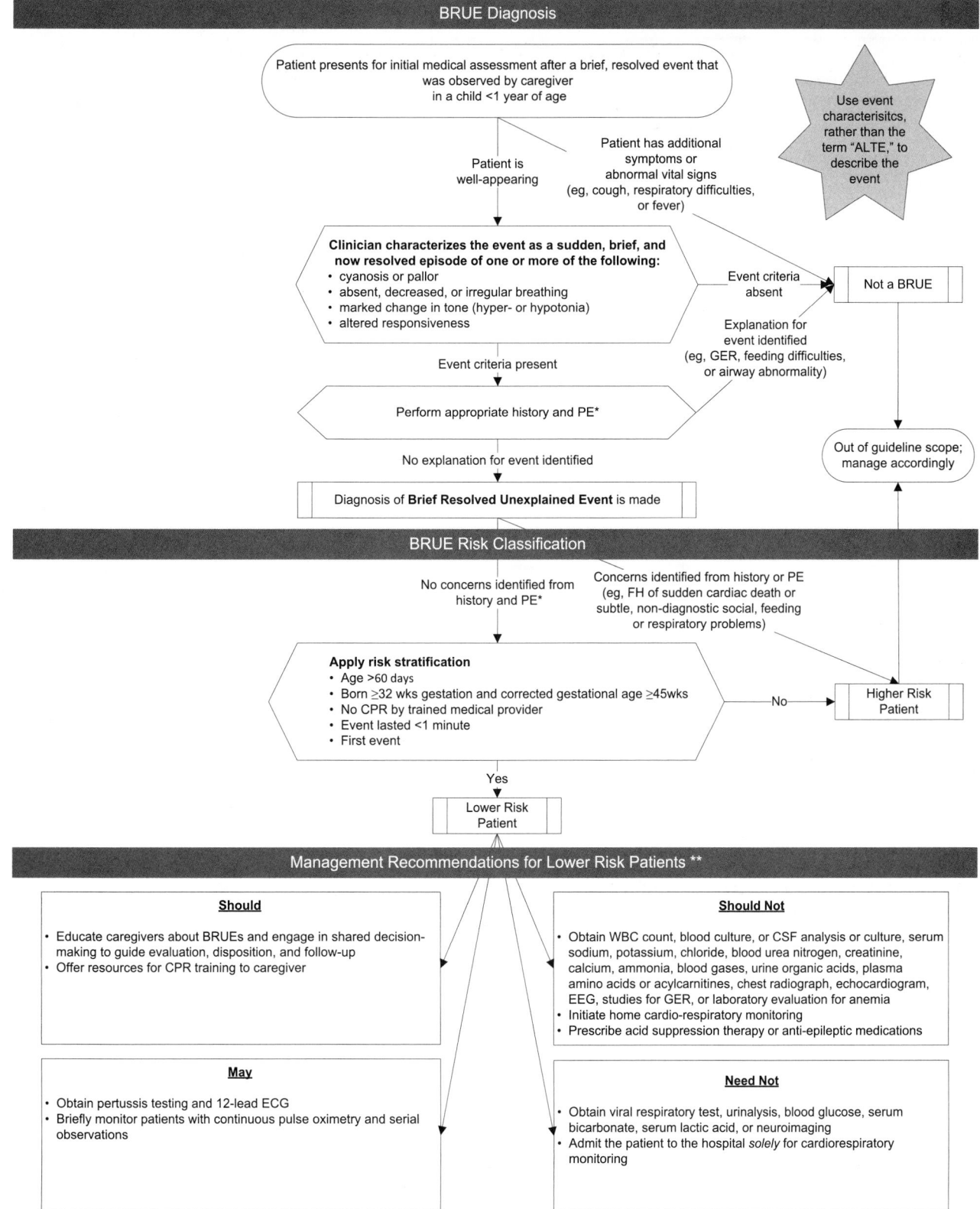

FIGURE 1

Diagnosis, risk classification, and recommended management of a BRUE. *See Tables 3 and 4 for the determination of an appropriate and negative FH and PE. **See Fig 2 for the AAP method for rating of evidence and recommendations. CSF, cerebrospinal fluid; FH, family history; PE, physical examination; WBC, white blood cell.

Figure 1, shown here, has been updated per the erratum at http://pediatrics.aappublications.org/content/138/2/e20161487.

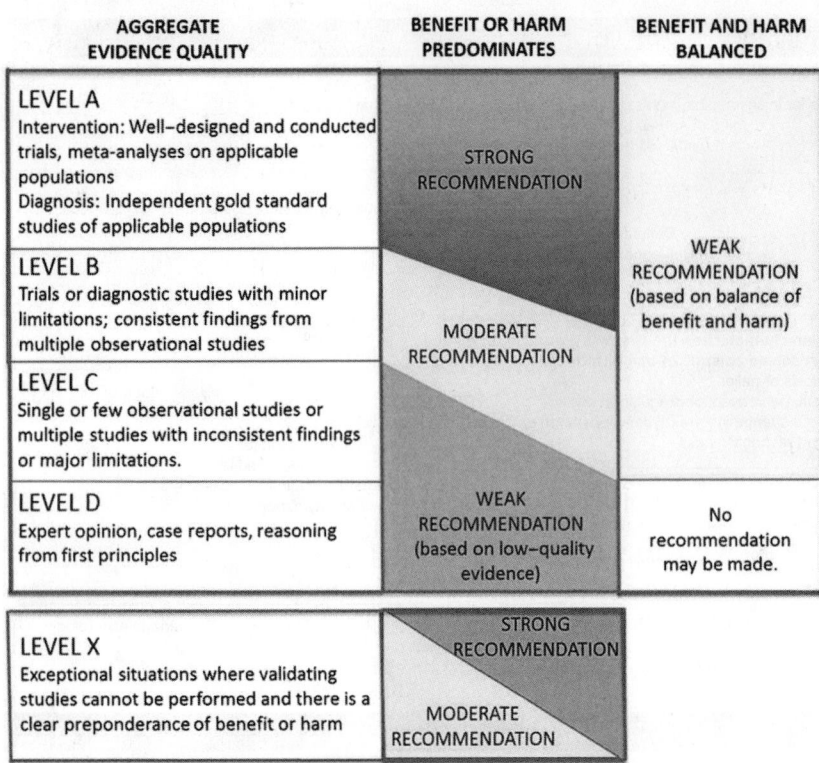

FIGURE 2
AAP rating of evidence and recommendations.

a systematic grading of the quality of evidence from the updated literature review by 2 independent reviewers and incorporation of the previous systematic review. Expert consensus was used when definitive data were not available. If committee members disagreed with the rest of the consensus, they were encouraged to voice their concern until full agreement was reached. If full agreement could not be reached, each committee member reserved the right to state concern or disagreement in the publication (which did not occur). Because the recommendations of this guideline were based on the ALTE literature, we relied on the studies and outcomes that could be attributable to the new definition of lower- or higher-risk BRUE patients.

Key action statements (summarized in Table 5) were generated by using BRIDGE-Wiz (Building Recommendations in a Developers Guideline Editor), an interactive software tool that leads guideline development teams through a series of questions that are intended to create clear, transparent, and actionable key action statements.[30] BRIDGE-Wiz integrates the quality of available evidence and a benefit-harm assessment into the final determination of the strength of each recommendation. Evidence-based guideline recommendations from the AAP may be graded as strong,

limitations, potential sources of bias, and stated conclusions. If at least 1 reviewer judged an article to be relevant on the basis of the full text, subsequently at least 2 reviewers critically appraised the article and determined by consensus what evidence, if any, should be cited in the systematic review. Selected articles used in the earlier review were also reevaluated for their quality. The final recommendations were based on articles identified in the updated (n = 18) and original (n = 37) systematic review (Supplemental Table 7).[6,7,13–28] The resulting systematic review was used to develop the guideline recommendations by following the policy statement from the AAP Steering Committee on Quality Improvement and Management, "Classifying Recommendations for Clinical Practice Guidelines."[29] Decisions and the strength of recommendations were based on

TABLE 4 Guideline Definitions for Key Action Statements

Statement	Definition	Implication
Strong recommendation	A particular action is favored because anticipated benefits clearly exceed harms (or vice versa) and quality of evidence is excellent or unobtainable.	Clinicians should follow a strong recommendation unless a clear and compelling rationale for an alternative approach is present.
Moderate recommendation	A particular action is favored because anticipated benefits clearly exceed harms (or vice versa) and the quality of evidence is good but not excellent (or is unobtainable).	Clinicians would be prudent to follow a moderate recommendation but should remain alert to new information and sensitive to patient preferences.
Weak recommendation (based on low-quality evidence)	A particular action is favored because anticipated benefits clearly exceed harms (or vice versa), but the quality of evidence is weak.	Clinicians would be prudent follow a weak recommendation but should remain alert to new information and very sensitive to patient preferences.
Weak recommendation (based on balance of benefits and harms)	Weak recommendation is provided when the aggregate database shows evidence of both benefit and harm that appear to be similar in magnitude for any available courses of action.	Clinicians should consider the options in their decision-making, but patient preference may have a substantial role.

TABLE 5 Summary of Key Action Statements for Lower-Risk BRUEs

When managing an infant aged >60 d and <1 y and who, on the basis of a thorough history and physical examination, meets criteria for having experienced a lower-risk BRUE, clinicians:	Evidence Quality; Strength of Recommendation
1. Cardiopulmonary evaluation	
1A. Need not admit infants to the hospital solely for cardiorespiratory monitoring.	B; Weak
1B. May briefly monitor patients with continuous pulse oximetry and serial observations.	D; Weak
1C. Should not obtain a chest radiograph.	B; Moderate
1D. Should not obtain a measurement of venous or arterial blood gas.	B; Moderate
1E. Should not obtain an overnight polysomnograph.	B; Moderate
1F. May obtain a 12-lead electrocardiogram.	C; Weak
1G. Should not obtain an echocardiogram.	C; Moderate
1H. Should not initiate home cardiorespiratory monitoring.	B; Moderate
2. Child abuse evaluation	
2A. Need not obtain neuroimaging (CT, MRI, or ultrasonography) to detect child abuse.	C; Weak
2B. Should obtain an assessment of social risk factors to detect child abuse.	C; Moderate
3. Neurologic evaluation	
3A. Should not obtain neuroimaging (CT, MRI, or ultrasonography) to detect neurologic disorders.	C; Moderate
3B. Should not obtain an EEG to detect neurologic disorders.	C; Moderate
3C. Should not prescribe antiepileptic medications for potential neurologic disorders.	C; Moderate
4. Infectious disease evaluation	
4A. Should not obtain a WBC count, blood culture, or cerebrospinal fluid analysis or culture to detect an occult bacterial infection.	B; Strong
4B. Need not obtain a urinalysis (bag or catheter).	C; Weak
4C. Should not obtain chest radiograph to assess for pulmonary infection.	B; Moderate
4D. Need not obtain respiratory viral testing if rapid testing is available.	C; Weak
4E. May obtain testing for pertussis.	B; Weak
5. Gastrointestinal evaluation	
5A. Should not obtain investigations for GER (eg, upper gastrointestinal tract series, pH probe, endoscopy, barium contrast study, nuclear scintigraphy, and ultrasonography).	C; Moderate
5B. Should not prescribe acid suppression therapy.	C; Moderate
6. IEM evaluation	
6A. Need not obtain measurement of serum lactic acid or serum bicarbonate.	C; Weak
6B. Should not obtain a measurement of serum sodium, potassium, chloride, blood urea nitrogen, creatinine, calcium, or ammonia.	C; Moderate
6C. Should not obtain a measurement of venous or arterial blood gases.	C; Moderate
6D. Need not obtain a measurement of blood glucose.	C; Weak
6E. Should not obtain a measurement of urine organic acids, plasma amino acids, or plasma acylcarnitines.	C; Moderate
7. Anemia evaluation	
7A. Should not obtain laboratory evaluation for anemia.	C; Moderate
8. Patient- and family-centered care	
8A. Should offer resources for CPR training to caregiver.	C; Moderate
8B. Should educate caregivers about BRUEs.	C; Moderate
8C. Should use shared decision-making.	C; Moderate

CPR, cardiopulmonary resuscitation; CT, computed tomography; GER, gastroesophageal reflux; WBC, white blood cell.

moderate, weak based on low-quality evidence, or weak based on balance between benefits and harms. Strong and moderate recommendations are associated with "should" and "should not" recommendation statements, whereas weak recommendation may be recognized by use of "may" or "need not" (Fig 2, Table 4).

A strong recommendation means that the committee's review of the evidence indicates that the benefits of the recommended approach clearly exceed the harms of that approach (or, in the case of a strong negative recommendation, that the

harms clearly exceed the benefits) and that the quality of the evidence supporting this approach is excellent. Clinicians are advised to follow such guidance unless a clear and compelling rationale for acting in a contrary manner is present. A moderate recommendation means that the committee believes that the benefits exceed the harms (or, in the case of a negative recommendation, that the harms exceed the benefits), but the quality of the evidence on which this recommendation is based is not as strong. Clinicians are also encouraged to follow such guidance

but also should be alert to new information and sensitive to patient preferences.

A weak recommendation means either that the evidence quality that exists is suspect or that well-designed, well-conducted studies have shown little clear advantage to one approach versus another. Weak recommendations offer clinicians flexibility in their decision-making regarding appropriate practice, although they may set boundaries on alternatives. Family and patient preference should have a substantial role in influencing clinical

1A. Clinicians Need Not Admit Infants Presenting With a Lower-Risk BRUE to the Hospital Solely for Cardiorespiratory Monitoring (Grade B, Weak Recommendation)

Aggregate Evidence Quality	Grade B
Benefits	Reduce unnecessary testing and caregiver/infant anxiety
	Avoid consequences of false-positive result, health care– associated infections, and other patient safety risks
Risks, harm, cost	May rarely miss a recurrent event or diagnostic opportunity for rare underlying condition
Benefit-harm assessment	The benefits of reducing unnecessary testing, nosocomial infections, and false-positive results, as well as alleviating caregiver and infant anxiety, outweigh the rare missed diagnostic opportunity for an underlying condition
Intentional vagueness	None
Role of patient preferences	Caregiver anxiety and access to quality follow-up care may be important considerations in determining whether a hospitalization for cardiovascular monitoring is indicated
Exclusions	None
Strength	Weak recommendation (because of equilibrium between benefits and harms)
Key references	31, 32

1B. Clinicians May Briefly Monitor Infants Presenting With a Lower-Risk BRUE With Continuous Pulse Oximetry and Serial Observations (Grade D, Weak Recommendation)

Aggregate Evidence Quality	Grade D
Benefits	Identification of hypoxemia
Risks, harm, cost	Increased costs due to monitoring over time and the use of hospital resources
	False-positive results may lead to subsequent testing and hospitalization
	False reassurance from negative test results
Benefit-harm assessment	The potential benefit of detecting hypoxemia outweighs the harm of cost and false results
Intentional vagueness	Duration of time to monitor patients with continuous pulse oximetry and the number and frequency of serial observations may vary
Role of patient preferences	Level of caregiver concern may influence the duration of oximetry monitoring
Exclusions	None
Strength	Weak recommendation (based on low quality of evidence)
Key references	33, 36

decision-making, particularly when recommendations are expressed as weak. Key action statements based on that evidence and expert consensus are provided. A summary is provided in Table 5.

The practice guideline underwent a comprehensive review by stakeholders before formal approval by the AAP, including AAP councils, committees, and sections; selected outside organizations; and individuals identified by the subcommittee as experts in the field.

All comments were reviewed by the subcommittee and incorporated into the final guideline when appropriate.

This guideline is intended for use primarily by clinicians providing care for infants who have experienced a BRUE and their families. This guideline may be of interest to parents and payers, but it is not intended to be used for reimbursement or to determine insurance coverage. This guideline is not intended as the sole source of guidance in the evaluation and

management of BRUEs but rather is intended to assist clinicians by providing a framework for clinical decision-making.

KEY ACTION STATEMENTS FOR LOWER-RISK BRUE

1. Cardiopulmonary

1A. Clinicians Need Not Admit Infants Presenting With a Lower-Risk BRUE to the Hospital Solely for Cardiorespiratory Monitoring (Grade B, Weak Recommendation)

Infants presenting with an ALTE often have been admitted for observation and testing. Observational data indicate that 12% to 14% of infants presenting with a diagnosis of ALTE had a subsequent event or condition that required hospitalization.[7,31] Thus, research has sought to identify risk factors that could be used to identify infants likely to benefit from hospitalization. A long-term follow-up study in infants hospitalized with an ALTE showed that no infants subsequently had SIDS but 11% were victims of child abuse and 4.9% had adverse neurologic outcomes (see 3. Neurology).[32] The ALTE literature supports that infants presenting with a lower-risk BRUE do not have an increased rate of cardiovascular or other events during admission and hospitalization may not be required, but close follow-up is recommended. Careful outpatient follow-up is advised (repeat clinical history and physical examination within 24 hours after the initial evaluation) to identify infants with ongoing medical concerns that would indicate further evaluation and treatment.

Al-Kindy et al[33] used documented monitoring in 54% of infants admitted for an ALTE (338 of 625) and identified 46 of 338 (13.6%) with "extreme" cardiovascular events (central apnea >30 seconds, oxygen saturation <80% for 10 seconds, decrease in heart rate <50–60/ minutes for 10 seconds on the basis of postconceptional age). However, no adverse outcomes were noted for any of their cohort (although whether there is a protective effect of observation alone is not known). Some of the infants with extreme events developed symptoms of upper respiratory infection 1 to 2 days after the ALTE presentation. The risk factors for "extreme" events were prematurity, postconceptional age <43 weeks, and (presence of) upper respiratory infection symptoms. Importantly, infants with a postconceptional age >48 weeks were not documented as having an extreme event in this cohort. A previous longitudinal study also identified "extreme" events that occurred with comparable frequency in otherwise normal term infants and that were not statistically increased in term infants with a history of ALTE.[34]

Preterm infants have been shown to have more serious events, although an ALTE does not further increase that risk compared with asymptomatic preterm infants without ALTE.[34] Claudius and Keens[31] performed an observational prospective study in 59 infants presenting with ALTE who had been born at >30 weeks' gestation and had no significant medical illness. They evaluated factors in the clinical history and physical examination that, according to the authors, would warrant hospital admission on the basis of adverse outcomes (including recurrent cardiorespiratory events, infection, child abuse, or any life-threatening condition). Among these otherwise well infants, those with multiple ALTEs or age <1 month experienced adverse outcomes necessitating hospitalization. Prematurity was also a risk factor predictive of subsequent adverse events after an ALTE. Paroxysmal decreases in oxygen saturation in infants immediately before and during viral illnesses have been

well documented.[33,35] However, the significance of these brief hypoxemic events has not been established.

1B. Clinicians May Briefly Monitor Infants Presenting With a Lower-Risk BRUE With Continuous Pulse Oximetry and Serial Observations (Grade D, Weak Recommendation)

A normal physical examination, including vital signs and oximetry, is needed for a patient who has experienced a BRUE to be considered lower-risk. An evaluation at a single point in time may not be as accurate as a longer interval of observation. Unfortunately, there are few data to suggest the optimal duration of this period, the value of repeat examinations, and the effect of false-positive evaluations on family-centered care. Several studies have documented intermittent episodes of hypoxemia after admission for ALTE.[7,31,33] Pulse oximetry identified more infants with concerning paroxysmal events than cardiorespiratory monitoring alone.[33] However, occasional oxygen desaturations are commonly observed in normal infants, especially during sleep.[36] Furthermore, normative oximetry data are dependent on the specific machine, averaging interval, altitude, behavioral state, and postconceptional age. Similarly, there may be considerable variability in the vital signs and the clinical appearance of an infant. Pending further research into this important issue, clinicians may choose to monitor and provide serial examinations of infants in the lower-risk group for a brief period of time, ranging from 1 to 4 hours, to establish that the vital signs, physical examination, and symptomatology remain stable.

1C. Clinicians Should Not Obtain a Chest Radiograph in Infants Presenting With a Lower-Risk BRUE (Grade B, Moderate Recommendation)

Infectious processes can precipitate apnea. In 1 ALTE study, more than 80% of these infections involved the

respiratory tract.[37] Most, but not all, infants with significant lower respiratory tract infections will be symptomatic at the time of ALTE presentation. However, 2 studies have documented pneumonia in infants presenting with ALTE and an otherwise noncontributory history and physical examination.[4,37] These rare exceptions have generally been in infants younger than 2 months and would have placed them in the higher-risk category for a BRUE in this guideline. Similarly, Davies and Gupta[38] reported that 9 of 65 patients (ages unknown) who had ALTEs had abnormalities on chest radiography (not fully specified) despite no suspected respiratory disorder on clinical history or physical examination. Some of the radiographs were performed up to 24 hours after presentation. Davies and Gupta further reported that 33% of infants with ALTEs that were ultimately associated with a respiratory disease had a normal initial respiratory examination.[38] Kant et al[18] reported that 2 of 176 infants discharged after admission for ALTE died within 2 weeks, both of pneumonia. One infant had a normal chest radiograph initially; the other, with a history of prematurity, had a "possible" infiltrate. Thus, most experience has shown that a chest radiograph in otherwise well-appearing infants rarely alters clinical management.[7] Careful follow-up within 24 hours is important in infants with a nonfocal clinical history and physical examination to identify those who will ultimately have a lower respiratory tract infection diagnosed.

1D. Clinicians Should Not Obtain Measurement of Venous or Arterial Blood Gases in Infants Presenting With a Lower-Risk BRUE (Grade B, Moderate Recommendation)

Blood gas measurements have not been shown to add significant clinical information in otherwise well-appearing infants presenting with an ALTE.[4] Although not part of

1C. Clinicians Should Not Obtain Chest Radiograph in Infants Presenting With a Lower-Risk BRUE (Grade B, Moderate Recommendation)

Aggregate Evidence Quality	Grade B
Benefits	Reduce costs, unnecessary testing, radiation exposure, and caregiver/infant anxiety
	Avoid consequences of false-positive results
Risks, harm, cost	May rarely miss diagnostic opportunity for early lower respiratory tract or cardiac disease
Benefit-harm assessment	The benefits of reducing unnecessary testing, radiation exposure, and false-positive results, as well as alleviating caregiver and infant anxiety, outweigh the rare missed diagnostic opportunity for lower respiratory tract or cardiac disease
Intentional vagueness	None
Role of patient preferences	Caregiver may express concern regarding a longstanding breathing pattern in his/her infant or a recent change in breathing that might influence the decision to obtain chest radiography
Exclusions	None
Strength	Moderate recommendation
Key references	4, 37

1D. Clinicians Should Not Obtain Measurement of Venous or Arterial Blood Gases in Infants Presenting With a Lower-Risk BRUE (Grade B, Moderate Recommendation)

Aggregate Evidence Quality	Grade B
Benefits	Reduce costs, unnecessary testing, pain, risk of thrombosis, and caregiver/infant anxiety
	Avoid consequences of false-positive results
Risks, harm, cost	May miss rare instances of hypercapnia and acid-base imbalances
Benefit-harm assessment	The benefits of reducing unnecessary testing and false-positive results, as well as alleviating caregiver and infant anxiety, outweigh the rare missed diagnostic opportunity for hypercapnia and acid-base imbalances
Intentional vagueness	None
Role of patient preferences	None
Exclusions	None
Strength	Moderate recommendation
Key reference	4

this guideline, future research may demonstrate that blood gases are helpful in select infants with a higher risk BRUE to support the diagnosis of pulmonary disease, control-of-breathing disorders, or inborn errors of metabolism (IEMs).

1E. Clinicians Should Not Obtain an Overnight Polysomnograph in Infants Presenting With a Lower-Risk BRUE (Grade B, Moderate Recommendation)

Polysomnography consists of 8 to 12 hours of documented monitoring, including EEG, electro-oculography, electromyography, nasal/oral airflow, electrocardiography, end-tidal carbon dioxide, chest/ abdominal excursion, and oximetry. Polysomnography is considered by many to be the gold standard for identifying obstructive sleep apnea (OSA), central sleep apnea, and periodic breathing and may identify seizures. Some data have suggested using polysomnography in infants presenting with ALTEs as a means to predict the likelihood of recurrent significant cardiorespiratory events. A study in which polysomnography was performed in a cohort of infants with ALTEs (including recurrent episodes) reported that polysomnography may reveal respiratory pauses of >20 seconds or brief episodes of bradycardia that are predictive of ensuing events over the next several months.[40] However, without a control population, the clinical significance of these events is uncertain, because respiratory pauses are frequently observed in otherwise normal infants.[35] Similarly, Kahn and Blum[41] reported that 10 of 71 infants with a clinical history of "benign" ALTEs had an abnormal polysomnograph, including periodic breathing (7 of 10) or obstructive apnea (4 of 100), but specific data were not presented. These events were not found in a control group of 181 infants. The severity of the periodic breathing (frequency of arousals and extent of oxygen desaturation) could not be evaluated from these data. Daniëls et al[42] performed polysomnography in 422 infants with ALTEs and identified 11 infants with significant bradycardia, OSA, and/or oxygen desaturation. Home monitoring revealed episodes of bradycardia (<50 per minute) in 7 of 11 infants and concluded that polysomnography is a useful modality. However, the clinical history, physical examination, and laboratory findings were not presented. GER has also been associated with specific episodes of severe bradycardia in monitored infants.[43] Overall, most polysomnography studies have shown minimal or nonspecific findings in infants presenting with ALTEs.[44,45] Polysomnography studies generally have not been predictive of ALTE recurrence and do not identify those infants at risk of SIDS.[46] Thus, the routine use of polysomnography in infants presenting with a lower-risk BRUE is likely to have a low diagnostic yield and is unlikely to lead to changes in therapy.

OSA has been occasionally associated with ALTEs in many series, but not all.[39,47–49] The use of overnight polysomnography to evaluate for OSA should be guided by an assessment of risk on the basis of a

1E. Clinicians Should Not Obtain an Overnight Polysomnograph in Infants Presenting With a Lower-Risk BRUE (Grade B, Moderate Recommendation)

Aggregate Evidence Quality	Grade B
Benefits	Reduce costs, unnecessary testing, and caregiver/infant anxiety
	Avoid consequences of false-positive results
Risks, harm, cost	May miss rare instances of hypoxemia, hypercapnia, and/or bradycardia that would be detected by polysomnography
Benefit-harm assessment	The benefits of reducing unnecessary testing and false-positive results, as well as alleviating caregiver and infant anxiety, outweigh the rare missed diagnostic opportunity for hypoxemia, hypercapnia, and/or bradycardia
Intentional vagueness	None
Role of patient preferences	Caregivers may report concern regarding some aspects of their infant's sleep pattern that may influence the decision to perform polysomnography
Exclusions	None
Strength	Moderate recommendation
Key reference	39

1F. Clinicians May Obtain a 12-Lead Electrocardiogram for Infants Presenting With Lower-Risk BRUE (Grade C, Weak Recommendation)

Aggregate Evidence Quality	Grade C
Benefits	May identify BRUE patients with channelopathies (long QT syndrome, short QT syndrome, and Brugada syndrome), ventricular pre-excitation (Wolff-Parkinson-White syndrome), cardiomyopathy, or other heart disease
Risks, harm, cost	False-positive results may lead to further workup, expert consultation, anxiety, and cost
	False reassurance from negative results
	Cost and availability of electrocardiography testing and interpretation
Benefit-harm assessment	The benefit of identifying patients at risk of sudden cardiac death outweighs the risk of cost and false results
Intentional vagueness	None
Role of patient preferences	Caregiver may decide not to have testing performed
Exclusions	None
Strength	Weak recommendation (because of equilibrium between benefits and harms)
Key references	4, 16

comprehensive clinical history and physical examination.[50] Symptoms of OSA, which may be subtle or absent in infants, include snoring, noisy respirations, labored breathing, mouth breathing, and profuse sweating.[51] Occasionally, infants with OSA will present with failure to thrive, witnessed apnea, and/or developmental delay.[52] Snoring may be absent in younger infants with OSA, including those with micrognathia. In addition, snoring in otherwise normal infants is present at least 2 days per week in 11.8% and at least 3 days per week in 5.3% of infants.[53] Some infants with OSA

may be asymptomatic and have a normal physical examination.[54] However, some studies have reported a high incidence of snoring in infants with (26%–44%) and without (22%–26%) OSA, making the distinction difficult.[55] Additional risk factors for infant OSA include prematurity, maternal smoking, bronchopulmonary dysplasia, obesity, and specific medical conditions including laryngomalacia, craniofacial abnormalities, neuromuscular weakness, Down syndrome, achondroplasia, Chiari malformations, and Prader-Willi syndrome.[34,56–58]

1F. Clinicians May Obtain a 12-Lead Electrocardiogram for Infants Presenting With Lower-Risk BRUE (Grade C, Weak Recommendation)

ALTE studies have examined screening electrocardiograms (ECGs). A study by Brand et al[4] found no positive findings on 24 ECGs performed on 72 patients (33%) without a contributory history or physical examination. Hoki et al[16] reported a 4% incidence of cardiac disease found in 485 ALTE patients; ECGs were performed in 208 of 480 patients (43%) with 3 of 5 abnormal heart rhythms identified by the ECG and the remaining 2 showing structural heart disease. Both studies had low positive-predictive values of ECGs (0% and 1%, respectively). Hoki et al had a negative predictive value of 100% (96%–100%), and given the low prevalence of disease, there is little need for further testing in patients with a negative ECG.

Some cardiac conditions that may present as a BRUE include channelopathies (long QT syndrome, short QT syndrome, Brugada syndrome, and catecholaminergic polymorphic ventricular tachycardia), ventricular pre-excitation (Wolff-Parkinson-White syndrome), and cardiomyopathy/myocarditis (hypertrophic cardiomyopathy, dilated cardiomyopathy). Resting ECGs are ineffective in identifying patients with catecholaminergic polymorphic ventricular tachycardia. Family history is important in identifying individuals with channelopathies.

Severe potential outcomes of any of these conditions, if left undiagnosed or untreated, include sudden death or neurologic injury.[59] However, many patients do not ever experience symptoms in their lifetime and adverse outcomes are uncommon. A genetic autopsy study in infants who died of SIDS in Norway showed an association between 9.5% and 13.0% of infants with abnormal

1G. Clinicians Should Not Obtain an Echocardiogram in Infants Presenting With Lower-Risk BRUE (Grade C, Moderate Recommendation)

Aggregate Evidence Quality	Grade C
Benefits	Reduce costs, unnecessary testing, caregiver/infant anxiety, and sedation risk
	Avoid consequences of false-positive results
Risks, harm, cost	May miss rare diagnosis of cardiac disease
Benefit-harm assessment	The benefits of reducing unnecessary testing and sedation risk, as well as alleviating caregiver and infant anxiety, outweigh the rare missed diagnostic opportunity for cardiac causes
Intentional vagueness	Abnormal cardiac physical examination reflects the clinical judgment of the clinician
Role of patient preferences	Some caregivers may prefer to have echocardiography performed
Exclusions	Patients with an abnormal cardiac physical examination
Strength	Moderate recommendation
Key references	4, 16

1H. Clinicians Should Not Initiate Home Cardiorespiratory Monitoring in Infants Presenting With a Lower-Risk BRUE (Grade B, Moderate Recommendation)

Aggregate Evidence Quality	Grade B
Benefits	Reduce costs, unnecessary testing, and caregiver/infant anxiety
	Avoid consequences of false-positive results
Risks, harm, cost	May rarely miss an infant with recurrent central apnea or cardiac arrhythmias
Benefit-harm assessment	The benefits of reducing unnecessary testing and false-positive results, as well as alleviating caregiver and infant anxiety, outweigh the rare missed diagnostic opportunity for recurrent apnea or cardiac arrhythmias
Intentional vagueness	None
Role of patient preferences	Caregivers will frequently request monitoring be instituted after an ALTE in their infant; a careful explanation of the limitations and disadvantages of this technology should be given
Exclusions	None
Strength	Moderate recommendation
Key reference	34

or novel gene findings at the long QT loci.[60] A syncopal episode, which could present as a BRUE, is strongly associated with subsequent sudden cardiac arrest in patients with long QT syndrome.[61] The incidence and risk in those with other channelopathies have not been adequately studied. The incidence of sudden cardiac arrest in patients with ventricular pre-excitation (Wolff-Parkinson-White syndrome) is 3% to 4% over the lifetime of the individual.[62]

1G. Clinicians Should Not Obtain an Echocardiogram in Infants Presenting With Lower-Risk BRUE (Grade C, Moderate Recommendation)

Cardiomyopathy (hypertrophic and dilated cardiomyopathy) and myocarditis could rarely present as a lower-risk BRUE and can be identified with echocardiography. The cost of an echocardiogram is high and accompanied by sedation risks.

In a study in ALTE patients, Hoki et al[16] did not recommend echocardiography as an initial cardiac test unless there are findings on examination or from an echocardiogram consistent with heart disease. The majority of abnormal echocardiogram findings in their study were not perceived to be life-threatening or related to a cause for the ALTE (eg, septal defects or mild valve abnormalities), and they would have been detected on echocardiogram or physical examination. Brand et al[4] reported

32 echocardiograms in 243 ALTE patients and found only 1 abnormal echocardiogram, which was suspected because of an abnormal history and physical examination (double aortic arch).

1H. Clinicians Should Not Initiate Home Cardiorespiratory Monitoring in Infants Presenting With a Lower-Risk BRUE (Grade B, Moderate Recommendation)

The use of ambulatory cardiorespiratory monitors in infants presenting with ALTEs has been proposed as a modality to identify subsequent events, reduce the risk of SIDS, and alert caregivers of the need for intervention. Monitors can identify respiratory pauses and bradycardia in many infants presenting with ALTE; however, these events are also occasionally observed in otherwise normal infants.[34,40] In addition, infant monitors are prone to artifact and have not been shown to improve outcomes or prevent SIDS or improve neurodevelopmental outcomes.[63] Indeed, caregiver anxiety may be exacerbated with the use of infant monitors and potential false alarms. The overwhelming majority of monitor-identified alarms, including many with reported clinical symptomatology, do not reveal abnormalities on cardiorespiratory recordings.[64–66] Finally, there are several studies showing a lack of correlation between ALTEs and SIDS.[24,32]

Kahn and Blum[41] monitored 50 infants considered at "high risk" of SIDS and reported that 80% had alarms at home. All infants with alarms had at least 1 episode of parental intervention motivated by the alarms, although the authors acknowledged that some cases of parental intervention may have been attributable to parental anxiety. Nevertheless, the stimulated infants did not die of SIDS or require rehospitalization and therefore it was concluded that monitoring resulted in successful resuscitation, but this was not firmly established. Côté et al[40] reported "significant events" involving central apnea and bradycardia with long-term monitoring. However, these events were later shown to be frequently present in otherwise well infants.[34] There are insufficient data to support the use of commercial infant monitoring devices marketed directly to parents for the purposes of SIDS prevention.[63] These monitors may be prone to false alarms, produce anxiety, and disrupt sleep. Furthermore, these machines are frequently used without a medical support system and in the absence of specific training to respond to alarms. Although it is beyond the scope of this clinical practice guideline, future research may show that home monitoring (cardiorespiratory and/ or oximetry) is appropriate for some infants with higher-risk BRUE.

2. Child Abuse

2A. Clinicians Need Not Obtain Neuroimaging (Computed Tomography, MRI, or Ultrasonography) To Detect Child Abuse in Infants Presenting With a Lower-Risk BRUE (Grade C, Weak Recommendation)

2B. Clinicians Should Obtain an Assessment of Social Risk Factors To Detect Child Abuse in Infants Presenting With a Lower-Risk BRUE (Grade C, Moderate Recommendation)

Child abuse is a common and serious cause of an ALTE. Previous research has suggested that this occurs in up to 10% of ALTE cohorts.[3,67] Abusive head trauma is the most common form of child maltreatment associated with an ALTE. Other forms of child abuse that can present as an ALTE, but would not be identified by radiologic evaluations, include caregiver-fabricated illness (formally known as Münchausen by proxy), smothering, and poisoning.

Children who have experienced child abuse, most notably abusive head trauma, may present with a

2A. Clinicians Need Not Obtain Neuroimaging (Computed Tomography, MRI, or Ultrasonography) To Detect Child Abuse in Infants Presenting With a Lower-Risk BRUE (Grade C, Weak Recommendation)

Aggregate Evidence Quality	Grade C
Benefits	Decrease cost
	Avoid sedation, radiation exposure, consequences of false-positive results
Risks, harm, cost	May miss cases of child abuse and potential subsequent harm
Benefit-harm assessment	The benefits of reducing unnecessary testing, sedation, radiation exposure, and false-positive results, as well as alleviating caregiver and infant anxiety, outweigh the rare missed diagnostic opportunity for child abuse
Intentional vagueness	None
Role of patient preferences	Caregiver concerns may lead to requests for CNS imaging
Exclusions	None
Strength	Weak recommendation (based on low quality of evidence)
Key references	3, 67

2B. Clinicians Should Obtain an Assessment of Social Risk Factors To Detect Child Abuse in Infants Presenting With a Lower-Risk BRUE (Grade C, Moderate Recommendation)

Aggregate Evidence Quality	Grade C
Benefits	Identification of child abuse
	May benefit the safety of other children in the home
	May identify other social risk factors and needs and help connect caregivers with appropriate resources (eg, financial distress)
Risks, harm, cost	Resource intensive and not always available, particularly for smaller centers
	Some social workers may have inadequate experience in child abuse assessment
	May decrease caregiver's trust in the medical team
Benefit-harm assessment	The benefits of identifying child abuse and identifying and addressing social needs outweigh the cost of attempting to locate the appropriate resources or decreasing the trust in the medical team
Intentional vagueness	None
Role of patient preferences	Caregivers may perceive social services involvement as unnecessary and intrusive
Exclusions	None
Strength	Moderate recommendation
Key reference	68

BRUE. Four studies reported a low incidence (0.54%–2.5%) of abusive head trauma in infants presenting to the emergency department with an ALTE.[22,37,67,69] If only those patients meeting lower-risk BRUE criteria were included, the incidence of abusive head trauma would have been <0.3%. Although missing abusive head trauma can result in significant morbidity and mortality, the yield of performing neuroimaging

to screen for abusive head trauma is extremely low and has associated risks of sedation and radiation exposure.[32,70]

Unfortunately, the subtle presentation of child abuse may lead to a delayed diagnosis of abuse and result in significant morbidity and mortality.[70] A thorough history and physical examination is the best way to identify infants at risk of these conditions.[67,71] Significant concerning features for child abuse (especially abusive head trauma) can include a developmentally inconsistent or discrepant history provided by the caregiver(s), a previous ALTE, a recent emergency service telephone call, vomiting, irritability, or bleeding from the nose or mouth.[67,71]

Clinicians and medical team members (eg, nurses and social workers) should obtain an assessment of social risk factors in infants with a BRUE, including negative attributions to and unrealistic expectations of the child, mental health problems, domestic violence/intimate partner violence, social service involvement, law enforcement involvement, and substance abuse.[68] In addition, clinicians and medical team members can help families identify and use resources that may expand and strengthen their network of social support.

In previously described ALTE cohorts, abnormal physical findings were associated with an increased risk of abusive head trauma. These findings include bruising, subconjunctival hemorrhage, bleeding from the nose or mouth, and a history of rapid head enlargement or head circumference >95th percentile.[67,70-74] It is important to perform a careful physical examination to identify subtle findings of child abuse, including a large or full/bulging anterior fontanel, scalp bruising or bogginess, oropharynx or frenula damage, or skin findings such as bruising or petechiae, especially on the trunk, face, or ears. A normal physical examination does not rule out the possibility of abusive head trauma. Although beyond the scope of this guideline, it is important for the clinician to note that according to the available evidence, brain neuroimaging is probably indicated in patients who qualify as higher-risk because of concerns about abuse resulting from abnormal history or physical findings.[67]

A social and environmental assessment should evaluate the risk of intentional poisoning, unintentional poisoning, and environmental exposure (eg, home environment), because these can be associated with the symptoms of ALTEs in infants.[75-78] In 1 study, 8.4% of children presenting to the emergency department after an ALTE were found to have a clinically significant, positive comprehensive toxicology screen.[76] Ethanol or other drugs have also been associated with ALTEs.[79] Pulmonary hemorrhage can be caused by environmental exposure to moldy, water-damaged homes; it would usually present with hemoptysis and thus probably would not qualify as a BRUE.[80]

3. Neurology

3A. Clinicians Should Not Obtain Neuroimaging (Computed Tomography, MRI, or Ultrasonography) To Detect Neurologic Disorders in Infants Presenting With a Lower-Risk BRUE (Grade C, Moderate Recommendation)

Epilepsy or an abnormality of brain structure can present as a lower-risk BRUE. CNS imaging is 1 method for evaluating whether underlying abnormalities of brain development or structure might have led to the BRUE. The long-term risk of a diagnosis of neurologic disorders ranges from 3% to 11% in historical cohorts of ALTE patients.[2,32] One retrospective study in 243 ALTE patients reported that CNS imaging contributed to a neurologic diagnosis in 3% to 7% of patients.[4] However, the study population included all ALTEs, including those with a significant past medical history, non–well-appearing infants, and those with tests ordered as part of the emergency department evaluation.

In a large study of ALTE patients, the utility of CNS imaging studies in potentially classifiable lower-risk BRUE patients was found to be low.[32] The cohort of 471 patients was followed both acutely and long-term

for the development of epilepsy and other neurologic disorders, and the sensitivity and positive-predictive value of abnormal CNS imaging for subsequent development of epilepsy was 6.7% (95% confidence interval [CI]: 0.2%–32%) and 25% (95% CI: 0.6%–81%), respectively.

The available evidence suggests minimal utility of CNS imaging to evaluate for neurologic disorders, including epilepsy, in lower-risk patients. This situation is particularly true for pediatric epilepsy, in which even if a patient is determined ultimately to have seizures/epilepsy, there is no evidence of benefit from starting therapy after the first seizure compared with starting therapy after a second seizure in terms of achieving seizure remission.[81-83] However, our recommendations for BRUEs are not based on any prospective studies and only on a single retrospective study. Future work should track both short- and long-term neurologic outcomes when considering this issue.

3B. Clinicians Should Not Obtain an EEG To Detect Neurologic Disorders in Infants Presenting With a Lower-Risk BRUE (Grade C, Moderate Recommendation)

Epilepsy may first present as a lower-risk BRUE. The long-term risk of epilepsy ranges from 3% to 11% in historical cohorts of ALTE patients.[2,32] EEG is part of the typical evaluation for diagnosis of seizure disorders. However, the utility of obtaining an EEG routinely was found to be low in 1 study.[32] In a cohort of 471 ALTE patients followed both acutely and long-term for the development of epilepsy, the sensitivity and positive-predictive value of an abnormal EEG for subsequent development of epilepsy was 15% (95% CI: 2%–45%) and 33% (95% CI: 4.3%–48%), respectively. In contrast, another retrospective study in 243 ALTE patients reported that EEG contributed to a neurologic diagnosis in 6% of patients.[4] This study

3A. Clinicians Should Not Obtain Neuroimaging (Computed Tomography, MRI, or Ultrasonography) To Detect Neurologic Disorders in Infants Presenting With a Lower-Risk BRUE (Grade C, Moderate Recommendation)

Aggregate Evidence Quality	Grade C
Benefits	Reduce unnecessary testing, radiation exposure, sedation, caregiver/infant anxiety, and costs
	Avoid consequences of false-positive results
Risks, harm, cost	May rarely miss diagnostic opportunity for CNS causes of BRUEs
	May miss unexpected cases of abusive head trauma
Benefit-harm assessment	The benefits of reducing unnecessary testing, radiation exposure, sedation, and false-positive results, as well as alleviating caregiver and infant anxiety, outweigh the rare missed diagnostic opportunity for CNS cause
Intentional vagueness	None
Role of patient preferences	Caregivers may seek reassurance from neuroimaging and may not understand the risks from radiation and sedation
Exclusions	None
Strength	Moderate recommendation
Key references	2, 32, 81

3B. Clinicians Should Not Obtain an EEG To Detect Neurologic Disorders in Infants Presenting With a Lower-Risk BRUE (Grade C, Moderate Recommendation)

Aggregate Evidence Quality	Grade C
Benefits	Reduce unnecessary testing, sedation, caregiver/infant anxiety, and costs
	Avoid consequences of false-positive or nonspecific results
Risks, harm, cost	Could miss early diagnosis of seizure disorder
Benefit-harm assessment	The benefits of reducing unnecessary testing, sedation, and false-positive results, as well as alleviating caregiver and infant anxiety, outweigh the rare missed diagnostic opportunity for epilepsy
Intentional vagueness	None
Role of patient preferences	Caregivers may seek reassurance from an EEG, but they may not appreciate study limitations and the potential of false-positive results
Exclusions	None
Strength	Moderate recommendation
Key references	32, 84, 85

population differed significantly from that of Bonkowsky et al[32] in that all ALTE patients with a significant past medical history and non–well-appearing infants were included in the analysis and that tests ordered in the emergency department evaluation were also included in the measure of EEG yield.

A diagnosis of seizure is difficult to make from presenting symptoms of an ALTE.[30] Although EEG is recommended by the American Academy of Neurology after a first-time nonfebrile seizure, the yield and sensitivity of an EEG after a first-time ALTE in a lower-risk child are low.[86] Thus, the evidence available suggests

no utility for routine EEG to evaluate for epilepsy in a lower-risk BRUE. However, our recommendations for BRUEs are based on no prospective studies and on only a single retrospective study. Future work should track both short- and long-term epilepsy when considering this issue.

Finally, even if a patient is determined ultimately to have seizures/epilepsy, the importance of an EEG for a first-time ALTE is low, because there is little evidence that shows a benefit from starting therapy after the first seizure compared with after a second seizure in terms of achieving seizure remission.[81–83,85]

3C. Clinicians Should Not Prescribe Antiepileptic Medications for Potential Neurologic Disorders in Infants Presenting With a Lower-Risk BRUE (Grade C, Moderate Recommendation)

Once epilepsy is diagnosed, treatment can consist of therapy with an antiepileptic medication. In a cohort of 471 ALTE patients followed both acutely and long-term for the development of epilepsy, most patients who developed epilepsy had a second event within 1 month of their initial presentation.[32,87] Even if a patient is determined ultimately to have seizures/epilepsy, there is no evidence of benefit from starting therapy after the first seizure compared with starting therapy after a second seizure in terms of achieving seizure remission.[81–83,85] Sudden unexpected death in epilepsy (SUDEP) has a frequency close to 1 in 1000 patient-years, but the risks of SUDEP are distinct from ALTEs/BRUEs and include adolescent age and presence of epilepsy for more than 5 years. These data do not support prescribing an antiepileptic medicine for a first-time possible seizure because of a concern for SUDEP. Thus, the evidence available for ALTEs suggests lack of benefit for starting an antiepileptic medication for a lower-risk BRUE. However, our recommendations for BRUEs are based on no prospective studies and on only a single retrospective study. Future work should track both short- and long-term epilepsy when considering this issue.

4. Infectious Diseases

4A. Clinicians Should Not Obtain a White Blood Cell Count, Blood Culture, or Cerebrospinal Fluid Analysis or Culture To Detect an Occult Bacterial Infection in Infants Presenting With a Lower-Risk BRUE (Grade B, Strong Recommendation)

Some studies reported that ALTEs are the presenting complaint of an invasive infection, including bacteremia and/or meningitis

3C. Clinicians Should Not Prescribe Antiepileptic Medications for Potential Neurologic Disorders in Infants Presenting With a Lower-Risk BRUE (Grade C, Moderate Recommendation)

Aggregate Evidence Quality	Grade C
Benefits	Reduce medication adverse effects and risks, avoid treatment with unproven efficacy, and reduce cost
Risks, harm, cost	Delay in treatment of epilepsy could lead to subsequent BRUE or seizure
Benefit-harm assessment	The benefits of reducing medication adverse effects, avoiding unnecessary treatment, and reducing cost outweigh the risk of delaying treatment of epilepsy
Intentional vagueness	None
Role of patient preferences	Caregivers may feel reassured by starting a medicine but may not understand the medication risks
Exclusions	None
Strength	Moderate recommendation
Key references	32, 85, 87

4A. Clinicians Should Not Obtain a White Blood Cell Count, Blood Culture, or Cerebrospinal Fluid Analysis or Culture To Detect an Occult Bacterial Infection in Infants Presenting With a Lower-Risk BRUE (Grade B, Strong Recommendation)

Aggregate Evidence Quality	Grade B
Benefits	Reduce unnecessary testing, pain, exposure, caregiver/infant anxiety, and costs
	Avoid unnecessary antibiotic use and hospitalization pending culture results
	Avoid consequences of false-positive results/contaminants
Risks, harm, cost	Could miss serious bacterial infection at presentation
Benefit-harm assessment	The benefits of reducing unnecessary testing, pain, exposure, costs, unnecessary antibiotic use, and false-positive results, as well as alleviating caregiver and infant anxiety, outweigh the rare missed diagnostic opportunity for a bacterial infection
Intentional vagueness	None
Role of patient preferences	Caregiver concerns over possible infectious etiology may lead to requests for antibiotic therapy
Exclusions	None
Strength	Strong recommendation
Key references	4, 37, 88

detected during the initial workup. However, on further review of such cases with serious bacterial infections, these infants did not qualify as lower-risk BRUEs, because they had risk factors (eg, age <2 months) and/or appeared ill and had abnormal findings on physical examination (eg, meningeal signs, nuchal rigidity, hypothermia, shock, respiratory failure) suggesting a possible severe bacterial infection. After eliminating those cases, it appears extremely unlikely that meningitis or sepsis will be the etiology of a lower-risk BRUE.[2-4,37,88,89] Furthermore,

performing these tests for bacterial infection may then lead the clinician to empirically treat with antibiotics with the consequent risks of medication adverse effects, intravenous catheters, and development of resistant organisms. Furthermore, false-positive blood cultures (eg, coagulase negative staphylococci, *Bacillus* species, *Streptococcus viridans)* are likely to occur at times, leading to additional testing, longer hospitalization and antibiotic use, and increased parental anxiety until they are confirmed as contaminants.

Thus, the available evidence suggests that a complete blood cell count,

blood culture, and lumbar puncture are not of benefit in infants with the absence of risk factors or findings from the patient's history, vital signs, and physical examination (ie, a lower-risk BRUE).

4B. Clinicians Need Not Obtain a Urinalysis (Bag or Catheter) in Infants Presenting With a Lower-Risk BRUE (Grade C, Weak Recommendation)

Case series of infants with ALTEs have suggested that a urinary tract infection (UTI) may be detected at the time of first ALTE presentation in up to 8% of cases.[3,4,37,88] Claudius et al[88] provided insight into 17 cases of certain (*n* = 13) or possible (*n* = 4) UTI. However, 14 of these cases would not meet the criteria for a lower-risk BRUE on the basis of age younger than 2 months or being ill-appearing and/or having fever at presentation.

Furthermore, these studies do not always specify the method of urine collection, urinalysis findings, and/or the specific organisms and colony-forming units per milliliter of the isolates associated with the reported UTIs that would confirm the diagnosis. AAP guidelines for the diagnosis and management of UTIs in children 2 to 24 months of age assert that the diagnosis of UTI requires "*both* urinalysis results that suggest infection (pyuria and/or bacteruria) *and* the presence of at least 50 000 colony-forming units/mL of a uropathogen cultured from a urine specimen obtained through catheterization or suprapubic aspirate."[90] Thus, it seems unlikely for a UTI to present as a lower-risk BRUE.

Pending more detailed studies that apply a rigorous definition of UTI to infants presenting with a lower-risk BRUE, a screening urinalysis need not be obtained routinely. If it is decided to evaluate the infant for a possible UTI, then a urinalysis can be obtained but should only be followed up with a culture if the urinalysis has

4B. Clinicians Need Not Obtain a Urinalysis (Bag or Catheter) in Infants Presenting With a Lower-Risk BRUE (Grade C, Weak Recommendation)

Aggregate Evidence Quality	Grade C
Benefits	Reduce unnecessary testing, pain, iatrogenic infection, caregiver/infant anxiety, and costs
	Avoid consequences of false-positive results
	Avoid delay from time it takes to obtain a bag urine
Risks, harm, cost	May delay diagnosis of infection
Benefit-harm assessment	The benefits of reducing unnecessary testing, iatrogenic infection, pain, costs, and false-positive results, as well as alleviating caregiver and infant anxiety, outweigh the rare missed diagnostic opportunity for a urinary tract infection
Intentional vagueness	None
Role of patient preferences	Caregiver concerns may lead to preference for testing
Exclusions	None
Strength	Weak recommendation (based on low quality of evidence)
Key references	4, 88

4C. Clinicians Should Not Obtain a Chest Radiograph To Assess for Pulmonary Infection in Infants Presenting With a Lower-Risk BRUE (Grade B, Moderate Recommendation)

Aggregate Evidence Quality	Grade B
Benefits	Reduce costs, unnecessary testing, radiation exposure, and caregiver/infant anxiety
	Avoid consequences of false-positive results
Risks, harm, cost	May miss early lower respiratory tract infection
Benefit-harm assessment	The benefits of reducing unnecessary testing, radiation exposure, and false-positive results, as well as alleviating caregiver and infant anxiety, outweigh the rare missed diagnostic opportunity for pulmonary infection
Intentional vagueness	None
Role of patient preferences	Caregiver concerns may lead to requests for a chest radiograph
Exclusions	None
Strength	Moderate recommendation
Key references	4, 18, 37

abnormalities suggestive of possible infection (eg, increased white blood cell count, positive nitrates, and/or leukocyte esterase).

4C. Clinicians Should Not Obtain a Chest Radiograph To Assess for Pulmonary Infection in Infants Presenting With a Lower-Risk BRUE (Grade B, Moderate Recommendation)

Chest radiography is unlikely to yield clinical benefit in a well-appearing infant presenting with a lower-risk BRUE. In the absence of abnormal respiratory findings (eg, cough, tachypnea, decreased oxygen saturation, auscultatory changes), lower respiratory tract infection is unlikely to be present.

Studies in children presenting with an ALTE have described occasional cases with abnormal findings on chest radiography in the absence of respiratory findings on history or physical examination.[4,37] However, the nature of the abnormalities and their role in the ALTE presentation in the absence of further details about the radiography results make it difficult to interpret the significance of these observations. For instance, descriptions of increased interstitial markings or small areas of atelectasis would not have the same implication as a focal consolidation or pleural effusion.

Kant et al,[18] in a follow-up of 176 children admitted for an ALTE, reported that 2 infants died within 2 weeks of discharge and both were found to have pneumonia on postmortem examination. This observation does not support the potential indication for an initial radiograph. In fact, one of the children had a normal radiograph during the initial evaluation. The finding of pneumonia on postmortem examination may reflect an agonal aspiration event. Brand et al[4] reported 14 cases of pneumonia identified at presentation in their analysis of 95 cases of ALTEs. However, in 13 of the patients, findings suggestive of lower respiratory infection, such as tachypnea, stridor, retractions, use of accessory muscles, or adventitious sounds on auscultation, were detected at presentation, leading to the request for chest radiography.

4D. Clinicians Need Not Obtain Respiratory Viral Testing If Rapid Testing Is Available in Infants Presenting With a Lower-Risk BRUE (Grade C, Weak Recommendation)

Respiratory viral infections (especially with respiratory syncytial virus [RSV]) have been reported as presenting with apnea or an ALTE, with anywhere from 9% to 82% of patients tested being positive for RSV.[2,4,37,88] However, this finding was observed predominantly in children younger than 2 months and/or those who were born prematurely. Recent data suggest that apnea or an ALTE presentation is not unique to RSV and may be seen with a spectrum of respiratory viral infections.[90] The data in ALTE cases do not address the potential role of other respiratory viruses in ALTEs or BRUEs.

In older children, respiratory viral infection would be expected to present with symptoms ranging from upper respiratory to lower respiratory tract infection rather than as an isolated BRUE. A history of respiratory symptoms and illness exposure; findings of congestion and/or cough, tachypnea, or lower respiratory tract abnormalities; and local epidemiology regarding currently circulating viruses are

4D. Clinicians Need Not Obtain Respiratory Viral Testing If Rapid Testing Is Available in Infants Presenting With a Lower-Risk BRUE (Grade C, Weak Recommendation)

Aggregate Evidence Quality	Grade C
Benefits	Reduce costs, unnecessary testing, and caregiver/infant discomfort
	Avoid false-negative result leading to missed diagnosis and false reassurance
Risks, harm, cost	Failure to diagnose a viral etiology
	Not providing expectant management for progression and appropriate infection control interventions for viral etiology
Benefit-harm assessment	The benefits of reducing unnecessary testing, pain, costs, false reassurance, and false-positive results, as well as alleviating caregiver and infant anxiety and challenges associated with providing test results in a timely fashion, outweigh the rare missed diagnostic opportunity for a viral infection
Intentional vagueness	"Rapid testing"; time to results may vary
Role of patient preferences	Caregiver may feel reassured by a specific viral diagnosis
Exclusions	None
Strength	Weak recommendation (based on low-quality evidence)
Key references	4, 37, 91

4E. Clinicians May Obtain Testing for Pertussis in Infants Presenting With a Lower-Risk BRUE (Grade B, Weak Recommendation)

Aggregate Evidence Quality	Grade B
Benefits	Identify a potentially treatable infection
	Monitor for progression of symptoms, additional apneic episodes
	Potentially prevent secondary spread and/or identify and treat additional cases
Risks, harm, cost	Cost of test
	Discomfort of nasopharyngeal swab
	False-negative results leading to missed diagnosis and false reassurance
	Rapid testing not always available
	False reassurance from negative results
Benefit-harm assessment	The benefits of identifying and treating pertussis and preventing apnea and secondary spread outweigh the cost, discomfort, and consequences of false test results and false reassurance; the benefits are greatest in at-risk populations (exposed, underimmunized, endemic, and during outbreaks)
Intentional vagueness	None
Role of patient preferences	Caregiver may feel reassured if a diagnosis is obtained and treatment can be implemented
Exclusions	None
Strength	Weak recommendation (based on balance of benefit and harm)
Key reference	93

considerations in deciding whether to order rapid testing for respiratory viruses. Because lower-risk BRUE patients do not have these symptoms, clinicians need not perform such testing.

In addition, until recently and in reports of ALTE patients to date, RSV testing was performed by using antigen detection tests. More recently, automated nucleic acid

amplification-based tests have entered clinical practice. These assays are more sensitive than antigen detection tests and can detect multiple viruses from a single nasopharyngeal swab. The use of these tests in future research may allow better elucidation of the role of respiratory viruses in patients presenting with an ALTE in general and whether they play a role in BRUEs.

As a cautionary note, detection of a virus in a viral multiplex assay may not prove causality, because some agents, such as rhinovirus and adenovirus, may persist for periods beyond the acute infection (up to 30 days) and may or may not be related to the present episode.[92] In a lower-risk BRUE without respiratory symptoms testing for viral infection may not be indicated, but in the presence of congestion and/or cough, or recent exposure to a viral respiratory infection, such testing may provide useful information regarding the cause of the child's symptoms and for infection control management. Anticipatory guidance and arranging close follow-up at the initial presentation could be helpful if patients subsequently develop symptoms of a viral infection.

4E. Clinicians May Obtain Testing for Pertussis in Infants Presenting With a Lower-Risk BRUE (Grade B, Weak Recommendation)

Pertussis infection has been reported to cause ALTEs in infants, because it can cause gagging, gasping, and color change followed by respiratory pause. Such infants can be afebrile and may not develop cough or lower respiratory symptoms for several days afterward.

The decision to test a lower-risk BRUE patient for pertussis should consider potential exposures, vaccine history (including intrapartum immunization of the mother as well as the infant's vaccination history), awareness of pertussis activity in the community, and turnaround time for results. Polymerase chain reaction testing for pertussis on a nasopharyngeal specimen, if available, offers the advantage of rapid turnaround time to results.[94] Culture for the organism requires selective media and will take days to yield results but may still be useful in the face of identified risk of exposure. In patients in whom there is a high index of suspicion on the basis of the aforementioned risk factors, clinicians may consider prolonging the observation period and starting empirical antibiotics while awaiting test results (more information is available from the Centers for Disease Control and Prevention).[95]

5. Gastroenterology

5A. Clinicians Should Not Obtain Investigations for GER (eg, Upper Gastrointestinal Series, pH Probe, Endoscopy, Barium Contrast Study, Nuclear Scintigraphy, and Ultrasonography) in Infants Presenting With a Lower-Risk BRUE (Grade C, Moderate Recommendation)

GER occurs in more than two-thirds of infants and is the topic of discussion with pediatricians at one-quarter of all routine 6-month infant visits.[96] GER can lead to airway obstruction, laryngospasm, or aspiration. Although ALTEs that can be attributed to GER symptoms (eg, choking after spitting up) qualify as an ALTE according to the National Institutes of Health definition, importantly, they do not qualify as a BRUE.

GER may still be a contributing factor to a lower-risk BRUE if the patient's GER symptoms were not witnessed or well described by caregivers. However, the available evidence suggests no utility of routine diagnostic testing to evaluate for GER in these patients. The brief period of observation that occurs during an upper gastrointestinal series is inadequate to rule out the occurrence of pathologic reflux at other times, and the high prevalence of nonpathologic reflux that often occurs during the study can encourage false-positive diagnoses. In addition, the observation of the reflux of a barium column into the esophagus during gastrointestinal contrast studies may not correlate with the severity of GER or the degree of esophageal mucosal inflammation in patients with reflux esophagitis. Routine performance

5A. Clinicians Should Not Obtain Investigations for GER (eg, Upper Gastrointestinal Series, pH Probe, Endoscopy, Barium Contrast Study, Nuclear Scintigraphy, and Ultrasonography) in Infants Presenting With a Lower-Risk BRUE (Grade C, Moderate Recommendation)

Aggregate Evidence Quality	Grade C
Benefits	Reduce unnecessary testing, procedural complications (sedation, intestinal perforation, bleeding), pain, radiation exposure, caregiver/infant anxiety, and costs
	Avoid consequences of false-positive results
Risks, harm, cost	Delay diagnosis of rare but serious gastrointestinal abnormalities (eg, tracheoesophageal fistula)
	Long-term morbidity of repeated events (eg, chronic lung disease)
Benefit-harm assessment	The benefits of reducing unnecessary testing, complications, radiation, pain, costs, and false-positive results, as well as alleviating caregiver and infant anxiety, outweigh the rare missed diagnostic opportunity for a gastrointestinal abnormality or morbidity from repeat events
Intentional vagueness	None
Role of patient preferences	Caregiver may be reassured by diagnostic evaluation of GER
Exclusions	None
Strength	Moderate recommendation
Key references	96, 97

of an upper gastrointestinal series to diagnose GER is not justified and should be reserved to screen for anatomic abnormalities associated with vomiting (which is a symptom that precludes the diagnosis of a lower-risk BRUE).[98] Gastroesophageal scintigraphy scans for reflux of ^{99m}Tc-labeled solids or liquids into the esophagus or lungs after the administration of the test material into the stomach. The lack of standardized techniques and age-specific normal values limits the usefulness of this test. Therefore, gastroesophageal scintigraphy is not recommended in the routine evaluation of pediatric patients with GER symptoms or a lower-risk BRUE.[97] Multiple intraluminal impedance (MII) is useful for detecting both acidic and nonacidic reflux, thereby providing a more detailed picture of esophageal events than pH monitoring. Combined pH/MII testing is evolving into the test of choice to detect temporal relationships between specific symptoms and the reflux of both acid and nonacid gastric contents. In particular, MII has been used in recent years to investigate how GER correlates with respiratory symptoms, such as apnea or

cough. Performing esophageal pH +/- impedance monitoring is not indicated in the routine evaluation of infants presenting with a lower-risk BRUE, although it may be considered in patients with recurrent BRUEs and GER symptoms even if these occur independently.

Problems with the coordination of feedings can lead to ALTEs and BRUEs. In a study in Austrian newborns, infants who experienced an ALTE had a more than twofold increase in feeding difficulties (multivariate relative risk: 2.5; 95% CI: 1.3–4.6).[99] In such patients, it is likely that poor suck-swallow-breathe coordination triggered choking or laryngospasm. A clinical speech therapy evaluation may help to evaluate any concerns for poor coordination swallowing with feeding.

5B. Clinicians Should Not Prescribe Acid Suppression Therapy for Infants Presenting With a Lower-Risk BRUE (Grade C, Moderate Recommendation)

The available evidence suggests no proven efficacy of acid suppression therapy for esophageal reflux in patients presenting with a lower-risk BRUE. Acid suppression therapy with H2-receptor antagonists or proton

5B. Clinicians Should Not Prescribe Acid Suppression Therapy for Infants Presenting With a Lower-Risk BRUE (Grade C, Moderate Recommendation)

Aggregate Evidence Quality	Grade C
Benefits	Reduce unnecessary medication use, adverse effects, and cost from treatment with unproven efficacy
Risks, harm, cost	Delay treatment of rare but undiagnosed gastrointestinal disease, which could lead to complications (eg, esophagitis)
Benefit-harm assessment	The benefits of reducing medication adverse effects, avoiding unnecessary treatment, and reducing cost outweigh the risk of delaying treatment of gastrointestinal disease
Intentional vagueness	None
Role of patient preferences	Caregiver concerns may lead to requests for treatment
Exclusions	None
Strength	Moderate recommendation
Key reference	98

pump inhibitors may be indicated in selected pediatric patients with GER disease (GERD), which is diagnosed in patients when reflux of gastric contents causes troublesome symptoms or complications.[98] Infants with spitting up or throat-clearing coughs that are not troublesome do not meet diagnostic criteria for GERD. Indeed, the inappropriate administration of acid suppression therapy may have harmful adverse effects because it exposes infants to an increased risk of pneumonia or gastroenteritis.[100]

GER leading to apnea is not always clinically apparent and can be the cause of a BRUE. Acid reflux into the esophagus has been shown to be temporally associated with oxygen desaturation and obstructive apnea, suggesting that esophageal reflux may be one of the underlying conditions in selected infants presenting with BRUEs.[101] Respiratory symptoms are more likely to be associated with GER when gross emesis occurs at the time of a BRUE, when episodes occur while the infant is awake and supine (sometimes referred to as "awake apnea"), and when a pattern of obstructive apnea is observed while the infant is making respiratory efforts without effective air movement.[102]

Wenzl et al[103] reported a temporal association between 30% of the nonpathologic, short episodes of central apnea and GER by analyzing combined data from simultaneous esophageal and cardiorespiratory monitoring. These findings cannot be extrapolated to pathologic infant apnea and may represent a normal protective cessation of breathing during regurgitation. Similarly, Mousa et al[104] analyzed data from 527 apneic events in 25 infants and observed that only 15.2% were temporally associated with GER. Furthermore, there was no difference in the linkage between apneic events and acid reflux (7.0%) and nonacid reflux (8.2%). They concluded that there is little evidence for an association between acid reflux or nonacid reflux and the frequency of apnea. Regression analysis revealed a significant association between apnea and reflux in 4 of 25 infants. Thus, in selected infants, a clear temporal relationship between apnea and ALTE can be shown. However, larger studies have not proven a causal relationship between pathologic apnea and GER.[105]

As outlined in the definition of a BRUE, when an apparent explanation for the event, such as GER, is evident at the time of initial evaluation, the patient should be managed as appropriate for the clinical situation. However, BRUEs can be caused by episodes of reflux-related laryngospasm (sometimes referred to as "silent reflux"), which may not be clinically apparent at the time of initial evaluation. Laryngospasm may also occur during feeding in the absence of GER. Measures that have been shown to be helpful in the nonpharmacologic management of GER in infants include avoiding overfeeding, frequent burping during feeding, upright positioning in the caregiver's arms after feeding, and avoidance of secondhand smoke.[106] Thickening feedings with commercially thickened formula for infants without milk-protein intolerance does not alter esophageal acid exposure detected by esophageal pH study but has been shown to decrease the frequency of regurgitation. Given the temporal association observed between GER and respiratory symptoms in selected infants, approaches that decrease the height of the reflux column, the volume of refluxate, and the frequency of reflux episodes may theoretically be beneficial.[98] Combined pH/MII testing has shown that, although the frequency of reflux events is unchanged with thickened formula, the height of the column of refluxate is decreased. Studies have shown that holding the infant on the caregiver's shoulders for 10 to 20 minutes to allow for adequate burping after a feeding before placing the infant in the "back to sleep position" can decrease the frequency of GER in infants. In contrast, placing an infant in a car seat or in other semisupine positions, such as in an infant carrier, exacerbates esophageal reflux and should be avoided.[98] The frequency of GER has been reported to be decreased in breastfed compared with formula-fed infants. Thus, the benefits of breastfeeding are preferred over the theoretical effect of thickened formula feeding, so exclusive breastfeeding should be encouraged whenever possible.

6. Inborn Errors of Metabolism

6A. Clinicians Need Not Obtain Measurement of Serum Lactic Acid or Serum Bicarbonate To Detect an IEM in Infants Presenting With a Lower-Risk BRUE (Grade C, Weak Recommendation)

6B. Clinicians Should Not Obtain a Measurement of Serum Sodium, Potassium, Chloride, Blood Urea Nitrogen, Creatinine, Calcium, or Ammonia To Detect an IEM on Infants Presenting With a Lower-Risk BRUE (Grade C, Moderate Recommendation)

6C. Clinicians Should Not Obtain a Measurement of Venous or Arterial Blood Gases To Detect an IEM in Infants Presenting With Lower-Risk BRUE (Grade C, Moderate Recommendation)

6D. Clinicians Need Not Obtain a Measurement of Blood Glucose To Detect an IEM in Infants Presenting With a Lower-Risk BRUE (Grade C, Weak Recommendation)

6E. Clinicians Should Not Obtain Measurements of Urine Organic Acids, Plasma Amino Acids, or Plasma Acylcarnitines To Detect an IEM in Infants Presenting With a Lower-Risk BRUE (Grade C, Moderate Recommendation)

IEMs are reported to cause an ALTE in 0% to 5% of cases.[2,27,38,99,107,108] On the basis of the information provided by the authors for these patients, it seems unlikely that events could have been classified as a lower-risk BRUE, either because the patient had a positive history or physical examination or a recurrent event. The most commonly reported disorders include fatty acid oxidation disorders or urea cycle disorders.[107,109] In cases of vague or resolved symptoms, a careful history can help determine whether the infant had not received previous treatment (eg, feeding after listlessness for suspected hypoglycemia). These rare circumstances could include milder or later-onset presentations of IEMs.

Infants may be classified as being at a higher risk of BRUE because

6A. Clinicians Need Not Obtain Measurement of Serum Lactic Acid or Serum Bicarbonate To Detect an IEM in Infants Presenting With a Lower-Risk BRUE (Grade C, Weak Recommendation)

Aggregate Evidence Quality	Grade C
Benefits	Reduce unnecessary testing, caregiver/infant anxiety, and costs
	Avoid consequences of false-positive or nonspecific results
Risks, harm, cost	May miss detection of an IEM
Benefit-harm assessment	The benefits of reducing unnecessary testing, cost, and false-positive results, as well as alleviating caregiver and infant anxiety, outweigh the rare missed diagnostic opportunity for an IEM
Intentional vagueness	Detection of higher lactic acid or lower bicarbonate levels should be considered to have a lower likelihood of being a false-positive result and may warrant additional investigation
Role of patient preferences	Caregiver concerns may lead to requests for diagnostic testing
Exclusions	None
Strength	Weak recommendation (based on low-quality evidence)
Key reference	38

6B. Clinicians Should Not Obtain a Measurement of Serum Sodium, Potassium, Chloride, Blood Urea Nitrogen, Creatinine, Calcium, or Ammonia To Detect an IEM on Infants Presenting With a Lower-Risk BRUE (Grade C, Moderate Recommendation)

Aggregate Evidence Quality	Grade C
Benefits	Reduce costs, unnecessary testing, pain, and caregiver/infant anxiety
	Avoid consequences of false-positive results
Risks, harm, cost	May miss detection of an IEM
Benefit-harm assessment	The benefits of reducing unnecessary testing, cost, and false-positive results, as well as alleviating caregiver and infant anxiety, outweigh the rare missed diagnostic opportunity for an IEM
Intentional vagueness	None
Role of patient preferences	Caregiver concerns may lead to requests for diagnostic testing
Exclusions	None
Strength	Moderate recommendation
Key reference	4

of a family history of an IEM, developmental disabilities, SIDS, or a medical history of abnormal newborn screening results, unexplained infant death, age younger than 2 months, a prolonged event (>1 minute), or multiple events without an explanation. Confirmation that a newborn screen is complete and is negative is an important aspect of the medical history, but the clinician must consider that not all potential disorders are included in current newborn screening panels in the United States.

Lactic Acid

Measurement of lactic acid can result in high false-positive rates if the sample is not collected properly, making the decision to check a lactic

acid problematic. In addition, lactic acid may be elevated because of metabolic abnormalities attributable to other conditions, such as sepsis, and are not specific for IEMs.

Only 2 studies evaluated the specific measurement of lactic acid.[27,38] Davies and Gupta[38] reported 65 infants with consistent laboratory evaluations and found that 54% of infants had a lactic acid >2 mmol/L but only 15% had levels >3 mmol/L. The latter percentage of infants are more likely to be clinically significant and less likely to reflect a false-positive result. Five of 7 infants with a lactic acid >3 mmol/L had a "specific, serious diagnosis," although the specifics of these diagnoses were not included and no IEM was

6C. Clinicians Should Not Obtain a Measurement of Venous or Arterial Blood Gases To Detect an IEM in Infants Presenting With Lower-Risk BRUE (Grade C, Moderate Recommendation)

Aggregate Evidence Quality	Grade C
Benefits	Reduce costs, unnecessary testing, pain, risk of thrombosis, and caregiver/infant anxiety
	Avoid consequences of false-positive results
Risks, harm, cost	May miss detection of an IEM
Benefit-harm assessment	The benefits of reducing unnecessary testing, cost, and false-positive results, as well as alleviating caregiver and infant anxiety, outweigh the rare missed diagnostic opportunity for an IEM
Intentional vagueness	None
Role of patient preferences	Caregiver concerns may lead to requests for diagnostic testing
Exclusions	None
Strength	Moderate recommendation
Key reference	4

6D. Clinicians Need Not Obtain a Measurement of Blood Glucose To Detect an IEM in Infants Presenting With a Lower-Risk BRUE (Grade C, Weak Recommendation)

Aggregate Evidence Quality	Grade C
Benefits	Reduce costs, unnecessary testing, pain, risk of thrombosis, and caregiver/infant anxiety
	Avoid consequences of false-positive results
Risks, harm, cost	May miss rare instances of hypoglycemia attributable to undiagnosed IEM
Benefit-harm assessment	The benefits of reducing unnecessary testing, cost, and false-positive results, as well as alleviating caregiver and infant anxiety, outweigh the rare missed diagnostic opportunity for an IEM
Intentional vagueness	Measurement of glucose is often performed immediately through a simple bedside test; no abnormalities have been reported in asymptomatic infants, although studies often do not distinguish between capillary or venous measurement
Role of patient preferences	Caregiver concerns may lead to requests for diagnostic testing
Exclusions	None
Strength	Weak recommendation (based on low-quality evidence)
Key reference	4

confirmed in this study. This study also reported a 20% positive yield of testing for a bicarbonate <20 mmol/L and commented that there was a trend for lower bicarbonate and higher lactic acid levels in those with a recurrent event or a definitive diagnosis. The second publication[27] found no elevations of lactate in 4 of 49 children who had an initial abnormal venous blood gas, of which all repeat blood gas measurements were normal.

Serum Bicarbonate

Abnormal serum bicarbonate levels have been studied in 11 infants, of whom 7 had a diagnosis of sepsis or seizures.[38] Brand et al[4] studied 215 infants who had bicarbonate measured and found only 9 abnormal results, and only 3 of these contributed to the final diagnosis. Although unknown, it is most likely that the event in those infants would not have been classified as a BRUE under the new classification, because those infants were most likely symptomatic on presentation.

Serum Glucose

Abnormal blood glucose levels were evaluated but not reported in 3 studies.[4,38,110] Although abnormalities of blood glucose can occur from various IEMs, such as medium-chain acyl–coenzyme A dehydrogenase deficiency or other fatty acid oxidation disorders, their prevalence has not been increased in SIDS and near-miss SIDS but could be considered as a cause of higher-risk BRUEs.[111] It is important to clarify through a careful medical history evaluation that the infant was not potentially hypoglycemic at discovery of the event and improved because of enteral treatment, because these disorders will not typically self-resolve without intervention (ie, feeding).

Serum Electrolytes and Calcium

ALTE studies evaluating the diagnostic value of electrolytes, including sodium, potassium, blood urea nitrogen, and creatinine, reported the rare occurrence of abnormalities, ranging from 0% to 4.3%.[4,38,110] Abnormal calcium levels have been reported in 0% to 1.5% of infants with ALTE, although these reports did not provide specific causes of hypocalcemia. Another study reported profound vitamin D deficiency with hypocalcemia in 5 of 25 infants with a diagnosis of an ALTE over a 2-year period in Saudi Arabia.[4,21,38,110] In lower-risk BRUE infants, clinicians should not obtain a calcium measurement unless the clinical history raises suspicion of hypocalcemia (eg, vitamin D deficiency or hypoparathyroidism).

Ammonia

Elevations of ammonia are typically associated with persistent symptoms and recurring events, and therefore testing would not be indicated in lower-risk BRUEs. Elevations of ammonia were reported in 11 infants (7 whom had an IEM) in a report of infants with recurrent ALTE and SIDS, limiting extrapolation to lower-risk BRUEs.[109] Elevations of ammonia >100 mmol/L were found in 4% of 65 infants, but this publication did not document a confirmed IEM.[38] Weiss et al[27] reported no abnormal elevations of ammonia in 4 infants with abnormal venous blood gas.

Venous or Arterial Blood Gas

Blood gas abnormalities leading to a diagnosis have not been reported in previous ALTE studies. Brand et al[4] reported 53 of 60 with positive findings, with none contributing to the final diagnosis. Weiss et al[27] reported 4 abnormal findings of 49 completed, all of which were normal on repeat measurements (along with normal lactate and ammonia levels). Blood gas detection is a routine test performed in acutely symptomatic patients who are being evaluated for suspected IEMs and may be considered in higher-risk BRUEs.

Urine Organic Acids, Plasma Amino Acids, Plasma Acylcarnitines

The role of advanced screening for IEMs has been reported in only 1 publication. Davies and Gupta[38] reported abnormalities of urine organic acids in 2% of cases and abnormalities of plasma amino acids in 4% of cases. Other reports have described an "unspecified metabolic screen" that was abnormal in 4.5% of cases but did not provide further description of specifics within that "screen."[4] Other reports have frequently included the descriptions of ALTEs with urea cycle disorders, organic acidemias, lactic acidemias, and fatty acid oxidation disorders such as medium chain acyl–coenzyme A dehydrogenase deficiency but did not distinguish between SIDS and near-miss SIDS.[107,109,111] Specific testing of urine organic acids, plasma amino acids, or plasma acylcarnitines may have a role in patients with a higher-risk BRUE.

6E. Clinicians Should Not Obtain Measurements of Urine Organic Acids, Plasma Amino Acids, or Plasma Acylcarnitines To Detect an IEM in Infants Presenting With a Lower-Risk BRUE (Grade C, Moderate Recommendation)

Aggregate Evidence Quality	Grade C
Benefits	Reduce costs, unnecessary testing, pain, risk of thrombosis, and caregiver/infant anxiety
	Avoid consequences of false-positive results
Risks, harm, cost	May miss detection of an IEM
Benefit-harm assessment	The benefits of reducing unnecessary testing, cost, and false-positive results, as well as alleviating caregiver and infant anxiety, outweigh the rare missed diagnostic opportunity for an IEM
Intentional vagueness	Lower-risk BRUEs will have a very low likelihood of disease, but these tests may be indicated in rare cases in which there is no documentation of a newborn screen being performed
Role of patient preferences	Caregiver concerns may lead to requests for diagnostic testing
Exclusions	None
Strength	Moderate recommendation
Key references	4, 38

7A. Clinicians Should Not Obtain Laboratory Evaluation for Anemia in Infants Presenting With a Lower-Risk BRUE (Grade C, Moderate Recommendation)

Aggregate Evidence Quality	Grade C
Benefits	Reduce costs, unnecessary testing, pain, risk of thrombosis, and caregiver/infant anxiety
	Avoid consequences of false-positive results
Risks, harm, cost	May miss diagnosis of anemia
Benefit-harm assessment	The benefits of reducing unnecessary testing, cost, and false-positive results, as well as alleviating caregiver and infant anxiety, outweigh the missed diagnostic opportunity for anemia
Intentional vagueness	None
Role of patient preferences	Caregivers may be reassured by testing
Exclusions	None
Strength	Moderate recommendation
Key reference	22

7. Anemia

7A. Clinicians Should Not Obtain Laboratory Evaluation for Anemia in Infants Presenting With a Lower-Risk BRUE (Grade C, Moderate Recommendation)

Anemia has been associated with ALTEs in infants, but the significance and causal association with the event itself are unclear.[38,112,113] Normal hemoglobin concentrations have also been reported in many other ALTE populations.[69,112,114] Brand et al[4] reported an abnormal hemoglobin in 54 of 223 cases, but in only 2 of 159 was the hemoglobin concentration associated with the final diagnosis (which was abusive head injury in both). Parker and Pitetti[22] also reported that infants who presented with ALTEs and ultimately were determined to be victims of child abuse were more likely to have a lower mean hemoglobin (10.6 vs 12.7 g/dL; $P = .02$).

8. Patient- and Family-Centered Care

8A. Clinicians Should Offer Resources for CPR Training to Caregivers (Grade C, Moderate Recommendation)

The majority of cardiac arrests in children result from a respiratory deterioration. Bystander CPR has been reported to have been conducted in 37% to 48% of pediatric out-of-hospital cardiac arrests and in 34% of respiratory arrests.[116] Bystander CPR results in significant improvement in 1-month survival rates in both cardiac and respiratory arrest.[117–119]

Although lower-risk BRUEs are neither a cardiac nor a respiratory arrest, the AAP policy statement on CPR recommends that pediatricians advocate for life-support training for caregivers and the general public.[115] A technical report that accompanies the AAP policy statement on CPR proposes that this can improve overall community health.[115] CPR training has not been shown to increase caregiver anxiety, and in fact, caregivers have reported a sense of empowerment.[120–122] There

are many accessible and effective methods for CPR training (eg, e-learning).

8B. Clinicians Should Educate Caregivers About BRUEs (Grade C, Moderate Recommendation)

Pediatric providers are an important source of this health information and can help guide important conversations around BRUEs. A study by Feudtner et al[123] identified 4 groups of attributes of a "good parent": (1) making sure the child feels loved, (2) focusing on the child's health, (3) advocating for the child and being informed, and (4) ensuring the child's spiritual well-being. Clinicians should be the source of information for caregivers.

Informed caregivers can advocate for their child in all of the attribute areas/domains, and regardless of health literacy levels, prefer being offered choices and being asked for information.[124] A patient- and family-centered care approach results in better health outcomes.[125,126]

8C. Clinicians Should Use Shared Decision-Making for Infants Presenting With a Lower-Risk BRUE (Grade C, Moderate Recommendation)

Shared decision-making is a partnership between the clinician and the patient and family.[125,126] The general principles of shared decision-making are as follows: (1) information sharing, (2) respect and honoring differences, (3) partnership and collaboration, (4) negotiation, and (5) care in the context of family and community.[125] The benefits include improved care and outcomes; improved patient, family, and clinician satisfaction; and better use of health resources.[126] It is advocated for by organizations such as the AAP and the Institute of Medicine.[126,127] The 5 principles can be applied to all aspects of the infant who has experienced a BRUE, through each step (assessment, stabilization, management, disposition, and follow-up). Shared decision-making will empower families and foster a stronger clinician-patient/family alliance as they make decisions together in the face of a seemingly uncertain situation.

DISSEMINATION AND IMPLEMENTATION

Dissemination and implementation efforts are needed to facilitate guideline use across pediatric medicine, family medicine, emergency medicine, research, and patient/family communities.[128] The following general approaches and a Web-based toolkit are proposed for the dissemination and implementation of this guideline.

8A. Clinicians Should Offer Resources for CPR Training to Caregivers (Grade C, Moderate Recommendation)

Aggregate Evidence Quality	Grade C
Benefits	Decrease caregiver anxiety and increase confidence
	Benefit to society
Risks, harm, cost	May increase caregiver anxiety
	Cost and availability of training
Benefit-harm assessment	The benefits of decreased caregiver anxiety and increased confidence, as well as societal benefits, outweigh the increase in caregiver anxiety, cost, and resources
Intentional vagueness	None
Role of patient preferences	Caregiver may decide not to seek out the training
Exclusions	None
Strength	Moderate recommendation
Key reference	115

8B. Clinicians Should Educate Caregivers About BRUEs (Grade C, Moderate Recommendation)

Aggregate Evidence Quality	Grade C
Benefits	Improve caregiver empowerment and health literacy and decrease anxiety
	May reduce unnecessary return visits
	Promotion of the medical home
Risks, harm, cost	Increase caregiver anxiety and potential for caregiver intimidation in voicing concerns
	Increase health care costs and length of stay
Benefit-harm assessment	The benefits of decreased caregiver anxiety and increased empowerment and health literacy outweigh the increase in cost, length of stay, and caregiver anxiety and intimidation
Intentional vagueness	None
Role of patient preferences	Caregiver may decide not to listen to clinician
Exclusions	None
Strength	Moderate recommendation
Key references	None

8C. Clinicians Should Use Shared Decision-Making for Infants Presenting With a Lower-Risk BRUE (Grade C, Moderate Recommendation)

Aggregate Evidence Quality	Grade C
Benefits	Improve caregiver empowerment and health literacy and decrease anxiety
	May reduce unnecessary return visits
	Promotion of the medical home
Risks, harm, cost	Increase cost, length of stay, and caregiver anxiety and intimidation in voicing concerns
Benefit-harm assessment	The benefits of decreased caregiver anxiety and unplanned return visits and increased empowerment, health, literacy, and medical home promotion outweigh the increase in cost, length of stay, and caregiver anxiety and information
Intentional vagueness	None
Role of patient preferences	Caregiver may decide not to listen to clinician
Exclusions	None
Strength	Moderate recommendation
Key references	None

1. Education

Education will be partially achieved through the AAP communication outlets and educational services (*AAP News, Pediatrics,* and PREP). Further support will be sought from stakeholder organizations (American Academy of Family Physicians, American College of Emergency Physicians, American Board of Pediatrics, Society of Hospital Medicine). A Web-based toolkit (to be published online) will include caregiver handouts and a shared decision-making tool to facilitate patient- and family-centered care. Efforts will address appropriate disease classification and diagnosis coding.

2. Integration of Clinical Workflow

An algorithm is provided (Fig 1) for diagnosis and management. Structured history and physical examination templates also are provided to assist in addressing all of the relevant risk factors for BRUEs (Tables 2 and 3). Order sets and modified documents will be hosted on a Web-based learning platform that promotes crowd-sourcing.

3. Administrative and Research

International Classification of Diseases, 9th Revision, and International Classification of Diseases, 10th Revision, diagnostic codes are used for billing, quality improvement, and research; and new codes for lower- and higher-risk BRUEs will need to be developed. In the interim, the current code for an ALTE (799.82) will need to be used for billing purposes. Efforts will be made to better reflect present knowledge and to educate clinicians and payers in appropriate use of codes for this condition.

4. Quality Improvement

Quality improvement initiatives that provide Maintenance of Certification credit, such as the AAP's PREP and EQIPP courses, or collaborative opportunities through the AAP's Quality Improvement Innovation Networks, will engage clinicians in the use and improvement of the guideline. By using proposed quality measures, adherence and outcomes can be assessed and benchmarked with others to inform continual improvement efforts. Proposed measures include process evaluation (use of definition and evaluation), outcome assessment (family experience and diagnostic outcomes), and balancing issues (cost and length of visit). Future research will need to be conducted to validate any measures.

FUTURE RESEARCH

The transition in nomenclature from the term ALTE to BRUE after 30 years reflects the expanded understanding of the etiology and consequences of this entity. Previous research has been largely retrospective or observational in nature, with little long-term follow-up data available. The more-precise definition, the classification of lower- and higher-risk groups, the recommendations for the lower-risk group, and the implementation toolkit will serve as the basis for future research. Important areas for future prospective research include the following.

1. Epidemiology

- Incidence of BRUEs in all infants (in addition to those seeking medical evaluation)
- Influence of race, gender, ethnicity, seasonality, environmental exposures, and socioeconomic status on incidence and outcomes

2. Diagnosis

- Use and effectiveness of the BRUE definition
- Screening tests and risk of UTI
- Quantify and better understand risk in higher- and lower-risk groups
- Risk and benefit of screening tests
- Risk and benefit and optimal duration of observation and monitoring periods
- Effect of prematurity on risk
- Appropriate indications for subspecialty referral
- Early recognition of child maltreatment
- Importance of environmental history taking
- Role of human psychology on accuracy of event characterization

- Type and length of monitoring in the acute setting

3. Pathophysiology

- Role of abnormalities of swallowing, laryngospasm, GER, and autonomic function

4. Outcomes

- Patient- and family-centered outcomes, including caregiver satisfaction, anxiety, and family dynamics (eg, risk of vulnerable child syndrome)

- Long-term health and cognitive consequences

5. Treatment

- Empirical GER treatment on recurrent BRUEs

- Caregiver education strategies, including basic life support, family-centered education, and postpresentation clinical visits

6. Follow-up

- Strategies for timely follow-up and surveillance

SUBCOMMITTEE ON BRIEF RESOLVED UNEXPLAINED EVENTS (FORMERLY REFERRED TO AS APPARENT LIFE THREATENING EVENTS) (OVERSIGHT BY THE COUNCIL ON QUALITY IMPROVEMENT AND PATIENT SAFETY)

Joel S. Tieder, MD, MPH, FAAP, Chair (no financial conflicts, published research related to BRUEs/ALTEs)

Joshua L. Bonkowsky, MD, PhD, FAAP, Pediatric Neurologist

Ruth A. Etzel, MD, PhD, FAAP, Pediatric Epidemiologist

Wayne H. Franklin, MD, MPH, MMM, FAAP, Pediatric Cardiologist

David A. Gremse, MD, FAAP, Pediatric Gastroenterologist

Bruce Herman, MD, FAAP, Child Abuse and Neglect

Eliot Katz, MD, FAAP, Pediatric Pulmonologist

Leonard R. Krilov, MD, FAAP, Pediatric Infectious Diseases

J. Lawrence Merritt II, MD, FAAP, Clinical Genetics and Biochemical Genetics

Chuck Norlin, MD, FAAP, Pediatrician

Robert E. Sapién, MD, MMM, FAAP, Pediatric Emergency Medicine

Richard Shiffman, MD, FAAP, Partnership for Policy Implementation Representative

Michael B.H. Smith, MB, FRCPCH, FAAP, Hospital Medicine

Jack Percelay, MD, MPH, FAAP, Liaison, Society for Hospital Medicine

STAFF

Kymika Okechukwu, MPA

ABBREVIATIONS

AAP: American Academy of Pediatrics

ALTE: apparent life-threatening event

BRUE: brief resolved unexplained event

CI: confidence interval

CNS: central nervous system

CPR: cardiopulmonary resuscitation

ECG: electrocardiogram

GER: gastroesophageal reflux

IEM: inborn error of metabolism

MII: multiple intraluminal impedance

OSA: obstructive sleep apnea

RSV: respiratory syncytial virus

SIDS: sudden infant death syndrome

SUDEP: sudden unexpected death in epilepsy

UTI: urinary tract infection

REFERENCES

1. National Institutes of Health Consensus Development Conference on Infantile Apnea and Home Monitoring, Sept 29 to Oct 1, 1986. *Pediatrics.* 1987;79(2):292–299

2. McGovern MC, Smith MB. Causes of apparent life threatening events in infants: a systematic review. *Arch Dis Child.* 2004;89(11):1043–1048

3. Tieder JS, Altman RL, Bonkowsky JL, et al Management of apparent life-threatening events in infants: a systematic review. *J Pediatr.* 2013;163(1):94–99, e91–e96

4. Brand DA, Altman RL, Purtill K, Edwards KS. Yield of diagnostic testing in infants who have had an apparent life-threatening event. *Pediatrics.* 2005;115(4):885–893

5. Green M. Vulnerable child syndrome and its variants. *Pediatr Rev.* 1986;8(3):75–80

6. Kaji AH, Claudius I, Santillanes G, et al. Apparent life-threatening event: multicenter prospective cohort study to develop a clinical decision rule for admission to the hospital. *Ann Emerg Med.* 2013;61(4):379–387.e4

7. Mittal MK, Sun G, Baren JM. A clinical decision rule to identify infants with apparent life-threatening event who can be safely discharged from the emergency department. *Pediatr Emerg Care.* 2012;28(7):599–605

8. Moher D, Liberati A, Tetzlaff J, Altman DG; PRISMA Group. Preferred reporting items for systematic reviews and meta-analyses: the PRISMA statement. *Ann Intern Med.* 2009;151(4):264–269, W64

9. Haynes RB, Cotoi C, Holland J, et al; McMaster Premium Literature Service (PLUS) Project. Second-order peer review of the medical literature for clinical practitioners. *JAMA.* 2006;295(15):1801–1808

10. Lokker C, McKibbon KA, McKinlay RJ, Wilczynski NL, Haynes RB. Prediction of citation counts for clinical articles at two years using data available within three weeks of publication: retrospective cohort study. *BMJ.* 2008;336(7645):655–657

11. Laupacis A, Wells G, Richardson WS, Tugwell P; Evidence-Based Medicine Working Group. Users' guides to the medical literature. V. How to use an article about prognosis. *JAMA.* 1994;272(3):234–237

12. Jaeschke R, Guyatt G, Sackett DL. Users' guides to the medical literature. III. How to use an article about a diagnostic test. A. Are the results of the study valid? Evidence-Based Medicine Working Group. *JAMA.* 1994;271(5):389–391

13. Anjos AM, Nunes ML. Prevalence of epilepsy and seizure disorders as causes of apparent life-threatening event (ALTE) in children admitted to a tertiary hospital. *Arq Neuropsiquiatr.* 2009;67(3a 3A):616–620

14. Doshi A, Bernard-Stover L, Kuelbs C, Castillo E, Stucky E. Apparent lifethreatening event admissions and gastroesophageal reflux disease: the value of hospitalization. *Pediatr Emerg Care*. 2012;28(1):17–21

15. Franco P, Montemitro E, Scaillet S, et al. Fewer spontaneous arousals in infants with apparent life-threatening event. *Sleep*. 2011;34(6):733–743

16. Hoki R, Bonkowsky JL, Minich LL, Srivastava R, Pinto NM. Cardiac testing and outcomes in infants after an apparent life-threatening event. *Arch Dis Child*. 2012;97(12):1034–1038

17. Kaji AH, Santillanes G, Claudius I, et al. Do infants less than 12 months of age with an apparent life-threatening event need transport to a pediatric critical care center? *Prehosp Emerg Care*. 2013;17(3):304–311

18. Kant S, Fisher JD, Nelson DG, Khan S. Mortality after discharge in clinically stable infants admitted with a firsttime apparent life-threatening event. *Am J Emerg Med*. 2013;31(4):730–733

19. Miano S, Castaldo R, Ferri R, et al. Sleep cyclic alternating pattern analysis in infants with apparent life-threatening events: a daytime polysomnographic study. *Clin Neurophysiol*. 2012;123(7):1346–1352

20. Mittal MK, Donda K, Baren JM. Role of pneumography and esophageal pH monitoring in the evaluation of infants with apparent life-threatening event: a prospective observational study. *Clin Pediatr (Phila)*. 2013;52(4):338–343

21. Mosalli RM, Elsayed YY, Paes BA. Acute life threatening events associated with hypocalcemia and vitamin D deficiency in early infancy: a single center experience from the Kingdom of Saudi Arabia. *Saudi Med J*. 2011;32(5):528–530

22. Parker K, Pitetti R. Mortality and child abuse in children presenting with apparent life-threatening events. *Pediatr Emerg Care*. 2011;27(7):591–595

23. Poets A, Urschitz MS, Steinfeldt R, Poets CF. Risk factors for early sudden deaths and severe apparent lifethreatening events.

Arch Dis Child Fetal Neonatal Ed. 2012;97(6):F395–F397

24. Semmekrot BA, van Sleuwen BE, Engelberts AC, et al. Surveillance study of apparent life-threatening events (ALTE) in the Netherlands. *Eur J Pediatr*. 2010;169(2):229–236

25. Tieder JS, Altman RL, Bonkowsky JL, et al. Management of apparent life-threatening events in infants: a systematic review. *J Pediatr*. 2013;163(1):94–9.e1, 6

26. Wasilewska J, Sienkiewicz-Szłapka E, Kuźbida E, Jarmołowska B, Kaczmarski M, Kostyra E. The exogenous opioid peptides and DPPIV serum activity in infants with apnoea expressed as apparent life threatening events (ALTE). *Neuropeptides*. 2011;45(3):189–195

27. Weiss K, Fattal-Valevski A, Reif S. How to evaluate the child presenting with an apparent life-threatening event? *Isr Med Assoc J*. 2010;12(3):154–157

28. Zimbric G, Bonkowsky JL, Jackson WD, Maloney CG, Srivastava R. Adverse outcomes associated with gastroesophageal reflux disease are rare following an apparent life-threatening event. *J Hosp Med*. 2012;7(6):476–481

29. American Academy of Pediatrics Steering Committee on Quality Improvement and Management. Classifying recommendations for clinical practice guidelines. *Pediatrics*. 2004;114(3):874–877

30. Shiffman RN, Michel G, Rosenfeld RM, Davidson C. Building better guidelines with BRIDGE-Wiz: development and evaluation of a software assistant to promote clarity, transparency, and implementability. *J Am Med Inform Assoc*. 2012;19(1):94–101

31. Claudius I, Keens T. Do all infants with apparent life-threatening events need to be admitted? *Pediatrics*. 2007;119(4):679–683

32. Bonkowsky JL, Guenther E, Filloux FM, Srivastava R. Death, child abuse, and adverse neurological outcome of infants after an apparent lifethreatening event. *Pediatrics*. 2008;122(1):125–131

33. Al-Kindy HA, Gelinas JF, Hatzakis G, Cote A. Risk factors for extreme events

in infants hospitalized for apparent life-threatening events. *J Pediatr*. 2009;154(3):332–337, 337.e1–337.e2

34. Ramanathan R, Corwin MJ, Hunt CE, et al; Collaborative Home Infant Monitoring Evaluation (CHIME) Study Group. Cardiorespiratory events recorded on home monitors: comparison of healthy infants with those at increased risk for SIDS. *JAMA*. 2001;285(17):2199–2207

35. Poets CF, Stebbens VA, Alexander JR, Arrowsmith WA, Salfield SA, Southall DP. Hypoxaemia in infants with respiratory tract infections. *Acta Paediatr*. 1992;81(6–7):536–541

36. Hunt CE, Corwin MJ, Lister G, et al; Collaborative Home Infant Monitoring Evaluation (CHIME) Study Group. Longitudinal assessment of hemoglobin oxygen saturation in healthy infants during the first 6 months of age. *J Pediatr*. 1999;135(5):580–586

37. Altman RL, Li KI, Brand DA. Infections and apparent life-threatening events. *Clin Pediatr (Phila)*. 2008;47(4):372–378

38. Davies F, Gupta R. Apparent life threatening events in infants presenting to an emergency department. *Emerg Med J*. 2002;19(1):11–16

39. Guilleminault C, Ariagno R, Korobkin R, et al. Mixed and obstructive sleep apnea and near miss for sudden infant death syndrome: 2. Comparison of near miss and normal control infants by age. *Pediatrics*. 1979;64(6):882–891

40. Côté A, Hum C, Brouillette RT, Themens M. Frequency and timing of recurrent events in infants using home cardiorespiratory monitors. *J Pediatr*. 1998;132(5):783–789

41. Kahn A, Blum D. Home monitoring of infants considered at risk for the sudden infant death syndrome: four years' experience (1977-1981). *Eur J Pediatr*. 1982;139(2):94–100

42. Daniëls H, Naulaers G, Deroost F, Devlieger H. Polysomnography and home documented monitoring of cardiorespiratory pattern. *Arch Dis Child*. 1999;81(5):434–436

43. Marcus CL, Hamer A. Significance of isolated bradycardia detected

by home monitoring. *J Pediatr*. 1999;135(3):321–326

44. Rebuffat E, Groswasser J, Kelmanson I, Sottiaux M, Kahn A. Polygraphic evaluation of night-to-night variability in sleep characteristics and apneas in infants. *Sleep*. 1994;17(4):329–332

45. Horemuzova E, Katz-Salamon M, Milerad J. Increased inspiratory effort in infants with a history of apparent life-threatening event. *Acta Paediatr*. 2002;91(3):280–286; discussion: 260–261

46. Schechtman VL, Harper RM, Wilson AJ, Southall DP. Sleep state organization in normal infants and victims of the sudden infant death syndrome. *Pediatrics*. 1992;89(5 Pt 1):865–870

47. Arad-Cohen N, Cohen A, Tirosh E. The relationship between gastroesophageal reflux and apnea in infants. *J Pediatr*. 2000;137(3):321–326

48. Harrington C, Kirjavainen T, Teng A, Sullivan CE. Altered autonomic function and reduced arousability in apparent life-threatening event infants with obstructive sleep apnea. *Am J Respir Crit Care Med*. 2002;165(8):1048–1054

49. Guilleminault C, Pelayo R, Leger D, Philip P. Apparent life-threatening events, facial dysmorphia and sleep-disordered breathing. *Eur J Pediatr*. 2000;159(6):444–449

50. Aurora RN, Zak RS, Karippot A, et al; American Academy of Sleep Medicine. Practice parameters for the respiratory indications for polysomnography in children. *Sleep*. 2011;34(3):379–388

51. Kahn A, Groswasser J, Sottiaux M, Rebuffat E, Franco P. Mechanisms of obstructive sleep apneas in infants. *Biol Neonate*. 1994;65(3–4):235–239

52. Leiberman A, Tal A, Brama I, Sofer S. Obstructive sleep apnea in young infants. *Int J Pediatr Otorhinolaryngol*. 1988;16(1):39–44

53. Montgomery-Downs HE, Gozal D. Sleep habits and risk factors for sleep-disordered breathing in infants and young toddlers in Louisville, Kentucky. *Sleep Med*. 2006;7(3):211–219

54. Brouillette RT, Fernbach SK, Hunt CE. Obstructive sleep apnea in infants and children. *J Pediatr*. 1982;100(1):31–40

55. Kahn A, Groswasser J, Sottiaux M, et al. Clinical symptoms associated with brief obstructive sleep apnea in normal infants. *Sleep*. 1993;16(5):409–413

56. Kahn A, Groswasser J, Sottiaux M, et al. Prenatal exposure to cigarettes in infants with obstructive sleep apneas. *Pediatrics*. 1994;93(5):778–783

57. Kahn A, Mozin MJ, Rebuffat E, et al. Sleep pattern alterations and brief airway obstructions in overweight infants. *Sleep*. 1989;12(5):430–438

58. Fajardo C, Alvarez J, Wong A, Kwiatkowski K, Rigatto H. The incidence of obstructive apneas in preterm infants with and without bronchopulmonary dysplasia. *Early Hum Dev*. 1993;32(2–3):197–206

59. Horigome H, Nagashima M, Sumitomo N, et al. Clinical characteristics and genetic background of congenital long-QT syndrome diagnosed in fetal, neonatal, and infantile life: a nationwide questionnaire survey in Japan. *Circ Arrhythm Electrophysiol*. 2010;3(1):10–17

60. Arnestad M, Crotti L, Rognum TO, et al. Prevalence of long-QT syndrome gene variants in sudden infant death syndrome. *Circulation*. 2007;115(3):361–367

61. Goldenberg I, Moss AJ, Peterson DR, et al. Risk factors for aborted cardiac arrest and sudden cardiac death in children with the congenital long-QT syndrome. *Circulation*. 2008;117(17):2184–2191

62. Munger TM, Packer DL, Hammill SC, et al. A population study of the natural history of Wolff-Parkinson-White syndrome in Olmsted County, Minnesota, 1953-1989. *Circulation*. 1993;87(3):866–873

63. American Academy of Pediatrics, Committee on Fetus and Newborn. Apnea, sudden infant death syndrome, and home monitoring. *Pediatrics*. 2003;111(4 pt 1):914–917

64. Krongrad E, O'Neill L. Near miss sudden infant death syndrome episodes? A clinical and electrocardiographic correlation. *Pediatrics*. 1986;77(6):811–815

65. Nathanson I, O'Donnell J, Commins MF. Cardiorespiratory patterns

during alarms in infants using apnea/ bradycardia monitors. *Am J Dis Child*. 1989;143(4):476–480

66. Weese-Mayer DE, Brouillette RT, Morrow AS, Conway LP, Klemka-Walden LM, Hunt CE. Assessing validity of infant monitor alarms with event recording. *J Pediatr*. 1989;115(5 pt 1):702–708

67. Guenther E, Powers A, Srivastava R, Bonkowsky JL. Abusive head trauma in children presenting with an apparent life-threatening event. *J Pediatr*. 2010;157(5):821–825

68. Pierce MC, Kaczor K, Thompson R. Bringing back the social history. *Pediatr Clin North Am*. 2014;61(5):889–905

69. Pitetti RD, Maffei F, Chang K, Hickey R, Berger R, Pierce MC. Prevalence of retinal hemorrhages and child abuse in children who present with an apparent life-threatening event. *Pediatrics*. 2002;110(3):557–562

70. Jenny C, Hymel KP, Ritzen A, Reinert SE, Hay TC. Analysis of missed cases of abusive head trauma. *JAMA*. 1999;281(7):621–626

71. Southall DP, Plunkett MC, Banks MW, Falkov AF, Samuels MP. Covert video recordings of life-threatening child abuse: lessons for child protection. *Pediatrics*. 1997;100(5):735–760

72. Sugar NF, Taylor JA, Feldman KW; Puget Sound Pediatric Research Network. Bruises in infants and toddlers: those who don't cruise rarely bruise. *Arch Pediatr Adolesc Med*. 1999;153(4):399–403

73. Harper NS, Feldman KW, Sugar NF, Anderst JD, Lindberg DM; Examining Siblings To Recognize Abuse Investigators. Additional injuries in young infants with concern for abuse and apparently isolated bruises. *J Pediatr*. 2014;165(2):383–388, e1

74. DeRidder CA, Berkowitz CD, Hicks RA, Laskey AL. Subconjunctival hemorrhages in infants and children: a sign of nonaccidental trauma. *Pediatr Emerg Care*. 2013;29(2):222–226

75. Buck ML, Blumer JL. Phenothiazine-associated apnea in two siblings. *DICP*. 1991;25(3):244–247

76. Hardoin RA, Henslee JA, Christenson CP, Christenson PJ, White M. Colic

medication and apparent life-threatening events. *Clin Pediatr (Phila)*. 1991;30(5):281–285

77. Hickson GB, Altemeier WA, Martin ED, Campbell PW. Parental administration of chemical agents: a cause of apparent life-threatening events. *Pediatrics*. 1989;83(5):772–776

78. Pitetti RD, Whitman E, Zaylor A. Accidental and nonaccidental poisonings as a cause of apparent life-threatening events in infants. *Pediatrics*. 2008;122(2). Available at: www.pediatrics.org/cgi/content/full/122/2/e359

79. McCormick T, Levine M, Knox O, Claudius I. Ethanol ingestion in two infants under 2 months old: a previously unreported cause of ALTE. *Pediatrics*. 2013;131(2). Available at: www.pediatrics.org/cgi/content/full/131/2/e604

80. Dearborn DG, Smith PG, Dahms BB, et al. Clinical profile of 30 infants with acute pulmonary hemorrhage in Cleveland. *Pediatrics*. 2002;110(3):627–637

81. Leone MA, Solari A, Beghi E; First Seizure Trial (FIRST) Group. Treatment of the first tonic-clonic seizure does not affect long-term remission of epilepsy. *Neurology*. 2006;67(12):2227–2229

82. Musicco M, Beghi E, Solari A, Viani F; First Seizure Trial (FIRST) Group. Treatment of first tonic-clonic seizure does not improve the prognosis of epilepsy. *Neurology*. 1997;49(4):991–998

83. Camfield P, Camfield C, Smith S, Dooley J, Smith E. Long-term outcome is unchanged by antiepileptic drug treatment after a first seizure: a 15-year follow-up from a randomized trial in childhood. *Epilepsia*. 2002;43(6):662–663

84. Gilbert DL, Buncher CR. An EEG should not be obtained routinely after first unprovoked seizure in childhood. *Neurology*. 2000;54(3):635–641

85. Arts WF, Geerts AT. When to start drug treatment for childhood epilepsy: the clinical-epidemiological evidence. *Eur J Paediatr Neurol*. 2009;13(2):93–101

86. Hirtz D, Ashwal S, Berg A, et al. Practice parameter: evaluating a first nonfebrile seizure in children: report of the Quality Standards Subcommittee of the American Academy of Neurology, The Child Neurology Society, and The American Epilepsy Society. *Neurology*. 2000;55(5):616–623

87. Bonkowsky JL, Guenther E, Srivastava R, Filloux FM. Seizures in children following an apparent life-threatening event. *J Child Neurol*. 2009;24(6):709–713

88. Claudius I, Mittal MK, Murray R, Condie T, Santillanes G. Should infants presenting with an apparent life-threatening event undergo evaluation for serious bacterial infections and respiratory pathogens? *J Pediatr*. 2014;164(5):1231–1233, e1

89. Mittal MK, Shofer FS, Baren JM. Serious bacterial infections in infants who have experienced an apparent life-threatening event. *Ann Emerg Med*. 2009;54(4):523–527

90. Roberts KB; Subcommittee on Urinary Tract Infection, Steering Committee on Quality Improvement and Management. Urinary tract infection: clinical practice guideline for the diagnosis and management of the initial UTI in febrile infants and children 2 to 24 months. *Pediatrics*. 2011;128(3):595–610

91. Schroeder AR, Mansbach JM, Stevenson M, et al. Apnea in children hospitalized with bronchiolitis. *Pediatrics*. 2013;132(5). Available at: www.pediatrics.org/cgi/content/full/132/5/e1194

92. Loeffelholz MJ, Trujillo R, Pyles RB, et al. Duration of rhinovirus shedding in the upper respiratory tract in the first year of life. *Pediatrics*. 2014;134(6):1144–1150

93. Crowcroft NS, Booy R, Harrison T, et al. Severe and unrecognised: pertussis in UK infants. *Arch Dis Child*. 2003;88(9):802–806

94. Centers for Disease Control and Prevention. Pertussis (whooping cough): diagnostic testing. Available at: www.cdc.gov/pertussis/clinical/diagnostic-testing/index.html. Accessed June 26, 2015

95. Centers for Disease Control and Prevention. Pertussis (whooping cough): treatment. Available at: www.cdc.gov/pertussis/clinical/treatment.html. Accessed June 26, 2015

96. Campanozzi A, Boccia G, Pensabene L, et al. Prevalence and natural history of gastroesophageal reflux: pediatric prospective survey. *Pediatrics*. 2009;123(3):779–783

97. Lightdale JR, Gremse DA; American Academy of Pediatrics, Section on Gastroenterology, Hepatology, and Nutrition. Gastroesophageal reflux: management guidance for the pediatrician. *Pediatrics*. 2013;131(5). Available at: www.pediatrics.org/cgi/content/full/131/5/e1684

98. Vandenplas Y, Rudolph CD, Di Lorenzo C, et al; North American Society for Pediatric Gastroenterology Hepatology and Nutrition; European Society for Pediatric Gastroenterology Hepatology and Nutrition. Pediatric gastroesophageal reflux clinical practice guidelines: joint recommendations of the North American Society for Pediatric Gastroenterology, Hepatology, and Nutrition (NASPGHAN) and the European Society for Pediatric Gastroenterology, Hepatology, and Nutrition (ESPGHAN). *J Pediatr Gastroenterol Nutr*. 2009;49(4):498–547

99. Kiechl-Kohlendorfer U, Hof D, Peglow UP, Traweger-Ravanelli B, Kiechl S. Epidemiology of apparent life threatening events. *Arch Dis Child*. 2005;90(3):297–300

100. Chung EY, Yardley J. Are there risks associated with empiric acid suppression treatment of infants and children suspected of having gastroesophageal reflux disease? *Hosp Pediatr*. 2013;3(1):16–23

101. Herbst JJ, Minton SD, Book LS. Gastroesophageal reflux causing respiratory distress and apnea in newborn infants. *J Pediatr*. 1979;95(5 pt 1):763–768

102. Orenstein SR. An overview of reflux-associated disorders in infants: apnea, laryngospasm, and aspiration. *Am J Med*. 2001;111(suppl 8A):60S–63S

103. Wenzl TG, Schenke S, Peschgens T, Silny J, Heimann G, Skopnik H. Association of

apnea and nonacid gastroesophageal reflux in infants: investigations with the intraluminal impedance technique. *Pediatr Pulmonol*. 2001;31(2):144–149

104. Mousa H, Woodley FW, Metheney M, Hayes J. Testing the association between gastroesophageal reflux and apnea in infants. *J Pediatr Gastroenterol Nutr*. 2005;41(2):169–177

105. Kahn A, Rebuffat E, Sottiaux M, Dufour D, Cadranel S, Reiterer F. Lack of temporal relation between acid reflux in the proximal oesophagus and cardiorespiratory events in sleeping infants. *Eur J Pediatr*. 1992;151(3):208–212

106. Orenstein SR, McGowan JD. Efficacy of conservative therapy as taught in the primary care setting for symptoms suggesting infant gastroesophageal reflux. *J Pediatr*. 2008;152(3):310–314

107. Kahn A; European Society for the Study and Prevention of Infant Death. Recommended clinical evaluation of infants with an apparent life-threatening event: consensus document of the European Society for the Study and Prevention of Infant Death, 2003. *Eur J Pediatr*. 2004;163(2):108–115

108. Veereman-Wauters G, Bochner A, Van Caillie-Bertrand M. Gastroesophageal reflux in infants with a history of near-miss sudden infant death. *J Pediatr Gastroenterol Nutr*. 1991;12(3):319–323

109. Arens R, Gozal D, Williams JC, Ward SL, Keens TG. Recurrent apparent life-threatening events during infancy: a manifestation of inborn errors of metabolism. *J Pediatr*. 1993;123(3):415–418

110. See CC, Newman LJ, Berezin S, et al. Gastroesophageal reflux-induced hypoxemia in infants with apparent life-threatening event(s). *Am J Dis Child*. 1989;143(8):951–954

111. Penzien JM, Molz G, Wiesmann UN, Colombo JP, Bühlmann R, Wermuth B. Medium-chain acyl-CoA dehydrogenase deficiency does not correlate with apparent life-threatening events and the sudden infant death syndrome: results from phenylpropionate loading tests and DNA analysis. *Eur J Pediatr*. 1994;153(5):352–357

112. Pitetti RD, Lovallo A, Hickey R. Prevalence of anemia in children presenting with apparent life-threatening events. *Acad Emerg Med*. 2005;12(10):926–931

113. Gray C, Davies F, Molyneux E. Apparent life-threatening events presenting to a pediatric emergency department. *Pediatr Emerg Care*. 1999;15(3):195–199

114. Poets CF, Samuels MP, Wardrop CA, Picton-Jones E, Southall DP. Reduced haemoglobin levels in infants presenting with apparent life-threatening events—a retrospective investigation. *Acta Paediatr*. 1992;81(4):319–321

115. Pyles LA, Knapp J; American Academy of Pediatrics Committee on Pediatric Emergency Medicine. Role of pediatricians in advocating life support training courses for parents and the public. *Pediatrics*. 2004;114(6). Available at: www.pediatrics.org/cgi/content/full/114/6/e761

116. Tunik MG, Richmond N, Treiber M, et al. Pediatric prehospital evaluation of NYC respiratory arrest survival (PHENYCS). *Pediatr Emerg Care*. 2012;28(9):859–863

117. Foltin GL, Richmond N, Treiber M, et al. Pediatric prehospital evaluation of NYC cardiac arrest survival (PHENYCS). *Pediatr Emerg Care*. 2012;28(9):864–868

118. Akahane M, Tanabe S, Ogawa T, et al. Characteristics and outcomes of pediatric out-of-hospital cardiac arrest by scholastic age category. *Pediatr Crit Care Med*. 2013;14(2):130–136

119. Atkins DL, Everson-Stewart S, Sears GK, et al; Resuscitation Outcomes Consortium Investigators. Epidemiology and outcomes from out-of-hospital cardiac arrest in children: the Resuscitation Outcomes Consortium Epistry-Cardiac Arrest. *Circulation*. 2009;119(11):1484–1491

120. McLauchlan CA, Ward A, Murphy NM, Griffith MJ, Skinner DV, Camm AJ. Resuscitation training for cardiac patients and their relatives—its effect on anxiety. *Resuscitation*. 1992;24(1):7–11

121. Higgins SS, Hardy CE, Higashino SM. Should parents of children with congenital heart disease and life-threatening dysrhythmias be taught cardiopulmonary resuscitation? *Pediatrics*. 1989;84(6):1102–1104

122. Dracup K, Moser DK, Taylor SE, Guzy PM. The psychological consequences of cardiopulmonary resuscitation training for family members of patients at risk for sudden death. *Am J Public Health*. 1997;87(9):1434–1439

123. Feudtner C, Walter JK, Faerber JA, et al. Good-parent beliefs of parents of seriously ill children. *JAMA Pediatr*. 2015;169(1):39–47

124. Yin HS, Dreyer BP, Vivar KL, MacFarland S, van Schaick L, Mendelsohn AL. Perceived barriers to care and attitudes towards shared decision-making among low socioeconomic status parents: role of health literacy. *Acad Pediatr*. 2012;12(2):117–124

125. Kuo DZ, Houtrow AJ, Arango P, Kuhlthau KA, Simmons JM, Neff JM. Family-centered care: current applications and future directions in pediatric health care. *Matern Child Health J*. 2012;16(2):297–305

126. American Academy of Pediatrics, Committee on Hospital Care; Institute for Patient- and Family-Centered Care. Patient- and family-centered care and the pediatrician's role. *Pediatrics*. 2012;129(2):394–404

127. Institute of Medicine. *Crossing the Quality Chasm: A New Health System for the 21st Century*. Washington, DC: Institute of Medicine, Committee on Quality Healthcare in America National Academies Press; 2001

128. Pronovost PJ. Enhancing physicians' use of clinical guidelines. *JAMA*. 2013;310(23):2501–2502

CLINICAL PRACTICE GUIDELINE   Guidance for the Clinician in Rendering Pediatric Care

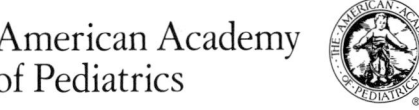

American Academy
of Pediatrics

DEDICATED TO THE HEALTH OF ALL CHILDREN™

Brief Resolved Unexplained Events (Formerly Apparent Life-Threatening Events) and Evaluation of Lower-Risk Infants: Executive Summary

Joel S. Tieder, MD, MPH, FAAP, Joshua L. Bonkowsky, MD, PhD, FAAP, Ruth A. Etzel, MD, PhD, FAAP, Wayne H. Franklin, MD, MPH, MMM, FAAP, David A. Gremse, MD, FAAP, Bruce Herman, MD, FAAP, Eliot S. Katz, MD, FAAP, Leonard R. Krilov, MD, FAAP, J. Lawrence Merritt II, MD, FAAP, Chuck Norlin, MD, FAAP, Jack Percelay, MD, MPH, FAAP, Robert E. Sapién, MD, MMM, FAAP, Richard N. Shiffman, MD, MCIS, FAAP, Michael B.H. Smith, MB, FRCPCH, FAAP, SUBCOMMITTEE ON APPARENT LIFE THREATENING EVENTS

EXECUTIVE SUMMARY

This clinical practice guideline has 2 primary objectives. First, it recommends the replacement of the term "apparent life-threatening event" (ALTE) with a new term, "brief resolved unexplained event" (BRUE). Second, it provides an approach to evaluation and management that is based on the risk that the infant will have a repeat event or has a serious underlying disorder.

Clinicians should use the term BRUE to describe an event occurring in an infant younger than 1 year when the observer reports a sudden, brief, and now resolved episode of ≥1 of the following: (1) cyanosis or pallor; (2) absent, decreased, or irregular breathing; (3) marked change in tone (hyper- or hypotonia); and (4) altered level of responsiveness. Moreover, clinicians should diagnose a BRUE only when there is no explanation for a qualifying event after conducting an appropriate history and physical examination (see Tables 2 and 3 in www.pediatrics.org/cgi/doi/10.1542/peds.2016-0590). Among infants who present for medical attention after a BRUE, the guideline identifies (1) lower-risk patients on the basis of history and physical examination, for whom evidence-based guidelines for evaluation and management are offered, and (2) higher-risk patients, whose history and physical examination suggest the need for further investigation, monitoring, and/or treatment, but for whom recommendations are not offered (because of insufficient evidence or the availability of guidance from other clinical practice guidelines specific to their presentation or diagnosis). Recommendations in this guideline apply only to lower-risk patients,

This document is copyrighted and is property of the American Academy of Pediatrics and its Board of Directors. All authors have filed conflict of interest statements with the American Academy of Pediatrics. Any conflicts have been resolved through a process approved by the Board of Directors. The American Academy of Pediatrics has neither solicited nor accepted any commercial involvement in the development of the content of this publication.

The guidance in this report does not indicate an exclusive course of treatment or serve as a standard of medical care. Variations, taking into account individual circumstances, may be appropriate.

All clinical practice guidelines from the American Academy of Pediatrics automatically expire 5 years after publication unless reaffirmed, revised, or retired at or before that time.

DOI: 10.1542/peds.2016-0591

PEDIATRICS (ISSN Numbers: Print, 0031-4005; Online, 1098-4275).

Copyright © 2016 by the American Academy of Pediatrics

To cite: Tieder JS, Bonkowsky JL, Etzel RA, et al. Brief Resolved Unexplained Events (Formerly Apparent Life-Threatening Events) and Evaluation of Lower-Risk Infants: Executive Summary. *Pediatrics.* 2016;137(5):e20160591

who are defined by (1) age >60 days; (2) gestational age ≥32 weeks and postconceptional age ≥45 weeks; (3) occurrence of only 1 BRUE (no prior BRUE ever and not occurring in clusters); (4) duration of BRUE <1 minute; (5) no cardiopulmonary resuscitation by trained medical provider required; (6) no concerning historical features; and (7) no concerning physical examination findings (Fig 1). This clinical practice guideline also provides implementation support and suggests directions for future research.

The term ALTE originated from a 1986 National Institutes of Health Consensus Conference on Infantile Apnea and was intended to replace the term "near-miss sudden infant death syndrome (SIDS)."[1] An ALTE was defined as "[a]n episode that is frightening to the observer and that is characterized by some combination of apnea (central or occasionally obstructive), color change (usually cyanotic or pallid but occasionally erythematous or plethoric), marked change in muscle tone (usually marked limpness), choking, or gagging. In some cases, the observer fears that the infant has died."[2] Although the definition of ALTE enabled researchers to establish over time that these events were a separate entity from SIDS, the clinical application of this classification, which describes a constellation of observed, subjective, and nonspecific symptoms, has raised significant challenges for clinicians and parents in the evaluation and care of these infants.[3] Although a broad range of disorders can present as an ALTE (eg, child abuse, congenital abnormalities, epilepsy, inborn errors of metabolism, and infections), for a majority of well-appearing infants, the risk of a recurrent event or a serious underlying disorder is extremely low.

ALTEs can create a feeling of uncertainty in both the caregiver and the clinician. Clinicians may feel compelled to perform tests and hospitalize the patient even though this may subject the patient to unnecessary risk and is unlikely to lead to a treatable diagnosis or prevent future events.[2,4,5] Understanding the risk of an adverse outcome for an infant who has experienced an ALTE has been difficult because of the nonspecific nature and variable application of the ALTE definition in research. A recent systematic review of nearly 1400 ALTE publications spanning 4 decades concluded that risk of a subsequent or underlying disorder could not be quantified because of the variability in case definitions across studies.[3] Although there are history and physical examination factors that can determine lower or higher risk, it is clear that the term ALTE must be replaced to advance the quality of care and improve research.

This guideline is intended for use primarily by clinicians providing care for infants who have experienced a BRUE, as well as their families. The guideline may be of interest to payers, but it is not intended to be used for reimbursement or to determine insurance coverage. This guideline is not intended as the sole source of guidance in the evaluation and management of BRUEs and specifically does not address higher-risk BRUE patients. Rather, it is intended to assist clinicians by providing a framework for clinical decision making. It is not intended to replace clinical judgment, and these recommendations may not provide the only appropriate approach to the management of this problem.

This guideline is intended to provide a patient- and family-centered approach to

care, reduce unnecessary and costly medical interventions, and improve patient outcomes. It includes recommendations for diagnosis, risk-based stratification, monitoring, disposition planning, effective communication with the patient and family, guideline implementation and evaluation, and future research. In addition, it aims to help clinicians determine the presence of a serious underlying cause and a safe disposition by alerting them to the most significant features of the clinical history and physical examination on which to base an approach for diagnostic testing and hospitalization. Key action statements are summarized in Table 1.

SUBCOMMITTEE ON BRIEF RESOLVED UNEXPLAINED EVENTS (FORMERLY REFERRED TO AS APPARENT LIFE THREATENING EVENTS); OVERSIGHT BY THE COUNCIL ON QUALITY IMPROVEMENT AND PATIENT SAFETY

Joel S. Tieder, MD, MPH, FAAP, Chair
Joshua L. Bonkowsky, MD, PhD, FAAP, Pediatric Neurologist
Ruth A. Etzel, MD, PhD, FAAP, Pediatric Epidemiologist
Wayne H. Franklin, MD, MPH, MMM, FAAP, Pediatric Cardiologist
David A. Gremse, MD, FAAP, Pediatric Gastroenterologist
Bruce Herman, MD, FAAP, Child Abuse and Neglect
Eliot Katz, MD, FAAP, Pediatric Pulmonologist
Leonard R. Krilov, MD, FAAP, Pediatric Infectious Diseases
J. Lawrence Merritt, II, MD, FAAP, Clinical Genetics and Biochemical Genetics
Chuck Norlin, MD, FAAP, Pediatrician
Robert E. Sapién, MD, MMM, FAAP, Pediatric Emergency Medicine
Richard Shiffman, MD, FAAP, Partnership for Policy Implementation Representative
Michael B.H. Smith, MB, FRCPCH, FAAP, Hospital Medicine

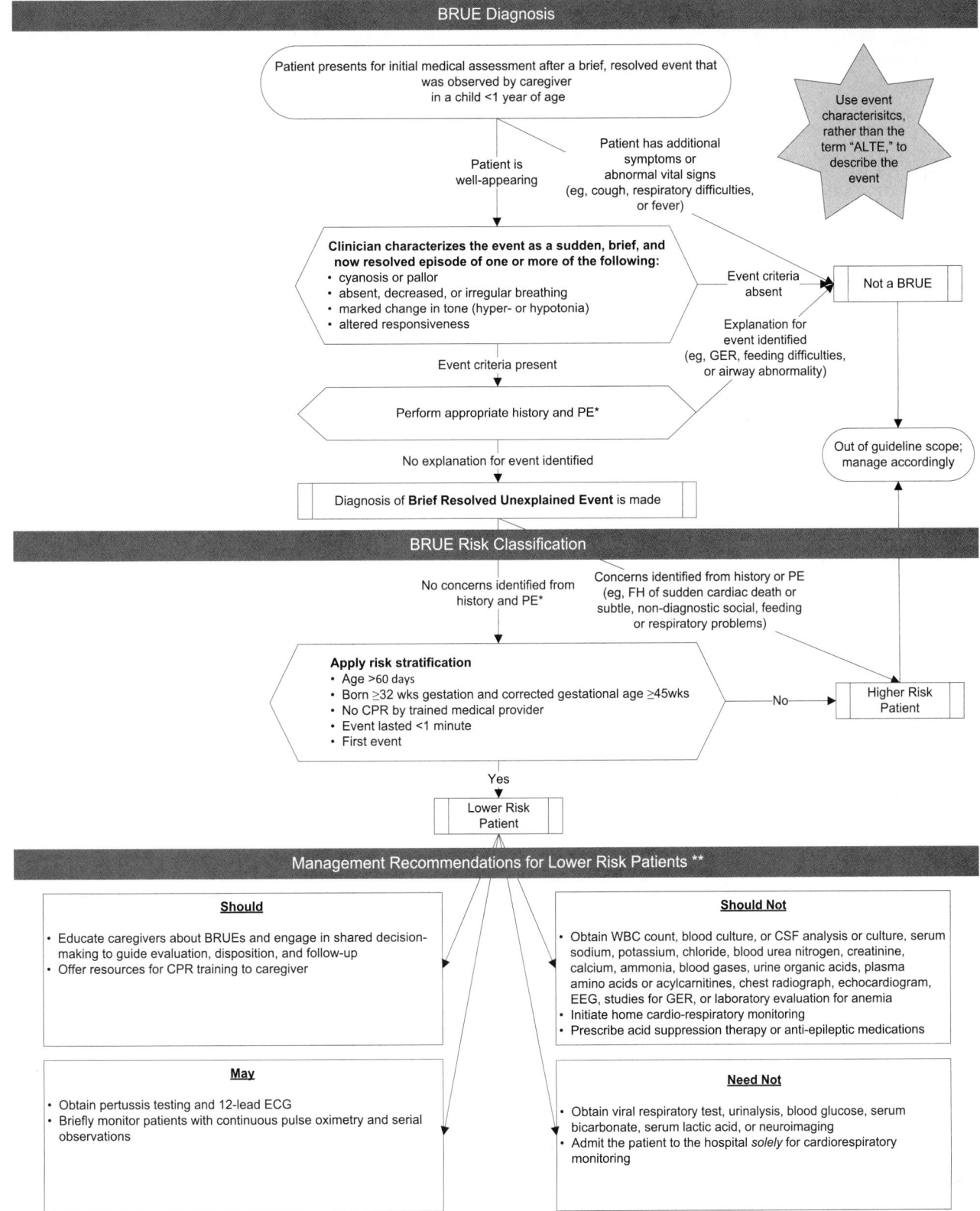

FIGURE 1

Diagnosis, risk classification, and recommended management of a BRUE. *Refer to Tables 3 and 4 in www.pediatrics.org/cgi/doi/10.1542/peds.2016-0591 for the determination of an appropriate and negative history and PE. **Refer to Figure 2 in www.pediatrics.org/cgi/doi/10.1542/peds.2016-0591 for the American Academy of Pediatrics method for rating of evidence and recommendations. CPR, cardiopulmonary resuscitation; CSF, cerebrospinal fluid; ECG, electrocardiogram; FH, family history; GER, gastroesophageal reflux; PE, physical examination; WBC, white blood cell.

Figure 1, shown here, has been updated per the erratum at http://pediatrics.aappublications.org/content/138/2/e20161488.

TABLE 1 Summary of Key Action Statements for Lower-Risk BRUEs

When managing an infant who is >60 d and <1 y of age and who, on the basis of a thorough history and physical examination, meets criteria for having experienced a lower-risk BRUE, clinicians:	Evidence Quality; Strength of Recommendation
1. Cardiopulmonary Evaluation	
1A. Need not admit infants to the hospital solely for cardiorespiratory monitoring.	B; Weak
1B. May briefly monitor patients with continuous pulse oximetry and serial observations.	D; Weak
1C. Should not obtain chest radiograph.	B; Moderate
1D. Should not obtain a measurement of venous or arterial blood gas.	B; Moderate
1E. Should not obtain an overnight polysomnograph.	B; Moderate
1F. May obtain a 12-lead electrocardiogram.	C; Weak
1G. Should not obtain an echocardiogram.	C; Moderate
1H. Should not initiate home cardiorespiratory monitoring.	B; Moderate
2. Child Abuse Evaluation	
2A. Need not obtain neuroimaging (CT, MRI, or ultrasonography) to detect child abuse.	C; Weak
2B. Should obtain an assessment of social risk factors to detect child abuse.	C; Moderate
3. Neurologic Evaluation	
3A. Should not obtain neuroimaging (CT, MRI, or ultrasonography) to detect neurologic disorders.	C; Moderate
3B. Should not obtain an EEG to detect neurologic disorders.	C; Moderate
3C. Should not prescribe antiepileptic medications for potential neurologic disorders.	C; Moderate
4. Infectious Disease Evaluation	
4A. Should not obtain a WBC count, blood culture, or cerebrospinal fluid analysis or culture to detect an occult bacterial infection.	B; Strong
4B. Need not obtain a urinalysis (bag or catheter).	C; Weak
4C. Should not obtain chest radiograph to assess for pulmonary infection.	B; Moderate
4D. Need not obtain respiratory viral testing if rapid testing is available.	C; Weak
4E. May obtain testing for pertussis.	B; Weak
5. Gastrointestinal Evaluation	
5A. Should not obtain investigations for GER (eg, upper gastrointestinal tract series, pH probe, endoscopy, barium contrast study, nuclear scintigraphy, and ultrasonography).	C; Moderate
5B. Should not prescribe acid suppression therapy.	C; Moderate
6. Inborn Error of Metabolism Evaluation	
6A. Need not obtain measurement of serum lactic acid or serum bicarbonate.	C; Weak
6B. Should not obtain a measurement of serum sodium, potassium, chloride, blood urea nitrogen, creatinine, calcium, or ammonia.	C; Moderate
6C. Should not obtain a measurement of venous or arterial blood gases.	C; Moderate
6D. Need not obtain a measurement of blood glucose.	C; Weak
6E. Should not obtain measurements of urine organic acids, plasma amino acids, or plasma acylcarnitines.	C; Moderate
7. Anemia Evaluation	
7A. Should not obtain laboratory evaluation for anemia.	C; Moderate
8. Patient- and Family-Centered Care	
8A. Should offer resources for CPR training to caregiver.	C; Moderate
8B. Should educate caregivers about BRUEs.	C; Moderate
8C. Should use shared decision making.	C; Moderate

CPR, cardiopulmonary resuscitation; CT, computed tomography; GER, gastroesophageal reflux; WBC, white blood cell.

Jack Percelay, MD, MPH, FAAP, Liaison, Society for Hospital Medicine

STAFF

Kymika Okechukwu, MPA

ABBREVIATIONS

ALTE: apparent life-threatening event
BRUE: brief resolved unexplained event
SIDS: sudden infant death syndrome

REFERENCES

1. National Institutes of Health Consensus Development Conference on Infantile Apnea and Home Monitoring, Sept 29 to Oct 1, 1986. *Pediatrics.* 1987;79(2). Available at: www.pediatrics.org/cgi/content/full/79/2/e292

2. McGovern MC, Smith MB. Causes of apparent life threatening events in infants: a systematic review. *Arch Dis Child.* 2004;89(11):1043–1048

3. Tieder JS, Altman RL, Bonkowsky JL, et al Management of apparent life-threatening events in infants: a systematic review. *J Pediatr.* 2013;163(1):94–99, e91–e96

4. Brand DA, Altman RL, Purtill K, Edwards KS. Yield of diagnostic testing in infants who have had an apparent life-threatening event. *Pediatrics.* 2005;115(4). Available at: www.pediatrics.org/cgi/content/full/115/4/e885

5. Green M. Vulnerable child syndrome and its variants. *Pediatr Rev.* 1986; 8(3):75–80

Brief Resolved Unexplained Events Clinical Practice Guideline Quick Reference Tools

· ·

- Action Statement Summary
  — Brief Resolved Unexplained Events (Formerly Apparent Life-Threatening Events) and Evaluation of Lower-Risk Infants
- *ICD-10-CM* Coding Quick Reference for Brief Resolved Unexplained Events
- AAP Patient Education Handout
  — *Brief Resolved Unexplained Event: What Parents and Caregivers Need to Know*

Action Statement Summary

Brief Resolved Unexplained Events (Formerly Apparent Life-Threatening Events) and Evaluation of Lower-Risk Infants

Key Action Statement 1
Cardiopulmonary

Key Action Statement 1A
Clinicians need not admit infants presenting with a lower-risk BRUE to the hospital solely for cardiorespiratory monitoring (grade B, weak recommendation)

Key Action Statement 1B
Clinicians may briefly monitor infants presenting with a lower-risk BRUE with continuous pulse oximetry and serial observations (grade D, weak recommendation)

Key Action Statement 1C
Clinicians should not obtain a chest radiograph in infants presenting with a lower-risk BRUE (grade B, moderate recommendation)

Key Action Statement 1D
Clinicians should not obtain measurement of venous or arterial blood gases in infants presenting with a lower-risk BRUE (grade B, moderate recommendation)

Key Action Statement 1E
Clinicians should not obtain an overnight polysomnograph in infants presenting with a lower-risk BRUE (grade B, moderate recommendation)

Key Action Statement 1F
Clinicians may obtain a 12-lead electrocardiogram for infants presenting with lower-risk BRUE (grade C, weak recommendation)

Key Action Statement 1G
Clinicians should not obtain an echocardiogram in infants presenting with lower-risk BRUE (grade C, moderate recommendation)

Key Action Statement 1H
Clinicians should not initiate home cardiorespiratory monitoring in infants presenting with a lower-risk BRUE (grade B, moderate recommendation)

Key Action Statement 2
Child abuse

Key Action Statement 2A
Clinicians need not obtain neuroimaging (computed tomography, MRI, or ultrasonography) to detect child abuse in infants presenting with a lower-risk BRUE (grade C, weak recommendation)

Key Action Statement 2B
Clinicians should obtain an assessment of social risk factors to detect child abuse in infants presenting with a lower-risk BRUE (grade C, moderate recommendation)

Key Action Statement 3
Neurology

Key Action Statement 3A
Clinicians should not obtain neuroimaging (computed tomography, MRI, or ultrasonography) to detect neurologic disorders in infants presenting with a lower-risk BRUE (grade C, moderate recommendation)

Key Action Statement 3B
Clinicians should not obtain an EEG to detect neurologic disorders in infants presenting with a lower-risk BRUE (grade C, moderate recommendation)

Key Action Statement 3C
Clinicians should not prescribe antiepileptic medications for potential neurologic disorders in infants presenting with a lower-risk BRUE (grade C, moderate recommendation)

Key Action Statement 4
Infectious diseases

Key Action Statement 4A
Clinicians should not obtain a white blood cell count, blood culture, or cerebrospinal fluid analysis or culture to detect an occult bacterial infection in infants presenting with a lower-risk BRUE (grade B, strong recommendation)

Key Action Statement 4B
Clinicians need not obtain a urinalysis (bag or catheter) in infants presenting with a lower-risk BRUE (grade C, weak recommendation)

Key Action Statement 4C

Clinicians should not obtain a chest radiograph to assess for pulmonary infection in infants presenting with a lower-risk BRUE (grade B, moderate recommendation)

Key Action Statement 4D

Clinicians need not obtain respiratory viral testing if rapid testing is available in infants presenting with a lower-risk BRUE (grade C, weak recommendation)

Key Action Statement 4E

Clinicians may obtain testing for pertussis in infants presenting with a lower-risk BRUE (grade B, weak recommendation)

Key Action Statement 5

Gastroenterology

Key Action Statement 5A

Clinicians should not obtain investigations for GER (eg, upper gastrointestinal series, pH probe, endoscopy, barium contrast study, nuclear scintigraphy, and ultrasonography) in infants presenting with a lower-risk BRUE (grade C, moderate recommendation)

Key Action Statement 5B

Clinicians should not prescribe acid suppression therapy for infants presenting with a lower-risk BRUE (grade C, moderate recommendation)

Key Action Statement 6

Inborn errors of metabolism

Key Action Statement 6A

Clinicians need not obtain measurement of serum lactic acid or serum bicarbonate to detect an IEM in infants presenting with a lower-risk BRUE (grade C, weak recommendation)

Key Action Statement 6B

Clinicians should not obtain a measurement of serum sodium, potassium, chloride, blood urea nitrogen, creatinine, calcium, or ammonia to detect an IEM in infants presenting with a lower-risk BRUE (grade C, moderate recommendation)

Key Action Statement 6C

Clinicians should not obtain a measurement of venous or arterial blood gases to detect an IEM in infants presenting with lower-risk BRUE (grade C, moderate recommendation)

Key Action Statement 6D

Clinicians need not obtain a measurement of blood glucose to detect an IEM in infants presenting with a lower-risk BRUE (grade C, weak recommendation)

Key Action Statement 6E

Clinicians should not obtain measurements of urine organic acids, plasma amino acids, or plasma acylcarnitines to detect an IEM in infants presenting with a lower-risk BRUE (grade C, moderate recommendation)

Key Action Statement 7

Anemia

Key Action Statement 7A

Clinicians should not obtain laboratory evaluation for anemia in infants presenting with a lower-risk BRUE (grade C, moderate recommendation)

Key Action Statement 8

Patient- and family-centered care

Key Action Statement 8A

Clinicians should offer resources for CPR training to caregivers (grade C, moderate recommendation)

Key Action Statement 8B

Clinicians should educate caregivers about BRUEs (grade C, moderate recommendation)

Key Action Statement 8C

Clinicians should use shared decision-making for infants presenting with a lower-risk BRUE (grade C, moderate recommendation)

Coding Quick Reference for Brief Resolved Unexplained Events
ICD-10-CM
R68.13 Apparent life threatening event (ALTE) in infant (includes brief resolved unexplained events [BRUE])

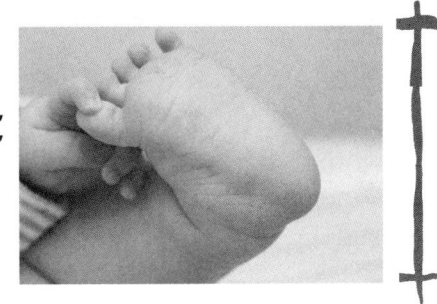

Brief Resolved Unexplained Event:
What Parents and Caregivers Need to Know

What is a brief resolved unexplained event?

A **b**rief **r**esolved **u**nexplained **e**vent (or BRUE for short) occurs suddenly and can be scary for parents and caregivers. A brief resolved unexplained event is a diagnosis made after your baby's doctor or health care professional has examined your baby and determined that there was no known concerning cause for the event.

When a brief resolved unexplained event occurs, babies may seem to stop breathing, their skin color may change to pale or blue, their muscles may relax or tighten, or they may seem to pass out. After a brief period of time, they recover (with or without any medical help) and are soon back to normal.

Though we can never say that a baby who has had a brief resolved unexplained event is at *no* risk for future problems, we can say that babies are at lower risk if

- They are older than 60 days.
- They were born on time (not premature).
- They did not need CPR (cardiopulmonary resuscitation) by a health care professional.
- The brief resolved unexplained event lasted less than 1 minute.
- This was their only such event.

Frequently asked questions after a brief resolved unexplained event

Q: Why did my baby have this event?

A: Your baby's doctor was unable to find a cause based on the results of your baby's examination and cannot tell you why this event happened. If it happens again or your baby develops additional problems, contact your baby's doctor or health care professional. The doctor may decide to have your baby return for another visit.

Q: Should my baby stay in the hospital?

A: Babies who are felt to be at lower risk by their doctors or health care professionals do not need to stay in the hospital. They are safe to go home without doing blood tests or imaging that uses x-rays, and they do not need home monitoring of their heart or lungs.

Q: Does having a brief resolved unexplained event increase my baby's risk for sudden infant death syndrome (SIDS)?

A: No—though the causes of SIDS are not known, events like these do not increase the risk of SIDS. For all babies, it is important to create a safe home and sleeping environment. Your baby should not be exposed to smoky

environments. Visit **www.HealthyChildren.org/safesleep** to learn more about how to create a safe sleeping environment for your baby.

Q: What should I do if it happens again?

A: If you are worried that this new event is life threatening, call 911 or your local emergency numbers. If not, call your baby's doctor if you have any questions or worries and to let the doctor know about the event.

Q: Does my baby need extra care after having a brief resolved unexplained event? Is my baby more delicate or weak?

A: No special care is needed. Continue to love and care for your baby as you normally do.

A few important reminders for parents and caregivers of healthy infants

- Remember to take your baby to regular well-child visits to help keep your child healthy and safe.
- Though your baby is not more likely to need it, it is a good idea for everyone who cares for an infant to learn CPR. If you know CPR, you may also use it one day to help someone else in need. For classes near you, contact your child's doctor, the American Red Cross, the American Heart Association, or a national or local organization that offers training.

Listing of resources does not imply an endorsement by the American Academy of Pediatrics (AAP). The AAP is not responsible for the content of external resources. Information was current at the time of publication.

The information contained in this publication should not be used as a substitute for the medical care and advice of your pediatrician. There may be variations in treatment that your pediatrician may recommend based on individual facts and circumstances.

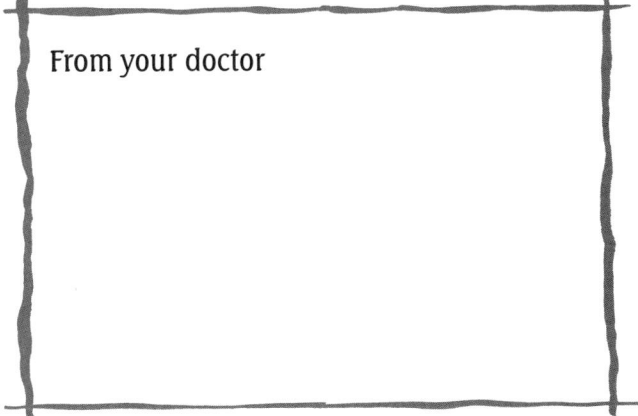

From your doctor

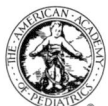

American Academy of Pediatrics

DEDICATED TO THE HEALTH OF ALL CHILDREN™

The American Academy of Pediatrics (AAP) is an organization of 64,000 primary care pediatricians, pediatric medical subspecialists, and pediatric surgical specialists dedicated to the health, safety, and well-being of all infants, children, adolescents, and young adults.

American Academy of Pediatrics
Web site—www.HealthyChildren.org

The Diagnosis, Management, and Prevention of Bronchiolitis

- *Clinical Practice Guideline*

    - *PPI: AAP Partnership for Policy Implementation*
    See Appendix 2 for more information.

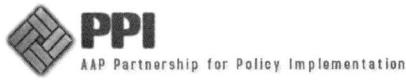

CLINICAL PRACTICE GUIDELINE

Clinical Practice Guideline: The Diagnosis, Management, and Prevention of Bronchiolitis

abstract

This guideline is a revision of the clinical practice guideline, "Diagnosis and Management of Bronchiolitis," published by the American Academy of Pediatrics in 2006. The guideline applies to children from 1 through 23 months of age. Other exclusions are noted. Each key action statement indicates level of evidence, benefit-harm relationship, and level of recommendation. Key action statements are as follows: *Pediatrics* 2014;134:e1474–e1502

DIAGNOSIS

1a. Clinicians should diagnose bronchiolitis and assess disease severity on the basis of history and physical examination (Evidence Quality: B; Recommendation Strength: Strong Recommendation).

1b. Clinicians should assess risk factors for severe disease, such as age less than 12 weeks, a history of prematurity, underlying cardiopulmonary disease, or immunodeficiency, when making decisions about evaluation and management of children with bronchiolitis (Evidence Quality: B; Recommendation Strength: Moderate Recommendation).

1c. When clinicians diagnose bronchiolitis on the basis of history and physical examination, radiographic or laboratory studies should not be obtained routinely (Evidence Quality: B; Recommendation Strength: Moderate Recommendation).

TREATMENT

2. Clinicians should not administer albuterol (or salbutamol) to infants and children with a diagnosis of bronchiolitis (Evidence Quality: B; Recommendation Strength: Strong Recommendation).

3. Clinicians should not administer epinephrine to infants and children with a diagnosis of bronchiolitis (Evidence Quality: B; Recommendation Strength: Strong Recommendation).

4a. Nebulized hypertonic saline should not be administered to infants with a diagnosis of bronchiolitis in the emergency department (Evidence Quality: B; Recommendation Strength: Moderate Recommendation).

4b. Clinicians may administer nebulized hypertonic saline to infants and children hospitalized for bronchiolitis (Evidence Quality: B; Recommendation Strength: Weak Recommendation [based on randomized controlled trials with inconsistent findings]).

Shawn L. Ralston, MD, FAAP, Allan S. Lieberthal, MD, FAAP, H. Cody Meissner, MD, FAAP, Brian K. Alverson, MD, FAAP, Jill E. Baley, MD, FAAP, Anne M. Gadomski, MD, MPH, FAAP, David W. Johnson, MD, FAAP, Michael J. Light, MD, FAAP, Nizar F. Maraqa, MD, FAAP, Eneida A. Mendonca, MD, PhD, FAAP, FACMI, Kieran J. Phelan, MD, MSc, Joseph J. Zorc, MD, MSCE, FAAP, Danette Stanko-Lopp, MA, MPH, Mark A. Brown, MD, Ian Nathanson, MD, FAAP, Elizabeth Rosenblum, MD, Stephen Sayles III, MD, FACEP, and Sinsi Hernandez-Cancio, JD

KEY WORDS
bronchiolitis, infants, children, respiratory syncytial virus, evidence-based, guideline

ABBREVIATIONS
AAP—American Academy of Pediatrics
AOM—acute otitis media
CI—confidence interval
ED—emergency department
KAS—Key Action Statement
LOS—length of stay
MD—mean difference
PCR—polymerase chain reaction
RSV—respiratory syncytial virus
SBI—serious bacterial infection

www.pediatrics.org/cgi/doi/10.1542/peds.2014-2742

doi:10.1542/peds.2014-2742

PEDIATRICS (ISSN Numbers: Print, 0031-4005; Online, 1098-4275).

Copyright © 2014 by the American Academy of Pediatrics

5. Clinicians should not administer systemic corticosteroids to infants with a diagnosis of bronchiolitis in any setting (Evidence Quality: A; Recommendation Strength: Strong Recommendation).

6a. Clinicians may choose not to administer supplemental oxygen if the oxyhemoglobin saturation exceeds 90% in infants and children with a diagnosis of bronchiolitis (Evidence Quality: D; Recommendation Strength: Weak Recommendation [based on low level evidence and reasoning from first principles]).

6b. Clinicians may choose not to use continuous pulse oximetry for infants and children with a diagnosis of bronchiolitis (Evidence Quality: D; Recommendation Strength: Weak Recommendation [based on low-level evidence and reasoning from first principles]).

7. Clinicians should not use chest physiotherapy for infants and children with a diagnosis of bronchiolitis (Evidence Quality: B; Recommendation Strength: Moderate Recommendation).

8. Clinicians should not administer antibacterial medications to infants and children with a diagnosis of bronchiolitis unless there is a concomitant bacterial infection, or a strong suspicion of one (Evidence Quality: B; Recommendation Strength: Strong Recommendation).

9. Clinicians should administer nasogastric or intravenous fluids for infants with a diagnosis of bronchiolitis who cannot maintain hydration orally (Evidence Quality: X; Recommendation Strength: Strong Recommendation).

PREVENTION

10a. Clinicians should not administer palivizumab to otherwise healthy infants with a gestational age of 29 weeks, 0 days or greater (Evidence Quality: B; Recommendation Strength: Strong Recommendation).

10b. Clinicians should administer palivizumab during the first year of life to infants with hemodynamically significant heart disease or chronic lung disease of prematurity defined as preterm infants <32 weeks 0 days' gestation who require >21% oxygen for at least the first 28 days of life (Evidence Quality: B; Recommendation Strength: Moderate Recommendation).

10c. Clinicians should administer a maximum 5 monthly doses (15 mg/kg/dose) of palivizumab during the respiratory syncytial virus season to infants who qualify for palivizumab in the first year of life (Evidence Quality: B; Recommendation Strength: Moderate Recommendation).

11a. All people should disinfect hands before and after direct contact with patients, after contact with inanimate objects in the direct vicinity of the patient, and after removing gloves (Evidence Quality: B; Recommendation Strength: Strong Recommendation).

11b. All people should use alcohol-based rubs for hand decontamination when caring for children with bronchiolitis. When alcohol-based rubs are not available, individuals should wash their hands with soap and water (Evidence Quality: B; Recommendation Strength: Strong Recommendation).

12a. Clinicians should inquire about the exposure of the infant or child to tobacco smoke when assessing infants and children for bronchiolitis (Evidence Quality: C; Recommendation Strength: Moderate Recommendation).

12b. Clinicians should counsel caregivers about exposing the infant or child to environmental tobacco smoke and smoking cessation when assessing a child for bronchiolitis (Evidence Quality: B; Recommendation Strength: Strong).

13. Clinicians should encourage exclusive breastfeeding for at least 6 months to decrease the morbidity of respiratory infections. (Evidence Quality: B; Recommendation Strength: Moderate Recommendation).

14. Clinicians and nurses should educate personnel and family members on evidence-based diagnosis, treatment, and prevention in bronchiolitis. (Evidence Quality: C; observational studies; Recommendation Strength: Moderate Recommendation).

INTRODUCTION

In October 2006, the American Academy of Pediatrics (AAP) published the clinical practice guideline "Diagnosis and Management of Bronchiolitis."[1] The guideline offered recommendations ranked according to level of evidence and the benefit-harm relationship. Since completion of the original evidence review in July 2004, a significant body of literature on bronchiolitis has been published. This update of the 2006 AAP bronchiolitis guideline evaluates published evidence, including that used in the 2006 guideline as well as evidence published since 2004. Key action statements (KASs) based on that evidence are provided.

The goal of this guideline is to provide an evidence-based approach to the diagnosis, management, and prevention of bronchiolitis in children from 1 month through 23 months of age. The guideline is intended for pediatricians, family physicians, emergency medicine specialists, hospitalists, nurse practitioners, and physician assistants who care for these children. The guideline does not apply to children with immunodeficiencies, including those with HIV infection or recipients of solid organ or hematopoietic stem cell transplants. Children with underlying respiratory illnesses, such as recurrent wheezing, chronic neonatal lung disease (also known as bronchopulmonary dysplasia), neuromuscular disease, or cystic fibrosis and those with hemodynamically significant congenital heart disease are excluded from the sections on management unless otherwise noted but are included in the discussion of prevention. This guideline will not address long-term sequelae of bronchiolitis, such as recurrent wheezing or risk of asthma, which is a field with a large and distinct literature.

Bronchiolitis is a disorder commonly caused by viral lower respiratory tract infection in infants. Bronchiolitis is characterized by acute inflammation, edema, and necrosis of epithelial cells lining small airways, and increased mucus production. Signs and symptoms typically begin with rhinitis and cough, which may progress to tachypnea, wheezing, rales, use of accessory muscles, and/or nasal flaring.[2]

Many viruses that infect the respiratory system cause a similar constellation of signs and symptoms. The most common etiology of bronchiolitis is respiratory syncytial virus (RSV), with the highest incidence of infection occurring between December and March in North America; however, regional variations occur[3] (Fig 1).[4] Ninety percent of children are infected with RSV in the first 2 years of life,[5] and up to 40% will experience lower respiratory tract infection during the initial infection.[6,7] Infection with RSV does not grant permanent or long-term immunity, with reinfections common throughout life.[8] Other viruses that cause bronchiolitis include human rhinovirus, human meta-

pneumovirus, influenza, adenovirus, coronavirus, human, and parainfluenza viruses. In a study of inpatients and outpatients with bronchiolitis,[9] 76% of patients had RSV, 39% had human rhinovirus, 10% had influenza, 2% had coronavirus, 3% had human metapneumovirus, and 1% had parainfluenza viruses (some patients had coinfections, so the total is greater than 100%).

Bronchiolitis is the most common cause of hospitalization among infants during the first 12 months of life. Approximately 100 000 bronchiolitis admissions occur annually in the United States at an estimated cost of $1.73 billion.[10] One prospective, population-based study sponsored by the Centers for Disease Control and Prevention reported the

average RSV hospitalization rate was 5.2 per 1000 children younger than 24 months of age during the 5-year period between 2000 and 2005.[11] The highest age-specific rate of RSV hospitalization occurred among infants between 30 days and 60 days of age (25.9 per 1000 children). For preterm infants (<37 weeks' gestation), the RSV hospitalization rate was 4.6 per 1000 children, a number similar to the RSV hospitalization rate for term infants of 5.2 per 1000. Infants born at <30 weeks' gestation had the highest hospitalization rate at 18.7 children per 1000, although the small number of infants born before 30 weeks' gestation make this number unreliable. Other studies indicate the RSV hospitalization rate in extremely

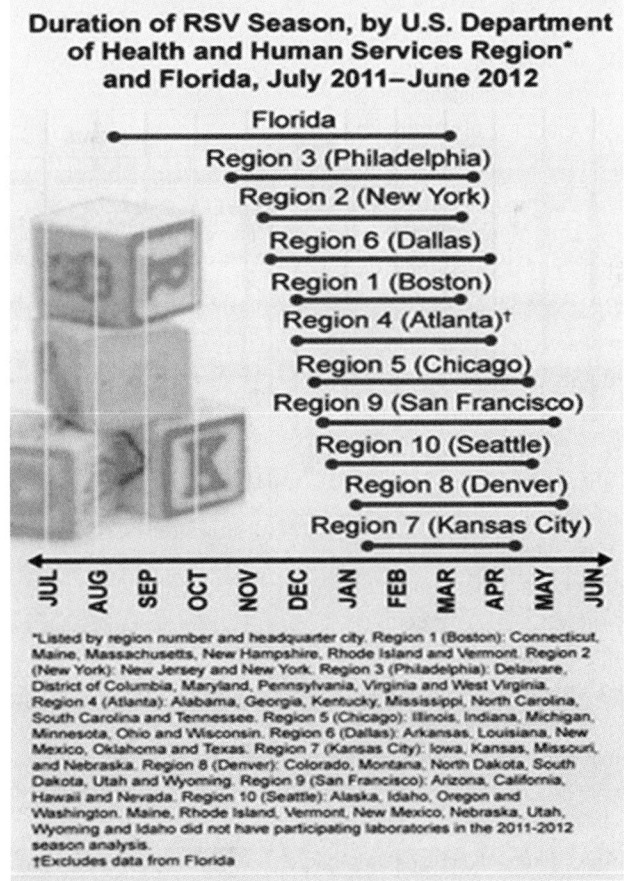

Duration of RSV Season, by U.S. Department of Health and Human Services Region* and Florida, July 2011–June 2012

*Listed by region number and headquarter city. Region 1 (Boston): Connecticut, Maine, Massachusetts, New Hampshire, Rhode Island and Vermont. Region 2 (New York): New Jersey and New York. Region 3 (Philadelphia): Delaware, District of Columbia, Maryland, Pennsylvania, Virginia and West Virginia. Region 4 (Atlanta): Alabama, Georgia, Kentucky, Mississippi, North Carolina, South Carolina and Tennessee. Region 5 (Chicago): Illinois, Indiana, Michigan, Minnesota, Ohio and Wisconsin. Region 6 (Dallas): Arkansas, Louisiana, New Mexico, Oklahoma and Texas. Region 7 (Kansas City): Iowa, Kansas, Missouri and Nebraska. Region 8 (Denver): Colorado, Montana, North Dakota, South Dakota, Utah and Wyoming. Region 9 (San Francisco): Arizona, California, Hawaii and Nevada. Region 10 (Seattle): Alaska, Idaho, Oregon and Washington. Maine, Rhode Island, Vermont, New Mexico, Nebraska, Utah, Wyoming and Idaho did not have participating laboratories in the 2011-2012 season analysis.
†Excludes data from Florida

FIGURE 1

RSV season by US regions. Centers for Disease Control and Prevention. RSV activity—United States, July 2011–Jan 2013. *MMWR Morb Mortal Wkly Rep.* 2013;62(8):141–144.

preterm infants is similar to that of term infants.[12,13]

METHODS

In June 2013, the AAP convened a new subcommittee to review and revise the 2006 bronchiolitis guideline. The subcommittee included primary care physicians, including general pediatricians, a family physician, and pediatric subspecialists, including hospitalists, pulmonologists, emergency physicians, a neonatologist, and pediatric infectious disease physicians. The subcommittee also included an epidemiologist trained in systematic reviews, a guideline methodologist/informatician, and a parent representative. All panel members reviewed the AAP Policy on Conflict of Interest and Voluntary Disclosure and were given an opportunity to declare any potential conflicts. Any conflicts can be found in the author listing at the end of this guideline. All funding was provided by the AAP, with travel assistance from the American Academy of Family Physicians, the American College of Chest Physicians, the American Thoracic Society, and the American College of Emergency Physicians for their liaisons.

The evidence search and review included electronic database searches in *The Cochrane Library*, Medline via Ovid, and CINAHL via EBSCO. The search strategy is shown in the Appendix. Related article searches were conducted in PubMed. The bibliographies of articles identified by database searches were also reviewed by 1 of 4 members of the committee, and references identified in this manner were added to the review. Articles included in the 2003 evidence report on bronchiolitis in preparation of the AAP 2006 guideline2 also were reviewed. In addition, the committee reviewed articles published after completion of the systematic review for these updated guidelines. The current literature re-

view encompasses the period from 2004 through May 2014.

The evidence-based approach to guideline development requires that the evidence in support of a policy be identified, appraised, and summarized and that an explicit link between evidence and recommendations be defined. Evidence-based recommendations reflect the quality of evidence and the balance of benefit and harm that is anticipated when the recommendation is followed. The AAP policy statement "Classifying Recommendations for Clinical Practice"[14] was followed in designating levels of recommendation (Fig 2; Table 1).

A draft version of this clinical practice guideline underwent extensive peer review by committees, councils, and sections within AAP; the American Thoracic Society, American College of Chest Physicians, American Academy

of Family Physicians, and American College of Emergency Physicians; other outside organizations; and other individuals identified by the subcommittee as experts in the field. The resulting comments were reviewed by the subcommittee and, when appropriate, incorporated into the guideline.

This clinical practice guideline is not intended as a sole source of guidance in the management of children with bronchiolitis. Rather, it is intended to assist clinicians in decision-making. It is not intended to replace clinical judgment or establish a protocol for the care of all children with bronchiolitis. These recommendations may not provide the only appropriate approach to the management of children with bronchiolitis.

All AAP guidelines are reviewed every 5 years.

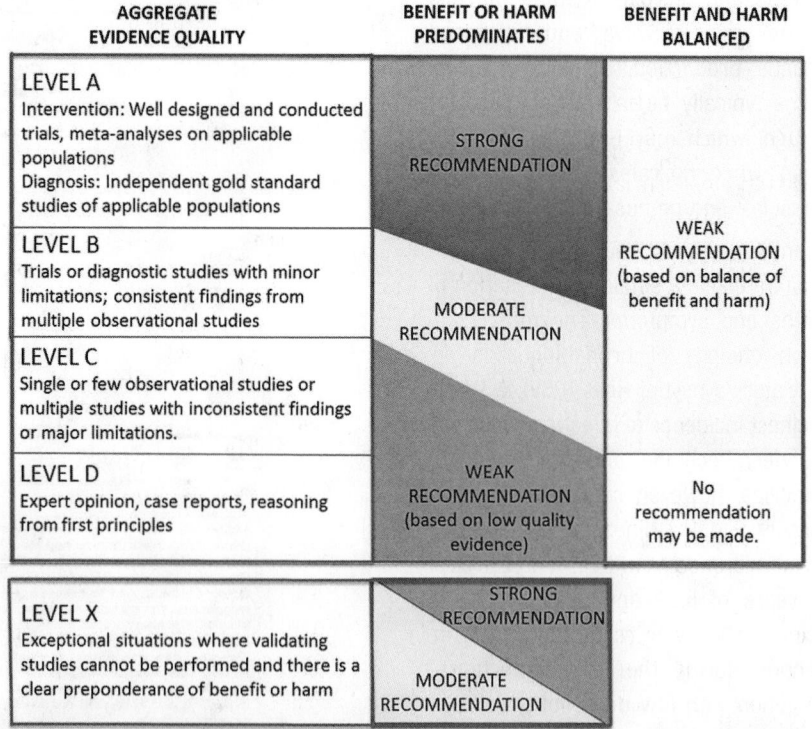

FIGURE 2

Integrating evidence quality appraisal with an assessment of the anticipated balance between benefits and harms leads to designation of a policy as a strong recommendation, moderate recommendation, or weak recommendation.

TABLE 1 Guideline Definitions for Evidence-Based Statements

Statement	Definition	Implication
Strong recommendation	A particular action is favored because anticipated benefits clearly exceed harms (or vice versa), and quality of evidence is excellent or unobtainable.	Clinicians should follow a strong recommendation unless a clear and compelling rationale for an alternative approach is present.
Moderate recommendation	A particular action is favored because anticipated benefits clearly exceed harms (or vice versa), and the quality of evidence is good but not excellent (or is unobtainable).	Clinicians would be prudent to follow a moderate recommendation but should remain alert to new information and sensitive to patient preferences.
Weak recommendation (based on low-quality evidence	A particular action is favored because anticipated benefits clearly exceed harms (or vice versa), but the quality of evidence is weak.	Clinicians would be prudent to follow a weak recommendation but should remain alert to new information and very sensitive to patient preferences.
Weak recommendation (based on balance of benefits and harms)	Weak recommendation is provided when the aggregate database shows evidence of both benefit and harm that appear similar in magnitude for any available courses of action	Clinicians should consider the options in their decision making, but patient preference may have a substantial role.

DIAGNOSIS

Key Action Statement 1a

Clinicians should diagnose bronchiolitis and assess disease severity on the basis of history and physical examination (Evidence Quality: B; Recommendation Strength: Strong Recommendation).

Action Statement Profile KAS 1a

Aggregate evidence quality	B
Benefits	Inexpensive, noninvasive, accurate
Risk, harm, cost	Missing other diagnoses
Benefit-harm assessment	Benefits outweigh harms
Value judgments	None
Intentional vagueness	None
Role of patient preferences	None
Exclusions	None
Strength	Strong recommendation
Differences of opinion	None

Key Action Statement 1b

Clinicians should assess risk factors for severe disease, such as age <12 weeks, a history of prematurity, underlying cardiopulmonary disease, or immunodeficiency, when making decisions about eval- uation and management of children with bronchiolitis (Evidence Quality: B; Recommendation Strength: Moderate Recommendation).

Action Statement Profile KAS 1b

Aggregate evidence quality	B
Benefits	Improved ability to predict course of illness, appropriate disposition
Risk, harm, cost	Possible unnecessary hospitalization parental anxiety
Benefit-harm assessment	Benefits outweigh harms
Value judgments	None
Intentional vagueness	"Assess" is not defined
Role of patient preferences	None
Exclusions	None
Strength	Moderate recommendation
Differences of opinion	None

Key Action Statement 1c

When clinicians diagnose bronchiolitis on the basis of history and physical examination, radiographic or laboratory studies should not be obtained routinely (Evidence Quality: B; Recommendation Strength: Moderate Recommendation).

Action Statement Profile KAS 1b

Aggregate evidence quality	B
Benefits	Decreased radiation exposure, noninvasive (less procedure-associated discomfort), decreased antibiotic use, cost savings, time saving
Risk, harm, cost	Misdiagnosis, missed diagnosis of comorbid condition
Benefit-harm assessment	Benefits outweigh harms
Value judgments	None
Intentional vagueness	None
Role of patient preferences	None
Exclusions	Infants and children with unexpected worsening disease
Strength	Moderate recommendation
Differences of opinion	None

The main goals in the history and physical examination of infants presenting with wheeze or other lower respiratory tract symptoms, particularly in the winter season, is to differentiate infants with probable viral bronchiolitis from those with other disorders. In addition, an estimate of disease severity (increased respiratory rate, retractions, decreased oxygen saturation) should be made. Most clinicians recognize bronchiolitis as a constellation of clinical signs and symptoms occurring in children younger than 2 years, including a viral upper respiratory tract prodrome followed by increased respiratory effort and wheezing. Clinical signs and symptoms of bronchiolitis consist of rhinorrhea, cough, tachypnea, wheezing, rales, and increased respiratory effort manifested as grunting, nasal flaring, and intercostal and/or subcostal retractions.

The course of bronchiolitis is variable and dynamic, ranging from transient events, such as apnea, to progressive respiratory distress from lower airway obstruction. Important issues to assess in the history include the effects of respiratory symptoms on mental status, feeding, and hydration. The clinician should assess the ability of the family to care for the child and to return for further evaluation if needed. History of underlying conditions, such as prematurity, cardiac disease, chronic pulmonary disease, immunodeficiency, or episodes of previous wheezing, should be identified. Underlying conditions that may be associated with an increased risk of progression to severe disease or mortality include hemodynamically significant congenital heart disease, chronic lung disease (bronchopulmonary dysplasia), congenital anomalies,[15–17] in utero smoke exposure,[18] and the presence of an immunocompromising state.[19,20] In addition, genetic abnormalities have been associated with more severe presentation with bronchiolitis.[21]

Assessment of a child with bronchiolitis, including the physical examination, can be complicated by variability in the disease state and may require serial observations over time to fully assess the child's status. Upper airway obstruction contributes to work of breathing. Suctioning and positioning may decrease the work of breathing and improve the quality of the examination. Respiratory

rate in otherwise healthy children changes considerably over the first year of life.[22–25] In hospitalized children, the 50th percentile for respiratory rate decreased from 41 at 0 to 3 months of age to 31 at 12 to 18 months of age.[26] Counting respiratory rate over the course of 1 minute is more accurate than shorter observations.[27] The presence of a normal respiratory rate suggests that risk of significant viral or bacterial lower respiratory tract infection or pneumonia in an infant is low (negative likelihood ratio approximately 0.5),[27–29] but the presence of tachypnea does not distinguish between viral and bacterial disease.[30,31]

The evidence relating the presence of specific findings in the assessment of bronchiolitis to clinical outcomes is limited. Most studies addressing this issue have enrolled children when presenting to hospital settings, including a large, prospective, multicenter study that assessed a variety of outcomes from the emergency department (ED) and varied inpatient settings.[18,32,33] Severe adverse events, such as ICU admission and need for mechanical ventilation, are uncommon among children with bronchiolitis and limit the power of these studies to detect clinically important risk factors associated with disease progression.[16,34,35] Tachypnea, defined as a respiratory rate $\geq$70 per minute, has been associated with increased risk of severe disease in some studies[35–37] but not others.[38] Many scoring systems have been developed in an attempt to objectively quantify respiratory distress, although none has achieved widespread acceptance and few have demonstrated any predictive validity, likely because of the substantial temporal variability in physical findings in infants with bronchiolitis.[39]

Pulse oximetry has been rapidly adopted into clinical assessment of children with bronchiolitis on the basis of data

suggesting that it reliably detects hypoxemia not suspected on physical examination[36,40]; however, few studies have assessed the effectiveness of pulse oximetry to predict clinical outcomes. Among inpatients, perceived need for supplemental oxygen on the basis of pulse oximetry has been associated with prolonged hospitalization, ICU admission, and mechanical ventilation.[16,34,41] Among outpatients, available evidence differs on whether mild reductions in pulse oximetry (<95% on room air) predict progression of disease or need for a return observational visit.[38]

Apnea has been reported to occur with a wide range of prevalence estimates and viral etiologies.[42,43] Retrospective, hospital-based studies have included a high proportion of infants with risk factors, such as prematurity or neuromuscular disease, that may have biased the prevalence estimates. One large study found no apnea events for infants assessed as low risk by using several risk factors: age >1 month for full-term infants or 48 weeks' postconceptional age for preterm infants, and absence of any previous apneic event at presentation to the hospital.[44] Another large multicenter study found no association between the specific viral agent and risk of apnea in bronchiolitis.[42]

The literature on viral testing for bronchiolitis has expanded in recent years with the availability of sensitive polymerase chain reaction (PCR) assays. Large studies of infants hospitalized for bronchiolitis have consistently found that 60% to 75% have positive test results for RSV, and have noted coinfections in up to one-third of infants.[32,33,45] In the event an infant receiving monthly prophylaxis is hospitalized with bronchiolitis, testing should be performed to determine if RSV is the etiologic agent. If a breakthrough RSV infection is determined to be present based on antigen detection or other assay, monthly palivizumab prophylaxis should be discontinued because of the very low likelihood of a second RSV infection in the same year. Apart from this setting, routine virologic testing is not recommended.

Infants with non-RSV bronchiolitis, in particular human rhinovirus, appear to have a shorter courses and may represent a different phenotype associated with repeated wheezing.[32] PCR assay results should be interpreted cautiously, given that the assay may detect prolonged viral shedding from an unrelated previous illness, particularly with rhinovirus. In contrast, RSV detected by PCR assay almost always is associated with disease. At the individual patient level, the value of identifying a specific viral etiology causing bronchiolitis has not been demonstrated.[33]

Current evidence does not support routine chest radiography in children with bronchiolitis. Although many infants with bronchiolitis have abnormalities on chest radiography, data are insufficient to demonstrate that chest radiography correlates well with disease severity. Atelectasis on chest radiography was associated with increased risk of severe disease in 1 outpatient study.[16] Further studies, including 1 randomized trial, suggest children with suspected lower respiratory tract infection who had radiography performed were more likely to receive antibiotics without any difference in outcomes.[46,47] Initial radiography should be reserved for cases in which respiratory effort is severe enough to warrant ICU admission or where signs of an airway complication (such as pneumothorax) are present.

TREATMENT

ALBUTEROL

Key Action Statement 2

Clinicians should not administer albuterol (or salbutamol) to infants

and children with a diagnosis of bronchiolitis (Evidence Quality: B; Recommendation Strength: Strong Recommendation).

Action Statement Profile KAS 2

Aggregate evidence quality	B
Benefits	Avoid adverse effects, avoid ongoing use of ineffective medication, lower costs
Risk, harm, cost	Missing transient benefit of drug
Benefit-harm assessment	Benefits outweigh harms
Value judgments	Overall ineffectiveness outweighs possible transient benefit
Intentional vagueness	None
Role of patient preferences	None
Exclusions	None
Strength	Strong recommendation
Differences of opinion	None
Notes	This guideline no longer recommends a trial of albuterol, as was considered in the 2006 AAP bronchiolitis guideline

Although several studies and reviews have evaluated the use of bronchodilator medications for viral bronchiolitis, most randomized controlled trials have failed to demonstrate a consistent benefit from α- or β-adrenergic agents. Several meta-analyses and systematic reviews[48–53] have shown that bronchodilators may improve clinical symptom scores, but they do not affect disease resolution, need for hospitalization, or length of stay (LOS). Because clinical scores may vary from one observer to the next[39,54] and do not correlate with more objective measures, such as pulmonary function tests,[55] clinical scores are not validated measures of the efficacy of bronchodilators. Although transient improvements in clinical score have been observed, most infants treated with bronchodilators will not benefit from their use.

A recently updated Cochrane systematic review assessing the impact of bronchodilators on oxygen saturation, the primary outcome measure, reported 30 randomized controlled trials involving 1992 infants in 12 countries.[56] Some studies included in this review evaluated agents other than albuterol/salbutamol (eg, ipratropium and metaproterenol) but did not include epinephrine. Small sample sizes, lack of standardized methods for outcome evaluation (eg, timing of assessments), and lack of standardized intervention (various bronchodilators, drug dosages, routes of administration, and nebulization delivery systems) limit the interpretation of these studies. Because of variable study designs as well as the inclusion of infants who had a history of previous wheezing in some studies, there was considerable heterogeneity in the studies. Sensitivity analysis (ie, including only studies at low risk of bias) significantly reduced heterogeneity measures for oximetry while having little effect on the overall effect size of oximetry (mean difference [MD] −0.38, 95% confidence interval [CI] −0.75 to 0.00). Those studies showing benefit[57–59] are methodologically weaker than other studies and include older children with recurrent wheezing. Results of the Cochrane review indicated no benefit in the clinical course of infants with bronchiolitis who received bronchodilators. The potential adverse effects (tachycardia and tremors) and cost of these agents outweigh any potential benefits.

In the previous iteration of this guideline, a trial of β-agonists was included as an option. However, given the greater strength of the evidence demonstrating no benefit, and that there is no well-established way to determine an "objective method of response" to bronchodilators in bronchiolitis, this option has been removed. Although it is true that a small subset of children with bronchiolitis may have reversible airway obstruction resulting from smooth muscle constriction, attempts to define a subgroup of responders have not been successful to date. If a clinical trial of bronchodilators is undertaken, clinicians should note that the variability of the disease process, the host's airway, and the clinical assessments, particularly scoring, would limit the clinician's ability to observe a clinically relevant response to bronchodilators.

Chavasse et al[60] reviewed the available literature on use of β-agonists for children younger than 2 years with recurrent wheezing. At the time of that review, there were 3 studies in the outpatient setting, 2 in the ED, and 3 in the pulmonary function laboratory setting. This review concluded there were no clear benefits from the use of β-agonists in this population. The authors noted some conflicting evidence, but further study was recommended only if the population could be clearly defined and meaningful outcome measures could be identified.

The population of children with bronchiolitis studied in most trials of bronchodilators limits the ability to make recommendations for all clinical scenarios. Children with severe disease or with respiratory failure were generally excluded from these trials, and this evidence cannot be generalized to these situations. Studies using pulmonary function tests show no effect of albuterol among infants hospitalized with bronchiolitis.[56,61] One study in a critical care setting showed a small decrease in inspiratory resistance after albuterol in one group and levalbuterol in another group, but therapy was accompanied by clinically significant tachycardia.[62] This small clinical change occurring with significant adverse effects does not justify recommending albuterol for routine care.

EPINEPHRINE

Key Action Statement 3

Clinicians should not administer epinephrine to infants and children with a diagnosis of bronchiolitis (Evidence Quality: B; Recommendation Strength: Strong Recommendation).

Action Statement Profile KAS 3

Aggregate evidence quality	B
Benefits	Avoiding adverse effects, lower costs, avoiding ongoing use of ineffective medication
Risk, harm, cost	Missing transient benefit of drug
Benefit-harm assessment	Benefits outweigh harms
Value judgments	The overall ineffectiveness outweighs possible transient benefit
Intentional vagueness	None
Role of patient preferences	None
Exclusions	Rescue treatment of rapidly deteriorating patients
Strength	Strong recommendation
Differences of opinion	None

Epinephrine is an adrenergic agent with both β- and α-receptor agonist activity that has been used to treat upper and lower respiratory tract illnesses both as a systemic agent and directly into the respiratory tract, where it is typically administered as a nebulized solution. Nebulized epinephrine has been administered in the racemic form and as the purified L-enantiomer, which is commercially available in the United States for intravenous use. Studies in other diseases, such as croup, have found no difference in efficacy on the basis of preparation,[63] although the comparison has not been specifically studied for bronchiolitis. Most studies have compared L-epinephrine to placebo or albuterol. A recent Cochrane meta-

analysis by Hartling et al[64] systematically evaluated the evidence on this topic and found no evidence for utility in the inpatient setting. Two large, multicenter randomized trials comparing nebulized epinephrine to placebo[65] or albuterol[66] in the hospital setting found no improvement in LOS or other inpatient outcomes. A recent, large multicenter trial found a similar lack of efficacy compared with placebo and further demonstrated longer LOS when epinephrine was used on a fixed schedule compared with an as-needed schedule.[67] This evidence suggests epinephrine should not be used in children hospitalized for bronchiolitis, except potentially as a rescue agent in severe disease, although formal study is needed before a recommendation for the use of epinephrine in this setting.

The role of epinephrine in the outpatient setting remains controversial. A major addition to the evidence base came from the Canadian Bronchiolitis Epinephrine Steroid Trial.[68] This multicenter randomized trial enrolled 800 patients with bronchiolitis from 8 EDs and compared hospitalization rates over a 7-day period. This study had 4 arms: nebulized epinephrine plus oral dexamethasone, nebulized epinephrine plus oral placebo, nebulized placebo plus oral dexamethasone, and nebulized placebo plus oral placebo. The group of patients who received epinephrine concomitantly with corticosteroids had a lower likelihood of hospitalization by day 7 than the double placebo group, although this effect was no longer statistically significant after adjusting for multiple comparisons.

The systematic review by Hartling et al[64] concluded that epinephrine reduced hospitalizations compared with placebo on the day of the ED visit but not overall. Given that epinephrine has a transient effect and home administration is not routine practice, discharging an infant after observing a response in a monitored setting raises concerns for subsequent progression of illness. Studies have not found a difference in revisit rates, although the numbers of revisits are small and may not be adequately powered for this outcome. In summary, the current state of evidence does not support a routine role for epinephrine for bronchiolitis in outpatients, although further data may help to better define this question.

HYPERTONIC SALINE

Key Action Statement 4a

Nebulized hypertonic saline should not be administered to infants with a diagnosis of bronchiolitis in the emergency department (Evidence Quality: B; Recommendation Strength: Moderate Recommendation).

Action Statement Profile KAS 4a

Aggregate evidence quality	B
Benefits	Avoiding adverse effects, such as wheezing and excess secretions, cost
Risk, harm, cost	None
Benefit-harm assessment	Benefits outweigh harms
Value judgments	None
Intentional vagueness	None
Role of patient preferences	None
Exclusions	None
Strength	Moderate recommendation
Differences of opinion	None

Key Action Statement 4b

Clinicians may administer nebulized hypertonic saline to infants and children hospitalized for bronchiolitis (Evidence Quality: B; Recommendation Strength: Weak

Recommendation [based on randomized controlled trials with inconsistent findings]).

Action Statement Profile KAS 4b

Aggregate evidence quality	B
Benefits	May shorten hospital stay if LOS is >72 h
Risk, harm, cost	Adverse effects such as wheezing and excess secretions; cost
Benefit-harm assessment	Benefits outweigh harms for longer hospital stays
Value judgments	Anticipating an individual child's LOS is difficult. Most US hospitals report an average LOS of <72 h for patients with bronchiolitis. This weak recommendation applies only if the average length of stay is >72 h
Intentional vagueness	This weak recommendation is based on an average LOS and does not address the individual patient.
Role of patient preferences	None
Exclusions	None
Strength	Weak
Differences of opinion	None

Nebulized hypertonic saline is an increasingly studied therapy for acute viral bronchiolitis. Physiologic evidence suggests that hypertonic saline increases mucociliary clearance in both normal and diseased lungs.[69–71] Because the pathology in bronchiolitis involves airway inflammation and resultant mucus plugging, improved mucociliary clearance should be beneficial, although there is only indirect evidence to support such an assertion. A more specific theoretical mechanism of action has been proposed on the basis of the concept of rehydration of the airway surface liquid, although again, evidence remains indirect.[72]

A 2013 Cochrane review[73] included 11 trials involving 1090 infants with mild to moderate disease in both inpatient and emergency settings. There were 6 studies involving 500 inpatients providing data

for the analysis of LOS with an aggregate 1-day decrease reported, a result largely driven by the inclusion of 3 studies with relatively long mean length of stay of 5 to 6 days. The analysis of effect on clinical scores included 7 studies involving 640 patients in both inpatient and outpatient settings and demonstrated incremental positive effect with each day posttreatment from day 1 to day 3 (−0.88 MD on day 1, −1.32 MD on day 2, and −1.51 MD on day 3). Finally, Zhang et al[73] found no effect on hospitalization rates in the pooled analysis of 1 outpatient and 3 ED studies including 380 total patients.

Several randomized trials published after the Cochrane review period further informed the current guideline recommendation. Four trials evaluated admission rates from the ED, 3 using 3% saline and 1 using 7% saline.[74–76] A single trial[76] demonstrated a difference in admission rates from the ED favoring hypertonic saline, although the other 4 studies were concordant with the studies included in the Cochrane review. However, contrary to the studies included in the Cochrane review, none of the more recent trials reported improvement in LOS and, when added to the older studies for an updated meta-analysis, they significantly attenuate the summary estimate of the effect on LOS.[76,77] Most of the trials included in the Cochrane review occurred in settings with typical LOS of more than 3 days in their usual care arms. Hence, the significant decrease in LOS noted by Zhang et al[73] may not be generalizable to the United States where the average LOS is 2.4 days.[10] One other ongoing clinical trial performed in the United States, unpublished except in abstract form, further supports the observation that hypertonic saline does not decrease LOS in settings where expected stays are less than 3 days.[78]

The preponderance of the evidence suggests that 3% saline is safe and effective at improving symptoms of mild to moderate bronchiolitis after 24 hours of use and reducing hospital LOS in settings in which the duration of stay typically exceeds 3 days. It has not been shown to be effective at reducing hospitalization in emergency settings or in areas where the length of usage is brief. It has not been studied in intensive care settings, and most trials have included only patients with mild to moderate disease. Most studies have used a 3% saline concentration, and most have combined it with bronchodilators with each dose; however, there is retrospective evidence that the rate of adverse events is similar without bronchodilators,[79] as well as prospective evidence extrapolated from 2 trials without bronchodilators.[79,80] A single study was performed in the ambulatory outpatient setting[81]; however, future studies in the United States should focus on sustained usage on the basis of pattern of effects discerned in the available literature.

CORTICOSTEROIDS

Key Action Statement 5

Clinicians should not administer systemic corticosteroids to infants with a diagnosis of bronchiolitis in any setting (Evidence Quality: A; Recommendation Strength: Strong Recommendation).

Action Statement Profile KAS 5

Aggregate evidence quality	A
Benefits	No clinical benefit, avoiding adverse effects
Risk, harm, cost	None
Benefit-harm assessment	Benefits outweigh harms
Value judgments	None
Intentional vagueness	None
Role of patient preferences	None
Exclusions	None
Strength	Strong recommendation
Differences of opinion	None

Although there is good evidence of benefit from corticosteroids in other respiratory diseases, such as asthma and croup,[82–84] the evidence on corticosteroid use in bronchiolitis is negative. The most recent Cochrane systematic review shows that corticosteroids do not significantly reduce outpatient admissions when compared with placebo (pooled risk ratio, 0.92; 95% CI, 0.78 to 1.08; and risk ratio, 0.86; 95% CI, 0.7 to 1.06, respectively) and do not reduce LOS for inpatients (MD −0.18 days; 95% CI −0.39 to 0.04).[85] No other comparisons showed relevant differences for either primary or secondary outcomes. This review contained 17 trials with 2596 participants and included 2 large ED-based randomized trials, neither of which showed reductions in hospital admissions with treatment with corticosteroids as compared with placebo.[69,86]

One of these large trials, the Canadian Bronchiolitis Epinephrine Steroid Trial, however, did show a reduction in hospitalizations 7 days after treatment with combined nebulized epinephrine and oral dexamethasone as compared with placebo.[69] Although an unadjusted analysis showed a relative risk for hospitalization of 0.65 (95% CI 0.45 to 0.95; $P = .02$) for combination therapy as compared with placebo, adjustment for multiple comparison rendered the result insignificant ($P = .07$). These results have generated considerable controversy.[87] Although there is no standard recognized rationale for why combination epinephrine and dexamethasone would be synergistic in infants with bronchiolitis, evidence in adults and children older than 6 years with asthma shows that adding inhaled long-acting β agonists to moderate/high doses of inhaled corticosteroids allows reduction of the corticosteroid dose by, on average, 60%.[88] Basic science studies focused on understanding the interaction between β agonists and corticosteroids have shown potential mechanisms for

why simultaneous administration of these drugs could be synergistic.[89–92] However, other bronchiolitis trials of corticosteroids administered by using fixed simultaneous bronchodilator regimens have not consistently shown benefit[93–97]; hence, a recommendation regarding the benefit of combined dexamethasone and epinephrine therapy is premature.

The systematic review of corticosteroids in children with bronchiolitis cited previously did not find any differences in short-term adverse events as compared with placebo.[86] However, corticosteroid therapy may prolong viral shedding in patients with bronchiolitis.[17]

In summary, a comprehensive systematic review and large multicenter randomized trials provide clear evidence that corticosteroids alone do not provide significant benefit to children with bronchiolitis. Evidence for potential benefit of combined corticosteroid and agents with both α- and β-agonist activity is at best tentative, and additional large trials are needed to clarify whether this therapy is effective.

Further, although there is no evidence of short-term adverse effects from corticosteroid therapy, other than prolonged viral shedding, in infants and children with bronchiolitis, there is inadequate evidence to be certain of safety.

OXYGEN

Key Action Statement 6a

Clinicians may choose not to administer supplemental oxygen if the oxyhemoglobin saturation exceeds 90% in infants and children with a diagnosis of bronchiolitis (Evidence Quality: D; Recommendation Strength: Weak Recommendation [based on low-level evidence and reasoning from first principles]).

Action Statement Profile KAS 6a

Benefits	Decreased hospitalizations, decreased LOS
Risk, harm, cost	Hypoxemia, physiologic stress, prolonged LOS, increased hospitalizations, increased LOS, cost
Benefit-harm assessment	Benefits outweigh harms
Value judgments	Oxyhemoglobin saturation >89% is adequate to oxygenate tissues; the risk of hypoxemia with oxyhemoglobin saturation >89% is minimal
Intentional vagueness	None
Role of patient preferences	Limited
Exclusions	Children with acidosis or fever
Strength	Weak recommendation (based on low-level evidence/ reasoning from first principles)
Differences of opinion	None

Key Action Statement 6b

Clinicians may choose not to use continuous pulse oximetry for infants and children with a diagnosis of bronchiolitis (Evidence Quality: C; Recommendation Strength: Weak Recommendation [based on lower-level evidence]).

Action Statement Profile KAS 6b

Aggregate evidence quality	C
Benefits	Shorter LOS, decreased alarm fatigue, decreased cost
Risk, harm, cost	Delayed detection of hypoxemia, delay in appropriate weaning of oxygen
Benefit-harm assessment	Benefits outweigh harms
Value judgments	None
Intentional vagueness	None
Role of patient preferences	Limited
Exclusions	None
Strength	Weak recommendation (based on lower level of evidence)
Differences of opinion	None

Although oxygen saturation is a poor predictor of respiratory distress, it is associated closely with a perceived need for hospitalization in infants with bronchiolitis.[98,99] Additionally, oxygen saturation has been implicated as a primary determinant of LOS in bronchiolitis.[40,100,101]

Physiologic data based on the oxyhemoglobin dissociation curve (Fig 3) demonstrate that small increases in arterial partial pressure of oxygen are associated with marked improvement in pulse oxygen saturation when the latter is less than 90%; with pulse oxygen saturation readings greater than 90% it takes very large elevations in arterial partial pressure of oxygen to affect further increases. In infants and children with bronchiolitis, no data exist to suggest such increases result in any clinically significant difference in physiologic function, patient symptoms, or clinical outcomes. Although it is well understood that acidosis, temperature, and 2,3-diphosphoglutarate influence the oxyhemoglobin dissociation curve, there has never been research to demonstrate how those influences practically affect infants with hypoxemia. The risk of hypoxemia must be weighed against the risk of hospitalization when making any decisions about site of care. One study of hospitalized children with bronchiolitis, for example, noted a 10% adverse error or near-miss rate for harm-causing interventions.[103] There are no studies on the effect of short-term, brief periods of hypoxemia such as may be seen in bronchiolitis. Transient hypoxemia is common in healthy infants.[104] Travel of healthy children even to moderate altitudes of 1300 m results in transient sleep desaturation to an average of 84% with no known adverse consequences.[105] Although children with chronic hypoxemia do incur developmental and behavioral problems, children who suffer intermittent hypoxemia from diseases such as asthma do not have impaired intellectual abilities or behavioral disturbance.[106–108]

Supplemental oxygen provided for infants not requiring additional respiratory support is best initiated with nasal prongs, although exact measurement of fraction of inspired oxygen is unreliable with this method.[109]

Pulse oximetry is a convenient method to assess the percentage of hemoglobin bound by oxygen in children. Pulse oximetry has been erroneously used in bronchiolitis as a proxy for respiratory distress. Accuracy of pulse oximetry is poor, especially in the 76% to 90% range.[110] Further, it has been well demonstrated that oxygen saturation has much less impact on respiratory drive than carbon dioxide concentrations in the blood.[111] There is very poor correlation between respiratory distress and oxygen saturations among infants with lower respiratory tract infections.[112] Other than cyanosis, no published clinical sign, model, or score accurately identifies hypoxemic children.[113]

Among children admitted for bronchiolitis, continuous pulse oximetry measurement is not well studied and potentially problematic for children who do not require oxygen. Transient desaturation is a normal phenomenon in healthy infants. In 1 study of 64 healthy infants between 2 weeks and 6 months of age, 60% of these infants exhibited a transient oxygen desaturation below 90%, to values as low as 83%.[105] A retrospective study of the role of continuous measurement of oxygenation in infants hospitalized with bronchiolitis found that 1 in 4 patients incur unnecessarily prolonged hospitalization as a result of a perceived need for oxygen outside of other symptoms[40] and no evidence of benefit was found.

Pulse oximetry is prone to errors of measurement. Families of infants hospitalized with continuous pulse oximeters are exposed to frequent alarms that

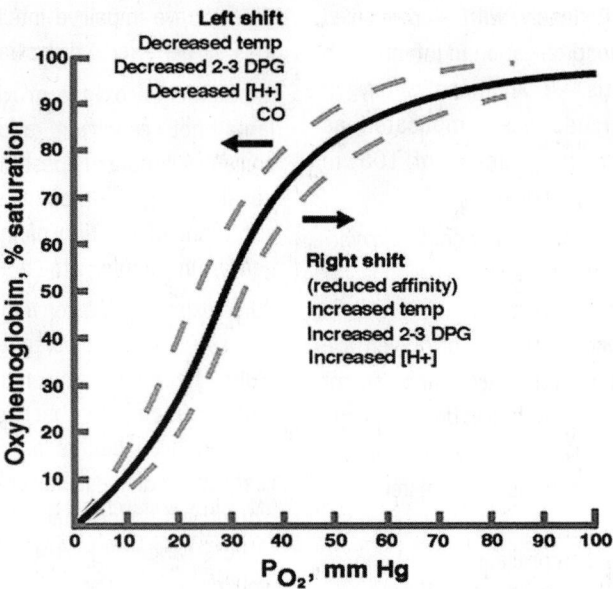

FIGURE 3
Oxyhemoglobin dissociation curve showing percent saturation of hemoglobin at various partial pressures of oxygen (reproduced with permission from the educational Web site www.anaesthesiauk.com).[102]

may negatively affect sleep. Alarm fatigue is recognized by The Joint Commission as a contributor toward in-hospital morbidity and mortality.[114] One adult study demonstrated very poor documentation of hypoxemia alerts by pulse oximetry, an indicator of alarm fatigue.[115] Pulse oximetry probes can fall off easily, leading to inaccurate measurements and alarms.[116] False reliance on pulse oximetry may lead to less careful monitoring of respiratory status. In one study, continuous pulse oximetry was associated with increased risk of minor adverse events in infants admitted to a general ward.[117] The pulse oximetry–monitored patients were found to have less-effective surveillance of their severity of illness when controlling for other variables.

There are a number of new approaches to oxygen delivery in bronchiolitis, 2 of which are home oxygen and high-frequency nasal cannula. There is emerging evidence for the role of home oxygen in reducing LOS or admission rate for infants with bronchiolitis, in-

cluding 2 randomized trials.[118,119] Most of the studies have been performed in areas of higher altitude, where prolonged hypoxemia is a prime determinant of LOS in the hospital.[120,121] Readmission rates may be moderately higher in patients discharged with home oxygen; however, overall hospital use may be reduced,[122] although not in all settings.[123] Concerns have been raised that home pulse oximetry may complicate care or confuse families.[124] Communication with follow-up physicians is important, because primary care physicians may have difficulty determining safe pulse oximetry levels for discontinuation of oxygen.[125] Additionally, there may be an increased demand for follow-up outpatient visits associated with home oxygen use.[124]

Use of humidified, heated, high-flow nasal cannula to deliver air-oxygen mixtures provides assistance to infants with bronchiolitis through multiple proposed mechanisms.[126] There is evidence that high-flow nasal cannula improves physiologic measures of respiratory effort and can generate

continuous positive airway pressure in bronchiolitis.[127–130] Clinical evidence suggests it reduces work of breathing[131,132] and may decrease need for intubation,[133–136] although studies are generally retrospective and small. The therapy has been studied in the ED[136,137] and the general inpatient setting,[134,138] as well as the ICU. The largest and most rigorous retrospective study to date was from Australia,[138] which showed a decline in intubation rate in the subgroup of infants with bronchiolitis (n = 330) from 37% to 7% after the introduction of high-flow nasal cannula, while the national registry intubation rate remained at 28%. A single pilot for a randomized trial has been published to date.[139] Although promising, the absence of any completed randomized trial of the efficacy of high-flow nasal cannula in bronchiolitis precludes specific recommendations on it use at present. Pneumothorax is a reported complication.

CHEST PHYSIOTHERAPY

Key Action Statement 7

Clinicians should not use chest physiotherapy for infants and children with a diagnosis of bronchiolitis (Evidence Quality: B; Recommendation Strength: Moderate Recommendation).

Action Statement Profile KAS 7

Aggregate evidence quality	B
Benefits	Decreased stress from therapy, reduced cost
Risk, harm, cost	None
Benefit-harm assessment	Benefits outweigh harms
Value judgments	None
Intentional vagueness	None
Role of patient preferences	None
Exclusions	None
Strength	Moderate recommendation
Differences of opinion	None

Airway edema, sloughing of respiratory epithelium into airways, and generalized hyperinflation of the lungs, coupled with poorly developed collateral ventilation, put infants with bronchiolitis at risk for atelectasis. Although lobar atelectasis is not characteristic of this disease, chest radiographs may show evidence of subsegmental atelectasis, prompting clinicians to consider ordering chest physiotherapy to promote airway clearance. A Cochrane Review[140] found 9 randomized controlled trials that evaluated chest physiotherapy in hospitalized patients with bronchiolitis. No clinical benefit was found by using vibration or percussion (5 trials)[141–144] or passive expiratory techniques (4 trials).[145–148] Since that review, a study[149] of the passive expiratory technique found a small, but significant reduction in duration of oxygen therapy, but no other benefits.

Suctioning of the nasopharynx to remove secretions is a frequent practice in infants with bronchiolitis. Although suctioning the nares may provide temporary relief of nasal congestion or upper airway obstruction, a retrospective study reported that deep suctioning[150] was associated with longer LOS in hospitalized infants 2 to 12 months of age. The same study also noted that lapses of greater than 4 hours in noninvasive, external nasal suctioning were also associated with longer LOS. Currently, there are insufficient data to make a recommendation about suctioning, but it appears that routine use of "deep" suctioning[151,153] may not be beneficial.

ANTIBACTERIALS

Key Action Statement 8

Clinicians should not administer antibacterial medications to infants and children with a diagnosis of bronchiolitis unless there is a concomitant bacterial infection, or a strong suspicion of one. (Evidence

Quality: B; Recommendation Strength: Strong Recommendation).

Action Statement Profile KAS 8

Aggregate evidence quality	B
Benefits	Fewer adverse effects, less resistance to antibacterial agents, lower cost
Risk, harm, cost	None
Benefit-harm assessment	Benefits outweigh harms
Value judgments	None
Intentional vagueness	Strong suspicion is not specifically defined and requires clinician judgment. An evaluation for the source of possible serious bacterial infection should be completed before antibiotic use
Role of patient preferences	None
Exclusions	None
Strength	Strong recommendation
Differences of opinion	None

Infants with bronchiolitis frequently receive antibacterial therapy because of fever,[152] young age,[153] and concern for secondary bacterial infection.[154] Early randomized controlled trials[155,156] showed no benefit from routine antibacterial therapy for children with bronchiolitis. Nonetheless, antibiotic therapy continues to be overused in young infants with bronchiolitis because of concern for an undetected bacterial infection. Studies have shown that febrile infants without an identifiable source of fever have a risk of bacteremia that may be as high as 7%. However, a child with a distinct viral syndrome, such as bronchiolitis, has a lower risk (much less than 1%) of bacterial infection of the cerebrospinal fluid or blood.[157]

Ralston et al[158] conducted a systematic review of serious bacterial infections (SBIs) occurring in hospitalized febrile infants between 30 and 90 days of age with bronchiolitis. Instances of bacteremia or meningitis were extremely rare.

Enteritis was not evaluated. Urinary tract infection occurred at a rate of approximately 1%, but asymptomatic bacteriuria may have explained this finding. The authors concluded routine screening for SBI among hospitalized febrile infants with bronchiolitis between 30 and 90 days of age is not justified. Limited data suggest the risk of bacterial infection in hospitalized infants with bronchiolitis younger than 30 days of age is similar to the risk in older infants. An abnormal white blood cell count is not useful for predicting a concurrent SBI in infants and young children hospitalized with RSV lower respiratory tract infection.[159] Several retrospective studies support this conclusion.[160–166] Four prospective studies of SBI in patients with bronchiolitis and/or RSV infections also demonstrated low rates of SBI.[167–171]

Approximately 25% of hospitalized infants with bronchiolitis have radiographic evidence of atelectasis, and it may be difficult to distinguish between atelectasis and bacterial infiltrate or consolidation.[169] Bacterial pneumonia in infants with bronchiolitis without consolidation is unusual.[170] Antibiotic therapy may be justified in some children with bronchiolitis who require intubation and mechanical ventilation for respiratory failure.[172,173]

Although acute otitis media (AOM) in infants with bronchiolitis may be attributable to viruses, clinical features generally do not permit differentiation of viral AOM from those with a bacterial component.[174] Two studies address the frequency of AOM in patients with bronchiolitis. Andrade et al[175] prospectively identified AOM in 62% of 42 patients who presented with bronchiolitis. AOM was present in 50% on entry to the study and developed in an additional 12% within 10 days. A subsequent report[176] followed 150 children hospitalized for bronchiolitis for the development of AOM. Seventy-nine (53%) developed AOM, two-thirds within the first 2 days of hospitalization. AOM did not influence the clinical course or laboratory findings of bronchiolitis. The current AAP guideline on AOM[177] recommends that a diagnosis of AOM should include bulging of the tympanic membrane. This is based on bulging being the best indicator for the presence of bacteria in multiple tympanocentesis studies and on 2 articles comparing antibiotic to placebo therapy that used a bulging tympanic membrane as a necessary part of the diagnosis.[178,179] New studies are needed to determine the incidence of AOM in bronchiolitis by using the new criterion of bulging of the tympanic membrane. Refer to the AOM guideline[180] for recommendations regarding the management of AOM.

NUTRITION AND HYDRATION

Key Action Statement 9

Clinicians should administer nasogastric or intravenous fluids for infants with a diagnosis of bronchiolitis who cannot maintain hydration orally (Evidence Quality: X; Recommendation Strength: Strong Recommendation).

Action Statement Profile KAS 9

Aggregate evidence quality	X
Benefits	Maintaining hydration
Risk, harm, cost	Risk of infection, risk of aspiration with nasogastric tube, discomfort, hyponatremia, intravenous infiltration, overhydration
Benefit-harm assessment	Benefits outweigh harms
Value judgments	None
Intentional vagueness	None
Role of patient preferences	Shared decision as to which mode is used
Exclusions	None
Strength	Strong recommendation
Differences of opinion	None

The level of respiratory distress attributable to bronchiolitis guides the indications for fluid replacement. Conversely, food intake in the previous 24 hours may be a predictor of oxygen saturation among infants with bron-

chiolitis. One study found that food intake at less than 50% of normal for the previous 24 hours is associated with a pulse oximetry value of <95%.[180] Infants with mild respiratory distress may require only observation, particularly if feeding remains unaffected. When the respiratory rate exceeds 60 to 70 breaths per minute, feeding may be compromised, particularly if nasal secretions are copious. There is limited evidence to suggest coordination of breathing with swallowing may be impaired among infants with bronchiolitis.[181] These infants may develop increased nasal flaring, retractions, and prolonged expiratory wheezing when fed and may be at increased risk of aspiration.[182]

One study estimated that one-third of infants hospitalized for bronchiolitis require fluid replacement.[183] One case series[184] and 2 randomized trials,[185,186] examined the comparative efficacy and safety of the intravenous and nasogastric routes for fluid replacement. A pilot trial in Israel that included 51 infants younger than 6 months demonstrated no significant differences in the duration of oxygen needed or time to full oral feeds between infants receiving intravenous 5% dextrose in normal saline solution or nasogastric breast milk or formula.[187] Infants in the intravenous group had a shorter LOS (100 vs 120 hours) but it was not statistically

significant. In a larger open randomized trial including infants between 2 and 12 months of age and conducted in Australia and New Zealand, there were no significant differences in rates of admission to ICUs, need for ventilatory support, and adverse events between 381 infants assigned to nasogastric hydration and 378 infants assigned to intravenous hydration.[188] There was a difference of 4 hours in mean LOS between the intravenous group (82.2 hours) and the nasogastric group (86.2 hours) that was not statistically significant. The nasogastric route had a higher success rate of insertion than the intravenous route. Parental satisfaction scores did not differ between the intravenous and nasogastric groups. These studies suggest that infants who have difficulty feeding safely because of respiratory distress can receive either intravenous or nasogastric fluid replacement; however, more evidence is needed to increase the strength of this recommendation.

The possibility of fluid retention related to production of antidiuretic hormone has been raised in patients with bronchiolitis.[187–189] Therefore, receipt of hypotonic fluid replacement and maintenance fluids may increase the risk of iatrogenic hyponatremia in these infants. A recent meta-analysis demonstrated that among hospitalized children requiring maintenance fluids, the use of hypotonic fluids was associated with significant hyponatremia compared with isotonic fluids in older children.[190] Use of isotonic fluids, in general, appears to be safer.

PREVENTION

Key Action Statement 10a

Clinicians should not administer palivizumab to otherwise healthy

infants with a gestational age of 29 weeks, 0 days or greater (Evidence Quality: B; Recommendation Strength: Strong Recommendation).

Action Statement Profile KAS 10a

Aggregate evidence quality	B
Benefits	Reduced pain of injections, reduced use of a medication that has shown minimal benefit, reduced adverse effects, reduced visits to health care provider with less exposure to illness
Risk, harm, cost	Minimal increase in risk of RSV hospitalization
Benefit-harm assessment	Benefits outweigh harms
Value judgments	None
Intentional vagueness	None
Role of patient preferences	Parents may choose to not accept palivizumab
Exclusions	Infants with chronic lung disease of prematurity and hemodynamically significant cardiac disease (as described in KAS 10b)
Strength	Recommendation
Differences of opinion	None
Notes	This KAS is harmonized with the AAP policy statement on palivizumab

Key Action Statement 10b

Clinicians should administer palivizumab during the first year of life to infants with hemodynamically significant heart disease or chronic lung disease of prematurity defined as preterm infants <32 weeks, 0 days' gestation who require >21% oxygen for at least the first 28 days of life (Evidence Quality: B; Recommendation Strength: Moderate Recommendation).

Action Statement Profile KAS 10b

Aggregate evidence quality	B
Benefits	Reduced risk of RSV hospitalization
Risk, harm, cost	Injection pain; increased risk of illness from increased visits to clinician office or clinic; cost; side effects from palivizumab
Benefit-harm assessment	Benefits outweigh harms
Value judgments	None
Intentional vagueness	None
Role of patient preferences	Parents may choose to not accept palivizumab
Exclusions	None
Strength	Moderate recommendation
Differences of opinion	None
Notes	This KAS is harmonized with the AAP policy statement on palivizumab[191,192]

Key Action Statement 10c

Clinicians should administer a maximum 5 monthly doses (15 mg/kg/dose) of palivizumab during the RSV season to infants who qualify for palivizumab in the first year of life (Evidence Quality: B, Recommendation Strength: Moderate Recommendation).

Action Statement Profile KAS 10c

Aggregate evidence quality	B
Benefits	Reduced risk of hospitalization; reduced admission to ICU
Risk, harm, cost	Injection pain; increased risk of illness from increased visits to clinician office or clinic; cost; adverse effects of palivizumab
Benefit-harm assessment	Benefits outweigh harms
Value judgments	None
Intentional vagueness	None
Role of patient preferences	None
Exclusions	Fewer doses should be used if the bronchiolitis season ends before the completion of 5 doses; if the child is hospitalized with a breakthrough RSV, monthly prophylaxis should be discontinued
Strength	Moderate recommendation
Differences of opinion	None
Notes	This KAS is harmonized with the AAP policy statement on palivizumab[191,192]

Detailed evidence to support the policy statement on palivizumab and this palivizumab section can be found in the technical report on palivizumab.[192]

Palivizumab was licensed by the US Food and Drug Administration in June 1998 largely on the basis of results of 1 clinical trial.[193] The results of a second clinical trial among children with congenital heart disease were reported in December 2003.[194] No other prospective, randomized, placebo-controlled trials have been conducted in any subgroup. Since licensure of palivizumab, new peer-reviewed publications provide greater insight into the epidemiology of disease caused by RSV.[195–197] As a result of new data, the Bronchiolitis Guideline Committee and the Committee on Infectious Diseases have updated recommendations for use of prophylaxis.

PREMATURITY

Monthly palivizumab prophylaxis should be restricted to infants born before 29 weeks, 0 days' gestation, except for infants who qualify on the basis of congenital heart disease or chronic lung disease of prematurity. Data show that infants born at or after 29 weeks, 0 days' gestation have an RSV hospitalization rate similar to the rate of full-term infants.[11,198] Infants with a gestational age of 28 weeks, 6 days or less who will be younger than 12 months at the start of the RSV season should receive a maximum of 5 monthly doses of palivizumab or until the end of the RSV season, whichever comes first. Depending on the month of birth, fewer than 5 monthly doses will provide protection for most infants for the duration of the season.

CONGENITAL HEART DISEASE

Despite the large number of subjects enrolled, little benefit from palivizumab prophylaxis was found in the industry-sponsored cardiac study among infants in the cyanotic group (7.9% in control group versus 5.6% in palivizumab group, or 23 fewer hospitalizations per1000 children; P = .285).[197] In the acyanotic group (11.8% vs 5.0%), there were 68 fewer RSV hospitalizations per 1000 prophylaxis recipients (P = .003).[197,199,200]

CHRONIC LUNG DISEASE OF PREMATURITY

Palivizumab prophylaxis should be administered to infants and children younger than 12 months who develop chronic lung disease of prematurity, defined as a requirement for 28 days of more than 21% oxygen beginning at birth. If a child meets these criteria and is in the first 24 months of life and continues to require supplemental oxygen, diuretic therapy, or chronic corticosteroid therapy within 6 months of the start of the RSV season, monthly prophylaxis should be administered for the remainder of the season.

NUMBER OF DOSES

Community outbreaks of RSV disease usually begin in November or December, peak in January or February, and end by late March or, at times, in April.[4] Figure 1 shows the 2011–2012 bronchiolitis season, which is typical of most years. Because 5 monthly doses will provide more than 24 weeks of protective serum palivizumab concentration, administration of more than 5 monthly doses is not recommended within the continental United States. For infants who qualify for 5 monthly doses, initiation of prophylaxis in November and continua-

tion for a total of 5 doses will provide protection into April.[201] If prophylaxis is initiated in October, the fifth and final dose should be administered in February, and protection will last into March for most children.

SECOND YEAR OF LIFE

Because of the low risk of RSV hospitalization in the second year of life, palivizumab prophylaxis is not recommended for children in the second year of life with the following exception. Children who satisfy the definition of chronic lung disease of infancy and continue to require supplemental oxygen, chronic corticosteroid therapy, or diuretic therapy within 6 months of the onset of the second RSV season may be considered for a second season of prophylaxis.

OTHER CONDITIONS

Insufficient data are available to recommend routine use of prophylaxis in children with Down syndrome, cystic fibrosis, pulmonary abnormality, neuromuscular disease, or immune compromise.

Down Syndrome

Routine use of prophylaxis for children in the first year of life with Down syndrome is not recommended unless the child qualifies because of cardiac disease or prematurity.[202]

Cystic Fibrosis

Routine use of palivizumab prophylaxis in patients with cystic fibrosis is not recommended.[203,204] Available studies indicate the incidence of RSV hospitalization in children with cystic fibrosis is low and unlikely to be different from children without cystic fibrosis. No evidence suggests a benefit from palivizumab prophylaxis in patients with cystic fibrosis. A randomized clinical trial involving 186 children with cystic

fibrosis from 40 centers reported 1 subject in each group was hospitalized because of RSV infection. Although this study was not powered for efficacy, no clinically meaningful differences in outcome were reported.[205] A survey of cystic fibrosis center directors published in 2009 noted that palivizumab prophylaxis is not the standard of care for patients with cystic fibrosis.[206] If a neonate is diagnosed with cystic fibrosis by newborn screening, RSV prophylaxis should not be administered if no other indications are present. A patient with cystic fibrosis with clinical evidence of chronic lung disease in the first year of life may be considered for prophylaxis.

Neuromuscular Disease and Pulmonary Abnormality

The risk of RSV hospitalization is not well defined in children with pulmonary abnormalities or neuromuscular disease that impairs ability to clear secretions from the lower airway because of ineffective cough, recurrent gastroesophageal tract reflux, pulmonary malformations, tracheoesophageal fistula, upper airway conditions, or conditions requiring tracheostomy. No data on the relative risk of RSV hospitalization are available for this cohort. Selected infants with disease or congenital anomaly that impairs their ability to clear secretions from the lower airway because of ineffective cough may be considered for prophylaxis during the first year of life.

Immunocompromised Children

Population-based data are not available on the incidence or severity of RSV hospitalization in children who undergo solid organ or hematopoietic stem cell transplantation, receive chemotherapy, or are immunocompromised because of other conditions. Prophylaxis may be considered for hematopoietic stem cell transplant patients who undergo transplantation and are profoundly immunosuppressed during the RSV season.[207]

MISCELLANEOUS ISSUES

Prophylaxis is not recommended for prevention of nosocomial RSV disease in the NICU or hospital setting.[208,209]

No evidence suggests palivizumab is a cost-effective measure to prevent recurrent wheezing in children. Prophylaxis should not be administered to reduce recurrent wheezing in later years.[210,211]

Monthly prophylaxis in Alaska Native children who qualify should be determined by locally generated data regarding season onset and end.

Continuation of monthly prophylaxis for an infant or young child who experiences breakthrough RSV hospitalization is not recommended.

HAND HYGIENE

Key Action Statement 11a

All people should disinfect hands before and after direct contact with patients, after contact with inanimate objects in the direct vicinity of the patient, and after removing gloves (Evidence Quality: B; Recommendation Strength: Strong Recommendation).

Action Statement Profile KAS 11a

Aggregate evidence quality	B
Benefits	Decreased transmission of disease
Risk, harm, cost	Possible hand irritation
Benefit-harm assessment	Benefits outweigh harms
Value judgments	None
Intentional vagueness	None
Role of patient preferences	None
Exclusions	None
Strength	Strong recommendation
Differences of opinion	None

Key Action Statement 11b

All people should use alcohol-based rubs for hand decontamination when caring for children with bronchiolitis. When alcohol-based rubs are not available, individuals should wash their hands with soap and water (Evidence Quality: B; Recommendation Strength: Strong Recommendation).

Action Statement Profile KAS 11b

Aggregate evidence quality	B
Benefits	Less hand irritation
Risk, harm, cost	If there is visible dirt on the hands, hand washing is necessary; alcohol-based rubs are not effective for *Clostridium difficile*, present a fire hazard, and have a slight increased cost
Benefit-harm assessment	Benefits outweigh harms
Value judgments	None
Intentional vagueness	None
Role of patient preferences	None
Exclusions	None
Strength	Strong recommendation
Differences of opinion	None

Efforts should be made to decrease the spread of RSV and other causative agents of bronchiolitis in medical settings, especially in the hospital. Secretions from infected patients can be found on beds, crib railings, tabletops, and toys.[12] RSV, as well as many other viruses, can survive better on hard surfaces than on porous surfaces or hands. It can remain infectious on counter tops for ≥6 hours, on gowns or paper tissues for 20 to 30 minutes, and on skin for up to 20 minutes.[212]

It has been shown that RSV can be carried and spread to others on the hands of caregivers.[213] Studies have shown that health care workers have acquired infection by performing activities such as feeding, diaper change, and playing with the RSV-infected infant. Caregivers who had contact only with surfaces contaminated with the infants' secretions or touched inanimate objects in patients' rooms also acquired RSV. In these studies, health care workers contaminated their hands (or gloves) with RSV and inoculated their oral or conjunctival mucosa.[214] Frequent hand washing by health care workers has been shown to reduce the spread of RSV in the health care setting.[215]

The Centers for Disease Control and Prevention published an extensive review of the hand-hygiene literature and made recommendations as to indications for hand washing and hand antisepsis.[216] Among the recommendations are that hands should be disinfected before and after direct contact with every patient, after contact with inanimate objects in the direct vicinity of the patient, and before putting on and after removing gloves. If hands are not visibly soiled, an alcohol-based rub is preferred. In guidelines published in 2009, the World Health Organization also recommended alcohol-based hand-rubs as the standard for hand hygiene in health care.[217] Specifically, systematic reviews show them to remove organisms more effectively, require less time, and irritate skin less often than hand washing with soap or other antiseptic agents and water. The availability of bedside alcohol-based solutions increased compliance with hand hygiene among health care workers.[214]

When caring for hospitalized children with clinically diagnosed bronchiolitis, strict adherence to hand decontamination and use of personal protective equipment (ie, gloves and gowns) can reduce the risk of cross-infection in the health care setting.[215]

Other methods of infection control in viral bronchiolitis include education of personnel and family members, surveillance for the onset of RSV season, and wearing masks when anticipating exposure to aerosolized secretions while performing patient care activities. Programs that implement the aforementioned principles, in conjunction with effective hand decontamination and cohorting of patients, have been shown to reduce the spread of RSV in the health care setting by 39% to 50%.[218,219]

TOBACCO SMOKE

Key Action Statement 12a

Clinicians should inquire about the exposure of the infant or child to tobacco smoke when assessing infants and children for bronchiolitis (Evidence Quality: C; Recommendation Strength: Moderate Recommendation).

Action Statement Profile KAS 12a

Aggregate evidence quality	C
Benefits	Can identify infants and children at risk whose family may benefit from counseling, predicting risk of severe disease
Risk, harm, cost	Time to inquire
Benefit-harm assessment	Benefits outweigh harms
Value judgments	None
Intentional vagueness	None
Role of patient preferences	Parent may choose to deny tobacco use even though they are, in fact, users
Exclusions	None
Strength	Moderate recommendation
Differences of opinion	None

Key Action Statement 12b

Clinicians should counsel caregivers about exposing the infant or child to environmental tobacco smoke and smoking cessation when assessing a child for bronchiolitis (Evidence Quality: B; Recommendation Strength: Strong Recommendation).

Action Statement Profile KAS 12b

Aggregate evidence quality	B
Benefits	Reinforces the detrimental effects of smoking, potential to decrease smoking
Risk, harm, cost	Time to counsel
Benefit-harm assessment	Benefits outweigh harms
Value judgments	None
Intentional vagueness	None
Role of patient preferences	Parents may choose to ignore counseling
Exclusions	None
Strength	Moderate recommendation
Differences of opinion	None
Notes	Counseling for tobacco smoke prevention should begin in the prenatal period and continue in family-centered care and at all well-infant visits

Tobacco smoke exposure increases the risk and severity of bronchiolitis. Strachan and Cook[220] first delineated the effects of environmental tobacco smoke on rates of lower respiratory tract disease in infants in a meta-analysis including 40 studies. In a more recent systematic review, Jones et al[221] found a pooled odds ratio of 2.51 (95% CI 1.96 to 3.21) for tobacco smoke exposure and bronchiolitis hospitalization among the 7 studies specific to the condition. Other investigators have consistently reported tobacco smoke exposure increases both severity of illness and risk of hospitalization for bronchioli-

tis.[222–225] The AAP issued a technical report on the risks of secondhand smoke in 2009. The report makes recommendations regarding effective ways to eliminate or reduce secondhand smoke exposure, including education of parents.[226]

Despite our knowledge of this important risk factor, there is evidence to suggest health care providers identify fewer than half of children exposed to tobacco smoke in the outpatient, inpatient, or ED settings.[227–229] Furthermore, there is evidence that counseling parents in these settings is well received and has a measurable impact. Rosen et al[230] performed a meta-analysis of the effects of interventions in pediatric settings on parental cessation and found a pooled risk ratio of 1.3 for cessation among the 18 studies reviewed.

In contrast to many of the other recommendations, protecting children from tobacco exposure is a recommendation that is primarily implemented outside of the clinical setting. As such, it is critical that parents are fully educated about the importance of not allowing smoking in the home and that smoke lingers on clothes and in the environment for prolonged periods.[231] It should be provided in plain language and in a respectful, culturally effective manner that is family centered, engages parents as partners in their child's health, and factors in their literacy, health literacy, and primary language needs.

BREASTFEEDING

Key Action Statement 13

Clinicians should encourage exclusive breastfeeding for at least 6 months to decrease the morbidity of respiratory infections (Evidence Quality: Grade B; Recommendation Strength: Moderate Recommendation).

Action Statement Profile KAS 13

Aggregate evidence quality	B
Benefits	May reduce the risk of bronchiolitis and other illnesses; multiple benefits of breastfeeding unrelated to bronchiolitis
Risk, harm, cost	None
Benefit-harm assessment	Benefits outweigh risks
Value judgments	None
Intentional vagueness	None
Role of patient preferences	Parents may choose to feed formula rather than breastfeed
Exclusions	None
Strength	Moderate recommendation
Notes	Education on breastfeeding should begin in the prenatal period

In 2012, the AAP presented a general policy on breastfeeding.[232] The policy statement was based on the proven benefits of breastfeeding for at least 6 months. Respiratory infections were shown to be significantly less common in breastfed children. A primary resource was a meta-analysis from the Agency for Healthcare Research and Quality that showed an overall 72% reduction in the risk of hospitalization secondary to respiratory diseases in infants who were exclusively breastfed for 4 or more months compared with those who were formula fed.[233]

The clinical evidence also supports decreased incidence and severity of illness in breastfed infants with bronchiolitis. Dornelles et al[234] concluded that the duration of exclusive breastfeeding was inversely related to the length of oxygen use and the length of hospital stay in previously healthy infants with acute bronchiolitis. In a large prospective study in Australia, Oddy et al[235] showed that breastfeeding for less than 6 months was associated with an increased risk for 2 or more medical visits and hospital admission for wheezing lower respiratory illness. In Japan, Nishimura et al[236] looked at 3 groups of RSV-positive infants defined as full, partial, or token breastfeeding. There were no significant differences in the hospitalization rate among the 3 groups; however, there were significant differences in the duration of hospitalization and the rate of requiring oxygen therapy, both favoring breastfeeding.

FAMILY EDUCATION

Key Action Statement 14

Clinicians and nurses should educate personnel and family members on evidence-based diagnosis, treatment, and prevention in bronchiolitis (Evidence Quality: C; observational studies; Recommendation Strength; Moderate Recommendation).

Action Statement Profile KAS 14

Aggregate evidence quality	C
Benefits	Decreased transmission of disease, benefits of breastfeeding, promotion of judicious use of antibiotics, risks of infant lung damage attributable to tobacco smoke
Risk, harm, cost	Time to educate properly
Benefit-harm assessment	Benefits outweigh harms
Value judgments	None
Intentional vagueness	Personnel is not specifically defined but should include all people who enter a patient's room
Role of patient preferences	None
Exclusions	None
Strength	Moderate recommendation
Differences of opinion	None

Shared decision-making with parents about diagnosis and treatment of bronchiolitis is a key tenet of patient-centered care. Despite the absence of effective therapies for viral bronchiolitis, caregiver education by clinicians may have a significant impact on care patterns in the disease. Children with bronchiolitis typically suffer from symptoms for 2 to 3 weeks, and parents often seek care in multiple settings during that time period.[237] Given that children with RSV generally shed virus for 1 to 2 weeks and from 30% to 70% of family members may become ill,[238,239] education about prevention of transmission of disease is key. Restriction of visitors to newborns during the respiratory virus season should be considered. Consistent evidence suggests that parental education is helpful in the promotion of judicious use of antibiotics and that clinicians may misinterpret parental expectations about therapy unless the subject is openly discussed.[240–242]

FUTURE RESEARCH NEEDS

- Better algorithms for predicting the course of illness
- Impact of clinical score on patient outcomes
- Evaluating different ethnic groups and varying response to treatments
- Does epinephrine alone reduce admission in outpatient settings?
- Additional studies on epinephrine in combination with dexamethasone or other corticosteroids
- Hypertonic saline studies in the outpatient setting and in in hospitals with shorter LOS
- More studies on nasogastric hydration
- More studies on tonicity of intravenous fluids

- Incidence of true AOM in bronchiolitis by using 2013 guideline definition
- More studies on deep suctioning and nasopharyngeal suctioning
- Strategies for monitoring oxygen saturation
- Use of home oxygen
- Appropriate cutoff for use of oxygen in high altitude
- Oxygen delivered by high-flow nasal cannula
- RSV vaccine and antiviral agents
- Use of palivizumab in special populations, such as cystic fibrosis, neuromuscular diseases, Down syndrome, immune deficiency
- Emphasis on parent satisfaction/patient-centered outcomes in all research (ie, not LOS as the only measure)

SUBCOMMITTEE ON BRONCHIOLITIS (OVERSIGHT BY THE COUNCIL ON QUALITY IMPROVEMENT AND PATIENT SAFETY, 2013–2014)

Shawn L. Ralston, MD, FAAP: Chair, Pediatric Hospitalist (no financial conflicts; published research related to bronchiolitis)

Allan S. Lieberthal, MD, FAAP: Chair, General Pediatrician with Expertise in Pulmonology (no conflicts)

Brian K. Alverson, MD, FAAP: Pediatric Hospitalist, AAP Section on Hospital Medicine Representative (no conflicts)

Jill E. Baley, MD, FAAP: Neonatal-Perinatal Medicine, AAP Committee on Fetus and Newborn Representative (no conflicts)

Anne M. Gadomski, MD, MPH, FAAP: General Pediatrician and Research Scientist (no financial conflicts; published research related to bronchiolitis including Cochrane review of bronchodilators)

David W. Johnson, MD, FAAP: Pediatric Emergency Medicine Physician (no financial conflicts; published research related to bronchiolitis)

Michael J. Light, MD, FAAP: Pediatric Pulmonologist, AAP Section on Pediatric Pulmonology Representative (no conflicts)

Nizar F. Maraqa, MD, FAAP: Pediatric Infectious Disease Physician, AAP Section on Infectious Diseases Representative (no conflicts)

H. Cody Meissner, MD, FAAP: Pediatric Infectious Disease Physician, AAP Committee on Infectious Diseases Representative (no conflicts)

Eneida A. Mendonca, MD, PhD, FAAP, FACMI: Informatician/Academic Pediatric Intensive Care Physician, Partnership for Policy Implementation Representative (no conflicts)

Kieran J. Phelan, MD, MSc: General Pediatrician (no conflicts)

Joseph J. Zorc, MD, MSCE, FAAP: Pediatric Emergency Physician, AAP Section on Emergency Medicine Representative (no financial conflicts; published research related to bronchiolitis)

Danette Stanko-Lopp, MA, MPH: Methodologist, Epidemiologist (no conflicts)

Mark A. Brown, MD: Pediatric Pulmonologist, American Thoracic Society Liaison (no conflicts)

Ian Nathanson, MD, FAAP: Pediatric Pulmonologist, American College of Chest Physicians Liaison (no conflicts)

Elizabeth Rosenblum, MD: Academic Family Physician, American Academy of Family Physicians liaison (no conflicts).

Stephen Sayles, III, MD, FACEP: Emergency Medicine Physician, American College of Emergency Physicians Liaison (no conflicts)

Sinsi Hernández-Cancio, JD: Parent/Consumer Representative (no conflicts)

STAFF

Caryn Davidson, MA
Linda Walsh, MAB

REFERENCES

1. American Academy of Pediatrics Subcommittee on Diagnosis and Management of Bronchiolitis. Diagnosis and management of bronchiolitis. *Pediatrics.* 2006;118 (4):1774–1793

2. Agency for Healthcare Research and Quality. Management of Bronchiolitis in Infants and Children. Evidence Report/Technology Assessment No. 69. Rockville, MD: Agency for Healthcare Research and Quality; 2003. AHRQ Publication No. 03-E014

3. Mullins JA, Lamonte AC, Bresee JS, Anderson LJ. Substantial variability in community respiratory syncytial virus season timing. *Pediatr Infect Dis J.* 2003; 22(10):857–862

4. Centers for Disease Control and Prevention. Respiratory syncytial virus activity—United States, July 2011-January 2013. *MMWR Morb Mortal Wkly Rep.* 2013; 62(8):141–144

5. Greenough A, Cox S, Alexander J, et al. Health care utilisation of infants with chronic lung disease, related to hospitalisation for RSV infection. *Arch Dis Child.* 2001;85(6):463–468

6. Parrott RH, Kim HW, Arrobio JO, et al. Epidemiology of respiratory syncytial virus infection in Washington, D.C. II. Infection and disease with respect to age, immunologic status, race and sex. *Am J Epidemiol.* 1973;98(4):289–300

7. Meissner HC. Selected populations at increased risk from respiratory syncytial virus infection. *Pediatr Infect Dis J.* 2003; 22(suppl 2):S40–S44, discussion S44–S45

8. Shay DK, Holman RC, Roosevelt GE, Clarke MJ, Anderson LJ. Bronchiolitis-associated mortality and estimates of respiratory syncytial virus-associated deaths among US children, 1979-1997. *J Infect Dis.* 2001; 183(1):16–22

9. Miller EK, Gebretsadik T, Carroll KN, et al. Viral etiologies of infant bronchiolitis, croup and upper respiratory illness during 4 consecutive years. *Pediatr Infect Dis J.* 2013;32(9):950–955

10. Hasegawa K, Tsugawa Y, Brown DF, Mansbach JM, Camargo CA Jr. Trends in bronchiolitis hospitalizations in the United States, 2000-2009. *Pediatrics.* 2013;132(1): 28–36

11. Hall CB, Weinberg GA, Blumkin AK, et al. Respiratory syncytial virus-associated hospitalizations among children less than 24 months of age. *Pediatrics.* 2013; 132(2). Available at: www.pediatrics.org/cgi/content/full/132/2/e341

12. Hall CB. Nosocomial respiratory syncytial virus infections: the "Cold War" has not ended. *Clin Infect Dis.* 2000;31(2): 590–596

13. Stevens TP, Sinkin RA, Hall CB, Maniscalco WM, McConnochie KM. Respiratory syncytial virus and premature infants born at 32 weeks' gestation or earlier: hospitalization and economic implications of prophylaxis. *Arch Pediatr Adolesc Med.* 2000; 154(1):55–61

14. American Academy of Pediatrics Steering Committee on Quality Improvement and Management. Classifying recommendations for clinical practice guidelines. *Pediatrics.* 2004;114(3):874–877

15. Ricart S, Marcos MA, Sarda M, et al. Clinical risk factors are more relevant than respiratory viruses in predicting bronchiolitis severity. *Pediatr Pulmonol.* 2013;48(5):456–463

16. Shaw KN, Bell LM, Sherman NH. Outpatient assessment of infants with bronchiolitis. *Am J Dis Child.* 1991;145(2):151–155

17. Hall CB, Powell KR, MacDonald NE, et al. Respiratory syncytial viral infection in children with compromised immune function. *N Engl J Med.* 1986;315(2):77–81

18. Mansbach JM, Piedra PA, Stevenson MD, et al; MARC-30 Investigators. Prospective multicenter study of children with bronchiolitis requiring mechanical ventilation. *Pediatrics.* 2012;130(3). Available at: www.pediatrics.org/cgi/content/full/130/3/e492

19. Prescott WA Jr, Hutchinson DJ. Respiratory syncytial virus prophylaxis in special populations: is it something worth considering in cystic fibrosis and immunosuppression? *J Pediatr Pharmacol Ther.* 2011;16(2):77–86

20. Armstrong D, Grimwood K, Carlin JB, et al. Severe viral respiratory infections in infants with cystic fibrosis. *Pediatr Pulmonol.* 1998;26(6):371–379

21. Alvarez AE, Marson FA, Bertuzzo CS, Arns CW, Ribeiro JD. Epidemiological and genetic characteristics associated with the severity of acute viral bronchiolitis by respiratory syncytial virus. *J Pediatr (Rio J).* 2013;89(6):531–543

22. Iliff A, Lee VA. Pulse rate, respiratory rate, and body temperature of children between two months and eighteen years of age. *Child Dev.* 1952;23(4):237–245

23. Rogers MC. Respiratory monitoring. In: Rogers MC, Nichols DG, eds. *Textbook of Pediatric Intensive Care.* Baltimore, MD: Williams & Wilkins; 1996:332–333

24. Berman S, Simoes EA, Lanata C. Respiratory rate and pneumonia in infancy. *Arch Dis Child.* 1991;66(1):81–84

25. Fleming S, Thompson M, Stevens R, et al. Normal ranges of heart rate and respiratory rate in children from birth to 18 years of age: a systematic review of observational studies. *Lancet.* 2011;377(9770):1011–1018

26. Bonafide CP, Brady PW, Keren R, Conway PH, Marsolo K, Daymont C. Development of heart and respiratory rate percentile curves for hospitalized children. *Pediatrics.* 2013;131(4). Available at: www.pediatrics.org/cgi/content/full/131/4/e1150

27. Margolis P, Gadomski A. The rational clinical examination. Does this infant have pneumonia? *JAMA.* 1998;279(4):308–313

28. Mahabee-Gittens EM, Grupp-Phelan J, Brody AS, et al. Identifying children with pneumonia in the emergency department. *Clin Pediatr (Phila).* 2005;44(5):427–435

29. Brooks AM, McBride JT, McConnochie KM, Aviram M, Long C, Hall CB. Predicting deterioration in previously healthy infants hospitalized with respiratory syncytial virus infection. *Pediatrics.* 1999;104(3 pt 1):463–467

30. Neuman MI, Monuteaux MC, Scully KJ, Bachur RG. Prediction of pneumonia in a pediatric emergency department. *Pediatrics.* 2011;128(2):246–253

31. Shah S, Bachur R, Kim D, Neuman MI. Lack of predictive value of tachypnea in the diagnosis of pneumonia in children. *Pediatr Infect Dis J.* 2010;29(5):406–409

32. Mansbach JM, McAdam AJ, Clark S, et al. Prospective multicenter study of the viral etiology of bronchiolitis in the emergency department. *Acad Emerg Med.* 2008;15(2):111–118

33. Mansbach JM, Piedra PA, Teach SJ, et al; MARC-30 Investigators. Prospective multicenter study of viral etiology and hospital length of stay in children with severe bronchiolitis. *Arch Pediatr Adolesc Med.* 2012;166(8):700–706

34. Navas L, Wang E, de Carvalho V, Robinson J; Pediatric Investigators Collaborative Network on Infections in Canada. Improved outcome of respiratory syncytial virus infection in a high-risk hospitalized population of Canadian children. *J Pediatr.* 1992;121(3):348–354

35. Wang EE, Law BJ, Stephens D. Pediatric Investigators Collaborative Network on Infections in Canada (PICNIC) prospective study of risk factors and outcomes in patients hospitalized with respiratory syncytial viral lower respiratory tract infection. *J Pediatr.* 1995;126(2):212–219

36. Chan PW, Lok FY, Khatijah SB. Risk factors for hypoxemia and respiratory failure in respiratory syncytial virus bronchiolitis. *Southeast Asian J Trop Med Public Health.* 2002;33(4):806–810

37. Roback MG, Baskin MN. Failure of oxygen saturation and clinical assessment to predict which patients with bronchiolitis discharged from the emergency department will return requiring admission. *Pediatr Emerg Care.* 1997;13(1):9–11

38. Lowell DI, Lister G, Von Koss H, McCarthy P. Wheezing in infants: the response to epinephrine. *Pediatrics.* 1987;79(6):939–945

39. Destino L, Weisgerber MC, Soung P, et al. Validity of respiratory scores in bronchiolitis. *Hosp Pediatr.* 2012;2(4):202–209

40. Schroeder AR, Marmor AK, Pantell RH, Newman TB. Impact of pulse oximetry and oxygen therapy on length of stay in bronchiolitis hospitalizations. *Arch Pediatr Adolesc Med.* 2004;158(6):527–530

41. Dawson KP, Long A, Kennedy J, Mogridge N. The chest radiograph in acute bronchiolitis. *J Paediatr Child Health.* 1990;26(4):209–211

42. Schroeder AR, Mansbach JM, Stevenson M, et al. Apnea in children hospitalized with bronchiolitis. *Pediatrics.* 2013;132(5). Available at: www.pediatrics.org/cgi/content/full/132/5/e1194

43. Ralston S, Hill V. Incidence of apnea in infants hospitalized with respiratory syncytial virus bronchiolitis: a systematic review. *J Pediatr.* 2009;155(5):728–733

44. Willwerth BM, Harper MB, Greenes DS. Identifying hospitalized infants who have bronchiolitis and are at high risk for apnea. *Ann Emerg Med.* 2006;48(4):441–447

45. García CG, Bhore R, Soriano-Fallas A, et al. Risk factors in children hospitalized with RSV bronchiolitis versus non-RSV bronchiolitis. *Pediatrics.* 2010;126(6). Available at: www.pediatrics.org/cgi/content/full/126/6/e1453

46. Swingler GH, Hussey GD, Zwarenstein M. Randomised controlled trial of clinical outcome after chest radiograph in ambulatory acute lower-respiratory infection in children. *Lancet.* 1998;351(9100):404–408

47. Schuh S, Lalani A, Allen U, et al. Evaluation of the utility of radiography in acute bronchiolitis. *J Pediatr.* 2007;150(4):429–433

48. Kellner JD, Ohlsson A, Gadomski AM, Wang EE. Efficacy of bronchodilator therapy in bronchiolitis. A meta-analysis. *Arch Pediatr Adolesc Med.* 1996;150(11):1166–1172

49. Flores G, Horwitz RI. Efficacy of beta2-agonists in bronchiolitis: a reappraisal and meta-analysis. *Pediatrics.* 1997;100(2 pt 1):233–239

50. Hartling L, Wiebe N, Russell K, Patel H, Klassen TP. A meta-analysis of randomized controlled trials evaluating the efficacy of epinephrine for the treatment of acute viral bronchiolitis. *Arch Pediatr Adolesc Med.* 2003;157(10):957–964

51. King VJ, Viswanathan M, Bordley WC, et al. Pharmacologic treatment of bronchiolitis in infants and children: a systematic review. *Arch Pediatr Adolesc Med.* 2004;158(2):127–137

52. Zorc JJ, Hall CB. Bronchiolitis: recent evidence on diagnosis and management. *Pediatrics.* 2010;125(2):342–349

53. Wainwright C. Acute viral bronchiolitis in children—a very common condition with few therapeutic options. *Paediatr Respir Rev.* 2010;11(1):39–45, quiz 45

54. Walsh P, Caldwell J, McQuillan KK, Friese S, Robbins D, Rothenberg SJ. Comparison of nebulized epinephrine to albuterol in bronchiolitis. *Acad Emerg Med.* 2008;15(4):305–313

55. Scarlett EE, Walker S, Rovitelli A, Ren CL. Tidal breathing responses to albuterol and normal saline in infants with viral bronchiolitis. *Pediatr Allergy Immunol Pulmonol.* 2012;25(4):220–225

56. Gadomski AM, Scribani MB. Bronchodilators for bronchiolitis. *Cochrane Database Syst Rev.* 2014;(6):CD001266

57. Mallol J, Barrueto L, Girardi G, et al. Use of nebulized bronchodilators in infants under 1 year of age: analysis of four forms of therapy. *Pediatr Pulmonol.* 1987;3(5):298–303

58. Lines DR, Kattampallil JS, Liston P. Efficacy of nebulized salbutamol in bronchiolitis. *Pediatr Rev Commun.* 1990;5(2):121–129

59. Alario AJ, Lewander WJ, Dennehy P, Seifer R, Mansell AL. The efficacy of nebulized metaproterenol in wheezing infants and young children. *Am J Dis Child.* 1992;146(4):412–418

60. Chavasse RJPG, Seddon P, Bara A, McKean MC. Short acting beta2-agonists for recurrent wheeze in children under two years of age. *Cochrane Database Syst Rev.* 2009;(2):CD002873

61. Totapally BR, Demerci C, Zureikat G, Nolan B. Tidal breathing flow-volume loops in bronchiolitis in infancy: the effect of albuterol [ISRCTN47364493]. *Crit Care.* 2002;6(2):160–165

62. Levin DL, Garg A, Hall LJ, Slogic S, Jarvis JD, Leiter JC. A prospective randomized controlled blinded study of three bronchodilators in infants with respiratory syncytial virus bronchiolitis on mechanical ventilation. *Pediatr Crit Care Med.* 2008;9(6):598–604

63. Bjornson C, Russell K, Vandermeer B, Klassen TP, Johnson DW. Nebulized epinephrine for croup in children. *Cochrane Database Syst Rev.* 2013;(10):CD006619

64. Hartling L, Fernandes RM, Bialy L, et al. Steroids and bronchodilators for acute bronchiolitis in the first two years of life: systematic review and meta-analysis. *BMJ.* 2011;342:d1714

65. Wainwright C, Altamirano L, Cheney M, et al. A multicenter, randomized, double-blind, controlled trial of nebulized epinephrine in infants with acute bronchiolitis. *N Engl J Med.* 2003;349(1):27–35

66. Patel H, Gouin S, Platt RW. Randomized, double-blind, placebo-controlled trial of oral albuterol in infants with mild-to-moderate acute viral bronchiolitis. *J Pediatr.* 2003;142(5):509–514

67. Skjerven HO, Hunderi JO, Brügmann-Pieper SK, et al. Racemic adrenaline and inhalation strategies in acute bronchiolitis. *N Engl J Med.* 2013;368(24):2286–2293

68. Plint AC, Johnson DW, Patel H, et al; Pediatric Emergency Research Canada (PERC). Epinephrine and dexamethasone in children with bronchiolitis. *N Engl J Med.* 2009;360(20):2079–2089

69. Wark PA, McDonald V, Jones AP. Nebulised hypertonic saline for cystic fibrosis. *Cochrane Database Syst Rev.* 2005;(3):CD001506

70. Daviskas E, Anderson SD, Gonda I, et al. Inhalation of hypertonic saline aerosol enhances mucociliary clearance in asthmatic and healthy subjects. *Eur Respir J.* 1996;9(4):725–732

71. Sood N, Bennett WD, Zeman K, et al. Increasing concentration of inhaled saline with or without amiloride: effect on mucociliary clearance in normal subjects. *Am J Respir Crit Care Med.* 2003;167(2):158–163

72. Mandelberg A, Amirav I. Hypertonic saline or high volume normal saline for viral bronchiolitis: mechanisms and rationale. *Pediatr Pulmonol.* 2010;45(1):36–40

73. Zhang L, Mendoza-Sassi RA, Wainwright C, Klassen TP. Nebulized hypertonic saline solution for acute bronchiolitis in infants. *Cochrane Database Syst Rev.* 2008;(4):CD006458

74. Jacobs JD, Foster M, Wan J, Pershad J. 7% Hypertonic saline in acute bronchiolitis: a randomized controlled trial. *Pediatrics.* 2014;133(1). Available at: www.pediatrics.org/cgi/content/full/133/1/e8

75. Wu S, Baker C, Lang ME, et al. Nebulized hypertonic saline for bronchiolitis: a randomized clinical trial. *JAMA Pediatr.* 2014;168(7):657–663

76. Florin TA, Shaw KN, Kittick M, Yakscoe S, Zorc JJ. Nebulized hypertonic saline for bronchiolitis in the emergency department: a randomized clinical trial. *JAMA Pediatr.* 2014;168(7):664–670

77. Sharma BS, Gupta MK, Rafik SP. Hypertonic (3%) saline vs 0.93% saline nebulization for acute viral bronchiolitis: a randomized controlled trial. *Indian Pediatr.* 2013;50(8):743–747

78. Silver AH. Randomized controlled trial of the efficacy of nebulized 3% saline without bronchodilators for infants admitted with bronchiolitis: preliminary data [abstr E-PAS2014:2952.685]. Paper presented at: Pediatric Academic Societies Annual Meeting; May 3–6, 2014; Vancouver, British Columbia, Canada

79. Ralston S, Hill V, Martinez M. Nebulized hypertonic saline without adjunctive bronchodilators for children with bronchiolitis. *Pediatrics.* 2010;126(3). Available at: www.pediatrics.org/cgi/content/full/126/3/e520

80. Luo Z, Liu E, Luo J, et al. Nebulized hypertonic saline/salbutamol solution treatment in hospitalized children with mild to moderate bronchiolitis. *Pediatr Int.* 2010;52(2):199–202

81. Sarrell EM, Tal G, Witzling M, et al. Nebulized 3% hypertonic saline solution treatment in ambulatory children with viral bronchiolitis decreases symptoms. *Chest.* 2002;122(6):2015–2020

82. Rowe BH, Spooner C, Ducharme FM, Bretzlaff JA, Bota GW. Early emergency department treatment of acute asthma with systemic corticosteroids. *Cochrane Database Syst Rev.* 2001;(1):CD002178

83. Smith M, Iqbal S, Elliott TM, Everard M, Rowe BH. Corticosteroids for hospitalised children with acute asthma. *Cochrane Database Syst Rev.* 2003;(2):CD002886

84. Russell KF, Liang Y, O'Gorman K, Johnson DW, Klassen TP. Glucocorticoids for croup. *Cochrane Database Syst Rev.* 2011;(1):CD001955

85. Fernandes RM, Bialy LM, Vandermeer B, et al. Glucocorticoids for acute viral bronchiolitis in infants and young children. *Cochrane Database Syst Rev.* 2013;(6):CD004878

86. Corneli HM, Zorc JJ, Mahajan P, et al; Bronchiolitis Study Group of the Pediatric Emergency Care Applied Research Network (PECARN). A multicenter, randomized, controlled trial of dexamethasone for bronchiolitis [published correction appears in *N Engl J Med* 2008;359(18):1972]. *N Engl J Med.* 2007;357(4):331–339

87. Frey U, von Mutius E. The challenge of managing wheezing in infants. *N Engl J Med.* 2009;360(20):2130–2133

88. Gibson PG, Powell H, Ducharme F. Long-acting beta2-agonists as an inhaled corticosteroid-sparing agent for chronic asthma in adults and children. *Cochrane Database Syst Rev.* 2005;(4):CD005076

89. Barnes PJ. Scientific rationale for using a single inhaler for asthma control. *Eur Respir J.* 2007;29(3):587–595

90. Giembycz MA, Kaur M, Leigh R, Newton R. A Holy Grail of asthma management: toward understanding how long-acting beta(2)-adrenoceptor agonists enhance the clinical efficacy of inhaled corticosteroids. *Br J Pharmacol.* 2008;153(6):1090–1104

91. Kaur M, Chivers JE, Giembycz MA, Newton R. Long-acting beta2-adrenoceptor agonists synergistically enhance glucocorticoid-dependent transcription in human airway

epithelial and smooth muscle cells. *Mol Pharmacol.* 2008;73(1):203–214

92. Holden NS, Bell MJ, Rider CF, et al. β2-Adrenoceptor agonist-induced RGS2 expression is a genomic mechanism of bronchoprotection that is enhanced by glucocorticoids. *Proc Natl Acad Sci U S A.* 2011;108(49):19713–19718

93. Schuh S, Coates AL, Binnie R, et al. Efficacy of oral dexamethasone in outpatients with acute bronchiolitis. *J Pediatr.* 2002;140(1):27–32

94. Bentur L, Shoseyov D, Feigenbaum D, Gorichovsky Y, Bibi H. Dexamethasone inhalations in RSV bronchiolitis: a double-blind, placebo-controlled study. *Acta Paediatr.* 2005;94(7):866–871

95. Kuyucu S, Unal S, Kuyucu N, Yilgor E. Additive effects of dexamethasone in nebulized salbutamol or L-epinephrine treated infants with acute bronchiolitis. *Pediatr Int.* 2004;46(5):539–544

96. Mesquita M, Castro-Rodríguez JA, Heinichen L, Fariña E, Iramain R. Single oral dose of dexamethasone in outpatients with bronchiolitis: a placebo controlled trial. *Allergol Immunopathol (Madr).* 2009;37(2):63–67

97. Alansari K, Sakran M, Davidson BL, Ibrahim K, Alrefai M, Zakaria I. Oral dexamethasone for bronchiolitis: a randomized trial. *Pediatrics.* 2013;132(4). Available at: www.pediatrics.org/cgi/content/full/132/4/e810

98. Mallory MD, Shay DK, Garrett J, Bordley WC. Bronchiolitis management preferences and the influence of pulse oximetry and respiratory rate on the decision to admit. *Pediatrics.* 2003;111(1). Available at: www.pediatrics.org/cgi/content/full/111/1/e45

99. Corneli HM, Zorc JJ, Holubkov R, et al; Bronchiolitis Study Group for the Pediatric Emergency Care Applied Research Network. Bronchiolitis: clinical characteristics associated with hospitalization and length of stay. *Pediatr Emerg Care.* 2012;28(2):99–103

100. Unger S, Cunningham S. Effect of oxygen supplementation on length of stay for infants hospitalized with acute viral bronchiolitis. *Pediatrics.* 2008;121(3):470–475

101. Cunningham S, McMurray A. Observational study of two oxygen saturation targets for discharge in bronchiolitis. *Arch Dis Child.* 2012;97(4):361–363

102. Anaesthesia UK. Oxygen dissociation curve. Available at: http://www.anaesthesiauk.com/SearchRender.aspx?DocId=1419&Index=D%3a\dtSearch\UserData\AUK&HitCount=19&hits=4+5+d+e+23+24+37+58+59+a7+a8+14a+14b+17e+180+181+1a9+1aa+1d4 Accessed July 15, 2014

103. McBride SC, Chiang VW, Goldmann DA, Landrigan CP. Preventable adverse events in infants hospitalized with bronchiolitis. *Pediatrics.* 2005;116(3):603–608

104. Hunt CE, Corwin MJ, Lister G, et al; Collaborative Home Infant Monitoring Evaluation (CHIME) Study Group. Longitudinal assessment of hemoglobin oxygen saturation in healthy infants during the first 6 months of age. *J Pediatr.* 1999;135(5):580–586

105. Gavlak JC, Stocks J, Laverty A, et al. The Young Everest Study: preliminary report of changes in sleep and cerebral blood flow velocity during slow ascent to altitude in unacclimatised children. *Arch Dis Child.* 2013;98(5):356–362

106. O'Neil SL, Barysh N, Setear SJ. Determining school programming needs of special population groups: a study of asthmatic children. *J Sch Health.* 1985;55(6):237–239

107. Bender BG, Belleau L, Fukuhara JT, Mrazek DA, Strunk RC. Psychomotor adaptation in children with severe chronic asthma. *Pediatrics.* 1987;79(5):723–727

108. Rietveld S, Colland VT. The impact of severe asthma on schoolchildren. *J Asthma.* 1999;36(5):409–417

109. Sung V, Massie J, Hochmann MA, Carlin JB, Jamsen K, Robertson CF. Estimating inspired oxygen concentration delivered by nasal prongs in children with bronchiolitis. *J Paediatr Child Health.* 2008;44(1-2):14–18

110. Ross PA, Newth CJL, Khemani RG. Accuracy of pulse oximetry in children. *Pediatrics.* 2014;133(1):22–29

111. Hasselbalch KA. Neutralitatsregulation und reizbarkeit des atemzentrums in ihren Wirkungen auf die koklensaurespannung des Blutes. *Biochem Ztschr.* 1912;46:403–439

112. Wang EE, Milner RA, Navas L, Maj H. Observer agreement for respiratory signs and oximetry in infants hospitalized with lower respiratory infections. *Am Rev Respir Dis.* 1992;145(1):106–109

113. Rojas MX, Granados Rugeles C, Charry-Anzola LP. Oxygen therapy for lower respiratory tract infections in children between 3 months and 15 years of age. *Cochrane Database Syst Rev.* 2009;(1):CD005975

114. Mitka M. Joint commission warns of alarm fatigue: multitude of alarms from monitoring devices problematic. *JAMA.* 2013;309(22):2315–2316

115. Bowton DL, Scuderi PE, Harris L, Haponik EF. Pulse oximetry monitoring outside the intensive care unit: progress or problem? *Ann Intern Med.* 1991;115(6):450–454

116. Groothuis JR, Gutierrez KM, Lauer BA. Respiratory syncytial virus infection in children with bronchopulmonary dysplasia. *Pediatrics.* 1988;82(2):199–203

117. Voepel-Lewis T, Pechlavanidis E, Burke C, Talsma AN. Nursing surveillance moderates the relationship between staffing levels and pediatric postoperative serious adverse events: a nested case-control study. *Int J Nurs Stud.* 2013;50(7):905–913

118. Bajaj L, Turner CG, Bothner J. A randomized trial of home oxygen therapy from the emergency department for acute bronchiolitis. *Pediatrics.* 2006;117(3):633–640

119. Tie SW, Hall GL, Peter S, et al. Home oxygen for children with acute bronchiolitis. *Arch Dis Child.* 2009;94(8):641–643

120. Halstead S, Roosevelt G, Deakyne S, Bajaj L. Discharged on supplemental oxygen from an emergency department in patients with bronchiolitis. *Pediatrics.* 2012;129(3). Available at: www.pediatrics.org/cgi/content/full/129/3/e605

121. Sandweiss DR, Mundorff MB, Hill T, et al. Decreasing hospital length of stay for bronchiolitis by using an observation unit and home oxygen therapy. *JAMA Pediatr.* 2013;167(5):422–428

122. Flett KB, Breslin K, Braun PA, Hambidge SJ. Outpatient course and complications associated with home oxygen therapy for mild bronchiolitis. *Pediatrics.* 2014;133(5):769–775

123. Gauthier M, Vincent M, Morneau S, Chevalier I. Impact of home oxygen therapy on hospital stay for infants with acute bronchiolitis. *Eur J Pediatr.* 2012;171(12):1839–1844

124. Bergman AB. Pulse oximetry: good technology misapplied. *Arch Pediatr Adolesc Med.* 2004;158(6):594–595

125. Sandweiss DR, Kadish HA, Campbell KA. Outpatient management of patients with bronchiolitis discharged home on oxygen: a survey of general pediatricians. *Clin Pediatr (Phila).* 2012;51(5):442–446

126. Dysart K, Miller TL, Wolfson MR, Shaffer TH. Research in high flow therapy: mechanisms of action. *Respir Med.* 2009;103(10):1400–1405

127. Milési C, Baleine J, Matecki S, et al. Is treatment with a high flow nasal cannula effective in acute viral bronchiolitis? A physiologic study [published correction appears in *Intensive Care Med.* 2013;39(6):1170]. *Intensive Care Med.* 2013;39(6):1088–1094

128. Arora B, Mahajan P, Zidan MA, Sethuraman U. Nasopharyngeal airway pressures in bronchiolitis patients treated with high-flow nasal cannula oxygen therapy. *Pediatr Emerg Care.* 2012;28(11):1179–1184

129. Spentzas T, Minarik M, Patters AB, Vinson B, Stidham G. Children with respiratory distress treated with high-flow nasal cannula. *J Intensive Care Med.* 2009;24(5):323–328

130. Hegde S, Prodhan P. Serious air leak syndrome complicating high-flow nasal cannula therapy: a report of 3 cases. *Pediatrics.* 2013;131(3). Available at: www.pediatrics.org/cgi/content/full/131/3/e939

131. Pham TM, O'Malley L, Mayfield S, Martin S, Schibler A. The effect of high flow nasal cannula therapy on the work of breathing in infants with bronchiolitis [published online ahead of print May 21, 2014]. *Pediatr Pulmonol.* doi:doi:10.1002/ppul.23060

132. Bressan S, Balzani M, Krauss B, Pettenazzo A, Zanconato S, Baraldi E. High-flow nasal cannula oxygen for bronchiolitis in a pediatric ward: a pilot study. *Eur J Pediatr.* 2013;172(12):1649–1656

133. Ganu SS, Gautam A, Wilkins B, Egan J. Increase in use of non-invasive ventilation for infants with severe bronchiolitis is associated with decline in intubation rates over a decade. *Intensive Care Med.* 2012;38(7):1177–1183

134. Wing R, James C, Maranda LS, Armsby CC. Use of high-flow nasal cannula support in the emergency department reduces the need for intubation in pediatric acute respiratory insufficiency. *Pediatr Emerg Care.* 2012;28(11):1117–1123

135. McKiernan C, Chua LC, Visintainer PF, Allen H. High flow nasal cannulae therapy in infants with bronchiolitis. *J Pediatr.* 2010;156(4):634–638

136. Schibler A, Pham TM, Dunster KR, et al. Reduced intubation rates for infants after introduction of high-flow nasal prong oxygen delivery. *Intensive Care Med.* 2011;37(5):847–852

137. Kelly GS, Simon HK, Sturm JJ. High-flow nasal cannula use in children with respiratory distress in the emergency department: predicting the need for subsequent intubation. *Pediatr Emerg Care.* 2013;29(8):888–892

138. Kallappa C, Hufton M, Millen G, Ninan TK. Use of high flow nasal cannula oxygen (HFNCO) in infants with bronchiolitis on a paediatric ward: a 3-year experience. *Arch Dis Child.* 2014;99(8):790–791

139. Hilliard TN, Archer N, Laura H, et al. Pilot study of vapotherm oxygen delivery in moderately severe bronchiolitis. *Arch Dis Child.* 2012;97(2):182–183

140. Roqué i Figuls M, Giné-Garriga M, Granados Rugeles C, Perrotta C. Chest physiotherapy for acute bronchiolitis in paediatric patients between 0 and 24 months old. *Cochrane Database Syst Rev.* 2012;(2):CD004873

141. Aviram M, Damri A, Yekutielli C, Bearman J, Tal A. Chest physiotherapy in acute bronchiolitis [abstract]. *Eur Respir J.* 1992;5(suppl 15):229–230

142. Webb MS, Martin JA, Cartlidge PH, Ng YK, Wright NA. Chest physiotherapy in acute bronchiolitis. *Arch Dis Child.* 1985;60(11):1078–1079

143. Nicholas KJ, Dhouieb MO, Marshal TG, Edmunds AT, Grant MB. An evaluation of chest physiotherapy in the management of acute bronchiolitis: changing clinical practice. *Physiotherapy.* 1999;85(12):669–674

144. Bohé L, Ferrero ME, Cuestas E, Polliotto L, Genoff M. Indications of conventional chest physiotherapy in acute bronchiolitis [in Spanish]. *Medicina (B Aires).* 2004;64(3):198–200

145. De Córdoba F, Rodrigues M, Luque A, Cadrobbi C, Faria R, Solé D. Fisioterapia respiratória em lactentes com bronquiolite: realizar ou não? *Mundo Saúde.* 2008;32(2):183–188

146. Gajdos V, Katsahian S, Beydon N, et al. Effectiveness of chest physiotherapy in infants hospitalized with acute bronchiolitis: a multicenter, randomized, controlled trial. *PLoS Med.* 2010;7(9):e1000345

147. Rochat I, Leis P, Bouchardy M, et al. Chest physiotherapy using passive expiratory techniques does not reduce bronchiolitis severity: a randomised controlled trial. *Eur J Pediatr.* 2012;171(3):457–462

148. Postiaux G, Louis J, Labasse HC, et al. Evaluation of an alternative chest physiotherapy method in infants with respiratory syncytial virus bronchiolitis. *Respir Care.* 2011;56(7):989–994

149. Sánchez Bayle M, Martín Martín R, Cano Fernández J, et al. Chest physiotherapy and bronchiolitis in the hospitalised infant. Double-blind clinical trial [in Spanish]. *An Pediatr (Barc).* 2012;77(1):5–11

150. Mussman GM, Parker MW, Statile A, Sucharew H, Brady PW. Suctioning and length of stay in infants hospitalized with bronchiolitis. *JAMA Pediatr.* 2013;167(5):414–421

151. Weisgerber MC, Lye PS, Li SH, et al. Factors predicting prolonged hospital stay for infants with bronchiolitis. *J Hosp Med.* 2011;6(5):264–270

152. Nichol KP, Cherry JD. Bacterial-viral interrelations in respiratory infections of children. *N Engl J Med.* 1967;277(13):667–672

153. Field CM, Connolly JH, Murtagh G, Slattery CM, Turkington EE. Antibiotic treatment of epidemic bronchiolitis—a double-blind trial. *BMJ.* 1966;1(5479):83–85

154. Antonow JA, Hansen K, McKinstry CA, Byington CL. Sepsis evaluations in hospitalized infants with bronchiolitis. *Pediatr Infect Dis J.* 1998;17(3):231–236

155. Friis B, Andersen P, Brenøe E, et al. Antibiotic treatment of pneumonia and bronchiolitis. A prospective randomised study. *Arch Dis Child.* 1984;59(11):1038–1045

156. Greenes DS, Harper MB. Low risk of bacteremia in febrile children with recognizable viral syndromes. *Pediatr Infect Dis J.* 1999;18(3):258–261

157. Spurling GK, Doust J, Del Mar CB, Eriksson L. Antibiotics for bronchiolitis in children. *Cochrane Database Syst Rev.* 2011;(6):CD005189

158. Ralston S, Hill V, Waters A. Occult serious bacterial infection in infants younger than 60 to 90 days with bronchiolitis: a systematic review. *Arch Pediatr Adolesc Med.* 2011;165(10):951–956

159. Purcell K, Fergie J. Lack of usefulness of an abnormal white blood cell count for predicting a concurrent serious bacterial infection in infants and young children hospitalized with respiratory syncytial virus lower respiratory tract infection. *Pediatr Infect Dis J.* 2007;26(4):311–315

160. Purcell K, Fergie J. Concurrent serious bacterial infections in 2396 infants and children hospitalized with respiratory syncytial virus lower respiratory tract infections. *Arch Pediatr Adolesc Med.* 2002;156(4):322–324

161. Purcell K, Fergie J. Concurrent serious bacterial infections in 912 infants and children hospitalized for treatment of respiratory syncytial virus lower respiratory tract infection. *Pediatr Infect Dis J.* 2004;23(3):267–269

162. Kuppermann N, Bank DE, Walton EA, Senac MO Jr, McCaslin I. Risks for bacteremia and urinary tract infections in young febrile children with bronchiolitis. *Arch Pediatr Adolesc Med.* 1997;151(12):1207–1214

163. Titus MO, Wright SW. Prevalence of serious bacterial infections in febrile infants with respiratory syncytial virus infection. *Pediatrics.* 2003;112(2):282–284

164. Melendez E, Harper MB. Utility of sepsis evaluation in infants 90 days of age or younger with fever and clinical bronchiolitis. *Pediatr Infect Dis J.* 2003;22(12):1053–1056

165. Hall CB, Powell KR, Schnabel KC, Gala CL, Pincus PH. Risk of secondary bacterial

infection in infants hospitalized with respiratory syncytial viral infection. *J Pediatr.* 1988;113(2):266–271

166. Hall CB. Respiratory syncytial virus: a continuing culprit and conundrum. *J Pediatr.* 1999;135(2 pt 2):2–7

167. Davies HD, Matlow A, Petric M, Glazier R, Wang EE. Prospective comparative study of viral, bacterial and atypical organisms identified in pneumonia and bronchiolitis in hospitalized Canadian infants. *Pediatr Infect Dis J.* 1996;15(4):371–375

168. Levine DA, Platt SL, Dayan PS, et al; Multicenter RSV-SBI Study Group of the Pediatric Emergency Medicine Collaborative Research Committee of the American Academy of Pediatrics. Risk of serious bacterial infection in young febrile infants with respiratory syncytial virus infections. *Pediatrics.* 2004;113(6):1728–1734

169. Kellner JD, Ohlsson A, Gadomski AM, Wang EE. Bronchodilators for bronchiolitis. *Cochrane Database Syst Rev.* 2000;(2): CD001266

170. Pinto LA, Pitrez PM, Luisi F, et al. Azithromycin therapy in hospitalized infants with acute bronchiolitis is not associated with better clinical outcomes: a randomized, double-blinded, and placebo-controlled clinical trial. *J Pediatr.* 2012; 161(6):1104–1108

171. McCallum GB, Morris PS, Chang AB. Antibiotics for persistent cough or wheeze following acute bronchiolitis in children. *Cochrane Database Syst Rev.* 2012;(12): CD009834

172. Levin D, Tribuzio M, Green-Wrzesinki T, et al. Empiric antibiotics are justified for infants with RSV presenting with respiratory failure. *Pediatr Crit Care.* 2010; 11(3):390–395

173. Thorburn K, Reddy V, Taylor N, van Saene HK. High incidence of pulmonary bacterial co-infection in children with severe respiratory syncytial virus (RSV) bronchiolitis. *Thorax.* 2006;61(7):611–615

174. Gomaa MA, Galal O, Mahmoud MS. Risk of acute otitis media in relation to acute bronchiolitis in children. *Int J Pediatr Otorhinolaryngol.* 2012;76(1):49–51

175. Andrade MA, Hoberman A, Glustein J, Paradise JL, Wald ER. Acute otitis media in children with bronchiolitis. *Pediatrics.* 1998;101(4 pt 1):617–619

176. Shazberg G, Revel-Vilk S, Shoseyov D, Ben-Ami A, Klar A, Hurvitz H. The clinical course of bronchiolitis associated with acute otitis media. *Arch Dis Child.* 2000;83 (4):317–319

177. Lieberthal AS, Carroll AE, Chonmaitree T, et al. The diagnosis and management of

acute otitis media [published correction appears in *Pediatrics.* 2014;133(2):346]. *Pediatrics.* 2013;131(3). Available at: www.pediatrics.org/cgi/content/full/131/3/e964

178. Hoberman A, Paradise JL, Rockette HE, et al. Treatment of acute otitis media in children under 2 years of age. *N Engl J Med.* 2011;364(2):105–115

179. Tähtinen PA, Laine MK, Huovinen P, Jalava J, Ruuskanen O, Ruohola A. A placebo-controlled trial of antimicrobial treatment for acute otitis media. *N Engl J Med.* 2011;364(2):116–126

180. Corrard F, de La Rocque F, Martin E, et al. Food intake during the previous 24 h as a percentage of usual intake: a marker of hypoxia in infants with bronchiolitis: an observational, prospective, multicenter study. *BMC Pediatr.* 2013;13:6

181. Pinnington LL, Smith CM, Ellis RE, Morton RE. Feeding efficiency and respiratory integration in infants with acute viral bronchiolitis. *J Pediatr.* 2000;137(4):523–526

182. Khoshoo V, Edell D. Previously healthy infants may have increased risk of aspiration during respiratory syncytial viral bronchiolitis. *Pediatrics.* 1999;104(6):1389–1390

183. Kennedy N, Flanagan N. Is nasogastric fluid therapy a safe alternative to the intravenous route in infants with bronchiolitis? *Arch Dis Child.* 2005;90(3):320–321

184. Sammartino L, James D, Goutzamanis J, Lines D. Nasogastric rehydration does have a role in acute paediatric bronchiolitis. *J Paediatr Child Health.* 2002;38(3):321–322

185. Kugelman A, Raibin K, Dabbah H, et al. Intravenous fluids versus gastric-tube feeding in hospitalized infants with viral bronchiolitis: a randomized, prospective pilot study. *J Pediatr.* 2013;162(3):640–642.e1

186. Oakley E, Borland M, Neutze J, et al; Paediatric Research in Emergency Departments International Collaborative (PREDICT). Nasogastric hydration versus intravenous hydration for infants with bronchiolitis: a randomised trial. *Lancet Respir Med.* 2013;1(2):113–120

187. Gozal D, Colin AA, Jaffe M, Hochberg Z. Water, electrolyte, and endocrine homeostasis in infants with bronchiolitis. *Pediatr Res.* 1990;27(2):204–209

188. van Steensel-Moll HA, Hazelzet JA, van der Voort E, Neijens HJ, Hackeng WH. Excessive secretion of antidiuretic hormone in infections with respiratory syncytial virus. *Arch Dis Child.* 1990;65(11):1237–1239

189. Rivers RP, Forsling ML, Olver RP. Inappropriate secretion of antidiuretic hormone

in infants with respiratory infections. *Arch Dis Child.* 1981;56(5):358–363

190. Wang J, Xu E, Xiao Y. Isotonic versus hypotonic maintenance IV fluids in hospitalized children: a meta-analysis. *Pediatrics.* 2014;133(1):105–113

191. American Academy of Pediatrics, Committee on Infectious Diseases and Bronchiolitis Guidelines Committee. Policy statement: updated guidance for palivizumab prophylaxis among infants and young children at increased risk of hospitalization for respiratory syncytial virus infection. *Pediatrics.* 2014;134(2):415–420

192. American Academy of Pediatrics; Committee on Infectious Diseases and Bronchiolitis Guidelines Committee. Technical report: updated guidance for palivizumab prophylaxis among infants and young children at increased risk of hospitalization for respiratory syncytial virus infection. *Pediatrics.* 2014;134(2):e620–e638.

193. IMpact-RSV Study Group. Palivizumab, a humanized respiratory syncytial virus monoclonal antibody, reduces hospitalization from respiratory syncytial virus infection in high-risk infants. The IMpact-RSV Study Group. *Pediatrics.* 1998;102(3): 531–537

194. Feltes TF, Cabalk AK, Meissner HC, et al. Palivizumab prophylaxis reduces hospitalization due to respiratory syncytial virus in young children with hemodynamically significant congenital heart disease. *J Pediatr.* 2003;143(4):532–540

195. Andabaka T, Nickerson JW, Rojas-Reyes MX, Rueda JD, Bacic VV, Barsic B. Monoclonal antibody for reducing the risk of respiratory syncytial virus infection in children. *Cochrane Database Syst Rev.* 2013;(4):CD006602

196. Wang D, Bayliss S, Meads C. Palivizumab for immunoprophylaxis of respiratory syncytial virus (RSV) bronchiolitis in high-risk infants and young children: a systematic review and additional economic modelling of subgroup analyses. *Health Technol Assess.* 2011;1(5):iii–iv, 1–124

197. Hampp C, Kauf TL, Saidi AS, Winterstein AG. Cost-effectiveness of respiratory syncytial virus prophylaxis in various indications. *Arch Pediatr Adolesc Med.* 2011;165(6): 498–505

198. Hall CB, Weinberg GA, Iwane MK, et al. The burden of respiratory syncytial virus infection in young children. *N Engl J Med.* 2009;360(6):588–598

199. Dupenthaler A, Ammann RA, Gorgievski-Hrisoho M, et al. Low incidence of respiratory syncytial virus hospitalisations in haemodynamically significant congenital

heart disease. *Arch Dis Child.* 2004;89:961–965

200. Geskey JM, Thomas NJ, Brummel GL. Palivizumab in congenital heart disease: should international guidelines be revised? *Expert Opin Biol Ther.* 2007;7(11):1615–1620

201. Robbie GJ, Zhao L, Mondick J, Losonsky G, Roskos LK. Population pharmacokinetics of palivizumab, a humanized anti-respiratory syncytial virus monoclonal antibody, in adults and children. *Antimicrob Agents Chemother.* 2012;56(9):4927–4936

202. Megged O, Schlesinger Y. Down syndrome and respiratory syncytial virus infection. *Pediatr Infect Dis J.* 2010;29(7):672–673

203. Robinson KA, Odelola OA, Saldanha IJ, Mckoy NA. Palivizumab for prophylaxis against respiratory syncytial virus infection in children with cystic fibrosis. *Cochrane Database Syst Rev.* 2012;(2):CD007743

204. Winterstein AG, Eworuke E, Xu D, Schuler P. Palivizumab immunoprophylaxis effectiveness in children with cystic fibrosis. *Pediatr Pulmonol.* 2013;48(9):874–884

205. Cohen AH, Boron ML, Dingivan C. A phase IV study of the safety of palivizumab for prophylaxis of RSV disease in children with cystic fibrosis [abstract]. *American Thoracic Society Abstracts*, 2005 International Conference; 2005. p. A178

206. Giusti R. North American synagis prophylaxis survey. *Pediatr Pulmonol.* 2009;44(1):96–98

207. El Saleeby CM, Somes GW, DeVincenzo HP, Gaur AH. Risk factors for severe respiratory syncytial virus disease in children with cancer: the importance of lymphopenia and young age. *Pediatrics.* 2008;121(2):235–243

208. Berger A, Obwegeser E, Aberle SW, Langgartner M, Popow-Kraupp T. Nosocomial transmission of respiratory syncytial virus in neonatal intensive care and intermediate care units. *Pediatr Infect Dis J.* 2010;29(7):669–670

209. Ohler KH, Pham JT. Comparison of the timing of initial prophylactic palivizumab dosing on hospitalization of neonates for respiratory syncytial virus. *Am J Health Syst Pharm.* 2013;70(15):1342–1346

210. Blanken MO, Robers MM, Molenaar JM, et al. Respiratory syncytial virus and recurrent wheeze in healthy preterm infants. *N Engl J Med.* 2013;368(19):1794–1799

211. Yoshihara S, Kusuda S, Mochizuki H, Okada K, Nishima S, Simões EAF; C-CREW Investigators. Effect of palivizumab prophylaxis on subsequent recurrent wheezing in preterm infants. *Pediatrics.* 2013;132(5):811–818

212. Hall CB, Douglas RG Jr, Geiman JM. Possible transmission by fomites of respiratory syncytial virus. *J Infect Dis.* 1980;141(1):98–102

213. Sattar SA, Springthorpe VS, Tetro J, Vashon R, Keswick B. Hygienic hand antiseptics: should they not have activity and label claims against viruses? *Am J Infect Control.* 2002;30(6):355–372

214. Picheansathian W. A systematic review on the effectiveness of alcohol-based solutions for hand hygiene. *Int J Nurs Pract.* 2004;10(1):3–9

215. Hall CB. The spread of influenza and other respiratory viruses: complexities and conjectures. *Clin Infect Dis.* 2007;45(3):353–359

216. Boyce JM, Pittet D; Healthcare Infection Control Practices Advisory Committee; HICPAC/SHEA/APIC/IDSA Hand Hygiene Task Force; Society for Healthcare Epidemiology of America/Association for Professionals in Infection Control/Infectious Diseases Society of America. Guideline for Hand Hygiene in Health-Care Settings. Recommendations of the Healthcare Infection Control Practices Advisory Committee and the HICPAC/SHEA/APIC/IDSA Hand Hygiene Task Force. *MMWR Recomm Rep.* 2002;51(RR-16):1–45, quiz CE1–CE4

217. World Health Organization. Guidelines on hand hygiene in health care. Geneva, Switzerland: World Health Organization; 2009. Available at: http://whqlibdoc.who.int/publications/2009/9789241597906_eng.pdf. Accessed July 15, 2014

218. Karanfil LV, Conlon M, Lykens K, et al. Reducing the rate of nosocomially transmitted respiratory syncytial virus. [published correction appears in Am J Infect Control. 1999;27(3):303] *Am J Infect Control.* 1999;27(2):91–96

219. Macartney KK, Gorelick MH, Manning ML, Hodinka RL, Bell LM. Nosocomial respiratory syncytial virus infections: the cost-effectiveness and cost-benefit of infection control. *Pediatrics.* 2000;106(3):520–526

220. Strachan DP, Cook DG. Health effects of passive smoking. 1. Parental smoking and lower respiratory illness in infancy and early childhood. *Thorax.* 1997;52(10):905–914

221. Jones LL, Hashim A, McKeever T, Cook DG, Britton J, Leonardi-Bee J. Parental and household smoking and the increased risk of bronchitis, bronchiolitis and other lower respiratory infections in infancy: systematic review and meta-analysis. *Respir Res.* 2011;12:5

222. Bradley JP, Bacharier LB, Bonfiglio J, et al. Severity of respiratory syncytial virus bronchiolitis is affected by cigarette smoke exposure and atopy. *Pediatrics.* 2005;115(1). Available at: www.pediatrics.org/cgi/content/full/115/1/e7

223. Al-Shawwa B, Al-Huniti N, Weinberger M, Abu-Hasan M. Clinical and therapeutic variables influencing hospitalisation for bronchiolitis in a community-based paediatric group practice. *Prim Care Respir J.* 2007;16(2):93–97

224. Carroll KN, Gebretsadik T, Griffin MR, et al. Maternal asthma and maternal smoking are associated with increased risk of bronchiolitis during infancy. *Pediatrics.* 2007;119(6):1104–1112

225. Semple MG, Taylor-Robinson DC, Lane S, Smyth RL. Household tobacco smoke and admission weight predict severe bronchiolitis in infants independent of deprivation: prospective cohort study. *PLoS ONE.* 2011;6(7):e22425

226. Best D; Committee on Environmental Health; Committee on Native American Child Health; Committee on Adolescence. From the American Academy of Pediatrics: Technical report—Secondhand and prenatal tobacco smoke exposure. *Pediatrics.* 2009;124(5). Available at: www.pediatrics.org/cgi/content/full/124/5/e1017

227. Wilson KM, Wesgate SC, Best D, Blumkin AK, Klein JD. Admission screening for secondhand tobacco smoke exposure. *Hosp Pediatr.* 2012;2(1):26–33

228. Mahabee-Gittens M. Smoking in parents of children with asthma and bronchiolitis in a pediatric emergency department. *Pediatr Emerg Care.* 2002;18(1):4–7

229. Dempsey DA, Meyers MJ, Oh SS, et al. Determination of tobacco smoke exposure by plasma cotinine levels in infants and children attending urban public hospital clinics. *Arch Pediatr Adolesc Med.* 2012;166(9):851–856

230. Rosen LJ, Noach MB, Winickoff JP, Hovell MF. Parental smoking cessation to protect young children: a systematic review and meta-analysis. *Pediatrics.* 2012;129(1):141–152

231. Matt GE, Quintana PJ, Destaillats H, et al. Thirdhand tobacco smoke: emerging evidence and arguments for a multidisciplinary research agenda. *Environ Health Perspect.* 2011;119(9):1218–1226

232. Section on Breastfeeding. Breastfeeding and the use of human milk. *Pediatrics.* 2012;129(3). Available at: www.pediatrics.org/cgi/content/full/129/3/e827

233. Ip S, Chung M, Raman G, et al. *Breastfeeding and Maternal and Infant Health Outcomes in Developed Countries.* Rockville,

MD: Agency for Healthcare Research and Quality; 2007

234. Dornelles CT, Piva JP, Marostica PJ. Nutritional status, breastfeeding, and evolution of infants with acute viral bronchiolitis. *J Health Popul Nutr.* 2007;25(3):336–343

235. Oddy WH, Sly PD, de Klerk NH, et al. Breast feeding and respiratory morbidity in infancy: a birth cohort study. *Arch Dis Child.* 2003;88(3):224–228

236. Nishimura T, Suzue J, Kaji H. Breastfeeding reduces the severity of respiratory syncytial virus infection among young infants: a multi-center prospective study. *Pediatr Int.* 2009;51(6):812–816

237. Petruzella FD, Gorelick MH. Duration of illness in infants with bronchiolitis evaluated in the emergency department. *Pediatrics.* 2010;126(2):285–290

238. von Linstow ML, Eugen-Olsen J, Koch A, Winther TN, Westh H, Hogh B. Excretion patterns of human metapneumovirus and respiratory syncytial virus among young children. *Eur J Med Res.* 2006;11(8):329–335

239. Sacri AS, De Serres G, Quach C, Boulianne N, Valiquette L, Skowronski DM. Transmission of acute gastroenteritis and respiratory illness from children to parents. *Pediatr Infect Dis J.* 2014;33(6):583–588

240. Taylor JA, Kwan-Gett TS, McMahon EM Jr. Effectiveness of an educational intervention in modifying parental attitudes about antibiotic usage in children. *Pediatrics.* 2003;111 (5 pt 1). Available at: www.pediatrics.org/cgi/content/full/111/5pt1/e548

241. Kuzujanakis M, Kleinman K, Rifas-Shiman S, Finkelstein JA. Correlates of parental antibiotic knowledge, demand, and reported use. *Ambul Pediatr.* 2003;3(4):203–210

242. Mangione-Smith R, McGlynn EA, Elliott MN, Krogstad P, Brook RH. The relationship between perceived parental expectations and pediatrician antimicrobial prescribing behavior. *Pediatrics.* 1999;103(4 pt 1):711–718

APPENDIX 1 SEARCH TERMS BY TOPIC

Introduction

MedLine

(("bronchiolitis"[MeSH]) OR ("respiratory syncytial viruses"[MeSH]) NOT "bronchiolitis obliterans"[All Fields])

1. and exp Natural History/
2. and exp Epidemiology/
3. and (exp economics/ or exp "costs and cost analysis"/ or exp "cost allocation"/ or exp cost-benefit analysis/ or exp "cost control"/ or exp "cost of illness"/ or exp "cost sharing"/ or exp health care costs/ or exp health expenditures/)
4. and exp Risk Factors/

Limit to English Language AND Humans AND ("all infant (birth to 23 months)" or "newborn infant (birth to 1 month)" or "infant (1 to 23 months)")

CINAHL

(MM "Bronchiolitis+") AND ("natural history" OR (MM "Epidemiology") OR (MM "Costs and Cost Analysis") OR (MM "Risk Factors"))

The Cochrane Library

Bronchiolitis AND (epidemiology OR risk factor OR cost)

Diagnosis/Severity

MedLine

exp BRONCHIOLITIS/di [Diagnosis] OR exp Bronchiolitis, Viral/di [Diagnosis]

limit to English Language AND ("all infant (birth to 23 months)" or "newborn infant (birth to 1 month)" or "infant (1 to 23 months)")

CINAHL

(MH "Bronchiolitis/DI")

The Cochrane Library

Bronchiolitis AND Diagnosis

*Upper Respiratory Infection Symptoms

MedLine

(exp Bronchiolitis/ OR exp Bronchiolitis, Viral/) AND exp *Respiratory Tract Infections/

Limit to English Language

Limit to "all infant (birth to 23 months)" OR "newborn infant (birth to 1 month)" OR "infant (1 to 23 months)")

CINAHL

(MM "Bronchiolitis+") AND (MM "Respiratory Tract Infections+")

The Cochrane Library

Bronchiolitis AND Respiratory Infection

Inhalation Therapies

*Bronchodilators & Corticosteroids

MedLine

(("bronchiolitis"[MeSH]) OR ("respiratory syncytial viruses"[MeSH]) NOT "bronchiolitis obliterans"[All Fields])

AND (exp Receptors, Adrenergic, β-2/ OR exp Receptors, Adrenergic, β/ OR exp Receptors, Adrenergic, β-1/ OR β adrenergic*.mp. OR exp ALBUTEROL/ OR levalbuterol.mp. OR exp EPINEPHRINE/ OR exp Cholinergic Antagonists/ OR exp IPRATROPIUM/ OR exp Anti-Inflammatory Agents/ OR ics.mp. OR inhaled corticosteroid*.mp. OR exp Adrenal Cortex Hormones/ OR exp Leukotriene Antagonists/ OR montelukast.mp. OR exp Bronchodilator Agents/)

Limit to English Language AND ("all infant (birth to 23 months)" or "newborn infant (birth to 1 month)" or "infant (1 to 23 months)")

CINAHL

(MM "Bronchiolitis+") AND (MM "Bronchodilator Agents")

The Cochrane Library

Bronchiolitis AND (bronchodilator OR epinephrine OR albuterol OR salbutamol OR corticosteroid OR steroid)

*Hypertonic Saline

MedLine

(("bronchiolitis"[MeSH]) OR ("respiratory syncytial viruses"[MeSH]) NOT "bronchiolitis obliterans"[All Fields])

AND (exp Saline Solution, Hypertonic/ OR (aerosolized saline.mp. OR (exp AEROSOLS/ AND exp Sodium Chloride/)) OR (exp Sodium Chloride/ AND exp "Nebulizers and Vaporizers"/) OR nebulized saline.mp.)

Limit to English Language

Limit to "all infant (birth to 23 months)" OR "newborn infant (birth to 1 month)" OR "infant (1 to 23 months)")

CINAHL

(MM "Bronchiolitis+") AND (MM "Saline Solution, Hypertonic")

The Cochrane Library

Bronchiolitis AND Hypertonic Saline

Oxygen

MedLine

(("bronchiolitis"[MeSH]) OR ("respiratory syncytial viruses"[MeSH]) NOT "bronchiolitis obliterans"[All Fields])

1. AND (exp Oxygen Inhalation Therapy/ OR supplemental oxygen.mp. OR oxygen saturation.mp. OR *Oxygen/ad, st [Administration & Dosage, Standards] OR oxygen treatment.mp.)
2. AND (exp OXIMETRY/ OR oximeters.mp.) AND (exp "Reproducibility of Results"/ OR reliability.mp. OR function.mp. OR technical specifications.mp.) OR (percutaneous measurement*.mp. OR exp Blood Gas Analysis/)

Limit to English Language

Limit to "all infant (birth to 23 months)" OR "newborn infant (birth to 1 month)" OR "infant (1 to 23 months)")

CINAHL

(MM "Bronchiolitis+") AND

((MM "Oxygen Therapy") OR (MM "Oxygen+") OR (MM "Oxygen Saturation") OR (MM "Oximetry+") OR (MM "Pulse Oximetry") OR (MM "Blood Gas Monitoring, Transcutaneous"))

The Cochrane Library

Bronchiolitis AND (oxygen OR oximetry)

Chest Physiotherapy and Suctioning

MedLine

(("bronchiolitis"[MeSH]) OR ("respiratory syncytial viruses"[MeSH]) NOT "bronchiolitis obliterans"[All Fields])

1. AND (Chest physiotherapy.mp. OR (exp Physical Therapy Techniques/ AND exp Thorax/))

2. AND (Nasal Suction.mp. OR (exp Suction/))

Limit to English Language

Limit to "all infant (birth to 23 months)" OR "newborn infant (birth to 1 month)" or "infant (1 to 23 months)")

CINAHL

(MM "Bronchiolitis+")

1. AND ((MH "Chest Physiotherapy (Saba CCC)") OR (MH "Chest Physical Therapy+") OR (MH "Chest Physiotherapy (Iowa NIC)"))

2. AND (MH "Suctioning, Nasopharyngeal")

The Cochrane Library

Bronchiolitis AND (chest physiotherapy OR suction*)

Hydration

MedLine

(("bronchiolitis"[MeSH]) OR ("respiratory syncytial viruses"[MeSH])

NOT "bronchiolitis obliterans"[All Fields])

AND (exp Fluid Therapy/ AND (exp infusions, intravenous OR exp administration, oral))

Limit to English Language

Limit to ("all infant (birth to 23 months)" or "newborn infant (birth to 1 month)" or "infant (1 to 23 months)")

CINAHL

(MM "Bronchiolitis+") AND

((MM "Fluid Therapy+") OR (MM "Hydration Control (Saba CCC)") OR (MM "Hydration (Iowa NOC)"))

The Cochrane Library

Bronchiolitis AND (hydrat* OR fluid*)

SBI and Antibacterials

MedLine

(("bronchiolitis"[MeSH]) OR ("respiratory syncytial viruses"[MeSH]) NOT "bronchiolitis obliterans"[All Fields])

AND

(exp Bacterial Infections/ OR exp Bacterial Pneumonia/ OR exp Otitis Media/ OR exp Meningitis/ OR exp *Anti-bacterial Agents/ OR exp Sepsis/ OR exp Urinary Tract Infections/ OR exp Bacteremia/ OR exp Tracheitis OR serious bacterial infection.mp.)

Limit to English Language

Limit to ("all infant (birth to 23 months)" or "newborn infant (birth to 1 month)" or "infant (1 to 23 months)")

CINAHL

(MM "Bronchiolitis+") AND

((MM "Pneumonia, Bacterial+") OR (MM "Bacterial Infections+") OR (MM "Otitis Media+") OR (MM "Meningitis, Bacterial+") OR (MM "Antiinfective Agents+") OR (MM "Sepsis+") OR (MM

"Urinary Tract Infections+") OR (MM "Bacteremia"))

The Cochrane Library

Bronchiolitis AND (serious bacterial infection OR sepsis OR otitis media OR meningitis OR urinary tract infection or bacteremia OR pneumonia OR antibacterial OR antimicrobial OR antibiotic)

Hand Hygiene, Tobacco, Breastfeeding, Parent Education

MedLine

(("bronchiolitis"[MeSH]) OR ("respiratory syncytial viruses"[MeSH]) NOT "bronchiolitis obliterans"[All Fields])

1. AND (exp Hand Disinfection/ OR hand decontamination.mp. OR handwashing.mp.)

2. AND exp Tobacco/

3. AND (exp Breast Feeding/ OR exp Milk, Human/ OR exp Bottle Feeding/)

Limit to English Language

Limit to ("all infant (birth to 23 months)" or "newborn infant (birth to 1 month)" or "infant (1 to 23 months)")

CINAHL

(MM "Bronchiolitis+")

1. AND (MH "Handwashing+")

2. AND (MH "Tobacco+")

3. AND (MH "Breast Feeding+" OR MH "Milk, Human+" OR MH "Bottle Feeding+")

The Cochrane Library

Bronchiolitis

1. AND (Breast Feeding OR breastfeeding)

2. AND tobacco

3. AND (hand hygiene OR handwashing OR hand decontamination)

Bronchiolitis Clinical Practice Guideline Quick Reference Tools

• •

- Action Statement Summary
  — The Diagnosis, Management, and Prevention of Bronchiolitis
- *ICD-10-CM* Coding Quick Reference for Bronchiolitis
- AAP Patient Education Handout
  — *Bronchiolitis and Your Young Child*

Action Statement Summary

The Diagnosis, Management, and Prevention of Bronchiolitis

Key Action Statement 1a

Clinicians should diagnose bronchiolitis and assess disease severity on the basis of history and physical examination (Evidence Quality: B; Recommendation Strength: Strong Recommendation).

Key Action Statement 1b

Clinicians should assess risk factors for severe disease, such as age <12 weeks, a history of prematurity, underlying cardiopulmonary disease, or immunodeficiency, when making decisions about evaluation and management of children with bronchiolitis (Evidence Quality: B; Recommendation Strength: Moderate Recommendation).

Key Action Statement 1c

When clinicians diagnose bronchiolitis on the basis of history and physical examination, radiographic or laboratory studies should not be obtained routinely (Evidence Quality: B; Recommendation Strength: Moderate Recommendation).

Key Action Statement 2

Clinicians should not administer albuterol (or salbutamol) to infants and children with a diagnosis of bronchiolitis (Evidence Quality: B; Recommendation Strength: Strong Recommendation).

Key Action Statement 3

Clinicians should not administer epinephrine to infants and children with a diagnosis of bronchiolitis (Evidence Quality: B; Recommendation Strength: Strong Recommendation).

Key Action Statement 4a

Nebulized hypertonic saline should not be administered to infants with a diagnosis of bronchiolitis in the emergency department (Evidence Quality: B; Recommendation Strength: Moderate Recommendation).

Key Action Statement 4b

Clinicians may administer nebulized hypertonic saline to infants and children hospitalized for bronchiolitis (Evidence Quality: B; Recommendation Strength: Weak Recommendation [based on randomized controlled trials with inconsistent findings]).

Key Action Statement 5

Clinicians should not administer systemic corticosteroids to infants with a diagnosis of bronchiolitis in any setting (Evidence Quality: A; Recommendation Strength: Strong Recommendation).

Key Action Statement 6a

Clinicians may choose not to administer supplemental oxygen if the oxyhemoglobin saturation exceeds 90% in infants and children with a diagnosis of bronchiolitis (Evidence Quality: D; Recommendation Strength: Weak Recommendation [based on low-level evidence and reasoning from first principles]).

Key Action Statement 6b

Clinicians may choose not to use continuous pulse oximetry for infants and children with a diagnosis of bronchiolitis (Evidence Quality: C; Recommendation Strength: Weak Recommendation [based on lower-level evidence]).

Key Action Statement 7

Clinicians should not use chest physiotherapy for infants and children with a diagnosis of bronchiolitis (Evidence Quality: B; Recommendation Strength: Moderate Recommendation).

Key Action Statement 8

Clinicians should not administer antibacterial medications to infants and children with a diagnosis of bronchiolitis unless there is a concomitant bacterial infection, or a strong suspicion of one. (Evidence Quality: B; Recommendation Strength: Strong Recommendation).

Key Action Statement 9

Clinicians should administer nasogastric or intravenous fluids for infants with a diagnosis of bronchiolitis who cannot maintain hydration orally (Evidence Quality: X; Recommendation Strength: Strong Recommendation).

Key Action Statement 10a

Clinicians should not administer palivizumab to otherwise healthy infants with a gestational age of 29 weeks, 0 days or greater (Evidence Quality: B; Recommendation Strength: Strong Recommendation).

Key Action Statement 10b

Clinicians should administer palivizumab during the first year of life to infants with hemodynamically significant heart disease or chronic lung disease of prematurity defined as preterm infants <32 weeks, 0 days' gestation who require >21% oxygen for at least the first 28 days of life (Evidence Quality: B; Recommendation Strength: Moderate Recommendation).

Key Action Statement 10c

Clinicians should administer a maximum 5 monthly doses (15 mg/kg/dose) of palivizumab during the RSV season to infants who qualify for palivizumab in the first year of life (Evidence Quality: B, Recommendation Strength: Moderate Recommendation).

Key Action Statement 11a

All people should disinfect hands before and after direct contact with patients, after contact with inanimate objects in the direct vicinity of the patient, and after removing gloves (Evidence Quality: B; Recommendation Strength: Strong Recommendation).

Key Action Statement 11b

All people should use alcohol-based rubs for hand decontamination when caring for children with bronchiolitis. When alcohol-based rubs are not available, individuals should wash their hands with soap and water (Evidence Quality: B; Recommendation Strength: Strong Recommendation).

Key Action Statement 12a

Clinicians should inquire about the exposure of the infant or child to tobacco smoke when assessing infants and children for bronchiolitis (Evidence Quality: C; Recommendation Strength: Moderate Recommendation).

Key Action Statement 12b

Clinicians should counsel caregivers about exposing the infant or child to environmental tobacco smoke and smoking cessation when assessing a child for bronchiolitis (Evidence Quality: B; Recommendation Strength: Strong Recommendation).

Key Action Statement 13

Clinicians should encourage exclusive breastfeeding for at least 6 months to decrease the morbidity of respiratory infections (Evidence Quality: Grade B; Recommendation Strength: Moderate Recommendation).

Key Action Statement 14

Clinicians and nurses should educate personnel and family members on evidence-based diagnosis, treatment, and prevention in bronchiolitis (Evidence Quality: C; observational studies; Recommendation Strength; Moderate Recommendation).

Coding Quick Reference for Bronchiolitis
ICD-10-CM
J21.0 Acute bronchiolitis due to syncytial virus
J21.8 Acute bronchiolitis due to other specified organisms

Bronchiolitis and Your Young Child

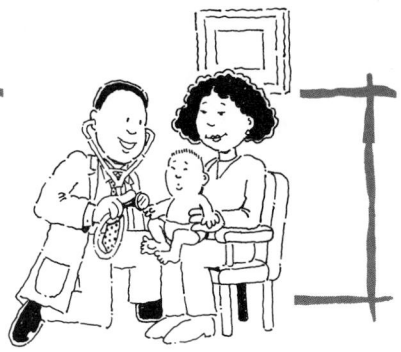

Bronchiolitis is a common respiratory illness among infants. One of its symptoms is trouble breathing, which can be scary for parents and young children. Read on for more information from the American Academy of Pediatrics about bronchiolitis, causes, signs and symptoms, how to treat it, and how to prevent it.

What is bronchiolitis?

Bronchiolitis is an infection that causes the small breathing tubes of the lungs (bronchioles) to swell. This blocks airflow through the lungs, making it hard to breathe. It occurs most often in infants because their airways are smaller and more easily blocked than in older children. Bronchiolitis is not the same as bronchitis, which is an infection of the larger, more central airways that typically causes problems in adults.

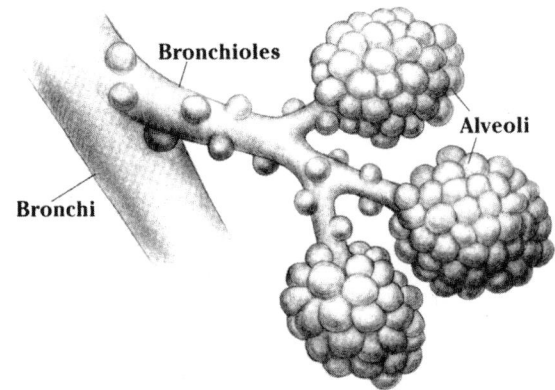

What causes bronchiolitis?

Bronchiolitis is caused by one of several respiratory viruses such as influenza, respiratory syncytial virus (RSV), parainfluenza, and human metapneumovirus. Other viruses can also cause bronchiolitis.

Infants with RSV infection are more likely to get bronchiolitis with wheezing and difficulty breathing. Most adults and many older children with RSV infection only get a cold. RSV is spread by contact with an infected person's mucus or saliva (respiratory droplets produced during coughing or wheezing). It often spreads through families and child care centers. (See "How can you prevent your baby from getting bronchiolitis?").

What are the signs and symptoms of bronchiolitis?

Bronchiolitis often starts with signs of a cold, such as a runny nose, mild cough, and fever. After 1 or 2 days, the cough may get worse and an infant will begin to breathe faster. Your child may become dehydrated if he cannot comfortably drink fluids

If your child shows any signs of troubled breathing or dehydration, call your child's doctor.

Signs of troubled breathing

- He may widen his nostrils and squeeze the muscles under his rib cage to try to get more air into and out of his lungs.
- When he breathes, he may grunt and tighten his stomach muscles.
- He will make a high-pitched whistling sound, called a wheeze, when he breathes out.
- He may have trouble drinking because he may have trouble sucking and swallowing.
- If it gets very hard for him to breathe, you may notice a bluish tint around his lips and fingertips. This tells you his airways are so blocked that there is not enough oxygen getting into his blood.

Signs of dehydration

- Drinking less than normal
- Dry mouth
- Crying without tears
- Urinating less often than normal

Bronchiolitis and children with severe chronic illness

Bronchiolitis may cause more severe illness in children who have a chronic illness. If you think your child has bronchiolitis and she has any of the following conditions, call her doctor:

- Cystic fibrosis
- Congenital heart disease
- Chronic lung disease (seen in some infants who were on breathing machines or respirators as newborns)
- Immune deficiency disease (eg, acquired immunodeficiency syndrome [AIDS])
- Organ or bone marrow transplant
- A cancer for which she is receiving chemotherapy

Can bronchiolitis be treated at home?

There is no specific treatment for RSV or other viruses that cause bronchiolitis. Antibiotics are not helpful because they treat illnesses caused by bacteria, not viruses. However, you can try to ease your child's symptoms.

To relieve a stuffy nose

- Thin the mucus using saline nose drops recommended by your child's doctor. Never use nonprescription nose drops that contain medicine.
- Clear your baby's nose with a suction bulb.

Squeeze the bulb first. Gently put the rubber tip into one nostril, and slowly release the bulb.

This suction will draw the clogged mucus out of the nose. This works best when your baby is younger than 6 months.

To relieve fever

Give your baby acetaminophen. (Follow the recommended dosage for your baby's age.) Do not give your baby aspirin because it has been associated with Reye syndrome, a disease that affects the liver and brain. Check with your child's doctor first before giving any other cold medicines.

To prevent dehydration

Make sure your baby drinks lots of fluid. She may want clear liquids rather than milk or formula. She may feed more slowly or not feel like eating because she is having trouble breathing.

How will your child's doctor treat bronchiolitis?

Your child's doctor will evaluate your child and advise you on nasal suctioning, fever control, and observation, as well as when to call back.

Some children with bronchiolitis need to be treated in a hospital for breathing problems or dehydration. Breathing problems may need to be treated with oxygen and medicine. Dehydration is treated with a special liquid diet or intravenous (IV) fluids.

In very rare cases when these treatments aren't working, an infant might have to be put on a respirator. This is usually only temporary until the infection is gone.

How can you prevent your baby from getting bronchiolitis?

The best steps you can follow to reduce the risk that your baby becomes infected with RSV or other viruses that cause bronchiolitis include

- Make sure everyone washes their hands before touching your baby.
- Keep your baby away from anyone who has a cold, fever, or runny nose.
- Avoid sharing eating utensils and drinking cups with anyone who has a cold, fever, or runny nose.

If you have questions about the treatment of bronchiolitis, call your child's doctor.

The information contained in this publication should not be used as a substitute for the medical care and advice of your pediatrician. There may be variations in treatment that your pediatrician may recommend based on individual facts and circumstances.

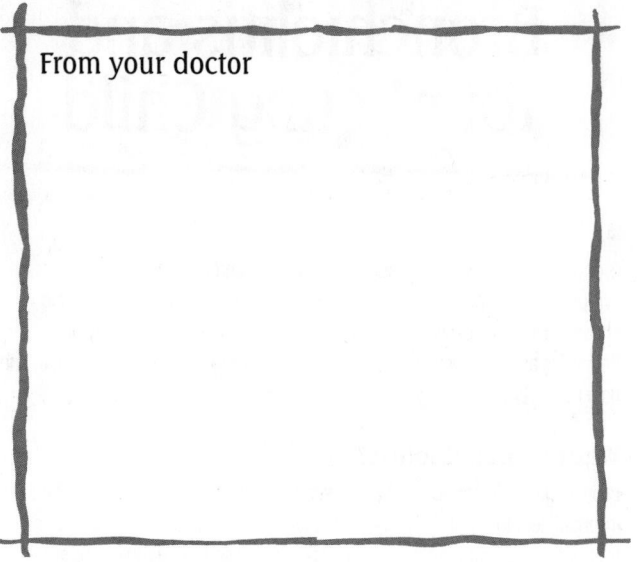

From your doctor

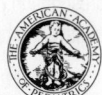

American Academy of Pediatrics

DEDICATED TO THE HEALTH OF ALL CHILDREN™

Management of Newly Diagnosed Type 2 Diabetes Mellitus (T2DM) in Children and Adolescents

- *Clinical Practice Guideline*
- *Technical Report*

    - *PPI: AAP Partnership for Policy Implementation*
    See Appendix 2 for more information.

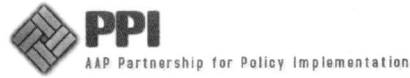

Readers of this clinical practice guideline are urged to review the technical report to enhance the evidence-based decision-making process. The full technical report is available following the clinical practice guideline and on the companion eBook.

CLINICAL PRACTICE GUIDELINE

Management of Newly Diagnosed Type 2 Diabetes Mellitus (T2DM) in Children and Adolescents

abstract

Over the past 3 decades, the prevalence of childhood obesity has increased dramatically in North America, ushering in a variety of health problems, including type 2 diabetes mellitus (T2DM), which previously was not typically seen until much later in life. The rapid emergence of childhood T2DM poses challenges to many physicians who find themselves generally ill-equipped to treat adult diseases encountered in children. This clinical practice guideline was developed to provide evidence-based recommendations on managing 10- to 18-year-old patients in whom T2DM has been diagnosed. The American Academy of Pediatrics (AAP) convened a Subcommittee on Management of T2DM in Children and Adolescents with the support of the American Diabetes Association, the Pediatric Endocrine Society, the American Academy of Family Physicians, and the Academy of Nutrition and Dietetics (formerly the American Dietetic Association). These groups collaborated to develop an evidence report that served as a major source of information for these practice guideline recommendations. The guideline emphasizes the use of management modalities that have been shown to affect clinical outcomes in this pediatric population. Recommendations are made for situations in which either insulin or metformin is the preferred first-line treatment of children and adolescents with T2DM. The recommendations suggest integrating lifestyle modifications (ie, diet and exercise) in concert with medication rather than as an isolated initial treatment approach. Guidelines for frequency of monitoring hemoglobin A1c (HbA1c) and finger-stick blood glucose (BG) concentrations are presented. Decisions were made on the basis of a systematic grading of the quality of evidence and strength of recommendation. The clinical practice guideline underwent peer review before it was approved by the AAP. This clinical practice guideline is not intended to replace clinical judgment or establish a protocol for the care of all children with T2DM, and its recommendations may not provide the only appropriate approach to the management of children with T2DM. Providers should consult experts trained in the care of children and adolescents with T2DM when treatment goals are not met or when therapy with insulin is initiated. The AAP acknowledges that some primary care clinicians may not be confident of their ability to successfully treat T2DM in a child because of the child's age, coexisting conditions, and/or other concerns. At any point at which a clinician feels he or she is not adequately trained or is uncertain about treatment, a referral to a pediatric medical subspecialist should be made. If a diagnosis of T2DM is made by a pediatric medical subspecialist, the primary care clinician should develop a comanagement strategy with the subspecialist to ensure that the child continues to receive appropriate care consistent with a medical home model in which the pediatrician partners with parents to ensure that all health needs are met. *Pediatrics* 2013;131:364–382

Kenneth C. Copeland, MD, Janet Silverstein, MD, Kelly R. Moore, MD, Greg E. Prazar, MD, Terry Raymer, MD, CDE, Richard N. Shiffman, MD, Shelley C. Springer, MD, MBA, Vidhu V. Thaker, MD, Meaghan Anderson, MS, RD, LD, CDE, Stephen J. Spann, MD, MBA, and Susan K. Flinn, MA

KEY WORDS
diabetes, type 2 diabetes mellitus, childhood, youth, clinical practice guidelines, comanagement, management, treatment

ABBREVIATIONS
AAP—American Academy of Pediatrics
AAFP—American Academy of Family Physicians
BG—blood glucose
FDA—US Food and Drug Administration
HbA1c—hemoglobin A1c
PES—Pediatric Endocrine Society
T1DM—type 1 diabetes mellitus
T2DM—type 2 diabetes mellitus
TODAY—Treatment Options for type 2 Diabetes in Adolescents and Youth

This document is copyrighted and is property of the American Academy of Pediatrics and its Board of Directors. All authors have filed conflict of interest statements with the American Academy of Pediatrics. Any conflicts have been resolved through a process approved by the Board of Directors. The American Academy of Pediatrics has neither solicited nor accepted any commercial involvement in the development of the content of this publication.

The recommendations in this report do not indicate an exclusive course of treatment or serve as a standard of medical care. Variations, taking into account individual circumstances, may be appropriate.

All clinical practice guidelines from the American Academy of Pediatrics automatically expire 5 years after publication unless reaffirmed, revised, or retired at or before that time.

www.pediatrics.org/cgi/doi/10.1542/peds.2012-3494

doi:10.1542/peds.2012-3494

PEDIATRICS (ISSN Numbers: Print, 0031-4005; Online, 1098-4275).

Key action statements are as follows:

1. Clinicians must ensure that insulin therapy is initiated for children and adolescents with T2DM who are ketotic or in diabetic ketoacidosis and in whom the distinction between types 1 and 2 diabetes mellitus is unclear and, in usual cases, should initiate insulin therapy for patients

   a. who have random venous or plasma BG concentrations ≥250 mg/dL; or

   b. whose HbA1c is >9%.

2. In all other instances, clinicians should initiate a lifestyle modification program, including nutrition and physical activity, and start metformin as first-line therapy for children and adolescents at the time of diagnosis of T2DM.

3. The committee suggests that clinicians monitor HbA1c concentrations every 3 months and intensify treatment if treatment goals for finger-stick BG and HbA1c concentrations are not being met (intensification is defined in the Definitions box).

4. The committee suggests that clinicians advise patients to monitor finger-stick BG (see Key Action Statement 4 in the guideline for further details) concentrations in patients who

   a. are taking insulin or other medications with a risk of hypoglycemia; or

   b. are initiating or changing their diabetes treatment regimen; or

   c. have not met treatment goals; or

   d. have intercurrent illnesses.

5. The committee suggests that clinicians incorporate the Academy of Nutrition and Dietetics' *Pediatric Weight Management Evidence-Based Nutrition Practice Guidelines* in their dietary or nutrition counseling of patients with T2DM at the time of diagnosis and as part of ongoing management.

6. The committee suggests that clinicians encourage children and adolescents with T2DM to engage in moderate-to-vigorous exercise for at least 60 minutes daily and to limit nonacademic "screen time" to less than 2 hours a day.

Definitions

Adolescent: an individual in various stages of maturity, generally considered to be between 12 and 18 years of age.

Childhood T2DM: disease in the child who typically

- is overweight or obese (BMI ≥85th–94th and >95th percentile for age and gender, respectively);

- has a strong family history of T2DM;

- has substantial residual insulin secretory capacity at diagnosis (reflected by normal or elevated insulin and C-peptide concentrations);

- has insidious onset of disease;

- demonstrates insulin resistance (including clinical evidence of polycystic ovarian syndrome or acanthosis nigricans);

- lacks evidence for diabetic autoimmunity (negative for autoantibodies typically associated with T1DM). These patients are more likely to have hypertension and dyslipidemia than are those with T1DM.

Clinician: any provider within his or her scope of practice; includes medical practitioners (including physicians and physician extenders), dietitians, psychologists, and nurses.

Diabetes: according to the American Diabetes Association criteria, defined as

1. HbA1c ≥6.5% (test performed in an appropriately certified laboratory); or

2. fasting (defined as no caloric intake for at least 8 hours) plasma glucose ≥126 mg/dL (7.0 mmol/L); or

3. 2-hour plasma glucose ≥200 mg/dL (11.1 mmol/L) during an oral glucose tolerance test performed as described by the World Health Organization by using a glucose load containing the equivalent of 75 g anhydrous glucose dissolved in water; or

4. a random plasma glucose ≥200 mg/dL (11.1 mmol/L) with symptoms of hyperglycemia.

(In the absence of unequivocal hyperglycemia, criteria 1–3 should be confirmed by repeat testing.)

Diabetic ketoacidosis: acidosis resulting from an absolute or relative insulin deficiency, causing fat breakdown and formation of β hydroxybutyrate. Symptoms include nausea, vomiting, dehydration, Kussmaul respirations, and altered mental status.

Fasting blood glucose: blood glucose obtained before the first meal of the day and after a fast of at least 8 hours.

Glucose toxicity: The effect of high blood glucose causing both insulin resistance and impaired β-cell production of insulin.

Intensification: Increase frequency of blood glucose monitoring and adjustment of the dose and type of medication in an attempt to normalize blood glucose concentrations.

Intercurrent illnesses: Febrile illnesses or associated symptoms severe enough to cause the patient to stay home from school and/or seek medical care.

Microalbuminuria: Albumin:creatinine ratio ≥30 mg/g creatinine but <300 mg/g creatinine.

Moderate hyperglycemia: blood glucose = 180–250 mg/dL.

Moderate-to-vigorous exercise: exercise that makes the individual breathe hard and perspire and that raises his or her heart rate. An easy way to define exercise intensity for patients is the "talk test": during moderate physical activity a person can talk, but not sing. During vigorous activity, a person cannot talk without pausing to catch a breath.

Obese: BMI ≥95th percentile for age and gender.

Overweight: BMI between the 85th and 94th percentile for age and gender.

Prediabetes: Fasting plasma glucose ≥100–125 mg/dL or 2-hour glucose concentration during an oral glucose tolerance test ≥126 but <200 mg/dL or an HbA1c of 5.7% to 6.4%.

Severe hyperglycemia: blood glucose >250 mg/dL.

Thiazolidinediones (TZDs): Oral hypoglycemic agents that exert their effect at least in part by activation of the peroxisome proliferator-activated receptor γ.

Type 1 diabetes mellitus (T1DM): Diabetes secondary to autoimmune destruction of β cells resulting in absolute (complete or near complete) insulin deficiency and requiring insulin injections for management.

Type 2 diabetes mellitus (T2DM): The investigators' designation of the diagnosis was used for the purposes of the literature review. The committee acknowledges the distinction between T1DM and T2DM in this population is not always clear cut, and clinical judgment plays an important role. Typically, this diagnosis is made when hyperglycemia is secondary to insulin resistance accompanied by impaired β-cell function resulting in inadequate insulin production to compensate for the degree of insulin resistance.

Youth: used interchangeably with "adolescent" in this document.

INTRODUCTION

Over the past 3 decades, the prevalence of childhood obesity has increased dramatically in North America,[1–5] ushering in a variety of health problems, including type 2 diabetes mellitus (T2DM), which previously was not typically seen until much later in life. Currently, in the United States, up to 1 in 3 new cases of diabetes mellitus diagnosed in youth younger than 18 years is T2DM (depending on the ethnic composition of the patient population),[6,7] with a disproportionate representation in ethnic minorities[8,9] and occurring most commonly among youth between 10 and 19 years of age.[5,10] This trend is not limited to the United States but is occurring internationally[11]; it is projected that by the year 2030, an estimated 366 million people worldwide will have diabetes mellitus.[12]

The rapid emergence of childhood T2DM poses challenges to many physicians who find themselves generally ill-equipped to treat adult diseases encountered in children. Most diabetes education materials designed for pediatric patients are directed primarily to families of children with type 1 diabetes mellitus (T1DM) and emphasize insulin treatment and glucose monitoring, which may or may not be appropriate for children with

T2DM.[13,14] The National Diabetes Education Program TIP sheets (which can be ordered or downloaded from www.yourdiabetesinfo.org or ndep.nih.gov) provide guidance on healthy eating, physical activity, and dealing with T2DM in children and adolescents, but few other resources are available that are directly targeted at youth with this disease.[15] Most medications used for T2DM have been tested for safety and efficacy only in people older than 18 years, and there is scant scientific evidence for optimal management of children with T2DM.[16,17] Recognizing the scarcity of evidence-based data, this report provides a set of guidelines for the management and treatment of children with T2DM that is based on a review of current medical literature covering a period from January 1, 1990, to July 1, 2008.

Despite these limitations, the practicing physician is likely to be faced with the need to provide care for children with T2DM. Thus, the American Academy of Pediatrics (AAP), the Pediatric Endocrine Society (PES), the American Academy of Family Physicians (AAFP), American Diabetes Association, and the Academy of Nutrition and Dietetics (formerly the American Dietetic Association) partnered to develop a set of guidelines that might benefit endocrinologists and generalists, including pediatricians and family physicians alike. This clinical practice guideline may not provide the only appropriate approach to the management of children with T2DM. It is not expected to serve as a sole source of guidance in the management of children and adolescents with T2DM, nor is it intended to replace clinical judgment or establish a protocol for the care of all children with this condition. Rather, it is intended to assist clinicians in decision-making.

Primary care providers should endeavor to obtain the requisite skills to care for children and adolescents with

T2DM, and should communicate and work closely with a diabetes team of subspecialists when such consultation is available, practical, and appropriate. The frequency of such consultations will vary, but should usually be obtained at diagnosis and then at least annually if possible. When treatment goals are not met, the committee encourages clinicians to consult with an expert trained in the care of children and adolescents with T2DM.[18,19] When first-line therapy (eg, metformin) fails, recommendations for intensifying therapy should be generally the same for pediatric and adult populations. The picture is constantly changing, however, as new drugs are introduced, and some drugs that initially appeared to be safe demonstrate adverse effects with wider use. Clinicians should, therefore, remain alert to new developments with regard to treatment of T2DM. Seeking the advice of an expert can help ensure that the treatment goals are appropriately set and that clinicians benefit from cutting-edge treatment information in this rapidly changing area.

The Importance of Family-Centered Diabetes Care

Family structure, support, and education help inform clinical decision-making and negotiations with the patient and family about medical preferences that affect medical decisions, independent of existing clinical recommendations. Because adherence is a major issue in any lifestyle intervention, engaging the family is critical not only to maintain needed changes in lifestyle but also to foster medication adherence.[20–22] The family's ideal role in lifestyle interventions varies, however, depending on the child's age. Behavioral interventions in younger children have shown a favorable effect. With adolescents, however, interventions based on target-age behaviors (eg, including phone or Internet-based

interventions as well as face-to-face or peer-enhanced activities) appear to foster better results, at least for weight management.[23]

Success in making lifestyle changes to attain therapeutic goals requires the initial and ongoing education of the patient and the entire family about healthy nutrition and exercise. Any behavior change recommendations must establish realistic goals and take into account the families' health beliefs and behaviors. Understanding the patient and family's perception of the disease (and overweight status) before establishing a management plan is important to dispel misconceptions and promote adherence.[24] Because T2DM disproportionately affects minority populations, there is a need to ensure culturally appropriate, family-centered care along with ongoing education.[25–28] Several observational studies cite the importance of addressing cultural issues within the family.[20–22]

Restrictions in Creating This Document

In developing these guidelines, the following restrictions governed the committee's work:

- Although the importance of diabetes detection and screening of at-risk populations is acknowledged and referenced, the guidelines are restricted to patients meeting the diagnostic criteria for diabetes (eg, this document focuses on treatment postdiagnosis). Specifically, this document and its recommendations do not pertain to patients with impaired fasting plasma glucose (100–125 mg/dL) or impaired glucose tolerance (2-hour oral glucose tolerance test plasma glucose: 140–200 mg/dL) or isolated insulin resistance.

- Although it is noted that the distinction between types 1 and 2 diabetes mellitus in children may be difficult,[29,30] these recommendations pertain specifically to patients 10 to less than 18 years of age with T2DM (as defined above).

- Although the importance of high-risk care and glycemic control in pregnancy, including pregravid glycemia, is affirmed, the evidence considered and recommendations contained in this document do not pertain to diabetes in pregnancy, including diabetes in pregnant adolescents.

- Recommended screening schedules and management tools for select comorbid conditions (hypertension, dyslipidemia, nephropathy, microalbuminuria, and depression) are provided as resources in the accompanying technical report.[31] These therapeutic recommendations were adapted from other recommended guideline documents with references, without an independent assessment of their supporting evidence.

METHODS

A systematic review was performed and is described in detail in the accompanying technical report.[31] To develop the clinical practice guideline on the management of T2DM in children and adolescents, the AAP convened the Subcommittee on Management of T2DM in Children and Adolescents with the support of the American Diabetes Association, the PES, the AAFP, and the Academy of Nutrition and Dietetics. The subcommittee was co-chaired by 2 pediatric endocrinologists preeminent in their field and included experts in general pediatrics, family medicine, nutrition, Native American health, epidemiology, and medical informatics/guideline methodology. All panel members reviewed the AAP policy on Conflict of Interest and Voluntary Disclosure and declared all potential conflicts (see conflicts statements in the Task Force member list).

These groups partnered to develop an evidence report that served as a major source of information for these practice guideline recommendations.[31] Specific clinical questions addressed in the evidence review were as follows: (1) the effectiveness of treatment modalities for T2DM in children and adolescents, (2) the efficacy of pharmaceutical therapies for treatment of children and adolescents with T2DM, (3) appropriate recommendations for screening for comorbidities typically associated with T2DM in children and adolescents, and (4) treatment recommendations for comorbidities of T2DM in children and adolescents. The accompanying technical report contains more information on comorbidities.[31]

Epidemiologic project staff searched Medline, the Cochrane Collaboration, and Embase. MESH terms used in various combinations in the search included diabetes, mellitus, type 2, type 1, treatment, prevention, diet, pediatric, T2DM, T1DM, NIDDM, metformin, lifestyle, RCT, meta-analysis, child, adolescent, therapeutics, control, adult, obese, gestational, polycystic ovary syndrome, metabolic syndrome, cardiovascular, dyslipidemia, men, and women. In addition, the Boolean operators NOT, AND, OR were included in various combinations. Articles addressing treatment of diabetes mellitus were prospectively limited to those that were published in English between January 1990 and June 2008, included abstracts, and addressed children between the ages of 120 and 215 months with an established diagnosis of T2DM. Studies in adults were considered for inclusion if >10% of the study population was 45 years of age or younger. The Medline search limits included the following: clinical trial; meta-analysis; randomized controlled trial; review; child: 6–12 years; and adolescent: 13–18 years. Additional articles were identified by review of reference lists of relevant articles and ongoing studies recommended by a technical expert advisory group. All articles were reviewed for compliance with the search limitations and appropriateness for inclusion in this document.

Initially, 199 abstracts were identified for possible inclusion, of which 52 were retained for systematic review. Results of the literature review were presented in evidence tables and published in the final evidence report. An additional literature search of Medline and the Cochrane Database of

Evidence Quality	Preponderance of Benefit or Harm	Balance of Benefit and Harm
A. Well-designed RCTs or diagnostic studies on relevant population	Strong Recommendation	
B. RCTs or diagnostic studies with minor limitations; overwhelmingly consistent evidence from observational studies		Option
C. Observational studies (case-control and cohort design)	Recommendation	
D. Expert opinion, case reports, reasoning from first principles	Option	No Rec
X. Exceptional situations where validating studies cannot be performed and there is a clear preponderance of benefit or harm	Strong Recommendation / Recommendation	

FIGURE 1

Evidence quality. Integrating evidence quality appraisal with an assessment of the anticipated balance between benefits and harms if a policy is carried out leads to designation of a policy as a strong recommendation, recommendation, option, or no recommendation.[32] RCT, randomized controlled trial; Rec, recommendation.

TABLE 1 Definitions and Recommendation Implications

Statement	Definition	Implication
Strong recommendation	A *strong recommendation* in favor of a particular action is made when the anticipated benefits of the recommended intervention clearly exceed the harms (as a strong recommendation against an action is made when the anticipated harms clearly exceed the benefits) and the quality of the supporting evidence is excellent. In some clearly identified circumstances, strong recommendations may be made when high-quality evidence is impossible to obtain and the anticipated benefits strongly outweigh the harms.	Clinicians should follow a strong recommendation unless a clear and compelling rationale for an alternative approach is present.
Recommendation	A *recommendation* in favor of a particular action is made when the anticipated benefits exceed the harms but the quality of evidence is not as strong. Again, in some clearly identified circumstances, recommendations may be made when high-quality evidence is impossible to obtain but the anticipated benefits outweigh the harms.	Clinicians would be prudent to follow a recommendation but should remain alert to new information and sensitive to patient preferences.
Option	*Options* define courses that may be taken when either the quality of evidence is suspect or carefully performed studies have shown little clear advantage to 1 approach over another.	Clinicians should consider the option in their decision-making, and patient preference may have a substantial role.
No recommendation	*No recommendation* indicates that there is a lack of pertinent published evidence and that the anticipated balance of benefits and harms is presently unclear.	Clinicians should be alert to new published evidence that clarifies the balance of benefit versus harm.

It should be noted that, because childhood T2DM is a relatively recent medical phenomenon, there is a paucity of evidence for many or most of the recommendations provided. In some cases, supporting references for a specific recommendation are provided that do not deal specifically with childhood T2DM, such as T1DM, childhood obesity, or childhood "prediabetes," or that were not included in the original comprehensive search. Committee members have made every effort to identify those references that did not affect or alter the level of evidence for specific recommendations.

Systematic Reviews was performed in July 2009 for articles discussing recommendations for screening and treatment of 5 recognized comorbidities of T2DM: cardiovascular disease, dyslipidemia, retinopathy, nephropathy, and peripheral vascular disease. Search criteria were the same as for the search on treatment of T2DM, with the inclusion of the term "type 1 diabetes mellitus." Search terms included, in various combinations, the following: diabetes, mellitus, type 2, type 1, pediatric, T2DM, T1DM, NIDDM, hyperlipidemia, retinopathy, microalbuminuria, comorbidities, screening, RCT, meta-analysis, child, and adolescent. Boolean operators and search limits mirrored those of the primary search.

An additional 336 abstracts were identified for possible inclusion, of which 26 were retained for systematic review. Results of this subsequent literature review were also presented in evidence tables and published in the final evidence report. An epidemiologist appraised the methodologic quality of the research before it was considered by the committee members.

The evidence-based approach to guideline development requires that the evidence in support of each key action statement be identified, appraised, and summarized and that an explicit link between evidence and recommendations be defined. Evidence-based recommendations reflect the quality of evidence and the balance of benefit and harm that is anticipated when the recommendation is followed. The AAP policy statement, "Classifying Recommendations for Clinical Practice Guidelines,"[32] was followed in designating levels of recommendation (see Fig 1 and Table 1).

To ensure that these recommendations can be effectively implemented, the Guidelines Review Group at Yale Center for Medical Informatics provided feedback on a late draft of these recommendations, using the GuideLine Implementability Appraisal.[33] Several potential obstacles to successful implementation were identified and resolved in the final guideline. Evidence was incorporated systematically into 6 key action statements about appropriate management facilitated by BRIDGE-Wiz software (Building Recommendations in a Developer's Guideline Editor; Yale Center for Medical Informatics).

A draft version of this clinical practice guideline underwent extensive peer review by 8 groups within the AAP, the American Diabetes Association, PES, AAFP, and the Academy of Nutrition and Dietetics. Members of the subcommittee were invited to distribute the draft to other representatives and committees within their specialty organizations. The resulting comments were reviewed by the subcommittee and incorporated into the guideline, as appropriate. All AAP guidelines are reviewed every 5 years.

KEY ACTION STATEMENTS

Key Action Statement 1

Clinicians must ensure that insulin therapy is initiated for children and adolescents with T2DM who are ketotic or in diabetic ketoacidosis and in whom the distinction between T1DM and T2DM is unclear; and, in usual cases, should initiate insulin therapy for patients:

a. **who have random venous or plasma BG concentrations ≥250 mg/dL; or**

b. **whose HbA1c is >9%.**

(Strong Recommendation: evidence quality X, validating studies cannot be performed, and C, observational studies and expert opinion; preponderance of benefit over harm.)

Action Statement Profile KAS 1

Aggregate evidence quality	X (validating studies cannot be performed)
Benefits	Avoidance of progression of diabetic ketoacidosis (DKA) and worsening metabolic acidosis; resolution of acidosis and hyperglycemia; avoidance of coma and/or death. Quicker restoration of glycemic control, potentially allowing islet β cells to "rest and recover," increasing long-term adherence to treatment; avoiding progression to DKA if T1DM. Avoiding hospitalization. Avoidance of potential risks associated with the use of other agents (eg, abdominal discomfort, bloating, loose stools with metformin; possible cardiovascular risks with sulfonylureas).
Harms/risks/cost	Potential for hypoglycemia, insulin-induced weight gain, cost, patient discomfort from injection, necessity for BG testing, more time required by the health care team for patient training.
Benefits-harms assessment	Preponderance of benefit over harm.
Value judgments	Extensive clinical experience of the expert panel was relied on in making this recommendation.
Role of patient preferences	Minimal.
Exclusions	None.
Intentional vagueness	None.
Strength	Strong recommendation.

The presentation of T2DM in children and adolescents varies according to the disease stage. Early in the disease, before diabetes diagnostic criteria are met, insulin resistance predominates with compensatory high insulin secretion, resulting in normoglycemia. Over time, β cells lose their ability to secrete adequate amounts of insulin to overcome insulin resistance, and hyperglycemia results. Early in this process, blood glucose (BG) concentrations may be normal much of the time and the patient likely will be asymptomatic. At this stage, the disease may only be detected by abnormal BG concentrations identified during screening. As insulin secretion declines further, the patient is likely to develop symptoms of hyperglycemia, occasionally with ketosis or frank ketoacidosis. High glucose concentrations can cause a reversible toxicity to islet β cells that contributes further to insulin deficiency. Of adolescents in whom T2DM is subsequently diagnosed, 5% to 25% present with ketoacidosis.[34]

Diabetic ketoacidosis must be treated with insulin and fluid and electrolyte replacement to prevent worsening metabolic acidosis, coma, and death. Children and adolescents with symptoms of hyperglycemia (polyuria, polydipsia, and polyphagia) who are diagnosed with diabetes mellitus should be evaluated for ketosis (serum or urine ketones) and, if positive, for ketoacidosis (venous pH), even if their phenotype and risk factor status (obesity, acanthosis nigricans, positive family history of T2DM) suggests T2DM. Patients in whom ketoacidosis is diagnosed require immediate treatment with insulin and fluid replacement in an inpatient setting under the supervision of a physician who is experienced in treating this complication.

Youth and adolescents who present with T2DM with poor glycemic control (BG concentrations ≥250 mg/dL or HbA1c >9%) but who lack evidence of ketosis or ketoacidosis may also benefit from initial treatment with insulin, at least on a short-term basis.[34] This allows for quicker restoration of glycemic control and, theoretically, may allow islet β cells to "rest and recover."[35,36] Furthermore, it has been noted that initiation of insulin may increase long-term adherence to treatment in children and adolescents with T2DM by enhancing the patient's perception of the seriousness of the disease.[7,37–40] Many patients with T2DM can be weaned gradually from insulin therapy and subsequently managed with metformin and lifestyle modification.[34]

As noted previously, in some children and adolescents with newly diagnosed diabetes mellitus, it may be difficult to distinguish between type 1 and type 2 disease (eg, an obese child presenting with ketosis).[39,41] These patients are best managed initially with insulin therapy while appropriate tests are performed to differentiate between T1DM and T2DM. The care of children and adolescents who have either newly diagnosed T2DM or undifferentiated-type diabetes and who require initial insulin treatment should be supervised by a physician experienced in treating diabetic patients with insulin.

Key Action Statement 2

In all other instances, clinicians should initiate a lifestyle modification program, including nutrition

and physical activity, and start metformin as first-line therapy for children and adolescents at the time of diagnosis of T2DM. (Strong recommendation: evidence quality B; 1 RCT showing improved outcomes with metformin versus lifestyle; preponderance of benefits over harms.)

Action Statement Profile KAS 2

Aggregate evidence quality	B (1 randomized controlled trial showing improved outcomes with metformin versus lifestyle combined with expert opinion).
Benefit	Lower HbA1c, target HbA1c sustained longer, less early deterioration of BG, less chance of weight gain, improved insulin sensitivity, improved lipid profile.
Harm (of using metformin)	Gastrointestinal adverse effects or potential for lactic acidosis and vitamin B_{12} deficiency, cost of medications, cost to administer, need for additional instruction about medication, self-monitoring blood glucose (SMBG), perceived difficulty of insulin use, possible metabolic deterioration if T1DM is misdiagnosed and treated as T2DM, potential risk of lactic acidosis in the setting of ketosis or significant dehydration. It should be noted that there have been no cases reported of vitamin B_{12} deficiency or lactic acidosis with the use of metformin in children.
Benefits-harms assessment	Preponderance of benefit over harm.
Value judgments	Committee members valued faster achievement of BG control over not medicating children.
Role of patient preferences	Moderate; precise implementation recommendations likely will be dictated by patient preferences regarding healthy nutrition, potential medication adverse reaction, exercise, and physical activity.
Exclusions	Although the recommendation to start metformin applies to all, certain children and adolescents with T2DM will not be able to tolerate metformin. In addition, certain older or more debilitated patients with T2DM may be restricted in the amount of moderate-to-vigorous exercise they can perform safely. Nevertheless, this recommendation applies to the vast majority of children and adolescents with T2DM.
Intentional vagueness	None.
Policy level	Strong recommendation.

Metformin as First-Line Therapy

Because of the low success rate with diet and exercise alone in pediatric patients diagnosed with T2DM, metformin should be initiated along with the promotion of lifestyle changes, unless insulin is needed to reverse glucose toxicity in the case of significant hyperglycemia or ketoacidosis (see Key Action Statement 1). Because gastrointestinal adverse effects are common with metformin therapy, the committee recommends starting the drug at a low dose of 500 mg daily, increasing by 500 mg every 1 to 2 weeks, up to an ideal and maximum dose of 2000 mg daily in divided doses.[41] It should be noted that the main gastrointestinal adverse effects (abdominal pain, bloating, loose stools) present at initiation of metformin often are transient and often disappear completely if medication is continued. Generally, doses higher than 2000 mg daily do not provide additional therapeutic benefit.[34,42,43] In addition, the use of extended-release metformin, especially with evening dosing, may be considered, although data regarding the frequency of adverse effects with this preparation are scarce. Metformin is generally better tolerated when taken with food. It is important to recognize the paucity of credible RCTs in adolescents with T2DM. The evidence to recommend initiating metformin at diagnosis along with lifestyle changes comes from 1 RCT, several observational studies, and consensus recommendations.

Lifestyle modifications (including nutrition interventions and increased physical activity) have long been the cornerstone of therapy for T2DM. Yet, medical practitioners recognize that effecting these changes is both challenging and often accompanied by regression over time to behaviors not conducive to maintaining the target range of BG concentrations. In pediatric patients, lifestyle change is most likely to be successful when a multidisciplinary approach is used and the entire family is involved. (Encouragement of healthy eating and physical exercise are discussed in Key Action Statements 5 and 6.) Unfortunately, efforts at lifestyle change often fail for a variety of reasons, including high rates of loss to follow-up; a high rate of depression in teenagers, which affects adherence; and peer pressure to participate in activities that often center on unhealthy eating.

Expert consensus is that fewer than 10% of pediatric T2DM patients will attain their BG goals through lifestyle interventions alone.[6,35,44] It is possible that the poor long-term success rates observed from lifestyle interventions stem from patients' perception that the intervention is not important because medications are not being prescribed. One might speculate that prescribing medications, particularly insulin therapy, may convey a greater degree of concern for the patient's health and the seriousness of the diagnosis, relative to that conveyed when medications are not needed, and that improved treatment adherence and follow-up may result from the use of medication. Indeed, 2 prospective observational studies revealed that treatment with lifestyle modification alone is associated with a higher rate of loss to follow-up than that found in patients who receive medication.[45]

Before initiating treatment with metformin, a number of important considerations must be taken into account. First, it is important to determine whether the child with a new diagnosis has T1DM or T2DM, and it is critical to err on the side of caution if there is any uncertainty. The 2009 *Clinical Practice Consensus Guidelines on Type 2 Diabetes in Children and Adolescents* from the International Society for Pediatric and Adolescent Diabetes provides more information on the classification of diabetes in children and adolescents with new diagnoses.[46] If the diagnosis is unclear (as may be the case when an obese child with diabetes presents also with ketosis), the adolescent must be treated with insulin until the T2DM diagnosis is confirmed.[47] Although it is recognized that some children with newly diagnosed T2DM may respond to metformin alone, the committee believes that the presence of either ketosis or ketoacidosis dictates an absolute initial requirement for insulin replacement. (This is addressed in Key Action Statement 1.)

Although there is little debate that a child presenting with significant hyperglycemia and/or ketosis requires insulin, children presenting with more modest levels of hyperglycemia (eg, random BG of 200–249 mg/dL) or asymptomatic T2DM present additional therapeutic challenges to the clinician. In such cases, metformin alone, insulin alone, or metformin with insulin all represent reasonable options. Additional agents are likely to become reasonable options for initial pharmacologic management in the near future. Although metformin and insulin are the only antidiabetic agents currently approved by the US Food and Drug Administration (FDA) for use in children, both thiazolidinediones and incretins are occasionally used in adolescents younger than 18 years.[48]

Metformin is recommended as the initial pharmacologic agent in adolescents presenting with mild hyperglycemia and without ketonuria or severe hyperglycemia. In addition to improving hepatic insulin sensitivity, metformin has a number of practical advantages over insulin:

- Potential weight loss or weight neutrality.[37,48]
- Because of a lower risk of hypoglycemia, less frequent finger-stick BG measurements are required with metformin, compared with insulin therapy or sulfonylureas.[37,42,49–51]
- Improves insulin sensitivity and may normalize menstrual cycles in females with polycystic ovary syndrome. (Because metformin may also improve fertility in patients with polycystic ovary syndrome, contraception is indicated for sexually active patients who wish to avoid pregnancy.)
- Taking pills does not have the discomfort associated with injections.
- Less instruction time is required to start oral medication, making it is easier for busy practitioners to prescribe.
- Adolescents do not always accept injections, so oral medication might enhance adherence.[52]

Potential advantages of insulin over metformin for treatment at diabetes onset include the following:

- Metabolic control may be achieved more rapidly with insulin compared with metformin therapy.[37]
- With appropriate education and targeting the regimen to the individual, adolescents are able to accept and use insulin therapy with improved metabolic outcomes.[53]

- Insulin offers theoretical benefits of improved metabolic control while preserving β-cell function or even reversing β-cell damage.[34,35]
- Initial use of insulin therapy may convey to the patient a sense of seriousness of the disease.[7,53]

Throughout the writing of these guidelines, the authors have been following the progress of the National Institute of Diabetes and Digestive and Kidney Diseases—supported Treatment Options for type 2 Diabetes in Adolescents and Youth (TODAY) trial,[54] designed to compare standard (metformin alone) therapy versus more aggressive therapy as the initial treatment of youth with recent-onset T2DM. Since the completion of these guidelines, results of the TODAY trial have become available and reveal that metformin alone is inadequate in effecting sustained glycemic control in the majority of youth with diabetes. The study also revealed that the addition of rosiglitazone to metformin is superior to metformin alone in preserving glycemic control. Direct application of these findings to clinical practice is problematic, however, because rosiglitazone is not FDA-approved for use in children, and its use, even in adults, is now severely restricted by the FDA because of serious adverse effects reported in adults. Thus, the results suggest that therapy that is more aggressive than metformin monotherapy may be required in these adolescents to prevent loss of glycemic control, but they do not provide specific guidance because it is not known whether the effect of the additional agent was specific to rosiglitazone or would be seen with the addition of other agents. Unfortunately, there are limited data for the use of other currently available oral or injected hypoglycemic agents in this age range, except for insulin. Therefore, the writing group for these guidelines continues to recommend metformin as first-line therapy in this age group but with close monitoring for glycemic deterioration and the early addition of insulin or another pharmacologic agent if needed.

Lifestyle Modification, Including Nutrition and Physical Activity

Although lifestyle changes are considered indispensable to reaching treatment goals in diabetes, no significant data from RCTs provide information on success rates with such an approach alone.

A potential downside for initiating lifestyle changes alone at T2DM onset is potential loss of patients to follow-up and worse health outcomes. The value of lifestyle modification in the management of adolescents with T2DM is likely forthcoming after a more detailed analysis of the lifestyle intervention arm of the multicenter TODAY trial becomes available.[54] As noted previously, although it was published after

plus-rosiglitazone intervention in maintaining glycemic control over time.[54]

Summary

As noted previously, metformin is a safe and effective agent for use at the time of diagnosis in conjunction with lifestyle changes. Although observational studies and expert opinion strongly support lifestyle changes as a key component of the regimen in addition to metformin, randomized trials are needed to delineate whether using lifestyle options alone is a reasonable first step in treating any select subgroups of children with T2DM.

Key Action Statement 3

The committee suggests that clinicians monitor HbA1c concentrations every 3 months and intensify treatment if treatment goals for BG and HbA1c concentrations are not being met. (Option: evidence quality D; expert opinion and studies in children with T1DM and in adults with T2DM; preponderance of benefits over harms.)

Action Statement Profile KAS 3

Aggregate evidence quality	D (expert opinion and studies in children with T1DM and in adults with T2DM; no studies have been performed in children and adolescents with T2DM).
Benefit	Diminishing the risk of progression of disease and deterioration resulting in hospitalization; prevention of microvascular complications of T2DM.
Harm	Potential for hypoglycemia from overintensifying treatment to reach HbA1c target goals; cost of frequent testing and medical consultation; possible patient discomfort.
Benefits-harms assessment	Preponderance of benefits over harms.
Value judgments	Recommendation dictated by widely accepted standards of diabetic care.
Role of patient preferences	Minimal; recommendation dictated by widely accepted standards of diabetic care.
Exclusions	None.
Intentional vagueness	Intentional vagueness in the recommendation as far as setting goals and intensifying treatment attributable to limited evidence.
Policy level	Option.

this guideline was developed, the TODAY trial indicated that results from the metformin-plus-lifestyle intervention were not significantly different from either metformin alone or the metformin-

HbA1c provides a measure of glycemic control in patients with diabetes mellitus and allows an estimation of the individual's average BG over the previous 8 to 12 weeks. No RCTs have

evaluated the relationship between glycemic control and the risk of developing microvascular and/or macrovascular complications in children and adolescents with T2DM. A number of studies of children with T1DM[55–57] and adults with T2DM have, however, shown a significant relationship between glycemic control (as measured by HbA1c concentration) and the risk of microvascular complications (eg, retinopathy, nephropathy, and neuropathy).[58,59] The relationship between HbA1c concentration and risk of microvascular complications appears to be curvilinear; the lower the HbA1c concentration, the lower the downstream risk of microvascular complications, with the greatest risk reduction seen at the highest HbA1c concentrations.[57]

It is generally recommended that HbA1c concentrations be measured every 3 months.[60] For adults with T1DM, the American Diabetes Association recommends target HbA1c concentrations of less than 7%; the American Association of Clinical Endocrinologists recommends target concentrations of less than 6.5%. Although HbA1c target concentrations for children and adolescents with T1DM are higher,[13] several review articles suggest target HbA1c concentrations of less than 7% for children and adolescents with T2DM.[40,61–63] The committee concurs that, ideally, target HbA1c concentration should be less than 7% but notes that specific goals must be achievable for the individual patient and that this concentration may not be applicable for all patients. For patients in whom a target concentration of less than 7% seems unattainable, individualized goals should be set, with the ultimate goal of reaching guideline target concentrations. In addition, in the absence of hypoglycemia, even lower HbA1c target concentrations can be considered on the basis of an absence of hypoglycemic events and other individual considerations.

When concentrations are found to be above the target, therapy should be intensified whenever possible, with the goal of bringing the concentration to target. Intensification activities may include, but are not limited to, increasing the frequency of clinic visits, engaging in more frequent BG monitoring, adding 1 or more antidiabetic agents, meeting with a registered dietitian and/or diabetes educator, and increasing attention to diet and exercise regimens. Patients whose HbA1c concentrations remain relatively stable may only need to be tested every 6 months. Ideally, real-time HbA1c concentrations should be available at the time of the patient's visit with the clinician to allow the physician and patient and/or parent to discuss intensification of therapy during the visit, if needed.

Key Action Statement 4

The committee suggests that clinicians advise patients to monitor finger-stick BG concentrations in those who

a. **are taking insulin or other medications with a risk of hypoglycemia; or**

b. **are initiating or changing their diabetes treatment regimen; or**

c. **have not met treatment goals; or**

d. **have intercurrent illnesses.**

(Option: evidence quality D; expert consensus. Preponderance of benefits over harms.)

Action Statement Profile KAS 4

Aggregate evidence quality	D (expert consensus).
Benefit	Potential for improved metabolic control, improved potential for prevention of hypoglycemia, decreased long-term complications.
Harm	Patient discomfort, cost of materials.
Benefits-harms assessment	Benefit over harm.
Value judgments	Despite lack of evidence, there were general committee perceptions that patient safety concerns related to insulin use or clinical status outweighed any risks from monitoring.
Role of patient preferences	Moderate to low; recommendation driven primarily by safety concerns.
Exclusions	None.
Intentional vagueness	Intentional vagueness in the recommendation about specific approaches attributable to lack of evidence and the need to individualize treatment.
Policy level	Option.

Glycemic control correlates closely with the frequency of BG monitoring in adolescents with T1DM.[64,65] Although studies evaluating the efficacy of frequent BG monitoring have not been conducted in children and adolescents with T2DM, benefits have been described in insulin-treated adults with T2DM who tested their BG 4 times per day, compared with adults following a less frequent monitoring regimen.[66] These data support the value of BG monitoring in adults treated with insulin, and likely are relevant to youth with T2DM as well, especially those treated with insulin, at the onset of the disease, when treatment goals are not met, and when the treatment regimen is changed. The committee believes that current (2011) ADA recommendations for finger-stick BG monitoring apply to most youth with T2DM[67]:

- Finger-stick BG monitoring should be performed 3 or more times daily for patients using multiple insulin injections or insulin pump therapy.

- For patients using less-frequent insulin injections, noninsulin therapies, or medical nutrition therapy alone, finger-stick BG monitoring may be useful as a guide to the success of therapy.

- To achieve postprandial glucose targets, postprandial finger-stick BG monitoring may be appropriate.

Recognizing that current practices may not always reflect optimal care, a 2004 survey of practices among members of the PES revealed that 36% of pediatric endocrinologists asked their pediatric patients with T2DM to monitor BG concentrations twice daily; 12% asked patients to do so once daily; 13% asked patients to do so 3 times per day; and 12% asked patients to do so 4 times daily.[61] The questionnaire provided to the pediatric endocrinologists did not ask about the frequency of BG monitoring in relationship to the diabetes regimen, however.

Although normoglycemia may be difficult to achieve in adolescents with T2DM, a fasting BG concentration of 70 to 130 mg/dL is a reasonable target for most. In addition, because postprandial hyperglycemia has been associated with increased risk of cardiovascular events in adults, postprandial BG testing may be valuable in select patients. BG concentrations obtained 2 hours after meals (and paired with pre-meal concentrations) provide an index of glycemic excursion, and may be useful in improving glycemic control, particularly for the patient whose fasting plasma glucose is normal but whose HbA1c is not at target.[68] Recognizing the limited evidence for benefit of FSBG testing in this population, the committee provides suggested guidance for testing frequency, tailored to the medication regimen, as follows:

BG Testing Frequency for Patients With Newly Diagnosed T2DM: Fasting, Premeal, and Bedtime Testing

The committee suggests that all patients with newly diagnosed T2DM, regardless of prescribed treatment plan, should perform finger-stick BG monitoring before meals (including a morning fasting concentration) and at bedtime until reasonable metabolic control is achieved.[69] Once BG concentrations are at target levels, the frequency of monitoring can be modified depending on the medication used, the regimen's intensity, and the patient's metabolic control. Patients who are prone to marked hyperglycemia or hypoglycemia or who are on a therapeutic regimen associated with increased risk of hypoglycemia will require continued frequent BG testing. Expectations for frequency and timing of BG monitoring should be clearly defined through shared goal-setting between the patient and clinician. The adolescent and family members should be given a written action plan stating the medication regimen, frequency and timing of expected BG monitoring, as well as follow-up instructions.

BG Testing Frequency for Patients on Single Insulin Daily Injections and Oral Agents

Single bedtime long-acting insulin: The simplest insulin regimen consists of a single injection of long-acting insulin at bedtime (basal insulin only). The appropriateness of the insulin dose for patients using this regimen is best defined by the fasting/prebreakfast BG test. For patients on this insulin regimen, the committee suggests daily fasting BG measurements. This regimen is associated with some risk of hypoglycemia (especially overnight or fasting hypoglycemia) and may not provide adequate insulin coverage for mealtime ingestions throughout the day, as reflected by fasting BG concentrations in target, but daytime readings above target. In such cases, treatment with meglitinide (Prandin [Novo Nordisk Pharmaceuticals] or Starlix [Novartis Pharmaceuticals]) or a short-acting insulin before meals (see below) may be beneficial.

Oral agents: Once treatment goals are met, the frequency of monitoring can be decreased; however, the committee recommends some continued BG testing for all youth with T2DM, at a frequency determined within the clinical context (e.g. medication regimen, HbA1c, willingness of the patient, etc.). For example, an infrequent or intermittent monitoring schedule may be adequate when the patient is using exclusively an oral agent associated with a low risk of hypoglycemia and if HbA1c concentrations are in the ideal or non-diabetic range. A more frequent monitoring schedule should be advised during times of illness or if symptoms of hyperglycemia or hypoglycemia develop.

Oral agent plus a single injection of a long-acting insulin: Some youth with T2DM can be managed successfully with a single injection of long-acting insulin in conjunction with an oral agent. Twice a day BG monitoring (fasting plus a second BG concentration — ideally 2-hour post prandial) often is recommended, as long as HbA1c and BG concentrations remain at goal and the patient remains asymptomatic.

BG Testing Frequency for Patients Receiving Multiple Daily Insulin Injections (eg, Basal Bolus Regimens): Premeal and Bedtime Testing

Basal bolus regimens are commonly used in children and youth with T1DM and may be appropriate for some youth with T2DM as well. They are the most labor intensive, providing both basal insulin plus bolus doses of short-acting insulin at meals. Basal insulin is provided through either the use of long-acting, relatively peak-free insulin (by needle) or via an insulin pump. Bolus insulin doses are given at meal-time, using one of the rapid-acting insulin analogs. The bolus dose is calculated by using a correction algorithm for the premeal BG concentration as well as a "carb ratio," in which 1 unit of

a rapid-acting insulin analog is given for "X" grams of carbohydrates ingested (see box below). When using this method, the patient must be willing and able to count the number of grams of carbohydrates in the meal and divide by the assigned "carb ratio (X)" to know how many units of insulin should be taken. In addition, the patient must always check BG concentrations before the meal to determine how much additional insulin should be given as a correction dose using an algorithm assigned by the care team if the fasting BG is not in target. Insulin pumps are based on this concept of "basal-bolus" insulin administration and have the capability of calculating a suggested bolus dosage, based on inputted grams of carbohydrates and BG concentrations. Because the BG value determines the amount of insulin to be given at each meal, the recommended testing frequency for patients on this regimen is before every meal.

Box 1 Example of Basal Bolus Insulin Regimen

If an adolescent has a BG of 250 mg/dL, is to consume a meal containing 60 g of carbohydrates, with a carbohydrate ratio of 1:10 and an assigned correction dose of 1:25>125 (with 25 being the insulin sensitivity and 125 mg/dL the target blood glucose level), the mealtime bolus dose of insulin would be as follows:

60 g/10 "carb ratio" =

6 units rapid-acting insulin for meal

plus

(250−125)/25 = 125/25 =

5 units rapid-acting insulin for correction

Thus, total bolus insulin coverage at mealtime is: **11 U** (6 + 5) of rapid-acting insulin.

Key Action Statement 5

The committee suggests that clinicians incorporate the Academy of Nutrition and Dietetics' *Pediatric Weight Management Evidence-Based Nutrition Practice Guidelines* **in the nutrition counseling of patients with T2DM both at the time of diagnosis and as part of ongoing management. (Option; evidence quality D; expert opinion; preponderance of benefits over harms. Role of patient preference is dominant.)**

Action Statement Profile KAS 5

Aggregate evidence quality	D (expert opinion).
Benefit	Promotes weight loss; improves insulin sensitivity; contributes to glycemic control; prevents worsening of disease; facilitates a sense of well-being; and improves cardiovascular health.
Harm	Costs of nutrition counseling; inadequate reimbursement of clinicians' time; lost opportunity costs vis-a-vis time and resources spent in other counseling activities.
Benefits-harms assessment	Benefit over harm.
Value judgments	There is a broad societal agreement on the benefits of dietary recommendations.
Role of patient preference	Dominant. Patients may have different preferences for how they wish to receive assistance in managing their weight-loss goals. Some patients may prefer a referral to a nutritionist while others might prefer accessing online sources of help. Patient preference should play a significant role in determining an appropriate weight-loss strategy.
Exclusions	None.
Intentional vagueness	Intentional vagueness in the recommendation about specific approaches attributable to lack of evidence and the need to individualize treatment.
Policy level	Option.

Consuming more calories than one uses results in weight gain and is a major contributor to the increasing incidence of T2DM in children and adolescents. Current literature is inconclusive about a single best meal plan for patients with diabetes mellitus, however, and studies specifically addressing the diet of children and adolescents with T2DM are limited. Challenges to making recommendations stem from the small sample size of these studies, limited specificity for children and adolescents, and difficulties in generalizing the data from dietary research studies to the general population.

Although evidence is lacking in children with T2DM, numerous studies have been conducted in overweight children and adolescents, because the great majority of children with T2DM are obese or overweight at diagnosis.[26] The committee suggests that clinicians encourage children and adolescents with T2DM to follow the Academy of Nutrition and Dietetics' recommendations for maintaining healthy weight to promote health and reduce obesity in this population. The committee recommends that clinicians refer patients to a registered dietitian who has expertise in the nutritional needs of youth with T2DM. Clinicians should incorporate the Academy of Nutrition and Dietetics' *Pediatric Weight Management Evidence-Based Nutrition Practice Guidelines*, which describe effective, evidence-based treatment options for weight management, summarized below (A complete list of these recommendations is accessible to health care professionals at: http://www.andevidencelibrary.com/topic.cfm?cat=4102&auth=1.)

According to the Academy of Nutrition and Dietetics' guidelines, when incorporated with lifestyle changes, balanced macronutrient diets at 900 to 1200 kcal per day are associated with both short- and long-term (eg, ≥ 1 year) improvements in weight status and body composition in children 6 to 12 years of age.[70] These calorie recommendations are to be incorporated with lifestyle changes, including increased activity and possibly medication. Restrictions of no less than 1200 kcal per day in adolescents 13 to 18 years old result in improved weight status and body composition as well.[71] The Diabetes Prevention Program demonstrated that participants assigned to the intensive lifestyle-intervention arm had a reduction in daily energy intake of 450 kcal and a 58% reduction in progression to diabetes at the 2.8-year follow-up.[71] At the study's end, 50% of the lifestyle-arm participants had achieved the goal weight loss of at least 7% after the 24-week curriculum and 38% showed weight loss of at least 7% at the time of their most recent visit.[72] The Academy of Nutrition and Dietetics recommends that protein-sparing, modified-fast (ketogenic) diets be restricted to children who are >120% of their ideal body weight and who have a serious medical complication that would benefit from rapid weight loss.[71] Specific recommendations are for the intervention to be short-term (typically 10 weeks) and to be conducted under the supervision of a multidisciplinary team specializing in pediatric obesity.

Regardless of the meal plan prescribed, some degree of nutrition education must be provided to maximize adherence and positive results. This education should encourage patients to follow healthy eating patterns, such as consuming 3 meals with planned snacks per day, not eating while watching television or using computers, using smaller plates to make portions appear larger, and leaving small amounts of food on the plate.[73] Common dietary recommendations to reduce calorie intake and to promote weight loss in children include the following: (1) eating regular meals and snacks; (2) reducing portion sizes; (3) choosing calorie-free beverages, except for milk; (4) limiting juice to 1 cup per day; (5) increasing consumption of fruits and vegetables; (6) consuming 3 or 4 servings of low-fat dairy products per day; (7) limiting intake of high-fat foods; (8) limiting frequency and size of snacks; and (9) reducing calories consumed in fast-food meals.[74]

Key Action Statement 6

The committee suggests that clinicians encourage children and adolescents with T2DM to engage in moderate-to-vigorous exercise for at least 60 minutes daily and to limit nonacademic screen time to less than 2 hours per day. (Option: evidence quality D, expert opinion and evidence from studies of metabolic syndrome and obesity; preponderance of benefits over harms. Role of patient preference is dominant.)

Action Statement Profile KAS 6

Aggregate evidence quality	D (expert opinion and evidence from studies of metabolic syndrome and obesity).
Benefit	Promotes weight loss; contributes to glycemic control; prevents worsening of disease; facilitates the ability to perform exercise; improves the person's sense of well-being; and fosters cardiovascular health.
Harm	Cost for patient of counseling, food, and time; costs for clinician in taking away time that could be spent on other activities; inadequate reimbursement for clinician's time.
Benefits-harms assessment	Preponderance of benefit over harm.
Value judgments	Broad consensus.
Role of patient preference	Dominant. Patients may seek various forms of exercise. Patient preference should play a significant role in creating an exercise plan.
Exclusions	Although certain older or more debilitated patients with T2DM may be restricted in the amount of moderate-to-vigorous exercise they can perform safely, this recommendation applies to the vast majority of children and adolescents with T2DM.
Intentional vagueness	Intentional vagueness on the sequence of follow-up contact attributable to the lack of evidence and the need to individualize care.
Policy level	Option.

Recommendations From the Academy of Nutrition and Dietetics

Pediatric Weight Management Evidence-Based Nutrition Practice Guidelines

Recommendation	Strength
Interventions to reduce pediatric obesity should be multicomponent and include diet, physical activity, nutritional counseling, and parent or caregiver participation.	Strong
A nutrition prescription should be formulated as part of the dietary intervention in a multicomponent pediatric weight management program.	Strong
Dietary factors that may be associated with an increased risk of overweight are increased total dietary fat intake and increased intake of calorically sweetened beverages.	Strong
Dietary factors that may be associated with a decreased risk of overweight are increased fruit and vegetable intake.	Strong
A balanced macronutrient diet that contains no fewer than 900 kcal per day is recommended to improve weight status in children aged 6–12 y who are medically monitored.	Strong
A balanced macronutrient diet that contains no fewer than 1200 kcal per day is recommended to improve weight status in adolescents aged 13–18 y who are medically monitored.	Strong
Family diet behaviors that are associated with an increased risk of pediatric obesity are parental restriction of highly palatable foods, consumption of food away from home, increased meal portion size, and skipping breakfast.	Fair

Engaging in Physical Activity

Physical activity is an integral part of weight management for prevention and treatment of T2DM. Although there is a paucity of available data from children and adolescents with T2DM, several well-controlled studies performed in obese children and adolescents at risk of metabolic syndrome and T2DM provide guidelines for physical activity. (See the Resources section for tools on this subject.) A summary of the references supporting the evidence for this guideline can be found in the technical report.[31]

At present, moderate-to-vigorous exercise of at least 60 minutes daily is recommended for reduction of BMI and improved glycemic control in patients with T2DM.[75] "Moderate to vigorous exercise" is defined as exercise that makes the individual breathe hard and perspire and that raises his or her heart rate. An easy way to define exercise intensity for patients is the "talk test"; during moderate physical activity a person can talk but not sing. During vigorous activity, a person cannot talk without pausing to catch a breath.[76]

Adherence may be improved if clinicians provide the patient with a written prescription to engage in physical activity, including a "dose" describing ideal duration, intensity, and frequency.[75] When prescribing physical exercise, clinicians are encouraged to be sensitive to the needs of children, adolescents, and their families. Routine, organized exercise may be beyond the family's logistical and/or financial means, and some families may not be able to provide structured exercise programs for their children. It is most helpful to recommend an individualized approach that can be incorporated into the daily routine, is tailored to the patients' physical abilities and preferences, and recognizes the families' circumstances.[77] For example, clinicians might recommend only daily walking, which has been shown to improve weight loss and insulin sensitivity in adults with T2DM[78] and may constitute "moderate to vigorous activity" for some children with T2DM. It is also important to recognize that the recommended 60 minutes of exercise do not have to be accomplished in 1 session but can be completed through several, shorter increments (eg, 10–15 minutes). Patients should be encouraged to identify a variety of forms of activity that can be performed both easily and frequently.[77] In addition, providers should be cognizant of the potential need to adjust the medication dosage, especially if the patient is receiving insulin, when initiating an aggressive physical activity program.

Reducing Screen Time

Screen time contributes to a sedentary lifestyle, especially when the child or adolescent eats while watching television or playing computer games. The US Department of Health and Human Services recommends that individuals limit "screen time" spent watching television and/or using computers and handheld devices to less than 2 hours per day unless the use is related to work or homework.[79] Physical activity may be gained either through structured games and sports or through everyday activities, such as walking, ideally with involvement of the parents as good role models.

Increased screen time and food intake and reduced physical activity are associated with obesity. There is good evidence that modifying these factors can help prevent T2DM by reducing the individual's rate of weight gain. The evidence profile in pediatric patients with T2DM is inadequate at this time, however. Pending new data, the committee suggests that clinicians follow the AAP Committee on Nutrition's guideline, *Prevention of Pediatric Overweight and Obesity.* The guideline recommends restricting nonacademic screen time to a maximum of 2 hours per day and discouraging the presence of video screens and television sets in children's bedrooms.[80–82] The American Medical Association's Expert Panel on Childhood Obesity has endorsed this guideline.

Valuable recommendations for enhancing patient health include the following:

- With patients and their families, jointly determining an individualized plan that includes specific goals to reduce sedentary behaviors and increase physical activity.
- Providing a written prescription for engaging in 60-plus minutes of moderate-to-vigorous physical activities per day that includes

dose, timing, and duration. It is important for clinicians to be sensitive to the needs of children, adolescents, and their families in encouraging daily physical exercise. Graded duration of exercise is recommended for those youth who cannot initially be active for 60 minutes daily, and the exercise may be accomplished through several, shorter increments (eg, 10–15 minutes).

- Incorporating physical activities into children's and adolescents' daily routines. Physical activity may be gained either through structured games and sports or through everyday activities, such as walking.
- Restricting nonacademic screen time to a maximum of 2 hours per day.
- Discouraging the presence of video screens and television sets in children's bedrooms.

Conversations pertaining to the Key Action Statements should be clearly documented in the patient's medical record.

AREAS FOR FUTURE RESEARCH

As noted previously, evidence for medical interventions in children in general is scant and is especially lacking for interventions directed toward children who have developed diseases not previously seen commonly in youth, such as childhood T2DM. Recent studies such as the Search for Diabetes in Youth Study (SEARCH)—an observational multicenter study in 2096 youth with T2DM funded by the Centers for Disease Control and Prevention and the National Institute of Diabetes and Digestive and Kidney Diseases—now provide a detailed description of childhood diabetes. Subsequent trials will describe the short-term and enduring effects of specific interventions on the progression of the disease with time.

Although it is likely that children and adolescents with T2DM have an aggressive form of diabetes, as reflected by the age of onset, future research should determine whether the associated comorbidities and complications of diabetes also are more aggressive in pediatric populations than in adults and if they are more or less responsive to therapeutic interventions. Additional research should explore whether early introduction of insulin or the use of particular oral agents will preserve β-cell function in these children, and whether recent technologic advances (such as continuous glucose monitoring and insulin pumps) will benefit this population. Additional issues that require further study include the following:

- To delineate whether using lifestyle options without medication is a reliable first step in treating selected children with T2DM.

- To determine whether BG monitoring should be recommended to all children and youth with T2DM, regardless of therapy used; what the optimal frequency of BG monitoring is for pediatric patients on the basis of treatment regimen; and which subgroups will be able to successfully maintain glycemic goals with less frequent monitoring.

- To explore the efficacy of school- and clinic-based diet and physical activity interventions to prevent and manage pediatric T2DM.

- To explore the association between increased "screen time" and reduced physical activity with respect to T2DM's risk factors.

RESOURCES

Several tools are available online to assist providers in improving patient adherence to lifestyle modifications, including examples of activities to be recommended for patients:

- The American Academy of Pediatrics:
  - www.healthychildren.org
  - www.letsmove.gov
  - Technical Report: Management of Type 2 Diabetes Mellitus in Children and Adolescents.[31]
    - Includes an overview and screening tools for a variety of comorbidities.
  - Gahagan S, Silverstein J; Committee on Native American Child Health and Section on Endocrinology. Clinical report: prevention and treatment of type 2 diabetes mellitus in children, with special emphasis on American Indian and Alaska Native Children. *Pediatrics.* 2003;112 (4):e328–e347. Available at: http://www.pediatrics.org/cgi/content/full/112/4/e328[63]
    - Fig 3 presents a screening tool for microalbumin.
  - Bright Futures: http://brightfutures.aap.org/
  - Daniels SR, Greer FR; Committee on Nutrition. Lipid screening and cardiovascular health in childhood. *Pediatrics.* 2008;122 (1):198–208. Available at:
- The American Diabetes Association: www.diabetes.org
  - Management of dyslipidemia in children and adolescents with diabetes. *Diabetes Care.* 2003;26(7):2194–2197. Available at: http://care.diabetesjournals. org/content/26/7/2194.full
- Academy of Nutrition and Dietetics:
  - http://www.eatright.org/childhoodobesity/
  - http://www.eatright.org/kids/
  - http://www.eatright.org/cps/rde/xchg/ada/hs.xsl/index.html

- Pediatric Weight Management Evidence-Based Nutrition Practice Guidelines: http://www.adaevidencelibrary.com/topic.cfm?cat=2721
- American Heart Association:
  - American Heart Association *Circulation.* 2006 Dec 12;114(24):2710-2738. Epub 2006 Nov 27. Review.
- Centers for Disease Control and Prevention:
  - http://www.cdc.gov/obesity/childhood/solutions.html
  - BMI and other growth charts can be downloaded and printed from the CDC Web site: http://www.cdc.gov/growth-charts.
  - Center for Epidemiologic Studies Depression Scale (CES-D): http://www.chcr.brown.edu/pcoc/cesdscale.pdf; see attachments
- *Diagnostic and Statistical Manual of Mental Disorders.* 4th ed. Washington, DC: American Psychiatric Association; 1994
- Let's Move Campaign: www.letsmove.gov
- The Reach Institute. *Guidelines for Adolescent Depression in Primary Care (GLAD-PC) Toolkit,* 2007. Contains a listing of the criteria for major depressive disorder as defined by the DSM-IV-TR. Available at: http://www.gladpc.org
- The National Heart, Lung, and Blood Institute (NHLBI) hypertension guidelines: http://www.nhlbi.nih.gov/guidelines/hypertension/child_tbl.htm
- The National Diabetes Education Program and TIP sheets (including tip sheets on youth transitioning to adulthood and adult providers, Staying Active, Eating Healthy, Ups and Downs of Diabetes, etc): www.ndep.nih.gov or www.yourdiabetesinfo.org

- National High Blood Pressure Education Program Working Group on High Blood Pressure in Children and Adolescents, The Fourth Report on the Diagnosis, Evaluation, and Treatment of High Blood Pressure in Children and Adolescents: *Pediatrics*. 2004;114:555–576. Available at: http://pediatrics.aappublications.org/content/114/Supplement_2/555.long

- National Initiative for Children's Healthcare Quality (NICHQ): childhood obesity section: http://www.nichq.org/childhood_obesity/index.html

- The National Institute of Child Health and Human Development (NICHD): www.NICHD.org

- President's Council on Physical Fitness and Sports: http://www.presidentchallenge.org/home_kids.aspx

- US Department of Agriculture's "My Pyramid" Web site:

- http://www.choosemyplate.gov/

- http://fnic.nal.usda.gov/life-cycle-nutrition/child-nutrition-and-health

SUBCOMMITTEE ON TYPE 2 DIABETES (OVERSIGHT BY THE STEERING COMMITTEE ON QUALITY IMPROVEMENT AND MANAGEMENT, 2008–2012)

Kenneth Claud Copeland, MD, FAAP: Co-chair—Endocrinology and Pediatric Endocrine Society Liaison (2009: Novo Nordisk, Genentech, Endo [National Advisory Groups]; 2010: Novo Nordisk [National Advisory Group]); published research related to type 2 diabetes

Janet Silverstein, MD, FAAP: Co-chair—Endocrinology and American Diabetes Association Liaison (small grants with Pfizer, Novo Nordisk, and Lilly; grant review committee for Genentech; was on an advisory committee for Sanofi Aventis, and Abbott Laboratories for a 1-time meeting); published research related to type 2 diabetes

Kelly Roberta Moore, MD, FAAP: General Pediatrics, Indian Health, AAP Committee on Native American Child Health Liaison (board member of the Merck Company Foundation Alliance to Reduce Disparities in Diabetes. Their national program office is the University of Michigan's Center for Managing Chronic Disease.)

Greg Edward Prazar, MD, FAAP: General Pediatrics (no conflicts)

Terry Raymer, MD, CDE: Family Medicine, Indian Health Service (no conflicts)

Richard N. Shiffman, MD, FAAP: Partnership for Policy Implementation Informatician, General Pediatrics (no conflicts)

Shelley C. Springer, MD, MBA, FAAP: Epidemiologist (no conflicts)

Meaghan Anderson, MS, RD, LD, CDE: Academy of Nutrition and Dietetics Liaison (formerly a Certified Pump Trainer for Animas)

Stephen J. Spann, MD, MBA, FAAFP: American Academy of Family Physicians Liaison (no conflicts)

Vidhu V. Thaker, MD, FAAP: QuIIN Liaison, General Pediatrics (no conflicts)

CONSULTANT

Susan K. Flinn, MA: Medical Writer (no conflicts)

STAFF

Caryn Davidson, MA

REFERENCES

1. Centers for Disease Control and Prevention. Data and Statistics. Obesity rates among children in the United States. Available at: www.cdc.gov/obesity/childhood/prevalence.html. Accessed August 13, 2012

2. Copeland KC, Chalmers LJ, Brown RD. Type 2 diabetes in children: oxymoron or medical metamorphosis? *Pediatr Ann*. 2005;34(9):686–697

3. Narayan KM, Boyle JP, Thompson TJ, Sorensen SW, Williamson DF. Lifetime risk for diabetes mellitus in the United States. *JAMA*. 2003;290(14):1884–1890

4. Chopra M, Galbraith S, Darnton-Hill I. A global response to a global problem: the epidemic of overnutrition. *Bull World Health Organ*. 2002;80(12):952–958

5. Liese AD, D'Agostino RB, Jr, Hamman RF, et al; SEARCH for Diabetes in Youth Study Group. The burden of diabetes mellitus among US youth: prevalence estimates from the SEARCH for Diabetes in Youth Study. *Pediatrics*. 2006;118(4):1510–1518

6. Silverstein JH, Rosenbloom AL. Type 2 diabetes in children. *Curr Diab Rep*. 2001;1(1):19–27

7. Pinhas-Hamiel O, Zeitler P. Clinical presentation and treatment of type 2 diabetes in children. *Pediatr Diabetes*. 2007;8(suppl 9):16–27

8. Dabelea D, Bell RA, D'Agostino RB Jr, et al; Writing Group for the SEARCH for Diabetes in Youth Study Group. Incidence of diabetes in youth in the United States. *JAMA*. 2007;297(24):2716–2724

9. Mayer-Davis EJ, Bell RA, Dabelea D, et al; SEARCH for Diabetes in Youth Study Group. The many faces of diabetes in American youth: type 1 and type 2 diabetes in five race and ethnic populations: the SEARCH for Diabetes in Youth Study. *Diabetes Care*. 2009;32(suppl 2):S99–S101

10. Copeland KC, Zeitler P, Geffner M, et al; TODAY Study Group. Characteristics of adolescents and youth with recent-onset type 2 diabetes: the TODAY cohort at baseline. *J Clin Endocrinol Metab*. 2011;96(1):159–167

11. Narayan KM, Williams R. Diabetes—a global problem needing global solutions. *Prim Care Diabetes*. 2009;3(1):3–4

12. Wild S, Roglic G, Green A, Sicree R, King H. Global prevalence of diabetes: estimates for the year 2000 and projections for 2030. *Diabetes Care*. 2004;27(5):1047–1053

13. Silverstein J, Klingensmith G, Copeland K, et al; American Diabetes Association. Care of children and adolescents with type 1 diabetes: a statement of the American Diabetes Association. *Diabetes Care*. 2005;28(1):186–212

14. Pinhas-Hamiel O, Zeitler P. Barriers to the treatment of adolescent type 2 diabetes—a survey of provider perceptions. *Pediatr Diabetes*. 2003;4(1):24–28

15. Moore KR, McGowan MK, Donato KA, Kollipara S, Roubideaux Y. Community resources for promoting youth nutrition and physical activity. *Am J Health Educ*. 2009;40(5):298–303

16. Zeitler P, Epstein L, Grey M, et al; The TODAY Study Group. Treatment Options for type 2 diabetes mellitus in Adolescents and Youth: a study of the comparative efficacy of metformin alone or in combination with rosiglitazone or lifestyle intervention in adolescents with type 2 diabetes mellitus. *Pediatr Diabetes*. 2007;8(2):74–87

17. Kane MP, Abu-Baker A, Busch RS. The utility of oral diabetes medications in type 2

diabetes of the young. *Curr Diabetes Rev.* 2005;1(1):83–92

18. De Berardis G, Pellegrini F, Franciosi M, et al. Quality of care and outcomes in type 2 diabetes patientes. *Diabetes Care.* 2004;27 (2):398–406

19. Ziemer DC, Miller CD, Rhee MK, et al. Clinical inertia contributes to poor diabetes control in a primary care setting. *Diabetes Educ.* 2005;31(4):564–571

20. Bradshaw B. The role of the family in managing therapy in minority children with type 2 diabetes mellitus. *J Pediatr Endocrinol Metab.* 2002;15(suppl 1):547–551

21. Pinhas-Hamiel O, Standiford D, Hamiel D, Dolan LM, Cohen R, Zeitler PS. The type 2 family: a setting for development and treatment of adolescent type 2 diabetes mellitus. *Arch Pediatr Adolesc Med.* 1999; 153(10):1063–1067

22. Mulvaney SA, Schlundt DG, Mudasiru E, et al. Parent perceptions of caring for adolescents with type 2 diabetes. *Diabetes Care.* 2006;29(5):993–997

23. Summerbell CD, Ashton V, Campbell KJ, Edmunds L, Kelly S, Waters E. Interventions for treating obesity in children. *Cochrane Database Syst Rev.* 2003;(3):CD001872

24. Skinner AC, Weinberger M, Mulvaney S, Schlundt D, Rothman RL. Accuracy of perceptions of overweight and relation to self-care behaviors among adolescents with type 2 diabetes and their parents. *Diabetes Care.* 2008;31(2):227–229

25. American Diabetes Association. Type 2 diabetes in children and adolescents. *Diabetes Care.* 2000;23(3):381–389

26. Pinhas-Hamiel O, Zeitler P. Type 2 diabetes in adolescents, no longer rare. *Pediatr Rev.* 1998;19(12):434–435

27. Fagot-Campagna A, Pettitt DJ, Engelgau MM, et al. Type 2 diabetes among North American children and adolescents: an epidemiologic review and a public health perspective. *J Pediatr.* 2000;136(5):664–672

28. Rothman RL, Mulvaney S, Elasy TA, et al. Self-management behaviors, racial disparities, and glycemic control among adolescents with type 2 diabetes. *Pediatrics.* 2008;121(4). Available at: www.pediatrics. org/cgi/content/full/121/4/e912

29. Scott CR, Smith JM, Cradock MM, Pihoker C. Characteristics of youth-onset noninsulin-dependent diabetes mellitus and insulin-dependent diabetes mellitus at diagnosis. *Pediatrics.* 1997;100(1):84–91

30. Libman IM, Pietropaolo M, Arslanian SA, LaPorte RE, Becker DJ. Changing prevalence of overweight children and adolescents at onset of insulin-treated diabetes. *Diabetes Care.* 2003;26(10):2871–2875

31. Springer SC, Copeland KC, Silverstein J, et al. Technical report: management of type 2 diabetes mellitus in children and adolescents. *Pediatrics.* 2012, In press

32. American Academy of Pediatrics Steering Committee on Quality Improvement and Management. Classifying recommendations for clinical practice guidelines. *Pediatrics.* 2004;114(3):874–877

33. Shiffman RN, Dixon J, Brandt C, et al. The GuideLine Implementability Appraisal (GLIA): development of an instrument to identify obstacles to guideline implementation. *BMC Med Inform Decis Mak.* 2005;5:23

34. Gungor N, Hannon T, Libman I, Bacha F, Arslanian S. Type 2 diabetes mellitus in youth: the complete picture to date. *Pediatr Clin North Am.* 2005;52(6):1579–1609

35. Daaboul JJ, Siverstein JH. The management of type 2 diabetes in children and adolescents. *Minerva Pediatr.* 2004;56(3):255–264

36. Kadmon PM, Grupposo PA. Glycemic control with metformin or insulin therapy in adolescents with type 2 diabetes mellitus. *J Pediatr Endocrinol.* 2004;17(9):1185–1193

37. Owada M, Nitadori Y, Kitagawa T. Treatment of NIDDM in youth. *Clin Pediatr (Phila).* 1998;37(2):117–121

38. Pinhas-Hamiel O, Zeitler P. Advances in epidemiology and treatment of type 2 diabetes in children. *Adv Pediatr.* 2005;52: 223–259

39. Jones KL, Haghi M. Type 2 diabetes mellitus in children and adolescence: a primer. *Endocrinologist.* 2000;10:389–396

40. Kawahara R, Amemiya T, Yoshino M, et al. Dropout of young non-insulin-dependent diabetics from diabetic care. *Diabetes Res Clin Pract.* 1994;24(3):181–185

41. Kaufman FR. Type 2 diabetes mellitus in children and youth: a new epidemic. *J Pediatr Endocrinol Metab.* 2002;15(suppl 2): 737–744

42. Garber AJ, Duncan TG, Goodman AM, Mills DJ, Rohlf JL. Efficacy of metformin in type II diabetes: results of a double-blind, placebo-controlled, dose-response trial. *Am J Med.* 1997;103(6):491–497

43. Dabelea D, Pettitt DJ, Jones KL, Arslanian SA. Type 2 diabetes mellitus in minority children and adolescents: an emerging problem. *Endocrinol Metabo Clin North Am.* 1999;28(4):709–729

44. Miller JL, Silverstein JH. The management of type 2 diabetes mellitus in children and adolescents. *J Pediatr Endocrinol Metab.* 2005;18(2):111–123

45. Reinehr T, Schober E, Roth CL, Wiegand S, Holl R; DPV-Wiss Study Group. Type 2 diabetes in children and adolescents in a 2-year

follow-up: insufficient adherence to diabetes centers. *Horm Res.* 2008;69(2):107–113

46. Rosenbloom AL, Silverstein JH, Amemiya S, Zeitler P, Klingensmith GJ. Type 2 diabetes in children and adolescents. *Pediatr Diabetes.* 2009;10(suppl 12):17–32

47. Zuhri-Yafi MI, Brosnan PG, Hardin DS. Treatment of type 2 diabetes mellitus in children and adolescents. *J Pediatr Endocrinol Metab.* 2002;15(suppl 1):541–546

48. Rapaport R, Silverstein JH, Garzarella L, Rosenbloom AL. Type 1 and type 2 diabetes mellitus in childhood in the United States: practice patterns by pediatric endocrinologists. *J Pediatr Endocrinol Metab.* 2004;17 (6):871–877

49. Glaser N, Jones KL. Non-insulin-dependent diabetes mellitus in children and adolescents. *Adv Pediatr.* 1996;43:359–396

50. Miller JL, Silverstein JH. The treatment of type 2 diabetes mellitus in youth: which therapies? *Treat Endocrinol.* 2006;5(4):201–210

51. Silverstein JH, Rosenbloom AL. Treatment of type 2 diabetes mellitus in children and adolescents. *J Pediatr Endocrinol Metab.* 2000;13(suppl 6):1403–1409

52. Dean H. Treatment of type 2 diabetes in youth: an argument for randomized controlled studies. *Paediatr Child Health (Oxford).* 1999;4(4):265–270

53. Sellers EAC, Dean HJ. Short-term insulin therapy in adolescents with type 2 diabetes mellitus. *J Pediatr Endocrinol Metab.* 2004; 17(11):1561–1564

54. Zeitler P, Hirst K, Pyle L, et al; TODAY Study Group. A clinical trial to maintain glycemic control in youth with type 2 diabetes. *N Engl J Med.* 2012;366(24):2247–2256

55. White NH, Cleary PA, Dahms W, Goldstein D, Malone J, Tamborlane WV; Diabetes Control and Complications Trial (DCCT)/Epidemiology of Diabetes Interventions and Complications (EDIC) Research Group. Beneficial effects of intensive therapy of diabetes during adolescence: outcomes after the conclusion of the Diabetes Control and Complications Trial (DCCT). *J Pediatr.* 2001;139(6):804–812

56. The Diabetes Control and Complications Trial Research Group. The effect of intensive treatment of diabetes on the development and progression of long-term complications in insulin-dependent diabetes mellitus. *N Engl J Med.* 1993;329(14):977–986

57. Orchard TJ, Olson JC, Erbey JR, et al. Insulin resistance-related factors, but not glycemia, predict coronary artery disease in type 1 diabetes: 10-year follow-up data from the Pittsburgh Epidemiology of Diabetes Complications Study. *Diabetes Care.* 2003;26(5):1374–1379

58. UK Prospective Diabetes Study Group. U.K. prospective diabetes study 16. Overview of 6 years' therapy of type II diabetes: a progressive disease. *Diabetes.* 1995;44(11):1249–1258

59. Shichiri M, Kishikawa H, Ohkubo Y, Wake N. Long-term results of the Kumamoto Study on optimal diabetes control in type 2 diabetic patients. *Diabetes Care.* 2000;23(suppl 2):B21–B29

60. Baynes JW, Bunn HF, Goldstein D, et al; National Diabetes Data Group. National Diabetes Data Group: report of the expert committee on glucosylated hemoglobin. *Diabetes Care.* 1984;7(6):602–606

61. Dabiri G, Jones K, Krebs J, et al. Benefits of rosiglitazone in children with type 2 diabetes mellitus [abstract]. *Diabetes.* 2005; A457

62. Ponder SW, Sullivan S, McBath G. Type 2 diabetes mellitus in teens. *Diabetes Spectrum.* 2000;13(2):95–119

63. Gahagan S, Silverstein J, and the American Academy of Pediatrics Committee on Native American Child Health. Prevention and treatment of type 2 diabetes mellitus in children, with special emphasis on American Indian and Alaska Native children. *Pediatrics.* 2003;112(4). Available at: www.pediatrics.org/cgi/content/full/112/4/e328

64. Levine BS, Anderson BJ, Butler DA, Antisdel JE, Brackett J, Laffel LM. Predictors of glycemic control and short-term adverse outcomes in youth with type 1 diabetes. *J Pediatr.* 2001;139(2):197–203

65. Haller MJ, Stalvey MS, Silverstein JH. Predictors of control of diabetes: monitoring may be the key. *J Pediatr.* 2004;144(5):660–661

66. Murata GH, Shah JH, Hoffman RM, et al; Diabetes Outcomes in Veterans Study (DOVES). Intensified blood glucose monitoring improves glycemic control in stable, insulin-treated veterans with type 2 diabetes: the Diabetes Outcomes in Veterans Study (DOVES). *Diabetes Care.* 2003;26(6):1759–1763

67. American Diabetes Association. Standards of medical care in diabetes—2011. *Diabetes Care.* 2011;34(suppl 1):S11–S61

68. Hanefeld M, Fischer S, Julius U, et al. Risk factors for myocardial infarction and death in newly detected NIDDM: the Diabetes Intervention Study, 11-year follow-up. *Diabetologia.* 1996;39(12):1577–1583

69. Franciosi M, Pellegrini F, De Berardis G, et al; QuED Study Group. The impact of blood glucose self-monitoring on metabolic control and quality of life in type 2 diabetic patients: an urgent need for better educational strategies. *Diabetes Care.* 2001;24(11):1870–1877

70. American Dietetic Association. Recommendations summary: pediatric weight management (PWM) using protein sparing modified fast diets for pediatric weight loss. Available at: www.adaevidencelibrary.com/template.cfm?template=guide_-summary&key=416. Accessed August 13, 2012

71. Knowler WC, Barrett-Connor E, Fowler SE, et al; Diabetes Prevention Program Research Group. Reduction in the incidence of type 2 diabetes with lifestyle intervention or metformin. *N Engl J Med.* 2002;346(6):393–403

72. Willi SM, Martin K, Datko FM, Brant BP. Treatment of type 2 diabetes in childhood using a very-low-calorie diet. *Diabetes Care.* 2004;27(2):348–353

73. Berry D, Urban A, Grey M. Management of type 2 diabetes in youth (part 2). *J Pediatr Health Care.* 2006;20(2):88–97

74. Loghmani ES. Nutrition therapy for overweight children and adolescents with type 2 diabetes. *Curr Diab Rep.* 2005;5(5):385–390

75. McGavock J, Sellers E, Dean H. Physical activity for the prevention and management of youth-onset type 2 diabetes mellitus: focus on cardiovascular complications. *Diab Vasc Dis Res.* 2007;4(4):305–310

76. Centers for Disease Control and Prevention. Physical activity for everyone: how much physical activity do you need? Atlanta, GA: Centers for Disease Control and Prevention; 2008. Available at: www.cdc.gov/physicalactivity/everyone/guidelines/children.html. Accessed August 13, 2012

77. Pinhas-Hamiel O, Zeitler P. A weighty problem: diagnosis and treatment of type 2 diabetes in adolescents. *Diabetes Spectrum.* 1997;10(4):292–298

78. Yamanouchi K, Shinozaki T, Chikada K, et al. Daily walking combined with diet therapy is a useful means for obese NIDDM patients not only to reduce body weight but also to improve insulin sensitivity. *Diabetes Care.* 1995;18(6):775–778

79. National Heart, Lung, and Blood Institute, US Department of Health and Human Services, National Institutes of Health. Reduce screen time. Available at: www.nhlbi.nih.gov/health/public/heart/obesity/wecan/reduce-screen-time/index.htm. Accessed August 13, 2012

80. Krebs NF, Jacobson MS; American Academy of Pediatrics Committee on Nutrition. Prevention of pediatric overweight and obesity. *Pediatrics.* 2003;112(2):424–430

81. American Academy of Pediatrics Committee on Public Education. American Academy of Pediatrics: children, adolescents, and television. *Pediatrics.* 2001;107(2):423–426

82. American Medical Association. Appendix. Expert Committee recommendations on the assessment, prevention, and treatment of child and adolescent overweight and obesity. Chicago, IL: American Medical Association; January 25, 2007. Available at: www.ama-assn.org/ama1/pub/upload/mm/433/ped_obesity_recs.pdf. Accessed August 13, 2012

ERRATA

Several inaccuracies occurred in the American Academy of Pediatrics "Clinical Practice Guideline: Management of Newly Diagnosed Type 2 Diabetes Mellitus (T2DM) in Children and Adolescents" published in the February 2013 issue of *Pediatrics* (2013;131[2]:364–382).

On page 366 in the table of definitions, "Prediabetes" should be defined as "Fasting plasma glucose ≥100–125 mg/dL or 2-hour glucose concentration during an oral glucose tolerance test of ≥140 but <200 mg/dL or an HbA1c of 5.7% to 6.4%."

On page 378, middle column, under "Reducing Screen Time," the second sentence should read as follows: "The US Department of Health and Human Services reflects the American Academy of Pediatrics policies by recommending that individuals limit "screen time" spent watching television and/or using computers and handheld devices to <2 hours per day unless the use is related to work or homework."[79–81,83]

Also on page 378, middle column, in the second paragraph under "Reducing Screen Time," the fourth sentence should read: "Pending new data, the committee suggests that clinicians follow the policy statement 'Children, Adolescents, and Television' from the AAP Council on Communications and Media (formerly the Committee on Public Education)." The references cited in the next sentence should be 80–83.

Reference 82 should be replaced with the following reference: Barlow SE; Expert Committee. Expert committee recommendations regarding the prevention, assessment, and treatment of child and adolescent overweight and obesity: summary report. *Pediatrics*. 2007;120(suppl 4):S164–S192

Finally, a new reference 83 should be added: American Academy of Pediatrics, Council on Communications and Media. Policy statement: children, adolescents, obesity, and the media. *Pediatrics*. 2011;128(1):201–208

doi:10.1542/peds.2013-0666

TECHNICAL REPORT

Management of Type 2 Diabetes Mellitus in Children and Adolescents

abstract

OBJECTIVE: Over the last 3 decades, the prevalence of childhood obesity has increased dramatically in North America, ushering in a variety of health problems, including type 2 diabetes mellitus (T2DM), which previously was not typically seen until much later in life. This technical report describes, in detail, the procedures undertaken to develop the recommendations given in the accompanying clinical practice guideline, "Management of Type 2 Diabetes Mellitus in Children and Adolescents," and provides in-depth information about the rationale for the recommendations and the studies used to make the clinical practice guideline's recommendations.

METHODS: A primary literature search was conducted relating to the treatment of T2DM in children and adolescents, and a secondary literature search was conducted relating to the screening and treatment of T2DM's comorbidities in children and adolescents. Inclusion criteria were prospectively and unanimously agreed on by members of the committee. An article was eligible for inclusion if it addressed treatment (primary search) or 1 of 4 comorbidities (secondary search) of T2DM, was published in 1990 or later, was written in English, and included an abstract. Only primary research inquiries were considered; review articles were considered if they included primary data or opinion. The research population had to constitute children and/or adolescents with an existing diagnosis of T2DM; studies of adult patients were considered if at least 10% of the study population was younger than 35 years. All retrieved titles, abstracts, and articles were reviewed by the consulting epidemiologist.

RESULTS: Thousands of articles were retrieved and considered in both searches on the basis of the aforementioned criteria. From those, in the primary search, 199 abstracts were identified for possible inclusion, 58 of which were retained for systematic review. Five of these studies were classified as grade A studies, 1 as grade B, 20 as grade C, and 32 as grade D. Articles regarding treatment of T2DM selected for inclusion were divided into 4 major subcategories on the basis of type of treatment being discussed: (1) medical treatments (32 studies); (2) nonmedical treatments (9 studies); (3) provider behaviors (8 studies); and (4) social issues (9 studies). From the secondary search, an additional 336 abstracts relating to comorbidities were identified for possible inclusion, of which 26 were retained for systematic review. These articles included the following: 1 systematic review of literature regarding comorbidities of T2DM in adolescents; 5 expert

Shelley C. Springer, MD, MBA, MSc, JD, Janet Silverstein, MD, Kenneth Copeland, MD, Kelly R. Moore, MD, Greg E. Prazar, MD, Terry Raymer, MD, CDE, Richard N. Shiffman, MD, Vidhu V. Thaker, MD, Meaghan Anderson, MS, RD, LD, CDE, Stephen J. Spann, MD, MBA, and Susan K. Flinn, MA

KEY WORDS
childhood, clinical practice guidelines, comanagement, diabetes, management, treatment, type 2 diabetes mellitus, youth

ABBREVIATIONS
AAP—American Academy of Pediatrics
ACE—angiotensin-converting enzyme
ADA—American Diabetes Association
AHA—American Heart Association
BG—blood glucose
CAM—complementary and alternative medicine
CES-D—Center for Epidemiologic Studies Depression Scale
CVD—cardiovascular disease
HbA1c—hemoglobin A1c
LDL-C—low-density lipoprotein cholesterol
PCP—primary care provider
QDS—Quality Data Set
RCT—randomized controlled trial
T1DM—type 1 diabetes mellitus
T2DM—type 2 diabetes mellitus

www.pediatrics.org/cgi/doi/10.1542/peds.2012-3496

doi:10.1542/peds.2012-3496

PEDIATRICS (ISSN Numbers: Print, 0031-4005; Online, 1098-4275).

opinions presenting global recommendations not based on evidence; 5 cohort studies reporting natural history of disease and comorbidities; 3 with specific attention to comorbidity patterns in specific ethnic groups (case-control, cohort, and clinical report using adult literature); 3 reporting an association between microalbuminuria and retinopathy (2 case-control, 1 cohort); 3 reporting the prevalence of nephropathy (cohort); 1 reporting peripheral vascular disease (case series); 2 discussing retinopathy (1 case-control, 1 position statement); and 3 addressing hyperlipidemia (American Heart Association position statement on cardiovascular risks; American Diabetes Association consensus statement; case series). A breakdown of grade of recommendation shows no grade A studies, 10 grade B studies, 6 grade C studies, and 10 grade D studies. With regard to screening and treatment recommendations for comorbidities, data in children are scarce, and the available literature is conflicting. Therapeutic recommendations for hypertension, dyslipidemia, retinopathy, microalbuminuria, and depression were summarized from expert guideline documents and are presented in detail in the guideline. The references are provided, but the committee did not independently assess the supporting evidence. Screening tools are provided in the Supplemental Information. *Pediatrics* 2013;131:e648–e664

INTRODUCTION

This technical report details the procedures undertaken to develop the recommendations given in the accompanying clinical practice guideline, "Management of Type 2 Diabetes Mellitus in Children and Adolescents." What follows is a description of the process, including the committee's objectives; methods of evidence identification, retrieval, review, and analysis; and summaries of the committee's conclusions.

Statement of the Issue

Over the last 3 decades, type 2 diabetes mellitus (T2DM), a disease previously confined to adult patients, has markedly increased in prevalence among children and adolescents. Currently, in the United States, approximately 1 in 3 new cases of diabetes mellitus diagnosed in patients younger than 18 years is T2DM,[1,2] with a disproportionate representation in ethnic minorities,[3,4] especially among adolescents.[5] This trend is not limited to the United States but is occurring internationally as well.[6]

The rapid emergence of childhood T2DM poses challenges to the physician who is unequipped to treat adult diseases encountered in children. Most diabetes training and educational materials designed for pediatric patients address type 1 diabetes mellitus (T1DM) and emphasize insulin treatment and glucose monitoring, which may or may not be appropriate for children with T2DM.[7,8] Most medications used for T2DM have been tested for safety and efficacy only in individuals older than 18 years, and there is scant scientific evidence for optimal management of children with T2DM.[9,10] Extrapolation of data from adult studies to pediatric populations may not be valid because the hormonal milieu of the prepubescent and pubescent patient with T2DM can affect treatment goals and modalities in ways heretofore unencountered in adult patients.[11]

The United States has a severe shortage of pediatric endocrinologists, making access to these specialists difficult or, in some cases, impossible.[12] Vast geographic areas lack a pediatric endocrinologist: in 2011, 3 states had no pediatric endocrinologists, and 22 had fewer than 10, and the situation is unlikely to improve in the near future.[13] In 2004, the National Association of Children's Hospitals and Related Institutions performed a workforce survey and found that patients had to wait almost 9 weeks for an appointment to see an endocrinologist.[14] Because the number of patients with T1DM and T2DM has increased since then, this situation is presumably worse today. Regardless of their age, most patients in the United States who have T2DM are cared for by primary care providers (PCPs).[15]

Furthermore, given the expected increases in the national and global incidence of T2DM and the near impossibility that the pediatric endocrine workforce will increase proportionately, PCPs must be prepared for and capable of managing children and adolescents who have uncomplicated T2DM.

Numerous experts have argued that the ideal care of a child with T2DM is provided through a team approach, with care shared among a pediatric endocrinologist, diabetes nurse educator, nutritionist, and behavioral specialist.[16–18] In areas of limited access to pediatric endocrinologists, however, contact with the pediatric endocrinology team might involve contact at diagnosis for initial diabetes education and intermittently thereafter; annually, with interval care by a PCP and interval communication with the pediatric endocrinology team; or at every visit, for those patients who are either doing poorly or are taking insulin.

In areas where access to subspecialists is hampered by geographic distances and/or professional shortages, care provided by local generalists who are skilled in treating children and youth with T2DM is likely to improve access to medical care. Although there are no pediatric studies evaluating this issue, the committee believes that this improved access to care might result in:

- Reduced wait times and increased timeliness of care.

- Reduced economic burden to the patient, including reduced need to travel and reduced time lost from work and/or school.

- Potentially improved patient retention. Kawahara et al[19] reported that 56.9% of patients with T2DM stopped coming to their hospital diabetes clinic appointments, most commonly because they were "too busy" to keep their appointments.

Recent advances in medical technology have the potential to ameliorate limited access to specialists. Reporting on the provision of clinical specialty diabetes care to remote locations using telemedicine, Malasanos et al[20] found that weekly telemedicine clinics were able to effectively replace quarterly face-to-face clinics after an initial face-to-face clinic visit. This more frequent contact provided by the telemedicine clinics resulted in improved hemoglobin A1c (HbA1c) concentrations, better patient satisfaction, fewer days missed from work or school, more time spent with the patient during clinic visits, and fewer subsequent hospitalizations and emergency department visits. Telemedicine is costly, however, and requires equipment to be in place at both the subspecialist's office and the remote clinic; it is, therefore, not appropriate for every practice. It is possible that a similar model of service could be provided by a generalist working locally and in close communication with a specialist.

For family physicians and others who care for adult patients, managing T2DM in children poses potential challenges. The first is that what works for adults may not work for children. Experiences and results observed in adults do not necessarily apply to children. Children (and even adolescents) are not small adults; they have a changing hormonal environment, have differences in physiology, and their growth can have effects on medication doses, toxicity, and responses.[11] As a result, generalists who are confident in caring for adults with diabetes may attempt to apply adult practice experiences to children, in whom these may not necessarily be appropriate. Kaufman cited data on various drugs' effects in children and argued that harm may occur if children with T2DM are treated like adults with T2DM.[11] The author called for treatment trials for children with T2DM, to "better define the risk-benefit ratio in children and youth, since this may differ substantially from that in the adult type 2 diabetic population." In contrast, others have noted that most adolescents with T2DM are similar to adults in terms of size and reproductive maturity and argued that, in the absence of studies specifically targeted to adolescents, treatment regimens can be extrapolated from studies of adults with T2DM; they do agree, however, that more randomized controlled trials (RCTs) are needed in the pediatric population.[1]

A second challenge is presented by the conflicting evidence regarding outcomes in patients with diabetes who are managed by generalists versus subspecialists. Some studies in adult patients indicate that generalists are capable of achieving outcomes similar to those of subspecialists. Greenfield et al[21] observed that physiologic and functional status (ie, physical, psychological, social functioning) were similar at both 2 and 4 years and mortality was similar at 7 years in adult hypertensive patients with diabetes treated in multispecialty groups versus health maintenance organization general practices. Other studies indicate that generalists may achieve outcomes similar to those of diabetes specialists, as long as they have input from subspecialists.

Indeed, unlike diseases in several other specialties, care for children with diabetes that is conducted by generalists without input from specialists may be inferior to that provided by specialists. Ziemer et al[22] used an RCT design to examine the effect of providing 5 minutes of direct feedback from an endocrinologist to a PCP every 2 weeks. Performance in the feedback group was sustained after 3 years, and performance decayed in a comparison group that received computer-generated decision support reminders, including a flow-sheet section showing previous clinical data and a recommendations section. Specialist feedback contributed independently to intensification of diabetes management. In addition, "clinical inertia" (defined as failure by providers to intensify pharmacologic therapy for hyperglycemia) was more likely in a primary care versus a diabetes clinic setting (91% vs 52%) and resulted in higher HbA1c concentrations among patients.[23]

How these observations might be applied to the child who has T2DM is not entirely clear, but they suggest that regular, direct contact between the generalist and a specialist can have a positive outcome on these patients. De Berardis et al[24] reported that, compared with adult patients with diabetes mellitus who were seen in general practice offices, patients cared for in diabetes clinics were more likely to conform with process-of-care measures, including HbA1c concentrations, blood pressure, total cholesterol and low-density lipoprotein cholesterol (LDL-C) levels, microalbuminuria testing, and foot and eye examinations and were more likely to have adequate concentrations of total cholesterol. No differences were found in glycemic, blood pressure, or LDL-C control, however. In that same study, all process-of-care measures improved when the patient was seen by a single physician as opposed to being seen by several different physicians. No similar studies have been performed in children, and it is therefore unknown whether similar outcomes can be achieved in the pediatric population.

A third challenge is presented by the fact that children with T2DM are overrepresented among racial and ethnic minority populations and are more likely to be living in poverty; therefore, they may face significant challenges in accessing specialists, even under the best situations.[25] Recognizing these barriers to care and patients' real-world needs, it is the committee's consensus that it is impractical to expect every patient with T2DM to be able to access a pediatric endocrinologist on a regular basis. It is also unreasonable to assume that these visits will be frequent enough to provide the level of care needed to maintain the best possible metabolic control. For this reason alone, PCPs must have a thorough knowledge of the management of T2DM, including its unique aspects related to childhood and adolescence.

The committee also believes it is the PCP's responsibility to obtain the requisite skills for such care and to communicate and work closely with a diabetes team of subspecialists whenever possible. For this reason, when treatment goals are not met, the committee encourages clinicians to consult with an expert trained in the care of children and adolescents with T2DM. When first-line therapy fails (eg, metformin), recommendations for intensifying therapy should be generally the same for pediatric and adult populations. The picture is constantly changing, however, as new drugs are being introduced, and some drugs that initially seemed to be safe exhibit adverse effects with wider use. Clinicians should, therefore, remain alert to new developments in this area. Seeking the advice of an expert can help ensure that the treatment goals are appropriately set and that clinicians benefit from cutting-edge treatment information in this rapidly changing area.

Stated Objective of the American Academy of Pediatrics

Because the PCP caring for children will likely encounter T2DM, the American Academy of Pediatrics (AAP), the Pediatric Endocrine Society, the American Academy of Family Physicians, the American Diabetes Association (ADA), and the American Dietetic Association undertook a cooperative effort to develop clinical guidelines for the treatment of T2DM in children and adolescents, for the benefit of subspecialists and generalists alike. Representatives from these groups collaborated on developing an evidence profile that served as a major source of information for the accompanying clinical practice guideline recommendations. This report, based on a review of the current medical literature covering a period from January 1, 1990, to July 1, 2009, provides a set of evidence-based guidelines for the management and treatment of T2DM in children and adolescents.

It should be noted that, because childhood T2DM is a relatively recent medical phenomenon, there is a paucity of evidence for many or most of the recommendations provided in the accompanying guideline. Committee members have made every effort to demarcate in the guideline those references that were not identified in the original literature search and are not included in this technical report. Although provided for the reader's information, these references not identified in the literature search did not affect or alter the level of evidence for specific recommendations.

Composition of the Committee

The ad hoc multidisciplinary committee was cochaired by 2 pediatric endocrinologists pre-eminent in their field and included experts in general pediatrics, family medicine, nutrition, Native American health, epidemiology, and medical informatics. All panel members reviewed the AAP Policy on Conflict of Interest and Voluntary Disclosure and declared all potential conflicts.

Definitions

- Children and adolescents: patients ≥ 10 and ≥ 18 years of age.

- Childhood T2DM: disease in the child who typically: is obese (BMI $\geq$85th to 94th percentile and >95th percentile for age and gender, respectively); has a strong family history of T2DM; has substantial residual insulin secretory capacity at diagnosis (reflected by normal or elevated insulin and C-peptide concentrations); has insidious onset of disease; demonstrates insulin resistance (including clinical evidence of polycystic ovarian syndrome or acanthosis nigricans); and lacks evidence of diabetic autoimmunity. These patients are more likely to have hypertension and dyslipidemia than those with T1DM.

- Hyperglycemia: definition as accepted by the ADA. Specifically: fasting blood glucose (BG) concentration >126 mg/dL, random or 2-hour post-Glucola (Ames Co, Elkhart, IN) BG concentration >200 mg/dL.

- Clinician: any provider within his or her scope of practice; includes medical practitioners (including physicians and physician extenders), dietitians, psychologists, and nurses.

- Comorbidities: specifically limited to cardiovascular disease (CVD), hypertension, dyslipidemias and hypercholesterolemias, atherosclerosis, peripheral neuropathy, retinopathy, and nephropathy (microvascular and macrovascular). Obesity was considered a prediabetic condition and was specifically excluded.

- Diabetes: according to the ADA criteria, defined as:

  1. HbA1c concentration $\geq$6.5% (test performed in an appropriately certified laboratory); or

  2. Fasting (defined as no caloric intake for at least 8 hours) plasma glucose concentration $\geq$126 mg/dL (7.0 mmol/L); or

  3. Two-hour plasma glucose concentration $\geq$200 mg/dL (11.1 mmol/L) during an oral glucose tolerance test (test performed as described by the World Health Organization by using a glucose load containing the equivalent of 75 g of anhydrous glucose dissolved in water); or

  4. A random plasma glucose concentration $\geq$200 mg/dL (11.1 mmol/L) with symptoms of hyperglycemia.

  (In the absence of unequivocal hyperglycemia, criteria 1–3 should be confirmed by repeat testing.)

- Diabetic ketoacidosis: the absolute or relative insulin deficiency resulting in fat breakdown with resultant formation of β-hydroxybutyrate and accompanying acidosis. Symptoms include nausea, vomiting, Kussmaul respirations, dehydration, and altered mental status.

- Fasting BG: BG concentration obtained before the first meal of the day and after a fast of at least 8 hours.

- Glucose toxicity: the effect of high BG causing both insulin resistance and impaired β-cell production of insulin.

- Intensification: increasing frequency of BG monitoring and adjustment of the dose and type of medication to decrease BG concentrations.

- Intercurrent illnesses: febrile illnesses or associated symptoms severe enough to cause the patient to stay home from school and/or seek medical care.

- Microalbuminuria: albumin-to-creatinine ratio $\geq$30 mg/g creatinine but <300 mg/g creatinine.

- Moderate hyperglycemia: BG concentration of 180 to 250 mg/dL.

- Moderate to vigorous exercise: exercise that makes the individual breathe hard and perspire and which raises his or her heart rate. An easy way to define exercise intensity for patients is the "talk test": during moderate physical activity a person can talk but not sing. During vigorous activity, a person cannot talk without pausing to catch a breath.

- Obese: BMI $\geq$95th percentile for age and gender.

- Overweight: BMI between 85th and 94th percentile for age and gender.

- Prediabetes: Fasting plasma glucose concentration $\geq$100 to 125 mg/dL or 2-hour glucose concentration during an oral glucose tolerance test $\geq$126 mg/dL but <200 mg/dL or HbA1c of 5.7% to 6.4%.

- Severe hyperglycemia: BG concentration >250 mg/dL.

- Thiazolidinediones: oral hypoglycemic agents that exert their effect at least in part by activation of the peroxisome proliferator-activated receptor-γ.

- T1DM: diabetes secondary to autoimmune destruction of β-cells resulting in absolute (complete or near complete) insulin deficiency and requiring insulin injections for management.

- T2DM: The investigators' designation of the diagnosis was used for the purposes of the literature review. The committee acknowledges that the distinction between T1DM and T2DM in this population is not always clear-cut, and clinical judgment plays an important role. Typically, this diagnosis is made when hyperglycemia is secondary to insulin resistance accompanied by impaired β-cell function, resulting in inadequate insulin production to compensate for the degree of insulin resistance.

- Youth: used interchangeably with "adolescent" in this document.

FORMULATION AND ARTICULATION OF THE QUESTION ADDRESSED BY THE COMMITTEE

The committee first formulated explicit questions for which evidence would be queried by the epidemiologist. Specific clinical questions addressed by the committee included: (1) the effectiveness of treatment modalities for T2DM in children and adolescents; (2) the efficacy of pharmaceutical therapies for treatment of children and adolescents with T2DM; (3) appropriate recommendations for screening for comorbidities typically associated with T2DM in children and adolescents; and (4) treatment recommendations for comorbidities of T2DM in children and adolescents.

These recommendations pertain specifically to patients at least 10 but younger than 18 years of age with T2DM. Although the distinction between T1DM and T2DM in children may be difficult,[26,27] for purposes of this report, the definition of childhood T2DM includes the child who typically is overweight or obese (defined as having a BMI $\geq$85th to 94th percentile and >95th percentile for age and gender, respectively); has a strong family history of T2DM; has substantial residual insulin secretory capacity at diagnosis (reflected by normal or elevated insulin and C-peptide concentrations); has insidious onset of disease; demonstrates insulin resistance (including clinical evidence of polycystic ovarian syndrome or acanthosis nigricans); and lacks evidence of diabetic autoimmunity (negative for autoantibodies typically associated with T1DM). Patients with T2DM are more likely to have hypertension and dyslipidemia than are those with T1DM.

Methods

Primary Literature Search: Treatment of T2DM

The committee unanimously agreed on the objectives of the guideline and scope of the evidence search. A primary literature search was conducted by the consulting epidemiologist, using the strategy as described in the following text.

An article was eligible for inclusion if it addressed treatment of T2DM, was published in 1990 or later, was written in English, and included an abstract. Only primary research inquiries were considered; review articles were considered if they included primary data or opinion. Children and/or adolescents with an existing diagnosis of T2DM were required to constitute the research population; studies of adult patients were considered if $\geq$10% of their population was younger than 35 years.

The electronic databases PubMed, Cochrane Collaboration, and Embase were searched using the following Medical Subject Headings, alone and in various combinations: diabetes, mellitus, type 2, type 1, treatment, prevention, insipidus, diet, pediatric, T2DM, T1DM, non–insulin dependent diabetes mellitus (NIDDM), metformin, lifestyle, RCT, meta-analysis, child, adolescent, therapeutics, control, adult, obese, gestational, polycystic ovary syndrome, metabolic syndrome, cardiovascular, dyslipidemia, men, and women. In addition, the Boolean operators NOT, AND, and OR were used with the aforementioned terms, also in various combinations. Search limits included clinical trial, meta-analysis, randomized controlled trial, review, child: 6–12 years, and adolescent: 13–18 years.

Reference lists of identified articles were searched for additional studies using the same criteria for inclusion enumerated earlier. Finally, articles personally known to members of the committee that were not identified by other means were submitted for consideration and were included if they fulfilled the inclusion criteria.

A total of 196 articles were identified by using these search criteria. Of those, 58 were accepted as evidence for the guideline, and 138 were rejected as not meeting all requirements. A summary evidence table for the accepted articles can be found in Supplemental Information A.

Secondary Literature Search: Comorbidities of T2DM

After completion of the primary literature review, at the request of the committee, a second literature review was conducted to identify evidence relating to screening, diagnosis, and treatment of comorbidities of T2DM in children and adolescents. Similar to inclusion criteria for the primary review, an article relating to comorbidities was eligible for inclusion if it was published in 1990 or later, was written in English, and included an abstract. Again, only primary research inquiries were considered; review articles were considered if they included primary data or opinion. Children and/or adolescents in whom either T1DM or T2DM was diagnosed were required to constitute the research population; studies of adult patients were considered if $\geq$10% of the population was younger than 35 years. The focus of the research article must be hyperlipidemia, microalbuminuria, retinopathy, or "comorbidities of diabetes mellitus."

The electronic databases PubMed, Cochrane Collaboration, and Embase were searched using the following Medical Subject Headings, alone and in various combinations: diabetes,

mellitus, type 2, type 1, pediatric, T2DM, T1DM, NIDDM, hyperlipidemia, retinopathy, microalbuminuria, comorbidities, screening, RCT, meta-analysis, child, and adolescent. In addition, the Boolean operators NOT, AND, and OR were used with the aforementioned terms, also in various combinations. Search limitations included clinical trial, meta-analysis, randomized controlled trial, review, child: 6–12 years, and adolescent: 13–18 years. Reference lists of identified articles were searched for additional studies, with the use of the same criteria for inclusion enumerated earlier. Finally, articles personally known to members of the committee that were not identified by other means were submitted for consideration and were included if they fulfilled the inclusion criteria.

A total of 75 articles were identified by using these search criteria. Of those, 26 were accepted as evidence for the guideline, and 49 were rejected as not meeting all requirements. A summary evidence table for the accepted comorbidity articles can be found in Supplemental Information B.

Analysis of Available Evidence

A strict evidence-based approach was used to extract data used to develop the recommendations presented in the accompanying clinical practice guideline. Individual articles meeting the prospective search criteria were critically appraised for strength of methodology, and they were assigned an evidence level grade on the basis of guidelines published by the University of Oxford's Centre for Evidence-based Medicine, which are synthesized in the next discussion.[28]

Levels of Evidence (Based on Methodology)

• Level 1A: Systematic review with homogeneity of included RCTs.

- Level 1B: Individual RCT with narrow CI and >80% follow-up.
- Level 2A: Systematic review with homogeneity of cohort studies.
- Level 2B: Individual cohort study, follow-up of untreated controls in an RCT, or low-quality RCT (ie, less than 80% follow-up).
- Level 2C: "Outcomes research."
- Level 3A: Systematic review with homogeneity of case-control studies.
- Level 3B: Individual case-control studies.
- Level 4: Case series; poor-quality cohort and/or case-control studies.
- Level 5: Expert opinion without explicit critical appraisal or based on physiology, bench research, or "first principles."

Grades of Evidence Supporting the Recommendations

The AAP policy statement, "Classifying Recommendations for Clinical Practice Guidelines," was followed in designating grades of recommendation (Fig 1, Table 1), based on the levels of available evidence. AAP policy stipulates that the evidence in support of each key action statement be prospectively identified, appraised, and summarized and that an explicit link between level of evidence and grade of recommendation be defined.

Possible grades of recommendations range from A to D, with A being the highest. Some qualification of the grade is further allowed on the basis of subtle characteristics of the level of supporting evidence. The AAP policy statement is consistent with the grading recommendations advanced by the University of Oxford's Centre for Evidence-based Medicine. The AAP policy statement "Classifying Recommendations for Clinical Practice Guidelines" offers further details.[29]

- Grade A: Consistent level 1 studies. (Examples include meta-analyses with appropriate adjustments for heterogeneity, well-designed RCTs, or high-quality diagnostic studies on relevant populations.)
- Grade B: Consistent level 2 or level 3 studies or extrapolations from level 1 studies. (Examples include RCTs or diagnostic studies with methodologic flaws or performed in less relevant populations; consistent and persuasive evidence from well-designed observational trials.)
- Grade C: Level 4 studies or extrapolations from level 2 or level 3 studies. (Examples include poor-quality observational studies, including case-control and cohort design methodologies, as well as case series.)
- Grade D: Level 5 evidence, or troublingly inconsistent or inconclusive studies of any level. (Examples include case reports, expert opinion, reasoning from first principles, or methodologically troubling studies with questionable validity.)
- Level X: Not an explicit level of evidence as outlined by the Centre for Evidence-based Medicine. Reserved for interventions that are unethical or impossible to test in a controlled or scientific fashion, in which the preponderance of benefit or harm is overwhelming, precluding rigorous investigation.

The relationship between grades of evidence supporting recommendations and recommended key action statements is depicted in Fig 1. Note that any given recommended key action statement may only be as strong as its supporting evidence will allow.

Recommended Key Action Statements

After considering the available levels of evidence and grades of recommendations, the committee formulated

FIGURE 1
Evidence quality. Integrating evidence quality appraisal with an assessment of the anticipated balance between benefits and harms if a policy is carried out leads to designation of a policy as a strong recommendation, recommendation, option, or no recommendation.

TABLE 1 Grades of Study According to Subdivision

Evidence Quality	Medical Treatment	Nonmedical Treatment	Provider Behaviors	Social Issues
A	4	1	0	0
B	0	1	0	0
C	4	3	7	6
D	24	4	1	3

several recommended key action statements, published in the companion clinical practice guideline. As discussed previously, recommended key action statements vary in strength on the basis of the quality of the supporting evidence.

- Strong recommendation: The highest level of recommendation, this category is reserved for recommendations supported by grade A or grade B evidence demonstrating a preponderance of benefit or harm. Interventions based on level X evidence may also be categorized as strong on the basis of their risk/benefit profile. A strong recommendation in favor of a particular action is made when the anticipated benefits of the recommended intervention clearly exceed the harms (as a strong recommendation against an action is made when the anticipated harms clearly exceed the benefits) and the quality of the supporting evidence is excellent. In some clearly identified circumstances, strong recommendations may be made when high-quality evidence is impossible to obtain and the anticipated benefits strongly outweigh the harms. The implication for clinicians is that they should follow a strong recommendation unless a clear and compelling rationale for an alternative approach is present.

- Recommendation: A recommended key action statement is made when the anticipated benefit exceeds the harms but the evidence is not as methodologically sound. Recommended key action statements must be supported by grade B or grade C evidence; level X evidence may also result in a recommendation depending on risk/benefit considerations. A recommendation in favor of a particular action is made when the anticipated benefits exceed

the harms, but the quality of evidence is not as strong. Again, in some clearly identified circumstances, recommendations may be made when high-quality evidence is impossible to obtain but the anticipated benefits outweigh the harms. The implication for clinicians is that they would be prudent to follow a recommendation but should remain alert to new information and sensitive to patient preferences.

- Option: Option statements are offered when the available evidence is grade D or the anticipated benefit is balanced with the potential harm. Options define courses that may be taken when either the quality of evidence is suspect or carefully performed studies have shown little clear advantage to 1 approach over another. The implication for clinicians is that they should consider the option in their decision-making, and patient preference may have a substantial role.

- No recommendation: When published evidence is lacking, and/or what little evidence is available demonstrates an equivocal risk/benefit profile, no recommended key action can be offered. No recommendation indicates that there is a lack of pertinent published evidence and that the anticipated balance of benefits and harms is presently unclear. The implication for clinicians is that they should be alert to new published evidence that clarifies the balance of benefit versus harm.

Implementation Strategy

Implementing the guideline's recommendations to improve care processes involves identifying potential barriers to the use of the knowledge, creating strategies to address those barriers, and selecting appropriate quality improvement methods (eg,

education, audit and feedback, computer-based decision support).

Computer-mediated decision support offers an implementation mode that has been demonstrated to be effective[30] and that is expected to be of increasing relevance to pediatricians with the adoption of electronic health records. To facilitate translation of the recommendations into computable statements, the guideline recommendations were transformed into declarative production rule (eg, IF-THEN) statements.[31] The Key Action Statements are displayed as production rules in Supplemental Information C. The concepts required to describe antecedent and consequent clauses in these rules were translated into the following standardized coding systems: SNOMED-CT,[32] RxNorm,[33] and LOINC.[34]

In addition, the concepts described in the guideline recommendations were translated, where possible, into elements of the National Quality Forum's Quality Data Set (QDS).[35] The QDS provides a framework from which performance measurement data can be derived. The QDS is intended to serve as a standard set of reusable data elements that can be used to promote quality measurement. Each QDS element includes a name, a quality data type that describes part of the clinical care process, quality data type specific attributes, a standard code set name, and a code listing. The Methods for Developing the Guidelines section displays the relevant decision variables and actions as well as coding information. A QDS listing of decision variables and actions is provided in Supplemental Information D.

RESULTS

Primary Literature Search: Treatment of T2DM

Thousands of articles were retrieved and considered on the basis of the aforementioned criteria. From those,

199 abstracts were identified for possible inclusion, and 58 were retained for systematic review. Results of the literature review are presented in the following text and listed in the evidence tables in the Supplemental Information.

Of the 58 articles retained for systematic review, 5 studies were classified as grade A studies, 1 as grade B, 20 as grade C, and 32 as grade D. Articles regarding the treatment of T2DM selected for inclusion were divided into 4 major subcategories on the basis of type of treatment being discussed: (1) medical treatments (32 studies); (2) nonmedical treatments (9 studies); (3) provider behaviors (8 studies); and (4) social issues (9 studies). Detailed information about these articles is presented in Supplemental Information A. A graphic depiction of the grades of study according to subdivision is given in Table 1.

Rejected Articles

Of the 257 articles meeting search criteria, 199 were rejected, categorized as follows:

- Comorbidities: 69 studies. (Note: these articles were rejected within the context of the primary search string relating to treatment of T2DM. A second prospective literature search was conducted solely addressing comorbidities, the results of which are presented in the next section.)
- Medical treatment: 99 articles.
- Nonmedical treatment: 16 articles.
- Social issues: 12 articles.
- Provider behaviors: 3 articles.

To view the recommendations related to management of T2DM, please see the accompanying clinical practice guideline.[36]

Secondary Literature Search: Comorbidities of T2DM

Evidence is sparse in children and adolescents regarding the risks for developing various comorbidities of diabetes that are well recognized in adult patients. Numerous reports have documented the occurrence of comorbidities in adolescents with T2DM, but no randomized clinical trials have examined the progression and treatment of comorbidities in youth with T2DM.[29] The evidence that does exist is contradictory with regard to both screening and treatment recommendations. After applying the previously described search criteria and screening to thousands of articles, an additional 336 abstracts relating to comorbidities were identified for possible inclusion, of which 26 were retained for systematic review. Results of this subsequent literature review are presented in Supplemental Information E.

Articles discussing comorbidities ran the gamut of study focus, type, level of evidence, and grade of recommendation. The 26 articles that met the revised objective criteria had the following characteristics:

- Expert opinion global recommendations not based on evidence (5 articles).
- Cohort studies reporting natural history of disease and comorbidities (5 articles).
- Specific attention to comorbidity patterns in specific ethnic groups (case-control, cohort, and clinical report by using adult literature: 3 articles).
- Association between microalbuminuria and retinopathy (2 case-control, 1 cohort: 3 articles).
- Prevalence of nephropathy (cohort: 3 articles).
- Hyperlipidemia (American Heart Association [AHA] position statement on cardiovascular risks, ADA consensus statement, case series: 3 articles).
- Retinopathy (1 case-control, 1 position statement: 2 articles).

- Peripheral vascular disease (case series: 1 article).
- Systematic review of literature regarding comorbidities of T2DM in adolescents (1 article).

A graphic depiction of the grades of recommendation is given in Table 2.

Rejected Articles

A total of 310 articles did not meet primary inclusion criteria and were rejected; details are presented in Supplemental Information F. Profiles of the rejected articles are:

- Articles relating to T1DM (125 articles); specifically on the following topics:
  - Retinopathy (42 articles).
  - Vascular complications (34 articles).
  - Nephropathy (29 articles).
  - Natural history and epidemiology of T1DM (8 articles).
  - Hyperlipidemia (5 articles).
  - Risk factors for comorbidities (ie, ethnicity, puberty: 4 articles).
  - Neuropathy (3 articles).
- Articles involving adults, practice management issues, and other nonpertinent topics (118 articles).
- Articles about nondiabetic subjects, prediabetic subjects, or adults, including recommendations for testing for conditions such as hyperlipidemias and CVD (36 articles).
- Reviews, published trials, guidelines, and position statements not meeting criteria (19 articles).
- Studies addressing methods of testing for comorbidities (12 articles).

The initial search strategy for comorbidities included patients diagnosed with T1DM. The committee thus assumed that (with the exception of initiating screening) the pattern of comorbidities—and the need to screen for and treat them—would be similar between T1DM and T2DM. It was also assumed that comorbidities would be similar between pediatric and adult patients, with length and severity of disease the driving factors. During the search, articles addressing the following themes were identified and reviewed:

- The pattern of comorbidities in T1DM versus T2DM and the role of puberty (9 articles).
- Differences in comorbidity patterns in children with T2DM compared with adults (8 articles).

Although not included in the final list of studies, these articles are included in the Supplemental Information because they resulted in an alteration to the original inclusion criteria. The results of these articles indicate that the pattern of comorbidities in children and adolescents with T2DM may not resemble that of either T1DM patients (possibly because of the influence of puberty) or adults, as was hypothesized by the committee when identifying the primary search parameters. Accordingly, the search string was modified to include only children and adolescents with the diagnosis of T2DM.

Recommendations Regarding Comorbidities

Unlike T2DM in adult patients, data are scarce in children and adolescents regarding the diagnosis, natural history, progression, screening recommendations, and treatment recommendations. Numerous reports have documented the occurrence of comorbidities in adolescents with T2DM, but no RCTs have examined the progression and treatment of comorbidities in youth with T2DM.

TABLE 2 Grades of Recommendation

Evidence Quality	No. of Studies
A	0
B	10
C	6
D	10

The available literature is conflicting regarding whether clinical signs of pathology in adults are variants of normal for adolescents, the role of puberty in diagnosis and progression of various comorbidities, the screening tests that should be performed and how they should be interpreted, when screenings should be initiated, how often screening should be performed and by whom, and how abnormal results should be treated. Medications commonly prescribed in adult patients have not been rigorously tested in children or adolescents for safety or efficacy. The peculiarities of the developing adolescent brain, typical lifestyle, and social issues confound issues of treatment effectiveness.

Despite the limited evidence available, the committee provides information on expert recommendations for the following selected comorbidities: hypertension, dyslipidemia, retinopathy, microalbuminuria, and depression. These therapeutic recommendations were summarized from expert guideline documents and are presented in detail in the following sections. The references are provided, but the committee did not independently assess the supporting evidence. Sample screening tools are provided in the Supplemental Information (see Supplemental Information H and I).

Hypertension

Hypertension is a significant comorbidity associated with endothelial dysfunction, vessel stiffness, and increased risk of future CVD and chronic kidney disease for the child with diabetes.[37,38] It is present in 36% of youth with T2DM within 1.3 years of diagnosis[39] and was present in 65% of youth with T2DM enrolled in the SEARCH for Diabetes in Youth Study (SEARCH study).[40] Because development of CVD is associated with hypertension, recognition and treatment of this comorbidity are essential, especially in youth with T2DM.

Unfortunately, health care providers underdiagnose hypertension in children and adolescents (both with and without diabetes), resulting in a lack of appropriate treatment.[41]

Screening:

- Blood pressure should be measured with an appropriate-sized cuff and reliable equipment, monitored at every clinic visit, and plotted against norms for age, gender, and height provided in tables available at the following Web site: http://www.nhlbi.nih.gov/guidelines/hypertension/child_tbl.htm[42] or in "The Fourth Report on the Diagnosis, Evaluation, and Treatment of High Blood Pressure in Children and Adolescents."[43] (See the Supplemental Information for the National Institutes of Health table.)

Treatment:

- Once a diagnosis of hypertension is established, the clinician can institute appropriate treatment, which might include lifestyle change and/or pharmacologic agents. Although a complete discussion of this topic is beyond the scope of these guidelines, rational treatment guidelines exist.[43,44] In adult patients with T2DM, concomitant treatment of hypertension has been shown to improve microvascular and macrovascular outcomes at least as much as control of BG concentrations.[45,46] Therefore, it is the consensus of this committee that similar benefits are likely with early recognition and treatment of hypertension in the child or adolescent with increased CVD risk secondary to T2DM.[47,48] The committee recommends appropriate surveillance and therapy as outlined in "The Fourth Report on the Diagnosis, Evaluation, and Treatment of High Blood Pressure in Children and Adolescents."[43]

- Initial treatment of blood pressure consistently at, or above, the 95th percentile on at least 3 occasions should consist of efforts at weight loss reduction, limitation of dietary salt, and increased activity.

- If, after 6 months, blood pressure is still above the 95th percentile for age, gender, and height, initiation of an angiotensin-converting enzyme (ACE) inhibitor should be considered to achieve blood pressure values that are less than the 90th percentile.

- If ACE inhibitors are not tolerated because of adverse effects (most commonly cough), an angiotensin receptor blocker should be used.

- If adequate control of hypertension is not achieved, referral to a physician specialist trained in the treatment of hypertension in youth is recommended.

Dyslipidemia

Long-term complications of T2DM in children and adolescents are not as well documented as those found in adults. It should be noted that the pediatric experience with niacin and fibrates is limited. In a review, however, Pinhas-Hamiel and Zeitler[49] noted the presence of dyslipidemia in a substantial proportion of young patients with T2DM in various populations worldwide. The SEARCH study found that 60% to 65% of 2096 youth with T2DM had hypertriglyceridemia, and 73% had a low high-density lipoprotein cholesterol level.[50] Thus, although variations exist in the criteria used for defining hyperlipidemia, there is unequivocal evidence that screening for dyslipidemia is imperative in pediatric patients with T2DM.[49,51,52] Hyperglycemia and insulin resistance may play a direct role in dyslipidemia, and cardiovascular risk is further enhanced by the presence of other risk factors, including obesity and a family

history of early CVD.[49,53] The AHA classifies T2DM as a tier 2 condition (moderate risk) in which accelerated atherosclerosis has been documented in patients younger than 30 years.[51] The presence of 2 other risk factors, including obesity, smoking, family history of CVD, and poor exercise history, can accelerate this status to tier 1 (high risk), which is relevant to many young patients with T2DM.

Screening:

- On the basis of current recommendations by the ADA and the AHA, at the initial evaluation, all patients with T2DM should have baseline lipid screening (after initial glycemic control has been established) consisting of a complete fasting lipid profile, with follow-up testing based on the findings or every 2 years thereafter, if initial results are normal.[51–53] (See the Supplemental Information for screening tools.)

Treatment:

The committee suggests following the AHA position statement, "Cardiovascular Risk Reduction in High-risk Pediatric Patients," for management of dyslipidemia.[51] This position statement recommends:

- Evaluation and dietary education by a registered dietitian for all patients, with initiation of intensive therapy and follow-up for patients with a BMI >95th percentile.

- Lipid targets:
  - LDL-C: Initial concentration ≥130 mg/dL: nutritionist training with diet <30% calories from fat, <7% calories from saturated fat, cholesterol intake <200 mg/day, and avoidance of trans fats. LDL measurements should be repeated after 6 months. If concentrations are still 130 to 160 mg/dL, statin therapy should be initiated,

with a goal of <130 mg/dL and an ideal target of <100 mg/dL.

  - Triglycerides: If initial concentrations are between 150 and 600 mg/dL, patients should decrease intake of simple carbohydrates and fat, with weight loss management for those who are overweight. If levels are >700 to 1000 mg/dL at initial or follow-up visit, fibrate or niacin should be considered if the patient is older than 10 years because of increased risk of pancreatitis at these concentrations.

- Control of hypertension, per guidelines referenced previously.

- Intensification of management of hyperglycemia.

- Assessment of parental smoking history and patient smoking history if the patient is older than 10 years; active antismoking counseling at every visit and referral to a smoking cessation program, if required.

- Assessment of family history of early CVD along with current family lifestyle habits; a positive family history increases the level of risk.

- Promotion of physical exercise and limitation of sedentary activities.

Retinopathy

The eye has been called a unique window into the neural and vascular health in patients with diabetes.[54] Retinopathy is well documented in adults, both alone and in association with other comorbidities,[55] but descriptions of its frequency and associations with other comorbidities in youth are limited. Some observational and case-control studies show that retinopathy in adolescents with T2DM is present earlier than in adults, whereas others indicate that it appears much later.[56–60]

The review by Pinhas-Hamiel and Zeitler[49] of complications of T2DM among adolescents cited studies in which the diagnosis of retinopathy appeared to occur strikingly early in the disease process. Two large studies in the Japanese population documented early development of retinopathy in young adults, some even before the diagnosis of diabetes mellitus. In a study of 1065 patients diagnosed with T2DM before 30 years of age, Okudaira et al[57] reported the presence of retinopathy in 99 patients (9.3%) before the first visit. One hundred thirty-five patients (12.7%) developed proliferative retinopathy before 35 years of age, and 32 (23.7%) of these patients were blind by a mean age of 32 years. Bronson-Castain et al[54] used sophisticated techniques to evaluate the neural and vascular health of the retina and reported a much higher incidence of focal retinal neuropathy, retinal thinning, and retinal venular dilation in a cohort of 15 adolescent patients with T2DM matched with 26 controls. Okudaira et al observed the development of retinopathy in 394 patients diagnosed with T2DM before 30 years of age. Of the 322 patients who were free of retinopathy at entry, 88 developed background diabetic retinopathy over 5.7 years, an incidence of 57.7 per 1000 person-years. Fifty of the 160 patients with background retinopathy developed proliferative retinopathy over 7.1 years, an incidence of 17.9 per 1000 person-years. Poor glycemic control, duration of disease, and high blood pressure seemed to be the primary risk factors.

Conversely, the study by Krakoff et al[58] of 178 youth that used the proportional hazards model showed a lower risk for retinopathy in Pima Indians (compared with the Japanese study cited previously), even after adjusting for glucose concentrations and blood pressure. Similar results were reported by Farah et al[59] in 40 African American and Hispanic youth and by Karabouta et al[60] in 7 adolescent patients. It is unclear whether these differences in results arise from variations in study design, population demographic characteristics, and/or techniques used in diagnosis. Given the variability in the results of epidemiologic studies and absence of long-term data, the committee considers it prudent for providers to follow the ADA "Standards of Medical Care in Diabetes" for identification and management of retinopathy in adolescents with T2DM, as follows[61]:

Screening:

- Patients with T2DM should have an initial dilated and comprehensive eye examination performed by an ophthalmologist or optometrist shortly after diabetes diagnosis.

- Subsequent examinations by an ophthalmologist should be repeated annually. Less frequent examinations may be considered (eg, every 2–3 years) after 1 or more normal eye examinations. More frequent examinations are required if retinopathy is progressing.

Treatment:

- Providers should promptly refer patients with any level of macular edema, severe nonproliferative diabetic retinopathy, or any proliferative diabetic retinopathy to an ophthalmologist who is knowledgeable and experienced in the management and treatment of diabetic retinopathy.

- Laser photocoagulation therapy is indicated to reduce the risk of vision loss in patients with high-risk proliferative diabetic retinopathy, clinically significant macular edema, and some cases of severe nonproliferative diabetic retinopathy.

Microalbuminuria

Microalbuminuria is a marker of vascular inflammation and a sign of early nephropathy; it has been found to be associated with CVD risk in adults. It may be present at diagnosis in youth with T2DM.[49] Higher rates of microalbuminuria have been reported among youth with T2DM than in their peers with T1DM.[39,59] Diabetic nephropathy may also be more frequent and severe among youth with T2DM.[62,63] According to the ADA statement "Care of Children and Adolescents with Type 1 Diabetes," the definition of microalbuminuria is either:

- "Albumin-to-creatinine ratio 30–299 mg/g in a spot urine sample; slightly higher values can be used in females because of the difference in creatinine excretion,"[7,64] or

- "Timed overnight or 24-hour collections: albumin excretion rate of 20–199 mcg/min."[7]

According to the ADA, "an abnormal value should be repeated as exercise, smoking, and menstruation can affect results and albumin excretion can vary from day to day. The diagnosis of persistent abnormal microalbumin excretion requires documentation of two of three consecutive abnormal values obtained on different days."[7,65] In addition, nondiabetes-related causes of renal disease should be excluded; consultation with specialists trained in the care of children with renal diseases should be considered as required. It should be noted that orthostatic proteinuria is not uncommon in adolescents and usually is considered benign. For that reason, all patients with documented microalbuminuria should have a first morning void immediately on arising to determine if this is the case. Orthostatic proteinuria does not require treatment with medication.

The committee considers it prudent for providers to follow the ADA "Standards of Medical Care in Diabetes" for the identification and management of microalbuminuria in adolescents with T2DM, as described here. Note that monitoring should always be done on a first morning void specimen:

Screening:

- Screening for microalbuminuria should begin at the time of T2DM diagnosis and be repeated annually.
- An annual random spot urine sample for microalbumin-to-creatinine ratio is recommended.[66]

Treatment:

- Treatment with an ACE inhibitor should be initiated in nonpregnant individuals with confirmed persistent microalbuminuria from 2 additional urine specimens, even if blood pressure is not elevated.
- If possible, treatment with an ACE inhibitor should be titrated to normalization of microalbumin excretion. "Microalbumin excretion should be monitored at three- to six-month intervals to assess both the patient's response to therapy and the disease progression, and therapy should be titrated to achieve as normal an albumin-to-creatinine ratio as possible."[7]

Additional relevant issues noted in the ADA statement "Care of Children and Adolescents with Type 1 Diabetes" include[7]:

- Concomitant hypertension should be addressed. If present, hypertension should be aggressively treated to achieve normotension for age, sex, and height.
- Patients should be educated about the importance of attention to glycemic control and avoidance or cessation of smoking in preventing and/or reversing diabetic nephropathy.
- If medical treatment is unsatisfactory, referral to a nephrologist should be considered.

Depression

Depression is a significant comorbidity that can complicate the medical management of diabetes and is associated with poor adherence. Longitudinal studies of the association between T2DM and depression among youth are not available. In a longitudinal study among youth with T1DM, however, Kovacs et al[67] estimated the rate of psychiatric disorders to be 3 times higher in youth with diabetes than in those without diabetes, with the increased morbidity primarily attributable to major depression.[7,67,68] In addition, cross-sectional data from the SEARCH study have shown the prevalence of depressed mood to be higher among males with T2DM than among males with T1DM.[67] Lawrence et al[68] also found higher levels of depressed mood to be associated with poor glycemic control and number of emergency department visits among participants with both T1DM and T2DM, compared with youth with T1DM and T2DM who had "minimal" levels of depressed mood.

Because depression is associated with poor adherence to diabetic treatment recommendations, its identification and proper management are essential for maximizing therapeutic success. Given the serious nature of this comorbidity and its propensity for poor metabolic control, the committee recommends that clinicians assess youth with T2DM for depression at diagnosis; perform periodic, routine screening for depression on all youth with T2DM, especially those with frequent emergency department visits or poor glycemic control; and promptly refer youth who have positive screenings to appropriate mental health care providers for treatment. Addressing a family history of diabetes and its effect on the family unit can be a major factor in depression as well as compliance with the disease management needs.

Screening:

- According to the American Psychiatric Association, a diagnosis of major depressive disorder requires[69]:
  - (a). The presence of 5 or more of the following symptoms within the same 2-week period and represents a change from previous functioning. At least 1 of the symptoms is either depressed mood or loss of interest or pleasure.
- Depressed mood most of the day, nearly every day, as indicated by either substantive report or observation made by others. (Note that in children and adolescents, this can be irritable mood.)
- Markedly diminished interest or pleasure in all, or nearly all, activities most of the day, nearly every day.
- Significant weight loss when not dieting or weight gain (eg, more than 5% of body weight in a month), or increased or decreased appetite nearly every day. (Note that in children and adolescents, this should include failure to make expected weight gains.)
- Insomnia or hypersomnia nearly every day.
- Psychomotor agitation or retardation nearly every day (observable by others, not merely the subject's feeling restless or slowed down).
- Fatigue or loss of energy nearly every day.
- Feelings of worthlessness or inappropriate guilt (which may be delusional) nearly every day.
- Diminished ability to think or to concentrate, or indecisiveness, nearly every day.
- Recurrent thoughts of death (not just fear of dying), recurrent suicidal ideation without a specific plan, or a suicide attempt, or a specific plan to commit suicide.

(b). The symptoms do not meet the criteria for a mixed episode (defined as a specific time period in which the individual experiences nearly daily fluctuations in mood that qualify for diagnoses of manic episode and major depressive episode).

(c). The symptoms cause clinically significant distress or impairment in social, occupational, or other important areas of functioning.

(d). The symptoms are not due to the direct physiologic effects of a substance (eg, a drug of abuse, medication) or a general medical condition (eg, hypothyroidism).

(e). The symptoms are not better accounted for by bereavement (ie, after the loss of a loved one), symptoms persist longer than 2 months, or symptoms are characterized by marked functional impairment, morbid preoccupation with worthlessness, suicidal ideation, psychotic symptoms, or psychomotor retardation.

- Another potentially valuable screening tool for depression is the Center for Epidemiologic Studies Depression Scale (CES-D), a 20-item scale originally developed for use in adults[70] but which has been used subsequently in studies of youth as young as 12 years.[71–74] (See Supplemental Information G for this scale.)

Treatment:

- Recognition of depression should trigger a referral to a mental health care provider skilled in addressing this condition in children and adolescents.

Other Comorbidities or Associated Medical Conditions

In addition to the comorbidities mentioned previously, T2DM is associated with other obesity-related medical conditions, many of which, when discovered, necessitate consultation with specialists who have specific expertise in the field. These associated conditions include:

- Nonalcoholic fatty liver disease: Baseline aspartate aminotransferase and alanine aminotransferase concentrations should be obtained, especially if treatment with lipid-lowering drugs is instituted. Referral to a pediatric or internal medicine gastroenterologist may be indicated.

- Obstructive sleep apnea: The diagnosis of obstructive sleep apnea can only be made reliably by using a sleep study. If the diagnosis is made, an electrocardiogram and possibly an echocardiogram should be obtained to rule out right ventricular hypertrophy. Referral to a pediatric cardiologist, internal medicine cardiologist, or sleep specialist may be indicated.

- Orthopedic problems: These comorbidities (especially slipped capital femoral epiphysis and Blount disease) require immediate referral to a specialist in orthopedics and will limit the physical activity that can be prescribed to the individual.

COMPLEMENTARY AND ALTERNATIVE MEDICINE

The clinical practice guidelines do not present any evidence-based recommendations for the use of complementary and alternative medicine (CAM) to treat T2DM in children and adolescents. Limited data are available on CAM, and none is specific to this age group. However, noting that adult patients with diabetes are 1.6 times more likely to use CAM than are individuals without diabetes, the committee believes it is important for clinicians to encourage their patients to communicate openly about the use of CAM (especially because the parents may have diabetes themselves) and, when acknowledged, to differentiate between coadministration with the prescribed therapy versus replacement of (and, thus, noncompliance with) the prescribed therapy.[75]

CAM is most likely to be used by West Indian, African, Indian, Latin American, and Asian subjects.[76] CAM is also more common in families with higher income and education levels and an increased interest in self-care. One multicenter study conducted in Germany found that, among 228 families with a T1DM diagnosis, 18.4% reported using at least 1 form of CAM.[77] Reported parental motivators for using CAM for their children included the hope of improving their well-being (92.1%); the desire to try every available treatment option (77.8%); and the assumption that CAM has fewer adverse effects than conventional therapy (55.2%). Many forms of CAM are used because of patient-perceived inadequacies of current treatments.[75]

A wide variety of CAM dietary supplements are targeted at patients with diabetes and promise to lower BG concentrations or prevent and/or treat complications associated with the disease. Common supplements used by individuals with diabetes include aloe, bitter melon, chromium, cinnamon, fenugreek, ginseng, gymnema, and nopal.[78] These products lack product standardization and are not regulated by the US Food and Drug Administration for either safety or possible complications. Although these supplements may or may not have proven beneficial effects on diabetes, many might have harmful adverse effects and/or lead to medication interactions. Adverse effects from dietary supplements can include gastrointestinal discomfort, hypoglycemia, favism, insomnia, and increased blood pressure.[78]

In addition to dietary supplements, patients may use forms of CAM that include prayer, acupuncture, massage, hot tub therapy, biofeedback, and yoga. The University of Chicago's Division of Pediatric Endocrinology interviewed 106 families with T1DM and found that 33% of children had tried CAM in the past year; the most common form used was faith-healing or prayer.[79] Parents who reported the use of CAM for their children were also more likely to report having experienced struggles with adherence to conventional medicine.

It is the committee's opinion that providers should question patients on their use of CAM and also educate patients on potential adverse effects, review evidence for efficacy, and discourage the use of potentially dangerous or ineffective products.

SUMMARY

The clinical practice guideline that this technical report accompanies provides evidence-based recommendations on the management of patients between 10 and 18 years of age who have been diagnosed with T2DM. The document does not pertain to patients with impaired glucose tolerance, isolated insulin resistance, or prediabetes, nor does it pertain to obese but nondiabetic youth. It emphasizes the use of management modalities that have been shown to affect clinical outcomes in this pediatric population. The clinical practice guideline addresses situations in which either insulin or metformin is the preferred first-line treatment of children and adolescents with T2DM. It suggests integrating lifestyle modifications (ie, diet and exercise) in concert with medication rather than as an isolated initial treatment approach. Guidelines for frequency of monitoring HbA1c and finger-stick BG concentrations are presented. The clinical practice guideline is intended to assist clinician decision-making rather than replace clinical judgment and/or establish a protocol for the care of all children with this condition. These recommendations may not provide the only appropriate approach to the management of children with T2DM. Providers should consult experts trained in the care of children and adolescents with T2DM when treatment goals are not met or when therapy with insulin is initiated.

ACKNOWLEDGMENTS

The committee acknowledges the work of Edwin Lomotan, MD, FAAP, and George Michel, MS, in creating the reports.

SUBCOMMITTEE ON TYPE 2 DIABETES (OVERSIGHT BY THE STEERING COMMITTEE ON QUALITY IMPROVEMENT AND MANAGEMENT, 2008–2012)

Kenneth Claud Copeland, MD, FAAP: Co-chair —Endocrinology and Pediatric Endocrine Society Liaison (2009: Novo Nordisk, Genentech, Endo [National Advisory Groups]; 2010: Novo Nordisk [National Advisory Group]); published research related to type 2 diabetes

Janet Silverstein, MD, FAAP: Co-chair—Endocrinology and American Diabetes Association Liaison (small grants with Pfizer, Novo Nordisk, and Lilly; grant review committee for Genentech; was on an advisory committee for Sanofi Aventis, and Abbott Laboratories for a 1-time meeting); published research related to type 2 diabetes

Kelly Roberta Moore, MD, FAAP: General Pediatrics, Indian Health, AAP Committee on Native American Child Health Liaison (board member of the Merck Company Foundation Alliance to Reduce Disparities in Diabetes. Their national program office is the University of Michigan's Center for Managing Chronic Disease.)

Greg Edward Prazar, MD, FAAP: General Pediatrics (no conflicts)

Terry Raymer, MD, CDE: Family Medicine, Indian Health Service (no conflicts)

Richard N. Shiffman, MD, FAAP: Partnership for Policy Implementation Informatician, General Pediatrics (no conflicts)

Shelley C. Springer, MD, MBA, MSc, JD, FAAP: Epidemiologist, neonatologist (no conflicts)

Meaghan Anderson, MS, RD, LD, CDE: Academy of Nutrition and Dietetics Liaison (formerly a Certified Pump Trainer for Animas)

Stephen J. Spann, MD, MBA, FAAFP: American Academy of Family Physicians Liaison (no conflicts)

Vidhu V. Thaker, MD, FAAP: QuIIN Liaison, General Pediatrics (no conflicts)

CONSULTANT

Susan K. Flinn, MA: Medical Writer (no conflicts)

STAFF

Caryn Davidson, MA

REFERENCES

1. Silverstein JH, Rosenbloom AL. Type 2 diabetes in children. *Curr Diab Rep.* 2001;1(1):19–27
2. Pinhas-Hamiel O, Zeitler P. Clinical presentation and treatment of type 2 diabetes in children. *Pediatr Diabetes.* 2007;8(9 suppl 9):16–27
3. Dabelea D, Bell RA, D'Agostino RB Jr, et al; Writing Group for the SEARCH for Diabetes in Youth Study Group. Incidence of diabetes in youth in the United States. *JAMA.* 2007; 297(24):2716–2724
4. Mayer-Davis EJ, Bell RA, Dabelea D, et al; SEARCH for Diabetes in Youth Study Group. The many faces of diabetes in American youth: type 1 and type 2 diabetes in five race and ethnic populations: the SEARCH for Diabetes in Youth Study. *Diabetes Care.* 2009;32(2 suppl 2):S99–S101
5. Liese AD, D'Agostino RB, Jr, Hamman RF, et al; SEARCH for Diabetes in Youth Study Group. The burden of diabetes mellitus among US youth: prevalence estimates from the SEARCH for Diabetes in Youth Study. *Pediatrics.* 2006;118(4):1510–1518
6. Narayan KM, Williams R. Diabetes— a global problem needing global solutions. *Prim Care Diabetes.* 2009;3(1):3–4
7. Silverstein J, Klingensmith G, Copeland K, et al; American Diabetes Association. Care of children and adolescents with type 1 diabetes: a statement of the American Diabetes Association. *Diabetes Care.* 2005;28 (1):186–212

8. Pinhas-Hamiel O, Zeitler P. Barriers to the treatment of adolescent type 2 diabetes—a survey of provider perceptions. *Pediatr Diabetes*. 2003;4(1):24–28

9. TODAY Study Group, Zeitler P, Epstein L, Grey M, et alTreatment options for type 2 diabetes in adolescents and youth: a study of the comparative efficacy of metformin alone or in combination with rosiglitazone or lifestyle intervention in adolescents with type 2 diabetes. *Pediatr Diabetes*. 2007;8(2):74–87

10. Kane MP, Abu-Baker A, Busch RS. The utility of oral diabetes medications in type 2 diabetes of the young. *Curr Diabetes Rev*. 2005;1(1):83–92

11. Kaufman FR. Type 2 diabetes mellitus in children and youth: a new epidemic. *J Pediatr Endocrinol Metab*. 2002;15(suppl 2):737–744

12. Silverstein JH. Workforce issues for pediatric endocrinology. *J Pediatr*. 2006;149(1):A3

13. American Board of Pediatrics. 2011 Endocrinology examination. Available at: https://www.abp.org/abpwebsite/stats/wrkfrc/endo.ppt. Accessed December 20, 2012

14. National Association of Children's Hospitals and Related Institutions. *Pediatric Subspecialists Survey Results*. Alexandria, VA: National Association of Children's Hospitals and Related Institutions; 2004

15. Saudek CD. The role of primary care professionals in managing diabetes. *Clin Diabetes*. 2002;20(2):65–66

16. Libman IM, Arslanian SA. Prevention and treatment of type 2 diabetes in youth. *Horm Res*. 2007;67(1):22–34

17. Gungor N, Hannon T, Libman I, Bacha F, Arslanian S. Type 2 diabetes mellitus in youth: the complete picture to date. *Pediatr Clin North Am*. 2005;52(6):1579–1609

18. Hannon TS, Rao G, Arslanian SA. Childhood obesity and type 2 diabetes mellitus. *Pediatrics*. 2005;116(2):473–480

19. Kawahara R, Amemiya T, Yoshino M, Miyamae M, Sasamoto K, Omori Y. Dropout of young non-insulin-dependent diabetics from diabetic care. *Diabetes Res Clin Pract*. 1994;24(3):181–185

20. Malasanos TH, Burlingame JB, Youngblade L, Patel BD, Muir AB. Improved access to subspecialist diabetes care by telemedicine: cost savings and care measures in the first two years of the FITE diabetes project. *J Telemed Telecare*. 2005;11(suppl 1):74–76

21. Greenfield S, Rogers W, Mangotich M, Carney MF, Tarlov AR. Outcomes of patients with hypertension and non-insulin dependent diabetes mellitus treated by different systems and specialties. Results from the medical outcomes study. *JAMA*. 1995;274(18):1436–1444

22. Ziemer DC, Tsui C, Caudle J, Barnes CS, Dames F, Phillips LS. An informatics-supported intervention improves diabetes control in a primary care setting. *AMIA Annu Symp Proc*. 2006:1160

23. Ziemer DC, Miller CD, Rhee MK, et al. Clinical inertia contributes to poor diabetes control in a primary care setting. *Diabetes Educ*. 2005;31(4):564–571

24. De Berardis G, Pellegrini F, Franciosi M, et al; QuED Study. Quality of care and outcomes in type 2 diabetic patients: a comparison between general practice and diabetes clinics. *Diabetes Care*. 2004;27(2):398–406

25. Copeland KC, Zeitler P, Geffner M, et al; TODAY Study Group. Characteristics of adolescents and youth with recent-onset type 2 diabetes: the TODAY cohort at baseline. *J Clin Endocrinol Metab*. 2011;96(1):159–167

26. Scott CR, Smith JM, Cradock MM, Pihoker C. Characteristics of youth-onset noninsulin-dependent diabetes mellitus and insulin-dependent diabetes mellitus at diagnosis. *Pediatrics*. 1997;100(1):84–91

27. Libman IM, Pietropaolo M, Arslanian SA, LaPorte RE, Becker DJ. Changing prevalence of overweight children and adolescents at onset of insulin-treated diabetes. *Diabetes Care*. 2003;26(10):2871–2875

28. Centre for Evidence-based Medicine. *Levels of Evidence*. Oxford, England: Centre for Evidence-based Medicine; March 2009

29. American Academy of Pediatrics Steering Committee on Quality Improvement and Management. Classifying recommendations for clinical practice guidelines. *Pediatrics*. 2004;114(3):874–877

30. Garg AX, Adhikari NK, McDonald H, et al. Effects of computerized clinical decision support systems on practitioner performance and patient outcomes: a systematic review. *JAMA*. 2005;293(10):1223–1238

31. Shiffman RN, Michel G, Essaihi A. Bridging the guideline implementation gap: a systematic, document-centered approach to guideline implementation. *J Am Med Inform Assoc*. 2004;11(5):418–426

32. National Library of Medicine. SNOMED clinical terms. Available at: www.nlm.nih.gov/research/umls/Snomed/snomed_main.html. Accessed August 13, 2012

33. National Library of Medicine. RxNorm. Available at: www.nlm.nih.gov/research/umls/rxnorm/. Accessed August 13, 2012

34. Regenstrief Institute. Logical observations identifiers names and codes. Available at: http://loinc.org/. Accessed August 13, 2012

35. National Quality Forum. *Health Information Technology Automation of Quality Measurement: Quality Data Set and Data Flow*. Washington, DC: National Quality Forum; 2009

36. American Academy of Pediatrics. Subcommittee on Type 2 Diabetes. Diabetes mellitus, type 2: clinical practice guideline for the management of newly diagnosed type 2 diabetes mellitus (T2DM) in children and adolescents. *Pediatrics*. 2013, In press

37. Shear CL, Burke GL, Freedman DS, Berenson GS. Value of childhood blood pressure measurements and family history in predicting future blood pressure status: results from 8 years of follow-up in the Bogalusa Heart Study. *Pediatrics*. 1986;77(6):862–869

38. Williams CL, Hayman LL, Daniels SR, et al; American Heart Association. Cardiovascular health in childhood: a statement for health professionals from the Committee on Atherosclerosis, Hypertension, and Obesity in the Young (AHOY) of the Council on Cardiovascular Disease in the Young, American Heart Association [published correction appears in *Circulation*. 2002;106(9):1178]. *Circulation*. 2002;106(1):143–160

39. Eppens MC, Craig ME, Cusumano J, et al. Prevalence of diabetes complications in adolescents with type 2 compared with type 1 diabetes. *Diabetes Care*. 2006;29(6):1300–1306

40. Mayer-Davis EJ, Ma B, Lawson A, et al; SEARCH for Diabetes in Youth Study Group. Cardiovascular disease risk factors in youth with type 1 and type 2 diabetes: implications of a factor analysis of clustering. *Metab Syndr Relat Disord*. 2009;7(2):89–95

41. Hansen ML, Gunn PW, Kaelber DC. Underdiagnosis of hypertension in children and adolescents. *JAMA*. 2007;298(8):874–879

42. National Heart, Lung and Blood Institute. Blood pressure tables for children and adolescents. Available at: www.nhlbi.nih.gov/guidelines/hypertension/child_tbl.htm. Accessed August 13, 2012

43. National High Blood Pressure Education Program Working Group on High Blood Pressure in Children and Adolescents. The fourth report on the diagnosis, evaluation, and treatment of high blood pressure in children and adolescents. *Pediatrics*. 2004;114(2 suppl 4th report):555–576

44. Brady TM, Feld LG. Pediatric approach to hypertension. *Semin Nephrol*. 2009;29(4):379–388

45. Hansson L, Zanchetti A, Carruthers SG, et al. Effects of intensive blood-pressure lowering and low-dose aspirin in patients

with hypertension: principal results of the Hypertension Optimal Treatment (HOT) randomised trial. *Lancet*. 1998;351(9118):1755–1762

46. UK Prospective Diabetes Study Group. Tight blood pressure control and risk of macrovascular and microvascular complications in type 2 diabetes: UKPDS 38. *BMJ*. 1998;317(7160):703–713

47. Yoon EY, Davis MM, Rocchini A, Kershaw D, Freed GL. Medical management of children with primary hypertension by pediatric subspecialists. *Pediatr Nephrol*. 2009;24(1):147–153

48. Zanchetti A, Hansson L, Ménard J, et al. Risk assessment and treatment benefit in intensively treated hypertensive patients of the Hypertension Optimal Treatment (HOT) study. *J Hypertens*. 2001;19(4):819–825

49. Pinhas-Hamiel O, Zeitler P. Acute and chronic complications of type 2 diabetes mellitus in children and adolescents. *Lancet*. 2007;369(9575):1823–1831

50. Rodriguez BL, Fujimoto WY, Mayer-Davis EJ, et al. Prevalence of cardiovascular disease risk factors in U.S. children and adolescents with diabetes: the SEARCH for Diabetes in Youth Study. *Diabetes Care*. 2006;29(8):1891–1896

51. Kavey RE, Allada V, Daniels SR, et al; American Heart Association Expert Panel on Population and Prevention Science; American Heart Association Council on Cardiovascular Disease in the Young; American Heart Association Council on Epidemiology and Prevention; American Heart Association Council on Nutrition, Physical Activity and Metabolism; American Heart Association Council on High Blood Pressure Research; American Heart Association Council on Cardiovascular Nursing; American Heart Association Council on the Kidney in Heart Disease; Interdisciplinary Working Group on Quality of Care and Outcomes Research. Cardiovascular risk reduction in high-risk pediatric patients: a scientific statement from the American Heart Association Expert Panel on Population and Prevention Science; the Councils on Cardiovascular Disease in the Young, Epidemiology and Prevention, Nutrition, Physical Activity and Metabolism, High Blood Pressure Research, Cardiovascular Nursing, and the Kidney in Heart Disease; and the Interdisciplinary Working Group on Quality of Care and Outcomes Research: endorsed by the American Academy of Pediatrics. *Circulation*. 2006;114(24):2710–2738

52. American Diabetes Association. Management of dyslipidemia in children and adolescents with diabetes. *Diabetes Care*. 2003;26(7):2194–2197

53. Taha D. Hyperlipidemia in children with type 2 diabetes mellitus. *J Pediatr Endocrinol Metab*. 2002;15(suppl 1):505–507

54. Bronson-Castain KW, Bearse MA, Jr, Neuville J, et al. Adolescents with type 2 diabetes: early indications of focal retinal neuropathy, retinal thinning, and venular dilation. *Retina*. 2009;29(5):618–626

55. Mokdad AH, Bowman BA, Ford ES, Vinicor F, Marks JS, Koplan JP. The continuing epidemics of obesity and diabetes in the United States. *JAMA*. 2001;286(10):1195–1200

56. Yokoyama H, Okudaira M, Otani T, et al. Existence of early-onset NIDDM Japanese demonstrating severe diabetic complications. *Diabetes Care*. 1997;20(5):844–847

57. Okudaira M, Yokoyama H, Otani T, Uchigata Y, Iwamoto Y. Slightly elevated blood pressure as well as poor metabolic control are risk factors for the progression of retinopathy in early-onset Japanese type 2 diabetes. *J Diabetes Complications*. 2000;14(5):281–287

58. Krakoff J, Lindsay RS, Looker HC, Nelson RG, Hanson RL, Knowler WC. Incidence of retinopathy and nephropathy in youth-onset compared with adult-onset type 2 diabetes. *Diabetes Care*. 2003;26(1):76–81

59. Farah SE, Wals KT, Friedman IB, Pisacano MA, DiMartino-Nardi J. Prevalence of retinopathy and microalbuminuria in pediatric type 2 diabetes mellitus. *J Pediatr Endocrinol Metab*. 2006;19(7):937–942

60. Karabouta Z, Barnett S, Shield JP, Ryan FJ, Crowne EC. Peripheral neuropathy is an early complication of type 2 diabetes in adolescence. *Pediatr Diabetes*. 2008;9(2):110–114

61. Executive summary: standards of medical care in diabetes—2009 [published correction appears in *Diabetes Care*. 2009;32(4):754]. *Diabetes Care*. 2009;32(suppl 1):S6–S12

62. Svensson M, Sundkvist G, Arnqvist HJ, et al; Diabetes Incidence Study in Sweden (DISS). Signs of nephropathy may occur early in young adults with diabetes despite modern diabetes management: results from the nationwide population-based Diabetes Incidence Study in Sweden (DISS). *Diabetes Care*. 2003;26(10):2903–2909

63. Yokoyama H, Okudaira M, Otani T, et al. Higher incidence of diabetic nephropathy in type 2 than in type 1 diabetes in early-onset diabetes in Japan. *Kidney Int*. 2000;58(1):302–311

64. Mogensen CE, Keane WF, Bennett PH, et al. Prevention of diabetic renal disease with special reference to microalbuminuria. *Lancet*. 1995;346(8982):1080–1084

65. Molitch ME, DeFronzo RA, Franz MJ, et al; American Diabetes Association. Nephropathy in diabetes. *Diabetes Care*. 2004;27(suppl 1):S79–S83

66. American Diabetes Association. Standards of medical care in diabetes—2010. *Diabetes Care*. 2010;33(suppl 1):S11–S61

67. Kovacs M, Goldston D, Obrosky DS, Bonar LK. Psychiatric disorders in youths with IDDM: rates and risk factors. *Diabetes Care*. 1997;20(1):36–44

68. Lawrence JM, Standiford DA, Loots B, et al; SEARCH for Diabetes in Youth Study. Prevalence and correlates of depressed mood among youth with diabetes: the SEARCH for Diabetes in Youth study. *Pediatrics*. 2006;117(4):1348–1358

69. American Psychiatric Association. *Diagnostic and Statistical Manual of Mental Disorders*. 4th ed. Washington, DC: American Psychiatric Association; 1994

70. Radloff LS. The CES-D scale: a self report depression scale for research in the general population. *Appl Psychol Meas*. 1977;1:385–401

71. Garrison CZ, Jackson KL, Marsteller F, McKeown R, Addy C. A longitudinal study of depressive symptomatology in young adolescents. *J Am Acad Child Adolesc Psychiatry*. 1990;29(4):581–585

72. Killen JD, Hayward C, Wilson DM, et al. Factors associated with eating disorder symptoms in a community sample of 6th and 7th grade girls. *Int J Eat Disord*. 1994;15(4):357–367

73. Roberts RE, Chen YW. Depressive symptoms and suicidal ideation among Mexican-origin and Anglo adolescents. *J Am Acad Child Adolesc Psychiatry*. 1995;34(1):81–90

74. Schoenbach VJ, Kaplan BH, Wagner EH, Grimson RC, Miller FT. Prevalence of self-reported depressive symptoms in young adolescents. *Am J Public Health*. 1983;73(11):1281–1287

75. Egede LE, Ye X, Zheng D, Silverstein MD. The prevalence and pattern of complementary and alternative medicine use in individuals with diabetes. *Diabetes Care*. 2002;25(2):324–329

76. Dham S, Shah V, Hirsch S, Banerji MA. The role of complementary and alternative medicine in diabetes. *Curr Diab Rep*. 2006;6(3):251–258

77. Dannemann K, Hecker W, Haberland H, et al. Use of complementary and alternative medicine in children with type 1 diabetes mellitus—prevalence, patterns of use, and costs. *Pediatr Diabetes*. 2008;9(3 pt 1):228–235

78. Geil P, Shane-McWhorter L. Dietary supplements in the management of diabetes: potential risks and benefits. *J Am Diet Assoc*. 2008;108(4 suppl 1):S59–S65

79. Miller JL, Cao D, Miller JG, Lipton RB. Correlates of complementary and alternative medicine (CAM) use in Chicago area children with diabetes (DM). *Prim Care Diabetes*. 2009;3(3):149–156

ERRATUM

An error occurred in the American Academy of Pediatrics "Technical Report: Management of Type 2 Diabetes Mellitus in Children and Adolescents" published in the February 2013 issue of *Pediatrics* (2013;131[2]:e648–e664).

On page e651, third column, under "Definitions," the first sentence should read as follows: "Children and adolescents: children <10 years of age; adolescents ≥ 10 years but ≤ 18 years of age."

doi:10.1542/peds.2013-0667

Diabetes Clinical Practice Guideline Quick Reference Tools

- Action Statement Summary
  — Management of Newly Diagnosed Type 2 Diabetes Mellitus (T2DM) in Children and Adolescents
- *ICD-10-CM* Coding Quick Reference for Type 2 Diabetes Mellitus
- AAP Patient Education Handout
  — *Type 2 Diabetes: Tips for Healthy Living*

Action Statement Summary

Management of Newly Diagnosed Type 2 Diabetes Mellitus (T2DM) in Children and Adolescents

Key Action Statement 1

Clinicians must ensure that insulin therapy is initiated for children and adolescents with T2DM who are ketotic or in diabetic ketoacidosis and in whom the distinction between T1DM and T2DM is unclear; and, in usual cases, should initiate insulin therapy for patients:
- who have random venous or plasma BG concentrations ≥250 mg/dL; or
- whose HbA1c is >9%.

(Strong Recommendation: evidence quality X, validating studies cannot be performed, and C, observational studies and expert opinion; preponderance of benefit over harm.)

Key Action Statement 2

In all other instances, clinicians should initiate a lifestyle modification program, including nutrition and physical activity, and start metformin as first-line therapy for children and adolescents at the time of diagnosis of T2DM. (Strong recommendation: evidence quality B; 1 RCT showing improved outcomes with metformin versus lifestyle; preponderance of benefits over harms.)

Key Action Statement 3

The committee suggests that clinicians monitor HbA1c concentrations every 3 months and intensify treatment if treatment goals for BG and HbA1c concentrations are not being met. (Option: evidence quality D; expert opinion and studies in children with T1DM and in adults with T2DM; preponderance of benefits over harms.)

Key Action Statement 4

The committee suggests that clinicians advise patients to monitor finger-stick BG concentrations in those who
- are taking insulin or other medications with a risk of hypoglycemia; or
- are initiating or changing their diabetes treatment regimen; or
- have not met treatment goals; or
- have intercurrent illnesses.

(Option: evidence quality D; expert consensus. Preponderance of benefits over harms.)

Key Action Statement 5

The committee suggests that clinicians incorporate the Academy of Nutrition and Dietetics' *Pediatric Weight Management Evidence-Based Nutrition Practice Guidelines* in the nutrition counseling of patients with T2DM both at the time of diagnosis and as part of ongoing management. (Option; evidence quality D; expert opinion; preponderance of benefits over harms. Role of patient preference is dominant.)

Key Action Statement 6

The committee suggests that clinicians encourage children and adolescents with T2DM to engage in moderate-to-vigorous exercise for at least 60 minutes daily and to limit nonacademic screen time to less than 2 hours per day. (Option: evidence quality D, expert opinion and evidence from studies of metabolic syndrome and obesity; preponderance of benefits over harms. Role of patient preference is dominant.)

Coding Quick Reference for Type 2 Diabetes Mellitus

ICD-10-CM

E11.649	Type 2 diabetes mellitus with hypoglycemia without coma
E11.65	Type 2 diabetes mellitus with hyperglycemia
E11.8	Type 2 diabetes mellitus with unspecified complications
E11.9	Type 2 diabetes mellitus without complications
E13.9	Other specified diabetes mellitus without complications

Use codes above (**E11.8–E13.9**). *ICD-10-CM* does not discern between controlled and uncontrolled.

Type 2 Diabetes: Tips for Healthy Living

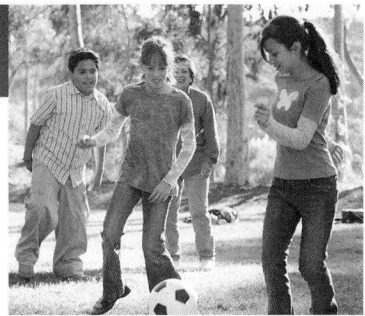

Children with type 2 diabetes can live a healthy life. If your child has been diagnosed with type 2 diabetes, your child's doctor will talk with you about the importance of lifestyle and medication in keeping your child's blood glucose (blood sugar) levels under control.

Read on for information from the American Academy of Pediatrics (AAP) about managing blood glucose and creating plans for healthy living.

What is blood glucose?

Glucose is found in the blood and is the body's main source of energy. The food your child eats is broken down by the body into glucose. Glucose is a type of sugar that gives energy to the cells in the body.

The cells need the help of insulin to take the glucose from the blood to the cells. Insulin is made by an organ called the pancreas.

In children with type 2 diabetes, the pancreas does not make enough insulin and the cells don't use the insulin very well.

Why is it important to manage blood glucose levels?

Glucose will build up in the blood if it cannot be used by the cells. High blood glucose levels can damage many parts of the body, such as the eyes, kidneys, nerves, and heart.

Your child's blood glucose levels may need to be checked on a regular schedule to make sure the levels do not get too high. Your child's doctor will tell you what your child's blood glucose level should be. You and your child will need to learn how to use a glucose meter. Blood glucose levels can be quickly and easily measured using a glucose meter. First, a lancet is used to prick the skin; then a drop of blood from your child's finger is placed on a test strip that is inserted into the meter.

Are there medicines for type 2 diabetes?

Insulin in a shot or another medicine by mouth may be prescribed by your child's doctor if needed to help control your child's blood glucose levels. If your child's doctor has prescribed a medicine, it's important that your child take it as directed. Side effects from certain medicines may include bloating or gassiness. Check with your child's doctor if you have questions.

Along with medicines, your child's doctor will suggest changes to your child's diet and encourage your child to be physically active.

Tips for healthy living

A healthy diet and staying active are especially important for children with type 2 diabetes. Your child's blood glucose levels are easier to manage when you child is at a healthy weight.

Create a plan for eating healthy

Talk with your child's doctor and registered dietitian about a meal plan that meets the needs of your child. The following tips can help you select foods that are healthy and contain a high content of nutrients (protein, vitamins, and minerals):

- Eat at least 5 servings of fruits and vegetables each day.
- Include high-fiber, whole-grain foods such as brown rice, whole-grain pasta, corns, peas, and breads and cereals at meals. Sweet potatoes are also a good choice.
- Choose lower-fat or fat-free toppings like grated low-fat parmesan cheese, salsa, herbed cottage cheese, nonfat/low-fat gravy, low-fat sour cream, low-fat salad dressing, or yogurt.
- Select lean meats such as skinless chicken and turkey, fish, lean beef cuts (round, sirloin, chuck, loin, lean ground beef—no more than 15% fat content), and lean pork cuts (tenderloin, chops, ham). Trim off all visible fat. Remove skin from cooked poultry before eating.
- Include healthy oils such as canola or olive oil in your diet. Choose margarine and vegetable oils without trans fats made from canola, corn, sunflower, soybean, or olive oils.
- Use nonstick vegetable sprays when cooking.
- Use fat-free cooking methods such as baking, broiling, grilling, poaching, or steaming when cooking meat, poultry, or fish.
- Serve vegetable- and broth-based soups, or use nonfat (skim) or low-fat (1%) milk or evaporated skim milk when making cream soups.
- Use the Nutrition Facts label on food packages to find foods with less saturated fat per serving. Pay attention to the serving size as you make choices. Remember that the percent daily values on food labels are based on portion sizes and calorie levels for adults.

Create a plan for physical activity

Physical activity, along with proper nutrition, promotes lifelong health. Following are some ideas on how to get fit:

- **Encourage your child to be active at least 1 hour a day.** Active play is the best exercise for younger children! Parents can join their children and have fun while being active too. School-aged child should participate every day in 1 hour or more of moderate to vigorous physical activity that is right for their age, is enjoyable, and involves a variety of activities.
- **Limit television watching and computer use.** The AAP discourages TV and other media use by children younger than 2 years and encourages interactive play. For older children, total entertainment screen time should be limited to less than 1 to 2 hours per day.
- **Keep an activity log.** The use of activity logs can help children and teens keep track of their exercise programs and physical activity. Online tools can be helpful.

- **Get the whole family involved.** It is a great way to spend time together. Also, children who regularly see their parents enjoying sports and physical activity are more likely to do so themselves.
- **Provide a safe environment.** Make sure your child's equipment and chosen site for the sport or activity are safe. Make sure your child's clothing is comfortable and appropriate.

For more information

National Diabetes Education Program

http://ndep.nih.gov

Listing of resources does not imply an endorsement by the American Academy of Pediatrics (AAP). The AAP is not responsible for the content of the resources mentioned in this publication. Web site addresses are as current as possible, but may change at any time.

The persons whose photographs are depicted in this publication are professional models. They have no relation to the issues discussed. Any characters they are portraying are fictional.

The information contained in this publication should not be used as a substitute for the medical care and advice of your pediatrician. There may be variations in treatment that your pediatrician may recommend based on individual facts and circumstances.

From your doctor

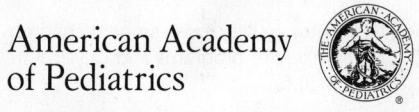

American Academy
of Pediatrics

DEDICATED TO THE HEALTH OF ALL CHILDREN™

The American Academy of Pediatrics is an organization of 60,000 primary care pediatricians, pediatric medical subspecialists, and pediatric surgical specialists dedicated to the health, safety, and well-being of infants, children, adolescents, and young adults.

American Academy of Pediatrics
Web site—www.HealthyChildren.org

Early Detection of Developmental Dysplasia of the Hip

- *Clinical Practice Guideline*
- *Technical Report Summary*

Readers of this clinical practice guideline are urged to review the technical report summary to enhance the evidence-based decision-making process.

AMERICAN ACADEMY OF PEDIATRICS

Committee on Quality Improvement, Subcommittee on Developmental Dysplasia of the Hip

Clinical Practice Guideline: Early Detection of Developmental Dysplasia of the Hip

ABSTRACT. *Developmental dysplasia of the hip* is the preferred term to describe the condition in which the femoral head has an abnormal relationship to the acetabulum. Developmental dysplasia of the hip includes frank dislocation (luxation), partial dislocation (subluxation), instability wherein the femoral head comes in and out of the socket, and an array of radiographic abnormalities that reflect inadequate formation of the acetabulum. Because many of these findings may not be present at birth, the term *developmental* more accurately reflects the biologic features than does the term *congenital*. The disorder is uncommon. The earlier a dislocated hip is detected, the simpler and more effective is the treatment. Despite newborn screening programs, dislocated hips continue to be diagnosed later in infancy and childhood,[1–11] in some instances delaying appropriate therapy and leading to a substantial number of malpractice claims. The objective of this guideline is to reduce the number of dislocated hips detected later in infancy and childhood. The target audience is the primary care provider. The target patient is the healthy newborn up to 18 months of age, excluding those with neuromuscular disorders, myelodysplasia, or arthrogryposis.

ABBREVIATIONS. DDH, developmental dysplasia of the hip; AVN, avascular necrosis of the hip.

BIOLOGIC FEATURES AND NATURAL HISTORY

Understanding the developmental nature of developmental dysplasia of the hip (DDH) and the subsequent spectrum of hip abnormalities requires a knowledge of the growth and development of the hip joint.[12] Embryologically, the femoral head and acetabulum develop from the same block of primitive mesenchymal cells. A cleft develops to separate them at 7 to 8 weeks' gestation. By 11 weeks' gestation, development of the hip joint is complete. At birth, the femoral head and the acetabulum are primarily cartilaginous. The acetabulum continues to develop postnatally. The growth of the fibrocartilaginous rim (the labrum) that surrounds

The recommendations in this statement do not indicate an exclusive course of treatment or serve as a standard of medical care. Variations, taking into account individual circumstances, may be appropriate.

The Practice Guideline, "Early Detection of Developmental Dysplasia of the Hip," was reviewed by appropriate committees and sections of the American Academy of Pediatrics (AAP) including the Chapter Review Group, a focus group of office-based pediatricians representing each AAP District: Gene R. Adams, MD; Robert M. Corwin, MD; Diane Fuquay, MD; Barbara M. Harley, MD; Thomas J. Herr, MD, Chair; Kenneth E. Matthews, MD; Robert D. Mines, MD; Lawrence C. Pakula, MD; Howard B. Weinblatt, MD; and Delosa A. Young, MD. The Practice Guideline was also reviewed by relevant outside medical organizations as part of the peer review process.

the bony acetabulum deepens the socket. Development of the femoral head and acetabulum are intimately related, and normal adult hip joints depend on further growth of these structures. Hip dysplasia may occur in utero, perinatally, or during infancy and childhood.

The acronym DDH includes hips that are unstable, subluxated, dislocated (luxated), and/or have malformed acetabula. A hip is *unstable* when the tight fit between the femoral head and the acetabulum is lost and the femoral head is able to move within (subluxated) or outside (dislocated) the confines of the acetabulum. A *dislocation* is a complete loss of contact of the femoral head with the acetabulum. Dislocations are divided into 2 types: teratologic and typical.[12] *Teratologic dislocations* occur early in utero and often are associated with neuromuscular disorders, such as arthrogryposis and myelodysplasia, or with various dysmorphic syndromes. The *typical dislocation* occurs in an otherwise healthy infant and may occur prenatally or postnatally.

During the immediate newborn period, laxity of the hip capsule predominates, and, if clinically significant enough, the femoral head may spontaneously dislocate and relocate. If the hip spontaneously relocates and stabilizes within a few days, subsequent hip development usually is normal. If subluxation or dislocation persists, then structural anatomic changes may develop. A deep concentric position of the femoral head in the acetabulum is necessary for normal development of the hip. When not deeply reduced (subluxated), the labrum may become everted and flattened. Because the femoral head is not reduced into the depth of the socket, the acetabulum does not grow and remodel and, therefore, becomes shallow. If the femoral head moves further out of the socket (dislocation), typically superiorly and laterally, the inferior capsule is pulled upward over the now empty socket. Muscles surrounding the hip, especially the adductors, become contracted, limiting abduction of the hip. The hip capsule constricts; once this capsular constriction narrows to less than the diameter of the femoral head, the hip can no longer be reduced by manual manipulative maneuvers, and operative reduction usually is necessary.

The hip is at risk for dislocation during 4 periods: 1) the 12th gestational week, 2) the 18th gestational week, 3) the final 4 weeks of gestation, and 4) the postnatal period. During the 12th gestational week, the hip is at risk as the fetal lower limb rotates medially. A dislocation at this time is termed teratologic. All elements of the hip joint develop abnormally. The hip muscles develop around the 18th gestational week. Neuromuscular problems at this time, such as myelodysplasia and arthrogryposis, also lead to teratologic dislocations. During the final 4 weeks of pregnancy, mechanical forces have a role. Conditions such as oligohydramnios or breech position predispose to DDH.[13] Breech position occurs in ~3% of births, and DDH occurs more frequently in breech presentations, reportedly in as many as 23%. The frank breech position of hip flexion and knee extension places a newborn or infant at the highest risk. Postnatally, infant positioning such as swaddling, combined with ligamentous laxity, also has a role.

The true incidence of dislocation of the hip can only be presumed. There is no "gold standard" for diagnosis during the newborn period. Physical examination, plane radiography, and ultrasonography all are fraught with false-positive and false-negative results. Arthrography (insertion of contrast medium into the hip joint) and magnetic resonance imaging, although accurate for determining the precise hip anatomy, are inappropriate methods for screening the newborn and infant.

The reported incidence of DDH is influenced by genetic and racial factors, diagnostic criteria, the experience and training of the examiner, and the age of the child at the time of the examination. Wynne-Davies[14] reported an increased risk to subsequent children in the presence of a diagnosed dislocation (6% risk with healthy parents and an affected child, 12% risk with an affected parent, and 36% risk with an affected parent and 1 affected child). DDH is not always detectable at birth, but some newborn screening surveys suggest an incidence as high as 1 in 100 newborns with evidence of instability, and 1 to 1.5 cases of dislocation per 1000 newborns. The incidence of DDH is higher in girls. Girls are especially susceptible to the maternal hormone relaxin, which may contribute to ligamentous laxity with the resultant instability of the hip. The left hip is involved 3 times as commonly as the right hip, perhaps related to the left occiput anterior positioning of most non-breech newborns. In this position, the left hip resides posteriorly against the mother's spine, potentially limiting abduction.

PHYSICAL EXAMINATION

DDH is an evolving process, and its physical findings on clinical examination change.[12,15,16] The newborn must be relaxed and preferably examined on a firm surface. Considerable patience and skill are required. The physical examination changes as the child grows older. No signs are pathognomonic for a dislocated hip. The examiner must look for asymmetry. Indeed, bilateral dislocations are more difficult to diagnose than unilateral dislocations because symmetry is retained. Asymmetrical thigh or gluteal folds, better observed when the child is prone, apparent limb length discrepancy, and restricted motion, especially abduction, are significant, albeit not pathognomonic signs. With the infant supine and the pelvis stabilized, abduction to 75° and adduction to 30° should occur readily under normal circumstances.

The 2 maneuvers for assessing hip stability in the newborn are the Ortolani and Barlow tests. The Ortolani elicits the sensation of the dislocated hip reducing, and the Barlow detects the unstable hip dislocating from the acetabulum. The Ortolani is performed with the newborn supine and the examiner's index and middle fingers placed along the greater trochanter with the thumb placed along the inner thigh. The hip is flexed to 90° but not more, and the leg is held in neutral rotation. The hip is gently abducted while lifting the leg anteriorly. With this maneuver, a "clunk" is felt as the dislocated femoral head reduces into the acetabulum. This is a positive Ortolani sign. The Barlow provocative test is performed with the newborn positioned supine and the hips flexed to 90°. The leg is then gently adducted while posteriorly directed pressure is placed on the knee. A palpable clunk or sensation of movement is felt as the femoral head exits the acetabulum posteriorly. This is a positive Barlow sign. The Ortolani and Barlow maneuvers are performed 1 hip at a time. Little force is required for the performance of either of these tests. The goal is not to prove that the hip can be dislocated. Forceful and repeated examinations can break the seal between the labrum and the femoral head. These strongly positive signs of Ortolani and Barlow are distinguished from a large array of soft or equivocal physical findings present during the newborn period. High-pitched clicks are commonly elicited with flexion and extension and are inconsequential. A dislocatable hip has a rather distinctive clunk, whereas a subluxable hip is characterized by a feeling of looseness, a sliding movement, but without the true Ortolani and Barlow clunks. Separating true dislocations (clunks) from a feeling of instability and from benign adventitial sounds (clicks) takes practice and expertise. This guideline recognizes the broad range of physical findings present in newborns and infants and the confusion of terminology generated in the literature. By 8 to 12 weeks of age, the capsule laxity decreases, muscle tightness increases, and the Barlow and Ortolani maneuvers are no longer positive regardless of the status of the femoral head. In the 3-month-old infant, limitation of abduction is the most reliable sign associated with DDH. Other features that arouse suspicion include asymmetry of thigh folds, a positive Allis or Galeazzi sign (relative shortness of the femur with the hips and knees flexed), and discrepancy of leg lengths. These physical findings alert the examiner that abnormal relationships of the femoral head to the acetabulum (dislocation and subluxation) *may* be present.

Maldevelopments of the acetabulum alone (acetabular dysplasia) can be determined only by imaging techniques. Abnormal physical findings may be absent in an infant with acetabular dysplasia but no subluxation or dislocation. Indeed, because of the confusion, inconsistencies, and misuse of language in the literature (eg, an Ortolani sign called a click by some and a clunk by others), this guideline uses the following definitions.

- A *positive examination* result for DDH is the Barlow or Ortolani sign. This is the clunk of dislocation or reduction.
- An *equivocal examination* or *warning signs* include an array of physical findings that may be found in children with DDH, in children with another orthopaedic disorder, or in children who are completely healthy. These physical findings include asymmetric thigh or buttock creases, an apparent or true short leg, and limited abduction. These signs, used singly or in combination, serve to raise the pediatrician's index of suspicion and act as a threshold for referral. Newborn soft tissue hip clicks are not predictive of DDH[17] but may be confused with the Ortolani and Barlow clunks by some screening physicians and thereby be a reason for referral.

IMAGING

Radiographs of the pelvis and hips have historically been used to assess an infant with suspected DDH. During the first few months of life when the femoral heads are composed entirely of cartilage, radiographs have limited value. Displacement and instability may be undetectable, and evaluation of acetabular development is influenced by the infant's position at the time the radiograph is performed. By 4 to 6 months of age, radiographs become more reliable, particularly when the ossification center develops in the femoral head. Radiographs are readily available and relatively low in cost.

Real-time ultrasonography has been established as an accurate method for imaging the hip during the first few months of life.[15,18–25] With ultrasonography, the cartilage can be visualized and the hip can be viewed while assessing the stability of the hip and the morphologic features of the acetabulum. In some clinical settings, ultrasonography can provide information comparable to arthrography (direct injection of contrast into the hip joint), without the need for sedation, invasion, contrast medium, or ionizing radiation. Although the availability of equipment for ultrasonography is widespread, accurate results in hip sonography require training and experience. Although expertise in pediatric hip ultrasonography is increasing, this examination may not always be available or obtained conveniently. Ultrasonographic techniques include *static evaluation* of the morphologic features of the hip, as popularized in Europe by Graf,[26] and a *dynamic evaluation*, as developed by Harcke[20] that assesses the hip for stability of the femoral head in the socket, as well as static anatomy. Dynamic ultrasonography yields more useful information. With both techniques, there is considerable interobserver variability, especially during the first 3 weeks of life.[7,27]

Experience with ultrasonography has documented its ability to detect abnormal position, instability, and dysplasia not evident on clinical examination. Ultrasonography during the first 4 weeks of life often reveals the presence of minor degrees of instability and acetabular immaturity. Studies[7,28,29] indicate that nearly all these mild early findings, which will not be apparent on physical examination, resolve spontaneously without treatment. Newborn screening with ultrasonography has required a high frequency of reexamination and results in a large number of hips being unnecessarily treated. One study[23] demonstrates that a screening process with higher false-positive results also yields increased prevention of late cases. Ultrasonographic screening of all infants at 4 to 6 weeks of age would be expensive, requiring considerable resources. This practice is yet to be validated by clinical trial. *Consequently, the use of ultrasonography is recommended as an adjunct to the clinical evaluation.* It is the technique of choice for clarifying a physical finding, assessing a high-risk infant, and monitoring DDH as it is observed or treated. Used in this selective capacity, it can guide treatment and may prevent overtreatment.

PRETERM INFANTS

DDH may be unrecognized in prematurely born infants. When the infant has cardiorespiratory problems, the diagnosis and management are focused on providing appropriate ventilatory and cardiovascular support, and careful examination of the hips may be deferred until a later date. The most complete examination the infant receives may occur at the time of discharge from the hospital, and this single examination may not detect subluxation or dislocation. Despite the medical urgencies surrounding the preterm infant, it is critical to examine the entire child.

METHODS FOR GUIDELINE DEVELOPMENT

Our goal was to develop a practice parameter by using a process that would be based whenever possible on available evidence. The methods used a combination of expert panel, decision modeling, and evidence synthesis[30] (see the Technical Report available on *Pediatrics electronic pages* at www.pediatrics.org). The predominant methods recommended for such evidence synthesis are generally of 2 types: a *data-driven* method and a *model-driven*[31,32] method. In data-driven methods, the analyst finds the best data available and induces a conclusion from these data. A model-driven method, in contrast, begins with an effort to define the context for evidence and then searches for the data as defined by that context. Data-driven methods are useful when the quality of evidence is high. A careful review of the medical literature revealed that the published evidence about DDH did not meet the criteria for high quality. There was a paucity of randomized clinical trials.[8] We decided, therefore, to use the model-driven method.

A decision model was constructed based on the perspective of practicing clinicians and determining the best strategy for screening and diagnosis. The target child was a full-term newborn with no obvious orthopaedic abnormalities. We focused on the various options available to the pediatrician* for the detection of DDH, including screening by physical examination, screening by ultrasonography, and episodic screening during health supervision. Because

---

*In this guideline, the term *pediatrician* includes the range of pediatric primary care providers, eg, family practitioners and pediatric nurse practitioners.

the detection of a dislocated hip usually results in referral by the pediatrician, and because management of DDH is not in the purview of the pediatrician's care, treatment options are not included. We also included in our model a wide range of options for detecting DDH during the first year of life if the results of the newborn screen are negative.

The outcomes on which we focused were a dislocated hip at 1 year of age as the major morbidity of the disease and avascular necrosis of the hip (AVN) as the primary complication of DDH treatment. AVN is a loss of blood supply to the femoral head resulting in abnormal hip development, distortion of shape, and, in some instances, substantial morbidity. Ideally, a gold standard would be available to define DDH at any point in time. However, as noted, no gold standard exists except, perhaps, arthrography of the hip, which is an inappropriate standard for use in a detection model. Therefore, we defined outcomes in terms of the *process of care*. We reviewed the literature extensively. The purpose of the literature review was to provide the probabilities required by the decision model since there were no randomized clinical trials. The article or chapter title and the abstracts were reviewed by 2 members of the methodology team and members of the subcommittee. Articles not rejected were reviewed, and data were abstracted that would provide evidence for the probabilities required by the decision model. As part of the literature abstraction process, the evidence quality in each article was assessed. A computer-based literature search, hand review of recent publications, or examination of the reference section for other articles ("ancestor articles") identified 623 articles; 241 underwent detailed review, 118 of which provided some data. Of the 100 ancestor articles, only 17 yielded useful articles, suggesting that our accession process was complete. By traditional epidemiologic standards,[33] the quality of the evidence in this set of articles was uniformly low. There were few controlled trials and few studies of the follow-up of infants for whom the results of newborn examinations were negative. When the evidence was poor or lacking entirely, extensive discussions among members of the committee and the expert opinion of outside consultants were used to arrive at a consensus. No votes were taken. Disagreements were discussed, and consensus was achieved.

The available evidence was distilled in 3 ways.

First, estimates were made of DDH at birth in infants without risk factors. These estimates constituted the baseline risk. Second, estimates were made of the rates of DDH in the children with risk factors. These numbers guide clinical actions: rates that are too high might indicate referral or different follow-up despite negative physical findings. Third, each screening strategy (pediatrician-based, orthopaedist-based, and ultrasonography-based) was scored for the estimated number of children given a diagnosis of DDH at birth, at mid-term (4–12 months of age), and at late-term (12 months of age and older) and for the estimated number of cases of AVN incurred, assuming that all children given a diagnosis of DDH would be treated. These numbers suggest the best strategy, balancing DDH detection with incurring adverse effects.

The baseline estimate of DDH based on orthopaedic screening was 11.5/1000 infants. Estimates from pediatric screening were 8.6/1000 and from ultrasonography were 25/1000. The 11.5/1000 rate translates into a rate for not-at-risk boys of 4.1/1000 boys and a rate for not-at-risk girls of 19/1000 girls. These numbers derive from the facts that the relative risk—the rate in girls divided by the rate in boys across several studies—is 4.6 and because infants are split evenly between boys and girls, so .5 × 4.1/1000 + .5 × 19/1000 = 11.5/1000.[34,35] We used these baseline rates for calculating the rates in other risk groups. Because the relative risk of DDH for children with a positive family history (first-degree relatives) is 1.7, the rate for boys with a positive family history is 1.7 × 4.1 = 6.4/1000 boys, and for girls with a positive family history, 1.7 × 19 = 32/1000 girls. Finally, the relative risk of DDH for breech presentation (of all kinds) is 6.3, so the risk for breech boys is 7.0 × 4.1 = 29/1000 boys and for breech girls, 7.0 × 19 = 133/1000 girls. These numbers are summarized in Table 1.

These numbers suggest that boys without risk or those with a family history have the lowest risk; girls without risk and boys born in a breech presentation have an intermediate risk; and girls with a positive family history, and especially girls born in a breech presentation, have the highest risks. Guidelines, considering the risk factors, should follow these risk profiles. Reports of newborn screening for DDH have included various screening techniques. In some, the screening clinician was an orthopaedist, in

TABLE 1.   Relative and Absolute Risks for Finding a Positive Examination Result at Newborn Screening by Using the Ortolani and Barlow Signs

Newborn Characteristics	Relative Risk of a Positive Examination Result	Absolute Risk of a Positive Examination Result per 1000 Newborns With Risk Factors
All newborns	. . .	11.5
Boys	1.0	4.1
Girls	4.6	19
Positive family history	1.7	
Boys	. . .	6.4
Girls	. . .	32
Breech presentation	7.0	
Boys	. . .	29
Girls	. . .	133

TABLE 2.   Newborn Strategy*

Outcome	Orthopaedist PE	Pediatrician PE	Ultrasonography
DDH in newborn	12	8.6	25
DDH at ~6 mo of age	.1	.45	.28
DDH at 12 mo of age or more	.16	.33	.1
AVN at 12 mo of age	.06	.1	.1

* PE indicates physical examination. Outcome per 1000 infants initially screened.

others, a pediatrician, and in still others, a physiotherapist. In addition, screening has been performed by ultrasonography. In assessing the expected effect of each strategy, we estimated the newborn DDH rates, the mid-term DDH rates, and the late-term DDH rates for each of the 3 strategies, as shown in Table 2. We also estimated the rate of AVN for DDH treated before 2 months of age (2.5/1000 treated) and after 2 months of age (109/1000 treated). We could not distinguish the AVN rates for children treated between 2 and 12 months of age from those treated later. Table 2 gives these data. The total cases of AVN per strategy are calculated, assuming that all infants with positive examination results are treated.

Table 2 shows that a strategy using pediatricians to screen newborns would give the lowest newborn rate but the highest mid- and late-term DDH rates. To assess how much better an ultrasonography-only screening strategy would be, we could calculate a cost-effectiveness ratio. In this case, the "cost" of ultrasonographic screening is the number of "extra" newborn cases that probably include children who do not need to be treated. (The cost from AVN is the same in the 2 strategies.) By using these cases as the cost and the number of later cases averted as the effect, a ratio is obtained of 71 children treated neonatally because of a positive ultrasonographic screen for each later case averted. Because this number is high, and because the presumption of better late-term efficacy is based on a single study, we do not recommend ultrasonographic screening at this time.

RECOMMENDATIONS AND NOTES TO ALGORITHM (Fig 1)

1. **All newborns are to be screened by physical examination**. The evidence† for this recommendation is good. The expert consensus‡ is strong. Although initial screening by orthopaedists§ would be optimal (Table 2), it is doubtful that if widely practiced, such a strategy would give the same good results as those published from pediatric orthopaedic research centers. **It is recommended that screening be done by a properly trained health care provider** (eg, physician, pediatric nurse practitioner, physician assistant, or physical therapist). (Evidence for this recommendation is strong.) A number of studies performed by properly trained nonphysicians report results

indistinguishable from those performed by physicians.[36] The examination after discharge from the neonatal intensive care unit should be performed as a newborn examination with appropriate screening. **Ultrasonography of all newborns is not recommended.** (Evidence is fair; consensus is strong.) Although there is indirect evidence to support the use of ultrasonographic screening of all newborns, it is not advocated because it is operator-dependent, availability is questionable, it increases the rate of treatment, and interobserver variability is high. There are probably some increased costs. We considered a strategy of "no newborn screening." This arm is politically indefensible because screening newborns is inherent in pediatrician's care. The technical report details this limb through decision analysis. Regardless of the screening method used for the newborn, DDH is detected in 1 in 5000 infants at 18 months of age.[3] The evidence and consensus for newborn screening remain strong.

Newborn Physical Examination and Treatment

2. **If a positive Ortolani or Barlow sign is found in the newborn examination, the infant should be referred to an orthopaedist**. Orthopaedic referral is recommended when the Ortolani sign is unequivocally positive (a clunk). Orthopaedic referral is not recommended for any softly positive finding in the examination (eg, hip click without dislocation). The precise time frame for the newborn to be evaluated by the orthopaedist cannot be determined from the literature. However, the literature suggests that the majority of "abnormal" physical findings of hip examinations at birth (clicks and clunks) will resolve by 2 weeks; therefore, consultation and possible initiation of treatment are recommended by that time. The data recommending that all those with a positive Ortolani sign be referred to an orthopaedist are limited, but expert panel consensus, nevertheless, was strong, because pediatricians do not have the training to take full responsibility and because true Ortolani clunks are rare and their management is more appropriately performed by the orthopaedist.

If the results of the physical examination at birth are "equivocally" positive (ie, soft click, mild asymmetry, but neither an Ortolani nor a Barlow sign is present), then a follow-up hip examination by the pediatrician in 2 weeks is recommended. (Evidence is good; consensus is strong.) The available data suggest that most clicks resolve by 2 weeks and that these "benign hip clicks" in the newborn period do

---

†In this guideline, evidence is listed as good, fair, or poor based on the methodologist's evaluation of the literature quality. (See the Technical Report.)

‡Opinion or consensus is listed as *strong* if opinion of the expert panel was unanimous or *mixed* if there were dissenting points of view.

§In this guideline, the term *orthopaedist* refers to an orthopaedic surgeon with expertise in pediatric orthopaedic conditions.

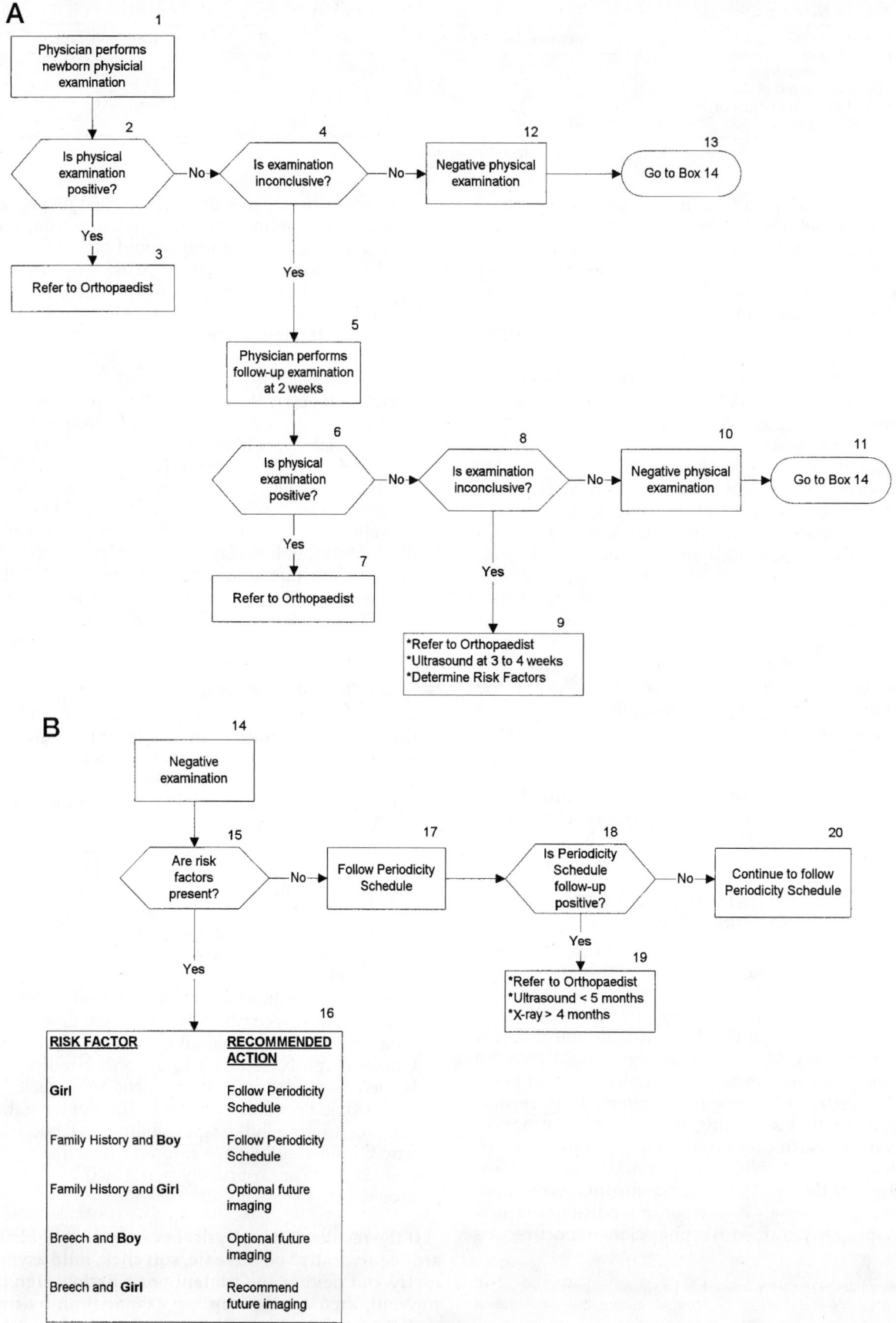

Fig 1. Screening for developmental hip dysplasia—clinical algorithm.

not lead to later hip dysplasia.[9,17,28,37] Thus, for an infant with softly positive signs, the pediatrician should reexamine the hips at 2 weeks before making referrals for orthopaedic care or ultrasonography. We recognize the concern of pediatricians about adherence to follow-up care regimens, but this concern regards all aspects of health maintenance and is not a reason to request ultrasonography or other diagnostic study of the newborn hips.

3. **If the results of the newborn physical examination are positive (ie, presence of an Ortolani or a Barlow sign), ordering an ultrasonographic examination of the newborn is not recommended.** (Evidence is poor; opinion is strong.) Treatment decisions are not influenced by the results of ultrasonography but are based on the results of the physical examination. The treating physician may use a variety of imaging studies during clinical management. **If the results of the newborn physical examination are positive, obtaining a radiograph of the newborn's pelvis and hips is not recommended** (evidence is poor; opinion is strong), because they are of limited value and do not influence treatment decisions.

The use of triple diapers when abnormal physical signs are detected during the newborn period is not recommended. (Evidence is poor; opinion is strong.) Triple diaper use is common practice despite the lack of data on the effectiveness of triple diaper use; and, in instances of frank dislocation, the use of triple diapers may delay the initiation of more appropriate treatment (such as with the Pavlik harness). Often, the primary care pediatrician may not have performed the newborn examination in the hospital. The importance of communication cannot be overemphasized, and triple diapers may aid in follow-up as a reminder that a possible abnormal physical examination finding was present in the newborn.

2-Week Examination

4. **If the results of the physical examination are positive (eg, positive Ortolani or Barlow sign) at 2 weeks, refer to an orthopaedist.** (Evidence is strong; consensus is strong.) Referral is urgent but is not an emergency. Consensus is strong that, as in the newborn, the presence of an Ortolani or Barlow sign at 2 weeks warrants referral to an orthopaedist. An Ortolani sign at 2 weeks may be a new finding or a finding that was not apparent at the time of the newborn examination.

5. **If at the 2-week examination the Ortolani and Barlow signs are absent but physical findings raise suspicions, consider referral to an orthopaedist or request ultrasonography at age 3 to 4 weeks.** Consensus is mixed about the follow-up for softly positive or equivocal findings at 2 weeks of age (eg, adventitial click, thigh asymmetry, and apparent leg length difference). Because it is necessary to confirm the status of the hip joint, the pediatrician can consider referral to an orthopaedist or for ultrasonography if the constellation of physical findings raises a high level of suspicion.

However, if the physical findings are minimal, continuing follow-up by the periodicity schedule with focused hip examinations is also an option, provided risk factors are considered. (See "Recommendations" 7 and 8.)

6. **If the results of the physical examination are negative at 2 weeks, follow-up is recommended at the scheduled well-baby periodic examinations.** (Evidence is good; consensus is strong.)

7. **Risk factors. If the results of the newborn examination are negative (or equivocally positive), risk factors may be considered.**[13,21,38–41] Risk factors are a study of thresholds to act.[42] Table 1 gives the risk of finding a positive Ortolani or Barlow sign at the time of the initial newborn screening. If this examination is negative, the absolute risk of there being a true dislocated hip is greatly reduced. Nevertheless, the data in Table 1 may influence the pediatrician to perform confirmatory evaluations. Action will vary based on the individual clinician. The following recommendations are made (evidence is strong; opinion is strong):

   • **Girl** (newborn risk of 19/1000). When the results of the newborn examination are negative or equivocally positive, hips should be reevaluated at 2 weeks of age. If negative, continue according to the periodicity schedule; if positive, refer to an orthopaedist or for ultrasonography at 3 weeks of age.

   • **Infants with a positive family history of DDH** (newborn risk for boys of 9.4/1000 and for girls, 44/1000). When the results of the newborn examination in boys are negative or equivocally positive, hips should be reevaluated at 2 weeks of age. If negative, continue according to the periodicity schedule; if positive, refer to an orthopaedist or for ultrasonography at 3 weeks of age. In girls, the absolute risk of 44/1000 may exceed the pediatrician's threshold to act, and imaging with an ultrasonographic examination at 6 weeks of age or a radiograph of the pelvis at 4 months of age is recommended.

   • **Breech presentation** (newborn risk for boys of 26/1000 and for girls, 120/1000). **For negative or equivocally positive newborn examinations, the infant should be reevaluated at regular intervals (according to the periodicity schedule) if the examination results remain negative.** Because an absolute risk of 120/1000 (12%) probably exceeds most pediatricians' threshold to act, imaging with an ultrasonographic examination at 6 weeks of age or with a radiograph of the pelvis and hips at 4 months of age is recommended. In addition, because some reports show a high incidence of hip abnormalities detected at an older age in children born breech, this imaging strategy remains an option for all children born breech, not just girls. These hip abnormalities are, for the most part, inadequate development of the acetabulum. Acetabular dysplasia is best found by a radiographic examination at 6 months of age or older. A suggestion of poorly formed acetabula may be observed at 6 weeks of age by ultrasonography, but the best study remains a radiograph performed closer to 6 months of age. Ultrasonographic newborn screening of all breech infants will not eliminate the possibility of later acetabular dysplasia.

8. **Periodicity. The hips must be examined at every well-baby visit according to the recommended periodicity schedule for well-baby examinations (2–4 days for newborns discharged in less than 48 hours after delivery, by 1 month, 2 months, 4 months, 6 months, 9 months, and 12 months of age).** If at any time during the follow-up period DDH is suspected because of an abnormal physical examination or by a parental complaint of difficulty diapering or abnormal appearing legs, the pediatrician must confirm that the hips are stable, in the sockets, and developing normally. Confirmation can be made by a focused physical examination when the infant is calm and relaxed, by consultation with another primary care pediatrician, by consultation with an orthopaedist, by ultrasonography if the infant is younger than 5 months of age, or by radiography if the infant is older than 4 months of age. (Between 4 and 6 months of age, ultrasonography and radiography seem to be equally effective diagnostic imaging studies.)

DISCUSSION

DDH is an important term because it accurately reflects the biologic features of the disorder and the susceptibility of the hip to become dislocated at various times. Dislocated hips always will be diagnosed later in infancy and childhood because not every dislocated hip is detectable at birth, and hips continue to dislocate throughout the first year of life. Thus, this guideline requires that the pediatrician follow *a process of care for the detection of DDH*. The process recommended for early detection of DDH includes the following:

- Screen all newborns' hips by physical examination.
- Examine all infants' hips according to a periodicity schedule and follow-up until the child is an established walker.
- Record and document physical findings.
- Be aware of the changing physical examination for DDH.
- If physical findings raise suspicion of DDH, or if parental concerns suggest hip disease, confirmation is required by expert physical examination, referral to an orthopaedist, or by an age-appropriate imaging study.

When this process of care is followed, the number of dislocated hips diagnosed at 1 year of age should be minimized. However, the problem of late detection of dislocated hips will not be eliminated. The results of screening programs have indicated that 1 in 5000 children have a dislocated hip detected at 18 months of age or older.[3]

TECHNICAL REPORT

The Technical Report is available from the American Academy of Pediatrics from several sources. The Technical Report is published in full-text on *Pediatrics electronic pages*. It is also available in a compendium of practice guidelines that contains guidelines and evidence reports together. The objective was to create a recommendation to pediatricians and other primary care providers about their role as screeners for detecting DDH. The patients are a theoretical cohort of newborns. A model-based method using decision analysis was the foundation. Components of the approach include:

- Perspective: primary care provider
- Outcomes: DDH and AVN
- Preferences: expected rates of outcomes
- Model: influence diagram assessed from the subcommittee and from the methodology team with critical feedback from the subcommittee
- Evidence sources: Medline and EMBase (detailed in "Methods" section)
- Evidence quality: assessed on a custom, subjective scale, based primarily on the fit of the evidence in the decision model

The results are detailed in the "Methods" section. Based on the raw evidence and Bayesian hierarchical meta-analysis,[34,35] estimates for the incidence of DDH based on the type of screener (orthopaedist vs pediatrician); the odds ratio for DDH given risk factors of sex, family history, and breech presentation; and estimates for late detection and AVN were determined and are detailed in the "Methods" section and in Tables 1 and 2.

The decision model (reduced based on available evidence) suggests that orthopaedic screening is optimal, but because orthopaedists in the published studies and in practice would differ in pediatric expertise, the supply of pediatric orthopaedists is relatively limited, and the difference between orthopaedists and pediatricians is statistically insignificant, we conclude that pediatric screening is to be recommended. The place for ultrasonography in the screening process remains to be defined because of the limited data available regarding late diagnosis in ultrasonography screening to permit definitive recommendations.

These data could be used by others to refine the conclusion based on costs, parental preferences, or physician style. Areas for research are well defined by our model-based method. All references are in the Technical Report.

RESEARCH QUESTIONS

The quality of the literature suggests many areas for research, because there is a paucity of randomized clinical trials and case-controlled studies. The following is a list of possibilities:

1. Minimum diagnostic abilities of a screener. Although there are data for pediatricians in general, few, if any, studies evaluated the abilities of an individual examiner. What should the minimum

sensitivity and specificity be, and how should they be assessed?

2. Intercurrent screening. There were few studies on systemic processes for screening after the newborn period.[2,43,44] Although several studies assessed postneonatal DDH, the data did not specify how many examinations were performed on each child before the abnormal result was found.

3. Trade-offs. Screening always results in false-positive results, and these patients suffer the adverse effects of therapy. How many unnecessary AVNs are we—families, physicians, and society—willing to tolerate from a screening program for every appropriately treated infant in whom late DDH was averted? This assessment depends on people's values and preferences and is not strictly an epidemiologic issue.

4. Postneonatal DDH after ultrasonographic screening. Although we concluded that ultrasonographic screening did not result in fewer diagnoses of postneonatal DDH, that conclusion was based on only 1 study.[36] Further study is needed.

5. Cost-effectiveness. If ultrasonographic screening reduces the number of postneonatal DDH diagnoses, then there will be a cost trade-off between the resources spent up front to screen everyone with an expensive technology, as in the case of ultrasonography, and the resources spent later to treat an expensive adverse event, as in the case of physical examination-based screening. The level at which the cost per case of postneonatal DDH averted is no longer acceptable is a matter of social preference, not of epidemiology.

ACKNOWLEDGMENTS

We acknowledge and appreciate the help of our methodology team, Richard Hinton, MD, Paola Morello, MD, and Jeanne Santoli, MD, who diligently participated in the literature review and abstracting the articles into evidence tables, and the subcommittee on evidence analysis.

We would also like to thank Robert Sebring, PhD, for assisting in the management of this process; Bonnie Cosner for managing the workflow; and Chris Kwiat, MLS, from the American Academy of Pediatrics Bakwin Library, who performed the literature searches.

COMMITTEE ON QUALITY IMPROVEMENT, 1999–2000
Charles J. Homer, MD, MPH, Chairperson
Richard D. Baltz, MD
Gerald B. Hickson, MD
Paul V. Miles, MD
Thomas B. Newman, MD, MPH
Joan E. Shook, MD
William M. Zurhellen, MD

Betty A. Lowe, MD, Liaison, National Association of Children's Hospitals and Related Institutions (NACHRI)
Ellen Schwalenstocker, MBA, Liaison, NACHRI
Michael J. Goldberg, MD, Liaison, Council on Sections
Richard Shiffman, MD, Liaison, Section on Computers and Other Technology
Jan Ellen Berger, MD, Liaison, Committee on Medical Liability
F. Lane France, MD, Committee on Practice and Ambulatory Medicine

SUBCOMMITTEE ON DEVELOPMENTAL DYSPLASIA OF THE HIP, 1999–2000
Michael J. Goldberg, MD, Chairperson
 Section on Orthopaedics
Theodore H. Harcke, MD
 Section on Radiology
Anthony Hirsch, MD
 Practitioner
Harold Lehmann, MD, PhD
 Section on Epidemiology
Dennis R. Roy, MD
 Section on Orthopaedics
Philip Sunshine, MD
 Section on Perinatology

CONSULTANT
Carol Dezateux, MB, MPH

REFERENCES

1. Bjerkreim I, Hagen O, Ikonomou N, Kase T, Kristiansen T, Arseth P. Late diagnosis of developmental dislocation of the hip in Norway during the years 1980–1989. *J Pediatr Orthop B*. 1993;2:112–114
2. Clarke N, Clegg J, Al-Chalabi A. Ultrasound screening of hips at risk for CDH: failure to reduce the incidence of late cases. *J Bone Joint Surg Br*. 1989;71:9–12
3. Dezateux C, Godward C. Evaluating the national screening programme for congenital dislocation of the hip. *J Med Screen*. 1995;2:200–206
4. Hadlow V. Neonatal screening for congenital dislocation of the hip: a prospective 21-year survey. *J Bone Joint Surg Br*. 1988;70:740–743
5. Krikler S, Dwyer N. Comparison of results of two approaches to hip screening in infants. *J Bone Joint Surg Br*. 1992;74:701–703
6. Macnicol M. Results of a 25-year screening programme for neonatal hip instability. *J Bone Joint Surg Br*. 1990;72:1057–1060
7. Marks DS, Clegg J, Al-Chalabi AN. Routine ultrasound screening for neonatal hip instability: can it abolish late-presenting congenital dislocation of the hip? *J Bone Joint Surg Br*. 1994;76:534–538
8. Rosendahl K, Markestad T, Lie R. Congenital dislocation of the hip: a prospective study comparing ultrasound and clinical examination. *Acta Paediatr*. 1992;81:177–181
9. Sanfridson J, Redlund-Johnell I, Uden A. Why is congenital dislocation of the hip still missed? Analysis of 96,891 infants screened in Malmo 1956–1987. *Acta Orthop Scand*. 1991;62:87–91
10. Tredwell S, Bell H. Efficacy of neonatal hip examination. *J Pediatr Orthop*. 1981;1:61–65
11. Yngve D, Gross R. Late diagnosis of hip dislocation in infants. *J Pediatr Orthop*. 1990;10:777–779
12. Aronsson DD, Goldberg MJ, Kling TF, Roy DR. Developmental dysplasia of the hip. *Pediatrics*. 1994;94:201–212
13. Hinderaker T, Daltveit AK, Irgens LM, Uden A, Reikeras O. The impact of intra-uterine factors on neonatal hip instability: an analysis of 1,059,479 children in Norway. *Acta Orthop Scand*. 1994;65:239–242
14. Wynne-Davies R. Acetabular dysplasia and familial joint laxity: two etiological factors in congenital dislocation of the hip: a review of 589 patients and their families. *J Bone Joint Surg Br*. 1970;52:704–716
15. De Pellegrin M. Ultrasound screening for congenital dislocation of the hip: results and correlations between clinical and ultrasound findings. *Ital J Orthop Traumatol*. 1991;17:547–553
16. Stoffelen D, Urlus M, Molenaers G, Fabry G. Ultrasound, radiographs, and clinical symptoms in developmental dislocation of the hip: a study of 170 patients. *J Pediatr Orthop B*. 1995;4:194–199
17. Bond CD, Hennrikus WL, Della Maggiore E. Prospective evaluation of newborn soft tissue hip clicks with ultrasound. *J Pediatr Orthop*. 1997;17:199–201
18. Bialik V, Wiener F, Benderly A. Ultrasonography and screening in developmental displacement of the hip. *J Pediatr Orthop B*. 1992;1:51–54
19. Castelein R, Sauter A. Ultrasound screening for congenital dysplasia of the hip in newborns: its value. *J Pediatr Orthop*. 1988;8:666–670
20. Clarke NMP, Harcke HT, McHugh P, Lee MS, Borns PF, MacEwen GP. Real-time ultrasound in the diagnosis of congenital dislocation and dysplasia of the hip. *J Bone Joint Surg Br*. 1985;67:406–412
21. Garvey M, Donoghue V, Gorman W, O'Brien N, Murphy J. Radiographic screening at four months of infants at risk for congenital hip dislocation. *J Bone Joint Surg Br*. 1992;74:704–707
22. Langer R. Ultrasonic investigation of the hip in newborns in the diagnosis of congenital hip dislocation: classification and results of a screening program. *Skeletal Radiol*. 1987;16:275–279

23. Rosendahl K, Markestad T, Lie RT. Ultrasound screening for developmental dysplasia of the hip in the neonate: the effect on treatment rate and prevalence of late cases. *Pediatrics*. 1994;94:47–52

24. Terjesen T. Ultrasound as the primary imaging method in the diagnosis of hip dysplasia in children aged <2 years. *J Pediatr Orthop B*. 1996;5: 123–128

25. Vedantam R, Bell M. Dynamic ultrasound assessment for monitoring of treatment of congenital dislocation of the hip. *J Pediatr Orthop*. 1995;15: 725–728

26. Graf R. Classification of hip joint dysplasia by means of sonography. *Arch Orthop Trauma Surg*. 1984;102:248–255

27. Berman L, Klenerman L. Ultrasound screening for hip abnormalities: preliminary findings in 1001 neonates. *Br Med J (Clin Res Ed)*. 1986;293: 719–722

28. Castelein R, Sauter A, de Vlieger M, van Linge B. Natural history of ultrasound hip abnormalities in clinically normal newborns. *J Pediatr Orthop*. 1992;12:423–427

29. Clarke N. Sonographic clarification of the problems of neonatal hip stability. *J Pediatr Orthop*. 1986;6:527–532

30. Eddy DM. The confidence profile method: a Bayesian method for assessing health technologies. *Operations Res*. 1989;37:210–228

31. Howard RA, Matheson JE. Influence diagrams. In: Matheson JE, ed. *Readings on the Principles and Applications of Decision Analysis*. Menlo Park, CA: Strategic Decisions Group; 1981:720–762

32. Nease RF, Owen DK. Use of influence diagrams to structure medical decisions. *Med Decis Making*. 1997;17:265–275

33. Guyatt GH, Sackett DL, Sinclair JC, Hayward R, Cook DJ, Cook RJ. Users' guide to the medical literature, IX: a method for grading health care recommendations. *JAMA*. 1995;274:1800–1804

34. Gelman A, Carlin JB, Stern HS, Rubin DB. *Bayesian Data Analysis*. London, UK: Chapman and Hall; 1997

35. Spiegelhalter D, Thomas A, Best N, Gilks W. *BUGS 0.5: Bayesian Inference Using Gibbs Sampling Manual, II*. Cambridge, MA: MRC Biostatistics Unit, Institute of Public Health; 1996. Available at: http://www.mrc-bsu.cam.ac.uk/bugs/software/software.html

36. Fiddian NJ, Gardiner JC. Screening for congenital dislocation of the hip by physiotherapists: results of a ten-year study. *J Bone Joint Surg Br*. 1994;76:458–459

37. Dunn P, Evans R, Thearle M, Griffiths H, Witherow P. Congenital dislocation of the hip: early and late diagnosis and management compared. *Arch Dis Child*. 1992;60:407–414

38. Holen KJ, Tegnander A, Terjesen T, Johansen OJ, Eik-Nes SH. Ultrasonographic evaluation of breech presentation as a risk factor for hip dysplasia. *Acta Paediatr*. 1996;85:225–229

39. Jones D, Powell N. Ultrasound and neonatal hip screening: a prospective study of "high risk" babies. *J Bone Joint Surg Br*. 1990;72:457–459

40. Teanby DN, Paton RW. Ultrasound screening for congenital dislocation of the hip: a limited targeted programme. *J Pediatr Orthop*. 1997;17: 202–204

41. Tonnis D, Storch K, Ulbrich H. Results of newborn screening for CDH with and without sonography and correlation of risk factors. *J Pediatr Orthop*. 1990;10:145–152

42. Pauker SG, Kassirer JP. The threshold approach to clinical decision making. *N Engl J Med*. 1980;302:1109–1117

43. Bower C, Stanley F, Morgan B, Slattery H, Stanton C. Screening for congenital dislocation of the hip by child-health nurses in western Australia. *Med J Aust*. 1989;150:61–65

44. Franchin F, Lacalendola G, Molfetta L, Mascolo V, Quagliarella L. Ultrasound for early diagnosis of hip dysplasia. *Ital J Orthop Traumatol*. 1992;18:261–269

ADDENDUM TO REFERENCES FOR THE DDH GUIDELINE

New information is generated constantly. Specific details of this report must be changed over time.

New articles (additional articles 1–7) have been published since the completion of our literature search and construction of this Guideline. These articles taken alone might seem to contradict some of the Guideline's estimates as detailed in the article and in the Technical Report. However, taken in context with the literature synthesis carried out for the construction of this Guideline, our estimates remain intact and no conclusions are obviated.

ADDITIONAL ARTICLES

1. Bialik V, Bialik GM, Blazer S, Sujov P, Wiener F, Berant M. Developmental dysplasia of the hip: a new approach to incidence. *Pediatrics*. 1999;103:93–99

2. Clegg J, Bache CE, Raut VV. Financial justification for routine ultrasound screening of the neonatal hip. *J Bone Joint Surg*. 1999;81-B:852–857

3. Holen KJ, Tegnander A, Eik-Nes SH, Terjesen T. The use of ultrasound in determining the initiation in treatment in instability of the hips in neonates. *J Bone Joint Surg*. 1999;81-B:846–851

4. Lewis K, Jones DA, Powell N. Ultrasound and neonatal hip screening: the five-year results of a prospective study in high risk babies. *J Pediatr Orthop*. 1999;19:760–762

5. Paton RW, Srinivasan MS, Shah B, Hollis S. Ultrasound screening for hips at risk in developmental dysplasia: is it worth it? *J Bone Joint Surg*. 1999;81-B:255–258

6. Sucato DJ, Johnston CE, Birch JG, Herring JA, Mack P. Outcomes of ultrasonographic hip abnormalities in clinically stable hips. *J Pediatr Orthop*. 1999;19:754–759

7. Williams PR, Jones DA, Bishay M. Avascular necrosis and the aberdeen splint in developmental dysplasia of the hip. *J Bone Joint Surg*. 1999;81-B:1023–1028

Technical Report Summary:
Developmental Dysplasia of the Hip Practice Guideline

Authors:

Harold P. Lehmann, MD, PhD; Richard Hinton, MD, MPH;
Paola Morello, MD; and Jeanne Santoli, MD
in conjunction with the
American Academy of Pediatrics
Subcommittee on Developmental
Dysplasia of the Hip

American Academy of Pediatrics
PO Box 927, 141 Northwest Point Blvd
Elk Grove Village, IL 60009-0927

ABSTRACT

Objective. To create a recommendation for pediatricians and other primary care providers about their role as screeners for detecting developmental dysplasia of the hip (DDH) in children.

Patients. Theoretical cohorts of newborns.

Method. Model-based approach using decision analysis as the foundation. Components of the approach include the following:

Perspective: Primary care provider.

Outcomes: DDH, avascular necrosis of the hip (AVN).

Options: Newborn screening by pediatric examination; orthopaedic examination; ultrasonographic examination; orthopaedic or ultrasonographic examination by risk factors. Intercurrent health supervision-based screening.

Preferences: 0 for bad outcomes, 1 for best outcomes.

Model: Influence diagram assessed by the Subcommittee and by the methodology team, with critical feedback from the Subcommittee.

Evidence Sources: Medline and EMBASE search of the research literature through June 1996. Hand search of sentinel journals from June 1996 through March 1997. Ancestor search of accepted articles.

Evidence Quality: Assessed on a custom subjective scale, based primarily on the fit of the evidence to the decision model.

Results. After discussion, explicit modeling, and critique, an influence diagram of 31 nodes was created. The computer-based and the hand literature searches found 534 articles, 101 of which were reviewed by 2 or more readers. Ancestor searches of these yielded a further 17 articles for evidence abstraction. Articles came from around the globe, although primarily Europe, British Isles, Scandinavia, and their descendants. There were 5 controlled trials, each with a sample size less than 40. The remainder were case series. Evidence was available for 17 of the desired 30 probabilities. Evidence quality ranged primarily between one third and two thirds of the maximum attainable score (median: 10–21; interquartile range: 8–14).

Based on the raw evidence and Bayesian hierarchical meta-analyses, our estimate for the incidence of DDH revealed by physical examination performed by pediatricians is 8.6 per 1000; for orthopaedic screening, 11.5; for ultrasonography, 25. The odds ratio for DDH, given breech delivery, is 5.5; for female sex, 4.1; for positive family history, 1.7, although this last factor is not statistically significant. Postneonatal cases of DDH were divided into mid-term (younger than 6 months of age) and late-term (older than 6 months of age). Our estimates for the mid-term rate for screening by pediatricians is 0.34/1000 children screened; for orthopaedists, 0.1; and for ultrasonography, 0.28. Our estimates for late-term DDH rates are 0.21/1000 newborns screened by pediatricians; 0.08, by orthopaedists; and 0.2 for ultrasonography. The rates of AVN for children referred before 6 months of age is estimated at 2.5/1000 infants referred. For those referred after 6 months of age, our estimate is 109/1000 referred infants.

The decision model (reduced, based on available evidence) suggests that orthopaedic screening is optimal, but because orthopaedists in the published studies and in practice would differ, the supply of orthopaedists is relatively limited, and the difference between orthopaedists and pediatricians is statistically insignificant, we conclude that pediatric screening is to be recommended. The place of ultrasonography in the screening process remains to be defined because there are too few data about postneonatal diagnosis by ultrasonographic screening to permit definitive recommendations. These data could be used by others to refine the conclusions based on costs, parental preferences, or physician style. Areas for research are well defined by our model-based approach. *Pediatrics* 2000;105(4). URL: http://www.pediatrics.org/cgi/content/full/105/4/e57; keywords: *developmental dysplasia of the hip, avascular necrosis of the hip, newborn.*

I. GUIDELINE METHODS

A. Decision Model

The steps required to build the model were taken with the Subcommittee as a whole, with individuals in the group, and with members of the methodology team. Agreement on the model was sought from the Subcommittee as a whole during face-to-face meetings.

1. Perspective

Although there are a number of perspectives to take in this problem (parental, child's, societal, and payer's), we opted for the view of the practicing clinician: What are the clinician's obligations, and what is the best strategy for the clinician? This choice of perspective meant that the focus would be on screening for developmental dysplasia of the hip (DDH) and obviated the need to review the evidence for efficacy or effectiveness of specific strategies.

2. Context

The target child is a full-term newborn with no obvious orthopaedic abnormalities. Children with such findings would be referred to an orthopaedist, obviating the need for a practice parameter.

3. Options

We focused on the following options: screening by physical examination (PE) at birth by a pediatrician, orthopaedist, or other care provider; ultrasonographic screening at birth; and episodic screening during health supervision. Treatment options are not included.

We also included in our model a wide range of options for managing the screening process during the first year of life when the newborn screening was negative.

4. Outcomes

Our focus is on dislocated hips at 1 year of age as the major morbidity of the disease and on avascular necrosis of the hip (AVN), as the primary sentinel complication of DDH therapy.

Ideally, we would have a "gold standard" that would define DDH at any point in time, much as cardiac output can be obtained from a pulmonary-artery catheter. However, no gold standard exists. Therefore, we defined our outcomes in terms of the process of care: a pediatrician and an ultrasonographer perform initial or confirmatory examinations and refer the patient, whereas the orthopaedist treats the patient. It is the treatment that has the greatest effect on postneonatal DDH or on complications, so we focus on that intermediate outcome, rather than the orthopaedist's stated diagnosis. We operationalized the definitions of these outcomes for use in abstracting the data from articles. A statement that a "click" was found on PE was considered to refer to an intermediate result, unless the authors defined their "click" in terms of our definition of a positive examination. Dynamic ultrasonographic examinations include those of Harcke et al, and static refers primarily to that of Graf. The radiologic focus switches from ultrasonography to plain radiographs after 4 months of age, in keeping with the development of the femoral head.

5. Decision Structure

We used an influence diagram to represent the decision model. In this representation, nodes refer to actions to be taken or to states of the world (the patient) about which we are uncertain. We devoted substantial effort to the construction of a model that balanced the need to represent the rich array of possible screening pathways with the need to be parsimonious. We constructed the master influence diagram and determined its construct validity through consensus by the Subcommittee before data abstraction. However, the available evidence could specify only a portion of the diagram. The missing components suggest research questions that need to be posed.

6. Probabilities

The purpose of the literature review was to provide the probabilities required by the decision model. The initial number of individual probabilities was 55. (Sensitivity and specificity for a single truth-indicator pair are counted as a single probability because they are garnered from the same table.) Although this is a large number of parameters, the structure of the model helped the team of readers. As 1 reader said, referring to the influence diagram, "Because we did the picture together, it was easy to find the parameters." What follows are some operational rules for matching the data to our parameters. The list is not complete. If an orthopaedic clinic worked at case finding, we used our judgment to determine whether to accept such reports as representing a population incidence.

Risk factors were included generally only if a true control group was used for comparison. For postneonatal diagnoses, no study we reviewed included the examination of all children without DDH, say, 1 year of age, so there is always the possibility of missed cases (false-negative diagnoses) in the screen, which leads to a falsely elevated estimate of the denominator. For studies originating in referral clinics, the data on the reasons for referrals were not usable for our purposes.

7. Preferences

Ideally, we would have cost data for the options, as well as patient data on the human burden of therapy and of DDH itself. We have deferred these assessments to later research. Therefore, we assigned a preference score of 0 to DDH at 1 year of age and 1 to its absence; for AVN, we assigned 0 for presence at 1 year of age and 1 for absence at 1 year of age.

B. Literature Review

For the literature through May 1995, the following sources were searched: Books in Print, CAT-LINE, Current Contents, EMBASE, Federal Research in Progress, Health Care Standards, Health Devices Alerts, Health Planning and Administration, Health Services/Technology Assessment, International Health Technology Assessment, and Medline. Medline and EMBASE were searched through June 1996. The search terms used in all databases included the following: hip dislocation, congenital; hip dysplasia; congenital hip dislocation; developmental dysplasia; ultrasonography/adverse effects; and osteonecrosis. Hand searches of leading orthopaedic journals were performed for the issues from June 1996 to March 1997. The bibliographies of journals accepted for use in formulating the practice parameter also were perused.

The titles and the abstracts were then reviewed by 2 members of the methodology team to determine whether to accept or reject the articles for use. Decisions were reviewed by the Subcommittee, and conflicts were adjudicated. Similarly, articles were read by pairs of reviewers; conflicts were resolved in discussion.

The focus of the data abstraction process was on data that would provide evidence for the probabilities required by the decision model.

As part of the literature abstraction process, the evidence quality in each article was assessed. The scoring process was based on our decision model and involved traditional epidemiologic concerns, like outcome definition and bias of ascertainment, as well as influence–diagram-based concerns, such as how well the data fit into the model.

Cohort definition: Does the cohort represented by the denominator in the study match a node in our influence diagram? Does the cohort represented by the numerator match a node in our influence diagram? The closer the match, the more confident we are that the reported data provide good evidence of the conditional probability implied by the arrow between the corresponding nodes in the influence diagram.

Path: Does the implied path from denominator to numerator lead through 1 or more nodes of the influence diagram? The longer the path, the more likely that uncontrolled biases entered into the study, making us less confident about accepting the raw data as a conditional probability in our model. Assignment and comparison: Was there a control group? How was assignment made to experimental or control arms? A randomized, controlled study provides the best quality evidence.

Follow-up: Were patients with positive and negative initial findings followed up? The best studies should have data on both.

Outcome definition: Did the language of the outcome definitions (PE, orthopaedic examination, ultrasonography, and radiography) match ours, and, in particular, were PE findings divided into 3 categories or 2? The closer the definition to ours, the more we could pool the data. Studies with only 2 categories do not help to distinguish clicks from "clunks."

Ascertainment: When the denominator represented more than 1 node, to what degree was the denominator a mix of nodes? The smaller the contamination, the more confident we were that the raw data represented a desired conditional probability.

Results: Did the results fill an entire table or were data missing? This is related to the follow-up category but is more general.

C. Synthesis of Evidence

There are 3 levels of evidence synthesis.

1. Listing evidence for individual probabilities
2. Summarizing evidence across probabilities
3. Integrating the pooled evidence for individual probabilities into the decision model

A list of evidence for an individual probability (or arc) is called an *evidence table* and provides the reader a look at the individual pieces of data. The probabilities are summarized in 3 ways: by averaging, by averaging weighted by sample size (pooled), and by meta-analysis. We chose Bayesian meta-analytic techniques, which allow the representation of *prior belief* in the evidence and provide an explicit portrayal of the uncertainty of our conclusions. The framework we used was that of a hierarchical Bayesian model, similar to the random effects model in traditional meta-analysis. In this hierarchical model, each study has its own parameter, which, in turn, is sampled from a wider population parameter. Because there are 2 stages (ie, population to sample and sample to observation), and, therefore, the population parameter of interest is more distant from the data, the computed estimates in the population parameters are, in general, less certain (wider confidence interval) than simply pooling the data across studies. This lower certainty is appropriate in the DDH content area because the studies vary so widely in their raw estimates because of the range in time and geography over which they were performed. In the Bayesian model, the observations were assumed to be Poisson distributed, given the study DDH rates. Those rates, in turn, were assumed to be Gamma distributed, given the population rate. The prior belief on that rate was set as Gamma ($\propto$, β), with mean $\propto/\beta$, and variance $\propto/\beta^2$ (as defined in the BUGS software). In this parameterization, $\propto$ has the semantics closest to that of location, and β has the semantics of certainty: the higher its value, the narrower the distribution and the more certain we are of the estimate. The parameter, $\propto$, was modeled as Exponential (1), and β, as Gamma (0.01, 1), with a mean of 0.01. Together, these correspond to a prior belief in the rate of a mean of 100 per

1000, and a standard deviation (SD) of 100, representing ignorance of the true rate.

As an example of interpretation, for pediatric newborn screening, the posterior $\propto$ was 1.46, and the posterior β was 0.17, to give a posterior rate of 8.6/1000, with a variance of 50, or an SD of 7.1. The value of β rose from 0.01 to 0.17, indicating a higher level of certainty.

The Bayesian confidence interval is the narrowest interval that contains 95% of the area under the posterior-belief curve. The confidence interval for the prior curve is 2.53 to 370. The confidence interval for the posterior curve is 0.25 to 27.5, a significant shrinking and increase in certainty but still broad.

The model for the odds ratios is more complicated and is based on the Oxford data set and analysis in the BUGS manual.

D. Thresholds

In the course of discussions about results, the Subcommittee was surveyed about the acceptable risks of DDH for different levels of interventions.

E. Recommendations

Once the evidence and thresholds were obtained, a decision tree was created from the evidence available and was reviewed by the Subcommittee. In parallel, a consensus guideline (flowchart) was created. The Subcommittee evaluated whether evidence was available for links within the guidelines, as well as their strength of consensus. The decision tree was evaluated to check consistency of the evidence with the conclusions.

F. "Cost"-Effectiveness Ratios

To integrate the results, we defined cost-effectiveness ratios, in which cost was excess neonatal referrals or excess cases of AVNs, and *effectiveness* was a decrease in the number of later cases. The decision tree from section E ("Recommendations") was used to calculate the expected outcomes for each of pediatric, orthopaedic, and ultrasonographic strategies. Pediatric strategy was used as the baseline, because its neonatal screening rate was the lowest. The cost-effectiveness ratios then were calculated as the quotient of the difference in cost and the difference in effect.

RESULTS

A. Articles

The peak number of articles is for 1992, with 10 articles. The articles are from sites all over the world, although the Nordic, Anglo-Saxon, and European communities and their descendants are the most represented.

B. Evidence

By traditional epidemiologic standards, the quality of evidence in this set of articles is uniformly low. There are few controlled trials and few studies in which infants with negative results on their newborn examinations are followed up. (A number of studies attempted to cover all possible places where an affected child might have been ascertained.)

We found data on all chance nodes, for a total of 298 distinct tables. *Decision* nodes were poorly represented: beyond the neonatal strategy, there were almost no data clarifying the paths for the diagnosis children after the newborn period. Thus, although communities like those in southeast Norway have a postnewborn screening program, it is unclear what the program was, and it was unclear how many examination results were normal before a child was referred to an orthopaedist.

The mode is a score of 10, achieved in 16 articles. The median is 9.9, with an interquartile range of 8 to 14, suggesting that articles with scores below 8 are poor sources of evidence. Note that the maximum achievable quality score is 21, so half the articles do not achieve half the maximum quality score.

Graphing evidence quality against publication year suggests an improvement in quality over time, as shown in Fig 9, but the linear fit through the data is statistically indistinguishable from a flat line. (A nonparametric procedure yields the same conclusion).

The studies include 5 in which a comparative arm was designed into the study. The remainder are divided between prospective and retrospective studies. Surprisingly, the evidence quality is not higher in the former than in the latter (data not shown).

Of the 298 data tables, half the data tables relate to the following:
• probabilities of DDH in different screening strategies
• relative risk of DDH, given risk factors
• the incidence of postneonatal DDH, and
• the incidence of AVN.

The remainder of our discussion will focus on these probabilities.

C. Evidence Tables

The evidence table details are found in the appendix of the full technical report.

1. Newborn Screening

a. Pediatric Screening

There were 51 studies, providing 57 arms, for pediatric screening. However, of these, 17 were unclear on how the intermediate examinations were handled, and, unsurprisingly, their observed rates of positivity (clicks) were much higher than the studies that distinguished 3 categories, as we had specified. Therefore, we included only the 34 studies that used 3 categories.

For pediatric screening, the rate is about 8 positive cases per 1000 examinations. The rates are distributed almost uniformly between 0 and 20 per 1000. All studies represent a large experience: a total of 2 149 972 subjects. Although their methods may not have been the best, the studies demand attention simply because of their size.

In looking for covariates or confounding variables, we studied the relationship between positivity rate and the independent variables, year of publication, evidence quality, and sample size. Year and evidence quality show a positive effect: the higher the year (slope: 0.2; P 5 .018) or evidence quality (slope: 0.6; P 5 .046), the higher the observed rate. A model with both factors has evidence that suggests that most of the effect is in the factor, year

(slope for year: 0.08; P 5 .038; slope for quality of evidence: 0.49; P 5 .09). Note that a regression using evidence quality is improper, because our evidence scale is not properly ratio (eg, the distance between 6 and 7 is not necessarily equivalent to the distance between 14 and 15), but the regression is a useful exploratory device.

b. Orthopaedic Screening

Evidence was found in 25 studies. Three studies provided 2 arms each.

The positivity rate for orthopaedic screening is between 7 and 11/1000. One outlier study, with an observed rate of more than 300/1000, skews the unweighted and meta-analytic averages. The estimate (between 7.1 and 11) is just below that of pediatric screening and is statistically indistinguishable. Note, however, that a fair number of studies have rates near 22/1000 or higher.

Unlike with pediatric screening, there are no correlations with other factors.

c. Ultrasonographic Screening

Evidence was found in 17 studies, each providing a single arm.

The rate for ultrasonographic screening is 20/1000 or more. Although the estimates are sensitive to pooling and to the outlier, the positivity rate is clearly higher than in either PE strategy. There are no correlating factors. In particular, studies that use the Graf method 2 or those that use the method of Harcke et al show comparable rates.

2. Postneonatal Cases

We initially were interested in all postneonatal diagnoses of DDH. However, the literature did not provide data within the narrow time frames initially specified for our model. Based on the data that were available, we considered 3 classes of postneonatal DDH: DDH diagnosed after 12 months of age ("late-term"), DDH diagnosed between 6 and 12 months of age ("mid-term"), and DDH diagnosed before 6 months of age. There were few data for the latter group, which often was combined with the newborn screening programs. Therefore, we collected data on only the first 2 groups.

a. After Pediatric Screening

Evidence was found in 24 studies. The study by Dunn and O'Riordan provided 2 arms. It is difficult to discern an estimate rate for mid-term DDH, because the study by Czeizel et al is such an outlier, with a rate of 3.73/1000, and because the weighted and unweighted averages also differ greatly. The meta-analytic estimate of 0.55/1000 seems to be an upper limit.

The late-term rate is easier to estimate at ~0.3/1000. Although it is intuitive that the late-term rate should be lower than the mid-term rate, our data do not allow us to draw that conclusion.

b. *After Orthopaedic Screening*

There were only 4 studies. The rates were comparable for mid- and late-term: 0.1/1000 newborns. A meta-analytic estimate was not calculated.

c. *After Ultrasonographic Screening*

Only 1 study, by Rosendahl et al is available; it reported rates for infants with and without initial risk factors (eg, family history and breech presentation). The mid-term rate was 0.28/1000 newborns in the non-risk group, and the late-term rate was 0/1000 in the same group.

3. *AVN After Treatment*

For these estimates, we grouped together all treatments, because from the viewpoint of the referring primary care provider, orthopaedic treatment is a "black box:" A literature synthesis that teased apart the success and complications of particular *therapeutic* strategies is beyond the scope of the present study.

The complication rate should depend only on the age of the patient at time of orthopaedic referral and on the type of treatment received. We report on the complication rates for children treated before and after 12 months of age.

a. *After Early Referral*

There were 17 studies providing evidence. Infants were referred to orthopaedists during the newborn period in each study except 2. In the study by Pool et al, infants were referred during the newborn period and before 2 months of age; in the study by Sochart and Paton, infants were referred between 2 weeks and 2 months of age.

The range of AVN rates per 1000 infants referred was huge, from 0 to 123. The largest rate occurred in the study by Pool et al, a sample-based study that included later referrals. Its evidence quality was 8, within the 7 to 13 interquartile range of the other studies in this group. As in earlier tables, the meta-analytic estimate lies between the average and weighted (pooled) average of the studies.

b. *After Later Referral*

Evidence was obtained from 6 studies. Some of the studies included children referred during the newborn period or during the 2-week to 2-month period, but even in these, the majority of infants were referred later during the first year of life.

There were no outlier rates, although the highest rate (216/1000 referred children) occurred in the study with the oldest referred children in the sample with children referred who were older than 12 months of age. One study contributed 5700 patients to the analysis, more than half of the 9270 total, so its AVN rate of 27/1000 brought the unweighted rate of 116/1000 to 54. A meta-analytic estimate was not computed.

4. *Risk Factors*

A number of factors are known to predispose infants to DDH. We sought evidence for 3 of these: sex, obstetrical position at birth, and family history. Studies were included in these analyses only if a control group could be ascertained from the available study data.

The key measure is the odds ratio, an estimate of the relative risk. The meaning of the odds ratio is that if the DDH rate for the control group is known, then the DDH rate for the at-risk group is the product of the control-group DDH rate and the odds ratio for the risk factor. An odds ratio statistically significantly greater than 1 indicates that the factor is a risk factor.

The Bayesian meta-analysis produces estimates between the average of the odds ratios and the pooled odds ratio and is, therefore, the estimate we used in our later analyses.

a. *Female*

The studies were uniform in discerning a risk to girls ~4 times that of boys for being diagnosed with DDH. This risk was seen in all 3 screening environments.

b. *Breech*

The studies for breech also were confident in finding a risk for breech presentation, on the order of fivefold. One study found breech presentation to be protective, but the study was relatively small and used ultrasonography rather than PE as its outcome measure.

c. *Family History*

Although some studies found family history to be a risk factor, the range was wide. The confidence intervals for the pooled odds ratio and for the Bayesian analysis contained 1.0, suggesting that family history is *not* an independent risk factor for DDH. However, because of traditional concern with this risk factor, we kept it in our further considerations.

D. Evidence Summary and Risk Implications

To bring all evidence tables together, we constructed a summary table, which contains the estimates we chose for our recommendations. The intervals are asymmetric, in keeping with the intuition that rates near zero cannot be negative, but certainly can be very positive.

Risk factors are based on the pediatrician population rate of 8.6 labeled cases of DDH per 1000 infants screened. In the Subcommittee's discussion, 50/1000 was a cutoff for automatic referral during the newborn period. Hence, girls born in the breech position are classified in a separate category for newborn strategies than infants with other risk factors.

If we use the orthopaedists' rate as our baseline, numbers suggest that boys without risks or those with a family history have the lowest risk; girls without risks and boys born in the breech presentation have an intermediate risk; and girls with a positive family history, and especially girls born in the breech presentation, have the highest risks. Guidelines that consider risk factors should follow these risk profiles.

E. Decision Recommendations

With the evidence synthesized, we can estimate the expected results of the target newborn strategies for postneonatal DDH and AVN.

If a case of DDH is observed in an infant with an initially negative result of screening by an orthopaedist in a newborn screening program, that case is "counted" against the orthopaedist strategy.

The numbers are combined using a simple decision tree, which is not the final tree represented by our influence diagram but is a tree that is supported by our evidence. The results show that pediatricians diagnose fewer newborns with DDH and perhaps have a higher postneonatal DDH rate than orthopaedists but one that is comparable to ultrasonography (acknowledging that our knowledge of postneonatal DDH revealed by ultrasonographic screening is limited). The AVN rates are comparable with pediatrician and ultrasonographic screening and less than with orthopaedist screening.

F. Cost-Effectiveness Ratios

In terms of excess neonatal referrals, the ratios suggest that there is a trade-off: for every case that these strategies detect beyond the pediatric strategy, they require more than 7000 or 16 000 extra referrals, respectively.

DISCUSSION

A. Summary

We derived 298 evidence tables from 118 studies culled from a larger set of 624 articles. Our literature review captured most in our model-based approach, if not all, of the past literature on DDH that was usable. The decision model (reduced based on available evidence) suggests that orthopaedic screening is optimal, but because orthopaedists in the published studies and in practice would differ, the supply of orthopaedists is relatively limited, and the difference between orthopaedists and pediatricians is relatively small, we conclude that pediatric screening is to be recommended. The place of ultrasonography in the screening process remains to be defined because there are too few data about postneonatal diagnosis by ultrasonographic screening to permit definitive recommendations.

Our conclusions are tempered by the uncertainties resulting from the wide range of the evidence. The confidence intervals are wide for the primary parameters. The uncertainties mean that, even with all the evidence collected from the literature, we are left with large doubts about the values of the different parameters.

Our data do not bear directly on the issue about the earliest point that any patient destined to have DDH will show signs of the disease. Our use of the terms *mid-term* and *late-term* DDH addresses that ignorance.

Our conclusions about other areas of the full decision model are more tentative because of the paucity of data about the effectiveness of periodicity examinations. Even the studies that gave data on mid-term and late-term case findings by pediatricians were sparse in their details about how the screening was instituted, maintained, or followed up.

Our literature search was weakest in addressing the European literature, where results about ultrasonography are more prevalent. We found, however, that many of the seminal articles were republished in English or in a form that we could assess.

B. Specific Issues

1. Evidence Quality

Our measure of evidence quality is unique, although it is based on solid principles of study design and decision modeling. In particular, our measure was based on the notion that if the data conform poorly to how we need to use it, we downgrade its value.

However, throughout the analyses, there was never a correlation with the results of a study (in terms of the values of outcomes) and with evidence quality, so we never needed to use the measure for weighting the values of the outcome or for culling articles from our review. Had this been so, the measures would have needed further scrutiny and validation.

2. Outliers

Perhaps the true surrogates for study quality were the outlying values of outcomes. In general, however, there were few cases in which the outliers were clearly the result of poor-quality studies. One example is that of the outcomes of pediatric screening (1⊠3), in which the DDH rates in studies using only 2 categories were generally higher than those that explicitly specified 3 levels of outcomes.

Our general justification for using estimates that excluded outliers is that the outliers so much drove the results that they dominated the conclusion out of proportion to their sample sizes. As it is, our estimates have wide ranges.

3. Newborn Screening

The set of studies labeled "pediatrician screening" includes studies with a variety of examiners. We could not estimate the sensitivity and specificity of pediatricians' examinations versus those of other primary care providers versus orthopaedists. There are techniques for extracting these measures from agreement studies, but they are beyond the scope of the present study. It is intuitive that the more cases that one examines, the better an examiner one will be, regardless of professional title.

We were surprised that the results did not show a clear difference in results between the Graf and Harcke et al ultrasonographic examinations. Our data make no statement about the relative advantages of these methods for following up children or in addressing treatment.

4. Postneonatal Cases

As mentioned, our data cannot say when a postneonatal case is established or, therefore, the best time to screen children. We established our initial age categories for postneonatal cases based on biology, treatment changes, and optimal imaging and examination strategies. It is frustrating that the data in the literature are not organized to match this pathophysiological way of thinking about DDH. Similarly, as mentioned, the lack of details by authors on the methods of intercurrent screening means that we cannot recommend a preferred method for mid-term or late-term screening.

5. *AVN*

We used AVN as our primary marker for treatment morbidity. We acknowledge that the studies we grouped together may reflect different philosophies and results of orthopaedic practice. The hierarchical meta-analysis treats every study as an individual case, and the wide range in our confidence intervals reflects the uncertainty that results in grouping disparate studies together.

C. Comments on Methods

This study is unique in its strong use of decision modeling at each step in the process. In the end, our results are couched in traditional terms (estimated rates of disease or morbidity outcomes), although the context is relatively nontraditional: attaching the estimates to strategies rather than to treatments. In this, our study is typical of an *effectiveness* study, which studied results in the real world, rather than of an *efficacy* study, which examines the biological effects of a treatment.

We made strong and recurrent use of the Bayesian hierarchical meta-analysis. A review of the tables will confirm that the Bayesian results were in the same "ballpark" as the average and pooled average estimates and had a more solid grounding.

The usual criticism of using Bayesian methods is that they depend on prior belief. The usual response is to show that the final estimates are relatively insensitive to the prior belief. In fact, for the screening strategies, a wide range of prior beliefs had no effect on the estimate. However, the prior belief used for the screening strategies—with a mean of 100 cases/1000 with a variance of 100—was too broad for the postneonatal case and AVN analyses; when data were sparse, the prior belief overwhelmed the data. For instance, in late-term DDH revealed by orthopaedic screening (53 30), in an analysis not shown, the posterior estimate from the 4 studies was a rate of 0.345 cases per 1000, despite an average and a pooled average on the order of 0.08. Four studies were insufficient to overpower a prior belief of 100.

D. Research Issues

The place of ultrasonography in DDH screening needs more attention, as does the issue of intercurrent pediatrician screening. In the latter case, society and health care systems must assess the effectiveness of education and the "return on investment" for educational programs. The place of preferences—of the parents, of the clinician—must be established.

We hope that the framework we have delineated—of a decision model and of data—can be useful in these future research endeavors.

Dysplasia of the Hip Clinical Practice Guideline
Quick Reference Tools

• •

- Recommendation Summary
  — Early Detection of Developmental Dysplasia of the Hip
- *ICD-10-CM* Coding Quick Reference for Dysplasia of the Hip
- AAP Patient Education Handout
  — *Hip Dysplasia (Developmental Dysplasia of the Hip)*

Recommendation Summary
Early Detection of Developmental Dysplasia of the Hip

Recommendation 1

A. All newborns are to be screened by physical examination. (The evidence for this recommendation is good. The expert consensus is strong.)

B. It is recommended that screening be done by a properly trained health care provider (eg, physician, pediatric nurse practitioner, physician assistant, or physical therapist). (Evidence for this recommendation is strong.)

C. Ultrasonography of all newborns is not recommended. (Evidence is fair; consensus is strong.)

Recommendation 2

A. If a positive Ortolani or Barlow sign is found in the newborn examination, the infant should be referred to an orthopaedist. (The data recommending that all those with a positive Ortolani sign be referred to an orthopaedist are limited, but expert panel consensus, nevertheless, was strong….)

B. If the results of the physical examination at birth are "equivocally" positive (ie, soft click, mild asymmetry, but neither an Ortolani nor a Barlow sign is present), then a follow-up hip examination by the pediatrician in 2 weeks is recommended. (Evidence is good; consensus is strong.)

Recommendation 3

A. If the results of the newborn physical examination are positive (ie, presence of an Ortolani or a Barlow sign), ordering an ultrasonographic examination of the newborn is not recommended. (Evidence is poor; opinion is strong.)

B. If the results of the newborn physical examination are positive, obtaining a radiograph of the newborn's pelvis and hips is not recommended. (Evidence is poor; opinion is strong.)

C. The use of triple diapers when abnormal physical signs are detected during the newborn period is not recommended. (Evidence is poor; opinion is strong.)

Recommendation 4

If the results of the physical examination are positive (eg, positive Ortolani or Barlow sign) at 2 weeks, refer to an orthopaedist. (Evidence is strong; consensus is strong.)

Recommendation 5

If at the 2-week examination the Ortolani and Barlow signs are absent but physical findings raise suspicions, consider referral to an orthopaedist or request ultrasonography at age 3 to 4 weeks.

Recommendation 6

If the results of the physical examination are negative at 2 weeks, follow-up is recommended at the scheduled well-baby periodic examinations. (Evidence is good; consensus is strong.)

Recommendation 7

Risk factors. If the results of the newborn examination are negative (or equivocally positive), risk factors may be considered. The following recommendations are made (evidence is strong; opinion is strong):

A. Girl (newborn risk of 19/1000). When the results of the newborn examination are negative or equivocally positive, hips should be reevaluated at 2 weeks of age. If negative, continue according to the periodicity schedule; if positive, refer to an orthopaedist or for ultrasonography at 3 weeks of age.

B. Infants with a positive family history of DDH (newborn risk for boys of 9.4/1000 and for girls, 44/1000). When the results of the newborn examination in boys are negative or equivocally positive, hips should be reevaluated at 2 weeks of age. If negative, continue according to the periodicity schedule; if positive, refer to an orthopaedist or for ultrasonography at 3 weeks of age. In girls, the absolute risk of 44/1000 may exceed the pediatrician's threshold to act, and imaging with an ultrasonographic examination at 6 weeks of age or a radiograph of the pelvis at 4 months of age is recommended.

C. Breech presentation (newborn risk for boys of 26/1000 and for girls, 120/1000). For negative or equivocally positive newborn examinations, the infant should be reevaluated at regular intervals (according to the periodicity schedule) if the examination results remain negative.

Recommendation 8

Periodicity. The hips must be examined at every well-baby visit according to the recommended periodicity schedule for well-baby examinations (2–4 days for newborns discharged in less than 48 hours after delivery, by 1 month, 2 months, 4 months, 6 months, 9 months, and 12 months of age).

Coding Quick Reference for Dysplasia of the Hip

ICD-10-CM

Q65.0- Congenital dislocation of hip, unilateral
Q65.1 Congenital dislocation of hip, bilateral
Q65.3- Congenital partial dislocation of hip, unilateral
Q65.4 Congenital partial dislocation of hip, bilateral
Q65.6 Congenital unstable hip (Congenital dislocatable hip)
Q65.89 Other specified congenital deformities of hip

Symbol "-" requires a fifth character; **1** = right; **2** = left.

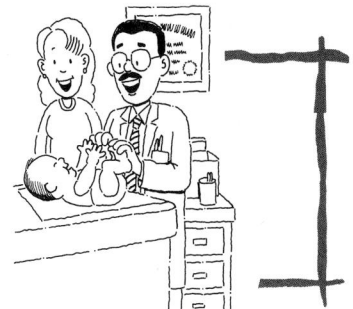

Hip Dysplasia

(Developmental Dysplasia of the Hip)

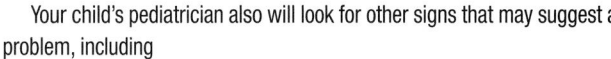

Hip dysplasia (developmental dysplasia of the hip) is a condition in which a child's upper thighbone is dislocated from the hip socket. It can be present at birth or develop during a child's first year of life.

Hip dysplasia is not always detectable at birth or even during early infancy. In spite of careful screening of children for hip dysplasia during regular well-child exams, a number of children with hip dysplasia are not diagnosed until after they are 1 year old.

Hip dysplasia is rare. However, if your baby is diagnosed with the condition, quick treatment is important.

What causes hip dysplasia?

No one is sure why hip dysplasia occurs (or why the left hip dislocates more often than the right hip). One reason may have to do with the hormones a baby is exposed to before birth. While these hormones serve to relax muscles in the pregnant mother's body, in some cases they also may cause a baby's joints to become too relaxed and prone to dislocation. This condition often corrects itself in several days, and the hip develops normally. In some cases, these dislocations cause changes in the hip anatomy that need treatment.

Who is at risk?

Factors that may increase the risk of hip dysplasia include

- Sex—more frequent in girls
- Family history—more likely when other family members have had hip dysplasia
- Birth position—more common in infants born in the breech position
- Birth order—firstborn children most at risk for hip dysplasia

Detecting hip dysplasia

Your pediatrician will check your newborn for hip dysplasia right after birth and at every well-child exam until your child is walking normally.

During the exam, your child's pediatrician will carefully flex and rotate your child's legs to see if the thighbones are properly positioned in the hip sockets. This does not require a great deal of force and will not hurt your baby.

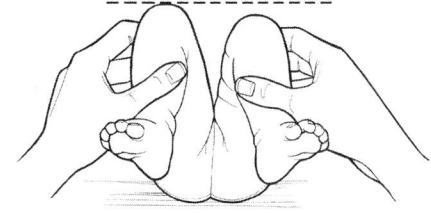

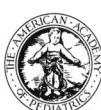

Your child's pediatrician also will look for other signs that may suggest a problem, including

- Limited range of motion in either leg
- One leg is shorter than the other
- Thigh or buttock creases appear uneven or lopsided

If your child's pediatrician suspects a problem with your child's hip, you may be referred to an orthopedic specialist who has experience treating hip dysplasia.

Treating hip dysplasia

Early treatment is important. The sooner treatment begins, the simpler it will be. In the past parents were told to double or triple diaper their babies to keep the legs in a position where dislocation was unlikely. *This practice is not recommended.* The diapering will not prevent hip dysplasia and will only delay effective treatment. Failure to treat this condition can result in permanent disability.

If your child is diagnosed with hip dysplasia before she is 6 months old, she will most likely be treated with a soft brace (such as the Pavlik harness) that holds the legs flexed and apart to allow the thighbones to be secure in the hip sockets.

The orthopedic consultant will tell you how long and when your baby will need to wear the brace. Your child also will be examined frequently during this time to make sure that the hips remain normal and stable.

In resistant cases or in older children, hip dysplasia may need to be treated with a combination of braces, casts, traction, or surgery. Your child will be admitted to the hospital if surgery is necessary. After surgery, your child will be placed in a hip spica cast for about 3 months. A hip

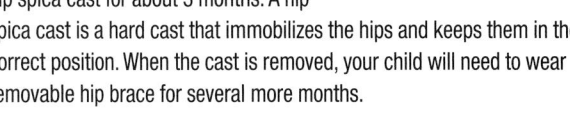

Pavlik Harness

spica cast is a hard cast that immobilizes the hips and keeps them in the correct position. When the cast is removed, your child will need to wear a removable hip brace for several more months.

Remember

If you have any concerns about your child's walking, talk with his pediatrician. If the cause is hip dysplasia, prompt treatment is important.

The information contained in this publication should not be used as a substitute for the medical care and advice of your pediatrician. There may be variations in treatment that your pediatrician may recommend based on individual facts and circumstances.

American Academy of Pediatrics

DEDICATED TO THE HEALTH OF ALL CHILDREN™

The American Academy of Pediatrics is an organization of 60,000 primary care pediatricians, pediatric medical subspecialists, and pediatric surgical specialists dedicated to the health, safety, and well-being of infants, children, adolescents, and young adults.

American Academy of Pediatrics
Web site—www.aap.org

Copyright © 2003
American Academy of Pediatrics

Febrile Seizures: Clinical Practice Guideline for the Long-term Management of the Child With Simple Febrile Seizures

• •

- *Clinical Practice Guideline*

CLINICAL PRACTICE GUIDELINE

Febrile Seizures: Clinical Practice Guideline for the Long-term Management of the Child With Simple Febrile Seizures

Steering Committee on Quality Improvement and Management, Subcommittee on Febrile Seizures

ABSTRACT

Febrile seizures are the most common seizure disorder in childhood, affecting 2% to 5% of children between the ages of 6 and 60 months. Simple febrile seizures are defined as brief (<15-minute) generalized seizures that occur once during a 24-hour period in a febrile child who does not have an intracranial infection, metabolic disturbance, or history of afebrile seizures. This guideline (a revision of the 1999 American Academy of Pediatrics practice parameter [now termed clinical practice guideline] "The Long-term Treatment of the Child With Simple Febrile Seizures") addresses the risks and benefits of both continuous and intermittent anticonvulsant therapy as well as the use of antipyretics in children with simple febrile seizures. It is designed to assist pediatricians by providing an analytic framework for decisions regarding possible therapeutic interventions in this patient population. It is not intended to replace clinical judgment or to establish a protocol for all patients with this disorder. Rarely will these guidelines be the only approach to this problem. *Pediatrics* 2008;121:1281–1286

www.pediatrics.org/cgi/doi/10.1542/peds.2008-0939

doi:10.1542/peds.2008-0939

All clinical reports from the American Academy of Pediatrics automatically expire 5 years after publication unless reaffirmed, revised, or retired at or before that time.

The guidance in this report does not indicate an exclusive course of treatment or serve as a standard of medical care. Variations, taking into account individual circumstances, may be appropriate.

Key Word
fever

Abbreviation
AAP—American Academy of Pediatrics

PEDIATRICS (ISSN Numbers: Print, 0031-4005; Online, 1098-4275). Copyright © 2008 by the American Academy of Pediatrics

The expected outcomes of this practice guideline include:

1. optimizing practitioner understanding of the scientific basis for using or avoiding various proposed treatments for children with simple febrile seizures;

2. improving the health of children with simple febrile seizures by avoiding therapies with high potential for adverse effects and no demonstrated ability to improve children's long-term outcomes;

3. reducing costs by avoiding therapies that will not demonstrably improve children's long-term outcomes; and

4. helping the practitioner educate caregivers about the low risks associated with simple febrile seizures.

The committee determined that with the exception of a high rate of recurrence, no long-term effects of simple febrile seizures have been identified. The risk of developing epilepsy in these patients is extremely low, although slightly higher than that in the general population. No data, however, suggest that prophylactic treatment of children with simple febrile seizures would reduce the risk, because epilepsy likely is the result of genetic predisposition rather than structural damage to the brain caused by recurrent simple febrile seizures. Although antipyretics have been shown to be ineffective in preventing recurrent febrile seizures, there is evidence that continuous anticonvulsant therapy with phenobarbital, primidone, or valproic acid and intermittent therapy with diazepam are effective in reducing febrile-seizure recurrence. The potential toxicities associated with these agents, however, outweigh the relatively minor risks associated with simple febrile seizures. As such, the committee concluded that, on the basis of the risks and benefits of the effective therapies, neither continuous nor intermittent anticonvulsant therapy is recommended for children with 1 or more simple febrile seizures.

INTRODUCTION

Febrile seizures are seizures that occur in febrile children between the ages of 6 and 60 months who do not have an intracranial infection, metabolic disturbance, or history of afebrile seizures. Febrile seizures are subdivided into 2 categories: simple and complex. Simple febrile seizures last for less than 15 minutes, are generalized (without a focal component), and occur once in a 24-hour period, whereas complex febrile seizures are prolonged (>15 minutes), are focal, or occur more than once in 24 hours.[1] Despite the frequency of febrile seizures (2%–5%), there is no unanimity of opinion about management options. This clinical practice guideline addresses potential therapeutic interventions in neurologically normal children with simple febrile seizures. It is not intended for patients with complex febrile seizures and does not pertain to children with previous neurologic insults, known central nervous system abnormalities, or a history of afebrile seizures. This clinical practice guideline is a revision of a 1999 American Academy of Pediatrics (AAP) clinical practice parameter, "The Long-term Treatment of the Child With Simple Febrile Seizures."[2]

For a child who has experienced a simple febrile seizure, there are potentially 4 adverse outcomes that theoretically may be altered by an effective therapeutic agent: (1) decline in IQ; (2) increased risk of epilepsy; (3) risk of recurrent febrile seizures; and (4) death. Neither a decline in IQ, academic performance or neurocognitive inattention nor behavioral abnormalities have been shown to be a consequence of recurrent simple febrile seizures.[3] Ellenberg and Nelson[4] studied 431 children who experienced febrile seizures and observed no significant difference in their learning compared with sibling controls. In a similar study by Verity et al,[5] 303 children with febrile seizures were compared with control children. No difference in learning was identified, except in those children who had neurologic abnormalities before their first seizure.

The second concern, increased risk of epilepsy, is more complex. Children with simple febrile seizures have approximately the same risk of developing epilepsy by the age of 7 years as does the general population (ie, 1%).[6] However, children who have had multiple simple febrile seizures, are younger than 12 months at the time of their first febrile seizure, and have a family history of epilepsy are at higher risk, with generalized afebrile seizures developing by 25 years of age in 2.4%.[7] Despite this fact, no study has demonstrated that successful treatment of simple febrile seizures can prevent this later development of epilepsy, and there currently is no evidence that simple febrile seizures cause structural damage to the brain. Indeed, it is most likely that the increased risk of epilepsy in this population is the result of genetic predisposition.

In contrast to the slightly increased risk of developing epilepsy, children with simple febrile seizures have a high rate of recurrence. The risk varies with age. Children younger than 12 months at the time of their first simple febrile seizure have an approximately 50% probability of having recurrent febrile seizures. Children older than 12 months at the time of their first event have an approximately 30% probability of a second febrile seizure; of those who do have a second febrile seizure, 50% have a chance of having at least 1 additional recurrence.[8]

Finally, there is a theoretical risk of a child dying during a simple febrile seizure as a result of documented injury, aspiration, or cardiac arrhythmia, but to the committee's knowledge, it has never been reported.

In summary, with the exception of a high rate of recurrence, no long-term adverse effects of simple febrile seizures have been identified. Because the risks associated with simple febrile seizures, other than recurrence, are so low and because the number of children who have febrile seizures in the first few years of life is so high, to be commensurate, a proposed therapy would need to be exceedingly low in risks and adverse effects, inexpensive, and highly effective.

METHODS

To update the clinical practice guideline on the treatment of children with simple febrile seizures, the AAP reconvened the Subcommittee on Febrile Seizures. The committee was chaired by a child neurologist and consisted of a neuroepidemiologist, 2 additional child neurologists, and a practicing pediatrician. All panel members reviewed and signed the AAP voluntary disclosure and conflict-of-interest form. The guideline was reviewed by members of the AAP Steering Committee on Quality Improvement and Management; members of the AAP Sections on Neurology, Pediatric Emergency Medicine, Developmental and Behavioral Pediatrics, and Epidemiology; members of the AAP Committees on Pediatric Emergency Medicine and Medical Liability and Risk Management; members of the AAP Councils on Children With Disabilities and Community Pediatrics; and members of outside organizations including the Child Neurology Society and the American Academy of Neurology.

A comprehensive review of the evidence-based literature published since 1998 was conducted with the aim of addressing possible therapeutic interventions in the management of children with simple febrile seizures. The review focused on both the efficacy and potential adverse effects of the proposed treatments. Decisions were made on the basis of a systematic grading of the quality of evidence and strength of recommendations.

The AAP established a partnership with the University of Kentucky (Lexington, KY) to develop an evidence report, which served as a major source of information for these practice-guideline recommendations. The specific issues addressed were (1) effectiveness of continuous anticonvulsant therapy in preventing recurrent febrile seizures, (2) effectiveness of intermittent anticonvulsant therapy in preventing recurrent febrile seizures, (3) effectiveness of antipyretics in preventing recurrent febrile seizures, and (4) adverse effects of either continuous or intermittent anticonvulsant therapy.

In the original practice parameter, more than 300 medical journal articles reporting studies of the natural history of simple febrile seizures or the therapy of these seizures were reviewed and abstracted.[2] An additional 65 articles were reviewed and abstracted for the update. Emphasis was placed on articles that differentiated simple febrile seizures from other types of seizures, that carefully matched treatment and control groups, and that described adherence to the drug regimen. Tables were constructed from the 65 articles that best fit these criteria. A more comprehensive review of the literature on which this report is based can be found in a forthcoming technical report (the initial technical report can be accessed at http://aappolicy.aappublications.org/cgi/content/full/pediatrics;103/6/e86). The technical report also will contain dosing information.

The evidence-based approach to guideline development requires that the evidence in support of a recommendation be identified, appraised, and summarized and that an explicit link between evidence and recommendations be defined. Evidence-based recommendations reflect the quality of evidence and the balance of benefit and harm that is

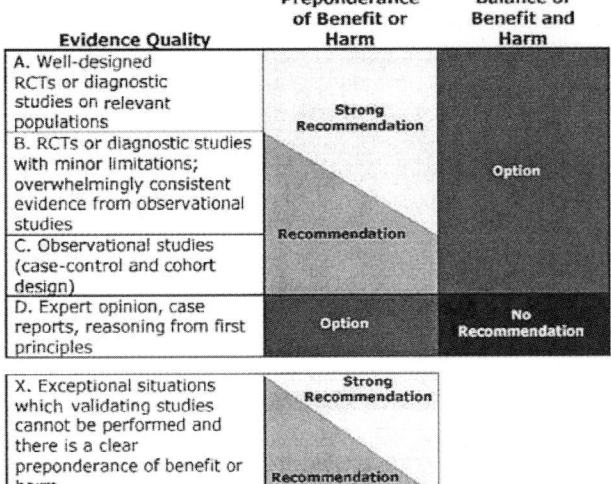

FIGURE 1
Integrating evidence-quality appraisal with an assessment of the anticipated balance between benefits and harms if a policy is conducted leads to designation of a policy as a strong recommendation, recommendation, option, or no recommendation. RCT indicates randomized, controlled trial.

anticipated when the recommendation is followed. The AAP policy statement "Classifying Recommendations for Clinical Practice Guidelines"[9] was followed in designating levels of recommendations (see Fig 1 and Table 1).

RECOMMENDATION

On the basis of the risks and benefits of the effective therapies, neither continuous nor intermittent anticonvulsant therapy is recommended for children with 1 or more simple febrile seizures.

- Aggregate evidence quality: B (randomized, controlled trials and diagnostic studies with minor limitations).

- Benefit: prevention of recurrent febrile seizures, which are not harmful and do not significantly increase the risk for development of future epilepsy.

- Harm: adverse effects including rare fatal hepatotoxicity (especially in children younger than 2 years who are also at greatest risk of febrile seizures), thrombocytopenia, weight loss and gain, gastrointestinal disturbances, and pancreatitis with valproic acid and hyperactivity, irritability, lethargy, sleep disturbances, and hypersensitivity reactions with phenobarbital; lethargy, drowsiness, and ataxia for intermittent diazepam as well as the risk of masking an evolving central nervous system infection.

- Benefits/harms assessment: preponderance of harm over benefit.

- Policy level: recommendation.

BENEFITS AND RISKS OF CONTINUOUS ANTICONVULSANT THERAPY

Phenobarbital

Phenobarbital is effective in preventing the recurrence of simple febrile seizures.[10] In a controlled double-blind study, daily therapy with phenobarbital reduced the rate of subsequent febrile seizures from 25 per 100 subjects per year to 5 per 100 subjects per year.[11] For the agent to be effective, however, it must be given daily and maintained in the therapeutic range. In a study by Farwell et al,[12] for example, children whose phenobarbital levels were in the therapeutic range had a reduction in recurrent seizures, but because noncompliance was so high, an overall benefit with phenobarbital therapy was not identified.

The adverse effects of phenobarbital include hyperactivity, irritability, lethargy, sleep disturbances, and hypersensitivity reactions. The behavioral adverse effects

TABLE 1   Guideline Definitions for Evidence-Based Statements

Statement	Definition	Implication
Strong recommendation	A strong recommendation in favor of a particular action is made when the anticipated benefits of the recommended intervention clearly exceed the harms (as a strong recommendation against an action is made when the anticipated harms clearly exceed the benefits) and the quality of the supporting evidence is excellent. In some clearly identified circumstances, strong recommendations may be made when high-quality evidence is impossible to obtain and the anticipated benefits strongly outweigh the harms.	Clinicians should follow a strong recommendation unless a clear and compelling rationale for an alternative approach is present.
Recommendation	A recommendation in favor of a particular action is made when the anticipated benefits exceed the harms but the quality of evidence is not as strong. Again, in some clearly identified circumstances, recommendations may be made when high-quality evidence is impossible to obtain but the anticipated benefits outweigh the harms.	Clinicians would be prudent to follow a recommendation but should remain alert to new information and sensitive to patient preferences.
Option	Options define courses that may be taken when either the quality of evidence is suspect or carefully performed studies have shown little clear advantage to 1 approach over another.	Clinicians should consider the option in their decision-making, and patient preference may have a substantial role.
No recommendation	No recommendation indicates that there is a lack of pertinent published evidence and that the anticipated balance of benefits and harms is presently unclear.	Clinicians should be alert to new published evidence that clarifies the balance of benefit versus harm.

may occur in up to 20% to 40% of patients and may be severe enough to necessitate discontinuation of the drug.[13-16]

Primidone

Primidone, in doses of 15 to 20 mg/kg per day, has also been shown to reduce the recurrence rate of febrile seizures.[17,18] It is of interest that the derived phenobarbital level in a Minigawa and Miura study[17] was below therapeutic (16 μg/mL) in 29 of the 32 children, suggesting that primidone itself may be active in preventing seizure recurrence. As with phenobarbital, adverse effects include behavioral disturbances, irritability, and sleep disturbances.[18]

Valproic Acid

In randomized, controlled studies, only 4% of children taking valproic acid, as opposed to 35% of control subjects, had a subsequent febrile seizure. Therefore, valproic acid seems to be at least as effective in preventing recurrent simple febrile seizures as phenobarbital and significantly more effective than placebo.[19-21]

Drawbacks to therapy with valproic acid include its rare association with fatal hepatotoxicity (especially in children younger than 2 years, who are also at greatest risk of febrile seizures), thrombocytopenia, weight loss and gain, gastrointestinal disturbances, and pancreatitis. In studies in which children received valproic acid to prevent recurrence of febrile seizures, no cases of fatal hepatotoxicity were reported.[15]

Carbamazepine

Carbamazepine has not been shown to be effective in preventing the recurrence of simple febrile seizures. Antony and Hawke[13] compared children who had been treated with therapeutic levels of either phenobarbital or carbamazepine, and 47% of the children in the carbamazepine-treated group had recurrent seizures compared with only 10% of those in the phenobarbital group. In another study, Camfield et al[22] treated children (whose conditions failed to improve with phenobarbital therapy) with carbamazepine. Despite good compliance, 13 of the 16 children treated with carbamazepine had a recurrent febrile seizure within 18 months. It is theoretically possible that these excessively high rates of recurrences might have been attributable to adverse effects of carbamazepine.

Phenytoin

Phenytoin has not been shown to be effective in preventing the recurrence of simple febrile seizures, even when the agent is in the therapeutic range.[23,24] Other anticonvulsants have not been studied for the continuous treatment of simple febrile seizures.

BENEFITS AND RISKS OF INTERMITTENT ANTICONVULSANT THERAPY

Diazepam

A double-blind controlled study of patients with a history of febrile seizures demonstrated that administration of oral diazepam (given at the time of fever) could reduce the recurrence of febrile seizures. Children with a history of febrile seizures were given either oral diazepam (0.33 mg/kg, every 8 hours for 48 hours) or a placebo at the time of fever. The risk of febrile seizures per person-year was decreased 44% with diazepam.[25] In a more recent study, children with a history of febrile seizures were given oral diazepam at the time of fever and then compared with children in an untreated control group. In the oral diazepam group, there was an 11% recurrence rate compared with a 30% recurrence rate in the control group.[26] It should be noted that all children for whom diazepam was considered a failure had been noncompliant with drug administration, in part because of adverse effects of the medication.

There is also literature that demonstrates the feasibility and safety of interrupting a simple febrile seizure lasting less than 5 minutes with rectal diazepam and with both intranasal and buccal midazolam.[27,28] Although these agents are effective in terminating the seizure, it is questionable whether they have any long-term influence on outcome. In a study by Knudsen et al,[29] children were given either rectal diazepam at the time of fever or only at the onset of seizure. Twelve-year follow-up found that the long-term prognosis of the children in the 2 groups did not differ regardless of whether treatment was aimed at preventing seizures or treating them.

A potential drawback to intermittent medication is that a seizure could occur before a fever is noticed. Indeed, in several of these studies, recurrent seizures were likely attributable to failure of method rather than failure of the agent.

Adverse effects of oral and rectal diazepam[26] and both intranasal and buccal midazolam include lethargy, drowsiness, and ataxia. Respiratory depression is extremely rare, even when given by the rectal route.[28,30] Sedation caused by any of the benzodiazepines, whether administered by the oral, rectal, nasal, or buccal route, have the potential of masking an evolving central nervous system infection. If used, the child's health care professional should be contacted.

BENEFITS AND RISKS OF INTERMITTENT ANTIPYRETICS

No studies have demonstrated that antipyretics, in the absence of anticonvulsants, reduce the recurrence risk of simple febrile seizures. Camfield et al[11] treated 79 children who had had a first febrile seizure with either a placebo plus antipyretic instruction (either aspirin or acetaminophen) versus daily phenobarbital plus antipyretic instruction (either aspirin or acetaminophen). Recurrence risk was significantly lower in the phenobarbital-treated group, suggesting that antipyretic instruction, including the use of antipyretics, is ineffective in preventing febrile-seizure recurrence.

Whether antipyretics are given regularly (every 4 hours) or sporadically (contingent on a specific body-temperature elevation) does not influence outcome. Acetaminophen was either given every 4 hours or only for temperature elevations of more than 37.9°C in 104 children. The incidence of febrile episodes did not differ significantly between the 2 groups, nor did the early recurrence of febrile seizures. The authors determined that administering prophylactic acetaminophen during febrile episodes was ineffective in preventing or reducing fever and in preventing febrile-seizure recurrence.[31]

In a randomized double-blind placebo-controlled trial, acetaminophen was administered along with low-dose oral diazepam.[32] Febrile-seizure recurrence was not reduced, compared with control groups. As with acetaminophen, ibuprofen also has been shown to be ineffective in preventing recurrence of febrile seizures.[33–35]

In general, acetaminophen and ibuprofen are considered to be safe and effective antipyretics for children. However, hepatotoxicity (with acetaminophen) and respiratory failure, metabolic acidosis, renal failure, and coma (with ibuprofen) have been reported in children after overdose or in the presence of risk factors.[36,37]

CONCLUSIONS

The subcommittee has determined that a simple febrile seizure is a benign and common event in children between the ages of 6 and 60 months. Nearly all children have an excellent prognosis. The committee concluded that although there is evidence that both continuous antiepileptic therapy with phenobarbital, primidone, or valproic acid and intermittent therapy with oral diazepam are effective in reducing the risk of recurrence, the potential toxicities associated with antiepileptic drugs outweigh the relatively minor risks associated with simple febrile seizures. As such, long-term therapy is not recommended. In situations in which parental anxiety associated with febrile seizures is severe, intermittent oral diazepam at the onset of febrile illness may be effective in preventing recurrence. Although antipyretics may improve the comfort of the child, they will not prevent febrile seizures.

SUBCOMMITTEE ON FEBRILE SEIZURES, 2002–2008

Patricia K. Duffner, MD, Chairperson
Robert J. Baumann, MD, Methodologist
Peter Berman, MD
John L. Green, MD
Sanford Schneider, MD

STEERING COMMITTEE ON QUALITY IMPROVEMENT AND MANAGEMENT, 2007–2008

Elizabeth S. Hodgson, MD, Chairperson
Gordon B. Glade, MD
Norman "Chip" Harbaugh, Jr, MD
Thomas K. McInerny, MD
Marlene R. Miller, MD, MSc
Virginia A. Moyer, MD, MPH
Xavier D. Sevilla, MD
Lisa Simpson, MB, BCh, MPH
Glenn S. Takata, MD

LIAISONS

Denise Dougherty, PhD
    Agency for Healthcare Research and Quality
Daniel R. Neuspiel, MD
    Section on Epidemiology

Ellen Schwalenstocker, MBA
    National Association of Children's Hospitals and
    Related Institutions

STAFF

Caryn Davidson, MA

REFERENCES

1. Nelson KB, Ellenberg JH. Prognosis in children with febrile seizures. *Pediatrics.* 1978;61(5):720–727
2. American Academy of Pediatrics, Committee on Quality Improvement, Subcommittee on Febrile Seizures. The long-term treatment of the child with simple febrile seizures. *Pediatrics.* 1999;103(6 pt 1):1307–1309
3. Chang YC, Guo NW, Huang CC, Wang ST, Tsai JJ. Neurocognitive attention and behavior outcome of school age children with a history of febrile convulsions: a population study. *Epilepsia.* 2000;41(4):412–420
4. Ellenberg JH, Nelson KB. Febrile seizures and later intellectual performance. *Arch Neurol.* 1978;35(1):17–21
5. Verity CM, Butler NR, Golding J. Febrile convulsions in a national cohort followed up from birth. II: medical history and intellectual ability at 5 years of age. *BMJ.* 1985;290(6478):1311–1315
6. Nelson KB, Ellenberg JH. Predictors of epilepsy in children who have experienced febrile seizures. *N Engl J Med.* 1976;295(19):1029–1033
7. Annegers JF, Hauser WA, Shirts SB, Kurland LT. Factors prognostic of unprovoked seizures after febrile convulsions. *N Engl J Med.* 1987;316(9):493–498
8. Berg AT, Shinnar S, Darefsky AS, et al. Predictors of recurrent febrile seizures: a prospective cohort study. *Arch Pediatr Adolesc Med.* 1997;151(4):371–378
9. American Academy of Pediatrics, Steering Committee on Quality Improvement and Management. Classifying recommendations for clinical practice guidelines. *Pediatrics.* 2004;114(3):874–877
10. Wolf SM, Carr A, Davis DC, Davidson S, et al. The value of phenobarbital in the child who has had a single febrile seizure: a controlled prospective study. *Pediatrics.* 1977;59(3):378–385
11. Camfield PR, Camfield CS, Shapiro SH, Cummings C. The first febrile seizure: antipyretic instruction plus either phenobarbital or placebo to prevent recurrence. *J Pediatr.* 1980;97(1):16–21
12. Farwell JR, Lee JY, Hirtz DG, Sulzbacher SI, Ellenberg JH, Nelson KB. Phenobarbital for febrile seizures: effects on intelligence and on seizure recurrence [published correction appears in *N Engl J Med.* 1992;326(2):144]. *N Engl J Med.* 1990;322(6):364–369
13. Antony JH, Hawke SHB. Phenobarbital compared with carbamazepine in prevention of recurrent febrile convulsions. *Am J Dis Child.* 1983;137(9):892–895
14. Knudsen Fu, Vestermark S. Prophylactic diazepam or phenobarbitone in febrile convulsions: a prospective, controlled study. *Arch Dis Child.* 1978;53(8):660–663
15. Lee K, Melchior JC. Sodium valproate versus phenobarbital in the prophylactic treatment of febrile convulsions in childhood. *Eur J Pediatr.* 1981;137(2):151–153
16. Camfield CS, Chaplin S, Doyle AB, Shapiro SH, Cummings C, Camfield PR. Side effects of phenobarbital in toddlers: behavioral and cognitive aspects. *J Pediatr.* 1979;95(3):361–365
17. Minagawa K, Miura H. Phenobarbital, primidone and sodium valproate in the prophylaxis of febrile convulsions. *Brain Dev.* 1981;3(4):385–393
18. Herranz JL, Armijo JA, Arteaga R. Effectiveness and toxicity of phenobarbital, primidone, and sodium valproate in the pre-

vention of febrile convulsions, controlled by plasma levels. *Epilepsia.* 1984;25(1):89–95

19. Wallace SJ, Smith JA. Successful prophylaxis against febrile convulsions with valproic acid or phenobarbitone. *BMJ.* 1980; 280(6211):353–354

20. Mamelle N, Mamelle JC, Plasse JC, Revol M, Gilly R. Prevention of recurrent febrile convulsions: a randomized therapeutic assay—sodium valproate, phenobarbitone and placebo. *Neuropediatrics.* 1984;15(1):37–42

21. Ngwane E, Bower B. Continuous sodium valproate or phenobarbitone in the prevention of "simple" febrile convulsions. *Arch Dis Child.* 1980;55(3):171–174

22. Camfield PR, Camfield CS, Tibbles JA. Carbamazepine does not prevent febrile seizures in phenobarbital failures. *Neurology.* 1982;32(3):288–289

23. Bacon CJ, Hierons AM, Mucklow JC, Webb JK, Rawlins MD, Weightman D. Placebo-controlled study of phenobarbitone and phenytoin in the prophylaxis of febrile convulsions. *Lancet.* 1981;2(8247):600–604

24. Melchior JC, Buchthal F, Lennox Buchthal M. The ineffectiveness of diphenylhydantoin in preventing febrile convulsions in the age of greatest risk, under 3 years. *Epilepsia.* 1971;12(1): 55–62

25. Rosman NP, Colton T, Labazzo J, et al. A controlled trial of diazepam administered during febrile illnesses to prevent recurrence of febrile seizures. *N Engl J Med.* 1993;329(2):79–84

26. Verrotti A, Latini G, di Corcia G, et al. Intermittent oral diazepam prophylaxis in febrile convulsions: its effectiveness for febrile seizure recurrence. *Eur J Pediatr Neurol.* 2004;8(3): 131–134

27. Lahat E, Goldman M, Barr J, Bistritzer T, Berkovitch M. Comparison of intranasal midazolam with intravenous diazepam for treating febrile seizures in children: prospective randomized study. *BMJ.* 2000;321(7253):83–86

28. McIntyre J, Robertson S, Norris E, et al. Safety and efficacy of buccal midazolam versus rectal diazepam for emergency treatment of seizures in children: a randomized controlled trial. *Lancet.* 2005;366(9481):205–210

29. Knudsen FU, Paerregaard A, Andersen R, Andresen J. Long term outcome of prophylaxis for febrile convulsions. *Arch Dis Child.* 1996;74(1):13–18

30. Pellock JM, Shinnar S. Respiratory adverse events associated with diazepam rectal gel. *Neurology.* 2005;64(10):1768–1770

31. Schnaiderman D, Lahat E, Sheefer T, Aladjem M. Antipyretic effectiveness of acetaminophen in febrile seizures: ongoing prophylaxis versus sporadic usage. *Eur J Pediatr.* 1993;152(9): 747–749

32. Uhari M, Rantala H, Vainionpaa L, Kurttila R. Effect of acetaminophen and of low dose intermittent doses of diazepam on prevention of recurrences of febrile seizures. *J Pediatr.* 1995; 126(6):991–995

33. van Stuijvenberg M, Derksen-Lubsen G, Steyerberg EW, Habbema JDF, Moll HA. Randomized, controlled trial of ibuprofen syrup administered during febrile illnesses to prevent febrile seizure recurrences. *Pediatrics.* 1998;102(5). Available at: www.pediatrics.org/cgi/content/full/102/5/e51

34. van Esch A, Van Steensel-Moll HA, Steyerberg EW, Offringa M, Habbema JDF, Derksen-Lubsen G. Antipyretic efficacy of ibuprofen and acetaminophen in children with febrile seizures. *Arch Pediatr Adolesc Med.* 1995;149(6):632–637

35. van Esch A, Steyerberg EW, Moll HA, et al. A study of the efficacy of antipyretic drugs in the prevention of febrile seizure recurrence. *Ambul Child Health.* 2000;6(1):19–26

36. Easley RB, Altemeier WA. Central nervous system manifestations of an ibuprofen overdose reversed by naloxone. *Pediatr Emerg Care.* 2000;16(1):39–41

37. American Academy of Pediatrics, Committee on Drugs. Acetaminophen toxicity in children. *Pediatrics.* 2001;108(4): 1020–1024

Febrile Seizures: Guideline for the Neurodiagnostic Evaluation of the Child With a Simple Febrile Seizure

- *Clinical Practice Guideline*

Clinical Practice Guideline—Febrile Seizures: Guideline for the Neurodiagnostic Evaluation of the Child With a Simple Febrile Seizure

SUBCOMMITTEE ON FEBRILE SEIZURES

KEY WORD

seizure

ABBREVIATIONS

AAP—American Academy of Pediatrics
Hib—*Haemophilus influenzae* type b
EEG—electroencephalogram
CT—computed tomography

www.pediatrics.org/cgi/doi/10.1542/peds.2010-3318

doi:10.1542/peds.2010-3318

All clinical practice guidelines from the American Academy of Pediatrics automatically expire 5 years after publication unless reaffirmed, revised, or retired at or before that time.

PEDIATRICS (ISSN Numbers: Print, 0031-4005; Online, 1098-4275).

abstract

OBJECTIVE: To formulate evidence-based recommendations for health care professionals about the diagnosis and evaluation of a simple febrile seizure in infants and young children 6 through 60 months of age and to revise the practice guideline published by the American Academy of Pediatrics (AAP) in 1996.

METHODS: This review included search and analysis of the medical literature published since the last version of the guideline. Physicians with expertise and experience in the fields of neurology and epilepsy, pediatrics, epidemiology, and research methodologies constituted a subcommittee of the AAP Steering Committee on Quality Improvement and Management. The steering committee and other groups within the AAP and organizations outside the AAP reviewed the guideline. The subcommittee member who reviewed the literature for the 1996 AAP practice guidelines searched for articles published since the last guideline through 2009, supplemented by articles submitted by other committee members. Results from the literature search were provided to the subcommittee members for review. Interventions of direct interest included lumbar puncture, electroencephalography, blood studies, and neuroimaging. Multiple issues were raised and discussed iteratively until consensus was reached about recommendations. The strength of evidence supporting each recommendation and the strength of the recommendation were assessed by the committee member most experienced in informatics and epidemiology and graded according to AAP policy.

CONCLUSIONS: Clinicians evaluating infants or young children after a simple febrile seizure should direct their attention toward identifying the cause of the child's fever. Meningitis should be considered in the differential diagnosis for any febrile child, and lumbar puncture should be performed if there are clinical signs or symptoms of concern. For any infant between 6 and 12 months of age who presents with a seizure and fever, a lumbar puncture is an option when the child is considered deficient in *Haemophilus influenzae* type b (Hib) or *Streptococcus pneumoniae* immunizations (ie, has not received scheduled immunizations as recommended), or when immunization status cannot be determined, because of an increased risk of bacterial meningitis. A lumbar puncture is an option for children who are pretreated with antibiotics. In general, a simple febrile seizure does not usually require further evaluation, specifically electroencephalography, blood studies, or neuroimaging. *Pediatrics* 2011;127:389–394

DEFINITION OF THE PROBLEM

This practice guideline provides recommendations for the neurodiagnostic evaluation of neurologically healthy infants and children 6 through 60 months of age who have had a simple febrile seizure and present for evaluation within 12 hours of the event. It replaces the 1996 practice parameter.[1] This practice guideline is not intended for patients who have had complex febrile seizures (prolonged, focal, and/or recurrent), and it does not pertain to children with previous neurologic insults, known central nervous system abnormalities, or history of afebrile seizures.

TARGET AUDIENCE AND PRACTICE SETTING

This practice guideline is intended for use by pediatricians, family physicians, child neurologists, neurologists, emergency physicians, nurse practitioners, and other health care providers who evaluate children for febrile seizures.

BACKGROUND

A febrile seizure is a seizure accompanied by fever (temperature $\geq$ 100.4°F or 38°C[2] by any method), without central nervous system infection, that occurs in infants and children 6 through 60 months of age. Febrile seizures occur in 2% to 5% of all children and, as such, make up the most common convulsive event in children younger than 60 months. In 1976, Nelson and Ellenberg,[3] using data from the National Collaborative Perinatal Project, further defined febrile seizures as being either simple or complex. Simple febrile seizures were defined as primary generalized seizures that lasted for less than 15 minutes and did not recur within 24 hours. Complex febrile seizures were defined as focal, prolonged ($\geq$15 minutes), and/or recurrent within 24 hours. Children who had simple febrile seizures had no evidence of increased mortality, hemiplegia, or mental retardation. During follow-up evaluation, the risk of epilepsy after a simple febrile seizure was shown to be only slightly higher than that of the general population, whereas the chief risk associated with simple febrile seizures was recurrence in one-third of the children. The authors concluded that simple febrile seizures are benign events with excellent prognoses, a conclusion reaffirmed in the 1980 consensus statement from the National Institutes of Health.[3,4]

The expected outcomes of this practice guideline include the following:

1. Optimize clinician understanding of the scientific basis for the neurodiagnostic evaluation of children with simple febrile seizures.

2. Aid the clinician in decision-making by using a structured framework.

3. Optimize evaluation of the child who has had a simple febrile seizure by detecting underlying diseases, minimizing morbidity, and reassuring anxious parents and children.

4. Reduce the costs of physician and emergency department visits, hospitalizations, and unnecessary testing.

5. Educate the clinician to understand that a simple febrile seizure usually does not require further evaluation, specifically electroencephalography, blood studies, or neuroimaging.

METHODOLOGY

To update the clinical practice guideline on the neurodiagnostic evaluation of children with simple febrile seizures,[1] the American Academy of Pediatrics (AAP) reconvened the Subcommittee on Febrile Seizures. The committee was chaired by a child neurologist and consisted of a neuroepidemiologist, 3 additional child neurologists, and a practicing pediatrician. All panel members reviewed and signed the AAP voluntary disclosure and conflict-of-interest form. No conflicts were reported. Participation in the guideline process was voluntary and not paid. The guideline was reviewed by members of the AAP Steering Committee on Quality Improvement and Management; members of the AAP Section on Administration and Practice Management, Section on Developmental and Behavioral Pediatrics, Section on Epidemiology, Section on Infectious Diseases, Section on Neurology, Section on Neurologic Surgery, Section on Pediatric Emergency Medicine, Committee on Pediatric Emergency Medicine, Committee on Practice and Ambulatory Medicine, Committee on Child Health Financing, Committee on Infectious Diseases, Committee on Medical Liability and Risk Management, Council on Children With Disabilities, and Council on Community Pediatrics; and members of outside organizations including the Child Neurology Society, the American Academy of Neurology, the American College of Emergency Physicians, and members of the Pediatric Committee of the Emergency Nurses Association.

A comprehensive review of the evidence-based literature published from 1996 to February 2009 was conducted to discover articles that addressed the diagnosis and evaluation of children with simple febrile seizures. Preference was given to population-based studies, but given the scarcity of such studies, data from hospital-based studies, groups of young children with febrile illness, and comparable groups were reviewed. Decisions were made on the basis of a systematic grading of the quality of evidence and strength of recommendations.

In the original practice parameter,[1] 203 medical journal articles were reviewed and abstracted. An additional 372 articles were reviewed and abstracted for this update. Emphasis was placed on articles that differentiated simple febrile seizures from other types of seizures. Tables were constructed from the 70 articles that best fit these criteria.

The evidence-based approach to guideline development requires that the evidence in support of a recommendation be identified, appraised, and summarized and that an explicit link between

Evidence Quality	Preponderance of Benefit or Harm	Balance of Benefit and Harm
A. Well-designed RCTs or diagnostic studies on relevant population	Strong	Option
B. RCTs or diagnostic studies with minor limitations; overwhelmingly consistent evidence from observational studies	Strong / Rec	Option
C. Observational studies (case-control and cohort design)	Rec	Option
D. Expert opinion, case reports, reasoning from first principles	Option	No Rec
X. Exceptional situations for which validating studies cannot be performed and there is a clear preponderance of benefit or harm	Strong / Rec	

FIGURE 1
Integrating evidence quality appraisal with an assessment of the anticipated balance between benefits and harms if a policy is carried out leads to designation of a policy as a strong recommendation, recommendation, option, or no recommendation. RCT indicates randomized controlled trial; Rec, recommendation.

evidence and recommendations be defined. Evidence-based recommendations reflect the quality of evidence and the balance of benefit and harm that is anticipated when the recommendation is followed. The AAP policy statement "Classifying Recommendations for Clinical Practice Guidelines"[5] was followed in designating levels of recommendations (see Fig 1).

KEY ACTION STATEMENTS

Action Statement 1

Action Statement 1a

A lumbar puncture should be performed in any child who presents with a seizure and a fever and has meningeal signs and symptoms (eg, neck stiffness, Kernig and/or Brudzinski signs) or in any child whose history or examination suggests the presence of meningitis or intracranial infection.

- Aggregate evidence level: B (overwhelming evidence from observational studies).
- Benefits: Meningeal signs and symptoms strongly suggest meningitis, which, if bacterial in etiology, will likely be fatal if left untreated.
- Harms/risks/costs: Lumbar puncture is an invasive and often painful procedure and can be costly.
- Benefits/harms assessment: Preponderance of benefit over harm.
- Value judgments: Observational data and clinical principles were used in making this judgment.
- Role of patient preferences: Although parents may not wish to have their child undergo a lumbar puncture, health care providers should explain that if meningitis is not diagnosed and treated, it could be fatal.
- Exclusions: None.
- Intentional vagueness: None.
- Policy level: Strong recommendation.

Action Statement 1b

In any infant between 6 and 12 months of age who presents with a seizure and fever, a lumbar puncture is an option when the child is considered deficient in *Haemophilus influenzae* type b (Hib) or *Streptococcus pneumoniae* immunizations (ie, has not received scheduled immunizations as recommended) or when immunization status cannot be determined because of an increased risk of bacterial meningitis.

- Aggregate evidence level: D (expert opinion, case reports).
- Benefits: Meningeal signs and symptoms strongly suggest meningitis, which, if bacterial in etiology, will likely be fatal or cause significant long-term disability if left untreated.
- Harms/risks/costs: Lumbar puncture is an invasive and often painful procedure and can be costly.
- Benefits/harms assessment: Preponderance of benefit over harm.
- Value judgments: Data on the incidence of bacterial meningitis from before and after the existence of immunizations against Hib and *S pneumoniae* were used in making this recommendation.
- Role of patient preferences: Although parents may not wish their child to undergo a lumbar puncture, health care providers should explain that in the absence of complete immunizations, their child may be at risk of having fatal bacterial meningitis.
- Exclusions: This recommendation applies only to children 6 to 12 months of age. The subcommittee felt that clinicians would recognize symptoms of meningitis in children older than 12 months.
- Intentional vagueness: None.
- Policy level: Option.

Action Statement 1c

A lumbar puncture is an option in the child who presents with a seizure and fever and is pretreated with antibiotics, because antibiotic treatment can mask the signs and symptoms of meningitis.

- Aggregate evidence level: D (reasoning from clinical experience, case series).
- Benefits: Antibiotics may mask meningeal signs and symptoms but may be insufficient to eradicate meningitis; a diagnosis of meningitis, if bacterial in etiology, will likely be fatal if left untreated.
- Harms/risks/costs: Lumbar puncture is an invasive and often painful procedure and can be costly.

- Benefits/harms assessment: Preponderance of benefit over harm.
- Value judgments: Clinical experience and case series were used in making this judgment while recognizing that extensive data from studies are lacking.
- Role of patient preferences: Although parents may not wish to have their child undergo a lumbar puncture, medical providers should explain that in the presence of pretreatment with antibiotics, the signs and symptoms of meningitis may be masked. Meningitis, if untreated, can be fatal.
- Exclusions: None.
- Intentional vagueness: Data are insufficient to define the specific treatment duration necessary to mask signs and symptoms. The committee determined that the decision to perform a lumbar puncture will depend on the type and duration of antibiotics administered before the seizure and should be left to the individual clinician.
- Policy level: Option.

The committee recognizes the diversity of past and present opinions regarding the need for lumbar punctures in children younger than 12 months with a simple febrile seizure. Since the publication of the previous practice parameter,[1] however, there has been widespread immunization in the United States for 2 of the most common causes of bacterial meningitis in this age range: Hib and S pneumoniae. Although compliance with all scheduled immunizations as recommended does not completely eliminate the possibility of bacterial meningitis from the differential diagnosis, current data no longer support routine lumbar puncture in well-appearing, fully immunized children who present with a simple febrile seizure.[6-8] Moreover, although approximately 25% of young children with meningitis have seizures as the presenting sign of the disease, some are ei-

ther obtunded or comatose when evaluated by a physician for the seizure, and the remainder most often have obvious clinical signs of meningitis (focal seizures, recurrent seizures, petechial rash, or nuchal rigidity).[9-11] Once a decision has been made to perform a lumbar puncture, then blood culture and serum glucose testing should be performed concurrently to increase the sensitivity for detecting bacteria and to determine if there is hypoglycorrhachia characteristic of bacterial meningitis, respectively.

Recent studies that evaluated the outcome of children with simple febrile seizures have included populations with a high prevalence of immunization.[7,8] Data for unimmunized or partially immunized children are lacking. Therefore, lumbar puncture is an option for young children who are considered deficient in immunizations or those in whom immunization status cannot be determined. There are also no definitive data on the outcome of children who present with a simple febrile seizure while already on antibiotics. The authors were unable to find a definition of "pretreated" in the literature, so they consulted with the AAP Committee on Infectious Diseases. Although there is no formal definition, pretreatment can be considered to include systemic antibiotic therapy by any route given within the days before the seizure. Whether pretreatment will affect the presentation and course of bacterial meningitis cannot be predicted but will depend, in part, on the antibiotic administered, the dose, the route of administration, the drug's cerebrospinal fluid penetration, and the organism causing the meningitis. Lumbar puncture is an option in any child pretreated with antibiotics before a simple febrile seizure.

Action Statement 2

An electroencephalogram (EEG) should not be performed in the evaluation of a neurologically healthy child with a simple febrile seizure.

- Aggregate evidence level: B (overwhelming evidence from observational studies).
- Benefits: One study showed a possible association with paroxysmal EEGs and a higher rate of afebrile seizures.[12]
- Harms/risks/costs: EEGs are costly and may increase parental anxiety.
- Benefits/harms assessment: Preponderance of harm over benefit.
- Value judgments: Observational data were used for this judgment.
- Role of patient preferences: Although an EEG might have limited prognostic utility in this situation, parents should be educated that the study will not alter outcome.
- Exclusions: None.
- Intentional vagueness: None.
- Policy level: Strong recommendation.

There is no evidence that EEG readings performed either at the time of presentation after a simple febrile seizure or within the following month are predictive of either recurrence of febrile seizures or the development of afebrile seizures/epilepsy within the next 2 years.[13,14] There is a single study that found that a paroxysmal EEG was associated with a higher rate of afebrile seizures.[12] There is no evidence that interventions based on this test would alter outcome.

Action Statement 3

The following tests should not be performed routinely for the sole purpose of identifying the cause of a simple febrile seizure: measurement of serum electrolytes, calcium, phosphorus, magnesium, or blood glucose or complete blood cell count.

- Aggregate evidence level: B (overwhelming evidence from observational studies).
- Benefits: A complete blood cell count may identify children at risk for bacte-

remia; however, the incidence of bacteremia in febrile children younger than 24 months is the same with or without febrile seizures.

- Harms/risks/costs: Laboratory tests may be invasive and costly and provide no real benefit.

- Benefits/harms assessment: Preponderance of harm over benefit.

- Value judgments: Observational data were used for this judgment.

- Role of patient preferences: Although parents may want blood tests performed to explain the seizure, they should be reassured that blood tests should be directed toward identifying the source of their child's fever.

- Exclusions: None.

- Intentional vagueness: None.

- Policy level: Strong recommendation.

There is no evidence to suggest that routine blood studies are of benefit in the evaluation of the child with a simple febrile seizure.[15–18] Although some children with febrile seizures have abnormal serum electrolyte values, their condition should be identifiable by obtaining appropriate histories and performing careful physical examinations. It should be noted that as a group, children with febrile seizures have relatively low serum sodium concentrations. As such, physicians and caregivers should avoid overhydration with hypotonic fluids.[18] Complete blood cell counts may be useful as a means of identifying young children at risk of bacteremia. It should be noted, however, that the incidence of bacteremia in children younger than 24 months with or without febrile seizures is the same. When fever is present, the decision regarding the need for laboratory testing should be directed toward identifying the source of the fever rather than as part of the routine evaluation of the seizure itself.

Action Statement 4

Neuroimaging should not be performed in the routine evaluation of the child with a simple febrile seizure.

- Aggregate evidence level: B (overwhelming evidence from observational studies).

- Benefits: Neuroimaging might provide earlier detection of fixed structural lesions, such as dysplasia, or very rarely, abscess or tumor.

- Harms/risks/costs: Neuroimaging tests are costly, computed tomography (CT) exposes children to radiation, and MRI may require sedation.

- Benefits/harms assessment: Preponderance of harm over benefit.

- Value judgments: Observational data were used for this judgment.

- Role of patient preferences: Although parents may want neuroimaging performed to explain the seizure, they should be reassured that the tests carry risks and will not alter outcome for their child.

- Exclusions: None.

- Intentional vagueness: None.

- Policy level: Strong recommendation.

The literature does not support the use of skull films in evaluation of the child with a febrile seizure.[15,19] No data have been published that either support or negate the need for CT or MRI in the evaluation of children with simple febrile seizures. Data, however, show that CT scanning is associated with radiation exposure that may escalate future cancer risk. MRI is associated with risks from required sedation and high cost.[20,21] Extrapolation of data from the literature on the use of CT in neurologically healthy children who have generalized epilepsy has shown that clinically important intracranial structural abnormalities in this patient population are uncommon.[22,23]

CONCLUSIONS

Clinicians evaluating infants or young children after a simple febrile seizure should direct their attention toward identifying the cause of the child's fever. Meningitis should be considered in the differential diagnosis for any febrile child, and lumbar puncture should be performed if the child is ill-appearing or if there are clinical signs or symptoms of concern. A lumbar puncture is an option in a child 6 to 12 months of age who is deficient in Hib and *S pneumoniae* immunizations or for whom immunization status is unknown. A lumbar puncture is an option in children who have been pretreated with antibiotics. In general, a simple febrile seizure does not usually require further evaluation, specifically EEGs, blood studies, or neuroimaging.

SUBCOMMITTEE ON FEBRILE SEIZURES, 2002–2010

Patricia K. Duffner, MD (neurology, no conflicts)
Peter H. Berman, MD (neurology, no conflicts)
Robert J. Baumann, MD (neuroepidemiology, no conflicts)
Paul Graham Fisher, MD (neurology, no conflicts)
John L. Green, MD (general pediatrics, no conflicts)
Sanford Schneider, MD (neurology, no conflicts)

STAFF

Caryn Davidson, MA

OVERSIGHT BY THE STEERING COMMITTEE ON QUALITY IMPROVEMENT AND MANAGEMENT, 2009–2011

REFERENCES

1. American Academy of Pediatrics, Provisional Committee on Quality Improvement and Subcommittee on Febrile Seizures. Practice parameter: the neurodiagnostic evaluation of a child with a first simple febrile seizure. *Pediatrics.* 1996;97(5):769–772; discussion 773–775

2. Michael Marcy S, Kohl KS, Dagan R, et al; Brighton Collaboration Fever Working Group. Fever as an adverse event following immunization: case definition and guidelines of data collection, analysis, and presentation. *Vaccine.* 2004;22(5–6):551–556

3. Nelson KB, Ellenberg JH. Predictors of epilepsy in children who have experienced febrile seizures. *N Engl J Med.* 1976;295(19):1029–1033

4. Consensus statement: febrile seizures—long-term management of children with fever-associated seizures. *Pediatrics.* 1980;66(6):1009–1012

5. American Academy of Pediatrics, Steering Committee on Quality Improvement and Management. Classifying recommendations for clinical practice guidelines. *Pediatrics.* 2004;114(3):874–877

6. Trainor JL, Hampers LC, Krug SE, Listernick R. Children with first-time simple febrile seizures are at low risk of serious bacterial illness. *Acad Emerg Med.* 2001;8(8):781–787

7. Shaked O, Peña BM, Linares MY, Baker RL. Simple febrile seizures: are the AAP guidelines regarding lumbar puncture being followed? *Pediatr Emerg Care.* 2009;25(1):8–11

8. Kimia AA, Capraro AJ, Hummel D, Johnston P, Harper MB. Utility of lumbar puncture for first simple febrile seizure among children 6 to 18 months of age. *Pediatrics.* 2009;123(1):6–12

9. Warden CR, Zibulewsky J, Mace S, Gold C, Gausche-Hill M. Evaluation and management of febrile seizures in the out-of-hospital and emergency department settings. *Ann Emerg Med.* 2003;41(2):215–222

10. Rutter N, Smales OR. Role of routine investigations in children presenting with their first febrile convulsion. *Arch Dis Child.* 1977;52(3):188–191

11. Green SM, Rothrock SG, Clem KJ, Zurcher RF, Mellick L. Can seizures be the sole manifestation of meningitis in febrile children? *Pediatrics.* 1993;92(4):527–534

12. Kuturec M, Emoto SE, Sofijanov N, et al. Febrile seizures: is the EEG a useful predictor of recurrences? *Clin Pediatr (Phila).* 1997;36(1):31–36

13. Frantzen E, Lennox-Buchthal M, Nygaard A. Longitudinal EEG and clinical study of children with febrile convulsions. *Electroencephalogr Clin Neurophysiol.* 1968;24(3):197–212

14. Thorn I. The significance of electroencephalography in febrile convulsions. In: Akimoto H, Kazamatsuri H, Seino M, Ward A, eds. *Advances in Epileptology: XIIIth International Epilepsy Symposium.* New York, NY: Raven Press; 1982:93–95

15. Jaffe M, Bar-Joseph G, Tirosh E. Fever and convulsions: indications for laboratory investigations. *Pediatrics.* 1981;67(5):729–731

16. Gerber MA, Berliner BC. The child with a "simple" febrile seizure: appropriate diagnostic evaluation. *Am J Dis Child.* 1981;135(5):431–443

17. Heijbel J, Blom S, Bergfors PG. Simple febrile convulsions: a prospective incidence study and an evaluation of investigations initially needed. *Neuropadiatrie.* 1980;11(1):45–56

18. Thoman JE, Duffner PK, Shucard JL. Do serum sodium levels predict febrile seizure recurrence within 24 hours? *Pediatr Neurol.* 2004;31(5):342–344

19. Nealis GT, McFadden SW, Ames RA, Ouellette EM. Routine skull roentgenograms in the management of simple febrile seizures. *J Pediatr.* 1977;90(4):595–596

20. Stein SC, Hurst RW, Sonnad SS. Meta-analysis of cranial CT scans in children: a mathematical model to predict radiation-induced tumors associated with radiation exposure that may escalate future cancer risk. *Pediatr Neurosurg.* 2008;44(6):448–457

21. Brenner DJ, Hall EJ. Computed tomography: an increasing source of radiation exposure. *N Engl J Med.* 2007;357(22):2277–2284

22. Yang PJ, Berger PE, Cohen ME, Duffner PK. Computed tomography and childhood seizure disorders. *Neurology.* 1979;29(8):1084–1088

23. Bachman DS, Hodges FJ, Freeman JM. Computerized axial tomography in chronic seizure disorders of childhood. *Pediatrics.* 1976;58(6):828–832

Febrile Seizures Clinical Practice Guidelines
Quick Reference Tools

• •

- Recommendation Summaries
  — Febrile Seizures: Clinical Practice Guideline for the Long-term Management of the Child With Simple Febrile Seizures
  — Febrile Seizures: Guidelines for the Neurodiagnostic Evaluation of the Child With a Simple Febrile Seizure
- *ICD-10-CM* Coding Quick Reference for Febrile Seizures
- AAP Patient Education Handout
  — *Febrile Seizures*

Recommendation Summaries

Febrile Seizures: Clinical Practice Guideline for the Long-term Management of the Child With Simple Febrile Seizures

On the basis of the risks and benefits of the effective therapies, neither continuous nor intermittent anticonvulsant therapy is recommended for children with 1 or more simple febrile seizures.

- Aggregate evidence quality: B (randomized, controlled trials and diagnostic studies with minor limitations).
- Benefit: prevention of recurrent febrile seizures, which are not harmful and do not significantly increase the risk for development of future epilepsy.
- Harm: adverse effects including rare fatal hepatotoxicity (especially in children younger than 2 years who are also at greatest risk of febrile seizures), thrombocytopenia, weight loss and gain, gastrointestinal disturbances, and pancreatitis with valproic acid and hyperactivity, irritability, lethargy, sleep disturbances, and hypersensitivity reactions with phenobarbital; lethargy, drowsiness, and ataxia for intermittent diazepam as well as the risk of masking an evolving central nervous system infection.
- Benefits/harms assessment: preponderance of harm over benefit.
- Policy level: recommendation.

Febrile Seizures: Guidelines for the Neurodiagnostic Evaluation of the Child With a Simple Febrile Seizure

Action Statement 1a

A lumbar puncture should be performed in any child who presents with a seizure and a fever and has meningeal signs and symptoms (eg, neck stiffness, Kernig and/or Brudzinski signs) or in any child whose history or examination suggests the presence of meningitis or intracranial infection.

Action Statement 1b

In any infant between 6 and 12 months of age who presents with a seizure and fever, a lumbar puncture is an option when the child is considered deficient in *Haemophilus influenzae* type b (Hib) or *Streptococcus pneumoniae* immunizations (ie, has not received scheduled immunizations as recommended) or when immunization status cannot be determined because of an increased risk of bacterial meningitis.

Action Statement 1c

A lumbar puncture is an option in the child who presents with a seizure and fever and is pretreated with antibiotics, because antibiotic treatment can mask the signs and symptoms of meningitis.

Action Statement 2

An electroencephalogram (EEG) should not be performed in the evaluation of a neurologically healthy child with a simple febrile seizure.

Action Statement 3

The following tests should not be performed routinely for the sole purpose of identifying the cause of a simple febrile seizure: measurement of serum electrolytes, calcium, phosphorus, magnesium, or blood glucose or complete blood cell count.

Action Statement 4

Neuroimaging should not be performed in the routine evaluation of the child with a simple febrile seizure.

Coding Quick Reference for Febrile Seizures
ICD-10-CM
R56.00 Simple febrile convulsions
R56.01 Complex febrile convulsions

Febrile Seizures

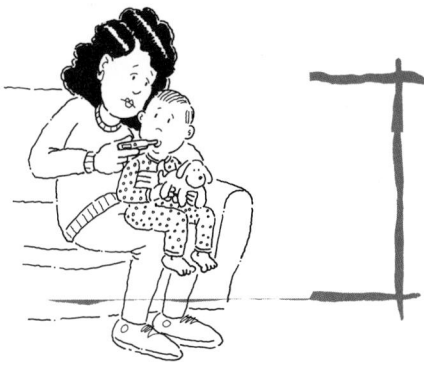

In some children, fevers can trigger seizures. Febrile seizures occur in 2% to 5% of all children between the ages of 6 months and 5 years. Seizures, sometimes called "fits" or "spells," are frightening, but they usually are harmless. Read on for information from the American Academy of Pediatrics that will help you understand febrile seizures and what happens if your child has one.

What is a febrile seizure?

A febrile seizure usually happens during the first few hours of a fever. The child may look strange for a few moments, then stiffen, twitch, and roll his eyes. He will be unresponsive for a short time, his breathing will be disturbed, and his skin may appear a little darker than usual. After the seizure, the child quickly returns to normal. Seizures usually last less than 1 minute but, although uncommon, can last for up to 15 minutes.

Febrile seizures rarely happen more than once within a 24-hour period. Other kinds of seizures (ones that are not caused by fever) last longer, can affect only one part of the body, and may occur repeatedly.

What do I do if my child has a febrile seizure?

If your child has a febrile seizure, act immediately to prevent injury.

- Place her on the floor or bed away from any hard or sharp objects.
- Turn her head to the side so that any saliva or vomit can drain from her mouth.
- Do not put anything into her mouth; she will not swallow her tongue.
- Call your child's doctor.
- If the seizure does not stop after 5 minutes, call 911 or your local emergency number.

Will my child have more seizures?

Febrile seizures tend to run in families. The risk of having seizures with other episodes of fever depends on the age of your child. Children younger than 1 year of age at the time of their first seizure have about a 50% chance of having another febrile seizure. Children older than 1 year of age at the time of their first seizure have only a 30% chance of having a second febrile seizure.

Will my child get epilepsy?

Epilepsy is a term used for multiple and recurrent seizures. Epileptic seizures are not caused by fever. Children with a history of febrile seizures are at only a slightly higher risk of developing epilepsy by age 7 than children who have not had febrile seizures.

Are febrile seizures dangerous?

While febrile seizures may be very scary, they are harmless to the child. Febrile seizures do not cause brain damage, nervous system problems, paralysis, intellectual disability (formerly called mental retardation), or death.

How are febrile seizures treated?

If your child has a febrile seizure, call your child's doctor right away. He or she will want to examine your child in order to determine the cause of your child's fever. It is more important to determine and treat the cause of the fever rather than the seizure. A spinal tap may be done to be sure your child does not have a serious infection like meningitis, especially if your child is younger than 1 year of age.

In general, doctors do not recommend treatment of a simple febrile seizure with preventive medicines. However, this should be discussed with your child's doctor. In cases of prolonged or repeated seizures, the recommendation may be different.

Medicines like acetaminophen and ibuprofen can help lower a fever, but they do not prevent febrile seizures. Your child's doctor will talk with you about the best ways to take care of your child's fever.

If your child has had a febrile seizure, do not fear the worst. These types of seizures are not dangerous to your child and do not cause long-term health problems. If you have concerns about this issue or anything related to your child's health, talk with your child's doctor.

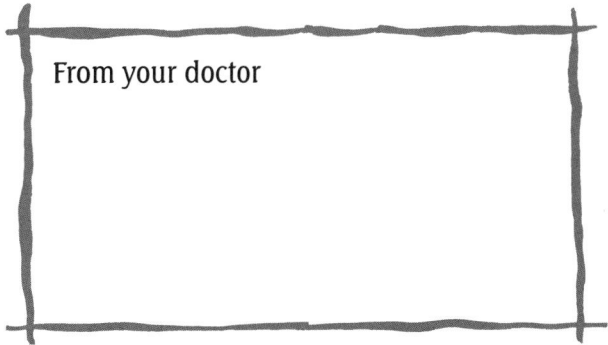

From your doctor

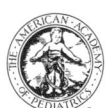

American Academy of Pediatrics

DEDICATED TO THE HEALTH OF ALL CHILDREN™

The American Academy of Pediatrics is an organization of 60,000 primary care pediatricians, pediatric medical subspecialists, and pediatric surgical specialists dedicated to the health, safety, and well-being of infants, children, adolescents, and young adults.

American Academy of Pediatrics
Web site — www.HealthyChildren.org

Management of Hyperbilirubinemia in the Newborn Infant 35 or More Weeks of Gestation

• •

- *Clinical Practice Guideline*
- *Technical Report Summary*
- *Technical Report*
- *2009 Commentaries*

Readers of this clinical practice guideline are urged to review the technical report and technical report summary to enhance the evidence-based decision-making process.

AMERICAN ACADEMY OF PEDIATRICS

CLINICAL PRACTICE GUIDELINE

Subcommittee on Hyperbilirubinemia

Management of Hyperbilirubinemia in the Newborn Infant 35 or More Weeks of Gestation

ABSTRACT. Jaundice occurs in most newborn infants. Most jaundice is benign, but because of the potential toxicity of bilirubin, newborn infants must be monitored to identify those who might develop severe hyperbilirubinemia and, in rare cases, acute bilirubin encephalopathy or kernicterus. The focus of this guideline is to reduce the incidence of severe hyperbilirubinemia and bilirubin encephalopathy while minimizing the risks of unintended harm such as maternal anxiety, decreased breastfeeding, and unnecessary costs or treatment. Although kernicterus should almost always be preventable, cases continue to occur. These guidelines provide a framework for the prevention and management of hyperbilirubinemia in newborn infants of 35 or more weeks of gestation. In every infant, we recommend that clinicians 1) promote and support successful breastfeeding; 2) perform a systematic assessment before discharge for the risk of severe hyperbilirubinemia; 3) provide early and focused follow-up based on the risk assessment; and 4) when indicated, treat newborns with phototherapy or exchange transfusion to prevent the development of severe hyperbilirubinemia and, possibly, bilirubin encephalopathy (kernicterus). *Pediatrics* 2004; 114:297–316; *hyperbilirubinemia, newborn, kernicterus, bilirubin encephalopathy, phototherapy.*

ABBREVIATIONS. AAP, American Academy of Pediatrics; TSB, total serum bilirubin; TcB, transcutaneous bilirubin; G6PD, glucose-6-phosphate dehydrogenase; $ETCO_c$, end-tidal carbon monoxide corrected for ambient carbon monoxide; B/A, bilirubin/albumin; UB, unbound bilirubin.

BACKGROUND

In October 1994, the Provisional Committee for Quality Improvement and Subcommittee on Hyperbilirubinemia of the American Academy of Pediatrics (AAP) produced a practice parameter dealing with the management of hyperbilirubinemia in the healthy term newborn.[1] The current guideline represents a consensus of the committee charged by the AAP with reviewing and updating the existing guideline and is based on a careful review of the evidence, including a comprehensive literature review by the New England Medical Center Evidence-Based Practice Center.[2] (See "An Evidence-Based Review of Important Issues Concerning Neonatal Hyperbilirubinemia"[3] for a description of the methodology, questions addressed, and conclusions of this report.) This guideline is intended for use by hospitals and pediatricians, neonatologists, family physicians, physician assistants, and advanced practice nurses who treat newborn infants in the hospital and as outpatients. A list of frequently asked questions and answers for parents is available in English and Spanish at www.aap.org/family/jaundicefaq. htm.

DEFINITION OF RECOMMENDATIONS

The evidence-based approach to guideline development requires that the evidence in support of a policy be identified, appraised, and summarized and that an explicit link between evidence and recommendations be defined. Evidence-based recommendations are based on the quality of evidence and the balance of benefits and harms that is anticipated when the recommendation is followed. This guideline uses the definitions for quality of evidence and balance of benefits and harms established by the AAP Steering Committee on Quality Improvement Management.[4] See Appendix 1 for these definitions.

The draft practice guideline underwent extensive peer review by committees and sections within the AAP, outside organizations, and other individuals identified by the subcommittee as experts in the field. Liaison representatives to the subcommittee were invited to distribute the draft to other representatives and committees within their specialty organizations. The resulting comments were reviewed by the subcommittee and, when appropriate, incorporated into the guideline.

BILIRUBIN ENCEPHALOPATHY AND KERNICTERUS

Although originally a pathologic diagnosis characterized by bilirubin staining of the brainstem nuclei and cerebellum, the term "kernicterus" has come to be used interchangeably with both the acute and chronic findings of bilirubin encephalopathy. Bilirubin encephalopathy describes the clinical central nervous system findings caused by bilirubin toxicity to the basal ganglia and various brainstem nuclei. To avoid confusion and encourage greater consistency in the literature, the committee recommends that in infants the term "acute bilirubin encephalopathy" be used to describe the acute manifestations of bilirubin toxicity seen in the first weeks after birth and that the term "kernicterus" be reserved for the chronic and permanent clinical sequelae of bilirubin toxicity.

See Appendix 1 for the clinical manifestations of acute bilirubin encephalopathy and kernicterus.

FOCUS OF GUIDELINE

The overall aim of this guideline is to promote an approach that will reduce the frequency of severe neonatal hyperbilirubinemia and bilirubin encephalopathy and minimize the risk of unintended harm such as increased anxiety, decreased breastfeeding, or unnecessary treatment for the general population and excessive cost and waste. Recent reports of kernicterus indicate that this condition, although rare, is still occurring.[2,5–10]

Analysis of these reported cases of kernicterus suggests that if health care personnel follow the recommendations listed in this guideline, kernicterus would be largely preventable.

These guidelines emphasize the importance of universal systematic assessment for the risk of severe hyperbilirubinemia, close follow-up, and prompt intervention when indicated. The recommendations apply to the care of infants at 35 or more weeks of gestation. These recommendations seek to further the aims defined by the Institute of Medicine as appropriate for health care:[11] safety, effectiveness, efficiency, timeliness, patient-centeredness, and equity. They specifically emphasize the principles of patient safety and the key role of timeliness of interventions to prevent adverse outcomes resulting from neonatal hyperbilirubinemia.

The following are the key elements of the recommendations provided by this guideline. Clinicians should:

1. Promote and support successful breastfeeding.
2. Establish nursery protocols for the identification and evaluation of hyperbilirubinemia.
3. Measure the total serum bilirubin (TSB) or transcutaneous bilirubin (TcB) level on infants jaundiced in the first 24 hours.
4. Recognize that visual estimation of the degree of jaundice can lead to errors, particularly in darkly pigmented infants.
5. Interpret all bilirubin levels according to the infant's age in hours.
6. Recognize that infants at less than 38 weeks' gestation, particularly those who are breastfed, are at higher risk of developing hyperbilirubinemia and require closer surveillance and monitoring.
7. Perform a systematic assessment on all infants before discharge for the risk of severe hyperbilirubinemia.
8. Provide parents with written and verbal information about newborn jaundice.
9. Provide appropriate follow-up based on the time of discharge and the risk assessment.
10. Treat newborns, when indicated, with phototherapy or exchange transfusion.

PRIMARY PREVENTION

In numerous policy statements, the AAP recommends breastfeeding for all healthy term and near-term newborns. This guideline strongly supports this general recommendation.

RECOMMENDATION 1.0: Clinicians should advise mothers to nurse their infants at least 8 to 12 times per day for the first several days[12] (evidence quality C: benefits exceed harms).

Poor caloric intake and/or dehydration associated with inadequate breastfeeding may contribute to the development of hyperbilirubinemia.[6,13,14] Increasing the frequency of nursing decreases the likelihood of subsequent significant hyperbilirubinemia in breastfed infants.[15–17] Providing appropriate support and advice to breastfeeding mothers increases the likelihood that breastfeeding will be successful.

Additional information on how to assess the adequacy of intake in a breastfed newborn is provided in Appendix 1.

RECOMMENDATION 1.1: The AAP recommends against routine supplementation of nondehydrated breastfed infants with water or dextrose water (evidence quality B and C: harms exceed benefits).

Supplementation with water or dextrose water will not prevent hyperbilirubinemia or decrease TSB levels.[18,19]

SECONDARY PREVENTION

RECOMMENDATION 2.0: Clinicians should perform ongoing systematic assessments during the neonatal period for the risk of an infant developing severe hyperbilirubinemia.

Blood Typing

RECOMMENDATION 2.1: All pregnant women should be tested for ABO and Rh (D) blood types and have a serum screen for unusual isoimmune antibodies (evidence quality B: benefits exceed harms).

RECOMMENDATION 2.1.1: If a mother has not had prenatal blood grouping or is Rh-negative, a direct antibody test (or Coombs' test), blood type, and an Rh (D) type on the infant's (cord) blood are strongly recommended (evidence quality B: benefits exceed harms).

RECOMMENDATION 2.1.2: If the maternal blood is group O, Rh-positive, it is an option to test the cord blood for the infant's blood type and direct antibody test, but it is not required provided that there is appropriate surveillance, risk assessment before discharge, and follow-up[20] (evidence quality C: benefits exceed harms).

Clinical Assessment

RECOMMENDATION 2.2: Clinicians should ensure that all infants are routinely monitored for the development of jaundice, and nurseries should have established protocols for the assessment of jaundice. Jaundice should be assessed whenever the infant's vital signs are measured but no less than every 8 to 12 hours (evidence quality D: benefits versus harms exceptional).

In newborn infants, jaundice can be detected by blanching the skin with digital pressure, revealing the underlying color of the skin and subcutaneous tissue. The assessment of jaundice must be per-

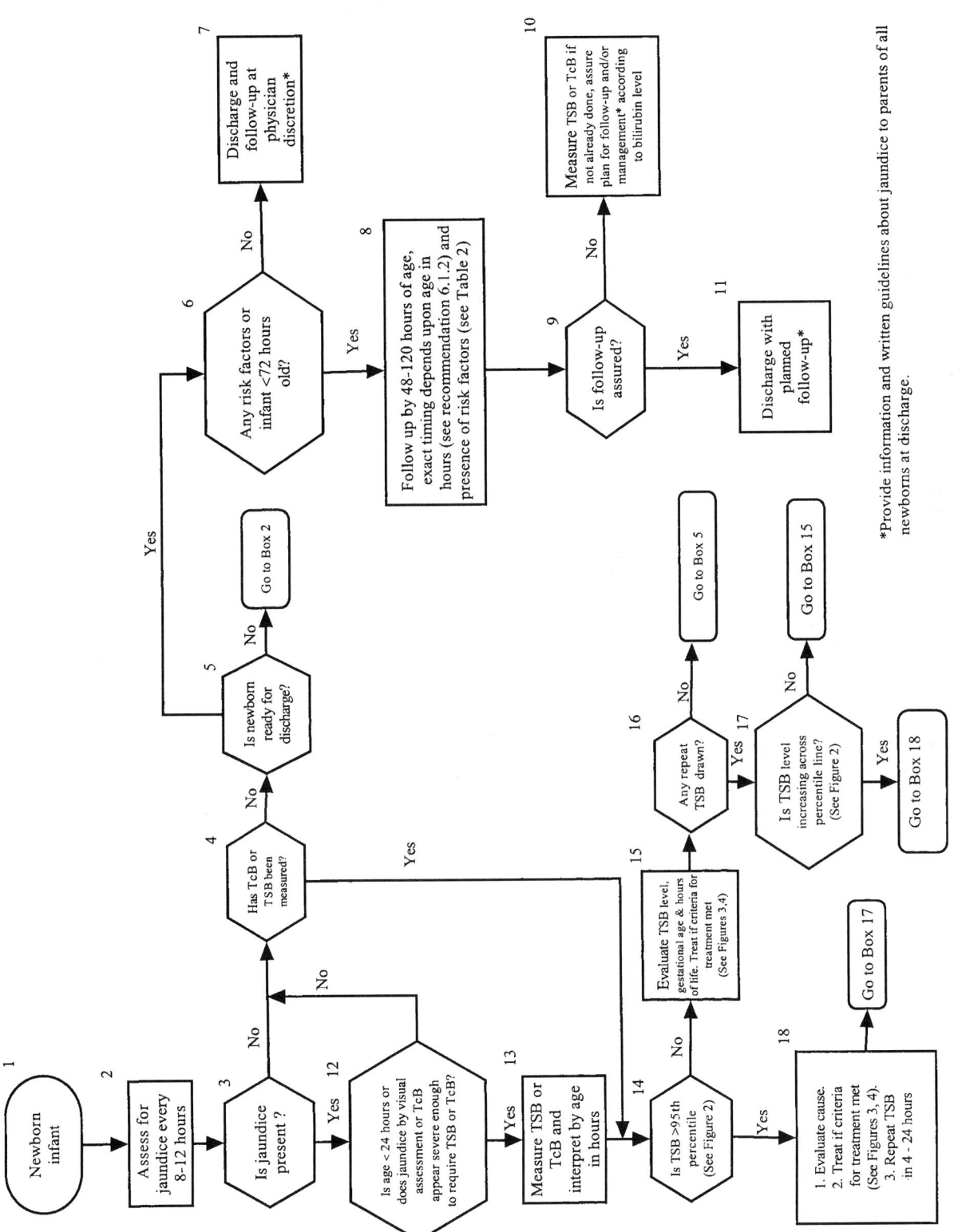

Fig 1. Algorithm for the management of jaundice in the newborn nursery.

*Provide information and written guidelines about jaundice to parents of all newborns at discharge.

formed in a well-lit room or, preferably, in daylight at a window. Jaundice is usually seen first in the face and progresses caudally to the trunk and extremities,[21] but visual estimation of bilirubin levels from the degree of jaundice can lead to errors.[22–24] In most infants with TSB levels of less than 15 mg/dL (257 μmol/L), noninvasive TcB-measurement devices can provide a valid estimate of the TSB level.[2,25–29] See Appendix 1 for additional information on the clinical evaluation of jaundice and the use of TcB measurements.

RECOMMENDATION 2.2.1: Protocols for the assessment of jaundice should include the circumstances in which nursing staff can obtain a TcB level or order a TSB measurement (evidence quality D: benefits versus harms exceptional).

Laboratory Evaluation

RECOMMENDATION 3.0: A TcB and/or TSB measurement should be performed on every infant who is jaundiced in the first 24 hours after birth (Fig 1 and Table 1)[30] (evidence quality C: benefits exceed harms). The need for and timing of a repeat TcB or TSB measurement will depend on the zone in which the TSB falls (Fig 2),[25,31] the age of the infant, and the evolution of the hyperbilirubinemia. Recommendations for TSB measurements after the age of 24 hours are provided in Fig 1 and Table 1.

See Appendix 1 for capillary versus venous bilirubin levels.

RECOMMENDATION 3.1: A TcB and/or TSB measurement should be performed if the jaundice appears excessive for the infant's age (evidence quality D: benefits versus harms exceptional). If there is any doubt about the degree of jaundice, the TSB or TcB should be measured. Visual estimation of bilirubin levels from the degree of jaundice can lead to errors, particularly in darkly pigmented infants (evidence quality C: benefits exceed harms).

RECOMMENDATION 3.2: All bilirubin levels should be interpreted according to the infant's age in hours (Fig 2) (evidence quality C: benefits exceed harms).

Cause of Jaundice

RECOMMENDATION 4.1: The possible cause of jaundice should be sought in an infant receiving phototherapy or whose TSB level is rising rapidly (ie, crossing percentiles [Fig 2]) and is not explained by the history and physical examination (evidence quality D: benefits versus harms exceptional).

RECOMMENDATION 4.1.1: Infants who have an elevation of direct-reacting or conjugated bilirubin should have a urinalysis and urine culture.[32] Additional laboratory evaluation for sepsis should be performed if indicated by history and physical examination (evidence quality C: benefits exceed harms).

See Appendix 1 for definitions of abnormal levels of direct-reacting and conjugated bilirubin.

RECOMMENDATION 4.1.2: Sick infants and those who are jaundiced at or beyond 3 weeks should have a measurement of total and direct or conjugated bilirubin to identify cholestasis (Table 1) (evidence quality D: benefit versus harms exceptional). The results of the newborn thyroid and galactosemia screen should also be checked in these infants (evidence quality D: benefits versus harms exceptional).

RECOMMENDATION 4.1.3: If the direct-reacting or conjugated bilirubin level is elevated, additional evaluation for the causes of cholestasis is recommended (evidence quality C: benefits exceed harms).

RECOMMENDATION 4.1.4: Measurement of the glucose-6-phosphate dehydrogenase (G6PD) level is recommended for a jaundiced infant who is receiving phototherapy and whose family history or ethnic or geographic origin suggest the likelihood of G6PD deficiency or for an infant in whom the response to phototherapy is poor (Fig 3) (evidence quality C: benefits exceed harms).

G6PD deficiency is widespread and frequently unrecognized, and although it is more common in the populations around the Mediterranean and in the Middle East, Arabian peninsula, Southeast Asia, and Africa, immigration and intermarriage have transformed G6PD deficiency into a global problem.[33,34]

TABLE 1. Laboratory Evaluation of the Jaundiced Infant of 35 or More Weeks' Gestation

Indications	Assessments
Jaundice in first 24 h	Measure TcB and/or TSB
Jaundice appears excessive for infant's age	Measure TcB and/or TSB
Infant receiving phototherapy or TSB rising rapidly (ie, crossing percentiles [Fig 2]) and unexplained by history and physical examination	Blood type and Coombs' test, if not obtained with cord blood
	Complete blood count and smear
	Measure direct or conjugated bilirubin
	It is an option to perform reticulocyte count, G6PD, and ETCO$_c$, if available
	Repeat TSB in 4–24 h depending on infant's age and TSB level
TSB concentration approaching exchange levels or not responding to phototherapy	Perform reticulocyte count, G6PD, albumin, ETCO$_c$, if available
Elevated direct (or conjugated) bilirubin level	Do urinalysis and urine culture. Evaluate for sepsis if indicated by history and physical examination
Jaundice present at or beyond age 3 wk, or sick infant	Total and direct (or conjugated) bilirubin level
	If direct bilirubin elevated, evaluate for causes of cholestasis
	Check results of newborn thyroid and galactosemia screen, and evaluate infant for signs or symptoms of hypothyroidism

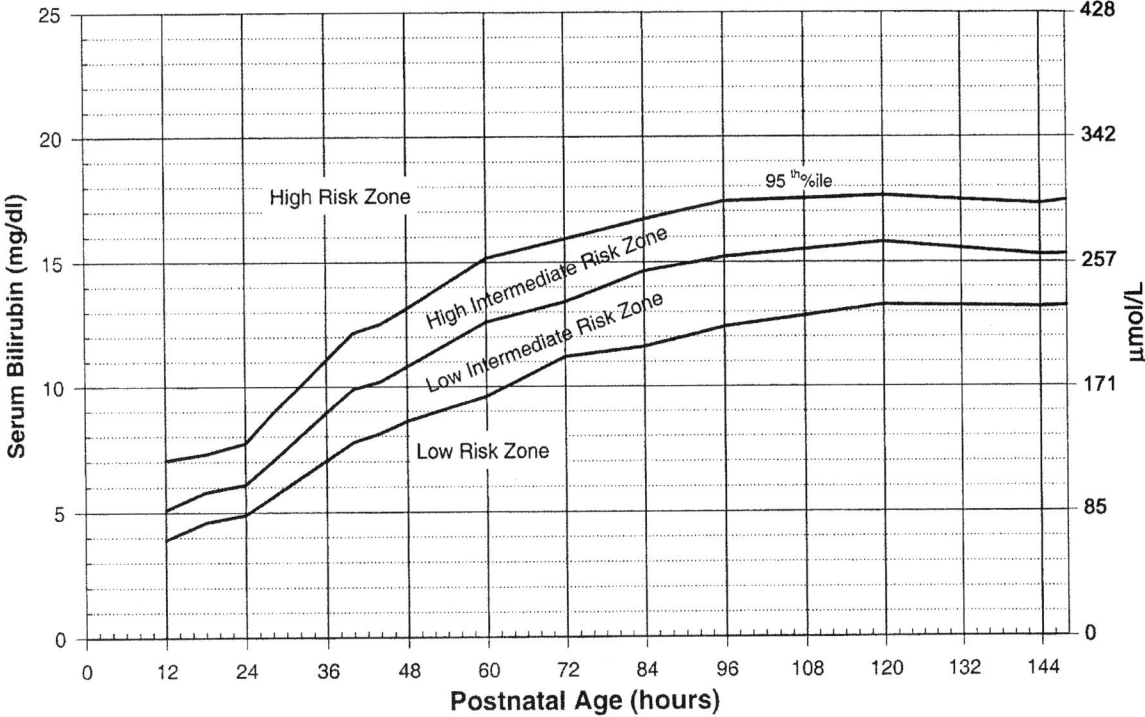

Fig 2. Nomogram for designation of risk in 2840 well newborns at 36 or more weeks' gestational age with birth weight of 2000 g or more or 35 or more weeks' gestational age and birth weight of 2500 g or more based on the hour-specific serum bilirubin values. The serum bilirubin level was obtained before discharge, and the zone in which the value fell predicted the likelihood of a subsequent bilirubin level exceeding the 95th percentile (high-risk zone) as shown in Appendix 1, Table 4. Used with permission from Bhutani et al.[31] See Appendix 1 for additional information about this nomogram, which should not be used to represent the natural history of neonatal hyperbilirubinemia.

Furthermore, G6PD deficiency occurs in 11% to 13% of African Americans, and kernicterus has occurred in some of these infants.[5,33] In a recent report, G6PD deficiency was considered to be the cause of hyperbilirubinemia in 19 of 61 (31.5%) infants who developed kernicterus.[5] (See Appendix 1 for additional information on G6PD deficiency.)

Risk Assessment Before Discharge

RECOMMENDATION 5.1: Before discharge, every newborn should be assessed for the risk of developing severe hyperbilirubinemia, and all nurseries should establish protocols for assessing this risk. Such assessment is particularly important in infants who are discharged before the age of 72 hours (evidence quality C: benefits exceed harms).

RECOMMENDATION 5.1.1: The AAP recommends 2 clinical options used individually or in combination for the systematic assessment of risk: predischarge measurement of the bilirubin level using TSB or TcB and/or assessment of clinical risk factors. Whether either or both options are used, appropriate follow-up after discharge is essential (evidence quality C: benefits exceed harms).

The best documented method for assessing the risk of subsequent hyperbilirubinemia is to measure the TSB or TcB level[25,31,35–38] and plot the results on a nomogram (Fig 2). A TSB level can be obtained at the time of the routine metabolic screen, thus obviating the need for an additional blood sample. Some authors have suggested that a TSB measurement should be part of the routine screening of all newborns.[5,31] An infant whose predischarge TSB is in the

low-risk zone (Fig 2) is at very low risk of developing severe hyperbilirubinemia.[5,38]

Table 2 lists those factors that are clinically signif-

TABLE 2. Risk Factors for Development of Severe Hyperbilirubinemia in Infants of 35 or More Weeks' Gestation (in Approximate Order of Importance)

Major risk factors
   Predischarge TSB or TcB level in the high-risk zone (Fig 2)[25,31]
   Jaundice observed in the first 24 h[30]
   Blood group incompatibility with positive direct antiglobulin test, other known hemolytic disease (eg, G6PD deficiency), elevated ETCO$_c$
   Gestational age 35–36 wk[39,40]
   Previous sibling received phototherapy[40,41]
   Cephalohematoma or significant bruising[39]
   Exclusive breastfeeding, particularly if nursing is not going well and weight loss is excessive[39,40]
   East Asian race[39]*
Minor risk factors
   Predischarge TSB or TcB level in the high intermediate-risk zone[25,31]
   Gestational age 37–38 wk[39,40]
   Jaundice observed before discharge[40]
   Previous sibling with jaundice[40,41]
   Macrosomic infant of a diabetic mother[42,43]
   Maternal age ≥25 y[39]
   Male gender[39,40]
Decreased risk (these factors are associated with decreased risk of significant jaundice, listed in order of decreasing importance)
   TSB or TcB level in the low-risk zone (Fig 2)[25,31]
   Gestational age ≥41 wk[39]
   Exclusive bottle feeding[39,40]
   Black race[38]*
   Discharge from hospital after 72 h[40,44]

* Race as defined by mother's description.

icant and most frequently associated with an increase in the risk of severe hyperbilirubinemia. But, because these risk factors are common and the risk of hyperbilirubinemia is small, individually the factors are of limited use as predictors of significant hyperbilirubinemia.[39] Nevertheless, if no risk factors are present, the risk of severe hyperbilirubinemia is extremely low, and the more risk factors present, the greater the risk of severe hyperbilirubinemia.[39] The important risk factors most frequently associated with severe hyperbilirubinemia are breastfeeding, gestation below 38 weeks, significant jaundice in a previous sibling, and jaundice noted before discharge.[39,40] A formula-fed infant of 40 or more weeks' gestation is at very low risk of developing severe hyperbilirubinemia.[39]

Hospital Policies and Procedures

RECOMMENDATION 6.1: *All hospitals should provide written and verbal information for parents at the time of discharge, which should include an explanation of jaundice, the need to monitor infants for jaundice, and advice on how monitoring should be done (evidence quality D: benefits versus harms exceptional).*

An example of a parent-information handout is available in English and Spanish at www.aap.org/family/jaundicefaq.htm.

Follow-up

RECOMMENDATION 6.1.1: *All infants should be examined by a qualified health care professional in the first few days after discharge to assess infant well-being and the presence or absence of jaundice. The timing and location of this assessment will be determined by the length of stay in the nursery, presence or absence of risk factors for hyperbilirubinemia (Table 2 and Fig 2), and risk of other neonatal problems (evidence quality C: benefits exceed harms).*

Timing of Follow-up

RECOMMENDATION 6.1.2: *Follow-up should be provided as follows:*

Infant Discharged	Should Be Seen by Age
Before age 24 h	72 h
Between 24 and 47.9 h	96 h
Between 48 and 72 h	120 h

For some newborns discharged before 48 hours, 2 follow-up visits may be required, the first visit between 24 and 72 hours and the second between 72 and 120 hours. Clinical judgment should be used in determining follow-up. Earlier or more frequent follow-up should be provided for those who have risk factors for hyperbilirubinemia (Table 2), whereas those discharged with few or no risk factors can be seen after longer intervals (evidence quality C: benefits exceed harms).

RECOMMENDATION 6.1.3: *If appropriate follow-up cannot be ensured in the presence of elevated risk for developing severe hyperbilirubinemia, it may be necessary to delay discharge either until appropriate follow-up can be ensured or the period of greatest risk has passed (72-96 hours) (evidence quality D: benefits versus harms exceptional).*

Follow-up Assessment

RECOMMENDATION 6.1.4: *The follow-up assessment should include the infant's weight and percent change from birth weight, adequacy of intake, the pattern of voiding and stooling, and the presence or absence of jaundice (evidence quality C: benefits exceed harms). Clinical judgment should be used to determine the need for a bilirubin measurement. If there is any doubt about the degree of jaundice, the TSB or TcB level should be measured. Visual estimation of bilirubin levels can lead to errors, particularly in darkly pigmented infants (evidence quality C: benefits exceed harms).*

See Appendix 1 for assessment of the adequacy of intake in breastfeeding infants.

TREATMENT

Phototherapy and Exchange Transfusion

RECOMMENDATION 7.1: *Recommendations for treatment are given in Table 3 and Figs 3 and 4 (evidence quality C: benefits exceed harms). If the TSB does not fall or continues to rise despite intensive phototherapy, it is very likely that hemolysis is occurring. The committee's recommendations for discontinuing phototherapy can be found in Appendix 2.*

RECOMMENDATION 7.1.1: *In using the guidelines for phototherapy and exchange transfusion (Figs 3 and 4), the direct-reacting (or conjugated) bilirubin level should not be subtracted from the total (evidence quality D: benefits versus harms exceptional).*

In unusual situations in which the direct bilirubin level is 50% or more of the total bilirubin, there are no good data to provide guidance for therapy, and consultation with an expert in the field is recommended.

RECOMMENDATION 7.1.2: *If the TSB is at a level at which exchange transfusion is recommended (Fig 4) or if the TSB level is 25 mg/dL (428 μmol/L) or higher at any time, it is a medical emergency and the infant should be admitted immediately and directly to a hospital pediatric service for intensive phototherapy. These infants should not be referred to the emergency department, because it delays the initiation of treatment[54] (evidence quality C: benefits exceed harms).*

RECOMMENDATION 7.1.3: *Exchange transfusions should be performed only by trained personnel in a neonatal intensive care unit with full monitoring and resuscitation capabilities (evidence quality D: benefits versus harms exceptional).*

RECOMMENDATION 7.1.4: *In isoimmune hemolytic disease, administration of intravenous γ-globulin (0.5-1 g/kg over 2 hours) is recommended if the TSB is rising despite intensive phototherapy or the TSB level is within 2 to 3 mg/dL (34-51 μmol/L) of the exchange level (Fig 4).[55] If necessary, this dose can be repeated in 12 hours (evidence quality B: benefits exceed harms).*

Intravenous γ-globulin has been shown to reduce the need for exchange transfusions in Rh and ABO hemolytic disease.[55–58] Although data are limited, it is reasonable to assume that intravenous γ-globulin will also be helpful in the other types of Rh hemolytic disease such as anti-C and anti-E.

TABLE 3. Example of a Clinical Pathway for Management of the Newborn Infant Readmitted for Phototherapy or Exchange Transfusion

Treatment
  Use intensive phototherapy and/or exchange transfusion as indicated in Figs 3 and 4 (see Appendix 2 for details of phototherapy use)
Laboratory tests
  TSB and direct bilirubin levels
  Blood type (ABO, Rh)
  Direct antibody test (Coombs')
  Serum albumin
  Complete blood cell count with differential and smear for red cell morphology
  Reticulocyte count
  $ETCO_c$ (if available)
  G6PD if suggested by ethnic or geographic origin or if poor response to phototherapy
  Urine for reducing substances
  If history and/or presentation suggest sepsis, perform blood culture, urine culture, and cerebrospinal fluid for protein, glucose, cell count, and culture
Interventions
  If TSB ≥25 mg/dL (428 μmol/L) or ≥20 mg/dL (342 μmol/L) in a sick infant or infant <38 wk gestation, obtain a type and crossmatch, and request blood in case an exchange transfusion is necessary
  In infants with isoimmune hemolytic disease and TSB level rising in spite of intensive phototherapy or within 2–3 mg/dL (34–51 μmol/L) of exchange level (Fig 4), administer intravenous immunoglobulin 0.5–1 g/kg over 2 h and repeat in 12 h if necessary
  If infant's weight loss from birth is >12% or there is clinical or biochemical evidence of dehydration, recommend formula or expressed breast milk. If oral intake is in question, give intravenous fluids.
For infants receiving intensive phototherapy
  Breastfeed or bottle-feed (formula or expressed breast milk) every 2–3 h
  If TSB ≥25 mg/dL (428 μmol/L), repeat TSB within 2–3 h
  If TSB 20–25 mg/dL (342–428 μmol/L), repeat within 3–4 h. If TSB <20 mg/dL (342 μmol/L), repeat in 4–6 h. If TSB continues to fall, repeat in 8–12 h
  If TSB is not decreasing or is moving closer to level for exchange transfusion or the TSB/albumin ratio exceeds levels shown in Fig 4, consider exchange transfusion (see Fig 4 for exchange transfusion recommendations)
  When TSB is <13–14 mg/dL (239 μmol/L), discontinue phototherapy
  Depending on the cause of the hyperbilirubinemia, it is an option to measure TSB 24 h after discharge to check for rebound

Serum Albumin Levels and the Bilirubin/Albumin Ratio

RECOMMENDATION 7.1.5: It is an option to measure the serum albumin level and consider an albumin level of less than 3.0 g/dL as one risk factor for lowering the threshold for phototherapy use (see Fig 3) (evidence quality D: benefits versus risks exceptional.).

RECOMMENDATION 7.1.6: If an exchange transfusion is being considered, the serum albumin level should be measured and the bilirubin/albumin (B/A) ratio used in conjunction with the TSB level and other factors in determining the need for exchange transfusion (see Fig 4) (evidence quality D: benefits versus harms exceptional).

The recommendations shown above for treating hyperbilirubinemia are based primarily on TSB levels and other factors that affect the risk of bilirubin encephalopathy. This risk might be increased by a prolonged (rather than a brief) exposure to a certain TSB level.[59,60] Because the published data that address this issue are limited, however, it is not possible to provide specific recommendations for intervention based on the duration of hyperbilirubinemia.

See Appendix 1 for the basis for recommendations 7.1 through 7.1.6 and for the recommendations provided in Figs 3 and 4. Appendix 1 also contains a discussion of the risks of exchange transfusion and the use of B/A binding.

Acute Bilirubin Encephalopathy

RECOMMENDATION 7.1.7: Immediate exchange transfusion is recommended in any infant who is jaun- diced and manifests the signs of the intermediate to advanced stages of acute bilirubin encephalopathy[61,62] *(hypertonia, arching, retrocollis, opisthotonos, fever, high-pitched cry) even if the TSB is falling (evidence quality D: benefits versus risks exceptional).*

Phototherapy

RECOMMENDATION 7.2: All nurseries and services treating infants should have the necessary equipment to provide intensive phototherapy (see Appendix 2) (evidence quality D: benefits exceed risks).

Outpatient Management of the Jaundiced Breastfed Infant

RECOMMENDATION 7.3: In breastfed infants who require phototherapy (Fig 3), the AAP recommends that, if possible, breastfeeding should be continued (evidence quality C: benefits exceed harms). It is also an option to interrupt temporarily breastfeeding and substitute formula. This can reduce bilirubin levels and/or enhance the efficacy of phototherapy[63–65] (evidence quality B: benefits exceed harms). In breastfed infants receiving phototherapy, supplementation with expressed breast milk or formula is appropriate if the infant's intake seems inadequate, weight loss is excessive, or the infant seems dehydrated.

IMPLEMENTATION STRATEGIES

The Institute of Medicine[11] recommends a dramatic change in the way the US health care system

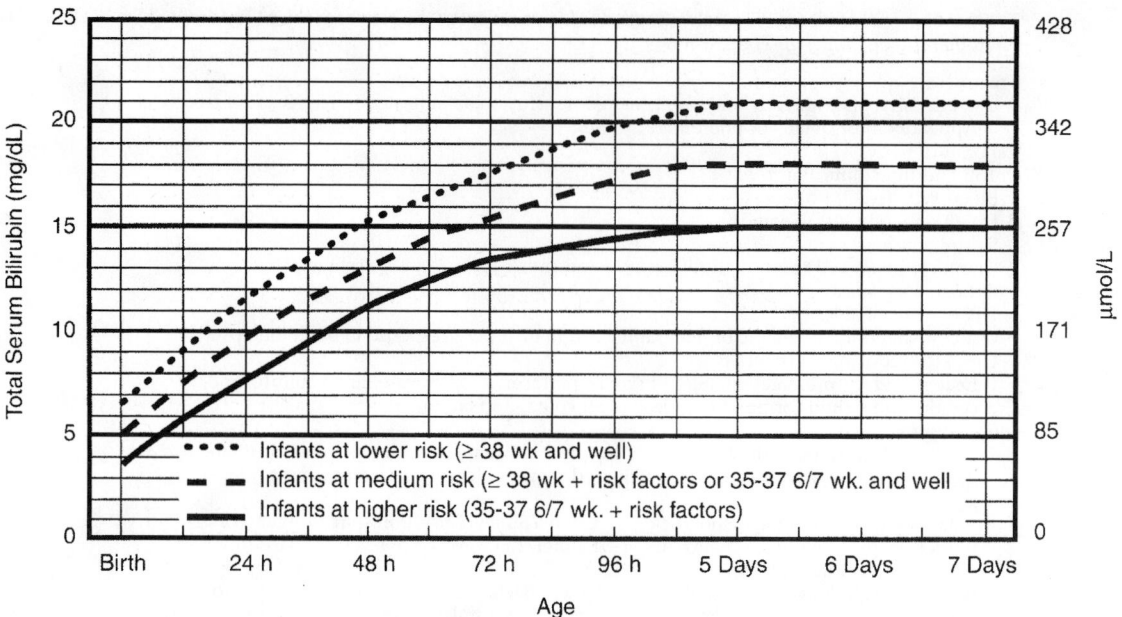

- Use total bilirubin. Do not subtract direct reacting or conjugated bilirubin.
- Risk factors = isoimmune hemolytic disease, G6PD deficiency, asphyxia, significant lethargy, temperature instability, sepsis, acidosis, or albumin < 3.0g/dL (if measured)
- For well infants 35-37 6/7 wk can adjust TSB levels for intervention around the medium risk line. It is an option to intervene at lower TSB levels for infants closer to 35 wks and at higher TSB levels for those closer to 37 6/7 wk.
- It is an option to provide conventional phototherapy in hospital or at home at TSB levels 2-3 mg/dL (35-50mmol/L) below those shown but home phototherapy should not be used in any infant with risk factors.

Fig 3. Guidelines for phototherapy in hospitalized infants of 35 or more weeks' gestation.

Note: These guidelines are based on limited evidence and the levels shown are approximations. The guidelines refer to the use of intensive phototherapy which should be used when the TSB exceeds the line indicated for each category. Infants are designated as "higher risk" because of the potential negative effects of the conditions listed on albumin binding of bilirubin,[45–47] the blood-brain barrier,[48] and the susceptibility of the brain cells to damage by bilirubin.[48]

"Intensive phototherapy" implies irradiance in the blue-green spectrum (wavelengths of approximately 430–490 nm) of at least 30 $\mu W/cm^2$ per nm (measured at the infant's skin directly below the center of the phototherapy unit) and delivered to as much of the infant's surface area as possible. Note that irradiance measured below the center of the light source is much greater than that measured at the periphery. Measurements should be made with a radiometer specified by the manufacturer of the phototherapy system.

See Appendix 2 for additional information on measuring the dose of phototherapy, a description of intensive phototherapy, and of light sources used. If total serum bilirubin levels approach or exceed the exchange transfusion line (Fig 4), the sides of the bassinet, incubator, or warmer should be lined with aluminum foil or white material.[50] This will increase the surface area of the infant exposed and increase the efficacy of phototherapy.[51]

If the total serum bilirubin does not decrease or continues to rise in an infant who is receiving intensive phototherapy, this strongly suggests the presence of hemolysis.

Infants who receive phototherapy and have an elevated direct-reacting or conjugated bilirubin level (cholestatic jaundice) may develop the bronze-baby syndrome. See Appendix 2 for the use of phototherapy in these infants.

ensures the safety of patients. The perspective of safety as a purely individual responsibility must be replaced by the concept of safety as a property of systems. Safe systems are characterized by a shared knowledge of the goal, a culture emphasizing safety, the ability of each person within the system to act in a manner that promotes safety, minimizing the use of memory, and emphasizing the use of standard procedures (such as checklists), and the involvement of patients/families as partners in the process of care.

These principles can be applied to the challenge of preventing severe hyperbilirubinemia and kernicterus. A systematic approach to the implementation of these guidelines should result in greater safety. Such approaches might include

- The establishment of standing protocols for nursing assessment of jaundice, including testing TcB and TSB levels, without requiring physician orders.

- Checklists or reminders associated with risk factors, age at discharge, and laboratory test results that provide guidance for appropriate follow-up.
- Explicit educational materials for parents (a key component of all AAP guidelines) concerning the identification of newborns with jaundice.

FUTURE RESEARCH

Epidemiology of Bilirubin-Induced Central Nervous System Damage

There is a need for appropriate epidemiologic data to document the incidence of kernicterus in the newborn population, the incidence of other adverse effects attributable to hyperbilirubinemia and its management, and the number of infants whose TSB levels exceed 25 or 30 mg/dL (428-513 μmol/L). Organizations such as the Centers for Disease Control and Prevention should implement strategies for appropriate data gathering to identify the number of

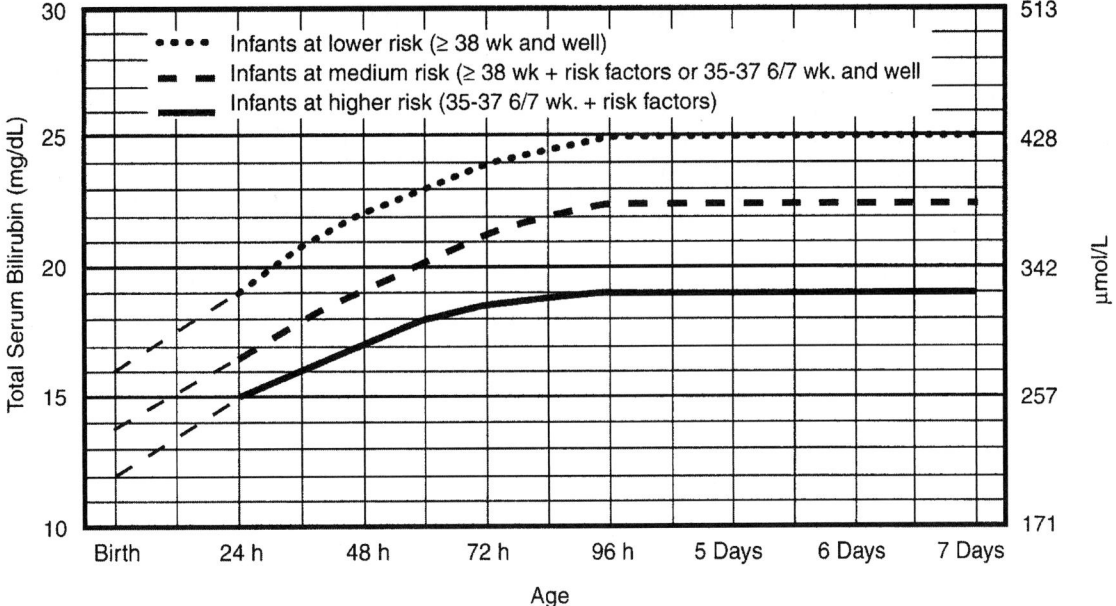

- The dashed lines for the first 24 hours indicate uncertainty due to a wide range of clinical circumstances and a range of responses to phototherapy.
- Immediate exchange transfusion is recommended if infant shows signs of acute bilirubin encephalopathy (hypertonia, arching, retrocollis, opisthotonos, fever, high pitched cry) or if TSB is ≥5 mg/dL (85 μmol/L) above these lines.
- Risk factors - isoimmune hemolytic disease, G6PD deficiency, asphyxia, significant lethargy, temperature instability, sepsis, acidosis.
- Measure serum albumin and calculate B/A ratio (See legend)
- Use total bilirubin. Do not subtract direct reacting or conjugated bilirubin
- If infant is well and 35-37 6/7 wk (median risk) can individualize TSB levels for exchange based on actual gestational age.

Fig 4. Guidelines for exchange transfusion in infants 35 or more weeks' gestation.

Note that these suggested levels represent a consensus of most of the committee but are based on limited evidence, and the levels shown are approximations. See ref. 3 for risks and complications of exchange transfusion. During birth hospitalization, exchange transfusion is recommended if the TSB rises to these levels despite intensive phototherapy. For readmitted infants, if the TSB level is above the exchange level, repeat TSB measurement every 2 to 3 hours and consider exchange if the TSB remains above the levels indicated after intensive phototherapy for 6 hours.

The following B/A ratios can be used together with but in not in lieu of the TSB level as an additional factor in determining the need for exchange transfusion[52]:

Risk Category	B/A Ratio at Which Exchange Transfusion Should be Considered	
	TSB mg/dL/Alb, g/dL	TSB μmol/L/Alb, μmol/L
Infants ≥38 0/7 wk	8.0	0.94
Infants 35 0/7–36 6/7 wk and well or ≥38 0/7 wk if higher risk or isoimmune hemolytic disease or G6PD deficiency	7.2	0.84
Infants 35 0/7–37 6/7 wk if higher risk or isoimmune hemolytic disease or G6PD deficiency	6.8	0.80

If the TSB is at or approaching the exchange level, send blood for immediate type and crossmatch. Blood for exchange transfusion is modified whole blood (red cells and plasma) crossmatched against the mother and compatible with the infant.[53]

infants who develop serum bilirubin levels above 25 or 30 mg/dL (428-513 μmol/L) and those who develop acute and chronic bilirubin encephalopathy. This information will help to identify the magnitude of the problem; the number of infants who need to be screened and treated to prevent 1 case of kernicterus; and the risks, costs, and benefits of different strategies for prevention and treatment of hyperbilirubinemia. In the absence of these data, recommendations for intervention cannot be considered definitive.

Effect of Bilirubin on the Central Nervous System

The serum bilirubin level by itself, except when it is extremely high and associated with bilirubin encephalopathy, is an imprecise indicator of long-term neurodevelopmental outcome.[2] Additional studies are needed on the relationship between central nervous system damage and the duration of hyperbilirubinemia, the binding of bilirubin to albumin, and changes seen in the brainstem auditory evoked response. These studies could help to better identify risk, clarify the effect of bilirubin on the central nervous system, and guide intervention.

Identification of Hemolysis

Because of their poor specificity and sensitivity, the standard laboratory tests for hemolysis (Table 1) are frequently unhelpful.[66,67] However, end-tidal carbon monoxide, corrected for ambient carbon monoxide (ETCO$_c$), levels can confirm the presence or absence of hemolysis, and measurement of ETCO$_c$ is the only clinical test that provides a direct measurement of the rate of heme catabolism and the rate of bilirubin production.[68,69] Thus, ETCO$_c$ may be helpful in determining the degree of surveillance needed and the timing of intervention. It is not yet known, however, how ETCO$_c$ measurements will affect management.

Nomograms and the Measurement of Serum and TcB

It would be useful to develop an age-specific (by hour) nomogram for TSB in populations of newborns that differ with regard to risk factors for hyperbilirubinemia. There is also an urgent need to improve the precision and accuracy of the measurement of TSB in the clinical laboratory.[70,71] Additional studies are also needed to develop and validate noninvasive (transcutaneous) measurements of serum bilirubin and to understand the factors that affect these measurements. These studies should also assess the cost-effectiveness and reproducibility of TcB measurements in clinical practice.[2]

Pharmacologic Therapy

There is now evidence that hyperbilirubinemia can be effectively prevented or treated with tin-mesoporphyrin,[72–75] a drug that inhibits the production of heme oxygenase. Tin-mesoporphyrin is not approved by the US Food and Drug Administration. If approved, tin-mesoporphyrin could find immediate application in preventing the need for exchange transfusion in infants who are not responding to phototherapy.[75]

Dissemination and Monitoring

Research should be directed toward methods for disseminating the information contained in this guideline to increase awareness on the part of physicians, residents, nurses, and parents concerning the issues of neonatal hyperbilirubinemia and strategies for its management. In addition, monitoring systems should be established to identify the impact of these guidelines on the incidence of acute bilirubin encephalopathy and kernicterus and the use of phototherapy and exchange transfusions.

CONCLUSIONS

Kernicterus is still occurring but should be largely preventable if health care personnel follow the recommendations listed in this guideline. These recommendations emphasize the importance of universal, systematic assessment for the risk of severe hyperbilirubinemia, close follow-up, and prompt intervention, when necessary.

SUBCOMMITTEE ON HYPERBILIRUBINEMIA
M. Jeffrey Maisels, MB, BCh, Chairperson
Richard D. Baltz, MD
Vinod K. Bhutani, MD
Thomas B. Newman, MD, MPH
Heather Palmer, MB, BCh
Warren Rosenfeld, MD
David K. Stevenson, MD
Howard B. Weinblatt, MD

CONSULTANT
Charles J. Homer, MD, MPH, Chairperson
    American Academy of Pediatrics Steering
    Committee on Quality Improvement and
    Management

STAFF
Carla T. Herrerias, MPH

ACKNOWLEDGMENTS

M.J.M. received grant support from Natus Medical, Inc, for multinational study of ambient carbon monoxide; WellSpring Pharmaceutical Corporation for study of Stannsoporfin (tin-mesoporphyrin); and Minolta, Inc, for study of the Minolta/Hill-Rom Air-Shields transcutaneous jaundice meter model JM-103. V.K.B. received grant support from WellSpring Pharmaceutical Corporation for study of Stannsoporfin (tin-mesoporphyrin) and Natus Medical, Inc, for multinational study of ambient carbon monoxide and is a consultant (volunteer) to SpectrX (BiliChek transcutaneous bilirubinometer). D.K.S. is a consultant to and holds stock options through Natus Medical, Inc.

The American Academy of Pediatrics Subcommittee on Hyperbilirubinemia gratefully acknowledges the help of the following organizations, committees, and individuals who reviewed drafts of this guideline and provided valuable criticisms and commentary: American Academy of Pediatrics Committee on Nutrition; American Academy of Pediatrics Committee on Practice and Ambulatory Medicine; American Academy of Pediatrics Committee on Child Health Financing; American Academy of Pediatrics Committee on Medical Liability; American Academy of Pediatrics Committee on Fetus and Newborn; American Academy of Pediatrics Section on Perinatal Pediatrics; Centers for Disease Control and Prevention; Parents of Infants and Children With Kernicterus (PICK); Charles Ahlfors, MD; Daniel Batton, MD; Thomas Bojko, MD; Sarah Clune, MD; Sudhakar Ezhuthachan, MD; Lawrence Gartner, MD; Cathy Hammerman, MD; Thor Hansen, MD; Lois Johnson, MD; Michael Kaplan, MB, ChB; Tony McDonagh, PhD; Gerald Merenstein, MD; Mary O'Shea, MD; Max Perlman, MD; Ronald Poland, MD; Alex Robertson, MD; Firmino Rubaltelli, MD; Steven Shapiro, MD; Stanford Singer, MD; Ann Stark, MD; Gautham Suresh, MD; Margot VandeBor, MD; Hank Vreman, PhD; Philip Walson, MD; Jon Watchko, MD; Richard Wennberg, MD; and Chap-Yung Yeung, MD.

REFERENCES

1. American Academy of Pediatrics, Provisional Committee for Quality Improvement and Subcommittee on Hyperbilirubinemia. Practice parameter: management of hyperbilirubinemia in the healthy term newborn. *Pediatrics*. 1994;94:558–562

2. Ip S, Glicken S, Kulig J, Obrien R, Sege R, Lau J. *Management of Neonatal Hyperbilirubinemia*. Rockville, MD: US Department of Health and Human Services, Agency for Healthcare Research and Quality; 2003. AHRQ Publication 03-E011

3. Ip S, Chung M, Kulig J. et al. An evidence-based review of important issues concerning neonatal hyperbilirubinemia. *Pediatrics*. 2004;113(6). Available at: www.pediatrics.org/cgi/content/full/113/6/e644

4. American Academy of Pediatrics, Steering Committee on Quality Improvement and Management. A taxonomy of recommendations. *Pediatrics*. 2004; In press

5. Johnson LH, Bhutani VK, Brown AK. System-based approach to management of neonatal jaundice and prevention of kernicterus. *J Pediatr*. 2002;140:396–403

6. Maisels MJ, Newman TB. Kernicterus in otherwise healthy, breast-fed term newborns. *Pediatrics.* 1995;96:730–733

7. MacDonald M. Hidden risks: early discharge and bilirubin toxicity due to glucose-6-phosphate dehydrogenase deficiency. *Pediatrics.* 1995;96: 734–738

8. Penn AA, Enzman DR, Hahn JS, Stevenson DK. Kernicterus in a full term infant. *Pediatrics.* 1994;93:1003–1006

9. Washington EC, Ector W, Abboud M, Ohning B, Holden K. Hemolytic jaundice due to G6PD deficiency causing kernicterus in a female newborn. *South Med J.* 1995;88:776–779

10. Ebbesen F. Recurrence of kernicterus in term and near-term infants in Denmark. *Acta Paediatr.* 2000;89:1213–1217

11. Institue of Medicine. *Crossing the Quality Chasm: A New Health System for the 21st Century.* Washington, DC: National Academy Press; 2001

12. American Academy of Pediatrics, American College of Obstetricians and Gynecologists. *Guidelines for Perinatal Care.* 5th ed. Elk Grove Village, IL: American Academy of Pediatrics; 2002:220–224

13. Bertini G, Dani C, Trochin M, Rubaltelli F. Is breastfeeding really favoring early neonatal jaundice? *Pediatrics.* 2001;107(3). Available at: www.pediatrics.org/cgi/content/full/107/3/e41

14. Maisels MJ, Gifford K. Normal serum bilirubin levels in the newborn and the effect of breast-feeding. *Pediatrics.* 1986;78:837–843

15. Yamauchi Y, Yamanouchi I. Breast-feeding frequency during the first 24 hours after birth in full-term neonates. *Pediatrics.* 1990;86:171–175

16. De Carvalho M, Klaus MH, Merkatz RB. Frequency of breastfeeding and serum bilirubin concentration. *Am J Dis Child.* 1982;136:737–738

17. Varimo P, Similä S, Wendt L, Kolvisto M. Frequency of breast feeding and hyperbilirubinemia [letter]. *Clin Pediatr (Phila).* 1986;25:112

18. De Carvalho M, Holl M, Harvey D. Effects of water supplementation on physiological jaundice in breast-fed babies. *Arch Dis Child.* 1981;56: 568–569

19. Nicoll A, Ginsburg R, Tripp JH. Supplementary feeding and jaundice in newborns. *Acta Paediatr Scand.* 1982;71:759–761

20. Madlon-Kay DJ. Identifying ABO incompatibility in newborns: selective vs automatic testing. *J Fam Pract.* 1992;35:278–280

21. Kramer LI. Advancement of dermal icterus in the jaundiced newborn. *Am J Dis Child.* 1969;118:454–458

22. Moyer VA, Ahn C, Sneed S. Accuracy of clinical judgment in neonatal jaundice. *Arch Pediatr Adolesc Med.* 2000;154:391–394

23. Davidson LT, Merritt KK, Weech AA. Hyperbilirubinemia in the newborn. *Am J Dis Child.* 1941;61:958–980

24. Tayaba R, Gribetz D, Gribetz I, Holzman IR. Noninvasive estimation of serum bilirubin. *Pediatrics.* 1998;102(3). Available at: www.pediatrics.org/cgi/content/full/102/3/e28

25. Bhutani V, Gourley GR, Adler S, Kreamer B, Dalman C, Johnson LH. Noninvasive measurement of total serum bilirubin in a multiracial predischarge newborn population to assess the risk of severe hyperbilirubinemia. *Pediatrics.* 2000;106(2). Available at: www.pediatrics.org/cgi/content/full/106/2/e17

26. Yasuda S, Itoh S, Isobe K, et al. New transcutaneous jaundice device with two optical paths. *J Perinat Med.* 2003;31:81–88

27. Maisels MJ, Ostrea EJ Jr, Touch S, et al. Evaluation of a new transcutaneous bilirubinometer. *Pediatrics.* 2004;113:1638–1645

28. Ebbesen F, Rasmussen LM, Wimberley PD. A new transcutaneous bilirubinometer, bilicheck, used in the neonatal intensive care unit and the maternity ward. *Acta Paediatr.* 2002;91:203–211

29. Rubaltelli FF, Gourley GR, Loskamp N, et al. Transcutaneous bilirubin measurement: a multicenter evaluation of a new device. *Pediatrics.* 2001;107:1264–1271

30. Newman TB, Liljestrand P, Escobar GJ. Jaundice noted in the first 24 hours after birth in a managed care organization. *Arch Pediatr Adolesc Med.* 2002;156:1244–1250

31. Bhutani VK, Johnson L, Sivieri EM. Predictive ability of a predischarge hour-specific serum bilirubin for subsequent significant hyperbilirubinemia in healthy term and near-term newborns. *Pediatrics.* 1999;103: 6–14

32. Garcia FJ, Nager AL. Jaundice as an early diagnostic sign of urinary tract infection in infancy. *Pediatrics.* 2002;109:846–851

33. Kaplan M, Hammerman C. Severe neonatal hyperbilirubinemia: a potential complication of glucose-6-phosphate dehydrogenase deficiency. *Clin Perinatol.* 1998;25:575–590

34. Valaes T. Severe neonatal jaundice associated with glucose-6-phosphate dehydrogenase deficiency: pathogenesis and global epidemiology. *Acta Paediatr Suppl.* 1994;394:58–76

35. Alpay F, Sarici S, Tosuncuk HD, Serdar MA, Inanç N, Gökçay E. The value of first-day bilirubin measurement in predicting the development of significant hyperbilirubinemia in healthy term newborns. *Pediatrics.*

2000;106(2). Available at: www.pediatrics.org/cgi/content/full/106/2/e16

36. Carbonell X, Botet F, Figueras J, Riu-Godo A. Prediction of hyperbilirubinaemia in the healthy term newborn. *Acta Paediatr.* 2001;90:166–170

37. Kaplan M, Hammerman C, Feldman R, Brisk R. Predischarge bilirubin screening in glucose-6-phosphate dehydrogenase-deficient neonates. *Pediatrics.* 2000;105:533–537

38. Stevenson DK, Fanaroff AA, Maisels MJ, et al. Prediction of hyperbilirubinemia in near-term and term infants. *Pediatrics.* 2001;108:31–39

39. Newman TB, Xiong B, Gonzales VM, Escobar GJ. Prediction and prevention of extreme neonatal hyperbilirubinemia in a mature health maintenance organization. *Arch Pediatr Adolesc Med.* 2000;154:1140–1147

40. Maisels MJ, Kring EA. Length of stay, jaundice, and hospital readmission. *Pediatrics.* 1998;101:995–998

41. Gale R, Seidman DS, Dollberg S, Stevenson DK. Epidemiology of neonatal jaundice in the Jerusalem population. *J Pediatr Gastroenterol Nutr.* 1990;10:82–86

42. Berk MA, Mimouni F, Miodovnik M, Hertzberg V, Valuck J. Macrosomia in infants of insulin-dependent diabetic mothers. *Pediatrics.* 1989; 83:1029–1034

43. Peevy KJ, Landaw SA, Gross SJ. Hyperbilirubinemia in infants of diabetic mothers. *Pediatrics.* 1980;66:417–419

44. Soskolne El, Schumacher R, Fyock C, Young ML, Schork A. The effect of early discharge and other factors on readmission rates of newborns. *Arch Pediatr Adolesc Med.* 1996;150:373–379

45. Ebbesen F, Brodersen R. Risk of bilirubin acid precipitation in preterm infants with respiratory distress syndrome: considerations of blood/brain bilirubin transfer equilibrium. *Early Hum Dev.* 1982;6:341–355

46. Cashore WJ, Oh W, Brodersen R. Reserve albumin and bilirubin toxicity index in infant serum. *Acta Paediatr Scand.* 1983;72:415–419

47. Cashore WJ. Free bilirubin concentrations and bilirubin-binding affinity in term and preterm infants. *J Pediatr.* 1980;96:521–527

48. Bratlid D. How bilirubin gets into the brain. *Clin Perinatol.* 1990;17: 449–465

49. Wennberg RP. Cellular basis of bilirubin toxicity. *N Y State J Med.* 1991;91:493–496

50. Eggert P, Stick C, Schroder H. On the distribution of irradiation intensity in phototherapy. Measurements of effective irradiance in an incubator. *Eur J Pediatr.* 1984;142:58–61

51. Maisels MJ. Why use homeopathic doses of phototherapy? *Pediatrics.* 1996;98:283–287

52. Ahlfors CE. Criteria for exchange transfusion in jaundiced newborns. *Pediatrics.* 1994;93:488–494

53. American Association of Blood Banks Technical Manual Committee. Perinatal issues in transfusion practice. In: Brecher M, ed. *Technical Manual.* Bethesda, MD: American Association of Blood Banks; 2002: 497–515

54. Garland JS, Alex C, Deacon JS, Raab K. Treatment of infants with indirect hyperbilirubinemia. Readmission to birth hospital vs nonbirth hospital. *Arch Pediatr Adolesc Med.* 1994;148:1317–1321

55. Gottstein R, Cooke R. Systematic review of intravenous immunoglobulin in haemolytic disease of the newborn. *Arch Dis Child Fetal Neonatal Ed.* 2003;88:F6–F10

56. Sato K, Hara T, Kondo T, Iwao H, Honda S, Ueda K. High-dose intravenous gammaglobulin therapy for neonatal immune haemolytic jaundice due to blood group incompatibility. *Acta Paediatr Scand.* 1991; 80:163–166

57. Rubo J, Albrecht K, Lasch P, et al. High-dose intravenous immune globulin therapy for hyperbilirubinemia caused by Rh hemolytic disease. *J Pediatr.* 1992;121:93–97

58. Hammerman C, Kaplan M, Vreman HJ, Stevenson DK. Intravenous immune globulin in neonatal ABO isoimmunization: factors associated with clinical efficacy. *Biol Neonate.* 1996;70:69–74

59. Johnson L, Boggs TR. Bilirubin-dependent brain damage: incidence and indications for treatment. In: Odell GB, Schaffer R, Simopoulos AP, eds. *Phototherapy in the Newborn: An Overview.* Washington, DC: National Academy of Sciences; 1974:122–149

60. Ozmert E, Erdem G, Topcu M. Long-term follow-up of indirect hyperbilirubinemia in full-term Turkish infants. *Acta Paediatr.* 1996;85: 1440–1444

61. Volpe JJ. *Neurology of the Newborn.* 4th ed. Philadelphia, PA: W. B. Saunders; 2001

62. Harris M, Bernbaum J, Polin J, Zimmerman R, Polin RA. Developmental follow-up of breastfed term and near-term infants with marked hyperbilirubinemia. *Pediatrics.* 2001;107:1075–1080

63. Osborn LM, Bolus R. Breast feeding and jaundice in the first week of life. *J Fam Pract.* 1985;20:475–480

64. Martinez JC, Maisels MJ, Otheguy L, et al. Hyperbilirubinemia in the breast-fed newborn: a controlled trial of four interventions. *Pediatrics.* 1993;91:470–473

65. Amato M, Howald H, von Muralt G. Interruption of breast-feeding versus phototherapy as treatment of hyperbilirubinemia in full-term infants. *Helv Paediatr Acta.* 1985;40:127–131

66. Maisels MJ, Gifford K, Antle CE, Leib GR. Jaundice in the healthy newborn infant: a new approach to an old problem. *Pediatrics.* 1988;81: 505–511

67. Newman TB, Easterling MJ. Yield of reticulocyte counts and blood smears in term infants. *Clin Pediatr (Phila).* 1994;33:71–76

68. Herschel M, Karrison T, Wen M, Caldarelli L, Baron B. Evaluation of the direct antiglobulin (Coombs') test for identifying newborns at risk for hemolysis as determined by end-tidal carbon monoxide concentration (ETCOc); and comparison of the Coombs' test with ETCOc for detecting significant jaundice. *J Perinatol.* 2002;22:341–347

69. Stevenson DK, Vreman HJ. Carbon monoxide and bilirubin production in neonates. *Pediatrics.* 1997;100:252–254

70. Vreman HJ, Verter J, Oh W, et al. Interlaboratory variability of bilirubin measurements. *Clin Chem.* 1996;42:869–873

71. Lo S, Doumas BT, Ashwood E. Performance of bilirubin determinations in US laboratories—revisited. *Clin Chem.* 2004;50:190–194

72. Kappas A, Drummond GS, Henschke C, Valaes T. Direct comparison of Sn-mesoporphyrin, an inhibitor of bilirubin production, and phototherapy in controlling hyperbilirubinemia in term and near-term newborns. *Pediatrics.* 1995;95:468–474

73. Martinez JC, Garcia HO, Otheguy L, Drummond GS, Kappas A. Control of severe hyperbilirubinemia in full-term newborns with the inhibitor of bilirubin production Sn-mesoporphyrin. *Pediatrics.* 1999;103:1–5

74. Suresh G, Martin CL, Soll R. Metalloporphyrins for treatment of unconjugated hyperbilirubinemia in neonates. *Cochrane Database Syst Rev.* 2003;2:CD004207

75. Kappas A, Drummond GS, Munson DP, Marshall JR. Sn-mesoporphyrin interdiction of severe hyperbilirubinemia in Jehovah's Witness newborns as an alternative to exchange transfusion. *Pediatrics.* 2001;108: 1374–1377

APPENDIX 1: Additional Notes

Definitions of Quality of Evidence and Balance of Benefits and Harms

The Steering Committee on Quality Improvement and Management categorizes evidence quality in 4 levels:

1. Well-designed, randomized, controlled trials or diagnostic studies on relevant populations
2. Randomized, controlled trials or diagnostic studies with minor limitations; overwhelming, consistent evidence from observational studies
3. Observational studies (case-control and cohort design)
4. Expert opinion, case reports, reasoning from first principles

The AAP defines evidence-based recommendations as follows:[1]

- Strong recommendation: the committee believes that the benefits of the recommended approach clearly exceed the harms of that approach and that the quality of the supporting evidence is either excellent or impossible to obtain. Clinicians should follow these recommendations unless a clear and compelling rationale for an alternative approach is present.
- Recommendation: the committee believes that the benefits exceed the harms, but the quality of evidence on which this recommendation is based is not as strong. Clinicians should also generally follow these recommendations but should be alert to new information and sensitive to patient prefer-

ences. In this guideline, the term "should" implies a recommendation by the committee.

- Option: either the quality of the evidence that exists is suspect or well-performed studies have shown little clear advantage to one approach over another. Patient preference should have a substantial role in influencing clinical decision-making when a policy is described as an option.
- No recommendation: there is a lack of pertinent evidence and the anticipated balance of benefits and harms is unclear.

Anticipated Balance Between Benefits and Harms

The presence of clear benefits or harms supports stronger statements for or against a course of action. In some cases, however, recommendations are made when analysis of the balance of benefits and harms provides an exceptional dysequilibrium and it would be unethical or impossible to perform clinical trials to "prove" the point. In these cases the balance of benefit and harm is termed "exceptional."

Clinical Manifestations of Acute Bilirubin Encephalopathy and Kernicterus

Acute Bilirubin Encephalopathy

In the early phase of acute bilirubin encephalopathy, severely jaundiced infants become lethargic and hypotonic and suck poorly.[2,3] The intermediate phase is characterized by moderate stupor, irritability, and hypertonia. The infant may develop a fever and high-pitched cry, which may alternate with drowsiness and hypotonia. The hypertonia is manifested by backward arching of the neck (retrocollis) and trunk (opisthotonos). There is anecdotal evidence that an emergent exchange transfusion at this stage, in some cases, might reverse the central nervous system changes.[4] The advanced phase, in which central nervous system damage is probably irreversible, is characterized by pronounced retrocollis-opisthotonos, shrill cry, no feeding, apnea, fever, deep stupor to coma, sometimes seizures, and death.[2,3,5]

Kernicterus

In the chronic form of bilirubin encephalopathy, surviving infants may develop a severe form of athetoid cerebral palsy, auditory dysfunction, dental-enamel dysplasia, paralysis of upward gaze, and, less often, intellectual and other handicaps. Most infants who develop kernicterus have manifested some or all of the signs listed above in the acute phase of bilirubin encephalopathy. However, occasionally there are infants who have developed very high bilirubin levels and, subsequently, the signs of kernicterus but have exhibited few, if any, antecedent clinical signs of acute bilirubin encephalopathy.[3,5,6]

Clinical Evaluation of Jaundice and TcB Measurements

Jaundice is usually seen in the face first and progresses caudally to the trunk and extremities,[7] but because visual estimation of bilirubin levels from the degree of jaundice can lead to errors,[8–10] a low threshold should be used for measuring the TSB.

Devices that provide a noninvasive TcB measurement have proven very useful as screening tools,[11] and newer instruments give measurements that provide a valid estimate of the TSB level.[12-17] Studies using the new TcB-measurement instruments are limited, but the data published thus far suggest that in most newborn populations, these instruments generally provide measurements within 2 to 3 mg/dL (34–51 μmol/L) of the TSB and can replace a measurement of serum bilirubin in many circumstances, particularly for TSB levels less than 15 mg/dL (257 μmol/L).[12-17] Because phototherapy "bleaches" the skin, both visual assessment of jaundice and TcB measurements in infants undergoing phototherapy are not reliable. In addition, the ability of transcutaneous instruments to provide accurate measurements in different racial groups requires additional study.[18,19] The limitations of the accuracy and reproducibility of TSB measurements in the clinical laboratory[20-22] must also be recognized and are discussed in the technical report.[23]

Capillary Versus Venous Serum Bilirubin Measurement

Almost all published data regarding the relationship of TSB levels to kernicterus or developmental outcome are based on capillary blood TSB levels. Data regarding the differences between capillary and venous TSB levels are conflicting.[24,25] In 1 study the capillary TSB levels were higher, but in another they were lower than venous TSB levels.[24,25] Thus, obtaining a venous sample to "confirm" an elevated capillary TSB level is not recommended, because it will delay the initiation of treatment.

Direct-Reacting and Conjugated Bilirubin

Although commonly used interchangeably, direct-reacting bilirubin is not the same as conjugated bilirubin. Direct-reacting bilirubin is the bilirubin that reacts directly (without the addition of an accelerating agent) with diazotized sulfanilic acid. Conjugated bilirubin is bilirubin made water soluble by binding with glucuronic acid in the liver. Depending on the technique used, the clinical laboratory will report total and direct-reacting or unconjugated and conjugated bilirubin levels. In this guideline and for clinical purposes, the terms may be used interchangeably.

Abnormal Direct and Conjugated Bilirubin Levels

Laboratory measurement of direct bilirubin is not precise,[26] and values between laboratories can vary widely. If the TSB is at or below 5 mg/dL (85 μmol/L), a direct or conjugated bilirubin of more than 1.0 mg/dL (17.1 μmol/L) is generally considered abnormal. For TSB values higher than 5 mg/dL (85 μmol/L), a direct bilirubin of more than 20% of the TSB is considered abnormal. If the hospital laboratory measures conjugated bilirubin using the Vitros (formerly Ektachem) system (Ortho-Clinical Diagnostics, Raritan, NJ), any value higher than 1 mg/dL is considered abnormal.

Assessment of Adequacy of Intake in Breastfeeding Infants

The data from a number of studies[27-34] indicate that unsupplemented, breastfed infants experience their maximum weight loss by day 3 and, on average, lose 6.1% ± 2.5% (SD) of their birth weight. Thus, ~5% to 10% of fully breastfed infants lose 10% or more of their birth weight by day 3, suggesting that adequacy of intake should be evaluated and the infant monitored if weight loss is more than 10%.[35] Evidence of adequate intake in breastfed infants also includes 4 to 6 thoroughly wet diapers in 24 hours and the passage of 3 to 4 stools per day by the fourth day. By the third to fourth day, the stools in adequately breastfed infants should have changed from meconium to a mustard yellow, mushy stool.[36] The above assessment will also help to identify breastfed infants who are at risk for dehydration because of inadequate intake.

Nomogram for Designation of Risk

Note that this nomogram (Fig 2) does not describe the natural history of neonatal hyperbilirubinemia, particularly after 48 to 72 hours, for which, because of sampling bias, the lower zones are spuriously elevated.[37] This bias, however, will have much less effect on the high-risk zone (95th percentile in the study).[38]

G6PD Dehydrogenase Deficiency

It is important to look for G6PD deficiency in infants with significant hyperbilirubinemia, because some may develop a sudden increase in the TSB. In addition, G6PD-deficient infants require intervention at lower TSB levels (Figs 3 and 4). It should be noted also that in the presence of hemolysis, G6PD levels can be elevated, which may obscure the diagnosis in the newborn period so that a normal level in a hemolyzing neonate does not rule out G6PD deficiency.[39] If G6PD deficiency is strongly suspected, a repeat level should be measured when the infant is 3 months old. It is also recognized that immediate laboratory determination of G6PD is generally not available in most US hospitals, and thus translating the above information into clinical practice is cur-

TABLE 4. Risk Zone as a Predictor of Hyperbilirubinemia[39]

TSB Before Discharge	Newborns (Total = 2840), n (%)	Newborns Who Subsequently Developed a TSB Level >95th Percentile, n (%)
High-risk zone (>95th percentile)	172 (6.0)	68 (39.5)
High intermediate-risk zone	356 (12.5)	46 (12.9)
Low intermediate-risk zone	556 (19.6)	12 (2.26)
Low-risk zone	1756 (61.8)	0

rently difficult. Nevertheless, practitioners are reminded to consider the diagnosis of G6PD deficiency in infants with severe hyperbilirubinemia, particularly if they belong to the population groups in which this condition is prevalent. This is important in the African American population, because these infants, as a group, have much lower TSB levels than white or Asian infants.[40,41] Thus, severe hyperbilirubinemia in an African American infant should always raise the possibility of G6PD deficiency.

Basis for the Recommendations 7.1.1 Through 7.1.6 and Provided in Figs 3 and 4

Ideally, recommendations for when to implement phototherapy and exchange transfusions should be based on estimates of when the benefits of these interventions exceed their risks and cost. The evidence for these estimates should come from randomized trials or systematic observational studies. Unfortunately, there is little such evidence on which to base these recommendations. As a result, treatment guidelines must necessarily rely on more uncertain estimates and extrapolations. For a detailed discussion of this question, please see "An Evidence-Based Review of Important Issues Concerning Neonatal Hyperbilirubinemia."[23]

The recommendations for phototherapy and exchange transfusion are based on the following principles:

- The main demonstrated value of phototherapy is that it reduces the risk that TSB levels will reach a level at which exchange transfusion is recommended.[42-44] Approximately 5 to 10 infants with TSB levels between 15 and 20 mg/dL (257–342 μmol/L) will receive phototherapy to prevent the TSB in 1 infant from reaching 20 mg/dL (the number needed to treat).[12] Thus, 8 to 9 of every 10 infants with these TSB levels will not reach 20 mg/dL (342 μmol/L) even if they are not treated. Phototherapy has proven to be a generally safe procedure, although rare complications can occur (see Appendix 2).
- Recommended TSB levels for exchange transfusion (Fig 4) are based largely on the goal of keeping TSB levels below those at which kernicterus has been reported.[12,45-48] In almost all cases, exchange transfusion is recommended only after phototherapy has failed to keep the TSB level below the exchange transfusion level (Fig 4).
- The recommendations to use phototherapy and exchange transfusion at lower TSB levels for infants of lower gestation and those who are sick are based on limited observations suggesting that sick infants (particularly those with the risk factors listed in Figs 3 and 4)[49-51] and those of lower gestation[51-54] are at greater risk for developing kernicterus at lower bilirubin levels than are well infants of more than 38 6/7 weeks' gestation. Nevertheless, other studies have not confirmed all of these associations.[52,55,56] There is no doubt, however, that infants at 35 to 37 6/7 weeks' gestation are at a much greater risk of developing very high

TSB levels.[57,58] Intervention for these infants is based on this risk as well as extrapolations from more premature, lower birth-weight infants who do have a higher risk of bilirubin toxicity.[52,53]
- For all newborns, treatment is recommended at lower TSB levels at younger ages because one of the primary goals of treatment is to prevent additional increases in the TSB level.

Subtle Neurologic Abnormalities Associated With Hyperbilirubinemia

There are several studies demonstrating measurable transient changes in brainstem-evoked potentials, behavioral patterns, and the infant's cry[59-63] associated with TSB levels of 15 to 25 mg/dL (257–428 μmol/L). In these studies, the abnormalities identified were transient and disappeared when the serum bilirubin levels returned to normal with or without treatment.[59,60,62,63]

A few cohort studies have found an association between hyperbilirubinemia and long-term adverse neurodevelopmental effects that are more subtle than kernicterus.[64-67] Current studies, however, suggest that although phototherapy lowers the TSB levels, it has no effect on these long-term neurodevelopmental outcomes.[68-70]

Risks of Exchange Transfusion

Because exchange transfusions are now rarely performed, the risks of morbidity and mortality associated with the procedure are difficult to quantify. In addition, the complication rates listed below may not be generalizable to the current era if, like most procedures, frequency of performance is an important determinant of risk. Death associated with exchange transfusion has been reported in approximately 3 in 1000 procedures,[71,72] although in otherwise well infants of 35 or more weeks' gestation, the risk is probably much lower.[71-73] Significant morbidity (apnea, bradycardia, cyanosis, vasospasm, thrombosis, necrotizing enterocolitis) occurs in as many as 5% of exchange transfusions,[71] and the risks associated with the use of blood products must always be considered.[74] Hypoxic-ischemic encephalopathy and acquired immunodeficiency syndrome have occurred in otherwise healthy infants receiving exchange transfusions.[73,75]

Serum Albumin Levels and the B/A Ratio

The legends to Figs 3 and 4 and recommendations 7.1.5 and 7.1.6 contain references to the serum albumin level and the B/A ratio as factors that can be considered in the decision to initiate phototherapy (Fig 3) or perform an exchange transfusion (Fig 4). Bilirubin is transported in the plasma tightly bound to albumin, and the portion that is unbound or loosely bound can more readily leave the intravascular space and cross the intact blood-brain barrier.[76] Elevations of unbound bilirubin (UB) have been associated with kernicterus in sick preterm newborns.[77,78] In addition, elevated UB concentrations are more closely associated than TSB levels with transient abnormalities in the audiometric brainstem response in term[79] and preterm[80] infants. Long-term studies relating B/A binding in infants to developmental outcome are limited and conflicting.[69,81,82] In addition, clinical laboratory measurement of UB is not currently available in the United States.

The ratio of bilirubin (mg/dL) to albumin (g/dL) does correlate with measured UB in newborns[83] and can be used as an approximate surrogate for the measurement of UB. It must be recognized, however, that both albumin levels and the ability of albumin to bind bilirubin vary significantly between newborns.[83,84] Albumin binding of bilirubin is impaired in sick infants,[84–86] and some studies show an increase in binding with increasing gestational[86,87] and postnatal[87,88] age, but others have not found a significant effect of gestational age on binding.[89] Furthermore, the risk of bilirubin encephalopathy is unlikely to be a simple function of the TSB level or the concentration of UB but is more likely a combination of both (ie, the total amount of bilirubin available [the miscible pool of bilirubin] as well as the tendency of bilirubin to enter the tissues [the UB concentration]).[83] An additional factor is the possible susceptibility of the cells of the central nervous system to damage by bilirubin.[90] It is therefore a clinical option to use the B/A ratio together with, but not in lieu of, the TSB level as an additional factor in determining the need for exchange transfusion[83] (Fig 4).

REFERENCES

1. American Academy of Pediatrics, Steering Committee on Quality Improvement and Management. Classification of recommendations for clinical practice guidelines. *Pediatrics.* 2004; In press

2. Johnson LH, Bhutani VK, Brown AK. System-based approach to management of neonatal jaundice and prevention of kernicterus. *J Pediatr.* 2002;140:396–403

3. Volpe JJ. *Neurology of the Newborn.* 4th ed. Philadelphia, PA: W. B. Saunders; 2001

4. Harris M, Bernbaum J, Polin J, Zimmerman R, Polin RA. Developmental follow-up of breastfed term and near-term infants with marked hyperbilirubinemia. *Pediatrics.* 2001;107:1075–1080

5. Van Praagh R. Diagnosis of kernicterus in the neonatal period. *Pediatrics.* 1961;28:870–876

6. Jones MH, Sands R, Hyman CB, Sturgeon P, Koch FP. Longitudinal study of incidence of central nervous system damage following erythroblastosis fetalis. *Pediatrics.* 1954;14:346–350

7. Kramer LI. Advancement of dermal icterus in the jaundiced newborn. *Am J Dis Child.* 1969;118:454–458

8. Moyer VA, Ahn C, Sneed S. Accuracy of clinical judgment in neonatal jaundice. *Arch Pediatr Adolesc Med.* 2000;154:391–394

9. Davidson LT, Merritt KK, Weech AA. Hyperbilirubinemia in the newborn. *Am J Dis Child.* 1941;61:958–980

10. Tayaba R, Gribetz D, Gribetz I, Holzman IR. Noninvasive estimation of serum bilirubin. *Pediatrics.* 1998;102(3). Available at: www.pediatrics.org/cgi/content/full/102/3/e28

11. Maisels MJ, Kring E. Transcutaneous bilirubinometry decreases the need for serum bilirubin measurements and saves money. *Pediatrics.* 1997;99:599–601

12. Ip S, Glicken S, Kulig J, Obrien R, Sege R, Lau J. *Management of Neonatal Hyperbilirubinemia.* Rockville, MD: US Department of Health and Human Services, Agency for Healthcare Research and Quality; 2003. AHRQ Publication 03-E011

13. Bhutani V, Gourley GR, Adler S, Kreamer B, Dalman C, Johnson LH. Noninvasive measurement of total serum bilirubin in a multiracial predischarge newborn population to assess the risk of severe hyperbilirubinemia. *Pediatrics.* 2000;106(2). Available at: www.pediatrics.org/cgi/content/full/106/2/e17

14. Yasuda S, Itoh S, Isobe K, et al. New transcutaneous jaundice device with two optical paths. *J Perinat Med.* 2003;31:81–88

15. Maisels MJ, Ostrea EJ Jr, Touch S, et al. Evaluation of a new transcutaneous bilirubinometer. *Pediatrics.* 2004;113:1638–1645

16. Ebbesen F, Rasmussen LM, Wimberley PD. A new transcutaneous bilirubinometer, bilicheck, used in the neonatal intensive care unit and the maternity ward. *Acta Paediatr.* 2002;91:203–211

17. Rubaltelli FF, Gourley GR, Loskamp N, et al. Transcutaneous bilirubin measurement: a multicenter evaluation of a new device. *Pediatrics.* 2001;107:1264–1271

18. Engle WD, Jackson GL, Sendelbach D, Manning D, Frawley W. Assessment of a transcutaneous device in the evaluation of neonatal hyperbilirubinemia in a primarily Hispanic population. *Pediatrics.* 2002;110:61–67

19. Schumacher R. Transcutaneous bilirubinometry and diagnostic tests: "the right job for the tool." *Pediatrics.* 2002;110:407–408

20. Vreman HJ, Verter J, Oh W, et al. Interlaboratory variability of bilirubin measurements. *Clin Chem.* 1996;42:869–873

21. Doumas BT, Eckfeldt JH. Errors in measurement of total bilirubin: a perennial problem. *Clin Chem.* 1996;42:845–848

22. Lo S, Doumas BT, Ashwood E. Performance of bilirubin determinations in US laboratories—revisited. *Clin Chem.* 2004;50:190–194

23. Ip S, Chung M, Kulig J. et al. An evidence-based review of important issues concerning neonatal hyperbilirubinemia. *Pediatrics.* 2004;113(6). Available at: www.pediatrics.org/cgi/content/full/113/6/e644

24. Leslie GI, Philips JB, Cassady G. Capillary and venous bilirubin values: are they really different? *Am J Dis Child.* 1987;141:1199–1200

25. Eidelman AI, Schimmel MS, Algur N, Eylath U. Capillary and venous bilirubin values: they are different—and how [letter]! *Am J Dis Child.* 1989;143:642

26. Watkinson LR, St John A, Penberthy LA. Investigation into paediatric bilirubin analyses in Australia and New Zealand. *J Clin Pathol.* 1982;35:52–58

27. Bertini G, Dani C, Trochin M, Rubaltelli F. Is breastfeeding really favoring early neonatal jaundice? *Pediatrics.* 2001;107(3). Available at: www.pediatrics.org/cgi/content/full/107/3/e41

28. De Carvalho M, Klaus MH, Merkatz RB. Frequency of breastfeeding and serum bilirubin concentration. *Am J Dis Child.* 1982;136:737–738

29. De Carvalho M, Holl M, Harvey D. Effects of water supplementation on physiological jaundice in breast-fed babies. *Arch Dis Child.* 1981;56:568–569

30. Nicoll A, Ginsburg R, Tripp JH. Supplementary feeding and jaundice in newborns. *Acta Paediatr Scand.* 1982;71:759–761

31. Butler DA, MacMillan JP. Relationship of breast feeding and weight loss to jaundice in the newborn period: review of the literature and results of a study. *Cleve Clin Q.* 1983;50:263–268

32. De Carvalho M, Robertson S, Klaus M. Fecal bilirubin excretion and serum bilirubin concentration in breast-fed and bottle-fed infants. *J Pediatr.* 1985;107:786–790

33. Gourley GR, Kreamer B, Arend R. The effect of diet on feces and jaundice during the first three weeks of life. *Gastroenterology.* 1992;103:660–667

34. Maisels MJ, Gifford K. Breast-feeding, weight loss, and jaundice. *J Pediatr.* 1983;102:117–118

35. Laing IA, Wong CM. Hypernatraemia in the first few days: is the incidence rising? *Arch Dis Child Fetal Neonatal Ed.* 2002;87:F158–F162

36. Lawrence RA. Management of the mother-infant nursing couple. In: *A Breastfeeding Guide for the Medical Profession.* 4th ed. St Louis, MO: Mosby-Year Book, Inc; 1994:215–277

37. Maisels MJ, Newman TB. Predicting hyperbilirubinemia in newborns: the importance of timing. *Pediatrics.* 1999;103:493–495

38. Bhutani VK, Johnson L, Sivieri EM. Predictive ability of a predischarge hour-specific serum bilirubin for subsequent significant hyperbilirubinemia in healthy term and near-term newborns. *Pediatrics.* 1999;103:6–14

39. Beutler E. Glucose-6-phosphate dehydrogenase deficiency. *Blood.* 1994;84:3613–3636

40. Linn S, Schoenbaum SC, Monson RR, Rosner B, Stubblefield PG, Ryan KJ. Epidemiology of neonatal hyperbilirubinemia. *Pediatrics.* 1985;75:770–774

41. Newman TB, Easterling MJ, Goldman ES, Stevenson DK. Laboratory evaluation of jaundiced newborns: frequency, cost and yield. *Am J Dis Child.* 1990;144:364–368

42. Martinez JC, Maisels MJ, Otheguy L, et al. Hyperbilirubinemia in the breast-fed newborn: a controlled trial of four interventions. *Pediatrics.* 1993;91:470–473

43. Maisels MJ. Phototherapy—traditional and nontraditional. *J Perinatol.* 2001;21(suppl 1):S93–S97

44. Brown AK, Kim MH, Wu PY, Bryla DA. Efficacy of phototherapy in prevention and management of neonatal hyperbilirubinemia. *Pediatrics.* 1985;75:393–400

45. Armitage P, Mollison PL. Further analysis of controlled trials of treatment of hemolytic disease of the newborn. *J Obstet Gynaecol Br Emp.* 1953;60:602–605

46. Mollison PL, Walker W. Controlled trials of the treatment of haemolytic disease of the newborn. *Lancet.* 1952;1:429–433

47. Hsia DYY, Allen FH, Gellis SS, Diamond LK. Erythroblastosis fetalis. VIII. Studies of serum bilirubin in relation to kernicterus. *N Engl J Med.* 1952;247:668–671

48. Newman TB, Maisels MJ. Does hyperbilirubinemia damage the brain of healthy full-term infants? *Clin Perinatol.* 1990;17:331–358

49. Ozmert E, Erdem G, Topcu M. Long-term follow-up of indirect hyperbilirubinemia in full-term Turkish infants. *Acta Paediatr.* 1996;85:1440–1444

50. Perlman JM, Rogers B, Burns D. Kernicterus findings at autopsy in 2 sick near-term infants. *Pediatrics.* 1997;99:612–615

51. Gartner LM, Snyder RN, Chabon RS, Bernstein J. Kernicterus: high incidence in premature infants with low serum bilirubin concentration. *Pediatrics.* 1970;45:906–917

52. Watchko JF, Oski FA. Kernicterus in preterm newborns: past, present, and future. *Pediatrics.* 1992;90:707–715

53. Watchko J, Claassen D. Kernicterus in premature infants: current prevalence and relationship to NICHD Phototherapy Study exchange criteria. *Pediatrics.* 1994;93(6 Pt 1):996–999

54. Stern L, Denton RL. Kernicterus in small, premature infants. *Pediatrics.* 1965;35:486–485

55. Turkel SB, Guttenberg ME, Moynes DR, Hodgman JE. Lack of identifiable risk factors for kernicterus. *Pediatrics.* 1980;66:502–506

56. Kim MH, Yoon JJ, Sher J, Brown AK. Lack of predictive indices in kernicterus. A comparison of clinical and pathologic factors in infants with or without kernicterus. *Pediatrics.* 1980;66:852–858

57. Newman TB, Xiong B, Gonzales VM, Escobar GJ. Prediction and prevention of extreme neonatal hyperbilirubinemia in a mature health maintenance organization. *Arch Pediatr Adolesc Med.* 2000;154:1140–1147

58. Newman TB, Escobar GJ, Gonzales VM, Armstrong MA, Gardner MN, Folck BF. Frequency of neonatal bilirubin testing and hyperbilirubinemia in a large health maintenance organization. *Pediatrics.* 1999;104:1198–1203

59. Vohr BR. New approaches to assessing the risks of hyperbilirubinemia. *Clin Perinatol.* 1990;17:293–306

60. Perlman M, Fainmesser P, Sohmer H, Tamari H, Wax Y, Pevsmer B. Auditory nerve-brainstem evoked responses in hyperbilirubinemic neonates. *Pediatrics.* 1983;72:658–664

61. Nakamura H, Takada S, Shimabuku R, Matsuo M, Matsuo T, Negishi H. Auditory and brainstem responses in newborn infants with hyperbilirubinemia. *Pediatrics.* 1985;75:703–708

62. Nwaesei CG, Van Aerde J, Boyden M, Perlman M. Changes in auditory brainstem responses in hyperbilirubinemic infants before and after exchange transfusion. *Pediatrics.* 1984;74:800–803

63. Wennberg RP, Ahlfors CE, Bickers R, McMurtry CA, Shetter JL. Abnormal auditory brainstem response in a newborn infant with hyperbilirubinemia: improvement with exchange transfusion. *J Pediatr.* 1982;100:624–626

64. Soorani-Lunsing I, Woltil H, Hadders-Algra M. Are moderate degrees of hyperbilirubinemia in healthy term neonates really safe for the brain? *Pediatr Res.* 2001;50:701–705

65. Grimmer I, Berger-Jones K, Buhrer C, Brandl U, Obladen M. Late neurological sequelae of non-hemolytic hyperbilirubinemia of healthy term neonates. *Acta Paediatr.* 1999;88:661–663

66. Seidman DS, Paz I, Stevenson DK, Laor A, Danon YL, Gale R. Neonatal hyperbilirubinemia and physical and cognitive performance at 17 years of age. *Pediatrics.* 1991;88:828–833

67. Newman TB, Klebanoff MA. Neonatal hyperbilirubinemia and long-term outcome: another look at the collaborative perinatal project. *Pediatrics.* 1993;92:651–657

68. Scheidt PC, Bryla DA, Nelson KB, Hirtz DG, Hoffman HJ. Phototherapy for neonatal hyperbilirubinemia: six-year follow-up of the National Institute of Child Health and Human Development clinical trial. *Pediatrics.* 1990;85:455–463

69. Scheidt PC, Graubard BI, Nelson KB, et al. Intelligence at six years in relation to neonatal bilirubin levels: follow-up of the National Institute of Child Health and Human Development Clinical Trial of Phototherapy. *Pediatrics.* 1991;87:797–805

70. Seidman DS, Paz I, Stevenson DK, Laor A, Danon YL, Gale R. Effect of phototherapy for neonatal jaundice on cognitive performance. *J Perinatol.* 1994;14:23–28

71. Keenan WJ, Novak KK, Sutherland JM, Bryla DA, Fetterly KL. Morbidity and mortality associated with exchange transfusion. *Pediatrics.* 1985;75:417–421

72. Hovi L, Siimes MA. Exchange transfusion with fresh heparinized blood is a safe procedure: Experiences from 1069 newborns. *Acta Paediatr Scand.* 1985;74:360–365

73. Jackson JC. Adverse events associated with exchange transfusion in healthy and ill newborns. *Pediatrics.* 1997;99(5):e7. Available at: www.pediatrics.org/cgi/content/full/99/5/e7

74. Schreiber GB, Busch MP, Kleinman SH, Korelitz JJ. The risk of transfusion-transmitted viral infections. *N Engl J Med.* 1996;334:1685–1690

75. Maisels MJ, Newman TB. Kernicterus in otherwise healthy, breast-fed term newborns. *Pediatrics.* 1995;96:730–733

76. Bratlid D. How bilirubin gets into the brain. *Clin Perinatol.* 1990;17:449–465

77. Cashore WJ, Oh W. Unbound bilirubin and kernicterus in low-birth-weight infants. *Pediatrics.* 1982;69:481–485

78. Nakamura H, Yonetani M, Uetani Y, Funato M, Lee Y. Determination of serum unbound bilirubin for prediction of kernicterus in low birth-weight infants. *Acta Paediatr Jpn.* 1992;34:642–647

79. Funato M, Tamai H, Shimada S, Nakamura H. Vigintiphobia, unbound bilirubin, and auditory brainstem responses. *Pediatrics.* 1994;93:50–53

80. Amin SB, Ahlfors CE, Orlando MS, Dalzell LE, Merle KS, Guillet R. Bilirubin and serial auditory brainstem responses in premature infants. *Pediatrics.* 2001;107:664–670

81. Johnson L, Boggs TR. Bilirubin-dependent brain damage: incidence and indications for treatment. In: Odell GB, Schaffer R, Simopoulos AP, eds. *Phototherapy in the Newborn: An Overview.* Washington, DC: National Academy of Sciences; 1974:122–149

82. Odell GB, Storey GNB, Rosenberg LA. Studies in kernicterus. 3. The saturation of serum proteins with bilirubin during neonatal life and its relationship to brain damage at five years. *J Pediatr.* 1970;76:12–21

83. Ahlfors CE. Criteria for exchange transfusion in jaundiced newborns. *Pediatrics.* 1994;93:488–494

84. Cashore WJ. Free bilirubin concentrations and bilirubin-binding affinity in term and preterm infants. *J Pediatr.* 1980;96:521–527

85. Ebbesen F, Brodersen R. Risk of bilirubin acid precipitation in preterm infants with respiratory distress syndrome: considerations of blood/brain bilirubin transfer equilibrium. *Early Hum Dev.* 1982;6:341–355

86. Cashore WJ, Oh W, Brodersen R. Reserve albumin and bilirubin toxicity index in infant serum. *Acta Paediatr Scand.* 1983;72:415–419

87. Ebbesen F, Nyboe J. Postnatal changes in the ability of plasma albumin to bind bilirubin. *Acta Paediatr Scand.* 1983;72:665–670

88. Esbjorner E. Albumin binding properties in relation to bilirubin and albumin concentrations during the first week of life. *Acta Paediatr Scand.* 1991;80:400–405

89. Robertson A, Sharp C, Karp W. The relationship of gestational age to reserve albumin concentration for binding of bilirubin. *J Perinatol.* 1988;8:17–18

90. Wennberg RP. Cellular basis of bilirubin toxicity. *N Y State J Med.* 1991;91:493–496

APPENDIX 2: Phototherapy

There is no standardized method for delivering phototherapy. Phototherapy units vary widely, as do the types of lamps used in the units. The efficacy of phototherapy depends on the dose of phototherapy administered as well as a number of clinical factors (Table 5).[1]

Measuring the Dose of Phototherapy

Table 5 shows the radiometric quantities used in measuring the phototherapy dose. The quantity most commonly reported in the literature is the spectral irradiance. In the nursery, spectral irradiance can be measured by using commercially available radiometers. These instruments take a single measurement across a band of wavelengths, typically 425 to 475 or 400 to 480 nm. Unfortunately, there is no standardized method for reporting phototherapy dosages in the clinical literature, so it is difficult to compare published studies on the efficacy of phototherapy and manufacturers' data for the irradiance produced by different systems.[2] Measurements of irradiance from the same system, using different radiometers,

TABLE 5.   Factors That Affect the Dose and Efficacy of Phototherapy

Factor	Mechanism/Clinical Relevance	Implementation and Rationale	Clinical Application
Spectrum of light emitted	Blue-green spectrum is most effective. At these wavelengths, light penetrates skin well and is absorbed maximally by bilirubin.	Special blue fluorescent tubes or other light sources that have most output in the blue-green spectrum and are most effective in lowering TSB.	Use special blue tubes or LED light source with output in blue-green spectrum for intensive PT.
Spectral irradiance (irradiance in certain wavelength band) delivered to surface of infant	↑ irradiance → ↑ rate of decline in TSB	Irradiance is measured with a radiometer as $\mu W/cm^2$ per nm. Standard PT units deliver 8–10 $\mu W/cm^2$ per nm (Fig 6). Intensive PT requires >30 $\mu W/cm^2$ per nm.	If special blue fluorescent tubes are used, bring tubes as close to infant as possible to increase irradiance (Fig 6). Note: This cannot be done with halogen lamps because of the danger of burn. Special blue tubes 10–15 cm above the infant will produce an irradiance of at least 35 $\mu W/cm^2$ per nm.
Spectral power (average spectral irradiance across surface area)	↑ surface area exposed → ↑ rate of decline in TSB	For intensive PT, expose maximum surface area of infant to PT.	Place lights above and fiber-optic pad or special blue fluorescent tubes* below the infant. For maximum exposure, line sides of bassinet, warmer bed, or incubator with aluminum foil.
Cause of jaundice	PT is likely to be less effective if jaundice is due to hemolysis or if cholestasis is present. (↑ direct bilirubin)		When hemolysis is present, start PT at lower TSB levels. Use intensive PT. Failure of PT suggests that hemolysis is the cause of jaundice. If ↑ direct bilirubin, watch for bronze baby syndrome or blistering.
TSB level at start of PT	The higher the TSB, the more rapid the decline in TSB with PT.		Use intensive PT for higher TSB levels. Anticipate a more rapid decrease in TSB when TSB >20 mg/dL (342 μmol/L).

PT indicates phototherapy; LED, light-emitting diode.
* Available in the Olympic BiliBassinet (Olympic Medical, Seattle, WA).

can also produce significantly different results. The width of the phototherapy lamp's emissions spectrum (narrow versus broad) will affect the measured irradiance. Measurements under lights with a very focused emission spectrum (eg, blue light-emitting diode) will vary significantly from one radiometer to another, because the response spectra of the radiometers vary from manufacturer to manufacturer. Broader-spectrum lights (fluorescent and halogen) have fewer variations among radiometers. Manufacturers of phototherapy systems generally recommend the specific radiometer to be used in measuring the dose of phototherapy when their system is used.

It is important also to recognize that the measured irradiance will vary widely depending on where the measurement is taken. Irradiance measured below the center of the light source can be more than double that measured at the periphery, and this dropoff at the periphery will vary with different phototherapy units. Ideally, irradiance should be measured at multiple sites under the area illuminated by the unit and the measurements averaged. The International Electrotechnical Commission[3] defines the "effective surface area" as the intended treatment surface that is illuminated by the phototherapy light. The commission uses 60 × 30 cm as the standard-sized surface.

Is It Necessary to Measure Phototherapy Doses Routinely?

Although it is not necessary to measure spectral irradiance before each use of phototherapy, it is important to perform periodic checks of phototherapy units to make sure that an adequate irradiance is being delivered.

The Dose-Response Relationship of Phototherapy

Figure 5 shows that there is a direct relationship between the irradiance used and the rate at which the serum bilirubin declines under phototherapy.[4] The data in Fig 5 suggest that there is a saturation point beyond which an increase in the irradiance produces no added efficacy. We do not know, however, that a saturation point exists. Because the conversion of bilirubin to excretable photoproducts is partly irreversible and follows first-order kinetics, there may not be a saturation point, so we do not know the maximum effective dose of phototherapy.

Effect on Irradiance of the Light Spectrum and the Distance Between the Infant and the Light Source

Figure 6 shows that as the distance between the light source and the infant decreases, there is a corresponding increase in the spectral irradiance.[5] Fig 6 also demonstrates the dramatic difference in irradi-

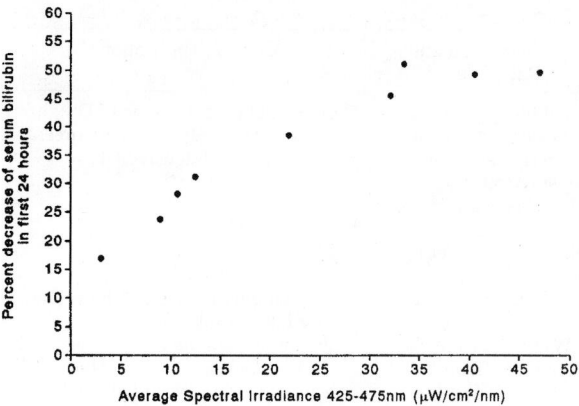

Fig 5. Relationship between average spectral irradiance and decrease in serum bilirubin concentration. Term infants with nonhemolytic hyperbilirubinemia were exposed to special blue lights (Phillips TL 52/20W) of different intensities. Spectral irradiance was measured as the average of readings at the head, trunk, and knees. Drawn from the data of Tan.[4] Source: *Pediatrics*. 1996;98: 283-287.

ance produced within the important 425- to 475-nm band by different types of fluorescent tubes.

What is Intensive Phototherapy?

Intensive phototherapy implies the use of high levels of irradiance in the 430- to 490-nm band (usually 30 $\mu W/cm^2$ per nm or higher) delivered to as much of the infant's surface area as possible. How this can be achieved is described below.

Using Phototherapy Effectively

Light Source

The spectrum of light delivered by a phototherapy unit is determined by the type of light source and

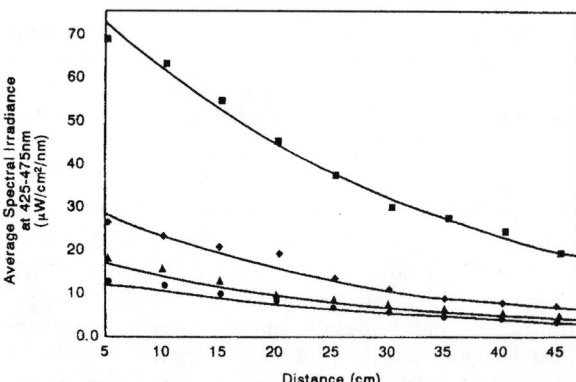

Fig 6. Effect of light source and distance from the light source to the infant on average spectral irradiance. Measurements were made across the 425- to 475-nm band by using a commercial radiometer (Olympic Bilimeter Mark II) and are the average of measurements taken at different locations at each distance (irradiance at the center of the light is much higher than at the periphery). The phototherapy unit was fitted with eight 24-in fluorescent tubes. ■ indicates special blue, General Electric 20-W F20T12/BB tube; ◆, blue, General Electric 20-W F20T12/B tube; ▲, daylight blue, 4 General Electric 20-W F20T12/B blue tubes and 4 Sylvania 20-W F20T12/D daylight tubes; •, daylight, Sylvania 20-W F20T12/D daylight tube. Curves were plotted by using linear curve fitting (True Epistat, Epistat Services, Richardson, TX). The best fit is described by the equation $y = Ae^{Bx}$. Source: *Pediatrics*. 1996;98:283-287.

any filters used. Commonly used phototherapy units contain daylight, cool white, blue, or "special blue" fluorescent tubes. Other units use tungsten-halogen lamps in different configurations, either free-standing or as part of a radiant warming device. Recently, a system using high-intensity gallium nitride light-emitting diodes has been introduced.[6] Fiber-optic systems deliver light from a high-intensity lamp to a fiber-optic blanket. Most of these devices deliver enough output in the blue-green region of the visible spectrum to be effective for standard phototherapy use. However, when bilirubin levels approach the range at which intensive phototherapy is recommended, maximal efficiency must be sought. The most effective light sources currently commercially available for phototherapy are those that use special blue fluorescent tubes[7] or a specially designed light-emitting diode light (Natus Inc, San Carlos, CA).[6] The special blue fluorescent tubes are labeled F20T12/BB (General Electric, Westinghouse, Sylvania) or TL52/20W (Phillips, Eindhoven, The Netherlands). It is important to note that special blue tubes provide much greater irradiance than regular blue tubes (labeled F20T12/B) (Fig 6). Special blue tubes are most effective because they provide light predominantly in the blue-green spectrum. At these wavelengths, light penetrates skin well and is absorbed maximally by bilirubin.[7]

There is a common misconception that ultraviolet light is used for phototherapy. The light systems used do not emit significant ultraviolet radiation, and the small amount of ultraviolet light that is emitted by fluorescent tubes and halogen bulbs is in longer wavelengths than those that cause erythema. In addition, almost all ultraviolet light is absorbed by the glass wall of the fluorescent tube and the Plexiglas cover of the phototherapy unit.

Distance From the Light

As can be seen in Fig 6, the distance of the light source from the infant has a dramatic effect on the spectral irradiance, and this effect is most significant when special blue tubes are used. To take advantage of this effect, the fluorescent tubes should be placed as close to the infant as possible. To do this, the infant should be in a bassinet, not an incubator, because the top of the incubator prevents the light from being brought sufficiently close to the infant. In a bassinet, it is possible to bring the fluorescent tubes within approximately 10 cm of the infant. Naked term infants do not become overheated under these lights. It is important to note, however, that the halogen spot phototherapy lamps cannot be positioned closer to the infant than recommended by the manufacturers without incurring the risk of a burn. When halogen lamps are used, manufacturers recommendations should be followed. The reflectors, light source, and transparent light filters (if any) should be kept clean.

Surface Area

A number of systems have been developed to provide phototherapy above and below the infant.[8,9] One commercially available system that does this is the BiliBassinet (Olympic Medical, Seattle, WA). This unit provides special blue fluorescent tubes above and below the infant. An alternative is to place fiber-optic pads below an infant with phototherapy lamps above. One disadvantage of fiber-optic pads is that they cover a relatively small surface area so that 2 or 3 pads may be needed.[5] When bilirubin levels are extremely high and must be lowered as rapidly as possible, it is essential to expose as much of the infant's surface area to phototherapy as possible. In these situations, additional surface-area exposure can be achieved by lining the sides of the bassinet with aluminum foil or a white cloth.[10]

In most circumstances, it is not necessary to remove the infant's diaper, but when bilirubin levels approach the exchange transfusion range, the diaper should be removed until there is clear evidence of a significant decline in the bilirubin level.

What Decline in the Serum Bilirubin Can You Expect?

The rate at which the bilirubin declines depends on the factors listed in Table 5, and different responses can be expected depending on the clinical circumstances. When bilirubin levels are extremely high (more than 30 mg/dL [513 μmol/L]), and intensive phototherapy is used, a decline of as much as 10 mg/dL (171 μmol/L) can occur within a few hours,[11] and a decrease of at least 0.5 to 1 mg/dL per hour can be expected in the first 4 to 8 hours.[12] On average, for infants of more than 35 weeks' gestation readmitted for phototherapy, intensive phototherapy can produce a decrement of 30% to 40% in the initial bilirubin level by 24 hours after initiation of phototherapy.[13] The most significant decline will occur in the first 4 to 6 hours. With standard phototherapy systems, a decrease of 6% to 20% of the initial bilirubin level can be expected in the first 24 hours.[8,14]

Intermittent Versus Continuous Phototherapy

Clinical studies comparing intermittent with continuous phototherapy have produced conflicting results.[15–17] Because all light exposure increases bilirubin excretion (compared with darkness), no plausible scientific rationale exists for using intermittent phototherapy. In most circumstances, however, phototherapy does not need to be continuous. Phototherapy may be interrupted during feeding or brief parental visits. Individual judgment should be exercised. If the infant's bilirubin level is approaching the exchange transfusion zone (Fig 4), phototherapy should be administered continuously until a satisfactory decline in the serum bilirubin level occurs or exchange transfusion is initiated.

Hydration

There is no evidence that excessive fluid administration affects the serum bilirubin concentration. Some infants who are admitted with high bilirubin levels are also mildly dehydrated and may need supplemental fluid intake to correct their dehydration. Because these infants are almost always breast-fed, the best fluid to use in these circumstances is a milk-based formula, because it inhibits the enterohepatic circulation of bilirubin and should help to lower the serum bilirubin level. Because the photo-products responsible for the decline in serum bilirubin are excreted in urine and bile,[18] maintaining adequate hydration and good urine output should help to improve the efficacy of phototherapy. Unless there is evidence of dehydration, however, routine intravenous fluid or other supplementation (eg, with dextrose water) of term and near-term infants receiving phototherapy is not necessary.

When Should Phototherapy Be Stopped?

There is no standard for discontinuing phototherapy. The TSB level for discontinuing phototherapy depends on the age at which phototherapy is initiated and the cause of the hyperbilirubinemia.[13] For infants who are readmitted after their birth hospitalization (usually for TSB levels of 18 mg/dL [308 μmol/L] or higher), phototherapy may be discontinued when the serum bilirubin level falls below 13 to 14 mg/dL (239-239 μmol/L). Discharge from the hospital need not be delayed to observe the infant for rebound.[13,19,20] If phototherapy is used for infants with hemolytic diseases or is initiated early and discontinued before the infant is 3 to 4 days old, a follow-up bilirubin measurement within 24 hours after discharge is recommended.[13] For infants who are readmitted with hyperbilirubinemia and then discharged, significant rebound is rare, but a repeat TSB measurement or clinical follow-up 24 hours after discharge is a clinical option.[13]

Home Phototherapy

Because the devices available for home phototherapy may not provide the same degree of irradiance or surface-area exposure as those available in the hospital, home phototherapy should be used only in infants whose bilirubin levels are in the "optional phototherapy" range (Fig 3); it is not appropriate for infants with higher bilirubin concentrations. As with hospitalized infants, it is essential that serum bilirubin levels be monitored regularly.

Sunlight Exposure

In their original description of phototherapy, Cremer et al[21] demonstrated that exposure of newborns to sunlight would lower the serum bilirubin level. Although sunlight provides sufficient irradiance in the 425- to 475-nm band to provide phototherapy, the practical difficulties involved in safely exposing a naked newborn to the sun either inside or outside (and avoiding sunburn) preclude the use of sunlight as a reliable therapeutic tool, and it therefore is not recommended.

Complications

Phototherapy has been used in millions of infants for more than 30 years, and reports of significant toxicity are exceptionally rare. Nevertheless, phototherapy in hospital separates mother and infant, and eye patching is disturbing to parents. The most important, but uncommon, clinical complication occurs in infants with cholestatic jaundice. When these infants are exposed to phototherapy, they may develop a dark, grayish-brown discoloration of the skin, serum, and urine (the bronze infant syndrome).[22] The pathogenesis of this syndrome is unknown, but it may be related to an accumulation of porphyrins and other metabolites in the plasma of infants who develop cholestasis.[22,23] Although it occurs exclusively in infants with cholestasis, not all infants with cholestatic jaundice develop the syndrome.

This syndrome generally has had few deleterious consequences, and if there is a need for phototherapy, the presence of direct hyperbilirubinemia should not be considered a contraindication to its use. This is particularly important in sick neonates. Because the products of phototherapy are excreted in the bile, the presence of cholestasis will decrease the efficacy of phototherapy. Nevertheless, infants with direct hyperbilirubinemia often show some response to phototherapy. In infants receiving phototherapy who develop the bronze infant syndrome, exchange transfusion should be considered if the TSB is in the intensive phototherapy range and phototherapy does not promptly lower the TSB. Because of the paucity of data, firm recommendations cannot be made. Note, however, that the direct serum bilirubin should not be subtracted from the TSB concentration in making decisions about exchange transfusions (see Fig 4).

Rarely, purpura and bullous eruptions have been described in infants with severe cholestatic jaundice receiving phototherapy,[24,25] and severe blistering and photosensitivity during phototherapy have occurred in infants with congenital erythropoietic porphyria.[26,27] Congenital porphyria or a family history of porphyria is an absolute contraindication to the use of phototherapy, as is the concomitant use of drugs or agents that are photosensitizers.[28]

REFERENCES

1. Maisels MJ. Phototherapy—traditional and nontraditional. *J Perinatol.* 2001;21(suppl 1):S93–S97
2. Fiberoptic phototherapy systems. *Health Devices.* 1995;24:132–153
3. International Electrotechnical Commission. Medical electrical equipment—part 2-50: particular requirements for the safety of infant phototherapy equipment. 2000. IEC 60601-2-50. Available at www.iec.ch. Accessed June 7, 2004
4. Tan KL. The pattern of bilirubin response to phototherapy for neonatal hyperbilirubinemia. *Pediatr Res.* 1982;16:670–674
5. Maisels MJ. Why use homeopathic doses of phototherapy? *Pediatrics.* 1996;98:283–287
6. Seidman DS, Moise J, Ergaz Z, et al. A new blue light-emitting phototherapy device: a prospective randomized controlled study. *J Pediatr.* 2000;136:771–774
7. Ennever JF. Blue light, green light, white light, more light: treatment of neonatal jaundice. *Clin Perinatol.* 1990;17:467–481
8. Garg AK, Prasad RS, Hifzi IA. A controlled trial of high-intensity double-surface phototherapy on a fluid bed versus conventional phototherapy in neonatal jaundice. *Pediatrics.* 1995;95:914–916
9. Tan KL. Phototherapy for neonatal jaundice. *Clin Perinatol.* 1991;18:423–439
10. Eggert P, Stick C, Schroder H. On the distribution of irradiation intensity in phototherapy. Measurements of effective irradiance in an incubator. *Eur J Pediatr.* 1984;142:58–61
11. Hansen TW. Acute management of extreme neonatal jaundice—the potential benefits of intensified phototherapy and interruption of enterohepatic bilirubin circulation. *Acta Paediatr.* 1997;86:843–846
12. Newman TB, Liljestrand P, Escobar GJ. Infants with bilirubin levels of 30 mg/dL or more in a large managed care organization. *Pediatrics.* 2003;111(6 Pt 1):1303–1311
13. Maisels MJ, Kring E. Bilirubin rebound following intensive phototherapy. *Arch Pediatr Adolesc Med.* 2002;156:669–672
14. Tan KL. Comparison of the efficacy of fiberoptic and conventional phototherapy for neonatal hyperbilirubinemia. *J Pediatr.* 1994;125:607–612
15. Rubaltelli FF, Zanardo V, Granati B. Effect of various phototherapy regimens on bilirubin decrement. *Pediatrics.* 1978;61:838–841
16. Maurer HM, Shumway CN, Draper DA, Hossaini AA. Controlled trial comparing agar, intermittent phototherapy, and continuous phototherapy for reducing neonatal hyperbilirubinemia. *J Pediatr.* 1973;82:73–76
17. Lau SP, Fung KP. Serum bilirubin kinetics in intermittent phototherapy of physiological jaundice. *Arch Dis Child.* 1984;59:892–894
18. McDonagh AF, Lightner DA. 'Like a shrivelled blood orange'—bilirubin, jaundice, and phototherapy. *Pediatrics.* 1985;75:443–455
19. Yetman RJ, Parks DK, Huseby V, Mistry K, Garcia J. Rebound bilirubin levels in infants receiving phototherapy. *J Pediatr.* 1998;133:705–707
20. Lazar L, Litwin A, Merlob P. Phototherapy for neonatal nonhemolytic hyperbilirubinemia. Analysis of rebound and indications for discontinuing therapy. *Clin Pediatr (Phila).* 1993;32:264–267
21. Cremer RJ, Perryman PW, Richards DH. Influence of light on the hyperbilirubinemia of infants. *Lancet.* 1958;1(7030):1094–1097
22. Rubaltelli FF, Jori G, Reddi E. Bronze baby syndrome: a new porphyrin-related disorder. *Pediatr Res.* 1983;17:327–330
23. Meisel P, Jahrig D, Theel L, Ordt A, Jahrig K. The bronze baby syndrome: consequence of impaired excretion of photobilirubin? *Photobiochem Photobiophys.* 1982;3:345–352
24. Mallon E, Wojnarowska F, Hope P, Elder G. Neonatal bullous eruption as a result of transient porphyrinemia in a premature infant with hemolytic disease of the newborn. *J Am Acad Dermatol.* 1995;33:333–336
25. Paller AS, Eramo LR, Farrell EE, Millard DD, Honig PJ, Cunningham BB. Purpuric phototherapy-induced eruption in transfused neonates: relation to transient porphyrinemia. *Pediatrics.* 1997;100:360–364
26. Tonz O, Vogt J, Filippini L, Simmler F, Wachsmuth ED, Winterhalter KH. Severe light dermatosis following phototherapy in a newborn infant with congenital erythropoietic urophyria [in German]. *Helv Paediatr Acta.* 1975;30:47–56
27. Soylu A, Kavukcu S, Turkmen M. Phototherapy sequela in a child with congenital erythropoietic porphyria. *Eur J Pediatr.* 1999;158:526–527
28. Kearns GL, Williams BJ, Timmons OD. Fluorescein phototoxicity in a premature infant. *J Pediatr.* 1985;107:796–798

All clinical practice guidelines from the American Academy of Pediatrics automatically expire 5 years after publication unless reaffirmed, revised, or retired at or before that time.

ERRATUM

Two errors appeared in the American Academy of Pediatrics clinical practice guideline, titled "Management of Hyperbilirubinemia in the Newborn Infant 35 or More Weeks of Gestation," that was published in the July 2004 issue of *Pediatrics* (2004;114:297–316). On page 107, Background section, first paragraph, the second sentence should read: "The current guideline represents a consensus of the committee charged by the AAP with reviewing and updating the existing guideline and is based on a careful review of the evidence, including a comprehensive literature review by the Agency for Healthcare Research and Quality and the New England Medical Center Evidence-Based Practice Center.[2]" On page 118, Appendix 1, first paragraph, the 4 levels of evidence quality should have been labeled A, B, C, and D rather than 1, 2, 3, and 4, respectively. The American Academy of Pediatrics regrets these errors.

PREFACE

Technical Report Summary:
An Evidence-Based Review of Important Issues Concerning Neonatal Hyperbilirubinemia

Authors:

Stanley Ip, MD; Mei Chung, MPH; John Kulig, MD, MPH; Rebecca O'Brien, MD; Robert Sege, MD, PhD; Stephan Glicken, MD; M. Jeffrey Maisels, MB, BCh; and Joseph Lau, MD, and the Subcommittee on Hyperbilirubinemia

American Academy of Pediatrics
PO Box 927, 141 Northwest Point Blvd
Elk Grove Village, IL 60009-0927

ABSTRACT. This article is adapted from a published evidence report concerning neonatal hyperbilirubinemia with an added section on the risk of blood exchange transfusion (BET). Based on a summary of multiple case reports that spanned more than 30 years, we conclude that kernicterus, although infrequent, has at least 10% mortality and at least 70% long-term morbidity. It is evident that the preponderance of kernicterus cases occurred in infants with a bilirubin level higher than 20 mg/dL. Given the diversity of conclusions on the relationship between peak bilirubin levels and behavioral and neurodevelopmental outcomes, it is apparent that the use of a single total serum bilirubin level to predict long-term outcomes is inadequate and will lead to conflicting results. Evidence for efficacy of treatments for neonatal hyperbilirubinemia was limited. Overall, the 4 qualifying studies showed that phototherapy had an absolute risk-reduction rate of 10% to 17% for prevention of serum bilirubin levels higher than 20 mg/dL in healthy infants with jaundice. There is no evidence to suggest that phototherapy for neonatal hyperbilirubinemia has any long-term adverse neurodevelopmental effects. Transcutaneous measurements of bilirubin have a linear correlation to total serum bilirubin and may be useful as screening devices to detect clinically significant jaundice and decrease the need for serum bilirubin determinations. Based on our review of the risks associated with BETs from 15 studies consisting mainly of infants born before 1970, we conclude that the mortality within 6 hours of BET ranged from 3 per 1000 to 4 per 1000 exchanged infants who were term and without serious hemolytic diseases. Regardless of the definitions and rates of BET-associated morbidity and the various pre-ex-change clinical states of the exchanged infants, in many cases the morbidity was minor (eg, postexchange anemia). Based on the results from the most recent study to report BET morbidity, the overall risk of permanent sequelae in 25 sick infants who survived BET was from 5% to 10%.

The American Academy of Pediatrics (AAP) requested an evidence report from the Agency for Healthcare Research and Quality (AHRQ) that would critically examine the available evidence regarding the effect of high levels of bilirubin on behavioral and neurodevelopmental outcomes, role of various comorbid effect modifiers (eg, sepsis and hemolysis) on neurodevelopment, efficacy of phototherapy, reliability of various strategies in predicting significant hyperbilirubinemia, and accuracy of transcutaneous bilirubin (TcB) measurements. The report was used by the AAP to update the 1994 AAP guidelines for the management of neonatal hyperbilirubinemia. This review focuses on otherwise healthy term or near-term (at least 34 weeks' estimated gestational age [EGA] or at least 2500 g birth weight) infants with hyperbilirubinemia. This article is adapted from that published report with an added section on the risk of blood exchange transfusion (BET).

Neither hyperbilirubinemia nor kernicterus are reportable diseases, and there are no reliable sources of information providing national annual estimates. Since the advent of effective prevention of rhesus (Rh) incompatibility and treatment of elevated bilirubin levels with phototherapy, kernicterus has become uncommon. When

laboratory records of a 1995–1996 birth cohort of more than 50 000 California infants were examined, Newman et al reported that 2% had total serum bilirubin (TSB) levels higher than 20 mg/dL, 0.15% had levels higher than 25 mg/dL, and only 0.01% had levels higher than 30 mg/dL. (These data were from infants with clinically identified hyperbilirubinemia and, as such, represent a minimum estimate of the true incidence of extreme hyperbilirubinemia.) This is undoubtedly the result of successful prevention of hemolytic anemia and the application of effective treatment of elevated serum bilirubin levels in accordance with currently accepted medical practice. Projecting the California estimates to the national birth rate of 4 million per year, one can predict 80 000, 6000, and 400 newborns per year with bilirubin levels of more than 20, 25, and 30 mg/dL, respectively.

Recently, concern has been expressed that the increase in early hospital discharges, coupled with a rise in breast-feeding rates, has led to a rise in the rate of preventable kernicterus resulting from "unattended to" hyperbilirubinemia. However, a report published in 2002, based on a national registry established since 1992, reported only 90 cases of kernicterus, although the efficiency of case ascertainment is not clear. Thus, there are no data to establish incidence trends reliably for either hyperbilirubinemia or kernicterus.

Despite these constraints, there has been substantial research on the neurodevelopmental outcomes of hyperbilirubinemia and its prediction and treatment. Subsequent sections of this review describe in more detail the precise study questions and the existing published work in this area.

METHODOLOGY

This evidence report is based on a systematic review of the medical literature. Our Evidence-Based Practice Center formed a review team consisting of pediatricians and Evidence-Based Practice Center methodologic staff to review the literature and perform data abstraction and analysis. For details regarding methodology, please see the original AHRQ report.

Key Questions

Question 1: What is the relationship between peak bilirubin levels and/or duration of hyperbilirubinemia and neurodevelopmental outcome?
Question 2: What is the evidence for effect modification of the results in question 1 by GA, hemolysis, serum albumin, and other factors? Question 3: What are the quantitative estimates of efficacy of treatment for 1) reducing peak bilirubin levels (eg, number needed to treat [NNT] at 20 mg/dL to keep TSB from rising); 2) reducing the duration of hyperbilirubinemia (eg, average number of hours by which time TSB is higher than 20 mg/dL may be shortened by treatment); and 3) improving neurodevelopmental outcomes?
Question 4: What is the efficacy of various strategies for predicting hyperbilirubinemia, including hour-specific bilirubin percentiles? Question 5: What is the accuracy of TcB measurements?

Search Strategies

We searched the Medline database on September 25, 2001, for publications from 1966 to the present using relevant medical subject heading terms ("hyperbilirubinemia"; "hyperbilirubinemia, hereditary"; "bilirubin"; "jaundice, neonatal"; and "kernicterus") and text words ("bilirubin,""hyperbilirubinemia,""jaundice," "kernicterus,"and "neonatal"). The abstracts were limited to human subjects and English-language studies focusing on newborns between birth and 1 month of age. In addition, the same text words used for the Medline search were used to search the Pre-Medline database. The strategy yielded 4280 Medline and 45 Pre-Medline abstracts. We consulted domain experts and examined relevant review articles for additional studies. A supplemental search for case reports of kernicterus in reference lists of relevant articles and reviews was performed also.

Screening and Selection Process

In our preliminary screening of abstracts, we identified more than 600 potentially relevant articles in total for questions 1, 2, and 3. To handle this large number of articles, we devised the following scheme to address the key questions and ensure that the report was completed within the time and resource constraints. We included only studies that measured neurodevelopmental or behavioral outcomes (except for question 3, part 1, for which we evaluated all studies addressing the efficacy of treatment). For the specific question of quantitative estimates of efficacy of treatment, all studies concerning therapies designed to prevent hyperbilirubinemia (generally bilirubin greater than or equal to 20 mg/dL) were included in the review.

Inclusion Criteria

The target population of this review was healthy, term infants. For the purpose of this review, we included articles concerning infants who were at least 34 weeks' EGA at the time of birth. From studies that reported birth weight rather than age, infants whose birth weight was greater than or equal to 2500 g were included. This cutoff was derived from findings of the National Institute of Child Health and Human Development (NICHD) hyperbilirubinemia study, in which none of the 1339 infants weighing greater than or equal to 2500 g were less than 34 weeks' EGA. Articles were selected for inclusion in the systematic review based on the following additional criteria:

Question 1 or 2 (Risk Association)

- Population: infants greater than or equal to 34 weeks' EGA or birth weight greater than or equal to 2500 g.
- Sample size: more than 5 subjects per arm
- Predictors: jaundice or hyperbilirubinemia
- Outcomes: at least 1 behavioral/neurodevelopmental outcome reported in the article
- Study design: prospective cohorts (more than 2 arms), prospective cross-sectional study, prospective longitudinal study, prospective single-arm study, or retrospective cohorts (more than 2 arms)

Case Reports of Kernicterus

- Population: kernicterus case
- Study design: case reports with kernicterus as a predictor or an outcome

Kernicterus, as defined by authors, included any of the following: acute phase of kernicterus (poor feeding, lethargy, high-pitched cry, increased tone, opisthotonos, or seizures), kernicterus sequelae (motor delay, sensorineural hearing loss, gaze palsy, dental dysplasia, cerebral palsy, or mental retardation), necropsy finding of yellow staining in the brain nuclei.

Question 3 (Efficacy of Treatment at Reducing Serum Bilirubin)

- Population: infants greater than or equal to 34 weeks' EGA or birth weight greater than or equal to 2500 g
- Sample size: more than 10 subjects per arm
- Treatments: any treatment for neonatal hyperbilirubinemia
- Outcomes: serum bilirubin level higher than or equal to 20 mg/dL or frequency of BET specifically for bilirubin level higher than or equal to 20 mg/dL
- Study design: randomized or nonrandomized, controlled trials

For All Other Issues

- Population: infants greater than or equal to 34 weeks' EGA or birth weight greater than or equal to 2500 g
- Sample size: more than 10 subjects per arm for phototherapy; any sample size for other treatments
- Treatments: any treatment for neonatal hyperbilirubinemia
- Outcomes: at least 1 neurodevelopmental outcome was reported in the article

Question 4 or 5 (Diagnosis)

- Population: infants greater than or equal to 34 weeks' EGA or birth weight greater than or equal to 2500 g
- Sample size: more than 10 subjects
- Reference standard: laboratory-based TSB

Exclusion Criteria

Case reports of kernicterus were excluded if they did not report serum bilirubin level or GA and birth weight.

Results of Screening of Titles and Abstracts

There were 158, 174, 99, 153, and 79 abstracts for questions 1, 2, 3, 4, and 5, respectively. Some articles were relevant to more than 1 question.

Results of Screening of Full-Text Articles

After full-text screening (according to the inclusion and exclusion criteria described previously), 138 retrieved articles were included in this report. There were 35 articles in the correlation section (questions 1 and 2), 28 articles of kernicterus case reports, 21 articles in the treatment section (question 3), and 54 articles in the diagnosis section (questions 4 and 5). There were inevitable overlaps, because treatment effects and assessment of neurodevelopmental outcomes were inherent in many study designs.

Reporting the Results

Articles that passed the full-text screening were grouped according to topic and analyzed in their entirety. Extracted data were synthesized into evidence tables.

Summarizing the Evidence of Individual Studies

Grading of the evidence can be useful for indicating the overall methodologic quality of a study. The evidence-grading scheme used here assesses 4 dimensions that are important for the proper interpretation of the evidence: study size, applicability, summary of results, and methodologic quality.

Definitions of Terminology

- Confounders (for question 1 only): 1) An ideal study design to answer question 1 would follow 2 groups, jaundiced and normal infants, without treating any infant for a current or consequent jaundice condition and observe their neurodevelopmental outcomes. Therefore, any treatment received by the subjects in the study was defined as a confounder. 2) If subjects had known risk factors for jaundice such as prematurity, breastfeeding, or low birth weight, the risk factors were defined as confounders. 3) Any disease condition other than jaundice was defined as a confounder. 4) Because bilirubin level is the essential predictor, if the study did not report or measure bilirubin levels for the subjects, lack of bilirubin measurements was defined as a confounder.
- Acute phase of kernicterus: poor feeding, lethargy, high-pitched cry, increased tone, opisthotonos, or seizures.
- Chronic kernicterus sequelae: motor delay, sensorineural hearing loss, gaze palsy, dental dysplasia, cerebral palsy, or mental retardation.

Statistical Analyses

In this report, 2 statistical analyses were performed in which there were sufficient data: the NNT and receiver operating characteristics (ROC) curve.

NNT

The NNT can be a clinically meaningful metric to assess the benefits of clinical trials. It is calculated by taking the inverse of the absolute risk difference. The absolute risk difference is the difference between the event rates between the treatment and control groups. For example, if the event rate is 15% in the control group and 10% in the treatment group, the absolute risk difference is 5% (an absolute risk reduction of 5%). The NNT then would be 20 (1 divided by 0.05), meaning that 20 patients will need to be treated to see 1 fewer event. In the setting of neonatal hyperbilirubinemia, NNT might be interpreted as the number of newborns needed to be treated (with phototherapy) at 13 to 15 mg/dL to prevent 1 newborn from reaching 20 mg/dL.

ROC Curve

ROC curves were developed for individual studies in question 4 if multiple thresholds of a diagnostic technology were reported. The areas under the curves (AUCs) were calculated to provide an assessment of the overall accuracy of the tests.

Meta-analyses of Diagnostic Test Performance

Meta-analyses were performed to quantify the TcB measurements for which the data were sufficient. We used 3 complementary methods for assessing diagnostic test performance: summary ROC analysis, independently combined sensitivity and specificity values, and meta-analysis of correlation coefficients.

RESULTS

Question 1. What Is the Relationship Between Peak Bilirubin Levels and/or Duration of Hyperbilirubinemia and Neurodevelopmental Outcome?

The first part of the results for this question deals with kernicterus; the second part deals with otherwise healthy term or near-term infants who had hyperbilirubinemia.

Case Reports of Kernicterus

Our literature search identified 28 case-report articles of infants with kernicterus that reported sufficient data for analysis. (The largest case series of 90 healthy term and near-term infants with kernicterus was reported by Johnson et al in 2002, but no individual data were available and therefore were not included in this analysis.

Those cases with available individual data previously reported were included in this analysis.) Most of the articles were identified in Medline and published since 1966. We retrieved additional articles published before 1966 based on review of references in articles published since 1966. Our report focuses on term and near-term infants (greater than or equal to 34 weeks' EGA). Only infants with measured peak bilirubin level and known GA or birth weight or with clinical or autop-sy-diagnosed kernicterus were included in the analysis. It is important to note that some of these peak levels were obtained more than 7 days after birth and therefore may not have represented true peak levels. Similarly, some of the diagnoses of kernicterus were made only at autopsies, and the measured bilirubin levels were obtained more than 24 hours before the infants died, and therefore the reported bilirubin levels may not have reported the true peak levels. Because of the small number of subjects, none of the following comparisons are statistically significant. Furthermore, because case reports in this section represent highly selected cases, interpreting these data must be done cautiously.

Demographics of Kernicterus Cases

Articles identified through the search strategy span from 1955 to 2001 with a total of 123 cases of kernicterus. Twelve cases in 2 studies were reported before 1960; however, some studies reported cases that spanned almost 2 decades. Data on subjects' birth years were reported in only 55 cases. Feeding status, gender, racial background, and ethnicity were not noted in most of the reports. Of those that were reported, almost all the subjects were breastfed and most were males.

Geographic Distribution of Reported Kernicterus Cases

The 28 case reports with a total of 123 cases are from 14 different countries. They are the United States, Singapore, Turkey, Greece, Taiwan, Denmark, Canada, Japan, United Kingdom, France, Jamaica, Norway, Scotland, and Germany. The number of kernicterus cases in each study ranged from 1 to 12.

Kernicterus has been defined by pathologic findings, acute clinical findings, and chronic sequelae (such as deafness or athetoid cerebral palsy). Because of the small number of subjects, all definitions of kernicterus have been included in the analysis. Exceptions will be noted in the following discussion.

Kernicterus Cases With Unknown Etiology

Among infants at greater than or equal to 34 weeks' GA or who weighed 2500 g or more at birth and had no known explanation for kernicterus, there were 35 infants with peak bilirubin ranging from 22.5 to 54 mg/dL. Fifteen had no information on gender, 14 were males, and 6 were females. Fourteen had no information on feeding,

20 were breastfed, and 1 was formula-fed. More than 90% of the infants with kernicterus had bilirubin higher than 25 mg/dL: 25% of the kernicterus cases had peak TSB levels up to 29.9 mg/dL, and 50% had peak TSB levels up to 34.9 mg/dL (Fig 2). There was no association between bilirubin level and birth weight.

Four infants died. Four infants who had acute clinical kernicterus had normal follow-up at 3 to 6 years by telephone. One infant with a peak bilirubin level of 44 mg/dL had a flat brainstem auditory evoked response (BAER) initially but normalized at 2 months of age; this infant had normal neurologic and developmental examinations at 6 months of age. Ten infants had chronic sequelae of kernicterus when followed up between 6 months and 7 years of age. Seven infants were noted to have neurologic findings consistent with kernicterus; however, the age at diagnosis was not provided. Nine infants had a diagnosis of kernicterus with no follow-up information provided. To summarize, 11% of this group of infants died, 14% survived with no sequelae, and at least 46% had chronic sequelae. The distribution of peak TSB levels was higher when only infants who died or had chronic sequelae were included.

Kernicterus Cases With Comorbid Factors

In the 88 term and near-term infants diagnosed with kernicterus and who had hemolysis, sepsis, and other neonatal complications, bilirubin levels ranged from 4.0 to 51.0 mg/dL (as previously mentioned, these may not represent true peak levels; the bilirubin level of 4 mg/dL was measured more than 24 hours before the infant died, the diagnosis of kernicterus was made by autopsy). Forty-two cases provided no information on gender, 25 were males, and 21 were females. Seventy-two cases had no information on feeding, 15 were breastfed, and 1 was formula-fed. Most infants with kernicterus had bilirubin levels higher than 20 mg/dL: 25% of the kernicterus cases had peak TSB levels up to 24.9 mg/dL, and 50% had peak TSB levels up to 29.9 mg/dL (Fig 4). In this group, there was no association between the bilirubin levels and birth weight.

Five infants without clinical signs of kernicterus were diagnosed with kernicterus by autopsy. Eight infants died of kernicterus. One infant was found to have a normal neurologic examination at 4 months of age. Another infant with galactosemia and a bilirubin level of 43.6 mg/dL who had acute kernicterus was normal at 5 months of age. Forty-nine patients had chronic sequelae ranging from hearing loss to athetoid cerebral palsy; the follow-up age reported ranged from 4 months to 14 years. Twenty-one patients were diagnosed with kernicterus, with no fol-low-up information. Not including the autopsy-diagnosed kernicterus, 10% of these infants died (8/82), 2% were found to be normal at 4 to 5 months of age, and

at least 60% had chronic sequelae. The distribution of peak TSB levels was slightly higher when only infants who died or had chronic sequelae were included.

Evidence Associating Bilirubin Exposures With Neurodevelopmental Outcomes in Healthy Term or Near-Term Infants

This section examines the evidence associating bilirubin exposures with neurodevelopmental outcomes primarily in subjects without kernicterus. Studies that were designed specifically to address the behavioral and neurodevelopmental outcomes in healthy infants at more than or equal to 34 weeks' GA will be discussed first. With the exception of the results from the Collaborative Perinatal Project (CPP) (CPP, with 54 795 subjects, has generated many follow-up studies with a smaller number of subjects, and those studies were discussed together in a separate section in the AHRQ summary report), the remainder of the studies that include mixed subjects (preterm and term, diseased and nondiseased) were categorized and discussed by outcome measures. These measures include behavioral and neurologic outcomes; hearing impairment, including sensorineural hearing loss; and intelligence measurements.

The CPP, with 54 795 live births between 1959 and 1966 from 12 centers in the United States, produced the largest database for the study of hyperbilirubinemia. Newman and Klebanoff, focusing only on black and white infants weighing 2500 g or more at birth, did a comprehensive analysis of 7-year outcome in 33 272 subjects. All causes of jaundice were included in the analysis. The study found no consistent association between peak bilirubin level and intelligence quotient (IQ). Sensorineural hearing loss was not related to bilirubin level. Only the frequency of abnormal or suspicious neurologic examinations was associated with bilirubin level. The specific neurologic examination items most associated with bilirubin levels were mild and nonspecific motor abnormalities.

In other studies stemming from the CPP population, there was no consistent evidence to suggest neurologic abnormalities in children with neonatal bilirubin higher than 20 mg/dL when followed up to 7 years of age.

A question that has concerned pediatricians for many years is whether moderate hyperbilirubinemia is associated with abnormalities in neurodevelopmental outcome in term healthy infants without perinatal or neonatal problems. Only 4 prospective studies and 1 retrospective study have the requisite subject characteristics to address this issue. Although there were some short-term (less than 12 months) abnormal neurologic or behavioral characteristics noted in infants with high bilirubin, the studies had methodologic problems and did not show consistent results.

Evidence Associating Bilirubin Exposures With Neurodevelopmental Outcomes in All Infants

These studies consist of subjects who, in addition to healthy term newborns, might include newborns less than 34 weeks' GA and neonatal complications such as sepsis, respiratory distress, hemolytic disorders, and other factors. Nevertheless, some of the conclusions drawn might be applicable to a healthy term population. In these studies, greater emphasis will be placed on the reported results for the group of infants who were at greater than or equal to 34 weeks' EGA or weighed 2500 g or more at birth.

Studies Measuring Behavioral and Neurologic Outcomes in Infants With Hyperbilirubinemia

A total of 9 studies in 11 publications examined primarily behavioral and neurologic outcomes in patients with hyperbilirubinemia. Of these 9 studies, 3 were of high methodologic quality. One short-term study showed a correlation between bilirubin level and decreased scores on newborn behavioral measurements. One study found no difference in prevalence of central nervous system abnormalities at 4 years old if bilirubin levels were less than 20 mg/dL, but infants with bilirubin levels higher than 20 mg/dL had a higher prevalence of central nervous system abnormalities. Another study that followed infants with bilirubin levels higher than 16 mg/dL found no relationship between bilirubin and neurovisuomotor testing at 61 to 82 months of age. Although data reported in the remainder of the studies are of lower methodologic quality, there is a suggestion of abnormalities in neurodevelopmental screening tests in infants with bilirubin levels higher than 20 mg/dL, at least by the Denver Developmental Screening Test, when infants were followed up at 1 year of age. It seems that bilirubin levels higher than 20 mg/dL may have short-term (up to 1 year of age) adverse effects at least by the Denver Developmental Screening Test, but there is no strong evidence to suggest neurologic abnormalities in children with neonatal bilirubin levels higher than 20 mg/dL when followed up to 7 years of age.

Effect of Bilirubin on Brainstem Auditory Evoked Potential (BAEP)

The following group of studies, in 14 publications, primarily examined the effect of bilirubin on BAEP or hearing impairment. Eight high-quality studies showed a significant relationship between abnormalities in BAEP and high bilirubin levels. Most reported resolution of abnormalities with treatment. Three studies reported hearing impairment associated with elevated bilirubin (higher than 16–20 mg/dL).

Effect of Bilirubin on Intelligence Outcomes

Eight studies looked primarily at the effect of bilirubin on intelligence outcomes. Four high-quality studies with follow-up ranging from 6.5 to 17 years reported no association between IQ and bilirubin level.

Question 2. What Is the Evidence for Effect Modification of the Results in Question 1 by GA, Hemolysis, Serum Albumin, and Other Factors?

There is only 1 article that directly addressed this question. Naeye, using the CPP population, found that at 4 years old the frequency of low IQ with increasing bilirubin levels increased more rapidly in infants with infected amniotic fluid. At 7 years old, neurologic abnormalities also were more prevalent in that subgroup of infants.

When comparing the group of term and near-term infants with comorbid factors who had kernicterus to the group of infants with idiopathic hyperbilirubinemia and kernicterus, the overall mean bilirubin was 31.6 ± 9 mg/dL in the former, versus 35.4 ± 8 mg/dL in the latter (difference not significant). Infants with glucose-6-phosphate dehydrogenase deficiency, sepsis, ABO incompatibility, or Rh incompatibility had similar mean bilirubin levels. Infants with more than 1 comorbid factor had a slightly lower mean bilirubin level of 29.1 ± 16.1 mg/dL.

Eighteen of 23 (78%) term infants with idiopathic hyperbilirubinemia and who developed acute kernicterus survived the neonatal period with chronic sequelae. Thirty-nine of 41 (95%) term infants with kernicterus and ABO or Rh incompatibility had chronic sequelae. Four of 5 (80%) infants with sepsis and kernicterus had chronic sequelae. All 4 infants with multiple comorbid factors had sequelae.

No firm conclusions can be drawn regarding co-morbid factors and kernicterus, because this is a small number of patients from a variety of case reports.

There was no direct study concerning serum albumin level as an effect modifier of neurodevelopmental outcome in infants with hyperbilirubinemia. One report found a significant association between reserve albumin concentration and latency to wave V in BAEP studies.

In addition, Ozmert et al noted that exchange transfusion and the duration that the infant's serum indirect bilirubin level remained higher than 20 mg/dL were important risk factors for prominent neurologic abnormalities.

Question 3. What Are the Quantitative Estimates of Efficacy of Treatment at 1) Reducing Peak Bilirubin Levels (eg, NNT at 20 mg/dL to Keep TSB From Rising); 2) Reducing the Duration of Hyperbilirubinemia (eg, Average Number of Hours by Which Time TSB Levels Higher Than 20 mg/dL May Be Shortened by Treatment); and 3) Improving Neurodevelopmental Outcomes?

Studies on phototherapy efficacy in terms of preventing TSB rising to the level that would require BET (and therefore would be considered "failure of phototherapy") were reviewed for the quantitative estimates of efficacy of phototherapy. Because trials evaluating the efficacy of phototherapy at improving neurodevelopmental outcomes by comparing 1 group of infants with treatment to an untreated group do not exist, the effects of treatment on neurodevelopmental outcomes could only be reviewed descriptively. Furthermore, all the reports primarily examined the efficacy of treatment at 15 mg/dL to prevent TSB from exceeding 20 mg/dL. There is no study to examine the efficacy of treatment at 20 mg/dL to prevent the TSB from rising.

Efficacy of Phototherapy for Prevention of TSB Levels Higher Than 20 mg/dL

Four publications examined the clinical efficacy of phototherapy for prevention of TSB levels higher than 20 mg/dL.

Two studies evaluated the same sample of infants. Both reports were derived from a randomized, controlled trial of phototherapy for neonatal hyperbilirubinemia commissioned by the NICHD between 1974 and 1976.

Because the phototherapy protocols differed significantly in the remaining studies, their results could not be statistically combined and are reported here separately. A total of 893 term or near-term jaundiced infants (325 in the treatment group and 568 in the control group) were evaluated in the current review.

The development, design, and sample composition of NICHD phototherapy trial were reported in detail elsewhere. The NICHD controlled trial of phototherapy for neonatal hyperbilirubinemia consisted of 672 infants who received phototherapy and 667 control infants. Brown et al evaluated the efficacy of phototherapy for prevention of the need for BET in the NICHD study population. For the purpose of current review, only the subgroup of 140 infants in the treatment groups and 136 in the control groups with birth weights 2500 g or more and greater than or equal to 34 weeks' GA were evaluated. The serum bilirubin level as criterion for BET in infants with birth weights of 2500 g or more was 20 mg/dL at standard risk and 18 mg/dL at high risk. It was found that infants with hyperbilirubinemia secondary to nonhemolytic causes who received phototherapy had a 14.3% risk reduction of BET than infants in no treatment group. NNT for prevention of the need for BET or for TSB levels higher than 20 mg/dL was 7 (95% confidence interval [CI]: 6–8). However, phototherapy did not reduce the need for BET for infants with hemolytic diseases or in the high-risk group. No therapeutic effect on reducing the BET rate in infants at greater than or equal to 34 weeks' GA with hemolytic disease was observed.

The same group of infants, 140 subjects in the treatment group and 136 controls with birth weights 2500 g or more and greater than or equal to 34 weeks' GA, were evaluated for the effect of phototherapy on the hyperbilirubinemia of Coombs' positive hemolytic disease in the study of Maurer et al. Of the 276 infants whose birth weights were 2500 g or more, 64 (23%) had positive Coombs' tests: 58 secondary to ABO incompatibility and 6 secondary to Rh incom-

patibility. Thirty-four of 64 in this group received phototherapy. The other 30 were placed in the control group. Of the 212 subjects who had negative Coombs' tests, 106 were in the treatment group and the same number was in the control group. No therapeutic effect on reducing the BET rate was observed in infants with Coombs' positive hemolytic disease, but there was a 9.4% absolute risk reduction in infants who had negative Coombs' tests. In this group of infants, the NNT for prevention of the need for BET, or a TSB higher than 20 mg/dL, was 11 (95% CI: 10–12).

A more recent randomized, controlled trial compared the effect of 4 different interventions on hyperbilirubinemia (serum bilirubin concentration greater than or equal to 291 µmol/L or 17 mg/dL) in 125 term breastfed infants. Infants with any congenital anomalies, neonatal complications, hematocrit more than 65%, significant bruising or large cephalohematomas, or hemolytic disease were excluded. The 4 interventions in the study were 1) continue breastfeeding and observe ($N = 25$); 2) discontinue breastfeeding and substitute formula ($N = 26$); 3) discontinue breastfeeding, substitute formula, and administer phototherapy ($N = 38$); and 4) continue breastfeeding and administer phototherapy ($N = 36$). The interventions were considered failures if serum bilirubin levels reached 324 µmol/L or 20 mg/dL. For the purpose of the current review, we regrouped the subjects into treatment group or phototherapy group and control group or no-phototherapy group. Therefore, the original groups 4 and 3 became the treatment groups I and II, and the original groups 1 and 2 were the corresponding control groups I and II. It was found that treatment I, phototherapy with continuation of breastfeeding, had a 10% absolute risk-reduction rate, and the NNT for prevention of a serum bilirubin level higher than 20 mg/dL was 10 (95% CI: 9–12). Compared with treatment I, treatment II (phototherapy with discontinuation of breastfeeding) was significantly more efficacious. The absolute risk-reduction rate was 17%, and the NNT for prevention of a serum bilirubin level exceeding 20 mg/dL was 6 (95% CI: 5–7).

John reported the effect of phototherapy in 492 term neonates born during 1971 and 1972 who developed unexplained jaundice with bilirubin levels higher than 15 mg/dL. One hundred eleven infants received phototherapy, and 381 did not. The author stated: "The choice of therapy was, in effect, random since two pediatricians approved of the treatment and two did not." The results showed that phototherapy had an 11% risk reduction of BET, performed in treatment and control groups when serum bilirubin levels exceeded 20 mg/dL. Therefore, the NNT for prevention of a serum bilirubin level higher than 20 mg/dL was 9 (95% CI: 8–10).

Regardless of different protocols for phototherapy, the NNT for prevention of serum bilirubin levels higher than 20 mg/dL ranged from 6 to 10 in healthy term or near-term infants. Evidence for the efficacy of treatments for neonatal hyperbilirubinemia was limited. Overall, the 4 qualifying studies showed that phototherapy had an absolute risk-reduction rate of 10% to 17% for prevention of serum bilirubin exceeding 20 mg/dL in healthy and jaundiced infants (TSB levels higher than or equal to 13 mg/dL) born at greater than or equal to 34 weeks' GA. Phototherapy combined with cessation of breastfeeding and substitution with formula was found to be the most efficient treatment protocol for healthy term or near-term infants with jaundice.

Effectiveness of Reduction in Bilirubin Level on BAER in Jaundiced Infants With Greater Than or Equal to 34 Weeks' EGA

Eight studies that compared BAER before and after treatments for neonatal hyperbilirubinemia are discussed in this section. Of the 8 studies, 3 studies treated jaundiced infants by administering phototherapy followed by BET according to different guidelines, 4 studies treated jaundiced infants with BET only, and 1 study did not specify what treatments jaundiced infants received. All the studies consistently showed that treatments for neonatal hyperbilirubinemia significantly improved abnormal BAERs in healthy jaundiced infants and jaundiced infants with hemolytic disease.

Effect of Phototherapy on Behavioral and Neurologic Outcomes and IQ

Five studies looked at the effect of hyperbilirubinemia and phototherapy on behavior. Of the 5 studies, 4 used the Brazelton Neonatal Behavioral Assessment Scale and 1 used the Vineland Social Maturity Scale. Three studies reported lower scores in the orientation cluster of the Brazelton Neonatal Behavioral Assessment Scale in the infants treated with phototherapy. The other 2 studies did not find behavioral changes in the phototherapy group. One study evaluated IQ at the age of 17 years. In 42 term infants with severe hyperbilirubinemia who were treated with phototherapy, 31 were also treated with BET. Forty-two infants who did not receive phototherapy were selected as controls. No significant difference in IQ between the 2 groups was found.

Effect of Phototherapy on Visual Outcomes

Three studies were identified that studied the effect of serum bilirubin and treatment on visual outcomes. All showed no short- or long-term (up to 36 months) effect on vision as a result of phototherapy when infants' eyes are protected properly during treatment.

Question 4. What Is the Accuracy of Various Strategies for Predicting Hyperbilirubinemia, Including Hour-Specific Bilirubin Percentiles?

Ten qualifying studies published from 1977 to 2001 examining 5 prediction methods of neonatal hyperbilirubinemia were included. A total of 8167 neonates, most healthy near-term or term infants, were subjects. These studies were conducted among multiple racial groups in multiple countries including China, Denmark, India, Israel, Japan, Spain, and the United States. Some studies included subjects with ABO incompatibility, and some did not. Four studies examined the accuracy of cord bilirubin level as a test for predicting the development of clinically significant neonatal jaundice. Four studies investigated the test performance of serum bilirubin levels before 48 hours of life to predict hyperbilirubinemia. Two studies further compared the test performances of cord bilirubin with that of early serum bilirubin levels. The accuracy of end-tidal carbon monoxide concentration as a predictor of the development of hyperbilirubinemia was examined in Okuyama et al and Stevenson et al. The study by Stevenson et al also examined the test performance of a combined strategy of end-tidal carbon monoxide concentration and early serum bilirubin levels. Finally, 2 studies tested the efficacy of predischarge risk assessment, determined by a risk index model and hour-specific bilirubin percentile, respectively, for predicting neonatal hyperbilirubinemia.

ROC curves were developed for 3 of the predictive strategies. The AUCs were calculated to provide an assessment of the overall accuracy of the tests. Hour-specific bilirubin percentiles had an AUC of 0.93, cord bilirubin levels had an AUC of 0.74, and predischarge risk index had an AUC of 0.80. These numbers should not be compared directly with each other, because the studies had different population characteristics and different defining parameters for hyperbilirubinemia.

Question 5. What Is the Accuracy of TcB Measurements?

A total of 47 qualifying studies in 50 publications examining the test performance of TcB measurements and/or the correlation of TcB measurements to serum bilirubin levels was reviewed in this section. Of the 47 studies, the Minolta Air-Shields jaundice meter (Air-Shields, Hatboro, PA) was used in 41 studies, the BiliCheck (SpectRx Inc, Norcross, GA) was used in 3 studies, the Ingram icterometer (Thomas A. Ingram and Co, Birmingham, England; distributed in the United States by Cascade Health Care Products, Salem, OR) was used in 4 studies, and the ColorMate III (Chromatics Color Sciences International Inc, New York, NY) was used in 1 study.

Based on the evidence from the systematic review, TcB measurements by each of the 4 devices described in the literature (the Minolta Air-Shields jaundice meter, Ingram icterometer, BiliCheck, and Chromatics ColorMate

III) have a linear correlation to TSB and may be useful as screening devices to detect clinically significant jaundice and decrease the need for serum bilirubin determinations.

Minolta Air-Shields Jaundice Meter

Generally, TcB readings from the forehead or sternum have correlated well with TSB but with a wide range of correlation coefficients, from a low of 0.52 for subgroup of infants less than 37 weeks' GA to as high as 0.96. Comparison of correlations across studies is difficult because of differences in study design and selection procedures. TcB indices that correspond to various TSB levels vary from institution to institution but seem to be internally consistent. Different TSB threshold levels were used across studies; therefore, there is limited ability to combine data across the studies. Most of the studies used TcB measurements taken at the forehead, several studies used multiple sites and combined results, 1 study used only the midsternum site, and 3 studies took the TcB measurement at multiple sites.

The Minolta Air-Shields jaundice meter seems to perform less well in black infants, compared with white infants, performs best when measurements are made at the sternum, and performs less well when infants have been exposed to phototherapy. This instrument requires daily calibration, and each institution must develop its own correlation curves of TcB to TSB. Eleven studies of the test performance of the Minolta Air-Shields jaundice meter measuring at forehead to predict a serum bilirubin threshold of higher than or equal to 13 mg/dL were included in the following analysis. A total of 1560 paired TcB and serum bilirubin measurements were evaluated. The cutoff points of Minolta AirShields TcB measurements (TcB index) ranged from 13 to 24 for predicting a serum bilirubin level higher than or equal to 13 mg/dL. As a screening test, it does not perform consistently across studies, as evidenced by the heterogeneity in the summary ROC curves not explained by threshold effect. The overall unweighted pooled estimates of sensitivity and specificity were 0.85 (0.77–0.91) and 0.77 (0.66–0.85).

Ingram Icterometer

The Ingram icterometer consists of a strip of transparent Plexiglas on which 5 yellow transverse stripes of precise and graded hue are painted. The correlation coefficients (r) in the 4 studies ranged from 0.63 to 0.97. The icterometer has the added limitation of lacking the objectivity of the other methods, because it depends on observer visualization of depth of yellow color of the skin.

BiliCheck

The recently introduced BiliCheck device, which uses reflectance data from multiple wavelengths, seems to be a significant improvement over the older devices (the Ingram icterometer and the Minolta Air-Shields jaundice meter) because of its ability to determine correction factors for the effect of melanin and hemoglobin. Three studies examined the accuracy of the BiliCheck TcB measurements to predict TSB ("gold standard"). All studies were rated as high quality. The correlation coefficient ranged from 0.83 to 0.91. In 1 study, the BiliCheck was shown to be as accurate as the laboratory measurement of TSB when compared with the reference gold-standard high-performance liquid chromatography (HPLC) measurement of TSB. Analysis of covariance found no differences in test performance by postnatal age, GA, birth weight, or race; however, 66.7% were white and only 4.3% were black.

Chromatics ColorMate III

One study that evaluated the performance of the ColorMate III transcutaneous bilirubinometer was reviewed. The correlation coefficient for the whole study group was 0.9563, and accuracy was not affected by race, weight, or phototherapy. The accuracy of the device is increased by the determination of an infant's underlying skin type before the onset of visual jaundice; thus, a drawback to the method when used as a screening device is that all infants would require an initial baseline measurement.

CONCLUSIONS AND DISCUSSION

Summarizing case reports of kernicterus from different investigators in different countries from different periods is problematic. First, definitions of kernicterus used in these reports varied greatly. They included gross yellow staining of the brain, microscopic neuronal degeneration, acute clinical neuromotor impairment, neuroauditory impairment, and chronic neuromotor impairment. In some cases, the diagnoses were not established until months or years after birth. Second, case reports without controls makes interpretation difficult, especially in infants with comorbid factors, and could very well lead to misinterpretation of the role of bilirubin in neurodevelopmental outcomes. Third, different reports used different outcome measures. "Normal at follow-up" may be based on parental reporting, physician assessment, or formal neuropsychologic testing. Fourth, time of reported follow-up ranged from days to years. Fifth, cases were reported from different countries at different periods and with different standards of practice managing hyperbilirubinemia. Some countries have a high prevalence of glucose-6-phosphate dehydrogenase deficiency. Some have cultural practices that predispose their infants to agents that cause hyperbilirubinemia (such as clothing stored in dressers with naphthalene moth balls). The effect of the differences on outcomes cannot be known for certain. Finally, it is difficult to infer from case reports the true incidence of this uncommon disorder.

To recap our findings, based on a summary of multiple case reports that spanned more than 30 years, we conclude that kernicterus, although infrequent, has significant mortality (at least 10%) and long-term morbidity (at least

70%). It is evident that the preponderance of kernicterus cases occurred in infants with high bilirubin (more than 20 mg/dL).

Of 26 (19%) term or near-term infants with acute manifestations of kernicterus and reported follow-up data, 5 survived without sequelae, whereas only 3 of 63 (5%) infants with acute kernicterus and comorbid factors were reported to be normal at follow-up. This result suggests the importance of comorbid factors in determining long-term outcome in infants initially diagnosed with kernicterus.

For future research, reaching a national consensus in defining this entity, as in the model suggested by Johnson et al, will help in formulating a valid comparison of different databases. It is also apparent that, without good prevalence and incidence data on hyperbilirubinemia and kernicterus, one would not be able to estimate the risk of kernicterus at a given bilirubin level. Making severe hyperbilirubinemia (eg, greater than or equal to 25 mg/dL) and kernicterus reportable conditions would be a first step in that direction. Also, because kernicterus is infrequent, doing a multicenter case-control study with kernicterus may help to delineate the role of bilirubin in the development of kernicterus.

Hyperbilirubinemia, in most cases, is a necessary but not sufficient condition to explain kernicterus. Factors acting in concert with bilirubin must be studied to seek a satisfactory explanation. Information from duration of exposure to bilirubin and albumin binding of bilirubin may yield a more useful profile of the risk of kernicterus.

Only a few prospective controlled studies looked specifically at behavioral and neurodevelopmental outcomes in healthy term infants with hyperbilirubinemia. Most of these studies have a small number of subjects. Two short-term studies with well-defined measurement of newborn behavioral organization and physiologic measurement of cry are of high methodologic quality; however, the significance of long-term abnormalities in newborn behavior scales and variations in cry formant frequencies are unknown. There remains little information on the long-term effects of hyperbilirubinemia in healthy term infants.

Among the mixed studies (combined term and preterm, nonhemolytic and hemolytic, nondiseased and diseased), the following observations can be made:

- Nine of 15 studies (excluding the CPP) addressing neuroauditory development and bilirubin level were of high quality. Six of them showed BAER abnormalities correlated with high bilirubin levels. Most reported resolution with treatment. Three studies reported hearing impairment associated with elevated bilirubin (more than 16 to more than 20 mg/dL). We conclude that a high bilirubin level does have an adverse effect on neuroauditory function, but the adverse effect on BAER is reversible.

- Of the 8 studies reporting intelligence outcomes in subjects with hyperbilirubinemia, 4 studies were considered high quality. These 4 studies reported no association between IQ and bilirubin level, with follow-up ranging from 6.5 to 17 years. We conclude that there is no evidence to suggest a linear association of bilirubin level and IQ.

- The analysis of the CPP population found no consistent association between peak bilirubin level and IQ. Sensorineural hearing loss was not related to bilirubin level. Only the frequency of abnormal or suspicious neurologic examinations was associated with bilirubin level. In the rest of the studies from the CPP population, there was no consistent evidence to suggest neurologic abnormalities in children with neonatal bilirubin levels more than 20 mg/dL when followed up to 7 years of age.

A large prospective study comprising healthy infants greater than or equal to 34 weeks' GA with hyperbilirubinemia, specifically looking at long-term neurodevelopmental outcomes, has yet to be done. The report of Newman and Klebanoff came closest to that ideal because of the large number of subjects and the study's analytic approach. However, a population born from 1959 to 1966 is no longer representative of present-day newborns: 1) there is now increased ethnic diversity in our newborn population; 2) breast milk jaundice has become more common than hemolytic jaundice; 3) phototherapy for hyperbilirubinemia has become standard therapy; and 4) hospital stays are shorter. These changes in biologic, cultural, and health care characteristics make it difficult to apply the conclusions from the CPP population to present-day newborns.

Although short-term studies, in general, have good methodologic quality, they use tools that have unknown long-term predictive abilities. Long-term studies suffer from high attrition rates of the study population and a nonuniform approach to defining "normal neurodevelopmental outcomes." The total bilirubin levels reported in all the studies mentioned were measured anywhere from the first day of life to more than 2 weeks of life. Definitions of significant hyperbilirubinemia ranged from greater than or equal to 12 mg/dL to greater than or equal to 20 mg/dL.

Given the diversity of conclusions reported, except in cases of kernicterus with sequelae, it is evident that the use of a single TSB level (within the range described in this review) to predict long-term behavioral or neurodevelopmental outcomes is inadequate and will lead to conflicting results.

Evidence for the efficacy of treatments for neonatal hyperbilirubinemia was limited. Overall, the 4 qualifying studies showed that phototherapy had an absolute risk-reduction rate of 10% to 17% for prevention of serum bilirubin exceeding 20 mg/dL in healthy jaundiced infants

(TSB higher than or equal to 13 mg/dL) of greater than or equal to 34 weeks' GA. Phototherapy combined with cessation of breastfeeding and substitution with formula was found to be the most efficient treatment protocol for healthy term or near-term infants with jaundice. There is no evidence to suggest that phototherapy for neonatal hyperbilirubinemia has any long-term adverse neuro-developmental effects in either healthy jaundiced infants or infants with hemolytic disease. It is also noted that in all the studies listed, none of the infants received what is currently known as "intensive phototherapy." Although phototherapy did not reduce the need for BET in infants with hemolytic disease in the NICHD phototherapy trial, it could be attributable to the low dose of phototherapy used. Proper application of "intensive phototherapy" should decrease the need for BET further.

It is difficult to draw conclusions regarding the accuracy of various strategies for prediction of neonatal hyperbilirubinemia. The first challenge is the lack of consistency in defining clinically significant neonatal hyperbilirubinemia. Not only did multiple studies use different levels of TSB to define neonatal hyperbilirubinemia, but the levels of TSB defined as significant also varied by age, but age at TSB determination varied by study as well. For example, significant levels of TSB were defined as more than 11.7, more than or equal to 15, more than 15, more than 16, more than 17, and more than or equal to 25 mg/dL.

A second challenge is the heterogeneity of the study populations. The studies were conducted in many racial groups in different countries including China, Denmark, India, Israel, Japan, Spain, and the United States. Although infants were defined as healthy term and near-term newborns, these studies included neonates with potential for hemolysis from ABO-incompatible pregnancies as well as breastfed and bottle-fed infants (often not specified). Therefore, it is not possible to directly compare the different predicting strategies. However, all the strategies provided strong evidence that early jaundice predicts late jaundice.

Hour-specific bilirubin percentiles had an AUC of 0.93, implying great accuracy of this strategy. In that study, 2976 of 13 003 eligible infants had a postdischarge TSB measurement, as discussed by Maisels and Newman. Because of the large number of infants who did not have a postdischarge TSB, the actual study sample would be deficient in study participants with low predischarge bilirubin levels, leading to false high-sensitivity estimates and false low-specificity estimates. Moreover, the population in the study is not representative of the entire US population. The strategy of using early hour-specific bilirubin percentiles to predict late jaundice looks promising, but a large multicenter study (with evaluation of potential differences by race and ethnicity as well as prenatal, natal, and postnatal factors) may need to be undertaken to produce more applicable data.

TcB measurements by each of the 3 devices described in the literature, the Minolta Air-Shields jaundice meter, the Ingram icterometer, and the Bili-Check, have a linear correlation to TSB and may be useful as screening devices to detect clinically significant jaundice and decrease the need for serum bilirubin determinations.

The recently introduced BiliCheck device, which uses reflectance data from multiple wavelengths, seems to be a significant improvement over the older devices (the Ingram icterometer and the Minolta Air-Shields jaundice meter) because of its ability to determine correction factors for the effect of melanin and hemoglobin. In 1 study, the BiliCheck was shown to be as accurate as laboratory measures of TSB when compared with the reference gold-standard HPLC measurement of TSB.

Future research should confirm these findings in larger samples of diverse populations and address issues that might affect performance, such as race, GA, age at measurement, phototherapy, sunlight exposure, feeding and accuracy as screening instruments, performance at higher levels of bilirubin, and ongoing monitoring of jaundice. Additionally, studies should address cost-effectiveness and reproducibility in actual clinical practice. Given the interlaboratory variability of measurements of TSB, future studies of noninvasive measures of bilirubin should use HPLC and routine laboratory methods of TSB as reference standards, because the transcutaneous measures may prove to be as accurate as the laboratory measurement when compared with HPLC as the gold standard.

Using correlation coefficients to determine the accuracy of TcB measurements should be interpreted carefully because of several limitations:

- The correlation coefficient does not provide any information about the clinical utility of the diagnostic test.
- Although correlation coefficients measure the association between TcB and "standard" serum bilirubin measurements, the correlation coefficient is highly dependent on the distribution of serum bilirubin in the study population selected.
- Correlation measures ignore bias and measure relative rather than absolute agreement.

ADDENDUM: THE RISK OF BET

At the suggestion of AAP technical experts, a review of the risks associated with BET was also undertaken after the original AHRQ report was published. Articles were obtained from an informal survey of studies published since 1960 dealing with large populations that permitted calculations of the risks of morbidity and mortality. Of 15 studies, 8 consisted of subjects born before 1970. One article published in 1997 consisted of subjects born in 1994 and 1995.

Fifteen studies that reported data on BET-related mortality and/or morbidity were included in this review. Three categories were created to describe the percentage of subjects who met the criteria of the target population of our evidence report (ie, term idiopathic jaundice infants). Category I indicates that more than 50% of the study subjects were term infants whose pre-exchange clinical state was vigorous or stable and without disease conditions other than jaundice. Category II indicates that between 10% and 50% of the study subjects had category I characteristics. Category III indicates that more than 90% of the study subjects were preterm infants and/or term infants whose pre-exchange clinical state was not stable or was critically ill and with other disease conditions.

BET Subject and Study Characteristics

Because BET is no longer the mainstay of treatment for hyperbilirubinemia, most infants who underwent BETs were born in the 1950s to 1970s. Two recent studies reported BET-related mortality and morbidity for infants born from 1981 to 1995. After 1970, there were more infants who were premature, low birth weight or very low birth weight, and/or had a clinical condition(s) other than jaundice who received BETs than those born in earlier years. Not all infants in this review received BETs for hyperbilirubinemia. Because of limited data on subjects' bilirubin levels when the BETs were performed, we could not exclude those nonjaundiced infants.

BET-Associated Mortality

For all infants, the reported BET-related mortality ranged from 0% to 7%. There were no consistent definitions for BET-related mortality in the studies. An infant who died within 6 hours after the BET was the first used to define a BET-related death by Boggs and Westphal in 1960. Including the study from Boggs and Westphal, there were 3 studies reporting the 6-hour mortality, and they ranged from 0% to 1.9%. It is difficult to isolate BET as the sole factor in explaining mortality, because most of the subjects have significant associated pre-exchange disease morbidities. Most of the infants who died from BET had blood incompatibility and sepsis or were premature, had kernicterus, and/or were critically ill before undergoing BET. When only term infants were counted, the 6-hour mortality ranged from 3 to 19 per 1000 exchanged. When those term infants with serious hemolytic diseases (such as Rh incompatibility) were excluded, the 6-hour mortality ranged from 3 to 4 per 1000 exchanged infants. All these infants were born before 1970, and their jaundice was primarily due to ABO incompatibility.

BET-Associated Morbidity

There is an extensive list of complications that have been associated with BETs. Complications include those related to the use of blood products (infection, hemolysis of transfused blood, thromboembolization, graft versus host reactions), metabolic derangements (acidosis and perturbation of the serum concentrations of potassium, sodium, glucose, and calcium), cardiorespiratory reactions (including arrhythmias, apnea, and cardiac arrest), complications related to umbilical venous and arterial catheterization, and other miscellaneous complications. As noted previously, the pre-exchange clinical state of the infants studied varied widely, as did the definitions and rates of BET-associated morbidity. In many cases, however, the morbidity was minor (eg, postexchange anemia).

In the NICHD cooperative phototherapy study, morbidity (apnea, bradycardia, cyanosis, vasospasm, thrombosis) was observed in 22 of 328 (6.7%) patients in whom BETs were performed (no data available in 3 BETs). Of the 22 adverse events, 6 were mild episodes of bradycardia associated with calcium infusion. If those infants are excluded, as well as 2 who experienced transient arterial spasm, the incidence of "serious morbidity" associated with the procedure itself was 5.22%.

The most recent study to report BET morbidity in the era of contemporary neonatal care provides data on infants cared for from 1980 to 1995 at the Children's Hospital and University of Washington Medical Center in Seattle. Of 106 infants receiving BET, 81 were healthy and there were no deaths; however, 1 healthy infant developed severe necrotizing enterocolitis requiring surgery. Of 25 sick infants (12 required mechanical ventilation), there were 5 deaths, and 3 developed permanent sequelae, including chronic aortic obstruction from BET via the umbilical artery, intraventricular hemorrhage with subsequent developmental delay, and sudden respiratory deterioration from a pulmonary hemorrhage and subsequent global developmental delay. The author classified the deaths as "possibly" (n =3) or "probably" (n = 2) and the complications as "possibly" (n = 2) or "probably" (n = 1) resulting from the BET. Thus in 25 sick infants, the overall risk of death or permanent sequelae ranged from 3 of 25 to 8 of 25 (12%–32%) and of permanent sequelae in survivors from 1 of 20 to 2 of 20 (5%–10%).

Most of the mortality and morbidity rates reported date from a time at which BET was a common procedure in nurseries. This is no longer the case, and newer phototherapy techniques are likely to reduce the need for BETs even further. Because the frequency of performance of any procedure is an important determinant of risk, the fact that BET is so rarely performed today could result in higher mortality and morbidity rates. However, none of the reports before 1986 included contemporary monitoring capabilities such as pulse oximetry, which should provide earlier identification of potential problems and might decrease morbidity and mortality. In addition, current standards for the monitoring of transfused blood products has significantly reduced the risk of transfusion-transmitted viral infections.

TECHNICAL REPORT

Phototherapy to Prevent Severe Neonatal Hyperbilirubinemia in the Newborn Infant 35 or More Weeks of Gestation

abstract

OBJECTIVE: To standardize the use of phototherapy consistent with the American Academy of Pediatrics clinical practice guideline for the management of hyperbilirubinemia in the newborn infant 35 or more weeks of gestation.

METHODS: Relevant literature was reviewed. Phototherapy devices currently marketed in the United States that incorporate fluorescent, halogen, fiber-optic, or blue light-emitting diode light sources were assessed in the laboratory.

RESULTS: The efficacy of phototherapy units varies widely because of differences in light source and configuration. The following characteristics of a device contribute to its effectiveness: (1) emission of light in the blue-to-green range that overlaps the in vivo plasma bilirubin absorption spectrum ($\sim$460–490 nm); (2) irradiance of at least 30 μW·cm^{-2}·nm^{-1} (confirmed with an appropriate irradiance meter calibrated over the appropriate wavelength range); (3) illumination of maximal body surface; and (4) demonstration of a decrease in total bilirubin concentrations during the first 4 to 6 hours of exposure.

RECOMMENDATIONS (SEE APPENDIX FOR GRADING DEFINITION): The intensity and spectral output of phototherapy devices is useful in predicting potential effectiveness in treating hyperbilirubinemia (group B recommendation). Clinical effectiveness should be evaluated before and monitored during use (group B recommendation). Blocking the light source or reducing exposed body surface should be avoided (group B recommendation). Standardization of irradiance meters, improvements in device design, and lower-upper limits of light intensity for phototherapy units merit further study. Comparing the in vivo performance of devices is not practical, in general, and alternative procedures need to be explored. *Pediatrics* 2011;128:e1046–e1052

Vinod K. Bhutani, MD, and THE COMMITTEE ON FETUS AND NEWBORN

KEY WORDS
phototherapy, newborn jaundice, hyperbilirubinemia, light treatment

ABBREVIATION
LED—light-emitting diode

This document is copyrighted and is property of the American Academy of Pediatrics and its Board of Directors. All authors have filed conflict of interest statements with the American Academy of Pediatrics. Any conflicts have been resolved through a process approved by the Board of Directors. The American Academy of Pediatrics has neither solicited nor accepted any commercial involvement in the development of the content of this publication.

The guidance in this report does not indicate an exclusive course of treatment or serve as a standard of medical care. Variations, taking into account individual circumstances, may be appropriate.

www.pediatrics.org/cgi/doi/10.1542/peds.2011-1494

doi:10.1542/peds.2011-1494

All technical reports from the American Academy of Pediatrics automatically expire 5 years after publication unless reaffirmed, revised, or retired at or before that time.

PEDIATRICS (ISSN Numbers: Print, 0031-4005; Online, 1098-4275).

INTRODUCTION

Clinical trials have validated the efficacy of phototherapy in reducing excessive unconjugated hyperbilirubinemia, and its implementation has drastically curtailed the use of exchange transfusions.[1] The initiation and duration of phototherapy is defined by a specific range of total bilirubin values based on an infant's postnatal age and the potential risk for bilirubin neurotoxicity.[1] Clinical response to phototherapy depends on the efficacy of the phototherapy device as well as the balance between an infant's rates of bilirubin production and elimination. The active agent in phototherapy is light delivered in measurable doses, which makes phototherapy conceptually similar to pharmacotherapy. This report standardizes the use of phototherapy consistent with the American Academy of Pediatrics clinical practice guideline for the management of hyperbilirubinemia in the newborn infant 35 or more weeks of gestation.

I. COMMERCIAL LIGHT SOURCES

A wide selection of commercial phototherapy devices is available in the United States. A complete discussion of devices is beyond the scope of this review; some are described in Tables 1 and 2. Phototherapy devices can be categorized according to their light source as follows: (1) fluorescent-tube devices that emit different colors (cool white daylight, blue [B], special blue [BB], turquoise, and green) and are straight (F20 T12, 60 cm, 20 W), U-shaped, or spiral-shaped; (2) metal halide bulbs, used in spotlights and incubator lights; (3) light-emitting diodes (LEDs) or metal halide bulbs, used with fiber-optic light guides in pads, blankets, or spotlights; and (4) high-intensity LEDs, used as over- and under-the-body devices.

TABLE 1 Phototherapy Devices Commonly Used in the United States and Their Performance Characteristics

Device	Manufacturer	Distance to Patient (cm)	% Treatable BSA	Spectrum, Total (nm)	Bandwidth* (nm)	Peak (nm)	Footprint Area (Length × Width, cm²)	Footprint Irradiance (μW/cm²/nm)		
								Min	Max	Mean ± SD
Light Emitting Diodes [LED]										
neoBLUE	Natus Medical, San Carlos, CA	30	100	420–540	20	462	1152 (48 × 24)	12	37	30 ± 7
PortaBed	Stanford University, Stanford, CA	≥5	100	425–540	27	463	1740 (30 × 58)	40	76	67 ± 8
Fluorescent										
BiliLite CW/BB	Olympic Medical, San Carlos, CA	45	100	380–720	69	578	2928 (48 × 61)	6	10	8 ± 1
BiliLite BB	Olympic Medical, San Carlos, CA	45	100	400–550	35	445	2928 (48 × 61)	11	22	17 ± 2
BiliLite TL52	Olympic Medical, San Carlos, CA	45	100	400–626	69	437	2928 (48 × 61)	13	23	19 ± 3
BiliBed	Medela, McHenry, IL	0	71	400–560	80	450	693 (21 × 33)	14	59	36 ± 2
Halogen										
MinBiliLite	Olympic Medical, San Carlos, CA	45	54	350–800	190	580	490 (25 diam)	<1	19	7 ± 5
Phototherapy Lite	Philips Inc, Andover, MA	45	54	370–850	200	590	490 (25 diam)	<1	17	5 ± 5
Halogen fiberoptic										
BiliBlanket	Ohmeda, Fairfield, CT	0	24	390–600	70	533	150 (10 × 15)	9	31	20 ± 6
Wallaby II Preterm	Philips, Inc, Andover, MA	0	19	400–560	45	513	117 (9 × 13)	8	30	16 ± 6
Wallaby II Term	Philips, Inc, Andover, MA	0	53	400–560	45	513	280 (8 × 35)	6	11	8 ± 1
SpotLight 1000	Philips, Inc, Andover, MA	45	54	400–560	45	513	490 (25 diam)	1	11	6 ± 3
PEP Model 2000	PEP, Fryeburg, ME	23	100	400–717	63	445	1530 (30 × 51)	12	49	28 ± 11
Bili Soft	GE Healthcare, Laurel, MD	0	71	400–670	40	453	825 (25 × 33)	1	52	25 ± 16

Data in Table 1 are expanded and updated from that previously reported by Vreman et al.[3] The definitions and standards for device assessment are explained below.

EMISSION SPECTRAL QUALITIES: Measured data of the light delivered by each of the light sources are presented as the minimum, maximum and range. Light source emission spectra within the range of 300–700 nm were recorded after the device had reached stable light emission, using a miniature fiberoptic radiometer (IRRAD2000, Ocean Optics, Inc, Dunedin, FL). For precision based device assessment, the spectral bandwidth (*), which is defined as the width of the emission spectrum in nm at 50% of peak light intensity, is the preferred method to distinguish and compare emission spectrum (data usually provided by manufacturers). Emission peak values are also used to characterize the quality of light emitted by a given light source.

IRRADIANCE: Measured data are presented as mean ± standard deviation (SD), representing the irradiance of blue light (including spectral bandwidth), for each device's light footprint at the manufacturer-recommended distance. To compare diverse devices, the spectral irradiance (μW/cm2/nm) measurements were made using calibrated BiliBlanket Meters I and II (Ohmeda, GE Healthcare, Fairfield, CT), which were found to yield identical results with stable output phototherapy devices. This type of meter was selected from the several devices with different photonic characteristics that are commercially available, because it has a wide sensitivity range (400–520 nm with peak sensitivity at 450 nm), which overlaps the bilirubin absorption spectrum and which renders it suitable for the evaluation of narrow and broad wavelength band light sources. The devices have been found exceptionally stable during several years of use and agree closely after each annual calibration.

FOOTPRINT: The minimum and maximum irradiance measured (at the intervals provided or defined) in the given irradiance footprint of the device (length × width). The footprint of a device is that area which is occupied by a patient to receive phototherapy. The irradiance footprint has greater dimensions than the emission surface, which is measured at the point where the light exits a phototherapy device. The minimum and maximum values are shown to indicate the range of irradiances encountered with a device and can be used as an indication of the uniformity of the emitted light. Most devices conform to an international standard to deliver a minimum/maximum footprint light ratio of no lower than 0.4.

BSA: BODY SURFACE AREA refers to percent (%) exposure of either the ventral or dorsal planar surface exposed to light and Irradiance measurements are accurate to ±0.5.

All of the reported devices are marketed in the United States except the PortaBed, which is a non-licensed Stanford-developed research device and the Dutch Crigler-Najjar Association (used by Crigler-Najjar patients).

TABLE 2 Maximum Spectral Irradiance of Phototherapy Devices (Using Commercial Light Meters at Manufacturer Recommended Distances) Compared to Clear-Sky Sunlight

Light Meter [Range, Peak]	Footprint Irradiance, (μW/cm^2/nm^a)							
	Halogen/Fiberoptic			Fluorescent		LED		Sunlight
	BiliBlanket	Wallaby (Neo)		PEP Bed	Martin/Philips BB	neoBLUE	PortaBed	@ Zenith on 8/31/05
		II	III					
	@ Contact	@ Contact		@ 10 cm	@ 25 cm	@ 30 cm	@ 10 cm	Level Ground
BiliBlanket Meter II [400–520, 450 nm]	34	28	34	40	69	34	76	144
Bili-Meter, Model 22 [425–475, 460 nm]	29	16	32	49	100	25	86	65**
Joey Dosimeter, JD-100 [420–550, 470 nm]	53	51	60	88	174	84	195	304**
PMA-2123 Bilirubin Detector^a [400–520, 460 nm]	24	24	37	35	70	38	73	81
GoldiLux UVA Photometer, GRP-1^b [315–400, 365 nm]	<0.04	<0.04	<0.04	<0.04	<0.04	<0.04	<0.04	2489

Data in Table 2 were tested and compiled by Hendrik J. Vreman (June 2007 and reverified December 2010).

** Irradiance presented to this meter exceeded its range. Measurement was made through a stainless-steel screen that attenuated the measured irradiance to 57%, which was subsequently corrected by this factor.

^{a} Solar Light Company, Inc., Glenside, PA 19038.

^{b} Oriel Instruments, Stratford, CT 06615 and SmartMeter GRP-1 with UV-A probe. GRP-1 measures UV-A light as μW/cm^2. No artificial light source delivered significant (<0.04 μW/cm^2) UV-A radiation at the distances measured.

II. STANDARDS FOR PHOTOTHERAPY DEVICES

Methods for reporting and measuring phototherapy doses are not standardized. Comparisons of commercially available phototherapy devices that use in vitro photodegradation techniques may not accurately predict clinical efficacy.[2] A recent report explored an approach to standardizing and quantifying the magnitude of phototherapy delivered by various devices.[3] Table 1 lists technical data for some of the devices marketed in the United States.[3] Factors to consider in prescribing and implementing phototherapy are (1) emission range of the light source, (2) the light intensity (irradiance), (3) the exposed ("treatable") body surface area illuminated, and (4) the decrease in total bilirubin concentration. A measure of the effectiveness of phototherapy to rapidly configure the bilirubin molecule to less toxic photoisomers (measured in seconds) is not yet clinically available.

A. Light Wavelength

The visible white light spectrum ranges from approximately 350 to 800 nm. Bilirubin absorbs visible light most strongly in the blue region of the spectrum (~460 nm). Absorption of light transforms unconjugated bilirubin molecules bound to human serum albumin in solution into bilirubin photoproducts (predominantly isomers of bilirubin).[2,4,5] Because of the photophysical properties of skin, the most effective light in vivo is probably in the blue-to-green region (~460–490 nm).[2] The first prototype phototherapy device to result in a clinically significant rate of bilirubin decrease used a blue (B) fluorescent-tube light source with 420- to 480-nm emission.[6,7] More effective narrow-band special blue bulbs (F20T12/BB [General Electric, Westinghouse, Sylvania] or TL52/20W [Phillips]) were subsequently used.[8,9] Most recently, commercial compact fluorescent-tube light sources and devices that use LEDs of narrow spectral bandwidth have been used.[9–14] Unless specified otherwise, plastic covers or optical filters need to be used to remove potentially harmful ultraviolet light.

Clinical Context

Devices with maximum emission within the 460- to 490-nm (blue-green) region of the visible spectrum are probably the most effective for treating hyperbilirubinemia.[2,4] Lights with broader emission also will work, although not as effectively. Special blue (BB) fluorescent lights are effective but should not be confused with white lights painted blue or covered with blue plastic sheaths, which should not be used. Devices that contain high-intensity gallium nitride LEDs with emission within the 460- to 490-nm regions are also effective and have a longer lifetime (>20 000 hours), lower heat output, low infrared emission, and no ultraviolet emission.

B. Measuring Light Irradiance

Light intensity or energy output is defined by irradiance and refers to the number of photons (spectral energy) that are delivered per unit area (cm^2) of exposed skin.[1] The dose of phototherapy is a measure of the irradiance delivered for a specific duration and adjusted to the exposed body surface area. Determination of an in vivo dose-response relationship is confounded by the optical properties of skin and the rates of bilirubin production and elimination.[1] Irradiance is measured with a radiometer (W·cm^{-2}) or spectroradiometer (μW·cm^{-2}·nm^{-1}) over a given wavelength band. Table 2 compares the spectral irradiance of some of the devices in the US market, as measured with different brands of meters. Often, radiometers measure wavelengths that do not penetrate skin well or that are far from optimal for phototherapy and, therefore, may be of little value for predicting the clinical efficacy of phototherapy units. A direct relationship between irradiance and the rate of in vivo total bilirubin concentration decrease was described in the report of a study of term "healthy" infants with nonhemolytic hyperbilirubinemia (peak values: 15–18 mg/dL) using fluorescent Philips daylight (TL20W/54, TL20W/52) and special blue (TLAK 40W/03) lamps.[15,16] The American Academy of Pediatrics has recommended that the irradiance for intensive phototherapy be at least 30 μW·cm^{-2}·nm^{-1} over the waveband interval 460 to 490 nm.[1] Devices that emit lower irradiance may be supplemented with auxiliary devices. Much higher doses (>65 μW·cm^{-2}·nm^{-1}) might have (as-yet-unidentified) adverse effects. Currently, no single method is in general use for measuring phototherapy dosages. In addition, the calibration methods, wavelength responses, and geometries of instruments are not standardized. Consequently, different radiometers may show different values for the same light source.[2]

Clinical Context

For routine measurements, clinicians are limited by reliance on irradiance meters supplied or recommended by the manufacturer. Visual estimations of brightness and use of ordinary photometric or colorimetric light meters are inappropriate.[1,2] Maximal irradiance can be achieved by bringing the light source close to the infant[1]; however, this should not be done with halogen or tungsten lights, because the heat generated can cause a burn. Furthermore, with some fixtures, increasing the proximity may reduce the exposed body surface area. Irradiance distribution in the illuminated area

(footprint) is rarely uniform; measurements at the center of the footprint may greatly exceed those at the periphery and are variable among phototherapy devices.[1] Thus, irradiance should be measured at several sites on the infant's body surface. The ideal distance and orientation of the light source should be maintained according to the manufacturer's recommendations. The irradiance of all lamps decreases with use; manufacturers may provide useful-lifetime estimates, which should not be exceeded.

C. Optimal Body Surface Area

An infant's total body surface area[17] can be influenced by the disproportionate head size, especially in the more preterm infant. Complete (100%) exposure of the total body surface to light is impractical and limited by use of eye masks and diapers. Circumferential illumination (total body surface exposure from multiple directions) achieves exposure of approximately 80% of the total body surface. In clinical practice, exposure is usually planar: ventral with overhead light sources and dorsal with lighted mattresses. Approximately 35% of the total body surface (ventral or dorsal) is exposed with either method. Changing the infant's posture every 2 to 3 hours may maximize the area exposed to light. Exposed body surface area treated rather than the number of devices (double, triple, etc) used is clinically more important. Maximal skin surface illumination allows for a more intensive exposure and may require combined use of more than 1 phototherapy device.[1]

Clinical Context

Physical obstruction of light by equipment, such as radiant warmers, head covers, large diapers, eye masks that enclose large areas of the scalp, tape, electrode patches, and insulating plastic covers, decrease the exposed skin

surface area. Circumferential phototherapy maximizes the exposed area. Combining several devices, such as fluorescent tubes with fiber-optic pads or LED mattresses placed below the infant or bassinet, will increase the surface area exposed. If the infant is in an incubator, the light rays should be perpendicular to the surface of the incubator to minimize reflectance and loss of efficacy.[1,2]

D. Rate of Response Measured by Decrease in Serum Bilirubin Concentration

The clinical impact of phototherapy should be evident within 4 to 6 hours of initiation with an anticipated decrease of more than 2 mg/dL (34 μmol/L) in serum bilirubin concentration.[1] The clinical response depends on the rates of bilirubin production, enterohepatic circulation, and bilirubin elimination; the degree of tissue bilirubin deposition[15,16,18]; and the rates of the photochemical reactions of bilirubin. Aggressive implementation of phototherapy for excessive hyperbilirubinemia, sometimes referred to as the "crash-cart" approach,[19,20] has been reported to reduce the need for exchange transfusion and possibly reduce the severity of bilirubin neurotoxicity.

Clinical Context

Serial measurements of bilirubin concentration are used to monitor the effectiveness of phototherapy, but the value of these measurements can be confounded by changes in bilirubin production or elimination and by a sudden increase in bilirubin concentration (rebound) if phototherapy is stopped. Periodicity of serial measurements is based on clinical judgment.

III. EVIDENCE FOR EFFECTIVE PHOTOTHERAPY

Light-emission characteristics of phototherapy devices help in predicting

TABLE 3 Practice Considerations for Optimal Administration of Phototherapy

Checklist	Recommendation	Implementation
Light source (nm)	Wavelength spectrum in ~460- 490-nm blue-green light region	Know the spectral output of the light source
Light irradiance (μW·cm^{-2}·nm^{-1})	Use optimal irradiance: >30 μW·cm^{-2}·nm^{-1} within the 460- to 490-nm waveband	Ensure uniformity over the light footprint area
Body surface area (cm^2)	Expose maximal skin area	Reduce blocking of light
Timeliness of implementation	Urgent or "crash-cart" intervention for excessive hyperbilirubinemia	May conduct procedures while infant is on phototherapy
Continuity of therapy	Briefly interrupt for feeding, parental bonding, nursing care	After confirmation of adequate bilirubin concentration decrease
Efficacy of intervention	Periodically measure rate of response in bilirubin load reduction	Degree of total serum/plasma bilirubin concentration decrease
Duration of therapy	Discontinue at desired bilirubin threshold; be aware of possible rebound increase	Serial bilirubin measurements based on rate of decrease

their effectiveness (group B recommendation) (see Appendix). The clinical effectiveness of the device should be known before and monitored during clinical application (group B recommendation). Local guidelines (instructions) for routine clinical use should be available. Important factors that need to be considered are listed in Table 3. Obstructing the light source and reducing the exposed body surface area must be avoided (group B recommendation).

These recommendations are appropriate for clinical care in high-resource settings. In low-resource settings the use of improvised technologies and affordable phototherapy device choices need to meet minimum efficacy and safety standards.

IV. SAFETY AND PROTECTIVE MEASURES

A clinician skilled in newborn care should assess the neonate's clinical status during phototherapy to ensure adequate hydration, nutrition, and temperature control. Clinical improvement or progression of jaundice should also be assessed, including signs suggestive of early bilirubin encephalopathy such as changes in sleeping pattern, deteriorating feeding pattern, or inability to be consoled while crying.[1] Staff should be educated regarding the importance of safely minimizing the distance of the phototherapy device from the infant. They should be aware that the intensity of light decreases at the outer perimeter of the light footprint and recognize the effects of physical factors that could impede or obstruct light exposure. Staff should be aware that phototherapy does not use ultraviolet light and that exposure to the lights is mostly harmless. Four decades of neonatal phototherapy use has revealed no serious adverse clinical effects in newborn infants 35 or more weeks of gestation. For more preterm infants, who are usually treated with prophylactic rather than therapeutic phototherapy, this may not be true. Informed staff should educate parents regarding the care of their newborn infant undergoing phototherapy. Devices must comply with general safety standards listed by the International Electrotechnical Commission.[21] Other clinical considerations include:

a. Interruption of phototherapy: After a documented decrease in bilirubin concentration, continuous exposure to the light source may be interrupted and the eye mask removed to allow for feeding and maternal-infant bonding.[1]

b. Use of eye masks: Eye masks to prevent retinal damage are used routinely, although there is no evidence to support this recommendation. Retinal damage has been documented in the unpatched eyes of newborn monkeys exposed to phototherapy, but there are no similar data available from human newborns, because eye patches have always been used.[22–24] Purulent eye discharge and conjunctivitis in term infants have been reported with prolonged use of eye patches.[25,26]

c. Use of diapers: Concerns for the long-term effects of continuous phototherapy exposure of the reproductive system have been raised but not substantiated.[27–29] Diapers may be used for hygiene but are not essential.

d. Other protective considerations: Devices used in environments with high humidity and oxygen must meet electrical and fire hazard safety standards.[21] Phototherapy is contraindicated in infants with congenital porphyria or those treated with photosensitizing drugs.[1] Prolonged phototherapy has been associated with increased oxidant stress and lipid peroxidation[30] and riboflavin deficiency.[31] Recent clinical reports of other adverse outcomes (eg, malignant melanoma, DNA damage, and skin changes) have yet to be validated.[1,2,32,33] Phototherapy does not exacerbate hemolysis.[34]

V. RESEARCH NEEDS

Among the gaps in knowledge that remain regarding the use of phototherapy to prevent severe neonatal hyperbilirubinemia, the following are among the most important:

1. The ability to measure the actual wavelength and irradiance delivered by a phototherapy device is urgently needed to assess the efficiency of

phototherapy in reducing total serum bilirubin concentrations.

2. The safety and efficacy of home phototherapy remains a research priority.

3. Further delineation of the short- and long-term consequences of exposing infants with conjugated and unconjugated hyperbilirubinemia to phototherapy is needed.

4. Whether use of phototherapy reduces the risk of bilirubin neurotoxicity in a timely and effective manner needs further exploration.

SUMMARY

Clinicians and hospitals should ensure that the phototherapy devices they use fully illuminate the patient's body surface area, have an irradiance level of $\geq 30\ \mu\text{W·cm}^{-2}\text{·nm}^{-1}$ (confirmed with accuracy with an appropriate spectral radiometer) over the waveband of approximately 460 to 490 nm, and are implemented in a timely manner. Standard procedures should be documented for their safe deployment.

LEAD AUTHOR
Vinod K. Bhutani, MD

COMMITTEE ON FETUS AND NEWBORN, 2010–2011
Lu-Ann Papile, MD, Chairperson
Jill E. Baley, MD
Vinod K. Bhutani, MD
Waldemar A. Carlo, MD
James J. Cummings, MD
Praveen Kumar, MD
Richard A. Polin, MD
Rosemarie C. Tan, MD, PhD
Kristi L. Watterberg, MD

FORMER COMMITTEE MEMBER
David H. Adamkin, MD

LIAISONS
CAPT Wanda Denise Barfield, MD, MPH – *Centers for Disease Control and Prevention*
William H. Barth Jr, MD – *American College of Obstetricians and Gynecologists*
Ann L. Jefferies, MD – *Canadian Paediatric Society*
Rosalie O. Mainous, PhD, RNC, NNP – *National Association of Neonatal Nurses*
Tonse N. K. Raju, MD, DCH – *National Institutes of Health*
Kasper S. Wang – *AAP Section on Surgery*

CONSULTANTS
M. Jeffrey Maisels, MBBCh, DSc
Antony F. McDonagh, PhD
David K. Stevenson, MD
Hendrik J. Vreman, PhD

STAFF
Jim Couto, MA

REFERENCES

1. American Academy of Pediatrics, Subcommittee on Hyperbilirubinemia. Management of hyperbilirubinemia in the newborn infant 35 or more weeks of gestation [published correction appears in *Pediatrics*. 2004;114(4):1138]. *Pediatrics*. 2004;114(1):297–316

2. McDonagh AF, Agati G, Fusi F, Pratesi R. Quantum yields for laser photocyclization of bilirubin in the presence of human serum albumin: dependence of quantum yield on excitation wavelength. *Photochem Photobiol*. 1989;50(3):305–319

3. Vreman HJ, Wong RJ, Murdock JR, Stevenson DK. Standardized bench method for evaluating the efficacy of phototherapy devices. *Acta Paediatr*. 2008;97(3):308–316

4. Maisels MJ, McDonagh AF. Phototherapy for neonatal jaundice. *N Engl J Med*. 2008;358(9):920–928

5. McDonagh AF, Lightner DA. Phototherapy and the photobiology of bilirubin. *Semin Liver Dis*. 1988;8(3):272–283

6. Cremer RJ, Perryman PW, Richards DH. Influence of light on the hyperbilirubinaemia of infants. *Lancet*. 1958;1(7030):1094–1097

7. Ennever JF, McDonagh AF, Speck WT. Phototherapy for neonatal jaundice: optimal wavelengths of light. *J Pediatr*. 1983;103(2):295–299

8. Ennever JF, Sobel M, McDonagh AF, Speck WT. Phototherapy for neonatal jaundice: in vitro comparison of light sources. *Pediatr Res*. 1984;18(7):667–670

9. Nakamura S, Fasol G. InGaN single-quantum-well LEDs. In: *The Blue Laser Diode*. Berlin, Germany: Springer-Verlag; 1997:201–221

10. Vreman HJ, Wong RJ, Stevenson DK, et al. Light-emitting diodes: a novel light source for phototherapy. *Pediatr Res*. 1998;44(5):804–809

11. Maisels MJ, Kring EA, DeRidder J. Randomized controlled trial of light-emitting diode phototherapy. *J Perinatol*. 2007;27(9):565–567

12. Seidman DS, Moise J, Ergaz Z, et al. A new blue light-emitting phototherapy device: a prospective randomized controlled study. *J Pediatr*. 2000;136(6):771–774

13. Martins BM, de Carvalho M, Moreira ME, Lopes JM. Efficacy of new microprocessed phototherapy system with five high intensity light emitting diodes (Super LED) [in Portuguese]. *J Pediatr (Rio J)*. 2007;83(3):253–258

14. Kumar P, Murki S, Malik GK, et al. Light-emitting diodes versus compact fluorescent tubes for phototherapy in neonatal jaundice: a multi-center randomized controlled trial. *Indian Pediatr*. 2010;47(2):131–137

15. Tan KL. The nature of the dose-response relationship of phototherapy for neonatal hyperbilirubinemia. *J Pediatr*. 1977;90(3):448–452

16. Tan KL. The pattern of bilirubin response to phototherapy for neonatal hyperbilirubinaemia. *Pediatr Res*. 1982;16(8):670–674

17. Mosteller RD. Simplified calculation of body-surface area. *N Engl J Med*. 1987;317(17):1098

18. Jährig K, Jährig D, Meisel P. Dependence of the efficiency of phototherapy on plasma bilirubin concentration. *Acta Paediatr Scand*. 1982;71(2):293–299

19. Johnson L, Bhutani VK, Karp K, Sivieri EM, Shapiro SM. Clinical report from the pilot USA Kernicterus Registry (1992 to 2004). *J Perinatol*. 2009;29(suppl 1):S25–S45

20. Hansen TW, Nietsch L, Norman E, et al. Reversibility of acute intermediate phase bilirubin encephalopathy. *Acta Paediatr*. 2009;98(10):1689–1694

21. International Electrotechnical Commission. International standard: medical electrical equipment part 2-50—particular requirements for the safety of infant phototherapy equipment 60601-2-50, ed2.0. (2009-03-24). Available at: http://webstore.iec.ch/webstore/webstore.nsf/Artnum_PK/42737. Accessed December 21, 2010

22. Ente G, Klein SW. Hazards of phototherapy. *N Engl J Med*. 1970;283(10):544–545

23. Messner KH, Maisels MJ, Leure-DuPree AE. Phototoxicity to the newborn primate retina. *Invest Ophthalmol Vis Sci*. 1978;17(2):178–182

24. Patz A, Souri EN. Phototherapy and other ocular risks to the newborn. *Sight Sav Rev*. 1972;42(1):29–33

25. Paludetto R, Mansi G, Rinaldi P, Saporito M, De Curtis M, Ciccimarra F. Effects of

different ways of covering the eyes on behavior of jaundiced infants treated with phototherapy. *Biol Neonate.* 1985;47(1): 1–8

26. Fok TF, Wong W, Cheung KL. Eye protection for newborns under phototherapy: comparison between a modified headbox and the conventional eyepatches. *Ann Trop Paediatr.* 1997;17(4):349–354

27. Koç H, Altunhan H, Dilsiz A, et al. Testicular changes in newborn rats exposed to phototherapy. *Pediatr Dev Pathol.* 1999;2(4): 333–336

28. Wurtman RJ. The effects of light on the human body. *Sci Am.* 1975;233(1):69–77

29. Cetinkursun S, Demirbag S, Cincik M, Baykal B, Gunal A. Effects of phototherapy on newborn rat testicles. *Arch Androl.* 2006;52(1): 61–70

30. Lightner DA, Linnane WP, Ahlfors CE. Bilirubin photooxidation products in the urine of jaundiced neonates receiving phototherapy. *Pediatr Res.* 1984;18(8):696–700

31. Sisson TR. Photodegradation of riboflavin in neonates. *Fed Proc.* 1987;46(5): 1883–1885

32. Bauer J, Büttner P, Luther H, Wiecker TS, Möhrle M, Garbe C. Blue light phototherapy of neonatal jaundice does not increase the risk for melanocytic nevus development. *Arch Dermatol.* 2004;140(4):493–494

33. Tatli MM, Minnet C, Kocyigit A, Karadag A. Phototherapy increases DNA damage in lymphocytes of hyperbilirubinemic neonates. *Mutat Res.* 2008;654(1):93–95

34. Maisels MJ, Kring EA. Does intensive phototherapy produce hemolysis in newborns of 35 or more weeks gestation? *J Perinatol.* 2006;26(8):498–500

APPENDIX Definition of Grades for Recommendation and Suggestion for Practice

Grade	Definition	Suggestion for Practice
A	This intervention is recommended. There is a high certainty that the net benefit is substantial	Offer and administer this intervention
B	This intervention is recommended. There is a moderate certainty that the net benefit is moderate to substantial	Offer and administer this intervention
C	This intervention is recommended. There may be considerations that support the use of this intervention in an individual patient. There is a moderate to high certainty that the net benefit is small	Offer and administer this intervention only if other considerations support this intervention in an individual patient
D	This intervention is not recommended. There is a moderate to high certainty that the intervention has no net benefit and that the harms outweigh the benefits	Discourage use of this intervention
I	The current evidence is insufficient to assess the balance of benefits against and harms of this intervention. There is a moderate to high certainty that the intervention has no net benefit and that the harms outweigh the benefits. Evidence is lacking, of poor quality, or conflicting, and the balance of benefits and harms cannot be determined	If this intervention is conducted, the patient should understand the uncertainty about the balance of benefits and harms

US Preventive Services Task Force Grade definitions, May, 2008 (available at www.uspreventiveservicestaskforce.org/3rduspstf/ratings.htm).

Hyperbilirubinemia in the Newborn Infant ≥35 Weeks' Gestation: An Update With Clarifications

AUTHORS: M. Jeffrey Maisels, MB, BCh, DSc,[a] Vinod K. Bhutani, MD,[b] Debra Bogen, MD,[c] Thomas B. Newman, MD, MPH,[d] Ann R. Stark, MD,[e] and Jon F. Watchko, MD[f]

[a]Department of Pediatrics, Oakland University William Beaumont School of Medicine and Division of Neonatology, Beaumont Children's Hospital, Royal Oak, Michigan; [b]Department of Neonatal and Developmental Medicine, Lucile Salter Packard Children's Hospital, Stanford University, Palo Alto, California; [c]Division of General Academic Pediatrics, Department of Pediatrics, University of Pittsburgh School of Medicine, Children's Hospital of Pittsburgh, Pittsburgh, Pennsylvania; [d]Department of Epidemiology and Biostatistics, Department of Pediatrics, University of California, San Francisco, California; [e]Department of Pediatrics and Section of Neonatology, Baylor College of Medicine and Texas Children's Hospital, Houston, Texas; and [f]Division of Newborn Medicine, Department of Pediatrics, University of Pittsburgh School of Medicine, Pittsburgh, Pennsylvania

ABBREVIATIONS

AAP—American Academy of Pediatrics
G6PD—glucose-6-phosphate dehydrogenase
TSB—total serum bilirubin
TcB—transcutaneous bilirubin

Opinions expressed in this commentary are those of the author and not necessarily those of the American Academy of Pediatrics or its Committees.

www.pediatrics.org/cgi/doi/10.1542/peds.2009-0329

doi:10.1542/peds.2009-0329

Accepted for publication Jun 3, 2009

Address correspondence to M. Jeffrey Maisels, MB, BCh, DSc, Beaumont Children's Hospital, 3601 W. 13 Mile Rd, Royal Oak, MI 48073. E-mail: JMaisels@beaumont.edu

PEDIATRICS (ISSN Numbers: Print, 0031-4005; Online, 1098-4275).

FINANCIAL DISCLOSURE: Dr Maisels is a consultant to and has received grant support from Draeger Medical Inc; the other authors have no financial relationships relevant to this article to disclose.

In July 2004, the Subcommittee on Hyperbilirubinemia of the American Academy of Pediatrics (AAP) published its clinical practice guideline on the management of hyperbilirubinemia in the newborn infant ≥35 weeks of gestation,[1] and a similar guideline was published in 2007 by the Canadian Paediatric Society.[2] Experience with implementation of the AAP guideline suggests that some areas require clarification. The 2004 AAP guideline also expressed hope that its implementation would "reduce the incidence of severe hyperbilirubinemia and bilirubin encephalopathy. . . ." We do not know how many practitioners are following the guideline, nor do we know the current incidence of bilirubin encephalopathy in the United States. We do know, however, that kernicterus is still occurring in the United States, Canada, and Western Europe.[3–7] In 2002, the National Quality Forum suggested that kernicterus should be classified as a "serious reportable event,"[8] sometimes termed a "never event,"[9] implying that with appropriate monitoring, surveillance, and intervention, this devastating condition can, or should, be eliminated. Although this is certainly a desirable objective, it is highly unlikely that it can be achieved given our current state of knowledge and practice.[10] In certain circumstances (notably, glucose-6-phosphate dehydrogenase [G6PD] deficiency, sepsis, genetic predisposition, or other unknown stressors), acute, severe hyperbilirubinemia can occur and can produce brain damage despite appropriate monitoring and intervention.

In addition to clarifying certain items in the 2004 AAP guideline, we recommend universal predischarge bilirubin screening using total serum bilirubin (TSB) or transcutaneous bilirubin (TcB) measurements, which help to assess the risk of subsequent severe hyperbilirubinemia. We also recommend a more structured approach to management and follow-up according to the predischarge TSB/TcB, gestational age, and other risk factors for hyperbilirubinemia. These recommendations represent a consensus of expert opinion based on the available evidence, and they are supported by several independent reviewers. Nevertheless, their efficacy in preventing kernicterus and their cost-effectiveness are unknown.

METHODS

We reviewed the report on screening for neonatal hyperbilirubinemia published by the Agency for Healthcare Research and Quality and prepared by the Tufts-New England Medical Center Evidence-Based Practice Center,[11] the current report by the US Preventive Services Task Force,[12] and other relevant literature.[1,3–10,13–26]

TABLE 1 Important Risk Factors for Severe Hyperbilirubinemia

Predischarge TSB or TcB measurement in the high-risk or high-intermediate–risk zone
Lower gestational age
Exclusive breastfeeding, particularly if nursing is not going well and weight loss is excessive
Jaundice observed in the first 24 h
Isoimmune or other hemolytic disease (eg, G6PD deficiency)
Previous sibling with jaundice
Cephalohematoma or significant bruising
East Asian race

TABLE 2 Hyperbilirubinemia Neurotoxicity
Risk Factors

Isoimmune hemolytic disease
G6PD deficiency
Asphyxia
Sepsis
Acidosis
Albumin <3.0 mg/dL

RISK FACTORS

The 2004 AAP guideline includes 2 categories of risk factors, but the distinction between these 2 categories has not been clear to all users of the guideline.

Laboratory and Clinical Factors That Help to Assess the Risk of Subsequent Severe Hyperbilirubinemia

These "risk factors for hyperbilirubinemia" are listed in Table 1. Understanding the predisposition to subsequent hyperbilirubinemia provides guidance for timely follow-up as well as the need for additional clinical and laboratory evaluation.

Laboratory and Clinical Factors That Might Increase the Risk of Brain Damage in an Infant Who Has Hyperbilirubinemia

These risk factors for bilirubin neurotoxicity are listed in the figures of the 2004 AAP guideline that provide recommendations for the use of phototherapy and exchange transfusion. These "neurotoxicity risk factors" encompass those that might increase the risk of brain damage in an infant who has severe hyperbilirubinemia[1] (see Fig 1 and Table 2). The neurotoxicity risk factors are used in making the decision to initiate phototherapy or perform an exchange transfusion. These interventions are recommended at a lower bilirubin level when any of the neurotoxicity risk factors is present. Some conditions are found in both risk-factor categories. For example, lower gestational age and isoimmune hemolytic disease increase the likelihood of subsequent severe hyperbilirubinemia as well as the risk of brain damage by bilirubin.

PREDISCHARGE RISK ASSESSMENT FOR SUBSEQUENT SEVERE HYPERBILIRUBINEMIA

The 2004 AAP guideline recommends a predischarge bilirubin measurement and/or assessment of clinical risk factors to evaluate the risk of subsequent severe hyperbilirubinemia.[1] New evidence suggests that combining a predischarge measurement of TSB or TcB with clinical risk factors might improve the prediction of the risk of subsequent hyperbilirubinemia.[13,14,23] In addition, when interpreted by using the hour-specific nomogram (Fig 2), measurement of TSB or TcB also provides a quantitative assessment of the degree of hyperbilirubinemia. This provides guidance regarding the need (or lack of need) for additional testing to identify a cause of the hyperbilirubinemia and for additional TSB measurements.[1]

The TSB can be measured from the same sample that is drawn for the

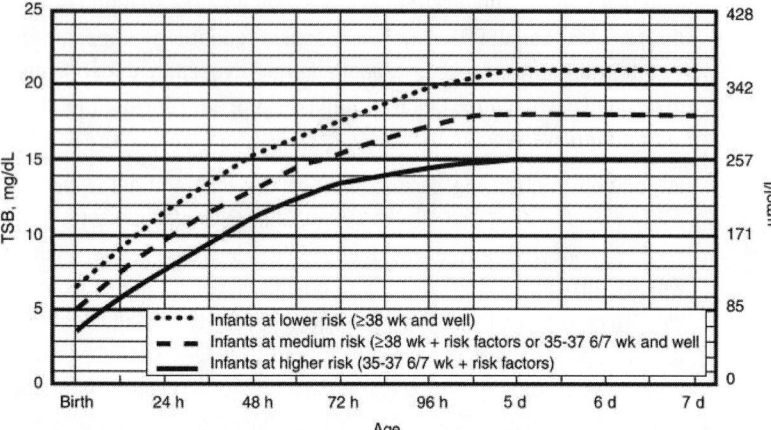

FIGURE 1
Guidelines for phototherapy in hospitalized infants ≥35 weeks' gestation. Note that these guidelines are based on limited evidence and that the levels shown are approximations. The guidelines refer to the use of intensive phototherapy, which should be used when the TSB level exceeds the line indicated for each category.

- Use total bilirubin. Do not subtract direct-reacting or conjugated bilirubin.
- Risk factors are isoimmune hemolytic disease, G6PD deficiency, asphyxia, significant lethargy, temperature instability, sepsis, acidosis, or an albumin level of <3.0 g/dL (if measured).
- For well infants at 35 to 37⁶/₇ weeks' gestation, one can adjust TSB levels for intervention around the medium-risk line. It is an option to intervene at lower TSB levels for infants closer to 35 weeks' gestation and at higher TSB levels for those closer to 37⁶/₇ weeks' gestation.
- It is an option to provide conventional phototherapy in the hospital or at home at TSB levels of 2 to 3 mg/dL (35–50 μmol/L) below those shown, but home phototherapy should not be used in any infant with risk factors.

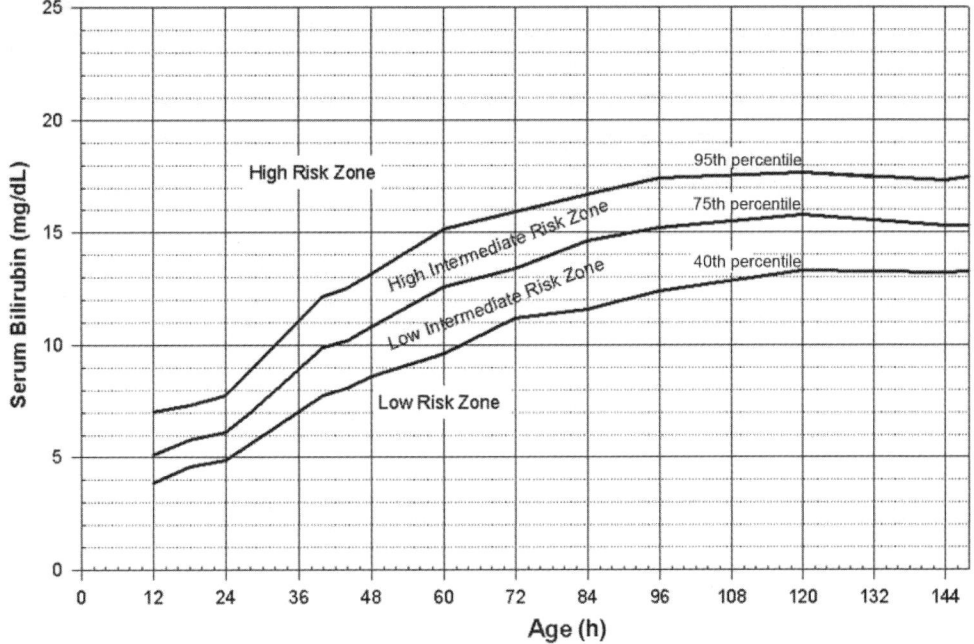

FIGURE 2
Nomogram for designation of risk in 2840 well newborns at ≥36 weeks' gestational age with birth weight of ≥2000 g or ≥35 weeks' gestational age and birth weight of ≥2500 g based on the hour-specific serum bilirubin values. (Reproduced with permission from Bhutani VK, Johnson L, Sivieri EM. *Pediatrics.* 1999;103[1]:6–14.)

metabolic screen. The risk zone (Fig 2) and the other clinical risk factors (Table 3) are then combined to assess the risk of subsequent hyperbilirubinemia and to formulate a plan for management and follow-up (Fig 3). When combined with the risk zone, the factors that are most predictive of hyperbilirubinemia risk are lower gestational age and exclusive breastfeeding.[13,14,23] The lower the gestational age, the greater the risk of developing hyperbilirubinemia.[13,14,23] For those infants from whom ≥2 successive TSB or TcB measurements are obtained, it is helpful to plot the data on the nomogram[15] to assess the rate of rise. Hemolysis is likely if the TSB/TcB is crossing percentiles on the nomogram and suggests the need for further testing and follow-up (see Table 1 in the 2004 AAP guideline).

Therefore, we recommend that a predischarge measurement of TSB or TcB be performed and the risk zone for hyperbilirubinemia determined[15] on the

basis of the infant's age in hours and the TSB or TcB measurement.

It should be noted that, even with a low predischarge TSB or TcB level, the risk of subsequent hyperbilirubinemia is not zero,[13,17] so appropriate follow-up should always be provided (Fig 3).

RESPONSE TO PREDISCHARGE TSB MEASUREMENTS

Figure 3 provides our recommendations for management and follow-up, according to predischarge screening. Note that this algorithm represents a consensus of the authors and is based on interpretation of limited evidence (see below).

FOLLOW-UP AFTER DISCHARGE

Most infants discharged at <72 hours should be seen within 2 days of discharge.

Earlier follow-up might be necessary for infants who have risk factors for severe hyperbilirubinemia,[1,13,14,23] whereas those in the lower risk zones with few or no risk factors can be seen later (Fig 3). Figure 3 also provides additional suggestions for evaluation and management at the first follow-up visit.

TcB MEASUREMENTS

TcB measurements are being used with increasing frequency in hospi-

TABLE 3 Other Risk Factors for Severe Hyperbilirubinemia to be Considered with the Gestational Age and the Pre-discharge TSB or TcB level (see Figure 3)

Exclusive breastfeeding, particularly if nursing is not going well and/or weight loss is excessive (>8 – 10%)
Isoimmune or other hemolytic disease (eg, G6PD deficiency, hereditary spherocytosis)
Previous sibling with jaundice
Cephalohematoma or significant bruising
East Asian race

The gestational age and the predischarge TSB or TcB level are the most important factors that help to predict the risk of hyperbilirubinemia. The risk increases with each decreasing week of gestation from 42–35 weeks (see Figure 3)

A

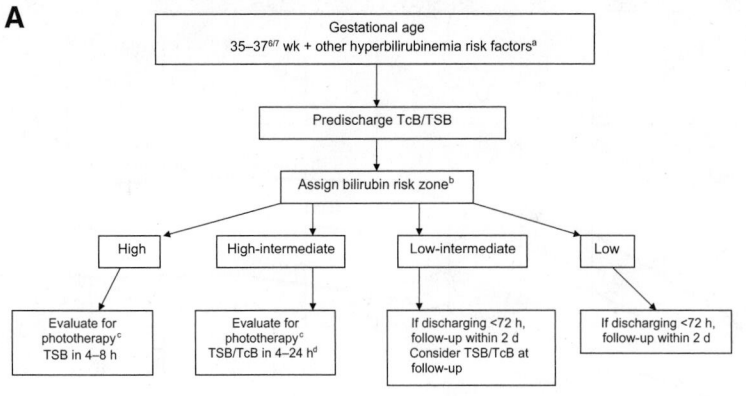

B

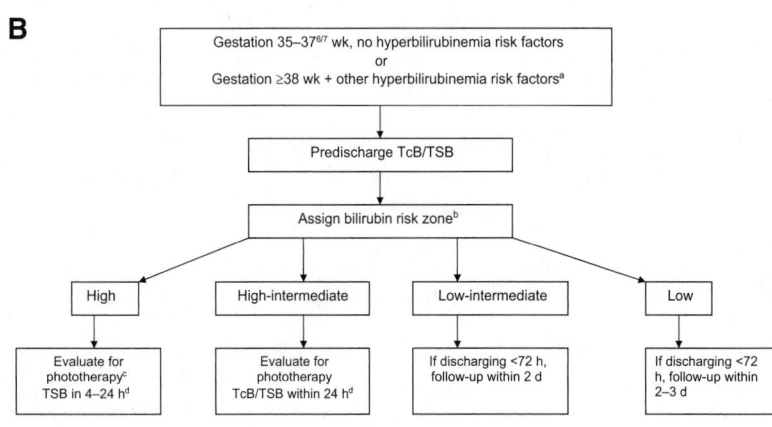

C

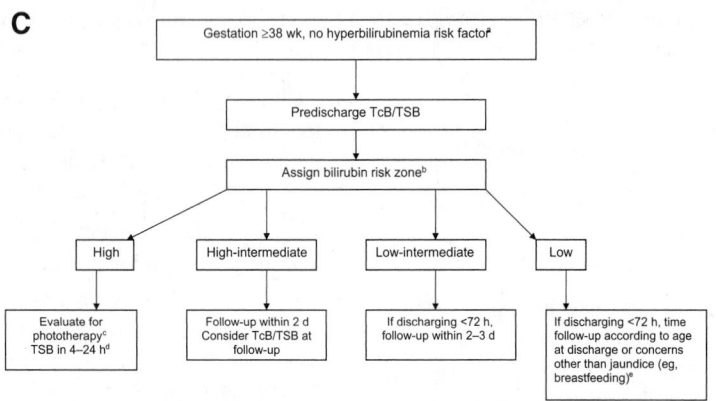

FIGURE 3

Algorithm providing recommendations for management and follow-up according to predischarge bilirubin measurements, gestation, and risk factors for subsequent hyperbilirubinemia.

- Provide lactation evaluation and support for all breastfeeding mothers.
- Recommendation for timing of repeat TSB measurement depends on age at measurement and how far the TSB level is above the 95th percentile (Fig 2). Higher and earlier initial TSB levels require an earlier repeat TSB measurement.
- Perform standard clinical evaluation at all follow-up visits.
- For evaluation of jaundice see 2004 AAP guideline.[1]
- [a] Table 3. [b] Fig 2. [c] Fig 1. [d] In hospital or as outpatient. [e] Follow-up recommendations can be modified according to level of risk for hyperbilirubinemia; depending on the circumstances in infants at low risk, later follow-up can be considered.

tal nurseries and in some outpatient settings. They have the advantage of providing instantaneous information and probably reduce the likelihood of missing a clinically significant TSB, making them particularly useful in outpatient practice. TcB measurements can significantly reduce the number of TSB measurements that are required, but as with any point-of-care test, regular monitoring for appropriate quality assurance by comparison with TSB measurements is necessary. Significant variation can occur among instruments, and the use of a new instrument should be compared with hospital laboratory measurements to ensure that the instrument is working properly; such checks should be performed periodically. TcB is a measurement of the yellow color of the blanched skin and subcutaneous tissue, not the serum, and should be used as a screening tool to help determine whether the TSB should be measured. Although TcB measurements provide a good estimate of the TSB level, they are not a substitute for TSB values, and a TSB level should always be obtained when therapeutic intervention is being considered.

Most studies in term and late-preterm infants have indicated that the TcB tends to underestimate the TSB, particularly at higher TSB levels.[18] Thus, investigators have adopted various techniques to avoid missing a high TSB level (ie, a false-negative TcB measurement). These techniques include measuring the TSB if

- the TcB value is at 70% of the TSB level recommended for the use of phototherapy[19];
- the TcB value is above the 75th percentile on the Bhutani nomogram (Fig 1)[15] or the 95th percentile on a TcB nomogram[16] (in 1 study, if the TcB was <75th percentile on the Bhutani nomogram, 0 of 349 infants

had a TSB level above the 95th percentile [a negative predictive value of 100%][20]; or

- at follow-up after discharge, the TcB value is >13 mg/dL (222 μmol/L)[21] (in this outpatient study, no infant who had a TcB value of ≤13 mg/dL had a TSB level of >17 mg/dL [291 μmol/L]).[21]

COSTS

The introduction of universal predischarge bilirubin screening, follow-up visits, and TSB/TcB measurements might increase costs. Ideally, a cost/benefit analysis should include the cost to prevent 1 case of kernicterus. The cost per case, however, highly depends on the incidence of kernicterus as well as its potential reduction resulting from the intervention. By using a strategy similar to that suggested in this guideline, and assuming an incidence of kernicterus of 1 in 100 000 live births and a relative risk reduction of 70%, the cost to prevent 1 case of kernicterus has been estimated as approximately $5.7 million.[22] Because we do not know the current incidence of kernicterus in the United States or the actual relative risk reduction (if these guidelines were implemented universally), we cannot calculate the true cost/benefit ratio. Taking into account the lifetime cost of an infant with kernicterus, it is possible that there could be savings.[22]

DISCUSSION

While endeavoring to clarify some areas addressed in the 2004 AAP guideline, we have also introduced new recommendations, both for the predis-

charge assessment of the risk of subsequent hyperbilirubinemia and for follow-up testing. We recognize that the quality of evidence for recommending universal predischarge screening and for the suggested management and follow-up (Fig 3) is limited and, in the absence of higher levels of evidence, our recommendations must, therefore, be based on expert opinion. As indicated in the reviews by the US Preventive Services Task Force[12] and Trikalinos et al[11] in this issue of *Pediatrics*, there are currently no good data to indicate that the implementation of these recommendations will reduce the risk of kernicterus, although published data suggest that predischarge screening can reduce the incidence of a TSB level of ≥25 mg/dL,[24,25] perhaps by increasing the use of phototherapy.[24] Nevertheless, because kernicterus is a devastating condition that leads to serious and permanent neurologic damage, and because published reports and our own review of cases in the medicolegal setting suggest that many of these cases could have been prevented, a reasonable argument can be made for implementing the suggested recommendations in the absence of better evidence. Because kernicterus is a rare condition, it is unlikely that we will be able to obtain adequate evidence in the short-term to support our recommendations. In their elegant polemic, Auerbach et al[26] discussed "the tension between needing to improve care and knowing how to do it." They noted that, in the absence of appropriate evidence, "bold efforts at improvement can consume tremendous resources yet confer only a small benefit."[26] We

also recognize that although predischarge testing is relatively inexpensive and convenient, measuring the TSB after discharge is more difficult. TcB measurement is quite easy but is not currently available in most primary care settings. In addition, more evidence is needed to support the cost and efficacy of these recommendations. There is certainly a risk that these recommendations could lead to additional testing and an increase in both appropriate and inappropriate use of phototherapy.[1,24] Nevertheless, it is our opinion that universal screening, when combined with the clinical risk factors (of which gestational age and exclusive breastfeeding are most important) and targeted follow-up, is a systems approach that is easy to implement and understand, and it provides a method of identifying infants who are at high or low risk for the development of severe hyperbilirubinemia. In addition to risk assessment, the measurement of TSB or TcB when interpreted by using the hour-specific nomogram provides the caregiver with an immediate and quantitative mechanism for assessing the degree of hyperbilirubinemia and the need for additional surveillance and testing. As such, it could play an important role in preventing acute bilirubin encephalopathy, although this has yet to be demonstrated.

ACKNOWLEDGMENTS

We are grateful for reviews and critiques of this commentary by neonatologists, bilirubinologists, pediatricians, and pediatric residents.

REFERENCES

1. American Academy of Pediatrics, Subcommittee on Hyperbilirubinemia. Management of hyperbilirubinemia in the newborn infant 35 or more weeks of gestation [published correction appears in *Pediatrics*. 2004;114(4):1138]. *Pediatrics*. 2004;114(1):297–316
2. Canadian Paediatric Society, Fetus and Newborn Committee. Guidelines for detection, manage-

ment and prevention of hyperbilirubinemia in term and late preterm newborn infants (35 or more weeks' gestation). *Paediatr Child Health.* 2007;12(5):1B–12B

3. Sgro M, Campbell DM, Fallah S, Shah V. Kernicterus, January 2007 to December 2009. Canadian Paediatric Surveillance Program 2008 Results. Available at: www.cps.ca/english/surveillance/CPSP/index.htm. Accessed July 30, 2009

4. Manning D, Todd P, Maxwell M, Platt MJ. Prospective surveillance study of severe hyperbilirubinaemia in the newborn in the UK and Ireland. *Arch Dis Child Fetal Neonatal Ed.* 2007;92(5):F342–F346

5. Bartmann P, Schaaff F. Kernicterus in Germany 2003–2005. *E-PAS.* 2007;617936.23

6. Ebbesen F. Recurrence of kernicterus in term and near-term infants in Denmark. *Acta Paediatr.* 2000;89(10):1213–1217

7. Ebbesen F, Andersson C, Verder H, et al. Extreme hyperbilirubinaemia in term and near-term infants in Denmark. *Acta Paediatr.* 2005;94(1):59–64

8. National Quality Forum. *Serious Reportable Events in Healthcare: A Consensus Report.* Washington, DC: National Quality Forum; 2002

9. Davidson L, Thilo EH. How to make kernicterus a "never event." *Neoreviews.* 2003;4(11):308–314

10. Watchko JF. Vigintiphobia revisited. *Pediatrics.* 2005;115(6):1747–1753

11. Trikalinos T, Chung M, Lau J, Ip S. Systematic review of screening for bilirubin encephalopathy in neonates. *Pediatrics.* 2009;124(4):1162–1171

12. US Preventive Services Task Force. Screening of infants for hyperbilirubinemia to prevent chronic bilirubin encephalopathy: recommendation statement. *Pediatrics.* 2009;124(4):1172–1177

13. Keren R, Luan X, Friedman S, Saddlemire S, Cnaan A, Bhutani V. A comparison of alternative risk-assessment strategies for predicting significant neonatal hyperbilirubinemia in term and near-term infants. *Pediatrics.* 2008;121(1). Available at: www.pediatrics.org/cgi/content/full/121/1/e170

14. Newman T, Liljestrand P, Escobar G. Combining clinical risk factors with bilirubin levels to predict hyperbilirubinemia in newborns. *Arch Pediatr Adolesc Med.* 2005;159(2):113–119

15. Bhutani VK, Johnson L, Sivieri EM. Predictive ability of a predischarge hour-specific serum bilirubin for subsequent significant hyperbilirubinemia in healthy-term and near-term newborns. *Pediatrics.* 1999;103(1):6–14

16. Maisels MJ, Kring E. Transcutaneous bilirubin levels in the first 96 hours in a normal newborn population of ≥35 weeks' of gestation. *Pediatrics.* 2006;117(4):1169–1173

17. Stevenson DK, Fanaroff AA, Maisels MJ, et al. Prediction of hyperbilirubinemia in near-term and term infants. *Pediatrics.* 2001;108(1):31–39

18. Maisels MJ. Transcutaneous bilirubinometry. *Neoreviews.* 2006;7(5):e217–e225

19. Ebbesen F, Rasmussen LM, Wimberley PD. A new transcutaneous bilirubinometer, BiliCheck, used in the neonatal intensive care unit and the maternity ward. *Acta Paediatr.* 2002;91(2):203–211

20. Bhutani V, Gourley GR, Adler S, Kreamer B, Dalman C, Johnson LH. Noninvasive measurement of total serum bilirubin in a multiracial predischarge newborn population to assess the risk of severe hyperbilirubinemia. *Pediatrics.* 2000;106(2). Available at: www.pediatrics.org/cgi/content/full/106/2/e17

21. Engle W, Jackson GC, Stehel EK, Sendelbach D, Manning MD. Evaluation of a transcutaneous jaundice meter following hospital discharge in term and near-term neonates. *J Perinatol.* 2005;25(7):486–490

22. Suresh G, Clark R. Cost-effectiveness of strategies that are intended to prevent kernicterus in newborn infants. *Pediatrics.* 2004;114(4):917–924

23. Maisels MJ, Deridder JM, Kring EA, Balasubramaniam M. Routine transcutaneous bilirubin measurements combined with clinical risk factors improve the prediction of subsequent hyperbilirubinemia. *J Perinatol.* 2009; In press

24. Kuzniewicz MW, Escobar GJ, Newman TB. The impact of universal bilirubin screening on severe hyperbilirubinemia and phototherapy use in a managed care organization. *Pediatrics.* 2009;124(4):1031–1039

25. Eggert L, Wiedmeier SE, Wilson J, Christensen R. The effect of instituting a prehospital-discharge newborn bilirubin screening program in an 18-hospital health system. *Pediatrics.* 2006;117(5). Available at: www.pediatrics.org/cgi/content/full/117/5/e855

26. Auerbach AD, Landefeld CS, Shojania K. The tension between needing to improve care and knowing how to do it. *N Engl J Med.* 2007;357(6):608–613

Universal Bilirubin Screening, Guidelines, and Evidence

AUTHOR: Thomas B. Newman, MD, MPH

Division of Clinical Epidemiology, Department of Epidemiology and Biostatistics, and Division of General Pediatrics, Department of Pediatrics, University of California, San Francisco, California; and Division of Research, Kaiser Permanente Medical Care Program, Oakland, California

ABBREVIATIONS
AAP—American Academy of Pediatrics
USPSTF—US Preventive Services Task Force
TSB—total serum bilirubin

Opinions expressed in these commentaries are those of the author and not necessarily those of the American Academy of Pediatrics or its Committees.

www.pediatrics.org/cgi/doi/10.1542/peds.2009-0412

doi:10.1542/peds.2009-0412

Accepted for publication Feb 17, 2009

Address correspondence to Thomas B. Newman, MD, MPH, University of California, Department of Epidemiology and Biostatistics, Box 0560, San Francisco, CA 94143. E-mail newman@epi.ucsf.edu

PEDIATRICS (ISSN Numbers: Print, 0031-4005; Online, 1098-4275).

FINANCIAL DISCLOSURE: *The author has indicated he has no financial relationships relevant to this article to disclose.*

In a commentary[1] and update of the 2004 American Academy of Pediatrics (AAP) guideline "Management of Hyperbilirubinemia in the Newborn Infant 35 or More Weeks of Gestation"[2] in this issue of *Pediatrics*, Maisels et al recommend that all newborns have a bilirubin measurement before discharge from their birth hospitalization. In contrast, a recommendation statement from the US Preventive Services Task Force (USPSTF),[3] supported by a systematic review,[4] concludes that evidence is insufficient to make that recommendation. As an author of the commentary[1] and the 2004 AAP jaundice guideline[2] who also has been critical of guidelines based on insufficient evidence,[5–11] I have felt particularly torn about this recommendation.

Perhaps partly because I have served as an expert consultant on dozens of heartbreaking kernicterus legal cases,[12] I find the argument in favor of universal bilirubin screening and systematic follow-up persuasive. We know kernicterus is devastating and that, although rare, cases are continuing to occur. Furthermore, anecdotal evidence suggests that many cases could have been prevented by earlier measurement of bilirubin levels, leading to closer follow-up and earlier initiation of appropriate therapy.[13,14] We have not had randomized trials to show that universal screening and systematic follow-up will lead to a reduction in kernicterus, but considerable research in the area of optimizing patient safety suggests that there is room for improvement in the 2004 guidelines. Specifically, we know that in the absence of universal screening, detection and management of clinically significant hyperbilirubinemia during the birth hospitalization relies on several imperfect steps: (1) nurses and doctors need to remember to examine the infant for jaundice; (2) they need to distinguish visually between jaundice that is and is not clinically significant for the infant's age in hours; and (3) they need to combine information from this visual assessment of jaundice and/or a total serum bilirubin (TSB) level with knowledge of the newborn's other risk factors to determine the need for and timing of bilirubin measurements, follow-up visits, and treatments. We also know that nurseries are busy places and that sometimes people may not do things that they should[15] or might do them under suboptimal conditions, such as assessing jaundice in the dim light found in many hospital rooms. Finally, compared with the devastating effects of kernicterus, the costs and risks of screening seem low, particularly with a transcutaneous bilirubinometer, which may actually decrease the number of serum bilirubin measurements obtained.[16]

On the other hand, as a proponent of evidence-based medicine, I recognize the insufficiency of the data to support the recommendation.[3,4] The rationale outlined above would apply whether the incidence of kernicterus were 1 in 10 000 or 1 in 1 million, but surely the potential benefits of screening depend on how much kernicterus there is to prevent, and this is not known. Even if we knew the incidence of kernicterus, the proportion that might be preventable by screening and systematic follow-up is unclear. Although plaintiffs in malpractice cases commonly assert that infants with bilirubin levels in the 40s at 4 or 5 days must have had proportionately high levels at the time of discharge (even if no or minimal jaundice was noted at that time), there is little evidence to support this assertion. Studies of the predictive value of early bilirubin levels have had much lower levels of hyperbilirubinemia (TSB of 17–20 mg/dL).[3] Because they may have different causes, such as glucose-6-phosphate dehydrogenase deficiency and infection, the very high levels that lead to kernicterus may be less predictable. Moreover, several studies have revealed that in the absence of any jaundice, a TSB level of ≥12 mg/dL is extremely unlikely.[17–20] As an experienced generalist who believes he can recognize at least some newborns who definitely are not jaundiced, I sympathize with colleagues who may question the cost-efficacy of measuring bilirubin (particularly if it involves an additional poke or trying to squeeze more blood out of a recalcitrant heel) in a light-skinned 2-day-old who has no hint of jaundice. Requiring a bilirubin measurement for every such infant because some clinicians may forget or be careless feels like keeping the whole class after school for the transgressions of a few.

After doing my best to reconcile these opposing viewpoints, I believe that universal predischarge bilirubin screening is a good idea but that the evidence is not sufficient to recommend it in an AAP guideline. This is consistent with AAP policy. In a 2004 statement, the Steering Committee on Quality Improvement and Management outlined levels of evidence and strengths of AAP guidelines.[21] The policy stated that ex-

cept in "exceptional situations where validating studies cannot be performed and there is a clear preponderance of benefit or harm," if the level of evidence is "expert opinion, case reports, and reasoning from first principles," a course of action should be designated an option rather than a recommendation. Because, as is explicitly acknowledged in the commentary, expert opinion, case reports, and reasoning from first principles are exactly the level of evidence that supports the recommendation for universal bilirubin screening, and because we wanted to make that recommendation, it needed to be published as a commentary rather than a guideline.

Is this AAP policy on evidence and guideline recommendations a good one? I believe it is. Practicing clinicians need and appreciate guidance from experts, but they also recognize the impossibility of following every guideline that an expert committee might recommend for them and need protection from well-meaning but sometimes paternalistic committees with their own agendas.[22] Guideline committees tend to be dominated by academics and subspecialists with special interest, expertise, and even emotional investment in the diseases for which they are producing guidelines.[23] Most of us authors of the hyperbilirubinemia commentary are no exception.[12,24] Although interest and expertise are invaluable, the career focus on a particular disease, with resulting close relationships with funders, patients, advocacy groups, industry, and each other, may lead to a narrow perspective in which heroic efforts at preventing or treating the target disease feel justified, even when a favorable balance of benefits over risks and costs is uncertain.[23] And, although slavishly adhering to evidence standards could lead to failure to recommend beneficial treatments[25,26] even what seem

like obvious, common-sense interventions can have unintended adverse consequences.[27,28]

The USPSTF uses a different model for producing guidelines, in which expertise at appraising and synthesizing evidence trumps disease-specific expertise.[29] Recommendations of the USPSTF are typically based on the results of systematic reviews of evidence, often performed by one of the Agency for Healthcare Research and Quality's evidence-based practice centers. Such thorough reviews are not within time, expertise, and budget constraints of most guideline committees. Ironically, however, the recommendation to measure a bilirubin level for every infant before discharge was the subject of just such a review,[4] which concluded that the evidence is insufficient to make a recommendation for or against universal bilirubin screening ("I" rating).[3]

The USPSTF statement comments not only on the lack of evidence that universal bilirubin screening will prevent bilirubin encephalopathy but also on the insufficiency of evidence regarding risks and efficacy of phototherapy.[3] This is important, because an unintended consequence of institution of universal bilirubin screening might be a greater focus on the danger of hyperbilirubinemia, leading to excessive use of phototherapy. There is evidence that this has occurred in the Northern California Kaiser Permanente Medical Care Program, in which increased bilirubin testing was associated with a decrease in bilirubin levels of >25 mg/dL and also an increase in use of phototherapy at levels lower than those recommended in the 2004 AAP guideline.[30] Thus, it is worth stressing that the recommendation for bilirubin screening should not be misinterpreted as suggesting the need for phototherapy at lower bilirubin levels.

The Maisels et al commentary on hyperbilirubinemia published in this issue came about because of a need to clarify the 2004 guideline and because the AAP had been asked for a statement that either recommended universal bilirubin screening or explained why not. I suspect that having the recommendation for universal screening come in the form of a commentary, rather than a guideline, will be disappointing to both advocates and opponents of universal screening. However, I believe it is the right decision. For now, it represents what some bilirubin experts believe is reasonable on the basis of limited evidence. With additional research, we hope to be able to make a stronger recommendation in the future.

ACKNOWLEDGMENT

This work was partially supported by National Institute of Child Health and Human Development grant R01 HD047557.

REFERENCES

1. Maisels MJ, Bhutani VK, Bogen D, Newman TB, Stark AR, Watchko JF. Management of hyperbilirubinemia in the newborn infant ≥35 weeks' gestation: an update with clarifications. *Pediatrics.* 2009;124(4):1193–1198

2. American Academy of Pediatrics, Subcommittee on Hyperbilirubinemia. Management of hyperbilirubinemia in the newborn infant 35 or more weeks of gestation [published correction appears in *Pediatrics.* 2004;114(4):1138]. *Pediatrics.* 2004;114(1):297–316

3. US Preventive Services Task Force. Screening of infants for hyperbilirubinemia to prevent chronic bilirubin encephalopathy: recommendation statement. *Pediatrics.* 2009;124(4):1172–1177

4. Trikalinos T, Chung M, Lau J, Ip S. Systematic review of screening for bilirubin encephalopathy in neonates. *Pediatrics.* 2009;124(4):1162–1171

5. Newman TB, Garber AM, Holtzman NA, Hulley SB. Problems with the report of the expert panel on blood cholesterol levels in children and adolescents. *Arch Pediatr Adolesc Med.* 1995;149(3): 241–247

6. Newman TB, Garber AM. Cholesterol screening in children and adolescents. *Pediatrics.* 2000;105(3 pt 1):637–638

7. Newman TB, Johnston BD, Grossman DC. Effects and costs of requiring child-restraint systems for young children traveling on commercial airplanes. *Arch Pediatr Adolesc Med.* 2003;157(10): 969–974

8. Newman TB. Evidence does not support American Academy of Pediatrics recommendation for routine imaging after a first urinary tract infection. *Pediatrics.* 2005;116(6):1613–1614

9. Newman TB. If it's not worth doing, it's not worth doing well. *Pediatrics.* 2005;115(1):196; author reply 196–197

10. Newman TB. Much pain, little gain from voiding cystourethrograms after urinary tract infection. *Pediatrics.* 2006;118(5):2251; author reply 2251–2252

11. Newman TB. Industry-sponsored "expert committee recommendations for acne management" promote expensive drugs on the basis of weak evidence. *Pediatrics.* 2007;119(3):650; author reply 650–651

12. Newman TB. The power of stories over statistics. *BMJ.* 2003;327(7429):1424–1427

13. Maisels MJ, Baltz RD, Bhutani VK, et al. Neonatal jaundice and kernicterus. *Pediatrics.* 2001;108(3): 763–765

14. Johnson LH, Bhutani VK, Brown AK. System-based approach to management of neonatal jaundice and prevention of kernicterus. *J Pediatr.* 2002;140(4):396–403

15. Newman TB, Liljestrand P, Escobar GJ. Jaundice noted in the first 24 hours after birth in a managed care organization. *Arch Pediatr Adolesc Med.* 2002;156(12):1244–1250

16. Maisels MJ, Kring E. Transcutaneous bilirubinometry decreases the need for serum bilirubin measurements and saves money. *Pediatrics.* 1997;99(4):599–601

17. Davidson L, Merritt K, Weech A. Hyperbilirubinemia in the newborn. *Am J Dis Child.* 1941;61(5): 958–980

18. Madlon-Kay DJ. Recognition of the presence and severity of newborn jaundice by parents, nurses, physicians, and icterometer. *Pediatrics.* 1997;100(3). Available at: www.pediatrics.org/cgi/content/full/100/3/e3

19. Moyer VA, Ahn C, Sneed S. Accuracy of clinical judgment in neonatal jaundice. *Arch Pediatr Adolesc Med.* 2000;154(4):391–394

20. Riskin A, Kuglman A, Abend-Weinger M, Green M, Hemo M, Bader D. In the eye of the beholder: how accurate is clinical estimation of jaundice in newborns? *Acta Paediatr.* 2003;92(5):574–576

21. American Academy of Pediatrics, Steering Committee on Quality Improvement and Management. Classifying recommendations for clinical practice guidelines. *Pediatrics.* 2004;114(3):874–877

22. Sanghavi D. Plenty of guidelines, but where's the evidence? *The New York Times*. December 9, 2008:D6

23. Hayward RA. Access to clinically-detailed patient information: a fundamental element for improving the efficiency and quality of healthcare. *Med Care*. 2008;46(3):229–231

24. Newman TB, Maisels MJ. Less aggressive treatment of neonatal jaundice and reports of kernicterus: lessons about practice guidelines. *Pediatrics*. 2000;105(1 pt 3):242–245

25. Smith GC, Pell JP. Parachute use to prevent death and major trauma related to gravitational challenge: systematic review of randomised controlled trials. *BMJ*. 2003;327(7429):1459–1461

26. Potts M, Prata N, Walsh J, Grossman A. Parachute approach to evidence based medicine. *BMJ*. 2006;333(7570):701–703

27. Auerbach AD, Landefeld CS, Shojania KG. The tension between needing to improve care and knowing how to do it. *N Engl J Med*. 2007;357(6):608–613

28. Shojania KG, Duncan BW, McDonald KM, Wachter RM. Safe but sound: patient safety meets evidence-based medicine. *JAMA*. 2002;288(4):508–513

29. Moyer VA, Nelson D; US Preventive Services Task Force. Pediatricians and the US Preventive Services Task Force: a natural partnership to enhance the health of children. *Pediatrics*. 2008;122(1):174–176

30. Kuzniewicz MW, Escobar GJ, Newman TB. The impact of universal bilirubin screening on severe hyperbilirubinemia and phototherapy use in a managed care organization. *Pediatrics*. 2009;124(4):1031–1039

Hyperbilirubinemia Clinical Practice Guideline Quick Reference Tools

- Recommendation Summary
  — Management of Hyperbilirubinemia in the Newborn Infant 35 or More Weeks of Gestation
- *ICD-10-CM* Coding Quick Reference for Hyperbilirubinemia
- AAP Patient Education Handout
  — *Jaundice and Your Newborn*

Recommendation Summary

Management of Hyperbilirubinemia in the Newborn Infant 35 or More Weeks of Gestation

The following are the key elements of the recommendations provided by this guideline. Clinicians should:

1. Promote and support successful breastfeeding.
2. Establish nursery protocols for the identification and evaluation of hyperbilirubinemia.
3. Measure the total serum bilirubin (TSB) or transcutaneous bilirubin (TcB) level on infants jaundiced in the first 24 hours.
4. Recognize that visual estimation of the degree of jaundice can lead to errors, particularly in darkly pigmented infants.
5. Interpret all bilirubin levels according to the infant's age in hours.
6. Recognize that infants at less than 38 weeks' gestation, particularly those who are breastfed, are at higher risk of developing hyperbilirubinemia and require closer surveillance and monitoring.
7. Perform a systematic assessment on all infants before discharge for the risk of severe hyperbilirubinemia.
8. Provide parents with written and verbal information about newborn jaundice.
9. Provide appropriate follow-up based on the time of discharge and the risk assessment.
10. Treat newborns, when indicated, with phototherapy or exchange transfusion.

Coding Quick Reference for Hyperbilirubinemia	
ICD-10-CM	
P59.0	Neonatal jaundice associated with preterm delivery
P59.3	Neonatal jaundice from breast milk inhibitor
P59.9	Neonatal jaundice, unspecified
R17	Unspecified jaundice

Jaundice and Your Newborn

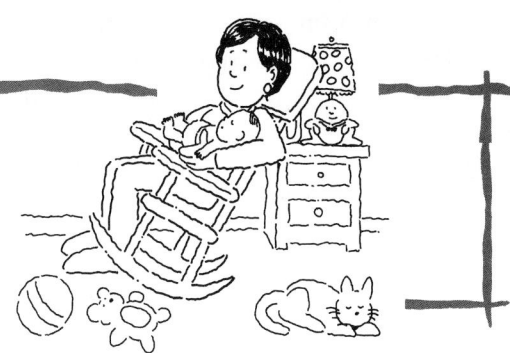

Congratulations on the birth of your new baby!

To make sure your baby's first week is safe and healthy, it is important that

1. You find a pediatrician you are comfortable with for your baby's ongoing care.
2. Your baby is checked for jaundice in the hospital.
3. If you are breastfeeding, you get the help you need to make sure it is going well.
4. Make sure your baby is seen by a doctor or nurse at 3 to 5 days of age.
5. If your baby is discharged before age 72 hours, your baby should be seen by a doctor or nurse within 2 days of discharge from the hospital.

Q: What is jaundice?

A: Jaundice is the yellow color seen in the skin of many newborns. It happens when a chemical called *bilirubin* builds up in the baby's blood. Jaundice can occur in babies of any race or color.

Q: Why is jaundice common in newborns?

A: Everyone's blood contains bilirubin, which is removed by the liver. Before birth, the mother's liver does this for the baby. Most babies develop jaundice in the first few days after birth because it takes a few days for the baby's liver to get better at removing bilirubin.

Q: How can I tell if my baby is jaundiced?

A: The skin of a baby with jaundice usually appears yellow. The best way to see jaundice is in good light, such as daylight or under fluorescent lights. Jaundice usually appears first in the face and then moves to the chest, abdomen, arms, and legs as the bilirubin level increases. The whites of the eyes may also be yellow. Jaundice may be harder to see in babies with darker skin color.

Q: Can jaundice hurt my baby?

A: Most babies have mild jaundice that is harmless, but in unusual situations the bilirubin level can get very high and might cause brain damage. This is why newborns should be checked carefully for jaundice and treated to prevent a high bilirubin level.

Q: How should my baby be checked for jaundice?

A: If your baby looks jaundiced in the first few days after birth, your baby's doctor or nurse may use a skin or blood test to check your baby's bilirubin level. However, because estimating the bilirubin level based on the baby's appearance can be difficult, some experts recommend that a skin or blood test be done even if your baby does not appear jaundiced. A bilirubin level is always needed if jaundice develops before the baby is 24 hours old. Whether a test is needed after that depends on the baby's age, the amount of jaundice, and whether the baby has other factors that make jaundice more likely or harder to see.

Q: Does breastfeeding affect jaundice?

A: Jaundice is more common in babies who are breastfed than babies who are formula-fed, but this occurs mainly in newborns who are not nursing well. If you are breastfeeding, you should nurse your baby at least 8 to 12 times a day for the first few days. This will help you produce enough milk and will help to keep the baby's bilirubin level down. If you are having trouble breastfeeding, ask your baby's doctor or nurse or a lactation specialist for help. Breast milk is the ideal food for your baby.

Q: When should my newborn get checked after leaving the hospital?

A: It is important for your baby to be seen by a nurse or doctor when the baby is between 3 and 5 days old, because this is usually when a baby's bilirubin level is highest. This is why, if your baby is discharged before age 72 hours, your baby should be seen within 2 days of discharge. The timing of this visit may vary depending on your baby's age when released from the hospital and other factors.

Q: Which babies require more attention for jaundice?

A: Some babies have a greater risk for high levels of bilirubin and may need to be seen sooner after discharge from the hospital. Ask your doctor about an early follow-up visit if your baby has any of the following:

- A high bilirubin level before leaving the hospital
- Early birth (more than 2 weeks before the due date)
- Jaundice in the first 24 hours after birth
- Breastfeeding that is not going well
- A lot of bruising or bleeding under the scalp related to labor and delivery
- A parent, brother, or sister who had high bilirubin and received light therapy

Q: When should I call my baby's doctor?

A: Call your baby's doctor if

- Your baby's skin turns more yellow.
- Your baby's abdomen, arms, or legs are yellow.
- The whites of your baby's eyes are yellow.
- Your baby is jaundiced and is hard to wake, fussy, or not nursing or taking formula well.

Q: How is harmful jaundice prevented?

A: Most jaundice requires no treatment. When treatment is necessary, placing your baby under special lights while he or she is undressed will lower the bilirubin level. Depending on your baby's bilirubin level, this can be done in the hospital or at home. Jaundice is treated at levels that are much lower than those at which brain damage is a concern. Treatment can prevent the harmful effects of jaundice. Putting your baby in sunlight is not recommended as a safe way of treating jaundice. Exposing your baby to sunlight might help lower the bilirubin level, but this will only work if the baby is completely undressed. This cannot be done safely inside your home because your baby will get cold, and newborns should never be put in direct sunlight outside because they might get sunburned.

Q: When does jaundice go away?

A: In breastfed babies, jaundice often lasts for more than 2 to 3 weeks. In formula-fed babies, most jaundice goes away by 2 weeks. If your baby is jaundiced for more than 3 weeks, see your baby's doctor.

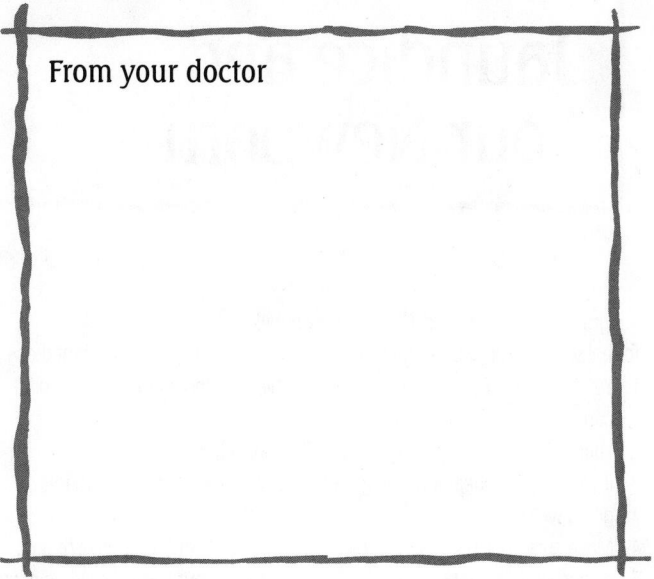

From your doctor

American Academy
of Pediatrics

DEDICATED TO THE HEALTH OF ALL CHILDREN™

The American Academy of Pediatrics is an organization of 60,000 primary care pediatricians, pediatric medical subspecialists, and pediatric surgical specialists dedicated to the health, safety, and well-being of infants, children, adolescents, and young adults.

American Academy of Pediatrics
Web site — www.aap.org

The Diagnosis and Management of Acute Otitis Media

• •

- *Clinical Practice Guideline*

CLINICAL PRACTICE GUIDELINE

The Diagnosis and Management of Acute Otitis Media

abstract

This evidence-based clinical practice guideline is a revision of the 2004 acute otitis media (AOM) guideline from the American Academy of Pediatrics (AAP) and American Academy of Family Physicians. It provides recommendations to primary care clinicians for the management of children from 6 months through 12 years of age with uncomplicated AOM.

In 2009, the AAP convened a committee composed of primary care physicians and experts in the fields of pediatrics, family practice, otolaryngology, epidemiology, infectious disease, emergency medicine, and guideline methodology. The subcommittee partnered with the Agency for Healthcare Research and Quality and the Southern California Evidence-Based Practice Center to develop a comprehensive review of the new literature related to AOM since the initial evidence report of 2000. The resulting evidence report and other sources of data were used to formulate the practice guideline recommendations.

The focus of this practice guideline is the appropriate diagnosis and initial treatment of a child presenting with AOM. The guideline provides a specific, stringent definition of AOM. It addresses pain management, initial observation versus antibiotic treatment, appropriate choices of antibiotic agents, and preventive measures. It also addresses recurrent AOM, which was not included in the 2004 guideline. Decisions were made on the basis of a systematic grading of the quality of evidence and benefit-harm relationships.

The practice guideline underwent comprehensive peer review before formal approval by the AAP.

This clinical practice guideline is not intended as a sole source of guidance in the management of children with AOM. Rather, it is intended to assist primary care clinicians by providing a framework for clinical decision-making. It is not intended to replace clinical judgment or establish a protocol for all children with this condition. These recommendations may not provide the only appropriate approach to the management of this problem. *Pediatrics* 2013;131:e964–e999

Allan S. Lieberthal, MD, FAAP, Aaron E. Carroll, MD, MS, FAAP, Tasnee Chonmaitree, MD, FAAP, Theodore G. Ganiats, MD, Alejandro Hoberman, MD, FAAP, Mary Anne Jackson, MD, FAAP, Mark D. Joffe, MD, FAAP, Donald T. Miller, MD, MPH, FAAP, Richard M. Rosenfeld, MD, MPH, FAAP, Xavier D. Sevilla, MD, FAAP, Richard H. Schwartz, MD, FAAP, Pauline A. Thomas, MD, FAAP, and David E. Tunkel, MD, FAAP, FACS

KEY WORDS
acute otitis media, otitis media, otoscopy, otitis media with effusion, watchful waiting, antibiotics, antibiotic prophylaxis, tympanostomy tube insertion, immunization, breastfeeding

ABBREVIATIONS
AAFP—American Academy of Family Physicians
AAP—American Academy of Pediatrics
AHRQ—Agency for Healthcare Research and Quality
AOM—acute otitis media
CI—confidence interval
FDA—US Food and Drug Administration
LAIV—live-attenuated intranasal influenza vaccine
MEE—middle ear effusion
MIC—minimum inhibitory concentration
NNT—number needed to treat
OM—otitis media
OME—otitis media with effusion
OR—odds ratio
PCV7—heptavalent pneumococcal conjugate vaccine
PCV13—13-valent pneumococcal conjugate vaccine
RD—rate difference
SNAP—safety-net antibiotic prescription
TIV—trivalent inactivated influenza vaccine
TM—tympanic membrane
WASP—wait-and-see prescription

(Continued on last page)

Key Action Statement 1A: Clinicians should diagnose acute otitis media (AOM) in children who present with moderate to severe bulging of the tympanic membrane (TM) *or* new onset of otorrhea not due to acute otitis externa. Evidence Quality: Grade B. Strength: Recommendation.

Key Action Statement 1B: Clinicians should diagnose AOM in children who present with mild bulging of the TM *and* recent (less than 48 hours) onset of ear pain (holding, tugging, rubbing of the ear in a nonverbal child) *or* intense erythema of the TM. Evidence Quality: Grade C. Strength: Recommendation.

Key Action Statement 1C: Clinicians should not diagnose AOM in children who do not have middle ear effusion (MEE) (based on pneumatic otoscopy and/or tympanometry). Evidence Quality: Grade B. Strength: Recommendation.

Key Action Statement 2: The management of AOM should include an assessment of pain. If pain is present, the clinician should recommend treatment to reduce pain. Evidence Quality: Grade B. Strength: Strong Recommendation.

Key Action Statement 3A: Severe AOM: The clinician should prescribe antibiotic therapy for AOM (bilateral or unilateral) in children 6 months and older with severe signs or symptoms (ie, moderate or severe otalgia or otalgia for at least 48 hours or temperature 39°C [102.2°F] or higher). Evidence Quality: Grade B. Strength: Strong Recommendation.

Key Action Statement 3B: Non-severe bilateral AOM in young children: The clinician should prescribe antibiotic therapy for bilateral AOM in children 6 months through 23 months of age without severe signs or symptoms (ie, mild otalgia for less than 48 hours and temperature less than 39°C [102.2°F]). Evidence Quality: Grade B. Strength: Recommendation.

Key Action Statement 3C: Non-severe unilateral AOM in young children: The clinician should either prescribe antibiotic therapy *or* offer observation with close follow-up based on joint decision-making with the parent(s)/caregiver for unilateral AOM in children 6 months to 23 months of age without severe signs or symptoms (ie, mild otalgia for less than 48 hours and temperature less than 39°C [102.2°F]). When observation is used, a mechanism must be in place to ensure follow-up and begin antibiotic therapy if the child worsens or fails to improve within 48 to 72 hours of onset of symptoms. Evidence Quality: Grade B. Strength: Recommendation.

Key Action Statement 3D: Nonsevere AOM in older children: The clinician should either prescribe antibiotic therapy *or* offer observation with close follow-up based on joint decision-making with the parent(s)/caregiver for AOM (bilateral or unilateral) in children 24 months or older without severe signs or symptoms (ie, mild otalgia for less than 48 hours and temperature less than 39°C [102.2°F]). When observation is used, a mechanism must be in place to ensure follow-up and begin antibiotic therapy if the child worsens or fails to improve within 48 to 72 hours of onset of symptoms. Evidence Quality: Grade B. Strength: Recommendation.

Key Action Statement 4A: Clinicians should prescribe amoxicillin for AOM when a decision to treat with antibiotics has been made *and* the child has not received amoxicillin in the past 30 days *or* the child does not have concurrent purulent conjunctivitis *or* the child is not allergic to penicillin. Evidence Quality: Grade B. Strength: Recommendation.

Key Action Statement 4B: Clinicians should prescribe an antibiotic with additional β-lactamase coverage for AOM when a decision to treat with antibiotics has been made, *and* the child has received amoxicillin in the last 30 days *or* has concurrent purulent conjunctivitis, *or* has a history of recurrent AOM unresponsive to amoxicillin. Evidence Quality: Grade C. Strength: Recommendation.

Key Action Statement 4C: Clinicians should reassess the patient if the caregiver reports that the child's symptoms have worsened or failed to respond to the initial antibiotic treatment within 48 to 72 hours and determine whether a change in therapy is needed. Evidence Quality: Grade B. Strength: Recommendation.

Key Action Statement 5A: Clinicians should not prescribe prophylactic antibiotics to reduce the frequency of episodes of AOM in children with recurrent AOM. Evidence Quality: Grade B. Strength: Recommendation.

Key Action Statement 5B: Clinicians may offer tympanostomy tubes for recurrent AOM (3 episodes in 6 months or 4 episodes in 1 year with 1 episode in the preceding 6 months). Evidence Quality: Grade B. Strength: Option.

Key Action Statement 6A: Clinicians should recommend pneumococcal conjugate vaccine to all children according to the schedule of the Advisory Committee on Immunization Practices of the Centers for Disease Control and Prevention, American Academy of Pediatrics (AAP), and American Academy of Family Physicians (AAFP). Evidence Quality: Grade B. Strength: Strong Recommendation.

Key Action Statement 6B: Clinicians should recommend annual influenza vaccine to all children according to the schedule of the Advisory Committee on Immunization Practices, AAP, and AAFP. Evidence Quality: Grade B. Strength: Recommendation.

2Key Action Statement 6C: Clinicians should encourage exclusive breast-feeding for at least 6 months. Evidence Quality: Grade B. Strength: Recommendation.

Key Action Statement 6D: Clinicians should encourage avoidance of tobacco smoke exposure. Evidence Quality: Grade C. Strength: Recommendation.

INTRODUCTION

In May 2004, the AAP and AAFP published the "Clinical Practice Guideline: Diagnosis and Management of Acute Otitis Media".[1] The guideline offered 8 recommendations ranked according to level of evidence and benefit-harm relationship. Three of the recommendations—diagnostic criteria, observation, and choice of antibiotics—led to significant discussion, especially among experts in the field of otitis media (OM). Also, at the time the guideline was written, information regarding the heptavalent pneumococcal conjugate vaccine (PCV7) was not yet published. Since completion of the guideline in November 2003 and its publication in May 2004, there has been a significant body of additional literature on AOM.

Although OM remains the most common condition for which antibacterial agents are prescribed for children in the United States[2,3] clinician visits for OM decreased from 950 per 1000 children in 1995–1996 to 634 per 1000 children in 2005–2006. There has been a proportional decrease in antibiotic prescriptions for OM from 760 per 1000 in 1995–1996 to 484 per 1000 in 2005–2006. The percentage of OM visits

resulting in antibiotic prescriptions remained relatively stable (80% in 1995–1996; 76% in 2005–2006).[2] Many factors may have contributed to the decrease in visits for OM, including financial issues relating to insurance, such as copayments, that may limit doctor visits, public education campaigns regarding the viral nature of most infectious diseases, use of the PCV7 pneumococcal vaccine, and increased use of the influenza vaccine. Clinicians may also be more attentive to differentiating AOM from OM with effusion (OME), resulting in fewer visits coded for AOM and fewer antibiotic prescriptions written.

Despite significant publicity and awareness of the 2004 AOM guideline, evidence shows that clinicians are hesitant to follow the guideline recommendations. Vernacchio et al[4] surveyed 489 primary care physicians as to their management of 4 AOM scenarios addressed in the 2004 guideline. No significant changes in practice were noted on this survey, compared with a survey administered before the 2004 AOM guideline. Coco[5] used the National Ambulatory Medical Care Survey from 2002 through 2006 to determine the frequency of AOM visits without antibiotics before and after publication of the 2004 guideline. There was no difference in prescribing rates. A similar response to otitis guidelines was found in Italy as in the United States.[6,7] These findings parallel results of other investigations regarding clinician awareness and adherence to guideline recommendations in all specialties, including pediatrics.[8] Clearly, for clinical practice guidelines to be effective, more must be done to improve their dissemination and implementation.

This revision and update of the AAP/AAFP 2004 AOM guideline[1] will evaluate published evidence on the diagnosis and management of uncomplicated AOM and make recommendations based on that evidence. The guideline is intended

for primary care clinicians including pediatricians and family physicians, emergency department physicians, otolaryngologists, physician assistants, and nurse practitioners. The scope of the guideline is the diagnosis and management of AOM, including recurrent AOM, in children 6 months through 12 years of age. It applies only to an otherwise healthy child without underlying conditions that may alter the natural course of AOM, including but not limited to the presence of tympanostomy tubes; anatomic abnormalities, including cleft palate; genetic conditions with craniofacial abnormalities, such as Down syndrome; immune deficiencies; and the presence of cochlear implants. Children with OME without AOM are also excluded.

Glossary of Terms

AOM—the rapid onset of signs and symptoms of inflammation in the middle ear[9,10]

Uncomplicated AOM—AOM without otorrhea[1]

Severe AOM—AOM with the presence of moderate to severe otalgia or fever equal to or higher than 39°C[9,10]

Nonsevere AOM—AOM with the presence of mild otalgia and a temperature below 39°C[9,10]

Recurrent AOM—3 or more well-documented and separate AOM episodes in the preceding 6 months or 4 or more episodes in the preceding 12 months with at least 1 episode in the past 6 months[11,12]

OME—inflammation of the middle ear with liquid collected in the middle ear; the signs and symptoms of acute infection are absent[9]

MEE—liquid in the middle ear without reference to etiology, pathogenesis, pathology, or duration[9]

Otorrhea—discharge from the ear, originating at 1 or more of the following sites: the external auditory canal, middle ear, mastoid, inner ear, or intracranial cavity

Otitis externa—an infection of the external auditory canal

Tympanometry—measuring acoustic immittance (transfer of acoustic energy) of the ear as a function of ear canal air pressure[13,14]

Number needed to treat (NNT)—the number of patients who need to be treated to prevent 1 additional bad outcome[15]

Initial antibiotic therapy—treatment of AOM with antibiotics that are prescribed at the time of diagnosis with the intent of starting antibiotic therapy as soon as possible after the encounter

Initial observation—initial management of AOM limited to symptomatic relief, with commencement of antibiotic therapy only if the child's condition worsens at any time or does not show clinical improvement within 48 to 72 hours of diagnosis; a mechanism must be in place to ensure follow-up and initiation of antibiotics if the child fails observation

METHODS

Guideline development using an evidence-based approach requires that all evidence related to the guideline is gathered in a systematic fashion, objectively assessed, and then described so readers can easily see the links between the evidence and recommendations made. An evidence-based approach leads to recommendations that are guided by both the quality of the available evidence and the benefit-to-harm ratio that results from following the recommendation. Figure 1 shows the relationship of evidence quality and benefit-harm balance in determining the level of recommendation. Table 1 presents the AAP definitions and implications of different levels of evidence-based recommendations.[16]

In preparing for the 2004 AAP guidelines, the Agency for Healthcare Research and Quality (AHRQ) funded and conducted an exhaustive review of the literature on diagnosis and management of AOM.[17–19] In 2008, the AHRQ and the Southern California Evidence-Based Practice Center began a similar process of reviewing the literature published since the 2001 AHRQ report. The AAP again partnered with AHRQ and the Southern California Evidence-Based Practice Center to develop the evidence report, which served as a major source of data for these practice guideline recommendations.[20,21] New key questions were determined by a technical expert panel. The scope of the new report went beyond the 2001 AHRQ report to include recurrent AOM. The key questions addressed by AHRQ in the 2010 report were as follows:

1. Diagnosis of AOM: What are the operating characteristics (sensitivity, specificity, and likelihood ratios) of clinical symptoms and otoscopic findings (such as bulging TM) to diagnose uncomplicated AOM and to distinguish it from OME?

2. What has been the effect of the use of heptavalent PCV7 on AOM microbial epidemiology, what organisms (bacterial and viral) are associated with AOM since the introduction of PCV7, and what are the patterns of antimicrobial resistance in AOM since the introduction of PCV7?

3. What is the comparative effectiveness of various treatment options for treating uncomplicated AOM in average risk children?

4. What is the comparative effectiveness of different management options for recurrent OM (uncomplicated) and persistent OM or relapse of AOM?

5. Do treatment outcomes in Questions 3 and 4 differ by characteristics of the condition (AOM), patient, environment, and/or health care delivery system?

6. What adverse effects have been observed for treatments for which outcomes are addressed in Questions 3 and 4?

For the 2010 review, searches of PubMed and the Cochrane Database of Systematic Reviews, Cochrane Central Register of Controlled Trials, and Education Resources Information Center were conducted by using the same search strategies used for the 2001 report for publications from 1998 through June 2010. Additional terms or conditions not considered in the 2001 review (recurrent OM, new drugs, and heptavalent pneumococcal vaccine) were also included. The Web of Science was also used to search for citations of the 2001 report and its peer-reviewed publications. Titles were screened independently by 2

Evidence Quality	Preponderance of Benefit or Harm	Balance of Benefit and Harm
A. Well designed RCTs or diagnostic studies on relevant population	Strong Recommendation	
B. RCTs or diagnostic studies with minor limitations; overwhelmingly consistent evidence from observational studies		
C. Observational studies (case-control and cohort design)	Recommendation	Option
D. Expert opinion, case reports, reasoning from first principles	Option	No Rec
X. Exceptional situations in which validating studies cannot be performed and there is a clear preponderance of benefit or harm	Strong Recommendation / Recommendation	

FIGURE 1
Relationship of evidence quality and benefit-harm balance in determining the level of recommendation. RCT, randomized controlled trial.

TABLE 1 Guideline Definitions for Evidence-Based Statements

Statement	Definition	Implication
Strong Recommendation	A strong recommendation in favor of a particular action is made when the anticipated benefits of the recommended intervention clearly exceed the harms (as a strong recommendation against an action is made when the anticipated harms clearly exceed the benefits) and the quality of the supporting evidence is excellent. In some clearly identified circumstances, strong recommendations may be made when high-quality evidence is impossible to obtain and the anticipated benefits strongly outweigh the harms.	Clinicians should follow a strong recommendation unless a clear and compelling rationale for an alternative approach is present.
Recommendation	A recommendation in favor of a particular action is made when the anticipated benefits exceed the harms, but the quality of evidence is not as strong. Again, in some clearly identified circumstances, recommendations may be made when high-quality evidence is impossible to obtain but the anticipated benefits outweigh the harms.	Clinicians would be prudent to follow a recommendation but should remain alert to new information and sensitive to patient preferences.
Option	Options define courses that may be taken when either the quality of evidence is suspect or carefully performed studies have shown little clear advantage to 1 approach over another.	Clinicians should consider the option in their decision-making, and patient preference may have a substantial role.
No Recommendation	No recommendation indicates that there is a lack of pertinent published evidence and that the anticipated balance of benefits and harms is presently unclear.	Clinicians should be alert to new published evidence that clarifies the balance of benefit versus harm.

pediatricians with experience in conducting systematic reviews.

For the question pertaining to diagnosis, efficacy, and safety, the search was primarily for clinical trials. For the question pertaining to the effect of PCV7 on epidemiology and microbiology, the group searched for trials that compared microbiology in the same populations before and after introduction of the vaccine or observational studies that compared microbiology across vaccinated and unvaccinated populations.

In total, the reviewers examined 7646 titles, of which 686 titles were identified for further review. Of those, 72 articles that met the predetermined inclusion and exclusion criteria were reviewed in detail. Investigators abstracted data into standard evidence tables, with accuracy checked by a second investigator. Studies were quality-rated by 2 investigators by using established criteria. For randomized controlled trials, the Jadad criteria were used.[22] QUADAS criteria[23] were used to evaluate the studies that pertained to diagnosis. GRADE criteria were applied to pooled analyses.[24] Data abstracted

included parameters necessary to define study groups, inclusion/exclusion criteria, influencing factors, and outcome measures. Some of the data for analysis were abstracted by a biostatistician and checked by a physician reviewer. A sequential resolution strategy was used to match and resolve the screening and review results of the 2 pediatrician reviewers.

For the assessment of treatment efficacy, pooled analyses were performed for comparisons for which 3 or more trials could be identified. Studies eligible for analyses of questions pertaining to treatment efficacy were grouped for comparisons by treatment options. Each comparison consisted of studies that were considered homogeneous across clinical practice. Because some of the key questions were addressed in the 2001 evidence report,[17] studies identified in that report were included with newly identified articles in the 2010 evidence report.[20]

Decisions were made on the basis of a systematic grading of the quality of evidence and strength of recommendations as well as expert consensus when

definitive data were not available. Results of the literature review were presented in evidence tables and published in the final evidence report.[20]

In June 2009, the AAP convened a new subcommittee to review and revise the May 2004 AOM guideline.[1] The subcommittee comprised primary care physicians and experts in the fields of pediatrics, family practice, otolaryngology, epidemiology, infectious disease, emergency medicine, and guideline methodology. All panel members reviewed the AAP policy on conflict of interest and voluntary disclosure and were given an opportunity to present any potential conflicts with the subcommittee's work. All potential conflicts of interest are listed at the end of this document. The project was funded by the AAP. New literature on OM is continually being published. Although the systematic review performed by AHRQ could not be replicated with new literature, members of the Subcommittee on Diagnosis and Management of Acute Otitis Media reviewed additional articles. PubMed was searched by using the single search term "acute otitis media," approximately every 6 months from June 2009 through October 2011 to obtain new articles. Subcommittee members evaluated pertinent articles for quality of methodology and importance of results. Selected articles used in the AHRQ review were also reevaluated for their quality. Conclusions were based on the consensus of the subcommittee after the review of newer literature and reevaluation of the AHRQ evidence. Key action statements were generated using BRIDGE-Wiz (Building Recommendations in a Developers Guideline Editor), an interactive software tool that leads guideline development through a series of questions that are intended to create a more actionable set of key action statements.[25] BRIDGE-Wiz also incorporates the quality of available evidence into the final determination of the strength of each recommendation.

After thorough review by the subcommittee for this guideline, a draft was reviewed by other AAP committees and sections, selected outside organizations, and individuals identified by the subcommittee as experts in the field. Additionally, members of the subcommittee were encouraged to distribute the draft to interested parties in their respective specialties. All comments were reviewed by the writing group and incorporated into the final guideline when appropriate.

This clinical practice guideline is not intended as a sole source of guidance in the management of children with AOM. Rather, it is intended to assist clinicians in decision-making. It is not intended to replace clinical judgment or establish a protocol for the care of all children with this condition. These recommendations may not provide the only appropriate approach to the management of children with AOM.

It is AAP policy to review and update evidence-based guidelines every 5 years.

KEY ACTION STATEMENTS
Key Action Statement 1A

Clinicians should diagnose AOM in children who present with moderate to severe bulging of the TM *or* new onset of otorrhea not due to acute otitis externa. (Evidence Quality: Grade B, Rec. Strength: Recommendation)

Key Action Statement Profile: KAS 1A

Aggregate evidence quality	Grade B
Benefits	• Identify a population of children most likely to benefit from intervention. • Avoid unnecessary treatment of those without highly certain AOM. • Promote consistency in diagnosis.
Risks, harms, cost	May miss AOM that presents with a combination of mild bulging, intense erythema, or otalgia that may not necessarily represent less severe disease and may also benefit from intervention.
Benefits-harms assessment	Preponderance of benefit.
Value judgments	Identification of a population of children with highly certain AOM is beneficial. Accurate, specific diagnosis is helpful to the individual patient. Modification of current behavior of overdiagnosis is a goal. Increased specificity is preferred even as sensitivity is lowered.
Intentional vagueness	By using stringent diagnostic criteria, the TM appearance of less severe illness that might be early AOM has not been addressed.
Role of patient preferences	None
Exclusions	None
Strength	**Recommendation**
Notes	Tympanocentesis studies confirm that using these diagnostic findings leads to high levels of isolation of pathogenic bacteria. Evidence is extrapolated from treatment studies that included tympanocentesis.

Key Action Statement 1B

Clinicians should diagnose AOM in children who present with mild bulging of the TM *and* recent (less than 48 hours) onset of ear pain (holding, tugging, rubbing of the ear in a nonverbal child) or intense erythema of the TM. (Evidence Quality: Grade C, Rec. Strength: Recommendation)

Key Action Statement Profile: KAS 1B

Aggregate evidence quality	Grade C
Benefits	Identify AOM in children when the diagnosis is not highly certain.
Risks, harms, cost	Overdiagnosis of AOM. Reduced precision in diagnosis.
Benefits-harms assessment	Benefits greater than harms.
Value judgments	None.
Intentional vagueness	Criteria may be more subjective.
Role of patient preferences	None
Exclusions	None
Strength	**Recommendation**
Notes	Recent onset of ear pain means within the past 48 hours.

Key Action Statement 1C

Clinicians should not diagnose AOM in children who do not have MEE (based on pneumatic otoscopy and/or tympanometry). (Evidence Quality: Grade B, Rec. Strength: Recommendation)

Key Action Statement Profile: KAS 1C

Aggregate evidence quality	Grade B
Benefits	Reduces overdiagnosis and unnecessary treatment. Increases correct diagnosis of other conditions with symptoms that otherwise might be attributed to AOM. Promotes the use of pneumatic otoscopy and tympanometry to improve diagnostic accuracy.
Risks, harms, cost	Cost of tympanometry. Need to acquire or reacquire skills in pneumatic otoscopy and tympanometry for some clinicians.
Benefits-harms assessment	Preponderance of benefit.
Value judgments	AOM is overdiagnosed, often without adequate visualization of the TM. Early AOM without effusion occurs, but the risk of overdiagnosis supersedes that concern.
Intentional vagueness	None
Role of patient preferences	None
Exclusions	Early AOM evidenced by intense erythema of the TM.
Strength	**Recommendation**

Purpose of This Section

There is no gold standard for the diagnosis of AOM. In fact, AOM has a spectrum of signs as the disease develops.[26] Therefore, the purpose of this section is to provide clinicians and researchers with a working clinical definition of AOM and to differentiate AOM from OME. The criteria were chosen to achieve high specificity recognizing that the resulting decreased sensitivity may exclude less severe presentations of AOM.

Changes From AAP/AAFP 2004 AOM Guideline

Accurate diagnosis of AOM is critical to sound clinical decision-making and high-quality research. The 2004 "Clinical Practice Guideline: Diagnosis and Management of AOM"[1] used a 3-part definition for AOM: (1) acute onset of symptoms, (2) presence of MEE, and (3) signs of acute middle ear inflammation. This definition generated extensive discussion and reanalysis of the AOM diagnostic evidence. The 2004 definition lacked precision to exclude cases of OME, and diagnoses of AOM could be made in children with acute onset of symptoms, including severe otalgia and MEE, without other otoscopic findings of inflammation.[27] Furthermore, the use of "uncertain diagnosis" in the 2004 AOM guideline may have permitted diagnoses of AOM without clear visualization of the TM. Earlier studies may have enrolled children who had OME rather than AOM, resulting in the possible classification of such children as improved because their nonspecific symptoms would have abated regardless of therapy.[28–30] Two studies, published in 2011, used stringent diagnostic criteria for diagnosing AOM with much less risk of conclusions based on data from mixed patients.[31,32]

Since publication of the 2004 AOM guideline, a number of studies have been conducted evaluating scales for the presence of symptoms. These studies did not show a consistent correlation of symptoms with the initial diagnosis of AOM, especially in preverbal children.[33–35]

Recent research has used precisely stated stringent criteria of AOM for purposes of the studies.[31,32] The current guideline endorses stringent otoscopic diagnostic criteria as a basis for management decisions (described later). As clinicians use the proposed stringent criteria to diagnose AOM, they should be aware that children with AOM may also present with recent onset of ear pain and intense erythema of the TM as the only otoscopic finding.

Symptoms

Older children with AOM usually present with a history of rapid onset of ear pain. However, in young preverbal children, otalgia as suggested by tugging/rubbing/holding of the ear, excessive crying, fever, or changes in the child's sleep or behavior pattern as noted by the parent are often relatively nonspecific symptoms. A number of studies have attempted to correlate symptom scores with diagnoses of AOM.

A systematic review[36] identified 4 articles that evaluated the accuracy of symptoms.[37–40] Ear pain appeared useful in diagnosing AOM (combined positive likelihood ratio 3.0–7.3, negative likelihood ratio 0.4–0.6); however, it was only present in 50% to 60% of children with AOM. Conclusions from these studies may be limited, because they (1) enrolled children seen by specialists, not likely to represent the whole spectrum of severity of illness; (2) used a clinical diagnosis of AOM based more on symptomatology rather than on tympanocentesis; and (3) included relatively older children.[37,40]

Laine et al[34] used a questionnaire administered to 469 parents who suspected their children, aged 6 to 35 months, had AOM. Of the children, 237 had AOM using strict otoscopic criteria, and 232 had upper respiratory tract infection without AOM. Restless sleep, ear rubbing, fever, and nonspecific respiratory or gastrointestinal tract symptoms did not differentiate children with or without AOM.

McCormick et al[30] used 2 symptom scores—a 3-item score (OM-3), consisting of symptoms of physical suffering such as ear pain or fever, emotional distress (irritability, poor appetite), and limitation in activity; and a 5-item score (Ear Treatment Group Symptom Questionnaire, 5 Items [ETG-5]), including fever, earache, irritability, decreased appetite, and sleep disturbance—to assess AOM symptoms at the time of diagnosis and daily during the 10-day treatment or observation period. They found both to be a responsive measure of changes in clinical symptoms. The same group[35] also tested a visual scale, Acute Otitis Media-Faces Scale (AOM-FS), with faces similar to the Wong-Baker pain scale.[41] None of the scales were adequately sensitive for making the diagnosis of AOM based on symptoms. The AOM-FS combined with an otoscopy score, OS-8,[30] were presented as a double-sided pocket card. The combination of AOM-FS and OS-8 was more responsive to change than either instrument alone.

Shaikh et al[33,42] validated a 7-item parent-reported symptom score (Acute Otitis Media Severity of Symptom Scale [AOM-SOS]) for children with AOM, following stringent guidance of the US Food and Drug Administration (FDA) on the development of patient-reported outcome scales. Symptoms included ear tugging/rubbing/holding, excessive crying, irritability, difficulty sleeping, decreased activity or appetite, and fever. AOM-SOS was correlated with otoscopic diagnoses (AOM, OME, and normal middle ear status). AOM-SOS changed appropriately in response to clinical change. Its day-to-day responsiveness supports its usefulness in following AOM symptoms over time.

Signs of AOM

Few studies have evaluated the relationship of otoscopic findings in AOM

and tympanocentesis. A study by Karma et al[43] is often cited as the best single study of otoscopic findings in AOM. However, the study uses only a symptom-based diagnosis of AOM plus the presence of MEE. Thus, children with acute upper respiratory tract infection symptoms and OME would have been considered to have AOM. There also were significant differences in findings at the 2 centers that participated in the study.

The investigators correlated TM color, mobility, and position with the presence of middle ear fluid obtained by tympanocentesis. At 2 sites in Finland (Tampere and Oulu), 2911 children were followed from 6 months to 2.5 years of age. A single otolaryngologist at Tampere and a single pediatrician at Oulu examined subjects. Color, position, and mobility were recorded. Myringotomy and aspiration were performed if MEE was suspected. AOM was diagnosed if MEE was found and the child had fever, earache, irritability, ear rubbing or tugging, simultaneous other acute respiratory tract symptoms, vomiting, or diarrhea. The presence or absence of MEE was noted, but no analyses of the fluid, including culture, were performed. Pneumatic otoscopic findings were classified as follows: color—hemorrhagic, strongly red, moderately red, cloudy or dull, slightly red, or normal; position—bulging, retracted, or normal; and mobility—distinctly impaired, slightly impaired, or normal.

For this analysis, 11 804 visits were available. For visits with acute symptoms, MEE was found in 84.9% and 81.8% at the 2 sites at which the study was performed. There were significant differences among the results at the 2 centers involved in the study. Table 2 shows specific data for each finding.

The combination of a "cloudy," bulging TM with impaired mobility was the

TABLE 2 Otoscopic Findings in Children With Acute Symptoms and MEE[a]

TM Finding in Acute Visits With MEE	Group I (Tampere, Finland), %	Group II (Oulo, Finland), %
Color		
Distinctly red	69.8	65.6
Hemorrhagic	81.3	62.9
Strongly red	87.7	68.1
Moderately red	59.8	66.0
Slightly red	39.4	16.7
Cloudy	95.7	80.0
Normal	1.7	4.9
Position		
Bulging	96.0	89
Retracted	46.8	48.6
Normal	32.1	22.2
Mobility		
Distinctly impaired	94.0	78.5
Slightly impaired	59.7	32.8
Normal	2.7	4.8

[a] Totals are greater than 100%, because each ear may have had different findings.[43]

best predictor of AOM using the symptom-based diagnosis in this study. Impaired mobility had the highest sensitivity and specificity (approximately 95% and 85%, respectively). Cloudiness had the next best combination of high sensitivity (~74%) and high specificity (~93%) in this study. Bulging had high specificity (~97%) but lower sensitivity (~51%). A TM that was hemorrhagic, strongly red, or moderately red also correlated with the presence of AOM, and a TM that was only "slightly red" was not helpful diagnostically.

McCormick et al reported that a bulging TM was highly associated with the presence of a bacterial pathogen, with or without a concomitant viral pathogen.[44] In a small study, 31 children (40 ears) underwent myringotomy.[45] Bulging TMs had positive bacterial cultures 75% of the time. The percentage of positive cultures for a pathogen increased to 80% if the color of the TM was yellow. The conclusion is that moderate to severe bulging of the TM represents the most important characteristic in the diagnosis of AOM—a finding that has implications for clinical care, research, and education.

The committee recognized that there is a progression from the presence of MEE to the bulging of the TM, and it is often difficult to differentiate this equivocal appearance from the highly certain AOM criteria advocated in this guideline.[26] As such, there is a role for individualized diagnosis and management decisions. Examples of normal, mild bulging, moderate bulging, and severe bulging can be seen in Fig 2.

Distinguishing AOM From OME

OME may occur either as the aftermath of an episode of AOM or as a consequence of eustachian tube dysfunction attributable to an upper respiratory tract infection.[46] However, OME may also precede and predispose to the development of AOM. These 2 forms of OM may be considered segments of a disease continuum.[47] However, because OME does not represent an acute infectious process that benefits from antibiotics, it is of utmost importance for clinicians to become proficient in distinguishing normal middle ear status from OME or AOM. Doing so will avoid unnecessary use of antibiotics, which leads to increased adverse effects of medication and facilitates the development of antimicrobial resistance.

Examination of the TM

Accurate diagnosis of AOM in infants and young children may be difficult. Symptoms may be mild or overlap with those of an upper respiratory tract illness. The TM may be obscured by cerumen, and subtle changes in the TM may be difficult to discern. Additional factors complicating diagnosis may include lack of cooperation from the child; less than optimal diagnostic equipment, including lack of a pneumatic bulb; inadequate instruments for clearing cerumen from the external auditory canal; inadequate assistance for restraining the child; and lack of experience in removing cerumen and performing pneumatic otoscopy.

The pneumatic otoscope is the standard tool used in diagnosing OM. Valuable also is a surgical head, which greatly facilitates cleaning cerumen from an infant's external auditory canal. Cerumen may be removed by using a curette, gentle suction, or irrigation.[48] The pneumatic otoscope should have a light source of sufficient brightness and an air-tight seal that permits application of positive and negative pressure. In general, nondisposable specula achieve a better seal with less pain because of a thicker, smoother edge and better light transmission properties. The speculum size should be chosen to gently seal at the outer portion of the external auditory canal.

Pneumatic otoscopy permits assessment of the contour of the TM (normal, retracted, full, bulging), its color (gray, yellow, pink, amber, white, red, blue), its translucency (translucent, semiopaque, opaque), and its mobility (normal, increased, decreased, absent). The normal TM is translucent, pearly gray, and has a ground-glass appearance (Fig 2A). Specific landmarks can be visualized. They include the short process and the manubrium of the malleus and the pars flaccida, located superiorly. These are easily observed and help to identify the position of the TM. Inward movement of the TM on positive pressure in the external canal and outward movement on negative pressure should occur, especially in the superior posterior quadrant. When the TM is retracted, the short process of the malleus becomes more prominent, and the manubrium appears shortened because of its change in position within the middle ear. Inward motion occurring with positive pressure is restricted or absent, because the TM is frequently as far inward as its range of motion allows. However, outward mobility can be visualized when negative pressure is applied. If the TM does not move perceptibly with applications of gentle positive or negative pressure, MEE is likely. Sometimes, the application of pressure will make an air-fluid interface behind the TM (which is diagnostic of MEE) more evident.[49]

Instruction in the proper evaluation of the child's middle ear status should begin with the first pediatric rotation in medical school and continue throughout postgraduate training.[50]

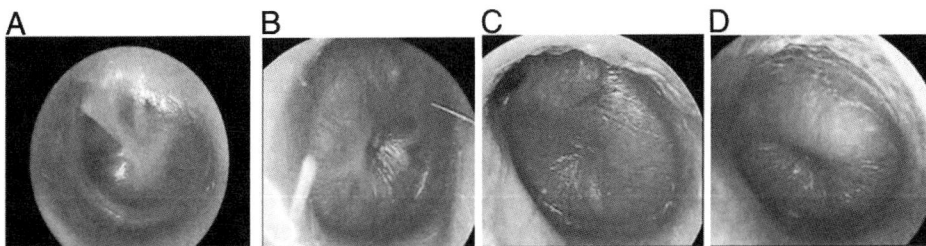

FIGURE 2
A, Normal TM. B, TM with mild bulging. C, TM with moderate bulging. D, TM with severe bulging. Courtesy of Alejandro Hoberman, MD.

Continuing medical education should reinforce the importance of, and retrain the clinician in, the use of pneumatic otoscopy.[51] Training tools include the use of a video-otoscope in residency programs, the use of Web-based educational resources,[49,52] as well as simultaneous or sequential examination of TMs with an expert otoscopist to validate findings by using a double headed or video otoscope. Tools for learning the ear examination can be found in a CD distributed by the Johns Hopkins University School of Medicine and the Institute for Johns

Hopkins Nursing,[53] also available at http://www2.aap.org/sections/infectdis/video.cfm,[54] and through a Web-based program, ePROM: Enhancing Proficiency in Otitis Media.[52]

Key Action Statement 2

The management of AOM should include an assessment of pain. If pain is present, the clinician should recommend treatment to reduce pain. (Evidence Quality: Grade B, Rec. Strength: Strong Recommendation)

Key Action Statement Profile: KAS 2

Aggregate evidence quality	Grade B
Benefits	Relieves the major symptom of AOM.
Risks, harms, cost	Potential medication adverse effects. Variable efficacy of some modes of treatment.
Benefits-harms assessment	Preponderance of benefit.
Value judgments	Treating pain is essential whether or not antibiotics are prescribed.
Intentional vagueness	Choice of analgesic is not specified.
Role of patient preferences	Parents may assist in the decision as to what means of pain relief they prefer.
Exclusions	Topical analgesics in the presence of a perforated TM.
Strength	**Strong Recommendation**

Purpose of This Section

Pain is the major symptom of AOM. This section addresses and updates the literature on treating otalgia.

Changes From AAP/AAFP 2004 AOM Guideline

Only 2 new articles directly address the treatment of otalgia. Both address topical treatment. The 2 new articles are consistent with the 2004 guideline statement. The text of the 2004 guideline is, therefore, reproduced here, with the addition of discussion of the 2 new articles. Table 3 has been updated to include the new references.

Treatment of Otalgia

Many episodes of AOM are associated with pain.[55] Some children with OME also have ear pain. Although pain is

a common symptom in these illnesses, clinicians often see otalgia as a peripheral concern not requiring direct attention.[56] Pain associated

with AOM can be substantial in the first few days of illness and often persists longer in young children.[57] Antibiotic therapy of AOM does not provide symptomatic relief in the first 24 hours[58–61] and even after 3 to 7 days, there may be persistent pain, fever, or both in 30% of children younger than 2 years.[62] In contrast, analgesics do relieve pain associated with AOM within 24 hours[63] and should be used whether antibiotic therapy is or is not prescribed; they should be continued as long as needed. The AAP published the policy statement "The Assessment and Management of Acute Pain in Infants, Children, and Adolescents"[64] to assist the clinician in addressing pain in the context of illness. The management of pain, especially during the first 24 hours of an episode of AOM, should be addressed regardless of the use of antibiotics.

Various treatments of otalgia have been used, but none has been well studied. The clinician should select a treatment on the basis of a consideration of benefits and risks and, wherever possible, incorporate parent/caregiver and patient preference (Table 3).

TABLE 3 Treatments for Otalgia in AOM

Treatment Modality	Comments
Acetaminophen, ibuprofen[63]	Effective analgesia for mild to moderate pain. Readily available. Mainstay of pain management for AOM.
Home remedies (no controlled studies that directly address effectiveness)	May have limited effectiveness.
Distraction	
External application of heat or cold	
Oil drops in external auditory canal	
Topical agents	
Benzocaine, procaine, lidocaine[65,67,70]	Additional, but brief, benefit over acetaminophen in patients older than 5 y.
Naturopathic agents[68]	Comparable to amethocaine/phenazone drops in patients older than 6 y.
Homeopathic agents[71,72]	No controlled studies that directly address pain.
Narcotic analgesia with codeine or analogs	Effective for moderate or severe pain. Requires prescription; risk of respiratory depression, altered mental status, gastrointestinal tract upset, and constipation.
Tympanostomy/myringotomy[73]	Requires skill and entails potential risk.

Since the 2004 guideline was published, there have been only 2 significant new articles.

Bolt et al reported in 2008 on a double-blind placebo-controlled trial at the Australia Children's Hospital emergency department conducted in 2003–2004.[65] They used a convenience sample of children 3 to 17 years of age diagnosed with AOM in the ED. They excluded children with perforation of the TM, pressure-equalizing tube, allergy to local anesthetic or paracetamol, epilepsy, or liver, renal, or cardiac disease. Sixty-three eligible children were randomized to receive aqueous lidocaine or normal saline ear drops up to 3 times in 24 hours. They demonstrated a statistically significant 50% reduction in reported pain at 10 and 30 minutes but not at 20 minutes after application of topical lidocaine, compared with normal saline. Complications were minimal: 3 children reported some dizziness the next day, and none reported tinnitus. A limitation was that some children had received oral acetaminophen before administration of ear drops.

A Cochrane review of topical analgesia for AOM[66] searched the Cochrane register of controlled trials, randomized controlled trials, or quasi-randomized controlled trials that compared otic preparations to placebo or that compared 2 otic preparations. It included studies of adults and children, without TM perforation.

It identified 5 trials in children 3 to 18 years of age. Two (including Bolt et al,[65] discussed above) compared anesthetic drops and placebo at diagnosis of AOM. In both studies, some children also received oral analgesics. Three studies compared anesthetic ear drops with naturopathic herbal drops. Naturopathic drops were favored 15 to 30 minutes after installation, and 1 to 3 days after diagnosis, but the difference was not statistically significant. The Cochrane group concluded that there is limited evidence that ear drops are effective at 30 minutes and unclear if results from these studies are a result of the natural course of illness, placebo effect of receiving treatment, soothing effect of any liquid in the ear, or the drops themselves. Three of the studies included in this review were cited in the 2004 AAP guideline[67–69] and the 1 new paper by Bolt et al.[65]

Key Action Statement 3A

Severe AOM

The clinician should prescribe antibiotic therapy for AOM (bilateral or unilateral) in children 6 months and older with severe signs or symptoms (ie, moderate or severe otalgia or otalgia for at least 48 hours, or temperature 39°C [102.2°F] or higher). (Evidence Quality: Grade B, Rec. Strength: Strong Recommendation)

Key Action Statement Profile: KAS 3A

Aggregate evidence quality	Grade B
Benefits	Increased likelihood of more rapid resolution of symptoms. Increased likelihood of resolution of AOM.
Risks, harms, cost	Adverse events attributable to antibiotics, such as diarrhea, diaper dermatitis, and allergic reactions. Overuse of antibiotics leads to increased bacterial resistance. Cost of antibiotics.
Benefits-harms assessment	Preponderance of benefit over harm.
Value judgments	None
Role of patient preference	None
Intentional vagueness	None
Exclusions	None
Strength	**Strong Recommendation**

Key Action Statement 3B

Nonsevere Bilateral AOM in Young Children

The clinician should prescribe antibiotic therapy for bilateral AOM in children younger than 24 months without severe signs or symptoms (ie, mild otalgia for less than 48 hours, temperature less than 39°C [102.2°F]). (Evidence Quality: Grade B, Rec. Strength: Recommendation)

Key Action Statement Profile: KAS 3B

Aggregate evidence quality	Grade B
Benefits	Increased likelihood of more rapid resolution of symptoms. Increased likelihood of resolution of AOM.
Risks, harms, cost	Adverse events attributable to antibiotics, such as diarrhea, diaper dermatitis, and allergic reactions. Overuse of antibiotics leads to increased bacterial resistance. Cost of antibiotics.
Benefits-harms assessment	Preponderance of benefit over harm.
Value judgments	None
Role of patient preference	None
Intentional vagueness	None
Exclusions	None
Strength	**Recommendation**

Key Action Statement 3C

Nonsevere Unilateral AOM in Young Children

The clinician should either prescribe antibiotic therapy *or* offer observation with close follow-up based on joint decision-making with the parent(s)/caregiver for unilateral AOM in children 6 months to 23 months of age without severe signs or symptoms (ie, mild otalgia for less than 48 hours, temperature less than 39°C [102.2°F]). When observation is used, a mechanism must be in place to ensure

follow-up and begin antibiotic therapy if the child worsens or fails to improve within 48 to 72 hours of **onset of symptoms. (Evidence Quality: Grade B, Rec. Strength: Recommendation)**

Key Action Statement Profile: KAS 3C

Aggregate evidence quality	Grade B
Benefits	Moderately increased likelihood of more rapid resolution of symptoms with initial antibiotics. Moderately increased likelihood of resolution of AOM with initial antibiotics.
Risks, harms, cost	Adverse events attributable to antibiotics, such as diarrhea, diaper dermatitis, and allergic reactions. Overuse of antibiotics leads to increased bacterial resistance. Cost of antibiotics.
Benefits-harms assessment	Moderate degree of benefit over harm.
Value judgments	Observation becomes an alternative as the benefits and harms approach balance.
Role of patient preference	Joint decision-making with the family is essential before choosing observation.
Intentional vagueness	Joint decision-making is highly variable from family to family
Exclusions	None
Strength	**Recommendation**
Note	In the judgment of 1 Subcommittee member (AH), antimicrobial treatment of these children is preferred because of a preponderance of benefit over harm. AH did not endorse Key Action Statement 3C

Key Action Statement 3D

Nonsevere AOM in Older Children

The clinician should either prescribe antibiotic therapy *or* offer observation with close follow-up based on joint decision-making with the parent(s)/caregiver for AOM (bilateral or unilateral) in children 24 months or older without severe signs or symptoms (ie, mild otalgia **for less than 48 hours, temperature less than 39°C [102.2°F]). When observation is used, a mechanism must be in place to ensure follow-up and begin antibiotic therapy if the child worsens or fails to improve within 48 to 72 hours of onset of symptoms. (Evidence Quality: Grade B, Rec Strength: Recommendation)**

Key Action Statement Profile: KAS 3D

Aggregate evidence quality	Grade B
Benefits	*Initial antibiotic treatment*: Slightly increased likelihood of more rapid resolution of symptoms; slightly increased likelihood of resolution of AOM. *Initial observation*: Decreased use of antibiotics; decreased adverse effects of antibiotics; decreased potential for development of bacterial resistance.
Risks, harms, cost	*Initial antibiotic treatment*: Adverse events attributable to antibiotics such as diarrhea, rashes, and allergic reactions. Overuse of antibiotics leads to increased bacterial resistance. *Initial observation*: Possibility of needing to start antibiotics in 48 to 72 h if the patient continues to have symptoms. Minimal risk of adverse consequences of delayed antibiotic treatment. Potential increased phone calls and doctor visits.
Benefits-harms assessment	Slight degree of benefit of initial antibiotics over harm.
Value judgments	Observation is an option as the benefits and harms approach balance.
Role of patient preference	Joint decision-making with the family is essential before choosing observation.
Intentional vagueness	Joint decision-making is highly variable from family to family.
Exclusions	None
Strength	**Recommendation.**

Purpose of This Section

The purpose of this section is to offer guidance on the initial management of AOM by helping clinicians choose between the following 2 strategies:

1. *Initial antibiotic therapy*, defined as treatment of AOM with antibiotics that are prescribed at the time of diagnosis with the intent of starting antibiotic therapy as soon as possible after the encounter.

2. *Initial observation*, defined as initial management of AOM limited to symptomatic relief, with commencement of antibiotic therapy only if the child's condition worsens at any time or does not show clinical improvement within 48 to 72 hours of diagnosis. A mechanism must be in place to ensure follow-up and initiation of antibiotics if the child fails observation.

This section assumes that the clinician has made an accurate diagnosis of AOM by using the criteria and strategies outlined earlier in this guideline. Another assumption is that a clear distinction is made between the role of analgesics and antibiotics in providing symptomatic relief for children with AOM.

Changes From Previous AOM Guideline

The AOM guideline published by the AAP and AAFP in 2004 proposed, for the first time in North America, an "observation option" for selected children with AOM, building on successful implementation of a similar policy in the state of New York[74] and the use of a similar paradigm in many countries in Europe. A common feature of both approaches was to prioritize initial antibiotic therapy according to diagnostic certainty, with greater reliance on observation when the diagnosis was uncertain. In response to criticism that allowing an "uncertain diagnosis" might condone incomplete visualization of the TM or allow inappropriate antibiotic use, this category has been eliminated with greater emphasis now placed on maximizing diagnostic accuracy for AOM.

Since the earlier AOM guideline was published, there has been substantial new research on initial management of AOM, including randomized controlled trials of antibiotic therapy versus placebo or no therapy,[31,32,75] immediate versus delayed antibiotic therapy,[30,76,77] or delayed antibiotic with or without a concurrent prescription.[78] The Hoberman and Tähtinen articles are especially important as they used stringent criteria for diagnosing AOM.[31,32] Systematic reviews have been published on delayed antibiotic therapy,[79] the natural history of AOM in untreated children,[57] predictive factors for antibiotic benefits,[62] and the effect of antibiotics on asymptomatic MEE after therapy.[80] Observational studies provide additional data on outcomes of initial observation with delayed antibiotic therapy, if needed,[81] and on the relationship of previous antibiotic therapy for AOM to subsequent acute mastoiditis.[82,83]

In contrast to the earlier AOM guideline,[1] which recommended antibiotic therapy for all children 6 months to 2 years of age with a certain diagnosis, the current guideline indicates a choice between initial antibiotic therapy or initial observation in this age group for children with unilateral AOM and mild symptoms but only after joint decision-making with the parent(s)/caregiver (Table 4). This change is supported by evidence on the safety of observation or delayed prescribing in young children.[30,31,32,75,76,81] A mechanism must be in place to ensure follow-up and begin antibiotics if the child fails observation.

Importance of Accurate Diagnosis

The recommendations for management of AOM assume an accurate diagnosis on the basis of criteria outlined in the diagnosis section of this guideline. Many of the studies since the 2004 AAP/AAFP AOM guideline[1] used more stringent and well-defined AOM diagnostic definitions than were previously used. Bulging of the TM was required for diagnosis of AOM for most of the children enrolled in the most recent studies.[31,32] By using the criteria in this guideline, clinicians will more accurately distinguish AOM from OME. The management of OME can be found in guidelines written by the AAP, AAFP, and American Academy of Otolaryngology-Head and Neck Surgery.[84,85]

Age, Severity of Symptoms, Otorrhea, and Laterality

Rovers et al[62] performed a systematic search for AOM trials that (1) used random allocation of children, (2) included children 0 to 12 years of age with AOM, (3) compared antibiotics with placebo or no treatment, and (4) had pain or fever as an outcome. The original investigators were asked for their original data.

Primary outcome was pain and/or fever (>38°C) at 3 to 7 days. The adverse effects of antibiotics were also analyzed. Baseline predictors were age <2 years versus ≥2 years, bilateral AOM versus unilateral AOM, and the presence versus absence of otorrhea. Statistical methods were used to assess heterogeneity and to analyze the data.

Of the 10 eligible studies, the investigators of 6 studies[30,75,86–89] provided the original data requested, and 4 did not. A total of 1642 patients were included in the 6 studies from which data were obtained. Of the cases submitted, the average age was 3 to 4 years, with 35% of children younger than 2 years. Bilateral AOM was present in 34% of children, and 42% of children had a bulging TM. Otorrhea was present in 21% of children. The antibiotic and control groups were comparable for all characteristics.

The rate difference (RD) for pain, fever, or both between antibiotic and control groups was 13% (NNT = 8). For children younger than 2 years, the RD was 15% (NNT = 7); for those ≥2 years, RD was 11% (NNT = 10). For unilateral AOM, the RD was 6% (NNT = 17); for bilateral AOM, the RD was 20% (NNT = 5). When unilateral AOM was broken into age groups, among those younger than 2 years, the RD was 5% (NNT = 20), and among those ≥2 years, the RD was 7% (NNT = 15). For bilateral AOM in children younger than 2 years, the RD was 25% (NNT = 4); for

TABLE 4 Recommendations for Initial Management for Uncomplicated AOM[a]

Age	Otorrhea With AOM[a]	Unilateral or Bilateral AOM[a] With Severe Symptoms[b]	Bilateral AOM[a] Without Otorrhea	Unilateral AOM[a] Without Otorrhea
6 mo to 2 y	Antibiotic therapy	Antibiotic therapy	Antibiotic therapy	Antibiotic therapy or additional observation
≥2 y	Antibiotic therapy	Antibiotic therapy	Antibiotic therapy or additional observation	Antibiotic therapy or additional observation[c]

[a] Applies only to children with well-documented AOM with high certainty of diagnosis (see Diagnosis section).

[b] A toxic-appearing child, persistent otalgia more than 48 h, temperature ≥39°C (102.2°F) in the past 48 h, or if there is uncertain access to follow-up after the visit.

[c] This plan of initial management provides an opportunity for shared decision-making with the child's family for those categories appropriate for additional observation. If observation is offered, a mechanism must be in place to ensure follow-up and begin antibiotics if the child worsens or fails to improve within 48 to 72 h of AOM onset.

bilateral AOM in children ≥ 2 years, the RD was 12% (NNT = 9). For otorrhea, the RD was 36% (NNT = 3). One child in the control group who developed meningitis had received antibiotics beginning on day 2 because of worsening status. There were no cases of mastoiditis.

In a Cochrane Review, Sanders et al[59] identified 10 studies that met the following criteria: (1) randomized controlled trial, (2) compared antibiotic versus placebo or antibiotic versus observation, (3) age 1 month to 15 years, (4) reported severity and duration of pain, (5) reported adverse events, and (6) reported serious complications of AOM, recurrent attacks, and hearing problems. Studies were analyzed for risk of bias and assessment of heterogeneity. The studies were the same as analyzed by Rovers et al[62] but included the 4 studies for which primary data were not available to Rovers.[60,61,90,91]

The authors' conclusions were that antibiotics produced a small reduction in the number of children with pain 2 to 7 days after diagnosis. They also concluded that most cases spontaneously remitted with no complications (NNT = 16). Antibiotics were most beneficial in children younger than 2 years with bilateral AOM and in children with otorrhea.

Two recent studies only included children younger than 3 years[32] or younger than 2 years.[31] Both included only subjects in whom the diagnosis of AOM was certain. Both studies used improvement of symptoms and improvement in the appearance of the TM in their definitions of clinical success or failure.

Hoberman et al[31] conducted a randomized, double-blind, placebo-controlled study of the efficacy of antimicrobial treatment on AOM. The criteria for AOM were acute symptoms with a score of at least 3 on the AOM-SOS,

a validated symptom scale[33,92]; MEE; and moderate or marked bulging of the TM or slight bulging accompanied by either otalgia or marked erythema of the TM. They chose to use high-dose amoxicillin-clavulanate (90 mg/kg/day) as active treatment, because it has the best oral antibiotic coverage for organisms causing AOM. Included in the study were 291 patients 6 to 23 months of age: 144 in the antibiotic group and 147 in the placebo group. The primary outcome measures were the time to resolution of symptoms and the symptom burden over time. The initial resolution of symptoms (ie, the first recording of an AOM-SOS score of 0 or 1) was recorded among the children who received amoxicillin-clavulanate in 35% by day 2, 61% by day 4, and 80% by day 7. Among children who received placebo, an AOM-SOS score of 0 or 1 was recorded in 28% by day 2, 54% by day 4, and 74% by day 7 (P = .14 for the overall comparison). For sustained resolution of symptoms (ie, the time to the second of 2 successive recordings of an AOM-SOS score of 0 or 1), the corresponding values were 20% at day 2, 41% at day 4, and 67% at day 7 with amoxicillin-clavulanate, compared with 14%, 36%, and 53% with placebo (P = .04 for the overall comparison). The symptom burden (ie, mean AOM-SOS scores) over the first 7 days were lower for the children treated with amoxicillin-clavulanate than for those who received placebo (P = .02). Clinical failure at or before the 4- to 5-day visit was defined as "either a lack of substantial improvement in symptoms, a worsening of signs on otoscopic examination, or both," and clinical failure at the 10- to 12-day visit was defined as "the failure to achieve complete or nearly complete resolution of symptoms and of otoscopic signs, without regard to the persistence or resolution of middle ear

effusion." Treatment failure occurred by day 4 to 5 in 4% of the antimicrobial treatment group versus 23% in the placebo group (P < .001) and at day 10 to 12 in 16% of the antimicrobial treatment group versus 51% in the placebo group (NNT = 2.9, P < .001). In a comparison of outcome in unilateral versus bilateral AOM, clinical failure rates by day 10 to 12 in children with unilateral AOM were 9% in those treated with amoxicillin-clavulanate versus 41% in those treated with placebo (RD, 32%; NNT = 3) and 23% vs 60% (RD, 37%; NNT = 3) in those with bilateral AOM. Most common adverse events were diarrhea (25% vs 15% in the treatment versus placebo groups, respectively; P = .05) and diaper dermatitis (51% vs 35% in the treatment versus placebo groups, respectively; P = .008). One placebo recipient developed mastoiditis. According to these results, antimicrobial treatment of AOM was more beneficial than in previous studies that used less stringent diagnostic criteria.

Tähtinen et al[32] conducted a randomized, double-blind, placebo-controlled, intention-to-treat study of amoxicillin-clavulanate (40 mg/kg/day) versus placebo. Three hundred nineteen patients from 6 to 35 months of age were studied: 161 in the antibiotic group and 158 in the placebo group. AOM definition was the presence of MEE, distinct erythema over a bulging or yellow TM, and acute symptoms such as ear pain, fever, or respiratory symptoms. Compliance was measured by using daily patient diaries and number of capsules remaining at the end of the study. Primary outcome was time to treatment failure defined as a composite of 6 independent components: no improvement in overall condition by day 3, worsening of the child's condition at any time, no improvement in otoscopic signs by day 8, perforation of the TM, development of severe infection (eg, pneumonia, mastoiditis), and any other reason for stopping the study drug/placebo.

Groups were comparable on multiple parameters. In the treatment group, 135 of 161 patients (84%) were younger than 24 months, and in the placebo group, 124 of 158 patients (78%) were younger than 24 months. Treatment failure occurred in 18.6% of the treatment group and 44.9% in the placebo group (NNT = 3.8, P < .001). Rescue treatment was needed in 6.8% of the treatment group and 33.5% of placebo patients (P < .001). Contralateral AOM developed in 8.2% and 18.6% of treatment and placebo groups, respectively (P = .007). There was no significant difference in use of analgesic or antipyretic medicine, which was used in 84.2% of the amoxicillin-clavulanate group and 85.9% of the placebo group.

Parents of child care attendees on placebo missed more days of work (P = .005). Clinical failure rates in children with unilateral AOM were 17.2% in those treated with amoxicillin-clavulanate versus 42.7% in those treated with placebo; for bilateral AOM, clinical failure rates were 21.7% for those treated with amoxicillin-clavulanate versus 46.3% in the placebo group. Reported rates of treatment failure by day 8 were 17.2% in the amoxicillin-clavulanate group versus 42.7% in the placebo group in children with unilateral AOM and 21.7% vs 46.3% among those with bilateral disease.

Adverse events, primarily diarrhea and/or rash, occurred in 52.8% of the treatment group and 36.1% of the placebo group (P = .003). Overall condition as evaluated by the parents and otoscopic appearance of the TM showed a benefit of antibiotics over placebo at the end of treatment visit (P < .001). Two placebo recipients

developed a severe infection; 1 developed pneumococcal bacteremia, and 1 developed radiographically confirmed pneumonia.

Most studies have excluded children with severe illness and all exclude those with bacterial disease other than AOM (pneumonia, mastoiditis, meningitis, streptococcal pharyngitis). Kaleida et al[91] compared myringotomy alone with myringotomy plus antibiotics. Severe AOM was defined as temperature >39°C (102.2°F) or the presence of severe otalgia. Patients with severe AOM in the group that received only myringotomy (without initial antibiotics) had much worse outcomes.

Initial Antibiotic Therapy

The rationale for antibiotic therapy in children with AOM is based on a high prevalence of bacteria in the accompanying MEE.[93] Bacterial and viral cultures of middle ear fluid collected by tympanocentesis from children with AOM showed 55% with bacteria only and 15% with bacteria and viruses. A beneficial effect of antibiotics on AOM was first demonstrated in 1968,[94] followed by additional randomized trials and a meta-analysis[95] showing a 14% increase in absolute rates of clinical improvement. Systematic reviews of the literature published before 2011[21,59,62] revealed increases of clinical improvement with initial antibiotics of 6% to 12%.

Randomized clinical trials using stringent diagnostic criteria for AOM in young children[31,32] show differences in clinical improvement of 26% to 35% favoring initial antibiotic treatment as compared with placebo. Greater benefit of immediate antibiotic therapy was observed for bilateral AOM[62,96] or AOM associated with otorrhea.[62] In most randomized trials,[30,75,77,88,89] antibiotic therapy also decreased the duration of pain, analgesic use, or

school absence and parent days missed from work.

Children younger than 2 years with AOM may take longer to improve clinically than older children,[57] and although they are more likely to benefit from antibiotics,[31,32] AOM in many children will resolve without antibiotics.[62] A clinically significant benefit of immediate antibiotic therapy is observed for bilateral AOM,[62,96] *Streptococcus pneumoniae* infection, or AOM associated with otorrhea.[62]

Initial Observation for AOM

In systematic reviews of studies that compare antibiotic therapy for AOM with placebo, a consistent finding has been the overall favorable natural history in control groups (NNT = 8–16).[12,59,62,95] However, randomized trials in these reviews had varying diagnostic criteria that would have permitted inclusion of some children with OME, viral upper respiratory infections, or myringitis, thereby limiting the ability to apply these findings to children with a highly certain AOM diagnosis. In more recent AOM studies[31,32] using stringent diagnostic criteria, approximately half of young children (younger than 2–3 years) experienced clinical success when given placebo, but the effect of antibiotic therapy was substantially greater than suggested by studies without precise diagnosis (NNT = 3–4).

Observation as initial management for AOM in properly selected children does not increase suppurative complications, provided that follow-up is ensured and a rescue antibiotic is given for persistent or worsening symptoms.[17] In contrast, withholding of antibiotics in all children with AOM, regardless of clinical course, would risk a return to the suppurative complications observed in the preantibiotic era. At the population level, antibiotics halve the risk of mastoiditis after AOM, but the high NNT of approximately 4800 patients to prevent 1 case of mastoiditis precludes a strategy of universal antibiotic therapy as a means to prevent mastoiditis.[83]

The favorable natural history of AOM makes it difficult to demonstrate significant differences in efficacy between antibiotic and placebo when a successful outcome is defined by relief or improvement of presenting signs and symptoms. In contrast, when otoscopic improvement (resolution of TM bulging, intense erythema, or both) is also required for a positive outcome,[31,32] the NNT is 3 to 4, compared with 8 to 16 for symptom improvement alone in older studies that used less precise diagnostic criteria. MEE, however, may persist for weeks or months after an AOM episode and is not a criterion for otoscopic failure.

National guidelines for initial observation of AOM in select children were first implemented in the Netherlands[97] and subsequently in Sweden,[98] Scotland,[99] the United States,[1] the United Kingdom,[100] and Italy.[101] All included observation as an initial treatment option under specified circumstances.

In numerous studies, only approximately one-third of children initially observed received a rescue antibiotic for persistent or worsening AOM,[30,32,76,81,89,102] suggesting that antibiotic use could potentially be reduced by 65% in eligible children. Given the high incidence of AOM, this reduction could help substantially in curtailing antibiotic-related adverse events.

McCormick et al[30] reported on 233 patients randomly assigned to receive immediate antibiotics (amoxicillin, 90 mg/kg/day) or to undergo watchful waiting. Criteria for inclusion were symptoms of ear infection, otoscopic evidence of AOM, and nonsevere AOM

based on a 3-item symptom score (OM-3) and TM appearance based on an 8-item scale (OS-8). Primary outcomes were parent satisfaction with AOM care, resolution of AOM symptoms after initial treatment, AOM failure and recurrence, and nasopharyngeal carriage of S pneumoniae strains resistant to antibiotics after treatment. The study was confounded by including patients who had received antibiotics in the previous 30 days.

In the watchful waiting group, 66% of children completed the study without antibiotics. There was no difference in parent satisfaction scores at day 12. A 5-item symptom score (ETG-5) was assessed at days 0 to 10 by using patient diaries. Subjects receiving immediate antibiotics resolved their symptoms faster than did subjects who underwent watchful waiting ($P = .004$). For children younger than 2 years, the difference was greater ($P = .008$). Otoscopic and tympanogram scores were also lower in the antibiotic group as opposed to the watchful waiting group ($P = .02$ for otoscopic score, $P = .004$ for tympanogram). Combining all ages, failure and recurrence rates were lower for the antibiotic group (5%) than for the watchful waiting group (21%) at 12 days. By day 30, there was no difference in failure or recurrence for the antibiotic and watchful waiting groups (23% and 24%, respectively). The association between clinical outcome and intervention group was not significantly different between age groups. Immediate antibiotics resulted in eradication of S pneumoniae carriage in the majority of children, but S pneumoniae strains cultured from children in the antibiotic group at day 12 were more likely to be multidrug resistant than were strains cultured from children in the watchful waiting group.

The decision not to give initial antibiotic treatment and observe should be

a joint decision of the clinician and the parents. In such cases, a system for close follow-up and a means of beginning antibiotics must be in place if symptoms worsen or no improvement is seen in 48 to 72 hours.

Initial observation of AOM should be part of a larger management strategy that includes analgesics, parent information, and provisions for a rescue antibiotic. Education of parents should include an explanation about the self-limited nature of most episodes of AOM, especially in children 2 years and older; the importance of pain management early in the course; and the potential adverse effects of antibiotics. Such an approach can substantially reduce prescription fill rates for rescue antibiotics.[103]

A critical component of any strategy involving initial observation for AOM is the ability to provide a rescue antibiotic if needed. This is often done by using a "safety net" or a "wait-and-see prescription,"[76,102] in which the parent/caregiver is given an antibiotic prescription during the clinical encounter but is instructed to fill the prescription only if the child fails to improve within 2 to 3 days or if symptoms worsen at any time. An alternative approach is not to provide a written prescription but to instruct the parent/caregiver to call or return if the child fails to improve within 2 to 3 days or if symptoms worsen.

In one of the first major studies of observation with a safety-net antibiotic prescription (SNAP), Siegel et al[102] enrolled 194 patients with protocol defined AOM, of whom 175 completed the study. Eligible patients were given a SNAP with instructions to fill the prescription only if symptoms worsened or did not improve in 48 hours. The SNAP was valid for 5 days. Pain medicine was recommended to be taken as needed. A phone interview was conducted 5 to 10 days after diagnosis.

One hundred twenty of 175 families did not fill the prescription. Reasons for filling the prescription (more than 1 reason per patient was acceptable) were as follows: continued pain, 23%; continued fever, 11%; sleep disruption, 6%; missed days of work, 3%; missed days of child care, 3%; and no reason given, 5%. One 16-month-old boy completed observation successfully but 6 weeks later developed AOM in the opposite ear, was treated with antibiotics, and developed postauricular cellulitis.

In a similar study of a "wait-and-see prescription" (WASP) in the emergency department, Spiro et al[76] randomly assigned 283 patients to either a WASP or standard prescription. Clinicians were educated on the 2004 AAP diagnostic criteria and initial treatment options for AOM; however, diagnosis was made at the discretion of the clinician. Patients were excluded if they did not qualify for observation per the 2004 guidelines. The primary outcome was whether the prescription was filled within 3 days of diagnosis. Prescriptions were not filled for 62% and 13% of the WASP and standard prescription patients, respectively ($P < .001$). Reasons for filling the prescription in the WASP group were fever (60%), ear pain (34%), or fussy behavior (6%). No serious adverse events were reported.

Strategies to observe children with AOM who are likely to improve on their own without initial antibiotic therapy reduces common adverse effects of antibiotics, such as diarrhea and diaper dermatitis. In 2 trials, antibiotic therapy significantly increased the absolute rates of diarrhea by 10% to 20% and of diaper rash or dermatitis by 6% to 16%.[31,32] Reduced antibiotic use may also reduce the prevalence of resistant bacterial pathogens. Multidrug-resistant *S pneumoniae* continues to be a significant concern for AOM, despite universal immunization of children in the United States with heptavalent pneumococcal conjugate vaccine.[104,105] In contrast, countries with low antibiotic use for AOM have a low prevalence of resistant nasopharyngeal pathogens in children.[106]

Key Action Statement 4A

Clinicians should prescribe amoxicillin for AOM when a decision to treat with antibiotics has been made *and* the child has not received amoxicillin in the past 30 days *or* the child does not have concurrent purulent conjunctivitis *or* the child is not allergic to penicillin. (Evidence Quality: Grade B, Rec. Strength: Recommendation)

Key Action Statement Profile: KAS 4A

Aggregate evidence quality	Grade B
Benefits	Effective antibiotic for most children with AOM. Inexpensive, safe, acceptable taste, narrow antimicrobial spectrum.
Risks, harms, cost	Ineffective against β-lactamase–producing organisms. Adverse effects of amoxicillin.
Benefits-harms assessment	Preponderance of benefit.
Value judgments	Better to use a drug that has reasonable cost, has an acceptable taste, and has a narrow antibacterial spectrum.
Intentional vagueness	The clinician must determine whether the patient is truly penicillin allergic.
Role of patient preferences	Should be considered if previous bad experience with amoxicillin.
Exclusions	Patients with known penicillin allergy.
Strength	**Recommendation.**

Key Action Statement 4B

Clinicians should prescribe an antibiotic with additional β-lactamase coverage for AOM when a decision to treat with antibiotics has been made *and* the child has received amoxicillin in the past 30 days *or* has concurrent purulent conjunctivitis *or* has a history of recurrent AOM unresponsive to amoxicillin. (Evidence Quality: Grade C, Rec. Strength: Recommendation)

Key Action Statement Profile: KAS 4B

Aggregate evidence quality	Grade C
Benefits	Successful treatment of β-lactamase–producing organisms.
Risks, harms, cost	Cost of antibiotic. Increased adverse effects.
Benefits-harms assessment	Preponderance of benefit.
Value judgments	Efficacy is more important than taste.
Intentional vagueness	None.
Role of patient preferences	Concern regarding side effects and taste.
Exclusions	Patients with known penicillin allergy.
Strength	**Recommendation**

Key Action Statement 4C

Clinicians should reassess the patient if the caregiver reports that the child's symptoms have worsened or failed to respond to the initial antibiotic treatment within 48 to 72 hours and determine whether a change in therapy is needed. (Evidence Quality: Grade B, Rec. Strength: Recommendation)

Key Action Statement Profile: KAS 4C

Aggregate evidence quality	Grade B
Benefits	Identify children who may have AOM caused by pathogens resistant to previous antibiotics.
Risks, harms, cost	Cost. Time for patient and clinician to make change. Potential need for parenteral medication.
Benefit-harm assessment	Preponderance of benefit.
Value judgments	None.
Intentional vagueness	"Reassess" is not defined. The clinician may determine the method of assessment.
Role of patient preferences	Limited.
Exclusions	Appearance of TM improved.
Strength	**Recommendation**

Purpose of This Section

If an antibiotic will be used for treatment of a child with AOM, whether as initial management or after a period of observation, the clinician must choose an antibiotic that will have a high likelihood of being effective against the most likely etiologic bacterial pathogens with considerations of cost, taste, convenience, and adverse effects. This section proposes first- and second-line antibiotics that best meet these criteria while balancing potential benefits and harms.

Changes From AAP/AAFP 2004 AOM Guideline

Despite new data on the effect of PCV7 and updated data on the in vitro susceptibility of bacterial pathogens most likely to cause AOM, the recommendations for the first-line antibiotic remains unchanged from 2004. The current guideline contains revised recommendations regarding penicillin allergy based on new data. The increase of multidrug-resistant strains of pneumococci is noted.

Microbiology

Microorganisms detected in the middle ear during AOM include pathogenic bacteria, as well as respiratory viruses.[107–110] AOM occurs most frequently as a consequence of viral upper respiratory tract infection,[111–113] which leads to eustachian tube inflammation/

dysfunction, negative middle ear pressure, and movement of secretions containing the upper respiratory tract infection causative virus and pathogenic bacteria in the nasopharynx into the middle ear cleft. By using comprehensive and sensitive microbiologic testing, bacteria and/or viruses can be detected in the middle ear fluid in up to 96% of AOM cases (eg, 66% bacteria and viruses together, 27% bacteria alone, and 4% virus alone).[114] Studies using less sensitive or less comprehensive microbiologic assays have yielded less positive results for bacteria and much less positive results for viruses.[115–117] The 3 most common bacterial pathogens in AOM are *S pneumoniae*, nontypeable *Haemophilus influenzae*, and *Moraxella catarrhalis*.[111] *Streptococcus pyogenes* (group A β-hemolytic streptococci) accounts for less than 5% of AOM cases. The proportion of AOM cases with pathogenic bacteria isolated from the middle ear fluids varies depending on bacteriologic techniques, transport issues, and stringency of AOM definition. In series of reports from the United States and Europe from 1952–1981 and 1985–1992, the mean percentage of cases with bacterial pathogens isolated from the middle ear fluids was 69% and 72%, respectively.[118] A large series from the University of Pittsburgh Otitis Media Study Group reported bacterial pathogens in 84% of the middle ear fluids

from 2807 cases of AOM.[118] Studies that applied more stringent otoscopic criteria and/or use of bedside specimen plating on solid agar in addition to liquid transport media have a reported rate of recovery of pathogenic bacteria from middle ear exudates ranging from 85% to 90%.[119–121] When using appropriate stringent diagnostic criteria, careful specimen handling, and sensitive microbiologic techniques, the vast majority of cases of AOM will involve pathogenic bacteria either alone or in concert with viral pathogens.

Among AOM bacterial pathogens, *S pneumoniae* was the most frequently cultured in earlier reports. Since the debut and routine use of PCV7 in 2000, the ordinal frequency of these 3 major middle ear pathogens has evolved.[105] In the first few years after PCV7 introduction, *H influenzae* became the most frequently isolated middle ear pathogen, replacing *S pneumoniae*.[122,123] Shortly thereafter, a shift to non-PCV7 serotypes of *S pneumoniae* was described.[124] Pichichero et al[104] later reported that 44% of 212 AOM cases seen in 2003–2006 were caused by *H influenzae*, and 28% were caused by *S pneumoniae*, with a high proportion of highly resistant *S pneumoniae*. In that study, a majority (77%) of cases involved recurrent disease or initial treatment failure. A later report[125] with data from 2007 to 2009, 6 to 8 years after the introduction of PCV7 in the United States, showed that PCV7 strains of *S pneumoniae* virtually disappeared from the middle ear fluid of children with AOM who had been vaccinated. However, the frequency of isolation of non-PCV7 serotypes of *S pneumoniae* from the middle ear fluid overall was increased; this has made isolation of *S pneumoniae* and *H influenzae* of children with AOM nearly equal.

In a study of tympanocentesis over 4 respiratory tract illness seasons in a private practice, the percentage of

S pneumoniae initially decreased relative to *H influenzae*. In 2005–2006 (*N* = 33), 48% of bacteria were *S pneumoniae*, and 42% were *H influenzae*. For 2006–2007 (*N* = 37), the percentages were equal at 41%. In 2007–2008 (*N* = 34), 35% were *S pneumoniae*, and 59% were *H influenzae*. In 2008–2009 (*N* = 24), the percentages were 54% and 38%, respectively, with an increase in intermediate and non-susceptible *S pneumoniae*.[126] Data on nasopharyngeal colonization from PCV7-immunized children with AOM have shown continued presence of *S pneumoniae* colonization. Revai et al[127] showed no difference in *S pneumoniae* colonization rate among children with AOM who have been unimmunized, underimmunized, or fully immunized with PCV7. In a study during a viral upper respiratory tract infection, including mostly PCV7-immunized children (6 months to 3 years of age), *S pneumoniae* was detected in 45.5% of 968 nasopharyngeal swabs, *H influenzae* was detected in 32.4%, and *M catarrhalis* was detected in 63.1%.[128] Data show that nasopharyngeal colonization of children vaccinated with PCV7 increasingly is caused by *S pneumoniae* serotypes not contained in the vaccine.[129–132] With the use of the recently licensed 13-valent pneumococcal conjugate vaccine (PCV13),[133] the patterns of nasopharyngeal colonization and infection with these common AOM bacterial pathogens will continue to evolve.

Investigators have attempted to predict the type of AOM pathogenic bacteria on the basis of clinical severity, but results have not been promising. *S pyogenes* has been shown to occur more commonly in older children[134] and to cause a greater degree of inflammation of the middle ear and TM, a greater frequency of spontaneous rupture of the TM, and more frequent progression to acute mastoiditis compared with other bacterial pathogens.[134–136] As for clinical findings in cases with *S pneumoniae* and nontypeable *H influenzae*, some studies suggest that signs and symptoms of AOM caused by *S pneumoniae* may be more severe (fever, severe earache, bulging TM) than those caused by other pathogens.[44,121,137] These findings were refuted by results of the studies that found AOM caused by nontypeable *H influenzae* to be associated with bilateral AOM and more severe inflammation of the TM.[96,138] Leibovitz et al[139] concluded, in a study of 372 children with AOM caused by *H influenzae* (*N* = 138), *S pneumoniae* (*N* = 64), and mixed *H influenzae* and *S pneumoniae* (*N* = 64), that clinical/otologic scores could not discriminate among various bacterial etiologies of AOM. However, there were significantly different clinical/otologic scores between bacterial culture negative and culture positive cases. A study of middle ear exudates of 82 cases of bullous myringitis has shown a 97% bacteria positive rate, primarily *S pneumoniae*. In contrast to the previous belief, mycoplasma is rarely the causative agent in this condition.[140] Accurate prediction of the bacterial cause of AOM on the basis of clinical presentation, without bacterial culture of the middle ear exudates, is not possible, but specific etiologies may be predicted in some situations. Published evidence has suggested that AOM associated with conjunctivitis (otitis-conjunctivitis syndrome) is more likely caused by nontypeable *H influenzae* than by other bacteria.[141–143]

Bacterial Susceptibility to Antibiotics

Selection of antibiotic to treat AOM is based on the suspected type of bacteria and antibiotic susceptibility pattern, although clinical pharmacology and clinical and microbiologic results and predicted compliance with the drug are also taken into account. Early studies of AOM patients show that 19% of children with *S pneumoniae* and 48% with *H influenzae* cultured on initial tympanocentesis who were not treated with antibiotic cleared the bacteria at the time of a second tympanocentesis 2 to 7 days later.[144] Approximately 75% of children infected with *M catarrhalis* experienced bacteriologic cure even after treatment with amoxicillin, an antibiotic to which it is not susceptible.[145,146]

Antibiotic susceptibility of major AOM bacterial pathogens continues to change, but data on middle ear pathogens have become scanty because tympanocentesis is not generally performed in studies of children with uncomplicated AOM. Most available data come from cases of persistent or recurrent AOM. Current US data from a number of centers indicates that approximately 83% and 87% of isolates of *S pneumoniae* from all age groups are susceptible to regular (40 mg/kg/day) and high-dose amoxicillin (80–90 mg/kg/day divided twice daily), respectively.[130,147–150] Pediatric isolates are smaller in number and include mostly ear isolates collected from recurrent and persistent AOM cases with a high percentage of multidrug-resistant *S pneumoniae*, most frequently nonvaccine serotypes that have recently increased in frequency and importance.[104]

High-dose amoxicillin will yield middle ear fluid levels that exceed the minimum inhibitory concentration (MIC) of all *S pneumoniae* serotypes that are intermediately resistant to penicillin (penicillin MICs, 0.12–1.0 µg/mL), and many but not all highly resistant serotypes (penicillin MICs, ≥2 µg/mL) for a longer period of the dosing interval and has been shown to improve bacteriologic and clinical efficacy compared with the regular dose.[151–153] Hoberman et al[154] reported superior efficacy of high-dose amoxicillin-clavulanate in eradication of *S pneumoniae* (96%) from the middle ear at days 4 to 6 of therapy compared with azithromycin.

The antibiotic susceptibility pattern for *S pneumoniae* is expected to continue to evolve with the use of PCV13, a conjugate vaccine containing 13 serotypes of *S pneumoniae*.[133,155,156] Widespread use of PCV13 could potentially reduce diseases caused by multidrug-resistant pneumococcal serotypes and diminish the need for the use of higher dose of amoxicillin or amoxicillin-clavulanate for AOM.

Some *H influenzae* isolates produce β-lactamase enzyme, causing the isolate to become resistant to penicillins. Current data from different studies with non-AOM sources and geographic locations that may not be comparable show that 58% to 82% of *H influenzae* isolates are susceptible to regular- and high-dose amoxicillin.[130,147,148,157,158] These data represented a significant decrease in β-lactamase–producing *H*

influenzae, compared with data reported in the 2004 AOM guideline.

Nationwide data suggest that 100% of *M catarrhalis* derived from the upper respiratory tract are β-lactamase–positive but remain susceptible to amoxicillin-clavulanate.[159] However, the high rate of spontaneous clinical resolution occurring in children with AOM attributable to *M catarrhalis* treated with amoxicillin reduces the concern for the first-line coverage for this microorganism.[145,146] AOM attributable to *M catarrhalis* rarely progresses to acute mastoiditis or intracranial infections.[102,160,161]

Antibiotic Therapy

High-dose amoxicillin is recommended as the first-line treatment in most patients, although there are a number of medications that are clinically effective (Table 5). The justification for the use of amoxicillin relates to its effectiveness against common AOM bacterial pathogens as well as its safety, low cost, acceptable taste, and narrow microbiologic spectrum.[145,151] In children who have taken amoxicillin in the previous 30 days, those with concurrent conjunctivitis, or those

for whom coverage for β-lactamase–positive *H influenzae* and *M catarrhalis* is desired, therapy should be initiated with high-dose amoxicillin-clavulanate (90 mg/kg/day of amoxicillin, with 6.4 mg/kg/day of clavulanate, a ratio of amoxicillin to clavulanate of 14:1, given in 2 divided doses, which is less likely to cause diarrhea than other amoxicillin-clavulanate preparations).[162]

Alternative initial antibiotics include cefdinir (14 mg/kg per day in 1 or 2 doses), cefuroxime (30 mg/kg per day in 2 divided doses), cefpodoxime (10 mg/kg per day in 2 divided doses), or ceftriaxone (50 mg/kg, administered intramuscularly). It is important to note that alternative antibiotics vary in their efficacy against AOM pathogens. For example, recent US data on in vitro susceptibility of *S pneumoniae* to cefdinir and cefuroxime are 70% to 80%, compared with 84% to 92% amoxicillin efficacy.[130,147–149] In vitro efficacy of cefdinir and cefuroxime against *H influenzae* is approximately 98%, compared with 58% efficacy of amoxicillin and nearly 100% efficacy of amoxicillin-clavulanate.[158] A multicenter double tympanocentesis open-label study of

TABLE 5 Recommended Antibiotics for (Initial or Delayed) Treatment and for Patients Who Have Failed Initial Antibiotic Treatment

Initial Immediate or Delayed Antibiotic Treatment		Antibiotic Treatment After 48–72 h of Failure of Initial Antibiotic Treatment	
Recommended First-line Treatment	Alternative Treatment (if Penicillin Allergy)	Recommended First-line Treatment	Alternative Treatment
Amoxicillin (80–90 mg/ kg per day in 2 divided doses)	Cefdinir (14 mg/kg per day in 1 or 2 doses)	Amoxicillin-clavulanate[a] (90 mg/kg per day of amoxicillin, with 6.4 mg/kg per day of clavulanate in 2 divided doses)	Ceftriaxone, 3 d Clindamycin (30–40 mg/kg per day in 3 divided doses), with or without third-generation cephalosporin
or	Cefuroxime (30 mg/kg per day in 2 divided doses)	or	Failure of second antibiotic
Amoxicillin-clavulanate[a] (90 mg/kg per day of amoxicillin, with 6.4 mg/kg per day of clavulanate [amoxicillin to clavulanate ratio, 14:1] in 2 divided doses)	Cefpodoxime (10 mg/kg per day in 2 divided doses)	Ceftriaxone (50 mg IM or IV for 3 d)	Clindamycin (30–40 mg/kg per day in 3 divided doses) plus third-generation cephalosporin
	Ceftriaxone (50 mg IM or IV per day for 1 or 3 d)		Tympanocentesis[b] Consult specialist[b]

IM, intramuscular; IV, intravenous.

[a] May be considered in patients who have received amoxicillin in the previous 30 d or who have the otitis-conjunctivitis syndrome.

[b] Perform tympanocentesis/drainage if skilled in the procedure, or seek a consultation from an otolaryngologist for tympanocentesis/drainage. If the tympanocentesis reveals multidrug-resistant bacteria, seek an infectious disease specialist consultation.

[c] Cefdinir, cefuroxime, cefpodoxime, and ceftriaxone are highly unlikely to be associated with cross-reactivity with penicillin allergy on the basis of their distinct chemical structures. See text for more information.

cefdinir in recurrent AOM attributable to H influenzae showed eradication of the organism in 72% of patients.[163]

For penicillin-allergic children, recent data suggest that cross-reactivity among penicillins and cephalosporins is lower than historically reported.[164–167] The previously cited rate of cross-sensitivity to cephalosporins among penicillin-allergic patients (approximately 10%) is likely an overestimate. The rate was based on data collected and reviewed during the 1960s and 1970s. A study analyzing pooled data of 23 studies, including 2400 patients with reported history of penicillin allergy and 39 000 with no penicillin allergic history concluded that many patients who present with a history of penicillin allergy do not have an immunologic reaction to penicillin.[166] The chemical structure of the cephalosporin determines the risk of cross-reactivity between specific agents.[165,168] The degree of cross-reactivity is higher between penicillins and first-generation cephalosporins but is negligible with the second- and third-generation cephalosporins. Because of the differences in the chemical structures, cefdinir, cefuroxime, cefpodoxime, and ceftriaxone are highly unlikely to be associated with cross-reactivity with penicillin.[165] Despite this, the Joint Task Force on Practice Parameters; American Academy of Allergy, Asthma and Immunology; American College of Allergy, Asthma and Immunology; and Joint Council of Allergy, Asthma and Immunology[169] stated that "cephalosporin treatment of patients with a history of penicillin allergy, selecting out those with severe reaction histories, show a reaction rate of 0.1%." They recommend a cephalosporin in cases without severe and/or recent penicillin allergy reaction history when skin test is not available.

Macrolides, such as erythromycin and azithromycin, have limited efficacy against both H influenzae and S pneumoniae.[130,147–149] Clindamycin lacks efficacy against H influenzae. Clindamycin alone (30–40 mg/kg per day in 3 divided doses) may be used for suspected penicillin-resistant S pneumoniae; however, the drug will likely not be effective for the multidrug-resistant serotypes.[130,158,166]

Several of these choices of antibiotic suspensions are barely palatable or frankly offensive and may lead to avoidance behaviors or active rejection by spitting out the suspension. Palatability of antibiotic suspensions has been compared in many studies.[170–172] Specific antibiotic suspensions such as cefuroxime, cefpodoxime, and clindamycin may benefit from adding taste-masking products, such as chocolate or strawberry flavoring agents, to obscure the initial bitter taste and the unpleasant aftertaste.[172,173] In the patient who is persistently vomiting or cannot otherwise tolerate oral medication, even when the taste is masked, ceftriaxone (50 mg/kg, administered intramuscularly in 1 or 2 sites in the anterior thigh, or intravenously) has been demonstrated to be effective for the initial or repeat antibiotic treatment of AOM.[174,175] Although a single injection of ceftriaxone is approved by the US FDA for the treatment of AOM, results of a double tympanocentesis study (before and 3 days after single dose ceftriaxone) by Leibovitz et al[175] suggest that more than 1 ceftriaxone dose may be required to prevent recurrence of the middle ear infection within 5 to 7 days after the initial dose.

Initial Antibiotic Treatment Failure

When antibiotics are prescribed for AOM, clinical improvement should be noted within 48 to 72 hours. During the 24 hours after the diagnosis of AOM, the child's symptoms may worsen slightly. In the next 24 hours, the patient's symptoms should begin to improve. If initially febrile, the temperature should decline within 48 to 72 hours. Irritability and fussiness should lessen or disappear, and sleeping and drinking patterns should normalize.[176,177] If the patient is not improved by 48 to 72 hours, another disease or concomitant viral infection may be present, or the causative bacteria may be resistant to the chosen therapy.

Some children with AOM and persistent symptoms after 48 to 72 hours of initial antibacterial treatment may have combined bacterial and viral infection, which would explain the persistence of ongoing symptoms despite appropriate antibiotic therapy.[109,178,179] Literature is conflicting on the correlation between clinical and bacteriologic outcomes. Some studies report good correlation ranging from 86% to 91%,[180,181] suggesting continued presence of bacteria in the middle ear in a high proportion of cases with persistent symptoms. Others report that middle ear fluid from children with AOM in whom symptoms are persistent is sterile in 42% to 49% of cases.[123,182] A change in antibiotic may not be required in some children with mild persistent symptoms.

In children with persistent, severe symptoms of AOM and unimproved otologic findings after initial treatment, the clinician may consider changing the antibiotic (Table 5). If the child was initially treated with amoxicillin and failed to improve, amoxicillin-clavulanate should be used. Patients who were given amoxicillin-clavulanate or oral third-generation cephalosporins may receive intramuscular ceftriaxone (50 mg/kg). In the treatment of AOM unresponsive to initial antibiotics, a 3-day course of ceftriaxone has been shown to be better than a 1-day regimen.[175]

Although trimethoprim-sulfamethoxazole and erythromycin-sulfisoxazole had been useful as therapy for patients with AOM, pneumococcal surveillance studies have indicated that resistance to these 2 combination agents is substantial.[130,149,183] Therefore, when patients fail to improve while receiving amoxicillin, neither trimethoprim-sulfamethoxazole[184] nor erythromycin-sulfisoxazole is appropriate therapy.

Tympanocentesis should be considered, and culture of middle ear fluid should be performed for bacteriologic diagnosis and susceptibility testing when a series of antibiotic drugs have failed to improve the clinical condition. If tympanocentesis is not available, a course of clindamycin may be used, with or without an antibiotic that covers nontypeable *H influenzae* and *M catarrhalis*, such as cefdinir, cefixime, or cefuroxime.

Because *S pneumoniae* serotype 19A is usually multidrug-resistant and may not be responsive to clindamycin,[104,149] newer antibiotics that are not approved by the FDA for treatment of AOM, such as levofloxacin or linezolid, may be indicated.[185–187] Levofloxacin is a quinolone antibiotic that is not approved by the FDA for use in children. Linezolid is effective against resistant Gram-positive bacteria. It is not approved by the FDA for AOM treatment and is expensive. In children with repeated treatment failures, every effort should be made for bacteriologic diagnosis by tympanocentesis with Gram stain, culture, and antibiotic susceptibility testing of the organism (s) present. The clinician may consider consulting with pediatric medical subspecialists, such as an otolaryngologist for possible tympanocentesis, drainage, and culture and an infectious disease expert, before use of unconventional drugs such as levofloxacin or linezolid.

When tympanocentesis is not available, 1 possible way to obtain information on the middle ear pathogens and their antimicrobial susceptibility is to obtain a nasopharyngeal specimen for bacterial culture. Almost all middle ear pathogens derive from the pathogens colonizing the nasopharynx, but not all nasopharyngeal pathogens enter the middle ear to cause AOM. The positive predictive value of nasopharyngeal culture during AOM (likelihood that bacteria cultured from the nasopharynx is the middle ear pathogen) ranges from 22% to 44% for *S pneumoniae*, 50% to 71% for nontypeable *H influenzae*, and 17% to 19% for *M catarrhalis*. The negative predictive value (likelihood that bacteria not found in the nasopharynx are not AOM pathogens) ranges from 95% to 99% for all 3 bacteria.[188,189] Therefore, if nasopharyngeal culture is negative for specific bacteria, that organism is likely not the AOM pathogen. A negative culture for *S pneumoniae*, for example, will help eliminate the concern for multidrug-resistant bacteria and the need for unconventional therapies, such as levofloxacin or linezolid. On the other hand, if *S pneumoniae* is cultured from the nasopharynx, the antimicrobial susceptibility pattern can help guide treatment.

Duration of Therapy

The optimal duration of therapy for patients with AOM is uncertain; the usual 10-day course of therapy was derived from the duration of treatment of streptococcal pharyngotonsillitis. Several studies favor standard 10-day therapy over shorter courses for children younger than 2 years.[162,190–194] Thus, for children younger than 2 years and children with severe symptoms, a standard 10-day course is recommended. A 7-day course of oral antibiotic appears to be equally effective in children 2 to 5 years of age with mild or moderate AOM. For children 6 years and older with mild to moderate

symptoms, a 5- to 7-day course is adequate treatment.

Follow-up of the Patient With AOM

Once the child has shown clinical improvement, follow-up is based on the usual clinical course of AOM. There is little scientific evidence for a routine 10- to 14-day reevaluation visit for all children with an episode of AOM. The physician may choose to reassess some children, such as young children with severe symptoms or recurrent AOM or when specifically requested by the child's parent.

Persistent MEE is common and can be detected by pneumatic otoscopy (with or without verification by tympanometry) after resolution of acute symptoms. Two weeks after successful antibiotic treatment of AOM, 60% to 70% of children have MEE, decreasing to 40% at 1 month and 10% to 25% at 3 months after successful antibiotic treatment.[177,195] The presence of MEE without clinical symptoms is defined as OME. OME must be differentiated clinically from AOM and requires infrequent additional monitoring but not antibiotic therapy. Assurance that OME resolves is particularly important for parents of children with cognitive or developmental delays that may be affected adversely by transient hearing loss associated with MEE. Detailed recommendations for the management of the child with OME can be found in the evidence-based guideline from the AAP/AAFP/American Academy of Otolaryngology-Head and Neck Surgery published in 2004.[84,85]

Key Action Statement 5A

Clinicians should *NOT* prescribe prophylactic antibiotics to reduce the frequency of episodes of AOM in children with recurrent AOM. (Evidence Quality: Grade B, Rec. Strength: Recommendation)

Key Action Statement Profile: KAS 5A

Aggregate evidence quality	Grade B
Benefits	No adverse effects from antibiotic. Reduces potential for development of bacterial resistance. Reduced costs.
Risks, harms, cost	Small increase in episodes of AOM.
Benefit-harm assessment	Preponderance of benefit.
Value judgments	Potential harm outweighs the potential benefit.
Intentional vagueness	None.
Role of patient preferences	Limited.
Exclusions	Young children whose only alternative would be tympanostomy tubes.
Strength	**Recommendation**

Key Action Statement 5B

Clinicians may offer tympanostomy tubes for recurrent AOM (3 episodes in 6 months or 4 episodes in 1 year, with 1 episode in the preceding 6 months). (Evidence Quality: Grade B, Rec. Strength: Option)

Key Action Statement Profile: KAS 5B

Aggregate evidence quality	Grade B
Benefits	Decreased frequency of AOM. Ability to treat AOM with topical antibiotic therapy.
Risks, harms, cost	Risks of anesthesia or surgery. Cost. Scarring of TM, chronic perforation, cholesteatoma. Otorrhea.
Benefits-harms assessment	Equilibrium of benefit and harm.
Value judgments	None.
Intentional vagueness	Option based on limited evidence.
Role of patient preferences	Joint decision of parent and clinician.
Exclusions	Any contraindication to anesthesia and surgery.
Strength	**Option**

Purpose of This Section

Recurrent AOM has been defined as the occurrence of 3 or more episodes of AOM in a 6-month period or the occurrence of 4 or more episodes of AOM in a 12-month period that includes at least 1 episode in the preceding 6 months.[20] These episodes should be well documented and separate acute infections.[11]

Winter season, male gender, and passive exposure to smoking have been associated with an increased likelihood of recurrence. Half of children younger than 2 years treated for AOM will experience a recurrence within 6 months. Symptoms that last more than 10 days may also predict recurrence.[196]

Changes From AAP/AAFP 2004 AOM Guideline

Recurrent AOM was not addressed in the 2004 AOM guideline. This section addresses the literature on recurrent AOM.

Antibiotic Prophylaxis

Long-term, low-dose antibiotic use, referred to as antibiotic prophylaxis or chemoprophylaxis, has been used to treat children with recurrent AOM to prevent subsequent episodes.[85] A 2006 Cochrane review analyzed 16 studies of long-term antibiotic use for AOM and found such use prevented 1.5 episodes of AOM per year, reducing in half the number of AOM episodes during the period of treatment.[197] Randomized placebo-controlled trials of prophylaxis reported a decrease of 0.09 episodes per month in the frequency of AOM attributable to therapy (approximately 0.5 to 1.5 AOM episodes per year for 95% of children). An estimated 5 children would need to be treated for 1 year to prevent 1 episode of OM. The effect may be more substantial for children with 6 or more AOM episodes in the preceding year.[12]

This decrease in episodes of AOM occurred only while the prophylactic antibiotic was being given. The modest benefit afforded by a 6-month course of antibiotic prophylaxis does not have longer-lasting benefit after cessation of therapy. Teele showed no differences between children who received prophylactic antibiotics compared with those who received placebo in AOM recurrences or persistence of OME.[198]

Antibiotic prophylaxis is not appropriate for children with long-term MEE or for children with infrequent episodes of AOM. The small reduction in frequency of AOM with long-term antibiotic prophylaxis must be weighed against the cost of such therapy; the potential adverse effects of antibiotics, principally allergic reaction and gastrointestinal tract consequences, such as diarrhea; and their contribution to the emergence of bacterial resistance.

Surgery for Recurrent AOM

The use of tympanostomy tubes for treatment of ear disease in general, and for AOM in particular, has been controversial.[199] Most published studies of surgical intervention for OM focus on children with persistent MEE with or without AOM. The literature on surgery for recurrent AOM as defined here is scant. A lack of consensus among otolaryngologists regarding the role of surgery for recurrent AOM was reported in a survey of Canadian otolaryngologists in which 40% reported they would "never," 30% reported they would "sometimes," and 30% reported they would "often or always" place tympanostomy tubes for a hypothetical 2-year-old child with frequent OM without persistent MEE or hearing loss.[200]

Tympanostomy tubes, however, remain widely used in clinical practice for both OME and recurrent OM.[201] Recurrent

AOM remains a common indication for referral to an otolaryngologist.

Three randomized controlled trials have compared the number of episodes of AOM after tympanostomy tube placement or no surgery.[202] Two found significant improvement in mean number of AOM episodes after tympanostomy tubes during a 6-month follow-up period.[203,204] One study randomly assigned children with recurrent AOM to groups receiving placebo, amoxicillin prophylaxis, or tympanostomy tubes and followed them for 2 years.[205] Although prophylactic antibiotics reduced the rate of AOM, no difference in number of episodes of AOM was noted between the tympanostomy tube group and the placebo group over 2 years. A Cochrane review of studies of tympanostomy tubes for recurrent AOM analyzed 2 studies[204,206] that met inclusion criteria and found that tympanostomy tubes reduced the number of episodes of AOM by 1.5 episodes in the 6 months after surgery.[207] Tympanostomy tube insertion has been shown to improve disease-specific quality-of-life measures in children with OM.[208] One multicenter, nonrandomized observational study showed large improvements in a disease-specific quality-of-life instrument that measured psychosocial domains of physical suffering, hearing loss, speech impairment, emotional distress, activity limitations, and caregiver concerns that are associated with ear infections.[209] These benefits of tympanostomy tubes have been demonstrated in mixed populations of children that include children with OME as well as recurrent AOM.

Beyond the cost, insertion of tympanostomy tubes is associated with a small but finite surgical and anesthetic risk. A recent review looking at protocols to minimize operative risk reported no major complications, such as sensorineural hearing loss, vascular injury, or ossicular chain disruption, in 10 000 tube insertions performed primarily by residents, although minor complications such as TM tears or displaced tubes in the middle ear were seen in 0.016% of ears.[210] Long-term sequelae of tympanostomy tubes include TM structural changes including focal atrophy, tympanosclerosis, retraction pockets, and chronic perforation. One meta-analysis found tympanosclerosis in 32% of patients after placement of tympanostomy tubes and chronic perforations in 2.2% of patients who had short-term tubes and 16.6% of patients with long-term tubes.[211]

Adenoidectomy, without myringotomy and/or tympanostomy tubes, did not reduce the number of episodes of AOM when compared with chemoprophylaxis or placebo.[212] Adenoidectomy alone should not be used for prevention of AOM but may have benefit when performed with placement of tympanostomy tubes or in children with previous tympanostomy tube placement in OME.[213]

Prevention of AOM: Key Action Statement 6A

Pneumococcal Vaccine

Clinicians should recommend pneumococcal conjugate vaccine to all children according to the schedule of the Advisory Committee on Immunization Practices, AAP, and AAFP. (Evidence Quality: Grade B, Rec. Strength: Strong Recommendation)

Key Action Statement Profile: KAS 6A

Aggregate evidence quality	Grade B
Benefits	Reduced frequency of AOM attributable to vaccine serotypes. Reduced risk of serious pneumococcal systemic disease.
Risks, harms, cost	Potential vaccine side effects. Cost of vaccine.
Benefits-harms assessment	Preponderance of benefit.
Value judgments	Potential vaccine adverse effects are minimal.
Intentional vagueness	None.
Role of patient preferences	Some parents may choose to refuse the vaccine.
Exclusions	Severe allergic reaction (eg, anaphylaxis) to any component of pneumococcal vaccine or any diphtheria toxoid-containing vaccine.
Strength	**Strong Recommendation**

Key Action Statement 6B

Influenza Vaccine: Clinicians should recommend annual influenza vaccine to all children according to the schedule of the Advisory Committee on Immunization Practices, AAP, and AAFP. (Evidence Quality: Grade B, Rec. Strength: Recommendation)

Key Action Statement Profile: KAS 6B

Aggregate evidence quality	Grade B
Benefits	Reduced risk of influenza infection. Reduction in frequency of AOM associated with influenza.
Risks, harms, cost	Potential vaccine adverse effects. Cost of vaccine. Requires annual immunization.
Benefits-harms assessment	Preponderance of benefit.
Value judgments	Potential vaccine adverse effects are minimal.
Intentional vagueness	None
Role of patient preferences	Some parents may choose to refuse the vaccine.
Exclusions	See CDC guideline on contraindications (http://www.cdc.gov/flu/professionals/acip/shouldnot.htm).
Strength	**Recommendation**

Key Action Statement 6C
Breastfeeding: Clinicians should encourage exclusive breastfeeding

for at least 6 months. (Evidence Quality: Grade B, Rec. Strength: Recommendation)

Key Action Statement Profile: KAS 6C

Aggregate evidence quality	Grade B
Benefits	May reduce the risk of early AOM. Multiple benefits of breastfeeding unrelated to AOM.
Risk, harm, cost	None
Benefit-harm assessment	Preponderance of benefit.
Value judgments	The intervention has value unrelated to AOM prevention.
Intentional vagueness	None
Role of patient preferences	Some parents choose to feed formula.
Exclusions	None
Strength	**Recommendation**

Key Action Statement 6D
Clinicians should encourage avoidance of tobacco smoke ex-

posure. (Evidence Quality: Grade C, Rec. Strength: Recommendation)

Key Action Statement Profile: KAS 6D

Aggregate evidence quality	Grade C
Benefits	May reduce the risk of AOM.
Risks, harms, cost	None
Benefits-harms assessment	Preponderance of benefit.
Value judgments	Avoidance of tobacco exposure has inherent value unrelated to AOM.
Intentional vagueness	None
Role of patient preferences	Many parents/caregivers choose not to stop smoking. Some also remain addicted, and are unable to quit smoking.
Exclusions	None
Strength	**Recommendation**

Purpose of This Section

The 2004 AOM guideline noted data on immunizations, breastfeeding, and lifestyle changes that would reduce the risk of acquiring AOM. This section addresses new data published since 2004.

Changes From AAP/AAFP 2004 AOM Guideline

PCV7 has been in use in the United States since 2000. PCV13 was introduced in the United States in 2010. The 10-valent pneumococcal nontypeable *H influenzae* protein D-conjugate vaccine was recently licensed in Europe for

prevention of diseases attributable to *S pneumoniae* and nontypeable *H influenzae*. Annual influenza immunization is now recommended for all children 6 months of age and older in the United States.[214,215] Updated information regarding these vaccines and their effect on the incidence of AOM is reviewed.

The AAP issued a new breastfeeding policy statement in February 2012.[216] This guideline also includes a recommendation regarding tobacco smoke exposure. Bottle propping, pacifier use, and child care are discussed, but no recommendations are made because of limited evidence. The use of

xylitol, a possible adjunct to AOM prevention, is discussed; however, no recommendations are made.

Pneumococcal Vaccine

Pneumococcal conjugate vaccines have proven effective in preventing OM caused by pneumococcal serotypes contained in the vaccines. A meta-analysis of 5 studies with AOM as an outcome determined that there is a 29% reduction in AOM caused by all pneumococcal serotypes among children who received PCV7 before 24 months of age.[217] Although the overall benefit seen in clinical trials for all causes of AOM is small (6%–7%),[218–221] observational studies have shown that medical office visits for otitis were reduced by up to 40% comparing years before and after introduction of PCV7.[222–224] Grijvala[223] reported no effect, however, among children first vaccinated at older ages. Poehling et al[225] reported reductions of frequent AOM and PE tube use after introduction of PCV7. The observations by some of greater benefit observed in the community than in clinical trials is not fully understood but may be related to effects of herd immunity or may be attributed to secular trends or changes in AOM diagnosis patterns over time.[223,226–229] In a 2009 Cochrane review,[221] Jansen et al found that the overall reduction in AOM incidence may only be 6% to 7% but noted that even that small rate may have public health relevance. O'Brien et al concurred and noted in addition the potential for cost savings.[230] There is evidence that serotype replacement may reduce the long-term efficacy of pneumococcal conjugate vaccines against AOM,[231] but it is possible that new pneumococcal conjugate vaccines may demonstrate an increased effect on reduction in AOM.[232–234] Data on AOM reduction secondary to the PCV13 licensed in the United States in 2010 are not yet available.

The *H influenzae* protein D-conjugate vaccine recently licensed in Europe has potential benefit of protection against 10 serotypes of *S pneumoniae* and nontypeable *H influenzae*.[221,234]

Influenza Vaccine

Most cases of AOM follow upper respiratory tract infections caused by viruses, including influenza viruses. As many as two-thirds of young children with influenza may have AOM.[235] Investigators have studied the efficacy of trivalent inactivated influenza vaccine (TIV) and live-attenuated intranasal influenza vaccine (LAIV) in preventing AOM. Many studies have demonstrated 30% to 55% efficacy of influenza vaccine in prevention of AOM during the respiratory illness season.[6,235–239] One study reported no benefit of TIV in reducing AOM burden; however, 1 of the 2 respiratory illness seasons during which this study was conducted had a relatively low influenza activity. A pooled analysis[240] of 8 studies comparing LAIV versus TIV or placebo[241–248] showed a higher efficacy of LAIV compared with both placebo and with TIV. Influenza vaccination is now recommended for all children 6 months of age and older in the United States.[214,215]

Breastfeeding

Multiple studies provide evidence that breastfeeding for at least 4 to 6 months reduces episodes of AOM and recurrent AOM.[249–253] Two cohort studies, 1 retrospective study[250] and 1 prospective study,[253] suggest a dose response, with some protection from partial breastfeeding and the greatest protection from exclusive breastfeeding through 6 months of age. In multivariate analysis controlling for exposure to child care settings, the risk of nonrecurrent otitis is 0.61 (95% confidence interval [CI]: 0.4–0.92) comparing exclusive breastfeeding through 6 months of age with no breastfeeding or breastfeeding less than 4 months. In a prospective cohort, Scariatti[253] found a significant dose-response effect. In this study, OM was self-reported by parents. In a systematic review, McNiel et al[254] found that when exclusive breastfeeding was set as the normative standard, the recalculated odds ratios (ORs) revealed the risks of any formula use. For example, any formula use in the first 6 months of age was significantly associated with increased incidence of OM (OR: 1.78; 95% CI: 1.19–2.70; OR: 4.55; 95% CI: 1.64–12.50 in the available studies; pooled OR for any formula in the first 3 months of age, 2.00; 95% CI: 1.40–2.78). A number of studies[255–259] addressed the association of AOM and other infectious illness in infants with duration and exclusivity of breastfeeding, but all had limitations and none had a randomized controlled design. However, taken together, they continue to show a protective effect of exclusive breastfeeding. In all studies, there has been a predominance of white subjects, and child care attendance and smoking exposure may not have been completely controlled. Also, feeding methods were self-reported.

The consistent finding of a lower incidence of AOM and recurrent AOM with increased breastfeeding supports the AAP recommendation to encourage exclusive breastfeeding for the first 6 months of life and to continue for at least the first year and beyond for as long as mutually desired by mother and child.[216]

Lifestyle Changes

In addition to its many other benefits,[260] eliminating exposure to passive tobacco smoke has been postulated to reduce the incidence of AOM in infancy.[252,261–264] Bottles and pacifiers have been associated with AOM. Avoiding supine bottle feeding ("bottle propping") and reducing or eliminating pacifier use in the second 6 months of life may reduce AOM incidence.[265–267] In a recent cohort study, pacifier use was associated with AOM recurrence.[268]

During infancy and early childhood, reducing the incidence of upper respiratory tract infections by altering child care-center attendance patterns can reduce the incidence of recurrent AOM significantly.[249,269]

Xylitol

Xylitol, or birch sugar, is chemically a pentitol or 5-carbon polyol sugar alcohol. It is available as chewing gum, syrup, or lozenges. A 2011 Cochrane review[270] examined the evidence for the use of xylitol in preventing recurrent AOM. A statistically significant 25% reduction in the risk of occurrence of AOM among healthy children at child care centers in the xylitol group compared with the control group (relative risk: 0.75; 95% CI: 0.65 to 0.88; RD: −0.07; 95% CI: −0.12 to −0.03) in the 4 studies met criteria for analysis.[271–274] Chewing gum and lozenges containing xylitol appeared to be more effective than syrup. Children younger than 2 years, those at the greatest risk of having AOM, cannot safely use lozenges or chewing gum. Also, xylitol needs to be given 3 to 5 times a day to be effective. It is not effective for treating AOM and it must be taken daily throughout the respiratory illness season to have an effect. Sporadic or as-needed use is not effective.

Future Research

Despite advances in research partially stimulated by the 2004 AOM guideline, there are still many unanswered clinical questions in the field. Following are possible clinical research questions that still need to be resolved.

Diagnosis

There will probably never be a gold standard for diagnosis of AOM because of the continuum from OME to AOM. Conceivably, new techniques that could be used on the small amount of fluid obtained during tympanocentesis could identify inflammatory markers in addition to the presence of bacteria or viruses. However, performing tympanocentesis studies on children with uncomplicated otitis is likely not feasible because of ethical and other considerations.

Devices that more accurately identify the presence of MEE and bulging that are easier to use than tympanometry during office visits would be welcome, especially in the difficult-to-examine infant. Additional development of inexpensive, easy-to-use video pneumatic otoscopes is still a goal.

Initial Treatment

The recent studies of Hoberman[31] and Tähtinen[32] have addressed clinical and TM appearance by using stringent diagnostic criteria of AOM. However, the outcomes for less stringent diagnostic criteria, a combination of symptoms, MEE, and TM appearance not completely consistent with OME can only be inferred from earlier studies that used less stringent criteria but did not specify outcomes for various grades of findings. Randomized controlled trials on these less certain TM appearances using scales similar to the OS-8 scale[35] could clarify the benefit of initial antibiotics and initial observation for these less certain diagnoses. Such studies must also specify severity of illness, laterality, and otorrhea.

Appropriate end points must be established. Specifically is the appearance of the TM in patients without clinical symptoms at the end of a study significant for relapse, recurrence, or persistent MEE. Such a study would require randomization of patients with unimproved TM appearance to continued observation and antibiotic groups.

The most efficient and acceptable methods of initial observation should continue to be studied balancing the convenience and benefits with the potential risks to the patient.

Antibiotics

Amoxicillin-clavulanate has a broader spectrum than amoxicillin and may be a better initial antibiotic. However, because of cost and adverse effects, the subcommittee has chosen amoxicillin as first-line AOM treatment. Randomized controlled trials comparing the 2 with adequate power to differentiate clinical efficacy would clarify this choice. Stringent diagnostic criteria should be the standard for these studies. Antibiotic comparisons for AOM should now include an observation arm for patients with nonsevere illness to ensure a clinical benefit over placebo. Studies should also have enough patients to show small but meaningful differences.

Although there have been studies on the likelihood of resistant S pneumoniae or H influenzae in children in child care settings and with siblings younger than 5 years, studies are still needed to determine whether these and other risk factors would indicate a need for different initial treatment than noted in the guideline.

New antibiotics that are safe and effective are needed for use in AOM because of the development of multidrug-resistant organisms. Such new antibiotics must be tested against the currently available medications.

Randomized controlled trials using different durations of antibiotic therapy in different age groups are needed to optimize therapy with the possibility of decreasing duration of antibiotic use. These would need to be performed initially with amoxicillin and amoxicillin-clavulanate but should also be performed for any antibiotic used in AOM. Again, an observation arm should be included in nonsevere illness.

Recurrent AOM

There have been adequate studies regarding prophylactic antibiotic use in recurrent AOM. More and better controlled studies of tympanostomy tube placement would help determine its benefit versus harm.

Prevention

There should be additional development of vaccines targeted at common organisms associated with AOM.[275] Focused epidemiologic studies on the benefit of breastfeeding, specifically addressing AOM prevention, including duration of breastfeeding and partial versus exclusive breastfeeding, would clarify what is now a more general database. Likewise, more focused studies of the effects of lifestyle changes would help clarify their effect on AOM.

Complementary and Alternative Medicine

There are no well-designed randomized controlled trials of the usefulness of complementary and alternative medicine in AOM, yet a large number of families turn to these methods. Although most alternative therapies are relatively inexpensive, some may be costly. Such studies should compare the alternative therapy to observation rather than antibiotics and only use an antibiotic arm if the alternative therapy is shown to be better than observation. Such studies should focus on children with less stringent criteria of AOM but using the same descriptive criteria for the patients as noted above.

DISSEMINATION OF GUIDELINES

An Institute of Medicine Report notes that "Effective multifaceted implementation strategies targeting both individuals and healthcare systems should be employed by implementers to promote adherence to trustworthy [clinical practice guidelines]."[230]

Many studies of the effect of clinical practice guidelines have been performed. In general, the studies show little overt change in practice after a guideline is published. However, as was seen after the 2004 AOM guideline, the number of visits for AOM and the number of prescriptions for antibiotics for AOM had decreased publication. Studies of educational and dissemination methods both at the practicing physician level and especially at the resident level need to be examined.

SUBCOMMITTEE ON DIAGNOSIS AND MANAGEMENT OF ACUTE OTITIS MEDIA

Allan S. Lieberthal, MD, FAAP (Chair, general pediatrician, no conflicts)

Aaron E. Carroll, MD, MS, FAAP (Partnership for Policy Implementation [PPI] Informatician, general academic pediatrician, no conflicts)

Tasnee Chonmaitree, MD, FAAP (pediatric infectious disease physician, no financial conflicts; published research related to AOM)

Theodore G. Ganiats, MD (family physician, American Academy of Family Physicians, no conflicts)

Alejandro Hoberman, MD, FAAP (general academic pediatrician, no financial conflicts; published research related to AOM)

Mary Anne Jackson, MD, FAAP (pediatric infectious disease physician, AAP Committee on Infectious Disease, no conflicts)

Mark D. Joffe, MD, FAAP (pediatric emergency medicine physician, AAP Committee/Section on Pediatric Emergency Medicine, no conflicts)

Donald T. Miller, MD, MPH, FAAP (general pediatrician, no conflicts)

Richard M. Rosenfeld, MD, MPH, FAAP (otolaryngologist, AAP Section on Otolaryngology, Head and Neck Surgery, American Academy of Otolaryngology-Head and Neck Surgery, no financial conflicts; published research related to AOM)

Xavier D. Sevilla, MD, FAAP (general pediatrics, Quality Improvement Innovation Network, no conflicts)

Richard H. Schwartz, MD, FAAP (general pediatrician, no financial conflicts; published research related to AOM)

Pauline A. Thomas, MD, FAAP (epidemiologist, general pediatrician, no conflicts)

David E. Tunkel, MD, FAAP, FACS (otolaryngologist, AAP Section on Otolaryngology, Head and Neck Surgery, periodic consultant to Medtronic ENT)

CONSULTANT

Richard N. Shiffman, MD, FAAP, FACMI (informatician, guideline methodologist, general academic pediatrician, no conflicts)

STAFF

Caryn Davidson, MA
Oversight by the Steering Committee on Quality Improvement and Management, 2009–2012

REFERENCES

1. American Academy of Pediatrics Subcommittee on Management of Acute Otitis Media. Diagnosis and management of acute otitis media. *Pediatrics.* 2004;113(5):1451–1465

2. Grijalva CG, Nuorti JP, Griffin MR. Antibiotic prescription rates for acute respiratory tract infections in US ambulatory settings. *JAMA.* 2009;302(7):758–766

3. McCaig LF, Besser RE, Hughes JM. Trends in antimicrobial prescribing rates for children and adolescents. *JAMA.* 2002;287(23):3096–3102

4. Vernacchio L, Vezina RM, Mitchell AA. Management of acute otitis media by primary care physicians: trends since the release of the 2004 American Academy of Pediatrics/American Academy of Family Physicians clinical practice guideline. *Pediatrics.* 2007;120(2):281–287

5. Coco A, Vernacchio L, Horst M, Anderson A. Management of acute otitis media after publication of the 2004 AAP and AAFP clinical practice guideline. *Pediatrics.* 2010;125(2):214–220

6. Marchisio P, Mira E, Klersy C, et al. Medical education and attitudes about acute otitis media guidelines: a survey of Italian pediatricians and otolaryngologists. *Pediatr Infect Dis J.* 2009;28(1):1–4

7. Arkins ER, Koehler JM. Use of the observation option and compliance with guidelines in treatment of acute otitis media. *Ann Pharmacother.* 2008;42(5):726–727

8. Flores G, Lee M, Bauchner H, Kastner B. Pediatricians' attitudes, beliefs, and practices regarding clinical practice guidelines: a national survey. *Pediatrics.* 2000;105(3 pt 1):496–501

9. Bluestone CD. Definitions, terminology, and classification. In: Rosenfeld RM, Bluestone CD, eds. *Evidence-Based Otitis Media.* Hamilton, Canada: BC Decker; 2003:120–135

10. Bluestone CD, Klein JO. Definitions, terminology, and classification. In: Bluestone CD, Klein JO, eds. *Otitis Media in Infants and Children.* 4th ed. Hamilton, Canada: BC Decker; 2007:1–19

11. Dowell SF, Marcy MS, Phillips WR, et al. Otitis media: principles of judicious use of antimicrobial agents. *Pediatrics.* 1998;101(suppl):165–171

12. Rosenfeld RM. Clinical pathway for acute otitis media. In: Rosenfeld RM, Bluestone CD, eds. *Evidence-Based Otitis Media.* 2nd ed. Hamilton, Canada: BC Decker; 2003:280–302

13. Carlson LH, Carlson RD. Diagnosis. In: Rosenfeld RM, Bluestone CD, eds. *Evidence-Based Otitis Media.* Hamilton, Canada: BC Decker; 2003:136–146

14. Bluestone CD, Klein JO. Diagnosis. In: *Otitis Media in Infants and Children.* 4th ed. Hamilton, Canada: BC Decker; 2007:147–212

15. University of Oxford, Centre for Evidence Based Medicine. Available at: www.cebm.net/index.aspx?o=1044. Accessed July 17, 2012

16. American Academy of Pediatrics Steering Committee on Quality Improvement and Management. Classifying recommendations for clinical practice guidelines. *Pediatrics.* 2004;114(3):874–877

17. Marcy M, Takata G, Shekelle P, et al. *Management of Acute Otitis Media.* Evidence Report/Technology Assessment No. 15. Rockville, MD: Agency for Healthcare Research and Quality; 2000

18. Chan LS, Takata GS, Shekelle P, Morton SC, Mason W, Marcy SM. Evidence assessment of management of acute otitis media: II. Research gaps and priorities for future research. *Pediatrics.* 2001;108(2):248–254

19. Takata GS, Chan LS, Shekelle P, Morton SC, Mason W, Marcy SM. Evidence assessment of management of acute otitis media: I. The role of antibiotics in treatment of uncomplicated acute otitis media. *Pediatrics.* 2001;108(2):239–247

20. Shekelle PG, Takata G, Newberry SJ, et al. *Management of Acute Otitis Media: Update.* Evidence Report/Technology Assessment No. 198. Rockville, MD: Agency for Healthcare Research and Quality; 2010

21. Coker TR, Chan LS, Newberry SJ, et al. Diagnosis, microbial epidemiology, and antibiotic treatment of acute otitis media in children: a systematic review. *JAMA.* 2010;304(19):2161–2169

22. Jadad AR, Moore RA, Carroll D, et al. Assessing the quality of reports of randomized clinical trials: is blinding necessary? *Control Clin Trials.* 1996;17(1):1–12

23. Whiting P, Rutjes AW, Reitsma JB, Bossuyt PM, Kleijnen J. The development of QUADAS: a tool for the quality assessment of studies of diagnostic accuracy included in systematic reviews. *BMC Med Res Methodol.* 2003;3:25

24. Guyatt GH, Oxman AD, Vist GE, et al; GRADE Working Group. GRADE: an emerging consensus on rating quality of evidence and strength of recommendations. *BMJ.* 2008;336(7650):924–926

25. Hoffman RN, Michel G, Rosenfeld RM, Davidson C. Building better guidelines with BRIDGE-Wiz: development and evaluation of a software assistant to promote clarity, transparency, and implementability. *J Am Med Inform Assoc.* 2012;19(1):94–101

26. Kalu SU, Ataya RS, McCormick DP, Patel JA, Revai K, Chonmaitree T. Clinical spectrum of acute otitis media complicating upper respiratory tract viral infection. *Pediatr Infect Dis J.* 2011;30(2):95–99

27. Block SL, Harrison CJ. *Diagnosis and Management of Acute Otitis Media.* 3rd ed. Caddo, OK: Professional Communications; 2005:48–50

28. Wald ER. Acute otitis media: more trouble with the evidence. *Pediatr Infect Dis J.* 2003;22(2):103–104

29. Paradise JL, Rockette HE, Colborn DK, et al. Otitis media in 2253 Pittsburgh-area infants: prevalence and risk factors during the first two years of life. *Pediatrics.* 1997;99(3):318–333

30. McCormick DP, Chonmaitree T, Pittman C, et al. Nonsevere acute otitis media: a clinical trial comparing outcomes of watchful waiting versus immediate antibiotic treatment. *Pediatrics.* 2005;115(6):1455–1465

31. Hoberman A, Paradise JL, Rockette HE, et al. Treatment of acute otitis media in children under 2 years of age. *N Engl J Med.* 2011;364(2):105–115

32. Tähtinen PA, Laine MK, Huovinen P, Jalava J, Ruuskanen O, Ruohola A. A placebo-controlled trial of antimicrobial treatment for acute otitis media. *N Engl J Med.* 2011;364(2):116–126

33. Shaikh N, Hoberman A, Paradise JL, et al. Development and preliminary evaluation of a parent-reported outcome instrument for clinical trials in acute otitis media. *Pediatr Infect Dis J.* 2009;28(1):5–8

34. Laine MK, Tähtinen PA, Ruuskanen O, Huovinen P, Ruohola A. Symptoms or symptom-based scores cannot predict acute otitis media at otitis-prone age. *Pediatrics.* 2010;125(5). Available at: www.pediatrics.org/cgi/content/full/125/5/e1154

35. Friedman NR, McCormick DP, Pittman C, et al. Development of a practical tool for assessing the severity of acute otitis media. *Pediatr Infect Dis J.* 2006;25(2):101–107

36. Rothman R, Owens T, Simel DL. Does this child have acute otitis media? *JAMA.* 2003;290(12):1633–1640

37. Niemela M, Uhari M, Jounio-Ervasti K, Luotonen J, Alho OP, Vierimaa E. Lack of specific symptomatology in children with acute otitis media. *Pediatr Infect Dis J.* 1994;13(9):765–768

38. Heikkinen T, Ruuskanen O. Signs and symptoms predicting acute otitis media. *Arch Pediatr Adolesc Med.* 1995;149(1):26–29

39. Ingvarsson L. Acute otalgia in children—findings and diagnosis. *Acta Paediatr Scand.* 1982;71(5):705–710

40. Kontiokari T, Koivunen P, Niemelä M, Pokka T, Uhari M. Symptoms of acute otitis media. *Pediatr Infect Dis J.* 1998;17(8):676–679

41. Wong DL, Baker CM. Pain in children: comparison of assessment scales. *Pediatr Nurs.* 1988;14(1):9–17

42. Shaikh N, Hoberman A, Paradise JL, et al. Responsiveness and construct validity of a symptom scale for acute otitis media. *Pediatr Infect Dis J.* 2009;28(1):9–12

43. Karma PH, Penttilä MA, Sipilä MM, Kataja MJ. Otoscopic diagnosis of middle ear effusion in acute and non-acute otitis media. I. The value of different otoscopic findings. *Int J Pediatr Otorhinolaryngol.* 1989;17(1):37–49

44. McCormick DP, Lim-Melia E, Saeed K, Baldwin CD, Chonmaitree T. Otitis media: can clinical findings predict bacterial or viral etiology? *Pediatr Infect Dis J.* 2000;19(3):256–258

45. Schwartz RH, Stool SE, Rodriguez WJ, Grundfast KM. Acute otitis media: toward a more precise definition. *Clin Pediatr (Phila).* 1981;20(9):549–554

46. Rosenfeld RM. Antibiotic prophylaxis for recurrent acute otitis media. In: Alper CM, Bluestone CD, eds. *Advanced Therapy of Otitis Media.* Hamilton, Canada: BC Decker; 2004

47. Paradise J, Bernard B, Colborn D, Smith C, Rockette H; Pittsburgh-area Child Development/Otitis Media Study Group. Otitis media with effusion: highly prevalent and often the forerunner of acute otitis media during the first year of life [abstract]. *Pediatr Res.* 1993;33:121A

48. Roland PS, Smith TL, Schwartz SR, et al. Clinical practice guideline: cerumen impaction. *Otolaryngol Head Neck Surg.* 2008;139(3 suppl 2):S1–S21

49. Shaikh N, Hoberman A, Kaleida PH, Ploof DL, Paradise JL. Videos in clinical medicine. Diagnosing otitis media—otoscopy and cerumen removal. *N Engl J Med.* 2010;362(20):e62

50. Pichichero ME. Diagnostic accuracy, tympanocentesis training performance, and antibiotic selection by pediatric residents in management of otitis media. *Pediatrics.* 2002;110(6):1064–1070

51. Kaleida PH, Ploof DL, Kurs-Lasky M, et al. Mastering diagnostic skills: Enhancing Proficiency in Otitis Media, a model for diagnostic skills training. *Pediatrics.* 2009;124(4). Available at: www.pediatrics.org/cgi/content/full/124/4/e714

52. Kaleida PH, Ploof D. ePROM: Enhancing Proficiency in Otitis Media. Pittsburgh, PA: University of Pittsburgh School of Medicine. Available at: http://pedsed.pitt.edu. Accessed December 31, 2011

53. Innovative Medical Education. *A View Through the Otoscope: Distinguishing Acute Otitis Media from Otitis Media with Effusion.* Paramus, NJ: Innovative Medical Education; 2000

54. American Academy of Pediatrics. Section on Infectious Diseases. A view through the otoscope: distinguishing acute otitis media from otitis media with effusion [video]. Available at: http://www2.aap.org/sections/infectdis/video.cfm. Accessed January 20, 2012

55. Hayden GF, Schwartz RH. Characteristics of earache among children with acute

otitis media. *Am J Dis Child.* 1985;139(7): 721–723

56. Schechter NL. Management of pain associated with acute medical illness. In: Schechter NL, Berde CB, Yaster M, eds. *Pain in Infants, Children, and Adolescents.* Baltimore, MD: Williams & Wilkins; 1993: 537–538

57. Rovers MM, Glasziou P, Appelman CL, et al. Predictors of pain and/or fever at 3 to 7 days for children with acute otitis media not treated initially with antibiotics: a meta-analysis of individual patient data. *Pediatrics.* 2007;119(3):579–585

58. Burke P, Bain J, Robinson D, Dunleavey J. Acute red ear in children: controlled trial of nonantibiotic treatment in children: controlled trial of nonantibiotic treatment in general practice. *BMJ.* 1991;303(6802): 558–562

59. Sanders S, Glasziou PP, DelMar C, Rovers M. Antibiotics for acute otitis media in children [review]. *Cochrane Database Syst Rev.* 2009;(2):1–43

60. van Buchem FL, Dunk JH, van't Hof MA. Therapy of acute otitis media: myringotomy, antibiotics, or neither? A double-blind study in children. *Lancet.* 1981;2(8252): 883–887

61. Thalin A, Densert O, Larsson A, et al. Is penicillin necessary in the treatment of acute otitis media? In: *Proceedings of the International Conference on Acute and Secretory Otitis Media. Part 1.* Amsterdam, Netherlands: Kugler Publications; 1986:441–446

62. Rovers MM, Glasziou P, Appelman CL, et al. Antibiotics for acute otitis media: an individual patient data meta-analysis. *Lancet.* 2006;368(9545):1429–1435

63. Bertin L, Pons G, d'Athis P, et al. A randomized, double-blind, multicentre controlled trial of ibuprofen versus acetaminophen and placebo for symptoms of acute otitis media in children. *Fundam Clin Pharmacol.* 1996;10(4):387–392

64. American Academy of Pediatrics. Committee on Psychosocial Aspects of Child and Family Health; Task Force on Pain in Infants, Children, and Adolescents. The assessment and management of acute pain in infants, children, and adolescents. *Pediatrics.* 2001;108(3): 793–797

65. Bolt P, Barnett P, Babl FE, Sharwood LN. Topical lignocaine for pain relief in acute otitis media: results of a double-blind placebo-controlled randomised trial. *Arch Dis Child.* 2008;93(1):40–44

66. Foxlee R, Johansson AC, Wejfalk J, Dawkins J, Dooley L, Del Mar C. Topical analgesia for acute otitis media. *Cochrane Database Syst Rev.* 2006;(3):CD005657

67. Hoberman A, Paradise JL, Reynolds EA, Urkin J. Efficacy of Auralgan for treating ear pain in children with acute otitis media. *Arch Pediatr Adolesc Med.* 1997; 151(7):675–678

68. Sarrell EM, Mandelberg A, Cohen HA. Efficacy of naturopathic extracts in the management of ear pain associated with acute otitis media. *Arch Pediatr Adolesc Med.* 2001;155(7):796–799

69. Sarrell EM, Cohen HA, Kahan E. Naturopathic treatment for ear pain in children. *Pediatrics.* 2003;111(5 pt 1):e574–e579

70. Adam D, Federspil P, Lukes M, Petrowicz O. Therapeutic properties and tolerance of procaine and phenazone containing ear drops in infants and very young children. *Arzneimittelforschung.* 2009;59(10):504–512

71. Barnett ED, Levatin JL, Chapman EH, et al. Challenges of evaluating homeopathic treatment of acute otitis media. *Pediatr Infect Dis J.* 2000;19(4):273–275

72. Jacobs J, Springer DA, Crothers D. Homeopathic treatment of acute otitis media in children: a preliminary randomized placebo-controlled trial. *Pediatr Infect Dis J.* 2001;20(2):177–183

73. Rosenfeld RM, Bluestone CD. Clinical efficacy of surgical therapy. In: Rosenfeld RM, Bluestone CD, eds. *Evidence-Based Otitis Media. 2003.* Hamilton, Canada: BC Decker; 2003:227–240

74. Rosenfeld RM. Observation option toolkit for acute otitis media. *Int J Pediatr Otorhinolaryngol.* 2001;58(1):1–8

75. Le Saux N, Gaboury I, Baird M, et al. A randomized, double-blind, placebo-controlled noninferiority trial of amoxicillin for clinically diagnosed acute otitis media in children 6 months to 5 years of age. *CMAJ.* 2005;172(3):335–341

76. Spiro DM, Tay KY, Arnold DH, Dziura JD, Baker MD, Shapiro ED. Wait-and-see prescription for the treatment of acute otitis media: a randomized controlled trial. *JAMA.* 2006;296(10):1235–1241

77. Neumark T, Mölstad S, Rosén C, et al. Evaluation of phenoxymethylpenicillin treatment of acute otitis media in children aged 2–16. *Scand J Prim Health Care.* 2007;25(3):166–171

78. Chao JH, Kunkov S, Reyes LB, Lichten S, Crain EF. Comparison of two approaches to observation therapy for acute otitis media in the emergency department. *Pediatrics.* 2008;121(5). Available at: www.pediatrics.org/cgi/content/full/121/5/e1352

79. Spurling GK, Del Mar CB, Dooley L, Foxlee R. Delayed antibiotics for respiratory infections. *Cochrane Database Syst Rev.* 2007;(3):CD004417

80. Koopman L, Hoes AW, Glasziou PP, et al. Antibiotic therapy to prevent the development of asymptomatic middle ear effusion in children with acute otitis media: a meta-analysis of individual patient data. *Arch Otolaryngol Head Neck Surg.* 2008;134(2):128–132

81. Marchetti F, Ronfani L, Nibali SC, Tamburlini G; Italian Study Group on Acute Otitis Media. Delayed prescription may reduce the use of antibiotics for acute otitis media: a prospective observational study in primary care. *Arch Pediatr Adolesc Med.* 2005; 159(7):679–684

82. Ho D, Rotenberg BW, Berkowitz RG. The relationship between acute mastoiditis and antibiotic use for acute otitis media in children. *Arch Otolaryngol Head Neck Surg.* 2008;34(1):45–48

83. Thompson PL, Gilbert RE, Long PF, Saxena S, Sharland M, Wong IC. Effect of antibiotics for otitis media on mastoiditis in children: a retrospective cohort study using the United Kingdom general practice research database. *Pediatrics.* 2009; 123(2):424–430

84. American Academy of Family Physicians; American Academy of Otolaryngology-Head and Neck Surgery; American Academy of Pediatrics Subcommittee on Otitis Media With Effusion. Otitis media with effusion. *Pediatrics.* 2004;113(5):1412–1429

85. Rosenfeld RM, Culpepper L, Doyle KJ, et al; American Academy of Pediatrics Subcommittee on Otitis Media with Effusion; American Academy of Family Physicians; American Academy of Otolaryngology—Head and Neck Surgery. Clinical practice guideline: otitis media with effusion. *Otolaryngol Head Neck Surg.* 2004;130(suppl 5): S95–S118

86. Appelman CL, Claessen JQ, Touw-Otten FW, Hordijk GJ, de Melker RA. Co-amoxiclav in recurrent acute otitis media: placebo controlled study. *BMJ.* 1991;303(6815): 1450–1452

87. Burke P, Bain J, Robinson D, Dunleavey J. Acute red ear in children: controlled trial of nonantibiotic treatment in children: controlled trial of nonantibiotic treatment in general practice. *BMJ.* 1991;303(6802): 558–562

88. van Balen FA, Hoes AW, Verheij TJ, de Melker RA. Primary care based randomized, double blind trial of amoxicillin versus placebo in children aged under 2 years. *BMJ.* 2000;320(7231):350–354

89. Little P, Gould C, Williamson I, Moore M, Warner G, Dunleavey J. Pragmatic randomised controlled trial of two prescribing strategies for childhood acute otitis media. *BMJ.* 2001;322(7282):336–342

90. Mygind N, Meistrup-Larsen K-I, Thomsen J, Thomsen VF, Josefsson K, Sørensen H. Penicillin in acute otitis media: a double-blind placebo-controlled trial. *Clin Otolaryngol Allied Sci.* 1981;6(1):5–13

91. Kaleida PH, Casselbrant ML, Rockette HE, et al. Amoxicillin or myringotomy or both for acute otitis media: results of a randomized clinical trial. *Pediatrics.* 1991;87(4):466–474

92. Shaikh N, Hoberman A, Paradise JL, et al. Responsiveness and construct validity of a symptom scale for acute otitis media. *Pediatr Infect Dis J.* 2009;28(1):9–12

93. Heikkinen T, Chonmaitree T. Importance of respiratory viruses in acute otitis media. *Clin Microbiol Rev.* 2003;16(2):230–241

94. Halsted C, Lepow ML, Balassanian N, Emmerich J, Wolinsky E. Otitis media. Clinical observations, microbiology, and evaluation of therapy. *Am J Dis Child.* 1968;115(5):542–551

95. Rosenfeld RM, Vertrees J, Carr J, et al. Clinical efficacy of antimicrobials for acute otitis media: meta-analysis of 5,400 children from 33 randomized trials. *J Pediatr.* 1994;124(3):355–367

96. McCormick DP, Chandler SM, Chonmaitree T. Laterality of acute otitis media: different clinical and microbiologic characteristics. *Pediatr Infect Dis J.* 2007;26(7):583–588

97. Appelman CLM, Bossen PC, Dunk JHM, Lisdonk EH, de Melker RA, van Weert HCPM. NHG Standard Otitis Media Acuta (Guideline on acute otitis media of the Dutch College of General Practitioners). *Huisarts Wet.* 1990;33:242–245

98. Swedish Medical Research Council. Treatment for acute inflammation of the middle ear: consensus statement. Stockholm, Sweden: Swedish Medical Research Council; 2000. Available at: http://soapimg.icecube.snowfall.se/strama/Konsensut_ora_eng.pdf. Accessed July 18, 2012

99. Scottish Intercollegiate Guideline Network. Diagnosis and management of childhood otitis media in primary care. Edinburgh, Scotland: Scottish Intercollegiate Guideline Network; 2000. Available at: www.sign.ac.uk/guidelines/fulltext/66/index.html. Accessed July 18, 2012

100. National Institute for Health and Clinical Excellence, Centre for Clinical Practice. Respiratory tract infections—antibiotic prescribing: prescribing of antibiotics for self-limiting respiratory tract infections in adults and children in primary care. NICE Clinical Guideline 69. London, United Kingdom: National Institute for Health and Clinical Excellence; July 2008. Available at: www.nice.org.uk/CG069. Accessed July 18, 2012

101. Marchisio P, Bellussi L, Di Mauro G, et al. Acute otitis media: from diagnosis to prevention. Summary of the Italian guideline. *Int J Pediatr Otorhinolaryngol.* 2010;74(11):1209–1216

102. Siegel RM, Kiely M, Bien JP, et al. Treatment of otitis media with observation and a safety-net antibiotic prescription. *Pediatrics.* 2003;112(3 pt 1):527–531

103. Pshetizky Y, Naimer S, Shvartzman P. Acute otitis media—a brief explanation to parents and antibiotic use. *Fam Pract.* 2003;20(4):417–419

104. Pichichero ME, Casey JR. Emergence of a multiresistant serotype 19A pneumococcal strain not included in the 7-valent conjugate vaccine as an otopathogen in children. *JAMA.* 2007;298(15):1772–1778

105. Pichichero ME, Casey JR. Evolving microbiology and molecular epidemiology of acute otitis media in the pneumococcal conjugate vaccine era. *Pediatr Infect Dis J.* 2007;26(suppl 10):S12–S16

106. Nielsen HUK, Konradsen HB, Lous J, Frimodt-Møller N. Nasopharyngeal pathogens in children with acute otitis media in a low-antibiotic use country. *Int J Pediatr Otorhinolaryngol.* 2004;68(9):1149–1155

107. Pitkäranta A, Virolainen A, Jero J, Arruda E, Hayden FG. Detection of rhinovirus, respiratory syncytial virus, and coronavirus infections in acute otitis media by reverse transcriptase polymerase chain reaction. *Pediatrics.* 1998;102(2 pt 1):291–295

108. Heikkinen T, Thint M, Chonmaitree T. Prevalence of various respiratory viruses in the middle ear during acute otitis media. *N Engl J Med.* 1999;340(4):260–264

109. Chonmaitree T. Acute otitis media is not a pure bacterial disease. *Clin Infect Dis.* 2006;43(11):1423–1425

110. Williams JV, Tollefson SJ, Nair S, Chonmaitree T. Association of human metapneumovirus with acute otitis media. *Int J Pediatr Otorhinolaryngol.* 2006;70(7):1189–1193

111. Chonmaitree T, Heikkinen T. Role of viruses in middle-ear disease. *Ann N Y Acad Sci.* 1997;830:143–157

112. Klein JO, Bluestone CD. Otitis media. In: Feigin RD, Cherry JD, Demmler-Harrison GJ, Kaplan SL, eds. *Textbook of Pediatric Infectious Diseases.* 6th ed. Philadelphia, PA: Saunders; 2009:216–237

113. Chonmaitree T, Revai K, Grady JJ, et al. Viral upper respiratory tract infection and otitis media complication in young children. *Clin Infect Dis.* 2008;46(6):815–823

114. Ruohola A, Meurman O, Nikkari S, et al. Microbiology of acute otitis media in children with tympanostomy tubes: prevalences of bacteria and viruses. *Clin Infect Dis.* 2006;43(11):1417–1422

115. Ruuskanen O, Arola M, Heikkinen T, Ziegler T. Viruses in acute otitis media: increasing evidence for clinical significance. *Pediatr Infect Dis J.* 1991;10(6):425–427

116. Chonmaitree T. Viral and bacterial interaction in acute otitis media. *Pediatr Infect Dis J.* 2000;19(suppl 5):S24–S30

117. Nokso-Koivisto J, Räty R, Blomqvist S, et al. Presence of specific viruses in the middle ear fluids and respiratory secretions of young children with acute otitis media. *J Med Virol.* 2004;72(2):241–248

118. Bluestone CD, Klein JO. Microbiology. In: Bluestone CD, Klein JO, eds. *Otitis Media in Infants and Children.* 4th ed. Hamilton, Canada: BC Decker; 2007:101–126

119. Del Beccaro MA, Mendelman PM, Inglis AF, et al. Bacteriology of acute otitis media: a new perspective. *J Pediatr.* 1992;120(1):81–84

120. Block SL, Harrison CJ, Hedrick JA, et al. Penicillin-resistant *Streptococcus pneumoniae* in acute otitis media: risk factors, susceptibility patterns and antimicrobial management. *Pediatr Infect Dis J.* 1995;14(9):751–759

121. Rodriguez WJ, Schwartz RH. *Streptococcus pneumoniae* causes otitis media with higher fever and more redness of tympanic membranes than *Haemophilus influenzae* or *Moraxella catarrhalis.* *Pediatr Infect Dis J.* 1999;18(10):942–944

122. Block SL, Hedrick J, Harrison CJ, et al. Community-wide vaccination with the heptavalent pneumococcal conjugate significantly alters the microbiology of acute otitis media. *Pediatr Infect Dis J.* 2004;23(9):829–833

123. Casey JR, Pichichero ME. Changes in frequency and pathogens causing acute otitis media in 1995–2003. *Pediatr Infect Dis J.* 2004;23(9):824–828

124. McEllistrem MC, Adams JM, Patel K, et al. Acute otitis media due to penicillin-nonsusceptible *Streptococcus pneumoniae* before and after the introduction of the pneumococcal conjugate vaccine. *Clin Infect Dis.* 2005;40(12):1738–1744

125. Casey JR, Adlowitz DG, Pichichero ME. New patterns in the otopathogens causing acute otitis media six to eight years after introduction of pneumococcal conjugate vaccine. *Pediatr Infect Dis J.* 2010;29(4):304–309

126. Grubb MS, Spaugh DC. Microbiology of acute otitis media, Puget Sound region, 2005–2009. *Clin Pediatr (Phila)*. 2010;49(8): 727–730

127. Revai K, McCormick DP, Patel J, Grady JJ, Saeed K, Chonmaitree T. Effect of pneumococcal conjugate vaccine on nasopharyngeal bacterial colonization during acute otitis media. *Pediatrics*. 2006;117(5): 1823–1829

128. Pettigrew MM, Gent JF, Revai K, Patel JA, Chonmaitree T. Microbial interactions during upper respiratory tract infections. *Emerg Infect Dis*. 2008;14(10):1584–1591

129. O'Brien KL, Millar EV, Zell ER, et al. Effect of pneumococcal conjugate vaccine on nasopharyngeal colonization among immunized and unimmunized children in a community-randomized trial. *J Infect Dis*. 2007;196(8):1211–1220

130. Jacobs MR, Bajaksouzian S, Windau A, Good C. Continued emergence of non-vaccine serotypes of *Streptococcus pneumoniae* in Cleveland. *Proceedings of the 49th Interscience Conference on Antimicrobial Agents and Chemotherapy*, 2009:G1-G1556

131. Hoberman A, Paradise JL, Shaikh N, et al. Pneumococcal resistance and serotype 19A in Pittsburgh-area children with acute otitis media before and after introduction of 7-valent pneumococcal polysaccharide vaccine. *Clin Pediatr (Phila)*. 2011;50(2): 114–120

132. Huang SS, Hinrichsen VL, Stevenson AE, et al. Continued impact of pneumococcal conjugate vaccine on carriage in young children. *Pediatrics*. 2009;124(1). Available at: www.pediatrics.org/cgi/content/full/124/1/e1

133. Centers for Disease Control and Prevention (CDC). Licensure of a 13-valent pneumococcal conjugate vaccine (PCV13) and recommendations for use among children—Advisory Committee on Immunization Practices (ACIP), 2010. *MMWR Morb Mortal Wkly Rep*. 2010;59(9):258–261

134. Segal N, Givon-Lavi N, Leibovitz E, Yagupsky P, Leiberman A, Dagan R. Acute otitis media caused by *Streptococcus pyogenes* in children. *Clin Infect Dis*. 2005;41(1):35–41

135. Luntz M, Brodsky A, Nusem S, et al. Acute mastoiditis—the antibiotic era: a multicenter study. *Int J Pediatr Otorhinolaryngol*. 2001;57(1):1–9

136. Nielsen JC. *Studies on the Aetiology of Acute Otitis Media*. Copenhagen, Denmark: Ejnar Mundsgaard Forlag; 1945

137. Palmu AA, Herva E, Savolainen H, Karma P, Mäkelä PH, Kilpi TM. Association of clinical signs and symptoms with bacterial findings in acute otitis media. *Clin Infect Dis*. 2004;38(2):234–242

138. Leibovitz E, Asher E, Piglansky L, et al. Is bilateral acute otitis media clinically different than unilateral acute otitis media? *Pediatr Infect Dis J*. 2007;26(7):589–592

139. Leibovitz E, Satran R, Piglansky L, et al. Can acute otitis media caused by *Haemophilus influenzae* be distinguished from that caused by *Streptococcus pneumoniae*? *Pediatr Infect Dis J*. 2003;22(6): 509–515

140. Palmu AA, Kotikoski MJ, Kaijalainen TH, Puhakka HJ. Bacterial etiology of acute myringitis in children less than two years of age. *Pediatr Infect Dis J*. 2001;20(6): 607–611

141. Bodor FF. Systemic antibiotics for treatment of the conjunctivitis-otitis media syndrome. *Pediatr Infect Dis J*. 1989;8(5): 287–290

142. Bingen E, Cohen R, Jourenkova N, Gehanno P. Epidemiologic study of conjunctivitis-otitis syndrome. *Pediatr Infect Dis J*. 2005;24(8):731–732

143. Barkai G, Leibovitz E, Givon-Lavi N, Dagan R. Potential contribution by nontypable *Haemophilus influenzae* in protracted and recurrent acute otitis media. *Pediatr Infect Dis J*. 2009;28(6):466–471

144. Howie VM, Ploussard JH. Efficacy of fixed combination antibiotics versus separate components in otitis media. Effectiveness of erythromycin estrolate, triple sulfonamide, ampicillin, erythromycin estolate-triple sulfonamide, and placebo in 280 patients with acute otitis media under two and one-half years of age. *Clin Pediatr (Phila)*. 1972;11(4):205–214

145. Klein JO. Microbiologic efficacy of antibacterial drugs for acute otitis media. *Pediatr Infect Dis J*. 1993;12(12): 973–975

146. Barnett ED, Klein JO. The problem of resistant bacteria for the management of acute otitis media. *Pediatr Clin North Am*. 1995;42(3):509–517

147. Tristram S, Jacobs MR, Appelbaum PC. Antimicrobial resistance in *Haemophilus influenzae*. *Clin Microbiol Rev*. 2007;20(2): 368–389

148. Critchley IA, Jacobs MR, Brown SD, Traczewski MM, Tillotson GS, Janjic N. Prevalence of serotype 19A *Streptococcus pneumoniae* among isolates from U.S. children in 2005≠2006 and activity of faropenem. *Antimicrob Agents Chemother*. 2008;52(7): 2639–2643

149. Jacobs MR, Good CE, Windau AR, et al. Activity of ceftaroline against emerging serotypes of Streptococcus pneumoniae. *Antimicrob Agents Chemother*. 2010;54(6): 2716–2719

150. Jacobs MR. Antimicrobial-resistant *Streptococcus pneumoniae*: trends and management. *Expert Rev Anti Infect Ther*. 2008;6(5):619–635

151. Piglansky L, Leibovitz E, Raiz S, et al. Bacteriologic and clinical efficacy of high dose amoxicillin for therapy of acute otitis media in children. *Pediatr Infect Dis J*. 2003;22(5):405–413

152. Dagan R, Johnson CE, McLinn S, et al. Bacteriologic and clinical efficacy of amoxicillin/clavulanate vs. azithromycin in acute otitis media. *Pediatr Infect Dis J*. 2000;19(2):95–104

153. Dagan R, Hoberman A, Johnson C, et al. Bacteriologic and clinical efficacy of high dose amoxicillin/clavulanate in children with acute otitis media. *Pediatr Infect Dis J*. 2001;20(9):829–837

154. Hoberman A, Dagan R, Leibovitz E, et al. Large dosage amoxicillin/clavulanate, compared with azithromycin, for the treatment of bacterial acute otitis media in children. *Pediatr Infect Dis J*. 2005;24 (6):525–532

155. De Wals P, Erickson L, Poirier B, Pépin J, Pichichero ME. How to compare the efficacy of conjugate vaccines to prevent acute otitis media? *Vaccine*. 2009;27(21): 2877–2883

156. Shouval DS, Greenberg D, Givon-Lavi N, Porat N, Dagan R. Serotype coverage of invasive and mucosal pneumococcal disease in Israeli children younger than 3 years by various pneumococcal conjugate vaccines. *Pediatr Infect Dis J*. 2009;28(4): 277–282

157. Jones RN, Farrell DJ, Mendes RE, Sader HS. Comparative ceftaroline activity tested against pathogens associated with community-acquired pneumonia: results from an international surveillance study. *J Antimicrob Chemother*. 2011;66(suppl 3): iii69–iii80

158. Harrison CJ, Woods C, Stout G, Martin B, Selvarangan R. Susceptibilities of Haemophilus influenzae, Streptococcus pneumoniae, including serotype 19A, and Moraxella catarrhalis paediatric isolates from 2005 to 2007 to commonly used antibiotics. *J Antimicrob Chemother*. 2009;63(3):511–519

159. Doern GV, Jones RN, Pfaller MA, Kugler K. *Haemophilus influenzae* and *Moraxella catarrhalis* from patients with community-acquired respiratory tract infections: antimicrobial susceptibility patterns from the SENTRY antimicrobial Surveillance Program (United States and Canada, 1997).

Antimicrob Agents Chemother. 1999;43(2): 385–389

160. Nussinovitch M, Yoeli R, Elishkevitz K, Varsano I. Acute mastoiditis in children: epidemiologic, clinical, microbiologic, and therapeutic aspects over past years. *Clin Pediatr (Phila).* 2004;43(3):261–267

161. Roddy MG, Glazier SS, Agrawal D. Pediatric mastoiditis in the pneumococcal conjugate vaccine era: symptom duration guides empiric antimicrobial therapy. *Pediatr Emerg Care.* 2007;23(11):779–784

162. Hoberman A, Paradise JL, Burch DJ, et al. Equivalent efficacy and reduced occurrence of diarrhea from a new formulation of amoxicillin/clavulanate potassium (Augmentin) for treatment of acute otitis media in children. *Pediatr Infect Dis J.* 1997;16(5):463–470

163. Arguedas A, Dagan R, Leibovitz E, Hoberman A, Pichichero M, Paris M. A multicenter, open label, double tympanocentesis study of high dose cefdinir in children with acute otitis media at high risk of persistent or recurrent infection. *Pediatr Infect Dis J.* 2006;25(3):211–218

164. Atanasković-Marković M, Velicković TC, Gavrović-Jankulović M, Vucković O, Nestorović B. Immediate allergic reactions to cephalosporins and penicillins and their cross-reactivity in children. *Pediatr Allergy Immunol.* 2005;16(4):341–347

165. Pichichero ME. Use of selected cephalosporins in penicillin-allergic patients: a paradigm shift. *Diagn Microbiol Infect Dis.* 2007;57(suppl 3):13S–18S

166. Pichichero ME, Casey JR. Safe use of selected cephalosporins in penicillin-allergic patients: a meta-analysis. *Otolaryngol Head Neck Surg.* 2007;136(3):340–347

167. DePestel DD, Benninger MS, Danziger L, et al. Cephalosporin use in treatment of patients with penicillin allergies. *J Am Pharm Assoc (2003).* 2008;48(4):530–540

168. Fonacier L, Hirschberg R, Gerson S. Adverse drug reactions to a cephalosporins in hospitalized patients with a history of penicillin allergy. *Allergy Asthma Proc.* 2005;26(2):135–141

169. Joint Task Force on Practice Parameters; American Academy of Allergy, Asthma and Immunology; American College of Allergy, Asthma and Immunology; Joint Council of Allergy, Asthma and Immunology. Drug allergy: an updated practice parameter. *Ann Allergy Asthma Immunol.* 2010;105(4): 259–273

170. Powers JL, Gooch WM, III, Oddo LP. Comparison of the palatability of the oral suspension of cefdinir vs. amoxicillin/clavulanate potassium, cefprozil and azithromycin in pediatric patients. *Pediatr Infect Dis J.* 2000; 19(suppl 12):S174–S180

171. Steele RW, Thomas MP, Bégué RE. Compliance issues related to the selection of antibiotic suspensions for children. *Pediatr Infect Dis J.* 2001;20(1):1–5

172. Steele RW, Russo TM, Thomas MP. Adherence issues related to the selection of antistaphylococcal or antifungal antibiotic suspensions for children. *Clin Pediatr (Phila).* 2006;45(3):245–250

173. Schwartz RH. Enhancing children's satisfaction with antibiotic therapy: a taste study of several antibiotic suspensions. *Curr Ther Res.* 2000;61(8):570–581

174. Green SM, Rothrock SG. Single-dose intramuscular ceftriaxone for acute otitis media in children. *Pediatrics.* 1993;91(1): 23–30

175. Leibovitz E, Piglansky L, Raiz S, Press J, Leiberman A, Dagan R. Bacteriologic and clinical efficacy of one day vs. three day intramuscular ceftriaxone for treatment of nonresponsive acute otitis media in children. *Pediatr Infect Dis J.* 2000;19(11): 1040–1045

176. Rosenfeld RM, Kay D. Natural history of untreated otitis media. *Laryngoscope.* 2003;113(10):1645–1657

177. Rosenfeld RM, Kay D. Natural history of untreated otitis media. In: Rosenfeld RM, Bluestone CD, eds. *Evidence-Based Otitis Media.* 2nd ed. Hamilton, Canada: BC Decker; 2003:180–198

178. Arola M, Ziegler T, Ruuskanen O. Respiratory virus infection as a cause of prolonged symptoms in acute otitis media. *J Pediatr.* 1990;116(5):697–701

179. Chonmaitree T, Owen MJ, Howie VM. Respiratory viruses interfere with bacteriologic response to antibiotic in children with acute otitis media. *J Infect Dis.* 1990; 162(2):546–549

180. Dagan R, Leibovitz E, Greenberg D, Yagupsky P, Fliss DM, Leiberman A. Early eradication of pathogens from middle ear fluid during antibiotic treatment of acute otitis media is associated with improved clinical outcome. *Pediatr Infect Dis J.* 1998;17(9):776–782

181. Carlin SA, Marchant CD, Shurin PA, Johnson CE, Super DM, Rehmus JM. Host factors and early therapeutic response in acute otitis media. *J Pediatr.* 1991;118(2):178–183

182. Teele DW, Pelton SI, Klein JO. Bacteriology of acute otitis media unresponsive to initial antimicrobial therapy. *J Pediatr.* 1981; 98(4):537–539

183. Doern GV, Pfaller MA, Kugler K, Freeman J, Jones RN. Prevalence of antimicrobial resistance among respiratory tract isolates of *Streptococcus pneumoniae* in North America: 1997 results from the SENTRY antimicrobial surveillance program. *Clin Infect Dis.* 1998;27(4):764–770

184. Leiberman A, Leibovitz E, Piglansky L, et al. Bacteriologic and clinical efficacy of trimethoprim-sulfamethoxazole for treatment of acute otitis media. *Pediatr Infect Dis J.* 2001;20(3):260–264

185. Humphrey WR, Shattuck MH, Zielinski RJ, et al. Pharmacokinetics and efficacy of linezolid in a gerbil model of *Streptococcus pneumoniae*-induced acute otitis media. *Antimicrob Agents Chemother.* 2003; 47(4):1355–1363

186. Arguedas A, Dagan R, Pichichero M, et al. An open-label, double tympanocentesis study of levofloxacin therapy in children with, or at high risk for, recurrent or persistent acute otitis media. *Pediatr Infect Dis J.* 2006;25(12):1102–1109

187. Noel GJ, Blumer JL, Pichichero ME, et al. A randomized comparative study of levofloxacin versus amoxicillin/clavulanate for treatment of infants and young children with recurrent or persistent acute otitis media. *Pediatr Infect Dis J.* 2008;27(6): 483–489

188. Howie VM, Ploussard JH. Simultaneous nasopharyngeal and middle ear exudate culture in otitis media. *Pediatr Digest.* 1971;13:31–35

189. Gehanno P, Lenoir G, Barry B, Bons J, Boucot I, Berche P. Evaluation of nasopharyngeal cultures for bacteriologic assessment of acute otitis media in children. *Pediatr Infect Dis J.* 1996;15(4): 329–332

190. Cohen R, Levy C, Boucherat M, Langue J, de La Rocque F. A multicenter, randomized, double-blind trial of 5 versus 10 days of antibiotic therapy for acute otitis media in young children. *J Pediatr.* 1998;133(5): 634–639

191. Pessey JJ, Gehanno P, Thoroddsen E, et al. Short course therapy with cefuroxime axetil for acute otitis media: results of a randomized multicenter comparison with amoxicillin/clavulanate. *Pediatr Infect Dis J.* 1999;18(10):854–859

192. Cohen R, Levy C, Boucherat M, et al. Five vs. ten days of antibiotic therapy for acute otitis media in young children. *Pediatr Infect Dis J.* 2000;19(5):458–463

193. Pichichero ME, Marsocci SM, Murphy ML, Hoeger W, Francis AB, Green JL. A prospective observational study of 5-, 7-, and 10-day antibiotic treatment for acute otitis media. *Otolaryngol Head Neck Surg.* 2001; 124(4):381–387

194. Kozyrskyj AL, Klassen TP, Moffatt M, Harvey K. Short-course antibiotics for acute otitis media. *Cochrane Database Syst Rev.* 2010;(9):CD001095

195. Shurin PA, Pelton SI, Donner A, Klein JO. Persistence of middle-ear effusion after acute otitis media in children. *N Engl J Med.* 1979;300(20):1121–1123

196. Damoiseaux RA, Rovers MM, Van Balen FA, Hoes AW, de Melker RA. Long-term prognosis of acute otitis media in infancy: determinants of recurrent acute otitis media and persistent middle ear effusion. *Fam Pract.* 2006;23(1):40–45

197. Leach AJ, Morris PS. Antibiotics for the prevention of acute and chronic suppurative otitis media in children. *Cochrane Database Syst Rev.* 2006;(4):CD004401

198. Teele DW, Klein JO, Word BM, et al; Greater Boston Otitis Media Study Group. Antimicrobial prophylaxis for infants at risk for recurrent acute otitis media. *Vaccine.* 2000;19(suppl 1):S140–S143

199. Paradise JL. On tympanostomy tubes: rationale, results, reservations, and recommendations. *Pediatrics.* 1977;60(1):86–90

200. McIsaac WJ, Coyte PC, Croxford R, Asche CV, Friedberg J, Feldman W. Otolaryngologists' perceptions of the indications for tympanostomy tube insertion in children. *CMAJ.* 2000;162(9):1285–1288

201. Casselbrandt ML. Ventilation tubes for recurrent acute otitis media. In: Alper CM, Bluestone CD, eds. *Advanced Therapy of Otitis Media.* Hamilton, Canada: BC Decker; 2004:113–115

202. Shin JJ, Stinnett SS, Hartnick CJ. Pediatric recurrent acute otitis media. In: Shin JJ, Hartnick CJ, Randolph GW, eds. *Evidence-Based Otolaryngology.* New York, NY: Springer; 2008:91–95

203. Gonzalez C, Arnold JE, Woody EA, et al. Prevention of recurrent acute otitis media: chemoprophylaxis versus tympanostomy tubes. *Laryngoscope.* 1986;96(12):1330–1334

204. Gebhart DE. Tympanostomy tubes in the otitis media prone child. *Laryngoscope.* 1981;91(6):849–866

205. Casselbrant ML, Kaleida PH, Rockette HE, et al. Efficacy of antimicrobial prophylaxis and of tympanostomy tube insertion for prevention of recurrent acute otitis media: results of a randomized clinical trial. *Pediatr Infect Dis J.* 1992;11(4):278–286

206. El-Sayed Y. Treatment of recurrent acute otitis media chemoprophylaxis versus ventilation tubes. *Aust J Otolaryngol.* 1996; 2(4):352–355

207. McDonald S, Langton Hewer CD, Nunez DA. Grommets (ventilation tubes) for recurrent acute otitis media in children. *Cochrane Database Syst Rev.* 2008;(4): CD004741

208. Rosenfeld RM, Bhaya MH, Bower CM, et al. Impact of tympanostomy tubes on child quality of life. *Arch Otolaryngol Head Neck Surg.* 2000;126(5):585–592

209. Witsell DL, Stewart MG, Monsell EM, et al. The Cooperative Outcomes Group for ENT: a multicenter prospective cohort study on the outcomes of tympanostomy tubes for children with otitis media. *Otolaryngol Head Neck Surg.* 2005;132(2):180–188

210. Isaacson G. Six Sigma tympanostomy tube insertion: achieving the highest safety levels during residency training. *Otolaryngol Head Neck Surg.* 2008;139(3):353–357

211. Kay DJ, Nelson M, Rosenfeld RM. Meta-analysis of tympanostomy tube sequelae. *Otolaryngol Head Neck Surg.* 2001;124(4):374–380

212. Koivunen P, Uhari M, Luotonen J, et al. Adenoidectomy versus chemoprophylaxis and placebo for recurrent acute otitis media in children aged under 2 years: randomised controlled trial. *BMJ.* 2004; 328(7438):487

213. Rosenfeld RM. Surgical prevention of otitis media. *Vaccine.* 2000;19(suppl 1):S134–S139

214. Centers for Disease Control and Prevention (CDC). Prevention and control of influenza with vaccines: recommendations of the Advisory Committee on Immunization Practices (ACIP), 2011. *MMWR Morb Mortal Wkly Rep.* 2011;60(33):1128–1132

215. American Academy of Pediatrics Committee on Infectious Diseases. Recommendations for prevention and control of influenza in children, 2011–2012. *Pediatrics.* 2011;128(4):813–825

216. Section on Breastfeeding. Breastfeeding and the use of human milk. *Pediatrics.* 2012;129(3). Available at: www.pediatrics.org/cgi/content/full/129/3/e827

217. Pavia M, Bianco A, Nobile CG, Marinelli P, Angelillo IF. Efficacy of pneumococcal vaccination in children younger than 24 months: a meta-analysis. *Pediatrics.* 2009; 123(6). Available at: www.pediatrics.org/cgi/content/full/123/6/e1103

218. Eskola J, Kilpi T, Palmu A, et al; Finnish Otitis Media Study Group. Efficacy of a pneumococcal conjugate vaccine against acute otitis media. *N Engl J Med.* 2001;344(6):403–409

219. Black S, Shinefield H, Fireman B, et al; Northern California Kaiser Permanente Vaccine Study Center Group. Efficacy, safety and immunogenicity of heptavalent pneumococcal conjugate vaccine in children. *Pediatr Infect Dis J.* 2000;19(3):187–195

220. Jacobs MR. Prevention of otitis media: role of pneumococcal conjugate vaccines in reducing incidence and antibiotic resistance. *J Pediatr.* 2002;141(2):287–293

221. Jansen AG, Hak E, Veenhoven RH, Damoiseaux RA, Schilder AG, Sanders EA. Pneumococcal conjugate vaccines for preventing otitis media. *Cochrane Database Syst Rev.* 2009;(2):CD001480

222. Fireman B, Black SB, Shinefield HR, Lee J, Lewis E, Ray P. Impact of the pneumococcal conjugate vaccine on otitis media. *Pediatr Infect Dis J.* 2003;22(1):10–16

223. Grijalva CG, Poehling KA, Nuorti JP, et al. National impact of universal childhood immunization with pneumococcal conjugate vaccine on otitis media. *Pediatr Infect Dis J.* 2006;118(3):865–873

224. Zhou F, Shefer A, Kong Y, Nuorti JP. Trends in acute otitis media-related health care utilization by privately insured young children in the United States, 1997–2004. *Pediatrics.* 2008;121(2):253–260

225. Poehling KA, Szilagyi PG, Grijalva CG, et al. Reduction of frequent otitis media and pressure-equalizing tube insertions in children after introduction of pneumococcal conjugate vaccine. *Pediatrics.* 2007; 119(4):707–715

226. Pelton SI. Prospects for prevention of otitis media. *Pediatr Infect Dis J.* 2007;26 (suppl 10):S20–S22

227. Pelton SI, Leibovitz E. Recent advances in otitis media. *Pediatr Infect Dis J.* 2009;28 (suppl 10):S133–S137

228. De Wals P, Erickson L, Poirier B, Pépin J, Pichichero ME. How to compare the efficacy of conjugate vaccines to prevent acute otitis media? *Vaccine.* 2009;27(21):2877–2883

229. Plasschaert AI, Rovers MM, Schilder AG, Verheij TJ, Hak E. Trends in doctor consultations, antibiotic prescription, and specialist referrals for otitis media in children: 1995–2003. *Pediatrics.* 2006;117(6):1879–1886

230. O'Brien MA, Prosser LA, Paradise JL, et al. New vaccines against otitis media: projected benefits and cost-effectiveness. *Pediatrics.* 2009;123(6):1452–1463

231. Hanage WP, Auranen K, Syrjänen R, et al. Ability of pneumococcal serotypes and clones to cause acute otitis media: implications for the prevention of otitis media by conjugate vaccines. *Infect Immun.* 2004; 72(1):76–81

232. Prymula R, Peeters P, Chrobok V, et al. Pneumococcal capsular polysaccharides

conjugated to protein D for prevention of acute otitis media caused by both Streptococcus pneumoniae and non-typable *Haemophilus influenzae*: a randomised double-blind efficacy study. *Lancet.* 2006; 367(9512):740–748

233. Prymula R, Schuerman L. 10-valent pneumococcal nontypeable *Haemophilus influenzae* PD conjugate vaccine: Synflorix. *Expert Rev Vaccines.* 2009;8(11):1479–1500

234. Schuerman L, Borys D, Hoet B, Forsgren A, Prymula R. Prevention of otitis media: now a reality? *Vaccine.* 2009;27(42):5748–5754

235. Heikkinen T, Ruuskanen O, Waris M, Ziegler T, Arola M, Halonen P. Influenza vaccination in the prevention of acute otitis media in children. *Am J Dis Child.* 1991;145(4):445–448

236. Clements DA, Langdon L, Bland C, Walter E. Influenza A vaccine decreases the incidence of otitis media in 6- to 30-month-old children in day care. *Arch Pediatr Adolesc Med.* 1995;149(10):1113–1117

237. Belshe RB, Gruber WC. Prevention of otitis media in children with live attenuated influenza vaccine given intranasally. *Pediatr Infect Dis J.* 2000;19(suppl 5):S66–S71

238. Marchisio P, Cavagna R, Maspes B, et al. Efficacy of intranasal virosomal influenza vaccine in the prevention of recurrent acute otitis media in children. *Clin Infect Dis.* 2002;35(2):168–174

239. Ozgur SK, Beyazova U, Kemaloglu YK, et al. Effectiveness of inactivated influenza vaccine for prevention of otitis media in children. *Pediatr Infect Dis J.* 2006;25(5): 401–404

240. Block SL, Heikkinen T, Toback SL, Zheng W, Ambrose CS. The efficacy of live attenuated influenza vaccine against influenza-associated acute otitis media in children. *Pediatr Infect Dis J.* 2011;30(3):203–207

241. Ashkenazi S, Vertruyen A, Aristegui J, et al; CAIV-T Study Group. Superior relative efficacy of live attenuated influenza vaccine compared with inactivated influenza vaccine in young children with recurrent respiratory tract infections. *Pediatr Infect Dis J.* 2006;25(10):870–879

242. Belshe RB, Edwards KM, Vesikari T, et al; CAIV-T Comparative Efficacy Study Group. Live attenuated versus inactivated influenza vaccine in infants and young children [published correction appears in *N Engl J Med.* 2007;356(12):1283]. *N Engl J Med.* 2007;356(7):685–696

243. Bracco Neto H, Farhat CK, Tregnaghi MW, et al; D153-P504 LAIV Study Group. Efficacy and safety of 1 and 2 doses of live attenuated influenza vaccine in vaccine-naive children. *Pediatr Infect Dis J.* 2009;28(5): 365–371

244. Tam JS, Capeding MR, Lum LC, et al; Pan-Asian CAIV-T Pediatric Efficacy Trial Network. Efficacy and safety of a live attenuated, cold-adapted influenza vaccine, trivalent against culture-confirmed influenza in young children in Asia. *Pediatr Infect Dis J.* 2007;26(7):619–628

245. Vesikari T, Fleming DM, Aristegui JF, et al; CAIV-T Pediatric Day Care Clinical Trial Network. Safety, efficacy, and effectiveness of cold-adapted influenza vaccine-trivalent against community-acquired, culture-confirmed influenza in young children attending day care. *Pediatrics.* 2006;118(6):2298–2312

246. Forrest BD, Pride MW, Dunning AJ, et al. Correlation of cellular immune responses with protection against culture-confirmed influenza virus in young children. *Clin Vaccine Immunol.* 2008;15(7): 1042–1053

247. Lum LC, Borja-Tabora CF, Breiman RF, et al. Influenza vaccine concurrently administered with a combination measles, mumps, and rubella vaccine to young children. *Vaccine.* 2010;28(6):1566–1574

248. Belshe RB, Mendelman PM, Treanor J, et al. The efficacy of live attenuated, cold-adapted, trivalent, intranasal influenzavirus vaccine in children. *N Engl J Med.* 1998;338(20): 1405–1412

249. Daly KA, Giebink GS. Clinical epidemiology of otitis media. *Pediatr Infect Dis J.* 2000; 19(suppl 5):S31–S36

250. Duncan B, Ey J, Holberg CJ, Wright AL, Martinez FD, Taussig LM. Exclusive breastfeeding for at least 4 months protects against otitis media. *Pediatrics.* 1993;91(5): 867–872

251. Duffy LC, Faden H, Wasielewski R, Wolf J, Krystofik D. Exclusive breastfeeding protects against bacterial colonization and day care exposure to otitis media. *Pediatrics.* 1997;100(4). Available at: www.pediatrics.org/cgi/content/full/100/4/e7

252. Paradise JL. Short-course antimicrobial treatment for acute otitis media: not best for infants and young children. *JAMA.* 1997;278(20):1640–1642

253. Scariati PD, Grummer-Strawn LM, Fein SB. A longitudinal analysis of infant morbidity and the extent of breastfeeding in the United States. *Pediatrics.* 1997;99(6). Available at: www.pediatrics.org/cgi/content/full/99/6/e5

254. McNiel ME, Labbok MH, Abrahams SW. What are the risks associated with formula feeding? A re-analysis and review. *Breastfeed Rev.* 2010;18(2):25–32

255. Chantry CJ, Howard CR, Auinger P. Full breastfeeding duration and associated decrease in respiratory tract infection in US children. *Pediatrics.* 2006;117(2):425–432

256. Hatakka K, Piirainen L, Pohjavuori S, Poussa T, Savilahti E, Korpela R. Factors associated with acute respiratory illness in day care children. *Scand J Infect Dis.* 2010;42(9):704–711

257. Ladomenou F, Kafatos A, Tselentis Y, Galanakis E. Predisposing factors for acute otitis media in infancy. *J Infect.* 2010;61(1):49–53

258. Ladomenou F, Moschandreas J, Kafatos A, Tselentis Y, Galanakis E. Protective effect of exclusive breastfeeding against infections during infancy: a prospective study. *Arch Dis Child.* 2010;95(12):1004–1008

259. Duijts L, Jaddoe VW, Hofman A, Moll HA. Prolonged and exclusive breastfeeding reduces the risk of infectious diseases in infancy. *Pediatrics.* 2010;126(1). Available at: www.pediatrics.org/cgi/content/full/126/1/e18

260. Best D; Committee on Environmental Health; Committee on Native American Child Health; Committee on Adolescence. From the American Academy of Pediatrics: technical report—secondhand and prenatal tobacco smoke exposure. *Pediatrics.* 2009;124(5). Available at: www.pediatrics.org/cgi/content/full/124/5/e1017

261. Etzel RA, Pattishall EN, Haley NJ, Fletcher RH, Henderson FW. Passive smoking and middle ear effusion among children in day care. *Pediatrics.* 1992;90(2 pt 1): 228–232

262. Ilicali OC, Keleş N, Değer K, Savaş I. Relationship of passive cigarette smoking to otitis media. *Arch Otolaryngol Head Neck Surg.* 1999;125(7):758–762

263. Wellington M, Hall CB. Pacifier as a risk factor for acute otitis media [letter]. *Pediatrics.* 2002;109(2):351–352, author reply 353

264. Kerstein R. Otitis media: prevention instead of prescription. *Br J Gen Pract.* 2008;58(550):364–365

265. Brown CE, Magnuson B. On the physics of the infant feeding bottle and middle ear sequela: ear disease in infants can be associated with bottle feeding. *Int J Pediatr Otorhinolaryngol.* 2000;54(1):13–20

266. Niemelä M, Pihakari O, Pokka T, Uhari M. Pacifier as a risk factor for acute otitis media: a randomized, controlled trial of parental counseling. *Pediatrics.* 2000;106(3): 483–488

267. Tully SB, Bar-Haim Y, Bradley RL. Abnormal tympanography after supine bottle feeding. *J Pediatr.* 1995;126(6):S105–S111

268. Rovers MM, Numans ME, Langenbach E, Grobbee DE, Verheij TJ, Schilder AG. Is pacifier use a risk factor for acute otitis media? A dynamic cohort study. *Fam Pract.* 2008;25(4):233–236

269. Adderson EE. Preventing otitis media: medical approaches. *Pediatr Ann.* 1998;27(2):101–107

270. Azarpazhooh A, Limeback H, Lawrence HP, Shah PS. Xylitol for preventing acute otitis media in children up to 12 years of age.

Cochrane Database Syst Rev. 2011;(11): CD007095

271. Hautalahti O, Renko M, Tapiainen T, Kontiokari T, Pokka T, Uhari M. Failure of xylitol given three times a day for preventing acute otitis media. *Pediatr Infect Dis J.* 2007;26(5):423–427

272. Tapiainen T, Luotonen L, Kontiokari T, Renko M, Uhari M. Xylitol administered only during respiratory infections failed to prevent acute otitis media. *Pediatrics.* 2002;109(2). Available at: www.pediatrics.org/cgi/content/full/109/2/e19

273. Uhari M, Kontiokari T, Koskela M, Niemelä M. Xylitol chewing gum in prevention of acute otitis media: double blind randomised trial. *BMJ.* 1996;313(7066):1180–1184

274. Uhari M, Kontiokari T, Niemelä M. A novel use of xylitol sugar in preventing acute otitis media. *Pediatrics.* 1998;102(4 pt 1): 879–884

275. O'Brien MA, Prosser LA, Paradise JL, et al. New vaccines against otitis media: projected benefits and cost-effectiveness. *Pediatrics.* 2009;123(6):1452–1463

(Continued from first page)

All clinical practice guidelines from the American Academy of Pediatrics automatically expire 5 years after publication unless reaffirmed, revised, or retired at or before that time.

www.pediatrics.org/cgi/doi/10.1542/peds.2012-3488

doi:10.1542/peds.2012-3488

PEDIATRICS (ISSN Numbers: Print, 0031-4005; Online, 1098-4275).

Otitis Media With Effusion

- *Clinical Practice Guideline*

AMERICAN ACADEMY OF PEDIATRICS

CLINICAL PRACTICE GUIDELINE

American Academy of Family Physicians, American Academy of Otolaryngology-Head and Neck Surgery, and American Academy of Pediatrics Subcommittee on Otitis Media With Effusion

Otitis Media With Effusion

ABSTRACT. The clinical practice guideline on otitis media with effusion (OME) provides evidence-based recommendations on diagnosing and managing OME in children. This is an update of the 1994 clinical practice guideline "Otitis Media With Effusion in Young Children," which was developed by the Agency for Healthcare Policy and Research (now the Agency for Healthcare Research and Quality). In contrast to the earlier guideline, which was limited to children 1 to 3 years old with no craniofacial or neurologic abnormalities or sensory deficits, the updated guideline applies to children aged 2 months through 12 years with or without developmental disabilities or underlying conditions that predispose to OME and its sequelae. The American Academy of Pediatrics, American Academy of Family Physicians, and American Academy of Otolaryngology-Head and Neck Surgery selected a subcommittee composed of experts in the fields of primary care, otolaryngology, infectious diseases, epidemiology, hearing, speech and language, and advanced-practice nursing to revise the OME guideline.

The subcommittee made a strong recommendation that clinicians use pneumatic otoscopy as the primary diagnostic method and distinguish OME from acute otitis media.

The subcommittee made recommendations that clinicians should 1) document the laterality, duration of effusion, and presence and severity of associated symptoms at each assessment of the child with OME, 2) distinguish the child with OME who is at risk for speech, language, or learning problems from other children with OME and more promptly evaluate hearing, speech, language, and need for intervention in children at risk, and 3) manage the child with OME who is not at risk with watchful waiting for 3 months from the date of effusion onset (if known) or diagnosis (if onset is unknown).

The subcommittee also made recommendations that 4) hearing testing be conducted when OME persists for 3 months or longer or at any time that language delay, learning problems, or a significant hearing loss is suspected in a child with OME, 5) children with persistent OME who are not at risk should be reexamined at 3- to 6-month intervals until the effusion is no longer present, significant hearing loss is identified, or structural abnormalities of the eardrum or middle ear are suspected, and 6) when a child becomes a surgical candidate (tympanostomy tube insertion is the preferred initial procedure). Adenoidectomy should not be performed unless a distinct indication exists (nasal obstruction, chronic adenoiditis); repeat surgery consists of adenoidectomy plus myringotomy with or without tubeinsertion. Tonsillectomy alone or myringotomy alone should not be used to treat OME.

The subcommittee made negative recommendations that 1) population-based screening programs for OME not be performed in healthy, asymptomatic children, and 2) because antihistamines and decongestants are ineffective for OME, they should not be used for treatment; antimicrobials and corticosteroids do not have long-term efficacy and should not be used for routine management.

The subcommittee gave as options that 1) tympanometry can be used to confirm the diagnosis of OME and 2) when children with OME are referred by the primary clinician for evaluation by an otolaryngologist, audiologist, or speech-language pathologist, the referring clinician should document the effusion duration and specific reason for referral (evaluation, surgery) and provide additional relevant information such as history of acute otitis media and developmental status of the child. The subcommittee made no recommendations for 1) complementary and alternative medicine as a treatment for OME, based on a lack of scientific evidence documenting efficacy, or 2) allergy management as a treatment for OME, based on insufficient evidence of therapeutic efficacy or a causal relationship between allergy and OME. Last, the panel compiled a list of research needs based on limitations of the evidence reviewed.

The purpose of this guideline is to inform clinicians of evidence-based methods to identify, monitor, and manage OME in children aged 2 months through 12 years. The guideline may not apply to children more than 12 years old, because OME is uncommon and the natural history is likely to differ from younger children who experience rapid developmental change. The target population includes children with or without developmental disabilities or underlying conditions that predispose to OME and its sequelae. The guideline is intended for use by providers of health care to children, including primary care and specialist physicians, nurses and nurse practitioners, physician assistants, audiologists, speech-language pathologists, and child-development specialists. The guideline is applicable to any setting in which children with OME would be identified, monitored, or managed.

This guideline is not intended as a sole source of guidance in evaluating children with OME. Rather, it is designed to assist primary care and other clinicians by providing an evidence-based framework for decision-making strategies. It is not intended to replace clinical judgment or establish a protocol for all children with this condition and may not provide the only appropriate approach to diagnosing and managing this problem. *Pediatrics* 2004;113:1412–1429; *acute otitis media, antibacterial, antibiotic.*

This document was approved by the American Academy of Otolaryngology–Head and Neck Surgery Foundation, Inc and the American Academy of Pediatrics, and is published in the May 2004 issue of *Otolaryngology-Head and Neck Surgery* and the May 2004 issue of *Pediatrics.*
PEDIATRICS (ISSN 0031 4005). Copyright © 2004 by the American Academy of Otolaryngology–Head and Neck Surgery Foundation, Inc and the American Academy of Pediatrics.

ABBREVIATIONS. OME, otitis media with effusion; AOM, acute otitis media; AAP, American Academy of Pediatrics; AHRQ, Agency for Healthcare Research and Quality; EPC, Southern California Evidence-Based Practice Center; CAM, complementary and alternative medicine; HL, hearing level.

Otitis media with effusion (OME) as discussed in this guideline is defined as the presence of fluid in the middle ear without signs or symptoms of acute ear infection.[1,2] OME is considered distinct from acute otitis media (AOM), which is defined as a history of acute onset of signs and symptoms, the presence of middle-ear effusion, and signs and symptoms of middle-ear inflammation. Persistent middle-ear fluid from OME results in decreased mobility of the tympanic membrane and serves as a barrier to sound conduction.[3] Approximately 2.2 million diagnosed episodes of OME occur annually in the United States, yielding a combined direct and indirect annual cost estimate of $4.0 billion.[2]

OME may occur spontaneously because of poor eustachian tube function or as an inflammatory response following AOM. Approximately 90% of children (80% of individual ears) have OME at some time before school age,[4] most often between ages 6 months and 4 years.[5] In the first year of life, >50% of children will experience OME, increasing to >60% by 2 years.[6] Many episodes resolve spontaneously within 3 months, but ~30% to 40% of children have recurrent OME, and 5% to 10% of episodes last 1 year or longer.[1,4,7]

The primary outcomes considered in the guideline include hearing loss; effects on speech, language, and learning; physiologic sequelae; health care utilization (medical, surgical); and quality of life.[1,2] The high prevalence of OME, difficulties in diagnosis and assessing duration, increased risk of conductive hearing loss, potential impact on language and cognition, and significant practice variations in management[8] make OME an important condition for the use of up-to-date evidence-based practice guidelines.

METHODS

General Methods and Literature Search

In developing an evidence-based clinical practice guideline on managing OME, the American Academy of Pediatrics (AAP), American Academy of Family Physicians, and American Academy of Otolaryngology-Head and Neck Surgery worked with the Agency for Healthcare Research and Quality (AHRQ) and other organizations. This effort included representatives from each partnering organization along with liaisons from audiology, speech-language pathology, informatics, and advanced-practice nursing. The most current literature on managing children with OME was reviewed, and research questions were developed to guide the evidence-review process.

The AHRQ report on OME from the Southern California Evidence-Based Practice Center (EPC) focused on key questions of natural history, diagnostic methods, and long-term speech, language, and hearing outcomes.[2] Searches were conducted through January 2000 in Medline, Embase, and the Cochrane Library. Additional articles were identified by review of reference listings in proceedings, reports, and other guidelines. The EPC accepted 970 articles for full review after screening 3200 abstracts. The EPC reviewed articles by using established quality criteria[9,10] and included randomized trials, prospective cohorts, and validations of diagnostic tests (validating cohort studies).

The AAP subcommittee on OME updated the AHRQ review with articles identified by an electronic Medline search through April 2003 and with additional material identified manually by subcommittee members. Copies of relevant articles were distributed to the subcommittee for consideration. A specific search for articles relevant to complementary and alternative medicine (CAM) was performed by using Medline and the Allied and Complementary Medicine Database through April 2003. Articles relevant to allergy and OME were identified by using Medline through April 2003. The subcommittee met 3 times over a 1-year period, ending in May 2003, with interval electronic review and feedback on each guideline draft to ensure accuracy of content and consistency with standardized criteria for reporting clinical practice guidelines.[11]

In May 2003, the Guidelines Review Group of the Yale Center for Medical Informatics used the Guideline Elements Model[12] to categorize content of the present draft guideline. Policy statements were parsed into component decision variables and actions and then assessed for decidability and executability. Quality appraisal using established criteria[13] was performed with Guideline Elements Model-Q Online.[14,15] Implementation issues were predicted by using the Implementability Rating Profile, an instrument under development by the Yale Guidelines Review Group (R. Shiffman, MD, written communication, May 2003). OME subcommittee members received summary results and modified an advanced draft of the guideline.

The final draft practice guideline underwent extensive peer review by numerous entities identified by the subcommittee. Comments were compiled and reviewed by the subcommittee cochairpersons. The recommendations contained in the practice guideline are based on the best available published data through April 2003. Where data are lacking, a combination of clinical experience and expert consensus was used. A scheduled review process will occur 5 years from publication or sooner if new compelling evidence warrants earlier consideration.

Classification of Evidence-Based Statements

Guidelines are intended to reduce inappropriate variations in clinical care, produce optimal health outcomes for patients, and minimize harm. The evidence-based approach to guideline development requires that the evidence supporting a policy be identified, appraised, and summarized and that an explicit link between evidence and statements be defined. Evidence-based statements reflect the quality of evidence and the balance of benefit and harm that is anticipated when the statement is followed. The AAP definitions for evidence-based statements[16] are listed in Tables 1 and 2.

Guidelines are never intended to overrule professional judgment; rather, they may be viewed as a relative constraint on individual clinician discretion in a particular clinical circumstance. Less frequent variation in practice is expected for a strong recommendation than might be expected with a recommendation. Options offer the most opportunity for practice variability.[17] All clinicians should always act and decide in a way that they believe will best serve their patients' interests and needs regardless of guideline recommendations. Guidelines represent the best judgment of a team of experienced clinicians and methodologists addressing the scientific evidence for a particular topic.[16]

Making recommendations about health practices involves value judgments on the desirability of various outcomes associated with management options. Value judgments applied by the OME subcommittee were made in an effort to minimize harm and diminish unnecessary therapy. Emphasis was placed on promptly identifying and managing children at risk for speech, language, or learning problems to maximize opportunities for beneficial outcomes. Direct costs also were considered in the statements concerning diagnosis and screening and to a lesser extent in other statements.

1A. PNEUMATIC OTOSCOPY: CLINICIANS SHOULD USE PNEUMATIC OTOSCOPY AS THE PRIMARY DIAGNOSTIC METHOD FOR OME, AND OME SHOULD BE DISTINGUISHED FROM AOM

This is a strong recommendation based on systematic review of cohort studies and the preponderance of benefit over harm.

TABLE 1.　Guideline Definitions for Evidence-Based Statements

Statement	Definition	Implication
Strong Recommendation	A strong recommendation means that the subcommittee believes that the benefits of the recommended approach clearly exceed the harms (or that the harms clearly exceed the benefits in the case of a strong negative recommendation) and that the quality of the supporting evidence is excellent (grade A or B).* In some clearly identified circumstances, strong recommendations may be made based on lesser evidence when high-quality evidence is impossible to obtain and the anticipated benefits strongly outweigh the harms.	Clinicians should follow a strong recommendation unless a clear and compelling rationale for an alternative approach is present.
Recommendation	A recommendation means that the subcommittee believes that the benefits exceed the harms (or that the harms exceed the benefits in the case of a negative recommendation), but the quality of evidence is not as strong (grade B or C).* In some clearly identified circumstances, recommendations may be made based on lesser evidence when high-quality evidence is impossible to obtain and the anticipated benefits outweigh the harms.	Clinicians also should generally follow a recommendation but should remain alert to new information and sensitive to patient preferences.
Option	An option means that either the quality of evidence that exists is suspect (grade D)* or that well-done studies (grade A, B, or C)* show little clear advantage to one approach versus another.	Clinicians should be flexible in their decision-making regarding appropriate practice, although they may set boundaries on alternatives; patient preference should have a substantial influencing role.
No Recommendation	No recommendation means that there is both a lack of pertinent evidence (grade D)* and an unclear balance between benefits and harms.	Clinicians should feel little constraint in their decision-making and be alert to new published evidence that clarifies the balance of benefit versus harm; patient preference should have a substantial influencing role.

* See Table 2 for the definitions of evidence grades.

TABLE 2.　Evidence Quality for Grades of Evidence

Grade	Evidence Quality
A	Well-designed, randomized, controlled trials or diagnostic studies performed on a population similar to the guideline's target population
B	Randomized, controlled trials or diagnostic studies with minor limitations; overwhelmingly consistent evidence from observational studies
C	Observational studies (case-control and cohort design)
D	Expert opinion, case reports, or reasoning from first principles (bench research or animal studies)

1B. TYMPANOMETRY: TYMPANOMETRY CAN BE USED TO CONFIRM THE DIAGNOSIS OF OME

This option is based on cohort studies and a balance of benefit and harm.

Diagnosing OME correctly is fundamental to proper management. Moreover, OME must be differentiated from AOM to avoid unnecessary antimicrobial use.[18,19]

OME is defined as fluid in the middle ear without signs or symptoms of acute ear infection.[2] The tympanic membrane is often cloudy with distinctly impaired mobility,[20] and an air-fluid level or bubble may be visible in the middle ear. Conversely, diagnosing AOM requires a history of acute onset of signs and symptoms, the presence of middle-ear effusion, and signs and symptoms of middle-ear inflammation. The critical distinguishing feature is that only AOM has acute signs and symptoms. Distinct redness of the tympanic membrane should not be a criterion for prescribing antibiotics, because it has poor predictive value for AOM and is present in ~5% of ears with OME.[20]

The AHRQ evidence report[2] systematically reviewed the sensitivity, specificity, and predictive values of 9 diagnostic methods for OME. Pneumatic otoscopy had the best balance of sensitivity and specificity, consistent with the 1994 guideline.[1] Meta-analysis revealed a pooled sensitivity of 94% (95% confidence interval: 91%–96%) and specificity of 80% (95% confidence interval: 75%–86%) for validated observers using pneumatic otoscopy versus myringotomy as the gold standard. Pneumatic otoscopy therefore should remain the primary method of OME diagnosis, because the instrument is readily available in practice settings, cost-effective, and accurate in experienced hands. Non–pneumatic otoscopy is not advised for primary diagnosis.

The accuracy of pneumatic otoscopy in routine clinical practice may be less than that shown in published results, because clinicians have varying training and experience.[21,22] When the diagnosis of OME is uncertain, tympanometry or acoustic reflectometry should be considered as an adjunct to pneumatic otoscopy. Tympanometry with a standard 226-Hz probe tone is reliable for infants 4 months old or older and has good interobserver agreement of curve patterns in routine clinical practice.[23,24] Younger infants require specialized equipment with a higher probe tone frequency. Tympanometry generates costs related to instrument purchase, annual calibration, and test administration. Acoustic reflectometry with spectral gradient analysis is a low-cost alternative to tympanometry that does not require an airtight seal in the ear canal; however, validation studies primarily have used children 2 years old or older with a high prevalence of OME.[25–27]

Although no research studies have examined whether pneumatic otoscopy causes discomfort, expert consensus suggests that the procedure does not have to be painful, especially when symptoms of acute infection (AOM) are absent. A nontraumatic examination is facilitated by using a gentle touch, restraining the child properly when necessary, and inserting the speculum only into the outer one third (cartilaginous portion) of the ear canal.[28] The pneumatic bulb should be compressed slightly before insertion, because OME often is associated with a negative middle-ear pressure, which can be assessed more accurately by releasing the already compressed bulb. The otoscope must be fully charged, the bulb (halogen or xenon) bright and luminescent,[29] and the insufflator bulb attached tightly to the head to avoid the loss of an air seal. The window must also be sealed.

Evidence Profile: Pneumatic Otoscopy

- Aggregate evidence quality: A, diagnostic studies in relevant populations.
- Benefit: improved diagnostic accuracy; inexpensive equipment.
- Harm: cost of training clinicians in pneumatic otoscopy.
- Benefits-harms assessment: preponderance of benefit over harm.
- Policy level: strong recommendation.

Evidence Profile: Tympanometry

- Aggregate evidence quality: B, diagnostic studies with minor limitations.
- Benefit: increased diagnostic accuracy beyond pneumatic otoscopy; documentation.
- Harm: acquisition cost, administrative burden, and recalibration.
- Benefits-harms assessment: balance of benefit and harm.
- Policy level: option.

1C. SCREENING: POPULATION-BASED SCREENING PROGRAMS FOR OME ARE NOT RECOMMENDED IN HEALTHY, ASYMPTOMATIC CHILDREN

This recommendation is based on randomized, controlled trials and cohort studies, with a preponderance of harm over benefit.

This recommendation concerns population-based screening programs of all children in a community or a school without regard to any preexisting symptoms or history of disease. This recommendation does not address hearing screening or monitoring of specific children with previous or recurrent OME.

OME is highly prevalent in young children. Screening surveys of healthy children ranging in age from infancy to 5 years old show a 15% to 40% point prevalence of middle-ear effusion.[5,7,30–36] Among children examined at regular intervals for a year, ~50% to 60% of child care center attendees[32] and 25% of school-aged children[37] were found to have a middle-ear effusion at some time during the examination period, with peak incidence during the winter months.

Population-based screening has not been found to influence short-term language outcomes,[33] and its long-term effects have not been evaluated in a randomized, clinical trial. Therefore, the recommendation against screening is based not only on the ability to identify OME but more importantly on a lack of demonstrable benefits from treating children so identified that exceed the favorable natural history of the disease. The New Zealand Health Technology Assessment[38] could not determine whether preschool screening for OME was effective. More recently, the Canadian Task Force on Preventive Health Care[39] reported that insufficient evidence was available to recommend including or excluding routine early screening for OME. Although screening for OME is not inherently harmful, potential risks include inaccurate diagnoses, overtreating self-limited disease, parental anxiety, and the costs of screening and unnecessary treatment.

Population-based screening is appropriate for conditions that are common, can be detected by a sensitive and specific test, and benefit from early detection and treatment.[40] The first 2 requirements are fulfilled by OME, which affects up to 80% of children by school entry[2,5,7] and can be screened easily with tympanometry (see recommendation 1B). Early detection and treatment of OME identified by screening, however, have not been shown to improve intelligence, receptive language, or expressive language.[2,39,41,42] Therefore, population-based screening for early detection of OME in asymptomatic children has not been shown to improve outcomes and is not recommended.

Evidence Profile: Screening

- Aggregate evidence quality: B, randomized, controlled trials with minor limitations and consistent evidence from observational studies.
- Benefit: potentially improved developmental outcomes, which have not been demonstrated in the best current evidence.

- Harm: inaccurate diagnosis (false-positive or false-negative), overtreating self-limited disease, parental anxiety, cost of screening, and/or unnecessary treatment.
- Benefits-harms assessment: preponderance of harm over benefit.
- Policy level: recommendation against.

2. DOCUMENTATION: CLINICIANS SHOULD DOCUMENT THE LATERALITY, DURATION OF EFFUSION, AND PRESENCE AND SEVERITY OF ASSOCIATED SYMPTOMS AT EACH ASSESSMENT OF THE CHILD WITH OME

This recommendation is based on observational studies and strong preponderance of benefit over harm.

Documentation in the medical record facilitates diagnosis and treatment and communicates pertinent information to other clinicians to ensure patient safety and reduce medical errors.[43] Management decisions in children with OME depend on effusion duration and laterality plus the nature and severity of associated symptoms. Therefore, these features should be documented at every medical encounter for OME. Although no studies have addressed documentation for OME specifically, there is room for improvement in documentation of ambulatory care medical records.[44]

Ideally, the time of onset and laterality of OME can be defined through diagnosis of an antecedent AOM, a history of acute onset of signs or symptoms directly referable to fluid in the middle ear, or the presence of an abnormal audiogram or tympanogram closely after a previously normal test. Unfortunately, these conditions are often lacking, and the clinician is forced to speculate on the onset and duration of fluid in the middle ear(s) in a child found to have OME at a routine office visit or school screening audiometry.

In ~40% to 50% of cases of OME, neither the affected children nor their parents or caregivers describe significant complaints referable to a middle-ear effusion.[45,46] In some children, however, OME may have associated signs and symptoms caused by inflammation or the presence of effusion (not acute infection) that should be documented, such as

- Mild intermittent ear pain, fullness, or "popping"
- Secondary manifestations of ear pain in infants, which may include ear rubbing, excessive irritability, and sleep disturbances
- Failure of infants to respond appropriately to voices or environmental sounds, such as not turning accurately toward the sound source
- Hearing loss, even when not specifically described by the child, suggested by seeming lack of attentiveness, behavioral changes, failure to respond to normal conversational-level speech, or the need for excessively high sound levels when using audio equipment or viewing television
- Recurrent episodes of AOM with persistent OME between episodes
- Problems with school performance
- Balance problems, unexplained clumsiness, or delayed gross motor development[47–50]
- Delayed speech or language development

The laterality (unilateral versus bilateral), duration of effusion, and presence and severity of associated symptoms should be documented in the medical record at each assessment of the child with OME. When OME duration is uncertain, the clinician must take whatever evidence is at hand and make a reasonable estimate.

Evidence Profile: Documentation

- Aggregate evidence quality: C, observational studies.
- Benefits: defines severity, duration has prognostic value, facilitates future communication with other clinicians, supports appropriate timing of intervention, and, if consistently unilateral, may identify a problem with specific ear other than OME (eg, retraction pocket or cholesteatoma).
- Harm: administrative burden.
- Benefits-harms assessment: preponderance of benefit over harm.
- Policy level: recommendation.

3. CHILD AT RISK: CLINICIANS SHOULD DISTINGUISH THE CHILD WITH OME WHO IS AT RISK FOR SPEECH, LANGUAGE, OR LEARNING PROBLEMS FROM OTHER CHILDREN WITH OME AND SHOULD EVALUATE HEARING, SPEECH, LANGUAGE, AND NEED FOR INTERVENTION MORE PROMPTLY

This recommendation is based on case series, the preponderance of benefit over harm, and ethical limitations in studying children with OME who are at risk.

The panel defines the child at risk as one who is at increased risk for developmental difficulties (delay or disorder) because of sensory, physical, cognitive, or behavioral factors listed in Table 3. These factors are not caused by OME but can make the child less tolerant of hearing loss or vestibular problems secondary to middle-ear effusion. In contrast the child with OME who is not at risk is otherwise healthy and does not have any of the factors shown in Table 3.

Earlier guidelines for managing OME have applied only to young children who are healthy and exhibit no developmental delays.[1] Studies of the relationship between OME and hearing loss or speech/language development typically exclude children with craniofacial anomalies, genetic syndromes, and other developmental disorders. Therefore, the available literature mainly applies to otherwise healthy children who meet inclusion criteria for randomized,

---

TABLE 3.   Risk Factors for Developmental Difficulties*

Permanent hearing loss independent of OME
Suspected or diagnosed speech and language delay or disorder
Autism-spectrum disorder and other pervasive developmental disorders
Syndromes (eg, Down) or craniofacial disorders that include cognitive, speech, and language delays
Blindness or uncorrectable visual impairment
Cleft palate with or without associated syndrome
Developmental delay

---

* Sensory, physical, cognitive, or behavioral factors that place children who have OME at an increased risk for developmental difficulties (delay or disorder).

controlled trials. Few, if any, existing studies dealing with developmental sequelae caused by hearing loss from OME can be generalized to children who are at risk.

Children who are at risk for speech or language delay would likely be affected additionally by hearing problems from OME,[51] although definitive studies are lacking. For example, small comparative studies of children or adolescents with Down syndrome[52] or cerebral palsy[53] show poorer articulation and receptive language associated with a history of early otitis media. Large studies are unlikely to be forthcoming because of methodologic and ethical difficulties inherent in studying children who are delayed or at risk for further delays. Therefore, clinicians who manage children with OME should determine whether other conditions coexist that put a child at risk for developmental delay (Table 3) and then take these conditions into consideration when planning assessment and management.

Children with craniofacial anomalies (eg, cleft palate; Down syndrome; Robin sequence; coloboma, heart defect, choanal atresia, retarded growth and development, genital anomaly, and ear defect with deafness [CHARGE] association) have a higher prevalence of chronic OME, hearing loss (conductive and sensorineural), and speech or language delay than do children without these anomalies.[54-57] Other children may not be more prone to OME but are likely to have speech and language disorders, such as those children with permanent hearing loss independent of OME,[58,59] specific language impairment,[60] autism-spectrum disorders,[61] or syndromes that adversely affect cognitive and linguistic development. Some retrospective studies[52,62,63] have found that hearing loss caused by OME in children with cognitive delays, such as Down syndrome, has been associated with lower language levels. Children with language delays or disorders with OME histories perform more poorly on speech-perception tasks than do children with OME histories alone.[64,65]

Children with severe visual impairments may be more susceptible to the effects of OME, because they depend on hearing more than children with normal vision.[51] Any decrease in their most important remaining sensory input for language (hearing) may significantly compromise language development and their ability to interact and communicate with others. All children with severe visual impairments should be considered more vulnerable to OME sequelae, especially in the areas of balance, sound localization, and communication.

Management of the child with OME who is at increased risk for developmental delays should include hearing testing and speech and language evaluation and may include speech and language therapy concurrent with managing OME, hearing aids or other amplification devices for hearing loss independent of OME, tympanostomy tube insertion,[54,63,66,67] and hearing testing after OME resolves to document improvement, because OME can mask a permanent underlying hearing loss and delay detection.[59,68,69]

Evidence Profile: Child at Risk

- Aggregate evidence quality: C, observational studies of children at risk; D, expert opinion on the ability of prompt assessment and management to alter outcomes.
- Benefits: optimizing conditions for hearing, speech, and language; enabling children with special needs to reach their potential; avoiding limitations on the benefits of educational interventions because of hearing problems from OME.
- Harm: cost, time, and specific risks of medications or surgery.
- Benefits-harms assessment: exceptional preponderance of benefits over harm based on subcommittee consensus because of circumstances to date precluding randomized trials.
- Policy level: recommendation.

4. WATCHFUL WAITING: CLINICIANS SHOULD MANAGE THE CHILD WITH OME WHO IS NOT AT RISK WITH WATCHFUL WAITING FOR 3 MONTHS FROM THE DATE OF EFFUSION ONSET (IF KNOWN) OR DIAGNOSIS (IF ONSET IS UNKNOWN)

This recommendation is based on systematic review of cohort studies and the preponderance of benefit over harm.

This recommendation is based on the self-limited nature of most OME, which has been well documented in cohort studies and in control groups of randomized trials.[2,70]

The likelihood of spontaneous resolution of OME is determined by the cause and duration of effusion.[70] For example, ~75% to 90% of residual OME after an AOM episode resolves spontaneously by 3 months.[71-73] Similar outcomes of defined onset during a period of surveillance in a cohort study are observed for OME.[32,37] Another favorable situation involves improvement (not resolution) of newly detected OME defined as change in tympanogram from type B (flat curve) to non-B (anything other than a flat curve). Approximately 55% of children so defined improve by 3 months,[70] but one third will have OME relapse within the next 3 months.[4] Although a type B tympanogram is an imperfect measure of OME (81% sensitivity and 74% specificity versus myringotomy), it is the most widely reported measure suitable for deriving pooled resolution rates.[2,70]

Approximately 25% of newly detected OME of unknown prior duration in children 2 to 4 years old resolves by 3 months when resolution is defined as a change in tympanogram from type B to type A/C1 (peak pressure >200 daPa).[2,70,74-77] Resolution rates may be higher for infants and young children in whom the preexisting duration of effusion is generally shorter, and particularly for those observed prospectively in studies or in the course of well-child care. Documented bilateral OME of 3 months' duration or longer resolves spontaneously after 6 to 12 months in ~30% of children primarily 2 years old or older, with only marginal benefits if observed longer.[70]

Any intervention for OME (medical or surgical) other than observation carries some inherent harm. There is little harm associated with a specified period of observation in the child who is not at risk for speech, language, or learning problems. When observing children with OME, clinicians should inform the parent or caregiver that the child may experience reduced hearing until the effusion resolves, especially if it is bilateral. Clinicians may discuss strategies for optimizing the listening and learning environment until the effusion resolves. These strategies include speaking in close proximity to the child, facing the child and speaking clearly, repeating phrases when misunderstood, and providing preferential classroom seating.[78,79]

The recommendation for a 3-month period of observation is based on a clear preponderance of benefit over harm and is consistent with the original OME guideline intent of avoiding unnecessary surgery.[1] At the discretion of the clinician, this 3-month period of watchful waiting may include interval visits at which OME is monitored by using pneumatic otoscopy, tympanometry, or both. Factors to consider in determining the optimal interval(s) for follow-up include clinical judgment, parental comfort level, unique characteristics of the child and/or his environment, access to a health care system, and hearing levels (HLs) if known.

After documented resolution of OME in all affected ears, additional follow-up is unnecessary.

Evidence Profile: Watchful Waiting

- Aggregate evidence quality: B, systematic review of cohort studies.
- Benefit: avoid unnecessary interventions, take advantage of favorable natural history, and avoid unnecessary referrals and evaluations.
- Harm: delays in therapy for OME that will not resolve with observation; prolongation of hearing loss.
- Benefits-harms assessment: preponderance of benefit over harm.
- Policy level: recommendation.

5. MEDICATION: ANTIHISTAMINES AND DECONGESTANTS ARE INEFFECTIVE FOR OME AND ARE NOT RECOMMENDED FOR TREATMENT; ANTIMICROBIALS AND CORTICOSTEROIDS DO NOT HAVE LONG-TERM EFFICACY AND ARE NOT RECOMMENDED FOR ROUTINE MANAGEMENT

This recommendation is based on systematic review of randomized, controlled trials and the preponderance of harm over benefit.

Therapy for OME is appropriate only if persistent and clinically significant benefits can be achieved beyond spontaneous resolution. Although statistically significant benefits have been demonstrated for some medications, they are short-term and relatively small in magnitude. Moreover, significant adverse events may occur with all medical therapies.

The prior OME guideline[1] found no data supporting antihistamine-decongestant combinations in treating OME. Meta-analysis of 4 randomized trials showed no significant benefit for antihistamines or decongestants versus placebo. No additional studies have been published since 1994 to change this recommendation. Adverse effects of antihistamines and decongestants include insomnia, hyperactivity, drowsiness, behavioral change, and blood-pressure variability.

Long-term benefits of antimicrobial therapy for OME are unproved despite a modest short-term benefit for 2 to 8 weeks in randomized trials.[1,80,81] Initial benefits, however, can become nonsignificant within 2 weeks of stopping the medication.[82] Moreover, ~7 children would need to be treated with antimicrobials to achieve one short-term response.[1] Adverse effects of antimicrobials are significant and may include rashes, vomiting, diarrhea, allergic reactions, alteration of the child's nasopharyngeal flora, development of bacterial resistance,[83] and cost. Societal consequences include direct transmission of resistant bacterial pathogens in homes and child care centers.[84]

The prior OME guideline[1] did not recommend oral steroids for treating OME in children. A later meta-analysis[85] showed no benefit for oral steroid versus placebo within 2 weeks but did show a short-term benefit for oral steroid plus antimicrobial versus antimicrobial alone in 1 of 3 children treated. This benefit became nonsignificant after several weeks in a prior meta-analysis[1] and in a large, randomized trial.[86] Oral steroids can produce behavioral changes, increased appetite, and weight gain.[1] Additional adverse effects may include adrenal suppression, fatal varicella infection, and avascular necrosis of the femoral head.[3] Although intranasal steroids have fewer adverse effects, one randomized trial[87] showed statistically equivalent outcomes at 12 weeks for intranasal beclomethasone plus antimicrobials versus antimicrobials alone for OME.

Antimicrobial therapy with or without steroids has not been demonstrated to be effective in long-term resolution of OME, but in some cases this therapy can be considered an option because of short-term benefit in randomized trials, when the parent or caregiver expresses a strong aversion to impending surgery. In this circumstance, a single course of therapy for 10 to 14 days may be used. The likelihood that the OME will resolve long-term with these regimens is small, and prolonged or repetitive courses of antimicrobials or steroids are strongly not recommended.

Other nonsurgical therapies that are discussed in the OME literature include autoinflation of the eustachian tube, oral or intratympanic use of mucolytics, and systemic use of pharmacologic agents other than antimicrobials, steroids, and antihistamine-decongestants. Insufficient data exist for any of these therapies to be recommended in treating OME.[3]

Evidence Profile: Medication

- Aggregate evidence quality: A, systematic review of well-designed, randomized, controlled trials.

- Benefit: avoid side effects and reduce cost by not administering medications; avoid delays in definitive therapy caused by short-term improvement then relapse.
- Harm: adverse effects of specific medications as listed previously; societal impact of antimicrobial therapy on bacterial resistance and transmission of resistant pathogens.
- Benefits-harms assessment: preponderance of harm over benefit.
- Policy level: recommendation against.

6. HEARING AND LANGUAGE: HEARING TESTING IS RECOMMENDED WHEN OME PERSISTS FOR 3 MONTHS OR LONGER OR AT ANY TIME THAT LANGUAGE DELAY, LEARNING PROBLEMS, OR A SIGNIFICANT HEARING LOSS IS SUSPECTED IN A CHILD WITH OME; LANGUAGE TESTING SHOULD BE CONDUCTED FOR CHILDREN WITH HEARING LOSS

This recommendation is based on cohort studies and the preponderance of benefit over risk.

Hearing Testing

Hearing testing is recommended when OME persists for 3 months or longer or at any time that language delay, learning problems, or a significant hearing loss is suspected. Conductive hearing loss often accompanies OME[1,88] and may adversely affect binaural processing,[89] sound localization,[90] and speech perception in noise.[91–94] Hearing loss caused by OME may impair early language acquisition,[95–97] but the child's home environment has a greater impact on outcomes[98]; recent randomized trials[41,99,100] suggest no impact on children with OME who are not at risk as identified by screening or surveillance.

Studies examining hearing sensitivity in children with OME report that average pure-tone hearing loss at 4 frequencies (500, 1000, 2000, and 4000 Hz) ranges from normal hearing to moderate hearing loss (0–55 dB). The 50th percentile is an ~25-dB HL, and ~20% of ears exceed 35-dB HL.[101,102] Unilateral OME with hearing loss results in overall poorer binaural hearing than in infants with normal middle-ear function bilaterally.[103,104] However, based on limited research, there is evidence that children experiencing the greatest conductive hearing loss for the longest periods may be more likely to exhibit developmental and academic sequelae.[1,95,105]

Initial hearing testing for children 4 years old or older can be done in the primary care setting.[106] Testing should be performed in a quiet environment, preferably in a separate closed or sound-proofed area set aside specifically for that purpose. Conventional audiometry with earphones is performed with a fail criterion of more than 20-dB HL at 1 or more frequencies (500, 1000, 2000, and 4000 Hz) in either ear.[106,107] Methods not recommended as substitutes for primary care hearing testing include tympanometry and pneumatic otoscopy,[102] caregiver judgment regarding hearing loss,[108,109] speech audiometry, and tuning forks, acoustic reflectometry, and behavioral observation.[1]

Comprehensive audiologic evaluation is recommended for children who fail primary care testing, are less than 4 years old, or cannot be tested in the primary care setting. Audiologic assessment includes evaluating air-conduction and bone-conduction thresholds for pure tones, speech-detection or speech-recognition thresholds,[102] and measuring speech understanding if possible.[94] The method of assessment depends on the developmental age of the child and might include visual reinforcement or conditioned orienting-response audiometry for infants 6 to 24 months old, play audiometry for children 24 to 48 months old, or conventional screening audiometry for children 4 years old and older.[106] The auditory brainstem response and otoacoustic emission are tests of auditory pathway structural integrity, not hearing, and should not substitute for behavioral pure-tone audiometry.[106]

Language Testing

Language testing should be conducted for children with hearing loss (pure-tone average more than 20-dB HL on comprehensive audiometric evaluation). Testing for language delays is important, because communication is integral to all aspects of human functioning. Young children with speech and language delays during the preschool years are at risk for continued communication problems and later delays in reading and writing.[110–112] In one study, 6% to 8% of children 3 years old and 2% to 13% of kindergartners had language impairment.[113] Language intervention can improve communication and other functional outcomes for children with histories of OME.[114]

Children who experience repeated and persistent episodes of OME and associated hearing loss during early childhood may be at a disadvantage for learning speech and language.[79,115] Although Shekelle et al[2] concluded that there was no evidence to support the concern that OME during the first 3 years of life was related to later receptive or expressive language, this meta-analysis should be interpreted cautiously, because it did not examine specific language domains such as vocabulary and the independent variable was OME and not hearing loss. Other meta-analyses[79,115] have suggested at most a small negative association of OME and hearing loss on children's receptive and expressive language through the elementary school years. The clinical significance of these effects for language and learning is unclear for the child not at risk. For example, in one randomized trial,[100] prompt insertion of tympanostomy tubes for OME did not improve developmental outcomes at 3 years old regardless of baseline hearing. In another randomized trial,[116] however, prompt tube insertion achieved small benefits for children with bilateral OME and hearing loss.

Clinicians should ask the parent or caregiver about specific concerns regarding their child's language development. Children's speech and language can be tested at ages 6 to 36 months by direct engagement of a child and interviewing the parent using the Early Language Milestone Scale.[117] Other approaches require interviewing only the child's parent or caregiver, such as the MacArthur Communicative Development Inventory[118] and the Language Development Survey.[119] For older children, the Denver Developmental Screening Test II[120] can be used to screen general development including speech and language. Comprehensive speech and language evaluation is recommended for children who fail testing or whenever the child's parent or caregiver expresses concern.[121]

Evidence Profile: Hearing and Language

- Aggregate evidence quality: B, diagnostic studies with minor limitations; C, observational studies.
- Benefit: to detect hearing loss and language delay and identify strategies or interventions to improve developmental outcomes.
- Harm: parental anxiety, direct and indirect costs of assessment, and/or false-positive results.
- Balance of benefit and harm: preponderance of benefit over harm.
- Policy level: recommendation.

7. SURVEILLANCE: CHILDREN WITH PERSISTENT OME WHO ARE NOT AT RISK SHOULD BE REEXAMINED AT 3- TO 6-MONTH INTERVALS UNTIL THE EFFUSION IS NO LONGER PRESENT, SIGNIFICANT HEARING LOSS IS IDENTIFIED, OR STRUCTURAL ABNORMALITIES OF THE EARDRUM OR MIDDLE EAR ARE SUSPECTED

This recommendation is based on randomized, controlled trials and observational studies with a preponderance of benefit over harm.

If OME is asymptomatic and is likely to resolve spontaneously, intervention is unnecessary even if OME persists for more than 3 months. The clinician should determine whether risk factors exist that would predispose the child to undesirable sequelae or predict nonresolution of the effusion. As long as OME persists, the child is at risk for sequelae and must be reevaluated periodically for factors that would prompt intervention.

The 1994 OME guideline[1] recommended surgery for OME persisting 4 to 6 months with hearing loss but requires reconsideration because of later data on tubes and developmental sequelae.[122] For example, selecting surgical candidates using duration-based criteria (eg, OME >3 months or exceeding a cumulative threshold) does not improve developmental outcomes in infants and toddlers who are not at risk.[41,42,99,100] Additionally, the 1994 OME guideline did not specifically address managing effusion without significant hearing loss persisting more than 6 months.

Asymptomatic OME usually resolves spontaneously, but resolution rates decrease the longer the effusion has been present,[36,76,77] and relapse is common.[123] Risk factors that make spontaneous resolution less likely include[124,125]:

- Onset of OME in the summer or fall season
- Hearing loss more than 30-dB HL in the better-hearing ear

- History of prior tympanostomy tubes
- Not having had an adenoidectomy

Children with chronic OME are at risk for structural damage of the tympanic membrane[126] because the effusion contains leukotrienes, prostaglandins, and arachidonic acid metabolites that invoke a local inflammatory response.[127] Reactive changes may occur in the adjacent tympanic membrane and mucosal linings. A relative underventilation of the middle ear produces a negative pressure that predisposes to focal retraction pockets, generalized atelectasis of the tympanic membrane, and cholesteatoma.

Structural integrity is assessed by carefully examining the entire tympanic membrane, which, in many cases, can be accomplished by the primary care clinician using a handheld pneumatic otoscope. A search should be made for retraction pockets, ossicular erosion, and areas of atelectasis or atrophy. If there is any uncertainty that all observed structures are normal, the patient should be examined by using an otomicroscope. All children with these tympanic membrane conditions, regardless of OME duration, should have a comprehensive audiologic evaluation.

Conditions of the tympanic membrane that generally mandate inserting a tympanostomy tube are posterosuperior retraction pockets, ossicular erosion, adhesive atelectasis, and retraction pockets that accumulate keratin debris. Ongoing surveillance is mandatory, because the incidence of structural damage increases with effusion duration.[128]

As noted in recommendation 6, children with persistent OME for 3 months or longer should have their hearing tested. Based on these results, clinicians can identify 3 levels of action based on HLs obtained for the better-hearing ear using earphones or in sound field using speakers if the child is too young for ear-specific testing.

1. HLs of ≥40 dB (at least a moderate hearing loss): A comprehensive audiologic evaluation is indicated if not previously performed. If moderate hearing loss is documented and persists at this level, surgery is recommended, because persistent hearing loss of this magnitude that is permanent in nature has been shown to impact speech, language, and academic performance.[129–131]
2. HLs of 21 to 39 dB (mild hearing loss): A comprehensive audiologic evaluation is indicated if not previously performed. Mild sensorineural hearing loss has been associated with difficulties in speech, language, and academic performance in school,[129,132] and persistent mild conductive hearing loss from OME may have a similar impact. Further management should be individualized based on effusion duration, severity of hearing loss, and parent or caregiver preference and may include strategies to optimize the listening and learning environment (Table 4) or surgery. Repeat hearing testing should be performed in 3 to 6 months if OME persists at follow-up evaluation or tympanostomy tubes have not been placed.
3. HLs of ≤20 dB (normal hearing): A repeat hearing test should be performed in 3 to 6 months if OME persists at follow-up evaluation.

TABLE 4. Strategies for Optimizing the Listening-Learning Environment for Children With OME and Hearing Loss*

Get within 3 feet of the child before speaking.
Turn off competing audio signals such as unnecessary music and television in the background.
Face the child and speak clearly, using visual clues (hands, pictures) in addition to speech.
Slow the rate, raise the level, and enunciate speech directed at the child.
Read to or with the child, explaining pictures and asking questions.
Repeat words, phrases, and questions when misunderstood.
Assign preferential seating in the classroom near the teacher.
Use a frequency-modulated personal- or sound-field-amplification system in the classroom.

* Modified with permission from Roberts et al.[78,79]

In addition to hearing loss and speech or language delay, other factors may influence the decision to intervene for persistent OME. Roberts et al[98,133] showed that the caregiving environment is more strongly related to school outcome than was OME or hearing loss. Risk factors for delays in speech and language development caused by a poor caregiving environment included low maternal educational level, unfavorable child care environment, and low socioeconomic status. In such cases, these factors may be additive to the hearing loss in affecting lower school performance and classroom behavior problems.

Persistent OME may be associated with physical or behavioral symptoms including hyperactivity, poor attention, and behavioral problems in some studies[134–136] and reduced child quality of life.[46] Conversely, young children randomized to early versus late tube insertion for persistent OME showed no behavioral benefits from early surgery.[41,100] Children with chronic OME also have significantly poorer vestibular function and gross motor proficiency when compared with non-OME controls.[48–50] Moreover, vestibular function, behavior, and quality of life can improve after tympanostomy tube insertion.[47,137,138] Other physical symptoms of OME that, if present and persistent, may warrant surgery include otalgia, unexplained sleep disturbance, and coexisting recurrent AOM. Tubes reduce the absolute incidence of recurrent AOM by ~1 episode per child per year, but the relative risk reduction is 56%.[139]

The risks of continued observation of children with OME must be balanced against the risks of surgery. Children with persistent OME examined regularly at 3- to 6-month intervals, or sooner if OME-related symptoms develop, are most likely at low risk for physical, behavioral, or developmental sequelae of OME. Conversely, prolonged watchful waiting of OME is not appropriate when regular surveillance is impossible or when the child is at risk for developmental sequelae of OME because of comorbidities (Table 3). For these children, the risks of anesthesia and surgery (see recommendation 9) may be less than those of continued observation.

Evidence Profile: Surveillance

- Aggregate evidence quality: C, observational studies and some randomized trials.

- Benefit: avoiding interventions that do not improve outcomes.
- Harm: allowing structural abnormalities to develop in the tympanic membrane, underestimating the impact of hearing loss on a child, and/or failing to detect significant signs or symptoms that require intervention.
- Balance of benefit and harm: preponderance of benefit over harm.
- Policy level: recommendation.

8. REFERRAL: WHEN CHILDREN WITH OME ARE REFERRED BY THE PRIMARY CARE CLINICIAN FOR EVALUATION BY AN OTOLARYNGOLOGIST, AUDIOLOGIST, OR SPEECH-LANGUAGE PATHOLOGIST, THE REFERRING CLINICIAN SHOULD DOCUMENT THE EFFUSION DURATION AND SPECIFIC REASON FOR REFERRAL (EVALUATION, SURGERY) AND PROVIDE ADDITIONAL RELEVANT INFORMATION SUCH AS HISTORY OF AOM AND DEVELOPMENTAL STATUS OF THE CHILD

This option is based on panel consensus and a preponderance of benefit over harm.

This recommendation emphasizes the importance of communication between the referring primary care clinician and the otolaryngologist, audiologist, and speech-language pathologist. Parents and caregivers may be confused and frustrated when a recommendation for surgery is made for their child because of conflicting information about alternative management strategies. Choosing among management options is facilitated when primary care physicians and advanced-practice nurses who best know the patient's history of ear problems and general medical status provide the specialist with accurate information. Although there are no studies showing improved outcomes from better documentation of OME histories, there is a clear need for better mechanisms to convey information and expectations from primary care clinicians to consultants and subspecialists.[140–142]

When referring a child for evaluation to an otolaryngologist, the primary care physician should explain the following to the parent or caregiver of the patient:

- Reason for referral: Explain that the child is seeing an otolaryngologist for evaluation, which is likely to include ear examination and audiologic testing, and not necessarily simply to be scheduled for surgery.
- What to expect: Explain that surgery may be recommended, and let the parent know that the otolaryngologist will explain the options, benefits, and risks further.
- Decision-making process: Explain that there are many alternatives for management and that surgical decisions are elective; the parent or caregiver should be encouraged to express to the surgeon any concerns he or she may have about the recommendations made.

When referring a child to an otolaryngologist, audiologist, or speech-language pathologist, the minimum information that should be conveyed in writing includes:

- Duration of OME: State how long fluid has been present.
- Laterality of OME: State whether one or both ears have been affected.
- Results of prior hearing testing or tympanometry.
- Suspected speech or language problems: State whether there had been a delay in speech and language development or whether the parent or a caregiver has expressed concerns about the child's communication abilities, school achievement, or attentiveness.
- Conditions that might exacerbate the deleterious effects of OME: State whether the child has conditions such as permanent hearing loss, impaired cognition, developmental delays, cleft lip or palate, or an unstable or nonsupportive family or home environment.
- AOM history: State whether the child has a history of recurrent AOM.

Additional medical information that should be provided to the otolaryngologist by the primary care clinician includes:

- Parental attitude toward surgery: State whether the parents have expressed a strong preference for or against surgery as a management option.
- Related conditions that might require concomitant surgery: State whether there have been other conditions that might warrant surgery if the child is going to have general anesthesia (eg, nasal obstruction and snoring that might be an indication for adenoidectomy or obstructive breathing during sleep that might mean tonsillectomy is indicated).
- General health status: State whether there are any conditions that might present problems for surgery or administering general anesthesia, such as congenital heart abnormality, bleeding disorder, asthma or reactive airway disease, or family history of malignant hyperthermia.

After evaluating the child, the otolaryngologist, audiologist, or speech-language pathologist should inform the referring physician regarding his or her diagnostic impression, plans for additional assessment, and recommendations for ongoing monitoring and management.

Evidence Profile: Referral

- Aggregate evidence quality: C, observational studies.
- Benefit: better communication and improved decision-making.
- Harm: confidentiality concerns, administrative burden, and/or increased parent or caregiver anxiety.
- Benefits-harms assessment: balance of benefit and harm.
- Policy level: option.

9. SURGERY: WHEN A CHILD BECOMES A SURGICAL CANDIDATE, TYMPANOSTOMY TUBE INSERTION IS THE PREFERRED INITIAL PROCEDURE; ADENOIDECTOMY SHOULD NOT BE PERFORMED UNLESS A DISTINCT INDICATION EXISTS (NASAL OBSTRUCTION, CHRONIC ADENOIDITIS). REPEAT SURGERY CONSISTS OF ADENOIDECTOMY PLUS MYRINGOTOMY, WITH OR WITHOUT TUBE INSERTION. TONSILLECTOMY ALONE OR MYRINGOTOMY ALONE SHOULD NOT BE USED TO TREAT OME

This recommendation is based on randomized, controlled trials with a preponderance of benefit over harm.

Surgical candidacy for OME largely depends on hearing status, associated symptoms, the child's developmental risk (Table 3), and the anticipated chance of timely spontaneous resolution of the effusion. Candidates for surgery include children with OME lasting 4 months or longer with persistent hearing loss or other signs and symptoms, recurrent or persistent OME in children at risk regardless of hearing status, and OME and structural damage to the tympanic membrane or middle ear. Ultimately, the recommendation for surgery must be individualized based on consensus between the primary care physician, otolaryngologist, and parent or caregiver that a particular child would benefit from intervention. Children with OME of any duration who are at risk are candidates for earlier surgery.

Tympanostomy tubes are recommended for initial surgery because randomized trials show a mean 62% relative decrease in effusion prevalence and an absolute decrease of 128 effusion days per child during the next year.[139,143-145] HLs improve by a mean of 6 to 12 dB while the tubes remain patent.[146,147] Adenoidectomy plus myringotomy (without tube insertion) has comparable efficacy in children 4 years old or older[143] but is more invasive, with additional surgical and anesthetic risks. Similarly, the added risk of adenoidectomy outweighs the limited, short-term benefit for children 3 years old or older without prior tubes.[148] Consequently, adenoidectomy is not recommended for initial OME surgery unless a distinct indication exists, such as adenoiditis, postnasal obstruction, or chronic sinusitis.

Approximately 20% to 50% of children who have had tympanostomy tubes have OME relapse after tube extrusion that may require additional surgery.[144,145,149] When a child needs repeat surgery for OME, adenoidectomy is recommended (unless the child has an overt or submucous cleft palate), because it confers a 50% reduction in the need for future operations.[143,150,151] The benefit of adenoidectomy is apparent at 2 years old,[150] greatest for children 3 years old or older, and independent of adenoid size.[143,151,152] Myringotomy is performed concurrent with adenoidectomy. Myringotomy plus adenoidectomy is effective for children 4 years old or older,[143] but tube insertion is advised for younger children, when potential relapse of effusion must be minimized (eg, children at risk) or pronounced inflammation of the tympanic membrane and middle-ear mucosa is present.

Tonsillectomy or myringotomy alone (without adenoidectomy) is not recommended to treat OME. Although tonsillectomy is either ineffective[152] or of limited efficacy,[148,150] the risks of hemorrhage (~2%) and additional hospitalization outweigh any potential benefits unless a distinct indication for tonsillectomy exists. Myringotomy alone, without tube placement or adenoidectomy, is ineffective for chronic OME,[144,145] because the incision closes within several days. Laser-assisted myringotomy extends the ventilation period several weeks,[153] but randomized trials with concurrent controls have not been conducted to establish efficacy. In contrast, tympanostomy tubes ventilate the middle ear for an average of 12 to 14 months.[144,145]

Anesthesia mortality has been reported to be ~1: 50 000 for ambulatory surgery,[154] but the current fatality rate may be lower.[155] Laryngospasm and bronchospasm occur more often in children receiving anesthesia than adults. Tympanostomy tube sequelae are common[156] but are generally transient (otorrhea) or do not affect function (tympanosclerosis, focal atrophy, or shallow retraction pocket). Tympanic membrane perforations, which may require repair, are seen in 2% of children after placement of short-term (grommet-type) tubes and 17% after long-term tubes.[156] Adenoidectomy has a 0.2% to 0.5% incidence of hemorrhage[150,157] and 2% incidence of transient velopharyngeal insufficiency.[148] Other potential risks of adenoidectomy, such as nasopharyngeal stenosis and persistent velopharyngeal insufficiency, can be minimized with appropriate patient selection and surgical technique.

There is a clear preponderance of benefit over harm when considering the impact of surgery for OME on effusion prevalence, HLs, subsequent incidence of AOM, and the need for reoperation after adenoidectomy. Information about adenoidectomy in children less than 4 years old, however, remains limited. Although the cost of surgery and anesthesia is nontrivial, it is offset by reduced OME and AOM after tube placement and by reduced need for reoperation after adenoidectomy. Approximately 8 adenoidectomies are needed to avoid a single instance of tube reinsertion; however, each avoided surgery probably represents a larger reduction in the number of AOM and OME episodes, including those in children who did not require additional surgery.[150]

Evidence Profile: Surgery

- Aggregate evidence quality: B, randomized, controlled trials with minor limitations.
- Benefit: improved hearing, reduced prevalence of OME, reduced incidence of AOM, and less need for additional tube insertion (after adenoidectomy).
- Harm: risks of anesthesia and specific surgical procedures; sequelae of tympanostomy tubes.
- Benefits-harms assessment: preponderance of benefit over harm.
- Policy level: recommendation.

10. CAM: NO RECOMMENDATION IS MADE REGARDING CAM AS A TREATMENT FOR OME

There is no recommendation based on lack of scientific evidence documenting efficacy and an uncertain balance of harm and benefit.

The 1994 OME guideline[1] made no recommendation regarding CAM as a treatment for OME, and no subsequent controlled studies have been published to change this conclusion. The current statement of "no recommendation" is based on the lack of scientific evidence documenting efficacy plus the balance of benefit and harm.

Evidence concerning CAM is insufficient to determine whether the outcomes achieved for OME differ from those achieved by watchful waiting and spontaneous resolution. There are no randomized, controlled trials with adequate sample sizes on the efficacy of CAM for OME. Although many case reports and subjective reviews on CAM treatment of AOM were found, little is published on OME treatment or prevention. Homeopathy[158] and chiropractic treatments[159] were assessed in pilot studies with small numbers of patients that failed to show clinically or statistically significant benefits. Consequently, there is no research base on which to develop a recommendation concerning CAM for OME.

The natural history of OME in childhood (discussed previously) is such that almost any intervention can be "shown" to have helped in an anecdotal, uncontrolled report or case series. The efficacy of CAM or any other intervention for OME can only be shown with parallel-group, randomized, controlled trials with valid diagnostic methods and adequate sample sizes. Unproved modalities that have been claimed to provide benefit in middle-ear disease include osteopathic and chiropractic manipulation, dietary exclusions (such as dairy), herbal and other dietary supplements, acupuncture, traditional Chinese medicine, and homeopathy. None of these modalities, however, have been subjected yet to a published, peer-reviewed, clinical trial.

The absence of any published clinical trials also means that all reports of CAM adverse effects are anecdotal. A systematic review of recent evidence[160] found significant serious adverse effects of unconventional therapies for children, most of which were associated with inadequately regulated herbal medicines. One report on malpractice liability associated with CAM therapies[161] did not address childhood issues specifically. Allergic reactions to echinacea occur but seem to be rare in children.[162] A general concern about herbal products is the lack of any governmental oversight into product quality or purity.[160,163,164] Additionally, herbal products may alter blood levels of allopathic medications, including anticoagulants. A possible concern with homeopathy is the worsening of symptoms, which is viewed as a positive, early sign of homeopathic efficacy. The adverse effects of manipulative therapies (such as chiropractic treatments and osteopathy) in children are difficult to assess because of scant evidence, but a case series of 332 children treated for AOM or OME with chiropractic manipulation did not mention any side effects.[165] Quadriplegia has been reported, however, after spinal manipulation in an infant with torticollis.[166]

Evidence Profile: CAM

- Aggregate evidence quality: D, case series without controls.
- Benefit: not established.
- Harm: potentially significant depending on the intervention.
- Benefits-harms assessment: uncertain balance of benefit and harm.
- Policy level: no recommendation.

11. ALLERGY MANAGEMENT: NO RECOMMENDATION IS MADE REGARDING ALLERGY MANAGEMENT AS A TREATMENT FOR OME

There is no recommendation based on insufficient evidence of therapeutic efficacy or a causal relationship between allergy and OME.

The 1994 OME guideline[1] made no recommendation regarding allergy management as a treatment for OME, and no subsequent controlled studies have been published to change this conclusion. The current statement of "no recommendation" is based on insufficient evidence of therapeutic efficacy or a causal relationship between allergy and OME plus the balance of benefit and harm.

A linkage between allergy and OME has long been speculated but to date remains unquantified. The prevalence of allergy among OME patients has been reported to range from less than 10% to more than 80%.[167] Allergy has long been postulated to cause OME through its contribution to eustachian tube dysfunction.[168] The cellular response of respiratory mucosa to allergens has been well studied. Therefore, similar to other parts of respiratory mucosa, the mucosa lining the middle-ear cleft is capable of an allergic response.[169,170] Sensitivity to allergens varies among individuals, and atopy may involve neutrophils in type I allergic reactions that enhance the inflammatory response.[171]

The correlation between OME and allergy has been widely reported, but no prospective studies have examined the effects of immunotherapy compared with observation alone or other management options. Reports of OME cure after immunotherapy or food-elimination diets[172] are impossible to interpret without concurrent control groups because of the favorable natural history of most untreated OME. The documentation of allergy in published reports has been defined inconsistently (medical history, physical examination, skin-prick testing, nasal smears, serum immunoglobulin E and eosinophil counts, inflammatory mediators in effusions). Study groups have been drawn primarily from specialist offices, likely lack heterogeneity, and are not representative of general medical practice.

Evidence Profile: Allergy Management

- Aggregate evidence quality: D, case series without controls.

- Benefit: not established.
- Harm: adverse effects and cost of medication, physician evaluation, elimination diets, and desensitization.
- Benefits-harms assessment: balance of benefit and harm.
- Policy level: no recommendation.

RESEARCH NEEDS

Diagnosis

- Further standardize the definition of OME.
- Assess the performance characteristics of pneumatic otoscopy as a diagnostic test for OME when performed by primary care physicians and advanced-practice nurses in the routine office setting.
- Determine the optimal methods for teaching pneumatic otoscopy to residents and clinicians.
- Develop a brief, reliable, objective method for diagnosing OME.
- Develop a classification method for identifying the presence of OME for practical use by clinicians that is based on quantifiable tympanometric characteristics.
- Assess the usefulness of algorithms combining pneumatic otoscopy and tympanometry for detecting OME in clinical practice.
- Conduct additional validating cohort studies of acoustic reflectometry as a diagnostic method for OME, particularly in children less than 2 years old.

Child At Risk

- Better define the child with OME who is at risk for speech, language, and learning problems.
- Conduct large, multicenter, observational cohort studies to identify the child at risk who is most susceptible to potential adverse sequelae of OME.
- Conduct large, multicenter, observational cohort studies to analyze outcomes achieved with alternative management strategies for OME in children at risk.

Watchful Waiting

- Define the spontaneous resolution of OME in infants and young children (existing data are limited primarily to children 2 years old or older).
- Conduct large-scale, prospective cohort studies to obtain current data on the spontaneous resolution of newly diagnosed OME of unknown prior duration (existing data are primarily from the late 1970s and early 1980s).
- Develop prognostic indicators to identify the best candidates for watchful waiting.
- Determine whether the lack of impact from prompt insertion of tympanostomy tubes on speech and language outcomes seen in asymptomatic young children with OME identified by screening or intense surveillance can be generalized to older children with OME or to symptomatic children with OME referred for evaluation.

Medication

- Clarify which children, if any, should receive antimicrobials, steroids, or both for OME.
- Conduct a randomized, placebo-controlled trial on the efficacy of antimicrobial therapy, with or without concurrent oral steroid, in avoiding surgery in children with OME who are surgical candidates and have not received recent antimicrobials.
- Investigate the role of mucosal surface biofilms in refractory or recurrent OME and develop targeted interventions.

Hearing and Language

- Conduct longitudinal studies on the natural history of hearing loss accompanying OME.
- Develop improved methods for describing and quantifying the fluctuations in hearing of children with OME over time.
- Conduct prospective controlled studies on the relation of hearing loss associated with OME to later auditory, speech, language, behavioral, and academic sequelae.
- Develop reliable, brief, objective methods for estimating hearing loss associated with OME.
- Develop reliable, brief, objective methods for estimating speech or language delay associated with OME.
- Evaluate the benefits and administrative burden of language testing by primary care clinicians.
- Agree on the aspects of language that are vulnerable to or affected by hearing loss caused by OME, and reach a consensus on the best tools for measurement.
- Determine whether OME and associated hearing loss place children from special populations at greater risk for speech and language delays.

Surveillance

- Develop better tools for monitoring children with OME that are suitable for routine clinical care.
- Assess the value of new strategies for monitoring OME, such as acoustic reflectometry performed at home by the parent or caregiver, in optimizing surveillance.
- Improve our ability to identify children who would benefit from early surgery instead of prolonged surveillance.
- Promote early detection of structural abnormalities in the tympanic membrane associated with OME that may require surgery to prevent complications.
- Clarify and quantify the role of parent or caregiver education, socioeconomic status, and quality of the caregiving environment as modifiers of OME developmental outcomes.
- Develop methods for minimizing loss to follow-up during OME surveillance.

Surgery

- Define the role of adenoidectomy in children 3 years old or younger as a specific OME therapy.
- Conduct controlled trials on the efficacy of tympanostomy tubes for developmental outcomes in children with hearing loss, other symptoms, or speech and language delay.
- Conduct randomized, controlled trials of surgery versus no surgery that emphasize patient-based outcome measures (quality of life, functional health status) in addition to objective measures (effusion prevalence, HLs, AOM incidence, reoperation).
- Identify the optimal ways to incorporate parent or caregiver preference into surgical decision-making.

CAM

- Conduct randomized, controlled trials on the efficacy of CAM modalities for OME.
- Develop strategies to identify parents or caregivers who use CAM therapies for their child's OME, and encourage surveillance by the primary care clinician.

Allergy Management

- Evaluate the causal role of atopy in OME.
- Conduct randomized, controlled trials on the efficacy of allergy therapy for OME that are generalizable to the primary care setting.

CONCLUSIONS

This evidence-based practice guideline offers recommendations for identifying, monitoring, and managing the child with OME. The guideline emphasizes appropriate diagnosis and provides options for various management strategies including observation, medical intervention, and referral for surgical intervention. These recommendations should provide primary care physicians and other health care providers with assistance in managing children with OME.

SUBCOMMITTEE ON OTITIS MEDIA WITH EFFUSION
Richard M. Rosenfeld, MD, MPH, Cochairperson
    American Academy of Pediatrics
    American Academy of Otolaryngology-Head and Neck Surgery
Larry Culpepper, MD, MPH, Cochairperson
    American Academy of Family Physicians
Karen J. Doyle, MD, PhD
    American Academy of Otolaryngology-Head and Neck Surgery
Kenneth M. Grundfast, MD
    American Academy of Otolaryngology-Head and Neck Surgery
Alejandro Hoberman, MD
    American Academy of Pediatrics
Margaret A. Kenna, MD
    American Academy of Otolaryngology-Head and Neck Surgery
Allan S. Lieberthal, MD
    American Academy of Pediatrics
Martin Mahoney, MD, PhD
    American Academy of Family Physicians
Richard A. Wahl, MD
    American Academy of Pediatrics
Charles R. Woods, Jr, MD, MS
    American Academy of Pediatrics

Barbara Yawn, MD, MSc
American Academy of Family Physicians

CONSULTANTS
S. Michael Marcy, MD
Richard N. Shiffman, MD

LIAISONS
Linda Carlson, MS, CPNP
National Association of Pediatric Nurse
Practitioners
Judith Gravel, PhD
American Academy of Audiology
Joanne Roberts, PhD
American Speech-Language-Hearing Association
STAFF
Maureen Hannley, PhD
American Academy of Otolaryngology-Head and
Neck Surgery
Carla T. Herrerias, MPH
American Academy of Pediatrics
Bellinda K. Schoof, MHA, CPHQ
American Academy of Family Physicians

ACKNOWLEDGMENTS

Dr Marcy serves as a consultant to Abbott Laboratories Glaxo-SmithKline (vaccines).

REFERENCES

1. Stool SE, Berg AO, Berman S, et al. *Otitis Media With Effusion in Young Children. Clinical Practice Guideline, Number 12.* AHCPR Publication No. 94-0622. Rockville, MD: Agency for Health Care Policy and Research, Public Health Service, US Department of Health and Human Services; 1994

2. Shekelle P, Takata G, Chan LS, et al. *Diagnosis, Natural History, and Late Effects of Otitis Media With Effusion. Evidence Report/Technology Assessment No. 55.* AHRQ Publication No. 03-E023. Rockville, MD: Agency for Healthcare Research and Quality; 2003

3. Williamson I. Otitis media with effusion. *Clin Evid.* 2002;7:469–476

4. Tos M. Epidemiology and natural history of secretory otitis. *Am J Otol.* 1984;5:459–462

5. Paradise JL, Rockette HE, Colborn DK, et al. Otitis media in 2253 Pittsburgh area infants: prevalence and risk factors during the first two years of life. *Pediatrics.* 1997;99:318–333

6. Casselbrant ML, Mandel EM. Epidemiology. In: Rosenfeld RM, Bluestone CD, eds. *Evidence-Based Otitis Media.* 2nd ed. Hamilton, Ontario: BC Decker; 2003:147–162

7. Williamson IG, Dunleavy J, Baine J, Robinson D. The natural history of otitis media with effusion—a three-year study of the incidence and prevalence of abnormal tympanograms in four South West Hampshire infant and first schools. *J Laryngol Otol.* 1994;108:930–934

8. Coyte PC, Croxford R, Asche CV, To T, Feldman W, Friedberg J. Physician and population determinants of rates of middle-ear surgery in Ontario. *JAMA.* 2001;286:2128–2135

9. Tugwell P. How to read clinical journals: III. To learn the clinical course and prognosis of disease. *Can Med Assoc J.* 1981;124:869–872

10. Jaeschke R, Guyatt G, Sackett DL. Users' guides to the medical literature. III. How to use an article about a diagnostic test. A. Are the results of the study valid? Evidence-Based Medicine Working Group. *JAMA.* 1994;271:389–391

11. Shiffman RN, Shekelle P, Overhage JM, Slutsky J, Grimshaw J, Deshpande AM. Standardized reporting of clinical practice guidelines: a proposal from the Conference on Guideline Standardization. *Ann Intern Med.* 2003;139:493–498

12. Shiffman RN, Karras BT, Agrawal A, Chen R, Marenco L, Nath S. GEM: a proposal for a more comprehensive guideline document model using XML. *J Am Med Inform Assoc.* 2000;7:488–498

13. Shaneyfelt TM, Mayo-Smith MF, Rothwangl J. Are guidelines following guidelines? The methodological quality of clinical practice guidelines in the peer-reviewed medical literature. *JAMA.* 1999;281:1900–1905

14. Agrawal A, Shiffman RN. Evaluation of guideline quality using GEM-Q. *Medinfo.* 2001;10:1097–1101

15. Yale Center for Medical Informatics. GEM: The Guideline Elements Model. Available at: http://ycmi.med.yale.edu/GEM/. Accessed December 8, 2003

16. American Academy of Pediatrics, Steering Committee on Quality Improvement and Management. A taxonomy of recommendations for clinical practice guidelines. *Pediatrics.* 2004; In press

17. Eddy DM. *A Manual for Assessing Health Practices and Designing Practice Policies: The Explicit Approach.* Philadelphia, PA: American College of Physicians; 1992

18. Dowell SF, Marcy MS, Phillips WR, Gerber MA, Schwartz B. Otitis media—principles of judicious use of antimicrobial agents. *Pediatrics.* 1998;101:165–171

19. Dowell SF, Butler JC, Giebink GS, et al. Acute otitis media: management and surveillance in an era of pneumococcal resistance—a report from the Drug-Resistant *Streptococcus pneumoniae* Therapeutic Working Group. *Pediatr Infect Dis J.* 1999;18:1–9

20. Karma PH, Penttila MA, Sipila MM, Kataja MJ. Otoscopic diagnosis of middle ear effusion in acute and non-acute otitis media. I. The value of different otoscopic findings. *Int J Pediatr Otorhinolaryngol.* 1989;17:37–49

21. Pichichero ME, Poole MD. Assessing diagnostic accuracy and tympanocentesis skills in the management of otitis media. *Arch Pediatr Adolesc Med.* 2001;155:1137–1142

22. Steinbach WJ, Sectish TC. Pediatric resident training in the diagnosis and treatment of acute otitis media. *Pediatrics.* 2002;109:404–408

23. Palmu A, Puhakka H, Rahko T, Takala AK. Diagnostic value of tympanometry in infants in clinical practice. *Int J Pediatr Otorhinolaryngol.* 1999;49:207–213

24. van Balen FA, Aarts AM, De Melker RA. Tympanometry by general practitioners: reliable? *Int J Pediatr Otorhinolaryngol.* 1999;48:117–123

25. Block SL, Mandel E, McLinn S, et al. Spectral gradient acoustic reflectometry for the detection of middle ear effusion by pediatricians and parents. *Pediatr Infect Dis J.* 1998;17:560–564, 580

26. Barnett ED, Klein JO, Hawkins KA, Cabral HJ, Kenna M, Healy G. Comparison of spectral gradient acoustic reflectometry and other diagnostic techniques for detection of middle ear effusion in children with middle ear disease. *Pediatr Infect Dis J.* 1998;17:556–559, 580

27. Block SL, Pichichero ME, McLinn S, Aronovitz G, Kimball S. Spectral gradient acoustic reflectometry: detection of middle ear effusion by pediatricians in suppurative acute otitis media. *Pediatr Infect Dis J.* 1999;18:741–744

28. Schwartz RH. A practical approach to the otitis prone child. *Contemp Pediatr.* 1987;4:30–54

29. Barriga F, Schwartz RH, Hayden GF. Adequate illumination for otoscopy. Variations due to power source, bulb, and head and speculum design. *Am J Dis Child.* 1986;140:1237–1240

30. Sorenson CH, Jensen SH, Tos M. The post-winter prevalence of middle-ear effusion in four-year-old children, judged by tympanometry. *Int J Pediatr Otorhinolaryngol.* 1981;3:119–128

31. Fiellau-Nikolajsen M. Epidemiology of secretory otitis media. A descriptive cohort study. *Ann Otol Rhinol Laryngol.* 1983;92:172–177

32. Casselbrant ML, Brostoff LM, Cantekin EI, et al. Otitis media with effusion in preschool children. *Laryngoscope.* 1985;95:428–436

33. Zielhuis GA, Rach GH, van den Broek P. Screening for otitis media with effusion in preschool children. *Lancet.* 1989;1:311–314

34. Poulsen G, Tos M. Repetitive tympanometric screenings of two-year-old children. *Scand Audiol.* 1980;9:21–28

35. Tos M, Holm-Jensen S, Sorensen CH. Changes in prevalence of secretory otitis from summer to winter in four-year-old children. *Am J Otol.* 1981;2:324–327

36. Thomsen J, Tos M. Spontaneous improvement of secretory otitis. A long-term study. *Acta Otolaryngol.* 1981;92:493–499

37. Lous J, Fiellau-Nikolajsen M. Epidemiology of middle ear effusion and tubal dysfunction. A one-year prospective study comprising monthly tympanometry in 387 non-selected seven-year-old children. *Int J Pediatr Otorhinolaryngol.* 1981;3:303–317

38. New Zealand Health Technology Assessment. *Screening Programmes for the Detection of Otitis Media With Effusion and Conductive Hearing Loss in Pre-School and New Entrant School Children: A Critical Appraisal of the Literature.* Christchurch, New Zealand: New Zealand Health Technology Assessment; 1998:61

39. Canadian Task Force on Preventive Health Care. Screening for otitis media with effusion: recommendation statement from the Canadian Task Force on Preventive Health Care. *CMAJ.* 2001;165:1092–1093

40. US Preventive Services Task Force. *Guide to Clinical Preventive Services.* 2nd ed. Baltimore, MD: Williams & Wilkins; 1995

41. Paradise JL, Feldman HM, Campbell TF, et al. Effect of early or delayed insertion of tympanostomy tubes for persistent otitis media on

developmental outcomes at the age of three years. *N Engl J Med.* 2001;344:1179–1187

42. Rovers MM, Krabble PF, Straatman H, Ingels K, van der Wilt GJ, Zielhuis GA. Randomized controlled trial of the effect of ventilation tubes (grommets) on quality of life at age 1–2 years. *Arch Dis Child.* 2001;84:45–49

43. Wood DL. Documentation guidelines: evolution, future direction, and compliance. *Am J Med.* 2001;110:332–334

44. Soto CM, Kleinman KP, Simon SR. Quality and correlates of medical record documentation in the ambulatory care setting. *BMC Health Serv Res.* 2002;2:22–35

45. Marchant CD, Shurin PA, Turczyk VA, Wasikowski DE, Tutihasi MA, Kinney SE. Course and outcome of otitis media in early infancy: a prospective study. *J Pediatr.* 1984;104:826–831

46. Rosenfeld RM, Goldsmith AJ, Tetlus L, Balzano A. Quality of life for children with otitis media. *Arch Otolaryngol Head Neck Surg.* 1997;123:1049–1054

47. Casselbrant ML, Furman JM, Rubenstein E, Mandel EM. Effect of otitis media on the vestibular system in children. *Ann Otol Rhinol Laryngol.* 1995;104:620–624

48. Orlin MN, Effgen SK, Handler SD. Effect of otitis media with effusion on gross motor ability in preschool-aged children: preliminary findings. *Pediatrics.* 1997;99:334–337

49. Golz A, Angel-Yeger B, Parush S. Evaluation of balance disturbances in children with middle ear effusion. *Int J Pediatr Otorhinolaryngol.* 1998;43:21–26

50. Casselbrant ML, Redfern MS, Furman JM, Fall PA, Mandel EM. Visual-induced postural sway in children with and without otitis media. *Ann Otol Rhinol Laryngol.* 1998;107:401–405

51. Ruben R. Host susceptibility to otitis media sequelae. In: Rosenfeld RM, Bluestone CD, eds. *Evidence-Based Otitis Media.* 2nd ed. Hamilton, ON, Canada: BC Decker; 2003:505–514

52. Whiteman BC, Simpson GB, Compton WC. Relationship of otitis media and language impairment on adolescents with Down syndrome. *Ment Retard.* 1986;24:353–356

53. van der Vyver M, van der Merwe A, Tesner HE. The effects of otitis media on articulation in children with cerebral palsy. *Int J Rehabil Res.* 1988;11:386–389

54. Paradise JL, Bluestone CD. Early treatment of the universal otitis media of infants with cleft palate. *Pediatrics.* 1974;53:48–54

55. Schwartz DM, Schwartz RH. Acoustic impedance and otoscopic findings in young children with Down's syndrome. *Arch Otolaryngol.* 1978;104:652–656

56. Corey JP, Caldarelli DD, Gould HJ. Otopathology in cranial facial dysostosis. *Am J Otol.* 1987;8:14–17

57. Schonweiler R, Schonweiler B, Schmelzeisen R. Hearing capacity and speech production in 417 children with facial cleft abnormalities [in German]. *HNO.* 1994;42:691–696

58. Ruben RJ, Math R. Serous otitis media associated with sensorineural hearing loss in children. *Laryngoscope.* 1978;88:1139–1154

59. Brookhouser PE, Worthington DW, Kelly WJ. Middle ear disease in young children with sensorineural hearing loss. *Laryngoscope.* 1993;103:371–378

60. Rice ML. Specific language impairments: in search of diagnostic markers and genetic contributions. *Ment Retard Dev Disabil Res Rev.* 1997;3:350–357

61. Rosenhall U, Nordin V, Sandstrom M, Ahlsen G, Gillberg C. Autism and hearing loss. *J Autism Dev Disord.* 1999;29:349–357

62. Cunningham C, McArthur K. Hearing loss and treatment in young Down's syndrome children. *Child Care Health Dev.* 1981;7:357–374

63. Shott SR, Joseph A, Heithaus D. Hearing loss in children with Down syndrome. *Int J Pediatr Otorhinolaryngol.* 2001;61:199–205

64. Clarkson RL, Eimas PD, Marean GC. Speech perception in children with histories of recurrent otitis media. *J Acoust Soc Am.* 1989;85:926–933

65. Groenen P, Crul T, Maassen B, van Bon W. Perception of voicing cues by children with early otitis media with and without language impairment. *J Speech Hear Res.* 1996;39:43–54

66. Hubbard TW, Paradise JL, McWilliams BJ, Elster BA, Taylor FH. Consequences of unremitting middle-ear disease in early life. Otologic, audiologic, and developmental findings in children with cleft palate. *N Engl J Med.* 1985;312:1529–1534

67. Nunn DR, Derkay CS, Darrow DH, Magee W, Strasnick B. The effect of very early cleft palate closure on the need for ventilation tubes in the first years of life. *Laryngoscope.* 1995;105:905–908

68. Pappas DG, Flexer C, Shackelford L. Otological and habilitative management of children with Down syndrome. *Laryngoscope.* 1994;104:1065–1070

69. Vartiainen E. Otitis media with effusion in children with congenital or early-onset hearing impairment. *J Otolaryngol.* 2000;29:221–223

70. Rosenfeld RM, Kay D. Natural history of untreated otitis media. *Laryngoscope.* 2003;113:1645–1657

71. Teele DW, Klein JO, Rosner BA. Epidemiology of otitis media in children. *Ann Otol Rhinol Laryngol Suppl.* 1980;89:5–6

72. Mygind N, Meistrup-Larsen KI, Thomsen J, Thomsen VF, Josefsson K, Sorensen H. Penicillin in acute otitis media: a double-blind, placebo-controlled trial. *Clin Otolaryngol.* 1981;6:5–13

73. Burke P, Bain J, Robinson D, Dunleavey J. Acute red ear in children: controlled trial of nonantibiotic treatment in general practice. *BMJ.* 1991;303:558–562

74. Fiellau-Nikolajsen M, Lous J. Prospective tympanometry in 3-year-old children. A study of the spontaneous course of tympanometry types in a nonselected population. *Arch Otolaryngol.* 1979;105:461–466

75. Fiellau-Nikolajsen M. Tympanometry in 3-year-old children. Type of care as an epidemiological factor in secretory otitis media and tubal dysfunction in unselected populations of 3-year-old children. *ORL J Otorhinolaryngol Relat Spec.* 1979;41:193–205

76. Tos M. Spontaneous improvement of secretory otitis and impedance screening. *Arch Otolaryngol.* 1980;106:345–349

77. Tos M, Holm-Jensen S, Sorensen CH, Mogensen C. Spontaneous course and frequency of secretory otitis in 4-year-old children. *Arch Otolaryngol.* 1982;108:4–10

78. Roberts JE, Zeisel SA. *Ear Infections and Language Development.* Rockville, MD: American Speech-Language-Hearing Association and the National Center for Early Development and Learning; 2000

79. Roberts JE, Rosenfeld RM, Zeisel SA. Otitis media and speech and language: a meta-analysis of prospective studies. *Pediatrics.* 2004;113(3). Available at: www.pediatrics.org/cgi/content/full/113/3/e238

80. Williams RL, Chalmers TC, Stange KC, Chalmers FT, Bowlin SJ. Use of antibiotics in preventing recurrent otitis media and in treating otitis media with effusion. A meta-analytic attempt to resolve the brouhaha. *JAMA.* 1993;270:1344–1351

81. Rosenfeld RM, Post JC. Meta-analysis of antibiotics for the treatment of otitis media with effusion. *Otolaryngol Head Neck Surg.* 1992;106:378–386

82. Mandel EM, Rockette HE, Bluestone CD, Paradise JL, Nozza RJ. Efficacy of amoxicillin with and without decongestant-antihistamine for otitis media with effusion in children. Results of a double-blind, randomized trial. *N Engl J Med.* 1987;316:432–437

83. McCormick AW, Whitney CG, Farley MM, et al. Geographic diversity and temporal trends of antimicrobial resistance in *Streptococcus pneumoniae* in the United States. *Nat Med.* 2003;9:424–430

84. Levy SB. *The Antibiotic Paradox. How the Misuse of Antibiotic Destroys Their Curative Powers.* Cambridge, MA: Perseus Publishing; 2002

85. Butler CC, van der Voort JH. Oral or topical nasal steroids for hearing loss associated with otitis media with effusion in children. *Cochrane Database Syst Rev.* 2002;4:CD001935

86. Mandel EM, Casselbrant ML, Rockette HE, Fireman P, Kurs-Lasky M, Bluestone CD. Systemic steroid for chronic otitis media with effusion in children. *Pediatrics.* 2002;110:1071–1080

87. Tracy JM, Demain JG, Hoffman KM, Goetz DW. Intranasal beclomethasone as an adjunct to treatment of chronic middle ear effusion. *Ann Allergy Asthma Immunol.* 1998;80:198–206

88. Joint Committee on Infant Hearing. Year 2000 position statement: principles and guidelines for early hearing detection and intervention programs. *Am J Audiol.* 2000;9:9–29

89. Pillsbury HC, Grose JH, Hall JW III. Otitis media with effusion in children. Binaural hearing before and after corrective surgery. *Arch Otolaryngol Head Neck Surg.* 1991;117:718–723

90. Besing J, Koehnke J A test of virtual auditory localization. *Ear Hear.* 1995;16:220–229

91. Jerger S, Jerger J, Alford BR, Abrams S. Development of speech intelligibility in children with recurrent otitis media. *Ear Hear.* 1983;4:138–145

92. Gravel JS, Wallace IF. Listening and language at 4 years of age: effects of early otitis media. *J Speech Hear Res.* 1992;35:588–595

93. Schilder AG, Snik AF, Straatman H, van den Broek P. The effect of otitis media with effusion at preschool age on some aspects of auditory perception at school age. *Ear Hear.* 1994;15:224–231

94. Rosenfeld RM, Madell JR, McMahon A. Auditory function in normal-hearing children with middle ear effusion. In: Lim DJ, Bluestone CD, Casselbrant M, Klein JO, Ogra PL, eds. *Recent Advances in Otitis Media: Proceedings of the 6th International Symposium.* Hamilton, ON, Canada: BC Decker; 1996:354–356

95. Friel-Patti S, Finitzo T. Language learning in a prospective study of otitis media with effusion in the first two years of life. *J Speech Hear Res.* 1990;33:188–194

96. Wallace IF, Gravel JS, McCarton CM, Stapells DR, Bernstein RS, Ruben RJ. Otitis media, auditory sensitivity, and language outcomes at one year. *Laryngoscope.* 1988;98:64–70

97. Roberts JE, Burchinal MR, Medley LP, et al. Otitis media, hearing sensitivity, and maternal responsiveness in relation to language during infancy. *J Pediatr.* 1995;126:481–489

98. Roberts JE, Burchinal MR, Zeisel SA. Otitis media in early childhood in relation to children's school-age language and academic skills. *Pediatrics.* 2002;110:696–706

99. Rovers MM, Straatman H, Ingels K, van der Wilt GJ, van den Broek P, Zielhuis GA. The effect of ventilation tubes on language development in infants with otitis media with effusion: a randomized trial. *Pediatrics.* 2000;106(3). Available at: www.pediatrics.org/cgi/content/full/106/3/e42

100. Paradise JL, Feldman HM, Campbell TF, et al. Early versus delayed insertion of tympanostomy tubes for persistent otitis media: developmental outcomes at the age of three years in relation to prerandomization illness patterns and hearing levels. *Pediatr Infect Dis J.* 2003;22:309–314

101. Kokko E. Chronic secretory otitis media in children. A clinical study. *Acta Otolaryngol Suppl.* 1974;327:1–44

102. Fria TJ, Cantekin EI, Eichler JA. Hearing acuity of children with otitis media with effusion. *Arch Otolaryngol.* 1985;111:10–16

103. Gravel JS, Wallace IF. Effects of otitis media with effusion on hearing in the first three years of life. *J Speech Lang Hear Res.* 2000;43:631–644

104. Roberts JE, Burchinal MR, Zeisel S, et al. Otitis media, the caregiving environment, and language and cognitive outcomes at 2 years. *Pediatrics.* 1998;102:346–354

105. Gravel JS, Wallace IF, Ruben RJ. Early otitis media and later educational risk. *Acta Otolaryngol.* 1995;115:279–281

106. Cunningham M, Cox EO; American Academy of Pediatrics, Committee on Practice and Ambulatory Medicine, Section on Otolaryngology and Bronchoesophagology. Hearing assessment in infants and children: recommendations beyond neonatal screening. *Pediatrics.* 2003;111:436–440

107. American Speech-Language-Hearing Association Panel on Audiologic Assessment. *Guidelines for Audiologic Screening.* Rockville, MD: American Speech-Language-Hearing Association; 1996

108. Rosenfeld RM, Goldsmith AJ, Madell JR. How accurate is parent rating of hearing for children with otitis media? *Arch Otolaryngol Head Neck Surg.* 1998;124:989–992

109. Brody R, Rosenfeld RM, Goldsmith AJ, Madell JR. Parents cannot detect mild hearing loss in children. *Otolaryngol Head Neck Surg.* 1999;121:681–686

110. Catts HW, Fey ME, Zhang X, Tomblin JB. Language basis of reading and reading disabilities: evidence from a longitudinal investigation. *Sci Stud Read.* 1999;3:331–362

111. Johnson CJ, Beitchman JH, Young A, et al. Fourteen-year follow-up of children with and without speech/language impairments: speech/language stability and outcomes. *J Speech Lang Hear Res.* 1999;42:744–760

112. Scarborough H, Dobrich W. Development of children with early language delay. *J Speech Hear Res.* 1990;33:70–83

113. Tomblin JB, Records NL, Buckwalter P, Zhang X, Smith E, O'Brien M. Prevalence of specific language impairment in kindergarten children. *J Speech Lang Hear Res.* 1997;40:1245–1260

114. Glade MJ. *Diagnostic and Therapeutic Technology Assessment: Speech Therapy in Patients With a Prior History of Recurrent Acute or Chronic Otitis Media With Effusion.* Chicago, IL: American Medical Association; 1996:1–14

115. Casby MW. Otitis media and language development: a meta-analysis. *Am J Speech Lang Pathol.* 2001;10:65–80

116. Maw R, Wilks J, Harvey I, Peters TJ, Golding J. Early surgery compared with watchful waiting for glue ear and effect on language development in preschool children: a randomised trial. *Lancet.* 1999;353:960–963

117. Coplan J. *Early Language Milestone Scale.* 2nd ed. Austin, TX: PRO-ED; 1983

118. Fenson L, Dale PS, Reznick JS, et al. *MacArthur Communicative Development Inventories. User's Guide and Technical Manual.* San Diego, CA: Singular Publishing Group; 1993

119. Rescoria L. The Language Development Survey: a screening tool for delayed language in toddlers. *J Speech Hear Dis.* 1989;54:587–599

120. Frankenburg WK, Dodds JA, Faucal A, et al. *Denver Developmental Screening Test II.* Denver, CO: University of Colorado Press; 1990

121. Klee T, Pearce K, Carson DK. Improving the positive predictive value of screening for developmental language disorder. *J Speech Lang Hear Res.* 2000;43:821–833

122. Shekelle PG, Ortiz E, Rhodes S, et al. Validity of the Agency for Healthcare Research and Quality clinical practice guidelines: how quickly do guidelines become outdated? *JAMA.* 2001;286:1461–1467

123. Zielhuis GA, Straatman H, Rach GH, van den Broek P. Analysis and presentation of data on the natural course of otitis media with effusion in children. *Int J Epidemiol.* 1990;19:1037–1044

124. MRC Multi-centre Otitis Media Study Group. Risk factors for persistence of bilateral otitis media with effusion. *Clin Otolaryngol.* 2001;26:147–156

125. van Balen FA, De Melker RA. Persistent otitis media with effusion: can it be predicted? A family practice follow-up study in children aged 6 months to 6 years. *J Fam Pract.* 2000;49:605–611

126. Sano S, Kamide Y, Schachern PA, Paparella MM. Micropathologic changes of pars tensa in children with otitis media with effusion. *Arch Otolaryngol Head Neck Surg.* 1994;120:815–819

127. Yellon RF, Doyle WJ, Whiteside TL, Diven WF, March AR, Fireman P. Cytokines, immunoglobulins, and bacterial pathogens in middle ear effusions. *Arch Otolaryngol Head Neck Surg.* 1995;121:865–869

128. Maw RA, Bawden R. Tympanic membrane atrophy, scarring, atelectasis and attic retraction in persistent, untreated otitis media with effusion and following ventilation tube insertion. *Int J Pediatr Otorhinolaryngol.* 1994;30:189–204

129. Davis JM, Elfenbein J, Schum R, Bentler RA. Effects of mild and moderate hearing impairment on language, educational, and psychosocial behavior of children. *J Speech Hear Disord.* 1986;51:53–62

130. Carney AE, Moeller MP. Treatment efficacy: hearing loss in children. *J Speech Lang Hear Res.* 1998;41:S61–S84

131. Karchmer MA, Allen TE. The functional assessment of deaf and hard of hearing students. *Am Ann Deaf.* 1999;144:68–77

132. Bess FH, Dodd-Murphy J, Parker RA. Children with minimal sensorineural hearing loss: prevalence, educational performance, and functional status. *Ear Hear.* 1998;19:339–354

133. Roberts JE, Burchinal MR, Jackson SC, et al. Otitis media in early childhood in relation to preschool language and school readiness skills among black children. *Pediatrics.* 2000;106:725–735

134. Haggard MP, Birkin JA, Browning GG, Gatehouse S, Lewis S. Behavior problems in otitis media. *Pediatr Infect Dis J.* 1994;13:S43–S50

135. Bennett KE, Haggard MP. Behaviour and cognitive outcomes from middle ear disease. *Arch Dis Child.* 1999;80:28–35

136. Bennett KE, Haggard MP, Silva PA, Stewart IA. Behaviour and developmental effects of otitis media with effusion into the teens. *Arch Dis Child.* 2001;85:91–95

137. Wilks J, Maw R, Peters TJ, Harvey I, Golding J. Randomised controlled trial of early surgery versus watchful waiting for glue ear: the effect on behavioural problems in pre-school children. *Clin Otolaryngol.* 2000;25:209–214

138. Rosenfeld RM, Bhaya MH, Bower CM, et al. Impact of tympanostomy tubes on child quality of life. *Arch Otolaryngol Head Neck Surg.* 2000;126:585–592

139. Rosenfeld RM, Bluestone CD. Clinical efficacy of surgical therapy. In: Rosenfeld RM, Bluestone CD, eds. *Evidence-Based Otitis Media.* 2nd ed. Hamilton, ON, Canada: BC Decker; 2003:227–240

140. Kuyvenhoven MM, De Melker RA. Referrals to specialists. An exploratory investigation of referrals by 13 general practitioners to medical and surgical departments. *Scand J Prim Health Care.* 1990;8:53–57

141. Haldis TA, Blankenship JC. Telephone reporting in the consultant-generalist relationship. *J Eval Clin Pract.* 2002;8:31–35

142. Reichman S. The generalist's patient and the subspecialist. *Am J Manag Care.* 2002;8:79–82

143. Gates GA, Avery CA, Prihoda TJ, Cooper JC Jr. Effectiveness of adenoidectomy and tympanostomy tubes in the treatment of chronic otitis media with effusion. *N Engl J Med.* 1987;317:1444–1451

144. Mandel EM, Rockette HE, Bluestone CD, Paradise JL, Nozza RJ. Myringotomy with and without tympanostomy tubes for chronic otitis media with effusion. *Arch Otolaryngol Head Neck Surg.* 1989;115:1217–1224

145. Mandel EM, Rockette HE, Bluestone CD, Paradise JL, Nozza RJ. Efficacy of myringotomy with and without tympanostomy tubes for chronic otitis media with effusion. *Pediatr Infect Dis J.* 1992;11:270–277

146. University of York Centre for Reviews and Dissemination. The treatment of persistent glue ear in children. *Eff Health Care.* 1992;4:1–16

147. Rovers MM, Straatman H, Ingels K, van der Wilt GJ, van den Broek P, Zielhuis GA. The effect of short-term ventilation tubes versus watchful waiting on hearing in young children with persistent otitis media with effusion: a randomized trial. *Ear Hear.* 2001;22:191–199

148. Paradise JL, Bluestone CD, Colborn DK, et al. Adenoidectomy and adenotonsillectomy for recurrent acute otitis media: parallel randomized clinical trials in children not previously treated with tympanostomy tubes. *JAMA.* 1999;282:945–953

149. Boston M, McCook J, Burke B, Derkay C. Incidence of and risk factors for additional tympanostomy tube insertion in children. *Arch Otolaryngol Head Neck Surg.* 2003;129:293–296

150. Coyte PC, Croxford R, McIsaac W, Feldman W, Friedberg J. The role of adjuvant adenoidectomy and tonsillectomy in the outcome of insertion of tympanostomy tubes. *N Engl J Med.* 2001;344:1188–1195

151. Paradise JL, Bluestone CD, Rogers KD, et al. Efficacy of adenoidectomy for recurrent otitis media in children previously treated with tympanostomy-tube placement. Results of parallel randomized and nonrandomized trials. *JAMA.* 1990;263:2066–2073

152. Maw AR. Chronic otitis media with effusion (glue ear) and adenotonsillectomy: prospective randomised controlled study. *Br Med J (Clin Res Ed).* 1983;287:1586–1588

153. Cohen D, Schechter Y, Slatkine M, Gatt N, Perez R. Laser myringotomy in different age groups. *Arch Otolaryngol Head Neck Surg.* 2001;127: 260–264

154. Holzman RS. Morbidity and mortality in pediatric anesthesia. *Pediatr Clin North Am.* 1994;41:239–256

155. Cottrell JE, Golden S. *Under the Mask: A Guide to Feeling Secure and Comfortable During Anesthesia and Surgery.* New Brunswick, NJ: Rutgers University Press; 2001

156. Kay DJ, Nelson M, Rosenfeld RM. Meta-analysis of tympanostomy tube sequelae. *Otolaryngol Head Neck Surg.* 2001;124:374–380

157. Crysdale WS, Russel D. Complications of tonsillectomy and adenoidectomy in 9409 children observed overnight. *CMAJ.* 1986;135: 1139–1142

158. Harrison H, Fixsen A, Vickers A. A randomized comparison of homeopathic and standard care for the treatment of glue ear in children. *Complement Ther Med.* 1999;7:132–135

159. Sawyer CE, Evans RL, Boline PD, Branson R, Spicer A. A feasibility study of chiropractic spinal manipulation versus sham spinal manipulation for chronic otitis media with effusion in children. *J Manipulative Physiol Ther.* 1999;22:292–298

160. Ernst E. Serious adverse effects of unconventional therapies for children and adolescents: a systematic review of recent evidence. *Eur J Pediatr.* 2003;162:72–80

161. Cohen MH, Eisenberg DM. Potential physician malpractice liability associated with complementary and integrative medical therapies. *Ann Intern Med.* 2002;136:596–603

162. Mullins RJ, Heddle R. Adverse reactions associated with echinacea: the Australian experience. *Ann Allergy Asthma Immunol.* 2002;88:42–51

163. Miller LG, Hume A, Harris IM, et al. White paper on herbal products. American College of Clinical Pharmacy. *Pharmacotherapy.* 2000;20: 877–891

164. Angell M, Kassirer JP. Alternative medicine—the risks of untested and unregulated remedies. *N Engl J Med.* 1998;339:839–841

165. Fallon JM. The role of chiropractic adjustment in the care and treatment of 332 children with otitis media. *J Clin Chiropractic Pediatr.* 1997;2:167–183

166. Shafrir Y, Kaufman BA. Quadriplegia after chiropractic manipulation in an infant with congenital torticollis caused by a spinal cord astrocytoma. *J Pediatr.* 1992;120:266–269

167. Corey JP, Adham RE, Abbass AH, Seligman I. The role of IgE-mediated hypersensitivity in otitis media with effusion. *Am J Otolaryngol.* 1994;15:138–144

168. Bernstein JM. Role of allergy in eustachian tube blockage and otitis media with effusion: a review. *Otolaryngol Head Neck Surg.* 1996;114: 562–568

169. Ishii TM, Toriyama M, Suzuki JI. Histopathological study of otitis media with effusion. *Ann Otol Rhinol Laryngol.* 1980;89(suppl):83–86

170. Hurst DS, Venge P. Evidence of eosinophil, neutrophil, and mast-cell mediators in the effusion of OME patients with and without atopy. *Allergy.* 2000;55:435–441

171. Hurst DS, Venge P. The impact of atopy on neutrophil activity in middle ear effusion from children and adults with chronic otitis media. *Arch Otolaryngol Head Neck Surg.* 2002;128:561–566

172. Hurst DS. Allergy management of refractory serous otitis media. *Otolaryngol Head Neck Surg.* 1990;102:664–669

Otitis Media Clinical Practice Guidelines
Quick Reference Tools

• •

- Action Statement Summary
  — The Diagnosis and Management of Acute Otitis Media
  — Otitis Media With Effusion
- *ICD-10-CM* Coding Quick Reference for Otitis Media
- Bonus Feature
  — Continuum Model for Otitis Media
- AAP Patient Education Handouts
  — *Acute Ear Infections and Your Child*
  — *Middle Ear Fluid and Your Child*

Action Statement Summary
The Diagnosis and Management of Acute Otitis Media

Key Action Statement 1A
Clinicians should diagnose acute otitis media (AOM) in children who present with moderate to severe bulging of the tympanic membrane (TM) *or* new onset of otorrhea not due to acute otitis externa. Evidence Quality: Grade B. Strength: Recommendation.

Key Action Statement 1B
Clinicians should diagnose AOM in children who present with mild bulging of the TM *and* recent (less than 48 hours) onset of ear pain (holding, tugging, rubbing of the ear in a nonverbal child) or intense erythema of the TM. Evidence Quality: Grade C. Strength: Recommendation.

Key Action Statement 1C
Clinicians should not diagnose AOM in children who do not have middle ear effusion (MEE) (based on pneumatic otoscopy and/or tympanometry). Evidence Quality: Grade B. Strength: Recommendation.

Key Action Statement 2
The management of AOM should include an assessment of pain. If pain is present, the clinician should recommend treatment to reduce pain. Evidence Quality: Grade B. Strength: Strong Recommendation.

Key Action Statement 3A
Severe AOM: The clinician should prescribe antibiotic therapy for AOM (bilateral or unilateral) in children 6 months and older with severe signs or symptoms (ie, moderate or severe otalgia or otalgia for at least 48 hours or temperature 39°C [102.2°F] or higher). Evidence Quality: Grade B. Strength: Strong Recommendation.

Key Action Statement 3B
Nonsevere bilateral AOM in young children: The clinician should prescribe antibiotic therapy for bilateral AOM in children 6 months through 23 months of age without severe signs or symptoms (ie, mild otalgia for less than 48 hours and temperature less than 39°C [102.2°F]). Evidence Quality: Grade B. Strength: Recommendation.

Key Action Statement 3C
Nonsevere unilateral AOM in young children: The clinician should either prescribe antibiotic therapy *or* offer observation with close follow-up based on joint decision-making with the parent(s)/caregiver for unilateral AOM in children 6 months to 23 months of age without severe signs or symptoms (ie, mild otalgia for less than 48 hours and temperature less than 39°C [102.2°F]). When observation is used, a mechanism must be in place to ensure follow-up and begin antibiotic therapy if the child worsens or fails to improve within 48 to 72 hours of onset of symptoms. Evidence Quality: Grade B. Strength: Recommendation.

Key Action Statement 3D
Nonsevere AOM in older children: The clinician should either prescribe antibiotic therapy *or* offer observation with close follow-up based on joint decision-making with the parent(s)/caregiver for AOM (bilateral or unilateral) in children 24 months or older without severe signs or symptoms (ie, mild otalgia for less than 48 hours and temperature less than 39°C [102.2°F]). When observation is used, a mechanism must be in place to ensure follow-up and begin antibiotic therapy if the child worsens or fails to improve within 48 to 72 hours of onset of symptoms. Evidence Quality: Grade B. Strength: Recommendation.

Key Action Statement 4A
Clinicians should prescribe amoxicillin for AOM when a decision to treat with antibiotics has been made *and* the child has not received amoxicillin in the past 30 days *or* the child does not have concurrent purulent conjunctivitis *or* the child is not allergic to penicillin. Evidence Quality: Grade B. Strength: Recommendation.

Key Action Statement 4B
Clinicians should prescribe an antibiotic with additional β-lactamase coverage for AOM when a decision to treat with antibiotics has been made, *and* the child has received amoxicillin in the last 30 days *or* has concurrent purulent conjunctivitis, *or* has a history of recurrent AOM unresponsive to amoxicillin. Evidence Quality: Grade C. Strength: Recommendation.

Key Action Statement 4C
Clinicians should reassess the patient if the caregiver reports that the child's symptoms have worsened or failed to respond to the initial antibiotic treatment within 48 to 72 hours and determine whether a change in therapy is needed. Evidence Quality: Grade B. Strength: Recommendation.

Key Action Statement 5A

Clinicians should not prescribe prophylactic antibiotics to reduce the frequency of episodes of AOM in children with recurrent AOM. Evidence Quality: Grade B. Strength: Recommendation.

Key Action Statement 5B

Clinicians may offer tympanostomy tubes for recurrent AOM (3 episodes in 6 months or 4 episodes in 1 year with 1 episode in the preceding 6 months). Evidence Quality: Grade B. Strength: Option.

Key Action Statement 6A

Clinicians should recommend pneumococcal conjugate vaccine to all children according to the schedule of the Advisory Committee on Immunization Practices of the Centers for Disease Control and prevention, American Academy of Pediatrics (AAP), and American Academy of Family Physicians (AAFP). Evidence Quality: Grade B. Strength: Strong Recommendation.

Otitis Media With Effusion

1A. Pneumatic Otoscopy

Clinicians should use pneumatic otoscopy as the primary diagnostic method for OME, and OME should be distinguished from AOM.

This is a strong recommendation based on systematic review of cohort studies and the preponderance of benefit over harm.

1B. Tympanometry

Tympanometry can be used to confirm the diagnosis a of OME.

This option is based on cohort studies and a balance of benefit and harm.

1C. Screening

Population-based screening programs for OME are not recommended in healthy, asymptomatic children.

This recommendation is based on randomized, controlled trials and cohort studies, with a preponderance of harm over benefit.

2. Documentation

Clinicians should document the laterality, duration of effusion, and presence and severity of associated symptoms at each assessment of the child with OME.

This recommendation is based on observational studies and strong preponderance of benefit over harm.

3. Child at Risk

Clinicians should distinguish the child with OME who is at risk for speech, language, or learning problems from other children with OME and should evaluate hearing, speech, language, and need for intervention more promptly.

This recommendation is based on case series, the preponderance of benefit over harm, and ethical limitations in studying children with OME who are at risk.

4. Watchful Waiting

Clinicians should manage the child with OME who is not at risk with watchful waiting for 3 months from the date of effusion onset (if known) or diagnosis (if onset is unknown).

This recommendation is based on systematic review of cohort studies and the preponderance of benefit over harm.

5. Medication

Antihistamines and decongestants are ineffective for OME and are not recommended for treatment; antimicrobials and corticosteroids do not have long-term efficacy and are not recommended for routine management.

This recommendation is based on systematic review of randomized, controlled trials and the preponderance of harm over benefit.

6. Hearing and Language

Hearing testing is recommended when OME persists for 3 months or longer or at any time that language delay, learning problems, or a significant hearing loss is suspected in a child with OME; language testing should be conducted for children with hearing loss.

This recommendation is based on cohort studies and the preponderance of benefit over risk.

7. Surveillance

Children with persistent OME who are not at risk should be reexamined at 3- to 6-month intervals until the effusion is no longer present, significant hearing loss is identified, or structural abnormalities of the eardrum or middle ear are suspected.

This recommendation is based on randomized, controlled trials and observational studies with a preponderance of benefit over harm.

8. Referral

When children with OME are referred by the primary care clinician for evaluation by an otolaryngologist, audiologist, or speech-language pathologist, the referring clinician should document the effusion duration and specific reason for referral (evaluation, surgery) and provide additional relevant information such as history of AOM and developmental status of the child.

This option is based on panel consensus and a preponderance of benefit over harm.

9. Surgery

When a child becomes a surgical candidate, tympanostomy tube insertion is the preferred initial procedure; adenoidectomy should not be performed unless a distinct indication exists (nasal obstruction, chronic adenoiditis). Repeat surgery consists of adenoidectomy plus myringotomy, with or without tube insertion. tonsillectomy alone or myringotomy alone should not be used to treat OME.

This recommendation is based on randomized, controlled trials with a preponderance of benefit over harm.

10. CAM

No recommendation is made regarding CAM as a treatment for OME.

There is no recommendation based on lack of scientific evidence documenting efficacy and an uncertain balance of harm and benefit.

11. Allergy Management

No recommendation is made regarding allergy management as a treatment for OME.

There is no recommendation based on insufficient evidence of therapeutic efficacy or a causal relationship between allergy and OME.

Coding Quick Reference for Otitis Media

ICD-10-CM

H65.01	Acute serous otitis media, right ear
H65.02	Left ear
H65.03	Bilateral
H65.04	Recurrent, right ear
H65.05	Recurrent, left ear
H65.06	Recurrent, bilateral

H65.21	Chronic serous otitis media, right ear
H65.22	Left ear
H65.23	Bilateral

H65.91	Unspecified nonsuppurative otitis media, right ear
H65.92	Left ear
H65.93	Bilateral

H66.001	Acute suppurative otitis media without spontaneous rupture of ear drum, right ear
H66.002	Left ear
H66.003	Bilateral
H66.004	Recurrent, right ear
H66.005	Recurrent, left ear
H66.006	Recurrent, bilateral

H66.011	Acute suppurative otitis media with spontaneous rupture of ear drum, right ear
H66.012	Left ear
H66.013	Bilateral
H66.014	Recurrent, right ear
H66.015	Recurrent, left ear
H66.016	Recurrent, bilateral

H67.1	Otitis media in diseases classified elsewhere, right ear
H67.2	Left ear
H67.3	Bilateral

H66.3X1	Other chronic suppurative otitis media, right ear
H66.3X2	Left ear
H66.3X3	Bilateral

Continuum Model for Otitis Media

The following continuum model from *Coding for Pediatrics 2017* has been devised to express the various levels of service for otitis media. This model demonstrates the cumulative effect of the key criteria for each level of service using a single diagnosis as the common denominator. It also shows the importance of other variables, such as patient age, duration and severity of illness, social contexts, and comorbid conditions, that often have key roles in pediatric cases.

Quick Reference for Codes Used in Continuum for Otitis Media—Established Patients				
E/M Code Level	**History**	**Examination**	**MDM**	**Time**
99211[a]	NA	NA	NA	5 minutes
99212	Problem-focused	Problem-focused	Straightforward	10 minutes
99213	Problem-focused	Expanded problem-focused	Low	15 minutes
99214	Detailed	Detailed	Moderate	25 minutes
99215	Detailed	Detailed	High	40 minutes

Abbreviations: E/M, evaluation and management; MDM; medical decision-making; NA, not applicable.

[a] Low level E/M service that may not require the presence of a physician.

Adapted from American Academy of Pediatrics. *Coding for Pediatrics 2017: A Manual for Pediatric Documentation and Payment.* 22nd ed. Elk Grove Village, IL: American Academy of Pediatrics; 2017.

Continuum Model for Otitis Media

CPT® Code Vignette	History	Physical Examination	Medical Decision-making
99211[a] Nursing evaluations Follow-up on serous fluid or hearing loss with tympanogram (Be sure to code tympanogram [**92567**] and/or audiogram [**92551** series] in addition to **99211**.)	1. Chief complaint 2. History of treatment		**Medical Decision-making** 1. Completion of medication 2. No need for further therapy 3. No need for further follow-up
99212 Follow-up otitis media, uncomplicated with primary examination being limited to ears	**Problem focused** 1. Chief complaint 2. History of treatment 3. Difficulties with medication 4. Hearing status	**Problem focused** 1. Ears	**Straightforward** 1. Completion of medication 2. No need for further therapy 3. No need for further follow-up

99213
2-year-old presents with tugging at her right ear. Afebrile. Mild upper respiratory infection symptoms and mild otitis media.
	Problem focused
	1. Chief complaint
	2. Brief HPI plus pertinent ROS
	  a. Symptoms
	  b. Duration of illness
	  c. Home management, including over-the-counter medications, and response
	  d. Additional symptoms from ROS
		Expanded problem focused
		1. Ears
		2. Nose
		3. Throat
		4. Conjunctiva
		5. Overall appearance
			Low complexity
			1. Observation and nonprescription analgesics

99214
Infant presents for suspected third episode within 2–3 months.
Infant presents with fever and cough.
	Detailed
	1. Chief complaint
	2. Detailed HPI plus pertinent ROS and pertinent PFSH
	  a. Symptoms of illness
	  b. Fever, other signs
	  c. Any other medications
	  d. Allergies
	  e. Frequency of similar infection in past and response to treatment
	  f. Environmental factors (eg, tobacco exposure, child care)
	  g. Immunization status
	  h. Feeding history
		Detailed
		1. Overall appearance
		2. Hydration status
		3. Eyes
		4. Ears
		5. Nose
		6. Throat
		7. Lungs
		8. Skin
			Moderate complexity
			1. Treatment including antibiotics and supportive care.
			2. Consider/discuss tympanocentesis (**69420** or **69421**).
			3. Hearing evaluation planned.
			4. Discuss possible referral to an allergist or otolaryngologist for tympanostomy.
			5. Discuss contributing environmental factors and supportive treatment.

Continuum Model for Otitis Media (*continued*)

CPT® Code Vignette	History	Physical Examination	Medical Decision-making

99215
 	
3-month-old presents with high fever, vomiting, irritability.
	Detailed
	1. Chief complaint
	2. Detailed HPI plus pertinent ROS and pertinent PFSH
	  a. Symptoms of illness
	  b. Fever, other signs
	  c. Any other medications
	  d. Allergies
	  e. Frequency of similar infection in past and response to treatment
	  f. Environmental factors (eg, tobacco exposure, child care)
	  g. Immunization status
	  h. Feeding history
		Detailed
		1. Overall appearance
		2. Hydration status
		3. Eyes
		4. Ears
		5. Nose
		6. Throat
		7. Lungs
		8. Skin
			High complexity
			1. Laboratory tests: Consider a complete blood cell count with differential, blood culture, blood urea nitrogen, creatinine, electrolytes, urinalysis with culture, chest radiograph, and possible lumbar puncture based on history and clinical findings.
			2. Antibiotic therapy: Consider parenteral antibiotics.
			3. Consider hospitalization based on history, physical findings, and laboratory studies.
			4. Determine need for follow-up (eg, reassess later in same day by phone or follow-up visit as well as later follow-up).
			5. Attempt oral rehydration in office.

99214 or 99215 **NOTE:** Depending on the variables (ie, time), this example could be reported as **99214** or **99215**. Extended evaluation of child with chronic or recurrent otitis media **NOTE:** Time is the key factor when counseling and/or coordination of care are more than 50% of the face-to-face time with the patient. For **99214**, the total visit time would be 25 minutes; for **99215**, the total time is 40 minutes. You must document time spent on counseling and/or coordination of care and list the areas discussed.	**Detailed** History with extended HPI as in **99214**, but complete ROS and PFSH	**Detailed** or **comprehensive** General or single organ system (ears, nose, mouth, and throat)	**Moderate** or **high complexity** Tests: audiometry and/or tympanometry Extensive discussion of treatment options, including, but not limited to, 1. Continued episodic treatment with antibiotics 2. Myringotomy and tube placement 3. Adenoidectomy 4. Allergy evaluation 5. Steroid therapy with weighing of risk-benefit ratio of various therapies

Abbreviations: CPT, Current Procedural Terminology; HPI, history of present illness; PFSH, past, family, and social history; ROS, review of systems.

[a] *There are no required key components for code 99211; however, the nurse must document his or her history, physical examination, and assessment to support medical necessity.*

Acute Ear Infections and Your Child

Next to the common cold, an ear infection is the most common childhood illness. In fact, most children have at least one ear infection by the time they are 3 years old. Many ear infections clear up without causing any lasting problems.

The following is information from the American Academy of Pediatrics about the symptoms, treatments, and possible complications of acute *otitis media*, a common infection of the middle ear.

How do ear infections develop?

The ear has 3 parts—the outer ear, middle ear, and inner ear. A narrow channel (eustachian tube) connects the middle ear to the back of the nose. When a child has a cold, nose or throat infection, or allergy, the mucus and fluid can enter the eustachian tube causing a buildup of fluid in the middle ear. If bacteria or a virus infects this fluid, it can cause swelling and pain in the ear. This type of ear infection is called *acute otitis media* (*middle ear inflammation*).

Often after the symptoms of acute otitis media clear up, fluid remains in the ear, creating another kind of ear problem called *otitis media with effusion* (*middle ear fluid*). This condition is harder to detect than acute otitis media because except for the fluid and usually some mild hearing loss, there is often no pain or other symptoms present. This fluid may last several months and, in most cases, disappears on its own. The child's hearing then returns to normal.

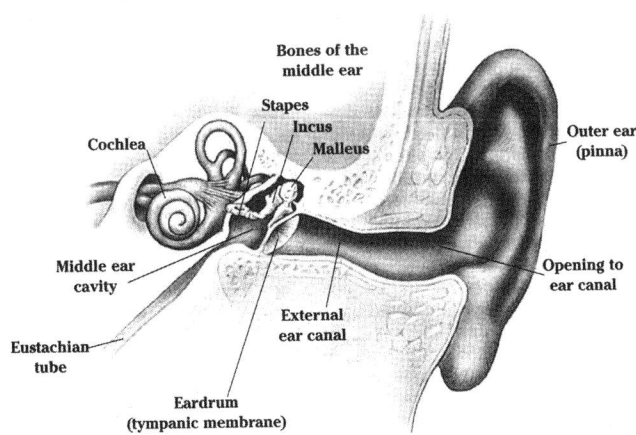

Cross-Section of the Ear

Is my child at risk for developing an ear infection?

Risk factors for developing childhood ear infections include

- **Age.** Infants and young children are more likely to get ear infections than older children. The size and shape of an infant's eustachian tube makes it easier for an infection to develop. Ear infections occur most often in children between 6 months and 3 years of age. Also, the younger a child is at the time of the first ear infection, the greater the chance he will have repeated infections.
- **Family history.** Ear infections can run in families. Children are more likely to have repeated middle ear infections if a parent or sibling also had repeated ear infections.
- **Colds.** Colds often lead to ear infections. Children in group child care settings have a higher chance of passing their colds to each other because they are exposed to more viruses from the other children.
- **Tobacco smoke.** Children who breathe in someone else's tobacco smoke have a higher risk of developing health problems, including ear infections.

How can I reduce the risk of an ear infection?

Some things you can do to help reduce your child's risk of getting an ear infection are

- Breastfeed instead of bottle-feed. Breastfeeding may decrease the risk of frequent colds and ear infections.
- Keep your child away from tobacco smoke, especially in your home or car.
- Throw away pacifiers or limit to daytime use, *if your child is older than 1 year*.
- Keep vaccinations up to date. Vaccines against bacteria (such as pneumococcal vaccine) and viruses (such as influenza vaccine) reduce the number of ear infections in children with frequent infections.

What are the symptoms of an ear infection?

Your child may have many symptoms during an ear infection. Talk with your pediatrician about the best way to treat your child's symptoms.

- **Pain.** The most common symptom of an ear infection is pain. Older children can tell you that their ears hurt. Younger children may only seem irritable and cry. You may notice this more during feedings because sucking and swallowing may cause painful pressure changes in the middle ear.
- **Loss of appetite.** Your child may have less of an appetite because of the ear pain.
- **Trouble sleeping.** Your child may have trouble sleeping because of the ear pain.
- **Fever.** Your child may have a temperature ranging from 100°F (normal) to 104°F.

- **Ear drainage.** You might notice yellow or white fluid, possibly blood-tinged, draining from your child's ear. The fluid may have a foul odor and will look different from normal earwax (which is orange-yellow or reddish-brown). Pain and pressure often decrease after this drainage begins, but this doesn't always mean that the infection is going away. If this happens it's not an emergency, but your child will need to see your pediatrician.
- **Trouble hearing.** During and after an ear infection, your child may have trouble hearing for several weeks. This occurs because the fluid behind the eardrum gets in the way of sound transmission. This is usually temporary and clears up after the fluid from the middle ear drains away.

Important: Your doctor *cannot* diagnose an ear infection over the phone; your child's eardrum must be examined by your doctor to confirm fluid buildup and signs of inflammation.

What causes ear pain?

There are other reasons why your child's ears may hurt besides an ear infection. The following can cause ear pain:

- An infection of the skin of the ear canal, often called "swimmer's ear"
- Reduced pressure in the middle ear from colds or allergies
- A sore throat
- Teething or sore gums
- Inflammation of the eardrum alone during a cold (without fluid buildup)

How are ear infections treated?

Because pain is often the first and most uncomfortable symptom of an ear infection, it's important to help comfort your child by giving her pain medicine. Acetaminophen and ibuprofen are over-the-counter (OTC) pain medicines that may help decrease much of the pain. Be sure to use the right dosage for your child's age and size. *Don't give aspirin to your child.* It has been associated with Reye syndrome, a disease that affects the liver and brain. There are also ear drops that may relieve ear pain for a short time. Ask your pediatrician whether these drops should be used. There is no need to use OTC cold medicines (decongestants and antihistamines), because they don't help clear up ear infections.

Not all ear infections require antibiotics. Some children who don't have a high fever and aren't severely ill may be observed without antibiotics. In most cases, pain and fever will improve in the first 1 to 2 days.

If your child is younger than 2 years, has drainage from the ear, has a fever higher than 102.5°F, seems to be in a lot of pain, is unable to sleep, isn't eating, or is acting ill, it's important to call your pediatrician. If your child is older than 2 years and your child's symptoms are mild, you may wait a couple of days to see if she improves.

Your child's ear pain and fever should improve or go away within 3 days of their onset. If your child's condition doesn't improve within 3 days, or worsens at any time, call your pediatrician. Your pediatrician may wish to see your child and may prescribe an antibiotic to take by mouth, if one wasn't given initially. If an antibiotic was already started, your child may need a different antibiotic. Be sure to follow your pediatrician's instructions closely.

If an antibiotic was prescribed, make sure your child finishes the entire prescription. If you stop the medicine too soon, some of the bacteria that caused the ear infection may still be present and cause an infection to start all over again.

As the infection starts to clear up, your child might feel a "popping" in the ears. This is a normal sign of healing. Children with ear infections don't need to stay home if they are feeling well, as long as a child care provider or someone at school can give them their medicine properly, if needed. If your child needs to travel in an airplane, or wants to swim, contact your pediatrician for specific instructions.

What are signs of hearing problems?

Because your child can have trouble hearing without other symptoms of an ear infection, watch for the following changes in behavior (especially during or after a cold):

- Talking more loudly or softly than usual
- Saying "huh?" or "what?" more than usual
- Not responding to sounds
- Having trouble understanding speech in noisy rooms
- Listening with the TV or radio turned up louder than usual

If you think your child may have difficulty hearing, call your pediatrician. Being able to hear and listen to others talk helps a child learn speech and language. This is especially important during the first few years of life.

Are there complications from ear infections?

Although it's very rare, complications from ear infections can develop, including the following:

- An infection of the inner ear that causes dizziness and imbalance (labyrinthitis)
- An infection of the skull behind the ear (mastoiditis)
- Scarring or thickening of the eardrum
- Loss of feeling or movement in the face (facial paralysis)
- Permanent hearing loss

It's normal for children to have several ear infections when they are young—even as many as 2 separate infections within a few months. Most ear infections that develop in children are minor. Recurring ear infections may be a nuisance, but they usually clear up without any lasting problems. With proper care and treatment, ear infections can usually be managed successfully. But, if your child has one ear infection after another for several months, you may want to talk about other treatment options with your pediatrician.

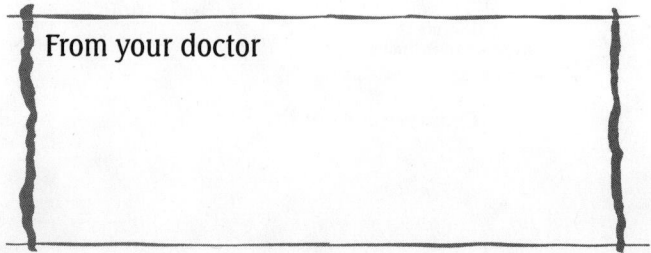

From your doctor

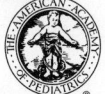

American Academy of Pediatrics

DEDICATED TO THE HEALTH OF ALL CHILDREN™

The American Academy of Pediatrics is an organization of 60,000 primary care pediatricians, pediatric medical subspecialists, and pediatric surgical specialists dedicated to the health, safety, and well-being of infants, children, adolescents, and young adults.

American Academy of Pediatrics
Web site — www.HealthyChildren.org

Middle Ear Fluid and Your Child

The *middle* ear is the space behind the eardrum that is usually filled with air. When a child has middle ear fluid (otitis media with effusion), it means that a watery or mucus-like fluid has collected in the middle ear. *Otitis media* means *middle ear inflammation*, and *effusion* means *fluid*.

Middle ear fluid is **not** the same as an ear infection. An ear infection occurs when middle ear fluid is infected with viruses, bacteria, or both, often during a cold. Children with middle ear fluid have no signs or symptoms of infection. Most children don't have fever or severe pain, but may have mild discomfort or trouble hearing. About 90% of children get middle ear fluid at some time before age 5.

The following is information from the American Academy of Pediatrics about the causes, symptoms, risk reduction, testing, and treatments for middle ear fluid, as well as how middle ear fluid may affect your child's learning.

What causes middle ear fluid?

There is no one cause for middle ear fluid. Often your child's doctor may not know the cause. Middle ear fluid could be caused by

- A past ear infection
- A cold or flu
- Blockage of the eustachian tube (a narrow channel that connects the middle ear to the back of the nose)

What are the symptoms of middle ear fluid?

Many healthy children with middle ear fluid have little or no problems. They usually get better on their own. Often middle ear fluid is found at a regular checkup. Ear discomfort, if present, is usually mild. Your child may be irritable, rub his ears, or have trouble sleeping. Other symptoms include hearing loss, irritability, sleep problems, clumsiness, speech or language problems, and poor school performance. You may notice your child sitting closer to the TV or turning the sound up louder than usual. Sometimes it may seem like your child isn't paying attention to you, especially when at the playground or in a noisy environment.

Talk with your child's doctor if you are concerned about your child's hearing. Keep a record of your child's ear problems. Write down your child's name, child's doctor's name and number, date and type of ear problem or infection, treatment, and results. This may help your child's doctor find the cause of the middle ear fluid.

Can middle ear fluid affect my child's learning?

Some children with middle ear fluid are at risk for delays in speaking or may have problems with learning or schoolwork, especially children with

- Permanent hearing loss not caused by middle ear fluid
- Speech and language delays or disorders
- Developmental delay of social and communication skills disorders (for example, autism spectrum disorders)
- Syndromes that affect cognitive, speech, and language delays (for example, Down syndrome)
- Craniofacial disorders that affect cognitive, speech, and language delays (for example, cleft palate)
- Blindness or visual loss that can't be corrected

If your child is at risk and has ongoing middle ear fluid, her hearing, speech, and language should be checked.

How can I reduce the risk of middle ear fluid?

Children who live with smokers, attend group child care, or use pacifiers have more ear infections. Because some children who have middle ear infections later get middle ear fluid, you may want to

- Keep your child away from tobacco smoke.
- Keep your child away from children who are sick.
- Throw away pacifiers or limit to daytime use, *if your child is older than 1 year*.

Are there special tests to check for middle ear fluid?

Two tests that can check for middle ear fluid are *pneumatic otoscopy* and *tympanometry*. A pneumatic otoscope is the recommended test for middle ear fluid. With this tool, the doctor looks at the eardrum and uses air to see how well the eardrum moves. Tympanometry is another test for middle ear fluid that uses sound to see how well the eardrum moves. An eardrum with fluid behind it doesn't move as well as a normal eardrum. Your child must sit still for both tests; the tests are painless.

Because these tests don't check hearing level, a hearing test may be given, if needed. Hearing tests measure how well your child hears. Although hearing tests don't test for middle ear fluid, they can measure if the fluid is affecting your child's hearing level. The type of hearing test given depends on your child's age and ability to participate.

How can middle ear fluid be treated?

Middle ear fluid can be treated in several ways. Treatment options include observation and tube surgery or adenoid surgery. Because a treatment that works for one child may not work for another, your child's doctor can help you decide which treatment is best for your child and when you should see an ear, nose, and throat (ENT) specialist. If one treatment doesn't work, another treatment can be tried. Ask your child's doctor or ENT specialist about the costs, advantages, and disadvantages of each treatment.

When should middle ear fluid be treated?

Your child is more likely to need treatment for middle ear fluid if she has any of the following:

- Conditions placing her at risk for developmental delays (see "Can middle ear fluid affect my child's learning?")
- Fluid in both ears, especially if present more than 3 months
- Hearing loss or other significant symptoms (see "What are the symptoms of middle ear fluid?")

What treatments are not recommended?

A number of treatments are **not** recommended for young children with middle ear fluid.

- **Medicines** not recommended include antibiotics, decongestants, antihistamines, and steroids (by mouth or in nasal sprays). All of these have side effects and do not cure middle ear fluid.
- **Surgical treatments** not recommended include myringotomy (draining of fluid without placing a tube) and tonsillectomy (removal of the tonsils). If your child's doctor or ENT specialist suggests one of these surgeries, it may be for another medical reason. Ask your doctor why your child needs the surgery.

What about other treatment options?

There is no evidence that complementary and alternative medicine treatments or that treatment for allergies works to decrease middle ear fluid. Some of these treatments may be harmful and many are expensive.

The information contained in this publication should not be used as a substitute for the medical care and advice of your pediatrician. There may be variations in treatment that your pediatrician may recommend based on individual facts and circumstances.

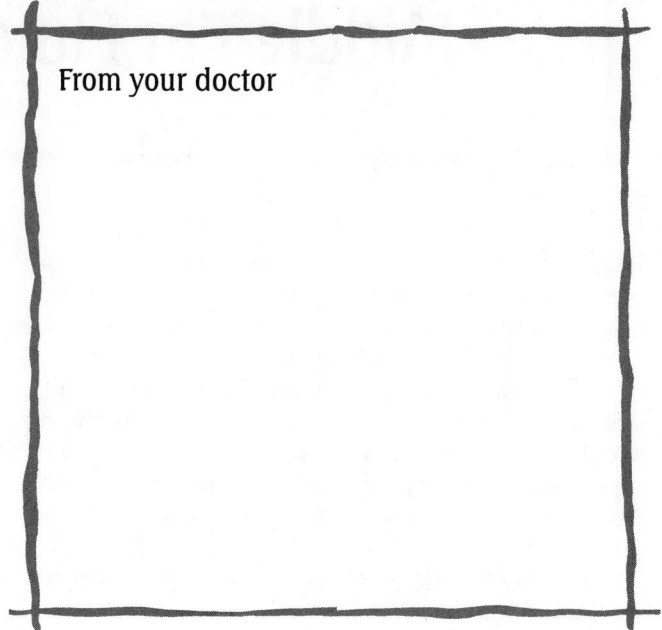

From your doctor

American Academy
of Pediatrics

DEDICATED TO THE HEALTH OF ALL CHILDREN™

The American Academy of Pediatrics is an organization of 60,000 primary care pediatricians, pediatric medical subspecialists, and pediatric surgical specialists dedicated to the health, safety, and well-being of infants, children, adolescents, and young adults.

American Academy of Pediatrics
Web site — www.healthychildren.org

Clinical Practice Guideline for the Diagnosis and Management of Acute Bacterial Sinusitis in Children Aged 1 to 18 Years

- *Clinical Practice Guideline*
  - *PPI: AAP Partnership for Policy Implementation*
    See Appendix 2 for more information.

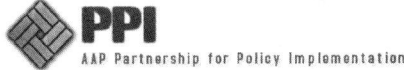

- *Technical Report*

Readers of this clinical practice guideline are urged to review the technical report to enhance the evidence-based decision-making process. The full technical report is available following the clinical practice guideline and on the companion eBook.

CLINICAL PRACTICE GUIDELINE

Clinical Practice Guideline for the Diagnosis and Management of Acute Bacterial Sinusitis in Children Aged 1 to 18 Years

abstract

OBJECTIVE: To update the American Academy of Pediatrics clinical practice guideline regarding the diagnosis and management of acute bacterial sinusitis in children and adolescents.

METHODS: Analysis of the medical literature published since the last version of the guideline (2001).

RESULTS: The diagnosis of acute bacterial sinusitis is made when a child with an acute upper respiratory tract infection (URI) presents with (1) persistent illness (nasal discharge [of any quality] or daytime cough or both lasting more than 10 days without improvement), (2) a worsening course (worsening or new onset of nasal discharge, daytime cough, or fever after initial improvement), or (3) severe onset (concurrent fever [temperature $\geq$39°C/102.2°F] and purulent nasal discharge for at least 3 consecutive days). Clinicians should not obtain imaging studies of any kind to distinguish acute bacterial sinusitis from viral URI, because they do not contribute to the diagnosis; however, a contrast-enhanced computed tomography scan of the paranasal sinuses should be obtained whenever a child is suspected of having orbital or central nervous system complications. The clinician should prescribe antibiotic therapy for acute bacterial sinusitis in children with severe onset or worsening course. The clinician should either prescribe antibiotic therapy or offer additional observation for 3 days to children with persistent illness. Amoxicillin with or without clavulanate is the first-line treatment of acute bacterial sinusitis. Clinicians should reassess initial management if there is either a caregiver report of worsening (progression of initial signs/symptoms or appearance of new signs/symptoms) or failure to improve within 72 hours of initial management. If the diagnosis of acute bacterial sinusitis is confirmed in a child with worsening symptoms or failure to improve, then clinicians may change the antibiotic therapy for the child initially managed with antibiotic or initiate antibiotic treatment of the child initially managed with observation.

CONCLUSIONS: Changes in this revision include the addition of a clinical presentation designated as "worsening course," an option to treat immediately or observe children with persistent symptoms for 3 days before treating, and a review of evidence indicating that imaging is not necessary in children with uncomplicated acute bacterial sinusitis. *Pediatrics* 2013;132:e262–e280

Ellen R. Wald, MD, FAAP, Kimberly E. Applegate, MD, MS, FAAP, Clay Bordley, MD, FAAP, David H. Darrow, MD, DDS, FAAP, Mary P. Glode, MD, FAAP, S. Michael Marcy, MD, FAAP, Carrie E. Nelson, MD, MS, Richard M. Rosenfeld, MD, FAAP, Nader Shaikh, MD, MPH, FAAP, Michael J. Smith, MD, MSCE, FAAP, Paul V. Williams, MD, FAAP, and Stuart T. Weinberg, MD, FAAP

KEY WORDS
acute bacterial sinusitis, sinusitis, antibiotics, imaging, sinus aspiration

ABBREVIATIONS
AAP—American Academy of Pediatrics
AOM—acute otitis media
CT—computed tomography
PCV-13—13-valent pneumococcal conjugate vaccine
RABS—recurrent acute bacterial sinusitis
RCT—randomized controlled trial
URI—upper respiratory tract infection

This document is copyrighted and is property of the American Academy of Pediatrics and its Board of Directors. All authors have filed conflict of interest statements with the American Academy of Pediatrics. Any conflicts have been resolved through a process approved by the Board of Directors. The American Academy of Pediatrics has neither solicited nor accepted any commercial involvement in the development of the content of this publication.

The recommendations in this report do not indicate an exclusive course of treatment or serve as a standard of medical care. Variations, taking into account individual circumstances, may be appropriate.

www.pediatrics.org/cgi/doi/10.1542/peds.2013-1071

doi:10.1542/peds.2013-1071

PEDIATRICS (ISSN Numbers: Print, 0031-4005; Online, 1098-4275).

Copyright © 2013 by the American Academy of Pediatrics

INTRODUCTION

Acute bacterial sinusitis is a common complication of viral upper respiratory infection (URI) or allergic inflammation. Using stringent criteria to define acute sinusitis, it has been observed that between 6% and 7% of children seeking care for respiratory symptoms has an illness consistent with this definition.[1–4]

This clinical practice guideline is a revision of the clinical practice guideline published by the American Academy of Pediatrics (AAP) in 2001.[5] It has been developed by a subcommittee of the Steering Committee on Quality Improvement and Management that included physicians with expertise in the fields of primary care pediatrics, academic general pediatrics, family practice, allergy, epidemiology and informatics, pediatric infectious diseases, pediatric otolaryngology, radiology, and pediatric emergency medicine. None of the participants had financial conflicts of interest, and only money from the AAP was used to fund the development of the guideline. The guideline will be reviewed in 5 years unless new evidence emerges that warrants revision sooner.

The guideline is intended for use in a variety of clinical settings (eg, office, emergency department, hospital) by clinicians who treat pediatric patients. The data on which the recommendations are based are included in a companion technical report, published in the electronic pages.[6] The Partnership for Policy Implementation has developed a series of definitions using accepted health information technology standards to assist in the implementation of this guideline in computer systems and quality measurement efforts. This document is available at: http://www2.aap.org/informatics/PPI.html.

This revision focuses on the diagnosis and management of acute sinusitis in children between 1 and 18 years of age. It does not apply to children with subacute or chronic sinusitis. Similar to the previous guideline, this document does not consider neonates and children younger than 1 year or children with anatomic abnormalities of the sinuses, immunodeficiencies, cystic fibrosis, or primary ciliary dyskinesia. The most significant areas of change from the 2001 guideline are in the addition of a clinical presentation designated as "worsening course," inclusion of new data on the effectiveness of antibiotics in children with acute sinusitis,[4] and a review of evidence indicating that imaging is not necessary to identify those children who will benefit from antimicrobial therapy.

METHODS

The Subcommittee on Management of Sinusitis met in June 2009 to identify research questions relevant to guideline revision. The primary goal was to update the 2001 report by identifying and reviewing additional studies of pediatric acute sinusitis that have been performed over the past decade.

Searches of PubMed were performed by using the same search term as in the 2001 report. All searches were limited to English-language and human studies. Three separate searches were performed to maximize retrieval of the most recent and highest-quality evidence for pediatric sinusitis. The first limited results to all randomized controlled trials (RCTs) from 1966 to 2009, the second to all meta-analyses from 1966 to 2009, and the third to all pediatric studies (limited to ages <18 years) published since the last technical report (1999–2009). Additionally, the Web of Science was queried to identify studies that cited the original AAP guidelines. This literature search was replicated in July 2010

Evidence Quality	Preponderance of Benefit or Harm	Balance of Benefit and Harm
A. Well-designed RCTs or diagnostic studies on relevant population	Strong Recommendation	Option
B. RCTs or diagnostic studies with minor limitations;overwhelmingly consistent evidence from observational studies	Strong Recommendation / Recommendation	Option
C. Observational studies (case-control and cohort design)	Recommendation	Option
D. Expert opinion, case reports, reasoning from first principles	Option	No Rec
X. Exceptional situations where validating studies cannot be performed and there is a clear preponderance of benefit or harm	Strong Recommendation / Recommendation	

FIGURE 1

Levels of recommendations. Rec, recommendation.

and November 2012 to capture recently published studies. The complete results of the literature review are published separately in the technical report.[6] In summary, 17 randomized studies of sinusitis in children were identified and reviewed. Only 3 trials met inclusion criteria. Because of significant heterogeneity among these studies, formal meta-analyses were not pursued.

The results from the literature review were used to guide development of the key action statements included in this document. These action statements were generated by using BRIDGE-Wiz (Building Recommendations in a Developers Guideline Editor, Yale School of Medicine, New Haven, CT), an interactive software tool that leads guideline development through a series of questions that are intended to create a more actionable set of key action statements.[7] BRIDGE-Wiz also incorporates the quality of available evidence into the final determination of the strength of each recommendation.

The AAP policy statement "Classifying Recommendations for Clinical Practice Guidelines" was followed in designating

levels of recommendations (Fig 1).[8] Definitions of evidence-based statements are provided in Table 1. This guideline was reviewed by multiple groups in the AAP and 2 external organizations. Comments were compiled and reviewed by the subcommittee, and relevant changes were incorporated into the guideline.

KEY ACTION STATEMENTS

Key Action Statement 1

Clinicians should make a presumptive diagnosis of acute bacterial sinusitis when a child with an acute URI presents with the following:

- **Persistent illness, ie, nasal discharge (of any quality) or daytime cough or both lasting more than 10 days without improvement;**

OR

- **Worsening course, ie, worsening or new onset of nasal discharge, daytime cough, or fever after initial improvement;**

OR

- **Severe onset, ie, concurrent fever (temperature ≥39°C/102.2°F) and purulent nasal discharge for at least 3 consecutive days (Evidence Quality: B; Recommendation).**

KAS Profile 1

Aggregate evidence quality: B	
Benefit	Diagnosis allows decisions regarding management to be made. Children likely to benefit from antimicrobial therapy will be identified.
Harm	Inappropriate diagnosis may lead to unnecessary treatment. A missed diagnosis may lead to persistent infection or complications
Cost	Inappropriate diagnosis may lead to unnecessary cost of antibiotics. A missed diagnosis leads to cost of persistent illness (loss of time from school and work) or cost of caring for complications.
Benefits-harm assessment	Preponderance of benefit.
Value judgments	None.
Role of patient preference	Limited.
Intentional vagueness	None.
Exclusions	Children aged <1 year or older than 18 years and with underlying conditions.
Strength	Recommendation.

TABLE 1 Guideline Definitions for Evidence-Based Statements

Statement	Definition	Implication
Strong recommendation	A strong recommendation in favor of a particular action is made when the anticipated benefits of the recommended intervention clearly exceed the harms (as a strong recommendation against an action is made when the anticipated harms clearly exceed the benefits) and the quality of the supporting evidence is excellent. In some clearly identified circumstances, strong recommendations may be made when high-quality evidence is impossible to obtain and the anticipated benefits strongly outweigh the harms.	Clinicians should follow a strong recommendation unless a clear and compelling rationale for an alternative approach is present.
Recommendation	A recommendation in favor of a particular action is made when the anticipated benefits exceed the harms but the quality of evidence is not as strong. Again, in some clearly identified circumstances, recommendations may be made when high-quality evidence is impossible to obtain but the anticipated benefits outweigh the harms.	Clinicians would be prudent to follow a recommendation, but should remain alert to new information and sensitive to patient preferences.
Option	Options define courses that may be taken when either the quality of evidence is suspect or carefully performed studies have shown little clear advantage to one approach over another.	Clinicians should consider the option in their decision-making, and patient preference may have a substantial role.
No recommendation	No recommendation indicates that there is a lack of pertinent published evidence and that the anticipated balance of benefits and harms is presently unclear.	Clinicians should be alert to new published evidence that clarifies the balance of benefit versus harm.

The purpose of this action statement is to guide the practitioner in making a diagnosis of acute bacterial sinusitis on the basis of stringent clinical criteria. To develop criteria to be used in distinguishing episodes of acute bacterial sinusitis from other common respiratory infections, it is helpful to describe the features of an uncomplicated viral URI. Viral URIs are usually characterized by nasal symptoms (discharge and congestion/obstruction) or cough or both. Most often, the nasal discharge begins as clear and watery. Often, however, the quality of nasal discharge changes during the course of the illness. Typically, the nasal discharge becomes thicker and more mucoid and may become purulent (thick, colored, and opaque) for several days. Then the situation reverses, with the purulent discharge becoming mucoid and then clear again or simply resolving. The transition from clear to purulent to clear again occurs in uncomplicated viral URIs without the use of antimicrobial therapy.

Fever, when present in uncomplicated viral URI, tends to occur early in the illness, often in concert with other constitutional symptoms such as headache and myalgias. Typically, the fever and constitutional symptoms disappear in the first 24 to 48 hours, and the respiratory symptoms become more prominent (Fig 2).

The course of most uncomplicated viral URIs is 5 to 7 days.[9–12] As shown in Fig 2, respiratory symptoms usually peak in severity by days 3 to 6 and then begin to improve; however, resolving symptoms and signs may persist in some patients after day 10.[9,10]

Symptoms of acute bacterial sinusitis and uncomplicated viral URI overlap considerably, and therefore it is their persistence without improvement that suggests a diagnosis of acute sinusitis.[9,10,13] Such symptoms include

nasal discharge (of any quality: thick or thin, serous, mucoid, or purulent) or daytime cough (which may be worse at night) or both. Bad breath, fatigue, headache, and decreased appetite, although common, are not specific indicators of acute sinusitis.[14] Physical examination findings are also not particularly helpful in distinguishing sinusitis from uncomplicated URIs. Erythema and swelling of the nasal turbinates are nonspecific findings.[14] Percussion of the sinuses is not useful. Transillumination of the sinuses is difficult to perform correctly in children and has been shown to be unreliable.[15,16] Nasopharyngeal cultures do not reliably predict the etiology of acute bacterial sinusitis.[14,16]

Only a minority (~6%–7%) of children presenting with symptoms of URI will meet criteria for persistence.[3,4,11] As a result, before diagnosing acute bacterial sinusitis, it is important for the practitioner to attempt to (1) differentiate between sequential episodes of uncomplicated viral URI (which may seem to coalesce in the mind of the patient or parent) from the onset of acute bacterial sinusitis with persistent symptoms and (2) establish whether the symptoms are clearly not improving.

A worsening course of signs and symptoms, termed "double sickening," in the context of a viral URI is another presentation of acute bacterial sinusitis.[13,17] Affected children experience substantial and acute worsening of

respiratory symptoms (nasal discharge or nasal congestion or daytime cough) or a new fever, often on the sixth or seventh day of illness, after initial signs of recovery from an uncomplicated viral URI. Support for this definition comes from studies in children and adults, for whom antibiotic treatment of worsening symptoms after a period of apparent improvement was associated with better outcomes.[4]

Finally, some children with acute bacterial sinusitis may present with severe onset, ie, concurrent high fever (temperature >39°C) and purulent nasal discharge. These children usually are ill appearing and need to be distinguished from children with uncomplicated viral infections that are unusually severe. If fever is present in uncomplicated viral URIs, it tends to be present early in the illness, usually accompanied by other constitutional symptoms, such as headache and myalgia.[9,13,18] Generally, the constitutional symptoms resolve in the first 48 hours and then the respiratory symptoms become prominent. In most uncomplicated viral infections, including influenza, purulent nasal discharge does not appear for several days. Accordingly, it is the concurrent presentation of high fever and purulent nasal discharge for the first 3 to 4 days of an acute URI that helps to define the severe onset of acute bacterial sinusitis.[13,16,18] This presentation in children is the corollary to acute onset of headache, fever, and facial pain in adults with acute sinusitis.

Allergic and nonallergic rhinitis are predisposing causes of some cases of acute bacterial sinusitis in childhood. In addition, at their onset, these conditions may be mistaken for acute bacterial sinusitis. A family history of atopic conditions, seasonal occurrences, or occurrences with exposure to common allergens and other

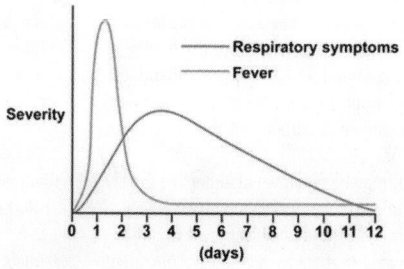

FIGURE 2
Uncomplicated viral URI.

allergic diatheses in the index patient (eczema, atopic dermatitis, asthma) may suggest the presence of non-infectious rhinitis. The patient may have complaints of pruritic eyes and nasal mucosa, which will provide a clue to the likely etiology of the condition. On physical examination, there may be a prominent nasal crease, allergic shiners, cobblestoning of the conjunctiva or pharyngeal wall, or pale nasal mucosa as other indicators of the diagnosis.

Key Action Statement 2A

Clinicians should not obtain imaging studies (plain films, contrast-enhanced computed tomography [CT], MRI, or ultrasonography) to distinguish acute bacterial sinusitis from viral URI (Evidence Quality: B; Strong Recommendation).

KAS Profile 2A

Aggregate evidence quality: B; overwhelmingly consistent evidence from observational studies.	
Benefit	Avoids exposure to radiation and costs of studies. Avoids unnecessary therapy for false-positive diagnoses.
Harm	None.
Cost	Avoids cost of imaging.
Benefits-harm assessment	Exclusive benefit.
Value judgments	Concern for unnecessary radiation and costs.
Role of patient preference	Limited. Parents may value a negative study and avoidance of antibiotics as worthy of radiation but panel disagrees.
Intentional vagueness	None.
Exclusions	Patients with complications of sinusitis.
Strength	Strong recommendation.

The purpose of this key action statement is to discourage the practitioner from obtaining imaging studies in children with uncomplicated acute bacterial sinusitis. As emphasized in Key Action Statement 1, acute bacterial sinusitis in children is a diagnosis that is made on the basis of stringent clinical criteria that describe signs, symptoms, and temporal patterns of a URI. Although historically imaging has been used as a confirmatory or diagnostic modality in children

suspected to have acute bacterial sinusitis, it is no longer recommended. The membranes that line the nose are continuous with the membranes (mucosa) that line the sinus cavities, the middle ear, the nasopharynx, and the oropharynx. When an individual experiences a viral URI, there is inflammation of the nasal mucosa and, often, the mucosa of the middle ear and paranasal sinuses as well. The continuity of the mucosa of the upper respiratory tract is responsible for the controversy regarding the usefulness of images of the paranasal sinuses in contributing to a diagnosis of acute bacterial sinusitis.

As early as the 1940s, observations were made regarding the frequency of abnormal sinus radiographs in healthy children without signs or symptoms of current respiratory disease.[19] In addition, several investigators in the 1970s and 1980s observed that children with uncomplicated viral URI had frequent abnormalities of the paranasal sinuses on plain radiographs.[20–22] These abnormalities were the same as those considered to be diagnostic of acute bacterial sinusitis (diffuse opacification, mucosal swelling of at least 4 mm, or an air-fluid level).[16]

As technology advanced and CT scanning of the central nervous system and skull became prevalent, several studies reported on incidental abnormalities of the paranasal sinuses that were observed in children.[23,24] Gwaltney et al[25] showed striking abnormalities (including air-fluid levels) in sinus CT scans of young adults with uncomplicated colds. Manning et al[26] evaluated children undergoing either CT or MRI of the head for indications other than respiratory complaints or suspected sinusitis. Each patient underwent rhinoscopy and otoscopy before imaging and each patient's parent was asked to fill out a questionnaire regarding recent symptoms of URI. Sixty-two percent of patients overall had physical findings or history consistent with an upper respiratory inflammatory process, and 55% of the total group showed some abnormalities on sinus imaging; 33% showed pronounced mucosal thickening or an air-fluid level. Gordts et al[27] made similar observations in children undergoing MRI. Finally, Kristo et al[28] performed MRI in children with URIs and confirmed the high frequency (68%) of major abnormalities seen in the paranasal sinuses.

In summary, when the paranasal sinuses are imaged, either with plain radiographs, contrast-enhanced CT, or MRI in children with uncomplicated URI, the majority of studies will be significantly abnormal with the same kind of findings that are associated with bacterial infection of the sinuses. Accordingly, although normal radiographs or CT or MRI results can ensure that a patient with respiratory symptoms does not have acute bacterial sinusitis, an abnormal image cannot confirm the diagnosis. Therefore, it is not necessary to perform imaging in children with uncomplicated episodes of clinical sinusitis. Similarly, the high likelihood of an abnormal imaging result in a child with an uncomplicated URI indicates that radiographic studies not be performed in an attempt to eliminate the diagnosis of sinusitis.

Key Action Statement 2B

Clinicians should obtain a contrast-enhanced CT scan of the paranasal sinuses and/or an MRI with contrast whenever a child is suspected of having orbital or central nervous system complications of acute bacterial sinusitis (Evidence Quality: B; Strong Recommendation).

KAS Profile 2B

Aggregate evidence quality: B; overwhelmingly consistent evidence from observational studies.	
Benefit	Determine presence of abscesses, which may require surgical intervention; avoid sequelae because of appropriate aggressive management.
Harm	Exposure to ionizing radiation for CT scans; need for sedation for MRI.
Cost	Direct cost of studies.
Benefits-harm assessment	Preponderance of benefit.
Value judgments	Concern for significant complication that may be unrecognized and, therefore, not treated appropriately.
Role of patient preference	Limited.
Intentional vagueness	None.
Exclusions	None.
Strength	Strong recommendation.

The purpose of this key action statement is to have the clinician obtain contrast-enhanced CT images when children are suspected of having serious complications of acute bacterial sinusitis. The most common complication of acute sinusitis involves the orbit in children with ethmoid sinusitis who are younger than 5 years.[29–31] Orbital complications should be suspected when the child presents with a swollen eye, especially if accompanied by proptosis or impaired function of the extraocular muscles. Orbital complications of acute sinusitis have been divided into 5 categories: sympathetic effusion, subperiosteal abscess, orbital cellulitis, orbital abscess, and cavernous sinus thrombosis.[32] Although sympathetic effusion (inflammatory edema) is categorized as an orbital complication, the site of infection remains confined to the sinus cavities; eye swelling is attributable to the impedance of venous drainage secondary to congestion within the ethmoid sinuses. Alternative terms for sympathetic effusion (inflammatory edema) are preseptal or periorbital cellulitis. The remaining "true" orbital complications are best visualized by contrast-enhanced CT scanning.

Intracranial complications of acute sinusitis, which are substantially less common than orbital complications, are more serious, with higher morbidity and mortality than those involving the orbit. Intracranial complications should be suspected in the patient who presents with a very severe headache, photophobia, seizures, or other focal neurologic findings. Intracranial complications include subdural empyema, epidural empyema, venous thrombosis, brain abscess, and meningitis.[29] Typically, patients with intracranial complications of acute bacterial sinusitis are previously healthy adolescent males with frontal sinusitis.[33,34]

There have been no head-to-head comparisons of the diagnostic accuracy of contrast-enhanced CT scanning to MRI with contrast in the evaluation of orbital and intracranial complications of sinusitis in children. In general, the contrast-enhanced CT scan has been the preferred imaging study when complications of sinusitis are suspected.[35,36] However, there are documented cases in which a contrast-enhanced CT scan has not revealed the abnormality responsible for the clinical presentation and the MRI with contrast has, especially for intracranial complications and rarely for orbital complications.[37,38] Accordingly, the most recent appropriateness criteria from the American College of Radiology endorse both MRI with contrast and contrast-enhanced CT as complementary examinations when evaluating potential complications of sinusitis.[35] The availability and speed of obtaining the contrast-enhanced CT are desirable; however, there is increasing concern regarding exposure to radiation. The MRI, although very sensitive, takes longer than the contrast-enhanced CT and often requires sedation in young children (which carries its own risks). In older children and adolescents who may not require sedation, MRI with contrast, if available, may be preferred when intracranial complications are likely. Furthermore, MRI with contrast should be performed when there is persistent clinical concern or incomplete information has been provided by the contrast-enhanced CT scan.

Key Action Statement 3

Initial Management of Acute Bacterial Sinusitis

3A: "Severe onset and worsening course" acute bacterial sinusitis. The clinician should prescribe antibiotic therapy for acute bacterial sinusitis in children with severe onset or worsening course (signs, symptoms, or both) (Evidence Quality: B; Strong Recommendation).

KAS Profile 3A

Aggregate evidence quality: B; randomized controlled trials with limitations.	
Benefit	Increase clinical cures, shorten illness duration, and may prevent suppurative complications in a high-risk patient population.
Harm	Adverse effects of antibiotics.
Cost	Direct cost of therapy.
Benefits-harm assessment	Preponderance of benefit.
Value judgments	Concern for morbidity and possible complications if untreated.
Role of patient preference	Limited.
Intentional vagueness	None.
Exclusions	None.
Strength	Strong recommendation.

3B: "Persistent illness." The clinician should either prescribe antibiotic therapy OR offer additional outpatient observation for 3 days to children with persistent illness (nasal discharge of any quality or cough or both for at least 10 days without evidence of improvement) (Evidence Quality: B; Recommendation).

The purpose of this section is to offer guidance on initial management of persistent illness sinusitis by helping clinicians choose between the following 2 strategies:

1. Antibiotic therapy, defined as initial treatment of acute bacterial sinusitis with antibiotics, with the intent of starting antibiotic therapy as soon as possible after the encounter.

2. Additional outpatient observation, defined as initial management of acute bacterial sinusitis limited to continued observation for 3 days, with commencement of antibiotic therapy if either the child does not improve clinically within several days of diagnosis or if there is clinical worsening of the child's condition at any time.

In contrast to the 2001 AAP guideline,[5] which recommended antibiotic therapy for all children diagnosed with acute bacterial sinusitis, this guideline allows for additional observation of children presenting with persistent illness (nasal discharge of any quality or daytime cough or both for at least 10 days without evidence of improvement). In both guidelines, however, children presenting with severe or worsening illness (which was not defined explicitly in the 2001 guideline[5]) are to receive antibiotic therapy. The rationale for this approach (Table 2) is discussed below.

Antibiotic Therapy for Acute Bacterial Sinusitis

In the United States, antibiotics are prescribed for 82% of children with acute sinusitis.[39] The rationale for antibiotic therapy of acute bacterial sinusitis is based on the recovery of bacteria in high density ($\geq 10^4$ colony-forming units/mL) in 70% of maxillary sinus aspirates obtained from children with a clinical syndrome characterized by persistent nasal discharge, daytime cough, or both.[16,40] Children who present with severe-onset acute bacterial sinusitis are presumed to have bacterial infection, because a temperature of at least 39°C/102.2°F coexisting for at least 3 consecutive days with purulent nasal discharge is not consistent with the well-documented pattern of acute viral URI. Similarly, children with worsening-course acute bacterial sinusitis have a clinical course that is also not consistent with the steady improvement that characterizes an uncomplicated viral URI.[9,10]

KAS Profile 3B

Aggregate evidence quality: B; randomized controlled trials with limitations.	
Benefit	Antibiotics increase the chance of improvement or cure at 10 to 14 days (number needed to treat, 3–5); additional observation may avoid the use of antibiotics with attendant cost and adverse effects.
Harm	Antibiotics have adverse effects (number needed to harm, 3) and may increase bacterial resistance. Observation may prolong illness and delay start of needed antibiotic therapy.
Cost	Direct cost of antibiotics as well as cost of adverse reactions; indirect costs of delayed recovery when observation is used.
Benefits-harm assessment	Preponderance of benefit (because both antibiotic therapy and additional observation with rescue antibiotic, if needed, are appropriate management).
Value judgments	Role for additional brief observation period for selected children with persistent illness sinusitis, similar to what is recommended for acute otitis media, despite the lack of randomized trials specifically comparing additional observation with immediate antibiotic therapy and longer duration of illness before presentation.
Role of patient preference	Substantial role in shared decision-making that should incorporate illness severity, child's quality of life, and caregiver values and concerns.
Intentional vagueness	None.
Exclusions	Children who are excluded from randomized clinical trials of acute bacterial sinusitis, as defined in the text.
Strength	Recommendation.

Three RCTs have compared antibiotic therapy with placebo for the initial management of acute bacterial sinusitis in children. Two trials by Wald et al[4,41] found an increase in cure or improvement after antibiotic therapy compared with placebo with a number needed to treat of 3 to 5 children. Most children in these studies had persistent acute bacterial sinusitis, but children with severe or worsening illness were also included. Conversely, Garbutt et al,[42] who studied only children with persistent acute bacterial sinusitis, found no difference in outcomes for antibiotic versus placebo. Another RCT by Kristo et al,[43] often cited as showing no benefit from antibiotics for acute bacterial sinusitis, will not be considered further because of methodologic flaws, including weak entry criteria and inadequate dosing of antibiotic treatment.

The guideline recommends antibiotic therapy for severe or worsening acute bacterial sinusitis because of the benefits revealed in RCTs[4,41] and a theoretically higher risk of suppurative complications than for children who present with persistent symptoms. Orbital and intracranial complications of acute bacterial sinusitis have not been observed in RCTs, even when placebo was administered; however, sample sizes have inadequate power to preclude an increased risk. This risk, however, has caused some investigators to exclude children with severe acute bacterial sinusitis from trial entry.[42]

Additional Observation for Persistent Onset Acute Bacterial Sinusitis

The guideline recommends either antibiotic therapy or an additional brief period of observation as initial management strategies for children with persistent acute bacterial sinusitis because, although there are benefits to antibiotic therapy (number needed to treat, 3–5), some children improve on their own, and the risk of suppurative

complications is low.[4,41] Symptoms of persistent acute bacterial sinusitis may be mild and have varying effects on a given child's quality of life, ranging from slight (mild cough, nasal discharge) to significant (sleep disturbance, behavioral changes, school or child care absenteeism). The benefits of antibiotic therapy in some trials[4,41] must also be balanced against an increased risk of adverse events (number need to harm, 3), most often self-limited diarrhea, but also including occasional rash.[4]

Choosing between antibiotic therapy or additional observation for initial management of persistent illness sinusitis presents an opportunity for shared decision-making with families (Table 2). Factors that might influence this decision include symptom severity, the child's quality of life, recent antibiotic use, previous experience or outcomes with acute bacterial sinusitis, cost of antibiotics, ease of administration, caregiver concerns about potential adverse effects of antibiotics, persistence of respiratory symptoms, or development of complications. Values and preferences expressed by the caregiver should be taken into consideration (Table 3).

Children with persistent acute bacterial sinusitis who received antibiotic therapy in the previous 4 weeks, those with concurrent bacterial infection (eg, pneumonia, suppurative cervical adenitis, group A streptococcal pharyngitis, or acute otitis media), those with actual or

suspected complications of acute bacterial sinusitis, or those with underlying conditions should generally be managed with antibiotic therapy. The latter group includes children with asthma, cystic fibrosis, immunodeficiency, previous sinus surgery, or anatomic abnormalities of the upper respiratory tract.

Limiting antibiotic use in children with persistent acute bacterial sinusitis who may improve on their own reduces common antibiotic-related adverse events, such as diarrhea, diaper dermatitis, and skin rash. The most recent RCT of acute bacterial sinusitis in children[4] found adverse events of 44% with antibiotic and 14% with placebo.

Limiting antibiotics may also reduce the prevalence of resistant bacterial pathogens. Although this is always a desirable goal, no increase in resistant bacterial species was observed within the group of children treated with a single course of antimicrobial agents (compared with those receiving placebo) in 2 recent large studies of antibiotic versus placebo for children with acute otitis media.[44,45]

Key Action Statement 4

Clinicians should prescribe amoxicillin with or without clavulanate as first-line treatment when a decision has been made to initiate antibiotic treatment of acute bacterial sinusitis (Evidence Quality: B; Recommendation).

KAS Profile 4

Aggregate evidence quality: B; randomized controlled trials with limitations.	
Benefit	Increase clinical cures with narrowest spectrum drug; stepwise increase in broadening spectrum as risk factors for resistance increase.
Harm	Adverse effects of antibiotics including development of hypersensitivity.
Cost	Direct cost of antibiotic therapy.
Benefits-harm assessment	Preponderance of benefit.
Value judgments	Concerns for not encouraging resistance if possible.
Role of patient preference	Potential for shared decision-making that should incorporate the caregiver's experiences and values.
Intentional vagueness	None.
Exclusions	May include allergy or intolerance.
Strength	Recommendation.

TABLE 2 Recommendations for Initial Use of Antibiotics for Acute Bacterial Sinusitis

Clinical Presentation	Severe Acute Bacterial Sinusitis[a]	Worsening Acute Bacterial Sinusitis[b]	Persistent Acute Bacterial Sinusitis[c]
Uncomplicated acute bacterial sinusitis without coexisting illness	Antibiotic therapy	Antibiotic therapy	Antibiotic therapy or additional observation for 3 days[d]
Acute bacterial sinusitis with orbital or intracranial complications	Antibiotic therapy	Antibiotic therapy	Antibiotic therapy
Acute bacterial sinusitis with coexisting acute otitis media, pneumonia, adenitis, or streptococcal pharyngitis	Antibiotic therapy	Antibiotic therapy	Antibiotic therapy

[a] Defined as temperature ≥39°C and purulent (thick, colored, and opaque) nasal discharge present concurrently for at least 3 consecutive days.

[b] Defined as nasal discharge or daytime cough with sudden worsening of symptoms (manifested by new-onset fever ≥38°C/100.4°F or substantial increase in nasal discharge or cough) after having experienced transient improvement of symptoms.

[c] Defined as nasal discharge (of any quality), daytime cough (which may be worse at night), or both, persisting for >10 days without improvement.

[d] Opportunity for shared decision-making with the child's family; if observation is offered, a mechanism must be in place to ensure follow-up and begin antibiotics if the child worsens at any time or fails to improve within 3 days of observation.

The purpose of this key action statement is to guide the selection of antimicrobial therapy once the diagnosis of acute bacterial sinusitis has been made. The microbiology of acute bacterial sinusitis was determined nearly 30 years ago through direct maxillary sinus aspiration in children with compatible signs and symptoms. The major bacterial pathogens recovered at that time were *Streptococcus pneumoniae* in approximately 30% of children and nontypeable *Haemophilus influenzae* and *Moraxella catarrhalis* in approximately 20% each.[16,40] Aspirates from the remaining 25% to 30% of children were sterile.

Maxillary sinus aspiration is rarely performed at the present time unless the course of the infection is unusually prolonged or severe. Although some authorities have recommended obtaining cultures from the middle meatus to determine the cause of a maxillary sinus infection, there are no data in children with acute bacterial sinusitis that have compared such cultures with cultures of a maxillary sinus aspirate. Furthermore, there are data indicating that the middle meatus in healthy children is commonly colonized with *S pneumoniae*, *H influenzae*, and *M catarrhalis*.[46]

Recent estimates of the microbiology of acute sinusitis have, of necessity, been based primarily on that of acute otitis media (AOM), a condition with relatively easy access to infective fluid through performance of tympanocentesis and one with a similar pathogenesis to acute bacterial sinusitis.[47,48] The 3 most common bacterial pathogens recovered from the middle ear fluid of children with AOM are the same as those that have been associated with acute bacterial sinusitis: *S pneumoniae*, nontypeable *H influenzae*, and *M catarrhalis*.[49] The proportion of each has varied from study to study depending on criteria used for diagnosis of AOM, patient characteristics, and bacteriologic techniques. Recommendations since the year 2000 for the routine use in infants of 7-valent and, more recently, 13-valent pneumococcal conjugate vaccine (PCV-13) have been associated with a decrease in recovery of *S pneumoniae* from ear fluid of children with AOM and a relative increase in the incidence of infections attributable to *H influenzae*.[50] Thus, on the basis of the proportions of bacteria

found in middle ear infections, it is estimated that *S pneumoniae* and *H influenzae* are currently each responsible for approximately 30% of cases of acute bacterial sinusitis in children, and *M catarrhalis* is responsible for approximately 10%. These percentages are contingent on the assumption that approximately one-quarter of aspirates of maxillary sinusitis would still be sterile, as reported in earlier studies. *Staphylococcus aureus* is rarely isolated from sinus aspirates in children with acute bacterial sinusitis, and with the exception of acute maxillary sinusitis associated with infections of dental origin,[51] respiratory anaerobes are also rarely recovered.[40,52] Although *S aureus* is a very infrequent cause of acute bacterial sinusitis in children, it is a significant pathogen in the orbital and intracranial complications of sinusitis. The reasons for this discrepancy are unknown.

Antimicrobial susceptibility patterns for *S pneumoniae* vary considerably from community to community. Isolates obtained from surveillance centers nationwide indicate that, at the present time, 10% to 15% of upper respiratory tract isolates of *S pneumoniae* are nonsusceptible to penicillin[53,54]; however, values for penicillin nonsusceptibility as high as 50% to 60% have been reported in some areas.[55,56] Of the organisms that are resistant, approximately half are highly resistant to penicillin and the remaining half are intermediate in resistance.[53,54,56–59] Between 10% and 42% of *H influenzae*[56–59] and close to 100% of *M catarrhalis* are likely to be β-lactamase positive and nonsusceptible to amoxicillin. Because of dramatic geographic variability in the prevalence of β-lactamase–positive *H influenzae*, it is extremely desirable for the practitioner to be familiar with local patterns of susceptibility. Risk factors for the presence of organisms likely to be resistant to amoxicillin include attendance at child care, receipt of antimicrobial treatment within the previous 30 days, and age younger than 2 years.[50,55,60]

Amoxicillin remains the antimicrobial agent of choice for first-line treatment of uncomplicated acute bacterial sinusitis in situations in which antimicrobial resistance is not suspected. This recommendation is based on amoxicillin's effectiveness, safety, acceptable taste, low cost, and relatively narrow microbiologic spectrum. For children aged 2 years or older with uncomplicated acute bacterial sinusitis that is mild to moderate in degree of severity who do not attend child care and who have not been treated with an antimicrobial agent within the last 4 weeks, amoxicillin is recommended at a standard dose of 45 mg/kg per day in 2 divided doses. In communities with a high prevalence of nonsusceptible *S pneumoniae* (>10%, including intermediate- and high-level resistance), treatment may be initiated at 80 to 90 mg/kg per day in 2 divided doses, with a maximum of 2 g per dose.[55] This high-dose amoxicillin therapy is likely to achieve sinus fluid concentrations that are adequate to overcome the resistance of *S pneumoniae*, which is attributable to alteration in penicillin-binding proteins on the basis of data derived from patients with AOM.[61] If, within the next several years after licensure of PCV-13, a continuing decrease in isolates of *S pneumoniae* (including a decrease in isolates of nonsusceptible *S pneumoniae*) and an increase in β-lactamase–producing *H influenzae* are observed, standard-dose amoxicillin-clavulanate (45 mg/kg per day) may be most appropriate.

Patients presenting with moderate to severe illness as well as those younger than 2 years, attending child care, or who have recently been treated with

an antimicrobial may receive high-dose amoxicillin-clavulanate (80–90 mg/kg per day of the amoxicillin component with 6.4 mg/kg per day of clavulanate in 2 divided doses with a maximum of 2 g per dose). The potassium clavulanate levels are adequate to inhibit all β-lactamase–producing *H influenzae* and *M catarrhalis*.[56,59]

A single 50-mg/kg dose of ceftriaxone, given either intravenously or intramuscularly, can be used for children who are vomiting, unable to tolerate oral medication, or unlikely to be adherent to the initial doses of antibiotic.[62–64] The 3 major bacterial pathogens involved in acute bacterial sinusitis are susceptible to ceftriaxone in 95% to 100% of cases.[56,58,59] If clinical improvement is observed at 24 hours, an oral antibiotic can be substituted to complete the course of therapy. Children who are still significantly febrile or symptomatic at 24 hours may require additional parenteral doses before switching to oral therapy.

The treatment of patients with presumed allergy to penicillin has been controversial. However, recent publications indicate that the risk of a serious allergic reaction to second- and third-generation cephalosporins in patients with penicillin or amoxicillin allergy appears to be almost nil and no greater than the risk among patients without such allergy.[65–67] Thus, patients allergic to amoxicillin with a non–type 1 (late or delayed, >72 hours) hypersensitivity reaction can safely be treated with cefdinir, cefuroxime, or cefpodoxime.[66–68] Patients with a history of a serious type 1 immediate or accelerated (anaphylactoid) reaction to amoxicillin can also safely be treated with cefdinir, cefuroxime, or cefpodoxime. In both circumstances, clinicians may wish to determine individual tolerance by referral to an allergist for penicillin

and/or cephalosporin skin-testing before initiation of therapy.[66–68] The susceptibility of *S pneumoniae* to cefdinir, cefpodoxime, and cefuroxime varies from 60% to 75%,[56–59] and the susceptibility of *H influenzae* to these agents varies from 85% to 100%.[56,58] In young children (<2 years) with a serious type 1 hypersensitivity to penicillin and moderate or more severe sinusitis, it may be prudent to use a combination of clindamycin (or linezolid) and cefixime to achieve the most comprehensive coverage against both resistant *S pneumoniae* and *H influenzae*. Linezolid has excellent activity against all *S pneumoniae*, including penicillin-resistant strains, but lacks activity against *H influenzae* and *M catarrhalis*. Alternatively, a quinolone, such as levofloxacin, which has a high level of activity against both *S pneumoniae* and *H influenzae*, may be prescribed.[57,58] Although the use of quinolones is usually restricted because of concerns for toxicity, cost, and emerging resistance, their use in this circumstance can be justified.

Pneumococcal and *H influenzae* surveillance studies have indicated that resistance of these organisms to trimethoprim-sulfamethoxazole and azithromycin is sufficient to preclude their use for treatment of acute bacterial sinusitis in patients with penicillin hypersensitivity.[56,58,59,69]

The optimal duration of antimicrobial therapy for patients with acute bacterial sinusitis has not received systematic study. Recommendations based on clinical observations have varied widely, from 10 to 28 days of treatment. An alternative suggestion has been made that antibiotic therapy be continued for 7 days after the patient becomes free of signs and symptoms.[5] This strategy has the advantage of individualizing the treatment of each patient, results in a minimum course of 10 days, and avoids prolonged antimicrobial therapy in patients who are asymptomatic and therefore unlikely to adhere to the full course of treatment.[5]

Patients who are acutely ill and appear toxic when first seen (see below) can be managed with 1 of 2 options. Consultation can be requested from an otolaryngologist for consideration of maxillary sinus aspiration (with appropriate analgesia/anesthesia) to obtain a sample of sinus secretions for Gram stain, culture, and susceptibility testing so that antimicrobial therapy can be adjusted precisely. Alternatively, inpatient therapy can be initiated with intravenous cefotaxime or ceftriaxone, with referral to an otolaryngologist if the patient's condition worsens or fails to show improvement within 48 hours. If a complication is suspected, management will differ depending on the site and severity.

A recent guideline was published by the Infectious Diseases Society of America for acute bacterial rhinosinusitis in children and adults.[70] Their recommendation for initial empirical antimicrobial therapy for acute bacterial sinusitis in children was amoxicillin-clavulanate based on the concern that there is an increasing prevalence of *H influenzae* as a cause of sinusitis since introduction of the pneumococcal conjugate vaccines and an increasing prevalence of β-lactamase production among these strains. In contrast, this guideline from the AAP allows either amoxicillin or amoxicillin-clavulanate as first-line empirical therapy and is therefore inclusive of the Infectious Diseases Society of America's recommendation. Unfortunately, there are scant data available regarding the precise microbiology of acute bacterial sinusitis in the post–PCV-13 era. Prospective surveillance of nasopharyngeal cultures may be helpful in completely

aligning these recommendations in the future.

Key Action Statement 5A

Clinicians should reassess initial management if there is either a caregiver report of worsening (progression of initial signs/symptoms or appearance of new signs/symptoms) OR failure to improve (lack of reduction in all presenting signs/symptoms) within 72 hours of initial management (Evidence Quality: C; Recommendation).

KAS Profile 5A

Aggregate evidence quality: C; observational studies	
Benefits	Identification of patients who may have been misdiagnosed, those at risk of complications, and those who require a change in management.
Harm	Delay of up to 72 hours in changing therapy if patient fails to improve.
Cost	Additional provider and caregiver time and resources.
Benefits-harm assessment	Preponderance of benefit.
Value judgments	Use of 72 hours to assess progress may result in excessive classification as treatment failures if premature; emphasis on importance of worsening illness in defining treatment failures.
Role of patient preferences	Caregivers determine whether the severity of the patient's illness justifies the report to clinician of the patient's worsening or failure to improve.
Intentional vagueness	None.
Exclusions	Patients with severe illness, poor general health, complicated sinusitis, immune deficiency, previous sinus surgery, or coexisting bacterial illness.
Strength	Recommendation.

The purpose of this key action statement is to ensure that patients with acute bacterial sinusitis who fail to improve symptomatically after initial management are reassessed to be certain that they have been correctly diagnosed and to consider initiation of alternate therapy to hasten resolution of symptoms and avoid complications. "Worsening" is defined as progression of presenting signs or symptoms of acute bacterial sinusitis or onset of new signs or symptoms. "Failure to improve" is lack of reduction in presenting signs or symptoms of acute

bacterial sinusitis by 72 hours after diagnosis and initial management; patients with persistent but improving symptoms do not meet this definition.

The rationale for using 72 hours as the time to assess treatment failure for acute bacterial sinusitis is based on clinical outcomes in RCTs. Wald et al[41] found that 18 of 35 patients (51%) receiving placebo demonstrated symptomatic improvement within 3 days of initiation of treatment; only an additional 3 patients receiving placebo (9%) improved between days 3 and 10. In the same study, 48 of 58 patients (83%) receiving antibiotics were cured or improved within 3 days; at 10 days, the overall rate of improvement was 79%, suggesting that no additional patients improved between days 3 and 10. In a more recent study, 17 of 19 children who ultimately failed initial therapy with either antibiotic or placebo demonstrated failure to improve within 72 hours.[4] Although Garbutt et al[42] did not report the percentage of patients who improved by day 3, they did demonstrate that the majority of improvement in symptoms occurred within the first 3 days of study entry whether they received active treatment or placebo.

Reporting of either worsening or failure to improve implies a shared responsibility between clinician and caregiver. Although the clinician should educate the caregiver regarding the anticipated reduction in symptoms within 3 days, it is incumbent on the caregiver to appropriately notify the clinician of concerns regarding worsening or failure to improve. Clinicians should emphasize the importance of reassessing those children whose symptoms are worsening whether or not antibiotic therapy was prescribed. Reassessment may be indicated before the 72-hour

process by which such reporting occurs should be discussed at the time the initial management strategy is determined.

Key Action Statement 5B

If the diagnosis of acute bacterial sinusitis is confirmed in a child with worsening symptoms or failure to improve in 72 hours, then clinicians may change the antibiotic therapy for the child initially managed with antibiotic OR initiate antibiotic treatment of the child initially managed with observation (Evidence Quality: D; Option based on expert opinion, case reports, and reasoning from first principles).

KAS Profile 5B

Aggregate evidence quality: D; expert opinion and reasoning from first principles.	
Benefit	Prevention of complications, administration of effective therapy.
Harm	Adverse effects of secondary antibiotic therapy.
Cost	Direct cost of medications, often substantial for second-line agents.
Benefits-harm assessment	Preponderance of benefit.
Value judgments	Clinician must determine whether cost and adverse effects associated with change in antibiotic is justified given the severity of illness.
Role of patient preferences	Limited in patients whose symptoms are severe or worsening, but caregivers of mildly affected children who are failing to improve may reasonably defer change in antibiotic.
Intentional vagueness	None.
Exclusions	None.
Strength	Option.

mark if the patient is substantially worse, because it may indicate the development of complications or a need for parenteral therapy. Conversely, in some cases, caregivers may think that symptoms are not severe enough to justify a change to an antibiotic with a less desirable safety profile or even the time, effort, and resources required for reassessment. Accordingly, the circumstances under which caregivers report back to the clinician and the

The purpose of this key action statement is to ensure optimal antimicrobial treatment of children with acute bacterial sinusitis whose symptoms worsen or fail to respond to the initial intervention to prevent complications and reduce symptom severity and duration (see Table 4).

Clinicians who are notified by a caregiver that a child's symptoms are worsening or failing to improve should confirm that the clinical diagnosis of acute bacterial sinusitis

corresponds to the patient's pattern of illness, as defined in Key Action Statement 1. If caregivers report worsening of symptoms at any time in a patient for whom observation was the initial intervention, the clinician should begin treatment as discussed in Key Action Statement 4. For patients whose symptoms are mild and who have failed to improve but have not worsened, initiation of antimicrobial agents or continued observation (for up to 3 days) is reasonable.

If caregivers report worsening of symptoms after 3 days in a patient initially treated with antimicrobial agents, current signs and symptoms should be reviewed to determine whether acute bacterial sinusitis is still the best diagnosis. If sinusitis is still the best diagnosis, infection with drug-resistant bacteria is probable, and an alternate antimicrobial agent may be administered. Face-to-face reevaluation of the patient is desirable. Once the decision is made to change medications, the clinician should consider the limitations of the initial antibiotic coverage, the anticipated susceptibility of residual bacterial pathogens, and the ability of antibiotics to adequately penetrate the site of infection. Cultures of sinus or nasopharyngeal secretions in patients with initial antibiotic failure have identified a large percentage of bacteria with resistance to the original antibiotic.[71,72] Furthermore, multidrug-resistant *S pneumoniae* and β-lactamase–positive *H influenzae* and *M catarrhalis* are more commonly isolated after previous antibiotic exposure.[73–78] Unfortunately, there are no studies in children that have investigated the microbiology of treatment failure in acute bacterial sinusitis or cure rates using second-line antimicrobial agents. As a result, the likelihood of adequate antibiotic coverage for resistant organisms must be addressed by extrapolations from studies of acute otitis media in children and sinusitis in adults and by using the results of data generated in vitro. A general guide to management of the child who worsens in 72 hours is shown in Table 4.

NO RECOMMENDATION

Adjuvant Therapy

Potential adjuvant therapy for acute sinusitis might include intranasal corticosteroids, saline nasal irrigation or lavage, topical or oral decongestants, mucolytics, and topical or oral antihistamines. A recent Cochrane review on decongestants, antihistamines, and nasal irrigation for acute sinusitis in children found no appropriately designed studies to determine the effectiveness of these interventions.[79]

Intranasal Steroids

The rationale for the use of intranasal corticosteroids in acute bacterial sinusitis is that an antiinflammatory agent may reduce the swelling around the sinus ostia and encourage drainage, thereby hastening recovery. However, there are limited data on how much inflammation is present, whether the inflammation is responsive to steroids, and whether there are differences in responsivity according to age. Nonetheless, there are several RCTs in adolescents and adults, most of which do show significant differences compared with placebo or active comparator that favor intranasal steroids in the reduction of symptoms and the patient's global assessment of overall improvement.[80–85] Several studies in adults with acute bacterial sinusitis provide data supporting the use of intranasal steroids as either monotherapy or adjuvant therapy to antibiotics.[81,86] Only one study did not show efficacy.[85]

There have been 2 trials of intranasal steroids performed exclusively in children: one comparing intranasal corticosteroids versus an oral decongestant[87] and the other comparing intranasal corticosteroids with placebo.[88] These studies showed a greater rate of complete resolution[87] or greater reduction in symptoms in patients receiving the steroid preparation, although the effects were modest.[88] It is important to note that nearly all of these studies (both those reported in children and adults) suffered from substantial methodologic problems. Examples of these methodologic problems are as follows: (1) variable inclusion criteria for sinusitis, (2) mixed populations of allergic and nonallergic subjects, and (3) different outcome criteria. All of these factors make deriving a clear conclusion difficult. Furthermore, the lack of stringent criteria in selecting the subject population increases the chance that the subjects had viral URIs or even persistent allergies rather than acute bacterial sinusitis.

The intranasal steroids studied to date include budesonide, flunisolide, fluticasone, and mometasone. There is no reason to believe that one steroid would be more effective than another, provided equivalent doses are used.

Potential harm in using nasal steroids in children with acute sinusitis includes the increased cost of therapy, difficulty in effectively administering nasal sprays in young children, nasal irritation and epistaxis, and potential systemic adverse effects of steroid use. Fortunately, no clinically significant steroid adverse effects have been discovered in studies in children.[89–96]

Saline Irrigation

Saline nasal irrigation or lavage (not saline nasal spray) has been used to remove debris from the nasal cavity and temporarily reduce tissue edema (hypertonic saline) to promote drainage from the sinuses. There have been very few RCTs using saline nasal irrigation or lavage in acute sinusitis, and these have had mixed results.[97,98] The 1 study in children showed greater improvement in nasal airflow and quality of life as well as a better rate of improvement in total symptom score when compared with placebo in patients treated with antibiotics and decongestants.[98] There are 2 Cochrane reviews published on the use of saline nasal irrigation in acute sinusitis in adults that showed variable results. One review published in 2007[99] concluded that it is a beneficial adjunct, but the other, published in 2010,[100] concluded that most trials were too small or contained too high a risk of bias to be confident about benefits.

Nasal Decongestants, Mucolytics, and Antihistamines

Data are insufficient to make any recommendations about the use of oral or topical nasal decongestants, mucolytics, or oral or nasal spray antihistamines as adjuvant therapy for acute bacterial sinusitis in children.[79] It is the opinion of the expert panel that antihistamines should not be used for the primary indication of acute bacterial sinusitis in any child, although such therapy might be helpful in reducing typical allergic symptoms in patients with atopy who also have acute sinusitis.

OTHER RELATED CONDITIONS

Recurrence of Acute Bacterial Sinusitis

Recurrent acute bacterial sinusitis (RABS) is an uncommon occurrence in healthy children and must be distinguished from recurrent URIs, exacerbations of allergic rhinitis, and chronic sinusitis. The former is defined by episodes of bacterial infection of the paranasal sinuses lasting fewer than 30 days and separated by intervals of

TABLE 3 Parent Information Regarding Initial Management of Acute Bacterial Sinusitis

How common are sinus infections in children?	Thick, colored, or cloudy mucus from your child's nose frequently occurs with a common cold or viral infection and does not by itself mean your child has sinusitis. In fact, fewer than 1 in 15 children get a true bacterial sinus infection during or after a common cold.
How can I tell if my child has bacterial sinusitis or simply a common cold?	Most colds have a runny nose with mucus that typically starts out clear, becomes cloudy or colored, and improves by about 10 d. Some colds will also include fever (temperature >38°C [100.4°F]) for 1 to 2 days. In contrast, acute bacterial sinusitis is likely when the pattern of illness is persistent, severe, or worsening.
	1. *Persistent* sinusitis is the most common type, defined as runny nose (of any quality), daytime cough (which may be worse at night), or both for at least 10 days without improvement.
	2. *Severe* sinusitis is present when fever (temperature ≥39°C [102.2°F]) lasts for at least 3 days in a row and is accompanied by nasal mucus that is thick, colored, or cloudy.
	3. *Worsening* sinusitis starts with a viral cold, which begins to improve but then worsens when bacteria take over and cause new-onset fever (temperature ≥38°C [100.4°F]) or a substantial increase in daytime cough or runny nose.
If my child has sinusitis, should he or she take an antibiotic?	Children with *persistent* sinusitis may be managed with either an antibiotic or with an additional brief period of observation, allowing the child up to another 3 days to fight the infection and improve on his or her own. The choice to treat or observe should be discussed with your doctor and may be based on your child's quality of life and how much of a problem the sinusitis is causing. In contrast, all children diagnosed with *severe* or *worsening* sinusitis should start antibiotic treatment to help them recover faster and more often.
Why not give all children with acute bacterial sinusitis an immediate antibiotic?	Some episodes of *persistent* sinusitis include relatively mild symptoms that may improve on their own in a few days. In addition, antibiotics can have adverse effects, which may include vomiting, diarrhea, upset stomach, skin rash, allergic reactions, yeast infections, and development of resistant bacteria (that make future infections more difficult to treat).

at least 10 days during which the patient is asymptomatic. Some experts require at least 4 episodes in a calendar year to fulfill the criteria for this condition. Chronic sinusitis is manifest as 90 or more uninterrupted days of respiratory symptoms, such as cough, nasal discharge, or nasal obstruction.

Children with RABS should be evaluated for underlying allergies, particularly allergic rhinitis; quantitative and functional immunologic defect(s), chiefly immunoglobulin A and immunoglobulin G deficiency; cystic fibrosis; gastroesophageal reflux disease; or dysmotile cilia syndrome.[101] Anatomic abnormalities obstructing one or more sinus ostia may be present. These include septal deviation, nasal polyps, or concha bullosa (pneumatization of the middle turbinate); atypical ethmoid cells with compromised drainage; a lateralized middle turbinate; and intrinsic ostiomeatal anomalies.[102]

Contrast-enhanced CT, MRI, or endoscopy or all 3 should be performed for detection of obstructive conditions, particularly in children with genetic or acquired craniofacial abnormalities.

The microbiology of RABS is similar to that of isolated episodes of acute bacterial sinusitis and warrants the same treatment.[72] It should be recognized that closely spaced sequential courses of antimicrobial therapy may foster the emergence of antibiotic-resistant bacterial species as the causative agent in recurrent episodes. There are no systematically evaluated options for prevention of RABS in children. In general, the use of prolonged prophylactic antimicrobial therapy should be avoided and is not usually recommended for children with recurrent acute otitis media. However, when there are no recognizable predisposing conditions to remedy in children with RABS, prophylactic antimicrobial agents may be used for several months during the respiratory season. Enthusiasm for this strategy is tempered by concerns regarding the encouragement of bacterial resistance. Accordingly, prophylaxis should only be considered in carefully selected children whose infections have been thoroughly documented.

Influenza vaccine should be administered annually, and PCV-13 should be administered at the recommended ages for all children, including those with RABS. Intranasal steroids and nonsedating antihistamines can be helpful for children with allergic rhinitis, as can antireflux medications for those with gastroesophageal reflux disease. Children with anatomic abnormalities may require endoscopic surgery for removal of or reduction in ostiomeatal obstruction.

The pathogenesis of chronic sinusitis is poorly understood and appears to be multifactorial; however, many of the conditions associated with RABS

TABLE 4 Management of Worsening or Lack of Improvement at 72 Hours

Initial Management	Worse in 72 Hours	Lack of Improvement in 72 Hours
Observation	Initiate amoxicillin with or without clavulanate	Additional observation or initiate antibiotic based on shared decision-making
Amoxicillin	High-dose amoxicillin-clavulanate	Additional observation or high-dose amoxicillin-clavulanate based on shared decision-making
High-dose amoxicillin-clavulanate	Clindamycin[a] and cefixime OR linezolid and cefixime OR levofloxacin	Continued high-dose amoxicillin-clavulanate OR clindamycin[a] and cefixime OR linezolid and cefixime OR levofloxacin

[a] Clindamycin is recommended to cover penicillin-resistant S pneumoniae. Some communities have high levels of clindamycin-resistant S pneumoniae. In these communities, linezolid is preferred.

have also been implicated in chronic sinusitis, and it is clear that there is an overlap between the 2 syndromes.[101,102] In some cases, there may be episodes of acute bacterial sinusitis superimposed on a chronic sinusitis, warranting antimicrobial therapy to hasten resolution of the acute infection.

Complications of Acute Bacterial Sinusitis

Complications of acute bacterial sinusitis should be diagnosed when the patient develops signs or symptoms of orbital and/or central nervous system (intracranial) involvement. Rarely, complicated acute bacterial sinusitis can result in permanent blindness, other neurologic sequelae, or death if not treated promptly and appropriately. Orbital complications have been classified by Chandler et al.[32] Intracranial complications include epidural or subdural abscess, brain abscess, venous thrombosis, and meningitis.

Periorbital and intraorbital inflammation and infection are the most common complications of acute sinusitis and most often are secondary to acute ethmoiditis in otherwise healthy young children. These disorders are commonly classified in relation to the orbital septum; periorbital or preseptal inflammation involves only the eyelid, whereas postseptal (intraorbital) inflammation involves structures of the orbit. Mild cases of preseptal cellulitis (eyelid <50% closed) may be treated on an outpatient basis with appropriate

oral antibiotic therapy (high-dose amoxicillin-clavulanate for comprehensive coverage) for acute bacterial sinusitis and daily follow-up until definite improvement is noted. If the patient does not improve within 24 to 48 hours or if the infection is progressive, it is appropriate to admit the patient to the hospital for antimicrobial therapy. Similarly, if proptosis, impaired visual acuity, or impaired and/or painful extraocular mobility is present on examination, the patient should be hospitalized, and a contrast-enhanced CT should be performed. Consultation with an otolaryngologist, an ophthalmologist, and an infectious disease expert is appropriate for guidance regarding the need for surgical intervention and the selection of antimicrobial agents.

Intracranial complications are most frequently encountered in previously healthy adolescent males with frontal sinusitis.[33,34] In patients with altered mental status, severe headache, or Pott's puffy tumor (osteomyelitis of the frontal bone), neurosurgical consultation should be obtained. A contrast-enhanced CT scan (preferably coronal thin cut) of the head, orbits, and sinuses is essential to confirm intracranial or intraorbital suppurative complications; in such cases, intravenous antibiotics should be started immediately. Alternatively, an MRI may also be desirable in some cases of intracranial abnormality. Appropriate antimicrobial therapy for intraorbital complications include vancomycin (to cover possible methicillin-resistant

S aureus or penicillin-resistant S pneumoniae) and either ceftriaxone, ampicillin-sulbactam, or piperacillin-tazobactam.[103] Given the polymicrobial nature of sinogenic abscesses, coverage for anaerobes (ie, metronidazole) should also be considered for intraorbital complications and should be started in all cases of intracranial complications if ceftriaxone is prescribed.

Patients with small orbital, subperiosteal, or epidural abscesses and minimal ocular and neurologic abnormalities may be managed with intravenous antibiotic treatment for 24 to 48 hours while performing frequent visual and mental status checks.[104] In patients who develop progressive signs and symptoms, such as impaired visual acuity, ophthalmoplegia, elevated intraocular pressure (>20 mm), severe proptosis (>5 mm), altered mental status, headache, or vomiting, as well as those who fail to improve within 24 to 48 hours while receiving antibiotics, prompt surgical intervention and drainage of the abscess should be undertaken.[104] Antibiotics can be tailored to the results of culture and sensitivity studies when they become available.

AREAS FOR FUTURE RESEARCH

Since the publication of the original guideline in 2001, only a small number of high-quality studies of the diagnosis and treatment of acute bacterial sinusitis in children have been published.[5] Ironically, the number of published guidelines on the topic (5) exceeds the number of prospective, placebo-controlled clinical trials of either antibiotics or ancillary treatments of acute bacterial sinusitis. Thus, as was the case in 2001, there are scant data on which to base recommendations. Accordingly, areas for future research include the following:

Etiology

1. Reexamine the microbiology of acute sinusitis in children in the postpneumococcal conjugate vaccine era and determine the value of using newer polymerase chain reaction–based respiratory testing to document viral, bacterial, and polymicrobial disease.

2. Correlate cultures obtained from the middle meatus of the maxillary sinus of infected children with cultures obtained from the maxillary sinus by puncture of the antrum.

3. Conduct more and larger studies to more clearly define and correlate the clinical findings with the various available diagnostic criteria of acute bacterial sinusitis (eg, sinus aspiration and treatment outcome).

4. Develop noninvasive strategies to accurately diagnose acute bacterial sinusitis in children.

5. Develop imaging technology that differentiates bacterial infection from viral infection or allergic inflammation, preferably without radiation.

Treatment

1. Determine the optimal duration of antimicrobial therapy for children with acute bacterial sinusitis.

2. Evaluate a "wait-and-see prescription" strategy for children with persistent symptom presentation of acute sinusitis.

3. Determine the optimal antimicrobial agent for children with acute bacterial sinusitis, balancing the incentives of choosing narrow-spectrum agents against the known microbiology of the disease and resistance patterns of likely pathogens.

4. Determine the causes and treatment of subacute, recurrent acute, and chronic bacterial sinusitis.

5. Determine the efficacy of prophylaxis with antimicrobial agents to prevent RABS.

6. Determine the effects of bacterial resistance among *S pneumoniae*, *H influenzae*, and *M catarrhalis* on outcome of treatment with antibiotics by the performance of randomized, double-blind, placebo-controlled studies in well-defined populations of patients.

7. Determine the role of adjuvant therapies (antihistamines, nasal corticosteroids, mucolytics, decongestants, nasal irrigation, etc) in patients with acute bacterial sinusitis by the performance of prospective, randomized clinical trials.

8. Determine whether early treatment of acute bacterial sinusitis prevents orbital or central nervous system complications.

9. Determine the role of complementary and alternative medicine strategies in patients with acute bacterial sinusitis by performing systematic, prospective, randomized clinical trials.

10. Develop new bacterial and viral vaccines to reduce the incidence of acute bacterial sinusitis.

SUBCOMMITTEE ON ACUTE SINUSITIS
Ellen R. Wald, MD, FAAP (Chair, Pediatric Infectious Disease Physician: no financial conflicts; published research related to sinusitis)
Kimberly E. Applegate, MD, MS, FAAP (Radiologist, AAP Section on Radiology: no conflicts)
Clay Bordley, MD, MPH, FAAP (Pediatric Emergency and Hospitalist Medicine physician: no conflicts)
David H. Darrow, MD, FAAP (Otolaryngologist, AAP Section on Otolaryngology–Head and Neck Surgery: no conflicts)
Mary P. Glode, MD, FAAP (Pediatric Infectious Disease Physician, AAP Committee on Infectious Disease: no conflicts)
S. Michael Marcy, MD, FAAP (General Pediatrician with Infectious Disease Expertise, AAP Section on Infectious Diseases: no conflicts)
Nader Shaikh, MD, FAAP (General Academic Pediatrician: no financial conflicts; published research related to sinusitis)
Michael J. Smith, MD, MSCE, FAAP (Epidemiologist, Pediatric Infectious Disease Physician: research funding for vaccine clinical trials from Sanofi Pasteur and Novartis)
Paul V. Williams, MD, FAAP (Allergist, AAP Section on Allergy, Asthma, and Immunology: no conflicts)
Stuart T. Weinberg, MD, FAAP (PPI Informatician, General Academic Pediatrician: no conflicts)
Carrie E. Nelson, MD, MS (Family Physician, American Academy of Family Physicians: employed by McKesson Health Solutions)
Richard M. Rosenfeld, MD, MPH, FAAP (Otolaryngologist, AAP Section on Otolaryngology–Head and Neck Surgery, American Academy of Otolaryngology–Head and Neck Surgery: no financial conflicts; published research related to sinusitis)

CONSULTANT
Richard N. Shiffman, MD, FAAP (Informatician, Guideline Methodologist, General Academic Pediatrician: no conflicts)

STAFF
Caryn Davidson, MA

REFERENCES
1. Aitken M, Taylor JA. Prevalence of clinical sinusitis in young children followed up by primary care pediatricians. *Arch Pediatr Adolesc Med.* 1998;152(3):244–248
2. Kakish KS, Mahafza T, Batieha A, Ekteish F, Daoud A. Clinical sinusitis in children attending primary care centers. *Pediatr Infect Dis J.* 2000;19(11):1071–1074
3. Ueda D, Yoto Y. The ten-day mark as a practical diagnostic approach for acute paranasal sinusitis in children. *Pediatr Infect Dis J.* 1996;15(7):576–579

4. Wald ER, Nash D, Eickhoff J. Effectiveness of amoxicillin/clavulanate potassium in the treatment of acute bacterial sinusitis in children. Pediatrics. 2009;124(1):9–15

5. American Academy of Pediatrics, Subcommittee on Management of Sinusitis and Committee on Quality Improvement. Clinical practice guideline: management of sinusitis. Pediatrics. 2001;108(3):798–808

6. Smith MJ. AAP technical report: evidence for the diagnosis and treatment of acute uncomplicated sinusitis in children: a systematic review. 2013, In press.

7. Shiffman RN, Michel G, Rosenfeld RM, Davidson C. Building better guidelines with BRIDGE-Wiz: development and evaluation of a software assistant to promote clarity, transparency, and implementability. J Am Med Inform Assoc. 2012;19(1):94–101

8. American Academy of Pediatrics, Steering Committee on Quality Improvement and Management. Classifying recommendations for clinical practice guidelines. Pediatrics. 2004;114(3):874–877

9. Gwaltney JM, Jr, Hendley JO, Simon G, Jordan WS Jr. Rhinovirus infections in an industrial population. II. Characteristics of illness and antibody response. JAMA. 1967;202(6):494–500

10. Pappas DE, Hendley JO, Hayden FG, Winther B. Symptom profile of common colds in school-aged children. Pediatr Infect Dis J. 2008;27(1):8–11

11. Wald ER, Guerra N, Byers C. Frequency and severity of infections in day care: three-year follow-up. J Pediatr. 1991;118(4 pt 1):509–514

12. Wald ER, Guerra N, Byers C. Upper respiratory tract infections in young children: duration of and frequency of complications. Pediatrics. 1991;87(2):129–133

13. Meltzer EO, Hamilos DL, Hadley JA, et al. Rhinosinusitis: establishing definitions for clinical research and patient care. J Allergy Clin Immunol. 2004;114(6 suppl):155–212

14. Shaikh N, Wald ER. Signs and symptoms of acute sinusitis in children. Pediatr Infect Dis J. 2013; in press

15. Wald ER. The diagnosis and management of sinusitis in children: diagnostic considerations. Pediatr Infect Dis. 1985;4(6 suppl):S61–S64

16. Wald ER, Milmoe GJ, Bowen A, Ledesma-Medina J, Salamon N, Bluestone CD. Acute maxillary sinusitis in children. N Engl J Med. 1981;304(13):749–754

17. Lindbaek M, Hjortdahl P, Johnsen UL. Use of symptoms, signs, and blood tests to diagnose acute sinus infections in primary care: comparison with computed tomography. Fam Med. 1996;28(3):183–188

18. Wald ER. Beginning antibiotics for acute rhinosinusitis and choosing the right treatment. Clin Rev Allergy Immunol. 2006;30(3):143–152

19. Maresh MM, Washburn AH. Paranasal sinuses from birth to late adolescence. II. Clinical and roentgenographic evidence of infection. Am J Dis Child. 1940;60:841–861

20. Glasier CM, Mallory GB, Jr, Steele RW. Significance of opacification of the maxillary and ethmoid sinuses in infants. J Pediatr. 1989;114(1):45–50

21. Kovatch AL, Wald ER, Ledesma-Medina J, Chiponis DM, Bedingfield B. Maxillary sinus radiographs in children with non-respiratory complaints. Pediatrics. 1984;73(3):306–308

22. Shopfner CE, Rossi JO. Roentgen evaluation of the paranasal sinuses in children. Am J Roentgenol Radium Ther Nucl Med. 1973;118(1):176–186

23. Diament MJ, Senac MO, Jr, Gilsanz V, Baker S, Gillespie T, Larsson S. Prevalence of incidental paranasal sinuses opacification in pediatric patients: a CT study. J Comput Assist Tomogr. 1987;11(3):426–431

24. Glasier CM, Ascher DP, Williams KD. Incidental paranasal sinus abnormalities on CT of children: clinical correlation. AJNR Am J Neuroradiol. 1986;7(5):861–864

25. Gwaltney JM, Jr, Phillips CD, Miller RD, Riker DK. Computed tomographic study of the common cold. N Engl J Med. 1994;330(1):25–30

26. Manning SC, Biavati MJ, Phillips DL. Correlation of clinical sinusitis signs and symptoms to imaging findings in pediatric patients. Int J Pediatr Otorhinolaryngol. 1996;37(1):65–74

27. Gordts F, Clement PA, Destryker A, Desprechins B, Kaufman L. Prevalence of sinusitis signs on MRI in a non-ENT paediatric population. Rhinology. 1997;35(4):154–157

28. Kristo A, Uhari M, Luotonen J, et al. Paranasal sinus findings in children during respiratory infection evaluated with magnetic resonance imaging. Pediatrics. 2003;111(5 pt 1):e586–e589

29. Brook I. Microbiology and antimicrobial treatment of orbital and intracranial complications of sinusitis in children and their management. Int J Pediatr Otorhinolaryngol. 2009;73(9):1183–1186

30. Sultesz M, Csakanyi Z, Majoros T, Farkas Z, Katona G. Acute bacterial rhinosinusitis and its complications in our pediatric otolaryngological department between 1997 and 2006. Int J Pediatr Otorhinolaryngol. 2009;73(11):1507–1512

31. Wald ER. Periorbital and orbital infections. Infect Dis Clin North Am. 2007;21(2):393–408

32. Chandler JR, Langenbrunner DJ, Stevens ER. The pathogenesis of orbital complications in acute sinusitis. Laryngoscope. 1970;80(9):1414–1428

33. Kombogiorgas D, Seth R, Modha J, Singh J. Suppurative intracranial complications of sinusitis in adolescence. Single institute experience and review of the literature. Br J Neurosurg. 2007;21(6):603–609

34. Rosenfeld EA, Rowley AH. Infectious intracranial complications of sinusitis, other than meningitis in children: 12 year review. Clin Infect Dis. 1994;18(5):750–754

35. American College of Radiology. Appropriateness criteria for sinonasal disease. 2009. Available at: www.acr.org/~/media/8172B4DE503149248E64856857674BB5.pdf. Accessed November 6, 2012

36. Triulzi F, Zirpoli S. Imaging techniques in the diagnosis and management of rhinosinusitis in children. Pediatr Allergy Immunol. 2007;18(suppl 18):46–49

37. McIntosh D, Mahadevan M. Failure of contrast enhanced computed tomography scans to identify an orbital abscess. The benefit of magnetic resonance imaging. J Laryngol Otol. 2008;122(6):639–640

38. Younis RT, Anand VK, Davidson B. The role of computed tomography and magnetic resonance imaging in patients with sinusitis with complications. Laryngoscope. 2002;112(2):224–229

39. Shapiro DJ, Gonzales R, Cabana MD, Hersh AL. National trends in visit rates and antibiotic prescribing for children with acute sinusitis. Pediatrics. 2011;127(1):28–34

40. Wald ER, Reilly JS, Casselbrant M, et al. Treatment of acute maxillary sinusitis in childhood: a comparative study of amoxicillin and cefaclor. J Pediatr. 1984;104(2):297–302

41. Wald ER, Chiponis D, Ledesma-Medina J. Comparative effectiveness of amoxicillin and amoxicillin-clavulanate potassium in acute paranasal sinus infections in children: a double-blind, placebo-controlled trial. Pediatrics. 1986;77(6):795–800

42. Garbutt JM, Goldstein M, Gellman E, Shannon W, Littenberg B. A randomized, placebo-controlled trial of antimicrobial treatment for children with clinically diagnosed acute sinusitis. Pediatrics. 2001;107(4):619–625

43. Kristo A, Uhari M, Luotonen J, Ilkko E, Koivunen P, Alho OP. Cefuroxime axetil versus placebo for children with acute respiratory infection and imaging evidence of sinusitis: a randomized, controlled trial. *Acta Paediatr.* 2005;94(9):1208–1213

44. Hoberman A, Paradise JL, Rockette HE, et al. Treatment of acute otitis media in children under 2 years of age. *N Engl J Med.* 2011;364(2):105–115

45. Tahtinen PA, Laine MK, Huovinen P, Jalava J, Ruuskanen O, Ruohola A. A placebo-controlled trial of antimicrobial treatment for acute otitis media. *N Engl J Med.* 2011;364(2):116–126

46. Gordts F, Abu Nasser I, Clement PA, Pierard D, Kaufman L. Bacteriology of the middle meatus in children. *Int J Pediatr Otorhinolaryngol.* 1999;48(2):163–167

47. Parsons DS, Wald ER. Otitis media and sinusitis: similar diseases. *Otolaryngol Clin North Am.* 1996;29(1):11–25

48. Revai K, Dobbs LA, Nair S, Patel JA, Grady JJ, Chonmaitree T. Incidence of acute otitis media and sinusitis complicating upper respiratory tract infection: the effect of age. *Pediatrics.* 2007;119(6). Available at: www.pediatrics.org/cgi/content/full/119/6/e1408

49. Klein JO, Bluestone CD. *Textbook of Pediatric Infectious Diseases.* 6th ed. Philadelphia, PA: Saunders; 2009

50. Casey JR, Adlowitz DG, Pichichero ME. New patterns in the otopathogens causing acute otitis media six to eight years after introduction of pneumococcal conjugate vaccine. *Pediatr Infect Dis J.* 2010;29(4):304–309

51. Brook I, Gober AE. Frequency of recovery of pathogens from the nasopharynx of children with acute maxillary sinusitis before and after the introduction of vaccination with the 7-valent pneumococcal vaccine. *Int J Pediatr Otorhinolaryngol.* 2007;71(4):575–579

52. Wald ER. Microbiology of acute and chronic sinusitis in children. *J Allergy Clin Immunol.* 1992;90(3 pt 2):452–456

53. Centers for Disease Control and Prevention. Effects of new penicillin susceptibility breakpoints for *Streptococcus pneumoniae*—United States, 2006-2007. *MMWR Morb Mortal Wkly Rep.* 2008;57(50):1353–1355

54. Centers for Disease Control and Prevention. Active Bacterial Core Surveillance (ABCs): Emerging Infections Program Network. 2011. Available at: www.cdc.gov/abcs/reports-findings/survreports/spneu09.html. Accessed November 6, 2012

55. Garbutt J, St Geme JW, III, May A, Storch GA, Shackelford PG. Developing community-specific recommendations for first-line treatment of acute otitis media: is high-dose amoxicillin necessary? *Pediatrics.* 2004;114(2):342–347

56. Harrison CJ, Woods C, Stout G, Martin B, Selvarangan R. Susceptibilities of *Haemophilus influenzae, Streptococcus pneumoniae,* including serotype 19A, and *Moraxella catarrhalis* paediatric isolates from 2005 to 2007 to commonly used antibiotics. *J Antimicrob Chemother.* 2009;63(3):511–519

57. Critchley IA, Jacobs MR, Brown SD, Traczewski MM, Tillotson GS, Janjic N. Prevalence of serotype 19A Streptococcus pneumoniae among isolates from U.S. children in 2005-2006 and activity of faropenem. *Antimicrob Agents Chemother.* 2008;52(7):2639–2643

58. Jacobs MR, Good CE, Windau AR, et al. Activity of ceftaroline against recent emerging serotypes of *Streptococcus pneumoniae* in the United States. *Antimicrob Agents Chemother.* 2010;54(6):2716–2719

59. Tristram S, Jacobs MR, Appelbaum PC. Antimicrobial resistance in *Haemophilus influenzae. Clin Microbiol Rev.* 2007;20(2):368–389

60. Levine OS, Farley M, Harrison LH, Lefkowitz L, McGeer A, Schwartz B. Risk factors for invasive pneumococcal disease in children: a population-based case-control study in North America. *Pediatrics.* 1999;103(3). Available at: www.pediatrics.org/cgi/content/full/103/3/e28

61. Seikel K, Shelton S, McCracken GH Jr. Middle ear fluid concentrations of amoxicillin after large dosages in children with acute otitis media. *Pediatr Infect Dis J.* 1997;16(7):710–711

62. Cohen R, Navel M, Grunberg J, et al. One dose ceftriaxone vs. ten days of amoxicillin/clavulanate therapy for acute otitis media: clinical efficacy and change in nasopharyngeal flora. *Pediatr Infect Dis J.* 1999;18(5):403–409

63. Green SM, Rothrock SG. Single-dose intramuscular ceftriaxone for acute otitis media in children. *Pediatrics.* 1993;91(1):23–30

64. Leibovitz E, Piglansky L, Raiz S, Press J, Leiberman A, Dagan R. Bacteriologic and clinical efficacy of one day vs. three day intramuscular ceftriaxone for treatment of nonresponsive acute otitis media in children. *Pediatr Infect Dis J.* 2000;19(11):1040–1045

65. DePestel DD, Benninger MS, Danziger L, et al. Cephalosporin use in treatment of patients with penicillin allergies. *J Am Pharm Assoc.* 2008;48(4):530–540

66. Pichichero ME. A review of evidence supporting the American Academy of Pediatrics recommendation for prescribing cephalosporin antibiotics for penicillin-allergic patients. *Pediatrics.* 2005;115(4):1048–1057

67. Pichichero ME, Casey JR. Safe use of selected cephalosporins in penicillin-allergic patients: a meta-analysis. *Otolaryngol Head Neck Surg.* 2007;136(3):340–347

68. Park MA, Koch CA, Klemawesch P, Joshi A, Li JT. Increased adverse drug reactions to cephalosporins in penicillin allergy patients with positive penicillin skin test. *Int Arch Allergy Immunol.* 2010;153(3):268–273

69. Jacobs MR. Antimicrobial-resistant Streptococcus pneumoniae: trends and management. *Expert Rev Anti Infect Ther.* 2008;6(5):619–635

70. Chow AW, Benninger MS, Brook I, et al; Infectious Diseases Society of America. IDSA clinical practice guideline for acute bacterial rhinosinusitis in children and adults. *Clin Infect Dis.* 2012;54(8):e72–e112

71. Brook I, Gober AE. Resistance to antimicrobials used for therapy of otitis media and sinusitis: effect of previous antimicrobial therapy and smoking. *Ann Otol Rhinol Laryngol.* 1999;108(7 pt 1):645–647

72. Brook I, Gober AE. Antimicrobial resistance in the nasopharyngeal flora of children with acute maxillary sinusitis and maxillary sinusitis recurring after amoxicillin therapy. *J Antimicrob Chemother.* 2004;53(2):399–402

73. Dohar J, Canton R, Cohen R, Farrell DJ, Felmingham D. Activity of telithromycin and comparators against bacterial pathogens isolated from 1,336 patients with clinically diagnosed acute sinusitis. *Ann Clin Microbiol Antimicrob.* 2004;3(3):15–21

74. Jacobs MR, Bajaksouzian S, Zilles A, Lin G, Pankuch GA, Appelbaum PC. Susceptibilities of *Streptococcus pneumoniae* and *Haemophilus influenzae* to 10 oral antimicrobial agents based on pharmacodynamic parameters: 1997 U.S. surveillance study. *Antimicrob Agents Chemother.* 1999;43(8):1901–1908

75. Jacobs MR, Felmingham D, Appelbaum PC, Gruneberg RN. The Alexander Project 1998-2000: susceptibility of pathogens isolated from community-acquired respiratory tract infection to commonly used antimicrobial agents. *J Antimicrob Chemother.* 2003;52(2):229–246

76. Lynch JP, III, Zhanel GG. *Streptococcus pneumoniae*: epidemiology and risk factors, evolution of antimicrobial resistance, and impact of vaccines. *Curr Opin Pulm Med.* 2010;16(3):217–225

77. Sahm DF, Jones ME, Hickey ML, Diakun DR, Mani SV, Thornsberry C. Resistance surveillance of *Streptococcus pneumoniae, Haemophilus influenzae* and *Moraxella catarrhalis* isolated in Asia and Europe, 1997-1998. *J Antimicrob Chemother.* 2000; 45(4):457–466

78. Sokol W. Epidemiology of sinusitis in the primary care setting: results from the 1999-2000 respiratory surveillance program. *Am J Med.* 2001;111(suppl 9A):19S–24S

79. Shaikh N, Wald ER, Pi M. Decongestants, antihistamines and nasal irrigation for acute sinusitis in children. *Cochrane Database Syst Rev.* 2010;(12):CD007909

80. Dolor RJ, Witsell DL, Hellkamp AS, Williams JW, Jr, Califf RM, Simel DL. Comparison of cefuroxime with or without intranasal fluticasone for the treatment of rhinosinusitis. The CAFFS Trial: a randomized controlled trial. *JAMA.* 2001;286(24):3097–3105

81. Meltzer EO, Bachert C, Staudinger H. Treating acute rhinosinusitis: comparing efficacy and safety of mometasone furoate nasal spray, amoxicillin, and placebo. *J Allergy Clin Immunol.* 2005;116(6):1289–1295

82. Meltzer EO, Charous BL, Busse WW, Zinreich SJ, Lorber RR, Danzig MR. Added relief in the treatment of acute recurrent sinusitis with adjunctive mometasone furoate nasal spray. The Nasonex Sinusitis Group. *J Allergy Clin Immunol.* 2000;106 (4):630–637

83. Meltzer EO, Orgel HA, Backhaus JW, et al. Intranasal flunisolide spray as an adjunct to oral antibiotic therapy for sinusitis. *J Allergy Clin Immunol.* 1993;92(6):812–823

84. Nayak AS, Settipane GA, Pedinoff A, et al. Effective dose range of mometasone furoate nasal spray in the treatment of acute rhinosinusitis. *Ann Allergy Asthma Immunol.* 2002;89(3):271–278

85. Williamson IG, Rumsby K, Benge S, et al. Antibiotics and topical nasal steroid for treatment of acute maxillary sinusitis: a randomized controlled trial. *JAMA.* 2007; 298(21):2487–2496

86. Zalmanovici A, Yaphe J. Intranasal steroids for acute sinusitis. *Cochrane Database Syst Rev.* 2009;(4):CD005149

87. Yilmaz G, Varan B, Yilmaz T, Gurakan B. Intranasal budesonide spray as an adjunct to oral antibiotic therapy for acute sinusitis in children. *Eur Arch Otorhinolaryngol.* 2000;257(5):256–259

88. Barlan IB, Erkan E, Bakir M, Berrak S, Basaran MM. Intranasal budesonide spray as an adjunct to oral antibiotic therapy for acute sinusitis in children. *Ann Allergy Asthma Immunol.* 1997;78(6):598–601

89. Bruni FM, De Luca G, Venturoli V, Boner AL. Intranasal corticosteroids and adrenal suppression. *Neuroimmunomodulation.* 2009;16 (5):353–362

90. Kim KT, Rabinovitch N, Uryniak T, Simpson B, O'Dowd L, Casty F. Effect of budesonide aqueous nasal spray on hypothalamic-pituitary-adrenal axis function in children with allergic rhinitis. *Ann Allergy Asthma Immunol.* 2004;93(1):61–67

91. Meltzer EO, Tripathy I, Maspero JF, Wu W, Philpot E. Safety and tolerability of fluticasone furoate nasal spray once daily in paediatric patients aged 6-11 years with allergic rhinitis: subanalysis of three randomized, double-blind, placebo-controlled, multicentre studies. *Clin Drug Investig.* 2009;29(2):79–86

92. Murphy K, Uryniak T, Simpson B, O'Dowd L. Growth velocity in children with perennial allergic rhinitis treated with budesonide aqueous nasal spray. *Ann Allergy Asthma Immunol.* 2006;96(5):723–730

93. Ratner PH, Meltzer EO, Teper A. Mometasone furoate nasal spray is safe and effective for 1-year treatment of children with perennial allergic rhinitis. *Int J Pediatr Otorhinolaryngol.* 2009;73(5):651–657

94. Skoner DP, Gentile DA, Doyle WJ. Effect on growth of long-term treatment with intranasal triamcinolone acetonide aqueous in children with allergic rhinitis. *Ann Allergy Asthma Immunol.* 2008;101(4): 431–436

95. Weinstein S, Qaqundah P, Georges G, Nayak A. Efficacy and safety of triamcinolone acetonide aqueous nasal spray in children aged 2 to 5 years with perennial allergic rhinitis: a randomized, double-blind, placebo-controlled study with an open-label extension. *Ann Allergy Asthma Immunol.* 2009;102(4):339–347

96. Zitt M, Kosoglou T, Hubbell J. Mometasone furoate nasal spray: a review of safety and systemic effects. *Drug Saf.* 2007;30(4): 317–326

97. Adam P, Stiffman M, Blake RL Jr. A clinical trial of hypertonic saline nasal spray in subjects with the common cold or rhinosinusitis. *Arch Fam Med.* 1998;7(1):39–43

98. Wang YH, Yang CP, Ku MS, Sun HL, Lue KH. Efficacy of nasal irrigation in the treatment of acute sinusitis in children. *Int J Pediatr Otorhinolaryngol.* 2009;73(12): 1696–1701

99. Harvey R, Hannan SA, Badia L, Scadding G. Nasal saline irrigations for the symptoms of chronic rhinosinusitis. *Cochrane Database Syst Rev.* 2007;(3):CD006394

100. Kassel JC, King D, Spurling GK. Saline nasal irrigation for acute upper respiratory tract infections. *Cochrane Database Syst Rev.* 2010;(3):CD006821

101. Shapiro GG, Virant FS, Furukawa CT, Pierson WE, Bierman CW. Immunologic defects in patients with refractory sinusitis. *Pediatrics.* 1991;87(3):311–316

102. Wood AJ, Douglas RG. Pathogenesis and treatment of chronic rhinosinusitis. *Postgrad Med J.* 2010;86(1016):359–364

103. Liao S, Durand ML, Cunningham MJ. Sinogenic orbital and subperiosteal abscesses: microbiology and methicillin-resistant Staphylococcus aureus incidence. *Otolaryngol Head Neck Surg.* 2010;143(3):392–396

104. Oxford LE, McClay J. Medical and surgical management of subperiosteal orbital abscess secondary to acute sinusitis in children. *Int J Pediatr Otorhinolaryngol.* 2006;70(11):1853–1861

TECHNICAL REPORT

Evidence for the Diagnosis and Treatment of Acute Uncomplicated Sinusitis in Children: A Systematic Review

abstract

In 2001, the American Academy of Pediatrics published clinical practice guidelines for the management of acute bacterial sinusitis (ABS) in children. The technical report accompanying those guidelines included 21 studies that assessed the diagnosis and management of ABS in children. This update to that report incorporates studies of pediatric ABS that have been performed since 2001. Overall, 17 randomized controlled trials of the treatment of sinusitis in children were identified and analyzed. Four randomized, double-blind, placebo-controlled trials of antimicrobial therapy have been published. The results of these studies varied, likely due to differences in inclusion and exclusion criteria. Because of this heterogeneity, formal meta-analyses were not performed. However, qualitative analysis of these studies suggests that children with greater severity of illness at presentation are more likely to benefit from antimicrobial therapy. An additional 5 trials compared different antimicrobial therapies but did not include placebo groups. Six trials assessed a variety of ancillary treatments for ABS in children, and 3 focused on subacute sinusitis. Although the number of pediatric trials has increased since 2001, there are still limited data to guide the diagnosis and management of ABS in children. Diagnostic and treatment guidelines focusing on severity of illness at the time of presentation have the potential to identify those children most likely to benefit from antimicrobial therapy and at the same time minimize unnecessary use of antibiotics. *Pediatrics* 2013;132:e284–e296

Michael J. Smith, MD, MSCE

KEY WORDS
acute bacterial sinusitis, antibiotics, ancillary treatment, diagnosis, systematic review

ABBREVIATIONS
AAP—American Academy of Pediatrics
CT—computed tomography

www.pediatrics.org/cgi/doi/10.1542/peds.2013-1072

doi:10.1542/peds.2013-1072

PEDIATRICS (ISSN Numbers: Print, 0031-4005; Online, 1098-4275).

INTRODUCTION

Acute bacterial sinusitis is reported as a complication of 5% to 10% of upper respiratory tract infections in children[1,2] and is 1 of the more common indications for antibiotic use in the United States. In 2001, the American Academy of Pediatrics (AAP) published clinical practice guidelines for the management of sinusitis in children.[3] The 2001 technical report that accompanied those guidelines included an analysis of 21 studies published from January 1966 through March 1999 which assessed the diagnosis and therapeutic management of acute sinusitis in children.[4] These included 5 randomized controlled trials involving 255 children and 8 case series involving 418 children. The primary goal of the current analysis was to update the 2001 technical report by identifying and reviewing additional studies of pediatric acute sinusitis that have been performed in the last decade to aid the revision of the AAP practice guidelines.

This technical report revisits the same questions as the original report: (1) What is the efficacy of various types of antimicrobial therapy in children with acute sinusitis? (2) What is the efficacy of nonantimicrobial ancillary treatments in children with acute sinusitis? (3) What is the concordance of various clinical, laboratory, and radiographic findings in the diagnosis of acute sinusitis? In addition, the Subcommittee on Management of Sinusitis met before the initial literature search for the current report and raised additional questions:

1. What is the incidence of adverse events in the treatment of sinusitis?

2. Are there data to support the clinical definitions of acute, subacute, and recurrent acute sinusitis?

3. Are there data to recommend a specific duration of symptoms that distinguishes bacterial from viral sinusitis?

4. How have the epidemiology and bacteriology of acute sinusitis changed in the pneumococcal conjugate vaccine era?

5. Is there evidence to support antimicrobial prophylaxis in children with recurrent sinusitis?

6. What other guidelines for the management of acute sinusitis in children exist?

METHODS

Searches of PubMed were performed by using the same search term as in the 2001 report ("sinusitis"). All searches were limited to English language and human studies. Three separate searches were performed to

maximize retrieval of the most recent and highest-quality evidence for pediatric sinusitis. The first search limited results to all randomized controlled trials from 1966 to 2009, the second to all meta-analyses from 1966 to 2009, and the third to all pediatric studies (age limit <18 years) published since the last technical report (1999–2009). In addition, Web of Science was used to search for additional studies that cited the 2001 technical report and guidelines as well as citations of each double-blind, randomized controlled pediatric trial identified. The Cochrane Database of Systematic Reviews was also reviewed. Finally, ClinicalTrials.gov was searched to identify results of unpublished and ongoing studies. The Jadad scale (Table 1) was used to assess the quality of randomized trials included in this analysis.[5] Additional literature updates using the same search strategies were performed in July 2010 and November 2012.

Whenever possible, data from randomized controlled trials (preferably placebo controlled) were used to answer the questions raised by the committee. When no such data were available, separate literature searches were performed.

TABLE 1 Criteria for Assessing Randomized Trials

Give 1 point for each of the following:
a. The study is described as randomized
b. The study is described as double-blind
c. There was a description of withdrawals and dropouts
Given 1 additional point if:
a. For randomized studies, the method of randomization was described and is appropriate
b. For double-blind studies, the method of blinding was described and is appropriate
Deduct 1 point if:
c. For randomized studies, the method of randomization was described and is inappropriate
d. For double-blind studies, the method of blinding was described and is inappropriate

Adapted from Jadad et al.[5]

RESULTS

In the initial search, 183 randomized trials were identified, 98 of which were published since 1998. Of these 98, a total of 62 were eliminated on the basis of titles indicating a focus on adults, chronic sinusitis, or post-surgical management. Inclusion criteria and results of the remaining 36 studies were reviewed. Seven studies included adolescents as young as 12 years, but they represented <2% of the study population, and no age-specific results were reported. Twenty-one additional studies included teenagers but did not report how many were included; average ages for these studies were in the third to fourth decade of life. The updated literature search in July 2010 identified 2 additional randomized controlled trials that focused on ancillary treatment of sinusitis in children. A final search performed in November 2012 did not identify any additional controlled trials.

Overall, 17 randomized studies of sinusitis in children were identified and included in the current analysis. The meta-analysis search identified 1 study that focused exclusively on children and 2 others that focused primarily on adults but also assessed and separately reported results of pediatric studies. A review of ClinicalTrials.gov identified 28 sinusitis studies including children aged <18 years, only 3 of which were limited exclusively to children. One of these (Wald et al[6]) has recently been published and is included in the analysis; the other 2 studies are not yet recruiting patients.

TREATMENT

Efficacy of Antimicrobial Therapy

Randomized Placebo-Controlled Trials

Four randomized, double-blind, placebo-controlled trials involving 392 children were identified (Table 2).[6–9] An additional study[10] that was included in the previous technical report was excluded because it included patients with chronic and subacute sinusitis. The results of these 4 studies varied. Two studies favored treatment, and the other 2 found no significant difference in clinical cure between the treatment and control groups.

Clinical improvement in children receiving placebo ranged from 14% to 79% across the 4 studies, suggesting significant heterogeneity. The outcomes in the treatment groups were less varied, ranging from 50% to 81%. However, the efficacies of specific treatments are difficult to compare directly because the studies were performed over a 25-year period, during which a universal conjugate pneumococcal vaccination program was introduced and the prevalence of penicillin-resistant *Streptococcus pneumoniae* and β-lactamase–producing *Moraxella* and *Haemophilus* species increased.

The disparity in outcomes in the placebo groups is likely explained by the different methods used in each study. Notably, the inclusion criteria differed between each of the 4 studies. For instance, the minimal duration of symptoms required for entry into the study by Kristo et al[9] was not specified and averaged between 8 and 9 days for the treatment and control groups, respectively. Furthermore, only 32% of subjects had symptoms lasting at least 10 days. Therefore, the results of this study are not generalizable to the AAP definition of sinusitis, which is 10 days of symptoms, and should not be considered in the revised guidelines. Inclusion criteria for persistent symptoms in the other 3 studies were similar. Each specified respiratory symptoms that persisted for at least 10 days but <30 days. Only the 1986 study by Wald et al[7] required an abnormal radiograph for study entry.

Another study by Wald et al (in 2009)[6] was the only trial to include a subgroup of children who met criteria for worsening (on or after day 6 with fever or increase in symptoms) or severe (temperature ≥102°F with purulent discharge for at least 3 consecutive days) symptoms of sinusitis.

Exclusion criteria for each of these 3 studies had some similarities. Allergy to study drug, recent receipt of antibiotics, and concurrent bacterial infection requiring treatment were exclusion criteria in all of the studies. Complications of sinusitis were also listed as exclusion criteria, although the definitions of this factor differed between the studies. For instance, Garbutt et al[8] excluded children with "fulminant sinusitis," including children with fever ≥39°C (102.2°F); this condition was a specific inclusion criterion for the severe group in the 2009 study by Wald et al.[6] In addition, underlying medical conditions were used to exclude children, but the specific diagnoses differed in the 3 studies. Wald et al[7] excluded children with a variety of underlying medical conditions, including history of asthma and allergic rhinitis. Garbutt et al[8] only excluded children with cystic fibrosis; children with asthma and allergic rhinitis were included. Wald et al[6] only excluded children with immunodeficiency or anatomic abnormality of the upper respiratory tract.

The 3 studies used similar randomization schemes: patients were stratified according to age group and clinical severity before randomization. However, the metrics of clinical severity differed. The 2 studies by Wald et al[6,7] used a 10-point questionnaire (Table 3), and the study by Garbutt et al[8] used the S5 score (Table 4), previously validated by the same author.[11] Although each of these 3 studies stratified patients according to clinical severity before randomization,

separate results stratified by severity are not reported. This information may be helpful in the identification of patients (on the basis of clinical grounds) who might benefit from antimicrobial therapy.

Another key methodologic difference is that the study by Wald et al (1986)[7] did not use intention-to-treat analysis. Fifteen (14%) of 108 children were excluded because of lack of compliance or drug toxicity, which may have introduced bias.

Because of these significant differences in study design, formal meta-analyses were not performed. However, qualitative analysis of these results suggests that there may be certain clinical characteristics that identify patients who benefit from antimicrobial therapy.

Randomized Controlled Comparison Trials

In addition to the 4 placebo-controlled studies described previously, there have been other randomized studies of acute sinusitis in children comparing different antimicrobial treatment courses (Table 5).[12–16] Three of these were included in the previous report, and 2 additional studies have been published since 1998. None of these studies demonstrated a clear advantage of 1 therapy over another, and rates of cure or improvement were well above 80%. Although these studies offer some insight into the relative efficacies of different treatments, they do not include a placebo group. This factor is important given that many of the children included in these studies may have improved spontaneously without any specific antimicrobial therapy. In addition, none of these studies was designed as noninferiority or equivalence studies and, therefore, may have been underpowered to detect true differences between competing treatments.

TABLE 2 Randomized, Placebo-Controlled Trials of Antimicrobial Treatment of Acute Sinusitis in Children

Variable	Wald et al[7]	Garbutt et al[8]	Kristo et al[9]	Wald et al[6]
Inclusion criteria	Nasal discharge of any quality	"Persistent upper respiratory symptoms"	Acute respiratory symptoms suggestive of sinusitis that were "not improving"	Persistent: nasal discharge of any quality and/or daytime cough persisting for >10 d without improvement
	and/or		Nasal discharge and obstruction, sneezing, cough	Worsening: worsening on or after day 6 with fever or increase in symptoms
	Cough			Severe: temperature ≥102°F with purulent nasal discharge for at least 3 consecutive days
	Symptoms present for 10–30 d	Symptoms present for 10–28 d	Symptoms present <3 wk, no lower bound	Symptoms present <30 d, lower bound per definitions above
	Age: 2–16 y	Age: 1–18 y	Age: 4–10 y	Age: 1–10 y
Exclusion criteria	Abnormal radiograph results	NA	Abnormal US	NA
	Penicillin allergy	Allergy	Allergy	Allergy
	Previous Rx within 3 d	Previous Rx within 2 wk	Previous Rx within 4 wk	Previous Rx within 15 d
	Underlying conditions (asthma, allergic rhinitis, CF, sickle cell anemia, congenital heart disease, immunodeficiency)	CF only	Previous sinus surgery	Underlying conditions (immunodeficiency or anatomic abnormality of upper respiratory tract)
	Otitis media, pneumonia, GAS pharyngitis (throat/NP culture performed at study enrollment)	"Fulminant sinusitis"	Current antimicrobial Rx	Concurrent bacterial infection
	Severe headache or periorbital swelling	(fever >39°C, facial swelling, facial pain)	"Complications of sinus disease"	Complication of sinusitis requiring hospitalization, IV antibiotics, or subspecialty evaluation.
	Normal radiograph of paranasal sinuses	NA	NA	NA
Source of patients	Primary or secondary care patients at an academic children's hospital	3 suburban primary care practices	1 private health care center	2 private practices, 1 hospital-based clinic
Randomization			Block randomization	Assigned to persistent or nonpersistent group then
	Stratified by age: (<6 and ≥6 y)	Stratified by age: (<7 and ≥7 y)		Stratified by age: (<6 and ≥6 y)
	And clinical severity	And clinical severity		And clinical severity
	Then randomized	Then randomized		Then randomized
Metric for severity	Clinical severity score: <8 is mild and ≥8 is severe	Clinical severity score using S5 score	8 acute symptoms, rated 0–4	Same as Wald et al[7]
Telephone follow-up	1, 2, 3, 5, and 7 d	3, 7, 10, 14, 21, 28, and 60 d	NA	1, 2, 3, 5, 7, 10, 20, and 30 d
Clinical visit	Day 10	Day 14	Day 14	Day 14
Primary outcome	Clinical outcome at 3 and 10 d	Change in sinus symptoms at day 14	% complete cure at 2 wk	Cure at day 14
Secondary outcomes	Not specified	Adverse events	Adverse effects	Adverse events
		Relapse	Improvement without complications	Proportion with treatment failure
		Change in functional status		
		Parental satisfaction with treatment	Days when analgesics, nasal decongestants or cough mixtures were given	
N placebo	35	55	41	28
N treatment group	30 amoxicillin (40 mg/kg per day) divided 3 times/d for 10 d	58 amoxicillin (40 mg/kg per day) divided 3 times/d for 14 d	41 cefuroxime 125 mg 2 times/d for 10 d	28 amoxicillin/clavulanate (90 mg/kg amoxicillin + 6.4 mg clavulanate) divided 2 times/d for 14 days
	28 amoxicillin/clavulanate	48 amoxicillin/clavulanate (45 mg/kg per day amoxicillin) divided 2 times/d for 14 d		
Adjuvant therapy	None were prescribed. Not formally studied	Prescription or over-the-counter symptomatic treatments allowed. Use recorded	Analgesics, nose drops, and cough mixtures allowed. Use recorded in diary	Use "discouraged"—not formally studied
Compliance	History and remaining medications at follow-up visit	Self-report at day 14	Residual drugs collected at day 14	History and remaining medications at follow-up visit

TABLE 2 Continued

Variable	Wald et al[7]	Garbutt et al[8]	Kristo et al[9]	Wald et al[6]
Adverse events	Children who developed rash and diarrhea were excluded from analysis	Assessed at day 14	Assessed at day 14	Assessed at day 14
Loss to follow-up	15 children excluded because of adverse events (8) and noncompliance (7)	None (typographic error in original manuscript)	3 children (2 placebo, 1 treatment) lost to follow-up	6 lost to follow-up in treatment group
Primary outcome	Cure at 10 d: Amoxicillin: 20/30 (67%); Amoxicillin/ clavulanate: 18/28 (64%); Placebo: 15/35 (43%) Total: Antibiotic: 38/58; Placebo: 15/35 (66% vs 43%; $P < .05$) Failure at 10 d: Amoxicillin: 5/30; Amoxicillin/clavulanate: 7/28; Placebo: 14/35 Total: Antibiotic: 12/58; Placebo: 15/35 (21% vs 43%; $P < .05$)	Improvement at 14 d: Amoxicillin: 79% (46/58); Amoxicillin/clavulanate: 81% (39/48); Placebo: 79% (43/55)	Cure at 14 d: 22/35 in experimental group vs 21/37 in placebo (63% vs 57%; $P = .64$)	Cure at 14 d: 14/28 in experimental group vs 4/28 in placebo (50% vs 14%' $P = .01$) Failure at 14 d: 4/28 in experimental group vs 19/28 in placebo (14% vs 68%; $P < .001$) If all subjects lost to follow-up were considered failures, therapy is still effective (35% vs 68%; $P = .032$)
Jadad score	3	5	4	4

CF, cystic fibrosis; GAS, group A streptococcal; IV, intravenous; NA, not applicable; NP, nasopharyngeal; Rx, prescription; US, ultrasonography.

In addition to these randomized comparator studies, Garbutt et al[8] and Wald et al[7] used amoxicillin and amoxicillin/ clavulanic acid treatments arms in their placebo-controlled studies. No significant differences between these 2 treatments were detected.

Adverse Events Associated With Antimicrobial Therapy

Randomized Placebo-Controlled Trials

Adverse effects of treatment were described in all 3 studies. In the first study by Wald et al,[7] rash developed in 1 child in the amoxicillin group and 1 in the placebo group. Diarrhea, requiring cessation of therapy, developed in 6 children in the amoxicillin/clavulanic acid group and 1 child in the placebo group. In the study by Garbutt et al,[8] one-half of all study participants reported an adverse effect; these events were equally distributed across the study groups. Diarrhea was reported by 20% to 22% of participants ($P = .97$ between the 3 groups). The only reported adverse effect that reached statistical significance was abdominal pain, which occurred in 29% of children in the amoxicillin group but only 15% and 9% of children in the amoxicillin/clavulanate and placebo groups, respectively ($P = .02$). In the most recent study by Wald et al,[6] 44% of children in the experimental group experienced an adverse event compared with 14% in the control group ($P = .014$). The incidences of specific adverse events were not described, but diarrhea was reportedly the most common. Although efficacy data from the study by Kristo et al[9] should not be considered in the guidelines, data can be used to compare adverse events associated with antimicrobial therapy compared with placebo. In this study, 3 children developed self-limited diarrhea (1 in the cefuroxime group and 2 in the placebo group).

Randomized Controlled Comparison Trials

Adverse events were reported in 4 of these studies.[12,14–16] The incidence of

TABLE 3 Scale Used in Studies by Wald et al[6,7]

Symptoms or Signs	Points
Abnormal nasal or postnasal discharge	
Minimal	1
Severe	2
Nasal congestion	1
Cough	2
Malodorous breath	1
Facial tenderness	3
Erythematous nasal mucosa	1
Fever	
<38.5°C	1
≥38.5°C	2
Headache (retro-orbital)	
Severe	3
Mild	1

Interpretation: <8 = mild, ≥8 = severe.

TABLE 4 Scale Used by Garbutt et al[11]

Symptom	Points			
	1	2	3	0
Blocked up or stuffy nose	Small	Medium	Large	Not a problem or do not know
Headaches or face pain	Small	Medium	Large	Not a problem or do not know
Coughing during the day	Small	Medium	Large	Not a problem or do not know
Coughing at night	Small	Medium	Large	Not a problem or do not know
Color of child's mucus			Yellow or green	None or clear

S5 score is obtained by averaging the scores for each symptom. In the clinical trial,[8] children were stratified into 2 groups before randomization: S5 score <2 or S5 score ≥2.

TABLE 5 Randomized Controlled Trials Comparing Different Antimicrobial Treatments for Acute Sinusitis

Author (Year)	Age (y)	Antimicrobial Agents	Duration	N	Cured (%)	Improved (%)	Failed (%)	Relapsed (%)	Recurred (%)	Jadad Score
Poachanukoon and Kitcharoensakkul (2008)[12]	1–15	Amoxicillin-clavulanate (80–90 mg/kg per day)	14 d	72	ND	85	ND	11	6	3
		Cefditoren (4–6 mg/kg) 2 times/d	14 d	66	ND	79	ND	9	3	
Simon (1999)[13]	0.5–17	Erythromycin (40 mg/kg per day)	14 d	50	96	ND	4	ND	10	1
		Ceftibuten (9 mg/kg per day)	10 d	50	92	ND	8	ND	12	
		Ceftibuten (9 mg/kg per day)	15 d	50	92	ND	8	ND	8	
		Ceftibuten (9 mg/kg per day)	20 d	50	100	ND	0	ND	8	
Ficnar et al (1997)[14]	0.5–12	Azithromycin (10 mg/kg per day)	3 d	27	96	ND	0	4	ND	1
		Azithromycin (10 mg/kg on day 1, then 5 mg/kg on days 2–5)	5 d	18	100	ND	0	0	ND	
Careddu et al (1993)[15]	2–14	Brodimoprim (10 mg/kg on day 1, then 5 mg/kg per day)	8 d	25	96	ND	4	ND	ND	1
		Amoxicillin-clavulanate (50 mg/kg per day)	NS	27	85	ND	15	ND	ND	
Wald et al (1984)[16]	1–16	Amoxicillin (40 mg/kg per day)	10 d	27	81	4	11	4	4	3
		Cefaclor (40 mg/kg per day)	10 d	23	78	9	4	11	17	

ND, not determined; NS, not specified.

adverse events did not differ between study groups for 3 of these studies. Poachanukoon and Kitcharoensakkul[12] reported a higher rate of diarrhea (18.1%) in children receiving amoxicillin/clavulanate compared with those receiving cefditoren (4.5% [P = .02]). However, diarrhea was self-limited and did not require termination of medication or study withdrawal.

ANCILLARY TREATMENTS

Six randomized-controlled trials have assessed a variety of ancillary treatments for acute sinusitis (Table 6)[17–20] and are summarized here.

Steroids

The 2001 technical report described 1 study that assessed the efficacy of intranasal steroids in children.[17] In that study, 89 children received amoxicillin/clavulanate (40 mg/kg per day) and were randomized to receive either budesonide nasal spray (n = 43) or placebo (n = 46) for 3 weeks. Although no difference in symptom improvement was noted between the groups at the end of therapy (3 weeks), children in the budesonide group had improved cough and nasal discharge at 2 weeks,

whereas children in the placebo group did not, suggesting that corticosteroids may lead to more rapid resolution of symptoms. Since then, there has been 1 other randomized controlled trial in children studying the efficacy of intranasal budesonide.[18] In this study, 52 children (mean age: 8 years; age range: 6–16 years) with acute maxillary sinusitis received cefaclor (40 mg/kg) for 10 days with either pseudoephedrine (2 × 30 mg daily) or intranasal budesonide (2 × 100 µg daily) for 10 days. There was no placebo group. Children with underlying allergy were excluded. Children in the budesonide group had statistically significantly better resolution of headache, cough, nasal stuffiness, and nasal drainage. There were no adverse events reported. However, these authors defined acute sinusitis as an infection that could take up to 12 weeks for complete resolution, and the results may therefore not be generalizable to AAP guidelines.

Decongestant-Antihistamine

No randomized controlled studies have been performed since a study cited in the 2001 report.[19] All children in that

study received 14 days of amoxicillin (37.5–50 mg/kg per day, divided 3 times per day). They were then randomized to receive either placebo or the combination of oxymetazoline nasal spray and an oral decongestant-antihistamine. Both groups had marked clinical improvement in symptoms 3 days into treatment. In addition, there were no significant differences in clinical or radiographic findings between the 2 groups at the end of treatment.

Nasal Spray

One randomized controlled trial compared the use of 14 days of treatment with Ems mineral salts versus xylometazoline (0.05% solution) nasal spray in children with acute sinusitis.[20] There was no placebo group, and antibiotic use was not permitted. The primary outcome was mucosal inflammation (rubescence, swelling, and discharge) at baseline, day 7, and day 14. There were no significant differences between the 2 groups at day 14. However, at day 7, the mineral salt group had less nasal discharge than the xylometazoline group (P = .0163), suggesting that the spray may lead to more

TABLE 6 Randomized Controlled Trials of Ancillary Therapies for Acute Sinusitis

Author (Year)	Age (y)	Inclusion Criteria	Primary Therapy	LOT	Other Treatments	N	Main Outcome	Jadad Score
Barlan et al (1997)[17]	1–15	2 major, or 1 major and 2 minor criteria. Duration >7 d; Major criteria: purulent nasal discharge, purulent pharyngeal drainage, cough; Minor criteria: periorbital edema, facial pain, tooth pain, earache, sore throat, wheeze, headache, foul breath, fever	Intranasal budesonide (50 µg each nostril) 2 times/day; Intranasal placebo bid	21 21	All received amoxicillin/clavulanate (40 mg/kg per day)	43 46	No difference in cough or nasal discharge scores at weeks 1 or 3. Budesonide scores statistically lower (less symptomatic) at week 2 for both outcomes	2
Yilmaz et al (2000)[18]	6–16	Specific symptoms not specified Duration: infection that could take up to 12 wk to resolve	Intranasal budesonide (2 × 100 µg) Oral pseudoephedrine (2 × 30 mg)	10 10	All received cefaclor (40 mg/kg per day)	26 26	Budesonide group statistically better improvement in headache, cough, nasal stuffiness, and nasal drainage at day 10	1
McCormick et al (1996)[19]	1–18	8–29 d of sinusitis symptoms	Oxymetazoline nasal spray (0.05%) plus syrup with decongestant-antihistamine Placebo nasal spray and syrup	14 14	All children received amoxicillin by age/weight: 10–12 kg, 150 mg tid; 12.1–15 kg, 200 mg tid; >15 kg, 250 mg tid Teenagers: 40 mg/kg per day (maximum: 500 tid)	34 34	No difference between groups in mean symptom score at enrollment, day 3, or day 14	4
Michel et al (2005)[20]	2–6	"Definition give[n] by the AAP"	Intranasal isotonic Ems mineral salts Intranasal xylometazoline (0.05%)	14 14	No additional treatment (including antibiotics) allowed	66[a]	No difference in symptoms at day 14. Ems group had statistically significant less inflammation at day 7	2
Wang et al (2009)[21]	3–12	(1) URI with purulent nasal discharge and/or cough >7 d (2) Abnormal findings of 1 or both maxillary sinuses by Water's projection	Standard therapy plus normal saline nasal irrigation, 15–20 mL per nostril 1–3 times/day Standard therapy alone	21 21	"Standard therapy" defined as systemic antibiotics, mucolytics, and nasal decongestants	30 39	Saline group had better scores for daytime rhinorrhea and nighttime nasal congestion. No statistically significant differences in quality of life score, nasal smear, or Water's projection	1
Unuvar et al (2010)[22]	3–12	(1) 10–30 d of URTI symptoms (2) Presence of severe symptoms of rhinosinusitis	Erdosteine syrup (5–8 mg/kg/day orally divided bid) Placebo	14 14	None	49 43	No significant difference in clinical improvement at 14 d between the 2 groups	4

bid, 2 times per day; LOT, length of therapy; tid, 3 times per day; URTI, upper respiratory tract infection.

[a] Sixty-six patients in trial; numbers in each treatment arm not specified.

rapid resolution of symptoms. Wang et al[21] randomized 69 children to receive standard therapy (systemic antibiotics, mucolytic agents, and nasal decongestants) or standard therapy plus nasal irrigation (15–20 mL of normal saline administered via syringe to each nostril 1–3 times per day). Outcomes included a daily nasal symptom score (summarized weekly), pediatric rhinoconjunctivitis quality of life questionnaire (at baseline and 3 weeks), weekly nasal peak expiratory flow rate, weekly nasal smear, and Water's projection (baseline and 3 weeks). The irrigation group had significantly better symptom scores for daytime (but not nighttime) rhinorrhea at weeks 1, 2, and 3 and nighttime (but not daytime) nasal congestion at weeks 1, 2, and 3. Children in the irrigation group also had better nasal peak expiratory flow rates and slightly better quality of life scores at 3 weeks. There were no statistically significant differences in nasal smear or Water's projections between the 2 groups after 3 weeks of treatment.

Mucolytic Agents

One randomized controlled trial assessed S5 scores in 49 children receiving the mucolytic erdosteine compared with 43 children who received placebo.[22] After 14 days of treatment, there was no significant difference in S5 scores between the 2 groups.

In addition to these studies, which were specifically designed to assess the efficacy of nonantimicrobial therapy, use of ancillary measures was measured and reported for 2 of the randomized trials of antimicrobial use. In the study by Garbutt et al,[8] there were no significant differences in the overall use of ancillary therapies between the treatment and placebo groups (52% vs 48% vs 49%; $P = .92$). Although individual-level data were not presented, this finding makes it unlikely that unbalanced use of adjuvant therapies contributed to the study outcomes. Among individual therapies, only use of combination products was reported more frequently in 1 group (10% of amoxicillin/ clavulanate vs 0% and 2% of amoxicillin and placebo, respectively; $P = .01$). In the study by Poachanukoon and Kitcharoensakkul,[12] use of concomitant intranasal corticosteroids (52%) and oral decongestants (22%) was common but did not differ between the study groups.

DIAGNOSIS

Although sinus aspiration remains the gold standard for diagnosis of acute sinusitis, it is rarely practiced outside of the research setting. Furthermore, few recent studies have used aspiration as a criterion for study entry or used bacteriologic cure as an outcome. Despite these microbiologic limitations, evidence from the trials summarized previously can answer a slightly different question: which (if any) clinical, laboratory, and/or radiologic findings are able to discriminate between children who are likely to benefit from antimicrobial therapy and those who are not?

CLINICAL FINDINGS
Duration of Symptoms

The most commonly used diagnostic criterion for acute bacterial sinusitis is persistent or prolonged duration of symptoms for 10 to 14 days.[23] This criterion is based on the observation that most viral upper respiratory tract infections last 5 to 7 days.[3] However, the study by Garbutt et al[8] demonstrated that duration of symptoms alone was not sufficient to warrant antimicrobial therapy. A minimum of 10 days of symptoms was required for study entry, and all 3 groups had a mean duration of symptoms greater than 2 weeks (amoxicillin: 15.8 days; amoxicillin/clavulanate: 18.5 days; placebo: 15.4 days).

Signs and Symptoms

Purulent rhinorrhea, nasal congestion, and headache are other common findings used to diagnose sinusitis.[23] The various clinical trials used different combinations of these findings in their inclusion criteria. The 3 placebo-controlled studies limited to children with at least 10 days of symptoms also used clinical severity scores based on these signs and symptoms Tables 2 and 3 stratify study participants before randomization. Because this stratification occurred before randomization, severity-specific results might help clarify which children are likely to benefit from antimicrobial therapy.

Imaging Studies

The 2001 guidelines recommended that radiologic studies should not be used to diagnose sinusitis in children 6 years or younger and that computed tomography (CT) should be considered only for children requiring surgery.[3] Ultrasonography has also been suggested as a potential diagnostic tool for acute sinusitis. The 2001 technical report cited 1 study that demonstrated good concordance between ultrasonographic findings and retrieval of fluid on sinus aspiration.[24] On the basis of that study, ultrasonographic findings (either mucosal thickening of ≥ 5 mm or fluid in at least 1 maxillary sinus) were used as entry criteria in the study by Kristo et al.[9] In that study, children also underwent occipitomental radiography, and the film results were defined as positive for sinusitis if there was mucosal thickening of at least 4 mm, an air-fluid level, or total opacification of at least 1 maxillary sinus. Eighty-nine percent of children in the treatment group and 92% of those in the placebo group met this criterion, suggesting good concordance between plain films and ultrasonography. However, these findings were not predictive of which children would benefit from antimicrobial therapy. Radiographic studies were not used in the other 2 recent placebo-controlled studies.[6,8]

Laboratory Studies

None of the studies required routine laboratory studies for study entry. Microbiologic samples were only obtained in 2 placebo-controlled studies and did not include direct sinus sampling. Wald et al[7] used results of throat and nasopharyngeal cultures to exclude patients with group A streptococcal pharyngitis from their study. Kristo et al[9] obtained nasopharyngeal cultures on all patients but only reported those with results positive for *Streptococcus pneumoniae* and *Haemophilus influenzae*, which occurred in 12.5% of study participants.

SUBACUTE SINUSITIS

Subacute sinusitis has been defined as infection that lasts between 30 and 90 days.[3] Three small randomized controlled trials assessing the efficacy of different treatment strategies for subacute sinusitis were identified (Table 7).[25–27] None of these studies included a placebo group. One compared empirical amoxicillin/clavulanate with culture-based (from nasal mucosa) antimicrobial treatment.[25] Culture of nasal specimens was not performed on the children in the empirical antibiotic group. Five (18.5%) of 27 culture results in the experimental group were positive for amoxicillin/clavulanate-resistant organisms (1 Pseudomonas species, 2 resistant to S pneumoniae, and 2 anaerobic streptococci), and appropriate therapy was initiated. Nasal obstruction at day 14 was unchanged or worse for 9 children (36%) in the empirical arm but only 4 children (15%) in the culture-based arm (P = .037, per authors). Another study compared azithromycin versus amoxicillin/clavulanate.[26] The third compared amoxicillin, amoxicillin/clavulanic acid, trimethoprim/sulfamethoxazole, and no antimicrobial therapy.[27] In these 2 studies, no advantage was detected in any treatment arm compared with others. However, the studies were small and were likely not powered to detect true differences.

CLINICAL QUESTIONS FOR WHICH HIGH-QUALITY DATA ARE LACKING

Definitions of Acute, Subacute, and Recurrent Acute Sinusitis

The definitions of acute, subacute, and recurrent acute sinusitis are outlined in the 2001 AAP guidelines.[3] Although logical and based on the presumed pathogenesis of these distinct clinical entities, there are few clinical or laboratory data to confirm these definitions in children. One study of subacute sinusitis included 52 sinus aspirations of 40 children with subacute (30–120 days of symptoms) sinusitis and found similar pathogens as in acute sinusitis.[28] The definition of subacute sinusitis used in this study and in the study be Ng et al[26] were derived from an expert consensus panel.[29] The study by El-Hennawi et al[23] cites the 2001 AAP guidelines, and the study by Dohlman et al[25] does not provide a reference for the study definition of subacute sinusitis.

Epidemiology of Sinusitis in the Pneumococcal Conjugate Vaccine Era

A separate literature search was performed to identify studies of sinusitis in the era of the pneumococcal conjugate vaccine. Although there are substantial data regarding the epidemiology of invasive pneumococcal disease and acute otitis media since implementation of pneumococcal immunization, no recent pediatric sinusitis studies that included microbiologic data were identified. Brook et al[30] compared culture results from sinuses of adults before and after introduction of the pneumococcal conjugate vaccine. There was a statistically significant decrease in the prevalence of S pneumoniae and a significant increase in the prevalence of H influenzae. In addition, there was a 12% decrease in penicillin resistance observed in pneumococcal

TABLE 7 Randomized Controlled Trials of Antimicrobial Therapy for Subacute Sinusitis

Author (Year)	Age (y)	Inclusion Criteria	Antimicrobial Agents	Length	Other Treatments	N	Better (%)	Worse or Same (%)	Jadad Score
El-Hennawi et al (2006)[25]	<2	Persistent nasal discharge and nasal obstruction for 30–90 d	Amoxicillin-clavulanate (40 mg/ kg per day)	14 d	All had therapeutic nasal suction every third day	30	64	36	2
			Culture-based (nasal suction)			30			
			Amoxicillin/clavulanate (40 mg/ kg per day)			12	83	17	
			Amoxicillin/clavulanate (90 mg/ kg per day)	14 d		6	100	0	
			Other antibiotics			5	100	0	
			No antibiotics (negative culture result)			4	50	50	
Ng et al (2000)[26]	5–16	Nasal discharge or blockage for 30–120 d and abnormal sinus radiograph	Azithromycin (10 mg/kg per day)	3 d	All received budesonide nasal spray 50 μg/nostril 2 times/ day for 91 d	20	ND[a]	30	3
			Amoxicillin/clavulanate (312 mg 3 times/day if aged ≤12 y or 375 mg 3 times/day if aged >12 y)	14 d		21	ND[a]	24	
Dohlman et al (1993)[27]	2–16	Mucoid nasal drainage, cough, or poorly controlled asthma for 3 wk–3 mo and abnormal sinus radiograph	Amoxicillin (30-40 mg/kg per day)	21 d	All received oral phenylephrine, phenylpropanolamine, and guaifenesin; all received saline nasal spray	25	72	28	3
			Amoxicillin-clavulanate (30-40 mg/kg per day)	21 d		26	73	27	
			TMP/SMX (8 mg/kg per day)	21 d		26	69	31	
			None			19	63	37	

ND, not determined; TMP/SMX, trimethoprim/sulfamethoxazole.
[a] This study only reported "failures."

isolates and a 6% increase in β-lactamase–producing *H influenzae,* but these findings did not reach statistical significance. The same authors also compared nasopharyngeal (but not sinus) cultures in children before and after licensure of the pneumococcal conjugate vaccine and found similar results.[31]

Antimicrobial Prophylaxis

One small, nonrandomized study of antimicrobial prophylaxis in children with chronic sinusitis was identified.[32] Twenty-six of 86 children with chronic sinusitis received prophylaxis for 1 year. There was a 50% reduction in the number of episodes of sinusitis in 19 (73%) subjects. Nearly 25% of the children in the cohort had an underlying immunologic defect, but this discovery did not predict efficacy of prophylaxis. A randomized controlled study of azithromycin prophylaxis for acute recurrent sinusitis in children was identified on ClinicalTrials.gov and began recruiting patients in August 2009.

Duration of Symptoms

As presented previously, data from randomized trials suggest that duration of symptoms alone is not predictive of necessity of antimicrobial therapy. A small case series of complications of rhinosinusitis (almost exclusively orbital cellulitis) in children was recently published.[33] The authors noted that only 3 of 20 children admitted to a single institution over a 10-year period had symptoms of sinusitis for >10 days before hospitalization. On the basis of these data, they concluded that prevention of complications should not be a justification for initiating treatment after 10 days of symptoms.

Imaging

Since publication of the guidelines, there have been additional studies of children undergoing CT of the head that have confirmed the poor specificity of CT for acute sinusitis.[34,35] In addition, several small observational studies have assessed the use of MRI to diagnose acute sinusitis.[36–38] In the first, MRI was performed on a group of children 4 to 7 years of age presenting to a primary care center with any sign of respiratory infection.[36] Forty-one (68%) of 60 children had a major abnormality on imaging. Twenty-six children underwent follow-up 2 weeks later. Of these, 18 (69%) still had abnormal MRI findings, although this finding did not correlate with clinical symptoms. Another study by the same authors compared MRI findings in a convenience sample of children without respiratory complaints. Eight of 19 asymptomatic children had abnormal MRI findings.[37] A similar study found abnormal sinuses in 14 (31%) of 45 asymptomatic children.[38]

OTHER PEDIATRIC SINUSITIS GUIDELINES

Published guidelines were identified during the primary literature search. In addition, the Guidelines International Network (www.g-i-n.net) database was searched but yielded no results. Recently published pediatric guidelines for acute bacterial sinusitis are presented in Table 8.[39–42] These include English-language, pediatric-specific guidelines and other English-language guidelines that included separate recommendations for children. These guidelines were in near-complete concordance with the 2001 AAP guidelines in terms of clinical diagnosis, choice of antimicrobial agents, avoidance of radiographic studies, and avoidance of adjuvant therapies. One exception was that the European position paper recommended topical corticosteroids (in addition to oral antibiotics) as a grade A recommendation.[39]

The American College of Radiology Appropriateness Criteria, last updated in 2009, are another set of professional recommendations relevant to the diagnosis of sinusitis in children.[43] In summary, no radiologic studies are recommended by the American College of Radiology for acute uncomplicated sinusitis. Coronal CT of the paranasal sinuses is recommended for children with symptoms that persist after 10 days of appropriate therapy. Cranial CT with contrast, including the sinuses and orbits, is recommended for suspected complications of sinusitis.

DISCUSSION

The 2001 technical report noted a paucity of high-quality evidence for establishing the diagnosis and management of acute sinusitis in children. Nearly a decade later, data are still limited. Overall, 17 randomized controlled trials of pediatric acute sinusitis were identified. Of these, only 10 studies scored 3 points or higher on the Jadad scale, which is considered indicative of good study design.[5] These findings are consistent with other recent systematic reviews of pediatric acute sinusitis. A 2002 Cochrane review included data from 6 randomized controlled trials involving 562 children.[44] However, 2 studies focused on chronic sinusitis and 1 focused on subacute sinusitis. In addition, a recently published meta-analysis of studies comparing antimicrobial therapy versus placebo in all age groups identified only 3 studies that included children, all of which were included in the current review.[45] The publication of another placebo-controlled trial in 2009 is a significant contribution; however, only 310 children with acute sinusitis (392 if the Kristo study is included) have been studied in placebo-controlled fashion, with inconsistent results. Although meta-analysis techniques are designed to increase sample size and power,

TABLE 8 Summary of Other Published Guidelines for the Management of Acute Sinusitis in Children

Guideline	Antimicrobial Guidelines for Acute Bacterial Sinusitis (Sinus and Allergy Health Partnership, 2004)[39]	Cincinnati Children's Hospital Evidence-Based Guideline (2006)[40]	European Position Paper on Primary Care Diagnosis and Management of Rhinosinusitis and Nasal Polyps (2007)[41]	Guidelines for Treatment of Acute and Subacute Rhinosinusitis in Children (Italy, 2008)[42]
Diagnosis	No resolution after 10 d or worsens after 5–7 d with any of the following: nasal drainage, nasal congestion, facial pressure/pain, postnasal drainage, hyposmia/anosmia, fever, cough, fatigue, maxillary dental pain, and ear pressure/fullness	Clinical: at least 10 d without improvement Specific note: character of nasal discharge is not useful	(1) Cold with nasal discharge, daytime cough worsening at night >10 d (2) Cold that seems more severe than usual (3) Cold that was improving but suddenly worsens	(1) URTI without improvement within 10 d (2) URTI with severe symptoms (high fever, purulent rhinorrhea, headache, facial pain) (3) URTI that completely recedes within 3–4 d but recurs within 10 d
Imaging	Not recommended routinely	Not routinely recommended For children with persistent findings or complications, imaging decisions should be made in consultation with consulting subspecialists	Not recommended	Not recommended CT when surgery being considered
Antimicrobials	Mild disease, no recent antibiotics: amoxicillin/clavulanate, amoxicillin, cefpodoxime, cefuroxime, cefdinir For allergies: TMP/SMX, macrolides Moderate disease or mild disease with recent antibiotics: amoxicillin/clavulanate (high-dose), ceftriaxone For allergies, same as above, plus clindamycin	First-line: high-dose amoxicillin or amoxicillin/clavulanate for 10–14 d Second-line: cefuroxime, cefpodoxime, cefdinir For allergies: second-line antibiotics if non-type I reaction Clarithromycin or azithromycin for type I reaction	Recommended: specific agents not discussed	Amoxicillin 50 mg/kg per day If recent antibiotic exposure, school-attendance, or suspicion of antibiotic-resistant pathogens: Amoxicillin/clavulanate (80-90 mg/kg per day),cefuroxime (30 mg/kg per day), or cefaclor (50 mg/kg per day)
Adjuvant therapies	NA	Not recommended (antitussives, mucolytics, inhaled steroids, β_2- agonists, antihistamines, decongestants)	Topical steroids (in addition to systemic antibiotics) listed as a level Ib recommendation (from at least 1 RCT)	Antihistamines, corticosteroids, decongestants, expectorants, mucolytics, and vasoconstrictors not recommended Antibiotic prophylaxis not recommended
Complications	NA	Consult otolaryngologist and/or ophthalmologist	Immediate referral/hospitalization	Prompt, aggressive, multidisciplinary intervention

This table incorporates pediatric-specific guidelines (Cincinnati, Italy) as well as general guidelines with pediatric-specific recommendations (Sinus and Allergy Health Partnership, European Position Paper). CT, computed tomography; NA; not applicable; RCT, randomized controlled trial; TMP/SMX, trimethoprim/sulfamethoxazole; URTI, upper respiratory tract infection.

these were not pursued given the significant heterogeneity between the studies.

There are no reliable diagnostic criteria to distinguish between children with acute viral and bacterial sinusitis. However, the inclusion and exclusion criteria used in the 2 randomized studies that demonstrated a benefit of antimicrobial therapy compared with placebo offer insight into criteria that may identify children who are likely to benefit from antimicrobial therapy. Qualitatively, greater severity of illness at the time of presentation seems to be associated with increased likelihood of antimicrobial efficacy.

No studies of the microbiology of acute sinusitis in children have been published since the introduction of the conjugate pneumococcal vaccine. It is reasonable to assume that the same pathogen shifts observed in acute otitis media are found in acute bacterial sinusitis. However, this assumption would not necessarily imply that the treatment outcomes for otitis and sinusitis are the same.

Although the need for and choice of antimicrobial therapy remains controversial, the short-term adverse effect profiles for common antibacterial agents used in the management of sinusitis seem to be fairly benign. Two studies found no significant differences in adverse events between placebo and antimicrobial therapy.[8,9] A third reported that, although adverse effects were more common in the treatment group, those events occuring in children who received high-dose amoxicillin/clavulanate were mostly mild and self-limited.[6] However, the long-term effects of antimicrobial use on resistance patterns at the population level remain unmeasured and need to be considered in the revised guidelines.

Evidence to support the use of ancillary measures in the management of acute sinusitis in children is limited. Two small, randomized controlled studies demonstrated that children treated with intranasal steroids had better outcomes compared with children treated with systemic decongestants plus antibiotics[18] or antibiotics alone.[17] One of these studies demonstrated that corticosteroids hastened resolution of symptoms, but cure at the end of the study was equivalent. The other

defined acute sinusitis as an infection lasting up to 12 weeks, which may not be applicable to the definition of acute sinusitis used in the AAP guidelines. The efficacy of decongestants and antihistamines for sinusitis has not been proven. Given recent concerns regarding their safety profile in young children, the use of these agents should be avoided.

CONCLUSIONS

There are limited data to guide the diagnosis and management of acute

bacterial sinusitis in children. Although there have been 4 placebo-controlled studies of antimicrobial therapy in children with acute sinusitis, the results of these studies varied. It is clear that some children with sinusitis benefit from antibiotic use and some do not. Diagnostic and treatment guidelines focusing on severity of illness at the time of presentation have the potential to identify children who will benefit from therapy and at the same time minimize unnecessary use of antibiotics.

REFERENCES

1. Aitken M, Taylor JA. Prevalence of clinical sinusitis in young children followed up by primary care pediatricians. *Arch Pediatr Adolesc Med.* 1998;152(3):244–248

2. Revai K, Dobbs LA, Nair S, Patel JA, Grady JJ, Chonmaitree T. Incidence of acute otitis media and sinusitis complicating upper respiratory tract infection: the effect of age. *Pediatrics.* 2007;119(6). Available at: www.pediatrics.org/cgi/content/full/119/6/e1408

3. Wald ER, Bordley WC, Darrow DH, et al. Clinical practice guideline: management of sinusitis. *Pediatrics.* 2001;108(3):798–808

4. Ioannidis JP, Lau J. Technical report: evidence for the diagnosis and treatment of acute uncomplicated sinusitis in children: a systematic overview. *Pediatrics.* 2001;108 (3). Available at: www.pediatrics.org/cgi/content/full/108/3/e57

5. Jadad AR, Moore RA, Carroll D, et al. Assessing the quality of reports of randomized clinical trials: is blinding necessary? *Control Clin Trials.* 1996;17(1):1–12

6. Wald ER, Nash D, Eickhoff J. Effectiveness of amoxicillin/clavulanate potassium in the treatment of acute bacterial sinusitis in children. *Pediatrics.* 2009;124(1):9–15

7. Wald ER, Chiponis D, Ledesmamedina J. Comparative effectiveness of amoxicillin and amoxicillin-clavulanate potassium in acute para-nasal sinus infections in children: a double-blind, placebo-controlled trial. *Pediatrics.* 1986;77(6):795–800

8. Garbutt JM, Goldstein M, Gellman E, Shannon W, Littenberg B. A randomized, placebo-

controlled trial of antimicrobial treatment for children with clinically diagnosed acute sinusitis. *Pediatrics.* 2001;107(4):619–625

9. Kristo A, Uhari M, Luotonen J, Ilkko E, Koivunen P, Alho OP. Cefuroxime axetil versus placebo for children with acute respiratory infection and imaging evidence of sinusitis: a randomized, controlled trial. *Acta Paediatr.* 2005;94(9):1208–1213

10. Jeppesen F, Illum P. Pivampicillin (Pondocillin) in treatment of maxillary sinusitis. *Acta Otolaryngol.* 1972;74(5):375–382

11. Garbutt JM, Gellman EF, Littenberg B. The development and validation of an instrument to assess acute sinus disease in children. *Qual Life Res.* 1999;8(3):225–233

12. Poachanukoon O, Kitcharoensakkul M. Efficacy of cefditoren pivoxil and amoxicillin/clavulanate in the treatment of pediatric patients with acute bacterial rhinosinusitis in Thailand: a randomized, investigator-blinded, controlled trial. *Clin Ther.* 2008;30 (10):1870–1879

13. Simon MW. Treatment of acute sinusitis in childhood with ceftibuten. *Clin Pediatr (Phila).* 1999;38(5):269–272

14. Ficnar B, Huzjak N, Oreskovic K, Matrapazovski M, Klinar I. Azithromycin: 3-day versus 5-day course in the treatment of respiratory tract infections in children. *J Chemother.* 1997;9(1):38–43

15. Careddu P, Bellosta C, Tonelli P, Boccazzi A. Efficacy and tolerability of brodimoprim in pediatric infections. *J Chemother.* 1993;5 (6):543–545

16. Wald ER, Reilly JS, Casselbrant M, et al. Treatment of acute maxillary sinusitis in childhood: a comparative study of amoxicillin and cefaclor. *J Pediatr.* 1984;104(2):297–302

17. Barlan IB, Erkan E, Bakir M, Berrak S, Basaran MM. Intranasal budesonide spray as an adjunct to oral antibiotic therapy for acute sinusitis in children. *Ann Allergy Asthma Immunol.* 1997;78(6):598–601

18. Yilmaz G, Varan B, Yilmaz T, Gurakan B. Intranasal budesonide spray as an adjunct to oral antibiotic therapy for acute sinusitis in children. *Eur Arch Otorhinolaryngol.* 2000;257(5):256–259

19. McCormick DP, John SD, Swischuk LE, Uchida T. A double-blind, placebo-controlled trial of decongestant-antihistamine for the treatment of sinusitis in children. *Clin Pediatr (Phila).* 1996;35(9):457–460

20. Michel O, Essers S, Heppt WJ, Johannssen V, Reuter W, Hommel G. The value of Ems mineral salts in the treatment of rhinosinusitis in children: prospective study on the efficacy of mineral salts versus xylometazoline in the topical nasal treatment of children. *Int J Pediatr Otorhinolaryngol.* 2005;69(10):1359–1365

21. Wang YH, Yang CP, Ku MS, Sun HL, Lue KH. Efficacy of nasal irrigation in the treatment of acute sinusitis in children. *Int J Pediatr Otorhinolaryngol.* 2009;73:1696–1701

22. Unuvar E, Tamay Z, Yildiz I, et al. Effectiveness of erdosteine, a second generation mucolytic agent, in children with acute rhinosinusitis: a randomized, placebo

controlled, double-blinded clinical study. *Acta Paediatr.* 2010;99(4):585–589

23. McQuillan L, Crane LA, Kempe A. Diagnosis and management of acute sinusitis by pediatricians. *Pediatrics.* 2009;123(2). Available at: www.pediatrics.org/cgi/content/full/123/2/e193

24. Revonta M, Suonpaa J. Diagnosis and follow-up of ultrasonographical sinus changes in children. *Int J Pediatr Otorhinolaryngol.* 1982;4(4):301–308

25. El-Hennawi DM, Abou-Halawa AS, Zaher SR. Management of clinically diagnosed subacute rhinosinusitis in children under the age of two years: a randomized, controlled study. *J Laryngol Otol.* 2006;120(10):845–848

26. Ng DK, Chow PY, Leung LC, Chau KW, Chan E, Ho JC. A randomized controlled trial of azithromycin and amoxycillin/clavulanate in the management of subacute childhood rhinosinusitis. *J Paediatr Child Health.* 2000;36(4):378–381

27. Dohlman AW, Hemstreet MPB, Odrezin GT, Bartolucci AA. Subacute sinusitis: are antimicrobials necessary? *J Allergy Clin Immunol.* 1993;91(5):1015–1023

28. Wald ER, Byers C, Guerra N, Casselbrant M, Beste D. Subacute sinusitis in children. *J Pediatr.* 1989;115(1):28–32

29. The diagnosis and management of sinusitis in children: proceedings of a closed conference. *Pediatr Infect Dis.* 1985;4(suppl 6):S49–S81

30. Brook I, Foote PA, Hausfeld JN. Frequency of recovery of pathogens causing acute maxillary sinusitis in adults before and after introduction of vaccination of children with the 7-valent pneumococcal vaccine. *J Med Microbiol.* 2006;55(7):943–946

31. Brook I, Gober AE. Frequency of recovery of pathogens from the nasopharynx of children with acute maxillary sinusitis before and after the introduction of vaccination with the 7-valent pneumococcal vaccine. *Int J Pediatr Otorhinolaryngol.* 2007;71(4):575–579

32. Gandhi A, Brodsky L, Ballow M. Benefits of antibiotic-prophylaxis in children with chronic sinusitis: assessment of outcome predictors. *Allergy Proc.* 1993;14(1):37–43

33. Kristo A, Uhari M. Timing of rhinosinusitis complications in children. *Pediatr Infect Dis J.* 2009;28(9):769–771

34. Cotter CS, Stringer S, Rust KR, Mancuso A. The role of computed tomography scans in evaluating sinus disease in pediatric patients. *Int J Pediatr Otorhinolaryngol.* 1999;50(1):63–68

35. Schwartz RH, Pitkaranta A, Winther B. Computed tomography imaging of the maxillary and ethmoid sinuses in children with short-duration purulent rhinorrhea. *Otolaryngol Head Neck Surg.* 2001;124(2):160–163

36. Kristo A, Uhari M, Luotonen J, et al. Paranasal sinus findings in children during respiratory infection evaluated with magnetic resonance imaging. *Pediatrics.* 2003;111(5). Available at: www.pediatrics.org/cgi/content/full/111/5/e586

37. Kristo A, Alho OP, Luotonen J, Koivunen P, Tervonen O, Uhari M. Cross-sectional survey of paranasal sinus magnetic resonance imaging findings in schoolchildren. *Acta Paediatr.* 2003;92(1):34–36

38. Lim WK, Ram B, Fasulakis S, Kane KJ. Incidental magnetic resonance image sinus abnormalities in asymptomatic Australian children. *J Laryngol Otol.* 2003;117(12):969–972

39. Anon JB, Jacobs MR, Roche R, et al. Antimicrobial treatment guidelines for acute bacterial rhinosinusitis: executive summary. *Otolaryngol Head Neck Surg.* 2004;130(1):1–45

40. Acute Bacterial Sinusitis Guideline Team, Cincinnati Children's Hospital Medical Center. Evidence-based care guideline for medical management of acute bacterial sinusitis in children 1 through 17 years of age. Available at: www.cincinnatichildrens.org/svc/alpha/h/health-policy/ev-based/sinus.htm. Accessed November 6, 2012

41. Fokkens W, Lund V, Mullol J. European position paper on rhinosinusitis and nasal polyps 2007. *Rhinol Suppl.* 2007;(20):1–136

42. Esposito S, Principi N. Guidelines for the diagnosis and treatment of acute and subacute rhinosinusitis in children. *J Chemother.* 2008;20(2):147–157

43. American College of Radiology. Appropriateness criteria for sinonasal disease. Available at: www.acr.org/~/media/8172B4DE503149248E64856857674BB5.pdf. Accessed November 6, 2012

44. Morris P, Leach A. Antibiotics for persistent nasal discharge (rhinosinusitis) in children. *Cochrane Database Syst Rev.* 2002;(4):CD001094

45. Falagas ME, Giannopoulou KP, Vardakas KZ, Dimopoulos G, Karageorgopoulos DE. Comparison of antibiotics with placebo for treatment of acute sinusitis: a meta-analysis of randomised controlled trials. *Lancet Infect Dis.* 2008;8(9):543–552

Sinusitis Clinical Practice Guideline Quick Reference Tools

- Action Statement Summary
  — Clinical Practice Guideline for the Diagnosis and Management of Acute Bacterial Sinusitis in Children Aged 1 to 18 Years
- *ICD-10-CM* Coding Quick Reference for Sinusitis
- AAP Patient Education Handout
  — *Sinusitis and Your Child*

Action Statement Summary

Clinical Practice Guideline for the Diagnosis and Management of Acute Bacterial Sinusitis in Children Aged 1 to 18 Years

Key Action Statement 1

Clinicians should make a presumptive diagnosis of acute bacterial sinusitis when a child with an acute URI presents with the following:
- Persistent illness, ie, nasal discharge (of any quality) or daytime cough or both lasting more than 10 days without improvement;

OR

- Worsening course, ie, worsening or new onset of nasal discharge, daytime cough, or fever after initial improvement;

OR

- Severe onset, ie, concurrent fever (temperature ≥39°C/102.2°F) and purulent nasal discharge for at least 3 consecutive days (Evidence Quality: B; Recommendation).

Key Action Statement 2A

Clinicians should not obtain imaging studies (plain films, contrast-enhanced computed tomography [CT], MRI, or ultrasonography) to distinguish acute bacterial sinusitis from viral URI (Evidence Quality: B; Strong Recommendation).

Key Action Statement 2B

Clinicians should obtain a contrast-enhanced CT scan of the paranasal sinuses and/or an MRI with contrast whenever a child is suspected of having orbital or central nervous system complications of acute bacterial sinusitis (Evidence Quality: B; Strong Recommendation).

Key Action Statement 3

Initial Management of Acute Bacterial Sinusitis

3A: "Severe onset and worsening course" acute bacterial sinusitis. The clinician should prescribe antibiotic therapy for acute bacterial sinusitis in children with severe onset or worsening course (signs, symptoms, or both) (Evidence Quality: B; Strong Recommendation).

3B: "Persistent illness." The clinician should either prescribe antibiotic therapy OR offer additional outpatient observation for 3 days to children with persistent illness (nasal discharge of any quality or cough or both for at least 10 days without evidence of improvement) (Evidence Quality: B; Recommendation).

Key Action Statement 4

Clinicians should prescribe amoxicillin with or without clavulanate as first-line treatment when a decision has been made to initiate antibiotic treatment of acute bacterial sinusitis (Evidence Quality: B; Recommendation).

Key Action Statement 5A

Clinicians should reassess initial management if there is either a caregiver report of worsening (progression of initial signs/symptoms or appearance of new signs/symptoms) OR failure to improve (lack of reduction in all presenting signs/symptoms) within 72 hours of initial management (Evidence Quality: C; Recommendation).

Key Action Statement 5B

If the diagnosis of acute bacterial sinusitis is confirmed in a child with worsening symptoms or failure to improve in 72 hours, then clinicians may change the antibiotic therapy for the child initially managed with antibiotic OR initiate antibiotic treatment of the child initially managed with observation (Evidence Quality: D; Option based on expert opinion, case reports, and reasoning from first principles).

Coding Quick Reference for Sinusitis
ICD-10-CM
J01.90 Acute sinusitis, unspecified **J01.91** Acute recurrent sinusitis, unspecified

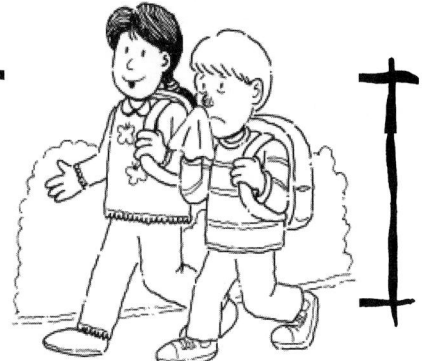

Sinusitis and Your Child

Sinusitis is an inflammation of the lining of the nose and sinuses. It is a very common infection in children.

Viral sinusitis usually accompanies a cold. Allergic sinusitis may accompany allergies such as hay fever. Bacterial sinusitis is a secondary infection caused by the trapping of bacteria in the sinuses during the course of a cold or allergy.

Fluid inside the sinuses

When your child has a viral cold or hay fever, the linings of the nose and sinus cavities swell up and produce more fluid than usual. This is why the nose gets congested and is "runny" during a cold.

Most of the time the swelling disappears by itself as the cold or allergy goes away. However, if the swelling does not go away, the openings that normally allow the sinuses to drain into the back of the nose get blocked and the sinuses fill with fluid. Because the sinuses are blocked and cannot drain properly, bacteria are trapped inside and grow there, causing a secondary infection. Although nose blowing and sniffing may be natural responses to this blockage, when excessive they can make the situation worse by pushing bacteria from the back of the nose into the sinuses.

Is it a cold or bacterial sinusitis?

It is often difficult to tell if an illness is just a viral cold or if it is complicated by a bacterial infection of the sinuses.

Generally viral colds have the following characteristics:

- Colds usually last only 5 to 10 days.
- Colds typically start with clear, watery nasal discharge. After a day or 2, it is normal for the nasal discharge to become thicker and white, yellow, or green. After several days, the discharge becomes clear again and dries.
- Colds include a daytime cough that often gets worse at night.
- If a fever is present, it is usually at the beginning of the cold and is generally low grade, lasting for 1 or 2 days.
- Cold symptoms usually peak in severity at 3 or 5 days, then improve and disappear over the next 7 to 10 days.

Signs and symptoms that your child may have bacterial sinusitis include:

- Cold symptoms (nasal discharge, daytime cough, or both) lasting more than 10 days *without improving*
- Thick yellow nasal discharge *and* a fever for at least 3 or 4 days in a row
- A severe headache behind or around the eyes that gets worse when bending over
- Swelling and dark circles around the eyes, especially in the morning
- Persistent bad breath along with cold symptoms (However, this also could be from a sore throat or a sign that your child is not brushing his teeth!)

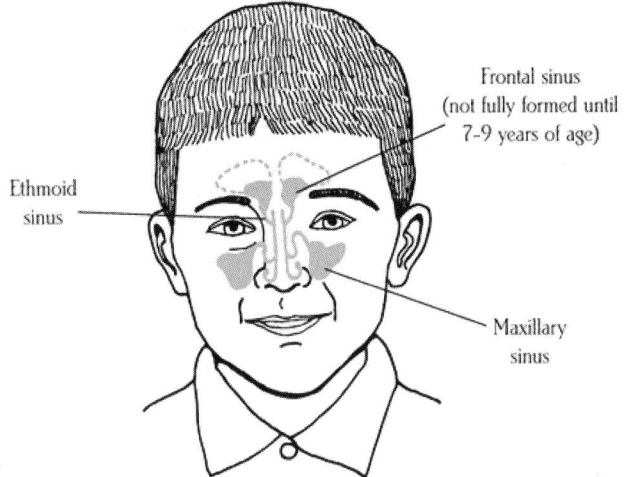

Frontal sinus (not fully formed until 7-9 years of age)

Ethmoid sinus

Maxillary sinus

The linings of the sinuses and the nose always produce some fluid (secretions). This fluid keeps the nose and sinus cavities from becoming too dry and adds moisture to the air that you breathe.

In very rare cases, a bacterial sinus infection may spread to the eye or the central nervous system (the brain). If your child has the following symptoms, call your pediatrician immediately:

- Swelling and/or redness around the eyes, not just in the morning but all day
- Severe headache and/or pain in the back of the neck
- Persistent vomiting
- Sensitivity to light
- Increasing irritability

Diagnosing bacterial sinusitis

It may be difficult to tell a sinus infection from an uncomplicated cold, especially in the first few days of the illness. Your pediatrician will most likely be able to tell if your child has bacterial sinusitis after examining your child and hearing about the progression of symptoms. In older children, when the diagnosis is uncertain, your pediatrician may order computed tomographic (CT) scans to confirm the diagnosis.

Treating bacterial sinusitis

If your child has bacterial sinusitis, your pediatrician may prescribe an antibiotic for at least 10 days. Once your child is on the medication, symptoms should start to go away over the next 2 to 3 days—the nasal discharge will clear and the cough will improve. *Even though your child may seem better, continue to give the antibiotics for the prescribed length of time. Ending the medications too early could cause the infection to return.*

When a diagnosis of sinusitis is made in children with cold symptoms lasting more than 10 days without improving, some doctors may choose to continue observation for another few days. If your child's symptoms worsen during this time or do not improve after 3 days, antibiotics should be started.

If your child's symptoms show no improvement 2 to 3 days after starting the antibiotics, talk with your pediatrician. Your child might need a different medication or need to be re-examined.

Treating related symptoms of bacterial sinusitis

Headache or sinus pain. To treat headache or sinus pain, try placing a warm washcloth on your child's face for a few minutes at a time. Pain medications such as acetaminophen or ibuprofen may also help. (However, do not give your child aspirin. It has been associated with a rare but potentially fatal disease called Reye syndrome.)

Nasal congestion. If the secretions in your child's nose are especially thick, your pediatrician may recommend that you help drain them with saline nose drops. These are available without a prescription or can be made at home by adding 1/4 teaspoon of table salt to an 8-ounce cup of water. Unless advised by your pediatrician, do not use nose drops that contain medications because they can be absorbed in amounts that can cause side effects.

Placing a cool-mist humidifier in your child's room may help keep your child more comfortable. Clean and dry the humidifier daily to prevent bacteria or mold from growing in it (follow the instructions that came with the humidifier). Hot water vaporizers are not recommended because they can cause scalds or burns.

Remember

If your child has symptoms of a bacterial sinus infection, see your pediatrician. Your pediatrician can properly diagnose and treat the infection and recommend ways to help alleviate the discomfort from some of the symptoms.

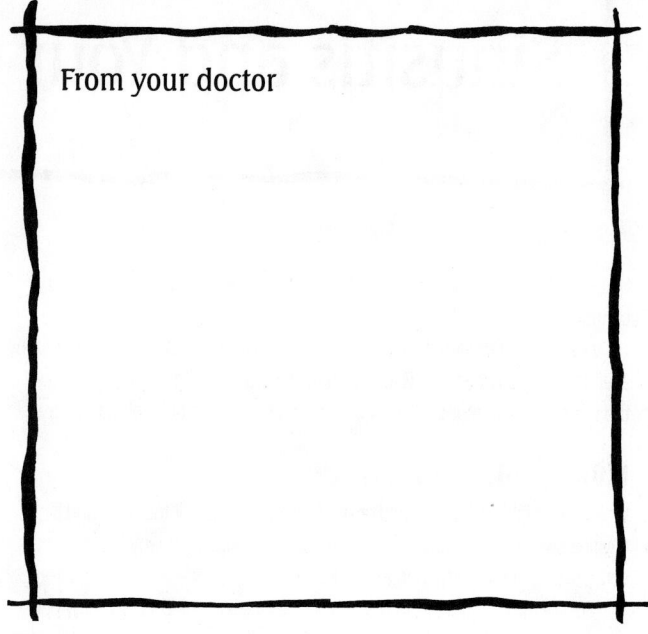

From your doctor

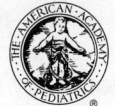

American Academy of Pediatrics

DEDICATED TO THE HEALTH OF ALL CHILDREN™

The American Academy of Pediatrics is an organization of 60,000 primary care pediatricians, pediatric medical subspecialists, and pediatric surgical specialists dedicated to the health, safety, and well-being of infants, children, adolescents, and young adults.

American Academy of Pediatrics
Web site — www.HealthyChildren.org

Diagnosis and Management of
Childhood Obstructive Sleep Apnea Syndrome

- *Clinical Practice Guideline*
- *Technical Report*

  - *PPI: AAP Partnership for Policy Implementation*
    See Appendix 2 for more information.

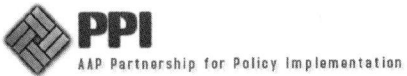

Readers of this clinical practice guideline are urged to review the technical report to enhance the evidence-based decision-making process. The full technical report is available following the clinical practice guideline and on the companion eBook.

CLINICAL PRACTICE GUIDELINE

Diagnosis and Management of Childhood Obstructive Sleep Apnea Syndrome

abstract

OBJECTIVES: This revised clinical practice guideline, intended for use by primary care clinicians, provides recommendations for the diagnosis and management of the obstructive sleep apnea syndrome (OSAS) in children and adolescents. This practice guideline focuses on uncomplicated childhood OSAS, that is, OSAS associated with adenotonsillar hypertrophy and/or obesity in an otherwise healthy child who is being treated in the primary care setting.

METHODS: Of 3166 articles from 1999–2010, 350 provided relevant data. Most articles were level II–IV. The resulting evidence report was used to formulate recommendations.

RESULTS AND CONCLUSIONS: The following recommendations are made. (1) All children/adolescents should be screened for snoring. (2) Polysomnography should be performed in children/adolescents with snoring and symptoms/signs of OSAS; if polysomnography is not available, then alternative diagnostic tests or referral to a specialist for more extensive evaluation may be considered. (3) Adenotonsillectomy is recommended as the first-line treatment of patients with adenotonsillar hypertrophy. (4) High-risk patients should be monitored as inpatients postoperatively. (5) Patients should be reevaluated postoperatively to determine whether further treatment is required. Objective testing should be performed in patients who are high risk or have persistent symptoms/signs of OSAS after therapy. (6) Continuous positive airway pressure is recommended as treatment if adenotonsillectomy is not performed or if OSAS persists postoperatively. (7) Weight loss is recommended in addition to other therapy in patients who are overweight or obese. (8) Intranasal corticosteroids are an option for children with mild OSAS in whom adenotonsillectomy is contraindicated or for mild postoperative OSAS. *Pediatrics* 2012;130:576–584

Carole L. Marcus, MBBCh, Lee Jay Brooks, MD, Kari A. Draper, MD, David Gozal, MD, Ann Carol Halbower, MD, Jacqueline Jones, MD, Michael S. Schechter, MD, MPH, Stephen Howard Sheldon, DO, Karen Spruyt, PhD, Sally Davidson Ward, MD, Christopher Lehmann, MD, Richard N. Shiffman, MD

KEY WORDS
snoring, sleep-disordered breathing, adenotonsillectomy, continuous positive airway pressure

ABBREVIATIONS
AAP—American Academy of Pediatrics
AHI—apnea hypopnea index
CPAP—continuous positive airway pressure
OSAS—obstructive sleep apnea syndrome

www.pediatrics.org/cgi/doi/10.1542/peds.2012-1671

doi:10.1542/peds.2012-1671

PEDIATRICS (ISSN Numbers: Print, 0031-4005; Online, 1098-4275).

INTRODUCTION

Obstructive sleep apnea syndrome (OSAS) is a common condition in childhood and can result in severe complications if left untreated. In 2002, the American Academy of Pediatrics (AAP) published a practice guideline for the diagnosis and management of childhood OSAS.[1] Since that time, there has been a considerable increase in publications and research on the topic; thus, the guidelines have been revised.

The purposes of this revised clinical practice guideline are to (1) increase the recognition of OSAS by primary care clinicians to minimize delay in diagnosis and avoid serious sequelae of OSAS; (2) evaluate diagnostic techniques; (3) describe treatment options; (4) provide guidelines for follow-up; and (5) discuss areas requiring further research. The recommendations in this statement do not indicate an exclusive course of treatment. Variations, taking into account individual circumstances, may be appropriate.

This practice guideline focuses on uncomplicated childhood OSAS—that is, the OSAS associated with adenotonsillar hypertrophy and/or obesity in an otherwise healthy child who is being treated in the primary care setting. This guideline specifically excludes infants younger than 1 year of age, patients with central apnea or hypoventilation syndromes, and patients with OSAS associated with other medical disorders, including but not limited to Down syndrome, craniofacial anomalies, neuromuscular disease (including cerebral palsy), chronic lung disease, sickle cell disease, metabolic disease, or laryngomalacia. These important patient populations are too complex to discuss within the scope of this article and require consultation with a pediatric subspecialist.

Additional information providing justification for the key action statements and a detailed review of the literature are provided in the accompanying technical report available online.[2]

METHODS OF GUIDELINE DEVELOPMENT

Details of the methods of guideline development are included in the accompanying technical report.[2] The AAP selected a subcommittee composed of pediatricians and other experts in the fields of sleep medicine, pulmonology, and otolaryngology, as well as experts

from epidemiology and pediatric practice to develop an evidence base of literature on this topic. The committee included liaison members from the AAP Section on Otolaryngology-Head and Neck Surgery, American Thoracic Society, American Academy of Sleep Medicine, American College of Chest Physicians, and the National Sleep Foundation. Committee members signed forms disclosing conflicts of interest.

An automated search of the literature on childhood OSAS from 1999 to 2008 was performed by using 5 scientific literature search engines.[2] The medical subject heading terms that were used in all fields were snoring, apnea, sleep-disordered breathing, sleep-related breathing disorders, upper airway resistance, polysomnography, sleep study, adenoidectomy, tonsillectomy, continuous positive airway pressure, obesity, adiposity, hypopnea, hypoventilation, cognition, behavior, and neuropsychology. Reviews, case reports, letters to the editor, and abstracts were not included. Non–English-language articles, animal studies, and studies relating to infants younger than 1 year and to special populations (eg, children with craniofacial anomalies or sickle cell disease) were excluded. In several steps, a total of 3166 hits was reduced to 350 articles, which underwent detailed review.[2] Committee members selectively updated this literature search for articles published from 2008 to 2011 specific to guideline categories. Details of the literature grading system are available in the accompanying technical report.

Since publication of the previous guidelines, there has been an improvement in the quality of OSAS studies in the literature; however, there remain few randomized, blinded, controlled studies. Most studies were questionnaire or polysomnography based. Many studies used standard definitions for pediatric polysomnography scoring, but

the interpretation of polysomnography (eg, the apnea hypopnea index [AHI] criterion used for diagnosis or to determine treatment) varied widely. The guideline notes the quality of evidence for each key action statement. Additional details are available in the technical report.

The evidence-based approach to guideline development requires that the evidence in support of each key action statement be identified, appraised, and summarized and that an explicit link between evidence and recommendations be defined. Evidence-based recommendations reflect the quality of evidence and the balance of benefit and harm that is anticipated when the recommendation is followed. The AAP policy statement, "Classifying Recommendations for Clinical Practice Guidelines,"[3] was followed in designating levels of recommendation (see Fig 1 and Table 1).

DEFINITION

This guideline defines OSAS in children as a "disorder of breathing during sleep characterized by prolonged partial upper airway obstruction and/or intermittent complete obstruction (obstructive apnea) that disrupts normal ventilation during sleep and normal sleep patterns,"[4] accompanied by symptoms or signs, as listed in Table 2. Prevalence rates based on level I and II studies range from 1.2% to 5.7%.[5–7] Symptoms include habitual snoring (often with intermittent pauses, snorts, or gasps), disturbed sleep, and daytime neurobehavioral problems. Daytime sleepiness may occur, but is uncommon in young children. OSAS is associated with neurocognitive impairment, behavioral problems, failure to thrive, hypertension, cardiac dysfunction, and systemic inflammation. Risk factors include adenotonsillar hypertrophy, obesity, craniofacial anomalies, and neuromuscular disorders. Only the first 2 risk factors are

Evidence Quality	Preponderance of Benefit or Harm	Balance of Benefit and Harm
A. Well designed RCTs or diagnostic studies on relevant population	Strong Recommendation	
B. RCTs or diagnostic studies with minor limitations;overwhelmingly consistent evidence from observational studies		Option
C. Observational studies (case-control and cohort design)	Recommendation	
D. Expert opinion, case reports, reasoning from first principles	Option	No Rec
X. Exceptional situations where validating studies cannot be performed and there is a clear preponderance of benefit or harm	Strong Recommendation / Recommendation	

FIGURE 1
Evidence quality. Integrating evidence quality appraisal with an assessment of the anticipated balance between benefits and harms if a policy is carried out leads to designation of a policy as a strong recommendation, recommendation, option, or no recommendation. RCT, randomized controlled trial; Rec, recommendation.

discussed in this guideline. In this guideline, obesity is defined as a BMI >95th percentile for age and gender.[8]

KEY ACTION STATEMENTS

Key Action Statement 1: Screening for OSAS

As part of routine health maintenance visits, clinicians should inquire whether the child or adolescent snores. If the answer is affirmative or if a child or adolescent presents with signs or symptoms of OSAS (Table 2), clinicians should perform a more focused evaluation. (Evidence Quality: Grade B, Recommendation Strength: Recommendation.)

Evidence Profile KAS 1

- Aggregate evidence quality: B
- Benefit: Early identification of OSAS is desirable, because it is a high-prevalence condition, and identification and treatment can result in alleviation of current symptoms, improved quality of life, prevention of sequelae, education of parents, and decreased health care utilization.

- Harm: Provider time, patient and parent time.
- Benefits-harms assessment: Preponderance of benefit over harm.
- Value judgments: Panelists believe that identification of a serious medical condition outweighs the time expenditure necessary for screening.
- Role of patient preferences: None.
- Exclusions: None.
- Intentional vagueness: None.
- Strength: Recommendation.

Almost all children with OSAS snore,[9–11] although caregivers frequently do not volunteer this information at medical visits.[12] Thus, asking about snoring at each health maintenance visit (as well as at other appropriate times, such as when evaluating for tonsillitis) is a sensitive, albeit nonspecific, screening measure that is quick and easy to perform. Snoring is common in children and adolescents; however, OSAS is less common. Therefore, an affirmative answer should be followed by a detailed history and examination to determine whether further evaluation for OSAS is needed (Table 2); this clinical evaluation alone

TABLE 1 Definitions and Recommendation Implications

Statement	Definition	Implication
Strong recommendation	A strong recommendation in favor of a particular action is made when the anticipated benefits of the recommended intervention clearly exceed the harms (as a strong recommendation against an action is made when the anticipated harms clearly exceed the benefits) and the quality of the supporting evidence is excellent. In some clearly identified circumstances, strong recommendations may be made when high-quality evidence is impossible to obtain and the anticipated benefits strongly outweigh the harms.	Clinicians should follow a strong recommendation unless a clear and compelling rationale for an alternative approach is present.
Recommendation	A recommendation in favor of a particular action is made when the anticipated benefits exceed the harms but the quality of evidence is not as strong. Again, in some clearly identified circumstances, recommendations may be made when high-quality evidence is impossible to obtain but the anticipated benefits outweigh the harms.	It would be prudent for clinicians to follow a recommendation, but they should remain alert to new information and sensitive to patient preferences.
Option	Options define courses that may be taken when either the quality of evidence is suspect or carefully performed studies have shown little clear advantage to one approach over another.	Clinicians should consider the option in their decision-making, and patient preference may have a substantial role.
No recommendation	No recommendation indicates that there is a lack of pertinent published evidence and that the anticipated balance of benefits and harms is presently unclear.	Clinicians should be alert to new published evidence that clarifies the balance of benefit versus harm.

TABLE 2 Symptoms and Signs of OSAS

History
    Frequent snoring (≥3 nights/wk)
    Labored breathing during sleep
    Gasps/snorting noises/observed
      episodes of apnea
    Sleep enuresis (especially secondary enuresis)[a]
    Sleeping in a seated position or with the neck
      hyperextended
    Cyanosis
    Headaches on awakening
    Daytime sleepiness
    Attention-deficit/hyperactivity disorder
    Learning problems
Physical examination
    Underweight or overweight
    Tonsillar hypertrophy
    Adenoidal facies
    Micrognathia/retrognathia
    High-arched palate
    Failure to thrive
    Hypertension

[a] Enuresis after at least 6 mo of continence.

does not establish the diagnosis (see technical report). Occasional snoring, for example, with an upper respiratory tract infection, is less of a concern than snoring that occurs at least 3 times a week and is associated with any of the symptoms or signs listed in Table 2.

Key Action Statement 2A: Polysomnography

If a child or adolescent snores on a regular basis and has any of the complaints or findings shown in Table 2, clinicians should either (1) obtain a polysomnogram (Evidence Quality A, Key Action strength: Recommendation) OR (2) refer the patient to a sleep specialist or otolaryngologist for a more extensive evaluation (Evidence quality D, Key Action strength: Option). (Evidence Quality: Grade A for polysomnography; Grade D for specialist referral, Recommendation Strength: Recommendation.)

Evidence Profile KAS 2A: Polysomnography

- Aggregate evidence quality: A
- Benefits: Establish diagnosis and determine severity of OSAS.

- Harm: Expense, time, anxiety/discomfort.
- Benefits-harms assessment: Preponderance of benefit over harm.
- Value judgments: Panelists weighed the value of establishing a diagnosis as more important than the minor potential harms listed.
- Role of patient preferences: Small because of preponderance of evidence that polysomnography is the most accurate way to make a diagnosis.
- Exclusions: See Key Action Statement 2B regarding lack of availability.
- Intentional vagueness: None.
- Strength: Recommendation.

Evidence Profile KAS 2A: Referral

- Aggregate evidence quality: D
- Benefits: Subspecialist may be better able to establish diagnosis and determine severity of OSAS.
- Harm: Expense, time, anxiety/discomfort.
- Benefits-harms assessment: Preponderance of benefit over harm.
- Value judgments: Panelists weighed the value of establishing a diagnosis as more important than the minor potential harms listed.
- Role of patient preferences: Large.
- Exclusions: None.
- Intentional vagueness: None.
- Strength: Option.

Although history and physical examination are useful to screen patients and determine which patients need further investigation for OSAS, the sensitivity and specificity of the history and physical examination are poor (see accompanying technical report). Physical examination when the child is awake may be normal, and the size of the tonsils cannot be used to predict the presence of OSAS in an individual child. Thus, objective testing is required. The gold standard test

is overnight, attended, in-laboratory polysomnography (sleep study). This is a noninvasive test involving the measurement of a number of physiologic functions overnight, typically including EEG; pulse oximetry; oronasal airflow, abdominal and chest wall movements, partial pressure of carbon dioxide (Pco_2); and video recording.[13] Specific pediatric measuring and scoring criteria should be used.[13] Polysomnography will demonstrate the presence or absence of OSAS. Polysomnography also demonstrates the severity of OSAS, which is helpful in planning treatment and in postoperative short- and long-term management.

Key Action Statement 2B: Alternative Testing

If polysomnography is not available, then clinicians may order alternative diagnostic tests, such as nocturnal video recording, nocturnal oximetry, daytime nap polysomnography, or ambulatory polysomnography. (Evidence Quality: Grade C, Recommendation Strength: Option.)

Evidence Profile KAS 2B

- Aggregate evidence quality: C
- Benefit: Varying positive and negative predictive values for establishing diagnosis.
- Harm: False-negative and false-positive results may underestimate or overestimate severity, expense, time, anxiety/discomfort.
- Benefits-harms assessment: Equilibrium of benefits and harms.
- Value judgments: Opinion of the panel that some objective testing is better than none. Pragmatic decision based on current shortage of pediatric polysomnography facilities (this may change over time).
- Role of patient preferences: Small, if choices are limited by availability;

families may choose to travel to centers where more extensive facilities are available.

- Exclusions: None.
- Intentional vagueness: None.
- Strength: Option.

Although polysomnography is the gold standard for diagnosis of OSAS, there is a shortage of sleep laboratories with pediatric expertise. Hence, polysomnography may not be readily available in certain regions of the country. Alternative diagnostic tests have been shown to have weaker positive and negative predictive values than polysomnography, but nevertheless, objective testing is preferable to clinical evaluation alone. If an alternative test fails to demonstrate OSAS in a patient with a high pretest probability, full polysomnography should be sought.

Key Action Statement 3: Adenotonsillectomy

If a child is determined to have OSAS, has a clinical examination consistent with adenotonsillar hypertrophy, and does not have a contraindication to surgery (see Table 3), the clinician should recommend adenotonsillectomy as the first line of treatment. If the child has OSAS but does not have adenotonsillar hypertrophy, other treatment should be considered (see Key Action Statement 6). Clinical judgment is required to determine the benefits of adenotonsillectomy compared with other treatments in obese children with varying degrees of adenotonsillar hypertrophy. (Evidence Quality: Grade B, Recommendation Strength: Recommendation.)

Evidence Profile KAS 3

- Aggregate evidence quality: B
- Benefit: Improve OSAS and accompanying symptoms and sequelae.

- Harm: Pain, anxiety, dehydration, anesthetic complications, hemorrhage, infection, postoperative respiratory difficulties, velopharyngeal incompetence, nasopharyngeal stenosis, death.
- Benefits-harms assessment: Preponderance of benefit over harm.
- Value judgments: The panel sees the benefits of treating OSAS as more beneficial than the low risk of serious consequences.
- Role of patient preferences: Low; continuous positive airway pressure (CPAP) is an option but involves prolonged, long-term treatment as compared with a single, relatively low-risk surgical procedure.
- Exclusions: See Table 3.
- Intentional vagueness: None.
- Strength: Recommendation.

Adenotonsillectomy is very effective in treating OSAS. Adenoidectomy or tonsillectomy alone may not be sufficient, because residual lymphoid tissue may contribute to persistent obstruction. In otherwise healthy children with adenotonsillar hypertrophy, adenotonsillectomy is associated with improvements in symptoms and sequelae of OSAS. Postoperative polysomnography typically shows a major decrease in the number of obstructive events, although some obstructions may still be present. Although obese children may have less satisfactory results, many will be adequately treated with

adenotonsillectomy; however, further research is needed to determine which obese children are most likely to benefit from surgery. In this population, the benefits of a 1-time surgical procedure, with a small but real risk of complications, need to be weighed against long-term treatment with CPAP, which is associated with discomfort, disruption of family lifestyle, and risks of poor adherence. Potential complications of adenotonsillectomy are shown in Table 4. Although serious complications (including death) may occur, the rate of these complications is low, and the risks of complications need to be weighed against the consequences of untreated OSAS. In general, a 1-time only procedure with a relatively low morbidity is preferable to lifelong treatment with CPAP; furthermore, the efficacy of CPAP is limited by generally suboptimal adherence. Other treatment options, such as anti-inflammatory medications, weight loss, or tracheostomy, are less effective, are difficult to achieve, or have higher morbidity, respectively.

Key Action Statement 4: High-Risk Patients Undergoing Adenotonsillectomy

Clinicians should monitor high-risk patients (Table 5) undergoing adenotonsillectomy as inpatients postoperatively. (Evidence Quality: Grade B, Recommendation Strength: Recommendation.)

TABLE 3 Contraindications for Adenotonsillectomy

Absolute contraindications
  No adenotonsillar tissue (tissue has been surgically removed)
Relative contraindications
  Very small tonsils/adenoid
  Morbid obesity and small tonsils/adenoid
  Bleeding disorder refractory to treatment
  Submucus cleft palate
  Other medical conditions making patient medically unstable for surgery

TABLE 4 Risks of Adenotonsillectomy

Minor
  Pain
  Dehydration attributable to postoperative nausea/vomiting and poor oral intake
Major
  Anesthetic complications
  Acute upper airway obstruction during induction or emergence from anesthesia
  Postoperative respiratory compromise
  Hemorrhage
  Velopharyngeal incompetence
  Nasopharyngeal stenosis
  Death

TABLE 5 Risk Factors for Postoperative Respiratory Complications in Children With OSAS Undergoing Adenotonsillectomy

Younger than 3 y of age
Severe OSAS on polysomnography[a]
Cardiac complications of OSAS
Failure to thrive
Obesity
Craniofacial anomalies[b]
Neuromuscular disorders[b]
Current respiratory infection

[a] It is difficult to provide exact polysomnographic criteria for severity, because these criteria will vary depending on the age of the child; additional comorbidities, such as obesity, asthma, or cardiac complications of OSAS; and other polysomnographic criteria that have not been evaluated in the literature, such as the level of hypercapnia and the frequency of desaturation (as compared with lowest oxygen saturation). Nevertheless, on the basis of published studies (primarily Level III, see Technical Report), it is recommended that all patients with a lowest oxygen saturation <80% (either on preoperative polysomnography or during observation in the recovery room postoperatively) or an AHI ≥24/h be observed as inpatients postoperatively as they are at increased risk for postoperative respiratory compromise. Additionally, on the basis of expert consensus, it is recommended that patients with significant hypercapnia on polysomnography (peak P_{CO_2} ≥60 mm Hg) be admitted postoperatively. The committee noted that that most published studies were retrospective and not comprehensive, and therefore these recommendations may change if higher-level studies are published. Clinicians may decide to admit patients with less severe polysomnographic abnormalities based on a constellation of risk factors (age, comorbidities, and additional polysomnographic factors) for a particular individual.

[b] Not discussed in these guidelines.

Evidence Profile KAS 4

- Aggregate evidence quality: B
- Benefit: Effectively manage severe respiratory compromise and avoid death.
- Harm: Expense, time, anxiety.
- Benefits-harms assessment: Preponderance of benefit over harm.
- Value judgments: The panel believes that early recognition of any serious adverse events is critically important.
- Role of patient preferences: Minimal; this is an important safety issue.
- Exclusions: None.
- Intentional vagueness: None.
- Strength: Recommendation.

Patients with OSAS may develop respiratory complications, such as worsening of OSAS or pulmonary edema, in the immediate postoperative period. Death attributable to respiratory complications in the immediate postoperative period has been reported in patients with severe OSAS. Identified risk factors are shown in Table 5. High-risk patients should undergo surgery in a center capable of treating complex pediatric patients. They should be hospitalized overnight for close monitoring postoperatively. Children with an acute respiratory infection on the day of surgery, as documented by fever, cough, and/or wheezing, are at increased risk of postoperative complications and, therefore, should be rescheduled or monitored closely postoperatively. Clinicians should decide on an individual basis whether these patients should be rescheduled, taking into consideration the severity of OSAS in the particular patient and keeping in mind that many children with adenotonsillar hypertrophy have chronic rhinorrhea and nasal congestion, even in the absence of viral infections.

Key Action Statement 5: Reevaluation

Clinicians should clinically reassess all patients with OSAS for persisting signs and symptoms after therapy to determine whether further treatment is required. (Evidence Quality: Grade B, Recommendation Strength: Recommendation.)

Evidence Profile KAS 5A

- Aggregate evidence quality: B
- Benefit: Determine effects of treatment.
- Harm: Expense, time.
- Benefits-harms assessment: Preponderance of benefit over harm.
- Value judgments: Data show that a significant proportion of children continue to have abnormalities postoperatively; therefore, the panel determined that the benefits of follow-up outweigh the minor inconveniences.
- Role of patient preferences: Minimal; follow-up is good clinical practice.
- Exclusions: None.
- Intentional vagueness: None.
- Strength: Recommendation.

Clinicians should reassess OSAS-related symptoms and signs (Table 2) after 6 to 8 weeks of therapy to determine whether further evaluation and treatment are indicated. Objective data regarding the timing of the postoperative evaluation are not available. Most clinicians recommend reevaluation 6 to 8 weeks after treatment to allow for healing of the operative site and to allow time for upper airway, cardiac, and central nervous system recovery. Patients who remain symptomatic should undergo objective testing (see Key Action Statement 2) or be referred to a sleep specialist for further evaluation.

Key Action Statement 5B: Reevaluation of High-Risk Patients

Clinicians should reevaluate high-risk patients for persistent OSAS after adenotonsillectomy, including those who had a significantly abnormal baseline polysomnogram, have sequelae of OSAS, are obese, or remain symptomatic after treatment, with an objective test (see Key Action Statement 2) or refer such patients to a sleep specialist. (Evidence Quality: Grade B, Recommendation Strength: Recommendation.)

Evidence Profile KAS 5B

- Aggregate evidence quality: B
- Benefit: Determine effects of treatment.
- Harm: Expense, time, anxiety/discomfort.
- Benefits-harms assessment: Preponderance of benefit over harm.

- Value judgments: Given the panel's concerns about the consequences of OSAS and the frequency of postoperative persistence in high-risk groups, the panel believes that the follow-up costs are outweighed by benefits of recognition of persistent OSAS. A minority of panelists believed that all children with OSAS should have follow-up polysomnography because of the high prevalence of persistent postoperative abnormalities on polysomnography, but most panelists believed that persistent polysomnographic abnormalities in uncomplicated children with mild OSAS were usually mild in patients who were asymptomatic after surgery.
- Role of patient preferences: Minimal. Further evaluation is needed to determine the need for further treatment.
- Exclusions: None.
- Intentional vagueness: None.
- Strength: Recommendation.

Numerous studies have shown that a large proportion of children at high risk continue to have some degree of OSAS postoperatively[10,13,14]; thus, objective evidence is required to determine whether further treatment is necessary.

Key Action Statement 6: CPAP

Clinicians should refer patients for CPAP management if symptoms/signs (Table 2) or objective evidence of OSAS persists after adenotonsillectomy or if adenotonsillectomy is not performed. (Evidence Quality: Grade B, Recommendation Strength: Recommendation.)

Evidence Profile KAS 6

- Aggregate evidence quality: B
- Benefit: Improve OSAS and accompanying symptoms and sequelae.

- Harm: Expense, time, anxiety; parental sleep disruption; nasal and skin adverse effects; possible midface remodeling; extremely rare serious pressure-related complications, such as pneumothorax; poor adherence.
- Benefits-harms assessment: Preponderance of benefit over harm.
- Value judgments: Panelists believe that CPAP is the most effective treatment of OSAS that persists postoperatively and that the benefits of treatment outweigh the adverse effects. Other treatments (eg, rapid maxillary expansion) may be effective in specially selected patients.
- Role of patient preferences: Other treatments may be effective in specially selected patients.
- Exclusions: Rare patients at increased risk of severe pressure complications.
- Intentional vagueness: None.
- Policy level: Recommendation.

CPAP therapy is delivered by using an electronic device that delivers air at positive pressure via a nasal mask, leading to mechanical stenting of the airway and improved functional residual capacity in the lungs. There is no clear advantage of using bilevel pressure over CPAP.[15] CPAP should be managed by an experienced and skilled clinician with expertise in its use in children. CPAP pressure requirements vary among individuals and change over time; thus, CPAP must be titrated in the sleep laboratory before prescribing the device and periodically readjusted thereafter. Behavioral modification therapy may be required, especially for young children or those with developmental delays. Objective monitoring of adherence, by using the equipment software, is important. If adherence is suboptimal, the clinician should institute measures to improve adherence (such as behavioral modification, or treating side effects of

CPAP) and institute alternative treatments if these measures are ineffective.

Key Action Statement 7: Weight Loss

Clinicians should recommend weight loss in addition to other therapy if a child/adolescent with OSAS is overweight or obese. (Evidence Quality: Grade C, Recommendation Strength: Recommendation.)

Evidence Profile KAS 7

- Aggregate evidence quality: C
- Benefit: Improve OSAS and accompanying symptoms and sequelae; non–OSAS-related benefits of weight loss.
- Harm: Hard to achieve and maintain weight loss.
- Benefits-harms assessment: Preponderance of benefit over harm.
- Value judgments: The panel agreed that weight loss is beneficial for both OSAS and other health issues, but clinical experience suggests that weight loss is difficult to achieve and maintain, and even effective weight loss regimens take time; therefore, additional treatment is required in the interim.
- Role of patient preferences: Strong role for patient and family preference regarding nutrition and exercise.
- Exclusions: None.
- Intentional vagueness: None.
- Strength: Recommendation.

Weight loss has been shown to improve OSAS,[16,17] although the degree of weight loss required has not been determined. Because weight loss is a slow and unreliable process, other treatment modalities (such as adenotonsillectomy or CPAP therapy) should be instituted until sufficient weight loss has been achieved and maintained.

Key Action Statement 8: Intranasal Corticosteroids

Clinicians may prescribe topical intranasal corticosteroids for children with mild OSAS in whom adenotonsillectomy is contraindicated or for children with mild postoperative OSAS. (Evidence Quality: Grade B, Recommendation Strength: Option.)

Evidence Profile KAS 8

- Aggregate evidence quality: B
- Benefit: Improves mild OSAS and accompanying symptoms and sequelae.
- Harm: Some subjects may not have an adequate response. It is not known whether therapeutic effect persists long-term; therefore, long-term observation is required. Low risk of steroid-related adverse effects.
- Benefits-harms assessment: Preponderance of benefit over harm.
- Value judgments: The panel agreed that intranasal steroids provide a less invasive treatment than surgery or CPAP and, therefore, may be preferred in some cases despite lower efficacy and lack of data on long-term efficacy.
- Role of patient preferences: Moderate role for patient and family preference if OSAS is mild.
- Exclusions: None.
- Intentional vagueness: None.
- Strength: Option.

Mild OSAS is defined, for this indication, as an AHI <5 per hour, on the basis of studies on intranasal corticosteroids described in the accompanying technical report.[2] Several studies have shown that the use of intranasal steroids decreases the degree of OSAS; however, although OSAS improves, residual OSAS may remain. Furthermore, there is individual variability in response to treatment, and long-term studies have not been performed to determine the duration of improvement. Therefore, nasal steroids are not recommended as a first-line therapy. The response to treatment should be measured objectively after a course of treatment of approximately 6 weeks. Because the long-term effect of this treatment is unknown, the clinician should continue to observe the patient for symptoms of recurrence and adverse effects of corticosteroids.

AREAS FOR FUTURE RESEARCH

A detailed list of research recommendations is provided in the accompanying technical report.[2] There is a great need for further research into the prevalence of OSAS, sequelae of OSAS, best treatment methods, and the role of obesity. In particular, well-controlled, blinded studies, including randomized controlled trials of treatment, are needed to determine the best care for children and adolescents with OSAS.

SUBCOMMITTEE ON OBSTRUCTIVE SLEEP APNEA SYNDROME*

Carole L. Marcus, MBBCh, Chairperson (Sleep Medicine, Pediatric Pulmonologist; Liaison, American Academy of Sleep Medicine; Research Support from Philips Respironics; Affiliated with an academic sleep center; Published research related to OSAS)

Lee J. Brooks, MD (Sleep Medicine, Pediatric Pulmonologist; Liaison, American College of Chest Physicians; No financial conflicts; Affiliated with an academic sleep center; Published research related to OSAS)

Sally Davidson Ward, MD (Sleep Medicine, Pediatric Pulmonologist; No financial conflicts; Affiliated with an academic sleep center; Published research related to OSAS)

Kari A. Draper, MD (General Pediatrician; No conflicts)

David Gozal, MD (Sleep Medicine, Pediatric Pulmonologist; Research support from AstraZeneca; Speaker for Merck Company; Affiliated with an academic sleep center; Published research related to OSAS)

Ann C. Halbower, MD (Sleep Medicine, Pediatric Pulmonologist; Liaison, American Thoracic Society; Research Funding from Resmed; Affiliated with an academic sleep center; Published research related to OSAS)

Jacqueline Jones, MD (Pediatric Otolaryngologist; AAP Section on Otolaryngology-Head and Neck Surgery; Liaison, American Academy of Otolaryngology-Head and Neck Surgery; No financial conflicts; Affiliated with an academic otolaryngologic practice)

Christopher Lehman, MD (Neonatologist, Informatician; No conflicts)

Michael S. Schechter, MD, MPH (Pediatric Pulmonologist; AAP Section on Pediatric Pulmonology; Consultant to Genentech, Inc and Gilead, Inc, not related to Obstructive Sleep Apnea; Research Support from Mpex Pharmaceuticals, Inc, Vertex Pharmaceuticals Incorporated, PTC Therapeutics, Bayer Healthcare, not related to Obstructive Sleep Apnea)

Stephen Sheldon, MD (Sleep Medicine, General Pediatrician; Liaison, National Sleep Foundation; No financial conflicts; Affiliated with an academic sleep center; Published research related to OSAS)

Richard N. Shiffman, MD, MCIS (General pediatrics, Informatician; No conflicts)

Karen Spruyt, PhD (Clinical Psychologist, Child Neuropsychologist, and Biostatistician/Epidemiologist; No financial conflicts; Affiliated with an academic sleep center)

Oversight from the Steering Committee on Quality Improvement and Management, 2009–2012

STAFF

Caryn Davidson, MA

*Areas of expertise are shown in parentheses after each name.

ACKNOWLEDGMENTS

The committee thanks Jason Caboot, June Chan, Mary Currie, Fiona Healy, Maureen Josephson, Sofia Konstantinopoulou, H. Madan Kumar, Roberta Leu, Darius Loghmanee, Rajeev Bhatia, Argyri Petrocheilou, Harsha Vardhan, and Colleen Walsh for assisting with evidence extraction.

REFERENCES

1. Section on Pediatric Pulmonology, Subcommittee on Obstructive Sleep Apnea Syndrome. American Academy of Pediatrics. Clinical practice guideline: diagnosis and management of childhood obstructive sleep apnea syndrome. *Pediatrics.* 2002;109(4):704–712

2. Marcus CL, Brooks LJ, Davidson C, et al; American Academy of Pediatrics, Subcommittee on Obstructive Sleep Apnea

Syndrome. Technical report: diagnosis and management of childhood obstructive sleep apnea syndrome. *Pediatrics*. 2012; 130(3):In press

3. American Academy of Pediatrics Steering Committee on Quality Improvement and Management. Classifying recommendations for clinical practice guidelines. *Pediatrics*. 2004;114(3):874–877

4. American Thoracic Society. Standards and indications for cardiopulmonary sleep studies in children. *Am J Respir Crit Care Med*. 1996;153(2):866–878

5. Bixler EO, Vgontzas AN, Lin HM, et al. Sleep disordered breathing in children in a general population sample: prevalence and risk factors. *Sleep*. 2009;32(6):731–736

6. Li AM, So HK, Au CT, et al. Epidemiology of obstructive sleep apnoea syndrome in Chinese children: a two-phase community study. *Thorax*. 2010;65(11):991–997

7. O'Brien LM, Holbrook CR, Mervis CB, et al. Sleep and neurobehavioral characteristics of 5- to 7-year-old children with parentally reported symptoms of attention-deficit/hyperactivity disorder. *Pediatrics*. 2003; 111(3):554–563

8. Himes JH, Dietz WH; The Expert Committee on Clinical Guidelines for Overweight in Adolescent Preventive Services. Guidelines for overweight in adolescent preventive services: recommendations from an expert committee. *Am J Clin Nutr*. 1994;59(2):307–316

9. Mitchell RB. Adenotonsillectomy for obstructive sleep apnea in children: outcome evaluated by pre- and postoperative polysomnography. *Laryngoscope*. 2007;117(10):1844–1854

10. Suen JS, Arnold JE, Brooks LJ. Adenotonsillectomy for treatment of obstructive sleep apnea in children. *Arch Otolaryngol Head Neck Surg*. 1995;121(5):525–530

11. Nieminen P, Tolonen U, Löppönen H. Snoring and obstructive sleep apnea in children: a 6-month follow-up study. *Arch Otolaryngol Head Neck Surg*. 2000;126(4):481–486

12. Blunden S, Lushington K, Lorenzen B, Wong J, Balendran R, Kennedy D. Symptoms of sleep breathing disorders in children are underreported by parents at general practice visits. *Sleep Breath*. 2003;7(4):167–176

13. Apostolidou MT, Alexopoulos EI, Chaidas K, et al. Obesity and persisting sleep apnea after adenotonsillectomy in Greek children. *Chest*. 2008;134(6):1149–1155

14. Mitchell RB, Kelly J. Outcome of adenotonsillectomy for severe obstructive sleep apnea in children. *Int J Pediatr Otorhinolaryngol*. 2004;68(11):1375–1379

15. Marcus CL, Rosen G, Ward SL, et al. Adherence to and effectiveness of positive airway pressure therapy in children with obstructive sleep apnea. *Pediatrics*. 2006; 117(3). Available at: www.pediatrics.org/cgi/content/full/117/3/e442

16. Verhulst SL, Franckx H, Van Gaal L, De Backer W, Desager K. The effect of weight loss on sleep-disordered breathing in obese teenagers. *Obesity (Silver Spring)*. 2009;17(6):1178–1183

17. Kalra M, Inge T. Effect of bariatric surgery on obstructive sleep apnoea in adolescents. *Paediatr Respir Rev*. 2006;7(4):260–267

TECHNICAL REPORT

Diagnosis and Management of Childhood Obstructive Sleep Apnea Syndrome

abstract 🄵🅁🄴🄴

OBJECTIVE: This technical report describes the procedures involved in developing recommendations on the management of childhood obstructive sleep apnea syndrome (OSAS).

METHODS: The literature from 1999 through 2011 was evaluated.

RESULTS AND CONCLUSIONS: A total of 3166 titles were reviewed, of which 350 provided relevant data. Most articles were level II through IV. The prevalence of OSAS ranged from 0% to 5.7%, with obesity being an independent risk factor. OSAS was associated with cardiovascular, growth, and neurobehavioral abnormalities and possibly inflammation. Most diagnostic screening tests had low sensitivity and specificity. Treatment of OSAS resulted in improvements in behavior and attention and likely improvement in cognitive abilities. Primary treatment is adenotonsillectomy (AT). Data were insufficient to recommend specific surgical techniques; however, children undergoing partial tonsillectomy should be monitored for possible recurrence of OSAS. Although OSAS improved postoperatively, the proportion of patients who had residual OSAS ranged from 13% to 29% in low-risk populations to 73% when obese children were included and stricter polysomnographic criteria were used. Nevertheless, OSAS may improve after AT even in obese children, thus supporting surgery as a reasonable initial treatment. A significant number of obese patients required intubation or continuous positive airway pressure (CPAP) postoperatively, which reinforces the need for inpatient observation. CPAP was effective in the treatment of OSAS, but adherence is a major barrier. For this reason, CPAP is not recommended as first-line therapy for OSAS when AT is an option. Intranasal steroids may ameliorate mild OSAS, but follow-up is needed. Data were insufficient to recommend rapid maxillary expansion. *Pediatrics* 2012;130:e714–e755

Carole L. Marcus, MBBCh, Lee J. Brooks, MD, Sally Davidson Ward, MD, Kari A. Draper, MD, David Gozal, MD, Ann C. Halbower, MD, Jacqueline Jones, MD, Christopher Lehmann, MD, Michael S. Schechter, MD, MPH, Stephen Sheldon, MD, Richard N. Shiffman, MD, MCIS, and Karen Spruyt, PhD

KEY WORDS
adenotonsillectomy, continuous positive airway pressure, sleep-disordered breathing, snoring

ABBREVIATIONS
AAP—American Academy of Pediatrics
ADHD—attention-deficit/hyperactivity disorder
AHI—apnea hypopnea index
AT—adenotonsillectomy
BP—blood pressure
BPAP—bilevel positive airway pressure
CBCL—Child Behavior Checklist
CPAP—continuous positive airway pressure
CRP—C-reactive protein
ECG—electrocardiography
HOMA—homeostatic model assessment
HS—habitual snoring
IL—interleukin
OSAS—obstructive sleep apnea syndrome
PAP—positive airway pressure
PSG—polysomnography
PT—partial tonsillectomy
QoL—quality of life
RDI—respiratory distress index
SDB—sleep-disordered breathing
SES—socioeconomic status
Spo2—oxygen saturation
URI—upper respiratory tract infection

(Continued on last page)

INTRODUCTION

This technical report describes in detail the procedures involved in developing the recommendations for the updated clinical practice guideline on childhood obstructive sleep apnea syndrome (OSAS).[1]

The clinical practice guideline is primarily aimed at pediatricians and other primary care clinicians (family physicians, nurse practitioners, and physician assistants) who treat children. The secondary audience for the guideline includes sleep medicine specialists, pediatric pulmonologists, neurologists, otolaryngologists, and developmental/behavioral pediatricians.

The primary focus of the committee was on OSAS in childhood.[2] The committee focused on otherwise healthy children who had adenotonsillar hypertrophy or obesity as underlying risk factors. Complex populations, including infants <1 year of age and children who had other medical conditions (eg, craniofacial anomalies, genetic or metabolic syndromes, neuromuscular disease, laryngomalacia, sickle cell disease), were excluded because these patients will typically require subspecialty referral.

Two professional studies recently published related guidelines: the American Academy of Otolaryngology–Head and Neck Surgery[3] and the American Academy of Sleep Medicine.[4] These guidelines have similar recommendations to many of the recommendations in the American Academy of Pediatrics (AAP) guideline.

The recommendations in this statement do not indicate an exclusive course of treatment. Variations, taking into account individual circumstances, may be appropriate.

METHODS

Literature Search

A literature search was performed that included English-language articles, children and adolescents aged 1 through 17.9 years, and publication between 1999 and 2008. Animal studies, abstracts, letters, case reports, and reviews were excluded. The Medical Subject Heading terms that were used in all fields were snoring, apnea, sleep-disordered breathing (SDB), sleep-related breathing disorders, upper airway resistance, polysomnography (PSG), sleep study, adenoidectomy, tonsillectomy, continuous positive airway pressure (CPAP), obesity, adiposity, hypopnea, hypoventilation, cognition, behavior, and neuropsychology. Search engines used were PubMed, Scopus, Ovid, PsycINFO, EBSCO (including Health Source [Nursing], Child Development and Adolescent Studies), and CINAHL. Articles covering special populations (eg, infants aged <1 year, those with craniofacial anomalies or syndromes) were excluded during the title and abstract reviews.

Titles and available abstracts of articles found by the literature search were reviewed by the committee members in several rounds (see Results). In the first round, duplicates and erroneous hits from the literature search were excluded. In the second round, titles were reviewed for relevancy by 2 committee members. Articles with relevant titles were then reviewed by 2 reviewers each, on the basis of the abstract. Because of the large number of remaining articles, text-mining (Statistica, StatSoft version 9; StatSoft, Inc, Tulsa, OK) was performed on the method section of the articles to reduce the large amount of articles for the final step of quality assessment. Text-mining is the combined, automated process of analyzing unstructured, natural language text to discover information and knowledge that are typically difficult to retrieve.[5]

Unfortunately, text-mining revealed that few articles reported research methods, such as the study design (eg, clinical case series, retrospective, observational, clinical experiment), blinding of the assessment, and recruitment and/or scoring, that could have been applied for further selection. A manual screening of the questionable articles after text-mining resulted in a pool of 605 articles. The committee decided on a final round of title selection; that is, each member was assigned a random batch of articles and selected titles based on relevance with respect to the guideline categories. These remaining articles were each reviewed and graded by a committee member, as detailed here. Because of the large volume of articles requiring detailed evaluation, some committee members recruited trainees and colleagues to assist them in the performance of these reviews, under their supervision. Jason Caboot, June Chan, Mary Currie, Fiona Healy, Maureen Josephson, Sofia Konstantinopoulou, H. Madan Kumar, Roberta Leu, Darius Loghmanee, Rajeev Bhatia, Argyri Petrocheilou, Harsha Vardhan, and Colleen Walsh participated. A literature search of more recent articles (2008–2011) was performed by individual committee members, per guideline category, and discussed during the committee meeting.

As would be expected from any panel of experts in a field, some of the citations were the work of the panel members. For this reason, a varied panel, including general pediatricians, pulmonologists, otolaryngologists, and sleep medicine physicians, was arranged to provide balance. For initial guideline drafts, committee members were assigned sections of the report that were not directly in their area of research, and the evidence, search results, and conclusions thereof were discussed by all committee members at a face-to-face meeting. Subsequent drafts of the guidelines and technical report were reviewed by all committee members.

Quality Assessment

The previous literature review form[6] was modified to include the evidence grading system developed by the American Academy of Neurology for the assessment of clinical utility of diagnostic tests (Table 1).[7] A specific customized software (OSA Taskforce;

TABLE 1 Evidence Grading System[7]

Level	Description
I	Evidence provided by a prospective study in a broad spectrum of persons who have the suspected condition, by using a reference (gold) standard for case definition, in which the test is applied in a blinded fashion, and enabling the assessment of appropriate test of diagnostic accuracy. All persons undergoing the diagnostic test have the presence or absence of the disease determined. Level I studies are judged to have a low risk of bias.
II	Evidence provided by a prospective study of a narrow spectrum of persons who have the suspected condition, or a well-designed retrospective study of a broad spectrum of persons who have an established condition (by gold standard) compared with a broad spectrum of controls, in which the test is applied in a blinded evaluation, and enabling the assessment of appropriate tests of diagnostic accuracy. Level II studies are judged to have a moderate risk of bias.
III	Evidence provided by a retrospective study in which either persons who have the established condition or controls are of a narrow spectrum, and in which the reference standard, if not objective, is applied by someone other than the person who performed (interpreted) the test. Level III studies are judged to have a moderate to high risk of bias.
IV	Any study design where the test is not applied in an independent evaluation or evidence is provided by expert opinion alone or in descriptive case series without controls. There is no blinding or there may be inadequate blinding. The spectrum of persons tested may be broad or narrow. Level IV studies are judged to have a very high risk of bias.

copyright Francesco Rundo and Karen Spruyt) was developed for the literature review form to standardize this part of the process. Of note, the quality assessment levels were comparable to the grading levels applied previously.[8,9] The quality assessment applied involved 4 tiers of evidence, with level I studies being judged to have a low risk of bias and level IV studies judged to have a very high level of bias. A weaker level of evidence indicates the need to integrate greater clinical judgment when applying results to clinical decision-making. The committee's quality assessment of data took into account not only the levels of evidence in relevant articles but also the number of articles identified, the magnitude and direction of various findings, and whether articles demonstrated convergent or divergent conclusions.

The evidence-based approach to guideline development requires that the evidence in support of each key action statement be identified, appraised, and summarized and that an explicit link between evidence and recommendations be defined. Evidence-based recommendations reflect the quality of evidence and the balance of benefit

and harm that is anticipated when the recommendation is followed. The AAP policy statement "Classifying Recommendations for Clinical Practice Guidelines"[10] was followed in designating levels of recommendations (Fig 1, Table 2).

RESULTS OF LITERATURE SEARCH

The automated Medical Subject Heading search resulted in 3166 hits. After duplicates and erroneous hits were excluded, 2395 hits fulfilled the criteria. After title review, 1091 articles were accepted, with a 0.70 interrater agreement between the 2 reviewers. These remaining articles were reviewed on the basis of the abstract, which resulted in 757 articles remaining, with a 0.60 agreement rate between reviewers. A final decision on those without agreement was made by the chairperson of the committee. Text-mining, although not helpful in reducing the number of articles for further evaluation, illustrated the spectrum of topics covered by the articles (Table 3). A manual screening of the questionable articles after text-mining resulted in a pool of 605 articles. The final round of title selection resulted in 397 articles for

detailed review. An additional 47 articles were found to not meet criteria during the detailed review. Thus, a total of 350 articles were included.

On the basis of the final 350 articles, one-third were epidemiologic studies, 26% were diagnostic studies, and 23% were treatment studies. Table 4 lists the type of study design; 34% of studies were descriptive and 32% were nonrandomized concurrent cohort series. PSG was the diagnostic method used for 57% of the articles, whereas 45% used questionnaires. The sample size varied from 9 to 6742 subjects. Figure 2 shows the level of evidence of the articles; 76% of studies were level III or IV. The majority of studies did not include a control group, which degraded the studies to level III or IV. Few studies applied any form of blinding.

Conclusion

There has been a large increase in the number of published studies since the initial guideline was published. However, there are few randomized, blinded, controlled studies. Most articles evaluated were level III or IV, and many studies were hampered by the lack of a control group. In most studies, blinding was not present or not reported. From a methodologic standpoint, a clear need for randomized clinical trials with blinding is evident.

TERMINOLOGY

OSAS in children is defined as a "disorder of breathing during sleep characterized by prolonged partial upper airway obstruction and/or intermittent complete obstruction (obstructive apnea) that disrupts normal ventilation during sleep and normal sleep patterns,"[2] accompanied by symptoms or signs as listed in Table 2 of the accompanying guideline. In this document, the term SDB is used to encompass both snoring and OSAS when studies did not distinguish between these entities.

PREVALENCE OF OSAS

The original clinical practice guideline found a prevalence of OSAS of 2% (3 studies) and a prevalence of habitual snoring (HS) of 3% to 12% (7 studies). Since publication of the original guideline, 10 studies (in 12 separate articles) used the gold standard of conventional overnight laboratory PSG to diagnose OSAS (Table 5). These studies were all levels I through IV, depending on the size and characteristics of the sample population, and represented many countries and age groups. They used various criteria, not all of which are standard, to diagnose OSAS. Many of the studies had a small sample size and/or studied only a selected high-risk sample of the population. Despite these limitations, the 10 studies found a prevalence of OSAS in the general pediatric population of 0% to 5.7%. Three studies to note were those of Bixler et al[11] from the United States, Li et al[12] from China, and O'Brien et al[13] from the United States. These 3 studies (levels I–II) had large sample sizes from the general pediatric population and reported OSAS prevalence rates of 1.2% to 5.7%. Six studies investigated the prevalence of OSAS by using various ambulatory studies rather than full, laboratory-based PSG (Table 6). Although the sample sizes were generally larger, home studies are not considered the gold standard of diagnosis and were thus level III. These studies found an OSAS prevalence of 0.8% to 24%. The 2 outliers (at 12% and 24%)[14,15] used more liberal criteria to diagnose OSAS. Excluding those studies, the OSAS prevalence was 0.8% to 2.8%.

Several studies attempted to discern variables associated with the presence of OSAS. Three studies found an equal prevalence between males and females,[16–18] and 2 studies found an increased prevalence in males.[12,15] Two studies reported an increased risk in children of ethnic minorities,[11,19] supporting older data.[20] Four studies found an increased risk in obese patients,[12,17,21,22] but 3 studies did

Evidence Quality	Preponderance of Benefit or Harm	Balance of Benefit and Harm
A. Well-designed RCTs or diagnostic studies in relevant population	Strong Recommendation	Option
B. RCTs or diagnostic studies with minor limitations; overwhelmingly consistent evidence from observational studies		
C. Observational studies (case-control and cohort design)	Recommendation	
D. Expert opinion, case reports, reasoning from first principles	Option	No Recommendation
X. Exceptional situations in which validating studies cannot be performed and there is a clear preponderance of benefit or harm	Strong Recommendation / Recommendation	

FIGURE 1
Evidence quality. Integrating evidence quality appraisal with an assessment of the anticipated balance between benefits and harms if a policy is carried out leads to designation of a policy as a strong recommendation, recommendation, option, or no recommendation. RCT, randomized controlled trial.

TABLE 2 Definitions and Recommendation Implications

Statement	Definition	Implication
Strong recommendation	A strong recommendation in favor of a particular action is made when the anticipated benefits of the recommended intervention clearly exceed the harms (as a strong recommendation against an action is made when the anticipated harms clearly exceed the benefits) and the quality of the supporting evidence is excellent. In some clearly identified circumstances, strong recommendations may be made when high-quality evidence is impossible to obtain and the anticipated benefits strongly outweigh the harms.	Clinicians should follow a strong recommendation unless a clear and compelling rationale for an alternative approach is present.
Recommendation	A recommendation in favor of a particular action is made when the anticipated benefits exceed the harms but the quality of evidence is not as strong. Again, in some clearly identified circumstances, recommendations may be made when high-quality evidence is impossible to obtain but the anticipated benefits outweigh the harms.	Clinicians would be prudent to follow a recommendation but should remain alert to new information and sensitive to patient preferences.
Option	Options define courses that may be taken when either the quality of evidence is suspect or carefully performed studies have shown little clear advantage to 1 approach over another.	Clinicians should consider the option in their decision-making, and patient preference may have a substantial role.
No recommendation	No recommendation indicates that there is a lack of pertinent published evidence and that the anticipated balance of benefits and harms is presently unclear.	Clinicians should be alert to new published evidence that clarifies the balance of benefit versus harm.

TABLE 3 Results of Text-Mining of the Methods Section of 757 Papers

Term Used for Text-Mining	Percentage of Papers
Snore/snoring	58.3
Polysomnography	53.6
Diagnosis	53.4
Medical management	51.6
Survey/questionnaire	38.8
Psychological	37.0
Surgery/surgical	35.9
Treatment	32.1
Design	27.8
Obese/obesity	25.0
BMI	24.6
Randomize	20.2
Blinding	16.4
Sampling	11.7
Control group	8.8
Actigraphy	2.6
Mortality	0.5

TABLE 4 Types of Studies in the Literature Based on 350 Articles

Type of Study	Percentage
Descriptive study	33.7
Nonrandomized concurrent cohort series	32.0
Descriptive study + other	10.8
Nonrandomized historical cohort series	7.8
Randomized clinical trial	4.6
Retrospective	3.6
Case-control study	1.3
Prospective consecutive cohort series	1.3
Cross-sectional population-based survey	1.0
Nonrandomized historical cohort series + other	1.0
Randomized + other	1.0
Undetermined	1.0
Nonrandomized concurrent cohort series + other	0.7
Experimental study	0.3

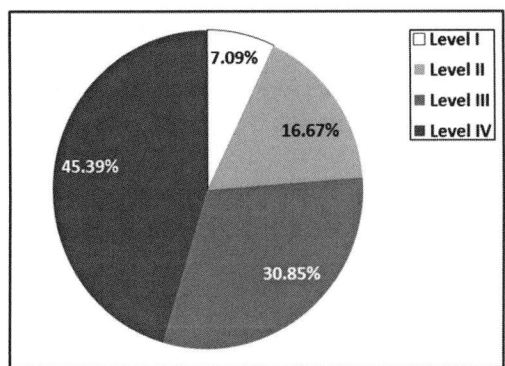

FIGURE 2
Levels of evidence of articles used for this report.

not.[15,16,23] Another study reported an increased risk of OSAS with increased waist circumference, a marker for obesity.[11] One study found an increased risk with nasal abnormalities,[11] 1 study found an increased risk with prematurity,[19] and 2 studies found increased risk with adenotonsillar hypertrophy.[12,22]

Multiple studies (levels II–IV) investigated the prevalence of HS, which is one of the most prominent manifestations of OSAS (Table 7). The presence of snoring was based on parental or personal questionnaires. Not all of the questionnaires used have been validated, and the data relied on subjective responses rather than objective clinical evaluations. The reported prevalence of HS varied widely, depending on the study and definition used, from 1.5% to 27.6%.

In summary, studies of OSAS and HS show varied prevalence rates, depending on the population studied, the methods used to measure breathing during sleep, and the definitions used for diagnosis. Nevertheless, the preponderance of evidence suggests a prevalence of OSAS in the range of 1% to 5%, making this a relatively common disease that would be encountered by most clinicians in primary practice.

Areas for Future Research

● Population-based studies on the gender and race distribution of OSAS among different age groups.

SEQUELAE OF OSAS

Neuropsychological and Cognitive Problems Associated With OSAS

Of the 350 articles related to this search over the last 10 years, 61 articles directly explored the relationship between SDB and cognitive or neuropsychological deficits. In total, 29 658 subjects were studied, including 2 level I studies[24,25] with a total of 174 subjects and 5 level II studies.[26–30] The diagnosis of SDB was based on clinical symptoms in 29 articles and on PSG in 32 articles.

Cognitive Deficits

All but 1 study (level IV)[31] demonstrated deficits in cognition or neuropsychological function in association with symptoms, signs, or diagnosis of SDB. The 1 exception examined children who had mild OSAS over a wide age range and did not include behavioral assessments. In this study, the mean IQ in the OSAS population was significantly above the standard mean. Some[32–34] but not all studies showed a correlation between the severity of obstructive apnea as measured on PSG and increasing neuropsychological morbidity. There are several reasons why correlations were not found for all studies. Standard PSG was developed to detect cardiorespiratory variations and may not be an adequate tool for detection of sleep changes that affect neuropsychological function. Another possibility is that any degree of SDB is associated with abnormal neuropsychological outcomes and might be affected variably by social, medical, environmental, or socioeconomic factors not measured by using PSG. This

TABLE 5 Prevalence of OSAS on the Basis of Laboratory PSG

Source	Year	No.	No. Undergoing PSG	Country	Age, y	OSASPrevalence	HSPrevalence	OSAS Criteria/Comments
Anuntaseree et al[201]	2001	1005	8	Thailand	6–13	0.69%	8.5%	AHI ≥1
Anuntaseree et al[202]	2005	755	Unclear, possibly 10			1.3%	6.9%	Note: 2 studies used same cohort
							"most nights"	
Beebe et al[21]	2007	60 obese 22 control	All	United States	10–16.9	0% normal 13% obese		AHI >5 ↑ in obese
Bixler et al[11]	2009	5740	700	United States	5–12	1.2%		AHI ≥5 ↑ in ↑ waist circumference ↑ with nasal abnormalities ↑ in minority race
Brunetti et al[203]	2001	895	34 home monitoring 12 PSG	Italy	3–11	1%–1.8%	4.9%	AHI >3
Brunetti et al[23]	2010						5.4%	Not ↑ in obese; Note: 2 studies used same cohort
							"always"	
Li et al[172]	2010	6447	619	China	5–13	4.8%	7.2%	Using ICSD-II criteria 4.8% ↑ in boys
Li et al[12]	2010						"frequently"	↑ in obese ↑ in ↑ tonsil size
Ng et al[204]	2002	200	16	Hong Kong	6.4 ± 4	1%	14.5%	AHI >1
O'Brien et al[13]	2003	5728	110	United States	5–7	5.7%	11.7%	AHI >5
							"frequent and loud"	Boys = girls Not ↑ in obese
Sogut et al[16]	2005	1198 total	28	Turkey	3–11	0.9%–1.3%	3.3% >3 times/week	Used AHI >3 Boys = girls Not ↑ in obese
Wing et al[17]	2003	46 obese, 44 control	All	China	7–15	2.3%–4.5% control; 26% to 32.6% obese		OAI ≥1 or RDI ≥5 Boys = girls ↑ in obese
Xu et al[22]	2008	99 obese, 99 control	All	China	Elementary school	0 if not obese and no ATH		AHI >5 or OAI >1 ↑ obese ↑ in ATH

ATH, adenotonsillar hypertrophy; ICSD, International Classification of Sleep Disorders; OAI, obstructive apnea index.

possibility is confirmed by a recent level I study showing that obesity, OSAS, and neurocognitive outcomes are all interdependent.[35] Furthermore, most studies were not controlled for socioeconomic status (SES), which is important because SES strongly affects the results of neurocognitive testing and because OSAS is associated with low SES.[36] Although some studies have shown abnormalities in snorers compared with nonsnoring controls, in many of these studies, data in snorers still fell within the normal range.[24] In addition, cutoffs for OSAS used in some studies resulted in a blurring of boundaries between the OSAS and snoring groups. For example, Chervin et al used an obstructive apnea index cutoff of only ≥0.5/hour to define OSAS, and the mean apnea index for the OSAS group was 2.9 events/hour, indicating that the study group had mild OSAS, which was not that different from the snorers.[37,38] A study with a wider spectrum of severity may have attained different results. Finally, most studies have not controlled for obesity, which has been associated with neurobehavioral and cognitive abnormalities.

Although most studies simply compared groups, others have looked at the correlation between polysomnographic indices and neurocognitive/behavioral outcomes and have shown a correlation between different polysomnographic factors and cognitive outcomes, behavioral outcomes, and sleepiness.[32–34,39]

Cognitive deficits associated with pediatric SDB include general intelligence level as well as processes measured by using IQ subtests (Table 8). Specific functions objectively measured by using neuropsychological assessments and included in the research studies include:

- Learning, memory, and visuospatial skills

TABLE 6 Prevalence of OSAS on the Basis of Ambulatory Monitoring

Source	Year	No.	No. Undergoing Ambulatory Monitoring	Country	Age, y	OSAS Prevalence, %	HS Prevalence	OSAS Criteria and Comments
Castronovo et al[14]	2003	595	265	Italy	3–6	12	34.5% "Often" or "Always"	OAI ≥5
Goodwin et al[15]	2005	480	All	United States	6–11	24	10.5% "Frequently"	RDI ≥1 ↑ in male Not ↑ in obese
Hultcrantz and Löfstrand Tideström[205]	2009	393	26	Sweden	12	0.8	6.9% "Regularly"	AHI ≥1 and/ or OAI ≥1
Rosen et al[19]	2003	850	All	United States	8–11	2.2		AHI ≥5 or OAI ≥1 ↑ in AA ↑ in premature infants
Sánchez-Armengol et al[18]	2001	101	All	Spain	12–16	1.9	14.8%	Based on RDI ≥10 and snoring, witnessed apneas, and/or excessive daytime sleepiness.
							"Often"	Girls = boys
Urschitz et al[206]	2010	1144	183	Germany	7.3–12.4	2.8		AHI ≥1

OAI, obstructive apnea index; AA, African American.

TABLE 7 Prevalence of HS

Source	Year	No.	Country	Age, y	HS Prevalence, %	HS Criteria
Akcay et al[207]	2006	1784	Turkey	4–17	4.1	"Often"
Alexopoulos et al[208]	2006	1821	Greece	5–14	7.4	>3 times/wk
Archbold et al[209]	2002	1038	United States	2–13.9	17.1	"More than half of the time"
Bidad et al[167]	2006	2900	Iran	11–17	7.9	≥3 times/wk
Chng et al[210]	2004	11 114	Singapore	4–7	6.0	>3 times/wk
Corbo et al[166]	2001	2209	Italy	10–15	5.6	"Often"
Ersu et al[211]	2004	2147	Turkey	5–13	7.0	"Often"
Goodwin et al[212]	2003	1494	United States	4–11	10.5	"Snoring frequently or almost always"
Gottlieb et al[213]	2003	3019	United States	5	12	≥3 times/week
Johnson and Roth[45]	2006	1014	United States	13–16	6	"Every or nearly every night"
Kuehni et al[214]	2008	6811	United Kingdom	1–4	7.9	"Almost always"
Liu et al[215]	2005	517 in China 494 in USA	China United States	Grade school	1.5 (China) 9.9 (United States)	Snoring loudly 5–7 times/wk
Liu et al[215]	2005	5979	China	2–12	5.6	"Frequent"
Löfstrand-Tideström and Hultcrantz[216]	2007	509	Sweden	4–6	5.3–6.9	"Snoring every night"
Lu et al[217]	2003	974	Australia	2–5	10.5	≥4 times/week
Montgomery–Downs et al[44]	2003	1010	United States	Preschool	HS and risk of SDB, 22	≥3 times/week
Nelson and Kulnis[218]	2001	405	United States	6–17	17	"Often"
Ng et al[219]	2005	3047	China	6–12	10.9	6–7 times/wk
Perez-Chada et al[220]	2007	2210	Argentina	9–17	9	"Frequent"
Petry et al[221]	2008	998	Brazil	9–14	27.6	"Frequently" or "always"
Sahin et al[222]	2009	1164	Turkey	7–13	3.5	"Frequently" or "almost every day"
Sogut et al[16]	2005	1030	Turkey	12–17	4.0	"Often" or "always"
Tafur et al[223]	2009	806	Ecuador	6–12	15.1	"Often" or "always"
Urschitz et al[164]	2004	1144	Germany	Primary school	9.6	"Always" or "frequently"
Zhang et al[224]	2004	996	Australia	4–12	15.2	>4 times/wk

- Language, verbal fluency, and phonological skills
- Concept formation, analytic thinking, and verbal and nonverbal comprehension
- School performance and mathematical abilities
- Executive functions

Executive functions were measured by using both objective testing and parent questionnaires. Executive functions are a network of skills and higher order functions that control and regulate other cognitive processes. These skills require mental flexibility, impulse control,

TABLE 8 Cognitive Deficits Associated With Pediatric SDB

Type of Deficit	Source	Level	No.	Findings/Comments
Cognition, general intelligence	Beebe et al[225] Blunden et al[226] Kaemingk et al[33] Kennedy et al[34] Kurnatowski et al[227]	IV	895	Deficits of general intelligence, sensorimotor integration by objective measurement; behavioral abnormalities included as well
	Carvalho et al[228] Montgomery-Downs et al[50] Suratt et al[43]	III	1332	Objective measures of general intelligence, verbal skills affected by SDB
	Friedman et al[26] Halbower et al[28] O'Brien et al[29] Kohler et al[30]	II	473	General intelligence, executive function, language all affected by SDB and measured objectively
	O'Brien et al[24] Suratt et al[25]	I	174	General conceptual ability, verbal and nonverbal reasoning, vocabulary affected by SDB (and time in bed[25])
Poor school performance	Chervin et al[42] Johnson and Roth[45] Kaemingk et al[33] Ng et al[219] Perez-Chada et al[220] Shin et al[47] Urschitz et al[229]	IV	11 110	Academic achievement measured either by parent or school grades Additive factors were SES and ethnicity[42-45] or BMI,[42-45-47] which contributed to findings of poor school performance in SDB
	Montgomery-Downs et al[44]	III	1010	Snoring associates with ethnicity, school performance in SES-challenged preschool-aged children
Executive function	Beebe et al[225] LeBourgeois et al[230] Karpinski et al[231]	IV	179	Mental flexibility, impulse control Objective testing performed
	Halbower et al[28] Kohler et al[30]	II	123	Response preparation, working memory, fluid and quantitative reasoning; objective testing performed by blinded tester
Learning, information processing, memory, visuospatial skills	Goodwin et al[212] Hamasaki Uema et al[232] Kaemingk et al[33] Kennedy et al[34] Kurnatowski et al[227] O'Brien et al[233] Spruyt et al[234] Giordani et al[38]	IV	1838	Objective testing performed in all but Goodwin et al[212] (questionnaire)
	Halbower et al[28] Tauman et al[46]	II	112	Race[28] and BMI may play an additive role in inflammation[46] and cognitive dysfunction in SDB
	O'Brien et al[24]	I	118	Primary snoring without gas exchange abnormalities associates with significantly lower learning and memory
Language/verbal skills	Kurnatowski et al[227] O'Brien et al[233] Perez-Chada et al[220] Honaker et al[235] Lundeborg et al[51]	IV	3304	Deficits of language or verbal skills in SDB Objective testing performed in all studies
	Suratt et al[43] Montgomery-Downs et al[50]	III	114	Race and time in bed may contribute to abnormal language associated with SDB
	O'Brien et al[24] Suratt et al[25]	I	118	Primary snoring without gas exchange abnormalities associated with significantly lower verbal skills; deficits of language or verbal skills in SDB
Attention	Beebe et al[225] Chervin et al[236] Galland et al[237] Gottlieb et al[213] Hamasaki Uema et al[232] Kaemingk et al[33] Li et al[238] Mulvaney et al[32] Urschitz et al[229]	IV	6411	Objective testing performed for attention except in refs 32,33,213,229, and 236 in which parent or teacher questionnaires were used
	Chervin et al[37]	I	105	
	O'Brien et al[24]	I	118	Visual and auditory attention

and working memory. Executive functions are required for optimal school performance and are acquired through adolescence in developing children.

Behavioral Abnormalities

The investigations on the cognitive effects of SDB in the 61 studies often included measures of neurobehavioral outcomes (Table 9). Hyperactivity was the most commonly studied and/or reported behavioral abnormality associated with SDB. It was reported as a frequent symptom of SDB in younger children, and in fact, in 1 study, snoring was found to be strongly predictive of a future diagnosis of hyperactivity over the long-term (level IV).[40] Attention-deficit/hyperactivity disorder (ADHD) or ADHD symptoms, hypersomnolence, somatization, depression, atypicality, aggression, and abnormal social behaviors were the other most frequently reported behavioral abnormalities associated with SDB in children. Most behavioral difficulties were defined by using parent or teacher questionnaires in unblinded level IV studies.

Sleepiness

Two studies (levels I–II) have shown a relationship between polysomnographic measures and objective measurement of daytime sleepiness on multiple sleep latency testing.[27,39]

Exacerbation of Neuropsychological Deficits by Other Factors Underlying Childhood SDB

Abnormal behavioral alterations associated with SDB might be modified or directly caused by other sleep disorders, such as coexistent periodic limb movement disorder.[41] In children with SDB displaying deficits of cognition, school performance, or behavioral functioning, there may be additive roles played by race,[28,42–44] decreased time in bed,[25,43] and low SES,[28,42,44,45] at least in part because of

the association between obesity and low SES.[42] Markers of inflammation and increased cardiovascular risk may point to 1 mechanism related to decreased cognitive function associated with OSAS,[46] seen also in children who are obese. BMI correlated with abnormal cognitive function in pediatric SDB,[42,45,47] although OSAS was found to be an independent risk factor for cognitive deficits. Finally, in 2 studies examining brain function, neuronal injury of the brain[28] and altered cerebral blood flow[48] were found in children who had SDB compared with normal controls and were associated with behavior and cognitive problems. These findings indicate the possibility of preexisting medical problems causing the development of OSAS or, alternatively, OSAS causing brain injury. Therefore, studies showing improved cognition and behavior after treatment of SDB are 1 key in the determination of causality (see the following discussion).

Neuropsychological and Cognitive Deficits in Children Who Have SDB Improve After Treatment

In the previous guideline, there were few before-and-after treatment studies of pediatric SDB focusing on objectively measured cognitive problems. In the last 10 years, 19 studies have examined changes in behavior and/or cognition after surgical treatment of OSAS. The majority of investigations demonstrated agreement about post-treatment improvement of behavior, quality of life (QoL), hyperactivity, ADHD, and impulsivity (Table 10). The exception was 1 study of exercise treatment (level IV),[49] in which snoring improved in obese children but behavior and sleepiness did not. Most studies used subjective questionnaire reports. Excessive daytime sleepiness improved in 1 study that measured this factor, as did depression, sleep quality, and aggressive behavior. Since

publication of the last guideline, 3 additional studies have demonstrated improved cognitive function (by using objective measurement) after treatment of OSAS, including measures of general intelligence, attention, memory, and analytic thinking, including level II,[26] level III,[50] and level IV[37] studies (Table 10). Of concern, however, is that some recent articles suggest that certain deficits of cognition measured by using objective testing may not improve to a large extent after treatment of childhood OSAS. Language, IQ, and executive function did not improve significantly in a well-designed, controlled study of 92 children (level II).[30] General intelligence in at-risk populations improved in 1 study (level III),[50] but phonologic processes and verbal fluency did not improve to normal (level III[50] and level IV[51]). QoL increases after treatment.[37,52–58] Three studies demonstrated long-term (≥1 year) behavioral or QoL improvements.[37,52,53] The majority of these studies suggest that in developing children who are dependent on executive function, cognition, and behavioral skills for daily function and school performance, treatment of childhood SDB has benefits.

Conclusion

In summary, these studies suggest that, in developing children, early diagnosis and treatment of pediatric OSAS may improve a child's long-term cognitive and social potential and school performance. These findings imply that the earlier a child is treated for OSAS, the higher the trajectory for academic and, therefore, economic success, but research is needed to support that implication. There is demonstrated benefit in terms of behavior, attention, and social interactions, as well as likely improvement in cognitive abilities with

TABLE 9 Behavioral Abnormalities Associated With Pediatric SDB

Type of Deficit	Source	Level	No.	Test Conditions
Hyperactivity and/or ADHD	Chervin et al[236]	IV	8101	Hyperactivity generally measured by using parent questionnaire
	Chervin et al[40]			
	Galland et al[237]			
	Golan et al[239]			
	Gottlieb et al[213]			
	Johnson and Roth[45]			
	LeBourgeois et al[230]			
	Mitchell and Kelly[240]			
	Owens et al[189]			
	Roemmich et al[191]			
	Urschitz et al[229]			
	Montgomery-Downs et al[44]	III	1010	Survey data
	Chervin et al[37]	I	105	ADHD assessed by using psychiatric interview and validated instrument
Somatization, depression	Galland et al[237]	IV	205	
	Mitchell and Kelly[240]			
	Mitchell and Kelly[241]			
	Rudnick and Mitchell[242]			
	Suratt et al[43]	III	114	
	O'Brien et al[24]	I	118	
Behavior problems, general	Goldstein et al[55]	IV	1946	Behavior generally measured by using parent questionnaire
	Goldstein et al[243]			
	Hogan et al[48]			
	Li et al[238]			
	Mitchell and Kelly[241]			
	Mulvaney et al[32]			
	Owens et al[189]			
	Roemmich et al[191]			
	Rosen et al[244]			
	Rudnick and Mitchell[242]			
	Tran et al[58]			
	Wei et al[245]			
Aggression, oppositional and social problems	Chervin et al[246]	IV	4407	
	Gottlieb et al[213]			
	Galland et al[237]			
	Mitchell and Kelly[240]			
	Mulvaney et al[32]			
	O'Brien et al[24]	I	118	
Excessive daytime sleepiness	Goodwin et al[212]	IV	9729	Sleepiness measured by using questionnaire
	Perez-Chada et al[220]			
	Shin et al[47]			
	Urschitz et al[229]			
	Johnson and Roth[45]			
	Gozal et al[27]	II	92	Sleepiness measured objectively by multiple sleep latency testing on PSG
	Chervin et al[37]	I	105	Sleepiness measured objectively by multiple sleep latency testing on PSG
Anxiety	O'Brien et al[24]	I	118	

the treatment of pediatric OSAS. However, more long-term studies are needed. The risks of treatment depend on the type of treatment but include risk of surgery, risk of medication, nonadherence to therapy, and cost.

The risks of not treating children who have OSAS include potentially affecting the child's trajectory of developmental gains dependent on intelligence, executive function, and proper social interactions, ultimately lowering lifetime

academic and social achievements. Therefore, the benefit of treating childhood OSAS outweighs the risk where treatment is feasible.

Areas for Future Research

● Further research is required to determine which domains of cognitive function will improve with treatment of OSAS. Reversibility of cognitive deficits associated with OSAS must be adjusted for the confounding effects of age, length of symptoms, SES, BMI, sleep duration, environment, and race and ethnicity.

Cardiovascular Effects of OSAS

A total of 24 studies related to cardiovascular effects of OSAS in childhood were identified since the last review. The levels of evidence were III and IV.

In a retrospective, level IV study of 271 clinical cases, only 1 child, who had congenital heart disease, had signs of cardiac failure preoperatively, and other cases had no evidence of left or right ventricular hypertrophy.[59] However, studies using more sophisticated, prospective techniques have found subclinical evidence of cardiac dysfunction. These studies are described in Table 11. Although postoperative adenotonsillectomy (AT) cardiac complications are rare (level IV),[59] left and right ventricular hypertrophy is significantly associated with postoperative respiratory complications (level III),[60] supporting the recommendation in the current and the previous guidelines that children who have cardiac abnormalities be monitored as inpatients postoperatively.

Blood pressure (BP) has also been shown to be affected by OSAS in children. There were 9 recent level III or IV studies, most of which showed a correlation between the presence/

TABLE 10 Cognitive, Behavioral, and QoL Abnormalities Improved After Treatment of Pediatric SBD

Deficit Measured	Source	Level	No.	Abnormalities Improved After SDB Treatment
Cognition/IQ	Chervin et al[37]	I	105	Attention measured on continuous performance test improved significantly after treatment
	Montgomery-Downs et al[50]	III	38	General conceptual ability improved (verbal fluency did not improve)
	Friedman et al[26]	II	59	Auditory-visual integration, auditory-motor memory, short-term memory, retention, analytic thinking, IQ/mental processing, attention all improved
Hyperactivity and/or ADHD	Galland et al[237] Li et al[238] Mitchell and Kelly[240] Mitchell and Kelly[241] Roemmich et al[191]	IV	247	Hyperactivity and/or diagnosis of ADHD improved
	Chervin et al[37]	I	105	Long-term improvement in hyperactivity
Somatization, depression	Galland et al[237] Mitchell and Kelly[240] Mitchell and Kelly[241]	IV	153	All showed improvement in depression and/or somatization
Behavior problems, general	Goldstein et al[55] Goldstein et al[243] Hogan et al[48] Li et al[238] Roemmich et al[191] Tran et al[58] Wei et al[245] Mitchell et al[53] Davis et al[49]	IV	450	All showed behavior improvement except Davis et al[49] Long-term behavior improvement in Mitchell et al[53]
Aggression, oppositional, and social problems	Galland et al[237] Mitchell and Kelly[240]	IV	113	Improvement in abnormal social behavior and aggression
Excessive daytime sleepiness	Chervin et al[37]	I	105	Sleepiness improved by 1 min, as measured by using multiple sleep latency testing on PSG
QoL	Colen et al[52] Constantin et al[54] Goldstein et al[55] Sohn et al[56] Silva and Leite[57] Tran et al[58]	IV	787	Includes disease-specific and emotional QoL[58] Long-term improvements ≥1 y[52,53]
	Chervin et al[37]	I	105	Long-term improvements at 1 y
Sleep quality	Constantin et al[54] Wei et al[245]	IV	590	Improved in both studies

severity of OSAS and indices of elevated BP (Table 12).

In a study by Kaditis et al,[61] overnight changes in brain natriuretic peptide levels were large in children who had an apnea hypopnea index (AHI) ≥5/hour when compared with those with milder OSAS and with controls (level III). This finding suggests the presence of nocturnal cardiac strain in children who have moderate to severe OSAS.

Two studies evaluated brain oxygenation and cerebral artery blood flow. Khadra et al[62] reported that male gender, arousal index, and amount of non–rapid eye movement sleep were associated with diminished cerebral oxygenation, whereas increasing mean arterial pressure, age, oxygen saturation (Sp_{O_2}), and amount of rapid eye movement sleep were associated with augmented cerebral oxygenation (level III). Hogan et al[48] found

a decrease in middle cerebral artery velocity postoperatively in patients treated for OSAS, whereas control subjects showed a slight increase over time (level IV).

Three studies evaluated autonomic variability in children who have OSAS. Constantin et al[63] reported resolution of tachycardia and diminished pulse rate variability after AT in children who had OSAS (diagnosis of OSAS based on oximetry plus questionnaire data) (level IV). Deng et al[64] studied heart rate variability and determined that heart rate chaos was modulated by OSAS as well as by sleep state (level IV). In a study of 28 children who had OSAS, O'Brien and Gozal[65] found evidence of altered autonomic nervous system regulation, as evidenced by increased sympathetic vascular reactivity, during wakefulness in these children (level III). These studies all suggest that OSAS places stress on the autonomic system.

In summary, a large number of studies, albeit primarily level III, found that cardiac changes occur in the presence of OSAS, with an effect on both the right and left ventricles. OSAS in childhood also has an effect on both systolic and diastolic BP. In addition, several studies suggest that childhood OSAS can affect autonomic regulation, brain oxygenation, and cerebral blood flow. These studies suggest that childhood OSAS may jeopardize long-term cardiovascular health.[66]

The association between left ventricular remodeling and 24-hour BP highlighted the role of SDB in increasing cardiovascular morbidity.

Areas for Future Research

- How reversible, after treatment, are cardiovascular changes in children who have OSAS?

- What are the long-term effects of OSAS on the cardiovascular system?

TABLE 11 Structural and Functional Cardiac Abnormalities in Children Who Have OSAS

Source	Level	No.	Findings
Left-sided cardiac dysfunction			
Amin et al[247]	III	28 OSAS 19 PS	Abnormalities of LV geometry in 39% of OSAS vs 15% of PS; OSAS associated with increased LV mass
Amin et al[248]	III	48 OSAS 15 PS	Dose-dependent decrease in LV diastolic function with increased severity of SDB
Right-sided cardiac dysfunction			
Duman et al[249]	III	21 children, ATH; 21 controls	Higher RV myocardial performance index in patient with adenotonsillar hypertrophy than in controls; this decreased significantly after AT, along with symptoms of OSAS
Ugur et al[250]	III	29 OSAS 26 PS	Improved RV diastolic function after AT, with postoperative values similar to controls
Biventricular cardiac dysfunction			
James et al[59]	IV	271	Case review of ECG and chest radiography results found only 1 case of cardiac failure, which occurred in a child who had congenital heart disease; most other cases showed no abnormalities
Weber et al[251]	III	30 OSAS 10 controls	Increased RV diameter and area during both systole and diastole; reduced LV diastolic diameter and ejection fraction

ATH, adenotonsillar hypertrophy; LV, left ventricle; PS, primary snoring; RV, right ventricle.

TABLE 12 BP in Children Who Have OSAS

Source	Level	No.	Findings
Kohyama et al[175]	IV	23 suspected OSAS	REM diastolic BP index correlated with AHI Age, BMI, and AHI were significant predictors of systolic BP index during REM
Kwok et al[66]	III	30 PS	Children with PS had increased daytime BP and reduced arterial distensibility
Leung et al[252]	III	96 suspected OSAS	Children with a higher AHI had higher wake systolic BP and sleep systolic and diastolic BP BMI, age, and desaturation index contributed to elevation of the diastolic BP during sleep, but only BMI contributed to the wake and sleeping systolic BP
Guilleminault et al[253]	III	Retrospective component: 301 suspected OSAS Prospective component: 78 OSAS	Some children who have OSAS have orthostatic hypotension
Li et al[176]	III	306 community sample	OSAS was associated with elevated daytime and nocturnal BP
Amin et al[177]	III	140 suspected OSAS	OSAS associated with an increase in morning BP surge, BP load, and 24-h BP. BP parameters predicted changes in left ventricular wall thickness
Amin et al[254]	III	39 OSAS 21 PS	OSAS was associated with 24-h BP dysregulation AHI, Spo2, and arousal contribute to abnormal BP control independent of obesity
Enright et al[255]	III	239 community sample	Obesity, sleep efficiency, and RDI were independently associated with elevated systolic BP
Kaditis et al[174]	IV	760 community sample	No difference in morning BP between habitual snorers and nonhabitual snorers

PS, primary snoring; REM, rapid eye movement.

Growth

The section on obesity contains a detailed review of obesity and OSAS, including the relationship between OSAS and the metabolic syndrome. The previous guideline documented many studies showing a relationship between OSAS and growth, and an increase in growth parameters after treatment of SDB by AT; this outcome has been confirmed by a number of more recent studies (as discussed in the recent meta-analysis by Bonuck et al[67]). In a confirmation of previous reports,[68,69] Selimoğlu et al[70] found a decreased level of serum insulin-like growth factor-I in children who have OSAS, which increased significantly 6 months after AT (level III).

Inflammation

Since the publication of the 2002 AAP guideline, there has been growing research on the role of OSAS in systemic inflammation. It has been postulated that OSAS results in intermittent hypoxemia, leading to production of reactive oxygen species. In addition, the hypoxemia and arousals from sleep lead to sympathetic activation. These factors may trigger inflammation or exacerbate obesity-related inflammation. However, the data on OSAS and markers of systemic inflammation in children are scarce and contradictory.

Eight studies (level II–III) measured levels of C-reactive protein (CRP) in children who had OSAS. Four studies (including 2 from the same center) showed no relationship between CRP and OSAS,[71–74] whereas 4 studies (2 from the same center) did show a relationship.[46,75–77] Part of the discrepancy between studies may be attributable to the varying proportions of obese subjects (because obesity is associated with high CRP levels) and varied age of subjects and definitions of OSAS in the different studies. Some studies controlled for obesity and degree of OSAS, whereas others did not. The studies showing a positive relationship indicated that OSAS was associated with elevated

CRP levels only above a certain threshold of severity. Thus, the relationship between OSAS and CRP seems to be complex and is affected by obesity and severity of OSAS.

A few level II and III studies have evaluated other circulating markers of inflammation in children who have OSAS. Two studies showed no difference in circulating intercellular adhesion molecule-1 between patients with OSAS and controls.[71,73] A single study found elevated p-selectin (a measure of platelet activation) in children who had OSAS compared with controls.[73] A single study showed elevated levels of interferon-γ in children who had OSAS.[74] One study showed increased interleukin (IL)-6 and lower IL-10 in those with OSAS,[78] whereas another study did not.[74] Another study reported no difference in cytokines IL-1β, IL-2, IL-4, IL-8, IL-12, and granulocyte macrophage colony-stimulating factor levels between children who had OSAS and controls.[74] Data on tumor necrosis factor-α are conflicting,[74,79] and differences in levels may be related to tumor necrosis factor-α gene polymorphisms.[80]

A pathology-based study found increased glucocorticoid receptors in adenotonsillar tissue from children who had OSAS compared with tissue from children who experienced chronic throat infections (level III)[81]; another study from the same group found elevated leukotriene receptors (level IV).[82] These findings provide a theoretical construct for the potential utility of antiinflammatory drugs as treatment of children who have OSAS, although possibly not for those who have already undergone AT.

In summary, the data on CRP are conflicting, but it may be that CRP levels increase above a certain threshold of severity of OSAS. Further research involving large samples of subjects who have varying degrees of OSAS severity,

with results controlled for BMI and age, are needed. There are too few data on other circulating markers of systemic inflammation to enable any recommendations.

Areas for Future Research

● Larger studies, stratified for the severity of OSAS and controlled for obesity, are required to determine whether OSAS is associated with systemic inflammation. If so, what are the long-term sequelae of this inflammation? Are inflammatory biomarkers potential good outcome measurements for OSAS treatment studies? Do they correlate with clinical outcomes or long-term prognosis?

METHODS OF DIAGNOSIS

The previous guideline discussed the diagnosis of OSAS in great detail. On the basis of published evidence at the time, it was concluded that the positive and predictive value of history and physical examination for the diagnosis of OSAS was 65% and 46%, respectively; that is, no better than chance. It was therefore recommended that objective testing be used for the diagnosis of OSAS. An evaluation of the literature regarding nocturnal pulse oximetry, video recording, nap PSG, and ambulatory PSG suggested that these methods tended to be helpful if results were positive but had a poor predictive value if results were negative. Thus, children who had negative study results should be referred for more comprehensive testing. These recommendations were based on only a few studies, most of which had a low level of evidence. Furthermore, it was recognized that these techniques were of limited use in evaluating the severity of OSAS (which is important in determining management, such as whether outpatient surgery can be performed safely). In

addition, the cost efficacy of these screening techniques had not been evaluated and would depend, in part, on how many patients eventually required full PSG. Since the publication of the initial guideline, there have been a number of new studies, but few are level I or II. Because few of the studies cited here included data that would enable calculation of overall sensitivity and specificity or positive and negative predictive values, an overall table could not be provided. For this section, PSG was considered the gold standard for diagnosis of OSAS.

Utility of History Alone for the Diagnosis of OSAS

Several level IV studies evaluated the use of history alone for the diagnosis of OSAS. Preutthipan et al[83] found overall poor sensitivity and specificity when evaluating various historical factors. The Pediatric Sleep Questionnaire published by Chervin et al[84] performed slightly better than other published questionnaires, with a sensitivity of 0.85 and a specificity of 0.87 by using a set cutoff. A follow-up study by the same group showed a sensitivity of 78% and a specificity of 72% for PSG-defined OSAS.[85] However, this is still a relatively low sensitivity and specificity for clinical purposes. By using this instrument, the same group also found that negative answers to only 2 questions on the Pediatric Sleep Questionnaire were helpful in identifying patients who had normal PSG results.[86] Taken together, the overall performance of questionnaire tools seems to support their use more as a screening tool than as a diagnostic tool, such that a negative score would be unlikely to mislabel a child with OSAS as being healthy, but a positive score would be unlikely to accurately diagnose a particular child with certainty.

Utility of Clinical Evaluation for the Diagnosis of OSAS

Similar to the data presented in the previous guideline, most studies found that clinical evaluation was not predictive of OSAS on PSG. Godwin et al[15] performed a large (N = 480), population-based study of 6- to 11-year-old children. The study included use of a standardized history, some clinical parameters, and ambulatory, full PSG (level II). They concluded that the sensitivity of any individual or combined clinical symptoms was poor. Certain parameters, such as snoring, excessive daytime sleepiness, and learning problems, had a high specificity.

In a level III study, van Someren et al[87] compared history and clinical examination by a pediatrician or otolaryngologist with abbreviated PSG (video recording, oximetry, and measurement of snoring). Both the sensitivity and specificity of the clinician's impression of moderate/severe OSAS were low (59% and 73%, respectively). In a similar number of cases, the clinicians underestimated (17%) and overestimated (16%) study results.

In a level III study, it was shown that waist circumference z score had a statistically significant but clinically poor correlation with symptoms of OSAS ($R = 0.32$, $P = .006$); BMI z score did not correlate with symptoms.[88]

Radiologic Studies

Several studies, all level III or IV, evaluated the utility of radiologic examinations in addition to clinical factors in establishing the diagnosis of OSAS (Table 13). Overall, these studies showed that the presence of airway narrowing on a lateral neck radiograph increased the probability of predicting OSAS on PSG. Cephalometric studies tended to show a small mandible in patients who had OSAS

compared with controls, although a study using an MRI did not confirm this.[89] None of the cephalometric studies provided sensitivity and specificity or positive and negative predictive values. Table 13 simplifies the cephalometric findings for the purpose of presentation. A level I study indicated that acoustic pharyngometry may be a useful screening technique for OSAS in older children, but approximately one-half of the children could not cooperate well with the testing.[90] One uncontrolled study (level IV) showed that nasal resistance, as measured by using rhinometry, had a high sensitivity and specificity for predicting polysomnographic OSAS.[91] This technique warrants further study and validation.

Snoring Evaluation

Two level IV studies found a weak association between objective snoring characteristics and the presence/severity of OSAS that was insufficient to assist in clinical diagnosis.[92,93]

Cardiovascular Parameters

Studies have evaluated the utility of screening tests based on heart rate or other vascular factors in predicting OSAS (Table 14). These studies ranged from studies of pulse rate alone to more sophisticated (and, hence, more expensive or time-consuming) studies, such as analyses of heart rate variability, pulse transit time, and peripheral arterial tonometry. Studies were level II through IV. Overall, the studies found changes in cardiovascular variables in children who had OSAS but with varying sensitivities and specificities. Thus, some of these measures may potentially be useful screening tests in the future if combined with other modalities that would increase the sensitivity and specificity but cannot

be recommended for clinical use at this point.

Nocturnal Oximetry

The previous AAP guideline, on the basis of a single study by Brouillette et al,[94] indicated that nocturnal pulse oximetry could provide an accurate screen for OSAS if the result was positive but that full PSG was needed if the oximetry result was negative. A need for further research in this area was indicated. Four additional studies were identified for the current report. Two of these did not compare oximetry versus PSG and therefore will not be discussed further.[95,96]

A follow-up study (level II) from the same group as the previous report by Brouillette et al[94] used overnight oximetry, primarily obtained in the home, to develop a scoring algorithm.[97] The subjects' median age was 4 years. The oximetry score correlated with the AHI obtained from PSG as well as with the presence of postoperative complications. However, the positive predictive value of oximetry for major postoperative respiratory compromise was only 13%. Of note, 80% of the 223 children had normal, inconclusive, or technically unsatisfactory oximetry results and were therefore referred for either repeat oximetry or PSG. In contrast, Kirk et al[98] compared overnight home oximetry (by using a system with an automated oximetry analysis algorithm that provided a desaturation index) with laboratory PSG in 58 children aged ≥4 years who had suspected OSAS (level III). They found poor agreement between the desaturation index on the basis of oximetry and the PSG-determined AHI. The sensitivity of oximetry for the identification of moderate OSAS (AHI >5/hour) was 67%, and specificity was 60%. The oximetry algorithm tended to overestimate the AHI at low levels and underestimate at high

TABLE 13 Relationship Between Airway Measurements and OSAS

Clinical Evaluation	Sleep Evaluation	Airway Evaluation	Source	Level	No.	Findings
Standardized history, clinical examination	PSG	Lateral neck radiography	Xu et al[256]	IV	50	Combinations of different predictor variables resulted in positive and negative predictor values ranging from 70% to 80%
Clinical examination	PSG	Lateral neck radiography	Jain and Sahni[257]	IV	40	Degree of OSAS correlated with adenoid size on radiography but not with tonsillar size on clinical examination
Clinical examination	PSG	Lateral neck radiography	Li et al[258]	IV	35	Tonsillar–pharyngeal ratio on radiography correlated with AHI but not clinical tonsil size. Clinical tonsil size did not correlate with AHI For a ratio of 0.479, the sensitivity and specificity in predicting moderately severe OSAS (AHI >10/h) was 96% and 82%, respectively
NA	PSG	Cephalometry	Kawashima et al[259]	III	15 OSAS 30 controls	Evidence of retrognathia in OSAS group
Clinical examination	Ambulatory abbreviated recordings	Cephalometry	Kawashima et al[260]	III	38 OSAS 31 controls	OSAS: retrognathia, long facies in those OSAS subjects who had large tonsils
NA	None	Cephalometry	Kikuchi et al[261]	IV	29 suspected OSAS 41 controls	OSAS: long facies
Questionnaire	None	Cephalometry	Kulnis et al[262]	IV	28 snorers 28 controls	Snorers: retrognathia, shorter maxilla and cranial base
Standardized history	Nap PSG	Cephalometry	Zucconi et al[263]	III	26 snorers 26 controls	Snorers: retrognathia, decreased nasopharyngeal space
NA	PSG	MRI	Schiffman et al[89]	III	24 OSAS 24 controls	No difference in mandibular size between OSAS and controls
Clinical assessment of tonsillar size	Ambulatory cardiorespiratory recordings	Acoustic pharyngometry Cephalometry	Monahan et al[90]	I	203	Degree of OSAS correlated with airway size on pharyngometry but not with tonsillar size Pharyngometric measures also correlated with mandibular length on cephalometry, only 78% of 8- to 11-y-old children could produce minimally acceptable data, and only 54% could produce high-quality data
Questionnaire, clinical examination	PSG	Rhinometry	Rizzi et al[91]	IV	73	Nasal resistance of 0.59 Pa/cm^3/s had a positive predictive value of 97% and a negative predictive value of 86%

levels. The authors concluded that oximetry alone was not adequate for the diagnosis of OSAS. On the basis of these limited studies, it seems as if oximetry alone is insufficient for the diagnosis of OSAS because of the high rate of inconclusive test results and the poor sensitivity and specificity compared with PSG, probably, in part, because children may have OSAS that results in arousals and sleep fragmentation but little desaturation. In addition, children tend to move a lot during sleep, which can result in movement artifact.

Ambulatory PSG

The term "ambulatory PSG" is used for unattended sleep studies conducted in the home. Frequently, ambulatory PSG consists of cardiorespiratory recordings alone. Although the use of ambulatory PSG is considered appropriate under certain circumstances in adults,[99] there is a paucity of studies evaluating ambulatory PSG in children. Zucconi et al[100] evaluated a home portable system comprising measurements of airflow (by using thermistry), snoring, chest and abdominal wall movements, electrocardiography (ECG), position, and oximetry (level II). However, the portable system was used in the sleep laboratory for the purpose of the study. A small sample of 12 children, 3 to 6 years of age, underwent routine PSG and in-laboratory portable testing

on a consecutive night with the portable system. The portable system had good sensitivity for detecting a respiratory distress index (RDI) >5/hour (78% with automated scoring; 89% with human scoring) but a specificity of zero. Rosen et al[19] reported on a study of 664 children aged 8 to 11 years who underwent abbreviated ambulatory study (by using inductance plethysmography, oximetry, heart rate, and position) (level III). Of these home studies, 94% were considered technically adequate. A subsample of 55 children also underwent full laboratory PSG. Few details were given regarding this subsample. However, it was reported that the ambulatory studies had a sensitivity

TABLE 14 Utility of Cardiovascular Parameters in Predicting OSAS

Measure	Sleep Evaluation	Source	Level	No.	Findings
Pulse rate	Oximetry	Constantin et al[63]	IV	25 OSAS	Pulse rate decreases in children who have OSAS after AT
Pulse rate	Home cardiorespiratory studies	Noehren et al[264]	III	5 OSAS 20 controls	Pulse rate changes poor at detecting differences between respiratory events and movements, and between central and obstructive apneas
Heart rate variability	PSG	Deng et al[64]	IV	34 OSAS 18 controls	Heart rate chaos intensity had sensitivity of 72% and specificity of 81% for OSAS
Pulse transit time	PSG	Katz et al[265]	III	24 SDB 10 controls	Depending on the severity of the event, 80%–91% of obstructive respiratory events were associated with pulse transit time changes. However, pulse transit time changes also occurred with spontaneous arousals from sleep
Heart rate, pulse transit time	PSG	Foo et al[266] (similar data published in Foo and Lim[267])	III	15 suspected OSAS	Pulse rate had 70% sensitivity and 89% specificity, and pulse transit time had 75% sensitivity and 92% specificity in identifying obstructive events
Peripheral arterial tonometry	PSG	Tauman et al[268]	II	40 OSAS 20 controls	Peripheral arterial tonometry had sensitivity of 95% and specificity of 35% in identifying EEG arousals

of 88% and specificity of 98% in diagnosing a laboratory PSG–based AHI >5/hour. It is not clear why the results of this study were so different from that of Zucconi et al but may possibly be related to the older age of the subjects. Goodwin et al[101] used a full PSG system, including EEG measurements, in the unattended home environment in 157 children aged 5 to 12 years (level IV). Adequate data were obtained from 91% of subjects on the first attempt and 97% when the test was repeated if needed. Data were reported as excellent in 61% of cases and good in 36%. In a small subsample of 5 subjects, data were similar to those with laboratory PSG. This study shows the feasibility of performing unattended full ambulatory PSG in older children, but results may not be the same for young children. In summary, ambulatory PSG seems to be technically feasible in school-aged children, although data are not available for younger children. Studies of differing levels, and studying different age groups, found widely discrepant specificities for diagnosing moderate OSAS. Clearly, additional studies are needed.

Nocturnal PSG

Nocturnal, attended, laboratory PSG is considered the gold standard for diagnosis of OSAS because it provides an objective, quantitative evaluation of disturbances in respiratory and sleep patterns. A recent review describes some of the relationships between PSG and sequelae of OSAS (see "Pediatric Issues" section in Redline et al[102]). PSG allows patients to be stratified in terms of severity, which helps determine which children are at risk for sequelae (thus alerting pediatricians to screen for complications of OSAS); which children are at risk for postoperative complications and would, therefore, benefit from inpatient observation postoperatively; and which children are at high risk of persistence of OSAS postoperatively, who may then need postoperative PSG to assess the need for further treatment (eg, CPAP).

Adult patients may sleep poorly the first time they are in a sleep laboratory because of anxiety, the unfamiliar environment, and the attached sensors. This "first night effect" can lead to altered sleep architecture and possible underestimation of the severity of OSAS. Five studies (levels I–IV) evaluated the night-to-night variability of PSG in children[101,103–106]; in one of these articles,[101] only a small subsample had night-to-night variability evaluated (Table 15). The time difference between PSGs varied from 24

hours to 4 weeks. Although some of the studies showed minor differences in respiratory parameters from night to night, the studies suggest that few children would have been clinically misclassified on the basis of a single night's PSG. Thus, 1 night of PSG seems to be adequate to establish the diagnosis of OSAS. All studies showed significant differences in sleep architecture from night to night. Therefore, research studies evaluating sleep architecture would require >1 night of PSG. For consistency, it is recommended that PSG be performed and scored by using the pediatric criteria from the American Academy of Sleep Medicine scoring manual.[107]

Other Tests

The shape of the maximal flow-volume loop on pulmonary function testing has been used to attempt to screen for OSAS in adults. Young children cannot perform standard maximal flow-volume loops. One small study of 10 subjects evaluated the relationship between tidal breathing flow-volume loops and PSG (level III).[108] The sensitivity was 37.5% and specificity was 100%, indicating that this method is of limited utility in screening for OSAS.

Two studies by the same group evaluated whether urinary/serum

TABLE 15 Night-to-Night Variability in Polysomnographic Respiratory Parameters

Time Between Evaluations	Source	Level	No.	Findings
1–4 wk	Katz et al[103]	I	30 suspected OSAS	No significant group difference in the AHI between nights. Those with the highest AHI had the most variability. However, no patient was reclassified as primary snoring versus OSAS on the basis of the second study
7–50 d	Goodwin et al[101]	IV	12	Used unattended home PSG. Studies were successful in 10. No difference in AHI between nights in this small sample
Consecutive nights	Scholle et al[105]	III	131 OSAS	No difference in AHI between nights
Consecutive nights	Li et al[104]	III	46 obese 44 controls	AHI was greater on night 2. The first night would have correctly identified 11 (85%) of the 13 cases of OSAS if the worst obstructive apnea index over any single night was used as the criterion. However, the 2 cases that would have been missed by the single PSG had only borderline OSAS
Consecutive nights	Verhulst et al[106]	I	70 suspected OSAS	First night classified OSAS correctly in 91% of subjects, if the worst AHI over any night was used as the diagnostic criterion. All but 1 of those who were missed had an AHI <5/h

proteinomic analysis could be used to screen for the presence of OSAS. In a level I study of urinary proteinomics, the investigators found that a combination of urinary proteins could predict OSAS with a sensitivity of 95% and a specificity of 100%.[109] Similarly, in a level III study from the same group, the investigators found that a different set of proteins could be used to identify 15 of 20 children who had OSAS and 18 of 20 children who were snorers.[110] The authors note that they studied a highly selected population matched for age, gender, ethnicity, BMI, and inflammatory respiratory disorders, such as allergic rhinitis or asthma. Thus, this technique, although promising, requires further validation in typical clinical cohorts and duplication in another laboratory.

Summary

In summary, few of the screening techniques mentioned here have a sensitivity and specificity high enough to be relied on for clinical diagnosis. In addition, it should be noted that many of the studies used an AHI >5/hour when determining sensitivity and specificity, although an AHI >1.5/hour is considered statistically abnormal in children.[111–113] Few studies used large study samples, and few were blinded. As a result, some of the studies of screening techniques resulted in contradictory evidence. On a pragmatic level, however, it is realized that current infrastructure is inadequate to provide PSG for all children with suspected OSAS. Therefore, the use of screening tests may be better than no objective testing at all. However, clinicians using these tests should familiarize themselves with the sensitivity and specificity of the test used and consider proceeding to full PSG if the test result is inconclusive.

Areas for Future Research

● Well-designed, large, controlled, blinded, multicenter, prospective studies are required to provide more definitive answers regarding the utility of screening tests for the diagnosis of OSAS. In particular, additional studies of ambulatory PSG in children of varying ages are needed.

TREATMENT OF OSAS

AT

Adenotonsillar hypertrophy is the most common cause of OSAS, and AT continues to be the primary treatment for this issue. Adenoidectomy alone may not be sufficient for children who have OSAS because it does not address oropharyngeal obstruction secondary to tonsillar hyperplasia. The previous guideline stated the importance of AT as the primary treatment for OSAS in children. No new literature is available to suggest a change to these recommendations. Table 3 in the guideline lists relative contraindications to AT. Note that whereas a submucus cleft palate is a relative contraindication to adenoidectomy, a partial adenoidectomy may be performed in such patients. However, postoperative PSG should be performed to ensure that OSAS has resolved.

AT in most children is associated with a low complication rate. Minor complications include pain and poor oral intake. More severe complications may include bleeding, infection, anesthetic complications, respiratory decompensation, velopharyngeal incompetence, subglottic stenosis, and, rarely, death.

Tarasiuk et al found that health care utilization costs were 226% higher in children with OSAS before diagnosis compared with control children[114] and that health care costs decreased by one-third in children who underwent AT, whereas there was no change in health care costs in control children or children who had untreated OSAS[115] (both studies were level IV).

Partial Tonsillectomy

Several newer techniques for tonsillectomy have gained increasing use since publication of the last guideline. The primary goal of these techniques is to decrease the morbidity associated with traditional tonsillectomy methods. One such technique is partial tonsillectomy (PT), in which a portion of tonsil tissue is left to cover the musculature of the tonsillar fossa. Multiple studies, ranging in level from II to IV, have evaluated recovery times and adverse effects from PT. However, only a few small, lower-level studies have specifically looked at the effect of PT on OSAS. In a level IV study, Tunkel et al[116] evaluated 14 children who underwent PSG before and after PT and found a cure rate (AHI $\leq$1/hour) of 93% postoperatively. In a retrospective study (level IV), Mangiardi et al[117] compared 15 children who underwent PT (of 45 eligible) with 15 children who underwent total tonsillectomy. This study had a number of technical limitations. A variety of techniques (overnight laboratory PSG, nap sleep studies, and limited-channel home sleep studies) were performed in subjects preoperatively, and limited-channel home sleep studies were performed in all patients postoperatively. These different monitoring techniques would be expected to provide varying results.[118,119] In both surgical groups, the authors found a higher rate of postoperative OSAS than typically reported in the literature, with a median (range) AHI of 7.5 $\pm$ 4.3/hour in the PT group and 8.8 $\pm$ 4.7/hour in the total tonsillectomy group (not significant).

PT carries an increased risk of regrowth of the tonsils, which occurred in 0.5% to 16% of patients in studies of varied duration. Celenk et al[120] performed a retrospective review of 42 children 1 to 10 years of age who underwent PT via radiofrequency ablation for symptoms of OSAS (level IV). Follow-up ranged from 6 to 32 months, with a mean follow-up of 14 months. They found tonsillar regrowth on physical examination in 7

(16.6%) patients; 5 of these were symptomatic and underwent completion tonsillectomy. The time frame for occurrence of regrowth ranged from 1 to 18 months. The authors noted that some episodes of regrowth occurred after episodes of tonsillitis. Zagólski[121] evaluated 374 children who underwent PT on the basis of clinical symptoms of OSAS (level IV). Patients underwent otolaryngology examinations annually for 4 years. Twenty-seven (7.2%) children had tonsillar regrowth; of those, 20 had clinical symptoms and, therefore, underwent completion tonsillectomy. Regrowth of the palatine tonsils was observed at a mean period of 3.8 years, suggesting the need for long-term follow-up. In a multicenter, retrospective case series of 870 children with a mean follow-up of 1.2 years, Solares et al[122] found an incidence of tonsillar regrowth of 0.5% (level III). The methods and criteria for assessing regrowth were not detailed in this article but may have been a clinical follow-up at 1 and 6 months postoperatively. The lower rate of regrowth in this study compared with the other studies may have been related to the shorter follow-up period. Eviatar et al[123] performed a long-term (10–14 years), retrospective, telephone survey comparing 33 children who had undergone PT for symptoms of OSAS versus 16 children who underwent tonsillectomy; children undergoing concomitant adenoidectomy were excluded (level III). They found similar rates of parent-reported snoring in the 2 groups (6.1% for PT, 12.5% for total tonsillectomy; not significant) but no cases of OSAS on the basis of symptoms.

PT for the treatment of adenotonsillar hypertrophy has shown some success in decreasing immediate postoperative pain. Derkay et al[124] prospectively evaluated 300 children undergoing

either PT or total tonsillectomy for adenotonsillar hypertrophy (level II). They found that children in the PT group had an earlier return to normal activity and were 3 times more likely not to need pain medication at 3 days compared with the total tonsillectomy group. There was no difference between groups in median return to a normal diet (3.0 vs 3.5 days). In a level III, retrospective study of 243 children undergoing PT versus 107 undergoing total tonsillectomy, Koltai et al[125] found less pain and quicker return to a normal diet in children undergoing PT. In a level II study, Sobol et al[126] prospectively evaluated 74 children who had adenotonsillar hypertrophy scheduled for AT. Their results showed a resumption to normal diet 1.7 days earlier in the PT group compared with children undergoing total tonsillectomy. There was no significant difference in the resolution of pain or return to normal activities between the 2 groups, but there was increased intraoperative blood loss in the PT group.

In summary, there are no level I studies comparing PT with total tonsillectomy in the pediatric population. Additional data are needed regarding the efficacy of PT for OSAS, by using objective outcome measurements. There is possibility of tonsillar regrowth after PT, with studies showing varied rates of regrowth. These studies are all limited by lack of blinding, lack of objective measures to quantitate tonsillar regrowth, and lack of polysomnographic data relating tonsillar regrowth to OSAS. Some studies found that patients who undergo PT have less pain and quicker recovery during the first few days compared with children undergoing total tonsillectomy. However, PT may be associated with greater intraoperative blood loss, and there is a risk of recurrent infections in the tonsillar remnants.[120,121,123] At this point, data are insufficient to recommend any particular surgical technique for tonsillectomy over another in terms of OSAS. However, children undergoing PT should be monitored carefully long-term to ensure that symptoms of OSAS related to tonsillar regrowth do not occur, and families should be warned about the possibility of recurrence of OSAS.

Postoperative Management After AT

Tonsillectomy and adenoidectomy can be safely performed in the vast majority of children on an outpatient basis. Risk factors that increase the risk of postoperative complications include age <3 years, severe OSAS, presence of cardiac complications, failure to thrive, obesity, and presence of upper respiratory tract infection (URI). Although there have been numerous publications regarding postoperative complications since publication of the last guideline, there have been no data to suggest a change in the previous recommendations. Children with medical comorbidities such as craniofacial anomalies, genetic syndromes, and neuromuscular disease are also high risk; these special populations are not covered by this guideline.

An important advantage of the objective documentation of the severity of OSAS by using PSG should be the ability to predict the need for overnight hospital stay after AT on the basis of a higher risk of postoperative complications. Severe OSAS has been proposed as a criterion for inpatient observation; the current evidence to define severe OSAS is derived primarily from level III retrospective studies. Although considerable physiologic information regarding the respiratory pattern and gas exchange during sleep is available from an overnight PSG, the available studies

have focused primarily on the AHI and, to a lesser degree, the nadir of the SpO_2. Relevant studies are listed in Table 16. Studies varied with regard to the type of patients included (proportion of obese patients; patients who had craniofacial and genetic syndromes) and severity of OSAS. Although the definition of postoperative respiratory compromise varied, most studies required that an intervention (eg, supplemental oxygen, nasopharyngeal tube, CPAP, intubation) be performed. Most studies found a high rate of postoperative respiratory complications. Different studies showed different PSG predictive factors for postoperative complications, and few studies developed receiver operating characteristic curves.[127] Nevertheless, studies were fairly consistent in indicating that an SpO_2 <80% and an AHI >24/hour were predictive of postoperative respiratory compromise. These criteria are more conservative than the recently published clinical practice guidelines from the American Academy of Otolaryngology–Head and Neck Surgery, which recommend that children who have an AHI ≥10/hour and/or an SpO_2 nadir <80% be admitted for overnight observation after AT.[3]

It is difficult to provide exact PSG criteria for OSAS severity because these criteria will vary depending on the age of the child; additional comorbidities, such as obesity, asthma, or cardiac complications of OSAS; and other PSG criteria that have not been evaluated in the literature, such as the level of hypercapnia and the frequency of desaturation (compared with SpO_2 nadir). Therefore, on the basis of published studies (Table 16), it is recommended that patients who have an SpO_2 nadir <80% (either on preoperative PSG or during observation in the recovery room postoperatively) or an AHI ≥24/hour be

observed as inpatients postoperatively because they are at increased risk of postoperative respiratory compromise. In addition, on the basis of expert consensus, it is recommended that patients with significant hypercapnia on PSG (peak P_{CO_2} ≥60 mm Hg) be admitted postoperatively. Clinicians may decide to admit patients who have less severe PSG abnormalities on the basis of a constellation of risk factors (age, comorbidities, and additional PSG factors) on an individual basis.

Data regarding URIs were based on studies of children undergoing general anesthesia for a variety of procedures. The committee could not identify any studies related specifically to URIs and AT. In a large, level III study, Tait et al[128] evaluated 1078 children 1 month to 18 years of age who were undergoing an elective surgical procedure. The presence of a URI was diagnosed by using a parental questionnaire. Data regarding perioperative respiratory events were recorded. There were no differences between children who had active URIs, recent URIs (within 4 weeks), and asymptomatic children with respect to the incidences of laryngospasm and bronchospasm. However, children who had active and recent URIs had significantly more episodes of breath-holding, desaturation <90%, and overall adverse respiratory events than children who had no URIs. Independent risk factors for the development of adverse respiratory events in children who had active URIs included use of an endotracheal tube (in those <5 years of age), preterm birth, history of reactive airway disease, paternal smoking, surgery involving the airway, the presence of copious secretions, and nasal congestion. In a large level III study of 831 children undergoing surgery with a laryngeal mask airway, von Ungern-Sternberg et al[129]

TABLE 16 Relationship Between PSG Parameters and Postoperative Respiratory Complications

Source	Level	Type of Study	No.	Study Group	Age, y	Special Populations Included[a]	Findings
Hill et al[269]	III	Retrospective	83	AHI >10	≤18	Yes	Major respiratory complication in 5%; minor in 20%
							Only age <2 y ($P < .01$) and AHI >24 ($P < .05$) significantly predicted postoperative airway complications
							Complication rate only 4% if special populations were excluded
							AHI >24 predicted 63% of complications
Jaryszak et al[270]	III	Retrospective	151	Any child who had a PSG	Not stated	Yes	Respiratory complication rate was 15%
							Children with complications had higher AHI (32 vs 14) and lower SpO_2 nadir (72% vs 84%) compared with those without complications
Koomson et al[271]	III	Retrospective	85	AHI >5	Not stated	Yes	Postoperative desaturation in 28%
							More likely to desaturate postoperatively if PSG SpO_2 nadir <80%
Ma et al[272]	III	Retrospective	86	Any child who had a PSG	1–16	Yes	Postoperative desaturation in 7%
							No difference in AHI between those with and without postoperative desaturation (11.6 ± 4.5 vs 14.7 ± 16.6)
Sanders et al[273]	I	Prospective	61	61 children who had OSAS vs 21 who had tonsillitis	2–16	No	Respiratory complication rate was 28%
							Subjects with RDI ≥30 were more likely to have laryngospasm and desaturation
							At an RDI ≥20, OSAS was more likely to have breath-holding on induction
Schroeder et al[274]	III	Retrospective	53	Severe OSAS (AHI >25)	Not stated	Yes	43% required oxygen or PAP
							Note: an additional 17 children were electively kept intubated postoperatively
Shine et al[196]	III	Retrospective	26	Obese OSAS	2–17	Obese; other comorbidities not stated	46% had respiratory complications
							Those requiring intervention for respiratory problems had a lower SpO_2 ($68 \pm 20\%$ vs $87 \pm 18\%$) but no difference in RDI (27 ± 44 vs 15 ± 28) than those who did not require intervention
							By using univariate analysis, a preoperative SpO_2 <70% was associated with postoperative respiratory compromise, but no threshold was found for RDI
Ye et al[127]	III	Retrospective	327	AHI ≥5	4–14	No	11% had respiratory complications
							An AHI of 26 had 74% sensitivity and 92% specificity for predicting postoperative respiratory complications

[a] Special populations include children with genetic syndromes and craniofacial abnormalities.

compared children who had a URI within 2 weeks of surgery versus those without a URI; 27% of children had a recent URI. They found a doubling of the incidence of laryngospasm, bronchospasm, and oxygen desaturation intraoperatively and in the recovery room in the children who had recent URIs, although the overall incidence of these events was low. The risk was highest in young children; those undergoing ear, nose, and throat surgery; and those in whom multiple attempts were made to insert the laryngeal mask airway. On the basis of data available regarding risk with general anesthesia,

the committee concluded that children who have an acute respiratory infection on the day of surgery, as documented by fever, cough, and/ or wheezing, are at increased risk for postoperative complications and, therefore, should be rescheduled or monitored closely postoperatively. Clinicians should decide on an individual basis whether these patients should be rescheduled, taking into consideration the severity of OSAS in the particular patient and keeping in mind that many children who have adenotonsillar hypertrophy exhibit chronic rhinorrhea and nasal congestion even in the absence of viral infections.

Postoperative Persistence of OSAS After AT

Although the majority of children have a marked improvement in OSAS after AT, OSAS may persist postoperatively. OSAS is especially likely to persist in children who have underlying illnesses such as craniofacial anomalies, Down syndrome, and neuromuscular disease; these special populations are not included in this review.

Over the years since the committee's first consensus report, a number of studies have been published discussing the impact of surgery on childhood OSAS. Most of these studies were omitted from consideration for this review because of their lack of preoperative and postoperative PSGs. Many other studies reported changes in group averages for polysomnographic and other measures postoperatively. All published articles found that AT leads to significant improvement in polysomnographic parameters in the majority of patients (although not in all). Studies providing data that could be interpreted to provide an estimate of the proportion of patients who were cured of their OSAS are shown in Table 17. Twenty original articles on the topic have been published since 2002, including 2 meta-analyses[130,131] of other articles included in the review. The lack of uniform agreement regarding the polysomnographic criteria for diagnosis of OSAS complicates this analysis of postoperative persistence of OSAS, as it does other aspects of this review, in part because the preoperative PSG criteria for surgery are not uniform across the different articles, but more importantly, because the postoperative prevalence of OSAS is highly dependent on the stringency of diagnostic criteria. In some cases, articles helpfully provided data on residual prevalence of OSAS by using different polysomnographic criteria (eg, AHI >1/hour and AHI >5/hour). At this point, it is generally accepted that AT has a higher success rate than isolated adenoidectomy or tonsillectomy, so although a few of the articles included some patients undergoing only adenoidectomy, only tonsillectomy, or ancillary procedures such as nasal turbinectomy, most focused exclusively on the impact of AT.

As shown in Table 17, a total of 11 articles were published, describing 10 general population cohorts referred either to a pediatric sleep specialist or otolaryngologist for OSAS, and 1 meta-analysis of articles dating back to 1980. Most of these were case

series of patients, with significant methodologic flaws, including non-blinding and incomplete follow-up for a high proportion of patients, and these issues were present even in the methodologically strongest articles.[132–134] The polysomnographic criteria for OSAS in each article may or may not have been the same as those used as an indication for AT, and these varied from an AHI ≥1/hour to AHI ≥5/hour and RDI >2 to 5/hour. Surprisingly, the overall estimate of postoperative persistence of OSAS did not seem to vary greatly by polysomnographic criteria for surgery. Conversely, the estimates of residual OSAS were clearly related to which polysomnographic criteria for OSAS were applied to the postoperative PSGs. When using an AHI ≥1/hour as the criterion for residual OSAS, estimates of persistence ranged from 19%[135] to 73%,[133] whereas when using an AHI ≥5/hour as the criterion, the estimate of persistence of OSAS ranged from 13%[134] to 29%.[132] It is important to recognize that there are clearly recognizable risk factors for postoperative persistence of OSAS and that the prevalence of these risk factors in the populations studied had an important impact on their estimates of postoperative persistence of OSAS. For example, >50% of patients in the multicenter study of Bhattacharjee et al[133] were obese, whereas 21% of the patients in the series by Ye et al[134] were obese, defined as 95th percentile for the Chinese population. It should be emphasized that although many of these studies showed a high proportion of patients with residual OSAS after AT, most patients exhibited a marked decrease in AHI postoperatively.

Risk Factors for Postoperative OSAS

1. Obesity

Five studies focused attention on obese patients (defined as 95th percentile for weight or BMI for age), and 1

meta-analysis[131] combined 4 of these studies. The meta-analysis reported that 88% of obese patients still had a postoperative AHI ≥1/hour, 75% had a postoperative AHI ≥2/hour, and 51% had a postoperative AHI ≥5/hour. Preoperative obesity was found to be a significant risk factor for postoperative residual OSAS in several other studies[133–135] as well, even when multivariable modeling was used to control for other factors such as age and preoperative AHI. The odds ratios of persistent OSAS in obese patients ranged in these models from 3.2[134] to 4.7.[136] One study found that the relationship of BMI to risk of persistent OSAS was no longer significant when adjusted for preoperative AHI.[137] In contrast to all of the studies that looked at this factor, a study of obese Greek children found no difference in the prevalence of residual OSAS in obese versus nonobese children; part of the reason for this finding might be that this study used a slightly less stringent criterion for obesity (1.645 SDs weight for age, which is the 90th percentile).[138]

2. Baseline Severity of OSAS

All studies that evaluated baseline AHI as a potential risk factor for persistent postoperative OSAS found it to be a significant risk factor, even when adjusted for other comorbidities such as obesity.[132–134,136,139]

3. Age

A series limited to children aged <3 years reported a high incidence (65%) of treatment failures in these younger children, but this cohort included a large proportion of children who have other risk factors, such as severe OSAS and chromosomal and craniofacial abnormalities.[140] In contrast, 2 studies reported that increasing age (especially 7 years and older) is a risk factor for persistent

TABLE 17 Studies Providing an Estimate of the Proportion of Patients Who Were Cured of OSAS With Surgery

Source	Year	Level	No.	Age, y	Population	Polysomnographic Criterion for Surgery	Operation	Follow-up Period, mo	Subjects Who Had OSAS at Follow-up	Miscellaneous
General population studies										
Chervin et al[37] Dillon et al[275]	2006	I	39	5.0–12.9		AHI ≥1	AT	13 ± 1.4	21%	2 articles documented findings in the same population
Guilleminault et al[135]	2004	III	56	1.25–12.5		AHI ≥1 or RDI >2	AT: 36 (some of whom also had nasal turbinectomy and/or tonsillar wound suturing); A: 8; T: 11	3	AT: 19.4%; A: 100%; T: 100%	Half of AT failures were in obese patients
Guilleminault et al[141]	2007	III	199	1.5–14		AHI ≥1	AT in 183; A or T in 19; nasal turbinectomy in 17.4%	3–5	46.2%	Increased nasal turbinate score, presence of deviated nasal septum and increased Mallampati score of relationship of tongue to uvula and retro position of the mandible were all predictive of higher failure rate
Guilleminault et al[276]	2004	IV	284	2–12.1		AHI >1.5	AT in 228; A or T inferior turbinectomy in 73	3–4	8.8% of those with preoperative AHI <10 and AT; 64.7% of those with preoperative AHI ≥10. No breakdown provided regarding results of AT versus other surgery	An additional 99 children had RDI >1.5 and AHI <1.5. Of this group, 100% had normal RDI after AT and 9.2% had residual abnormal RDI after A or T. Difficult to interpret findings because of inconsistent reporting of data
Mitchell[132]	2007	III	79	3–14		AHI ≥5	AT	1–9.3	16% (AHI ≥5); 29% (AHI >1.5)	Severity of preoperative AHI predicted response: preoperative 5–10, 0% ≥5; preoperative 10–20, postoperative 12% ≥5; preoperative >20, postoperative 36% ≥5; 13/22 with postoperative snoring had AHI ≥5; 0/57 without postoperative snoring had AHI ≥5
Tal et al[277]	2003	IV	36	1.8–12.6		RDI >1	AT	4.6 (1–16)	11.11% had RDI >5	In logistic regression, AHI before surgery and family history of OSAS were significant predictors of AHI >5 postoperative
Tauman et al[137]	2006	III	110	6.4 ± 3.9		AHI ≥1	AT	1–15	46% AHI 1–5, 29% with AHI >5	
Walker et al[278]	2008	IV	34	0.93–5		RDI >5 in REM sleep	AT	9.8	35% with RDI >5	Treatment failures limited to those with preoperative RDI in REM >30
Bhattacharjee et al[133]	2010	III	578	6.9 ± 3.8		AHI ≥1	AT	1–24	72.8% with AHI ≥1; 21.6% >5	Large multicenter study. Age >7 y, increased BMI, presence of asthma, and high preoperative AHI were independent predictors of persistent postoperative OSAS

TABLE 17 Continued

Source	Year	Level	No.	Age, y	Population	Polysomnographic Criterion for Surgery	Operation	Follow-up Period, mo	Subjects Who Had OSAS at Follow-up	Miscellaneous
Brietzke and Gallagher[130]	2006	III	325	4.9	Various	AHI ≥1	AT	3.3	17.1% (depended on OSAS criteria for each study)	Meta-analysis of 11 case series published between 1980 and 2004
Ye et al[134]	2010	IV	84	7.1 ± 3.2	Chinese	AHI ≥5	AT	18–23	31% with AHI ≥1; 13.1% with AHI ≥5	Obesity and high preoperative AHI were significant independent predictors of treatment failure
Focus on obese populations										
Mitchell and Kelly[279]	2004	III	30	3.0–17.2	Obese (BMI > 95th percentile)	AHI >5	AT	5.6	54%	
Mitchell and Kelly[139]	2007	III	72	3–18	Comparison of obese (BMI >95th percentile) with nonobese	AHI ≥2: AHI 2–5 mild, AHI 5–15 moderate AHI ≥15 severe	AT	5–6	Obese: 76%: (46% mild; 15% moderate; 15% severe). Nonobese: 28%: (18% mild; 10% moderate).	Preoperative AHI and obesity were independent risk factors for postoperative OSAS. OR for persistent OSAS in obese, adjusted for preoperative AHI, was 3.7 (95% CI: 1.3–10.8)
O'Brien et al[136]	2006	III	69	7.1 ± 4.2	Obese (weight >2 SDs from mean for age)	RDI ≥5	AT	20.4 ± 16.8	Nonobese: 22.5%; Obese: 55%	Preoperative AHI and obesity were independent risk factors for postoperative OSAS. OR for persistent OSAS in obese, adjusted for preoperative AHI, was 4.7 (95% CI: 1.7–11.2)
Shine et al[194]	2006	IV	19	6.5 ± 4.4	Obese (BMI >95th percentile)	RDI>5	18 AT (1 with UPPP), 1 T	2–6	63%	Missing data
Costa and Mitchell[131]	2009	III	110	7.3–9.3	Obese	Various	AT	3–5.7	88% had postoperative AHI ≥1; 75% had postoperative AHI ≥2; 51% had postoperative AHI ≥5	Meta-analysis of 4 obesity studies included here
Apostolidou et al[138]	2008	IV	70	6.5 ± 2.2	Greek; obese defined as >1.645 SDs from mean weight for age	OAHI ≥1	AT	2–14	Overall: 75.7% with AHI ≥1 (77.3% obese, 75% nonobese). Among children with a preoperative OAHI ≥5: 9% with AHI ≥5 (8% obese, 10% nonobese)	
Focus on other special populations										
Mitchell and Kelly[140]	2005	III	20	1.1–3.0	Children <3 y	RDI >5	AT	4.1–20.4	65%: 25% RDI 5–10; 25% RDI 10–20; 15% RDI >20	Included comorbidities (Down syndrome, cardiac disease, cerebral palsy) excluded from this guideline. 60% of patients were severe, with RDI >20 at baseline
Mitchell and Kelly[280]	2004	III	29	1.4–17	Severe OSAS	RDI >5; severe: RDI ≥30	AT	6	69% with postoperative RDI >5	48% were obese

A, adenoidectomy; CI, confidence interval; OAHI, obstructive AHI; OR, odds ratio; T, tonsillectomy; REM, rapid eye movement; UPPP, uvulopharyngopalatoplasty.

OSAS, even when controlling for obesity.[132,133]

4. Other Potential Risk Factors

Individual studies have noted that nasal abnormalities or craniofacial disproportion,[141] family history of OSAS,[137] and presence of asthma[133] were all predictive of higher failure rate, but these findings were not substantiated by other studies. Of note, Mitchell[132] found that 13 of 22 patients in the cohort who had postoperative snoring had an AHI ≥5/hour, whereas none of the 57 patients who did not exhibit postoperative snoring had an AHI ≥5/hour. This supports the findings of older studies reviewed in the previous technical report that found absence of snoring to have a 100% negative predictive value for postoperative OSAS.[6] However, in the Chinese cohort, 2 of 11 patients who have persistent AHI ≥5/hour reportedly did not snore; it is unclear whether cultural considerations might have affected parental report of snoring.[134]

Summary

AT is the most effective surgical therapy for pediatric patients, leading to an improvement in polysomnographic parameters in the vast majority of patients. Despite this improvement, a significant proportion of patients are left with persistent OSAS after AT. The estimate of this proportion in a relatively low-risk population ranges from a low of 13% to 29% when using an AHI ≥5/hour as the criterion to a high of 73% when including obese children and adolescents and a conservative AHI ≥1/hour. Children at highest risk of persistent OSAS are those who are obese and those with a high preoperative AHI, especially those with an AHI ≥20/hour, as well as children >7 years of age. Absence of snoring postoperatively is

reassuring but may not be 100% specific; it may therefore be advisable to obtain a postoperative PSG in very-high-risk children even in the absence of reported persistent snoring.

Areas for Future Research

- What are the risks of persistence of OSAS and long-term recurrence of OSAS after PT versus total tonsillectomy? Large, prospective, randomized trials with objective outcome measures including PSG are needed.

- Better delineation of which patients would benefit from postoperative PSG.

- How well does resolution of OSAS correlate with resolution of complications of OSAS?

- Are some of the newer surgical techniques for AT equally effective in resolving OSAS?

- What are the risks of performing AT in a patient with a URI?

- What are the PSG parameters that predict postoperative respiratory compromise? Future research should focus on refining the AHI and Sp_{O2} nadir cutoffs for severe OSAS. In addition, it may be possible to glean other predictive information from the PSG, such as the extent of hypoventilation, the percent sleep time spent with Sp_{O2} <90%, the frequency of desaturation events, the length of apneas and hypopneas, and the presence of central apneas, to create formulae for risk scores.

CPAP

At the time of the previous report, there were few prospective studies on CPAP use in children, although several retrospective studies indicated that CPAP was efficacious in the treatment of pediatric OSAS. Since that time, there have been at least 7 recent

studies evaluating the use of positive airway pressure (PAP) in children and adolescents who have OSAS. One of these was a randomized trial with low power (level II),[142] and others were case series without controls (level IV). A descriptive study examined the use of behavioral intervention in improving CPAP adherence.[143] In addition, a level III study described use of a high-flow nasal cannula as an alternative to CPAP.[144] In contrast to the previous guidelines, several of the current studies obtained objective evaluation of CPAP adherence by downloading usage data from the CPAP device. In most studies, CPAP therapy was instituted for persistent OSAS after AT; in many cases, the patients had additional risk factors for OSAS, such as obesity or craniofacial anomalies.

A multicenter study (level II) evaluated PAP in 29 children who were randomly assigned either CPAP or bilevel positive airway pressure (BPAP).[142] Patients demonstrated significant improvement in sleepiness, snoring, AHI, and oxyhemoglobin saturation while using PAP during the 6-month follow-up period. However, approximately one-third of patients dropped out, and of those who used PAP, objective adherence was 5.3 ± 2.5 hours/night. Parents overestimated the hours of PAP use compared with the devices' actual objective recordings of use. There was no significant difference in adherence between the CPAP and BPAP groups. A retrospective chart review of 46 children started on PAP for OSAS that persisted after AT also showed significant improvement in symptoms of OSAS as well as in polysomnographic parameters (level IV).[145] Seventy percent of patients were considered adherent. Parental report of adherence was most divergent from the machines' recording in the least adherent patients. More than one-half of the children had complicating factors, such as Down syndrome and Prader-Willi syndrome.[145] Another study of a heterogeneous group of patients displayed varying CPAP adherence, with 31 of 79 children showing continued CPAP use (level IV).[146] A small, nonblinded retrospective study (level IV) suggested that adherence to CPAP could be improved with behavioral techniques if the family accepted the interventions.[143]

A retrospective review described 9 children who successfully used BPAP in the intensive care setting because of respiratory compromise after AT.[147] Another retrospective review described the successful use of CPAP in 9 patients of a heterogeneous group of 18 children aged <2 years.[148] A nonrandomized, prospective level III study of 12 children who had OSAS treated in the sleep laboratory with a high-flow open nasal cannula system as an alternative to formal CPAP demonstrated an improvement in oxyhemoglobin saturation and arousals, but not AHI, compared with baseline.[144] There was a decrease in sleep efficiency with the cannula compared with baseline. Long-term use and use in the home situation were not assessed.

In summary, several studies (levels II–IV) have confirmed earlier data demonstrating that nasal CPAP is effective in the treatment of both symptoms and polysomnographic evidence of OSAS, even in young children. However, adherence can be a major barrier to effective CPAP use. For this reason, CPAP is not recommended as first-line therapy for OSAS when AT is an option. However, it is useful in children who do not respond adequately to surgery or in whom surgery is contraindicated. Patient and family preference may also be a consideration (eg, in families with

religious beliefs against surgery or blood transfusions). Objective assessment of CPAP adherence is important because parental estimates of use are often inaccurate. If the patient is nonadherent, then attempts should be made to improve adherence (eg, by addressing adverse effects, by using behavior modification techniques), or the patient should be treated with alternative methods. A study described in the previous report noted that CPAP pressures change over time in children, presumably because of growth and development.[149] Therefore, it is recommended that CPAP pressures be periodically reassessed in children.

At this time, data are insufficient to make a recommendation on the use of high-flow, open nasal cannula systems.

Areas for Future Research

- Efficacy of CPAP use as a first-line treatment of obese children.
- Determinants of CPAP adherence and ways to improve adherence.
- Long-term effects of CPAP, particularly on the development of the face, jaw, and teeth.
- Changes in CPAP pressure over time, and the frequency with which this needs to be monitored.
- Development of pediatric-specific devices and interfaces.

Medications

There have been several studies evaluating the use of corticosteroids and leukotriene antagonists in the treatment of OSAS. An older study showed no therapeutic effect of systemic steroids on OSAS.[150] Since then, 3 studies (1 level I, 1 level II, and 1 level III) have evaluated topical nasal steroids as treatment of OSAS, 1 level II study has evaluated montelukast, and 1 level IV study has evaluated a combination thereof. An additional

level I study evaluated the effect of intranasal steroids on adenoidal size and symptoms related to adenoidal hypertrophy but did not include PSG in the evaluation.[151]

A small, level II, randomized, double-blind trial,[152] a level I, randomized, double-blind trial of 62 children,[153] and a nonrandomized, open-label level III study of intranasal steroids[154] all showed a moderate improvement in patients who had mild OSAS. However, significant residual OSAS remained in 2 of the studies. Berlucchi et al[151] reported an improvement in symptoms of adenoidal hypertrophy, including snoring and observed apnea, but did not obtain objective evidence of improvement in OSAS. Two studies showed shrinkage of adenoidal tissue.[151,153] All studies were short term (2–6 weeks), although 1 study showed persistent improvement 8 weeks after discontinuation of the steroids (Table 18).[153]

An open-label, nonrandomized, 16-week level IV study of montelukast in children who had mild OSAS found a statistically significant but small change in the AHI (AHI decreased from 3.0 ± 0.2 to 2.0 ± 0.3; $P = .017$).[82] Another small, open-label, nonrandomized, 12-week level IV study of combined montelukast and nasal steroids found a mild but statistically significant improvement in AHI in children who had mild OSAS (AHI decreased from 3.9 ± 1.2/hour to 0.3 ± 0.3/hour; $P < .001$).[155]

In summary, several small level I through IV studies suggest that topical steroids may ameliorate mild OSAS. However, the clinical effects are small. On the basis of these studies, intranasal steroids may be considered for treatment of mild OSAS (defined, for this indication, as an AHI <5/hour, on the basis of studies described in Table 18). Steroids should not be used as the primary treatment of moderate

TABLE 18 Studies of Antiinflammatory Medications for the Treatment of OSAS

Medication	Source	Level	No.	Duration, wk	Randomized	Placebo-Controlled	Baseline AHI (per h)	AHI on Treatment (per h)	P
Intranasal steroids	Brouillette et al[152]	II	13 OSAS 12 controls	6	Yes	Yes	10.7 ± 9.4	5.8 ± 7.9	.04
Intranasal steroids	Alexopoulos et al[154]	III	27 OSAS	4	No	No	5.2 ± 2.2	3.2 ± 1.5	<.001
Intranasal steroids	Kheirandish-Gozal and Gozal[153]	I	62 OSAS	6; crossover	Yes	Yes	3.7 ± 0.3	1.3 ± 0.2	<.001
Montelukast	Goldbart et al[82]	IV	24 OSAS 16 controls	16	No	No	3.0 ± 0.2	2.0 ± 0.3	.017
Intranasal steroids + montelukast	Kheirandish et al[155]	IV	22 OSAS 14 controls	12	No	No	3.9 ± 1.2	0.3 ± 0.3	<.001

or severe OSAS. Because the long-term effects of intranasal steroids are not known, follow-up evaluation is needed to ensure that the OSAS does not recur and to monitor for adverse effects. Of note, no studies specifically evaluated children who had atopy or chronic rhinitis, although 1 study mentioned that similar improvements were seen in children who had a history of allergic symptoms compared with those without.[153] Further study to determine whether children who have atopy are more likely to respond to this therapy is needed. Data are insufficient at this time to recommend treatment of OSAS with montelukast.

Areas for Future Research

● What is the optimal duration of intranasal steroid use? All trials have been short-term with a short-term follow-up. Does the OSAS recur on discontinuation of therapy? How often should objective assessment of treatment effects be performed?

● What is the efficacy of intranasal steroids in children who have chronic or atopic rhinitis?

● How do the benefits and adverse effects of long-term nasal steroids compare with surgery?

● Larger studies, stratified for severity of OSAS and controlled for obesity, to determine whether OSAS is associated with systemic inflammation

● Will these biomarkers be good outcome measurements for treatment studies? Do they correlate with clinical outcomes or long-term prognosis?

Rapid Maxillary Expansion

Rapid maxillary expansion has recently been used to treat OSAS in select pediatric populations. It is an orthodontic procedure designed to increase the transverse diameter of the hard palate by reopening the midpalatal suture. It does this by means of a fixed appliance with an expansion screw anchored on selected teeth. After 3 to 4 months of expansion, a normal mineralized suture is built up again. The procedure is typically used only in children with maxillary constriction and dental malocclusion. Two case series without controls (level IV) have evaluated this procedure as a treatment of OSAS in children. One study described 31 patients selected from an orthodontic clinic; 4 months after surgery, all patients had normalized AHI.[156] Another screened 260 patients in a sleep center to find 35 that were eligible; only 14 were studied.[157] There was a significant improvement in signs and symptoms of OSAS as well as polysomnographic parameters. In summary, rapid maxillary expansion is an orthodontic technique that holds promise as an alternative treatment of OSAS in children. However, data are insufficient to recommend its use at this time.

Areas for Future Research

● A randomized controlled trial to assess the efficacy of rapid maxillary expansion in the treatment of OSAS in children.

Positional Therapy

Several level IV, retrospective studies evaluated the effect of body position during sleep on OSAS. The studies had conflicting results. One study found that young children had an increased AHI in the supine position,[158] and another study found that young children did not have a positional change in AHI but older children did.[159] Another study found an increased obstructive apnea index but not AHI (except in the obese subgroup) in the supine position,[160] whereas a study of obese and nonobese children, which controlled for sleep stage in each position, found that AHI was lowest when children were prone.[161] No study evaluated the effect of changing body positions or the feasibility of maintaining a child in a certain position overnight. Therefore, at this point, no recommendations can be made with regard to positional therapy for OSAS in children.

Other Treatment Options

Specific craniofacial procedures, such as mandibular distraction osteogenesis, are appropriate for select children with craniofacial anomalies. However, a discussion of these children is beyond the scope of this guideline. Minimal experience is available regarding intraoral appliances in children.[162] A tracheotomy is extremely effective at treating OSAS but is associated with much morbidity and is typically a last resort if CPAP and other treatments fail to offer improvement for a child who has severe OSAS.

OBESITY AND OSAS

This section reviews the evidence regarding the relationships between obesity and SDB (this term is used to encompass both snoring and OSAS, especially in studies that did not distinguish between these entities) in the pediatric population. The prevalence of childhood obesity is increasing,[163] and many studies on obesity and OSAS have been published since the last guideline. Because childhood obesity has a major impact on OSAS, it is described in detail in this report. Obesity is defined as BMI >95th percentile for age and gender.

Epidemiology: Obesity as a Risk Factor for Snoring and OSAS

A number of large, cross-sectional, community-based studies including more than 21 500 children have examined the risk of SDB conferred by overweight and obesity (Table 19). The majority of these studies obtained information regarding potential SDB from questionnaires, but some included objective measurements such as oximetry or overnight PSG. Similarly, many studies based the determination of BMI on data from questionnaires. The ages ranged from 6 to 17 years, consistent with recruitment strategies using local schools. Countries from around the world are represented, including North America, Asia, Europe, and the Middle East. Taken together, these studies indicate that the risk of snoring in children is increased

twofold to fourfold with obesity (defined as BMI ≥90th or 95th percentile). When analyzed, BMI was found to be an independent risk factor for snoring.

Several studies based on surveys of thousands of children, in some cases supplemented by use of physical examinations, showed that overweight/obesity was associated with an increased prevalence of snoring (Table 19).[47,164–167] Fewer studies that included objective measurements to identify SDB were available. Two population-based studies using PSG demonstrated a relationship between overweight/obesity and OSAS.[11,12] In contrast to the findings of the majority of studies, Brunetti et al[23] found that although HS was more prevalent in obese children in a sample of schoolchildren, there was no difference in the incidence of OSAS on PSG among the subset of normal-weight, overweight, and obese children who have HS who had abnormal overnight oximetry results. Similar to the population-based studies, studies using case series or subjects recruited from sleep disorders programs (some of which use PSG and some of which use surveys) also showed a relationship between weight and SDB.[168,169]

From these studies, it can be concluded that obesity is an independent risk factor for snoring and OSAS. The range of evidence from individual studies was II to III (Table 19) and on the aggregate rise to level I. The studies reported on large numbers of children recruited from community-based samples, some of whom had face-to-face examinations and measurements. Data obtained in different settings yielded similar results. The impact of race, if any, is not yet clear. Population-based studies of Hispanic children, a group at high risk of obesity and related comorbidities, are not

yet available.[163] For the clinician, it is recommended that particular attention is needed for screening obese and overweight children for signs and symptoms of OSAS, with a low threshold for ordering diagnostic tests. Future research should focus on population-based studies, with objective measurements of both measures of adiposity and PSG, and should include larger numbers of African American and Hispanic youth.

Predictors of Obesity-Related SDB

A number of program-based studies provide information regarding the predictors for SDB in obese children. Carotenuto et al[88] reported via data gathered from parental questionnaires that in obese subjects referred for obesity evaluation and nonobese controls randomly selected from schools, the waist circumference z score correlated with symptoms of SDB ($R = 0.37$, $P < .006$) but BMI and subcutaneous fat did not (level III). Verhulst et al[170] examined 91 consecutive overweight or obese children referred for PSG and found that OSAS was not related to indices of obesity, including bioelectric impedance analysis fat mass (level III). Central apnea was significantly predicted by using BMI score, waist circumference, waist-to-hip circumference ratio, and percent fat mass. Tonsillar size was the only significant correlate in their model for moderate to severe OSAS. In a retrospective review of 482 Chinese children referred for PSG and evaluated by using BMI and a tonsillar grading scale, the group of 111 obese children had a significantly higher median AHI and percentage with AHI >1.5/hour than did the nonobese group (level III).[171] In a regression analysis of log AHI as dependent variable, BMI and tonsil grade were predictors, but age and gender were not. In a large study of schoolchildren in

TABLE 19 Risk of SDB Conferred by Overweight and Obesity

Source	Level	Type of Study	No.	Duration	Diagnostic Technique	Other Features	Findings	P for Obesity as a Risk Factor
Urschitz et al[164]	II	Community-based sample of third graders	1144	1 y	Parental report of snoring, BMI, SES, risk factors for rhinitis, asthma	Habitual snorers reassessed at 1 y, with 49% continuing to snore	BMI ≥90% conferred a 4 times higher risk of HS versus a BMI <75%; 25% of obese subjects had HS	
Corbo et al[166]	II	Community-based sample of 10- to 15-y-old children from 10 schools	2439	2 y	Parental questionnaire and nasal examination and BMI by physician		Snoring increased significantly with BMI >90% and was >2 times for BMI >95% vs <75%	.000
Shin et al[47]	IV	Cross-sectional community-based sample of high school students	3871	NA	Questionnaire (tested for reliability) completed by subject, caretakers, and sleep partner	Korean children; 81% response rate to survey	Snoring frequency was significantly associated with increasing BMI	<.001
Bidad et al[167]	II	Cross-sectional study of 11- to 17-y-old children	3300	NA	Scripted face-to-face interview and measurements of BMI and tonsil size by physician	7.9% of sample with HS (≥3 nights per week when well)	>Twofold risk of snoring in overweight or obesity	
Stepanski et al[168]	III	Case series; mean age: 5.9 ± 3.7 y	190	NA	Clinical interview, PSG	68% with SDB (≥5 AHI, <90% SpO_2, sleep fragmentation, ECG changes)	BMI was higher in the SDB group	<.01
Rudnick et al[169]	III	Compared children scheduled for AT with control group from same urban setting	170 SDB 129 controls	NA	BMI, ethnicity		African American children who had SDB were more likely to be obese than African American children who did not have SDB	<.02
Li et al[12]	II	Cross-sectional study of 13 primary schools	6447 by questionnaire 410 high risk and 209 low risk with exam and PSG	NA	Questionnaire in all with PSG and examination in high-risk group and low-risk subset for comparison		Male gender, BMI, and AT size were independently associated with OSA	
Li et al[172]	II	Cross-sectional study of 13 primary schools; same population as previous study	6349	NA	Questionnaire	Designed to determine prevalence of HS and associated symptoms.	Prevalence of HS was 7.2%; male gender, BMI, parental HS, nasal allergies, asthma were associated with snoring	<.0001
Brunetti et al[23]	II	Cross-sectional; mean age 7.3 y	1207 screened, 809 eligible	NA	Questionnaire in all followed by oximetry in the 44 who had HS; PSG in subset who had abnormal oximetry results	Southern Italy	HS more common in the obese group; no difference in OSA by PSG across weight groups	.02
Bixler et al[11]	II	Cross-sectional study of grades K–5	5740 had questionnaire 700 randomly selected for PSG, 490 completed	NA	Questionnaire followed by PSG in subset	Prevalence of AHI >5 1.2%. Strong linear relationship between waist circumference and BMI with SDB	Waist circumference associated with all levels of SDB, also nasal complaints and minority race	
Urschitz et al[165]	III	Cross-sectional community-based of primary schoolchildren	995	NA	Overnight oximetry		Overweight, smoke exposure, respiratory allergies were independent risk factors for sleep hypoxemia	

AT, adenotonsillar; K, kindergarten; NA, not available; OSA, obstructive sleep apnea.

Hong Kong, Li et al reported that male gender, BMI score, and tonsillar size were independently associated with OSAS (level II).[12,172] In 490 US schoolchildren studied by using overnight PSG, Bixler et al[11] found waist circumference to be an independent risk factor for all levels of severity of OSAS (level II). Urschitz et al[165] studied 995 children in a cross-sectional, program-based study in Germany and divided those with SDB into mild (SpO_2 nadir 91%–93%), moderate (<90%), and recurrent hypoxemia (>3.9 episodes of desaturation per hour of sleep) groups (level III). Overweight (BMI >75th percentile) was found to be an independent risk factor for mild, moderate, and recurrent hypoxemia during sleep.

From these studies, it is observed that the distribution of body fat may be more important in predicting SDB than BMI alone. In addition, tonsillar size is important in predicting SDB, even in obese children. The authors of these articles comment that SDB is likely more complicated in obese children, with obesity contributing to gas exchange and respiratory pattern abnormalities. Obesity can result in decreased lung volumes, abnormal central nervous system ventilatory responses, decreased upper airway caliber, a potential impact of leptin on ventilation, and other factors. Taken together, the strength of the evidence for these study findings is level II. Findings are limited by the fact that controls were drawn from different populations than subjects and that the studies did not all reach the same conclusions regarding the importance of body fat distribution. The latter may have been affected by the use of different measurement techniques. Anthropomorphic measurement thresholds that indicate increased risk for SDB in children would be of use to clinicians. It is recommended that

clinicians consider fat distribution (eg, waist circumference) and not just BMI in their assessment of the risk of SDB.

Comorbidities: Interactions Between Obesity and SDB

Cardiovascular

Adults who have SDB and are obese are at increased risk of cardiovascular disease, including systemic hypertension and blunting of the normal decrease in BP during sleep (nocturnal dipping). This section deals with the evidence that children and adolescents who are obese and have SDB may be similarly at risk. Six studies evaluating SDB, obesity, and cardiovascular complications in children are available. Reade et al[173] retrospectively evaluated 130 patients referred for PSG and described 56 obese subjects (BMI >95th percentile), of whom 70% had hypertension and 54% had OSAS (level IV). Among the 34 nonobese subjects, only 8% ($P < .0005$) had hypertension and 29% had OSAS ($P < .05$). The authors concluded that BMI was a significant determinant of both SDB and diastolic BP, with the number of hypopneas predictive of diastolic BP in both weight categories. In a community-based sample of 760 Greek children evaluated by using morning BP measurements, BMI, and a questionnaire regarding sleep habits, Kaditis et al[174] identified 50 children who had HS (level IV). They found that 28% of the children in the HS group were obese versus 15% of nonsnoring children (significance not reported). They reported that HS had no impact on BP, but that age, gender, and BMI were significant covariates in predicting systolic BP; inclusion of HS in this analysis did not affect these relationships. Similar findings were identified for diastolic BP, with the exception that age had no effect. This study compared absolute BP

measurements rather than the variance from normal values on the basis of race, age, gender, and body size. Because children from 4 to 14 years of age were included, this may have affected the results and conclusions. Kohyama et al[175] examined 32 Asian subjects referred for PSG and measured overnight BP every 15 minutes. In this study, obstructive apneas and hypopneas were identified indirectly and, thus, could have been underestimated or overestimated compared with studies with more direct measurements of airflow (level IV). Subjects were divided into low (<10 obstructive events per hour; 16 subjects) and high AHI (>10 obstructive events per hour; 7 subjects). Of the total, 23 subjects tolerated the BP measurements. Three subjects were obese. BMI predicted the systolic BP during rapid eye movement sleep ($P < .001$) but did not predict any of the diastolic BP indices. Li et al[176] performed a population-based study of 306 Asian children 6 to 13 years of age who had overnight PSG and ambulatory day and night BP measurements (level III). Children who had primary snoring were excluded, and those who had OSAS were divided into normal, mild, and moderate (AHI >5) groups. Multiple linear regression analysis revealed significant associations for the severity of hypoxemia and AHI with day and night BP, respectively, independent of obesity. Although BP levels both awake and asleep increased with the severity of OSAS, obesity and waist circumference partially accounted for elevations in sleep systolic BP and sleep mean arterial pressure but not for diastolic BP measurements. Amin et al[177] studied 88 children who had OSAS ranging in severity from mild to severe and 52 controls matched for age and gender. They used PSG, ambulatory BP measurements, and actigraphy (level III). The obese SDB group, compared with the nonobese SDB group, had higher waking systolic BP ($P < .001$) and sleeping systolic BP ($P = .02$) after adjusting for severity of SDB. They concluded that there was no difference between the effects of SDB and obesity on waking systolic or diastolic BP or sleeping systolic BP but did find that SDB had a greater contribution to sleeping diastolic BP than did obesity.

In summary, this group of articles demonstrates that both obesity and SDB are associated with increased day and night BP in children, although hypertension per se is rare (aggregate evidence level III). It seems that after controlling for obesity, significant independent effects of SDB remain and that hypoxemia and the frequency of obstructive events, perhaps via sleep disruption or intrathoracic fluid shifts, are important. Practitioners should be aware that children and adolescents who have OSAS are at increased risk of elevated BP. Future studies would benefit from a treatment arm to determine whether BP improves with resolution of sleep apnea, as well as longitudinal studies to determine the impact of pediatric obesity related– SDB on adult hypertension.

Metabolic

Obesity is a risk factor for impaired glucose tolerance, liver disease, abnormal lipid profiles, and other metabolic derangements. OSAS has been explored as a possible contributor to these metabolic abnormalities. Ten articles were reviewed. Verhulst et al[178] studied 104 overweight/obese children and adolescents with Tanner staging, overnight PSG, oral glucose tolerance testing, lipid profile, and BP measurements (level IV). The subjects were divided into normal, mild, and moderate/severe SDB groups. Findings consistent with the metabolic syndrome were present in 37%. Those who had a moderate degree of SDB had a higher BMI z score than the

normal group, and the waist-to-hip circumference ratio increased across the 3 SDB groups. The severity of SDB was independently correlated with impaired glucose homeostasis and worse lipid profile. Mean Sp_{O_2} and Sp_{O_2} nadir during sleep were significant predictors of the metabolic syndrome ($P = .04$ for both). A community-based cohort of 270 adolescents was studied by Redline et al[179] using PSG, oral glucose tolerance testing, homeostatic model assessment (HOMA [a measure of insulin sensitivity]), BMI, waist circumference, BP measurements, Tanner stage, sleep diary, SES, and birth history (level II). Metabolic syndrome was defined as having at least 3 of the following 5 features: (1) waist circumference >75% of normal; (2) mean BP or diastolic BP >90% of normal or receiving current therapy for hypertension; (3) elevated triglycerides; (4) low high-density lipoprotein; or (5) abnormal oral glucose tolerance or fasting glucose test results. Twenty-five percent of the sample was overweight, and 19% were deemed to have metabolic syndrome. The authors found that children who had metabolic syndrome had more severe hypoxemia and decreased sleep efficiency and that as AHI severity increased, there was a progressive increase in the number of children who had metabolic syndrome ($P < .001$). Both overweight children and those who had metabolic syndrome were more prevalent in the SDB group ($P < .001$) and more were male. Age, race, birth history, and SES did not vary with SDB. With adjustment for BMI, the SDB group had higher BP, fasting insulin, and more abnormal HOMA and lipid profile. They concluded that adolescents who experience SDB are at a sevenfold increased risk of metabolic syndrome and that the relationship is not explained by gender, race, or SES and,

furthermore, persists with adjustment for BMI percentile.

A study by Kaditis et al[180] of 110 children (2–13 years of age) referred for snoring did not find an impact of SDB on glucose homeostasis in nonobese children. The subjects were divided into AHI ≥5/h and <5/h; the authors found no difference in HOMA, insulin, glucose, or lipid concentrations between the 2 groups (level III). There was no relationship identified between PSG indices and HOMA or fasting insulin. BMI, age, and gender were significant predictors for fasting insulin and HOMA in multiple linear regression analysis. They speculated that OSAS may have more detrimental effects in obese than in nonobese young subjects. Similarly, Tauman et al[181] studied 116 subjects referred for PSG, one-half of whom were obese, and 19 nonsnoring controls. The authors found no impact of SDB indices on metabolic parameters (level III). Only BMI and age were important, and there was no relationship between SDB and surrogate measures of insulin resistance. They concluded that obesity was the major determinant of insulin resistance and dyslipidemia. In obese children, data from de la Eva et al[182] demonstrated that the severity of OSAS correlated with fasting insulin levels, independent of BMI (level III). Of note, the study by Redline et al[179] included children older than those in the studies by Kaditis et al[180] and Tauman et al[181]; thus, the variation in the findings may be a function of the length of time SDB had been present or perhaps attributable to the strong influence puberty has on glucose homeostasis. Kelly et al[183] compared 37 prepubertal and 98 pubertal children in a study by using PSG, HOMA, adiponectin (an insulin-sensitizing hormone secreted by adipose tissue) measurements, as well as urinary catecholamine metabolites (level III).

Tanner stage was determined by self-attestation. In the prepubertal children, they found no association between polysomnographic parameters and metabolic measurements after correcting for BMI. Elevated fasting insulin ($\geq$20 μU/mL) was significantly more common in the OSAS group (P = .03), even when corrected for BMI. When pubertal obese subjects were considered separately, the risk of elevated fasting insulin (P = .04) and impaired HOMA was greater in the OSAS group (P = .05). Pubertal children who had OSAS also had lower adiponectin and higher urinary catecholamine levels, even when controlled for BMI. Kelly et al concluded that OSAS further predisposes obese children to metabolic syndrome, likely through multiple mechanisms involving adipose tissue and the sympathetic nervous system.

In a study that included pretreatment and posttreatment measurements in 62 prepubertal children who had moderate to severe OSAS, Gozal et al[184] found that although nonobese children had no change in measures of glucose homeostasis after treatment of OSAS, obese children had a significant improvement even while BMI remained stable (P < .001) (level II). Similar effects were not seen in nonobese children. Treatment (AT) improved the lipid profile and inflammatory markers in both obese and nonobese children.

Other studies have examined different aspects of altered metabolism in obesity-related OSAS. Kheirandish-Gozal et al[185] found elevated alanine transaminase (a marker for fatty liver) in a large sample of obese children who had OSAS (level IV). Verhulst et al[186] found elevated serum uric acid (a marker of oxidative stress) in 62 overweight children who had OSAS, with a significant relationship between the severity of OSAS and

serum uric acid independent of abdominal adiposity (P = .01) (level IV). Verhulst et al[187] demonstrated that, in a group of 95 obese and overweight children, total white blood cell and neutrophil counts increased with hypoxemia, and they speculated that inflammation may contribute to cardiovascular morbidity in obesity-related SDB (level IV).

In summary, as expected, this group of studies confirms that obesity increases the risk of insulin resistance, dyslipidemia, and other metabolic abnormalities in children. The role that OSAS plays in altering glucose metabolism is still not entirely clear but is likely less important in younger children and in lean children. Conflicting studies exist regarding the independent effect of OSAS on metabolic measures when it coexists with obesity in children. Puberty has an important role in this relationship. Screening of obese children who have OSAS for markers of metabolic syndrome should be considered, especially in the adolescent age group. Individual studies were level II through IV, with an aggregate level of III.

Neurobehavioral

The neurobehavioral complications of OSAS are discussed in detail elsewhere in this technical report. However, 6 studies have explored the potential contribution of obesity to behavior and cognition in children with OSAS and will be discussed in this section. A subanalysis of the Tucson Children's Assessment of Sleep Apnea Study evaluating parent-rated behavioral problems in overweight children before and after controlling for OSAS was performed by Mulvaney et al (level II).[188] They analyzed data from 402 subjects, 15% of whom were overweight; data were derived from home overnight PSG, the Conners scale, and the Child Behavior Checklist

(CBCL). They found that, after controlling for OSAS, behaviors such as withdrawal and social problems were higher in obese children compared with nonobese children. This finding emphasizes the need to control for obesity when designing studies evaluating neurobehavioral issues in children with OSAS. Chervin et al[42] evaluated students in the second and fifth grades in 6 elementary schools (level IV). Only 146 of 806 surveys were returned. Parental survey of health, race, BMI, Pediatric Sleep Questionnaire, teacher-rated performance, and SES were collected. SDB was associated with African American race, SES, and poor teacher ratings (P < .01), but only SES was independently associated with school performance. Low SES was not associated with SDB when controlled for BMI. The authors concluded that future studies evaluating the relationship between school performance and SDB should incorporate direct measurements of SES and obesity. Owens et al[189] examined all children evaluated at a tertiary center for sleep problems between 1999 and 2005; they used PSG, BMI, the Children's Sleep Health Questionnaire, and a mental health history, including the CBCL (level IV). In this study of 235 participants, 56% had a BMI >85th percentile and were thus considered overweight. They found modest correlations between measures of SDB and both somatic complaints and social problems but not with other behavioral complaints. Increased BMI was associated with total CBCL score, internalizing, social, thought, withdrawn, anxious, somatic, and aggressive behavior domains in a dose-response fashion (P = .03), thus emphasizing the need to control for obesity in future studies. Short sleep also correlated with a number of subscales on the CBCL (P < .001). Additional sleep disorders added to the risk of behavior problems ($P < .001$). BMI predicted both total and internalizing CBCL scores, and sleep duration predicted externalizing scores. The presence of an additional sleep diagnosis was the strongest predictor of all 3 CBCL scores. They concluded that overweight, insufficient sleep, and other sleep disorders should be considered when evaluating and treating behavioral problems associated with SDB. Beebe et al[21] studied 60 obese subjects recruited from a weight-management program compared with 22 controls; tools used included BMI; parent- and self-reported validated sleep, behavior, and mood questionnaires; actigraphy; and PSG (level IV). They reported that the obese group had later bedtimes ($P < .05$), shorter ($P < .01$) and more disrupted sleep ($P < .05$), more symptoms of OSAS ($P < .001$), sleepiness ($P = .009$), parasomnias ($P = .007$), higher AHI ($P < .01$), and poorer school performance. Another study by Beebe et al[190] of 263 overweight subjects enrolled in a hospital-based weight-management program found a negative relationship between the severity of OSAS and school performance and parent- and teacher-reported behaviors that persisted with adjustment for gender, race, SES, sleep duration, and BMI (level IV). Interestingly, Roemmich et al[191] found a relationship between a decrease in motor activity and increasing weight in overweight children after surgical treatment of OSAS by using AT ($P = .03$) (level IV). They hypothesized that a decrease in physical activity and "fidgeting" energy expenditure were responsible for the weight gain. However, because obese controls without surgery were not studied, it is unclear whether the degree of weight gain was greater than typically seen in obese children.

In summary, these studies point to obesity as a potential important factor in childhood performance, mood, and behavior (aggregate level III). Clinicians should be aware that children who are obese and have OSAS might continue to have difficulties in these domains after treatment of OSAS. It is recommended that sleep habits and nonrespiratory sleep complaints be included in the evaluation and treatment of obesity-related OSAS. The relationship between SES, obesity, and OSAS is complex and adds further emphasis to the premise that studies of behavior and cognition must be carefully designed and controlled.

QoL

Both obesity and OSAS can affect health-related QoL. Two studies have examined measures of QoL in children who are obese and have OSAS. In a study of 151 overweight children by Carno et al[192] that used surveys of QoL and SDB and PSG, overweight youth who have OSAS were found to have lower self- and parent-related QoL (level IV). Neither objective measures of OSAS by PSG nor BMI correlated with QoL, whereas reported symptoms of OSAS did ($P < .05$). Similarly, Crabtree et al[193] compared 85 children 8 to 12 years of age who had been referred for OSAS and who underwent PSG, BMI, QoL ascertainment, and the Children's Depression Inventory with a control group with previously documented normal PSG (level IV). They found that OSAS did not differ between obese and nonobese children and that there was no difference in QoL between children who snore and have OSAS. The referred SDB group had lower QoL scores than the control group ($P < .001$), but the authors found no difference between obese and nonobese SDB subjects or in those with OSAS versus snoring. They concluded that children who snore have a lower QoL than nonsnoring controls, and that this finding was not related to obesity of the severity of SDB.

In summary, QoL is an important outcome measure that may be more related to perceived symptoms of OSAS than measured physiologic disturbances of sleep and breathing, even in the obese patient (aggregate level IV). The impact of obesity on QoL in children with SDB is yet to be determined by using population-based studies and is an important outcome measure to be included in longitudinal and treatment studies.

Surgical Treatment of OSAS in the Obese Child

Surgical treatment of OSAS in general is discussed in detail in the technical report, but 5 studies have examined this area in obesity-related OSAS and are discussed here. Shine et al[194] evaluated 19 obese patients treated with AT (level IV). Although OSAS improved significantly ($P < .01$), only 37% of patients were deemed cured (defined as a postoperative AHI <5/hour), and 10 (53%) subjects needed CPAP postoperatively. A level IV retrospective review by Spector et al[195] included 14 patients who were morbidly obese who were electively sent to the ICU after AT (per policy). One patient needed intubation, and 2 patients required BPAP. Another retrospective review of 26 morbidly obese patients, all of whom were sent to the ICU after AT as per routine, found that 14 patients (54%) had an uncomplicated postoperative course, and 12 (45%) required respiratory intervention, including 1 requiring intubation and 2 requiring BPAP.[196] Costa and Mitchell[131] evaluated the response to AT in a meta-analysis of 4 studies that included 110 obese children who had OSAS (level III). They found that OSAS improved but did not resolve after AT, with 88% of children having an AHI >1/hour and 51% of children having an AHI >5/hour post-operatively. Apostolidou et al[138] reported on 70 snoring children with a mean age of 5.8 ± 1.8 years who underwent AT; 22 (31%) were obese (level IV). PSG was performed both preoperatively and postoperatively. They found no difference in cure rates between obese and nonobese subjects who had OSAS, by using an AHI <1/hour as the definition of cure. However, there was an improvement in AHI in both groups, and approximately 90% of all subjects had an AHI <5/hour postoperatively.

In summary, few studies have evaluated the effects of AT in the obese child who has OSAS, and studies have been of a low level of evidence (aggregate level IV). Studies suggest that the AHI may improve significantly after AT, even in obese children, supporting the idea that surgery may be a reasonable first-line treatment, even in obese patients. However, better-level studies are needed to assess the effects of AT in obese children and adolescents, including evaluation of subgroups such as adolescents and the morbidly obese. A significant number of children required intubation or CPAP postoperatively, which reinforces the need for inpatient observation in obese children postoperatively. Studies have not been performed to determine whether children at high risk who are obese and have OSAS, such as those with pulmonary or systemic hypertension, waking hypoventilation, or pathologic daytime sleepiness, may benefit from stabilization with BPAP therapy before undergoing AT to decrease the risk of postoperative complications.

Weight Loss and Other Nonsurgical Treatments

There is a paucity of data regarding the effects of weight loss on OSAS in children and adolescents. Verhulst et al[197] found that weight loss was a successful treatment of OSAS in a group of 61 adolescents being cared for in a residential weight loss treatment program (level IV). Davis et al[49] studied the effects of exercise in 100 overweight children by administering the Pediatric Sleep Questionnaire before and after enrollment in a no-exercise group, a low-dose aerobic exercise program, or a high-dose aerobic exercise program for 3 months (level IV). They found no change in BMI, but 50% of children who screened positive for SDB improved to a negative screening result after intervention. They found their results to be consistent with a dose-response effect of exercise on improvement in SDB ($P < .001$). Academic achievement did not improve in concert with changes in the Pediatric Sleep Questionnaire. Kalra et al[198] showed a significant improvement in OSAS after bariatric surgery, in association with a mean weight loss of 58 kg (level IV). In summary, along with many other health-related benefits, achieving weight loss and increasing exercise seem to be beneficial for OSAS and should be recommended along with other interventions for OSAS in obese children and adolescents (aggregate level IV). However, it should be noted that the 2 weight loss studies involved treatment regimens that are not commonly available to the majority of obese children. The effects of more modest weight loss regimens require further evaluation.

Pulmonary Disease and Obesity-Related SDB

Two studies addressed the relationship between obesity-related SDB and pulmonary disease. This has been described in adults as the "overlap syndrome," when chronic obstructive pulmonary disease and OSAS are present in the same individual. As part of the Cleveland Children's Sleep and Health Study, Sulit et al[199] evaluated parent-reported wheeze and asthma, history of snoring, and PSG in 788 participants (level III). They found that children who experienced wheeze and asthma were more likely to be obese ($P = .0097$) and concluded that SDB may partially explain this finding. They speculated that obesity changes airway mechanics and that SDB may increase gastroesophageal reflux, leptin levels, and cytokines and, thus, increase lower airways inflammation. Dubern et al[200] studied 54 children who had BMI z scores >3, 74% of whom were pubertal, by using history, physical examination, assessment of body fat mass, Tanner stage, HOMA, lipid profile, leptin, pulmonary function tests, and PSG (level IV). They confirmed the presence of OSAS, lower functional residual capacity, increased airways resistance, lower airways obstruction, and insulin resistance in this group of morbidly obese children. Snoring and AHI correlated with BMI ($P = .01$) and neck/height ratio ($P = .03$) (adjusted for age, gender, Tanner stage, and ethnicity). Airways resistance correlated with snoring index and AHI after adjustment. These studies remind us that the upper airway is part of the respiratory system and that its function is affected by lung mechanics. Abnormalities of pulmonary mechanics related to obesity affect OSAS and may add to abnormalities of gas exchange during sleep. It is suggested that evaluation of the child who is obese and has OSAS should include a history and physical examination directed at the entire respiratory system, and pulmonary function testing may be indicated.

Areas for Future Research

- What threshold of easily obtained anthropomorphic measurements predicts a significant risk of OSAS?

Overweight as well as obese children should be included in future studies.

- Are there additive or multiplicative effects of OSAS and obesity on BP? How do these relationships evolve over time, and what is the impact of genetic and racial background? Does treatment of OSAS improve hypertension in obese children and adolescents?

- The effect of OSAS on metabolic syndrome in children and adolescents remains controversial. Future research should include treatment arms with careful measurements before and after interventions. Longitudinal studies that track changes during puberty and into adulthood would be of interest.

- Further research is needed to clarify the effects of AT on OSAS, including evaluation of subgroups such as adolescents and morbidly obese patients. There should also be studies evaluating the use of CPAP or BPAP before surgery in the obese population, as a way of stabilizing the cardiopulmonary system and reducing operative risk.

- What is the effect of modest weight loss on OSAS in children and adolescents? Research should be directed at identifying strategies to effectively implement weight loss and exercise programs in this population.

SUBCOMMITTEE ON OBSTRUCTIVE SLEEP APNEA SYNDROME*

Carole L. Marcus, MBBCh, Chairperson (sleep medicine, pediatric pulmonologist; liaison, American Academy of Sleep Medicine; research support from Philips Respironics; affiliated with an academic sleep center; published research related to OSAS)

Lee J. Brooks, MD (sleep medicine, pediatric pulmonologist; liaison, American College of Chest Physicians; no conflicts; affiliated with an academic sleep center; published research related to OSAS)

Sally Davidson Ward, MD (sleep medicine, pediatric pulmonologist; no conflicts; affiliated with an academic sleep center; published research related to OSAS)

Kari A. Draper, MD (general pediatrician; no conflicts)

David Gozal, MD (sleep medicine, pediatric pulmonologist; research support from Astra-Zeneca; speaker for Merck Company; affiliated with an academic sleep center; published research related to OSAS)

Ann C. Halbower, MD (sleep medicine, pediatric pulmonologist; liaison, American Thoracic Society; research funding from ResMed; affiliated with an academic sleep center; published research related to OSAS)

Jacqueline Jones, MD (pediatric otolaryngologist; AAP Section on Otolaryngology–Head and Neck Surgery; liaison, American Academy of Otolaryngology–Head and Neck Surgery; no conflicts; affiliated with an academic otolaryngologic practice)

Christopher Lehmann, MD (neonatologist, informatician; no conflicts)

Michael S. Schechter, MD, MPH (pediatric pulmonologist; AAP Section on Pediatric Pulmonology; consultant to Genentech, Inc and Gilead, Inc, not related to obstructive sleep apnea; research support from Mpex Pharmaceuticals, Inc, Vertex Pharmaceuticals Incorporated, PTC Therapeutics, and Bayer Healthcare, not related to obstructive sleep apnea)

Stephen Sheldon, MD (sleep medicine, general pediatrician; liaison, National Sleep Foundation; no conflicts; affiliated with an academic sleep center; published research related to OSAS)

Richard N. Shiffman, MD, MCIS (general pediatrics, informatician; no conflicts)

Karen Spruyt, PhD (clinical psychologist, child neuropsychologist, and biostatistician/epidemiologist; no conflicts; affiliated with an academic sleep center)

OVERSIGHT FROM THE STEERING COMMITTEE ON QUALITY IMPROVEMENT AND MANAGEMENT, 2009--2011

STAFF
Caryn Davidson, MA

*Areas of expertise are shown in parentheses after each name.

ACKNOWLEDGMENT
The Committee thanks Christopher Hickey for administrative assistance.

REFERENCES

1. American Academy of Pediatrics. Obstructive sleep apnea syndrome: clinical practice guideline for the diagnosis and management of childhood obstructive sleep apnea syndrome. *Pediatrics.* 2012; 130(3): In press

2. American Thoracic Society. Standards and indications for cardiopulmonary sleep studies in children. *Am J Respir Crit Care Med.* 1996;153(2):866–878

3. Roland PS, Rosenfeld RM, Brooks LJ, et al; American Academy of Otolaryngology–Head and Neck Surgery Foundation. Clinical practice guideline: Polysomnography for sleep-disordered breathing prior to tonsillectomy in children. *Otolaryngol Head Neck Surg.* 2011;145(suppl 1):S1–S15

4. Aurora RN, Zak RS, Karippot A, et al; American Academy of Sleep Medicine. Practice parameters for the respiratory indications for polysomnography in children. *Sleep.* 2011;34(3):379–388

5. Hearst MA. Untangling Text Data Mining. In: Proceedings of the 37th Annual Meeting of the Association for Computational Linguistics. Stroudsburg, PA: Association for Computational Linguistics; 1999:3–10

6. Schechter MS; Section on Pediatric Pulmonology, Subcommittee on Obstructive Sleep Apnea Syndrome. Technical report: diagnosis and management of childhood obstructive sleep apnea syndrome. *Pediatrics.* 2002;109(4). Available at: www.pediatrics.org/cgi/content/full/109/4/e69

7. Edlund W, Gronseth G, So Y, Franklin G. *Clinical Practice Guideline Process Manual.* 4th ed. St Paul, MN: American Academy of Neurology; 2005

8. Sackett DL. Rules of evidence and clinical recommendations for the management of patients. *Can J Cardiol.* 1993;9(6):487–489

9. Centre for Evidence-Based Medicine. *Levels of Evidence and Grades of Recommendations.* Oxford, United Kingdom: Headington; 2001

10. American Academy of Pediatrics Steering Committee on Quality Improvement and

Management. Classifying recommendations for clinical practice guidelines. *Pediatrics.* 2004;114(3):874–877

11. Bixler EO, Vgontzas AN, Lin HM, et al. Sleep disordered breathing in children in a general population sample: prevalence and risk factors. *Sleep.* 2009;32(6):731–736

12. Li AM, So HK, Au CT, et al. Epidemiology of obstructive sleep apnoea syndrome in Chinese children: a two-phase community study. *Thorax.* 2010;65(11):991–997

13. O'Brien LM, Holbrook CR, Mervis CB, et al. Sleep and neurobehavioral characteristics of 5- to 7-year-old children with parentally reported symptoms of attention-deficit/hyperactivity disorder. *Pediatrics.* 2003; 111(3):554–563

14. Castronovo V, Zucconi M, Nosetti L, et al. Prevalence of habitual snoring and sleep-disordered breathing in preschool-aged children in an Italian community. *J Pediatr.* 2003;142(4):377–382

15. Goodwin JL, Kaemingk KL, Mulvaney SA, Morgan WJ, Quan SF. Clinical screening of school children for polysomnography to detect sleep-disordered breathing—the Tucson Children's Assessment of Sleep Apnea study (TuCASA). *J Clin Sleep Med.* 2005;1(3):247–254

16. Sogut A, Altin R, Uzun L, et al. Prevalence of obstructive sleep apnea syndrome and associated symptoms in 3–11-year-old Turkish children. *Pediatr Pulmonol.* 2005; 39(3):251–256

17. Wing YK, Hui SH, Pak WM, et al. A controlled study of sleep related disordered breathing in obese children. *Arch Dis Child.* 2003;88(12):1043–1047

18. Sánchez-Armengol A, Fuentes-Pradera MA, Capote-Gil F, et al. Sleep-related breathing disorders in adolescents aged 12 to 16 years: clinical and polygraphic findings. *Chest.* 2001;119(5):1393–1400

19. Rosen CL, Larkin EK, Kirchner HL, et al. Prevalence and risk factors for sleep-disordered breathing in 8- to 11-year-old children: association with race and prematurity. *J Pediatr.* 2003;142(4):383–389

20. Redline S, Tishler PV, Schluchter M, Aylor J, Clark K, Graham G. Risk factors for sleep-disordered breathing in children. Associations with obesity, race, and respiratory problems. *Am J Respir Crit Care Med.* 1999;159(5 pt 1):1527–1532

21. Beebe DW, Lewin D, Zeller M, et al. Sleep in overweight adolescents: shorter sleep, poorer sleep quality, sleepiness, and sleep-disordered breathing. *J Pediatr Psychol.* 2007;32(1):69–79

22. Xu Z, Jiaqing A, Yuchuan L, Shen K. A case-control study of obstructive sleep

apnea-hypopnea syndrome in obese and nonobese Chinese children. *Chest.* 2008; 133(3):684–689

23. Brunetti L, Tesse R, Miniello VL, et al. Sleep-disordered breathing in obese children: the southern Italy experience. *Chest.* 2010; 137(5):1085–1090

24. O'Brien LM, Mervis CB, Holbrook CR, et al. Neurobehavioral implications of habitual snoring in children. *Pediatrics.* 2004;114 (1):44–49

25. Suratt PM, Barth JT, Diamond R, et al. Reduced time in bed and obstructive sleep-disordered breathing in children are associated with cognitive impairment. *Pediatrics.* 2007;119(2):320–329

26. Friedman BC, Hendeles-Amitai A, Kozminsky E, et al. Adenotonsillectomy improves neurocognitive function in children with obstructive sleep apnea syndrome. *Sleep.* 2003;26(8):999–1005

27. Gozal D, Wang M, Pope DW Jr. Objective sleepiness measures in pediatric obstructive sleep apnea. *Pediatrics.* 2001; 108(3):693–697

28. Halbower AC, Degaonkar M, Barker PB, et al. Childhood obstructive sleep apnea associates with neuropsychological deficits and neuronal brain injury. *PLoS Med.* 2006;3(8):e301

29. O'Brien LM, Mervis CB, Holbrook CR, et al. Neurobehavioral correlates of sleep-disordered breathing in children. *J Sleep Res.* 2004;13(2):165–172

30. Kohler MJ, Lushington K, van den Heuvel CJ, Martin J, Pamula Y, Kennedy D. Adenotonsillectomy and neurocognitive deficits in children with sleep disordered breathing. *PLoS ONE.* 2009;4(10):e7343

31. Calhoun SL, Mayes SD, Vgontzas AN, Tsaoussoglou M, Shifflett LJ, Bixler EO. No relationship between neurocognitive functioning and mild sleep disordered breathing in a community sample of children. *J Clin Sleep Med.* 2009;5(3):228–234

32. Mulvaney SA, Goodwin JL, Morgan WJ, Rosen GR, Quan SF, Kaemingk KL. Behavior problems associated with sleep disordered breathing in school-aged children —the Tucson Children's Assessment of Sleep Apnea Study. *J Pediatr Psychol.* 2006;31(3):322–330

33. Kaemingk KL, Pasvogel AE, Goodwin JL, et al. Learning in children and sleep disordered breathing: findings of the Tucson Children's Assessment of Sleep Apnea (tuCASA) prospective cohort study. *J Int Neuropsychol Soc.* 2003;9(7):1016–1026

34. Kennedy JD, Blunden S, Hirte C, et al. Reduced neurocognition in children who

snore. *Pediatr Pulmonol.* 2004;37(4):330–337

35. Spruyt K, Gozal D. A mediation model linking body weight, cognition, and sleep-disordered breathing. *Am J Respir Crit Care Med.* 2012;185(2):199–205

36. Spilsbury JC, Storfer-Isser A, Kirchner HL, et al. Neighborhood disadvantage as a risk factor for pediatric obstructive sleep apnea. *J Pediatr.* 2006;149(3):342–347

37. Chervin RD, Ruzicka DL, Giordani BJ, et al. Sleep-disordered breathing, behavior, and cognition in children before and after adenotonsillectomy. *Pediatrics.* 2006;117 (4). Available at: www.pediatrics.org/cgi/content/full/117/4/e769

38. Giordani B, Hodges EK, Guire KE, et al. Neuropsychological and behavioral functioning in children with and without obstructive sleep apnea referred for tonsillectomy. *J Int Neuropsychol Soc.* 2008;14(4):571–581

39. Chervin RD, Weatherly RA, Ruzicka DL, et al. Subjective sleepiness and polysomnographic correlates in children scheduled for adenotonsillectomy vs other surgical care. *Sleep.* 2006;29(4):495–503

40. Chervin RD, Ruzicka DL, Archbold KH, Dillon JE. Snoring predicts hyperactivity four years later. *Sleep.* 2005;28(7):885–890

41. Chervin RD, Archbold KH. Hyperactivity and polysomnographic findings in children evaluated for sleep-disordered breathing. *Sleep.* 2001;24(3):313–320

42. Chervin RD, Clarke DF, Huffman JL, et al. School performance, race, and other correlates of sleep-disordered breathing in children. *Sleep Med.* 2003;4(1):21–27

43. Suratt PM, Peruggia M, D'Andrea L, et al. Cognitive function and behavior of children with adenotonsillar hypertrophy suspected of having obstructive sleep-disordered breathing. *Pediatrics.* 2006; 118(3). Available at: www.pediatrics.org/cgi/content/full/118/3/e771

44. Montgomery-Downs HE, Jones VF, Molfese VJ, Gozal D. Snoring in preschoolers: associations with sleepiness, ethnicity, and learning. *Clin Pediatr (Phila).* 2003;42 (8):719–726

45. Johnson EO, Roth T. An epidemiologic study of sleep-disordered breathing symptoms among adolescents. *Sleep.* 2006;29(9): 1135–1142

46. Tauman R, Ivanenko A, O'Brien LM, Gozal D. Plasma C-reactive protein levels among children with sleep-disordered breathing. *Pediatrics.* 2004;113(6). Available at: www.pediatrics.org/cgi/content/full/113/6/e564

47. Shin C, Joo S, Kim J, Kim T. Prevalence and correlates of habitual snoring in high school students. *Chest.* 2003;124(5):1709–1715

48. Hogan AM, Hill CM, Harrison D, Kirkham FJ. Cerebral blood flow velocity and cognition in children before and after adenotonsillectomy. *Pediatrics.* 2008;122(1):75–82

49. Davis CL, Tkacz J, Gregoski M, Boyle CA, Lovrekovic G. Aerobic exercise and snoring in overweight children: a randomized controlled trial. *Obesity (Silver Spring).* 2006;14(11):1985–1991

50. Montgomery-Downs HE, Crabtree VM, Gozal D. Cognition, sleep and respiration in at-risk children treated for obstructive sleep apnoea. *Eur Respir J.* 2005;25(2):336–342

51. Lundeborg I, McAllister A, Samuelsson C, Ericsson E, Hultcrantz E. Phonological development in children with obstructive sleep-disordered breathing. *Clin Linguist Phon.* 2009;23(10):751–761

52. Colen TY, Seidman C, Weedon J, Goldstein NA. Effect of intracapsular tonsillectomy on quality of life for children with obstructive sleep-disordered breathing. *Arch Otolaryngol Head Neck Surg.* 2008;134(2):124–127

53. Mitchell RB, Kelly J, Call E, Yao N. Long-term changes in quality of life after surgery for pediatric obstructive sleep apnea. *Arch Otolaryngol Head Neck Surg.* 2004;130(4):409–412

54. Constantin E, Kermack A, Nixon GM, Tidmarsh L, Ducharme FM, Brouillette RT. Adenotonsillectomy improves sleep, breathing, and quality of life but not behavior. *J Pediatr.* 2007;150:540–546, 546.e1

55. Goldstein NA, Fatima M, Campbell TF, Rosenfeld RM. Child behavior and quality of life before and after tonsillectomy and adenoidectomy. *Arch Otolaryngol Head Neck Surg.* 2002;128(7):770–775

56. Sohn H, Rosenfeld RM. Evaluation of sleep-disordered breathing in children. *Otolaryngol Head Neck Surg.* 2003;128(3):344–352

57. Silva VC, Leite AJ. Quality of life in children with sleep-disordered breathing: evaluation by OSA-18. *Braz J Otorhinolaryngol.* 2006;72(6):747–756

58. Tran KD, Nguyen CD, Weedon J, Goldstein NA. Child behavior and quality of life in pediatric obstructive sleep apnea. *Arch Otolaryngol Head Neck Surg.* 2005;131(1):52–57

59. James AL, Runciman M, Burton MJ, Freeland AP. Investigation of cardiac function in children with suspected obstructive sleep apnea. *J Otolaryngol.* 2003;32(3):151–154

60. Kalra M, Kimball TR, Daniels SR, et al. Structural cardiac changes as a predictor of respiratory complications after adenotonsillectomy for obstructive breathing during sleep in children. *Sleep Med.* 2005;6(3):241–245

61. Kaditis AG, Alexopoulos EI, Hatzi F, et al. Overnight change in brain natriuretic peptide levels in children with sleep-disordered breathing. *Chest.* 2006;130(5):1377–1384

62. Khadra MA, McConnell K, VanDyke R, et al. Determinants of regional cerebral oxygenation in children with sleep-disordered breathing. *Am J Respir Crit Care Med.* 2008;178(8):870–875

63. Constantin E, McGregor CD, Cote V, Brouillette RT. Pulse rate and pulse rate variability decrease after adenotonsillectomy for obstructive sleep apnea. *Pediatr Pulmonol.* 2008;43(5):498–504

64. Deng ZD, Poon CS, Arzeno NM, Katz ES. Heart rate variability in pediatric obstructive sleep apnea. *Conf Proc IEEE Eng Med Biol Soc.* 2006;1:3565–3568

65. O'Brien LM, Gozal D. Autonomic dysfunction in children with sleep-disordered breathing. *Sleep.* 2005;28(6):747–752

66. Kwok KL, Ng DK, Cheung YF. BP and arterial distensibility in children with primary snoring. *Chest.* 2003;123(5):1561–1566

67. Bonuck KA, Freeman K, Henderson J. Growth and growth biomarker changes after adenotonsillectomy: systematic review and meta-analysis. *Arch Dis Child.* 2009;94(2):83–91

68. Bar A, Tarasiuk A, Segev Y, Phillip M, Tal A. The effect of adenotonsillectomy on serum insulin-like growth factor-I and growth in children with obstructive sleep apnea syndrome. *J Pediatr.* 1999;135(1):76–80

69. Nieminen P, Löppönen T, Tolonen U, Lanning P, Knip M, Löppönen H. Growth and biochemical markers of growth in children with snoring and obstructive sleep apnea. *Pediatrics.* 2002;109(4). Available at: www.pediatrics.org/cgi/content/full/109/4/e55

70. Selimoğlu E, Selimoğlu MA, Orbak Z. Does adenotonsillectomy improve growth in children with obstructive adenotonsillar hypertrophy? *J Int Med Res.* 2003;31(2):84–87

71. Apostolidou MT, Alexopoulos EI, Damani E, et al. Absence of blood pressure, metabolic, and inflammatory marker changes after adenotonsillectomy for sleep apnea in Greek children. *Pediatr Pulmonol.* 2008;43(6):550–560

72. Kaditis AG, Alexopoulos EI, Kalampouka E, et al. Morning levels of C-reactive protein in children with obstructive sleep-disordered breathing. *Am J Respir Crit Care Med.* 2005;171(3):282–286

73. O'Brien LM, Serpero LD, Tauman R, Gozal D. Plasma adhesion molecules in children with sleep-disordered breathing. *Chest.* 2006;129(4):947–953

74. Tam CS, Wong M, McBain R, Bailey S, Waters KA. Inflammatory measures in children with obstructive sleep apnoea. *J Paediatr Child Health.* 2006;42(5):277–282

75. Gozal D, Crabtree VM, Sans Capdevila O, Witcher LA, Kheirandish-Gozal L. C-reactive protein, obstructive sleep apnea, and cognitive dysfunction in school-aged children. *Am J Respir Crit Care Med.* 2007;176(2):188–193

76. Li AM, Chan MH, Yin J, et al. C-reactive protein in children with obstructive sleep apnea and the effects of treatment. *Pediatr Pulmonol.* 2008;43(1):34–40

77. Larkin EK, Rosen CL, Kirchner HL, et al. Variation of C-reactive protein levels in adolescents: association with sleep-disordered breathing and sleep duration. *Circulation.* 2005;111(15):1978–1984

78. Gozal D, Serpero LD, Sans Capdevila O, Kheirandish-Gozal L. Systemic inflammation in non-obese children with obstructive sleep apnea. *Sleep Med.* 2008;9(3):254–259

79. Gozal D, Serpero LD, Kheirandish-Gozal L, Capdevila OS, Khalyfa A, Tauman R. Sleep measures and morning plasma TNF-alpha levels in children with sleep-disordered breathing. *Sleep.* 2010;33(3):319–325

80. Khalyfa A, Serpero LD, Kheirandish-Gozal L, Capdevila OS, Gozal D. TNF-α gene polymorphisms and excessive daytime sleepiness in pediatric obstructive sleep apnea. *J Pediatr.* 2011;158(1):77–82

81. Goldbart AD, Veling MC, Goldman JL, Li RC, Brittian KR, Gozal D. Glucocorticoid receptor subunit expression in adenotonsillar tissue of children with obstructive sleep apnea. *Pediatr Res.* 2005;57(2):232–236

82. Goldbart AD, Goldman JL, Veling MC, Gozal D. Leukotriene modifier therapy for mild sleep-disordered breathing in children. *Am J Respir Crit Care Med.* 2005;172(3):364–370

83. Preutthipan A, Chantarojanasiri T, Suwanjutha S, Udomsubpayakul U. Can parents predict the severity of childhood obstructive sleep apnoea? *Acta Paediatr.* 2000;89(6):708–712

84. Chervin RD, Hedger K, Dillon JE, Pituch KJ. Pediatric sleep questionnaire (PSQ):

validity and reliability of scales for sleep-disordered breathing, snoring, sleepiness, and behavioral problems. *Sleep Med.* 2000;1(1):21–32

85. Chervin RD, Weatherly RA, Garetz SL, et al. Pediatric sleep questionnaire: prediction of sleep apnea and outcomes. *Arch Otolaryngol Head Neck Surg.* 2007;133(3): 216–222

86. Weatherly RA, Ruzicka DL, Marriott DJ, Chervin RD. Polysomnography in children scheduled for adenotonsillectomy. *Otolaryngol Head Neck Surg.* 2004;131(5): 727–731

87. van Someren V, Burmester M, Alusi G, Lane R. Are sleep studies worth doing? *Arch Dis Child.* 2000;83(1):76–81

88. Carotenuto M, Bruni O, Santoro N, Del Giudice EM, Perrone L, Pascotto A. Waist circumference predicts the occurrence of sleep-disordered breathing in obese children and adolescents: a questionnaire-based study. *Sleep Med.* 2006;7(4):357–361

89. Schiffman PH, Rubin NK, Dominguez T, et al. Mandibular dimensions in children with obstructive sleep apnea syndrome. *Sleep.* 2004;27(5):959–965

90. Monahan KJ, Larkin EK, Rosen CL, Graham G, Redline S. Utility of noninvasive pharyngometry in epidemiologic studies of childhood sleep-disordered breathing. *Am J Respir Crit Care Med.* 2002;165(11): 1499–1503

91. Rizzi M, Onorato J, Andreoli A, et al. Nasal resistances are useful in identifying children with severe obstructive sleep apnea before polysomnography. *Int J Pediatr Otorhinolaryngol.* 2002;65(1):7–13

92. Brietzke SE, Mair EA. Acoustical analysis of pediatric snoring: what can we learn? *Otolaryngol Head Neck Surg.* 2007;136(4): 644–648

93. Rembold CM, Suratt PM. Children with obstructive sleep-disordered breathing generate high-frequency inspiratory sounds during sleep. *Sleep.* 2004;27(6): 1154–1161

94. Brouillette RT, Morielli A, Leimanis A, Waters KA, Luciano R, Ducharme FM. Nocturnal pulse oximetry as an abbreviated testing modality for pediatric obstructive sleep apnea. *Pediatrics.* 2000; 105(2):405–412

95. Patel A, Watson M, Habibi P. Unattended home sleep studies for the evaluation of suspected obstructive sleep apnoea syndrome in children. *J Telemed Telecare.* 2005;11(suppl 1):100–102

96. Saito H, Araki K, Ozawa H, et al. Pulse-oximetery is useful in determining the indications for adeno-tonsillectomy in pediatric sleep-disordered breathing. *Int J Pediatr Otorhinolaryngol.* 2007;71(1):1–6

97. Nixon GM, Kermack AS, Davis GM, Manoukian JJ, Brown KA, Brouillette RT. Planning adenotonsillectomy in children with obstructive sleep apnea: the role of overnight oximetry. *Pediatrics.* 2004;113(1 pt 1):e19–e25

98. Kirk VG, Bohn SG, Flemons WW, Remmers JE. Comparison of home oximetry monitoring with laboratory polysomnography in children. *Chest.* 2003;124(5):1702–1708

99. Collop NA, Anderson WM, Boehlecke B, et al; Portable Monitoring Task Force of the American Academy of Sleep Medicine. Clinical guidelines for the use of unattended portable monitors in the diagnosis of obstructive sleep apnea in adult patients. *J Clin Sleep Med.* 2007;3(7): 737–747

100. Zucconi M, Calori G, Castronovo V, Ferini-Strambi L. Respiratory monitoring by means of an unattended device in children with suspected uncomplicated obstructive sleep apnea: a validation study. *Chest.* 2003;124(2):602–607

101. Goodwin JL, Enright PL, Kaemingk KL, et al. Feasibility of using unattended polysomnography in children for research—report of the Tucson Children's Assessment of Sleep Apnea study (TuCASA). *Sleep.* 2001;24(8):937–944

102. Redline S, Budhiraja R, Kapur V, et al. The scoring of respiratory events in sleep: reliability and validity. *J Clin Sleep Med.* 2007;3(2):169–200

103. Katz ES, Greene MG, Carson KA, et al. Night-to-night variability of polysomnography in children with suspected obstructive sleep apnea. *J Pediatr.* 2002;140(5):589–594

104. Li AM, Wing YK, Cheung A, et al. Is a 2-night polysomnographic study necessary in childhood sleep-related disordered breathing? *Chest.* 2004;126(5):1467–1472

105. Scholle S, Scholle HC, Kemper A, et al. First night effect in children and adolescents undergoing polysomnography for sleep-disordered breathing. *Clin Neurophysiol.* 2003;114(11):2138–2145

106. Verhulst SL, Schrauwen N, De Backer WA, Desager KN. First night effect for polysomnographic data in children and adolescents with suspected sleep disordered breathing. *Arch Dis Child.* 2006;91(3): 233–237

107. Iber C. *The AASM Manual for the Scoring of Sleep and Associated Events: Rules, Terminology and Technical Specification.* Westchester, FL: American Academy of Sleep Medicine; 2007

108. Sritippayawan S, Desudchit T, Prapphal N, Harnruthakorn C, Deerojanawong J, Samransamruajkit R. Validity of tidal breathing flow volume loops in diagnosing obstructive sleep apnea in young children with adenotonsillar hypertrophy: a preliminary study. *J Med Assoc Thai.* 2004;87(suppl 2):S45–S49

109. Gozal D, Jortani S, Snow AB, et al. Two-dimensional differential in-gel electrophoresis proteomic approaches reveal urine candidate biomarkers in pediatric obstructive sleep apnea. *Am J Respir Crit Care Med.* 2009;180(12):1253–1261

110. Shah ZA, Jortani SA, Tauman R, Valdes R, Jr;Gozal D. Serum proteomic patterns associated with sleep-disordered breathing in children. *Pediatr Res.* 2006;59(3): 466–470

111. Uliel S, Tauman R, Greenfeld M, Sivan Y. Normal polysomnographic respiratory values in children and adolescents. *Chest.* 2004;125(3):872–878

112. Traeger N, Schultz B, Pollock AN, Mason T, Marcus CL, Arens R. Polysomnographic values in children 2-9 years old: additional data and review of the literature. *Pediatr Pulmonol.* 2005;40(1):22–30

113. Witmans MB, Keens TG, Davidson Ward SL, Marcus CL. Obstructive hypopneas in children and adolescents: normal values. *Am J Respir Crit Care Med.* 2003;168(12): 1540

114. Reuveni H, Simon T, Tal A, Elhayany A, Tarasiuk A. Health care services utilization in children with obstructive sleep apnea syndrome. *Pediatrics.* 2002;110(1 pt 1):68–72

115. Tarasiuk A, Simon T, Tal A, Reuveni H. Adenotonsillectomy in children with obstructive sleep apnea syndrome reduces health care utilization. *Pediatrics.* 2004; 113(2):351–356

116. Tunkel DE, Hotchkiss KS, Carson KA, Sterni LM. Efficacy of powered intracapsular tonsillectomy and adenoidectomy. *Laryngoscope.* 2008;118(7):1295–1302

117. Mangiardi J, Graw-Panzer KD, Weedon J, Regis T, Lee H, Goldstein NA. Polysomnography outcomes for partial intracapsular versus total tonsillectomy. *Int J Pediatr Otorhinolaryngol.* 2010;74(12): 1361–1366

118. Marcus CL, Keens TG, Ward SL. Comparison of nap and overnight polysomnography in children. *Pediatr Pulmonol.* 1992;13(1): 16–21

119. Saeed MM, Keens TG, Stabile MW, Bolokowicz J, Davidson Ward SL. Should children with suspected obstructive sleep apnea syndrome and normal nap sleep studies have overnight sleep studies? *Chest.* 2000;118 (2):360–365

120. Celenk F, Bayazit YA, Yilmaz M, et al. Tonsillar regrowth following partial tonsillectomy with radiofrequency. *Int J Pediatr Otorhinolaryngol.* 2008;72(1):19–22

121. Zagólski O. Why do palatine tonsils grow back after partial tonsillectomy in children? *Eur Arch Otorhinolaryngol.* 2010;267 (10):1613–1617

122. Solares CA, Koempel JA, Hirose K, et al. Safety and efficacy of powered intracapsular tonsillectomy in children: a multicenter retrospective case series. *Int J Pediatr Otorhinolaryngol.* 2005;69(1):21–26

123. Eviatar E, Kessler A, Shlamkovitch N, Vaiman M, Zilber D, Gavriel H. Tonsillectomy vs. partial tonsillectomy for OSAS in children—10 years post-surgery follow-up. *Int J Pediatr Otorhinolaryngol.* 2009;73(5):637–640

124. Derkay CS, Darrow DH, Welch C, Sinacori JT. Post-tonsillectomy morbidity and quality of life in pediatric patients with obstructive tonsils and adenoid: microdebrider vs electrocautery. *Otolaryngol Head Neck Surg.* 2006;134(1):114–120

125. Koltai PJ, Solares CA, Koempel JA, et al. Intracapsular tonsillar reduction (partial tonsillectomy): reviving a historical procedure for obstructive sleep disordered breathing in children. *Otolaryngol Head Neck Surg.* 2003;129(5):532–538

126. Sobol SE, Wetmore RF, Marsh RR, Stow J, Jacobs IN. Postoperative recovery after microdebrider intracapsular or monopolar electrocautery tonsillectomy: a prospective, randomized, single-blinded study. *Arch Otolaryngol Head Neck Surg.* 2006;132(3): 270–274

127. Ye J, Liu H, Zhang G, Huang Z, Huang P, Li Y. Postoperative respiratory complications of adenotonsillectomy for obstructive sleep apnea syndrome in older children: prevalence, risk factors, and impact on clinical outcome. *J Otolaryngol Head Neck Surg.* 2009;38(1):49–58

128. Tait AR, Malviya S, Voepel-Lewis T, Munro HM, Seiwert M, Pandit UA. Risk factors for perioperative adverse respiratory events in children with upper respiratory tract infections. *Anesthesiology.* 2001;95(2): 299–306

129. von Ungern-Sternberg BS, Boda K, Schwab C, Sims C, Johnson C, Habre W. Laryngeal mask airway is associated with an increased incidence of adverse respiratory events in children with recent upper respiratory tract infections. *Anesthesiology.* 2007;107(5):714–719

130. Brietzke SE, Gallagher D. The effectiveness of tonsillectomy and adenoidectomy in the treatment of pediatric obstructive sleep apnea/hypopnea syndrome: a meta-analysis.

Otolaryngol Head Neck Surg. 2006;134(6): 979–984

131. Costa DJ, Mitchell R. Adenotonsillectomy for obstructive sleep apnea in obese children: a meta-analysis. *Otolaryngol Head Neck Surg.* 2009;140(4):455–460

132. Mitchell RB. Adenotonsillectomy for obstructive sleep apnea in children: outcome evaluated by pre- and postoperative polysomnography. *Laryngoscope.* 2007;117 (10):1844–1854

133. Bhattacharjee R, Kheirandish-Gozal L, Spruyt K, et al. Adenotonsillectomy outcomes in treatment of obstructive sleep apnea in children: a multicenter retrospective study. *Am J Respir Crit Care Med.* 2010;182(5):676–683

134. Ye J, Liu H, Zhang GH, et al. Outcome of adenotonsillectomy for obstructive sleep apnea syndrome in children. *Ann Otol Rhinol Laryngol.* 2010;119(8):506–513

135. Guilleminault C, Li K, Quo S, Inouye RN. A prospective study on the surgical outcomes of children with sleep-disordered breathing. *Sleep.* 2004;27(1):95–100

136. O'Brien LM, Sitha S, Baur LA, Waters KA. Obesity increases the risk for persisting obstructive sleep apnea after treatment in children. *Int J Pediatr Otorhinolaryngol.* 2006;70(9):1555–1560

137. Tauman R, Gulliver TE, Krishna J, et al. Persistence of obstructive sleep apnea syndrome in children after adenotonsillectomy. *J Pediatr.* 2006;149(6):803–808

138. Apostolidou MT, Alexopoulos EI, Chaidas K, et al. Obesity and persisting sleep apnea after adenotonsillectomy in Greek children. *Chest.* 2008;134(6):1149–1155

139. Mitchell RB, Kelly J. Outcome of adenotonsillectomy for obstructive sleep apnea in obese and normal-weight children. *Otolaryngol Head Neck Surg.* 2007;137(1): 43–48

140. Mitchell RB, Kelly J. Outcome of adenotonsillectomy for obstructive sleep apnea in children under 3 years. *Otolaryngol Head Neck Surg.* 2005;132(5):681–684

141. Guilleminault C, Huang YS, Glamann C, Li K, Chan A. Adenotonsillectomy and obstructive sleep apnea in children: a prospective survey. *Otolaryngol Head Neck Surg.* 2007; 136(2):169–175

142. Marcus CL, Rosen G, Ward SL, et al. Adherence to and effectiveness of positive airway pressure therapy in children with obstructive sleep apnea. *Pediatrics.* 2006; 117(3). Available at: www.pediatrics.org/ cgi/content/full/117/3/e442

143. Koontz KL, Slifer KJ, Cataldo MD, Marcus CL. Improving pediatric compliance with

positive airway pressure therapy: the impact of behavioral intervention. *Sleep.* 2003;26(8):1010–1015

144. McGinley B, Halbower A, Schwartz AR, Smith PL, Patil SP, Schneider H. Effect of a high-flow open nasal cannula system on obstructive sleep apnea in children. *Pediatrics.* 2009;124(1):179–188

145. Uong EC, Epperson M, Bathon SA, Jeffe DB. Adherence to nasal positive airway pressure therapy among school-aged children and adolescents with obstructive sleep apnea syndrome. *Pediatrics.* 2007;120(5). Available at: www.pediatrics.org/cgi/content/full/120/5/e1203

146. O'Donnell AR, Bjornson CL, Bohn SG, Kirk VG. Compliance rates in children using noninvasive continuous positive airway pressure. *Sleep.* 2006;29(5):651–658

147. Friedman O, Chidekel A, Lawless ST, Cook SP. Postoperative bilevel positive airway pressure ventilation after tonsillectomy and adenoidectomy in children—a preliminary report. *Int J Pediatr Otorhinolaryngol.* 1999;51(3):177–180

148. Downey R, III, Perkin RM, MacQuarrie J. Nasal continuous positive airway pressure use in children with obstructive sleep apnea younger than 2 years of age. *Chest.* 2000;117(6):1608–1612

149. Marcus CL, Ward SL, Mallory GB, et al. Use of nasal continuous positive airway pressure as treatment of childhood obstructive sleep apnea. *J Pediatr.* 1995;127(1): 88–94

150. Al-Ghamdi SA, Manoukian JJ, Morielli A, Oudjhane K, Ducharme FM, Brouillette RT. Do systemic corticosteroids effectively treat obstructive sleep apnea secondary to adenotonsillar hypertrophy? *Laryngoscope.* 1997;107(10):1382–1387

151. Berlucchi M, Salsi D, Valetti L, Parrinello G, Nicolai P. The role of mometasone furoate aqueous nasal spray in the treatment of adenoidal hypertrophy in the pediatric age group: preliminary results of a prospective, randomized study. *Pediatrics.* 2007;119(6). Available at: www.pediatrics. org/cgi/content/full/119/6/e1392

152. Brouillette RT, Manoukian JJ, Ducharme FM, et al. Efficacy of fluticasone nasal spray for pediatric obstructive sleep apnea. *J Pediatr.* 2001;138(6):838–844

153. Kheirandish-Gozal L, Gozal D. Intranasal budesonide treatment for children with mild obstructive sleep apnea syndrome. *Pediatrics.* 2008;122(1). Available at: www.pediatrics.org/cgi/content/full/122/ 1/e149

154. Alexopoulos EI, Kaditis AG, Kalampouka E, et al. Nasal corticosteroids for children

with snoring. *Pediatr Pulmonol.* 2004;38 (2):161–167

155. Kheirandish L, Goldbart AD, Gozal D. Intranasal steroids and oral leukotriene modifier therapy in residual sleep-disordered breathing after tonsillectomy and adenoidectomy in children. *Pediatrics.* 2006;117(1). Available at: www.pediatrics.org/cgi/content/full/117/1/e61

156. Pirelli P, Saponara M, Guilleminault C. Rapid maxillary expansion in children with obstructive sleep apnea syndrome. *Sleep.* 2004;27(4):761–766

157. Villa MP, Malagola C, Pagani J, et al. Rapid maxillary expansion in children with obstructive sleep apnea syndrome: 12-month follow-up. *Sleep Med.* 2007;8(2):128–134

158. Pereira KD, Roebuck JC, Howell L. The effect of body position on sleep apnea in children younger than 3 years. *Arch Otolaryngol Head Neck Surg.* 2005;131(11): 1014–1016

159. Zhang XW, Li Y, Zhou F, Guo CK, Huang ZT. Association of body position with sleep architecture and respiratory disturbances in children with obstructive sleep apnea. *Acta Otolaryngol.* 2007;127(12):1321–1326

160. Dayyat E, Maarafeya MM, Capdevila OS, Kheirandish-Gozal L, Montgomery-Downs HE, Gozal D. Nocturnal body position in sleeping children with and without obstructive sleep apnea. *Pediatr Pulmonol.* 2007;42(4):374–379

161. Fernandes do Prado LB, Li X, Thompson R, Marcus CL. Body position and obstructive sleep apnea in children. *Sleep.* 2002;25(1): 66–71

162. Villa MP, Bernkopf E, Pagani J, Broia V, Montesano M, Ronchetti R. Randomized controlled study of an oral jaw-positioning appliance for the treatment of obstructive sleep apnea in children with malocclusion. *Am J Respir Crit Care Med.* 2002;165 (1):123–127

163. Ogden CL, Carroll MD, Curtin LR, McDowell MA, Tabak CJ, Flegal KM. Prevalence of overweight and obesity in the United States, 1999-2004. *JAMA.* 2006;295(13): 1549–1555

164. Urschitz MS, Guenther A, Eitner S, et al. Risk factors and natural history of habitual snoring. *Chest.* 2004;126(3):790–800

165. Urschitz MS, Eitner S, Wolff J, et al. Risk factors for sleep-related hypoxia in primary school children. *Pediatr Pulmonol.* 2007;42(9):805–812

166. Corbo GM, Forastiere F, Agabiti N, et al. Snoring in 9- to 15-year-old children: risk factors and clinical relevance. *Pediatrics.* 2001;108(5):1149–1154

167. Bidad K, Anari S, Aghamohamadi A, Gholami N, Zadhush S, Moaieri H. Prevalence and correlates of snoring in adolescents. *Iran J Allergy Asthma Immunol.* 2006;5(3):127–132

168. Stepanski E, Zayyad A, Nigro C, Lopata M, Basner R. Sleep-disordered breathing in a predominantly African-American pediatric population. *J Sleep Res.* 1999;8(1):65–70

169. Rudnick EF, Walsh JS, Hampton MC, Mitchell RB. Prevalence and ethnicity of sleep-disordered breathing and obesity in children. *Otolaryngol Head Neck Surg.* 2007;137(6):878–882

170. Verhulst SL, Schrauwen N, Haentjens D, et al. Sleep-disordered breathing in overweight and obese children and adolescents: prevalence, characteristics and the role of fat distribution. *Arch Dis Child.* 2007;92(3):205–208

171. Lam YY, Chan EY, Ng DK, et al. The correlation among obesity, apnea-hypopnea index, and tonsil size in children. *Chest.* 2006;130(6):1751–1756

172. Li AM, Au CT, So HK, Lau J, Ng PC, Wing YK. Prevalence and risk factors of habitual snoring in primary school children. *Chest.* 2010;138(3):519–527

173. Reade EP, Whaley C, Lin JJ, McKenney DW, Lee D, Perkin R. Hypopnea in pediatric patients with obesity hypertension. *Pediatr Nephrol.* 2004;19(9):1014–1020

174. Kaditis AG, Alexopoulos EI, Kostadima E, et al. Comparison of blood pressure measurements in children with and without habitual snoring. *Pediatr Pulmonol.* 2005;39(5):408–414

175. Kohyama J, Ohinata JS, Hasegawa T. Blood pressure in sleep disordered breathing. *Arch Dis Child.* 2003;88(2):139–142

176. Li AM, Au CT, Sung RY, et al. Ambulatory blood pressure in children with obstructive sleep apnoea: a community based study. *Thorax.* 2008;63(9):803–809

177. Amin R, Somers VK, McConnell K, et al. Activity-adjusted 24-hour ambulatory blood pressure and cardiac remodeling in children with sleep disordered breathing. *Hypertension.* 2008;51(1):84–91

178. Verhulst SL, Schrauwen N, Haentjens D, et al. Sleep-disordered breathing and the metabolic syndrome in overweight and obese children and adolescents. *J Pediatr.* 2007;150(6):608–612

179. Redline S, Storfer-Isser A, Rosen CL, et al. Association between metabolic syndrome and sleep-disordered breathing in adolescents. *Am J Respir Crit Care Med.* 2007; 176(4):401–408

180. Kaditis AG, Alexopoulos EI, Damani E, et al. Obstructive sleep-disordered breathing

and fasting insulin levels in nonobese children. *Pediatr Pulmonol.* 2005;40(6): 515–523

181. Tauman R, O'Brien LM, Ivanenko A, Gozal D. Obesity rather than severity of sleep-disordered breathing as the major determinant of insulin resistance and altered lipidemia in snoring children. *Pediatrics.* 2005;116(1). Available at: www.pediatrics. org/cgi/content/full/116/1/e66

182. de la Eva RC, Baur LA, Donaghue KC, Waters KA. Metabolic correlates with obstructive sleep apnea in obese subjects. *J Pediatr.* 2002;140(6):654–659

183. Kelly A, Dougherty S, Cucchiara A, Marcus CL, Brooks LJ. Catecholamines, adiponectin, and insulin resistance as measured by HOMA in children with obstructive sleep apnea. *Sleep.* 2010;33(9):1185–1191

184. Gozal D, Capdevila OS, Kheirandish-Gozal L. Metabolic alterations and systemic inflammation in obstructive sleep apnea among nonobese and obese prepubertal children. *Am J Respir Crit Care Med.* 2008; 177(10):1142–1149

185. Kheirandish-Gozal L, Sans Capdevila O, Kheirandish E, Gozal D. Elevated serum aminotransferase levels in children at risk for obstructive sleep apnea. *Chest.* 2008;133(1):92–99

186. Verhulst SL, Van Hoeck K, Schrauwen N, et al. Sleep-disordered breathing and uric acid in overweight and obese children and adolescents. *Chest.* 2007;132(1):76–80

187. Verhulst SL, Schrauwen N, Haentjens D, et al. Sleep-disordered breathing and systemic inflammation in overweight children and adolescents. *Int J Pediatr Obes.* 2008;3(4):234–239

188. Mulvaney SA, Kaemingk KL, Goodwin JL, Quan SF. Parent-rated behavior problems associated with overweight before and after controlling for sleep disordered breathing. *BMC Pediatr.* 2006;6:34

189. Owens JA, Mehlenbeck R, Lee J, King MM. Effect of weight, sleep duration, and comorbid sleep disorders on behavioral outcomes in children with sleep-disordered breathing. *Arch Pediatr Adolesc Med.* 2008; 162(4):313–321

190. Beebe DW, Ris MD, Kramer ME, Long E, Amin R. The association between sleep disordered breathing, academic grades, and cognitive and behavioral functioning among overweight subjects during middle to late childhood. *Sleep.* 2010;33(11):1447–1456

191. Roemmich JN, Barkley JE, D'Andrea L, et al. Increases in overweight after

adenotonsillectomy in overweight children with obstructive sleep-disordered breathing are associated with decreases in motor activity and hyperactivity. *Pediatrics.* 2006;117(2). Available at: www.pediatrics.org/cgi/content/full/117/2/e200

192. Carno MA, Ellis E, Anson E, et al. Symptoms of sleep apnea and polysomnography as predictors of poor quality of life in overweight children and adolescents. *J Pediatr Psychol.* 2008;33(3):269–278

193. Crabtree VM, Varni JW, Gozal D. Health-related quality of life and depressive symptoms in children with suspected sleep-disordered breathing. *Sleep.* 2004;27 (6):1131–1138

194. Shine NP, Lannigan FJ, Coates HL, Wilson A. Adenotonsillectomy for obstructive sleep apnea in obese children: effects on respiratory parameters and clinical outcome. *Arch Otolaryngol Head Neck Surg.* 2006;132(10):1123–1127

195. Spector A, Scheid S, Hassink S, Deutsch ES, Reilly JS, Cook SP. Adenotonsillectomy in the morbidly obese child. *Int J Pediatr Otorhinolaryngol.* 2003;67(4):359–364

196. Shine NP, Coates HL, Lannigan FJ, Duncan AW. Adenotonsillar surgery in morbidly obese children: routine elective admission of all patients to the intensive care unit is unnecessary. *Anaesth Intensive Care.* 2006;34(6):724–730

197. Verhulst SL, Franckx H, Van Gaal L, De Backer W, Desager K. The effect of weight loss on sleep-disordered breathing in obese teenagers. *Obesity (Silver Spring).* 2009;17(6):1178–1183

198. Kalra M, Inge T, Garcia V, et al. Obstructive sleep apnea in extremely overweight adolescents undergoing bariatric surgery. *Obes Res.* 2005;13(7):1175–1179

199. Sulit LG, Storfer-Isser A, Rosen CL, Kirchner HL, Redline S. Associations of obesity, sleep-disordered breathing, and wheezing in children. *Am J Respir Crit Care Med.* 2005;171(6):659–664

200. Dubern B, Tounian P, Medjadhi N, Maingot L, Girardet JP, Boulé M. Pulmonary function and sleep-related breathing disorders in severely obese children. *Clin Nutr.* 2006;25 (5):803–809

201. Anuntaseree W, Rookkapan K, Kuasirikul S, Thongsuksai P. Snoring and obstructive sleep apnea in Thai school-age children: prevalence and predisposing factors. *Pediatr Pulmonol.* 2001;32(3):222–227

202. Anuntaseree W, Kuasirikul S, Suntornlohanakul S. Natural history of snoring and obstructive sleep apnea in Thai school-age children. *Pediatr Pulmonol.* 2005; 39(5):415–420

203. Brunetti L, Rana S, Lospalluti ML, et al. Prevalence of obstructive sleep apnea syndrome in a cohort of 1,207 children of southern Italy. *Chest.* 2001;120(6):1930–1935

204. Ng DK, Kwok KL, Poon G, Chau KW. Habitual snoring and sleep bruxism in a paediatric outpatient population in Hong Kong. *Singapore Med J.* 2002;43(11): 554–556

205. Hultcrantz E, Löfstrand Tideström B. The development of sleep disordered breathing from 4 to 12 years and dental arch morphology. *Int J Pediatr Otorhinolaryngol.* 2009;73(9):1234–1241

206. Urschitz MS, Brockmann PE, Schlaud M, Poets CF. Population prevalence of obstructive sleep apnoea in a community of German third graders. *Eur Respir J.* 2010; 36(3):556–568

207. Akcay A, Kara CO, Dagdeviren E, Zencir M. Variation in tonsil size in 4- to 17-year-old schoolchildren. *J Otolaryngol.* 2006;35(4): 270–274

208. Alexopoulos EI, Kostadima E, Pagonari I, Zintzaras E, Gourgoulianis K, Kaditis AG. Association between primary nocturnal enuresis and habitual snoring in children. *Urology.* 2006;68(2):406–409

209. Archbold KH, Pituch KJ, Panahi P, Chervin RD. Symptoms of sleep disturbances among children at two general pediatric clinics. *J Pediatr.* 2002;140(1):97–102

210. Chng SY, Goh DY, Wang XS, Tan TN, Ong NB. Snoring and atopic disease: a strong association. *Pediatr Pulmonol.* 2004;38(3): 210–216

211. Ersu R, Arman AR, Save D, et al. Prevalence of snoring and symptoms of sleep-disordered breathing in primary school children in Istanbul. *Chest.* 2004;126(1): 19–24

212. Goodwin JL, Babar SI, Kaemingk KL, et al; Tucson Children's Assessment of Sleep Apnea Study. Symptoms related to sleep-disordered breathing in white and Hispanic children: the Tucson Children's Assessment of Sleep Apnea Study. *Chest.* 2003;124(1): 196–203

213. Gottlieb DJ, Vezina RM, Chase C, et al. Symptoms of sleep-disordered breathing in 5-year-old children are associated with sleepiness and problem behaviors. *Pediatrics.* 2003;112(4):870–877

214. Kuehni CE, Strippoli MP, Chauliac ES, Silverman M. Snoring in preschool children: prevalence, severity and risk factors. *Eur Respir J.* 2008;31(2):326–333

215. Liu X, Liu L, Owens JA, Kaplan DL. Sleep patterns and sleep problems among schoolchildren in the United States and China. *Pediatrics.* 2005;115(suppl 1):241–249

216. Löfstrand-Tideström B, Hultcrantz E. The development of snoring and sleep related breathing distress from 4 to 6 years in a cohort of Swedish children. *Int J Pediatr Otorhinolaryngol.* 2007;71(7):1025–1033

217. Lu LR, Peat JK, Sullivan CE. Snoring in preschool children: prevalence and association with nocturnal cough and asthma. *Chest.* 2003;124(2):587–593

218. Nelson S, Kulnis R. Snoring and sleep disturbance among children from an orthodontic setting. *Sleep Breath.* 2001;5(2): 63–70

219. Ng DK, Kwok KL, Cheung JM, et al. Prevalence of sleep problems in Hong Kong primary school children: a community-based telephone survey. *Chest.* 2005;128 (3):1315–1323

220. Perez-Chada D, Perez-Lloret S, Videla AJ, et al. Sleep disordered breathing and daytime sleepiness are associated with poor academic performance in teenagers. A study using the Pediatric Daytime Sleepiness Scale (PDSS). *Sleep.* 2007;30 (12):1698–1703

221. Petry C, Pereira MU, Pitrez PM, Jones MH, Stein RT. The prevalence of symptoms of sleep-disordered breathing in Brazilian schoolchildren. *J Pediatr (Rio J).* 2008;84 (2):123–129

222. Sahin U, Ozturk O, Ozturk M, Songur N, Bircan A, Akkaya A. Habitual snoring in primary school children: prevalence and association with sleep-related disorders and school performance. *Med Princ Pract.* 2009;18(6):458–465

223. Tafur A, Chérrez-Ojeda I, Patiño C, et al. Rhinitis symptoms and habitual snoring in Ecuadorian children. *Sleep Med.* 2009;10 (9):1035–1039

224. Zhang G, Spickett J, Rumchev K, Lee AH, Stick S. Snoring in primary school children and domestic environment: a Perth school based study. *Respir Res.* 2004;5:19

225. Beebe DW, Wells CT, Jeffries J, Chini B, Kalra M, Amin R. Neuropsychological effects of pediatric obstructive sleep apnea. *J Int Neuropsychol Soc.* 2004;10(7): 962–975

226. Blunden S, Lushington K, Lorenzen B, Martin J, Kennedy D. Neuropsychological and psychosocial function in children with a history of snoring or behavioral sleep problems. *J Pediatr.* 2005;146(6):780–786

227. Kurnatowski P, Putyński L, Lapienis M, Kowalska B. Neurocognitive abilities in children with adenotonsillar hypertrophy. *Int J Pediatr Otorhinolaryngol.* 2006;70(3): 419–424

228. Carvalho LB, Prado LF, Silva L, et al. Cognitive dysfunction in children with sleep-disordered breathing. *J Child Neurol.* 2005;20(5):400–404

229. Urschitz MS, Eitner S, Guenther A, et al. Habitual snoring, intermittent hypoxia, and impaired behavior in primary school children. *Pediatrics.* 2004;114(4):1041–1048

230. LeBourgeois MK, Avis K, Mixon M, Olmi J, Harsh J. Snoring, sleep quality, and sleepiness across attention-deficit/hyperactivity disorder subtypes. *Sleep.* 2004;27(3):520–525

231. Karpinski AC, Scullin MH, Montgomery-Downs HE. Risk for sleep-disordered breathing and executive function in preschoolers. *Sleep Med.* 2008;9(4):418–424

232. Hamasaki Uema SF, Nagata Pignatari SS, Fujita RR, Moreira GA, Pradella-Hallinan M, Weckx L. Assessment of cognitive learning function in children with obstructive sleep breathing disorders. *Braz J Otorhinolaryngol.* 2007;73(3):315–320

233. O'Brien LM, Tauman R, Gozal D. Sleep pressure correlates of cognitive and behavioral morbidity in snoring children. *Sleep.* 2004;27(2):279–282

234. Spruyt K, Capdevila OS, Kheirandish-Gozal L, Gozal D. Inefficient or insufficient encoding as potential primary deficit in neurodevelopmental performance among children with OSA. *Dev Neuropsychol.* 2009;34(5):601–614

235. Honaker SM, Gozal D, Bennett J, Capdevila OS, Spruyt K. Sleep-disordered breathing and verbal skills in school-aged community children. *Dev Neuropsychol.* 2009;34(5):588–600

236. Chervin RD, Archbold KH, Dillon JE, et al. Inattention, hyperactivity, and symptoms of sleep-disordered breathing. *Pediatrics.* 2002;109(3):449–456

237. Galland BC, Dawes PJ, Tripp EG, Taylor BJ. Changes in behavior and attentional capacity after adenotonsillectomy. *Pediatr Res.* 2006;59(5):711–716

238. Li HY, Huang YS, Chen NH, Fang TJ, Lee LA. Impact of adenotonsillectomy on behavior in children with sleep-disordered breathing. *Laryngoscope.* 2006;116(7):1142–1147

239. Golan N, Shahar E, Ravid S, Pillar G. Sleep disorders and daytime sleepiness in children with attention-deficit/hyperactive disorder. *Sleep.* 2004;27(2):261–266

240. Mitchell RB, Kelly J. Child behavior after adenotonsillectomy for obstructive sleep apnea syndrome. *Laryngoscope.* 2005;115(11):2051–2055

241. Mitchell RB, Kelly J. Behavioral changes in children with mild sleep-disordered breathing or obstructive sleep apnea after adenotonsillectomy. *Laryngoscope.* 2007;117(9):1685–1688

242. Rudnick EF, Mitchell RB. Behavior and obstructive sleep apnea in children: is obesity a factor? *Laryngoscope.* 2007;117(8):1463–1466

243. Goldstein NA, Post JC, Rosenfeld RM, Campbell TF. Impact of tonsillectomy and adenoidectomy on child behavior. *Arch Otolaryngol Head Neck Surg.* 2000;126(4):494–498

244. Rosen CL, Storfer-Isser A, Taylor HG, Kirchner HL, Emancipator JL, Redline S. Increased behavioral morbidity in school-aged children with sleep-disordered breathing. *Pediatrics.* 2004;114(6):1640–1648

245. Wei JL, Mayo MS, Smith HJ, Reese M, Weatherly RA. Improved behavior and sleep after adenotonsillectomy in children with sleep-disordered breathing. *Arch Otolaryngol Head Neck Surg.* 2007;133(10):974–979

246. Chervin RD, Dillon JE, Archbold KH, Ruzicka DL. Conduct problems and symptoms of sleep disorders in children. *J Am Acad Child Adolesc Psychiatry.* 2003;42(2):201–208

247. Amin RS, Kimball TR, Bean JA, et al. Left ventricular hypertrophy and abnormal ventricular geometry in children and adolescents with obstructive sleep apnea. *Am J Respir Crit Care Med.* 2002;165(10):1395–1399

248. Amin RS, Kimball TR, Kalra M, et al. Left ventricular function in children with sleep-disordered breathing. *Am J Cardiol.* 2005;95(6):801–804

249. Duman D, Naiboglu B, Esen HS, Toros SZ, Demirtunc R. Impaired right ventricular function in adenotonsillar hypertrophy. *Int J Cardiovasc Imaging.* 2008;24(3):261–267

250. Ugur MB, Dogan SM, Sogut A, et al. Effect of adenoidectomy and/or tonsillectomy on cardiac functions in children with obstructive sleep apnea. *ORL J Otorhinolaryngol Relat Spec.* 2008;70(3):202–208

251. Weber SA, Montovani JC, Matsubara B, Fioretto JR. Echocardiographic abnormalities in children with obstructive breathing disorders during sleep. *J Pediatr (Rio J).* 2007;83(6):518–522

252. Leung LC, Ng DK, Lau MW, et al. Twenty-four-hour ambulatory BP in snoring children with obstructive sleep apnea syndrome. *Chest.* 2006;130(4):1009–1017

253. Guilleminault C, Khramsov A, Stoohs RA, et al. Abnormal blood pressure in prepubertal children with sleep-disordered breathing. *Pediatr Res.* 2004;55(1):76–84

254. Amin RS, Carroll JL, Jeffries JL, et al. Twenty-four-hour ambulatory blood pressure in children with sleep-disordered breathing. *Am J Respir Crit Care Med.* 2004;169(8):950–956

255. Enright PL, Goodwin JL, Sherrill DL, Quan JR, Quan SF; Tucson Children's Assessment of Sleep Apnea study. Blood pressure elevation associated with sleep-related breathing disorder in a community sample of white and Hispanic children: the Tucson Children's Assessment of Sleep Apnea study. *Arch Pediatr Adolesc Med.* 2003;157(9):901–904

256. Xu Z, Cheuk DK, Lee SL. Clinical evaluation in predicting childhood obstructive sleep apnea. *Chest.* 2006;130(6):1765–1771

257. Jain A, Sahni JK. Polysomnographic studies in children undergoing adenoidectomy and/or tonsillectomy. *J Laryngol Otol.* 2002;116(9):711–715

258. Li AM, Wong E, Kew J, Hui S, Fok TF. Use of tonsil size in the evaluation of obstructive sleep apnoea. *Arch Dis Child.* 2002;87(2):156–159

259. Kawashima S, Niikuni N, Chia-hung L, et al. Cephalometric comparisons of craniofacial and upper airway structures in young children with obstructive sleep apnea syndrome. *Ear Nose Throat J.* 2000;79(7):499–502, 505–506

260. Kawashima S, Peltomäki T, Sakata H, Mori K, Happonen RP, Rönning O. Craniofacial morphology in preschool children with sleep-related breathing disorder and hypertrophy of tonsils. *Acta Paediatr.* 2002;91(1):71–77

261. Kikuchi M, Higurashi N, Miyazaki S, Itasaka Y, Chiba S, Nezu H. Facial pattern categories of sleep breathing-disordered children using Ricketts analysis. *Psychiatry Clin Neurosci.* 2002;56(3):329–330

262. Kulnis R, Nelson S, Strohl K, Hans M. Cephalometric assessment of snoring and nonsnoring children. *Chest.* 2000;118(3):596–603

263. Zucconi M, Caprioglio A, Calori G, et al. Craniofacial modifications in children with habitual snoring and obstructive sleep apnoea: a case-control study. *Eur Respir J.* 1999;13(2):411–417

264. Noehren A, Brockmann PE, Urschitz MS, Sokollik C, Schlaud M, Poets CF. Detection of respiratory events using pulse rate in children with and without obstructive sleep apnea. *Pediatr Pulmonol.* 2010;45(5):459–468

265. Katz ES, Lutz J, Black C, Marcus CL. Pulse transit time as a measure of arousal and

respiratory effort in children with sleep-disordered breathing. *Pediatr Res.* 2003; 53(4):580–588

266. Foo JY, Bradley AP, Wilson SJ, Williams GR, Dakin C, Cooper DM. Screening of obstructive and central apnoea/hypopnoea in children using variability: a preliminary study. *Acta Paediatr.* 2006;95(5): 561–564

267. Foo JY, Lim CS. Development of a home screening system for pediatric respiratory sleep studies. *Telemed J E Health.* 2006; 12(6):698–701

268. Tauman R, O'Brien LM, Mast BT, Holbrook CR, Gozal D. Peripheral arterial tonometry events and electroencephalographic arousals in children. *Sleep.* 2004;27(3):502–506

269. Hill CA, Litvak A, Canapari C, et al. A pilot study to identify pre- and peri-operative risk factors for airway complications following adenotonsillectomy for treatment of severe pediatric OSA. *Int J Pediatr Otorhinolaryngol.* 2011;75(11):1385–1390

270. Jaryszak EM, Shah RK, Vanison CC, Lander L, Choi SS. Polysomnographic variables predictive of adverse respiratory events after pediatric adenotonsillectomy. *Arch Otolaryngol Head Neck Surg.* 2011;137(1): 15–18

271. Koomson A, Morin I, Brouillette R, Brown KA. Children with severe OSAS who have adenotonsillectomy in the morning are less likely to have postoperative desaturation than those operated in the afternoon. *Can J Anaesth.* 2004;51(1):62–67

272. Ma AL, Lam YY, Wong SF, Ng DK, Chan CH. Risk factors for post-operative complications in Chinese children with tonsillectomy and adenoidectomy for obstructive sleep apnea syndrome [published online ahead of print July 30, 2011]. *Sleep Breath.*

273. Sanders JC, King MA, Mitchell RB, Kelly JP. Perioperative complications of adenotonsillectomy in children with obstructive sleep apnea syndrome. *Anesth Analg.* 2006;103(5):1115–1121

274. Schroeder JW, Jr;Anstead AS, Wong H. Complications in children who electively remain intubated after adenotonsillectomy for severe obstructive sleep apnea. *Int J Pediatr Otorhinolaryngol.* 2009;73(8):1095–1099

275. Dillon JE, Blunden S, Ruzicka DL, et al. DSM-IV diagnoses and obstructive sleep apnea in children before and 1 year after adenotonsillectomy. *J Am Acad Child Adolesc Psychiatry.* 2007;46(11):1425–1436

276. Guilleminault C, Li KK, Khramtsov A, Pelayo R, Martinez S. Sleep disordered breathing: surgical outcomes in prepubertal children. *Laryngoscope.* 2004;114(1):132–137

277. Tal A, Bar A, Leiberman A, Tarasiuk A. Sleep characteristics following adenotonsillectomy in children with obstructive sleep apnea syndrome. *Chest.* 2003;124(3): 948–953

278. Walker P, Whitehead B, Gulliver T. Polysomnographic outcome of adenotonsillectomy for obstructive sleep apnea in children under 5 years old. *Otolaryngol Head Neck Surg.* 2008;139 (1):83–86

279. Mitchell RB, Kelly J. Adenotonsillectomy for obstructive sleep apnea in obese children. *Otolaryngol Head Neck Surg.* 2004;131(1):104–108

280. Mitchell RB, Kelly J. Outcome of adenotonsillectomy for severe obstructive sleep apnea in children. *Int J Pediatr Otorhinolaryngol.* 2004;68(11):1375–1379

(Continued from first page)

www.pediatrics.org/cgi/doi/10.1542/peds.2012-1672

doi:10.1542/peds.2012-1672

PEDIATRICS (ISSN Numbers: Print, 0031-4005; Online, 1098-4275).

Sleep Apnea Clinical Practice Guideline
Quick Reference Tools

- Action Statement Summary
  — Diagnosis and Management of Childhood Obstructive Sleep Apnea Syndrome
- *ICD-10-CM* Coding Quick Reference for Sleep Apnea
- AAP Patient Education Handout
  — *Sleep Apnea and Your Child*

Action Statement Summary

Diagnosis and Management of Childhood Obstructive Sleep Apnea Syndrome

Key Action Statement 1: Screening for OSAS

As part of routine health maintenance visits, clinicians should inquire whether the child or adolescent snores. If the answer is affirmative or if a child or adolescent presents with signs or symptoms of OSAS (Table 2), clinicians should perform a more focused evaluation. (Evidence Quality: Grade B, Recommendation Strength: Recommendation.)

Key Action Statement 2A: Polysomnography

If a child or adolescent snores on a regular basis and has any of the complaints or findings shown in Table 2, clinicians should either (1) obtain a polysomnogram (Evidence Quality A, Key Action strength: Recommendation) OR (2) refer the patient to a sleep specialist or otolaryngologist for a more extensive evaluation (Evidence quality D, Key Action strength: Option). (Evidence Quality: Grade A for polysomnography; Grade D for specialist referral, Recommendation Strength: Recommendation.)

Key Action Statement 2B: Alternative Testing

If polysomnography is not available, then clinicians may order alternative diagnostic tests, such as nocturnal video recording, nocturnal oximetry, daytime nap polysomnography, or ambulatory polysomnography. (Evidence Quality: Grade C, Recommendation Strength: Option.)

Key Action Statement 3: Adenotonsillectomy

If a child is determined to have OSAS, has a clinical examination consistent with adenotonsillar hypertrophy, and does not have a contraindication to surgery (see Table 3), the clinician should recommend adenotonsillectomy as the first line of treatment. If the child has OSAS but does not have adenotonsillar hypertrophy, other treatment should be considered (see Key Action Statement 6). Clinical judgment is required to determine the benefits of adenotonsillectomy compared with other treatments in obese children with varying degrees of adenotonsillar hypertrophy. (Evidence Quality: Grade B, Recommendation Strength: Recommendation.)

Key Action Statement 4: High-Risk Patients Undergoing Adenotonsillectomy

Clinicians should monitor high-risk patients (Table 5) undergoing adenotonsillectomy as inpatients postoperatively. (Evidence Quality: Grade B, Recommendation Strength: Recommendation.)

Key Action Statement 5: Reevaluation

Clinicians should clinically reassess all patients with OSAS for persisting signs and symptoms after therapy to determine whether further treatment is required. (Evidence Quality: Grade B, Recommendation Strength: Recommendation.)

Key Action Statement 5B: Reevaluation of High-Risk Patients

Clinicians should reevaluate high-risk patients for persistent OSAS after adenotonsillectomy, including those who had a significantly abnormal baseline polysomnogram, have sequelae of OSAS, are obese, or remain symptomatic after treatment, with an objective test (see Key Action Statement 2) or refer such patients to a sleep specialist. (Evidence Quality: Grade B, Recommendation Strength: Recommendation.)

Key Action Statement 6: CPAP

Clinicians should refer patients for CPAP management if symptoms/signs (Table 2) or objective evidence of OSAS persists after adenotonsillectomy or if adenotonsillectomy is not performed. (Evidence Quality: Grade B, Recommendation Strength: Recommendation.)

Key Action Statement 7: Weight Loss

Clinicians should recommend weight loss in addition to other therapy if a child/adolescent with OSAS is overweight or obese. (Evidence Quality: Grade C, Recommendation Strength: Recommendation.)

Key Action Statement 8: Intranasal Corticosteroids

Clinicians may prescribe topical intranasal corticosteroids for children with mild OSAS in whom adenotonsillectomy is contraindicated or for children with mild postoperative OSAS. (Evidence Quality: Grade B, Recommendation Strength: Option.)

Coding Quick Reference for Sleep Apnea
ICD-10-CM
G47.30 Sleep apnea, unspecified
G47.31 Primary central sleep apnea
G47.33 Obstructive sleep apnea (adult) (pediatric)   _____(Code additional underlying conditions.)
J35.3   Hypertrophy of tonsils with hypertrophy of adenoids
E66.01 Morbid (severe) obesity due to excess calories   **E66.09** Other obesity due to excess calories   **E66.3**   Overweight   **E66.8**   Other obesity   **E66.9**   Obesity, unspecified

Sleep Apnea and Your Child

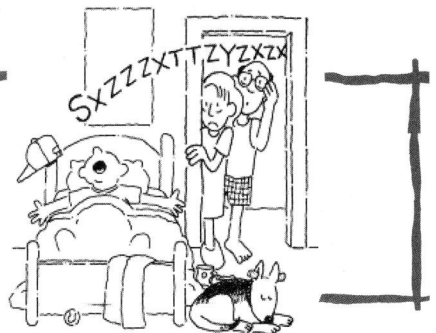

Does your child snore a lot? Does he sleep restlessly? Does he have difficulty breathing, or does he gasp or choke, while he sleeps?

If your child has these symptoms, he may have a condition known as sleep apnea.

Sleep apnea is a common problem that affects an estimated 2% of all children, including many who are undiagnosed.

If not treated, sleep apnea can lead to a variety of problems. These include heart, behavior, learning, and growth problems.

How do I know if my child has sleep apnea?

Symptoms of sleep apnea include

- Frequent snoring
- Problems breathing during the night
- Sleepiness during the day
- Difficulty paying attention
- Behavior problems

If you notice any of these symptoms, let your pediatrician know as soon as possible. Your pediatrician may recommend an overnight sleep study called a *polysomnogram.* Overnight polysomnograms are conducted at hospitals and major medical centers. During the study, medical staff will watch your child sleep. Several sensors will be attached to your child to monitor breathing, oxygenation, and brain waves. An electroencephalogram (EEG) is a test that measures brain waves.

The results of the study will show whether your child suffers from sleep apnea. Other specialists, such as pediatric pulmonologists, otolaryngologists, neurologists, and pediatricians with specialty training in sleep disorders, may help your pediatrician make the diagnosis.

What causes sleep apnea?

Many children with sleep apnea have larger tonsils and adenoids.

Tonsils are the round, reddish masses on each side of your child's throat. They help fight infections in the body. You can only see the adenoid with an x-ray or special mirror. It lies in the space between the nose and throat.

Large tonsils and adenoid may block a child's airway while she sleeps. This causes her to snore and wake up often during the night. However, not every child with large tonsils and adenoid has sleep

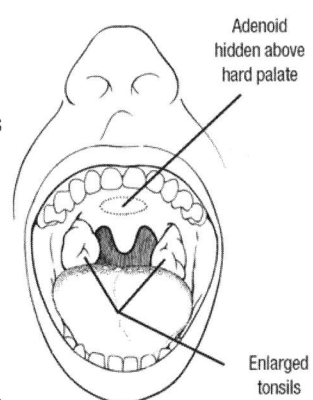

Adenoid hidden above hard palate

Enlarged tonsils

apnea. A sleep study can tell your doctor whether your child has sleep apnea or if she is simply snoring.

Children born with other medical conditions, such as Down syndrome, cerebral palsy, or craniofacial (skull and face) abnormalities, are at higher risk for sleep apnea. Overweight children are also more likely to suffer from sleep apnea.

How is sleep apnea treated?

The most common way to treat sleep apnea is to remove your child's tonsils and adenoid. This surgery is called a tonsillectomy and adenoidectomy. It is highly effective in treating sleep apnea.

Another effective treatment is nasal continuous positive airway pressure (CPAP), which requires the child to wear a mask while he sleeps. The mask delivers steady air pressure through the child's nose, allowing him to breathe comfortably. Continuous positive airway pressure is usually used in children who do not improve after tonsillectomy and adenoidectomy, or who are not candidates for tonsillectomy and adenoidectomy.

Children who may need additional treatment include children who are overweight or suffering from another complicating condition. Overweight children will improve if they lose weight, but may need to use CPAP until the weight is lost.

Remember

A good night's sleep is important to good health. If your child suffers from the symptoms of sleep apnea, talk with your pediatrician. A proper diagnosis and treatment can mean restful nights and restful days for your child and your family.

From your doctor

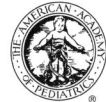

American Academy of Pediatrics

DEDICATED TO THE HEALTH OF ALL CHILDREN™

The American Academy of Pediatrics is an organization of 60,000 primary care pediatricians, pediatric medical subspecialists, and pediatric surgical specialists dedicated to the health, safety, and well-being of infants, children, adolescents, and young adults.

American Academy of Pediatrics
Web site — www.HealthyChildren.org

Reaffirmation of AAP Clinical Practice Guideline: The Diagnosis and Management of the Initial Urinary Tract Infection in Febrile Infants and Young Children 2–24 Months of Age

- *Reaffirmation of AAP Clinical Practice Guideline*

- *Clinical Practice Guideline*
  - *PPI: AAP Partnership for Policy Implementation See Appendix 2 for more information.*

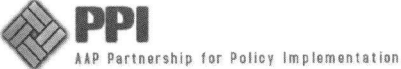

- *Technical Report*
  - *PPI: AAP Partnership for Policy Implementation See Appendix 2 for more information.*

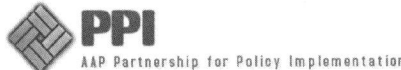

- *2011 Commentary*

Readers of this clinical practice guideline are urged to review the technical report to enhance the evidence-based decision-making process. The full technical report is available following the clinical practice guideline and on the companion eBook.

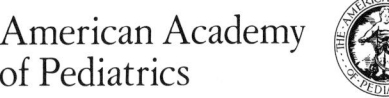

CLINICAL PRACTICE GUIDELINE   Guidance for the Clinician in Rendering Pediatric Care

American Academy
of Pediatrics

DEDICATED TO THE HEALTH OF ALL CHILDREN™

Reaffirmation of AAP Clinical Practice Guideline: The Diagnosis and Management of the Initial Urinary Tract Infection in Febrile Infants and Young Children 2–24 Months of Age

SUBCOMMITTEE ON URINARY TRACT INFECTION

It is the policy of the American Academy of Pediatrics to reassess clinical practice guidelines (CPGs) every 5 years and retire, revise, or reaffirm them. The members of the urinary tract infection (UTI) subcommittee who developed the 2011 UTI CPG[1] have reviewed the literature published since 2011 along with unpublished manuscripts and the status of some clinical trials still in progress. With this article, we reaffirm the 2011 UTI CPG and provide an updated review of the supporting evidence. For the convenience of the reader, we reiterate the 7 Key Action Statements here to obviate the need to consult the 2011 UTI CPG, although interested readers may want to review the text of the guideline[1] and/or its accompanying technical report.[2]

ACTION STATEMENT 1

If a clinician decides that a febrile infant with no apparent source for the fever requires antimicrobial therapy to be administered because of ill appearance or another pressing reason, the clinician should ensure that a urine specimen is obtained for both culture and urinalysis before an antimicrobial is administered; the specimen needs to be obtained through catheterization or suprapubic aspiration (SPA), because the diagnosis of UTI cannot be established reliably through culture of urine collected in a bag (evidence quality: A; strong recommendation).

Comment

A key to an accurate diagnosis of UTI is obtaining a sample of urine for culture with minimal contamination before starting antimicrobial

This document is copyrighted and is property of the American Academy of Pediatrics and its Board of Directors. All authors have filed conflict of interest statements with the American Academy of Pediatrics. Any conflicts have been resolved through a process approved by the Board of Directors. The American Academy of Pediatrics has neither solicited nor accepted any commercial involvement in the development of the content of this publication.

The recommendations in this practice guideline do not indicate an exclusive course of treatment or serve as a standard of medical care. Variations, taking into account individual circumstances, may be appropriate.

All clinical practice guidelines from the American Academy of Pediatrics automatically expire 5 years after publication unless reaffirmed, revised, or retired at or before that time.

DOI: 10.1542/peds.2016-3026

PEDIATRICS (ISSN Numbers: Print, 0031-4005; Online, 1098-4275).

Copyright © 2016 by the American Academy of Pediatrics

FINANCIAL DISCLOSURE: The authors have indicated they do not have a financial relationship relevant to this article to disclose.

FUNDING: No external funding.

POTENTIAL CONFLICT OF INTEREST: The authors have indicated they have no potential conflicts of interest to disclose.

To cite: AAP SUBCOMMITTEE ON URINARY TRACT INFECTION. Reaffirmation of AAP Clinical Practice Guideline: The Diagnosis and Management of the Initial Urinary Tract Infection in Febrile Infants and Young Children 2–24 Months of Age. *Pediatrics.* 2016;138(6):e20163026

agents. Urine collected in a bag or via a clean catch method is suitable for urinalysis (see Action Statement 2, Option 2), but such specimens (especially urine collected in a bag) are less appropriate for culture. If a culture obtained by bag is positive, the likelihood of a false positive is extremely high, so the result must be confirmed by culturing urine obtained by a more reliable method; if an antimicrobial agent is present in the urine, the opportunity for confirmation is likely to be lost.

Although samples of urine obtained by transurethral catheterization may be contaminated by urethral flora, meticulous technique can reduce this possibility. To avoid contamination, 2 practical steps should be implemented: (1) the first few milliliters obtained by catheter should be discarded (allowed to fall outside of the sterile collecting vessel) and only the subsequent urine cultured; and (2) if the attempt at catheterization is unsuccessful, a new, clean catheter should be used (aided, in girls, by leaving the initial catheter in place as a marker).

ACTION STATEMENT 2

If a clinician assesses a febrile infant with no apparent source for the fever as not being so ill as to require immediate antimicrobial therapy, then the clinician should assess the likelihood of UTI.

Action Statement 2a. If the clinician determines the febrile infant to have a low likelihood of UTI (see text), then clinical follow-up monitoring without testing is sufficient (evidence quality: A; strong recommendation).

Action Statement 2b. If the clinician determines that the febrile infant is not in a low-risk group (see below), then there are 2 choices (evidence quality: A; strong recommendation).

Option 1 is to obtain a urine specimen through catheterization or SPA for culture and urinalysis.

Option 2 is to obtain a urine specimen through the most convenient means and to perform a urinalysis. If the urinalysis results suggest a UTI (positive leukocyte esterase test results or nitrite test or microscopic analysis results for leukocytes or bacteria), then a urine specimen should be obtained through catheterization or SPA and cultured; if urinalysis of fresh (less than 1 hour since void) urine yields negative leukocyte esterase and nitrite results, then it is reasonable to monitor the clinical course without initiating antimicrobial therapy, recognizing that a negative urinalysis does not rule out a UTI with certainty.

Comment

When the patient's degree of illness does not warrant immediate antimicrobial treatment and the risk of UTI is extremely low, the patient may be observed without assessing the urine. (The risk assessment tables in the 2011 UTI CPG have been simplified into algorithm form.[3]) If there is a low but real risk of infection, then either the best possible specimen should be obtained for urinalysis and culture, or a sample of urine obtained by a convenient method and a judgment made about culturing the urine dependent on the findings of the urinalysis or dipstick. A positive urinalysis provides sufficient concern to mandate a properly obtained urine specimen. This 2-step process (Option 2) is not only suitable for office practice but has been demonstrated to be feasible and beneficial in a busy pediatric emergency department, with the catheterization rate decreasing from

63% to fewer than 30% without increasing length of stay or missing UTIs.[4]

ACTION STATEMENT 3

To establish the diagnosis of UTI, clinicians should require both urinalysis results that suggest infection (pyuria and/or bacteriuria) and the presence of at least 50 000 colony-forming units (cfu) per milliliter of a uropathogen cultured from a urine specimen obtained through transurethral catheterization or SPA (evidence quality: C; recommendation).

Comment

The thrust of this key action statement is that the diagnosis of UTI in febrile infants is signaled by the presence of both bacteriuria and pyuria. In general, pyuria without bacteriuria is insufficient to make a diagnosis of UTI because it is nonspecific and occurs in the absence of infection (eg, Kawasaki disease, chemical urethritis, streptococcal infections). Likewise, bacteriuria, without pyuria is attributable to external contamination, asymptomatic bacteriuria, or, rarely, very early infection (before the onset of inflammation). Non–*Escherichia coli* isolates are less frequently associated with pyuria than *E coli*,[5] but the significance of this association is not clear at present. Non–*E coli* uropathogens are of concern because they are more likely to result in scarring than *E coli*,[6] but animal studies demonstrate the host inflammatory response to be what causes scarring rather than the presence of organisms.[7] Moreover, the rate of asymptomatic bacteriuria is sufficient to account for the lack of association with pyuria.

The remaining question is what constitutes "significant" bacteriuria and "significant" pyuria. In 1994, by using single versus multiple organisms to distinguish true UTI from contamination, 50 000 cfu/mL was proposed as the appropriate threshold for specimens obtained by catheterization,[8] recommended in the 2011 UTI CPG and implemented in the Randomized Intervention for Children with Vesicoureteral Reflux (RIVUR) trial.[9] Lower colony counts are sufficient if the urine specimen is obtained by SPA and, thus, less likely to be contaminated, but most (80%) cases of UTI documented with urine obtained by SPA have 10^5 cfu/mL or more. Colony counts lower than 50 000 cfu/mL are currently being considered for the diagnosis of UTI.[10] If 10 000 cfu/mL coupled with symptoms (eg, fever) and evidence of inflammation (pyuria) proves both sensitive and specific, this threshold would be of particular assistance to clinicians who use laboratories that do not specify colony counts between 10 000 and 100 000 cfu/mL and, thereby, make the criterion of 50 000 cfu/mL difficult to use.

Significant pyuria is ≥10 white blood cells/mm^3 on an "enhanced urinalysis" or ≥5 white blood cells per high power field on a centrifuged specimen of urine or any leukocyte esterase on a dipstick.

ACTION STATEMENT 4

Action Statement 4a. When initiating treatment, the clinician should base the choice of route of administration on practical considerations: initiating treatment orally or parenterally is equally efficacious. The clinician should base the choice of agent on local antimicrobial sensitivity patterns (if available) and should adjust the choice according to sensitivity testing of the isolated uropathogen (evidence quality: A; strong recommendation).

Action Statement 4b. The clinician should choose 7 to 14 days as the duration of antimicrobial therapy (evidence quality B; recommendation).

Comment

Basing the choice of an initial antimicrobial agent on local sensitivity patterns can be difficult because applicable information may not be available. Whether the child has received antimicrobial therapy in the recent past should be considered. This exposure constitutes a risk factor for resistance to the recently prescribed antimicrobial. Further delineation of treatment duration has not been forthcoming, but a randomized controlled trial is currently under way comparing the effectiveness of 5 days versus 10 days of treatment.[11]

Note: The dose of ceftriaxone in Table 2 should be 50 mg/kg, every 24 h.

ACTION STATEMENT 5

Febrile infants with UTIs should undergo renal and bladder ultrasonography (RBUS) (evidence quality: C; recommendation).

Comment

As noted in the 2011 CPG, it is important that the study be a renal and bladder ultrasonogram, not a limited renal ultrasonogram. Ideally, the patient should be well-hydrated for the examination and the bladder should be evaluated while distended. Concern has been raised that RBUS is not effective to detect vesicoureteral reflux (VUR), as it is frequently normal in infants with low-grade VUR and even in some who have high-grade VUR. Moreover, nonspecific RBUS findings, such as mild renal pelvic or ureteral distention, are common and are not necessarily associated with reflux. However, low-grade VUR is generally not considered of concern for renal damage, and most studies (other than the RIVUR trial[9]) have demonstrated continuous antimicrobial prophylaxis

(CAP) to lack benefit in this group.[1,2] Although RBUS is not invariably abnormal in infants with grades IV and V VUR, it does identify most, and, of particular importance, an abnormal RBUS is a major risk factor for scarring.[6]

ACTION STATEMENT 6

Action Statement 6a. Voiding cystourethrography (VCUG) should not be performed routinely after the first febrile UTI; VCUG is indicated if RBUS reveals hydronephrosis, scarring, or other findings that would suggest either high-grade VUR or obstructive uropathy, as well as in other atypical or complex clinical circumstances (evidence quality B; recommendation).

Action Statement 6b. Further evaluation should be conducted if there is a recurrence of febrile UTI (evidence quality: X; recommendation).

Comment

For decades, UTIs in infants were considered harbingers of underlying anatomic and/or physiologic abnormalities, so RBUS and VCUG were recommended to be performed routinely. VUR was a particular concern; CAP was assumed to be effective in preventing UTI and became standard practice when VUR was discovered. In the years leading up to the 2011 guideline, randomized controlled trials of CAP were performed. Authors of the 6 studies published in 2006-2010 graciously provided data to the guideline committee, permitting a meta-analysis of data specifically targeting febrile infants 2 to 24 months of age. CAP was not demonstrated to be effective, so the need to identify VUR by routine voiding cystourethrography was discouraged.[1,2] A recent large trial in the United States, the RIVUR trial, concluded that CAP was of benefit, but, to prevent 1 UTI recurrence required 5840 doses of antimicrobial and did not reduce the rate of renal scarring.[9]

Since the publication of the 2011 guideline, multiple studies have demonstrated that abnormalities are missed by the selective imaging recommended in the guideline; however, there is no evidence that identifying these missed abnormalities is of sufficient clinical benefit to offset the cost, discomfort, and radiation.[12] Compared with performing the full array of imaging tests, the radiation burden incurred with the application of the guideline has been calculated to be reduced by 93%.[13] Moreover, in population studies, the significance of VUR and the value of treating VUR have been questioned.[14,15]

The authors of the RIVUR trial and its companion study, Careful Urinary Tract Infection Evaluation, have called attention to bowel/bladder dysfunction (BBD) as a major risk factor for UTI recurrences and recognize that, in children who have a UTI recurrence, evaluation for BBD (ie, constipation), rather than for VUR, can be performed by nonspecialists and does not incur high cost, cause discomfort, or require radiation.[16] BBD has long been underappreciated and deserves greater consideration.

ACTION STATEMENT 7

After confirmation of UTI, the clinician should instruct parents or guardians to seek prompt medical evaluation (ideally within 48 hours) for future febrile illnesses to ensure that recurrent infections can be detected and treated promptly (evidence quality: C; recommendation).

Comment

Prompt treatment is of clinical benefit to the child with the acute infection. What has been controversial is the definition of "prompt" and the relationship to renal scarring. A recent study identified that the median time to treatment was shorter in infants who did not incur a scar than in those who did (48 vs 72 hours). The study also noted that the rate of scarring increased minimally between days 1 and 2 and between days 2 and 3 but was much higher thereafter.[17]

SUBCOMMITTEE ON URINARY TRACT INFECTION, 2009-2011

Kenneth B. Roberts, MD, FAAP Chair
Stephen M. Downs, MD, MS, FAAP
S. Maria E. Finnell, MD, MS, FAAP
*Stanley Hellerstein, MD (deceased)
Linda D. Shortliffe, MD
Ellen R. Wald, MD, FAAP, Vice-Chair
J. Michael Zerin, MD

STAFF

Kymika Okechukwu, MPA, Manager, Evidence-Based Practice Initiatives

---

ABBREVIATIONS

BBD: bowel/bladder dysfunction
CAP: continuous antimicrobial prophylaxis
cfu: colony-forming units
CPG: clinical practice guideline
RBUS: renal and bladder ultrasonography
RIVUR: Randomized Intervention for Children with Vesicoureteral Reflux
SPA: suprapubic aspiration
UTI: urinary tract infection
VCUG: voiding cystourethrography
VUR: vesicoureteral reflux

REFERENCES

1. Roberts KB; Subcommittee on Urinary Tract Infection, Steering Committee on Quality Improvement and Management. Urinary tract infection: clinical practice guideline for the diagnosis and management of the initial UTI in febrile infants and children 2 to 24 months. *Pediatrics*. 2011;128(3):595–610

2. Finnell SM, Carroll AE, Downs SM; Subcommittee on Urinary Tract Infection. Technical report—Diagnosis and management of an initial UTI in febrile infants and young children. *Pediatrics*. 2011;128(3). Available at: www.pediatrics.org/cgi/content/full/128/3/e749 PubMed

3. Roberts KB. Revised AAP Guideline on UTI in Febrile Infants and Young Children. *Am Fam Physician*. 2012;86(10):940–946

4. Lavelle JM, Blackstone MM, Funari MK, et al. Two-step process for ED UTI screening in febrile young children: reducing catheterization rates. *Pediatrics*. 2016;138(1):e20153023

5. Shaikh N, Shope TR, Hoberman A, Vigliotti A, Kurs-Lasky M, Martin JM. Association between uropathogen and pyuria. *Pediatrics*. 2016;138(1):e20160087

6. Shaikh N, Craig JC, Rovers MM, et al. Identification of children and adolescents at risk for renal scarring after a first urinary tract infection: a meta-analysis with individual patient data. *JAMA Pediatr*. 2014;168(10):893–900

7. Glauser MP, Meylan P, Bille J. The inflammatory response and tissue damage. The example of renal scars following acute renal infection. *Pediatr Nephrol*. 1987;1(4):615–622

8. Hoberman A, Wald ER, Reynolds EA, Penchansky L, Charron M. Pyuria and bacteriuria in urine specimens obtained by catheter from young children with fever. *J Pediatr*. 1994;124(4):513–519

9. Hoberman A, Greenfield SP, Mattoo TK, et al; RIVUR Trial Investigators. Antimicrobial prophylaxis for children with vesicoureteral reflux. *N Engl J Med*. 2014;370(25):2367–2376

10. Tullus K. Low urinary bacterial counts: do they count? *Pediatr Nephrol*. 2016;31(2):171–174

11. Hoberman A. The SCOUT study: short course therapy for urinary tract infections in children. Available at: https://clinicaltrials.gov/ct2/show/

NCT01595529. Accessed October 14, 2016

12. Narchi H, Marah M, Khan AA, et al Renal tract abnormalities missed in a historical cohort of your children with UTI if the NICE and AAP imaging guidelines were applied. *J Pediatr Urol*. 2015;11(5):252.e1–7

13. La Scola C, De Mutiis C, Hewitt IK, et al. Different guidelines for imaging after first UTI in febrile infants: yield, cost, and radiation. *Pediatrics*. 2013;131(3).

Available at: www.pediatrics.org/cgi/content/full/131/3/e665 PubMed

14. Salo J, Ikäheimo R, Tapiainen T, Uhari M. Childhood urinary tract infections as a cause of chronic kidney disease. *Pediatrics*. 2011;128(5):840–847

15. Craig JC, Williams GJ. Denominators do matter: it's a myth—urinary tract infection does not cause chronic kidney disease. *Pediatrics*. 2011;128(5):984–985

16. Shaikh N, Hoberman A, Keren R, et al. Recurrent urinary tract infections in children with bladder and bowel dysfunction. *Pediatrics*. 2016;137(1):e20152982

17. Shaikh N, Mattoo TK, Keren R, et al. Early antibiotic treatment for pediatric febrile urinary tract infection and renal scarring. *JAMA Pediatr*. 2016;170(9):848–854

CLINICAL PRACTICE GUIDELINE

Urinary Tract Infection: Clinical Practice Guideline for the Diagnosis and Management of the Initial UTI in Febrile Infants and Children 2 to 24 Months

SUBCOMMITTEE ON URINARY TRACT INFECTION, STEERING COMMITTEE ON QUALITY IMPROVEMENT AND MANAGEMENT

KEY WORDS
urinary tract infection, infants, children, vesicoureteral reflux, voiding cystourethrography

ABBREVIATIONS
SPA—suprapubic aspiration
AAP—American Academy of Pediatrics
UTI—urinary tract infection
RCT—randomized controlled trial
CFU—colony-forming unit
VUR—vesicoureteral reflux
WBC—white blood cell
RBUS—renal and bladder ultrasonography
VCUG—voiding cystourethrography

www.pediatrics.org/cgi/doi/10.1542/peds.2011-1330

doi:10.1542/peds.2011-1330

PEDIATRICS (ISSN Numbers: Print, 0031-4005; Online, 1098-4275).

COMPANION PAPERS: Companions to this article can be found on pages 572 and e749, and online at www.pediatrics.org/cgi/doi/10.1542/peds.2011-1818 and www.pediatrics.org/cgi/doi/10.1542/peds.2011-1332.

abstract

OBJECTIVE: To revise the American Academy of Pediatrics practice parameter regarding the diagnosis and management of initial urinary tract infections (UTIs) in febrile infants and young children.

METHODS: Analysis of the medical literature published since the last version of the guideline was supplemented by analysis of data provided by authors of recent publications. The strength of evidence supporting each recommendation and the strength of the recommendation were assessed and graded.

RESULTS: Diagnosis is made on the basis of the presence of both pyuria and at least 50 000 colonies per mL of a single uropathogenic organism in an appropriately collected specimen of urine. After 7 to 14 days of antimicrobial treatment, close clinical follow-up monitoring should be maintained to permit prompt diagnosis and treatment of recurrent infections. Ultrasonography of the kidneys and bladder should be performed to detect anatomic abnormalities. Data from the most recent 6 studies do not support the use of antimicrobial prophylaxis to prevent febrile recurrent UTI in infants without vesicoureteral reflux (VUR) or with grade I to IV VUR. Therefore, a voiding cystourethrography (VCUG) is not recommended routinely after the first UTI; VCUG is indicated if renal and bladder ultrasonography reveals hydronephrosis, scarring, or other findings that would suggest either high-grade VUR or obstructive uropathy and in other atypical or complex clinical circumstances. VCUG should also be performed if there is a recurrence of a febrile UTI. The recommendations in this guideline do not indicate an exclusive course of treatment or serve as a standard of care; variations may be appropriate. Recommendations about antimicrobial prophylaxis and implications for performance of VCUG are based on currently available evidence. As with all American Academy of Pediatrics clinical guidelines, the recommendations will be reviewed routinely and incorporate new evidence, such as data from the Randomized Intervention for Children With Vesicoureteral Reflux (RIVUR) study.

CONCLUSIONS: Changes in this revision include criteria for the diagnosis of UTI and recommendations for imaging. *Pediatrics* 2011;128:595–610

INTRODUCTION

Since the early 1970s, occult bacteremia has been the major focus of concern for clinicians evaluating febrile infants who have no recognizable source of infection. With the introduction of effective conjugate vaccines against *Haemophilus influenzae* type b and *Streptococcus pneumoniae* (which have resulted in dramatic decreases in bacteremia and meningitis), there has been increasing appreciation of the urinary tract as the most frequent site of occult and serious bacterial infections. Because the clinical presentation tends to be nonspecific in infants and reliable urine specimens for culture cannot be obtained without invasive methods (urethral catheterization or suprapubic aspiration [SPA]), diagnosis and treatment may be delayed. Most experimental and clinical data support the concept that delays in the institution of appropriate treatment of pyelonephritis increase the risk of renal damage.[1,2]

This clinical practice guideline is a revision of the practice parameter published by the American Academy of Pediatrics (AAP) in 1999.[3] It was developed by a subcommittee of the Steering Committee on Quality Improvement and Management that included physicians with expertise in the fields of academic general pediatrics, epidemiology and informatics, pediatric infectious diseases, pediatric nephrology, pediatric practice, pediatric radiology, and pediatric urology. The AAP funded the development of this guideline; none of the participants had any financial conflicts of interest. The guideline was reviewed by multiple groups within the AAP (7 committees, 1 council, and 9 sections) and 5 external organizations in the United States and Canada. The guideline will be reviewed and/or revised in 5 years, unless new evidence emerges that warrants revision sooner. The guideline is intended

for use in a variety of clinical settings (eg, office, emergency department, or hospital) by clinicians who treat infants and young children. This text is a summary of the analysis. The data on which the recommendations are based are included in a companion technical report.[4]

Like the 1999 practice parameter, this revision focuses on the diagnosis and management of initial urinary tract infections (UTIs) in febrile infants and young children (2–24 months of age) who have no obvious neurologic or anatomic abnormalities known to be associated with recurrent UTI or renal damage. (For simplicity, in the remainder of this guideline the phrase "febrile infants" is used to indicate febrile infants and young children 2–24 months of age.) The lower and upper age limits were selected because studies on infants with unexplained fever generally have used these age limits and have documented that the prevalence of UTI is high (~5%) in this age group. In those studies, fever was defined as temperature of at least 38.0°C (≥100.4°F); accordingly, this definition of fever is used in this guideline. Neonates and infants less than 2 months of age are excluded, because there are special considerations in this age group that may limit the application of evidence derived from the studies of 2- to 24-month-old children. Data are insufficient to determine whether the evidence generated from studies of infants 2 to 24 months of age applies to children more than 24 months of age.

METHODS

To provide evidence for the guideline, 2 literature searches were conducted, that is, a surveillance of Medline-listed literature over the past 10 years for significant changes since the guideline was published and a systematic review of the literature on the effective-

ness of prophylactic antimicrobial therapy to prevent recurrence of febrile UTI/pyelonephritis in children with vesicoureteral reflux (VUR). The latter was based on the new and growing body of evidence questioning the effectiveness of antimicrobial prophylaxis to prevent recurrent febrile UTI in children with VUR. To explore this particular issue, the literature search was expanded to include trials published since 1993 in which antimicrobial prophylaxis was compared with no treatment or placebo treatment for children with VUR. Because all except 1 of the recent randomized controlled trials (RCTs) of the effectiveness of prophylaxis included children more than 24 months of age and some did not provide specific data according to grade of VUR, the authors of the 6 RCTs were contacted; all provided raw data from their studies specifically addressing infants 2 to 24 months of age, according to grade of VUR. Meta-analysis of these data was performed.

Results from the literature searches and meta-analyses were provided to committee members. Issues were raised and discussed until consensus was reached regarding recommendations. The quality of evidence supporting each recommendation and the strength of the recommendation were assessed by the committee member most experienced in informatics and epidemiology and were graded according to AAP policy[5] (Fig 1).

The subcommittee formulated 7 recommendations, which are presented in the text in the order in which a clinician would use them when evaluating and treating a febrile infant, as well as in algorithm form in the Appendix. This clinical practice guideline is not intended to be a sole source of guidance for the treatment of febrile infants with UTIs. Rather, it is intended to assist clinicians in decision-making. It is not intended to replace clinical judgment or to

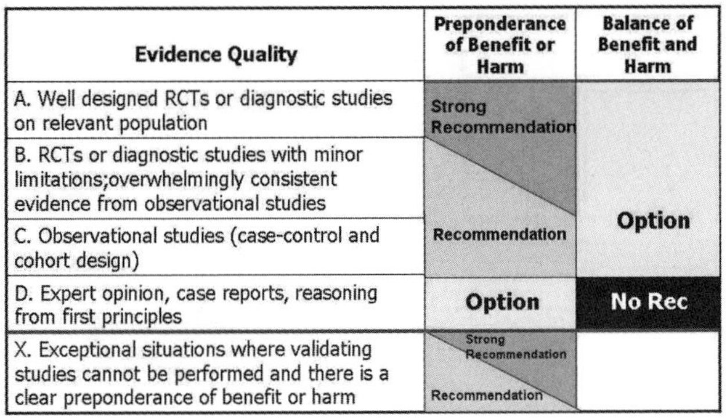

FIGURE 1
AAP evidence strengths.

establish an exclusive protocol for the care of all children with this condition.

DIAGNOSIS

Action Statement 1

If a clinician decides that a febrile infant with no apparent source for the fever requires antimicrobial therapy to be administered because of ill appearance or another pressing reason, the clinician should ensure that a urine specimen is obtained for both culture and urinalysis before an antimicrobial agent is administered; the specimen needs to be obtained through catheterization or SPA, because the diagnosis of UTI cannot be established reliably through culture of urine collected in a bag (evidence quality: A; strong recommendation).

When evaluating febrile infants, clinicians make a subjective assessment of the degree of illness or toxicity, in addition to seeking an explanation for the fever. This clinical assessment determines whether antimicrobial therapy should be initiated promptly and affects the diagnostic process regarding UTI. If the clinician determines that the degree of illness warrants immediate antimicrobial therapy, then a urine specimen suitable for culture should be obtained through catheterization or SPA before antimicrobial agents are administered, because the antimicrobial agents commonly prescribed in such situations would almost certainly obscure the diagnosis of UTI.

SPA has been considered the standard method for obtaining urine that is uncontaminated by perineal flora. Variable success rates for obtaining urine have been reported (23%–90%).[6–8] When ultrasonographic guidance is used, success rates improve.[9,10] The technique has limited risks, but technical expertise and experience are required, and many parents and physicians perceive the procedure as unacceptably invasive, compared with catheterization. However, there may be no acceptable alternative to SPA for boys with moderate or severe phimosis or girls with tight labial adhesions.

Urine obtained through catheterization for culture has a sensitivity of 95% and a specificity of 99%, compared with that obtained through SPA.[7,11,12] The techniques required for catheterization and SPA are well described.[13] When catheterization or SPA is being attempted, the clinician should have a sterile container ready to collect a urine specimen, because the preparation for the procedure may stimulate the child to void. Whether the urine is obtained through catheterization or is voided, the first few drops should be allowed to fall outside the sterile container, because they may be contaminated by bacteria in the distal urethra.

Cultures of urine specimens collected in a bag applied to the perineum have an unacceptably high false-positive rate and are valid only when they yield negative results.[6,14–16] With a prevalence of UTI of 5% and a high rate of false-positive results (specificity: ~63%), a "positive" culture result for urine collected in a bag would be a false-positive result 88% of the time. For febrile boys, with a prevalence of UTI of 2%, the rate of false-positive results is 95%; for circumcised boys, with a prevalence of UTI of 0.2%, the rate of false-positive results is 99%. Therefore, in cases in which antimicrobial therapy will be initiated, catheterization or SPA is required to establish the diagnosis of UTI.

- Aggregate quality of evidence: A (diagnostic studies on relevant populations).

- Benefits: A missed diagnosis of UTI can lead to renal scarring if left untreated; overdiagnosis of UTI can lead to overtreatment and unnecessary and expensive imaging. Once antimicrobial therapy is initiated, the opportunity to make a definitive diagnosis is lost; multiple studies of antimicrobial therapy have shown that the urine may be rapidly sterilized.

- Harms/risks/costs: Catheterization is invasive.

- Benefit-harms assessment: Preponderance of benefit over harm.

- Value judgments: Once antimicrobial therapy has begun, the opportunity to make a definitive diagnosis is lost. Therefore, it is important to have the most-accurate test for UTI performed initially.

- Role of patient preferences: There is no evidence regarding patient preferences for bag versus catheterized urine. However, bladder tap has been shown to be more painful than urethral catheterization.

- Exclusions: None.

- Intentional vagueness: The basis of the determination that antimicrobial therapy is needed urgently is not specified, because variability in clinical judgment is expected; considerations for individual patients, such as availability of follow-up care, may enter into the decision, and the literature provides only general guidance.

- Policy level: Strong recommendation.

Action Statement 2

If a clinician assesses a febrile infant with no apparent source for the fever as not being so ill as to require immediate antimicrobial therapy, then the clinician should assess the likelihood of UTI (see below for how to assess likelihood).

Action Statement 2a

If the clinician determines the febrile infant to have a low likelihood of UTI (see text), then clinical follow-up monitoring without testing is sufficient (evidence quality: A; strong recommendation).

Action Statement 2b

If the clinician determines that the febrile infant is not in a low-risk group (see below), then there are 2 choices (evidence quality: A; strong recommendation). Option 1 is to obtain a urine specimen through catheterization or SPA for culture and urinalysis. Option 2 is to obtain a urine specimen through the most convenient means and to perform a urinalysis. If the urinalysis results suggest a UTI (positive leukocyte esterase test results or nitrite test or microscopic analysis results positive for leukocytes or bacteria), then a urine specimen should

Individual Risk Factors: Girls
White race Age < 12 mo Temperature ≥ 39°C Fever ≥ 2 d Absence of another source of infection

Probability of UTI	No. of Factors Present
≤1%	No more than 1
≤2%	No more than 2

Individual Risk Factors: Boys
Nonblack race Temperature ≥ 39°C Fever > 24 h Absence of another source of infection

Probability of UTI	No. of Factors Present	
	Uncircumcised	Circumcised
≤1%	a	No more than 2
≤2%	None	No more than 3

FIGURE 2

Probability of UTI Among Febrile Infant Girls[28] and Infant Boys[30] According to Number of Findings Present. [a]Probability of UTI exceeds 1% even with no risk factors other than being uncircumcised.

be obtained through catheterization or SPA and cultured; if urinalysis of fresh (<1 hour since void) urine yields negative leukocyte esterase and nitrite test results, then it is reasonable to monitor the clinical course without initiating antimicrobial therapy, recognizing that negative urinalysis results do not rule out a UTI with certainty.

If the clinician determines that the degree of illness does not require immediate antimicrobial therapy, then the likelihood of UTI should be assessed. As noted previously, the overall prevalence of UTI in febrile infants who have no source for their fever evident on the basis of history or physical examination results is approximately 5%,[17,18] but it is possible to identify groups with higher-than-average likelihood and some with lower-than-average likelihood. The prevalence of UTI among febrile infant girls is more than twice that among febrile infant boys (relative risk: 2.27). The rate for uncircumcised boys is 4 to 20 times higher than that for circumcised boys, whose rate of UTI is only 0.2% to 0.4%.[19–24] The presence of another, clinically obvious source of infection reduces the likelihood of UTI by one-half.[25]

In a survey asking, "What yield is required to warrant urine culture in febrile infants?," the threshold was less than 1% for 10.4% of academicians and 11.7% for practitioners[26]; when the threshold was increased to 1% to 3%, 67.5% of academicians and 45.7% of practitioners considered the yield sufficiently high to warrant urine culture. Therefore, attempting to operationalize "low likelihood" (ie, below a threshold that warrants a urine culture) does not produce an absolute percentage; clinicians will choose a threshold depending on factors such as their confidence that contact will be maintained through the illness (so that a specimen can be obtained at a later time) and comfort with diagnostic uncertainty. Fig 2 indicates the number of risk factors associated with threshold probabilities of UTI of at least 1% and at least 2%.

In a series of studies, Gorelick, Shaw, and colleagues[27–29] derived and validated a prediction rule for febrile infant girls on the basis of 5 risk factors, namely, white race, age less than 12 months, temperature of at least 39°C, fever for at least 2 days, and absence of another source of infection. This prediction rule, with sensitivity of 88% and specificity of 30%, permits some infant girls to be considered in a low-likelihood group (Fig 2). For example, of girls with no identifiable source of infection, those who are nonwhite and more than 12 months of age with a recent onset (<2 days) of low-grade fever (<39°C) have less than a 1% probability of UTI; each additional risk factor increases the probability. It should be noted, however, that some of the factors (eg, duration of fever) may change during the course of the illness, excluding the infant from a low-likelihood designation and prompting testing as described in action statement 2a.

As demonstrated in Fig 2, the major risk factor for febrile infant boys is whether they are circumcised. The probability of UTI can be estimated on the basis of 4 risk factors, namely, nonblack race, temperature of at least 39°C, fever for more than 24 hours, and absence of another source of infection.[4,30]

If the clinician determines that the infant does not require immediate antimicrobial therapy and a urine specimen is desired, then often a urine collection bag affixed to the perineum is used. Many clinicians think that this collection technique has a low contamination rate under the following circumstances: the patient's perineum is properly cleansed and rinsed before application of the collection bag, the urine bag is removed promptly after urine is voided into the bag, and the specimen is refrigerated or processed immediately. Even if contamination from the perineal skin is minimized, however, there may be significant contamination from the vagina in girls or the prepuce in uncircumcised boys, the 2 groups at highest risk of UTI. A "positive" culture result from a specimen collected in a bag cannot be used to document a UTI; confirmation requires culture of a specimen collected through catheterization or SPA. Because there may be substantial delay waiting for the infant to void and a second specimen, obtained through catheterization, may be necessary if the urinalysis suggests the possibility of UTI, many clinicians prefer to obtain a

TABLE 1 Sensitivity and Specificity of Components of Urinalysis, Alone and in Combination

Test	Sensitivity (Range), %	Specificity (Range), %
Leukocyte esterase test	83 (67–94)	78 (64–92)
Nitrite test	53 (15–82)	98 (90–100)
Leukocyte esterase or nitrite test positive	93 (90–100)	72 (58–91)
Microscopy, WBCs	73 (32–100)	81 (45–98)
Microscopy, bacteria	81 (16–99)	83 (11–100)
Leukocyte esterase test, nitrite test, or microscopy positive	99.8 (99–100)	70 (60–92)

definitive urine specimen through catheterization initially.

- Aggregate quality of evidence: A (diagnostic studies on relevant populations).

- Benefits: Accurate diagnosis of UTI can prevent the spread of infection and renal scarring; avoiding overdiagnosis of UTI can prevent overtreatment and unnecessary and expensive imaging.

- Harms/risks/costs: A small proportion of febrile infants, considered at low likelihood of UTI, will not receive timely identification and treatment of their UTIs.

- Benefit-harms assessment: Preponderance of benefit over harm.

- Value judgments: There is a risk of UTI sufficiently low to forestall further evaluation.

- Role of patient preferences: The choice of option 1 or option 2 and the threshold risk of UTI warranting obtaining a urine specimen may be influenced by parents' preference to avoid urethral catheterization (if a bag urine sample yields negative urinalysis results) versus timely evaluation (obtaining a definitive specimen through catheterization).

- Exclusions: Because it depends on a range of patient- and physician-specific considerations, the precise threshold risk of UTI warranting obtaining a urine specimen is left to the clinician but is below 3%.

- Intentional vagueness: None.

- Policy level: Strong recommendation.

Action Statement 3

To establish the diagnosis of UTI, clinicians should require *both* urinalysis results that suggest infection (pyuria and/or bacteriuria) *and* the presence of at least 50 000 colony-forming units (CFUs) per mL of a uropathogen cultured from a urine specimen obtained through catheterization or SPA (evidence quality: C; recommendation).

Urinalysis

General Considerations

Urinalysis cannot substitute for urine culture to document the presence of UTI but needs to be used in conjunction with culture. Because urine culture results are not available for at least 24 hours, there is considerable interest in tests that may predict the results of the urine culture and enable presumptive therapy to be initiated at the first encounter. Urinalysis can be performed on any specimen, including one collected from a bag applied to the perineum. However, the specimen must be fresh (<1 hour after voiding with maintenance at room temperature or <4 hours after voiding with refrigeration), to ensure sensitivity and specificity of the urinalysis. The tests that have received the most attention are biochemical analyses of leukocyte esterase and nitrite through a rapid dipstick method and urine microscopic examination for white blood cells (WBCs) and bacteria (Table 1).

Urine dipsticks are appealing, because they provide rapid results, do not require microscopy, and are eligible for a waiver under the Clinical Laboratory Improvement Amendments. They indicate the presence of leukocyte esterase (as a surrogate marker for pyuria) and urinary nitrite (which is converted from dietary nitrates in the presence of most Gram-negative enteric bacteria in the urine). The conversion of dietary nitrates to nitrites by bacteria requires approximately 4 hours in the bladder.[31] The performance characteristics of both leukocyte esterase and nitrite tests vary according to the definition used for positive urine culture results, the age and symptoms of the population being studied, and the method of urine collection.

Nitrite Test

A nitrite test is not a sensitive marker for children, particularly infants, who empty their bladders frequently. Therefore, negative nitrite test results have little value in ruling out UTI. Moreover, not all urinary pathogens reduce nitrate to nitrite. The test is helpful when the result is positive, however, because it is highly specific (ie, there are few false-positive results).[32]

Leukocyte Esterase Test

The sensitivity of the leukocyte esterase test is 94% when it used in the context of clinically suspected UTI. Overall, the reported sensitivity in various studies is lower (83%), because the results of leukocyte esterase tests were related to culture results without exclusion of individuals with asymptomatic bacteriuria. The absence of leukocyte esterase in the urine of individuals with asymptomatic bacteriuria is an advantage of the test, rather than a limitation, because it distinguishes individuals with asymptomatic bacteriuria from those with true UTI.

The specificity of the leukocyte esterase test (average: 72% [range:

64%–92%]) generally is not as good as the sensitivity, which reflects the nonspecificity of pyuria in general. Accordingly, positive leukocyte esterase test results should be interpreted with caution, because false-positive results are common. With numerous conditions other than UTI, including fever resulting from other conditions (eg, streptococcal infections or Kawasaki disease), and after vigorous exercise, WBCs may be found in the urine. Therefore, a finding of pyuria by no means confirms that an infection of the urinary tract is present.

The absence of pyuria in children with true UTIs is rare, however. It is theoretically possible if a febrile child is assessed before the inflammatory response has developed, but the inflammatory response to a UTI produces both fever and pyuria; therefore, children who are being evaluated because of fever should already have WBCs in their urine. More likely explanations for significant bacteriuria in culture in the absence of pyuria include contaminated specimens, insensitive criteria for pyuria, and asymptomatic bacteriuria. In most cases, when true UTI has been reported to occur in the absence of pyuria, the definition of pyuria has been at fault. The standard method of assessing pyuria has been centrifugation of the urine and microscopic analysis, with a threshold of 5 WBCs per high-power field (~25 WBCs per μL). If a counting chamber is used, however, the finding of at least 10 WBCs per μL in uncentrifuged urine has been demonstrated to be more sensitive[33] and performs well in clinical situations in which the standard method does not, such as with very young infants.[34]

An important cause of bacteriuria in the absence of pyuria is asymptomatic bacteriuria. Asymptomatic bacteriuria often is associated with school-aged and older girls,[35] but it can be present

during infancy. In a study of infants 2 to 24 months of age, 0.7% of afebrile girls had 3 successive urine cultures with 10^5 CFUs per mL of a single uropathogen.[26] Asymptomatic bacteriuria can be easily confused with true UTI in a febrile infant but needs to be distinguished, because studies suggest that antimicrobial treatment may do more harm than good.[36] The key to distinguishing true UTI from asymptomatic bacteriuria is the presence of pyuria.

Microscopic Analysis for Bacteriuria

The presence of bacteria in a fresh, Gram-stained specimen of uncentrifuged urine correlates with 10^5 CFUs per mL in culture.[37] An "enhanced urinalysis," combining the counting chamber assessment of pyuria noted previously with Gram staining of drops of uncentrifuged urine, with a threshold of at least 1 Gram-negative rod in 10 oil immersion fields, has greater sensitivity, specificity, and positive predictive value than does the standard urinalysis[33] and is the preferred method of urinalysis when appropriate equipment and personnel are available.

Automated Urinalysis

Automated methods to perform urinalysis are now being used in many hospitals and laboratories. Image-based systems use flow imaging analysis technology and software to classify particles in uncentrifuged urine specimens rapidly.[38] Results correlate well with manual methods, especially for red blood cells, WBCs, and squamous epithelial cells. In the future, this may be the most common method by which urinalysis is performed in laboratories.

Culture

The diagnosis of UTI is made on the basis of quantitative urine culture results in addition to evidence of pyuria and/or bacteriuria. Urine specimens should be processed as expediently as possible. If the specimen is not processed promptly, then it should be refrigerated to prevent the growth of organisms that can occur in urine at room temperature; for the same reason, specimens that require transportation to another site for processing should be transported on ice. A properly collected urine specimen should be inoculated on culture medium that will allow identification of urinary tract pathogens.

Urine culture results are considered positive or negative on the basis of the number of CFUs that grow on the culture medium.[36] Definition of significant colony counts with regard to the method of collection considers that the distal urethra and periurethral area are commonly colonized by the same bacteria that may cause UTI; therefore, a low colony count may be present in a specimen obtained through voiding or catheterization when bacteria are not present in bladder urine. Definitions of positive and negative culture results are operational and not absolute. The time the urine resides in the bladder (bladder incubation time) is an important determinant of the magnitude of the colony count. The concept that more than 100 000 CFUs per mL indicates a UTI was based on morning collections of urine from adult women, with comparison of specimens from women without symptoms and women considered clinically to have pyelonephritis; the transition range, in which the proportion of women with pyelonephritis exceeded the proportion of women without symptoms, was 10 000 to 100 000 CFUs per mL.[39] In most instances, an appropriate threshold to consider bacteriuria "significant" in infants and children is the presence of at least 50 000 CFUs per mL of a single urinary pathogen.[40] (Organisms such as *Lactobacillus* spp, coagulase-negative staphylococci, and *Corynebacterium*

spp are not considered clinically relevant urine isolates for otherwise healthy, 2- to 24-month-old children.) Reducing the threshold from 100 000 CFUs per mL to 50 000 CFUs per mL would seem to increase the sensitivity of culture at the expense of decreased specificity; however, because the proposed criteria for UTI now include evidence of pyuria in addition to positive culture results, infants with "positive" culture results alone will be recognized as having asymptomatic bacteriuria rather than a true UTI. Some laboratories report growth only in the following categories: 0 to 1000, 1000 to 10 000, 10 000 to 100 000, and more than 100 000 CFUs per mL. In such cases, results in the 10 000 to 100 000 CFUs per mL range need to be evaluated in context, such as whether the urinalysis findings support the diagnosis of UTI and whether the organism is a recognized uropathogen.

Alternative culture methods, such as dipslides, may have a place in the office setting; sensitivity is reported to be in the range of 87% to 100%, and specificity is reported to be 92% to 98%, but dipslides cannot specify the organism or antimicrobial sensitivities.[41] Practices that use dipslides should do so in collaboration with a certified laboratory for identification and sensitivity testing or, in the absence of such results, may need to perform "test of cure" cultures after 24 hours of treatment.

- Aggregate quality of evidence: C (observational studies).
- Benefits: Accurate diagnosis of UTI can prevent the spread of infection and renal scarring; avoiding overdiagnosis of UTI can prevent overtreatment and unnecessary and expensive imaging. These criteria reduce the likelihood of overdiagnosis of UTI in infants with asymptomatic bacteriuria or contaminated specimens.

- Harms/risks/costs: Stringent diagnostic criteria may miss a small number of UTIs.
- Benefit-harms assessment: Preponderance of benefit over harm.
- Value judgments: Treatment of asymptomatic bacteriuria may be harmful.
- Role of patient preferences: We assume that parents prefer no action in the absence of a UTI (avoiding false-positive results) over a very small chance of missing a UTI.
- Exclusions: None.
- Intentional vagueness: None.
- Policy level: Recommendation.

MANAGEMENT

Action Statement 4

Action Statement 4a

When initiating treatment, the clinician should base the choice of route of administration on practical considerations. Initiating treatment orally or parenterally is equally efficacious. The clinician should base the choice of agent on local antimicrobial sensitivity patterns (if available) and should adjust the choice according to sensitivity testing of the isolated uropathogen (evidence quality: A; strong recommendation).

Action Statement 4b

The clinician should choose 7 to 14 days as the duration of antimicrobial therapy (evidence quality: B; recommendation).

The goals of treatment of acute UTI are to eliminate the acute infection, to prevent complications, and to reduce the likelihood of renal damage. Most children can be treated orally.[42–44] Patients whom clinicians judge to be "toxic" or who are unable to retain oral intake (including medications) should receive an antimicrobial agent parenter-

TABLE 2 Some Empiric Antimicrobial Agents for Parenteral Treatment of UTI

Antimicrobial Agent	Dosage
Ceftriaxone	75 mg/kg, every 24 h
Cefotaxime	150 mg/kg per d, divided every 6–8 h
Ceftazidime	100–150 mg/kg per d, divided every 8 h
Gentamicin	7.5 mg/kg per d, divided every 8 h
Tobramycin	5 mg/kg per d, divided every 8 h
Piperacillin	300 mg/kg per d, divided every 6–8 h

TABLE 3 Some Empiric Antimicrobial Agents for Oral Treatment of UTI

Antimicrobial Agent	Dosage
Amoxicillin-clavulanate	20–40 mg/kg per d in 3 doses
Sulfonamide	
Trimethoprim-sulfamethoxazole	6–12 mg/kg trimethoprim and 30-60 mg/kg sulfamethoxazole per d in 2 doses
Sulfisoxazole	120–150 mg/kg per d in 4 doses
Cephalosporin	
Cefixime	8 mg/kg per d in 1 dose
Cefpodoxime	10 mg/kg per d in 2 doses
Cefprozil	30 mg/kg per d in 2 doses
Cefuroxime axetil	20–30 mg/kg per d in 2 doses
Cephalexin	50–100 mg/kg per d in 4 doses

ally (Table 2) until they exhibit clinical improvement, generally within 24 to 48 hours, and are able to retain orally administered fluids and medications. In a study of 309 febrile infants with UTIs, only 3 (1%) were deemed too ill to be assigned randomly to either parenteral or oral treatment.[42] Parenteral administration of an antimicrobial agent also should be considered when compliance with obtaining an antimicrobial agent and/or administering it orally is uncertain. The usual choices for oral treatment of UTIs include a cephalosporin, amoxicillin plus clavulanic acid, or trimethoprim-sulfamethoxazole (Table 3). It is essential to know local patterns of susceptibility of coliforms to antimicrobial agents, particularly trimethoprim-sulfamethoxazole and cephalexin, because there is substantial geographic variability that needs to be taken into account during selection of an antimicrobial agent before sensitivity results are available. Agents that are excreted in the urine but do not achieve therapeutic concentrations in the bloodstream, such as nitrofurantoin, should not be used to treat febrile infants with UTIs, because parenchymal and serum antimicrobial concentrations may be insufficient to treat pyelonephritis or urosepsis.

Whether the initial route of administration of the antimicrobial agent is oral or parenteral (then changed to oral),

the total course of therapy should be 7 to 14 days. The committee attempted to identify a single, preferred, evidence-based duration, rather than a range, but data comparing 7, 10, and 14 days directly were not found. There is evidence that 1- to 3-day courses for febrile UTIs are inferior to courses in the recommended range; therefore, the minimal duration selected should be 7 days.

- Aggregate quality of evidence: A/B (RCTs).

- Benefits: Adequate treatment of UTI can prevent the spread of infection and renal scarring. Outcomes of short courses (1–3 d) are inferior to those of 7- to 14-d courses.

- Harms/risks/costs: There are minimal harm and minor cost effects of antimicrobial choice and duration of therapy.

- Benefit-harms assessment: Preponderance of benefit over harm.

- Value judgments: Adjusting antimicrobial choice on the basis of available data and treating according to best evidence will minimize cost and consequences of failed or unnecessary treatment.

- Role of patient preferences: It is assumed that parents prefer the most-effective treatment and the least amount of medication that ensures effective treatment.

- Exclusions: None.

- Intentional vagueness: No evidence

distinguishes the benefit of treating 7 vs 10 vs 14 days, and the range is allowable.

- Policy level: Strong recommendation/recommendation.

Action Statement 5

Febrile infants with UTIs should undergo renal and bladder ultrasonography (RBUS) (evidence quality: C; recommendation).

The purpose of RBUS is to detect anatomic abnormalities that require further evaluation, such as additional imaging or urologic consultation. RBUS also provides an evaluation of the renal parenchyma and an assessment of renal size that can be used to monitor renal growth. The yield of actionable findings is relatively low.[45,46] Widespread application of prenatal ultrasonography clearly has reduced the prevalence of previously unsuspected obstructive uropathy in infants, but the consequences of prenatal screening with respect to the risk of renal abnormalities in infants with UTIs have not yet been well defined. There is considerable variability in the timing and quality of prenatal ultrasonograms, and the report of "normal" ultrasonographic results cannot necessarily be relied on to dismiss completely the possibility of a structural abnormality unless the study was a detailed anatomic survey (with measurements), was performed during the third trimester, and was performed and interpreted by qualified individuals.[47]

The timing of RBUS depends on the clinical situation. RBUS is recommended during the first 2 days of treatment to identify serious complications, such as renal or perirenal abscesses or pyonephrosis associated with obstructive uropathy when the clinical illness is unusually severe or substantial clinical improvement is not occurring. For febrile infants with UTIs who demonstrate substantial clinical improvement, however, imaging does not need to occur early during the acute infection and can even be misleading; animal studies demonstrate that *Escherichia coli* endotoxin can produce dilation during acute infection, which could be confused with hydronephrosis, pyonephrosis, or obstruction.[48] Changes in the size and shape of the kidneys and the echogenicity of renal parenchyma attributable to edema also are common during acute infection. The presence of these abnormalities makes it inappropriate to consider RBUS performed early during acute infection to be a true baseline study for later comparisons in the assessment of renal growth.

Nuclear scanning with technetium-labeled dimercaptosuccinic acid has greater sensitivity for detection of acute pyelonephritis and later scarring than does either RBUS or voiding cystourethrography (VCUG). The scanning is useful in research, because it ensures that all subjects in a study have pyelonephritis to start with and it permits assessment of later renal scarring as an outcome measure. The findings on nuclear scans rarely affect acute clinical management, however, and are not recommended as part of routine evaluation of infants with their first febrile UTI. The radiation dose to the patient during dimercaptosuccinic acid scanning is generally low ($\sim$1 mSv),[49] although it may be increased in

children with reduced renal function. The radiation dose from dimercaptosuccinic acid is additive with that of VCUG when both studies are performed.[50] The radiation dose from VCUG depends on the equipment that is used (conventional versus pulsed digital fluoroscopy) and is related directly to the total fluoroscopy time. Moreover, the total exposure for the child will be increased when both acute and follow-up studies are obtained. The lack of exposure to radiation is a major advantage of RBUS, even with recognition of the limitations of this modality that were described previously.

- Aggregate quality of evidence: C (observational studies).

- Benefits: RBUS in this population will yield abnormal results in $\sim$15% of cases, and 1% to 2% will have abnormalities that would lead to action (eg, additional evaluation, referral, or surgery).

- Harms/risks/costs: Between 2% and 3% will be false-positive results, leading to unnecessary and invasive evaluations.

- Benefit-harms assessment: Preponderance of benefit over harm.

- Value judgments: The seriousness of the potentially correctable abnormalities in 1% to 2%, coupled with the absence of physical harm, was judged sufficiently important to tip the scales in favor of testing.

- Role of patient preferences: Because ultrasonography is noninvasive and poses minimal risk, we assume that parents will prefer RBUS over taking even a small risk of missing a serious and correctable condition.

- Exclusions: None.

- Intentional vagueness: None.

- Policy level: Recommendation.

Action Statement 6

Action Statement 6a

VCUG should not be performed routinely after the first febrile UTI; VCUG is indicated if RBUS reveals hydronephrosis, scarring, or other findings that would suggest either high-grade VUR or obstructive uropathy, as well as in other atypical or complex clinical circumstances (evidence quality B; recommendation).

Action Statement 6b

Further evaluation should be conducted if there is a recurrence of febrile UTI (evidence quality: X; recommendation).

For the past 4 decades, the strategy to protect the kidneys from further damage after an initial UTI has been to detect childhood genitourinary abnormalities in which recurrent UTI could increase renal damage. The most common of these is VUR, and VCUG is used to detect this. Management included continuous antimicrobial administration as prophylaxis and surgical intervention if VUR was persistent or recurrences of infection were not prevented with an antimicrobial prophylaxis regimen; some have advocated surgical intervention to correct high-grade reflux even when infection has not recurred. However, it is clear that there are a significant number of infants who develop pyelonephritis in whom VUR cannot be demonstrated, and the effectiveness of antimicrobial prophylaxis for patients who have VUR has been challenged in the past decade. Several studies have suggested that prophylaxis does not confer the desired benefit of preventing recurrent febrile UTI.[51–55] If prophylaxis is, in fact, not beneficial and VUR is not required for development of pyelonephritis, then the rationale for performing VCUG routinely after an initial febrile UTI must be questioned.

RCTs of the effectiveness of prophylaxis performed to date generally included children more than 24 months of age, and some did not provide complete data according to grade of VUR. These 2 factors have compromised meta-analyses. To ensure direct comparisons, the committee contacted the 6 researchers who had conducted the most recent RCTs and requested raw data from their studies.[51–56] All complied, which permitted the creation of a data set with data for 1091 infants 2 to 24 months of age according to grade of VUR. A χ^2 analysis (2-tailed) and a formal meta-analysis did not detect a statistically significant benefit of prophylaxis in preventing recurrence of febrile UTI/pyelonephritis in infants without reflux or those with grades I, II, III, or IV VUR (Table 4 and Fig 3). Only 5 infants with grade V VUR were included in the RCTs; therefore, data for those infants are not included in Table 4 or Fig 3.

The proportion of infants with high-grade VUR among all infants with febrile UTIs is small. Data adapted from current studies (Table 5) indicate that, of a hypothetical cohort of 100 infants with febrile UTIs, only 1 has grade V VUR; 99 do not. With a practice of waiting for a second UTI to perform VCUG, only 10 of the 100 would need to undergo the procedure and the 1 with grade V VUR would be identified. (It also is possible that the 1 infant with grade V VUR might have been identified after the first UTI on the basis of abnormal RBUS results that prompted VCUG to be performed.) Data to quantify additional potential harm to an infant who is not revealed to have high-grade VUR until a second UTI are not precise but suggest that the increment is insufficient to justify routinely subjecting all infants with an initial febrile UTI to VCUG (Fig 4). To minimize any harm incurred by that infant, attempts have been made to identify, at the time of

TABLE 4 Recurrences of Febrile UTI/Pyelonephritis in Infants 2 to 24 Months of Age With and Without Antimicrobial Prophylaxis, According to Grade of VUR

Reflux Grade	Prophylaxis		No Prophylaxis		P
	No. of Recurrences	Total N	No. of Recurrences	Total N	
None	7	210	11	163	.15
I	2	37	2	35	1.00
II	11	133	10	124	.95
III	31	140	40	145	.29
IV	16	55	21	49	.14

the initial UTI, those who have the greatest likelihood of having high-grade VUR. Unfortunately, there are no clinical or laboratory indicators that have been demonstrated to identify infants with high-grade VUR. Indications for VCUG have been proposed on the basis of consensus in the absence of data[57]; the predictive value of any of the indications for VCUG proposed in this manner is not known.

The level of evidence supporting routine imaging with VCUG was deemed insufficient at the time of the 1999 practice parameter to receive a recommendation, but the consensus of the subcommittee was to "strongly encourage" imaging studies. The position of the current subcommittee reflects the new evidence demonstrating antimicrobial prophylaxis not to be effective as presumed previously. Moreover, prompt diagnosis and effective treatment of a febrile UTI recurrence may be of greater importance regardless of whether VUR is present or the child is receiving antimicrobial prophylaxis. A national study (the Randomized Intervention for Children With Vesicoureteral Reflux study) is currently in progress to identify the effects of a prophylactic antimicrobial regimen for children 2 months to 6 years of age who have experienced a UTI, and it is anticipated to provide additional important data[58] (see Areas for Research).

Action Statement 6a

- Aggregate quality of evidence: B (RCTs).

- Benefits: This avoids, for the vast majority of febrile infants with UTIs, radiation exposure (of particular concern near the ovaries in girls), expense, and discomfort.

- Harms/risks/costs: Detection of a small number of cases of high-grade reflux and correctable abnormalities is delayed.

- Benefit-harms assessment: Preponderance of benefit over harm.

- Value judgments: The risks associated with radiation (plus the expense and discomfort of the procedure) for the vast majority of infants outweigh the risk of delaying the detection of the few with correctable abnormalities until their second UTI.

- Role of patient preferences: The judgment of parents may come into play, because VCUG is an uncomfortable procedure involving radiation exposure. In some cases, parents may prefer to subject their children to the procedure even when the chance of benefit is both small and uncertain. Antimicrobial prophylaxis seems to be ineffective in preventing recurrence of febrile UTI/pyelonephritis for the vast majority of infants. Some parents may want to avoid VCUG even after the second UTI. Because the benefit of identifying high-grade reflux is still in some doubt, these preferences should be considered. It is the judgment of the committee that VCUG is indicated after the second UTI.

- Exclusions: None.

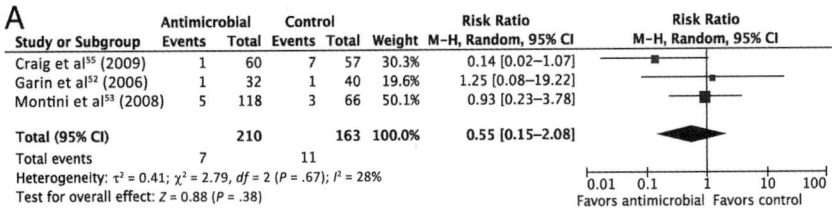

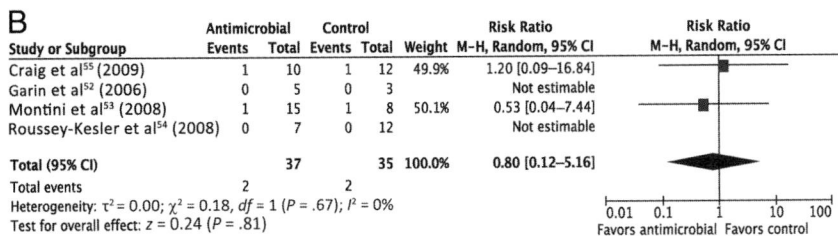

FIGURE 3

A, Recurrences of febrile UTI/pyelonephritis in 373 infants 2 to 24 months of age without VUR, with and without antimicrobial prophylaxis (based on 3 studies; data provided by Drs Craig, Garin, and Montini). B, Recurrences of febrile UTI/pyelonephritis in 72 infants 2 to 24 months of age with grade I VUR, with and without antimicrobial prophylaxis (based on 4 studies; data provided by Drs Craig, Garin, Montini, and Roussey-Kesler). C, Recurrences of febrile UTI/pyelonephritis in 257 infants 2 to 24 months of age with grade II VUR, with and without antimicrobial prophylaxis (based on 5 studies; data provided by Drs Craig, Garin, Montini, Pennesi, and Roussey-Kesler). D, Recurrences of febrile UTI/ pyelonephritis in 285 infants 2 to 24 months of age with grade III VUR, with and without antimicrobial prophylaxis (based on 6 studies; data provided by Drs Brandström, Craig, Garin, Montini, Pennesi, and Roussey-Kesler). E, Recurrences of febrile UTI/pyelonephritis in 104 infants 2 to 24 months of age with grade IV VUR, with and without antimicrobial prophylaxis (based on 3 studies; data provided by Drs Brandström, Craig, and Pennesi). M-H indicates Mantel-Haenszel; CI, confidence interval.

TABLE 5 Rates of VUR According to Grade in Hypothetical Cohort of Infants After First UTI and After Recurrence

	Rate, %	
	After First UTI (N = 100)	After Recurrence (N = 10)
No VUR	65	26
Grades I–III VUR	29	56
Grade IV VUR	5	12
Grade V VUR	1	6

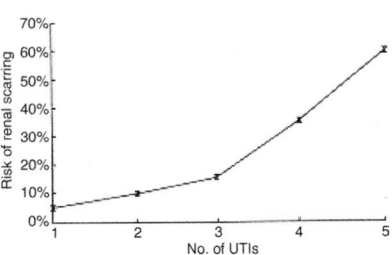

FIGURE 4

Relationship between renal scarring and number of bouts of pyelonephritis. Adapted from Jodal.[59]

- Intentional vagueness: None.
- Policy level: Recommendation.

Action Statement 6b

- Aggregate quality of evidence: X (exceptional situation).
- Benefits: VCUG after a second UTI should identify infants with very high-grade reflux.
- Harms/risks/costs: VCUG is an uncomfortable, costly procedure that involves radiation, including to the ovaries of girls.
- Benefit-harms assessment: Preponderance of benefit over harm.
- Value judgments: The committee judged that patients with high-grade reflux and other abnormalities may benefit from interventions to prevent further scarring. Further studies of treatment for grade V VUR are not underway and are unlikely in the near future, because the condition is uncommon and randomization of treatment in this group generally has been considered unethical.

- Role of patient preferences: As mentioned previously, the judgment of parents may come into play, because VCUG is an uncomfortable procedure involving radiation exposure. In some cases, parents may prefer to subject their children to the procedure even when the chance of benefit is both small and uncertain. The benefits of treatment of VUR remain unproven, but the point estimates suggest a small potential benefit. Similarly, parents may want to avoid VCUG even after the second UTI. Because the benefit of identifying high-grade reflux is still in some doubt, these preferences should be considered. It is the judgment of the committee that VCUG is indicated after the second UTI.
- Exclusions: None.
- Intentional vagueness: Further evaluation will likely start with VCUG but may entail additional studies depending on the findings. The details of further evaluation are beyond the scope of this guideline.
- Policy level: Recommendation.

Action Statement 7

After confirmation of UTI, the clinician should instruct parents or guardians to seek prompt medical evaluation (ideally within 48 hours) for future febrile illnesses, to ensure that recurrent infections can be detected and treated promptly (evidence quality: C; recommendation).

Early treatment limits renal damage better than late treatment,[1,2] and the risk of renal scarring increases as the number of recurrences increase (Fig 4).[59] For these reasons, all infants who have sustained a febrile UTI should have a urine specimen obtained at the onset of subsequent febrile illnesses, so that a UTI can be diagnosed and treated promptly.

- Aggregate quality of evidence: C (observational studies).
- Benefits: Studies suggest that early treatment of UTI reduces the risk of renal scarring.
- Harms/risks/costs: There may be additional costs and inconvenience to parents with more-frequent visits to the clinician for evaluation of fever.
- Benefit-harms assessment: Preponderance of benefit over harm.
- Value judgments: None.
- Role of patient preferences: Parents will ultimately make the judgment to seek medical care.
- Exclusions: None.
- Intentional vagueness: None.
- Policy level: Recommendation.

CONCLUSIONS

The committee formulated 7 key action statements for the diagnosis and treatment of infants and young children 2 to 24 months of age with UTI and unexplained fever. Strategies for diagnosis and treatment depend on whether the clinician determines that antimicrobial therapy is warranted immediately or can be delayed safely until urine culture and urinalysis results are available. Diagnosis is based on the presence of pyuria and at least 50 000 CFUs per mL of a single uropathogen in an appropriately collected specimen of urine; urinalysis alone does not provide a definitive diagnosis. After 7 to 14 days of antimicrobial treatment, close clinical follow-up monitoring should be maintained, with evaluation of the urine during subsequent febrile episodes to permit prompt diagnosis and treatment of recurrent infections. Ultrasonography of the kidneys and bladder should be performed to detect anatomic abnormalities that require further evaluation (eg, additional imaging or urologic consultation). Routine VCUG after the

first UTI is not recommended; VCUG is indicated if RBUS reveals hydronephrosis, scarring, or other findings that would suggest either high-grade VUR or obstructive uropathy, as well as in other atypical or complex clinical circumstances. VCUG also should be performed if there is a recurrence of febrile UTI.

AREAS FOR RESEARCH

One of the major values of a comprehensive literature review is the identification of areas in which evidence is lacking. The following 8 areas are presented in an order that parallels the previous discussion.

1. The relationship between UTIs in infants and young children and reduced renal function in adults has been established but is not well characterized in quantitative terms. The ideal prospective cohort study from birth to 40 to 50 years of age has not been conducted and is unlikely to be conducted. Therefore, estimates of undesirable outcomes in adulthood, such as hypertension and end-stage renal disease, are based on the mathematical product of probabilities at several steps, each of which is subject to bias and error. Other attempts at decision analysis and thoughtful literature review have recognized the same limitations. Until recently, imaging tools available for assessment of the effects of UTIs have been insensitive. With the imaging techniques now available, it may be possible to identify the relationship of scarring to renal impairment and hypertension.

2. The development of techniques that would permit an alternative to invasive sampling and culture would be valuable for general use. Special attention should be given to infant girls and uncircumcised boys, because urethral catheterization may

be difficult and can produce contaminated specimens and SPA now is not commonly performed. Incubation time, which is inherent in the culture process, results in delayed treatment or presumptive treatment on the basis of tests that lack the desired sensitivity and specificity to replace culture.

3. The role of VUR (and therefore of VCUG) is incompletely understood. It is recognized that pyelonephritis (defined through cortical scintigraphy) can occur in the absence of VUR (defined through VCUG) and that progressive renal scarring (defined through cortical scintigraphy) can occur in the absence of demonstrated VUR.[52,53] The presumption that antimicrobial prophylaxis is of benefit for individuals with VUR to prevent recurrences of UTI or the development of renal scars is not supported by the aggregate of data from recent studies and currently is the subject of the Randomized Intervention for Children With Vesicoureteral Reflux study.[58]

4. Although the effectiveness of antimicrobial prophylaxis for the prevention of UTI has not been demonstrated, the concept has biological plausibility. Virtually all antimicrobial agents used to treat or to prevent infections of the urinary tract are excreted in the urine in high concentrations. Barriers to the effectiveness of antimicrobial prophylaxis are adherence to a daily regimen, adverse effects associated with the various agents, and the potential for emergence of anti-microbial resistance. To overcome these issues, evidence of effectiveness with a well-tolerated, safe product would be required, and parents would need sufficient education to understand the value and importance of adherence. A urinary antiseptic, rather than an antimicrobial agent, would be particularly desirable, because it could be taken indefinitely without concern that bacteria would develop resistance. Another possible strategy might be the use of probiotics.

5. Better understanding of the genome (human and bacterial) may provide insight into risk factors (VUR and others) that lead to increased scarring. Blood specimens will be retained from children enrolled in the Randomized Intervention for Children With Vesicoureteral Reflux study, for future examination of genetic determinants of VUR, recurrent UTI, and renal scarring.[58] VUR is recognized to "run in families,"[60,61] and multiple investigators are currently engaged in research to identify a genetic basis for VUR. Studies may also be able to distinguish the contribution of congenital dysplasia from acquired scarring attributable to UTI.

6. One of the factors used to assess the likelihood of UTI in febrile infants is race. Data regarding rates among Hispanic individuals are limited and would be useful for prediction rules.

7. This guideline is limited to the initial management of the first UTI in febrile infants 2 to 24 months of age. Some of the infants will have recurrent UTIs; some will be identified as having VUR or other abnormalities. Further research addressing the optimal course of management in specific situations would be valuable.

8. The optimal duration of antimicrobial treatment has not been determined. RCTs of head-to-head comparisons of various duration would be valuable, enabling clinicians to limit antimicrobial exposure to what is needed to eradicate the offending uropathogen.

LEAD AUTHOR

Kenneth B. Roberts, MD

SUBCOMMITTEE ON URINARY TRACT INFECTION, 2009–2011

Kenneth B. Roberts, MD, Chair
Stephen M. Downs, MD, MS
S. Maria E. Finnell, MD, MS
Stanley Hellerstein, MD
Linda D. Shortliffe, MD
Ellen R. Wald, MD
J. Michael Zerin, MD

OVERSIGHT BY THE STEERING COMMITTEE ON QUALITY IMPROVEMENT AND MANAGEMENT, 2009–2011

STAFF

Caryn Davidson, MA

ACKNOWLEDGMENTS

The committee gratefully acknowledges the generosity of the researchers who graciously shared their data to permit the data set with data for 1091 infants aged 2 to 24 months according to grade of VUR to be compiled, that is, Drs Per Brandström, Jonathan Craig, Eduardo Garin, Giovanni Montini, Marco Pennesi, and Gwenaelle Roussey-Kesler.

REFERENCES

1. Winter AL, Hardy BE, Alton DJ, Arbus GS, Churchill BM. Acquired renal scars in children. *J Urol.* 1983;129(6):1190–1194

2. Smellie JM, Poulton A, Prescod NP. Retrospective study of children with renal scarring associated with reflux and urinary infection. *BMJ.* 1994;308(6938):1193–1196

3. American Academy of Pediatrics, Committee on Quality Improvement, Subcommittee on Urinary Tract Infection. Practice parameter: the diagnosis, treatment, and evaluation of the initial urinary tract infection in febrile infants and young children. *Pediatrics.* 1999;103(4):843–852

4. Finnell SM, Carroll AE, Downs SM, et al. Technical report: diagnosis and management of an initial urinary tract infection in febrile infants and young children. *Pediatrics.* 2011;128(3):e749

5. American Academy of Pediatrics, Steering Committee on Quality Improvement and Management. Classifying recommenda-

tions for clinical practice guidelines. *Pediatrics*. 2004;114(3):874–877

6. Leong YY, Tan KW. Bladder aspiration for diagnosis of urinary tract infection in infants and young children. *J Singapore Paediatr Soc*. 1976;18(1):43–47

7. Pryles CV, Atkin MD, Morse TS, Welch KJ. Comparative bacteriologic study of urine obtained from children by percutaneous suprapubic aspiration of the bladder and by catheter. *Pediatrics*. 1959;24(6):983–991

8. Djojohadipringgo S, Abdul Hamid RH, Thahir S, Karim A, Darsono I. Bladder puncture in newborns: a bacteriological study. *Paediatr Indones*. 1976;16(11–12):527–534

9. Gochman RF, Karasic RB, Heller MB. Use of portable ultrasound to assist urine collection by suprapubic aspiration. *Ann Emerg Med*. 1991;20(6):631–635

10. Buys H, Pead L, Hallett R, Maskell R. Suprapubic aspiration under ultrasound guidance in children with fever of undiagnosed cause. *BMJ*. 1994;308(6930):690–692

11. Kramer MS, Tange SM, Drummond KN, Mills EL. Urine testing in young febrile children: a risk-benefit analysis. *J Pediatr*. 1994;125(1):6–13

12. Bonadio WA. Urine culturing technique in febrile infants. *Pediatr Emerg Care*. 1987;3(2):75–78

13. Lohr J. *Pediatric Outpatient Procedures*. Philadelphia, PA: Lippincott; 1991

14. Taylor CM, White RH. The feasibility of screening preschool children for urinary tract infection using dipslides. *Int J Pediatr Nephrol*. 1983;4(2):113–114

15. Sørensen K, Lose G, Nathan E. Urinary tract infections and diurnal incontinence in girls. *Eur J Pediatr*. 1988;148(2):146–147

16. Shannon F, Sepp E, Rose G. The diagnosis of bacteriuria by bladder puncture in infancy and childhood. *Aust Pediatr J*. 1969;5(2):97–100

17. Hoberman A, Chao HP, Keller DM, Hickey R, Davis HW, Ellis D. Prevalence of urinary tract infection in febrile infants. *J Pediatr*. 1993;123(1):17–23

18. Haddon RA, Barnett PL, Grimwood K, Hogg GG. Bacteraemia in febrile children presenting to a paediatric emergency department. *Med J Aust*. 1999;170(10):475–478

19. Wiswell TE, Roscelli JD. Corroborative evidence for the decreased incidence of urinary tract infections in circumcised male infants. *Pediatrics*. 1986;78(1):96–99

20. To T, Agha M, Dick PT, Feldman W. Cohort study on circumcision of newborn boys and subsequent risk of urinary-tract infection. *Lancet*. 1998;352(9143):1813–1816

21. Wiswell TE, Hachey WE. Urinary tract infections and the uncircumcised state: an update. *Clin Pediatr (Phila)*. 1993;32(3):130–134

22. Wiswell TE, Smith FR, Bass JW. Decreased incidence of urinary tract infections in circumcised male infants. *Pediatrics*. 1985;75(5):901–903

23. Ginsburg CM, McCracken GH Jr. Urinary tract infections in young infants. *Pediatrics*. 1982;69(4):409–412

24. Craig JC, Knight JF, Sureshkumar P, Mantz E, Roy LP. Effect of circumcision on incidence of urinary tract infection in preschool boys. *J Pediatr*. 1996;128(1):23–27

25. Levine DA, Platt SL, Dayan PS, et al. Risk of serious bacterial infection in young febrile infants with respiratory syncytial virus infections. *Pediatrics*. 2004;113(6):1728–1734

26. Roberts KB, Charney E, Sweren RJ, et al. Urinary tract infection in infants with unexplained fever: a collaborative study. *J Pediatr*. 1983;103(6):864–867

27. Gorelick MH, Hoberman A, Kearney D, Wald E, Shaw KN. Validation of a decision rule identifying febrile young girls at high risk for urinary tract infection. *Pediatr Emerg Care*. 2003;19(3):162–164

28. Gorelick MH, Shaw KN. Clinical decision rule to identify febrile young girls at risk for urinary tract infection. *Arch Pediatr Adolesc Med*. 2000;154(4):386–390

29. Shaw KN, Gorelick M, McGowan KL, Yakscoe NM, Schwartz JS. Prevalence of urinary tract infection in febrile young children in the emergency department. *Pediatrics*. 1998;102(2). Available at: www.pediatrics.org/cgi/content/full/102/2/e16

30. Shaikh N, Morone NE, Lopez J, et al. Does this child have a urinary tract infection? *JAMA*. 2007;298(24):2895–2904

31. Powell HR, McCredie DA, Ritchie MA. Urinary nitrite in symptomatic and asymptomatic urinary infection. *Arch Dis Child*. 1987;62(2):138–140

32. Kunin CM, DeGroot JE. Sensitivity of a nitrite indicator strip method in detecting bacteriuria in preschool girls. *Pediatrics*. 1977;60(2):244–245

33. Hoberman A, Wald ER, Reynolds EA, Penchansky L, Charron M. Is urine culture necessary to rule out urinary tract infection in young febrile children? *Pediatr Infect Dis J*. 1996;15(4):304–309

34. Herr SM, Wald ER, Pitetti RD, Choi SS. Enhanced urinalysis improves identification of febrile infants ages 60 days and younger at low risk for serious bacterial illness. *Pediatrics*. 2001;108(4):866–871

35. Kunin C. A ten-year study of bacteriuria in schoolgirls: final report of bacteriologic, urologic, and epidemiologic findings. *J Infect Dis*. 1970;122(5):382–393

36. Kemper K, Avner E. The case against screening urinalyses for asymptomatic bacteriuria in children. *Am J Dis Child*. 1992;146(3):343–346

37. Wald E. Genitourinary tract infections: cystitis and pyelonephritis. In: Feigin R, Cherry JD, Demmler GJ, Kaplan SL, eds. *Textbook of Pediatric Infectious Diseases*. 5th ed. Philadelphia, PA: Saunders; 2004:541–555

38. Mayo S, Acevedo D, Quiñones-Torrelo C, Canós I, Sancho M. Clinical laboratory automated urinalysis: comparison among automated microscopy, flow cytometry, two test strips analyzers, and manual microscopic examination of the urine sediments. *J Clin Lab Anal*. 2008;22(4):262–270

39. Kass E. Asymptomatic infections of the urinary tract. *Trans Assoc Am Phys*. 1956;69:56–64

40. Hoberman A, Wald ER, Reynolds EA, Penchansky L, Charron M. Pyuria and bacteriuria in urine specimens obtained by catheter from young children with fever. *J Pediatr*. 1994;124(4):513–519

41. Downs SM. Technical report: urinary tract infections in febrile infants and young children. *Pediatrics*. 1999;103(4). Available at: www.pediatrics.org/cgi/content/full/103/4/e54

42. Hoberman A, Wald ER, Hickey RW, et al. Oral versus initial intravenous therapy for urinary tract infections in young febrile children. *Pediatrics*. 1999;104(1):79–86

43. Hodson EM, Willis NS, Craig JC. Antibiotics for acute pyelonephritis in children. *Cochrane Database Syst Rev*. 2007;(4):CD003772

44. Bloomfield P, Hodson EM, Craig JC. Antibiotics for acute pyelonephritis in children. *Cochrane Database Syst Rev*. 2005;(1):CD003772

45. Hoberman A, Charron M, Hickey RW, Baskin M, Kearney DH, Wald ER. Imaging studies after a first febrile urinary tract infection in young children. *N Engl J Med*. 2003;348(3):195–202

46. Jahnukainen T, Honkinen O, Ruuskanen O, Mertsola J. Ultrasonography after the first febrile urinary tract infection in children. *Eur J Pediatr*. 2006;165(8):556–559

47. Economou G, Egginton J, Brookfield D. The importance of late pregnancy scans for renal tract abnormalities. *Prenat Diagn*. 1994;14(3):177–180

48. Roberts J. Experimental pyelonephritis in the monkey, part III: pathophysiology of ure-

teral malfunction induced by bacteria. *Invest Urol.* 1975;13(2):117–120

49. Smith T, Evans K, Lythgoe MF, Anderson PJ, Gordon I. Radiation dosimetry of technetium-99m-DMSA in children. *J Nucl Med.* 1996;37(8):1336–1342

50. Ward VL. Patient dose reduction during voiding cystourethrography. *Pediatr Radiol.* 2006;36(suppl 2):168–172

51. Pennesi M, Travan L, Peratoner L, et al. Is antibiotic prophylaxis in children with vesicoureteral reflux effective in preventing pyelonephritis and renal scars? A randomized, controlled trial. *Pediatrics.* 2008; 121(6). Available at: www.pediatrics.org/cgi/content/full/121/6/e1489

52. Garin EH, Olavarria F, Garcia Nieto V, Valenciano B, Campos A, Young L. Clinical significance of primary vesicoureteral reflux and urinary antibiotic prophylaxis after acute pyelonephritis: a multicenter, randomized, controlled study. *Pediatrics.* 2006;117(3): 626–632

53. Montini G, Rigon L, Zucchetta P, et al. Prophylaxis after first febrile urinary tract infection in children? A multicenter, randomized, controlled, noninferiority trial. *Pediatrics.* 2008;122(5):1064–1071

54. Roussey-Kesler G, Gadjos V, Idres N, et al. Antibiotic prophylaxis for the prevention of recurrent urinary tract infection in children with low grade vesicoureteral reflux: results from a prospective randomized study. *J Urol.* 2008;179(2):674–679

55. Craig J, Simpson J, Williams G. Antibiotic prophylaxis and recurrent urinary tract infection in children. *N Engl J Med.* 2009; 361(18):1748–1759

56. Brandström P, Esbjorner E, Herthelius M, Swerkersson S, Jodal U, Hansson S. The Swedish Reflux Trial in Children, part III: urinary tract infection pattern. *J Urol.* 2010; 184(1):286–291

57. National Institute for Health and Clinical Excellence. *Urinary Tract Infection in Children: Diagnosis, Treatment, and Long-term Management: NICE Clinical Guideline 54.* London, England: National Institute for Health and Clinical Excellence; 2007. Available at: www.nice.org.uk/nicemedia/live/11819/36032/36032.pdf. Accessed March 14, 2011

58. Keren R, Carpenter MA, Hoberman A, et al. Rationale and design issues of the Randomized Intervention for Children With Vesicoureteral Reflux (RIVUR) study. *Pediatrics.* 2008;122(suppl 5):S240–S250

59. Jodal U. The natural history of bacteriuria in childhood. *Infect Dis Clin North Am.* 1987; 1(4):713–729

60. Eccles MR, Bailey RR, Abbott GD, Sullivan MJ. Unravelling the genetics of vesicoureteric reflux: a common familial disorder. *Hum Mol Genet.* 1996;5(Spec No.):1425–1429

61. Scott JE, Swallow V, Coulthard MG, Lambert HJ, Lee RE. Screening of newborn babies for familial ureteric reflux. *Lancet.* 1997; 350(9075):396–400

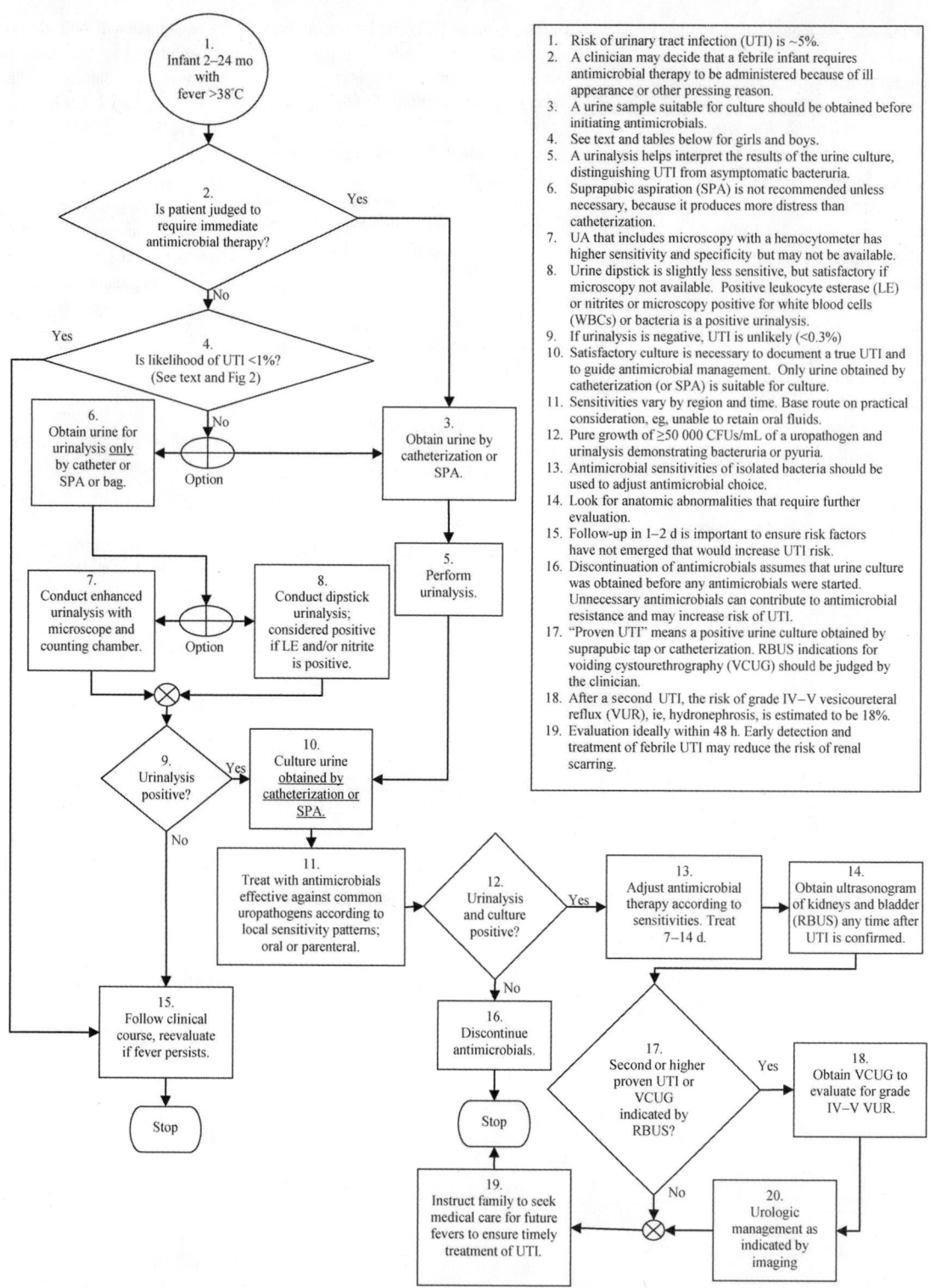

APPENDIX
Clinical practice guideline algorithm.

Technical Report—Diagnosis and Management of an Initial UTI in Febrile Infants and Young Children

S. Maria E. Finnell, MD, MS, Aaron E. Carroll, MD, MS, Stephen M. Downs, MD, MS, and the Subcommittee on Urinary Tract Infection

KEY WORDS
urinary tract infection, infants, children, vesicoureteral reflux, voiding cystourethrography, antimicrobial, prophylaxis, antibiotic prophylaxis, pyelonephritis

ABBREVIATIONS
UTI—urinary tract infection
VUR—vesicoureteral reflux
VCUG—voiding cystourethrography
CI—confidence interval
RR—risk ratio
RCT—randomized controlled trial
LR—likelihood ratio
SPA—suprapubic aspiration

www.pediatrics.org/cgi/doi/10.1542/peds.2011-1332

doi:10.1542/peds.2011-1332

All technical reports from the American Academy of Pediatrics automatically expire 5 years after publication unless reaffirmed, revised, or retired at or before that time.

PEDIATRICS (ISSN Numbers: Print, 0031-4005; Online, 1098-4275).

Copyright © 2011 by the American Academy of Pediatrics

COMPANION PAPERS: Companions to this article can be found on pages 572 and 595, and online at www.pediatrics.org/cgi/doi/10.1542/peds.2011-1330, www.pediatrics.org/cgi/doi/10.1542/peds.2011-1818, and www.pediatrics.org/cgi/doi/10.1542/peds.2011-1330.

abstract

OBJECTIVES: The diagnosis and management of urinary tract infections (UTIs) in young children are clinically challenging. This report was developed to inform the revised, evidence-based, clinical guideline regarding the diagnosis and management of initial UTIs in febrile infants and young children, 2 to 24 months of age, from the American Academy of Pediatrics Subcommittee on Urinary Tract Infection.

METHODS: The conceptual model presented in the 1999 technical report was updated after a comprehensive review of published literature. Studies with potentially new information or with evidence that reinforced the 1999 technical report were retained. Meta-analyses on the effectiveness of antimicrobial prophylaxis to prevent recurrent UTI were performed.

RESULTS: Review of recent literature revealed new evidence in the following areas. Certain clinical findings and new urinalysis methods can help clinicians identify febrile children at very low risk of UTI. Oral antimicrobial therapy is as effective as parenteral therapy in treating UTI. Data from published, randomized controlled trials do not support antimicrobial prophylaxis to prevent febrile UTI when vesicoureteral reflux is found through voiding cystourethrography. Ultrasonography of the urinary tract after the first UTI has poor sensitivity. Early antimicrobial treatment may decrease the risk of renal damage from UTI.

CONCLUSIONS: Recent literature agrees with most of the evidence presented in the 1999 technical report, but meta-analyses of data from recent, randomized controlled trials do not support antimicrobial prophylaxis to prevent febrile UTI. This finding argues against voiding cystourethrography after the first UTI. *Pediatrics* 2011;128:e749–e770

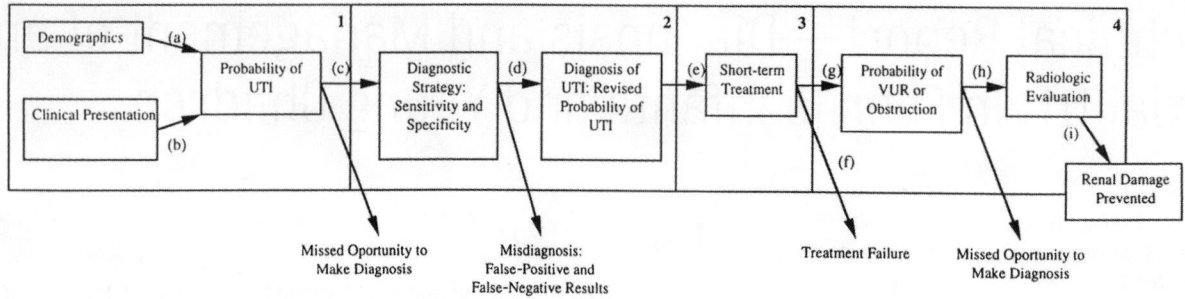

FIGURE 1
Evidence model from the 1999 technical report on the diagnosis and treatment of infants and children with UTIs.

In 1999, the Subcommittee on Urinary Tract Infection of the American Academy of Pediatrics released its guideline on detection, diagnosis, and management for children between 2 and 24 months of age with febrile urinary tract infections (UTIs).[1] The guideline was supported by a technical report[2] that included a critical review of the relevant literature and a cost-effectiveness analysis. Consistent with the policies of the American Academy of Pediatrics, the subcommittee has undertaken a revision of the guideline. This technical report was developed to support the guideline.[3]

The revised technical report was to be based on a selective review of the literature, focusing on changes in the evidence regarding detection, diagnosis, and management of UTIs in these children. The original technical report was designed around an evidence model (Fig 1). Each cell (numbered 1–4) corresponded to a stage in the recognition, diagnosis, or management of UTI. The boxes represented steps the clinician must follow, and the arrows represented the process of moving from one step to the next. Downward arrows represented undesirable consequences in management.[4]

In cell 1, the clinician must combine patient demographic data and other presenting clinical data to arrive at an assessment of the risk of UTI. Failure to do so results in a missed opportunity to make the diagnosis. In cell 2, the cli-

nician must undertake a diagnostic strategy, primarily involving laboratory testing, to arrive at a posterior (posttest) probability of UTI, ruling the diagnosis in or out. Poor test choices or interpretation of results can lead to misdiagnosis. In cell 3, the clinician must choose a treatment for acute UTI; in cell 4, the clinician must consider the possibility of structural or functional anomalies of the urinary tract and diagnose them appropriately to avoid ongoing renal damage.

Implicit in cell 4 is the idea that anomalies of the urinary tract, such as vesicoureteral reflux (VUR) and obstructions, may, if left untreated, lead to significant renal damage, resulting in hypertension or end-stage renal disease. Furthermore, it is assumed that treatment with medical or surgical therapies can prevent these consequences successfully.

The conclusions of the 1999 technical report were that there were high-quality data regarding the prevalence of UTI among febrile infants, the performance of standard diagnostic tests for UTI, and the prevalence of urinary tract abnormalities among children with UTI. The evidence indicating that certain patient characteristics (age, gender, and circumcision status) affected the probability of UTI was weaker. The evidence supporting the relationship between urinary tract abnormalities and future complications, such as hypertension or renal failure,

was considered very poor, and the effectiveness of treatments to prevent these complications was not addressed directly but was assumed.

The cost-effectiveness analysis using these data led to the conclusion that diagnosis and treatment of UTI and evaluation for urinary tract anomalies had borderline cost-effectiveness, costing approximately $700 000 per case of hypertension or end-stage renal disease prevented. On the basis of these results, the subcommittee recommended testing all children between 2 and 24 months of age with fever with no obvious source for UTI, by culturing urine obtained through bladder tap or catheterization. As an option for children who were not going to receive immediate antimicrobial treatment, the committee recommended ruling out UTI through urinalysis of urine obtained with any convenient method. The committee concluded that children found to have a UTI should undergo renal ultrasonography and voiding cystourethrography (VCUG) for evaluation for urinary tract abnormalities, most frequently VUR.

Ten years later, the subcommittee has undertaken a review of the technical analysis for a revised guideline. The strategy for this technical report was to survey the medical literature published in the past 10 years for studies of UTIs in young children. The literature was examined for any data that varied significantly from those analyzed in the first technical report. This survey found an emerging body of literature addressing the effectiveness of antimicrobial agents to prevent recurrent UTI. Therefore, the authors conducted a critical literature review and meta-analysis focused on that specific issue.

METHODS

Surveillance of Recent Literature

The authors searched Medline for articles published in the past 10 years with the medical subject headings "urinary tract infection" and "child (all)." The original search was conducted in 2007, but searches were repeated at intervals (approximately every 3 months) to identify new reports as the guideline was being developed. Titles were reviewed by 2 authors (Drs Downs and Carroll) to identify all articles that were potentially relevant and seemed to contain original data. All titles that were considered potentially relevant by either reviewer were retained. Abstracts of selected articles were reviewed, again to identify articles that were relevant to the guideline and that seemed to contain original data. Review articles that were relevant also were retained for review. Again, all abstracts that were considered potentially relevant by either reviewer were retained. In addition, members of the subcommittee submitted articles that they thought were relevant to be included in the review.

Selected articles were reviewed and summarized by 2 reviewers (Drs Finnell and Downs). The summaries were reviewed, and articles presenting potentially new information were retained. In addition, representative articles reinforcing evidence in the 1999 technical report were retained.

The most significant area of change in the UTI landscape was a new and growing body of evidence regarding the effectiveness of antimicrobial prophylaxis to prevent recurrent infections in

children with VUR. To explore this particular issue, a second, systematic, targeted literature search and formal meta-analysis were conducted to estimate the effectiveness of antimicrobial prophylaxis to prevent renal damage in children with VUR. In addition, 1 author (Dr Finnell) and the chairperson of the guideline committee (Dr Roberts) contacted the authors of those studies to obtain original data permitting subgroup analyses.

Targeted Literature Search and Meta-analysis

To examine specifically the effectiveness of antimicrobial prophylaxis to prevent recurrent UTI and pyelonephritis in children with VUR, a formal meta-analysis of randomized controlled trials (RCTs) was conducted. First, a systematic literature review focused on RCTs, including studies in press, was performed.

Inclusion Criteria

RCTs published in the past 15 years (1993–2009) that compared antimicrobial treatment versus no treatment or placebo treatment for the prevention of recurrent UTI and included a minimum of 6 months of follow-up monitoring were included. Published articles, articles in press, and published abstracts were included. There were no language restrictions. To be included, studies needed to enroll children who had undergone VCUG for determination of the presence and grade of VUR. Studies that examined antibiotic prophylaxis versus no treatment or placebo treatment were included.

Outcome Measures

The primary outcome was the number of episodes of pyelonephritis or febrile UTI diagnosed on the basis of the presence of fever and bacterial growth in urine cultures. A secondary outcome was an episode of any type of UTI, including cystitis, nonfebrile UTI, and

asymptomatic bacteriuria in addition to the cases of pyelonephritis or febrile UTI.

Search Methods

The initial literature search was conducted on June 24, 2008, and the search was repeated on April 14, 2009. Studies were obtained from the following databases: Medline (1993 to June 2008), Embase (1993 to June 2008), Cochrane Central Register for Controlled Trials, bibliographies of identified relevant articles and reviews, and the Web site www.ClinicalTrials.gov.

The search terms "vesico-ureteral reflux," "VUR," "vesicoureter*," "vesico ureter*," "vesicourethral," or "vesico urethral" and "antibiotic," "anti biotic," "antibacterial," "anti bacterial," "antimicrobial," "anti microbial," "antiinfective," or "anti infective" were used. The asterisk represents the truncation or wild card symbol, which indicates that all suffixes and variants were included. The search was limited to the publication types and subject headings for all clinical trials and included all keyword variants for "random" in Medline and Embase.[5] In addition, the Web site www.ClinicalTrials.gov was searched on May 20, 2010.

The search strategy and the screening of the titles for selection of potentially relevant abstracts were completed by 1 reviewer (Dr Finnell). Two reviewers (Drs Finnell and Downs) screened selected abstracts to identify appropriate articles. Published articles and abstracts that met the inclusion criteria were included in the meta-analysis. Additional information was sought from authors whose articles or abstracts did not contain the information needed for a decision regarding inclusion. The selection process is summarized in Fig 2.

Assessment of Studies

The quality of selected articles and abstracts was assessed with the scoring

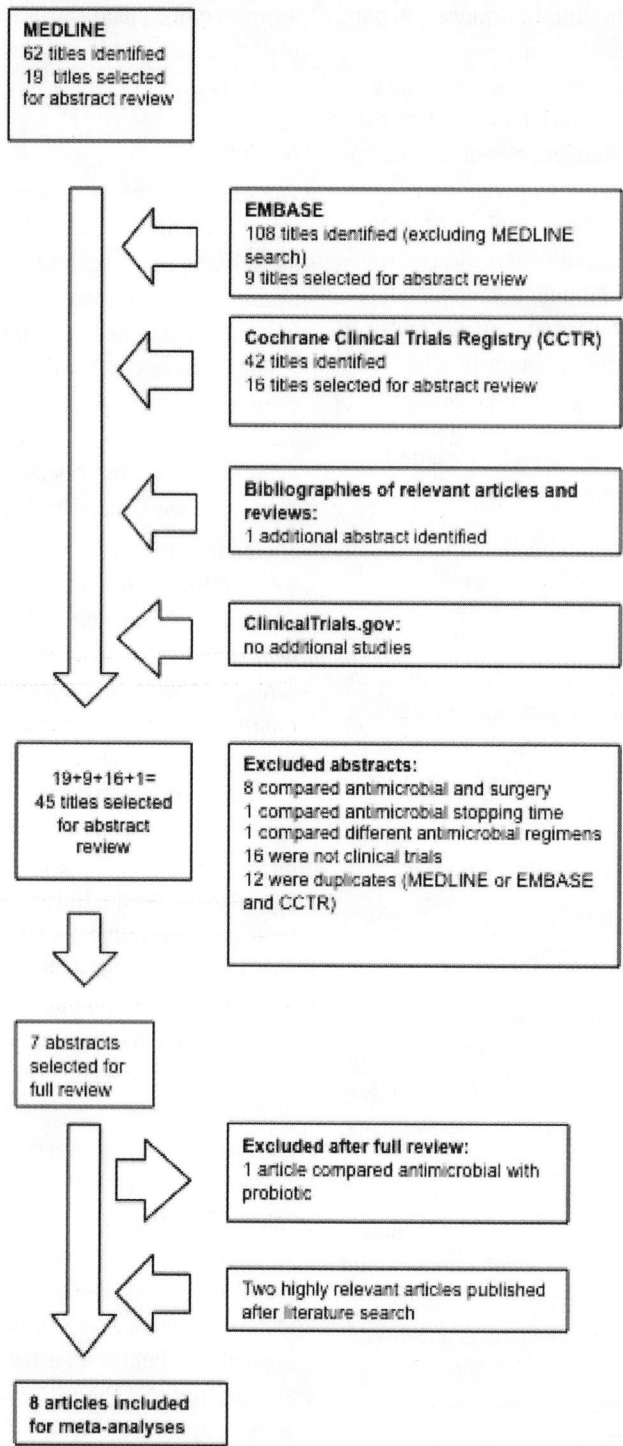

FIGURE 2
Study selection for meta-analyses.

Meta-analyses

All statistical tests were performed by using Review Manager 5.1 (Nordic Cochrane Centre, Copenhagen, Denmark). The following settings were used for the analyses: dichotomous outcome and Mantel-Haenzel statistical method. Data were analyzed with a random-effects model. When no statistically significant effect and no statistical heterogeneity were detected, data also were analyzed with a fixed-effects model, because that type of analysis is more likely to detect a difference. The effect measure was presented as a risk ratio (RR). The results for the primary outcome (pyelonephritis or febrile UTI) and the secondary outcome (any type of UTI, including cystitis, nonfebrile UTI, and asymptomatic bacteriuria) were calculated as point estimates with corresponding 95% confidence intervals (CIs). Heterogeneity was analyzed by using the Q statistic with a threshold of $P < .05$. The number of studies was insufficient for assessment of publication bias with a funnel plot.

Meta-analyses of Data According to VUR Grade and for Children 2 to 24 Months of Age

The published data on which the meta-analyses were based did not contain subgroup data relevant to the practice guideline. Specifically, some studies did not report outcomes according to the severity of VUR, and some did not report outcomes specific to the age range of interest (2–24 months). Therefore, the committee chairperson contacted the authors of the reports included in the meta-analysis, to obtain original data. Data on recurrence according to VUR grade and for the subgroup of children 2 to 24 months of age were received from the authors, and these data were analyzed in separate meta-analyses.

system described by Downs and Black in 1998.[6] Each study received scores (from 2 assessors) on a scale from 0 to 32. Six of the articles and abstracts were included in a first meta-analysis, which evaluated febrile UTI or pyelonephritis as the outcome. A second meta-analysis, which included all studies with the outcome "all UTI," also was conducted.

RESULTS

Surveillance of Recent Literature

The surveillance of recent literature yielded 1308 titles. Of those, 297 abstracts were selected for review. From among the abstracts, 159 articles were selected for full review. The results of this surveillance, as well as the full review and meta-analyses, are organized according to the evidence diagram in Fig 1.

Box 1: Prevalence and Risk Factors for UTI

The Presence of UTI Should Be Considered for Any Child 2 Months to 2 Years of Age With Unexplained Fever

The previous technical report described a very consistent UTI prevalence of 5% among children 2 to 24 months of age with a fever without obvious source. In 1996, Hoberman et al[7] conducted a study of urine diagnostic tests with a cohort of 4253 infants with fever and found a prevalence of 5%. Similarly, in a 1999 cohort study of 534 children 3 to 36 months of age with a temperature of more than 39°C and no apparent source of fever, UTI prevalence was determined to be 5%.[8] In a 1998 cohort study of 2411 children (boys and girls <12 months of age and girls 12–24 months of age) seen in the emergency department with a temperature of more than 38.5°C, Shaw et al[9] determined the prevalence of UTI to be 3.3%. Because 84% of those children were black, this estimate may be low for the general population (see below). In a meta-analysis of 14 studies, the pooled prevalence of UTI was 7% (95% CI: 5.5%–8.4%) among febrile children 0 to 24 months of age, of both genders, with or without additional symptoms of UTI.[10] In the 6- to 12-month age group, however, the prevalence was 5.4%; in the 12- to 24-month age group, the prevalence was 4.5%. Taken to-

gether, these estimates are consistent with a pooled prevalence of 5% determined in earlier studies.

The previous technical report examined the effects of age, gender, and circumcision status on the prevalence of UTI. The conclusion was that boys more than 1 year of age who had been circumcised were at sufficiently low risk of UTI (<1%) that evaluation of this subpopulation would not be cost-effective. New work confirms an approximately threefold to fourfold decreased risk of UTI among circumcised boys.[10] The difference seems to be greater for younger children.[11] Additional clinical characteristics were shown more recently to affect the risk of UTI among febrile infants and children. From a study by Shaikh et al,[12] a set of likelihood ratios (LRs) for various risk factors for UTI was derived (Table 1).

A simplified way to examine the data on boys from Shaikh et al[12] is first to ex-

clude boys with a history of UTI, because the guideline addresses only first-time UTIs, and to exclude those with ill appearance, because they are likely to require antimicrobial agents, in which case a urine specimen would be required. Finally, boys with and without circumcision should be considered separately. This leaves 4 risk factors for boys who present with fever, namely, temperature above 39°C, fever for more than 24 hours, no apparent fever source, and nonblack race. All 4 have similar LRs. If 2 assumptions are made, then the decision rule can be simplified. The first assumption is that, as a first approximation, each risk factor has a positive LR of 1.4 and a negative LR of 0.7. The second assumption is that the presence of each risk factor is conditionally independent of the others, given the presence or absence of UTI. With these reasonable assumptions, Table 2 applies to boys with no previous history of UTI

TABLE 1 LRs and Posttest Probabilities of UTI for Infant Boys According to Number of Findings Present

Finding	LR		Posttest Probability, %					
			All Boys		Circumcised Boys		Uncircumcised Boys	
	Positive	Negative	After Positive Results	After Negative Results	After Positive Results	After Negative Results	After Positive Results	After Negative Results
Uncircumcised	2.8	0.33	5.9	0.7	—	—	—	—
History of UTI	2.6	0.96	5.5	2.1	1.8	0.7	14.0	5.7
Temperature of >39°C	1.4	0.76	3.1	1.7	1.0	0.5	8.1	4.5
Fever without apparent source	1.4	0.69	3.1	1.5	1.0	0.5	8.1	4.1
Ill appearance	1.9	0.68	4.1	1.5	1.3	0.5	10.6	4.1
Fever for >24 h	2.0	0.9	4.3	2.0	1.4	0.6	11.1	5.3
Nonblack race	1.4	0.52	3.1	1.2	1.0	0.4	8.1	3.2

TABLE 2 LRs and Posttest Probabilities of UTI for Febrile Infant Boys According to Number of Findings Present

No. of Risk Factors	LR	Posttest Probability, %		
		All Boys	Uncircumcised	Circumcised
0	0.34	0.8	2.1	0.2
1	0.69	1.5	4.1	0.5
2	1.37	3.0	7.9	1.0
3	2.74	5.8	14.7	1.9
4	5.49	11.0	25.6	3.7

Risk factors: temperature above 39°C, fever for more than 24 hours, no apparent fever source, and nonblack race.

TABLE 3 LRs and Posttest Probabilities of UTI for Febrile Infant Girls According to Number of Findings Present (Prospective Original Study)

Cutoff Value, No. of Factors	LR		Posttest Probability, %	
	Positive	Negative (Approximate)	Below Cutoff Value	At or Above Cutoff Value
1	1.04	0.20	0.8	5.1
2	1.35	0.17	0.8	6.5
3	2.5	0.42	2.1	11.4
4	9.4	0.79	3.9	33.0
5	15.8	0.95	4.7	45.0

Risk factors: less than 12 months of age, white race, temperature > 39°C, fever for at least 2 days, and absence of another source of infection.

TABLE 4 LRs and Posttest Probabilities of UTI for Febrile Infant Girls According to Number of Findings Present (Retrospective Validation Study)

No. of Findings	LR	Posttest Probability, %
0 or 1	1.02	0.8
2	1.10	0.9
3	1.26	1.0
4	3.04	2.4
5	2.13	1.7

Risk factors: less than 12 months of age, white race, temperature > 39°C, fever for at least 2 days, and absence of another source of infection.

and do not appear ill. The LR is calculated as LR = $(1.4)^p \times (0.7)^n$, where p is the number of positive findings and n is the number of negative findings. This assumes that the clinician has assessed all 4 risk factors. It should be noted that, for uncircumcised boys, the risk of UTI never decreases below 2%. For circumcised boys, the probability exceeds 1% if there are 2 or more risk factors.

Other studies have shown that the presence of another, clinically obvious source of infection,[13] particularly documented viral infections,[14] such as respiratory syncytial virus infections,[15] reduces the risk of UTI by one-half. In a series of studies conducted by Gorelick, Shaw, and others,[9,16,17] male gender, black race, and no history of UTI were all found to reduce the risk. The authors derived a prediction rule specifically for girls, with 95% sensitivity and 31% specificity. In a subsequent validation study, they confirmed that these findings had predictive power, but the validation study used a weaker, retrospective, case-control design, compared with the more-robust, prospective, cohort design of the original derivation study. On the basis of the earlier cohort study and starting with a baseline risk of 5%, a child scoring low on the prediction rule would have a slightly less than 1% risk of UTI. To score this low on the prediction rule, a young girl would have to exhibit no more than 1 of the following features: less than 12 months of age, white race, temperature of more than 39°C, fever for at least 2 days, or absence of another source of infection.

However, those authors evaluated their decision rule with several different cutoff points, to determine the score below which the risk of UTI decreased below a test threshold of 1%. Unfortunately, the published article did not include the set of negative LRs needed to reproduce the posterior probabilities.[17] However, it was possible to approximate them through extrapolation from the receiver operating characteristic curve presented. On the basis of these estimated negative LRs and the positive LRs provided in the article,[17] Table 3 was derived. For each cutoff value in the number of risk factors, Table 3 shows the posterior probability for children with fewer than that number of risk factors (below the cutoff value) and for those with that number of risk factors *or more*. Therefore, the posttest probability is not the risk of UTI for children with exactly that

number of risk factors. Similar results could be derived from the validation study and are shown in Table 4. However, because the second study had a weaker design, the values in Table 3 are more reliable.

These studies provide criteria for practical decision rules that clinicians can use to select patients who need urine samples for analysis and/or culture. They do not establish a threshold or maximal risk of UTI above which a urine sample is needed. However, in surveys of pediatricians, Roberts et al[18] found that only 10% of clinicians thought that a urine culture is indicated if the probability of UTI is less than 1%. In addition, the cost-effectiveness analysis published in the 1999 technical report set a threshold of 1%. However, circumstances such as risk of loss to follow-up monitoring or other clinician concerns may shift this threshold up or down.

TABLE 5 List of Test Characteristics of Diagnostic Tests for UTI Reported in 1999 Technical Report[2]

Test	Sensitivity, %			Specificity, %		
	Range	Median	Mean	Range	Median	Mean
Leukocyte esterase test	67–94	84	83	64–92	77	78
Nitrite test	15–82	58	53	90–100	99	98
Blood assessment	25–64	53	47	60–89	85	78
Protein assessment	40–55	53	50	67–84	77	76
Microscopy, leukocytes	32–100	*78*	73	45–98	87	81
Microscopy, bacteria	16–99	88	81	11–100	93	83
Leukocyte esterase or nitrite test	90–100	92	93	58–91	70	72
Any positive test results in urinalysis	99–100	100	99.8	60–92	63	70

TABLE 6 Test Characteristics of Laboratory Tests for UTI in Children

Study	Test	Population	n	Sensitivity, %	Specificity, %
Lockhart et al[19] (1995)	Leukocyte esterase or nitrite test results positive	Prospective sample, <6 mo of age, ED	207	67	79
	Any bacteria with Gram-staining				
Hoberman et al[7] (1996)	>10 white blood cells per counting chamber or any bacteria per 10 oil emersion fields	<2 y of age, 95% febrile, ED	4253	96	93
Shaw et al[9] (1998)	Enhanced urinalysis	Infants <12 mo of age and girls	3873	94	84
	Dipslide or standard urinalysis	<2 y of age, ≥38.5°C, ED		83	87
Lin et al[20] (2000)	Hemocytometer, ≥10 cells per μL	Systematic review, febrile infants hospitalized, febrile UTI	NA	83	89

ED indicates emergency department; NA, not applicable.

Box 2: Diagnostic Tests for UTI

The 1999 technical report reviewed a large number of studies that described diagnostic tests for UTI. The results are summarized in Table 5. This updated review of the literature largely reinforced the findings of the original technical report.

More-recent work compared microscopy, including the use of hemocytometers and counting chambers (enhanced urinalysis), with routine urinalysis or dipslide reagents (Table 6). Lockhart et al[19] found that the observation of any visible bacteria in an uncentrifuged, Gram-stained, urine sample had better sensitivity and specificity than did combined dipslide leukocyte esterase and nitrite test results. Hoberman et al[7] in 1996 and Shaw et al[20] in 1998 both evaluated enhanced urinalysis, consisting of more than 10 white blood cells in a counting chamber or any bacteria seen in 10 oil emersion fields; they found sensitivity of 94% to 96% and specificity of 84% to 93%. In 2000, Lin et al[21] found that a count of at least 10 white blood cells per μL in a hemocytometer was less sensitive (83%) but quite specific (89%). Given the sensitivity of enhanced urinalysis, the probability of UTI for a typical febrile infant with a previous likelihood of UTI of 5% would be reduced to 0.2% to 0.4% with negative enhanced urinalysis results.

Obtaining a Urine Sample

In the UTI practice parameters from 1999, the subcommittee defined the gold standard of a UTI to be growth of bacteria on a culture of urine obtained through suprapubic aspiration (SPA). In the previous technical report, SPA was reported to have success rates ranging from 23% to 90%,[22–24] although higher success rates have been achieved when SPA is conducted under ultrasonographic guidance.[25,26] SPA is considered more invasive than catheterization and, in RCTs from 2006[27] and 2010,[28] pain scores associated with SPA were significantly higher than those associated with catheterization. This result was found for both boys and girls. Similar to previous studies, these RCTs also revealed lower success rates for SPA (66% and 60%), compared with catheterization (83% and 78%).[27,28] In comparison with SPA results, cultures of urine specimens obtained through catheterization are 95% sensitive and 99% specific.[7,11,12]

Cultures of bag specimens are difficult to interpret. In the original technical report, sensitivity was assumed to be 100% but the specificity of bag cultures was shown to range between 14% and 84%.[2] Our updated surveillance of the literature did not show that these numbers have improved.[29–33] One article suggested that a new type of collection bag may result in improved specificity,[34] but that study was not controlled. With a prevalence of 5% and specificity of 70%,

the positive predictive value of a positive culture result for urine obtained in a bag would be 15%. This means that, of all positive culture results for urine obtained in a bag, 85% would be false-positive results.

Box 3: Short-term Treatment of UTIs

General Principles of Treatment

Published evidence regarding the short-term treatment of UTIs supports 4 main points. First, complications, such as bacteremia or renal scarring, are sufficiently common to necessitate early, thorough treatment of febrile UTIs in infants.[35] Second, treatment with orally administered antimicrobial agents is as effective as parenteral therapy.[36,37] Third, bacterial sensitivity to antimicrobial agents is highly variable across time and geographic areas, which suggests that therapy should be guided initially by local sensitivity patterns and should be adjusted on the basis of sensitivities of isolated pathogens.[38,39] Fourth, meta-analyses have suggested that shorter durations of oral therapy may not have a disadvantage over longer courses for UTIs. However, those studies largely excluded febrile UTI and pyelonephritis.[40]

Experimental and Clinical Data Support the Concept That Delays in the Institution of Appropriate Treatment for Pyelonephritis Increase the Risk of Renal Damage

The 1999 technical report cited evidence that febrile UTIs in children less

TABLE 7 Recent Studies Documenting the Prevalence of VUR Among Children With UTI

Study	Description	n	Prevalence, %
Sargent and Stringer[50] (1995)	Retrospective study of first VCUG for UTI in children 1 wk to 15 y of age	309	30
Craig et al[51] (1997)	Cross-sectional study of children <5 y of age with first UTI	272	28
McDonald et al[52] (2000)	Retrospective chart review of children with VCUG after UTI	176	19
Oostenbrink et al[53] (2000)	Cross-sectional study of children <5 y of age with first UTI	140	26
Mahant et al[54] (2001)	Retrospective chart review of children with VCUG after UTI	162	22
Mahant et al[55] (2002)	Retrospective review of VCUG in children <5 y of age admitted with first UTI	162	22
Chand et al[56] (2003)	Retrospective review of VCUG or radionuclide cystogram in children <7 y of age	15 504	35
Fernandez-Menendez et al[44] (2003)	Prospective cohort study of 158 children <5 y of age (85% < 2 y) with first UTI	158	22
Camacho et al[41] (2004)	Prospective cohort study of children 1 mo to 12 y of age (mean age: 20 mo) with first febrile UTI	152	21
Hansson et al[57] (2004)	Retrospective cross-sectional study of children <2 y of age with first UTI	303	26
Pinto[58] (2004)	Retrospective chart review of first VCUG for UTI in children 1 mo to 14 y of age	341	30
Zamir et al[59] (2004)	Cohort study of children 0–5 y of age hospitalized with first UTI	255	18

than 2 years of age are associated with bacterial sepsis in 10% of cases.[35] Furthermore, renal scarring is common among children who have febrile UTIs. The risk is higher among those with higher grades of VUR[41] but occurs with all grades, even when there is no VUR. Although it was not confirmed in all studies,[42,43] older work[2] and newer studies[44] demonstrated an increased risk of scarring with delayed treatment. Children whose treatment is delayed more than 48 hours after onset of fever may have a more than 50% higher risk of acquiring a renal scar.

Oral Versus Intravenous Therapy

In a RCT from 1999, Hoberman et al[36] studied children 1 to 24 months of age with febrile UTIs. They compared 14 days of oral cefixime treatment with 3 days of intravenous cefotaxime treatment followed by oral cefixime treatment to complete a 14-day course. The investigators found no difference in outcomes between children who were treated with an orally administered, third-generation cephalosporin alone and those who received intravenous treatment.

In a Cochrane review, Hodson et al[37] evaluated studies with children 0 to 18 years of age, examining oral versus intravenous therapy. No significant differences were found in duration of fever (2 studies; mean difference: 2.05 hours [95% CI: −0.84 to 4.94 hours]) or

renal parenchymal damage at 6 to 12 months (3 studies; RR: 0.80 [95% CI: 0.50–1.26]) between oral antimicrobial therapy (10–14 days) and intravenous antimicrobial treatment (3 days) followed by oral antimicrobial treatment (11 days).

Duration of Therapy

In the 1999 technical report, data slightly favoring longer-duration (7–10 days) over shorter-duration (1 dose to 3 days) antimicrobial therapy for pediatric patients with UTIs were presented.[2] Since then, several meta-analyses with different conclusions have been published on this topic.[40,45,46] A 2003 Cochrane review addressing the question analyzed studies that examined the difference in rates of recurrence for positive urine cultures after treatment.[40] It compared short (2–4 days) and standard (7–14 days) duration of treatment for UTIs and found no significant difference in the frequency of bacteriuria after completion of treatment (8 studies; RR: 1.06 [95% CI: 0.64–1.76]). Although the authors of the review did not exclude studies of children with febrile UTIs or pyelonephritis, each individual study included in the meta-analysis had already excluded such children. To date, there are no conclusive data on the duration of therapy for children with febrile UTIs or pyelonephritis.

Proof of Cure

Data supporting routine repeat cultures of urine during or after completion of antimicrobial therapy were not available for the 1999 technical report. Retrospective studies did not show "proof of bacteriologic cure" cultures to be beneficial.[47,48] Studies demonstrating that clinical response alone *ensures* bacteriologic cure are not available.

Box 4: Evaluation and Management of Urinary Tract Abnormalities

Prevalence of VUR

Several cohort studies published since the 1999 technical report provide estimates of the prevalence of VUR of various grades among infants and children with UTIs (Table 7). Overall, these estimates are reasonably consistent with those reported in earlier studies, although the grades of reflux are now reported more consistently, by using the international system of radiographic grading of VUR.[49]

The prevalence of VUR among children in these studies varies between 18% and 35%. The weighted average prevalence is 34%, but this is largely driven by the enormous retrospective study by Chand et al.[56] Most studies report a rate of 24% or less, which is less than the estimate of VUR prevalence in the 1999 technical report.

Data on the prevalence of VUR among children *without* a history of UTI do not

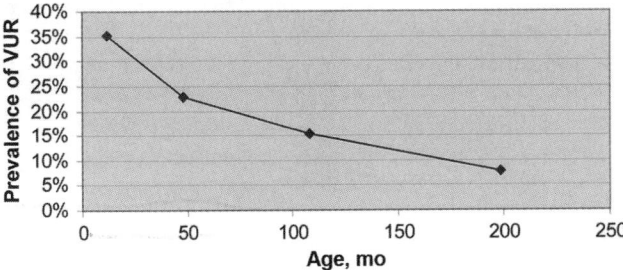

FIGURE 3
Prevalence of VUR as a function of the midpoint of each age stratum, as reported by Chand et al.[56]

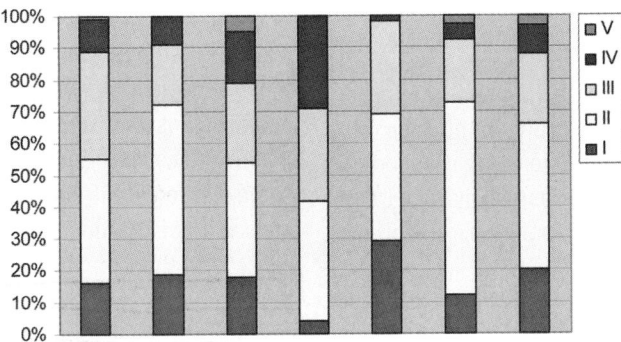

FIGURE 4
Distribution of reflux grades among children with VUR.[41,44,51,56,57,62,63]

exist. Using a retrospective approach and existing urine culture data, Hannula and Ventola and colleagues,[60,61] in 2 separate publications, found similar rates of prevalence of any grade of VUR among children with proven (37.4%) or certain (36%) UTI versus false (34.8%) or improbable (36%) UTI. These results suggest that VUR is prevalent even among children without a history of UTI.

The prevalence of VUR decreases with age. This was approximated by analysis across studies in the 1999 technical report. Since then, Chand et al[56] reported the prevalence VUR within age substrata of their cohort. Figure 3 shows the prevalence of VUR plotted as a function of the midpoint of each age stratum.

Seven studies reported the prevalence of different grades of reflux, by using the international grading system.[41,44,51,56,57,62,63] The distributions of different reflux grades among children who had VUR are shown in Fig 4. There is significant variability in the relative

predominance of each reflux grade, but grades II and III consistently are the most common. With the exception of the study by Camacho et al,[41] all studies showed grades IV and V to be the least frequent, and grade V accounted for 0% to 5% (weighted average: 3%) of reflux. With that value multiplied by the prevalence of VUR among young children with a first UTI, we

would expect grade V reflux to be present in <1% of children with a first UTI.

It has been suggested that the risk of VUR and, more specifically, high-grade VUR may be higher for children with recurrent UTI than for children with a first UTI. Although it was not tested directly in the studies reviewed, this idea can be tested and the magnitude of the effect can be estimated from the data found in the literature search for this meta-analysis.[64–70] These data clearly demonstrate that the risk of UTI recurrence is associated with VUR (Fig 5). Furthermore, this relationship allows the likelihood of each grade of reflux (given that a UTI recurrence has occurred) to be estimated by using Bayes' theorem, as follows:

$$p(VUR_i|UTI)$$
$$= \frac{p(UTI|VUR_i) \times p(VUR_i)}{\sum_{i=0}^{V} p(UTI|VUR_i) \times p(VUR_i)},$$

where $p(UTI|VUR_i)$ refers to the probability of VUR of grade i given the recurrence of UTI. If it is assumed that the conditional probabilities remain the same with second or third UTIs, then Bayes' theorem can be reapplied for a third UTI as well.

By using estimates of $p(UTI|VUR)$ (Fig 5) and the previously determined distri-

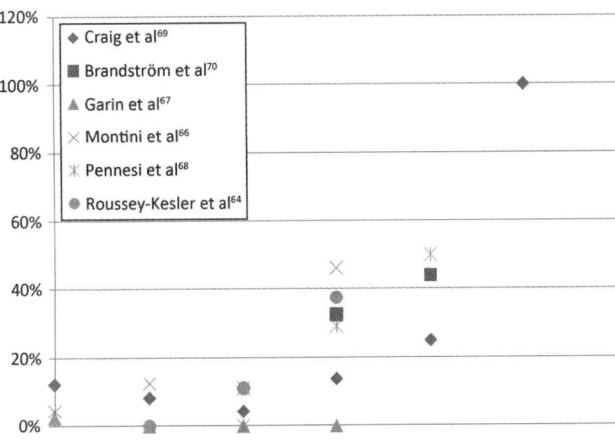

FIGURE 5
Probability of a recurrent febrile UTI as a function of VUR grade among infants 2 to 24 months of age in the control groups of the studies included in meta-analyses.[64,66–70]

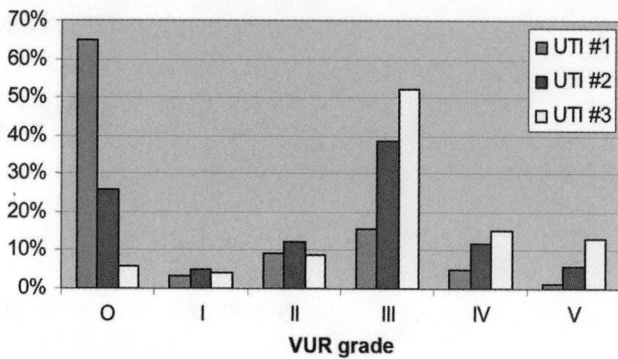

FIGURE 6
Distribution of VUR grades after different numbers of UTIs.

butions of VUR grades (Fig 4), a very approximate estimate of the distribution of VUR grades after the first, second, and third UTI can be made (Fig 6). The likelihood that there is no VUR decreases rapidly. Conversely, the likelihood of VUR grades III to V increases rapidly. The risk of grades I and II changes little.

Ultrasonography

Ultrasonography is used as a noninvasive technique to identify renal abnormalities in children after UTI. The sensitivity of the test varies greatly and has been reported to be as low as 5% for detection of renal scarring[71–73] and 10% for detection of VUR.[74] However, most studies report moderate specificity.

One possible reason for a decrease in specificity is that, in animal models, *Escherichia coli* endotoxin has been shown to produce temporary dilation of the urinary tract during acute infection.[75] Therefore, use of routine ultrasonography for children with UTIs during acute infection may increase the false-positive rate. However, no human data are available to confirm this hypothesis.

Ultrasonography is used during acute infection to identify renal or perirenal abscesses or pyonephrosis in children who fail to experience clinical improvement despite antimicrobial therapy. The sensitivity of ultrasonography for such complications is thought to be

very high, approaching 100%.[76] Therefore, ultrasonography in the case of a child with a UTI who is not responding to therapy as expected can be very helpful in ruling out these infectious complications.

Ultrasonography also is advocated for screening for renal abnormalities such as hydronephrosis, suggesting posterior urethral valves, ureteropelvic junction obstruction, or ureteroceles. The evidence model illustrates the expected outcomes from routine ultrasonography of the kidneys, ureters, and bladder after the first febrile UTI in infants and young children (Fig 7). The model is based on the study results documented in Tables 8 and 9 and a strategy of performing kidney and bladder ultrasonography for all infants with UTIs. The numbers are not exact for 2 reasons, namely, (1) study populations vary and do not always precisely meet the definitions of 2 to 24 months of age and febrile without an-

other fever source and, (2) even within similar populations, reported rates vary widely.

Ultrasonography yields ~15% positive results. However, it has a ~70% false-negative rate for reflux, scarring, and other abnormalities. Limited data exist regarding the false-negative rate for high-grade VUR (grade IV and V), but the studies reviewed presented 0% to 40% false-negative rates for detection of grade IV reflux through ultrasonography.[59,74] Among the 15% of results that are positive, between 1% and 24% are false-positive results. Of the true-positive results, ~40% represent some dilation of the collecting system, such as would be found on a VCUG; 10% represent abnormalities that are potentially surgically correctable (eg, ureteroceles or ureteropelvic junction obstruction). Approximately one-half represent findings such as horseshoe kidneys or renal scarring, for which there is no intervention but which might lead to further evaluations, such as technetium-99m–labeled dimercaptosuccinic acid renal scintigraphy. The 40% with dilation of the collecting system are problematic. This represents only a small fraction of children ($15\% \times 88\% \times 40\% = 5\%$) with first UTIs who would be expected to have VUR before ultrasonography. Ultrasonography does not seem to be enriching for this population (although ultrasonography might identify a population with higher-grade VUR).

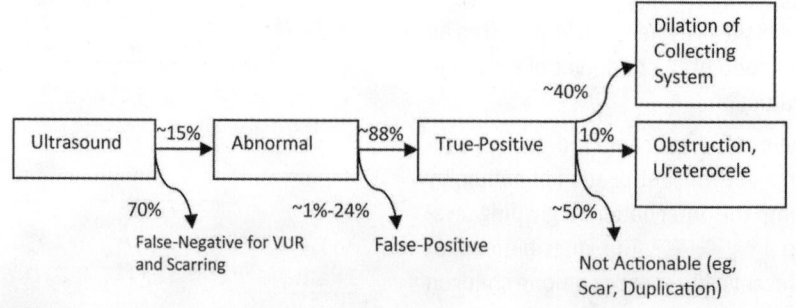

FIGURE 7
Evidence model for ultrasonography after a first UTI.

TABLE 8 Summary of Ultrasonography Literature

Study	n/N (%)	Comments
False-negative rate		
Scarring		
Smellie et al[73] (1995)	7/20 (35)	
Barry et al[77] (1998)	23/170 (14)	
Moorthy et al[71] (2004)	219/231 (95)	
Sinha et al[78] (2007)	61/79 (77)	Reported as renal units
Montini et al[79] (2009)	33/45 (73)	
VUR		
Smellie et al[73] (1995)	21/36 (58)	
Mahant et al[55] (2002)	14/35 (40)	
Hoberman et al[74] (2003)	104/117 (90)	
Zamir et al[59] (2004)	38/47 (81)	
Montini et al[79] (2009)	48/66 (73)	
Other		
Smellie et al[74] (1995)	5/5 (100)	Duplex kidney
False-positive rate		
Scarring		
Barry et al[77] (1998)	11/478 (2)	
Moorthy et al[71] (2004)	12/699 (1.7)	
Sinha et al[78] (2007)	9/870 (1)	
Monitini et al[79] (2009)	26/255 (10)	
VUR		
Smellie et al[73] (1995)	2/12 (17)	Normal VCUG, DMSA, and IVU results
Mahant et al[55] (2002)	30/127 (24)	
Hoberman et al[74] (2003)	17/185 (10)	
Zamir et al[59] (2004)	27/208 (13)	
Other		
Giorgi et al[80] (2005)	21/203 (10)	

IVU indicates intravenous urography; DMSA, dimercaptosuccinic acid.

Prenatal Ultrasonography

Urinary tract abnormalities also may be identified during prenatal ultrasonography,[85–87] which theoretically would decrease the number of new abnormalities found through later ultrasonography.[81] However, the extent to which normal prenatal ultrasonographic findings decrease the need for later studies remains in doubt.

Miron et al[88] studied 209 children who underwent ultrasonography prenatally and again after a UTI. They found that, among 9 children with abnormal ultrasonographic results after UTI, 7 had normal prenatal ultrasonographic results. These cases included 3 cases of hydronephrosis, 3 cases of moderate dilation, and 1 case of double collecting system. Similarly, in a study by Lakhoo et al[89] in 1996, 22 of 39 children with UTIs had normal prenatal ultrasonographic results but "abnormal" post-UTI ultrasonographic results; the abnormalities were not described. These studies suggest that normal prenatal ultrasonographic findings may not be sufficient to obviate the need for additional studies if a UTI occurs in infancy.

Results of Targeted Literature Review and Meta-analysis on Prophylaxis to Prevent Recurrent UTI

Study Identification

For the meta-analysis of studies on the effectiveness of antimicrobial agents to prevent recurrent UTI in children with VUR, we reviewed a total of 213 titles from our primary literature search. Of those, 45 were retained for abstract review on the basis of the title, of which 7 were selected for full review. Six of the studies met the inclusion criteria. Figure 2 summarizes the selection process.

Thirty-eight abstracts were excluded before full review (Fig 2). Eight of those studies were RCTs comparing prophylactic antimicrobial agent use with some type of surgical intervention. None of those studies included a placebo arm.[90–97] One study compared different lengths of antimicrobial prophylaxis.[98] Another study compared different antimicrobial regimens but did not include a placebo arm.[99] Sixteen studies were determined, on closer inspection, to be not clinical trials but prospective cohort studies, reviews, systematic reviews, or meta-analyses. Twelve studies were found twice, either in Medline or Embase and the Cochrane Clinical Trials Registry.

One article was excluded after full review (Fig 2). That study compared prophylactic antimicrobial agent use with probiotic use.[65] The study was not included in the meta-analysis, but the results are described separately.

There are RCTs of antimicrobial prophylaxis that are older than 15 years. In 4 studies from the 1970s, a total of 179 children were enrolled.[100–103] Less than 20% of those children had VUR. Because of limited reporting of results in that subgroup, those older studies were not included in the analyses.

Two additional RCTs comparing antimicrobial prophylaxis and placebo treatment for children were published in October 2009.[69,70] The first trial enrolled children 0 to 18 years of age after a first UTI, with 2% of enrolled children (12 of 576 children) being more than 10 years of age. The second trial enrolled children diagnosed as having VUR after a first UTI (194 [96%] of 203 children) or after prenatal ultrasonography (9 [4%] of 203 children), who were then assigned randomly to receive antimicrobial prophylaxis, surveillance, or endoscopic therapy, at 1 to 2 years of age. The majority of these children (132 children [65%]) had been diagnosed as having VUR before 1

TABLE 9 Distribution of Positive Ultrasonographic Findings

Study	n/N (%)
Alon and Ganapathy[62] (1999)	19/124 (15)
Minimal unilateral changes	
VUR	2 (1.6)
Normal VCUG findings	2 (1.6)
Resolved on repeat study	2 (1.6)
Not monitored further	3 (2.4)
Major changes	8 (6.5)
VUR	1 (1.6)
Normal findings	1 (1.6)
Posterior urethral valve	1 (1.6)
Hydroureternephrosis	1 (1.6)
Gelfand et al[81] (2000)	141/844 (16.7)
Bladder wall thickening	31 (3.7)
Hydroureter	6 (0.7)
Parenchymal abnormalities	42 (5.0)
Pelvocalyceal dilation	27 (3.2)
Renal calculus	1 (0.1)
Simple renal cyst	1 (0.1)
Urethelial thickening	31 (3.7)
Jothilakshmi et al[82] (2001)	42/262 (16)
Duplex kidney	3 (1)
Crossed renal ectopia	1 (0.38)
Horseshoe kidney	1 (0.38)
Hydronephrosis	5 (1.9)
Megaureter	6 (2.3)
Polycystic kidney	1 (0.38)
Pelviureteric junction obstruction	1 (0.38)
Posterior urethral valve	2 (0.76)
Renal calculus	3 (0.01)
Rotated kidney	2 (0.76)
Ureterocele	2 (0.76)
VUR	7 (2.7)
Hoberman et al[74] (2003)	37/309 (12)
Dilated pelvis	13 (4.2)
Pelvocaliectasis	12 (3.9)
Hydronephrosis	2 (0.6)
Dilated ureter	9 (2.9)
Double collecting system	3 (1.0)
Extrarenal pelvis	1 (0.3)
Calculus	1 (0.3)
Zamir et al[59] (2004)	36/255 (14.1)
Mild unilateral pelvis dilation	32 (12.5)
Moderate unilateral pelvis dilation	1 (0.04)
Enlargement kidney	1 (0.04)
Small renal cyst	1 (0.04)
Double collecting system and severe hydronephrosis	1 (0.04)
Jahnukainen et al[83] (2006)[a]	23/155 (14.8)
Hydronephrosis	8 (5)
Double collecting system	11 (7)
Multicystic dysplasia	1 (0.6)
Renal hypoplasia	1 (0.6)
Solitary kidney	1 (0.6)
Horseshoe kidney	1 (0.6)
Huang et al[84] (2008)	112/390 (28.7)
Nephromegaly	46 (11.8)
Isolated hydronephrosis	20 (5.1)
Intermittent hydronephrosis	3 (0.8)
Hydroureter	8 (2.1)
Hydroureter and hydronephrosis	3 (0.8)
Thickened bladder wall	11 (2.8)
Small kidneys	8 (2.1)
Simple ureterocele	5 (1.3)
Double collecting systems	4 (1.0)
Increased echogenicity	3 (0.8)
Horseshoe kidney	1 (0.3)
Montini et al[79] (2009)	38/300 (13)
Dilated pelvis, ureter, or pelvis and calyces	12 (4)
Renal swelling or local parenchymal changes	10 (3.3)
Increased bladder wall or pelvic mucosa, thickness	6 (2)
Other	10 (3.3)

[a] Hospitalized children with UTI.

year of age and thus had been receiving prophylaxis before random assignment. These studies were included in the meta-analysis.

Description of Included Studies

Table 10 presents characteristics of the 8 included studies.[64,66–70,104,105] Four studies enrolled children after diagnosis of a first episode of pyelonephritis.[64,66–68] In those 4 studies, pyelonephritis was described as fever of more than 38°C or 38.5°C and positive urine culture results. In 1 of those studies,[67] dimercaptosuccinic acid scanning results consistent with acute pyelonephritis represented an additional requirement for inclusion. The remaining studies had slightly different inclusion criteria. In the study by Craig et al[71] from 2009, symptoms consistent with UTI and positive urine culture results were required for inclusion. Fever was documented for 79% of enrolled children (454 of 576 children). In the study by Brandström et al,[70] 96% of enrolled children (194 of 203 children) had pyelonephritis, defined in a similar manner as in the 6 initial studies. The remaining patients were enrolled after prenatal diagnosis of VUR. The 2 included abstracts described studies that enrolled any child with VUR and not only children who had had pyelonephritis.[104,105] Seven of the 8 studies (all except the study by Reddy et al[108]) reported a gender ratio. Among those studies, there were 67% girls and 33% boys. Six studies compared antimicrobial treatment with no treatment. Only 2 studies were placebo controlled, and those 2 were the only blinded studies.[69,105] The grade of VUR among the enrolled children varied from 0 to V, but few of the children had grade V VUR.

The ages of children included in the initial meta-analyses were 0 to 18 years; therefore, some children were included who were outside the target

TABLE 10 Studies Included in Meta-analysis

Study	Study Sites	n		Age	VUR Grade	Antimicrobial Agents	Control	Follow-up Period, mo	Outcome
		VUR	No VUR						
Craig et al[105] (2002)	Australia	46	0	0–3 mo	I–V	TMP-SMX	Placebo	36	UTI and renal damage
Craig et al[69] (2009)	Australia	243	234	0–18 y	I–V	TMP-SMX	Placebo	12	Symptomatic UTI, febrile UTI, hospitalization, and renal scarring
Garin et al[67] (2006)	Chile, Spain, United States	113	105	3 mo to 18 y	0–III	TMP-SMX/ nitrofurantoin	No treatment	12	Asymptomatic UTI, cystitis, pyelonephritis, and renal scarring
Brandström et al[70] (2010)	Sweden	203	0	1–2 y	III–IV	TMP-SMX/cefadroxil, nitrofurantoin	No treatment	48	Febrile UTI, reflux status, and renal scarring
Montini et al[66] (2008)	Italy	128	210	2 mo to 7 y	0–III	TMP-SMX/amoxicillin-clavulanate	No treatment	12	Febrile UTI and renal scarring
Pennesi et al[68] (2008)	Italy	100	0	0–30 mo	II–IV	TMP-SMX	No treatment	48	UTI and renal scarring
Reddy et al[104] (1997)	United States	29	0	1–10 y	I–V	TMP-SMX/ nitrofurantoin	No treatment	24	UTI, progression of disease, need for surgery, parental compliance
Roussey-Kesler et al[64] (2008)	France	225	0	1–36 m	I–III	TMP-SMX	No treatment	18	Febrile and afebrile UTI

TMP-SMX indicates trimethoprim-sulfamethoxazole.

age range for this report and for whom other factors (eg, voiding and bowel habits) might have played a role. The median age of the included children, however, was not above 3 years in any of the included studies in which it was reported. Separate meta-analyses were subsequently performed for the subgroup of children who were 2 to 24 months of age. The duration of antimicrobial treatment and follow-up monitoring ranged from 12 to 48 months. The antimicrobial agents used were trimethoprim-sulfamethoxazole (1–2 or 5–10 mg/kg),[64,68,69,105] trimethoprim-sulfamethoxazole or amoxicillin-clavulanic acid (15 mg/kg),[66] trimethoprim-sulfamethoxazole or nitrofurantoin,[67,104] or trimethoprim-sulfamethoxazole, cefadroxil, or nitrofurantoin.[70] Urine collection methods differed among studies. Bag specimens were reported for 3 studies.[64,66,70] In an additional 4 studies, the description of the urine collection methods did not exclude the use of bag specimens.[67,68,104,105] Recurrent UTI was described as (1) asymptomatic bacteriuria (diagnosed through screening cultures), (2) cystitis, (3) febrile UTI, and (4) pyelonephritis (diagnosed on the basis of focal or diffuse uptake on di-

mercaptosuccinic acid scans) in the different articles.

Quality Assessment

The included studies received scores (from 2 assessors) from 7 to 26 (scale range: 0–32) with the scoring system described by Downs and Black,[6] with a median score of 16. Score deductions resulted from lack of blinding of patients (all except 2 studies[69,105]), lack of blinding of assessors (all except 2 studies[69,105]), limited or no information about patients lost to follow-up monitoring (3 studies[64,67,104]), lack of reporting of adverse effects (all except 2 studies[66,69]), and small sample sizes. The lowest scores, 7 and 12, were received by the 2 abstracts because of lack of details in the descriptions of the methods.[104,105]

Antimicrobial Therapy Versus No Treatment

Overview of Findings

Described here are the results of several meta-analyses, subdivided according to type of recurrence (pyelonephritis versus UTI), degree of VUR (none to grade V), and patient age. In summary, antimicrobial prophylaxis does not seem to reduce significantly the

rates of recurrence of pyelonephritis, regardless of age or degree of reflux. Although prophylaxis seems to reduce significantly but only slightly the risk of UTI when all forms are included, most of this effect is attributable to reductions in rates of cystitis or asymptomatic bacteriuria, which would not be expected to lead to ongoing renal damage.

Recurrence of Pyelonephritis/Febrile UTI Among All Studied Children With VUR of Any Grade

Recurrence of pyelonephritis was reported in 6 of the 8 studies. The study by Pennesi et al[68] presented the results as recurrence of pyelonephritis, but recurrence was defined as episodes of fever or "symptoms of UTI." When contacted, this author confirmed that all reported recurrences were characterized by fever above 38.5°C. Therefore, the article was included in the meta-analysis. With a random-effects model, there was no significant difference in rates of recurrence of pyelonephritis for children who received antimicrobial therapy and those who did not. This meta-analysis yielded a RR of 0.77 (95% CI: 0.47–1.24) (Fig 8). Heterogeneity test-

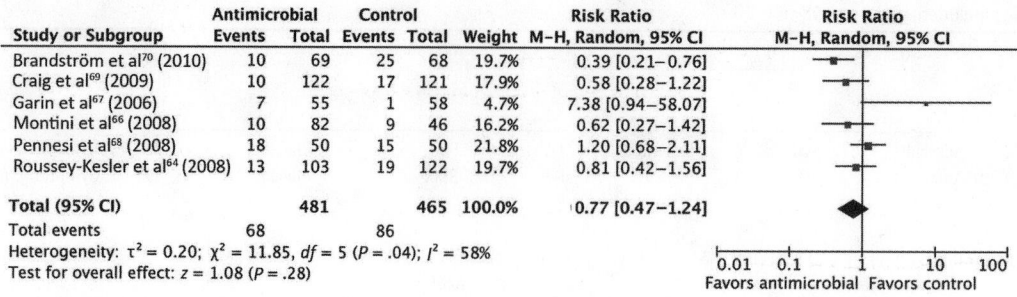

| Study or Subgroup | Antimicrobial | | Control | | Weight | Risk Ratio | Risk Ratio |
	Events	Total	Events	Total		M–H, Random, 95% CI	M–H, Random, 95% CI
Brandström et al[70] (2010)	10	69	25	68	19.7%	0.39 [0.21–0.76]	
Craig et al[69] (2009)	10	122	17	121	17.9%	0.58 [0.28–1.22]	
Garin et al[67] (2006)	7	55	1	58	4.7%	7.38 [0.94–58.07]	
Montini et al[66] (2008)	10	82	9	46	16.2%	0.62 [0.27–1.42]	
Pennesi et al[68] (2008)	18	50	15	50	21.8%	1.20 [0.68–2.11]	
Roussey-Kesler et al[64] (2008)	13	103	19	122	19.7%	0.81 [0.42–1.56]	
Total (95% CI)		**481**		**465**	**100.0%**	**0.77 [0.47–1.24]**	
Total events	68		86				

Heterogeneity: $\tau^2 = 0.20$; $\chi^2 = 11.85$, $df = 5$ $(P = .04)$; $I^2 = 58\%$
Test for overall effect: $z = 1.08$ $(P = .28)$

FIGURE 8
Combined estimates of the effect of antimicrobial prophylaxis on prevention of pyelonephritis in children with VUR, from random-effects modeling. RRs and 95% CIs are shown. M-H indicates Mantel-Haenszel.

| Study or Subgroup | Antimicrobial | | Control | | Weight | Risk Ratio | Risk Ratio |
	Events	Total	Events	Total		M–H, Random, 95% CI	M–H, Random, 95% CI
Craig et al[69] (2009)	6	119	14	115	60.2%	0.41 [0.16–1.04]	
Garin et al[67] (2006)	2	45	2	60	13.8%	1.33 [0.20–9.11]	
Montini et al[66] (2008)	5	129	3	81	25.9%	1.05 [0.26–4.26]	
Total (95% CI)		**293**		**256**	**100.0%**	**0.62 [0.30–1.27]**	
Total events	13		19				

Heterogeneity: $\tau^2 = 0.00$; $\chi^2 = 1.88$, $df = 2$ $(P = .39)$; $I^2 = 0\%$
Test for overall effect: $z = 1.31$ $(P = .19)$

FIGURE 9
Combined estimates of the effect of antimicrobial prophylaxis on prevention of pyelonephritis in children without VUR, from random-effects modeling. RRs and 95% CIs are shown. M-H indicates Mantel-Haenszel.

ing results were significant $(P = .04)$, which indicated statistical heterogeneity between studies.

Recurrence of Pyelonephritis/ Febrile UTI Among Children of All Ages Without VUR

There was no significant difference in rates of recurrence of pyelonephritis for children without VUR who received antimicrobial therapy and those who did not. With random-effects modeling, the meta-analysis yielded a RR of 0.62 (95% CI: 0.30–1.27) (Fig 9). Heterogeneity testing results were not significant $(P = .39)$. Because no difference was detected with a random-effects model and there was no statistical heterogeneity in this analysis, analysis also was conducted with a fixed-effects model. With fixed-effects modeling, the meta-analysis yielded a RR of 0.61 (95% CI: 0.31–1.23).

Recurrence of Pyelonephritis/Febrile UTI Among Children of All Ages With VUR, According to Grade

Table 11 summarizes the results of separate meta-analyses of subpopula-

TABLE 11 Combined Estimates of Effect of Antimicrobial Prophylaxis on Prevention of Pyelonephritis for All Children According to Grade of VUR

VUR Grade	No. of Children	No. of Studies	RR (95% CI)[a]
0	549	3	0.62 (0.30–1.27)
I–II	455	5	0.94 (0.49–1.80)
III	347	6	0.74 (0.42–1.29)
IV	122	3	0.69 (0.39–1.20)
V	5	1	0.40 (0.08–1.90)

[a] From random-effects model.

tions from each study with different grades of VUR. None of those analyses showed a statistically significant difference in rates of recurrence with random- or fixed-effects modeling. Random-effects modeling results are presented.

Recurrence of Pyelonephritis/Febrile UTI Among Children 2 to 24 Months of Age With VUR of Any Grade

There was no significant difference in rates of recurrence of pyelonephritis for children 2 to 24 months of age with VUR who received antimicrobial agents and those who did not. With random-effects modeling, the meta-analysis yielded a RR of 0.78

(95% CI: 0.48–1.26) (Fig 10). Heterogeneity testing results were not significant $(P = .07)$. With fixed-effects modeling, the meta-analysis yielded a RR of 0.79 (95% CI: 0.58–1.07). Heterogeneity testing results were not significant $(P = .07)$.

Recurrence of Pyelonephritis/Febrile UTI Among Children 2 to 24 Months of Age With No VUR

There was no significant difference in rates of recurrence of pyelonephritis for children 2 to 24 months of age without VUR who received antimicrobial agents and those who did not. With random-effects modeling, the meta-analysis yielded a RR of 0.55 (95% CI:

Study or Subgroup	Antimicrobial Events	Total	Control Events	Total	Weight	Risk Ratio M–H, Random, 95% CI
Brandström et al[70] (2010)	10	69	25	68	21.3%	0.39 [0.21–0.76]
Craig et al[69] (2009)	6	75	9	73	14.3%	0.65 [0.24–1.73]
Garin et al[67] (2006)	5	25	0	25	2.7%	11.00 [0.64–188.95]
Montini et al[66] (2008)	10	68	9	39	17.6%	0.64 [0.28–1.43]
Pennesi et al[68] (2008)	18	50	15	50	23.7%	1.20 [0.68–2.11]
Roussey-Kesler et al[64] (2008)	12	82	16	99	20.4%	0.91 [0.45–1.80]
Total (95% CI)		369		354	100.0%	0.78 [0.48–1.26]
Total events	61		74			

Heterogeneity: $\tau^2 = 0.17$; $\chi^2 = 10.36$, $df = 5$ ($P = .07$); $I^2 = 52\%$
Test for overall effect: $z = 1.03$ ($P = .30$)

Risk Ratio M–H, Random, 95% CI — scale 0.01 0.1 1 10 100; Favors antimicrobial / Favors control

FIGURE 10
Combined estimates of the effect of antimicrobial prophylaxis on prevention of pyelonephritis in children 2 to 24 months of age with any grade of VUR, from random-effects modeling. RRs and 95% CIs are shown. M-H indicates Mantel-Haenszel.

Study or Subgroup	Antimicrobial Events	Total	Control Events	Total	Weight	Risk Ratio M–H, Random, 95% CI
Craig et al[69] (2009)	1	60	7	57	30.3%	0.14 [0.02–1.07]
Garin et al[67] (2006)	1	32	1	40	19.6%	1.25 [0.08–19.22]
Montini et al[66] (2008)	5	118	3	66	50.1%	0.93 [0.23–3.78]
Total (95% CI)		210		163	100.0%	0.55 [0.15–2.08]
Total events	7		11			

Heterogeneity: $\tau^2 = 0.41$; $\chi^2 = 2.79$, $df = 2$ ($P = .25$); $I^2 = 28\%$
Test for overall effect: $z = 0.88$ ($P = .38$)

FIGURE 11
Combined estimates of the effect of antimicrobial prophylaxis on prevention of pyelonephritis in children 2 to 24 months of age without VUR, from random-effects modeling. RRs and 95% CIs are shown. M-H indicates Mantel-Haenszel.

Study or Subgroup	Antimicrobial Events	Total	Control Events	Total	Weight	Risk Ratio M–H, Random, 95% CI
Craig et al[69] (2009)	1	10	1	12	49.9%	1.20 [0.09–16.84]
Garin et al[67] (2006)	0	5	0	3		Not estimable
Montini et al[66] (2008)	1	15	1	8	50.1%	0.53 [0.04–7.44]
Roussey-Kesler et al[64] (2008)	0	7	0	12		Not estimable
Total (95% CI)		37		35	100.0%	0.80 [0.12–5.16]
Total events	2		2			

Heterogeneity: $\tau^2 = 0.00$; $\chi^2 = .18$, $df = 1$ ($P = .67$); $I^2 = 0\%$
Test for overall effect: $z = 0.24$ ($P = .81$)

FIGURE 12
Combined estimates of the effect of antimicrobial prophylaxis on prevention of pyelonephritis in children 2 to 24 months of age with grade I VUR, from random-effects modeling. RRs and 95% CIs are shown. M-H indicates Mantel-Haenszel.

0.15–2.08) (Fig 11). Heterogeneity testing results were not significant ($P = .25$). With fixed-effects modeling, the meta-analysis yielded a RR of 0.48 (95% CI: 0.18–1.27). Heterogeneity testing results were not significant ($P = .25$).

Recurrence of Pyelonephritis/Febrile UTI Among Children 2 to 24 Months of Age According to Grade of VUR

When results were analyzed according to VUR grade, there was no significant difference in rates of recurrence of pyelonephritis for children 2 to 24 months of age who received antimicrobial agents and those who did not in any of the analyses, with

random- or fixed-effects modeling. Results of random-effects modeling are presented in Figs 12 through 16. Heterogeneity testing results were not significant in any of the analyses.

Recurrence of Any Type of UTI Among Children of All Ages With VUR of Any Grade

In this meta-analysis, in which the 2 published abstracts that never resulted in published articles were included, there was a statistically significant difference in rates of recurrence of any type of UTI for children with VUR who received antimicrobial agents and those who did not. With random-effects modeling, the meta-analysis yielded a

RR of 0.70 (95% CI: 0.51–0.96) (Fig 17). Heterogeneity testing results were not significant ($P = .20$).

The inclusion of the published abstracts[104,105] in these meta-analyses can be criticized, because the investigators in those studies enrolled all children with VUR and not just those who had been diagnosed as having UTI; therefore, *recurrent* UTIs were not measured. With exclusion of the 2 abstracts from the meta-analyses for prevention of any UTI, the RR with random-effects modeling would be 0.73 (95% CI: 0.53–1.01). Heterogeneity testing results were not significant ($P = .16$).

Study or Subgroup	Antimicrobial Events	Total	Control Events	Total	Weight	Risk Ratio M-H, Random, 95% CI	Risk Ratio M-H, Random, 95% CI
Craig et al[69] (2009)	0	27	1	23	6.3%	0.29 [0.01–6.69]	
Garin et al[67] (2006)	1	12	0	10	6.5%	2.54 [0.11–56.25]	
Montini et al[66] (2008)	3	31	2	18	21.7%	0.87 [0.16–4.73]	
Pennesi et al[68] (2008)	1	11	0	10	6.5%	2.75 [0.12–60.70]	
Roussey-Kesler et al[64] (2008)	6	52	7	63	59.0%	1.04 [0.37–2.90]	
Total (95% CI)		**133**		**124**	**100.0%**	**1.04 [0.47–2.29]**	
Total events	11		10				

Heterogeneity: $\tau^2 = 0.00$; $\chi^2 = 1.38$, $df = 4$ ($P = .85$); $I^2 = 0\%$
Test for overall effect: $z = 0.10$ ($P = .92$)

0.01 0.1 1 10 100
Favors antimicrobial Favors control

FIGURE 13

Combined estimates of the effect of antimicrobial prophylaxis on prevention of pyelonephritis in children 2 to 24 months of age with grade II VUR, from random-effects modeling. RRs and 95% CIs are shown. M-H indicates Mantel-Haenszel.

Study or Subgroup	Antimicrobial Events	Total	Control Events	Total	Weight	Risk Ratio M-H, Random, 95% CI	Risk Ratio M-H, Random, 95% CI
Brandström et al[70] (2010)	5	41	14	43	20.9%	0.37 [0.15–0.95]	
Craig et al[69] (2009)	1	24	4	29	7.1%	0.30 [0.04–2.53]	
Garin et al[67] (2006)	4	8	0	12	4.5%	13.00 [0.79–212.80]	
Montini et al[66] (2008)	6	22	6	13	21.5%	0.59 [0.24–1.45]	
Pennesi et al[68] (2008)	9	22	7	24	23.6%	1.40 [0.63–3.12]	
Roussey-Kesler et al[64] (2008)	6	23	9	24	22.3%	0.70 [0.29–1.64]	
Total (95% CI)		**140**		**145**	**100.0%**	**0.75 [0.40–1.40]**	
Total events	31		40				

Heterogeneity: $\tau^2 = 0.27$; $\chi^2 = 9.54$, $df = 5$ ($P = .09$); $I^2 = 48\%$
Test for overall effect: $z = 0.90$ ($P = .37$)

0.01 0.1 1 10 100
Favors antimicrobial Favors control

FIGURE 14

Combined estimates of the effect of antimicrobial prophylaxis on prevention of pyelonephritis in children 2 to 24 months of age with grade III VUR, from random-effects modeling. RRs and 95% CIs are shown. M-H indicates Mantel-Haenszel.

Study or Subgroup	Antimicrobial Events	Total	Control Events	Total	Weight	Risk Ratio M-H, Random, 95% CI	Risk Ratio M-H, Random, 95% CI
Brandström et al[70] (2010)	5	28	11	25	35.0%	0.41 [0.16–1.01]	
Craig et al[69] (2009)	3	10	2	8	14.8%	1.20 [0.26–5.53]	
Pennesi et al[68] (2008)	8	17	8	16	50.2%	0.94 [0.47–1.90]	
Total (95% CI)		**55**		**49**	**100.0%**	**0.73 [0.39–1.35]**	
Total events	16		21				

Heterogeneity: $\tau^2 = 0.07$; $\chi^2 = 2.57$, $df = 2$ ($P = .28$); $I^2 = 22\%$
Test for overall effect: $z = 1.01$ ($P = .31$)

0.01 0.1 1 10 100
Favors antimicrobial Favors control

FIGURE 15

Combined estimates of the effect of antimicrobial prophylaxis on prevention of pyelonephritis in children 2 to 24 months of age with grade IV VUR, from random-effects modeling. RRs and 95% CIs are shown. M-H indicates Mantel-Haenszel.

Study or Subgroup	Antimicrobial Events	Total	Control Events	Total	Weight	Risk Ratio M-H, Random, 95% CI	Risk Ratio M-H, Random, 95% CI
Craig et al[69] (2009)	1	4	1	1	100.0%	0.40 [0.08–1.90]	
Total (95% CI)		**4**		**1**	**100.0%**	**0.40 [0.08–1.90]**	
Total events	1		1				

Heterogeneity: Not applicable
Test for overall effect: $z = 1.15$ ($P = .25$)

0.01 0.1 1 10 100
Favors antimicrobial Favors control

FIGURE 16

Estimate of the effect of antimicrobial prophylaxis on prevention of pyelonephritis in children 2 to 24 months of age with grade V VUR, from random-effects modeling. RRs and 95% CIs are shown. M-H indicates Mantel-Haenszel.

Recurrence of Any Type of UTI Among Children of All Ages Without VUR

There was no significant difference in rates of recurrence of any type of UTI for children without VUR who received antimicrobial agents and those who did not. With random-effects modeling, the meta-analysis yielded a RR of 0.72 (95% CI: 0.43–1.20) (Fig 18). Heterogeneity testing results were not significant ($P = .37$).

Effect on Studies of Inclusion of Bag Specimens

With the exception of the study by Craig et al,[69] no studies reported that bag urine specimens were excluded. The inclusion of such specimens might

Study or Subgroup	Antimicrobial Events	Total	Control Events	Total	Weight	Risk Ratio M-H, Random, 95% CI	Risk Ratio M-H, Random, 95% CI
Brandström et al[70] (2010)	10	69	25	68	15.4%	0.39 [0.21–0.76]	
Craig et al[105] (2002)	0	23	2	23	1.1%	0.20 [0.01–3.95]	
Craig et al[69] (2009)	14	122	21	121	16.2%	0.66 [0.35–1.24]	
Garin et al[67] (2006)	13	55	13	58	14.8%	1.05 [0.54–2.07]	
Montini et al[66] (2008)	10	82	9	46	11.1%	0.62 [0.27–1.42]	
Pennesi et al[68] (2008)	18	50	15	50	18.6%	1.20 [0.68–2.11]	
Reddy et al[104] (1997)	1	13	5	16	2.3%	0.25 [0.03–1.85]	
Roussey-Kesler et al[64] (2008)	18	103	32	121	20.6%	0.66 [0.40–1.11]	
Total (95% CI)		**517**		**503**	**100.0%**	**0.70 [0.51–0.96]**	
Total events	84		122				

Heterogeneity: $\tau^2 = 0.06$; $\chi^2 = 9.88$, $df = 7$ ($P = .20$); $I^2 = 29\%$
Test for overall effect: $z = 2.22$ ($P = .03$)

0.01 0.1 1 10 100
Favors antimicrobial   Favors control

FIGURE 17

Combined estimates of the effect of antimicrobial prophylaxis on prevention of any UTI in children with any grade of VUR, from random-effects modeling. RRs and 95% CIs are shown. M-H indicates Mantel-Haenszel.

Study or Subgroup	Antimicrobial Events	Total	Control Events	Total	Weight	Risk Ratio M-H, Random, 95% CI	Risk Ratio M-H, Random, 95% CI
Craig et al[69] (2009)	15	119	17	115	62.7%	0.85 [0.45–1.63]	
Garin et al[67] (2006)	4	45	14	60	24.1%	0.38 [0.13–1.08]	
Montini et al[66] (2008)	5	129	3	81	13.2%	1.05 [0.26–4.26]	
Total (95% CI)		**293**		**256**	**100.0%**	**0.72 [0.43–1.20]**	
Total events	24		34				

Heterogeneity: $\tau^2 = 0.00$; $\chi^2 = 1.98$, $df = 2$ ($P = .37$); $I^2 = 0\%$
Test for overall effect: $z = 1.25$ ($P = .21$)

0.01 0.1 1 10 100
Favors antimicrobial   Favors control

FIGURE 18

Combined estimates of the effect of antimicrobial prophylaxis on prevention of any UTI in children without VUR, from random-effects modeling. RRs and 95% CIs are shown. M-H indicates Mantel-Haenszel.

have resulted in increased numbers of false-positive urine culture results in both the antimicrobial prophylaxis and control groups, yielding a bias toward the null hypothesis in those studies.

Results of Excluded Study

The study by Lee et al[65] was excluded from the meta-analysis because it compared antimicrobial prophylaxis with probiotic treatment. A total of 120 children 13 to 36 months of age with a history of UTI and VUR of grade I to V who had been receiving trimethoprim-sulfamethoxazole once daily for 1 year were again assessed for VUR; if VUR persisted, then children were assigned randomly either to continue to receive trimethoprim-sulfamethoxazole or to receive *Lactobacillus acidophilus* twice daily for 1 additional year. The study showed no statistical difference in recurrent UTI rates between the 2 groups during the second year of follow-up monitoring.

Antimicrobial Prophylaxis and Antimicrobial Resistance

The antimicrobial resistance patterns of the pathogens isolated during UTI recurrences were assessed in 5 of the RCTs included in the meta-analyses.[64,66,68–70] All authors concluded that UTI recurrences with antimicrobial-resistant bacteria were more common in the groups of children assigned randomly to receive antimicrobial prophylaxis. In the placebo/surveillance groups, the proportions of resistant bacteria ranged from 0% to 39%; in the antimicrobial prophylaxis groups, the proportions of resistant bacteria ranged from 53% to 100%. These results are supported by other studies in which antimicrobial prophylaxis has been shown to promote resistant organisms.[106,107]

Surgical Intervention Versus Antimicrobial Prophylaxis

Data on the effectiveness of surgical interventions for VUR are quite limited.

To date, only 1 RCT has compared surgical intervention (only endoscopic therapy) for VUR with placebo treatment.[70] In that study, there was a statistically significant difference in the rates of recurrence of febrile UTI for girls treated with endoscopic therapy and those under surveillance (10 of 43 vs 24 of 42 girls; $P = .0014$). No such difference was noted among boys, for whom the results trended in the opposite direction (4 of 23 vs 1 of 26 boys). A meta-analysis examined the outcomes of UTIs and febrile UTIs in children assigned randomly to either reflux correction plus antimicrobial therapy or antimicrobial therapy alone.[108] By 2 years, the authors found no significant reduction in the risk of UTI in the surgery plus antimicrobial therapy group, compared with the antimicrobial therapy-only group (4 studies; RR: 1.07 [95% CI: 0.55–2.09]). The frequency of febrile UTIs was reported in only 2 studies. Children in the surgery plus antimicrobial therapy group had significantly fewer febrile UTIs than did children in the antimicrobial therapy-only group between 0 and 5 years after intervention (RR: 0.43 [95% CI: 0.27–0.70]). Although there may be some promise in endoscopic interventions for children with VUR, to date there are insufficient data to show whether and for whom such interventions may be helpful.

Long-term Consequences of VUR

The link between VUR discovered after the first UTI and subsequent hypertension and end-stage renal disease remains tenuous at best. There have been no longitudinal studies monitoring children long enough to quantify these outcomes. Retrospective studies evaluated highly selected populations, and their findings might not apply to otherwise healthy children with a first UTI.[109–112] Ecologic data from Australia demonstrated no changes in the rates of hypertension and renal failure since the widespread introduction of antimicrobial prophylaxis and ureteric reimplantation surgery for VUR in the 1960s.[113]

DISCUSSION

Review of the evidence regarding diagnosis and management of UTIs in 2- to 24-month-old children yields the following. First, the prevalence of UTI in febrile infants remains about the same, at ~5%. Studies have provided demographic features (age, race, and gender) and clinical characteristics (height and duration of fever, other causes of fever, and circumcision) that can help clinicians identify febrile infants whose low risk of UTI obviates the need for further evaluation.

Among children who do not receive immediate antimicrobial therapy, UTI can be ruled out on the basis of completely negative urinalysis results. For this purpose, enhanced urinalysis is preferable. However, facilities for urine microscopy with counting chambers and Gram staining may not be available in

all settings. A urine reagent strip with negative nitrite and leukocyte esterase reaction results is sufficient to rule out UTI if the pretest risk is moderate (~5%). Diagnosis of UTI is best achieved with a combination of culture and urinalysis. Cultures of urine collected through catheterization, compared with SPA, are nearly as sensitive and specific but have higher success rates and the process is less painful. Cultures of urine collected in bags have unacceptably high false-positive rates.

The previous guideline recommended VCUG after the first UTI for children between 2 and 24 months of age. The rationale for this recommendation was that antimicrobial prophylaxis among children with VUR could reduce subsequent episodes of pyelonephritis and additional renal scarring. However, evidence does not support antimicrobial prophylaxis to prevent UTI when VUR is found through VCUG. The only statistically significant effect of antimicrobial prophylaxis was in preventing UTI that included cystitis and asymptomatic bacteriuria. Statistically significant differences in the rates of febrile UTI or pyelonephritis were not seen. Moreover, VCUG is one of the most uncomfortable radiologic procedures performed with children.[114–116]

Even if additional studies were to show a statistically significant effect of prophylaxis in preventing pyelonephritis, our point estimates suggest that the RR would be ~0.80, corresponding to a reduction in RR of 20%. If we take into account the prevalence of VUR, the risk of recurrent UTI in those children, and this modest *potential* effect, we can determine that ~100 children would need to undergo VCUG for prevention of 1 UTI in the first year. Even more striking is the fact that the evidence of benefit is the same (or better) for children with *no* VUR, which makes the benefit of VCUG more dubious. Taken in light of the marginal cost-effectiveness of the procedure found under the more-optimistic as-

sumptions in the 1999 technical report, these data argue against VCUG after the first UTI. VCUG after a second or third UTI would have a higher yield of higher grades of reflux, but the optimal care for infants with higher-grade reflux is still not clear. Ultrasonography of the kidneys, ureters, and bladder after a first UTI has poor sensitivity and only a modest yield of "actionable" findings. However, the procedure is less invasive, less uncomfortable, and less risky (in terms of radiation) than is VCUG.

There is a significant risk of renal scarring among children with febrile UTI, and some evidence suggests that early antimicrobial treatment mitigates that risk. It seems prudent to recommend early evaluation (in the 24- to 48-hour time frame) of subsequent fevers and prompt treatment of UTI to minimize subsequent renal scarring.

LEAD AUTHORS

S. Maria E. Finnell, MD, MS
Aaron E. Carroll, MD, MS
Stephen M. Downs, MD, MS

SUBCOMMITTEE ON URINARY TRACT INFECTION, 2009–2011

Kenneth B. Roberts, MD, Chair
Stephen M. Downs, MD, MS
S. Maria E. Finnell, MD, MS
Stanley Hellerstein, MD
Linda D. Shortliffe, MD
Ellen R. Wald, MD
J. Michael Zerin, MD

OVERSIGHT BY THE STEERING COMMITTEE ON QUALITY IMPROVEMENT AND MANAGEMENT, 2009–2011

STAFF

Caryn Davidson, MA

ACKNOWLEDGMENTS

The committee gratefully acknowledges the generosity of the researchers who graciously shared their data to permit the data set with data for 1096 infants 2 to 24 months of age according to grade of VUR to be compiled, that is, Drs Per Brandström, Jonathan Craig, Eduardo Garin, Giovanni Montini, Marco Pennesi, and Gwenaelle Roussey-Kesler.

REFERENCES

1. American Academy of Pediatrics, Committee on Quality Improvement, Subcommittee on Urinary Tract Infection. Practice parameter: the diagnosis, treatment, and evaluation of the initial urinary tract infection in febrile infants and young children. *Pediatrics.* 1999;103(4):843–852

2. Downs SM. Technical report: urinary tract infections in febrile infants and young children. *Pediatrics.* 1999;103(4). Available at: www.pediatrics.org/cgi/content/full/103/4/e54

3. American Academy of Pediatrics, Committee on Quality Improvement, Subcommittee on Urinary Tract Infection. Urinary tract infection: clinical practice guideline for the diagnosis and management of initial urinary tract infections in febrile infants and children 2 to 24 months of age. *Pediatrics.* 2011;128(3):595–610

4. Eddy DM. Clinical decision making: from theory to practice: guidelines for policy statements: the explicit approach. *JAMA.* 1990;263(16):2239–2242

5. Haynes RB, McKibbon KA, Wilczynski NL, Walter SD, Werre SR; Hedge Team. Optimal search strategies for retrieving scientifically strong studies of treatment from Medline: analytical survey. *BMJ.* 2005; 330(7501):1179

6. Downs S, Black N. The feasibility of creating a checklist for the assessment of the methodological quality both of randomised and non-randomised studies of health care interventions. *J Epidemiol Community Health.* 1998;52(6):377–384

7. Hoberman A, Wald ER, Reynolds EA, Penchansky L, Charron M. Is urine culture necessary to rule out urinary tract infection in young febrile children? *Pediatr Infect Dis J.* 1996;15(4):304–309

8. Haddon RA, Barnett PL, Grimwood K, Hogg GG. Bacteraemia in febrile children presenting to a paediatric emergency department. *Med J Aust.* 1999;170(10):475–478

9. Shaw KN, Gorelick M, McGowan KL, Yakscoe NM, Schwartz JS. Prevalence of urinary tract infection in febrile young children in the emergency department. *Pediatrics.* 1998;102(2). Available at: www.pediatrics.org/cgi/content/full/102/2/e16

10. Shaikh N, Morone NE, Bost JE, Farrell MH. Prevalence of urinary tract infection in childhood: a meta-analysis. *Pediatr Infect Dis J.* 2008;27(4):302–308

11. To T, Agha M, Dick PT, Feldman W. Cohort study on circumcision of newborn boys and subsequent risk of urinary-tract infection. *Lancet.* 1998;352(9143):1813–1816

12. Shaikh N, Morone NE, Lopez J, et al. Does this child have a urinary tract infection? *JAMA.* 2007;298(24):2895–2904

13. Pantell RH, Newman TB, Bernzweig J, et al. Management and outcomes of care of fever in early infancy. *JAMA.* 2004;291(10):1203–1212

14. Byington CL, Enriquez FR, Hoff C, et al. Serious bacterial infections in febrile infants 1 to 90 days old with and without viral infections. *Pediatrics.* 2004;113(6):1662–1666

15. Levine DA, Platt SL, Dayan PS, et al. Risk of serious bacterial infection in young febrile infants with respiratory syncytial virus infections. *Pediatrics.* 2004;113(6):1728–1734

16. Gorelick MH, Hoberman A, Kearney D, Wald E, Shaw KN. Validation of a decision rule identifying febrile young girls at high risk for urinary tract infection. *Pediatr Emerg Care.* 2003;19(3):162–164

17. Gorelick MH, Shaw KN. Clinical decision rule to identify febrile young girls at risk for urinary tract infection. *Arch Pediatr Adolesc Med.* 2000;154(4):386–390

18. Roberts KB, Charney E, Sweren RJ, et al. Urinary tract infection in infants with unexplained fever: a collaborative study. *J Pediatr.* 1983;103(6):864–867

19. Lockhart GR, Lewander WJ, Cimini DM, Josephson SL, Linakis JG. Use of urinary Gram stain for detection of urinary tract infection in infants. *Ann Emerg Med.* 1995;25(1):31–35

20. Shaw KN, McGowan KL, Gorelick MH, Schwartz JS. Screening for urinary tract infection in infants in the emergency department: which test is best? *Pediatrics.* 1998;101(6). Available at: www.pediatrics.org/cgi/content/full/101/6/e1

21. Lin DS, Huang FY, Chiu NC, et al. Comparison of hemocytometer leukocyte counts and standard urinalyses for predicting urinary tract infections in febrile infants. *Pediatr Infect Dis J.* 2000;19(3):223–227

22. Leong YY, Tan KW. Bladder aspiration for diagnosis of urinary tract infection in infants and young children. *J Singapore Paediatr Soc.* 1976;18(1):43–47

23. Pryles CV, Atkin MD, Morse TS, Welch KJ. Comparative bacteriologic study of urine obtained from children by percutaneous suprapubic aspiration of the bladder and by catheter. *Pediatrics.* 1959;24(6):983–991

24. Djojohadipringgo S, Abdul Hamid RH, Thahir S, Karim A, Darsono I. Bladder puncture in newborns: a bacteriological study. *Paediatr Indones.* 1976;16(11–12):527–534

25. Gochman RF, Karasic RB, Heller MB. Use of portable ultrasound to assist urine collection by suprapubic aspiration. *Ann Emerg Med.* 1991;20(6):631–635

26. Buys H, Pead L, Hallett R, Maskell R. Suprapubic aspiration under ultrasound guidance in children with fever of undiagnosed cause. *BMJ.* 1994;308(6930):690–692

27. Kozer E, Rosenbloom E, Goldman D, Lavy G, Rosenfeld N, Goldman M. Pain in infants who are younger than 2 months during suprapubic aspiration and transurethral bladder catheterization: a randomized, controlled study. *Pediatrics.* 2006;118(1). Available at: www.pediatrics.org/cgi/content/full/118/1/e51

28. El-Naggar W, Yiu A, Mohamed A, et al. Comparison of pain during two methods of urine collection in preterm infants. *Pediatrics.* 2010;125(6):1224–1229

29. Al-Orifi F, McGillivray D, Tange S, Kramer MS. Urine culture from bag specimens in young children: are the risks too high? *J Pediatr.* 2000;137(2):221–226

30. Etoubleau C, Reveret M, Brouet D, et al. Moving from bag to catheter for urine collection in non-toilet-trained children suspected of having urinary tract infection: a paired comparison of urine cultures. *J Pediatr.* 2009;154(6):803–806

31. Alam M, Coulter J, Pacheco J, et al. Comparison of urine contamination rates using three different methods of collection: clean-catch, cotton wool pad and urine bag. *Ann Trop Paediatr.* 2005;25(1):29–34

32. Li PS, Ma LC, Wong SN. Is bag urine culture useful in monitoring urinary tract infection in infants? *J Paediatr Child Health.* 2002;38(4):377–381

33. Karacan C, Erkek N, Senel S, Akin Gunduz S, Catli G, Tavil B. Evaluation of urine collection methods for the diagnosis of urinary tract infection in children. *Med Princ Pract.* 2010;19(3):188–191

34. Perlhagen M, Forsberg T, Perlhagen J, Nivesjö M. Evaluating the specificity of a new type of urine collection bag for infants. *J Pediatr Urol.* 2007;3(5):378–381

35. Ginsburg CM, McCracken GH Jr. Urinary tract infections in young infants. *Pediatrics.* 1982;69(4):409–412

36. Hoberman A, Wald ER, Hickey RW, et al. Oral versus initial intravenous therapy for urinary tract infections in young febrile children. *Pediatrics.* 1999;104(1):79–86

37. Hodson EM, Willis NS, Craig JC. Antibiotics

for acute pyelonephritis in children. *Cochrane Database Syst Rev.* 2007;(4): CD003772

38. Zhanel GG, Hisanaga TL, Laing NM, et al. Antibiotic resistance in outpatient urinary isolates: final results from the North American Urinary Tract Infection Collaborative Alliance (NAUTICA). *Int J Antimicrob Agents.* 2005;26(5):380–388

39. Gaspari RJ, Dickson E, Karlowsky J, Doern G. Antibiotic resistance trends in paediatric uropathogens. *Int J Antimicrob Agents.* 2005;26(4):267–271

40. Michael M, Hodson EM, Craig JC, Martin S, Moyer VA. Short versus standard duration oral antibiotic therapy for acute urinary tract infection in children. *Cochrane Database Syst Rev.* 2003;(1):CD003966

41. Camacho V, Estorch M, Fraga G, et al. DMSA study performed during febrile urinary tract infection: a predictor of patient outcome? *Eur J Nucl Med Mol Imaging.* 2004; 31(6):862–866

42. Hewitt IK, Zucchetta P, Rigon L, et al. Early treatment of acute pyelonephritis in children fails to reduce renal scarring: data from the Italian Renal Infection Study Trials. *Pediatrics.* 2008;122(3):486–490

43. Doganis D, Siafas K, Mavrikou M, et al. Does early treatment of urinary tract infection prevent renal damage? *Pediatrics.* 2007; 120(4). Available at: www.pediatrics.org/cgi/content/full/120/4/e922

44. Fernández-Menéndez JM, Málaga S, Matesanz JL, Solís G, Alonso S, Pérez-Méndez C. Risk factors in the development of early technetium-99m dimercaptosuccinic acid renal scintigraphy lesions during first urinary tract infection in children. *Acta Paediatr.* 2003;92(1):21–26

45. Keren R, Chan E. A meta-analysis of randomized, controlled trials comparing short- and long-course antibiotic therapy for urinary tract infections in children. *Pediatrics.* 2002;109(5). Available at: www.pediatrics.org/cgi/content/full/109/5/e70

46. Tran D, Muchant DG, Aronoff SC. Short-course versus conventional length antimicrobial therapy for uncomplicated lower urinary tract infections in children: a meta-analysis of 1279 patients. *J Pediatr.* 2001;139(1):93–99

47. Oreskovic NM, Sembrano EU. Repeat urine cultures in children who are admitted with urinary tract infections. *Pediatrics.* 2007; 119(2). Available at: www.pediatrics.org/cgi/content/full/119/2/e325

48. Currie ML, Mitz L, Raasch CS, Greenbaum LA. Follow-up urine cultures and fever in children with urinary tract infection. *Arch Pediatr Adolesc Med.* 2003;157(12): 1237–1240

49. Lebowitz RL, Olbing H, Parkkulainen KV, Smellie JM, Tamminen-Mobius TE. International system of radiographic grading of vesicoureteric reflux. *Pediatr Radiol.* 1985; 15(2):105–109

50. Sargent MA, Stringer DA. Voiding cystourethrography in children with urinary tract infection: the frequency of vesicoureteric reflux is independent of the specialty of the physician requesting the study. *AJR.* 1995;164(5):1237–1241

51. Craig JC, Knight JF, Sureshkumar P, Lam A, Onikul E, Roy LP. Vesicoureteric reflux and timing of micturating cystourethrography after urinary tract infection. *Arch Dis Child.* 1997;76(3):275–277

52. McDonald A, Scranton M, Gillespie R, Mahajan V, Edwards GA. Voiding cystourethrograms and urinary tract infections: how long to wait? *Pediatrics.* 2000;105(4). Available at: www.pediatrics.org/cgi/content/full/105/4/e50

53. Oostenbrink R, van der Heijden AJ, Moons KG, Moll HA. Prediction of vesico-ureteric reflux in childhood urinary tract infection: a multivariate approach. *Acta Paediatr.* 2000;89(7):806–810

54. Mahant S, To T, Friedman J. Timing of voiding cystourethrogram in the investigation of urinary tract infections in children. *J Pediatr.* 2001;139(4):568–571

55. Mahant S, Friedman J, MacArthur C. Renal ultrasound findings and vesicoureteral reflux in children hospitalised with urinary tract infection. *Arch Dis Child.* 2002;86(6): 419–420

56. Chand DH, Rhoades T, Poe SA, Kraus S, Strife CF. Incidence and severity of vesicoureteral reflux in children related to age, gender, race and diagnosis. *J Urol.* 2003;170(4):1548–1550

57. Hansson S, Dhamey M, Sigström O, et al. Dimercapto-succinic acid scintigraphy instead of voiding cystourethrography for infants with urinary tract infection. *J Urol.* 2004;172(3):1071–1073

58. Pinto K. Vesicoureteral reflux in the Hispanic child with urinary tract infection. *J Urol.* 2004;171(3):1266–1267

59. Zamir G, Sakran W, Horowitz Y, Koren A, Miron D. Urinary tract infection: is there a need for routine renal ultrasonography? *Arch Dis Child.* 2004;89(5):466–468

60. Hannula A, Venhola M, Renko M, Pokka T, Huttunen NP, Uhari M. Vesicoureteral reflux in children with suspected and proven urinary tract infection. *Pediatr Nephrol.* 2010;25(8):1463–1469

61. Venhola M, Hannula A, Huttunen NP, Renko M, Pokka T, Uhari M. Occurrence of vesicoureteral reflux in children. *Acta Paediatr.* 2010;99(12):1875–1878

62. Alon US, Ganapathy S. Should renal ultrasonography be done routinely in children with first urinary tract infection? *Clin Pediatr (Phila).* 1999;38(1):21–25

63. Greenfield SP, Ng M, Wan J. Experience with vesicoureteral reflux in children: clinical characteristics. *J Urol.* 1997;158(2): 574–577

64. Roussey-Kesler G, Gadjos V, Idres N, et al. Antibiotic prophylaxis for the prevention of recurrent urinary tract infection in children with low grade vesicoureteral reflux: results from a prospective randomized study. *J Urol.* 2008;179(2):674–679

65. Lee SJ, Shim YH, Cho SJ, Lee JW. Probiotics prophylaxis in children with persistent primary vesicoureteral reflux. *Pediatr Nephrol.* 2007;22(9):1315–1320

66. Montini G, Rigon L, Zucchetta P, et al. Prophylaxis after first febrile urinary tract infection in children? A multicenter, randomized, controlled, noninferiority trial. *Pediatrics.* 2008;122(5):1064–1071

67. Garin EH, Olavarria F, Garcia Nieto V, Valenciano B, Campos A, Young L. Clinical significance of primary vesicoureteral reflux and urinary antibiotic prophylaxis after acute pyelonephritis: a multicenter, randomized, controlled study. *Pediatrics.* 2006;117(3):626–632

68. Pennesi M, Travan L, Peratoner L, et al. Is antibiotic prophylaxis in children with vesicoureteral reflux effective in preventing pyelonephritis and renal scars? A randomized, controlled trial. *Pediatrics.* 2008; 121(6). Available at: www.pediatrics.org/cgi/content/full/121/6/e1489

69. Craig J, Simpson J, Williams G. Antibiotic prophylaxis and recurrent urinary tract infection in children. *N Engl J Med.* 2009; 361(18):1748–1759

70. Brandström P, Esbjorner E, Herthelius M, Swerkersson S, Jodal U, Hansson S. The Swedish Reflux Trial in Children, part III: urinary tract infection pattern. *J Urol.* 2010;184(1):286–291

71. Moorthy I, Wheat D, Gordon I. Ultrasonography in the evaluation of renal scarring using DMSA scan as the gold standard. *Pediatr Nephrol.* 2004;19(2):153–156

72. Biggi A, Dardanelli L, Pomero G, et al. Acute renal cortical scintigraphy in children with a first urinary tract infection. *Pediatr Nephrol.* 2001;16(9):733–738

73. Smellie JM, Rigden SP, Prescod NP. Urinary tract infection: a comparison of four

methods of investigation. *Arch Dis Child.* 1995;72(3):247–260

74. Hoberman A, Charron M, Hickey RW, Baskin M, Kearney DH, Wald ER. Imaging studies after a first febrile urinary tract infection in young children. *N Engl J Med.* 2003;348(3):195–202

75. Roberts J. Experimental pyelonephritis in the monkey, part III: pathophysiology of ureteral malfunction induced by bacteria. *Invest Urol.* 1975;13(2):117–120

76. Wippermann CF, Schofer O, Beetz R, et al. Renal abscess in childhood: diagnostic and therapeutic progress. *Pediatr Infect Dis J.* 1991;10(6):446–450

77. Barry BP, Hall N, Cornford E, Broderick NJ, Somers JM, Rose DH. Improved ultrasound detection of renal scarring in children following urinary tract infection. *Clin Radiol.* 1998;53(10):747–751

78. Sinha MD, Gibson P, Kane T, Lewis MA. Accuracy of ultrasonic detection of renal scarring in different centres using DMSA as the gold standard. *Nephrol Dial Transplant.* 2007;22(8):2213–2216

79. Montini G, Zucchetta P, Tomasi L, et al. Value of imaging studies after a first febrile urinary tract infection in young children: data from Italian Renal Infection Study 1. *Pediatrics.* 2009;123(2). Available at: www.pediatrics.org/cgi/content/full/123/2/e239

80. Giorgi LJ Jr, Bratslavsky G, Kogan BA. Febrile urinary tract infections in infants: renal ultrasound remains necessary. *J Urol.* 2005;173(2):568–570

81. Gelfand MJ, Barr LL, Abunku O. The initial renal ultrasound examination in children with urinary tract infection: the prevalence of dilated uropathy has decreased. *Pediatr Radiol.* 2000;30(10):665–670

82. Jothilakshmi K, Vijayaraghavan B, Paul S, Matthai J. Radiological evaluation of the urinary tract in children with urinary infection. *Indian J Pediatr.* 2001;68(12):1131–1133

83. Jahnukainen T, Honkinen O, Ruuskanen O, Mertsola J. Ultrasonography after the first febrile urinary tract infection in children. *Eur J Pediatr.* 2006;165(8):556–559

84. Huang HP, Lai YC, Tsai IJ, Chen SY, Tsau YK. Renal ultrasonography should be done routinely in children with first urinary tract infections. *Urology.* 2008;71(3):439–443

85. Economou G, Egginton J, Brookfield D. The importance of late pregnancy scans for renal tract abnormalities. *Prenat Diagn.* 1994;14(3):177–180

86. Rosendahl H. Ultrasound screening for fetal urinary tract malformations: a prospective study in general population. *Eur J Obstet Gynecol Reprod Biol.* 1990;36(1–2):27–33

87. Paduano L, Giglio L, Bembi B, Peratoner L, Benussi, G. Clinical outcome of fetal uropathy, part II: sensitivity of echography for prenatal detection of obstructive pathology. *J Urol.* 1991;146(4):1097–1098

88. Miron D, Daas A, Sakran W, Lumelsky D, Koren A, Horovitz Y. Is omitting post urinary-tract-infection renal ultrasound safe after normal antenatal ultrasound? An observational study. *Arch Dis Child.* 2007;92(6):502–504

89. Lakhoo K, Thomas DF, Fuenfer M, D'Cruz AJ. Failure of pre-natal ultrasonography to prevent urinary infection associated with underlying urological abnormalities. *Br J Urol.* 1996;77(6):905–908

90. Scholtmeijer RJ. Treatment of vesicoureteric reflux: results of a prospective study. *Br J Urol.* 1993;71(3):346–349

91. Smellie JM, Barratt TM, Chantler C, et al. Medical versus surgical treatment in children with severe bilateral vesicoureteric reflux and bilateral nephropathy: a randomised trial. *Lancet.* 2001;357(9265):1329–1333

92. Jodal U, Smellie JM, Lax H, Hoyer PF. Ten-year results of randomized treatment of children with severe vesicoureteral reflux: final report of the International Reflux Study in Children. *Pediatr Nephrol.* 2006;21(6):785–792

93. Capozza N, Caione P. Dextranomer/hyaluronic acid copolymer implantation for vesico-ureteral reflux: a randomized comparison with antibiotic prophylaxis. *J Pediatr.* 2002;140(2):230–234

94. Wingen AM, Koskimies O, Olbing H, Seppanen J, Tamminen-Mobius T. Growth and weight gain in children with vesicoureteral reflux receiving medical versus surgical treatment: 10-year results of a prospective, randomized study. *Acta Paediatr.* 1999;88(1):56–61

95. Smellie JM, Tamminen-Möbius T, Olbing H, et al. Radiologic findings in the kidney of children with severe reflux: five-year comparative study of conservative and surgical treatment [in German]. *Urologe A.* 1993;32(1):22–29

96. Olbing H, Smellie JM, Jodal U, Lax H. New renal scars in children with severe VUR: a 10-year study of randomized treatment. *Pediatr Nephrol.* 2003;18(11):1128–1131

97. Olbing H, Hirche H, Koskimies O, et al. Renal growth in children with severe vesicoureteral reflux: 10-year prospective study of medical and surgical treatment. *Radiology.* 2000;216(3):731–737

98. Al-Sayyad AJ, Pike JG, Leonard MP. Can prophylactic antibiotics safely be discontinued in children with vesicoureteral reflux? *J Urol.* 2005;174(4):1587–1589

99. Kaneko K, Ohtomo Y, Shimizu T, Yamashiro Y, Yamataka A, Miyano T. Antibiotic prophylaxis by low-dose cefaclor in children with vesicoureteral reflux. *Pediatr Nephrol.* 2003;18(5):468–470

100. Lohr JA, Nunley DH, Howards SS, Ford RF. Prevention of recurrent urinary tract infections in girls. *Pediatrics.* 1977;59(4):562–565

101. Smellie JM, Katz G, Grüneberg RN. Controlled trial of prophylactic treatment in childhood urinary-tract infection. *Lancet.* 1978;2(8082):175–178

102. Savage DC, Howie G, Adler K, Wilson MI. Controlled trial of therapy in covert bacteriuria of childhood. *Lancet.* 1975;1(7903):358–361

103. Stansfeld JM. Duration of treatment for urinary tract infections in children. *Br Med J.* 1975;3(5975):65–66

104. Reddy PP, Evans MT, Hughes PA, et al. Antimicrobial prophylaxis in children with vesicoureteral reflux: a randomized prospective study of continuous therapy vs intermittent therapy vs surveillance. *Pediatrics.* 1997;100(3 suppl):555–556

105. Craig J, Roy L, Sureshkumar P, Burke J, Powell H. Long-term antibiotics to prevent urinary tract infection in children with isolated vesicoureteric reflux: a placebo-controlled randomized trial. *J Am Soc Nephrol.* 2002;13(3):3A

106. Bitsori M, Maraki S, Kalmanti M, Galanakis E. Resistance against broad-spectrum β-lactams among uropathogens in children. *Pediatr Nephrol.* 2009;24(12):2381–2386

107. Conway PH, Cnaan A, Zaoutis T, Henry BV, Grundmeier RW, Keren R. Recurrent urinary tract infections in children: risk factors and association with prophylactic antimicrobials. *JAMA.* 2007;298(2):179–186

108. Hodson EM, Wheeler DM, Vimalchandra D, Smith GH, Craig JC. Interventions for primary vesicoureteric reflux. *Cochrane Database Syst Rev.* 2007;(3):CD001532

109. xWilliams DI, Kenawi MM. The prognosis of pelviureteric obstruction in childhood: a review of 190 cases. *Eur Urol.* 1976;2(2):57–63

110. Mihindukulasuriya JC, Maskell R, Polak A. A study of fifty-eight patients with renal scarring associated with urinary tract infection. *Q J Med.* 1980;49(194):165–178

111. McKerrow W, Davidson-Lamb N, Jones PF. Urinary tract infection in children. *Br Med J (Clin Res Ed)*. 1984;289(6440):299–303

112. Jacobson SH, Eklof O, Lins LE, Wikstad I, Winberg J. Long-term prognosis of post-infectious renal scarring in relation to radiological findings in childhood: a 27-year follow-up. *Pediatr Nephrol*. 1992;6(1): 19–24

113. Craig JC, Irwig LM, Knight JF, Roy LP. Does treatment of vesicoureteric reflux in childhood prevent end-stage renal disease attributable to reflux nephropathy? *Pediatrics*. 2000;105(6):1236–1241

114. Phillips D, Watson AR, Collier J. Distress and radiological investigations of the urinary tract in children. *Eur J Pediatr*. 1996; 155(8):684–687

115. Phillips DA, Watson AR, MacKinlay D. Distress and the micturating cystourethrogram: does preparation help? *Acta Paediatr*. 1998;87(2): 175–179

116. Robinson M, Savage J, Stewart M, Sweeney L. The diagnostic value, parental and patient acceptability of micturating cystourethrography in children. *Ir Med J*. 1999; 92(5):366–368

The New American Academy of Pediatrics Urinary Tract Infection Guideline

This issue of *Pediatrics* includes a long-awaited update[1] of the American Academy of Pediatrics (AAP) 1999 urinary tract infection (UTI) practice parameter.[2] The new guideline is accompanied by a technical report[3] that provides a comprehensive literature review and also a new meta-analysis, for which the authors obtained individual-level data from investigators. The result is an exceptionally evidence-based guideline that differs in important ways from the 1999 guideline and sets a high standard for transparency and scholarship.

The guideline and technical report address a logical sequence of questions that arise clinically, including (1) Which children should have their urine tested? (2) How should the sample be obtained? (3) How should UTIs be treated? (4) What imaging and follow-up are recommended after a diagnosis of UTI? and (5) How should children be followed after a UTI has been diagnosed? I will follow that same sequence in this commentary. I will mention some important areas of agreement and make other suggestions when I believe alternative recommendations are supported by available evidence.

WHICH CHILDREN SHOULD HAVE THEIR URINE TESTED?

Unlike the 1999 practice parameter, which recommended urine testing for all children aged 2 months to 2 years with unexplained fever,[2] the new guideline recommends selective urine testing based on the prior probability of UTI, which is an important improvement. The guideline and technical report do an admirable job summarizing the main factors that determine that prior probability (summarized in Table 1 in the clinical report). This table will help clinicians estimate whether the probability of UTI is ≥1% or ≥2%, values that the authors suggest are reasonable thresholds for urine testing.

The guideline appropriately states that the threshold probability for urine testing is not known and that "clinicians will choose a threshold depending on factors such as their confidence that contact will be maintained through the illness… and comfort with diagnostic uncertainty." However, the authors assert that this threshold is below 3%, which indicates that it is worth performing urine tests on more than 33 febrile children to identify a single UTI. This is puzzling, because the only study cited to support a specific testing threshold found that 33% of academicians and 54% of practitioners had a urine culture threshold higher than 3%.[4]

An evidence-based urine-testing threshold probability would be based on the risks and costs of urine testing compared with the benefits of diagnosing a UTI. These benefits are not known and probably are not uniform; the younger and sicker an infant is and the longer he or she has been febrile, the greater the likely benefit of diagnosing and treating a UTI. Because acute symptoms of most UTIs seem to resolve un-

AUTHOR: Thomas B. Newman, MD, MPH

Division of Clinical Epidemiology, Department of Epidemiology and Biostatistics, and Division of General Pediatrics, Department of Pediatrics, University of California, San Francisco, California

ABBREVIATIONS
AAP—American Academy of Pediatrics
UTI—urinary tract infection
VCUG—voiding cystourethrogram
VUR—vesicoureteral reflux

Opinions expressed in these commentaries are those of the author and not necessarily those of the American Academy of Pediatrics or its Committees.

www.pediatrics.org/cgi/doi/10.1542/peds.2011-1818

doi:10.1542/peds.2011-1818

Accepted for publication Jun 28, 2011

Address correspondence to Thomas B. Newman, MD, MPH, Department of Epidemiology and Biostatistics, UCSF Box 0560, San Francisco, CA 94143. E-mail: newman@epi.ucsf.edu

PEDIATRICS (ISSN Numbers: Print, 0031-4005; Online, 1098-4275).

FINANCIAL DISCLOSURE: *The author has indicated he has no financial relationships relevant to this article to disclose.*

COMPANION PAPERS: Companions to this article can be found on pages 595 and e749, and online at www.pediatrics.org/cgi/doi/10.1542/peds.2011-1330 and www.pediatrics.org/cgi/doi/10.1542/peds.2011-1332.

eventfully, even without treatment,[5,6] some of the impetus for diagnosing UTIs rests on the belief that doing so will reduce the risk of renal scarring and associated sequelae.[7] This belief needs to be proven, and the benefit quantified, if a urine-testing threshold is to be evidence-based. Until then, rather than automatically testing urine on the basis of the risk factors and the 1% or 2% threshold suggested in Table 1, clinicians should continue to individualize. It seems reasonable, for example, to defer urine tests on the large number of febrile infants for whom, if their parents had called for advice, we would have estimated their probability of UTI or other serious illness to be low enough that they could be safely initially watched at home.

A potential source of confusion is that Table 1 lists "absence of another source of infection" as a risk factor, and the technical report indicates that this factor has a likelihood ratio of ~1.4 for UTI. However, the inclusion of this risk factor in the table is inconsistent with the text of the guideline, which directs clinicians to assess the likelihood of UTI in febrile infants with no apparent source for the fever. If children with an apparent source for their fever are included, the use of Table 1 could lead to excessive urine testing (eg, among infants with colds). For example, even using the 2% testing threshold, according to Table 1 all non-black uncircumcised boys younger than 24 months with any fever of any duration, even with an apparent source, would need their urine tested. I doubt that this level of urine testing is necessary or was intended by the authors of the guideline.

HOW SHOULD THE SAMPLE BE OBTAINED?

I am glad the new guideline continues to offer the option of obtaining urine for urinalyses noninvasively, but I am not convinced that the bag urine can never be used for culture. If the urinalysis is used to select urine for culture, the prior probability may sometimes be in a range where the bag culture will be useful. For example, the technical report calculates that "with a prevalence of 5% and specificity of 70%, the positive predictive value of a positive culture obtained by bag would be 15%." However, with the same 5% pretest probability, a positive nitrite test would raise the probability of UTI to ~75% (using the median sensitivity [58%] and specificity [99%] in the technical report). This is high enough to make the positive culture on bag urine convincing (and perhaps unnecessary).

Although bag urine cultures can lead to errors, catheterized urine cultures are not perfect[1] and urethral catheterization is painful,[8] frightening,[9] and risks introducing infection.[10] Fortunately, if other recommendations in the guideline are followed (including the elimination of routine voiding cystourethrograms [VCUGs] and outpatient rather than inpatient antimicrobial therapy; see below), the adverse consequences of falsely positive bag cultures will be markedly attenuated.

HOW SHOULD UTIs BE TREATED?

The guideline recognizes regional variation in antimicrobial susceptibility patterns and appropriately suggests that they dictate the choice of initial treatment. However, I would adjust the choice on the basis of the clinical course rather than on sensitivity testing of the isolated uropathogen, as recommended in the guideline. At the University of California at San Francisco we have the option of a "screening" urine culture, which provides only the colony count and Gram-stain results for positive cultures (eg, "10^5 Gram-negative rods"). We can later add identification and sensitivities of the organism in the rare instances in which obtaining them is clinically indicated. Use of screening cultures can lead to considerable savings, because identification of organisms and antimicrobial susceptibility testing are expensive and unnecessary in the majority of cases in which patients are better within 24 hours of starting treatment.

The guideline and technical report cite good evidence that oral antimicrobial treatment is as effective as parenteral treatment and state that the choice of route of administration should be based on "practical considerations." However, the examples they cite for when parenteral antibiotics are reasonable (eg, toxic appearance and inability to retain oral medications) seem more like clinical than practical considerations. Given equivalent estimates of efficacy and the dramatic differences in cost, the guideline could have more forcefully recommended oral treatment in the absence of clinical contraindications.

WHAT IMAGING IS INDICATED AFTER UTI?

As in the 1999 AAP guideline, the current guideline recommends a renal/bladder ultrasound examination after a first febrile UTI to rule out anatomic abnormalities (particularly obstruction) that warrant further evaluation. Although the yield of this test is low, particularly if there has been a normal third-trimester prenatal ultrasound scan, the estimated 1% to 2% yield of actionable abnormalities was believed to be sufficient to justify this noninvasive test. This may be so, but it is important to note that it is not just the yield of abnormalities but also the evidence of an advantage of early detection and cost-effectiveness that must be considered when deciding whether an ultrasound scan is indicated after the first febrile UTI, and this evidence was not reviewed.

The recommendation most dramatically different from the 1999 guideline is that a VCUG not be routinely performed after a first febrile UTI. The main reason for this change is the accumulation of evidence casting doubt on the benefit of making a diagnosis of vesicoureteral reflux (VUR). To put these data in historical perspective, operative ureteral reimplantation was standard treatment for VUR until randomized trials found it to be no better than prophylactic antibiotics at preventing renal scarring.[11–13] Although, as one commentator put it, "It is psychologically difficult to accept results that suggest that time-honored methods that are generally recommended and applied are of no or doubtful value,"[14] ureteral reimplantation was gradually replaced with prophylactic antibiotics as standard treatment for VUR. This was not because of evidence of benefit of antibiotics but because their use was easier and less invasive than ureteral reimplantation. Finally, in the last few years, several randomized trials have investigated the efficacy of prophylactic antibiotics for children with reflux and have found little, if any, benefit.[1,3] Thus, the risks, costs, and discomfort of the VCUG are hard to justify, because there is no evidence that patients benefit from having their VUR diagnosed.[15–18]

The recommendation not to perform a VCUG after the first UTI is consistent with a guideline published by the United Kingdom's National Institute for Health and Clinical Excellence (NICE).[19] However, unlike the AAP, the NICE does not recommend that VCUGs be performed routinely for recurrent UTIs in infants older than 6 months, which makes sense; the arguments against VCUGs after a first UTI still hold after a second UTI. The AAP recommendation to perform a VCUG after the second UTI is based on the increasing likelihood of detecting higher grades of reflux in children with recurrent UTIs and the belief that detecting grade V reflux is beneficial. However, the guideline appropriately recognizes that grade V reflux is rare and that the benefits of diagnosing it are still in some doubt. Therefore, the guideline suggests that parent preferences be considered in making these imaging decisions.

HOW SHOULD CHILDREN BE FOLLOWED AFTER A UTI HAS BEEN DIAGNOSED?

The guideline recommends that parents or guardians of children with confirmed UTI "seek prompt (ideally within 48 hours) medical evaluation for future febrile illnesses to ensure that recurrent infections can be detected and treated promptly." As pointed out in the guideline, parents will ultimately make the judgment to seek medical care, and there is room for judgment here. After-hours or weekend visits would not generally be required for infants who appear well, and the necessity and urgency of the visit would be expected to increase with the discomfort of the child, the height and duration of the fever, the absence of an alternative source, and the number of previous UTIs.

It should be noted that the guideline does not recommend prophylactic antibiotics to prevent UTI recurrences. This was a good decision; meta-analyses[3,20] have revealed no significant reduction in symptomatic UTI from such prophylaxis regardless of whether VUR was present. Even in the study that showed a benefit,[21] the absolute risk reduction for symptomatic UTI over the 1-year follow-up period was only ~6%, and there was no reduction in hospitalizations for UTI or in renal scarring. Thus, as one colleague put it, if UTI prophylaxis worked, it would offer the opportunity to "treat 16 children with antibiotics for a year to prevent treating one child with antibiotics for a week." (A. R. Schroeder, MD, written communication, June 24, 2011).

CONCLUSIONS

I salute the authors of the new AAP UTI guideline and the accompanying technical report. Both publications represent a significant advance that should be helpful to clinicians and families dealing with this common problem.

REFERENCES

1. American Academy of Pediatrics, Subcommittee on Urinary Tract Infection, Steering Committee on Quality Improvement and Management. Diagnosis and management of initial UTIs in febrile infants and children aged 2 to 24 months. *Pediatrics.* 2011;128(3):595–610

2. American Academy of Pediatrics, Committee on Quality Improvement, Subcommittee on Urinary Tract Infection. Practice parameter: the diagnosis, treatment, and evaluation of the initial urinary tract infection in febrile infants and young children [published corrections appear in *Pediatrics.* 1999;103(5 pt 1):1052 and *Pediatrics.* 1999;104(1 pt 1):118]. *Pediatrics.* 1999; 103(4 pt 1):843–852

3. American Academy of Pediatrics, Subcommittee on Urinary Tract Infection, Steering Committee on Quality Improvement and Management. The diagnosis and management of the initial urinary tract infection in febrile infants and young children. *Pediatrics.* 2011;128(3). Available at: www. pediatrics.org/cgi/content/full/128/3/e749

4. Roberts KB, Charney E, Sweren RJ, et al. Urinary tract infection in infants with unexplained fever: a collaborative study. *J Pediatr.* 1983;103(6):864–867

5. Newman TB, Bernzweig JA, Takayama JI, Finch SA, Wasserman RC, Pantell RH. Urine testing and urinary tract infections in febrile infants seen in office settings: the Pediatric Research in Office Settings' Febrile Infant Study. *Arch Pediatr Adolesc Med.* 2002;156(1):44–54

6. Craig JC, Williams GJ, Jones M, et al. The accuracy of clinical symptoms and signs for the diagnosis of serious bacterial infection in young febrile children: prospective cohort study of 15 781 febrile illnesses. *BMJ.* 2010;340:c1594

7. Roberts KB. Urinary tract infections in

young febrile infants: is selective testing acceptable? *Arch Pediatr Adolesc Med.* 2002; 156(1):6–7

8. Mularoni PP, Cohen LL, DeGuzman M, Mennuti-Washburn J, Greenwald M, Simon HK. A randomized clinical trial of lidocaine gel for reducing infant distress during urethral catheterization. *Pediatr Emerg Care.* 2009;25(7):439–443

9. Merritt KA, Ornstein PA, Spicker B. Children's memory for a salient medical procedure: implications for testimony. *Pediatrics.* 1994;94(1):17–23

10. Lohr JA, Downs SM, Dudley S, Donowitz LG. Hospital-acquired urinary tract infections in the pediatric patient: a prospective study. *Pediatr Infect Dis J.* 1994;13(1):8–12

11. Birmingham Reflux Study Group. Prospective trial of operative versus non-operative treatment of severe vesicoureteric reflux in children: five years' observation. *Br Med J (Clin Res Ed).* 1987;295(6592):237–241

12. Weiss R, Duckett J, Spitzer A. Results of a randomized clinical trial of medical versus surgical management of infants and children with grades III and IV primary vesicoureteral reflux (United States). The International Reflux Study in Children. *J Urol.* 1992;148(5 pt 2):1667–1673

13. Smellie JM, Tamminen-Mobius T, Olbing H, et al. Five-year study of medical or surgical treatment in children with severe reflux: radiological renal findings. The International Reflux Study in Children. *Pediatr Nephrol.* 1992;6(3):223–230

14. Winberg J. Management of primary vesicoureteric reflux in children: operation ineffective in preventing progressive renal damage. *Infection.* 1994;22(suppl 1):S4–S7

15. Ortigas A, Cunningham A. Three facts to know before you order a VCUG. *Contemp Pediatr.* 1997;14(9):69–79

16. Craig JC, Irwig LM, Knight JF, Roy LP. Does treatment of vesicoureteric reflux in childhood prevent end-stage renal disease attributable to reflux nephropathy? *Pediatrics.* 2000;105(6):1236–1241

17. Verrier Jones K. Time to review the value of imaging after urinary tract infection in infants. *Arch Dis Child.* 2005;90(7):663–664

18. Newman TB. Much pain, little gain from voiding cystourethrograms after urinary tract infection. *Pediatrics.* 2006;118(5):2251

19. National Collaborating Centre for Women's and Children's Health. *Urinary Tract Infection in Children: Diagnosis, Treatment and Long-term Management.* National Institute for Health and Clinical Excellence Clinical Guideline. London, United Kingdom: RCOG Press; 2007

20. Dai B, Liu Y, Jia J, Mei C. Long-term antibiotics for the prevention of recurrent urinary tract infection in children: a systematic review and meta-analysis. *Arch Dis Child.* 2010;95(7):499–508

21. Craig JC, Simpson JM, Williams GJ, et al; Prevention of Recurrent Urinary Tract Infection in Children With Vesicoureteric Reflux and Normal Renal Tracts (PRIVENT) Investigators. Antibiotic prophylaxis and recurrent urinary tract infection in children. *N Engl J Med.* 2009;361(18):1748–1759

Urinary Tract Infection Clinical Practice Guideline Quick Reference Tools

• •

- Action Statement Summary
  — Urinary Tract Infection: Clinical Practice Guideline for the Diagnosis and Management of the Initial UTI in Febrile Infants and Children 2 to 24 Months
- *ICD-10-CM* Coding Quick Reference for Urinary Tract Infection
- AAP Patient Education Handout
  — *Urinary Tract Infections in Young Children*

Action Statement Summary

Urinary Tract Infection: Clinical Practice Guideline for the Diagnosis and Management of the Initial UTI in Febrile Infants and Children 2 to 24 Months

Action Statement 1

If a clinician decides that a febrile infant with no apparent source for the fever requires antimicrobial therapy to be administered because of ill appearance or another pressing reason, the clinician should ensure that a urine specimen is obtained for both culture and urinalysis before an antimicrobial agent is administered; the specimen needs to be obtained through catheterization or SPA, because the diagnosis of UTI cannot be established reliably through culture of urine collected in a bag (evidence quality: A; strong recommendation).

Action Statement 2

If a clinician assesses a febrile infant with no apparent source for the fever as not being so ill as to require immediate antimicrobial therapy, then the clinician should assess the likelihood of UTI (see below for how to assess likelihood).

Action Statement 2a

If the clinician determines the febrile infant to have a low likelihood of UTI (see text), then clinical follow-up monitoring without testing is sufficient (evidence quality: A; strong recommendation).

Action Statement 2b

If the clinician determines that the febrile infant is not in a low-risk group (see below), then there are 2 choices (evidence quality: A; strong recommendation). Option 1 is to obtain a urine specimen through catheterization or SPA for culture and urinalysis. Option 2 is to obtain a urine specimen through the most convenient means and to perform a urinalysis. If the urinalysis results suggest a UTI (positive leukocyte esterase test results or nitrite test or microscopic analysis results positive for leukocytes or bacteria), then a urine specimen should be obtained through catheterization or SPA and cultured; if urinalysis of fresh (<1 hour since void) urine yields negative leukocyte esterase and nitrite test results, then it is reasonable to monitor the clinical course without initiating antimicrobial therapy, recognizing that negative urinalysis results do not rule out a UTI with certainty.

Action Statement 3

To establish the diagnosis of UTI, clinicians should require *both* urinalysis results that suggest infection (pyuria and/or bacteriuria) *and* the presence of at least 50 000 colony-forming units (CFUs) per mL of a uropathogen cultured from a urine specimen obtained through catheterization or SPA (evidence quality: C; recommendation).

Action Statement 4a

When initiating treatment, the clinician should base the choice of route of administration on practical considerations. Initiating treatment orally or parenterally is equally efficacious. The clinician should base the choice of agent on local antimicrobial sensitivity patterns (if available) and should adjust the choice according to sensitivity testing of the isolated uropathogen (evidence quality: A; strong recommendation).

Action Statement 4b

The clinician should choose 7 to 14 days as the duration of antimicrobial therapy (evidence quality: B; recommendation).

Action Statement 5

Febrile infants with UTIs should undergo renal and bladder ultrasonography (RBUS) (evidence quality: C; recommendation).

Action Statement 6a

VCUG should not be performed routinely after the first febrile UTI; VCUG is indicated if RBUS reveals hydronephrosis, scarring, or other findings that would suggest either high-grade VUR or obstructive uropathy, as well as in other atypical or complex clinical circumstances (evidence quality B; recommendation).

Action Statement 6b

Further evaluation should be conducted if there is a recurrence of febrile UTI (evidence quality: X; recommendation).

Action Statement 7

After confirmation of UTI, the clinician should instruct parents or guardians to seek prompt medical evaluation (ideally within 48 hours) for future febrile illnesses, to ensure that recurrent infections can be detected and treated promptly (evidence quality: C; recommendation).

Coding Quick Reference for Urinary Tract Infection

ICD-10-CM

N39.0 Urinary tract infection, site not specified

P39.3 Neonatal urinary tract infection

Urinary Tract Infections in Young Children

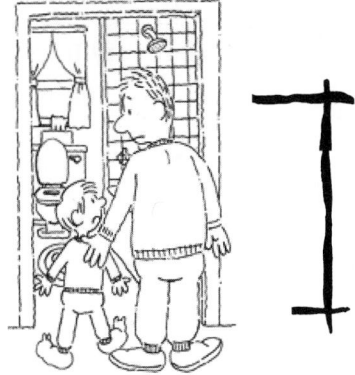

Urinary tract infections (UTIs) are common in young children. These infections can lead to serious health problems. UTIs may go untreated because the symptoms may not be obvious to the child or the parents. The following is information from the American Academy of Pediatrics about UTIs—what they are, how children get them, and how they are treated.

The urinary tract

The urinary tract makes and stores urine. It is made up of the kidneys, ureters, bladder, and urethra (see illustration on the next page). The kidneys produce urine. Urine travels from the kidneys down 2 narrow tubes called the ureters to the bladder. The bladder is a thin muscular bag that stores urine until it is time to empty urine out of the body. When it is time to empty the bladder, a muscle at the bottom of the bladder relaxes. Urine then flows out of the body through a tube called the urethra. The opening of the urethra is at the end of the penis in boys and above the vaginal opening in girls.

Urinary tract infections

Normal urine has no germs (bacteria). However, bacteria can get into the urinary tract from 2 sources: (1) the skin around the rectum and genitals and (2) the bloodstream from other parts of the body. Bacteria may cause infections in any or all parts of the urinary tract, including the following:

- Urethra (called urethritis)
- Bladder (called cystitis)
- Kidneys (called pyelonephritis)

UTIs are common in infants and young children. The frequency of UTIs in girls is much greater than in boys. About 3% of girls and 1% of boys will have a UTI by 11 years of age. A young child with a high fever and no other symptoms has a 1 in 20 chance of having a UTI. Uncircumcised boys have more UTIs than those who have been circumcised.

Symptoms

Symptoms of UTIs may include the following:

- Fever
- Pain or burning during urination
- Need to urinate more often, or difficulty getting urine out
- Urgent need to urinate, or wetting of underwear or bedding by a child who knows how to use the toilet
- Vomiting, refusal to eat
- Abdominal pain
- Side or back pain
- Foul-smelling urine
- Cloudy or bloody urine
- Unexplained and persistent irritability in an infant
- Poor growth in an infant

Diagnosis

If your child has symptoms of a UTI, your child's doctor will do the following:

- Ask about your child's symptoms.
- Ask about any family history of urinary tract problems.
- Ask about what your child has been eating and drinking.
- Examine your child.
- Get a urine sample from your child.

Your child's doctor will need to test your child's urine to see if there are bacteria or other abnormalities.

Ways urine is collected

Urine must be collected and analyzed to determine if there is a bacterial infection. Older children are asked to urinate into a container.

There are 3 ways to collect urine from a young child:

1. The preferred method is to place a small tube, called a catheter, through the urethra into the bladder. Urine flows through the tube into a special urine container.
2. Another method is to insert a needle through the skin of the lower abdomen to draw urine from the bladder. This is called needle aspiration.
3. If your child is very young or not yet toilet trained, the child's doctor may place a plastic bag over the genitals to collect the urine. Since bacteria on the skin can contaminate the urine and give a false test result, this method is used only to screen for infection. If an infection seems to be present, the doctor will need to collect urine through 1 of the first 2 methods in order to determine if bacteria are present.

Your child's doctor will discuss with you the best way to collect your child's urine.

Treatment

UTIs are treated with antibiotics. The way your child receives the antibiotic depends on the severity and type of infection. Antibiotics are usually given by mouth, as liquid or pills. If your child has a fever or is vomiting and is unable to keep fluids down, the antibiotics may be put directly into a vein or injected into a muscle.

UTIs need to be treated right away to

- Get rid of the infection.
- Prevent the spread of the infection outside of the urinary tract.
- Reduce the chances of kidney damage.

Infants and young children with UTIs usually need to take antibiotics for 7 to 14 days, sometimes longer. Make sure your child takes all the medicine your child's doctor prescribes. Do not stop giving your child the medicine until the child's doctor says the treatment is finished, even if your child feels better. UTIs can return if not fully treated.

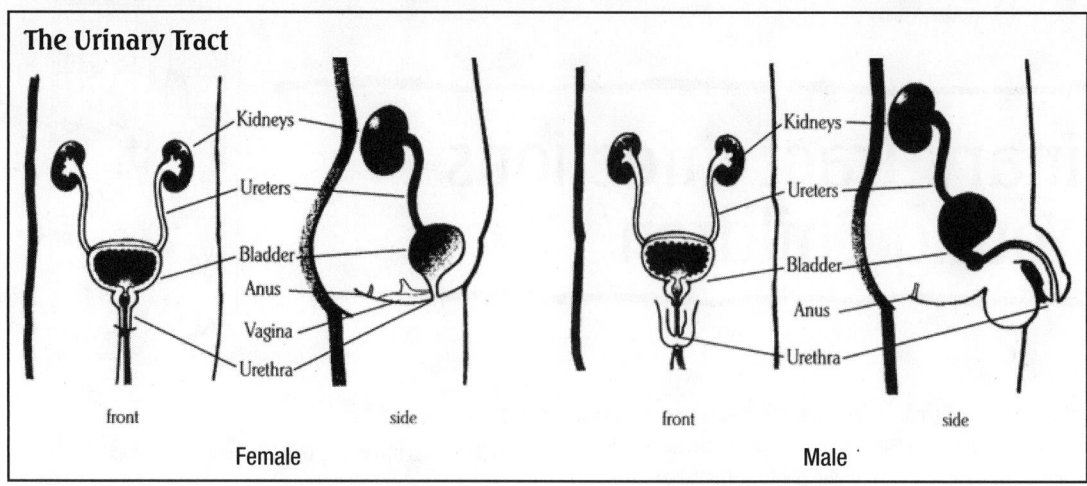

The Urinary Tract

Kidneys
Ureters
Bladder
Anus
Vagina
Urethra

front   side
Female

Kidneys
Ureters
Bladder
Anus
Urethra

front   side
Male

Follow-up

If the UTI occurs early in life, your child's doctor will probably want to make sure the urinary tract is normal with a kidney and bladder ultrasound. This test uses sound waves to examine the bladder and kidneys.

In addition, your child's doctor may want to make sure that the urinary tract is functioning normally and is free of any damage. Several tests are available to do this, including the following:

Voiding cystourethrogram (VCUG). A catheter is placed into the urethra and the bladder is filled with a liquid that can be seen on x-rays. This test shows whether the urine is flowing back from the bladder toward the kidneys instead of all of it coming out through the urethra as it should.

Nuclear scans. Radioactive material is injected into a vein to see if the kidneys are normal. There are many kinds of nuclear scans, each giving different information about the kidneys and bladder. The radioactive material gives no more radiation than any other kind of x-ray.

Remember

UTIs are common and most are easy to treat. Early diagnosis and prompt treatment are important because untreated or repeated infections can cause long-term medical problems. Children who have had one UTI are more likely to have another. Be sure to see your child's doctor early if your child has had a UTI in the past and has fever. Talk with your child's doctor if you suspect that your child might have a UTI.

The information contained in this publication should not be used as a substitute for the medical care and advice of your pediatrician. There may be variations in treatment that your pediatrician may recommend based on individual facts and circumstances.

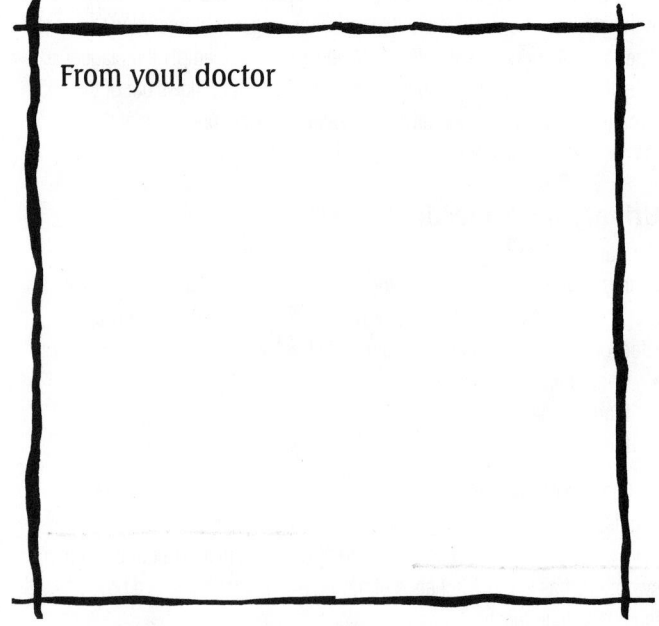

From your doctor

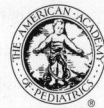

American Academy of Pediatrics

DEDICATED TO THE HEALTH OF ALL CHILDREN™

Section 2

Endorsed Clinical Practice Guidelines

The American Academy of Pediatrics endorses and accepts as its policy the following guidelines from other organizations.

AUTISM SPECTRUM DISORDER
Screening and Diagnosis of Autism
Quality Standards Subcommittee of the American Academy of Neurology and the Child Neurology Society

ABSTRACT. Autism is a common disorder of childhood, affecting 1 in 500 children. Yet, it often remains unrecognized and undiagnosed until or after late preschool age because appropriate tools for routine developmental screening and screening specifically for autism have not been available. Early identification of children with autism and intensive, early intervention during the toddler and preschool years improves outcome for most young children with autism. This practice parameter reviews the available empirical evidence and gives specific recommendations for the identification of children with autism. This approach requires a dual process: (1) routine developmental surveillance and screening specifically for autism to be performed on all children to first identify those at risk for any type of atypical development, and to identify those specifically at risk for autism; and (2) to diagnose and evaluate autism, to differentiate autism from other developmental disorders. (8/00)

CEREBRAL PALSY
Diagnostic Assessment of the Child With Cerebral Palsy
Quality Standards Subcommittee of the American Academy of Neurology and the Practice Committee of the Child Neurology Society

ABSTRACT. *Objective.* The Quality Standards Subcommittee of the American Academy of Neurology and the Practice Committee of the Child Neurology Society develop practice parameters as strategies for patient management based on analysis of evidence. For this parameter the authors reviewed available evidence on the assessment of a child suspected of having cerebral palsy (CP), a nonprogressive disorder of posture or movement due to a lesion of the developing brain.

Methods. Relevant literature was reviewed, abstracted, and classified. Recommendations were based on a four-tiered scheme of evidence classification.

Results. CP is a common problem, occurring in about 2 to 2.5 per 1,000 live births. In order to establish that a brain abnormality exists in children with CP that may, in turn, suggest an etiology and prognosis, neuroimaging is recommended with MRI preferred to CT (Level A). Metabolic and genetic studies should not be routinely obtained in the evaluation of the child with CP (Level B). If the clinical history or findings on neuroimaging do not determine a specific structural abnormality or if there are additional and atypical features in the history or clinical examination, metabolic and genetic testing should be considered (Level C). Detection of a brain malformation in a child with CP warrants consideration of an underlying genetic or metabolic etiology. Because the incidence of cerebral infarction is high in children with hemiplegic CP, diagnostic testing for coagulation disorders should be considered (Level B). However, there is insufficient evidence at present to be precise as to what studies should be ordered. An EEG is not recommended unless there are features suggestive of epilepsy or a specific epileptic syndrome (Level A). Because children with CP may have associated deficits of mental retardation, ophthalmologic and hearing impairments, speech and language disorders, and oral-motor dysfunction, screening for these conditions should be part of the initial assessment (Level A).

Conclusions. Neuroimaging results in children with CP are commonly abnormal and may help determine the etiology. Screening for associated conditions is warranted as part of the initial evaluation. (3/04)

COMMUNITY-ACQUIRED PNEUMONIA
The Management of Community-Acquired Pneumonia (CAP) in Infants and Children Older Than 3 Months of Age
Pediatric Infectious Diseases Society and Infectious Diseases Society of America

ABSTRACT. Evidenced-based guidelines for management of infants and children with community-acquired pneumonia (CAP) were prepared by an expert panel comprising clinicians and investigators representing community pediatrics, public health, and the pediatric specialties of critical care, emergency medicine, hospital medicine, infectious diseases, pulmonology, and surgery. These guidelines are intended for use by primary care and subspecialty providers responsible for the management of otherwise healthy infants and children with CAP in both outpatient and inpatient settings. Site-of-care management, diagnosis, antimicrobial and adjunctive surgical therapy, and prevention are discussed. Areas that warrant future investigations are also highlighted. (10/11)

CONGENITAL ADRENAL HYPERPLASIA
Congenital Adrenal Hyperplasia Due to Steroid 21-hydroxylase Deficiency: An Endocrine Society Clinical Practice Guideline
The Endocrine Society

CONCLUSIONS. We recommend universal newborn screening for severe steroid 21-hydroxylase deficiency followed by confirmatory tests. We recommend that prenatal treatment of CAH continue to be regarded as experimental. The diagnosis rests on clinical and hormonal data; genotyping is reserved for equivocal cases and genetic counseling. Glucocorticoid dosage should be minimized to avoid iatrogenic Cushing's syndrome. Mineralocorticoids and, in infants, supplemental sodium are recommended in classic CAH patients. We recommend against the routine use of experimental therapies to promote growth and delay puberty; we suggest patients avoid adrenalectomy. Surgical guidelines emphasize early single-stage genital repair for severely virilized girls, performed by experienced surgeons. Clinicians should consider patients' quality of life, consulting mental health professionals as appropriate. At the transition to adulthood, we recommend monitoring for potential complications of CAH. Finally, we recommend judicious use of medication during pregnancy and in symptomatic patients with nonclassic CAH. (9/10)

CONGENITAL MUSCULAR DYSTROPHY

Evidence-based Guideline Summary: Evaluation, Diagnosis, and Management of Congenital Muscular Dystrophy. Report of the Guideline Development Subcommittee of the American Academy of Neurology and the Practice Issues Review Panel of the American Association of Neuromuscular & Electrodiagnostic Medicine

American Academy of Neurology and American Association of Neuromuscular & Electrodiagnostic Medicine

ABSTRACT. *Objective.* To delineate optimal diagnostic and therapeutic approaches to congenital muscular dystrophy (CMD) through a systematic review and analysis of the currently available literature.

Methods. Relevant, peer-reviewed research articles were identified using a literature search of the MEDLINE, EMBASE, and Scopus databases. Diagnostic and therapeutic data from these articles were extracted and analyzed in accordance with the American Academy of Neurology classification of evidence schemes for diagnostic, prognostic, and therapeutic studies. Recommendations were linked to the strength of the evidence, other related literature, and general principles of care.

Results. The geographic and ethnic backgrounds, clinical features, brain imaging studies, muscle imaging studies, and muscle biopsies of children with suspected CMD help predict subtype-specific diagnoses. Genetic testing can confirm some subtype-specific diagnoses, but not all causative genes for CMD have been described. Seizures and respiratory complications occur in specific subtypes. There is insufficient evidence to determine the efficacy of various treatment interventions to optimize respiratory, orthopedic, and nutritional outcomes, and more data are needed regarding complications.

Recommendations. Multidisciplinary care by experienced teams is important for diagnosing and promoting the health of children with CMD. Accurate assessment of clinical presentations and genetic data will help in identifying the correct subtype-specific diagnosis in many cases. Multi-organ system complications occur frequently; surveillance and prompt interventions are likely to be beneficial for affected children. More research is needed to fill gaps in knowledge regarding this category of muscular dystrophies. (3/15)

DEPRESSION

Guidelines for Adolescent Depression in Primary Care (GLAD-PC): I. Identification, Assessment, and Initial Management
Rachel A. Zuckerbrot, MD; Amy H. Cheung, MD; Peter S. Jensen, MD; Ruth E. K. Stein, MD; Danielle Laraque, MD; and GLAD-PC Steering Group

ABSTRACT. *Objectives.* To develop clinical practice guidelines to assist primary care clinicians in the management of adolescent depression. This first part of the guidelines addresses identification, assessment, and initial management of adolescent depression in primary care settings.

Methods. By using a combination of evidence- and consensus-based methodologies, guidelines were developed by an expert steering committee in 5 phases, as informed by (1) current scientific evidence (published and unpublished), (2) a series of focus groups, (3) a formal survey, (4) an expert consensus workshop, and (5) draft revision and iteration among members of the steering committee.

Results. Guidelines were developed for youth aged 10 to 21 years and correspond to initial phases of adolescent depression management in primary care, including identification of at-risk youth, assessment and diagnosis, and initial management. The strength of each recommendation and its evidence base are summarized. The identification, assessment, and initial management section of the guidelines includes recommendations for (1) identification of depression in youth at high risk, (2) systematic assessment procedures using reliable depression scales, patient and caregiver interviews, and Diagnostic and Statistical Manual of Mental Disorders, Fourth Edition criteria, (3) patient and family psychoeducation, (4) establishing relevant links in the community, and (5) the establishment of a safety plan.

Conclusions. This part of the guidelines is intended to assist primary care clinicians in the identification and initial management of depressed adolescents in an era of great clinical need and a shortage of mental health specialists but cannot replace clinical judgment; these guidelines are not meant to be the sole source of guidance for adolescent depression management. Additional research that addresses the identification and initial management of depressed youth in primary care is needed, including empirical testing of these guidelines. (11/07)

Guidelines for Adolescent Depression in Primary Care (GLAD-PC): II. Treatment and Ongoing Management
Amy H. Cheung, MD; Rachel A. Zuckerbrot, MD; Peter S. Jensen, MD; Kareem Ghalib, MD; Danielle Laraque, MD; Ruth E. K. Stein, MD; and GLAD-PC Steering Group

ABSTRACT. *Objectives.* To develop clinical practice guidelines to assist primary care clinicians in the management of adolescent depression. This second part of the guidelines addresses treatment and ongoing management of adolescent depression in the primary care setting.

Methods. Using a combination of evidence- and consensus-based methodologies, guidelines were developed in 5 phases as informed by (1) current scientific evidence (published and unpublished), (2) a series of focus groups, (3) a formal survey, (4) an expert consensus workshop, and (5) revision and iteration among members of the steering committee.

Results. These guidelines are targeted for youth aged 10 to 21 years and offer recommendations for the management of adolescent depression in primary care, including (1) active monitoring of mildly depressed youth, (2) details for the specific application of evidence-based medication and psychotherapeutic approaches in cases of moderate-to-severe depression, (3) careful monitoring of adverse effects, (4) consultation and coordination of care with mental health specialists, (5) ongoing tracking of outcomes, and (6) specific steps to be taken in instances of partial or no improvement after an initial treatment has begun. The strength of each recommendation and its evidence base are summarized.

Conclusions. These guidelines cannot replace clinical judgment, and they should not be the sole source of guidance for adolescent depression management. Nonetheless, the guidelines may assist primary care clinicians in the management of depressed adolescents in an era of great clinical need and a shortage of mental health specialists. Additional research concerning the management of youth with depression in primary care is needed, including the usability, feasibility, and sustainability of guidelines and determination of the extent to which the guidelines actually improve outcomes of youth with depression. (11/07)

DIALYSIS
Shared Decision-Making in the Appropriate Initiation of and Withdrawal from Dialysis, 2nd Edition
Renal Physicians Association (10/10)

DUCHENNE MUSCULAR DYSTROPHY
Practice Guideline Update Summary: Corticosteroid Treatment of Duchenne Muscular Dystrophy
David Gloss, MD, MPH&TM; Richard T. Moxley III, MD; Stephen Ashwal, MD; and Maryam Oskoui, MD, for the American Academy of Neurology Guideline Development Subcommittee

ABSTRACT. *Objective.* To update the 2005 American Academy of Neurology (AAN) guideline on corticosteroid treatment of Duchenne muscular dystrophy (DMD).

Methods. We systematically reviewed the literature from January 2004 to July 2014 using the AAN classification scheme for therapeutic articles and predicated recommendations on the strength of the evidence.

Results. Thirty-four studies met inclusion criteria.

Recommendations. In children with DMD, prednisone should be offered for improving strength (Level B) and pulmonary function (Level B). Prednisone may be offered for improving timed motor function (Level C), reducing the need for scoliosis surgery (Level C), and delaying cardiomyopathy onset by 18 years of age (Level C). Deflazacort may be offered for improving strength and timed motor function and delaying age at loss of ambulation by 1.4–2.5 years (Level C). Deflazacort may be offered for improving pulmonary function, reducing the need for scoliosis surgery, delaying cardiomyopathy onset, and increasing survival at 5–15 years of follow-up (Level C for each). Deflazacort and prednisone may be equivalent in improving motor function (Level C). Prednisone may be associated with greater weight gain in the first years of treatment than deflazacort (Level C). Deflazacort may be associated with a greater risk of cataracts than prednisone (Level C). The preferred dosing regimen of prednisone is 0.75 mg/kg/d (Level B). Over 12 months, prednisone 10 mg/kg/weekend is equally effective (Level B), with no long-term data available. Prednisone 0.75 mg/kg/d is associated with significant risk of weight gain, hirsutism, and cushingoid appearance (Level B). *Neurology®* 2016;86:465–472 (2/16)

DYSPLASIA OF THE HIP
Guideline on Detection and Nonoperative Management of Pediatric Developmental Dysplasia of the Hip in Infants up to Six Months of Age: Evidence-based Clinical Practice Guideline
American Academy of Orthopaedic Surgeons

OVERVIEW. This clinical practice guideline is based upon a systematic review of published articles related to the detection and early management of hip instability and dysplasia in typically developing children less than 6 months of age. This guideline provides practice recommendations for the early screening and detection of hip instability and dysplasia and also highlights gaps in the published literature that should stimulate additional research. This guideline is intended towards appropriately trained practitioners involved in the early examination and assessment of typically developing children for hip instability and dysplasia. (9/14)

EMERGENCY MEDICAL SERVICES
National Model EMS Clinical Guidelines
National Association of State EMS Officials

ABSTRACT. These guidelines will be maintained by NASEMSO to facilitate the creation of state and local EMS system clinical guidelines, protocols or operating procedures. System medical directors and other leaders are invited to harvest content as will be useful. These guidelines are either evidence-based or consensus-based and have been formatted for use by field EMS professionals. (10/14)

ENDOCARDITIS
Prevention of Infective Endocarditis: Guidelines From the American Heart Association
Walter Wilson, MD, Chair; Kathryn A. Taubert, PhD, FAHA; Michael Gewitz, MD, FAHA; Peter B. Lockhart, DDS; Larry M. Baddour, MD; Matthew Levison, MD; Ann Bolger, MD, FAHA; Christopher H. Cabell, MD, MHS; Masato Takahashi, MD, FAHA; Robert S. Baltimore, MD; Jane W. Newburger, MD, MPH, FAHA; Brian L. Strom, MD; Lloyd Y. Tani, MD; Michael Gerber, MD; Robert O. Bonow, MD, FAHA; Thomas Pallasch, DDS, MS; Stanford T. Shulman, MD, FAHA; Anne H. Rowley, MD; Jane C. Burns, MD; Patricia Ferrieri, MD; Timothy Gardner, MD, FAHA; David Goff, MD, PhD, FAHA; David T. Durack, MD, PhD

ABSTRACT. *Background.* The purpose of this statement is to update the recommendations by the American Heart Association (AHA) for the prevention of infective endocarditis that were last published in 1997.

Methods and Results. A writing group was appointed by the AHA for their expertise in prevention and treatment of infective endocarditis, with liaison members representing the American Dental Association, the Infectious Diseases Society of America, and the American Academy of Pediatrics. The writing group reviewed input from national and international experts on infective endocarditis. The recommendations in this document reflect analyses of relevant literature regarding procedure-related bacteremia and infective endocarditis, in vitro susceptibility data of the most common microorganisms that cause infective endocarditis, results of prophylactic studies in animal models of experimental endocarditis, and retrospective and prospective studies of prevention of infective endocarditis. MEDLINE database searches from 1950 to 2006 were done for English-language papers using the following search terms: endocarditis, infective endocarditis, prophylaxis, prevention, antibiotic, antimicrobial, pathogens, organisms, dental, gastrointestinal, genitourinary, streptococcus, enterococcus, staphylococcus, respiratory, dental surgery, pathogenesis, vaccine, immunization, and bacteremia. The reference lists of the identified papers were also searched. We also searched the AHA online library. The American College of Cardiology/AHA classification of recommendations and levels of evidence for practice guidelines were used. The paper was subsequently reviewed by outside experts not affiliated with the writing group and by the AHA Science Advisory and Coordinating Committee.

Conclusions. The major changes in the updated recommendations include the following: (1) The Committee concluded that only an extremely small number of cases of infective endocarditis might be prevented by antibiotic prophylaxis for dental procedures even if such prophylactic therapy were 100% effective. (2) Infective endocarditis prophylaxis for dental procedures should be recommended only for patients with underlying cardiac conditions associated with the highest risk of adverse outcome from infective endocarditis. (3) For patients with these underlying cardiac conditions, prophylaxis is recommended for all dental procedures that involve manipulation of gingival tissue or the periapical region of teeth or perforation of the oral mucosa. (4) Prophylaxis is not recommended based solely on an increased lifetime risk of acquisition of infective endocarditis. (5) Administration of antibiotics solely to prevent endocarditis is not recommended for patients who undergo a genitourinary or gastrointestinal tract procedure. These changes are intended to define more clearly when infective endocarditis prophylaxis is or is not recommended and to provide more uniform and consistent global recommendations. (*Circulation*. 2007;116:1736–1754.) (5/07)

FLUORIDE

Recommendations for Using Fluoride to Prevent and Control Dental Caries in the United States
Centers for Disease Control and Prevention (8/01)

FOOD ALLERGY

Guidelines for the Diagnosis and Management of Food Allergy in the United States: Report of the NIAID-Sponsored Expert Panel
National Institute of Allergy and Infectious Diseases

ABSTRACT. Food allergy is an important public health problem that affects children and adults and may be increasing in prevalence. Despite the risk of severe allergic reactions and even death, there is no current treatment for food allergy: the disease can only be managed by allergen avoidance or treatment of symptoms. The diagnosis and management of food allergy also may vary from one clinical practice setting to another. Finally, because patients frequently confuse nonallergic food reactions, such as food intolerance, with food allergies, there is an unfounded belief among the public that food allergy prevalence is higher than it truly is. In response to these concerns, the National Institute of Allergy and Infectious Diseases, working with 34 professional organizations, federal agencies, and patient advocacy groups, led the development of clinical guidelines for the diagnosis and management of food allergy. These Guidelines are intended for use by a wide variety of health care professionals, including family practice physicians, clinical specialists, and nurse practitioners. The Guidelines include a consensus definition for food allergy, discuss comorbid conditions often associated with food allergy, and focus on both IgE-mediated and non-IgE-mediated reactions to food. Topics addressed include the epidemiology, natural history, diagnosis, and management of food allergy, as well as the management of severe symptoms and anaphylaxis. These Guidelines provide 43 concise clinical recommendations and additional guidance on points of current controversy in patient management. They also identify gaps in the current scientific knowledge to be addressed through future research. (12/10)

GASTROENTERITIS

Managing Acute Gastroenteritis Among Children: Oral Rehydration, Maintenance, and Nutritional Therapy
Centers for Disease Control and Prevention (11/03)

GASTROESOPHAGEAL REFLUX

Guidelines for Evaluation and Treatment of Gastroesophageal Reflux in Infants and Children
North American Society for Pediatric Gastroenterology, Hepatology, and Nutrition

ABSTRACT. Gastroesophageal reflux (GER), defined as passage of gastric contents into the esophagus, and GER disease (GERD), defined as symptoms or complications of GER, are common pediatric problems encountered by both primary and specialty medical providers. Clinical manifestations of GERD in children include vomiting, poor weight gain, dysphagia, abdominal or substernal pain, esophagitis and respiratory disorders. The GER Guideline Committee of the North American Society for Pediatric Gastroenterology and Nutrition has formulated a clinical practice guideline for the management of pediatric GER. The GER Guideline Committee, consisting of a primary care pediatrician, two clinical epidemiologists (who also practice primary care pediatrics) and five pediatric gastroenterologists, based its recommendations on an integration of a comprehensive and systematic review of the medical literature combined with expert opinion. Consensus was achieved through Nominal Group Technique, a structured quantitative method.

The Committee examined the value of diagnostic tests and treatment modalities commonly used for the management of GERD, and how those interventions can be applied to clinical situations in the infant and older child. The guideline provides recommendations for management by the primary care provider, including evaluation, initial treatment, follow-up management and indications for consultation by a specialist. The guideline also provides recommendations for management by the pediatric gastroenterologist.

This document represents the official recommendations of the North American Society for Pediatric Gastroenterology and Nutrition on the evaluation and treatment of gastroesophageal reflux in infants and children. The American Academy of Pediatrics has also endorsed these recommendations. The recommendations are summarized in a synopsis within the article. This review and recommendations are a general guideline and are not intended as a substitute for clinical judgment or as a protocol for the management of all patients with this problem. (2001)

GROUP B STREPTOCOCCAL DISEASE

Prevention of Perinatal Group B Streptococcal Disease: Revised Guidelines from CDC, 2010
Centers for Disease Control and Prevention

SUMMARY. Despite substantial progress in prevention of perinatal group B streptococcal (GBS) disease since the 1990s, GBS remains the leading cause of early-onset neonatal sepsis in the United States. In 1996, CDC, in collaboration with relevant professional societies, published guidelines for the prevention of perinatal group B streptococcal disease (CDC. Prevention of perinatal group B streptococcal disease: a public health perspective. *MMWR* 1996;45[No. RR-7]); those guidelines were updated and republished in 2002 (CDC. Prevention of perinatal group B streptococcal disease: revised guidelines from CDC. *MMWR* 2002;51[No. RR-11]). In June 2009, a meeting of clinical and public health representatives was held to reevaluate prevention strategies on the basis of data collected after the issuance of the 2002 guidelines. This report presents CDC's updated guidelines, which have been endorsed by the American College of Obstetricians and Gynecologists, the American Academy of Pediatrics, the American College of Nurse-Midwives, the American Academy of Family Physicians, and the American Society for Microbiology. The recommendations were made on the basis of available evidence when such evidence was sufficient and on expert opinion when available evidence was insufficient. The key changes in the 2010 guidelines include the following:

- expanded recommendations on laboratory methods for the identification of GBS,

- clarification of the colony-count threshold required for reporting GBS detected in the urine of pregnant women,

- updated algorithms for GBS screening and intrapartum chemoprophylaxis for women with preterm labor or preterm premature rupture of membranes,

- a change in the recommended dose of penicillin-G for chemoprophylaxis,

- updated prophylaxis regimens for women with penicillin allergy, and

- a revised algorithm for management of newborns with respect to risk for early-onset GBS disease.

Universal screening at 35–37 weeks' gestation for maternal GBS colonization and use of intrapartum antibiotic prophylaxis has resulted in substantial reductions in the burden of early-onset GBS disease among newborns. Although early-onset GBS disease has become relatively uncommon in recent years, the rates of maternal GBS colonization (and therefore the risk for early-onset GBS disease in the absence of intrapartum antibiotic prophylaxis) remain unchanged since the 1970s. Continued efforts are needed to sustain and improve on the progress achieved in the prevention of GBS disease. There also is a need to monitor for potential adverse consequences of intrapartum antibiotic prophylaxis (e.g., emergence of bacterial antimicrobial resistance or increased incidence or severity of non-GBS neonatal pathogens). In the absence of a licensed GBS vaccine, universal screening and intrapartum antibiotic prophylaxis continue to be the cornerstones of early-onset GBS disease prevention. (11/10)

HELICOBACTER PYLORI INFECTION

Helicobacter pylori Infection in Children: Recommendations for Diagnosis and Treatment
North American Society for Pediatric Gastroenterology, Hepatology, and Nutrition (11/00)

HEMATOPOIETIC STEM CELL TRANSPLANT

Guidelines for Preventing Opportunistic Infections Among Hematopoietic Stem Cell Transplant Recipients
Centers for Disease Control and Prevention, Infectious Diseases Society of America, and American Society of Blood and Marrow Transplantation (10/00)

HEMORRHAGE

An Evidence-based Prehospital Guideline for External Hemorrhage Control
American College of Surgeons Committee on Trauma

ABSTRACT. This report describes the development of an evidence-based guideline for external hemorrhage control in the prehospital setting. This project included a systematic review of the literature regarding the use of tourniquets and hemostatic agents for management of life-threatening extremity and junctional hemorrhage. Using the GRADE methodology to define the key clinical questions, an expert panel then reviewed the results of the literature review, established the quality of the evidence and made recommendations for EMS care. A clinical care guideline is proposed for adoption by EMS systems. (3/14)

HUMAN IMMUNODEFICIENCY VIRUS

Guidelines for the Prevention and Treatment of Opportunistic Infections in HIV-Exposed and HIV-Infected Children
US Department of Health and Human Services

SUMMARY. This report updates the last version of the Guidelines for the Prevention and Treatment of Opportunistic Infections (OIs) in HIV-Exposed and HIV-Infected Children, published in 2009. These guidelines are intended for use by clinicians and other health-care workers providing medical care for HIV-exposed and HIV-infected children in the United States. The guidelines discuss opportunistic pathogens that occur in the United States and ones that might be acquired during international travel, such as malaria. Topic areas covered for each OI include a brief description of the epidemiology, clinical presentation, and diagnosis of the OI in children; prevention of exposure; prevention of first episode of disease; discontinuation of primary prophylaxis after immune reconstitution; treatment of disease; monitoring for adverse effects during treatment, including immune reconstitution inflammatory syndrome (IRIS); management of treatment failure; prevention of disease recurrence; and discontinuation of secondary prophylaxis after immune reconstitution. A separate document providing recommendations for prevention and treatment of OIs among HIV-infected adults and post-pubertal adolescents (*Guidelines for the Prevention and Treatment of Opportunistic Infections in HIV-Infected Adults and Adolescents*) was prepared by a panel of adult HIV and infectious disease specialists (see http://aidsinfo.nih.gov/guidelines).

These guidelines were developed by a panel of specialists in pediatric HIV infection and infectious diseases (the Panel on Opportunistic Infections in HIV-Exposed and HIV-Infected Children) from the U.S. government and academic institutions. For each OI, one or more pediatric specialists with subject-matter expertise reviewed the literature for new information since the last guidelines were published and then proposed revised recommendations for review by the full Panel. After these reviews and discussions, the guidelines underwent further revision, with review and approval by the Panel, and final endorsement by the National Institutes of Health (NIH), Centers for Disease Control and Prevention (CDC), the HIV Medicine Association (HIVMA) of the Infectious Diseases Society of America (IDSA), the Pediatric Infectious Disease Society (PIDS), and the American Academy of Pediatrics (AAP). So that readers can ascertain how best to apply the recommendations in their practice environments, the recommendations are rated by a letter that indicates the strength of the recommendation, a Roman numeral that indicates the quality of the evidence supporting the recommendation, and where applicable, a * notation that signifies a hybrid of higher-quality adult study evidence and consistent but lower-quality pediatric study evidence.

More detailed methodologic considerations are listed in Appendix 1 (Important Guidelines Considerations), including a description of the make-up and organizational structure of the Panel, definition of financial disclosure and management of conflict of interest, funding sources for the guidelines, methods of collecting and synthesizing evidence and formulating recommendations, public commentary, and plans for updating the guidelines. The names and financial disclosures for each of the Panel members are listed in Appendices 2 and 3, respectively.

An important mode of childhood acquisition of OIs and HIV infection is from infected mothers. HIV-infected women may be more likely to have coinfections with opportunistic pathogens (e.g., hepatitis C) and more likely than women who are not HIV-infected to transmit these infections to their infants. In addition, HIV-infected women or HIV-infected family members coinfected with certain opportunistic pathogens may be more likely to transmit these infections horizontally to their children, resulting in increased likelihood of primary acquisition of such infections in young children. Furthermore, transplacental transfer of antibodies that protect infants against serious infections may be lower in HIV-infected women than in women who are HIV-uninfected. Therefore, infections with opportunistic pathogens may affect not just HIV-infected infants but also HIV-exposed, uninfected infants. These guidelines for treating OIs in children, therefore, consider treatment of infections in all children—HIV-infected and HIV-uninfected—born to HIV-infected women.

In addition, HIV infection increasingly is seen in adolescents with perinatal infection who are now surviving into their teens and in youth with behaviorally acquired HIV infection. Guidelines for postpubertal adolescents can be found in the adult OI guidelines, but drug pharmacokinetics (PK) and response to treatment may differ in younger prepubertal or pubertal adolescents. Therefore, these guidelines also apply to treatment of HIV-infected youth who have not yet completed pubertal development.

Major changes in the guidelines from the previous version in 2009 include:

- Greater emphasis on the importance of antiretroviral therapy (ART) for prevention and treatment of OIs, especially those OIs for which no specific therapy exists;

- Increased information about diagnosis and management of IRIS;

- Information about managing ART in children with OIs, including potential drug-drug interactions;

- Updated immunization recommendations for HIV-exposed and HIV-infected children, including pneumococcal, human papillomavirus, meningococcal, and rotavirus vaccines;

- Addition of sections on influenza, giardiasis, and isosporiasis;

- Elimination of sections on aspergillosis, bartonellosis, and HHV-6 and HHV-7 infections; and

- Updated recommendations on discontinuation of OI prophylaxis after immune reconstitution in children.

The most important recommendations are highlighted in boxed major recommendations preceding each section, and a table of dosing recommendations appears at the end of each section. The guidelines conclude with summary tables that display dosing recommendations for all of the conditions, drug toxicities and drug interactions, and 2 figures describing immunization recommendations for children aged 0 to 6 years and 7 to 18 years.

The terminology for describing use of antiretroviral (ARV) drugs for treatment of HIV infection has been standardized to ensure consistency within the sections of these guidelines and with the *Guidelines for the Use of Antiretroviral Agents in Pediatric HIV Infection*. Combination antiretroviral therapy (cART) indicates use of multiple (generally 3 or more) ARV drugs as part of an HIV treatment regimen that is designed to achieve virologic suppression; highly active antiretroviral therapy (HAART), synonymous with cART, is no longer used and has been replaced by cART; the term ART has been used when referring to use of ARV drugs for HIV treatment more generally, including (mostly historical) use of one- or two-agent ARV regimens that do not meet criteria for cART.

Because treatment of OIs is an evolving science, and availability of new agents or clinical data on existing agents may change therapeutic options and preferences, these recommendations will be periodically updated and will be available at http://AIDSinfo.nih.gov. (11/13)

IMMUNOCOMPROMISED HOST

2013 Infectious Diseases Society of America Clinical Practice Guidelines for the Immunization of the Immunocompromised Host
Infectious Diseases Society of America

EXECUTIVE SUMMARY. These guidelines were created to provide primary care and specialty clinicians with evidence-based guidelines for active immunization of patients with altered immunocompetence and their household contacts in order to safely prevent vaccine-preventable infections. They do not represent the only approach to vaccination. Recommended immunization schedules for normal adults and children as well as certain adults and children at high risk for vaccine-preventable infections are updated and published annually by the Centers for Disease Control and Prevention (CDC) and partner organizations. Some recommendations have not been addressed by the Advisory Committee on Immunization Practices (ACIP) to the CDC or they deviate from recommendations. The goal of presenting these guidelines is to decrease morbidity and mortality from vaccine-preventable infections in immunocompromised patients. Summarized below are the recommendations made by the panel. Supporting tables that provide additional information are available in the electronic version. The panel followed a process used in the development of other Infectious Diseases Society of America guidelines, which included a systematic weighting of the quality of the evidence and the grade of the recommendation. The key clinical questions and recommendations are summarized in this executive summary. A detailed description of the methods, background, and evidence summaries that support each recommendation can be found in the full text of the guidelines. (1/14)

INFLUENZA

Seasonal Influenza in Adults and Children—Diagnosis, Treatment, Chemoprophylaxis, and Institutional Outbreak Management: Clinical Practice Guidelines of the Infectious Diseases Society of America
Infectious Diseases Society of America

EXECUTIVE SUMMARY. *Background.* Influenza virus infection causes significant morbidity and mortality in the United States each year. The majority of persons infected with influenza virus exhibit self-limited, uncomplicated, acute febrile respiratory symptoms or are asymptomatic. However, severe disease and complications due to infection, including hospitalization and death, may occur in elderly persons, in very young persons, in persons with underlying medical conditions (including pulmonary and cardiac disease, diabetes, and immunosuppression), and in previously healthy persons. Early treatment with antiviral medications may reduce the severity and duration of symptoms, hospitalizations, and complications (otitis media, bronchitis, pneumonia), and may reduce the use of outpatient services and antibiotics, extent and quantity of viral shedding, and possibly mortality in certain populations. Vaccination is the best method for preventing influenza, but antivirals may also be used as primary or secondary means of preventing influenza transmission in certain settings.

The Centers for Disease Control and Prevention's (CDC's) Advisory Committee on Immunization Practices and the American Academy of Pediatrics provide recommendations on the appropriate use of trivalent inactivated and live, attenuated influenza vaccines, as well as information on diagnostics and antiviral use for treatment and chemoprophylaxis. The CDC's influenza Web site (http://www.cdc.gov/flu) also summarizes up-to-date information on current recommendations for influenza diagnostic testing and antiviral use. The Infectious Diseases Society of America's (IDSA's) influenza guideline provides an evidence-based set of recommendations and background on influenza with contributions from many sources, including the CDC, the American Academy of Pediatrics, the American College of Physicians, the American Academy of Family Physicians, the Pediatric Infectious Diseases Society, the Society for Healthcare Epidemiology of America, practicing clinicians, and the IDSA, to guide decision-making on these issues. The current guideline development process included a systematic weighting of the quality of the evidence and the grade of recommendation. These guidelines apply to seasonal (interpandemic) influenza and not to avian or pandemic disease. Clinical management guidelines for sporadic human infections due to avian A (H5N1) viruses have been published by the World Health Organization. (4/09)

INTRAVASCULAR CATHETER-RELATED INFECTIONS

Guidelines for the Prevention of Intravascular Catheter-Related Infections
Society of Critical Care Medicine, Infectious Diseases Society of America, Society for Healthcare Epidemiology of America, Surgical Infection Society, American College of Chest Physicians, American Thoracic Society, American Society of Critical Care Anesthesiologists, Association for Professionals in Infection Control and Epidemiology, Infusion Nurses Society, Oncology Nursing Society, Society of Cardiovascular and Interventional Radiology, American Academy of Pediatrics, and the Healthcare Infection Control Practices Advisory Committee of the Centers for Disease Control and Prevention

ABSTRACT. These guidelines have been developed for practitioners who insert catheters and for persons responsible for surveillance and control of infections in hospital, outpatient, and home health-care settings. This report was prepared by a working group comprising members from professional organizations representing the disciplines of critical care medicine, infectious diseases, health-care infection control, surgery, anesthesiology, interventional radiology, pulmonary medicine, pediatric medicine, and nursing. The working group was led by the Society of Critical Care Medicine (SCCM), in collaboration with the Infectious Disease Society of America (IDSA), Society for Healthcare Epidemiology of America (SHEA), Surgical Infection Society (SIS), American College of Chest Physicians (ACCP), American Thoracic Society (ATS), American Society of Critical Care Anesthesiologists (ASCCA), Association for Professionals in Infection Control and Epidemiology (APIC), Infusion Nurses Society (INS), Oncology Nursing Society (ONS), Society of Cardiovascular and Interventional Radiology (SCVIR), American Academy of Pediatrics (AAP), and the Healthcare Infection Control Practices Advisory Committee (HICPAC) of the Centers for Disease Control and Prevention (CDC) and is intended to replace the *Guideline for Prevention of Intravascular Device-Related Infections* published in 1996. These guidelines are intended to provide evidence-based recommendations for preventing catheter-related infections. Major areas of emphasis include (1) educating and training health-care providers who insert and maintain catheters; (2) using maximal sterile barrier precautions during central venous catheter insertion; (3) using a 2% chlorhexidine preparation for skin antisepsis; (4) avoiding routine replacement of central venous catheters as a strategy to prevent infection; and (5) using antiseptic/antibiotic impregnated short-term central venous catheters if the rate of infection is high despite adherence to other strategies (ie, education and training, maximal sterile barrier precautions, and 2% chlorhexidine for skin antisepsis). These guidelines also identify performance indicators that can be used locally by health- care institutions or organizations to monitor their success in implementing these evidence-based recommendations. (11/02)

JAUNDICE

Guideline for the Evaluation of Cholestatic Jaundice in Infants

North American Society for Pediatric Gastroenterology, Hepatology, and Nutrition

ABSTRACT. For the primary care provider, cholestatic jaundice in infancy, defined as jaundice caused by an elevated conjugated bilirubin, is an uncommon but potentially serious problem that indicates hepatobiliary dysfunction. Early detection of cholestatic jaundice by the primary care physician and timely, accurate diagnosis by the pediatric gastroenterologist are important for successful treatment and a favorable prognosis. The Cholestasis Guideline Committee of the North American Society for Pediatric Gastroenterology, Hepatology and Nutrition has formulated a clinical practice guideline for the diagnostic evaluation of cholestatic jaundice in the infant. The Cholestasis Guideline Committee, consisting of a primary care pediatrician, a clinical epidemiologist (who also practices primary care pediatrics), and five pediatric gastroenterologists, based its recommendations on a comprehensive and systematic review of the medical literature integrated with expert opinion. Consensus was achieved through the Nominal Group Technique, a structured quantitative method.

The Committee examined the value of diagnostic tests commonly used for the evaluation of cholestatic jaundice and how those interventions can be applied to clinical situations in the infant. The guideline provides recommendations for management by the primary care provider, indications for consultation by a pediatric gastroenterologist, and recommendations for management by the pediatric gastroenterologist.

The Cholestasis Guideline Committee recommends that any infant noted to be jaundiced at 2 weeks of age be evaluated for cholestasis with measurement of total and direct serum bilirubin. However, breast-fed infants who can be reliably monitored and who have an otherwise normal history (no dark urine or light stools) and physical examination may be asked to return at 3 weeks of age and, if jaundice persists, have measurement of total and direct serum bilirubin at that time.

This document represents the official recommendations of the North American Society for Pediatric Gastroenterology, Hepatology and Nutrition on the evaluation of cholestatic jaundice in infants. The American Academy of Pediatrics has also endorsed these recommendations. These recommendations are a general guideline and are not intended as a substitute for clinical judgment or as a protocol for the care of all patients with this problem. (8/04)

METHICILLIN-RESISTANT *STAPHYLOCOCCUS AUREUS*

Clinical Practice Guidelines by the Infectious Diseases Society of America for the Treatment of Methicillin-Resistant *Staphylococcus aureus* Infections in Adults and Children

Infectious Diseases Society of America

ABSTRACT. Evidence-based guidelines for the management of patients with methicillin-resistant *Staphylococcus aureus* (MRSA) infections were prepared by an Expert Panel of the Infectious Diseases Society of America (IDSA). The guidelines are intended for use by health care providers who care for adult and pediatric patients with MRSA infections. The guidelines discuss the management of a variety of clinical syndromes associated with MRSA disease, including skin and soft tissue infections (SSTI), bacteremia and endocarditis, pneumonia, bone and joint infections, and central nervous system (CNS) infections. Recommendations are provided regarding vancomycin dosing and monitoring, management of infections due to MRSA strains with reduced susceptibility to vancomycin, and vancomycin treatment failures. (2/11)

MIGRAINE HEADACHE

Pharmacological Treatment of Migraine Headache in Children and Adolescents

Quality Standards Subcommittee of the American Academy of Neurology and the Practice Committee of the Child Neurology Society (12/04)

PALLIATIVE CARE

Clinical Practice Guidelines for Quality Palliative Care, Third Edition

National Consensus Project for Quality Palliative Care (2013)

RADIOLOGY

Neuroimaging of the Neonate

Quality Standards Subcommittee of the American Academy of Neurology and the Practice Committee of the Child Neurology Society

ABSTRACT. *Objective.* The authors reviewed available evidence on neonatal neuroimaging strategies for evaluating both very low birth weight preterm infants and encephalopathic term neonates.

Imaging for the Preterm Neonate. Routine screening cranial ultrasonography (US) should be performed on all infants of <30 weeks' gestation once between 7 and 14 days of age and should be optimally repeated between 36 and 40 weeks' postmenstrual age. This strategy detects lesions such as intraventricular hemorrhage, which influences clinical care, and those such as periventricular leukomalacia and low-pressure ventriculomegaly, which provide information about long-term neurodevelopmental outcome. There is insufficient evidence for routine MRI of all very low birth weight preterm infants with abnormal results of cranial US.

Imaging for the Term Infant. Noncontrast CT should be performed to detect hemorrhagic lesions in the encephalopathic term infant with a history of birth trauma, low hematocrit, or coagulopathy. If CT findings are inconclusive, MRI should be performed between days 2 and 8 to assess the location and extent of injury. The pattern of injury identified with conventional MRI may provide diagnostic and prognostic information for term infants with evidence of encephalopathy. In particular, basal ganglia and thalamic lesions detected by conventional MRI are associated with poor neurodevelopmental outcome. Diffusion-weighted imaging may allow earlier detection of these cerebral injuries.

Recommendations. US plays an established role in the management of preterm neonates of <30 weeks' gestation. US also provides valuable prognostic information when the infant reaches 40 weeks' postmenstrual age. For encephalopathic term infants, early CT should be used to exclude hemorrhage; MRI should be performed later in the first postnatal week to establish the pattern of injury and predict neurologic outcome. (6/02)

SEDATION AND ANALGESIA

Clinical Policy: Evidence-based Approach to Pharmacologic Agents Used in Pediatric Sedation and Analgesia in the Emergency Department
American College of Emergency Physicians (10/04)

SEIZURE

Evaluating a First Nonfebrile Seizure in Children
Quality Standards Subcommittee of the American Academy of Neurology, the Child Neurology Society, and the American Epilepsy Society

ABSTRACT. *Objective.* The Quality Standards Subcommittee of the American Academy of Neurology develops practice parameters as strategies for patient management based on analysis of evidence. For this practice parameter, the authors reviewed available evidence on evaluation of the first nonfebrile seizure in children in order to make practice recommendations based on this available evidence. *Methods.* Multiple searches revealed relevant literature and each article was reviewed, abstracted, and classified. Recommendations were based on a three-tiered scheme of classification of the evidence. *Results.* Routine EEG as part of the diagnostic evaluation was recommended; other studies such as laboratory evaluations and neuroimaging studies were recommended as based on specific clinical circumstances. *Conclusions.* Further studies are needed using large, well-characterized

samples and standardized data collection instruments. Collection of data regarding appropriate timing of evaluations would be important. (8/00)

Treatment of the Child With a First Unprovoked Seizure
Quality Standards Subcommittee of the American Academy of Neurology and the Practice Committee of the Child Neurology Society

ABSTRACT. The Quality Standards Subcommittee of the American Academy of Neurology and the Practice Committee of the Child Neurology Society develop practice parameters as strategies for patient management based on analysis of evidence regarding risks and benefits. This parameter reviews published literature relevant to the decision to begin treatment after a child or adolescent experiences a first unprovoked seizure and presents evidence-based practice recommendations. Reasons why treatment may be considered are discussed. Evidence is reviewed concerning risk of recurrence as well as effect of treatment on prevention of recurrence and development of chronic epilepsy. Studies of side effects of anticonvulsants commonly used to treat seizures in children are also reviewed. Relevant articles are classified according to the Quality Standards Subcommittee classification scheme. Treatment after a first unprovoked seizure appears to decrease the risk of a second seizure, but there are few data from studies involving only children. There appears to be no benefit of treatment with regard to the prognosis for long-term seizure remission. Antiepileptic drugs (AED) carry risks of side effects that are particularly important in children. The decision as to whether or not to treat children and adolescents who have experienced a first unprovoked seizure must be based on a risk–benefit assessment that weighs the risk of having another seizure against the risk of chronic AED therapy. The decision should be individualized and take into account both medical issues and patient and family preference. (1/03)

STATUS EPILEPTICUS

Diagnostic Assessment of the Child With Status Epilepticus (An Evidence-based Review)
Quality Standards Subcommittee of the American Academy of Neurology and the Practice Committee of the Child Neurology Society

ABSTRACT. *Objective.* To review evidence on the assessment of the child with status epilepticus (SE).

Methods. Relevant literature were reviewed, abstracted, and classified. When data were missing, a minimum diagnostic yield was calculated. Recommendations were based on a four-tiered scheme of evidence classification.

Results. Laboratory studies (Na^{++} or other electrolytes, Ca^{++}, glucose) were abnormal in approximately 6% and are generally ordered as routine practice. When blood or spinal fluid cultures were done on these children, blood cultures were abnormal in at least 2.5% and a CNS infection was found in at least 12.8%. When antiepileptic drug (AED) levels were ordered in known epileptic children already taking AEDs, the levels were low in 32%. A total of 3.6% of children had evidence of ingestion. When studies for inborn errors of metabolism were done, an abnormality was found in 4.2%. Epileptiform abnormalities occurred in 43% of EEGs of children with SE and helped determine the nature and location of precipitating electroconvulsive events (8% generalized, 16% focal, and 19% both). Abnormalities on neuroimaging studies that may explain the etiology of SE were found in at least 8% of children.

Recommendations. Although common clinical practice is that blood cultures and lumbar puncture are obtained if there is a clinical suspicion of a systemic or CNS infection, there are insufficient data to support or refute recommendations as to whether blood cultures or lumbar puncture should be done on a routine basis in children in whom there is no clinical suspicion of a systemic or CNS infection (Level U). AED levels should be considered when a child with treated epilepsy develops SE (Level B). Toxicology studies and metabolic studies for inborn errors of metabolism may be considered in children with SE when there are clinical indicators for concern or when the initial evaluation reveals no etiology (Level C). An EEG may be considered in a child with SE as it may be helpful in determining whether there are focal or generalized epileptiform abnormalities that may guide further testing for the etiology of SE, when there is a suspicion of pseudostatus epilepticus (nonepileptic SE), or nonconvulsive SE, and may guide treatment (Level C). Neuroimaging may be considered after the child with SE has been stabilized if there are clinical indications or if the etiology is unknown (Level C). There is insufficient evidence to support or refute routine neuroimaging in a child presenting with SE (Level U). (11/06)

TOBACCO USE

Treating Tobacco Use and Dependence: 2008 Update
US Department of Health and Human Services

ABSTRACT. *Treating Tobacco Use and Dependence: 2008 Update*, a Public Health Service-sponsored Clinical Practice Guideline, is a product of the Tobacco Use and Dependence Guideline Panel ("the Panel"), consortium representatives, consultants, and staff. These 37 individuals were charged with the responsibility of identifying effective, experimentally validated tobacco dependence treatments and practices. The updated Guideline was sponsored by a consortium of eight Federal Government and nonprofit organizations: the Agency for Healthcare Research and Quality (AHRQ); Centers for Disease Control and Prevention (CDC); National Cancer Institute (NCI); National Heart, Lung, and Blood Institute (NHLBI); National Institute on Drug Abuse (NIDA); American Legacy Foundation; Robert Wood Johnson Foundation (RWJF); and University of Wisconsin School of Medicine and Public Health's Center for Tobacco Research and Intervention (UW-CTRI). This Guideline is an updated version of the 2000 *Treating Tobacco Use and Dependence: Clinical Practice Guideline* that was sponsored by the U.S. Public Health Service, U. S. Department of Health and Human Services.

An impetus for this Guideline update was the expanding literature on tobacco dependence and its treatment. The original 1996 Guideline was based on some 3,000 articles on tobacco treatment published between 1975 and 1994.

The 2000 Guideline entailed the collection and screening of an additional 3,000 articles published between 1995 and 1999. The 2008 Guideline update screened an additional 2,700 articles; thus, the present Guideline update reflects the distillation of a literature base of more than 8,700 research articles. Of course, this body of research was further reviewed to identify a much smaller group of articles that served as the basis for focused Guideline data analyses and review.

This Guideline contains strategies and recommendations designed to assist clinicians; tobacco dependence treatment specialists; and health care administrators, insurers, and purchasers in delivering and supporting effective treatments for tobacco use and dependence. The recommendations were made as a result of a systematic review and meta-analysis of 11 specific topics identified by the Panel (proactive quitlines; combining counseling and medication relative to either counseling or medication alone; varenicline; various medication combinations; long-term medications; cessation interventions for individuals with low socioeconomic status/limited formal education; cessation interventions for adolescent smokers; cessation interventions for pregnant smokers; cessation interventions for individuals with psychiatric disorders, including substance use disorders; providing cessation interventions as a health benefit; and systems interventions, including provider training and the combination of training and systems interventions). The strength of evidence that served as the basis for each recommendation is indicated clearly in the Guideline update. A draft of the Guideline update was peer reviewed prior to publication, and the input of 81 external reviewers was considered by the Panel prior to preparing the final document. In addition, the public had an opportunity to comment through a *Federal Register* review process. The key recommendations of the updated Guideline, *Treating Tobacco Use and Dependence: 2008 Update*, based on the literature review and expert Panel opinion, are as follows:

Ten Key Guideline Recommendations

The overarching goal of these recommendations is that clinicians strongly recommend the use of effective tobacco dependence counseling and medication treatments to their patients who use tobacco, and that health systems, insurers, and purchasers assist clinicians in making such effective treatments available.

1. Tobacco dependence is a chronic disease that often requires repeated intervention and multiple attempts to quit. Effective treatments exist, however, that can significantly increase rates of long-term abstinence.

2. It is essential that clinicians and health care delivery systems consistently identify and document tobacco use status and treat every tobacco user seen in a health care setting.

3. Tobacco dependence treatments are effective across a broad range of populations. Clinicians should encourage every patient willing to make a quit attempt to use the counseling treatments and medications recommended in this Guideline.

4. Brief tobacco dependence treatment is effective. Clinicians should offer every patient who uses tobacco at least the brief treatments shown to be effective in this Guideline.

5. Individual, group, and telephone counseling are effective, and their effectiveness increases with treatment intensity. Two components of counseling are especially effective, and clinicians should use these when counseling patients making a quit attempt:

   • Practical counseling (problem solving/skills training)

   • Social support delivered as part of treatment

6. Numerous effective medications are available for tobacco dependence, and clinicians should encourage their use by all patients attempting to quit smoking—except when medically contraindicated or with specific populations for which there is insufficient evidence of effectiveness (i.e., pregnant women, smokeless tobacco users, light smokers, and adolescents).

   • Seven first-line medications (5 nicotine and 2 nonnicotine) reliably increase long-term smoking abstinence rates:

     – Bupropion SR

     – Nicotine gum

     – Nicotine inhaler

     – Nicotine lozenge

     – Nicotine nasal spray

     – Nicotine patch

     – Varenicline

   • Clinicians also should consider the use of certain combinations of medications identified as effective in this Guideline.

7. Counseling and medication are effective when used by themselves for treating tobacco dependence. The combination of counseling and medication, however, is more effective than either alone. Thus, clinicians should encourage all individuals making a quit attempt to use both counseling and medication.

8. Telephone quitline counseling is effective with diverse populations and has broad reach. Therefore, both clinicians and health care delivery systems should ensure patient access to quitlines and promote quitline use.

9. If a tobacco user currently is unwilling to make a quit attempt, clinicians should use the motivational treatments shown in this Guideline to be effective in increasing future quit attempts.

10. Tobacco dependence treatments are both clinically effective and highly cost-effective relative to interventions for other clinical disorders. Providing coverage for these treatments increases quit rates. Insurers and purchasers should ensure that all insurance plans include the counseling and medication identified as effective in this Guideline as covered benefits.

The updated Guideline is divided into seven chapters that provide an overview, including methods (Chapter 1); information on the assessment of tobacco use (Chapter 2); clinical interventions, both for patients willing and unwilling to make a quit attempt at this time (Chapter 3); intensive interventions (Chapter 4); systems interventions for health care administrators, insurers, and purchasers (Chapter 5); the scientific evidence supporting the Guideline recommendations (Chapter 6); and information relevant to specific populations and other topics (Chapter 7).

A comparison of the findings of the updated Guideline with the 2000 Guideline reveals the considerable progress made in tobacco research over the brief period separating these two publications. Tobacco dependence increasingly is recognized as a chronic disease, one that typically requires ongoing assessment and repeated intervention. In addition, the updated Guideline offers the clinician many more effective treatment strategies than were identified in the original Guideline. There now are seven different first-line effective agents in the smoking cessation pharmacopoeia, allowing the clinician and patient many different medication options. In addition, recent evidence provides even stronger support for counseling (both when used alone and with other treatments) as an effective tobacco cessation strategy; counseling adds to the effectiveness of tobacco cessation medications, quitline counseling is an effective intervention with a broad reach, and counseling increases tobacco cessation among adolescent smokers.

Finally, there is increasing evidence that the success of any tobacco dependence treatment strategy cannot be divorced from the health care system in which it is embedded. The updated Guideline contains new evidence that health care policies significantly affect the likelihood that smokers will receive effective tobacco dependence treatment and successfully stop tobacco use. For instance, making tobacco dependence treatment a covered benefit of insurance plans increases the likelihood that a tobacco user will receive treatment and quit successfully. Data strongly indicate that effective tobacco interventions require coordinated interventions. Just as the clinician must intervene with his or her patient, so must the health care administrator, insurer, and purchaser foster and support tobacco intervention as an integral element of health care delivery. Health care administrators and insurers should ensure that clinicians have the training and support to deliver consistent, effective intervention to tobacco users.

One important conclusion of this Guideline update is that the most effective way to move clinicians to intervene is to provide them with information regarding multiple effective treatment options and to ensure that they have ample institutional support to use these options. Joint actions by clinicians, administrators, insurers, and purchasers can encourage a culture of health care in which failure to intervene with a tobacco user is inconsistent with standards of care. (5/08)

VESICOURETERAL REFLUX
Report on the Management of Primary Vesicoureteral Reflux in Children
American Urological Association (5/97)

SECTION 3

Affirmation of Value Clinical Practice Guidelines

These guidelines are not endorsed as policy of the American Academy of Pediatrics (AAP). Documents that lack a clear description of the process for identifying, assessing, and incorporating research evidence are not eligible for AAP endorsement as practice guidelines. However, such documents may be of educational value to members of the AAP.

ASTHMA

Environmental Management of Pediatric Asthma: Guidelines for Health Care Providers
National Environmental Education Foundation

INTRODUCTION (EXCERPT). These guidelines are the product of a new Pediatric Asthma Initiative aimed at integrating environmental management of asthma into pediatric health care. This document outlines competencies in environmental health relevant to pediatric asthma that should be mastered by primary health care providers, and outlines the environmental interventions that should be communicated to patients.

These environmental management guidelines were developed for pediatricians, family physicians, internists, pediatric nurse practitioners, pediatric nurses, and physician assistants. In addition, these guidelines should be integrated into respiratory therapists' and licensed case/care (LICSW) management professionals' education and training.

The guidelines contain three components:

- Competencies: An outline of the knowledge and skills that health care providers and health professional students should master and demonstrate in order to incorporate management of environmental asthma triggers into pediatric practice.
- Environmental History Form: A quick, easy, user-friendly document that can be utilized as an intake tool by the health care provider to help determine pediatric patients' environmental asthma triggers.
- Environmental Intervention Guidelines: Follow-up questions and intervention solutions to environmental asthma triggers. (8/05)

PALLIATIVE CARE AND HOSPICE

Standards of Practice for Pediatric Palliative Care and Hospice
National Hospice and Palliative Care Organization (2/09)

SLEEP APNEA

Practice Guidelines for the Perioperative Management of Patients with Obstructive Sleep Apnea
American Society of Anesthesiologists (5/06)

TURNER SYNDROME

Care of Girls and Women With Turner Syndrome: A Guideline of the Turner Syndrome Study Group
Turner Syndrome Consensus Study Group

ABSTRACT. *Objectives.* The objective of this work is to provide updated guidelines for the evaluation and treatment of girls and women with Turner syndrome (TS).

Participants. The Turner Syndrome Consensus Study Group is a multidisciplinary panel of experts with relevant clinical and research experience with TS that met in Bethesda, Maryland, April 2006. The meeting was supported by the National Institute of Child Health and unrestricted educational grants from pharmaceutical companies.

Evidence. The study group used peer-reviewed published information to form its principal recommendations. Expert opinion was used where good evidence was lacking.

Consensus. The study group met for 3 d to discuss key issues. Breakout groups focused on genetic, cardiological, auxological, psychological, gynecological, and general medical concerns and drafted recommendations for presentation to the whole group. Draft reports were available for additional comment on the meeting web site. Synthesis of the section reports and final revisions were reviewed by e-mail and approved by whole-group consensus.

Conclusions. We suggest that parents receiving a prenatal diagnosis of TS be advised of the broad phenotypic spectrum and the good quality of life observed in TS in recent years. We recommend that magnetic resonance angiography be used in addition to echocardiography to evaluate the cardiovascular system and suggest that patients with defined cardiovascular defects be cautioned in regard to pregnancy and certain types of exercise. We recommend that puberty should not be delayed to promote statural growth. We suggest a comprehensive educational evaluation in early childhood to identify potential attention-deficit or nonverbal learning disorders. We suggest that caregivers address the prospect of premature ovarian failure in an open and sensitive manner and emphasize the critical importance of estrogen treatment for feminization and for bone health during the adult years. All individuals with TS require continued monitoring of hearing and thyroid function throughout the lifespan. We suggest that adults with TS be monitored for aortic enlargement, hypertension, diabetes, and dyslipidemia. (1/07)

Section 4

2016 Policies

From the American Academy of Pediatrics
. . . .

- *Policy Statements*
  ORGANIZATIONAL PRINCIPLES TO GUIDE AND DEFINE THE CHILD HEALTH CARE SYSTEM
  AND TO IMPROVE THE HEALTH OF ALL CHILDREN

- *Clinical Reports*
  GUIDANCE FOR THE CLINICIAN IN RENDERING PEDIATRIC CARE

- *Technical Reports*
  BACKGROUND INFORMATION TO SUPPORT AMERICAN ACADEMY OF PEDIATRICS POLICY

*Includes policy statements, clinical reports, and technical reports
published between January 1, 2016, and December 31, 2016.*

INTRODUCTION

This section of *Pediatric Clinical Practice Guidelines & Policies: A Compendium of Evidence-based Research for Pediatric Practice* is composed of policy statements, clinical reports, and technical reports issued by the American Academy of Pediatrics (AAP) and is designed as a quick reference tool for AAP members, AAP staff, and other interested parties. Section 4 includes the full text of all AAP policies published in 2016. Section 5 is a compilation of all active AAP statements (through December 31, 2016) arranged alphabetically, with abstracts where applicable. A committee index (Appendix 1) and subject index are also available. These materials should help answer questions that arise about the AAP position on child health care issues. **However, remember that AAP policy statements, clinical reports, and technical reports do not indicate an exclusive course of treatment or serve as a standard of medical care. Variations, taking into account individual circumstances, may be appropriate.**

Policy statements have been written by AAP committees, councils, task forces, or sections and approved by the AAP Board of Directors. Most of these statements have appeared previously in *Pediatrics*, *AAP News*, or *News & Comments* (the forerunner of *AAP News*).

This section does not contain all AAP policies. It does not include
- Press releases.
- Motions and resolutions that were approved by the Board of Directors. These can be found in the Board of Directors' minutes.
- Policies in manuals, pamphlets, booklets, or other AAP publications. These items can be ordered through the AAP. To order, visit http://shop.aap.org/books or call toll-free 888/227-1770.
- Testimony before Congress or government agencies.

All policy statements, clinical reports, and technical reports from the American Academy of Pediatrics automatically expire 5 years after publication unless reaffirmed, revised, or retired at or before that time. Please check the American Academy of Pediatrics Web site at www.aap.org for up-to-date reaffirmations, revisions, and retirements.

Achieving Quality Health Services for Adolescents

• *Policy Statement*

POLICY STATEMENT Organizational Principles to Guide and Define the Child Health Care System and/or Improve the Health of all Children

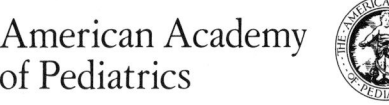

American Academy of Pediatrics

DEDICATED TO THE HEALTH OF ALL CHILDREN™

Achieving Quality Health Services for Adolescents

COMMITTEE ON ADOLESCENCE

abstract

This update of the 2008 statement from the American Academy of Pediatrics redirects the discussion of quality health care from the theoretical to the practical within the medical home. This statement reviews the evolution of the medical home concept and challenges to the provision of quality adolescent health care within the patient-centered medical home. Areas of attention for quality adolescent health care are reviewed, including developmentally appropriate care, confidentiality, location of adolescent care, providers who offer such care, the role of research in advancing care, and the transition to adult care.

DOI: 10.1542/peds.2016-1347

PEDIATRICS (ISSN Numbers: Print, 0031-4005; Online, 1098-4275).

FINANCIAL DISCLOSURE: The author has indicated he does not have a financial relationship relevant to this article to disclose.

FUNDING: No external funding.

POTENTIAL CONFLICT OF INTEREST: The author has indicated he has no potential conflicts of interest to disclose.

To cite: AAP COMMITTEE ON ADOLESCENCE. Achieving Quality Health Services for Adolescents. *Pediatrics.* 2016;138(2): e20161347

INTRODUCTION

The American Academy of Pediatrics (AAP)-endorsed patient-centered medical home (PCMH) model has transformed the delivery of primary care in the United States and offers newly defined measures of quality.[1] Coupled with *Bright Futures*,[2] an evidence- and expert opinion-based guide on how best to provide clinical care for adolescents, a new blueprint for quality health services has emerged. Advanced and open-access models of care delivery have improved efficiency and decreased wait time for patients. Continuity of care with a primary care provider, electronic health record use for population management, and implementation of evidence-based guidelines for preventive care have significantly progressed. Focus on preventive care with attention to specific quality measures, such as those within the Healthcare Effectiveness Data and Information Set (HEDIS),[3] which consists of 81 measures across 5 domains of care, allow for an objective measurement of quality care delivery. A renewed attention to patient satisfaction strengthens the provider-patient relationship. In addition, greater attention to transition of care may allow the opportunity for an easier move from adolescent to adult care. Despite these significant advances, unique challenges to achieving quality health care for adolescents remain in areas such as access to care, provider availability, confidentiality, the electronic health record, and adult transitions for adolescents with chronic health conditions.

EVOLUTION OF THE MEDICAL HOME AS QUALITY HEALTH CARE

The conceptual framework by which a primary care practice intends to improve the quality, efficiency, and patient experience of care has evolved since the middle of the 20th century. The AAP first introduced the term "medical home" in 1967 to describe the need for a central location of archiving a child's medical records. This medical home primarily focused on children with special health care needs.[4] By 1992, the AAP broadened the concept of a medical home to include an identifiable, well-trained primary care physician to promote quality care for all children and adolescents. In the 2002 revision of its 1992 statement, the AAP reiterated and enhanced its explanation of care under this model known as the medical home, retaining the 1992 principles of medical care that is accessible, family-centered, continuous, comprehensive, coordinated, compassionate, and culturally effective, and then expanded an operational definition to include 37 specific activities that should occur within a medical home.[5] Similar models of adult primary care were concurrently proposed by other medical organizations.

In 2007, the AAP joined the American Academy of Family Physicians, the American College of Physicians, and the American Osteopathic Association to endorse the "Joint Principals of the Patient-Centered Medical Home,"[1] which describes 7 core characteristics:

1. Personal physician for every patient.

2. Physician-directed medical practice.

3. Whole-person orientation.

4. Care is coordinated and/or integrated.

5. Quality and safety are hallmarks of PCMH care.

6. Enhanced access to care.

7. Appropriate payment for providing PCMH care.

The PCMH, a physician-led, team-based model of whole-person primary care intended to improve quality and efficiency of care, has been adopted by many stakeholders in addition to professional associations, including payers and policy makers.[6] The Agency for Healthcare Research and Quality defines the PCMH as a way to improve health care in America by transforming how primary care is organized and delivered.[7] Increased focus on improving the quality of health services in the United States through the PCMH model has led to a directed effort toward improving access to care, with more timely delivery of services, continuity of care with a primary care provider, patient satisfaction with care, and positive measurable outcomes resulting from care.[8-15] The PCMH uses these quality elements as its cornerstone and is a widely accepted means of achieving quality health service reform.[1,5] Voluntary certification of PCMH status assesses practice structural capabilities to meet the requirements of PCMHs. Certification is provided by a number of organizations, including the National Committee on Quality Assurance,[16] The Joint Commission,[17] the United States Military Health System,[18] and other certifying organizations.

THE PCMH SHIFTS FOCUS FROM QUANTITY TO QUALITY

Traditional productivity measures of quantity of care focus on business outcomes, which, in a fee-for-service system, assist in measuring revenue generation and complexity of care delivered. In such a model,

the health care system is rewarded when providing a high volume of care, particularly face-to-face care, because those visits generate the most revenue. From the patient's vantage point, this model promotes brief, episodic, discontinuous, acute illness-centric care. The result can be care that is not cost-effective, efficient, or guided by published recommendations, without sufficient regard for quality in the context of the whole patient. Access to care, continuity of care, and satisfaction with care are potentially excluded. This system may perpetuate a health and wellness trajectory in a negative direction.[19]

In contrast, the PCMH revolves around the patient-physician relationship. In this model, patient-based outcomes are at the forefront: access to care, continuity of care, confidentiality of care, preventive care, and measurable health outcomes, such as HEDIS quality measures. The PCMH reorients outcome measures of care away from provider- and system-based metrics of quantity of care and toward patient-centered metrics of quality of care. This model of care, if it includes appropriate payment by private-sector and government payers, encourages continuous, comprehensive, and preventive care that promotes wellness. This system rewards cost-effective care and promotes improvement in patient health to promote high-quality health care at reduced costs. This model transforms a health care system to a system of health.[19]

EFFECTIVENESS OF THE PCMH

The nascent research on the effectiveness of PCMH for child and adult health care is promising.[20] PCMHs with open-access scheduling have been shown, in multiple managed care systems, to increase access and continuity of care; improve outcomes; increase productivity, with relative value unit gains of as much as 17% per encounter; raise total revenue per visit; increase physician compensation; provide more efficient clinic operations, with decreased use of urgent-care services; and improve patient and provider satisfaction, all while reducing health care costs.[21-26] Not all studies have found short-term cost-savings, however.[27,28] By using claims data, one study found that participation in a multipayer medical home pilot of National Committee for Quality Assurance–certified adult practices was associated with limited improvements in quality and was not associated with reductions in utilization of hospital, emergency department, or ambulatory care services or total costs over 3 years. The authors suggested that there may be a need for continued refinement of PCMH practice models within complex health systems.[29] This study reveals the complexity of evaluating PCMH interventions in large multipayer systems and may support the lack of uniformity of success among PCMH practices or a variable latency period between initiating quality improvements and reaching desired outcomes.[30] Transition toward a fully operational PCMH has inherent challenges, and it may take several years to reach maturity and reduce costs in a managed care system.[31-33]

The future direction and modifications of PCMHs will rely on continued research and rigorous evaluation, particularly for health care outcomes for adolescents within PCMHs, for whom little research exists to date. Consistent with lack of research in this area, the ability of the medical home to address the unique health service needs of adolescents is not well defined, and there remain differing approaches to the care of adolescents, such as length of appointment times; availability of confidential time with the pediatric provider; access to confidential

services, including confidentiality within the electronic health record and explanation of benefits; and access to adolescent medicine specialists within the PCMH and neighborhood.

Medical organizations recommend that health services provided to adolescents be adolescent oriented, comprehensive, and coordinated and that they promote healthful behavior, manage chronic health conditions, and focus on prevention.[34-36] *Bright Futures* contains evidence-based and expert-informed practice guidelines for adolescent health care providers.[2] However, health services in the United States often are not designed around the adolescent, nor do they usually take into account the unique issues of adolescence that affect their health. As a result, some adolescents face gaps in care, fragmented services, less-than-ideal medical management, missed opportunities for health promotion and disease prevention, and challenges in transition to adult care for young people with chronic health conditions.[37]

ISSUES SPECIFIC TO ADOLESCENCE

Adolescents engage in high-risk behaviors that cause significant morbidity and mortality. Adolescents and young adults have higher incidences of reckless driving, substance abuse, unprotected sex, and violent behavior, compared with adults. Unintentional injuries are the leading cause of death for children, adolescents, and young adults, and alcohol use plays a role in many injuries. Homicide and suicide are the next leading causes of death for adolescents. Recent US high school data reveal that 4 in 10 high school students text or E-mail while driving. Thirty-five percent of high school students drink alcohol, and 23% have used marijuana. In the past year, nearly 15% of high school students were electronically bullied,

nearly 20% were bullied on school property, and 8% attempted suicide. Nearly half (46.8%) of US high school students have had sexual intercourse, 34% are currently sexually active, and 15% had sexual intercourse with 4 or more persons during their life. Among currently sexually active students, 59% used a condom during their last sexual intercourse.[38]

Risky and healthy behaviors that are associated with adult morbidity, such as cardiovascular disease, cancer, and diabetes, also have their origins during the adolescent years. Fifteen percent of high school students smoke cigarettes, and nearly 9% have used smokeless tobacco. Few adolescents consume the recommended amount of daily fruits and vegetables, and in the past week, 5% had not consumed any fruit or 100% fruit juice, and 6.6% had not eaten any vegetables. Forty-one percent had played video or computer games or used a computer for something not related to school work for 3 or more hours per day on an average school day.[38] In the context of these and other health behaviors, the PCMH, centered on the patient-pediatrician relationship, may have a significant impact on adolescent and young adult health.

Within the PCMH model of care as well as other health systems, adolescents receive care within a variety of delivery systems with varying access to comprehensive care, specialty care, and coordination of care and from a variety of providers with varied levels of training in adolescent care. The consequences of these variations are largely unknown for the adolescent population.[10] Issues unique to adolescence that are either incompletely or nonspecifically addressed with the PCMH model include developmentally appropriate care, confidentiality, location where adolescents receive care, providers who offer such care, the role of research in advancing care, and transition to adult care. These measures need to exist within the PCMH to address adolescent care effectively.

The AAP, American Academy of Family Physicians, and American College of Physicians purport that optimal health care is achieved when each person, at every age, receives developmentally appropriate care.[39] Providing quality health care for adolescents requires that pediatricians maintain relationships with families and with community institutions, such as schools or youth development organizations, while maintaining the relationship with each patient.[34,40] In providing quality care for adolescents, pediatricians help patients develop autonomy, responsibility, and an adult identity, and therefore, care should be developmentally appropriate. Developmentally appropriate care for adolescents may require longer appointment times, which may be a challenge to accommodate within a PCMH that serves a broad age spectrum.[13]

Confidentiality, both in determining whether youth receive what they need and whether there are opportunities for private one-on-one time during health care visits, is a major factor that determines the extent to which adolescents receive appropriate care.[41] Confidentiality and privacy issues can pose significant barriers to successful screening, assessment, compliance, and follow-up for adolescents and, therefore, is inextricably intertwined with quality health care for this population.[42–45] Moreover, lack of confidential billing for patients with commercial health insurance provides an obstacle to recommended screening and treatment, particularly for sexually transmitted infections and contraception care.[46]

Even within certified PCMHs, a range of providers may care for adolescents. A common clinical management approach within PCMH is for teenagers to be assigned advanced clinical practitioners, such as nurse practitioners and physician assistants, as primary care providers, because of relatively low utilization rates and generally well health status of this population overall to maximally leverage open- and advanced-access model systems of clinical care.[21,47] With the advent of excellent guidelines for provision of adolescent health care, such as *Bright Futures*, and use of validated quality measures, such as data from HEDIS, this may be an appropriate delivery model for well teenagers, presuming providers are adequately trained in provision of adolescent health care, but research on this topic is lacking. A primary concern is that elements necessary for highest-quality adolescent preventive health care, including additional time for confidential interview and discussion, may not be available in a medical home model focused on short-term cost benefits, when such care limits enrollment numbers and the number of patients available to be seen per day, further limiting access to preventive care in a population that often fails to receive preventive care.[48]

Supporting the health care transition from adolescence to adulthood in the medical home is another challenge for quality adolescent health care. In 2011, a clinical report authored by the AAP, American Academy of Family Physicians, and American College of Physicians reviewed the importance of supporting and facilitating the transition of adolescents with special health care needs into adulthood.[49] Despite renewed attention and effort, widespread implementation of health transition supports as a basic standard of high-quality care has not been realized and has not yet been incorporated into routine adolescent health care in the PCMH.[39]

Within the medical home model of care, and in comparison with other age groups, little research exists regarding adolescent health care. As a result, the impact of the medical home in delivery of quality adolescent health care is still unclear, because it is largely unstudied. Although more research is clearly needed, concerns also exist regarding the ability for the medical home to maintain clinical research activities to produce the types of outcomes data helpful in optimization of the model for adolescents.[50] Addressing these issues now is critical for the future success of adolescent care within the medical home, which remains early in its implementation in the United States.

PRIMARY CARE ACCESS AND UTILIZATION

Adolescents and young adults are among those least likely to have access to preventive health care, and they historically have the lowest rate of primary care use of any age group in the United States.[48,51] One analysis based on claims data from a 700 000-member health plan in Minnesota revealed that one-third of adolescents with 4 or more years of continuous enrollment had no preventive care visits from age 13 through 17 years, and another 40% had only a single preventive care visit.[52] National surveys with past-year preventive visit measures show significant variation across adolescents (43% to 81%) and young adults (26% to 58%).[53] Those with behavioral health diagnoses are especially lacking in access to care, as fewer than half of all adolescents with psychiatric disorders received care within the past year.[54] In 2012, more than 8% of adolescents lacked insurance, and as of 2014, 18.3% of 18- to 24-year-olds are uninsured in the United States.[55] Health disparities are well described among subgroups of adolescents, including those who are homeless or in the state child welfare or juvenile justice systems.[56,57] Lesbian, gay, bisexual, and transgender adolescents are at highest risk of lacking access to primary care and behavioral health services.[58] Further access challenges exist for adolescents in more rural areas, as well as those who have difficulty negotiating the health care system or live in poverty and lack insurance coverage.[57] The Patient Protection and Affordable Care Act[59] shows promise in improving preventive care of young adults and adolescents.[60] Among those 10 to 17 years old, Healthy People 2020 data reveal that the proportion of adolescents who have had a well-patient visit in the past 12 months increased by 9.6% from 2008 to 2013.[61] The Affordable Care Act may continue to improve access to preventive health care for many adolescents, but its implementation and access to services provided vary by state.

School-based health centers (SBHCs) provide convenient preventive health services for a small number of adolescents and young adults. They serve as a model for improving the linkage between health and education and community systems to improve preventive and primary care. SBHCs may further provide an entry point and source of primary care, with ongoing connections to a medical home, for children who do not otherwise have access to consistent care.[62] There are more than 130 000 schools in the United States serving students in kindergarten through 12th grade. According to the School-Based Health Alliance 2013–2014 census report, there are 2315 SBHCs that serve US students and communities in 49 of 50 states and the District of Columbia. Eighty percent of SBHCs provide care for students in grade 6 and above. More than half of SBHCs serve populations in addition to students in the school, such as students from other schools, family members of student users, out-of-school youth, school faculty and staff, and other people in the community. Although half of SBHCs are in urban areas, the largest growth of SBHCs has been in rural areas, accounting for nearly 60% of new SBHCs since 2010, and addressing unique challenges to rural youth access to quality primary, behavioral, and oral health care.[63]

Although household surveys indicate that most adolescents receive their primary care in a doctor's office or clinic, approximately 10% of adolescents rely on the hospital or emergency department as their usual source of care.[10] Among adolescents who received care, studies using national compliance rates data from the Medical Expenditures Panel Survey have shown that rates of preventive counseling, health promotion, and screening were low. Only half of adolescents received care that followed recommended guidelines, such as those for annual well-patient visits, confidential and comprehensive health screening, and immunizations.[48,64,65]

Adolescents with chronic medical needs face additional challenges within the medical home model.[39] The ability of primary care providers within a medical home to effectively manage chronic disease, considering time requirements, has been questioned.[66] Models of care encouraged in PCMH that address chronic health care needs include dedicated care coordinators and patient-care teams,[14] as well as population health registries, such as chronic disease, high-risk, high-utilizer, and transition registries. Solutions within the medical home for adults who have complex health needs and require both medical and social services and support from a wide variety of providers and caregivers have been proposed, but the feasibility for smaller practices, including those that care for pediatric and adolescent patients with complex needs, remain unclear.[67]

A further complicating factor is that adolescents and young adults, especially those living in poverty, are more likely to be uninsured than any other age group. Beginning in 2014, the Affordable Care Act required state Medicaid programs to cover adolescents 16 through 18 years of age in families with incomes up to 133% of the federal poverty level. States can also choose to expand their Medicaid programs to 133% of the federal poverty level for late adolescents and young adults starting at 19 years of age. Even under the Affordable Care Act, which provides this extended eligibility for Medicaid and access to private coverage through state exchanges, people living in poverty may remain uninsured, particularly in states that opt to not expand Medicaid.

ELECTRONIC HEALTH RECORDS AND HEALTH INFORMATION TECHNOLOGY

The electronic health record offers remarkable opportunity to improve the quality of care for adolescents within a PCMH and also offers unique challenges. The AAP, among other organizations, recommends standards for health information technology to help protect adolescent privacy.[68–70] Challenges to privacy for adolescents posed by commercial health information technology systems require the creation and implementation of electronic health record systems that do not impede access, continuity, privacy/confidentiality, or quality of care for adolescents. The AAP also offers specific recommendations for health information and the medical home to promote confidentiality, continuity of care, patient-care transitions, and overall quality of care. These include criteria for electronic health records that encompass flexibility and specific technological capabilities and are compatible with state-specific laws as well as billing systems.[69] Requirements regarding explanations of benefits add additional confidentiality concerns relevant to the medical visit for the privately insured adolescent, and strategies to address or mitigate the potential for inadvertent confidentiality breeches associated with explanations of benefits vary widely by state.[71] Current electronic health record and billing systems afford an opportunity to prompt providers to address adolescent-specific needs of the patient, to document adolescent health care compatible with current recommendations, and to provide data for process improvement in care for adolescents. Electronic health record and billing systems also allow for meaningful use of data, portals for patients to access their own electronic health records, secure messaging systems to expand access for adolescents to their health care team, and the opportunity for improved patient education through patient instruction sheets and other electronic means. Despite many systems in place, these opportunities are, as yet, not fully realized, and their effectiveness has not been well studied.[70-72]

QUALITY MEASURES FOR ADOLESCENT HEALTH CARE

Although multiple data sets and measures currently exist in the United States, there is no robust national information system that can provide timely, comprehensive, and valid and reliable indicators of health and health care quality specifically for adolescents. The health of adolescents is influenced by multiple factors, including biology, behavior, and social and physical environments. It is also influenced by the availability, use, and quality of health care services, especially for those with life-threatening conditions or special health care needs who require frequent interactions with health care providers. Therefore, understanding the health status of adolescents is closely intertwined with understanding the quality of

health care they receive. Health and health care measures can be used to assess the effects of many variables and inform improvements to adolescent health quality. In response to a mandate in the Children's Health Insurance Program Reauthorization Act of 2009 (Pub L No. 111-3), the Institute of Medicine and the National Research Council of the National Academies, under contract with the US Department of Health and Human Services, conducted an 18-month study concluding that, although multiple and independent federal, state, and private data sources exist that include measures of health and health care quality of children and adolescents, the existing data sources are fragmented, not timely, and insufficiently robust as a whole; lack standardization in measurements; and reveal an absence of common definitions.[73] The recommendations of that study included setting goals for child and adolescent quality measures, including adolescent measures in annual reports; standardizing measurement disparities in health and health care quality; improving data collection, reporting, and analysis; and improving public and private capacities to use and report data.

HEDIS outcomes within an adolescent medical home–enrolled population allow a practice to monitor the preventive health status for specific disease elements deemed important to the practice. HEDIS provides objective measurement of patient-centered quality care delivery. Limitations of HEDIS measures as markers of quality adolescent care are that they are relatively few in number, disease specific, and dependent on the practice to record and track the data. Similarly, a set of quality health care measures for Medicaid and the Children's Health Insurance Program, known as the child core set, allow for states to voluntarily report their quality metrics and may

serve as reasonable early measures for a practice to adopt (http://www.medicaid.gov/medicaid-chip-program-information/by-topics/quality-of-care/downloads/2015-child-core-set.pdf).

One area for improvement of quality measures includes using adolescents themselves as sources of measurement data. Adolescents have been found to be more valid and reliable than chart review and other data sources in reporting their experiences with preventive care.[74-76] However, even health systems that measure patient satisfaction with care do not directly query adolescents younger than 18 years. Although standardization of clinical care and the process of care within the medical home may provide much progress toward the goals outlined in this policy statement, it is important that this process be accompanied by similarly standardized and rigorous research methods in measures of quality and quality services for adolescents.[23,77]

RECOMMENDATIONS

The AAP recommends the following:

1. Adolescents should receive comprehensive, appropriately confidential, developmentally appropriate primary care, as recommended by AAP guidelines (*Bright Futures*), within a medical home.

2. Feasible, valid, and reliable quality measures should be developed and implemented that use adolescent self-reported data to help assess the quality of preventive care provided to youth. In addition, existing measures that were developed in association with initiatives designed to improve the care delivered to adolescent patients should be cataloged and improved for use by external quality-measurement organizations.

3. Research on the effectiveness of the PCMH to achieve specific adolescent quality outcome measures is necessary to gauge the impact, and guide the future direction, of the medical home on the health of adolescents.

4. Adolescent access to care, continuity of care, confidentiality of care, preventive care, and desired measurable health outcomes should be rewarded by private-sector and government payers to promote high-quality adolescent health care.

5. Electronic health records and associated billing and notification systems should protect the confidentiality of care for adolescents. Electronic health records should be configured with templates that are compliant with *Bright Futures* and HEDIS measures.

6. PCMHs that care for adolescents should plan for a well-timed and well-executed transition to adult care, especially for adolescents with chronic health conditions.

7. Pediatricians and other adolescent health care providers from multiple disciplines should receive professional education about effective strategies for delivery of high-quality adolescent primary care, in accordance with *Bright Futures* guidelines. Educational opportunities currently exist to improve quality through Maintenance of Certification part IV activities as offered by the American Board of Pediatrics.

LEAD AUTHORS

William Adelman, MD

COMMITTEE ON ADOLESCENCE, 2014–2015

Paula K. Braverman, MD, Chairperson
Elizabeth M. Alderman, MD, FSAHM
Cora C. Breuner, MD, MPH
David A. Levine, MD
Arik V. Marcell, MD, MPH
Rebecca Flynn O'Brien, MD

LIAISONS

Laurie L. Hornberger, MD, MPH – *Section on Adolescent Health*
Margo Lane, MD – *Canadian Pediatric Society*
Julie Strickland, MD – *American College of Obstetricians and Gynecologists*
Benjamin Shain, MD, PhD – *American Academy of Child and Adolescent Psychiatry*

STAFF

Karen Smith
James Baumberger, MPP

ABBREVIATIONS

AAP: American Academy of Pediatrics
HEDIS: Healthcare Effectiveness Data and Information Set
PCMH: patient-centered medical home
SBHC: school-based health centers

REFERENCES

1. American Academy of Family Physicians, American Academy of Pediatrics, American College of Physicians, American Osteopathic Association. Joint principles of the patient-centered medical home. Washington, DC: Patient-Centered Primary Care Collaborative; 2007. Available at: www.aafp.org/dam/AAFP/documents/practice_management/pcmh/initiatives/PCMHJoint.pdf. Accessed June 1, 2016

2. Hagan JF, Shaw JS, Duncan PM, eds. *Bright Futures: Guidelines for Health Supervision of Infants, Children and Adolescents*, 3rd ed. Elk Grove Village, IL: American Academy of Pediatrics; 2008

3. National Committee for Quality Assurance. HEDIS and quality measurement. Available at: www.ncqa.org/tabid/59/default.aspx. Accessed June 1, 2016

4. Sia C, Tonniges TF, Osterhus E, Taba S. History of the medical home concept. *Pediatrics*. 2004;113(suppl 5):1473–1478

5. Medical Home Initiatives for Children With Special Needs Project Advisory Committee. American Academy of Pediatrics. The medical home. *Pediatrics*. 2002;110(1 pt 1):184–186

6. Patient-Centered Primary Care Collaborative. Statements of support. Available at: https://www.acponline.org/system/files/documents/running_practice/delivery_and_payment_models/pcmh/demonstrations/jointprinc_05_17.pdf. Accessed June 1, 2016

7. Agency for Healthcare Research and Quality, US Department of Health and Human Services. Patient-centered medical home resource center. Available at: www.pcmh.ahrq.gov/page/defining-pcmh. Accessed June 1, 2016

8. Institute of Medicine, Committee on Quality of Health Care in America; Kohn LT, Corrigan JM, Donaldson MS, eds. *To Err is Human: Building a Safer Health System*. Washington, DC: National Academies Press; 2000

9. Institute of Medicine, Committee on Quality of Health Care in America. *Crossing the Quality Chasm: A New Health System for the 21st Century*. Washington, DC: National Academies Press; 2001

10. National Research Council and Institute of Medicine. *Challenges in Adolescent Health Care: Workshop Report. Committee on Adolescent Health Care Services and Models of Care for Treatment, Prevention and Healthy Development*. Washington, DC: National Academies Press; 2007

11. National Committee for Quality Assurance. Standards and guidelines for physician practice connections—patient centered medical home (PPC-PCMH). 2011. Available at: http://ncqa.org/Portals/0/Programs/Recognition/PCMH_Overview_Apr01.pdf. Accessed June 1, 2016

12. Institute of Medicine and National Research Council. *Improving the Health, Safety, and Well-Being of Young Adults: Workshop Summary*. Washington, DC: National Academies Press; 2013

13. Agency for Healthcare Research and Quality. 2006 National Healthcare Quality Report. AHRQ publication 7-0013. Rockville, MD: US Department of Health and Human Services, Agency for Healthcare Research and Quality; 2006

14. Wagner EH. The role of patient care teams in chronic disease management. *BMJ.* 2000;320(7234):569–572

15. Yu SM, Bellamy HA, Kogan MD, Dunbar JL, Schwalberg RH, Schuster MA. Factors that influence receipt of recommended preventive pediatric health and dental care. *Pediatrics.* 2002;110(6). Available at: www.pediatrics.org/cgi/content/full/110/6/e73

16. National Committee for Quality Assurance. Patient-centered medical home recognition. Available at: https://www.ncqa.org/Programs/Recognition.aspx. Accessed June 1, 2016

17. The Joint Commission. Primary care medical home. Available at: www.jointcommission.org/accreditation/pchi.aspx. Accessed June 1, 2016

18. Military Health System and the Defense Health Agency. Patient safety. Available at: www.tricare.mil/tma/ocmo/download/MHSPCMHGuide.pdf. Accessed June 1, 2016

19. Nathan ML. The patient-centered medical home in the transformation from healthcare to health. *Mil Med.* 2013;178(2):126–127

20. Peikes D, Zutshi A, Genevro JL, Parchman ML, Meyers DS. Early evaluations of the medical home: building on a promising start. *Am J Manag Care.* 2012;18(2):105–116

21. O'Hare CD, Corlett J. The outcomes of open-access scheduling. *Fam Pract Manag.* 2004;11(2):35–38

22. Hudak RP, Julian R, Kugler J, et al. The patient-centered medical home: a case study in transforming the military health system. *Mil Med.* 2013;178(2):146–152

23. Cooley WC, McAllister JW, Sherrieb K, Kuhlthau K. Improved outcomes associated with medical home implementation in pediatric primary care. *Pediatrics.* 2009;124(1):358–364

24. Christensen EW, Dorrance KA, Ramchandani S, et al. Impact of a patient-centered medical home on access, quality, and cost. *Mil Med.* 2013;178(2):135–141

25. Gilfillan RJ, Tomcavage J, Rosenthal MB, et al. Value and the medical home: effects of transformed primary care. *Am J Manag Care.* 2010;16(8):607–614

26. Savage AI, Lauby T, Burkard JF. Examining selected patient outcomes and staff satisfaction in a primary care clinic at a military treatment facility after implementation of the patient-centered medical home. *Mil Med.* 2013;178(2):128–134

27. Jackson GL, Powers BJ, Chatterjee R, et al. Improving patient care. The patient centered medical home. A systematic review. *Ann Intern Med.* 2013;158(3):169–178

28. Hoff T, Weller W, DePuccio M. The patient-centered medical home: a review of recent research. *Med Care Res Rev.* 2012;69(6):619–644

29. Friedberg MW, Schneider EC, Rosenthal MB, Volpp KG, Werner RM. Association between participation in a multipayer medical home intervention and changes in quality, utilization, and costs of care. *JAMA.* 2014;311(8):815–825

30. Valko G, Wender R. Evaluating a multipayer medical home intervention. *JAMA.* 2014;312(4):434–435

31. Reid RJ, Coleman K, Johnson EA, et al. The Group Health medical home at year two: cost savings, higher patient satisfaction, and less burnout for providers. *Health Aff (Millwood).* 2010;29(5):835–843

32. Jaen CR, Crabtree BF, Palmer RF, et al. Patient outcomes at 26 months in the patient-centered medical home national demonstration project. *Ann Fam Med.* 2010;8(1):510–520

33. Dorrance KA, Ramchandani S, LaRochelle J, Mael F, Lynch S, Grundy P. Protecting the culture of a patient-centered medical home. *Mil Med.* 2013;178(2):153–158

34. Committee on Adolescence American Academy of Pediatrics. Achieving quality health services for adolescents. *Pediatrics.* 2008;121(6):1263–1270

35. Society for Adolescent Medicine. Access to health care for adolescents and young adults. *J Adolesc Health.* 2004;35(4):342–344

36. Adelman WP. Adolescent preventive counseling [monograph]. BMJ Best Pract. Updated 2015. Available at: http://us.bestpractice.bmj.com/best-practice/monograph/881.html. Accessed June 1, 2016

37. National Research Council. *Adolescent Health Services: Missing Opportunities.* Washington, DC: National Academies Press; 2009

38. Kann L, Kinchen S, Shanklin SL, et al; Centers for Disease Control and Prevention (CDC). Youth risk behavior surveillance--United States, 2013. *MMWR Suppl.* 2014;63(4):1–168

39. American Academy of Pediatrics; American Academy of Family Physicians; American College of Physicians; Transitions Clinical Report Authoring Group, Cooley WC, Sagerman PJ. Supporting the health care transition from adolescence to adulthood in the medical home. *Pediatrics.* 2011;128(1):182–200

40. Centers for Disease Control and Prevention. *School Connectedness: Strategies for Increasing Protective Factors Among Youth.* Atlanta, GA: US Department of Health and Human Services; 2009

41. Britto MT, Tivorsak TL, Slap GB. Adolescents' needs for health care privacy. *Pediatrics.* 2010;126(6). Available at: www.pediatrics.org/cgi/content/full/126/6/e1469

42. Cullen E. *Adolescent Health: Coverage and Access to Care.* Menlo Park, CA: The Henry J. Kaiser Family Foundation; 2011

43. Ford C, English A, Sigman G. Confidential health care for adolescents: position paper for the society for adolescent medicine. *J Adolesc Health.* 2004;35(2):160–167

44. Ford CA, Millstein SG, Halpern-Felsher BL, Irwin CE Jr. Influence of physician confidentiality assurances on adolescents' willingness to disclose information and seek future health care. A randomized controlled trial. *JAMA.* 1997;278(12):1029–1034

45. Thrall JS, McCloskey L, Ettner SL, Rothman E, Tighe JE, Emans SJ. Confidentiality and adolescents' use of providers for health information and for pelvic examinations. *Arch Pediatr Adolesc Med.* 2000;154(9):885–892

46. American Academy of Pediatrics, Committee on Medical Liability and Risk Management. Adolescent health care. In: Donn SM, McAbee GN, eds. *Medicolegal Issues in Pediatrics.* 7th

ed. Elk Grove Village, IL: American Academy of Pediatrics; 2012:131–140

47. Murray M, Berwick DM. Advanced access: reducing waiting and delays in primary care. *JAMA.* 2003;289(8):1035–1040

48. Irwin CE Jr, Adams SH, Park MJ, Newacheck PW. Preventive care for adolescents: few get visits and fewer get services. *Pediatrics.* 2009;123(4). Available at: www.pediatrics.org/cgi/content/full/123/4/e565

49. American Academy of Pediatrics; American Academy of Family Physicians; American College of Physicians-American Society of Internal Medicine. A consensus statement on health care transitions for young adults with special health care needs. *Pediatrics.* 2002;110(6 pt 2):1304–1306

50. Jones WS. Military Graduate Medical Education: are the king's clothes tattered? *Mil Med.* 2013;178(11):1154–1156

51. Klein JD, Wilson KM, McNulty M, Kapphahn C, Collins KS. Access to medical care for adolescents: results from the 1997 Commonwealth Fund Survey of the Health of Adolescent Girls. *J Adolesc Health.* 1999;25(2):120–130

52. Nordin JD, Solberg LI, Parker ED. Adolescent primary care visit patterns. *Ann Fam Med.* 2010;8(6):511–516

53. Adams SH, Park MJ, Irwin CE Jr. Adolescent and young adult preventive care. comparing national survey rates. *Am J Prev Med.* 2015;49(2):238–247

54. Costello EJ, He JP, Sampson NA, Kessler RC, Merikangas KR. Services for adolescents with psychiatric disorders: 12-month data from the National Comorbidity Survey-Adolescent. *Psychiatr Serv.* 2014;65(3):359–366

55. Martinez ME, Cohen RA. Health insurance coverage: early release of estimates from the National Health Interview Survey, January–June 2014. Available at: www.cdc.gov/nchs/data/nhis/earlyrelease/insur201412.pdf. Accessed June 1, 2016

56. Bloom B, Jones LI, Freeman G; National Center for Health Statistics. Summary health statistics for US children:

National Health Interview Survey, 2012. *Vital Health Stat 10.* 2013;(258):1–81

57. US Interagency Council on Homelessness. Opening Doors: Federal Strategic Plan to Prevent and End Homelessness. Executive Summary. Washington, DC: US Interagency Council on Homelessness; 2010. Available at: https://www.usich.gov/resources/uploads/asset_library/USICH_OpeningDoors_Amendment2015_FINAL.pdf. Accessed June 1, 2016

58. Mustanski BS, Garofalo R, Emerson EM. Mental health disorders, psychological distress, and suicidality in a diverse sample of lesbian, gay, bisexual, and transgender youths. *Am J Public Health.* 2010;100(12):2426–2432

59. Patient Protection and Affordable Care Act. Pub L No. 111-148 (2010)

60. Lau JS, Adams SH, Park MJ, Boscardin WJ, Irwin CE Jr. Improvement in preventive care of young adults after the Affordable Care Act: the Affordable Care Act is helping. *JAMA Pediatr.* 2014;168(12):1101–1106

61. Healthy People 2020. Access to health services. Available at: https://www.healthypeople.gov/2020/topics-objectives/topic/Adolescent-Health/objectives. Accessed June 1, 2016

62. Keeton V, Soleimanpour S, Brindis CD. School-based health centers in an era of health care reform: building on history. *Curr Probl Pediatr Adolesc Health Care.* 2012;42(6):132–156, discussion 157–158

63. School-Based Health Alliance. 2013-14 Digital census report. Available at: http://censusreport.sbh4all.org/. Accessed June 1, 2016

64. Selden TM. Compliance with well-child visit recommendations: evidence from the Medical Expenditure Panel Survey, 2000-2002. *Pediatrics.* 2006;118(6). Available at: www.pediatrics.org/cgi/content/full/118/6/e1766

65. Agency for Healthcare Research and Quality. Medical expenditure panel survey. Available at: http://meps.ahrq.gov/mepsweb/data_stats/MEPS_topics.jsp?topicid=42Z-1&startAt=21. Accessed June 1, 2016

66. Østbye T, Yarnall KSH, Krause KM, Pollak KI, Gradison M, Michener JL. Is

there time for management of patients with chronic diseases in primary care? *Ann Fam Med.* 2005;3(3):209–214

67. Rich E, Lipson D, Libersky J, Parchman M. *Coordinating Care for Adults with Complex Care Needs in the Patient-Centered Medical Home: Challenges and Solutions. White Paper.* Prepared for Agency for Healthcare Research and Quality. AHRQ Publication No. 12-0010. Princeton, NJ: Mathematica Policy Research; 2012

68. Blythe MJ, Del Beccaro MA; Committee on Adolescence; Council on Clinical and Information Technology. Standards for health information technology to ensure adolescent privacy. *Pediatrics.* 2012;130(5):987–990

69. Council on Clinical Information Technology. Health information technology and the medical home. *Pediatrics.* 2011;127(5):978–982

70. Anoshiravani A, Gaskin GL, Groshek MR, Kuelbs C, Longhurst CA. Special requirements for electronic medical records in adolescent medicine. *J Adolesc Health.* 2012;51(5):409–414

71. Tebb KP, Sedlander E, Pica G, Diaz A, Peake K, Brindis CD. Protecting Adolescent Confidentiality Under Health Care Reform: The Special Case Regarding Explanation of Benefits (EOBs): Philip R. Lee Institute for Health Policy Studies and Division of Adolescent and Young Adult Medicine, Department of Pediatrics, University of California, San Francisco; June 2014. Available at: http://nahic.ucsf.edu/wp-content/uploads/2014/06/639265-0-000-00-020EOB-Policy-Brief-Final-June-2014.pdf. Accessed June 1, 2016

72. Council on Clinical Information Technology. Policy Statement—Using personal health records to improve the quality of health care for children. *Pediatrics.* 2009;124(1):403–409

73. National Research Council. *Child and Adolescent Health and Health Care Quality: Measuring What Matters.* Washington, DC: The National Academies Press; 2011

74. Santelli J, Klein J, Graff C, Allan M, Elster A. Reliability in adolescent reporting of clinician counseling, health care use, and health behaviors. *Med Care.* 2002;40(1):26–37

75. Klein JD, Graff CA, Santelli JS, Hedberg VA, Allan MJ, Elster AB. Developing quality measures for adolescent care: validity of adolescents' self-reported receipt of preventive services. *Health Serv Res*. 1999;34(1 pt 2):391–404

76. Klein JD, McNulty M, Flatau CN. Adolescents' access to care: teenagers' self-reported use of services and perceived access to confidential care. *Arch Pediatr Adolesc Med*. 1998;152(7):676–682

77. Chen EH, Thom DH, Hessler DM, et al. Using the Teamlet Model to improve chronic care in an academic primary care practice. *J Gen Intern Med*. 2010;25(suppl 4): S610–S614

Addressing Early Childhood Emotional and Behavioral Problems

• •

- *Policy Statement*

POLICY STATEMENT Organizational Principles to Guide and Define the Child Health
Care System and/or Improve the Health of all Children

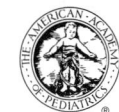

American Academy
of Pediatrics

DEDICATED TO THE HEALTH OF ALL CHILDREN™

Addressing Early Childhood Emotional and Behavioral Problems

COUNCIL ON EARLY CHILDHOOD, COMMITTEE ON PSYCHOSOCIAL ASPECTS OF CHILD AND
FAMILY HEALTH, SECTION ON DEVELOPMENTAL AND BEHAVIORAL PEDIATRICS

abstract

Emotional, behavioral, and relationship problems can develop in very young
children, especially those living in high-risk families or communities. These
early problems interfere with the normative activities of young children and
their families and predict long-lasting problems across multiple domains.
A growing evidence base demonstrates the efficacy of specific family-
focused therapies in reducing the symptoms of emotional, behavioral,
and relationship symptoms, with effects lasting years after the therapy
has ended. Pediatricians are usually the primary health care providers
for children with emotional or behavioral difficulties, and awareness of
emerging research about evidence-based treatments will enhance this
care. In most communities, access to these interventions is insufficient.
Pediatricians can improve the care of young children with emotional,
behavioral, and relationship problems by calling for the following: increased
access to care; increased research identifying alternative approaches,
including primary care delivery of treatments; adequate payment for
pediatric providers who serve these young children; and improved education
for pediatric providers about the principles of evidence-based interventions.

DOI: 10.1542/peds.2016-3023

PEDIATRICS (ISSN Numbers: Print, 0031-4005; Online, 1098-4275).

To cite: AAP COUNCIL ON EARLY CHILDHOOD, AAP COMMITTEE
ON PSYCHOSOCIAL ASPECTS OF CHILD AND FAMILY HEALTH, AAP
SECTION ON DEVELOPMENTAL AND BEHAVIORAL PEDIATRICS.
Addressing Early Childhood Emotional and Behavioral
Problems. *Pediatrics.* 2016;138(6):e20163023

INTRODUCTION

Emotional, relationship, and behavioral problems affect nearly as
many preschoolers as older children, with prevalence rates of 7% to
10%.[1-3] Emotional, behavioral, and relationship problems, including
disorders of attachment, disruptive behavior disorders, attention-
deficit/hyperactivity disorder (ADHD), anxiety and mood disorders,
and disorders of self-regulation of sleep and feeding in children younger
than 6 years, interfere with development across multiple domains,
including social interactions, parent–child relationships, physical safety,
ability to participate in child care, and school readiness.[4-6] Importantly,
if untreated, these problems can persist and have long-lasting effects,
including measurable abnormalities in brain functioning and persistent
emotional and behavioral problems.[7-10] In short, early emotional,

behavioral, and relationship problems in preschool-aged children interfere with their current well-being, jeopardize the foundations of emotional and behavioral health, and have the potential for long-term consequences.[11]

Pediatricians and other child health care providers can reduce the risk of childhood emotional and behavioral problems by reducing exposure to toxic stress, promoting protective factors, and systematically screening for risk factors for emerging clinical problems.[12,13] Existing policy statements address universal approaches, early identification, and strategies for children at risk. The present policy statement focuses on clinical interventions for children with clinical disorders that warrant targeted treatment. Treatment planning is guided by a comprehensive assessment of the clinical presentation with attention to the child, the parent–child relationships, and community stressors. Beyond assessment, effective treatment of clinical disorders requires the following: (1) access to evidence-based treatments; and (2) primary care providers' sufficient familiarity with evidence-based treatments to implement first-line approaches, make informed and effective referrals, and collaborate with specialty providers who have expertise in early childhood emotional and behavioral well-being.[14] Currently, most young children with an emotional, relationship, or behavioral problem receive no interventions for their disorder. This policy statement provides a summary of empirically supported approaches, describes readily identifiable barriers to accessing quality evidence-based interventions, and proposes recommendations to enhance the care of young children. This statement has been endorsed by Zero to Three and the American Academy of Child and Adolescent Psychiatry.

EVIDENCE-BASED TREATMENTS

Awareness of the relative levels of evidence supporting pharmacologic and nonpharmacologic therapies for emotional, behavioral, and relationship problems can guide clinical decisions in the primary care setting. The evidence base related to psychopharmacologic agents in children younger than 6 years is limited and has only addressed ADHD.[15] Only 2 rigorous trials have examined the safety and efficacy of medications in this age group. Both the trial of methylphenidate and the study of atomoxetine for moderate to severe ADHD demonstrated that the trial medication was more effective than placebo but was less effective for younger children than for older children and produced higher rates of adverse effects in younger children.[16,17] Other medications have been less rigorously evaluated in preschool-aged children, although the rates of prescriptions for atypical antipsychotic agents, with their potential for substantial metabolic morbidity, have increased steadily in this age group.[18-20]

Nonpharmacologic treatments have more durable effects than medications, with documented effects lasting for years.[21-23] A first step in reducing the barriers to evidence-based treatments is to ensure that primary care pediatricians are familiar with these approaches, which should be available to young children with emotional, behavioral, or relationship problems.[24]

For infants and toddlers with clinical-level emotional, behavioral, or relationship concerns, dyadic interventions promote attachment security and child emotional regulation and can promote regulation of stress hormones. Examples of these interventions include infant–parent psychotherapy, video feedback to promote positive parenting, and attachment biobehavioral catch-up. These interventions often use real-time infant–parent interactions to support positive interactions, enhance parents' capacity to reflect on their parenting patterns, and promote sensitivity and an understanding of the infant's needs.[25]

For preschool-aged children, parent management training models, including parent–child interaction therapy (PCIT), the Incredible Years series, the New Forest Program, Triple P (Positive Parenting Program), and Helping the Noncompliant Child,[26] are effective in decreasing symptoms of ADHD and disruptive behavior disorders. Parents are actively involved in all of these interventions, sometimes without the child and sometimes in parent–child interactions. All share similar behavioral principles, most consistently engaging parents as partners to: (1) reinforce positive behaviors; (2) ignore low-level provocative behaviors; and (3) provide clear, consistent, safe responses to unacceptable behaviors. Table 1 presents some of the characteristics of the best-supported programs for disruptive behavior disorders and ADHD.[25,27]

Posttraumatic stress disorder can be treated effectively with cognitive behavioral therapy and child–parent psychotherapy in very young children. In cognitive behavioral therapy for posttraumatic stress disorder, preschool-aged children learn relaxation techniques and are gradually exposed to their frightening memories while using these techniques. Child–parent psychotherapy focuses on supporting parents to create a safe, consistent relationship with the child through helping them understand the child's emotional experiences and needs.[33] Cognitive behavioral therapy is also effective for other common anxiety disorders, and recent promising studies report effectiveness of modified PCIT for selective mutism and depression.[34-36] Adaptations for use in primary care, including

TABLE 1 Characteristics of the Best-Supported Programs for Disruptive Behavior Disorders and ADHD

Program	Ages	Formal Psychoeducation for Parents?	Real-Time Observed Parent–Child Interactions?	Special Characteristics	Duration	Evidence Suggesting Effective for ADHD? (Effect Size)	Evidence Suggesting Effective for Disruptive Behavior Disorders? (Effect Size)
New Forest[28]	30–77 mo	Yes	Yes	Parent–child tasks are specifically intended to require attention Occurs in the home Explicit attention to parental depression	5 weekly sessions	Yes (very large, 1.9)	Yes (moderate, 0.7)
Incredible Years Parent Training and Child Training[29,30] (incredibleyearsseries.org)	24 mo–8 y	Yes	No	Separate parent and child groups Parental training uses video vignettes for discussion Child training includes circle time learning and coached free play	20 weekly 2-h sessions	Yes	Yes
Triple P[31] (triplep.org)	Birth–12 y	Yes (primary)	Yes	Multiple levels of intervention Primarily training parents with some opportunities to observe parent–child interactions Handouts and homework supplement the treatment	Primary care, four 15-min sessions Standard treatment is 10 sessions	No	Yes
PCIT[32] (pcit.org)	24 mo–7 y	Yes, minimal	Yes	Through a 1-way mirror, therapist coaches parent during in vivo interactions with child Homework requires parent child interactions Progress through therapy determined by parents' skill development	Duration depends on parental skill development	Modest	Yes
Helping the Noncomplaint Child[26]	3–8 y	Yes	Yes	Involves 2 phases: (1) differential attention; (2) compliance training using demonstration, role plays, and in-office and at home practice	8–10 average (depends on demonstrated progress)	Yes (1.24 parent report; .23 [NS] teacher report)	Yes

Triple P, the Incredible Years series, and PCIT, similarly show positive outcomes, although further research is warranted.[37–39]

Ensuring that parents have access to appropriate support or clinical care is often an important component of clinical intervention for children.

Effective parental treatment (eg, for depression) may reduce child symptoms substantially.[40]

SYSTEMIC BARRIERS
Despite the strong empirical support for these interventions, most young children with emotional, behavioral, and relationship problems do not receive nonpharmacologic treatments.[41] Physical separation, challenges coordinating across systems, stigma, parental beliefs, and provider beliefs about mental health services may interfere with identification of concerns and success of referrals. New models

such as co-located care, in which mental health professionals work together with medical care providers in the same space, improve care coordination and referral success, decrease stigma, and reduce symptoms compared with traditional referrals.[42–44] There are insufficient numbers of skilled providers to meet the emotional, behavioral, and relationship needs of children (and young children in particular) who require developmentally specialized interventions.[45,46] Therefore, when a primary care pediatrician identifies an emotional, relationship, or behavioral problem in a young child, it is often difficult to identify a professional (eg, social worker, psychologist, child and adolescent psychiatrist, developmental-behavioral pediatrician) with expertise in early childhood to accept the referral and provide evidence-based treatments.

Mental health coverage systems may also reduce access to care.[47] Although mental health parity regulations took effect in 2014, there are still "carved out" mental health programs that prohibit payment to primary care pediatricians for care of a child with an emotional, relationship, or behavioral health diagnosis and may limit access to trained specialists.[48] Even when a trained provider of an evidence-based treatment is identified, communication, coordination of care with primary care pediatricians, and adequate payment can be challenges.[14,49] Many health care systems do not pay for, or underpay for, necessary components of early childhood care such as care conferences, school observations, discussions with additional caregivers, same-day services, care coordination, and appointments that do not include face-to-face treatment of the child.

RECOMMENDATIONS

1. In the context of the focus of the American Academy of Pediatrics on early child and brain development, pediatricians have the opportunity to advocate for legislative and research approaches that will increase access to evidence-based treatments for very young children with emotional, behavioral, and relationship problems.

1a. At the legislative level, pediatricians should advocate for: (1) funding programs that increase dissemination and implementation of evidence-based treatments, especially in areas with limited resources; (2) addressing the early childhood mental health workforce shortage by providing incentives for training in these professions; (3) decreasing third-party payer barriers to accessing mental health services to very young children; and (4) promoting accountable care organization regulations that protect early childhood mental health services.

1b. In collaboration with other child-focused organizations, pediatricians should advocate for prioritization of research that will enhance the evidence base for treatment of very young children with emotional, behavioral, and relationship problems. Comparative effectiveness studies between psychopharmacologic and psychotherapeutic interventions and comparison of mental health service delivery approaches (eg, co-located models, community-based consultation, targeted referrals to specialists) are needed to guide management and policy decisions. In addition, studies that examine moderators of treatment effects, including family, social, and biological factors, are warranted. Studies of interventions adapted to treat young children with mild symptoms in the primary care setting could decrease barriers to care.

2. At the community and organizational levels, pediatricians should collaborate with local governmental and private agencies to identify local and national clinical services that can serve young children and explore opportunities for innovative service delivery models such as consultation or co-location.

3. Primary care pediatricians and developmental-behavioral pediatricians, together with early childhood mental health providers, including child and adolescent psychiatrists, and developmental specialists, can create educational materials for trainees and providers to enhance the care young children receive.

4. Without adequate payment for screening and assessment by primary care providers and management by specialty providers with expertise in early childhood mental health, treatment of very young children with emotional and behavioral problems will likely remain inaccessible for many children. Given existing knowledge regarding the importance of early childhood brain development on lifelong health, adequate payment for early childhood preventive services will benefit not only the patients but society as well and should be supported. Mental health carve-outs should be eliminated because they provide a significant barrier to access to mental health care for children. Additional steps toward equal access to mental health and physical health care include efficient prior authorization processes; adequate panels of early childhood mental health providers; payment to all providers, including primary care providers, for mental health

diagnoses; sustainable payment for co-located mental health providers and care coordination; payment for evidence-based approaches focused on parents; and payment for the necessary collection of information from children's many caregivers and for same-day services. Advocacy for true mental health parity must continue.

5. To ensure that all providers caring for children are knowledgeable participants and partners in the care of young children with emotional, behavioral, and relationship problems, graduate medical education and continuing medical education should include opportunities for training that ensure that pediatric providers: (1) are competent to identify young children with emotional, behavioral, and relationship problems as well as risk and protective factors; (2) are aware that common early childhood emotional, behavioral, and relationship problems can be treated with evidence-based treatments; (3) recognize the limitations in the data supporting use of medications in very young children, even for ADHD; (4) are prepared to identify and address parental factors that influence early child development; and (5) can collaborate and refer across disciplines and specialties, including developmental-behavioral pediatrics, child and adolescent psychiatry, psychology, and other mental health services.

LEAD AUTHORS

Mary Margaret Gleason, MD, FAAP
Edward Goldson, MD, FAAP
Michael W. Yogman, MD, FAAP

COUNCIL ON EARLY CHILDHOOD EXECUTIVE COMMITTEE, 2015–2016

Dina Lieser, MD, FAAP, Chairperson
Beth DelConte, MD, FAAP
Elaine Donoghue, MD, FAAP

Marian Earls, MD, FAAP
Danette Glassy, MD, FAAP
Terri McFadden, MD, FAAP
Alan Mendelsohn, MD, FAAP
Seth Scholer, MD, FAAP
Jennifer Takagishi, MD, FAAP
Douglas Vanderbilt, MD, FAAP
Patricia Gail Williams, MD, FAAP

LIAISONS

Lynette M. Fraga, PhD – *Child Care Aware*
Abbey Alkon, RN, PNP, PhD, MPH – *National Association of Pediatric Nurse Practitioners*
Barbara U. Hamilton, MA – *Maternal and Child Health Bureau*
David Willis, MD, FAAP – *Maternal and Child Health Bureau*
Claire Lerner, LCSW – *Zero to Three*

STAFF

Charlotte Zia, MPH, CHES

COMMITTEE ON PSYCHOSOCIAL ASPECTS OF CHILD AND FAMILY HEALTH, 2015–2016

Michael Yogman, MD, FAAP, Chairperson
Nerissa Bauer, MD, MPH, FAAP
Thresia B. Gambon, MD, FAAP
Arthur Lavin, MD, FAAP
Keith M. Lemmon, MD, FAAP
Gerri Mattson, MD, FAAP
Jason Richard Rafferty, MD, MPH, EdM
Lawrence Sagin Wissow, MD, MPH, FAAP

LIAISONS

Sharon Berry, PhD, LP – *Society of Pediatric Psychology*
Terry Carmichael, MSW – *National Association of Social Workers*
Edward Christophersen, PhD, FAAP – *Society of Pediatric Psychology*
Norah Johnson, PhD, RN, CPNP-BC – *National Association of Pediatric Nurse Practitioners*
Leonard Read Sulik, MD, FAAP – *American Academy of Child and Adolescent Psychiatry*

CONSULTANT

George J. Cohen, MD, FAAP

STAFF

Stephanie Domain, MS, CHES

SECTION ON DEVELOPMENTAL AND BEHAVIORAL PEDIATRICS EXECUTIVE COMMITTEE, 2015–2016

Nathan J. Blum, MD, FAAP, Chairperson
Michelle M. Macias, MD, FAAP, Immediate Past Chairperson
Nerissa S. Bauer, MD, MPH, FAAP
Carolyn Bridgemohan, MD, FAAP

Edward Goldson, MD, FAAP
Peter J. Smith, MD, MA, FAAP
Carol Cohen Weitzman, MD, FAAP
Stephen H. Contompasis, MD, FAAP, Web site Editor
Damon R. Korb, MD, FAAP, Discussion Board Moderator
Michael I. Reiff, MD, FAAP, Newsletter Editor
Robert G. Voigt, MD, FAAP, Program Chairperson

LIAISONS

Beth Ellen Davis, MD, MPH, FAAP – *Council on Children with Disabilities*
Pamela C. High, MD, MS, FAAP – *Society for Developmental and Behavioral Pediatrics*

STAFF

Linda Paul, MPH

ABBREVIATIONS

ADHD: attention-deficit/hyperactivity disorder
PCIT: parent–child interaction therapy

REFERENCES

1. Egger HL, Angold A. Common emotional and behavioral disorders in preschool children: presentation, nosology, and epidemiology. *J Child Psychol Psychiatry*. 2006;47(3–4):313–337

2. Wichstrøm L, Berg-Nielsen TS, Angold A, Egger HL, Solheim E, Sveen TH. Prevalence of psychiatric disorders in preschoolers. *J Child Psychol Psychiatry*. 2012;53(6):695–705

3. Gudmundsson OO, Magnusson P, Saemundsen E, et al. Psychiatric disorders in an urban sample of preschool children. *Child Adolesc Ment Health*. 2013;18(4):210–217

4. Schwebel DC, Speltz ML, Jones K, Bardina P. Unintentional injury in preschool boys with and without early onset of disruptive behavior. *J Pediatr Psychol*. 2002;27(8):727–737

5. Pagliaccio D, Luby J, Gaffrey M, et al. Anomalous functional brain activation following negative mood induction in children with pre-school onset major depression. *Dev Cogn Neurosci*. 2012;2(2):256–267

6. Briggs-Gowan MJ, Carter AS. Social-emotional screening status in early childhood predicts elementary

school outcomes. *Pediatrics.*
2008;121(5):957–962

7. Gaffrey MS, Luby JL, Belden AC, Hirshberg JS, Volsch J, Barch DM. Association between depression severity and amygdala reactivity during sad face viewing in depressed preschoolers: an fMRI study. *J Affect Disord.* 2011;129(1–3):364–370

8. Scheeringa MS, Zeanah CH, Myers L, Putnam F. Heart period and variability findings in preschool children with posttraumatic stress symptoms. *Biol Psychiatry.* 2004;55(7):685–691

9. Lahey BB, Pelham WE, Loney J, et al. Three-year predictive validity of DSM-IV attention deficit hyperactivity disorder in children diagnosed at 4-6 years of age. *Am J Psychiatry.* 2004;161(11):2014–2020

10. Barch DM, Gaffrey MS, Botteron KN, Belden AC, Luby JL. Functional brain activation to emotionally valenced faces in school-aged children with a history of preschool-onset major depression. *Biol Psychiatry.* 2012;72(12):1035–1042

11. Garner AS, Shonkoff JP; Committee on Psychosocial Aspects of Child and Family Health; Committee on Early Childhood, Adoption, and Dependent Care; Section on Developmental and Behavioral Pediatrics. Early childhood adversity, toxic stress, and the role of the pediatrician: translating developmental science into lifelong health. *Pediatrics.* 2012;129(1). Available at: www.pediatrics.org/cgi/content/full/129/1/e224

12. Shonkoff JP, Garner AS; Committee on Psychosocial Aspects of Child and Family Health; Committee on Early Childhood, Adoption, and Dependent Care; Section on Developmental and Behavioral Pediatrics. The lifelong effects of early childhood adversity and toxic stress. *Pediatrics.* 2012;129(1). Available at: www.pediatrics.org/cgi/content/full/129/1/e232

13. Weitzman C, Wegner L. American Academy of Pediatrics, Section on Developmental and Behavioral Pediatrics, Committee on Psychosocial Aspects of Child and Family Health, Council on Early Childhood; Society for Developmental and Behavioral Pediatrics. Promoting optimal development: screening for behavioral and emotional problems. *Pediatrics.* 2015;135(2):384–395

14. Horwitz SM, Kelleher KJ, Stein REK, et al. Barriers to the identification and management of psychosocial issues in children and maternal depression. *Pediatrics.* 2007;119(1). Available at: www.pediatrics.org/cgi/content/full/119/1/e208

15. Zito JM; American Society of Clinical Psychopharmacology. Pharmacoepidemiology: recent findings and challenges for child and adolescent psychopharmacology. *J Clin Psychiatry.* 2007;68(6):966–967

16. Kratochvil CJ, Vaughan BS, Stoner JA, et al. A double-blind, placebo-controlled study of atomoxetine in young children with ADHD. *Pediatrics.* 2011;127(4). Available at: www.pediatrics.org/cgi/content/full/127/4/e862

17. Greenhill L, Kollins S, Abikoff H, et al. Efficacy and safety of immediate-release methylphenidate treatment for preschoolers with ADHD. *J Am Acad Child Adolesc Psychiatry.* 2006;45(11):1284–1293

18. Correll CU, Carlson HE. Endocrine and metabolic adverse effects of psychotropic medications in children and adolescents. *J Am Acad Child Adolesc Psychiatry.* 2006;45(7):771–791

19. Olfson M, Crystal S, Huang C, Gerhard T. Trends in antipsychotic drug use by very young, privately insured children. *J Am Acad Child Adolesc Psychiatry.* 2010;49(1):13–23

20. Zito JM, Safer DJ, Valluri S, Gardner JF, Korelitz JJ, Mattison DR. Psychotherapeutic medication prevalence in Medicaid-insured preschoolers. *J Child Adolesc Psychopharmacol.* 2007;17(2):195–203

21. Pediatric OCD Treatment Study (POTS) Team. Cognitive-behavior therapy, sertraline, and their combination for children and adolescents with obsessive-compulsive disorder: the Pediatric OCD Treatment Study (POTS) randomized controlled trial. *JAMA.* 2004;292(16):1969–1976

22. Webster-Stratton C, Rinaldi J, Jamila MR. Long-term outcomes of Incredible Years parenting program: predictors of adolescent adjustment. *Child Adolesc Ment Health.* 2011;16(1):38–46

23. Hood KK, Eyberg SM. Outcomes of parent-child interaction therapy: mothers' reports of maintenance three to six years after treatment. *J Clin Child Adolesc Psychol.* 2003;32(3):419–429

24. Foy JM; American Academy of Pediatrics Task Force on Mental Health. Enhancing pediatric mental health care: algorithms for primary care. *Pediatrics.* 2010;125(suppl 3):S109–S125

25. Substance Abuse and Mental Health Services Administration. *National Registry of Evidence-based Programs and Practices.* Washington, DC: Substance Abuse and Mental Health Services Administration; 2013

26. Abikoff HB, Thompson MJ, Laver-Bradbury C, et al. Parent training for preschool ADHD: a randomized controlled trial of specialized and generic programs. *J Child Psychol Psychiatry.* 2015;56(6):618–631

27. Charach A, Dahshti B, Carson P, et al. *Attention Deficit Hyperactivity Disorder: Effectiveness of Treatment in At-Risk Preschoolers; Long-Term Effectiveness in All Ages; and Variability in Prevalence, Diagnosis, and Treatment.* Rockville, MD: Agency for Healthcare Research and Quality; 2012

28. Thompson MJ, Laver-Bradbury C, Ayres M, et al. A small-scale randomized controlled trial of the revised New Forest parenting programme for preschoolers with attention deficit hyperactivity disorder. *Eur Child Adolesc Psychiatry.* 2009;18(10):605–616

29. Webster-Stratton CH, Reid MJ, Beauchaine T. Combining parent and child training for young children with ADHD. *J Clin Child Adolesc Psychol.* 2011;40(2):191–203

30. Webster-Stratton C, Reid J. The Incredible Years parents, teachers, and children training series: a multifaceted treatment approach for young children with conduct disorders. In: Kazdin AE, ed. *Evidence-based Psychotherapies for Children and Adolescents.* 2nd ed. New York, NY: Guilford Press; 2010:194–210

31. Bodenmann G, Cina A, Ledermann T, Sanders MR. The efficacy of the Triple P-Positive Parenting Program in improving parenting and child behavior: a comparison with two other treatment conditions. *Behav Res Ther.* 2008;46(4):411–427

32. Eyberg SM, Funderburk BW, Hembree-Kigin TL, McNeil CB, Querido JG, Hood KK. Parent-child interaction therapy with behavior problem children: one and two year maintenance of treatment effects in the family. *Child Fam Behav Ther.* 2001;23(4):1–20

33. Lieberman AF, Ghosh Ippen C, Van Horn P. Child-parent psychotherapy: 6-month follow-up of a randomized controlled trial. *J Am Acad Child Adolesc Psychiatry.* 2006;45(8):913–918

34. Choate ML, Pincus DB, Eyberg SM. Parent-child interaction therapy for treatment of separation anxiety disorder in young children: a pilot study. *Cogn Behav Ther.* 2005;12(1):136–145

35. Donovan CL, March S. Online CBT for preschool anxiety disorders: a randomised control trial. *Behav Res Ther.* 2014;58:24–35

36. Hirshfeld-Becker DR, Masek B, Henin A, et al. Cognitive behavioral therapy for 4- to 7-year-old children with anxiety disorders: a randomized clinical trial. *J Consult Clin Psychol.* 2010;78(4):498–510

37. Markie-Dadds C, Sanders MR. Self-Directed Triple P (Positive Parenting Program) for mothers with children at-risk of developing conduct problems. *Behav Cogn Psychother.* 2006;34(03):259–275

38. Berkovits MD, O'Brien KA, Carter CG, Eyberg SM. Early identification and intervention for behavior problems in primary care: a comparison of two abbreviated versions of parent-child interaction therapy. *Behav Ther.* 2010;41(3):375–387

39. Perrin EC, Sheldrick RC, McMenamy JM, Henson BS, Carter AS. Improving parenting skills for families of young children in pediatric settings: a randomized clinical trial. *JAMA Pediatr.* 2014;168(1):16–24

40. Gunlicks ML, Weissman MM. Change in child psychopathology with improvement in parental depression: a systematic review. *J Am Acad Child Adolesc Psychiatry.* 2008;47(4):379–389

41. Luby JL, Stalets MM, Belden AC. Psychotropic prescriptions in a sample including both healthy and mood and disruptive disordered preschoolers: relationships to diagnosis, impairment, prescriber type, and assessment methods. *J Child Adolesc Psychopharmacol.* 2007;17(2):205–215

42. Kolko DJ, Campo JV, Kelleher K, Cheng Y. Improving access to care and clinical outcome for pediatric behavioral problems: a randomized trial of a nurse-administered intervention in primary care. *J Dev Behav Pediatr.* 2010;31(5):393–404

43. Sarvet B, Gold J, Bostic JQ, et al. Improving access to mental health care for children: the Massachusetts Child Psychiatry Access Project. *Pediatrics.* 2010;126(6):1191–1200

44. Kolko DJ, Campo JV, Kilbourne AM, Kelleher K. Doctor-office collaborative care for pediatric behavioral problems: a preliminary clinical trial. *Arch Pediatr Adolesc Med.* 2012;166(3):224–231

45. Thomas CR, Holzer CE III. The continuing shortage of child and adolescent psychiatrists. *J Am Acad Child Adolesc Psychiatry.* 2006;45(9):1023–1031

46. Kautz C, Mauch D, Smith SA. *Reimbursement of Mental Health Services in Primary Care Settings.* Rockville, MD: Center for Mental Health Services, Substance Abuse; 2008

47. Committee on Child Health Financing. Scope of health care benefits for children from birth through age 26. *Pediatrics.* 2012;129(1):185–189

48. Kelleher KJ, Campo JV, Gardner WP. Management of pediatric mental disorders in primary care: where are we now and where are we going? *Curr Opin Pediatr.* 2006;18(6):649–653

49. American Academy of Child and Adolescent Psychiatry. Policy Statements: Collaboration with Pediatric Medical Professionals. Washington, DC: American Academy of Child and Adolescent Psychiatry; 2008. Available at: http://www.aacap.org/aacap/policy_statements/2008/Collaboration_with_Pediatric_Medical_Professionals.aspx. Accessed October 17, 2016

Addressing Early Childhood Emotional and Behavioral Problems

• •

- *Technical Report*

TECHNICAL REPORT

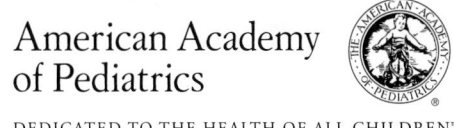

American Academy
of Pediatrics

DEDICATED TO THE HEALTH OF ALL CHILDREN™

Addressing Early Childhood Emotional and Behavioral Problems

Mary Margaret Gleason, MD, FAAP, Edward Goldson, MD, FAAP, Michael W. Yogman, MD, FAAP, COUNCIL ON EARLY CHILDHOOD, COMMITTEE ON PSYCHOSOCIAL ASPECTS OF CHILD AND FAMILY HEALTH, SECTION ON DEVELOPMENTAL AND BEHAVIORAL PEDIATRICS

abstract

More than 10% of young children experience clinically significant mental health problems, with rates of impairment and persistence comparable to those seen in older children. For many of these clinical disorders, effective treatments supported by rigorous data are available. On the other hand, rigorous support for psychopharmacologic interventions is limited to 2 large randomized controlled trials. Access to psychotherapeutic interventions is limited. The pediatrician has a critical role as the leader of the medical home to promote well-being that includes emotional, behavioral, and relationship health. To be effective in this role, pediatricians promote the use of safe and effective treatments and recognize the limitations of psychopharmacologic interventions. This technical report reviews the data supporting treatments for young children with emotional, behavioral, and relationship problems and supports the policy statement of the same name.

DOI: 10.1542/peds.2016-3025

PEDIATRICS (ISSN Numbers: Print, 0031-4005; Online, 1098-4275).

FINANCIAL DISCLOSURE: The authors have indicated they have no financial relationships relevant to this article to disclose.

FUNDING: No external funding.

POTENTIAL CONFLICT OF INTEREST: The authors have indicated they have no potential conflicts of interest to disclose.

To cite: Gleason MM, Goldson E, Yogman MW, AAP COUNCIL ON EARLY CHILDHOOD. Addressing Early Childhood Emotional and Behavioral Problems. *Pediatrics.* 2016;138(6):e20163025

At least 8% to 10% of children younger than 5 years experience clinically significant and impairing mental health problems, which include emotional, behavioral, and social relationship problems.[1] An additional 1.5% of children have an autism spectrum disorder, the management of which has been reviewed in a separate report from the American Academy of Pediatrics (AAP).[2] Children with emotional, behavioral, and social relationship problems ("mental health problems"), as well as their families, experience distress and can suffer substantially because of these problems. These children may demonstrate impairment across multiple domains, including social interactions, problematic parent–child relationships, physical safety, inability to participate in child care without expulsion, delayed school readiness, school problems, and physical health problems in adulthood.[3–13] These clinical presentations can be distinguished from the emotional and behavioral patterns of typically developing children by their symptoms, family history, and level of impairment and, in some disorders, physiologic signs.[14–17] Emotional, behavioral, and relationship disorders rarely are transient and often have lasting effects, including measurable differences in brain functioning in school-aged children and a high risk of later mental health problems.[18-24] Exposure to toxic stressors, such as maltreatment or violence, and individual, family, or community stressors can increase the risk of early-onset mental health problems, although such stressors are not necessary for the development of these problems. Early exposure to adversity also has notable effects on the hypothalamic–pituitary–adrenal axis and epigenetic processes, with short-term and long-term consequences in physical and mental health, including adult cardiovascular disease and obesity.[25] In short, young children's early emotional, behavioral, and social relationship problems can cause suffering for young children and families, weaken the developing foundation of emotional and behavioral health, and have the potential for long-term adverse consequences.[26,27] This technical report reviews the data supporting treatment of children with identified clinical disorders, including the efficacy, safety, and accessibility of both pharmacologic and psychotherapeutic approaches.

PREVENTION APPROACHES

Although not the focus of this report, a full system of care includes primary and secondary preventive approaches, which are addressed in separate AAP reports.[28,29] Many family, individual, and community risk factors for adverse emotional, behavioral, and relationship health outcomes, including low-income status, exposure to toxic stressors, and parental mental health problems, can be identified early using systematic surveillance and screening. An extensive review of established prevention programs for the general population and identified children at high risk are described in the Substance

Abuse and Mental Health Services Administration (SAMHSA)'s National Report of Evidence-Based Programs and Practices (http://www.nrepp.samhsa.gov/AdvancedSearch.aspx). Outcomes of these programs highlight the value of early intervention and the potential to improve parenting skills using universal or targeted approaches for children at risk. The programs use a variety of approaches, including home visiting, parent groups, targeted addressing of basic needs, and videos to enhance parental self-reflection skills and have demonstrated a range of outcomes related to positive emotional, behavioral, and relationship development. One model developed specifically for the pediatric primary care setting is the Video Interaction Project, in which parents are paired with a bachelor's-level or master's-level developmental specialist who uses video and educational techniques to support parents' awareness of their child's developmental needs.[30]

Acknowledging that early preventive interventions are an important component of a system of care, the body of this technical report focuses on treatment of identified clinical problems rather than children at risk because of family or community factors.

PSYCHOSOCIAL TREATMENT APPROACHES

The evidence supporting family-focused therapeutic interventions for children with clinical-level concerns is robust, and these are the first-line approaches for young children with significant emotional and behavioral problems in most practice guidelines.[31-35]

Generally, these interventions take an approach that focuses on enhancing emotional and behavioral regulation through specialized parenting tools and approaches. The interventions

are implemented by clinicians with training in the specific treatment modality, following manuals and with fidelity to the treatment model. Primary care providers can be trained in these interventions but more often lead a medical home management approach that includes ongoing primary care management and support and concurrent comanagement with a clinician trained in implementing an evidence-based treatment (EBT).

Effective treatments exist to address early clinical concerns, including relationship disturbances, attention-deficit/hyperactivity disorder (ADHD), disruptive behavior disorders, anxiety, and posttraumatic stress disorder. Measured outcomes include improved attachment relationships, symptom reduction, diagnostic remission, enhanced functioning, and in one study, normalization of diurnal cortisol release patterns, which are known to be related to stress regulation and mood disorders.[31,33-35] Psychotherapies, including treatments that involve cognitive, psychological, and behavioral approaches, have substantially more lasting effects than do medications. Some preschool treatments have been shown to be effective for years after the treatment ended, a finding not matched in longitudinal pharmacologic studies.[36-38] It is for this reason that the recent ADHD treatment guidelines from the AAP emphasize that first-line treatment of preschoolers with well-established ADHD should be family-focused psychotherapy.[39]

EXAMPLES OF EVIDENCE-BASED TREATMENTS FOR EXISTING DIAGNOSES IN YOUNG CHILDREN

Infants and Toddlers

This report focuses on programs that target current diagnoses or clear clinical problems (rather than risk) in infants and toddlers and includes only those with rigorous randomized controlled empirical support. Because the parent–child relationship is a central force in the early emotional and behavioral well-being of children, a number of empirically supported treatments focus on enhancing that relationship to promote child well-being. Each intervention focuses on enhancing parents' ability to identify and respond to the infant's cues and to meet the infant's emotional needs. All interventions use infant–parent interactions in vivo or through video to demonstrate the infant's cues and opportunities to meet them. Some explicitly focus on enhancing parents' self-reflection and increasing awareness of how their own upbringing may influence their parenting approach.

Child Parent Psychotherapy and its partner Infant Parent Psychotherapy are derived from attachment theory and address the parent–child relationship through emotional support for parents, modeling protective behaviors, reflective developmental guidance, and addressing parental traumatic memories as they intrude into parent–child interactions.[40,41] This therapy is flexible in its delivery and can be implemented in the office, at home, or in other locations convenient for the family. On average, child–parent psychotherapy lasts approximately 32 sessions. In infants and toddlers, the empirically supported therapy enhances parent–child relationships, attachment security, child cognitive functioning, and normalization of cortisol regulation.[42-44]

For infants and toddlers who have been adopted internationally, those in foster care, or those thought to be at high risk of maltreatment because of exposure to domestic violence, homelessness, or parental substance abuse, the Attachment and Biobehavioral Catch-Up caregiver training supports

caregivers in developing sensitive, nurturing, nonfrightening parenting behaviors. In 10 sessions, caregivers receive parenting skills training, psychoeducation, and support in understanding the needs of infants and young children. This intervention model is associated with decreased rates of disorganized attachment, the attachment status most closely linked to psychopathology, and is associated with increased caregiver sensitivity and, notably, normalized diurnal cortisol patterns.[45-47]

In the Video Feedback to Promote Positive Parenting program, mothers with low levels of sensitivity to their child's needs review video feedback about their own parent–child interactions, with a focus on supporting sensitive discipline, reading a child's cues, and developing empathy for a child who is frustrated or angry. In the most stressed families, this intervention is associated with decreased infant behavioral difficulties and increased parental sensitivity.[48]

Treatments focused on mother–infant dyads affected by postpartum depression show promising effects on relationships and infant regulation.[49] Data in older children suggest effective treatment of maternal depression may result in reduction of child symptoms or an increase in caregiving quality.[50-52]

Preschoolers (2–6 Years)

ADHD and disruptive behavior disorders (eg, oppositional defiant disorder and conduct disorder) are the most common group of early childhood mental health problems, and a number of parent management training models have been shown to be effective. It should be noted that the criteria for these disorders have been shown to have validity in young children,[22,53] although the validity is dependent on a systematic assessment process that is most easily conducted in specialty settings. All of these parent training

models share similar behavioral principles, most consistently teaching parents: (1) to implement positive reinforcement to promote positive behaviors; (2) to ignore low-level provocative behaviors; and (3) to respond in a clear, consistent, and safe manner to unacceptable behaviors. The specific approaches to sharing these principles with parents vary across interventions. Table 1 presents some of the characteristics of the best-supported programs, all of which are featured on SAMHSA's national registry of evidence-based programs and practices.[34,54] The New Forrest Therapy, Triple P (Positive Parenting Practices), the Incredible Years Series (IYS), Helping the Noncompliant Child, and Parent Child Interaction Therapy (PCIT) all have shown efficacy in reducing clinically significant disruptive behavior symptoms in toddlers, preschoolers, and early school-aged children. The New Forrest Therapy, Helping the Noncompliant Child, and IYS also have proven efficacy in treating ADHD.[35,55-57]

In the New Forrest Therapy, sessions include parent–child activities that require sustained attention, concentration, turn-taking, working memory, and delay of gratification, all followed by positive reinforcement when the child is successful.[32,35] This model has been shown to decrease ADHD symptoms substantially and to decrease parents' negative statements about their children.[35] Triple P is a multilevel intervention that includes targeted treatment of children with disruptive behaviors.[55] The 3 highest levels of care include teaching parents about the causes of disruptive behaviors and effective strategies as well as specific problem solving about the child's individual patterns. The child is included in some sessions to create opportunities to implement the new strategies and for the therapist to model the behaviors. IYS includes a parent-focused treatment approach,

TABLE 1 Evidence-Based Interventions Shown To Reduce Existing Disruptive Problems in Preschoolers

Program	Age Range Supported by Data	Patient Population	No. of Children in Randomized Controlled Trials	Formal Psychoeducation for Parents	Real-Time Observed Parent–Child Interactions	Special Characteristics	Duration	Follow-up Duration (If Applicable)	Evidence Reflecting Efficacy for ADHD (Effect Size)	Evidence Demonstrating Efficacy for ODD and CD (Effect Size)
New Forest[32,35]	30–77 mo	Children with ADHD	202	Yes	Yes	• Parent–child tasks are specifically intended to require attention • Occurs in the home • Explicit attention to parental depression	5 weekly sessions	n/a	Yes (1.9)	Yes (0.7)
IYS parent training, teacher training, and child training[32,53,57–59]	3–8 y	Children with CD, ODD, and ADHD	677	Yes	No	• Separate parent and child groups • Parent training uses video vignettes for discussion • Child training includes circle time learning and coached free play	20 weekly 2-h sessions		Yes (0.8)	Yes (home behavior, 0.4–0.7; school behavior, 0.7–1.25)
Triple P,[55,60,61] (levels 3 and 4)	36–48 mo	Children at high risk with parental concerns about behavioral difficulties (level 4)	330	Yes	Yes	• Multiple levels of intervention • Primarily training parents with some opportunities to observe parent–child interactions • Handouts and homework supplement the treatment	• Primary care = 4 sessions of 15 min • Standard treatment is 10 sessions	6 and 12 mo: effect size, 0.66 for children <4 y, 0.65 for children >4 y[62]	No	Yes (level 3: 0.69, level 4: 0.96; lower for children <4 y)[63]
Triple P online[59]	2–9 y	Children with CD and ODD	116	No	No	• Interactive self-directed program delivered via the internet • Instruction in 17 core positive parenting skills	8 modules (45–75 min)	6 mo: effect size from baseline, 0.6–0.7 on ECBI, no effect on SDQ	No effect	Yes (1.0; by parent report)

TABLE 1 Continued

Program	Age Range Supported by Data	Patient Population	No. of Children in Randomized Controlled Trials	Formal Psychoeducation for Parents	Real-Time Observed Parent–Child Interactions	Special Characteristics	Duration	Follow-up Duration (If Applicable)	Evidence Reflecting Efficacy for ADHD (Effect Size)	Evidence Demonstrating Efficacy for ODD and CD (Effect Size)
PCIT[37,64,65]	2–7 y	Children with clinical level disruptive behavior symptoms	358	Yes, minimal	Yes	• Through a 1-way mirror, therapist coaches parent during in vivo interactions with child • Homework requires parent–child interactions • Progress through therapy determined by parents' skill development	Depends on parent skill development	Up to 6 y after treatment, fewer signs of disruptive behavior disorder than baseline	Minimal	Yes (1.45)[38]
Helping the Noncompliant Child[57]	3–8 y	Children with noncompliant behaviors	350	Yes	Yes	Involves two phases 1) Differential Attention 2) Compliance training using demonstration, role plays, and in-office and at home practice	Depends on parent skill development	6.8 mo	Effect size 1.24; inattention 1.09; hyperactivity/impulsivity: 1.21	Yes (but no ES reported)

n/a, not available; ECBI, Eyberg Child Behavior Inventory; SDQ, Strengths and Difficulties Questionnaire; CD, conduct disorder; ODD, oppositional defiant disorder.

in which groups of parents learn effective strategies, practice with each other, and discuss clinical vignettes presented on videos.[56] The child group treatment can occur concurrently with the parent training and focuses on emotional recognition and problem solving. This treatment initially was developed to treat oppositional defiant disorder and conduct disorder, for which a large body of evidence demonstrates its efficacy. Recent studies also have demonstrated effectiveness in treating inattention and hyperactivity.[66] An unintended yet measureable benefit is promoting language.[67] In PCIT, parents are coached in positive interactions and safe discipline with their child by the therapist, who is behind a one-way mirror and communicates to a parent via a small microphone in the parent's ear ("bug in the ear"). This treatment is unique because parents' achievement of specific skills determines the pace of the therapy, allowing movement from the first phase, focused on positive reinforcement, to the second phase, focused on safe, consistent consequences. PCIT has been shown to have large effects on child behavior problems and parent negative behaviors in real time. Importantly, it is also effective in reducing recidivism of maltreating parents.[68] Helping the Noncompliant Child also provides 2 portions of the treatment, with the first focused on differential attention and the second focused on compliance training. Parents move through the therapy based on observed skill acquisition, learning by demonstration, role plays, and practice at home and in the office with their child. Helping the Noncompliant Child has been shown to have similar effectiveness as NFP in treating ADHD in children 3 to 4 years old and those wtih comorbid ODD.[69]

Anxiety disorders also are common in very young children, with nearly

10% of children meeting criteria for at least 1 anxiety disorder. Cognitive behavioral therapy and child–parent psychotherapy, both of which also are listed on the SAMHSA registry of EBTs, are effective in reducing anxiety in very young children. When cognitive behavioral therapy is modified to match young children's developmental levels, children as young as 4 years can learn the necessary skills, including relaxation strategies, naming their feelings, and learning to rate the intensity of the feelings.[31] In cognitive behavioral therapy, children are exposed to the story of their trauma in a systematic, graduated fashion, using the coping strategies and measuring feeling intensity skills that they practice simultaneously throughout the intervention. Two randomized studies have examined cognitive behavioral therapy in trauma-exposed preschoolers, and both have shown that children in the cognitive behavioral therapy treatment arm showed fewer posttraumatic stress symptoms as well as fewer symptoms of disruptive behavior disorders than did children in supportive treatment.[70,71] Effects are sustained for up to a year after treatment.[71,72] Child–parent psychotherapy is similarly effective in treating children exposed to trauma. Child–parent psychotherapy is an attachment-focused treatment that supports the parent in creating a safe, consistent relationship with the child through helping the parent understand the child's emotional experiences and needs as well as parental reactions.[40] Child–parent psychotherapy is more effective in reducing child and parent trauma symptoms than supportive case management and community referral.[73] Importantly, child–parent psychotherapy shows treatment durability with sustained results at least 6 months after treatment.

Other more common anxiety disorders and mood disorders have received less research attention.

CBT has been shown effective in addressing mixed anxiety disorders including selective mutism, generalized anxiety disorders, separation anxiety disorder, and social phobia.[62,63] A randomized controlled trial demonstrated that modified PCIT was effective in helping parents recognize emotions, although not better than parent education in reducing depressive symptoms.[74] Significant controversy and limited data about the validity of diagnostic criteria for bipolar disorder remain, and no rigorous studies of nonpharmacologic interventions in this age group exist.[75]

Although the studies described previously show positive effects of parent management training approaches, limitations are notable. Attrition of up to 30% is not uncommon among these approaches, suggesting that there is a significant proportion of the population for whom these treatments do not seem to be a good fit, whether because of the frequency of appointments, the content, the therapeutic relationship, stigma about mental health care, or other barriers.[60,76,77]

PSYCHOPHARMACOLOGIC TREATMENT APPROACHES

As highlighted in both the professional and lay press, an increasing number of publicly and privately insured preschool and even younger children are receiving prescriptions for psychotropic medications.[78–81] After increasing drastically in the 1990s, claims data indicate that rates of stimulant prescriptions have plateaued in recent years, but the rates of prescriptions of atypical antipsychotic agents continue to increase.[78,81–83] Although prescribing data are limited, it appears that pediatric providers are the primary prescribers for psychopharmacologic treatment in children younger

than 5 years, as they are for older children.[84,85]

The evidence base related to psychopharmacologic medications in young children is limited, and clinical practice has far outpaced the evidence supporting safety or efficacy, especially for children in foster care.[33,81] Specifically, 2 rigorous randomized controlled trials have examined the safety and efficacy of medications in young children. Both studies found that treatment of ADHD in young children with medication, specifically methylphenidate and atomoxetine, was more effective than placebo but less effective than documented in older children.[36,86,87] Both also reported that young children had higher rates of adverse effects, especially negative emotionality and appetite and sleep problems, than did older children.[86,87] Less rigorously studied are the atypical antipsychotic agents, such as risperidone, olanzapine, and aripiprazole, for which prescription rates have increased substantially.[33,88] These agents have known metabolic risks, including obesity, hyperlipidemia, glucose intolerance, and hyperprolactinemia, as well the potential for extrapyramidal effects.[89,90] Long-term safety data regarding use of these medications in humans, including the effects on the brain during its most rapid development, are not available.

ACCESS TO EVIDENCE-BASED TREATMENTS

The balance of risks and benefits of treatment of early childhood emotional, behavioral, or relationship problems strongly favors the safety and established efficacy of the EBTs over the potential for medical risks and lower levels of evidence supporting the medication. Fewer than 50% of young children with emotional, behavioral, or relationship disturbances, even those with severity sufficient to warrant medication trials, receive any treatment, especially nonpharmacologic treatments.[11,78,91,92] A number of barriers limit access to nonpharmacological EBTs.

Residency training and continuing medical education has traditionally provided limited opportunities for collaboration between pediatric and child psychiatry residents and with other mental health providers, including doctoral level and master's level clinicians, although there are calls to increase these opportunities.[93,94] The limited opportunities for collaboration in training and limited supervised opportunities to assess young children with mental health problems likely result in graduating residents having limited experience in early childhood mental health as they enter the primary care workforce. The AAP has worked to address this gap by developing practice transformation approaches, including educational modules and anticipatory guidance approaches that promote emotional, behavioral, and relationship wellness (see the AAP Early Brain and Child Development Web site at http://www.aap.org/en-us/advocacy-and-policy/aap-health-initiatives/EBCD), and around the country, there appears to be an increase in collaborative training opportunities for pediatric residents with developmental–behavioral pediatrics faculty and fellows, triple board residents, child and adolescent psychiatry trainees, and other mental health professionals.

Many of these barriers are not specific to early childhood emotional, behavioral, and relationship health but are quite apparent in this area. Although representative epidemiologic data examining the rates of psychotherapeutic treatment of preschoolers are not available, only 1 in 5 older children with a mental health problem receives treatment,[95] and it seems likely that

the rate is lower among preschool-aged children. A major challenge is the workforce shortage among child psychiatrists, child mental health professionals, and pediatric specialists trained to meet the specialized emotional, behavioral, and relationship needs of very young children and their families.[96-99] Anecdotally, it seems that many therapists trained in EBTs remain close to academic centers, further exacerbating the shortage in regions without such a center. Promising statewide initiatives, such as "PCIT of the Carolinas" learning collaborative, which promote organizational readiness and capacity within agencies, clinician competence, and treatment fidelity and consultation with therapists, may begin to foster access to EBTs. Such models are promising approaches to improving access to clinicians trained to evaluate a very young child or to implement EBTs.

Even in communities with early childhood experts who are trained in EBTs, third-party payment systems traditionally have rewarded brief medication-focused visits.[28] When emotional and behavioral health services are "carved out" of health insurance, important barriers to accessing care include limitations on primary care physicians' ability to bill for "mental health" diagnoses, limits on numbers of visits, payer restriction of mental health providers, and low payment rates.[98,100-102] Until 2013, the *Current Procedural Terminology* coding system did not recognize the extended time needed for early childhood emotional and behavioral assessment and treatment (and the payment for the new code tends to be minimal), and many payers will not reimburse for services without the patient present or for phone consultation or case conferences. Lastly, the billing and coding system does not recognize relationship-focused therapy, requiring the

individual participants to have an *International Classification of Diseases*–codable diagnosis, and only a few states accept developmentally specific diagnoses, such as the Diagnostic Criteria: 0-5, as reimbursable conditions.[103]

Finally, stigma and parental beliefs may interfere with referrals to EBTs for very young children with emotional, behavioral, and relationship problems.[104-108] Parents' interest in treatment may be influenced by perceived stigma related to the mental health problem or their own experiences with the mental health system.[109] Provider stigma about mental health and concerns about a child being "labeled" may reduce referrals as well. Some parents also may be concerned that involvement with a mental or behavioral health specialist may increase their risk of referral to child protection services.

INNOVATIVE MODELS OF ACCESS THROUGH THE MEDICAL HOME

For children with emotional, behavioral, or relationship problems, the pediatric medical home remains the hub of a child's care, just as it is for other children with special health care needs.[110] Even without a comprehensive diagnostic assessment or knowledge of the details of each EBT, use of specific communication strategies, the "common factors" approach, has been shown to improve outcomes in older children. Specifically, implementation of the common factors approach was associated with reduced impairment from symptoms and reduced parent symptoms in a randomized controlled trial of 58 providers.[111] Subsequently, the mnemonic "HELP" was introduced by the AAP Task Force on Mental Health to prompt clinicians in key elements of the model, including offering **h**ope, demonstrating **e**mpathy, demonstrating **l**oyalty, using the language the family uses about the concerns, and **p**artnering with the family to develop a clearly stated **p**lan, with the parents' **p**ermission.[112] Because of the stigma related to mental health issues, "hope" and "loyalty" are especially powerful first steps.

Innovative and successful adaptations of EBTs have been developed for the primary care setting.[55,64,65] Triple P has been implemented successfully in primary care settings using nurse visits to provide the psychoeducation for parents and also has been studied as a self-directed intervention for parents of children with clinically significant disruptive behavior symptoms, with modest but sustained effects up to 6 months.[61] A pilot PCIT adaptation for primary care showed promising results, although larger studies are needed.[113] Most recently, a randomized controlled trial demonstrated that the Incredible Years Series can be implemented effectively in the pediatric medical home for children with mild to moderate behavior problems. In this study, parent-reported behavioral problems decreased significantly compared with the group on the wait list, as did observed negative parent–child interactions.[114]

The strategy for identifying providers of EBTs varies state to state. However, all but 3 states have an Early Childhood Comprehensive Services grant from the Human Resources and Service Administration (http://mchb.hrsa. gov/programs/earlychildhood/ comprehensivesystems/grantees/) and are developing systems of care for young children. EBTs tend to be concentrated around academic settings, so contacting local developmental–behavioral pediatric divisions and child and adolescent psychiatry and psychology divisions often helps, and the originator of the model often knows providers trained in the intervention (eg, www.pcit.

org). Innovative practice models, such as consultation or colocated mental health professionals, can be effective approaches to ensuring children have access to care.[115]

In areas with more trained EBT providers, opportunities for colocated care seem promising. In such models, a clinician, who is often a master's level clinician or psychologist, works in the practice as part of the team to provide short-term mental health interventions, such as skills-training in behavioral management. In older children, such interventions are effective in decreasing ADHD and oppositional defiant disorder, although not conduct disorder or anxiety, and in increasing the likelihood of treatment completion.[116] Models of consultation that support primary care providers in the management of children who have been referred for EBT or who have no access to an EBT are under development, often through federally funded projects, such as SAMHSA's Linking Actions to Unmet Needs in Child Health Project (http://media.samhsa.gov/ samhsaNewsletter/Volume_18_ Number_3/PromotingWellness.aspx).

COMPREHENSIVE TREATMENT PLAN

Clinical emotional, behavioral, or relationship problems commonly cooccur with other developmental delays, especially speech problems. For example, in one mental health program for toddlers, 77% of children also had a developmental delay.[117] A comprehensive treatment plan includes attention to any comorbid conditions, although such combined or serial treatments have not been studied explicitly. Similarly, family mental health problems, such as maternal depression, can reduce the efficacy of parent management training approaches. In older children, effective treatment of maternal depression is effective in reducing child symptoms and fewer diagnoses.[51]

SUMMARY

Very young children can experience significant and impairing mental health problems at rates comparable to older children. Early adversity, including abuse and neglect, increases the risk of early childhood emotional, behavioral, and relationship problems and is associated with developmental, medical, and mental health problems through the lifespan. EBTs can address early childhood mental health problems effectively, reducing symptoms and impairment and even normalizing biological markers. By contrast, the research base examining safety and efficacy of pharmacologic interventions is sparse and inadequate. Systems issues, including graduate medical education systems, access to trained providers of EBTs for very young children, and coding, billing, and payment structures all interfere with access to effective interventions. Not insignificantly, social stigma related to mental health held by parents, primary care providers, and the greater society likely work against access to care for children.

CONCLUSIONS

The existing data demonstrate strong empirical support for family-focused interventions for young children with emotional, behavioral, and relationship problems, especially disruptive behavior disorders and anxiety or trauma exposure. By contrast, the empirical literature examining psychopharmacologic treatment is limited and highlights risks of adverse effects. A number of workforce and other barriers may contribute to the limited access.

LEAD AUTHORS

Mary Margaret Gleason, MD, FAAP
Edward Goldson, MD, FAAP
Michael W. Yogman, MD, FAAP

COUNCIL ON EARLY CHILDHOOD EXECUTIVE COMMITTEE, 2015–2016

Dina Lieser, MD, FAAP, Chairperson
Beth DelConte, MD, FAAP
Elaine Donoghue, MD, FAAP
Marian Earls, MD, FAAP
Danette Glassy, MD, FAAP
Terri McFadden, MD, FAAP
Alan Mendelsohn, MD, FAAP
Seth Scholer, MD, FAAP
Jennifer Takagishi, MD, FAAP
Douglas Vanderbilt, MD, FAAP
Patricia Gail Williams, MD, FAAP

LIAISONS

Lynette M. Fraga, PhD – *Child Care Aware*
Abbey Alkon, RN, PNP, PhD, MPH – *National Association of Pediatric Nurse Practitioners*
Barbara U. Hamilton, MA – *Maternal and Child Health Bureau*
David Willis, MD, FAAP – *Maternal and Child Health Bureau*
Claire Lerner, LCSW – *Zero to Three*

STAFF

Charlotte Zia, MPH, CHES

COMMITTEE ON PSYCHOSOCIAL ASPECTS OF CHILD AND FAMILY HEALTH, 2015–2016

Michael Yogman, MD, FAAP, Chairperson
Nerissa Bauer, MD, MPH, FAAP
Thresia B Gambon, MD, FAAP
Arthur Lavin, MD, FAAP
Keith M. Lemmon, MD, FAAP
Gerri Mattson, MD, FAAP
Jason Richard Rafferty, MD, MPH, EdM
Lawrence Sagin Wissow, MD, MPH, FAAP

LIAISONS

Sharon Berry, PhD, LP – *Society of Pediatric Psychology*
Terry Carmichael, MSW – *National Association of Social Workers*
Edward Christophersen, PhD, FAAP – *Society of Pediatric Psychology*
Norah Johnson, PhD, RN, CPNP-BC – *National Association of Pediatric Nurse Practitioners*
Leonard Read Sulik, MD, FAAP – *American Academy of Child and Adolescent Psychiatry*

CONSULTANT

George J. Cohen, MD, FAAP

STAFF

Stephanie Domain, MS

SECTION ON DEVELOPMENTAL AND BEHAVIORAL PEDIATRICS EXECUTIVE COMMITTEE, 2015–2016

Nathan J. Blum, MD, FAAP, Chairperson
Michelle M. Macias, MD, FAAP, Immediate Past Chairperson

Nerissa S. Bauer, MD, MPH, FAAP
Carolyn Bridgemohan, MD, FAAP
Edward Goldson, MD, FAAP
Peter J. Smith, MD, MA, FAAP
Carol C. Weitzman, MD, FAAP
Stephen H. Contompasis, MD, FAAP, Web Site Editor
Damon Russell Korb, MD, FAAP, Discussion Board Moderator
Michael I. Reiff, MD, FAAP, Newsletter Editor
Robert G. Voigt, MD, FAAP, Program Chairperson

LIAISONS

Beth Ellen Davis, MD, MPH, FAAP, *Council on Children with Disabilities*
Pamela C. High, MD, MS, FAAP, *Society for Developmental and Behavioral Pediatrics*

STAFF

Linda Paul, MPH

ABBREVIATIONS

AAP: American Academy of Pediatrics
ADHD: attention-deficit/hyperactivity disorder
EBT: evidence-based treatment
IYS: Incredible Years Series
PCIT: Parent Child Interaction Therapy
SAMHSA: Substance Abuse and Mental Health Services Administration

---

REFERENCES

1. Egger HL, Angold A. Common emotional and behavioral disorders in preschool children: presentation, nosology, and epidemiology. *J Child Psychol Psychiatry.* 2006;47(3-4):313–337

2. Myers SM, Johnson CP; American Academy of Pediatrics Council on Children With Disabilities. Management of children with autism spectrum disorders. *Pediatrics.* 2007;120(5):1162–1182

3. Kim-Cohen J, Arseneault L, Caspi A, Tomás MP, Taylor A, Moffitt TE. Validity of DSM-IV conduct disorder in 41/2-5-year-old children: a longitudinal epidemiological study. *Am J Psychiatry.* 2005;162(6):1108–1117

4. Harvey EA, Youngwirth SD, Thakar DA, Errazuriz PA. Predicting attention-deficit/hyperactivity disorder and oppositional defiant disorder from preschool diagnostic assessments. *J Consult Clin Psychol.* 2009;77(2):349–354

5. Wilens TE, Biederman J, Brown S, et al. Psychiatric comorbidity and functioning in clinically referred preschool children and school-age youths with ADHD. *J Am Acad Child Adolesc Psychiatry.* 2002;41(3):262–268

6. Schwebel DC, Speltz ML, Jones K, Bardina P. Unintentional injury in preschool boys with and without early onset of disruptive behavior. *J Pediatr Psychol.* 2002;27(8):727–737

7. Pagliaccio D, Luby J, Gaffrey M, et al. Anomalous functional brain activation following negative mood induction in children with pre-school onset major depression. *Dev Cogn Neurosci.* 2012;2(2):256–267

8. Luby JL, Si X, Belden AC, Tandon M, Spitznagel E. Preschool depression: homotypic continuity and course over 24 months. *Arch Gen Psychiatry.* 2009;66(8):897–905

9. Briggs-Gowan MJ, Carter AS, Bosson-Heenan J, Guyer AE, Horwitz SM. Are infant-toddler social-emotional and behavioral problems transient? *J Am Acad Child Adolesc Psychiatry.* 2006;45(7):849–858

10. Briggs-Gowan MJ, Carter AS. Social-emotional screening status in early childhood predicts elementary school outcomes. *Pediatrics.* 2008;121(5):957–962

11. Lavigne JV, Arend R, Rosenbaum D, Binns HJ, Christoffel KK, Gibbons RD. Psychiatric disorders with onset in the preschool years: I. Stability of diagnoses. *J Am Acad Child Adolesc Psychiatry.* 1998;37(12):1246–1254

12. Leblanc N, Boivin M, Dionne G, et al. The development of hyperactive-impulsive behaviors during the preschool years: the predictive validity of parental assessments. *J Abnorm Child Psychol.* 2008;36(7):977–987

13. Gaffrey MS, Luby JL, Belden AC, Hirshberg JS, Volsch J, Barch DM. Association between depression severity and amygdala reactivity during sad face viewing in depressed preschoolers: an fMRI study. *J Affect Disord.* 2011;129(1-3):364–370

14. Wakschlag LS, Leventhal BL, Briggs-Gowan MJ, et al. Defining the "disruptive" in preschool behavior: what diagnostic observation can teach us. *Clin Child Fam Psychol Rev.* 2005;8(3):183–201

15. Luby JL, Mrakotsky C, Heffelfinger A, Brown K, Hessler M, Spitznagel E. Modification of DSM-IV criteria for depressed preschool children. *Am J Psychiatry.* 2003;160(6):1169–1172

16. Scheeringa MS, Zeanah CH, Myers L, Putnam F. Heart period and variability findings in preschool children with posttraumatic stress symptoms. *Biol Psychiatry.* 2004;55(7):685–691

17. Lahey BB, Applegate B. Validity of DSM-IV ADHD. *J Am Acad Child Adolesc Psychiatry.* 2001;40(5):502–504

18. Luby JL, Belden AC, Pautsch J, Si X, Spitznagel E. The clinical significance of preschool depression: impairment in functioning and clinical markers of the disorder. *J Affect Disord.* 2009;112(1-3):111–119

19. Tyrka AR, Burgers DE, Philip NS, Price LH, Carpenter LL. The neurobiological correlates of childhood adversity and implications for treatment. *Acta Psychiatr Scand.* 2013;128(6):434–447

20. Luking KR, Repovs G, Belden AC, et al. Functional connectivity of the amygdala in early-childhood-onset depression. *J Am Acad Child Adolesc Psychiatry.* 2011;50(10):1027–41.e3

21. Felitti VJ, Anda RF, Nordenberg D, et al. Relationship of childhood abuse and household dysfunction to many of the leading causes of death in adults. The Adverse Childhood Experiences (ACE) Study. *Am J Prev Med.* 1998;14(4):245–258

22. Lahey BB, Pelham WE, Loney J, et al. Three-year predictive validity of DSM-IV attention deficit hyperactivity disorder in children diagnosed at 4-6 years of age. *Am J Psychiatry.* 2004;161(11):2014–2020

23. Wakschlag LS, Leventhal BL, Thomas J, et al. Disruptive behavior disorders and ADHD in preschool children: Characterizing heterotypic continuities for a developmentally informed nosology for DSM-V. In: Rieger D, First MB, Narrow WE, eds. *Age and gender considerations in psychiatric diagnosis: A research agenda for DSM-V.* Arlington, VA: American Psychiatric Publishing, Inc.; 2007:243–258

24. Scheeringa MS. Post -Traumatic Stress Disorder. In: DelCarmen-Wiggins R, Carter A, eds. *Handbook of Infant, Toddler, and Preschool Mental Health Assessment USA.* Oxford, United Kingdom: Oxford Univeristy Press; 2004:377–397

25. Dong M, Giles WH, Felitti VJ, et al. Insights into causal pathways for ischemic heart disease: adverse childhood experiences study. *Circulation.* 2004;110(13):1761–1766

26. Shonkoff JP, Phillips D. *From neurons to neighborhoods: The science of early childhood development.* Washington, D.C.: National Academy Press; 2000

27. Garner AS, Shonkoff JP; Committee on Psychosocial Aspects of Child and Family Health; Committee on Early Childhood, Adoption, and Dependent Care; Section on Developmental and Behavioral Pediatrics. Early childhood adversity, toxic stress, and the role of the pediatrician: translating developmental science into lifelong health. *Pediatrics.* 2012;129(1). Available at: http://pediatrics.aappublications.org/content/129/1/e224

28. Committee On Child Health Financing. Scope of health care benefits for children from birth through age 26. *Pediatrics.* 2012;129(1):185–189

29. Weitzman C, Wegner L; American Academy of Pediatrics, Section on Developmental and Behavioral Pediatrics; Committee on Psychosocial Aspects of Child and Family Health; Council on Early Childhood; Society for Developmental and Behavioral Pediatrics. Promoting optimal development: screening for behavioral and emotional problems. *Pediatrics.* 2015;135(2):384–395

30. Mendelsohn AL, Valdez PT, Flynn V, et al. Use of videotaped interactions during pediatric well-child care: impact at 33 months on parenting and on child development. *J Dev Behav Pediatr.* 2007;28(3):206–212

31. Scheeringa MS, Salloum A, Arnberger RA, Weems CF, Amaya-Jackson L, Cohen JA. Feasibility and effectiveness of cognitive-behavioral therapy for posttraumatic stress disorder in preschool children: two case reports. *J Trauma Stress.* 2007;20(4):631–636

32. Sonuga-Barke EJ, Daley D, Thompson M, Laver-Bradbury C, Weeks A. Parent-based therapies for preschool attention-deficit/hyperactivity disorder: a randomized, controlled trial with a community sample. *J Am Acad Child Adolesc Psychiatry.* 2001;40(4):402–408

33. Gleason MM, Egger HL, Emslie GJ, et al. Psychopharmacological treatment for very young children: contexts and guidelines. *J Am Acad Child Adolesc Psychiatry.* 2007;46(12):1532–1572

34. Charach A, Dashti B, Carson P, et al; Agency for Healthcare Research and Quality. Attention deficit hyperactivity disorder: effectiveness of treatment in at-risk preschoolers; long-term effectiveness in all ages; and variability in prevalence, diagnosis, and treatment. *Comparitive Effectiveness Review.* 2011;44: AHRQ Publication No. 12-EHC003-EF. Available at: www.effectivehealthcare.ahrq.gov/ehc/products/191/818/CER44-ADHD_20111021.pdf. Accessed October 17, 2016

35. Thompson MJ, Laver-Bradbury C, Ayres M, et al. A small-scale randomized controlled trial of the revised new forest parenting programme for preschoolers with attention deficit hyperactivity disorder. *Eur Child Adolesc Psychiatry.* 2009;18(10):605–616

36. Riddle MA, Yershova K, Lazzaretto D, Paykina N, Yenokyan G, Greenhill L, et al The preschool attention-deficit/hyperactivity disorder treatment study (PATS) 6-year follow-up. *J Am Acad Child Adolesc Psychiatry.* 2013;52(3):264–278.e2

37. Hood KK, Eyberg SM. Outcomes of parent-child interaction therapy: mothers' reports of maintenance three to six years after treatment. *J Clin Child Adolesc Psychol.* 2003;32(3):419–429

38. Pediatric OCD Treatment Study (POTS) Team. Cognitive-behavior therapy, sertraline, and their combination for children and adolescents with obsessive-compulsive disorder: the Pediatric OCD Treatment Study (POTS) randomized controlled trial. *JAMA.* 2004;292(16):1969–1976

39. Wolraich M, Brown L, Brown RT, et al; Subcommittee on Attention-Deficit/Hyperactivity Disorder; Steering Committee on Quality Improvement and Management. ADHD: clinical practice guideline for the diagnosis, evaluation, and treatment of attention-deficit/hyperactivity disorder in children and adolescents. *Pediatrics.* 2011;128(5):1007–1022

40. Lieberman AF, Van Horn P, Ippen CG. Toward evidence-based treatment: child-parent psychotherapy with preschoolers exposed to marital violence. *J Am Acad Child Adolesc Psychiatry.* 2005;44(12):1241–1248

41. Fraiberg S, Adelson E, Shapiro V. Ghosts in the nursery. A psychoanalytic approach to the problems of impaired infant-mother relationships. *J Am Acad Child Psychiatry.* 1975;14(3):387–421

42. Cicchetti D, Rogosch FA, Toth SL, Sturge-Apple ML. Normalizing the development of cortisol regulation in maltreated infants through preventive interventions. *Dev Psychopathol.* 2011;23(3):789–800

43. Toth SL, Rogosch FA, Manly JT, Cicchetti D. The efficacy of toddler-parent psychotherapy to reorganize attachment in the young offspring of mothers with major depressive disorder: a randomized preventive trial. *J Consult Clin Psychol.* 2006;74(6):1006–1016

44. Lieberman AF, Weston DR, Pawl JH. Preventive intervention and outcome with anxiously attached dyads. *Child Dev.* 1991;62(1):199–209

45. Dozier M, Peloso E, Lewis E, Laurenceau JP, Levine S. Effects of an attachment-based intervention on the cortisol production of infants and toddlers in foster care. *Dev Psychopathol.* 2008;20(3):845–859

46. Bernard K, Dozier M, Bick J, Lewis-Morrarty E, Lindhiem O, Carlson E. Enhancing attachment organization among maltreated children: results of a randomized clinical trial. *Child Dev.* 2012;83(2):623–636

47. Fisher PA, Burraston B, Pears K. The early intervention foster care program: permanent placement outcomes from a randomized trial. *Child Maltreat.* 2005;10(1):61–71

48. Van Zeijl J, Mesman J, Van IJzendoorn MH, et al. Attachment-based intervention for enhancing sensitive discipline in mothers of 1- to 3-year-old children at risk for externalizing behavior problems: a randomized controlled trial. *J Consult Clin Psychol.* 2006;74(6):994–1005

49. Murray L, Cooper PJ, Wilson A, Romaniuk H. Controlled trial of the short- and long-term effect of psychological treatment of post-partum depression: 2. Impact on the mother-child relationship and child outcome. *Br J Psychiatry.* 2003;182(5):420–427

50. Gunlicks ML, Weissman MM. Change in child psychopathology with improvement in parental depression: a systematic review. *J Am Acad Child Adolesc Psychiatry.* 2008;47(4):379–389

51. Weissman MM, Pilowsky DJ, Wickramaratne PJ, et al; STAR*D-Child Team. Remissions in maternal depression and child psychopathology: a STAR*D-child report. *JAMA.* 2006;295(12):1389–1398

52. Beardslee WR, Ayoub C, Avery MW, Watts CL, O'Carroll KL. Family Connections: an approach for strengthening early care systems in facing depression and adversity. *Am J Orthopsychiatry.* 2010;80(4):482–495

53. Keenan K, Wakschlag LS. Can a valid diagnosis of disruptive behavior disorder be made in preschool children? *Am J Psychiatry.* 2002;159(3):351–358

54. SAMHSA. National registry of evidence-based programs and practices. Available at: http://www.samhsa.gov/nrepp. Accessed October 17, 2016

55. Bodenmann G, Cina A, Ledermann T, Sanders MR. The efficacy of the Triple P-Positive Parenting Program in improving parenting and child behavior: a comparison with two other treatment conditions. *Behav Res Ther.* 2008;46(4):411–427

56. Webster-Stratton CH, Reid MJ, Beauchaine T. Combining parent and child training for young children with ADHD. *J Clin Child Adolesc Psychol.* 2011;40(2):191–203

57. Abikoff HB, Thompson MJ, Laver-Bradbury C, et al. Parent training for preschool ADHD: A randomized controlled trial of specialized and generic programs. *J Child Psychol Psychiatry.* 2015;56(6):618–631

58. Thomas R, Zimmer-Gembeck MJ. Behavioral outcomes of Parent-Child Interaction Therapy and Triple P-Positive Parenting Program: a review and meta-analysis. *J Abnorm Child Psychol.* 2007;35(3):475–495

59. Sanders MR, Baker S, Turner KM. A randomized controlled trial evaluating the efficacy of Triple P Online with parents of children with early-onset conduct problems. *Behav Res Ther.* 2012;50(11):675–684

60. Bor W, Sanders MR, Markie-Dadds C. The effects of the Triple P-positive Parenting Program on preschool children with co-occurring disruptive behavior and attentional/hyperactive difficulties. *J Abnorm Child Psychol.* 2002;30(6):571–587

61. Markie-Dadds C, Sanders MR. Self-directed Triple P (Positive Parenting Program) for mothers with children at-risk of developing conduct problems. *Behav Cogn Psychother.* 2006;34(3):259–275

62. Comer JS, Puliafico AC, Aschenbrand SG, et al. A pilot feasibility evaluation of the CALM Program for anxiety disorders in early childhood. *J Anxiety Disord.* 2012;26(1):40–49

63. Hirshfeld-Becker DR, Masek B, Henin A, et al. Cognitive behavioral therapy for 4- to 7-year-old children with anxiety disorders: a randomized clinical trial. *J Consult Clin Psychol.* 2010;78:498–510

64. Matos M, Bauermeister JJ, Bernal G. Parent-child interaction therapy for Puerto Rican preschool children with ADHD and behavior problems: a pilot efficacy study. *Fam Process.* 2009;48(2):232–252

65. Fernandez MA, Butler AM, Eyberg SM. Treatment outcome for low socioeconomic status African American families in parent-child interaction therapy: A pilot study. *Child Fam Behav Ther.* 2011;33(1):32–48

66. Webster-Stratton C, Rinaldi J, Jamila MR. Long-term outcomes of Incredible Years parenting program: Predictors of adolescent adjustment. *Child Adolesc Ment Health.* 2011;16(1):38–46

67. Gridley N, Hutchings J, Baker-Henningham H. The Incredible Years Parent-Toddler Programme and parental language: a randomised controlled trial. *Child Care Health Dev.* 2015;41(1):103–111

68. Chaffin M, Funderburk B, Bard D, Valle LA, Gurwitch R. A combined motivation and parent-child interaction therapy package reduces child welfare recidivism in a randomized dismantling field trial. *J Consult Clin Psychol.* 2011;79(1):84–95

69. Forehand R, Parent J, Sonuga-Barke E, Peisch VD, Long N, Abikoff HB. Which type of parent training works best for preschoolers with comorbid ADHD and ODD? A secondary analysis of a randomized controlled trial comparing generic and specialized programs. *J Abnorm Child Psychol.* 2016;44(8):1503–1513

70. Cohen JA, Mannarino AP. A treatment outcome study for sexually abused preschool children: initial findings. *J Am Acad Child Adolesc Psychiatry.* 1996;35(1):42–50

71. Scheeringa MS, Weems CF, Cohen JA, Amaya-Jackson L, Guthrie D. Trauma-focused cognitive-behavioral therapy for posttraumatic stress disorder in three-through six year-old children: a randomized clinical trial. *J Child Psychol Psychiatry.* 2011;52(8):853–860

72. Cohen JA, Mannarino AP. A treatment study for sexually abused preschool children: outcome during a one-year follow-up. *J Am Acad Child Adolesc Psychiatry.* 1997;36(9):1228–1235

73. Lieberman AF, Ghosh Ippen C, VAN Horn P. Child-parent psychotherapy: 6-month follow-up of a randomized controlled trial. *J Am Acad Child Adolesc Psychiatry.* 2006;45(8):913–918

74. Luby J, Lenze S, Tillman R. A novel early intervention for preschool depression: findings from a pilot randomized controlled trial. *J Child Psychol Psychiatry.* 2012;53(3):313–322

75. Connolly SD, Bernstein GA; Work Group on Quality Issues. Practice parameter for the assessment and treatment of children and adolescents with anxiety disorders. *J Am Acad Child Adolesc Psychiatry.* 2007;46(2):267–283

76. Shepard SA, Dickstein S. Preventive intervention for early childhood behavioral problems: an ecological perspective. *Child Adolesc Psychiatr Clin N Am.* 2009;18(3):687–706

77. Nock MK, Ferriter C. Parent management of attendance and adherence in child and adolescent therapy: a conceptual and empirical review. *Clin Child Fam Psychol Rev.* 2005;8(2):149–166

78. Olfson M, Crystal S, Huang C, Gerhard T. Trends in antipsychotic drug use by very young, privately insured children. *J Am Acad Child Adolesc Psychiatry.* 2010;49(1):13–23

79. Wilson DO. Child's ordeal shows risks of psychosis drugs for young. *New York Times.* September 2, 2010:A1.

80. Zuvekas SH, Vitiello B, Norquist GS. Recent trends in stimulant medication use among U.S. children. *Am J Psychiatry.* 2006;163(4):579–585

81. Zito JM, Safer DJ, Valluri S, Gardner JF, Korelitz JJ, Mattison DR. Psychotherapeutic medication prevalence in Medicaid-insured preschoolers. *J Child Adolesc Psychopharmacol.* 2007;17(2):195–203

82. Cooper WO, Hickson GB, Fuchs C, Arbogast PG, Ray WA. New users of antipsychotic medications among children enrolled in TennCare. *Arch Pediatr Adolesc Med.* 2004;158(8):753–759

83. Fontanella CA, Hiance DL, Phillips GS, Bridge JA, Campo J. Trends in psychotropic medication utilization for medicaid-enrolled preschool children. *J Child Fam Stud.* 2014;23(4):617–631

84. Rappley MD, Mullan PB, Alvarez FJ, Eneli IU, Wang J, Gardiner JC. Diagnosis of attention-deficit/hyperactivity disorder and use of psychotropic medication in very young children. *Arch Pediatr Adolesc Med.* 1999;153(10):1039–1045

85. Rappley MD, Eneli IU, Mullan PB, et al. Patterns of psychotropic medication use in very young children with attention-deficit hyperactivity disorder. *J Dev Behav Pediatr.* 2002;23(1):23–30

86. Greenhill L, Kollins S, Abikoff H, et al. Efficacy and safety of immediate-release methylphenidate treatment for preschoolers with ADHD. *J Am Acad Child Adolesc Psychiatry.* 2006;45(11):1284–1293

87. Kratochvil CJ, Vaughan BS, Stoner JA, et al. A double-blind, placebo-controlled study of atomoxetine in young children with ADHD. *Pediatrics.* 2011;127(4). Available at: http://pediatrics.aappublications.org/content/127/4/e862

88. Egger H. A perilous disconnect: antipsychotic drug use in very young children. *J Am Acad Child Adolesc Psychiatry.* 2010;49(1):3–6

89. Correll CU, Carlson HE. Endocrine and metabolic adverse effects of psychotropic medications in children and adolescents. *J Am Acad Child Adolesc Psychiatry.* 2006;45(7):771–791

90. Luby J, Mrakotsky C, Stalets MM, et al. Risperidone in preschool children with autistic spectrum disorders: an investigation of safety and efficacy. *J Child Adolesc Psychopharmacol.* 2006;16(5):575–587

91. Horwitz SM, Leaf PJ, Leventhal JM. Identification of psychosocial problems in pediatric primary care: do family attitudes make a difference? *Arch Pediatr Adolesc Med.* 1998;152(4):367–371

92. Horwitz SM, Gary LC, Briggs-Gowan MJ, Carter AS; Do Needs Drive Services Use in Young Children. Do needs drive services use in young children? *Pediatrics.* 2003;112(6 Pt 1):1373–1378

93. Accreditation Council for Graduate Medical Education. ACGME program requirements for graduate medical education in Pediatrics. Available at: www.acgme.org/Portals/0/PFAssets/ProgramRequirements/320_pediatrics_2016.pdf. Accessed October 17, 2016

94. Committee on Psychosocial Aspects of Child and Family Health and Task Force on Mental Health. Policy statement--The future of pediatrics: mental health competencies for pediatric primary care. *Pediatrics.* 2009;124(1):410–421

95. Jensen PS, Goldman E, Offord D, et al. Overlooked and underserved: "action signs" for identifying children with unmet mental health needs. *Pediatrics.* 2011;128(5):970–979

96. Cohen J, Oser C, Quigley K Making it happen: overcoming barriers to

providing infant-early childhood mental health. Available at: www.zerotothree.org/resources/511-making-it-happen-overcoming-barriers-to-providing-infant-early-childhood-mental-health

97. Thomas CR, Holzer CE III. The continuing shortage of child and adolescent psychiatrists. *J Am Acad Child Adolesc Psychiatry.* 2006;45(9):1023–1031

98. Kautz C, Mauch D, Smith SA. *Reimbursement of Mental Health Services in Primary Care Settings.* Rockville, MD: Center for Mental Health Services, Substance Abuse and Mental Health Services Administration; 2008

99. The Lewin Group. *Accessing Children's Mental Health Services in Massachusetts: Workforce Capacity Assessment.* Boston, MA: Blue Cross; 2009

100. Jellinek M, Little M. Supporting child psychiatric services using current managed care approaches: you can't get there from here. *Arch Pediatr Adolesc Med.* 1998;152(4):321–326

101. Kelleher KJ, Campo JV, Gardner WP. Management of pediatric mental disorders in primary care: where are we now and where are we going? *Curr Opin Pediatr.* 2006;18(6):649–653

102. American Academy of Child and Adolescent Psychiatry Committee on Health Care Access and Economics Task Force on Mental Health. Improving mental health services in primary care: reducing administrative and financial barriers to access and collaboration. *Pediatrics.* 2009;123(4):1248–1251

103. Zero to Three. *Diagnostic Classification of Mental Health and Developmental Disorders in Infants and Young Children.* Washington, DC: Zero to Three; in press

104. dosReis S, Barksdale CL, Sherman A, Maloney K, Charach A. Stigmatizing experiences of parents of children with a new diagnosis of ADHD. *Psychiatric Services.* 2010;61(6):811–816

105. Harwood MD, O'Brien KA, Carter CG, Eyberg SM. Mental health services for preschool children in primary care: a survey of maternal attitudes and beliefs. *J Pediatr Psychol.* 2009;34(7):760–768

106. Pescosolido BA. Culture, children, and mental health treatment: special section on the national stigma study-children. *Psychiatr Serv.* 2007;58(5):611–612

107. Pescosolido BA, Jensen PS, Martin JK, Perry BL, Olafsdottir S, Fettes D. Public knowledge and assessment of child mental health problems: findings from the National Stigma Study-Children. *J Am Acad Child Adolesc Psychiatry.* 2008;47(3):339–349

108. Sayal K, Tischler V, Coope C, et al. Parental help-seeking in primary care for child and adolescent mental health concerns: qualitative study. *Br J Psychiatry.* 2010;197(6):476–481

109. Steele MM, Lochrie AS, Roberts MC. Physician identification and management of psychosocial problems in primary care. *J Clin Psychol Med Settings.* 2010;17(2):103–115

110. American Academy of Pediatrics Council on Children with Disabilities. Care coordination in the medical home: integrating health and related systems of care for children with special health care needs. *Pediatrics.* 2005;116(5):1238–1244

111. Wissow L, Anthony B, Brown J, et al. A common factors approach to improving the mental health capacity of pediatric primary care. *Adm Policy Ment Health.* 2008;35(4):305–318

112. Foy JM, Kelleher KJ, Laraque D; American Academy of Pediatrics Task Force on Mental Health. Enhancing pediatric mental health care: strategies for preparing a primary care practice. *Pediatrics.* 2010;125(suppl 3):S87–S108

113. Berkovits MD, O'Brien KA, Carter CG, Eyberg SM. Early identification and intervention for behavior problems in primary care: a comparison of two abbreviated versions of parent-child interaction therapy. *Behav Ther.* 2010;41(3):375–387

114. Perrin EC, Sheldrick RC, McMenamy JM, Henson BS, Carter AS. Improving parenting skills for families of young children in pediatric settings: a randomized clinical trial. *JAMA Pediatr.* 2014;168(1):16–24

115. Hilt RJ, McDonell MG, Thompson J, et al. Telephone consultation assisting primary care child mental health. In: *55th National Meeting of the American Academy of Child and Adolescent Psychiatry;* October 28–November 2, 2008; Chicago, IL.

116. Kolko DJ, Campo JV, Kilbourne AM, Kelleher K. Doctor-office collaborative care for pediatric behavioral problems: a preliminary clinical trial. *Arch Pediatr Adolesc Med.* 2012;166(3):224–231

117. Fox RA, Keller KM, Grede PL, Bartosz AM. A mental health clinic for toddlers with developmental delays and behavior problems. *Res Dev Disabil.* 2007;28(2):119–129

Bone Densitometry in Children and Adolescents

• *Clinical Report*

CLINICAL REPORT Guidance for the Clinician in Rendering Pediatric Care

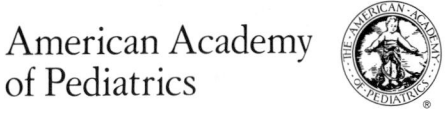

American Academy
of Pediatrics

DEDICATED TO THE HEALTH OF ALL CHILDREN™

Bone Densitometry in Children and Adolescents

Laura K. Bachrach, MD, Catherine M. Gordon, MD, MS, SECTION ON ENDOCRINOLOGY

abstract

Concerns about bone health and potential fragility in children and adolescents have led to a high interest in bone densitometry. Pediatric patients with genetic and acquired chronic diseases, immobility, and inadequate nutrition may fail to achieve expected gains in bone size, mass, and strength, leaving them vulnerable to fracture. In older adults, bone densitometry has been shown to predict fracture risk and reflect response to therapy. The role of densitometry in the management of children at risk of bone fragility is less clear. This clinical report summarizes current knowledge about bone densitometry in the pediatric population, including indications for its use, interpretation of results, and risks and costs. The report emphasizes updated consensus statements generated at the 2013 Pediatric Position Development Conference of the International Society of Clinical Densitometry by an international panel of bone experts. Some of these recommendations are evidence-based, whereas others reflect expert opinion, because data are sparse on many topics. The statements from this and other expert panels provide general guidance to the pediatrician, but decisions about ordering and interpreting bone densitometry still require clinical judgment. The interpretation of bone densitometry results in children differs from that in older adults. The terms "osteopenia" and "osteoporosis" based on bone densitometry findings alone should not be used in younger patients; instead, bone mineral content or density that falls >2 SDs below expected is labeled "low for age." Pediatric osteoporosis is defined by the Pediatric Position Development Conference by using 1 of the following criteria: ≥1 vertebral fractures occurring in the absence of local disease or high-energy trauma (without or with densitometry measurements) or low bone density for age and a significant fracture history (defined as ≥2 long bone fractures before 10 years of age or ≥3 long bone fractures before 19 years of age). Ongoing research will help define the indications and best methods for assessing bone strength in children and the clinical factors that contribute to fracture risk. The Pediatric Endocrine Society affirms the educational value of this publication.

DOI: 10.1542/peds.2016-2398

PEDIATRICS (ISSN Numbers: Print, 0031-4005; Online, 1098-4275).

FINANCIAL DISCLOSURE: The authors have indicated they do not have a financial relationship relevant to this article to disclose.

FUNDING: No external funding.

POTENTIAL CONFLICT OF INTEREST: The authors have indicated they have no potential conflicts of interest to disclose.

To cite: Bachrach LK, Gordon CM, AAP SECTION ON ENDOCRINOLOGY. Bone Densitometry in Children and Adolescents. *Pediatrics*. 2016;138(4):e20162398

INTRODUCTION

Threats to bone health are increasingly a pediatric concern. Genetic or acquired disorders can compromise gains in bone quantity and quality, leading to skeletal fragility early in life.[1] Recurrent fractures in otherwise healthy children may also indicate underlying bone fragility.[2-5] Children with forearm fractures have been shown to have lower bone mass, a greater percentage of body fat, and less calcium intake than their peers without a history of fracture.[3,4] The documented increase of 35% to 65% in childhood fractures over the past 4 decades has raised concern that current lifestyles are compromising early bone health.[5] Vitamin D insufficiency and deficiency are widespread, calcium intake often falls below recommended levels, and physical inactivity is common among American youth, all of which may increase a child's fracture risk.[6,7] These observations have led to greater demands for diagnostic and therapeutic tools to address bone fragility in children and adolescents. The efficacy, cost-effectiveness, and safety of pharmacologic agents used to treat osteoporosis in older patients have not been fully established in pediatric patients. The limited treatment options make it all the more important to predict accurately who will have fractures and who might recover without drug therapy. Bone densitometry is a valuable part of a comprehensive bone health assessment. Guidelines for densitometry were updated in 2013 by a group of pediatric bone experts at the Pediatric Position Development Conference (PDC) of the International Society of Clinical Densitometry.[8] The report by the PDC reviewed current bone densitometry methods, indications for ordering densitometry, and the role for densitometry in choosing and monitoring therapy. The Pediatric

Endocrine Society affirms the educational value of this publication.

BONE DENSITOMETRY METHODS

The pediatric skeleton can be assessed by using dual-energy radiograph absorptiometry (DXA), quantitative computed tomography (QCT), peripheral QCT (pQCT), high-resolution pQCT (HR-pQCT), quantitative ultrasonography, MRI, or plain films (radiogrammetry). Each modality offers distinct advantages and disadvantages, as previously reviewed.[9] DXA remains the preferred method for clinical measurements of bone density in children because of its availability, reproducibility, speed, low exposure to ionizing radiation, and robust pediatric reference data.[10] Three-dimensional densitometry methods (QCT, pQCT, HR-pQCT, and MRI) offer valuable insights into volumetric bone mineral density (BMD) as well as micro- and macroarchitecture. These tools may provide more information about bone strength and fracture risk than traditional DXA measures, but their use in clinical practice is limited in large part by the lack of standardized scanning protocols and pediatric normative data.[8]

FOR WHOM SHOULD BONE DENSITOMETRY BE CONSIDERED?

The general goals of bone densitometry are to identify patients at greatest risk of skeletal fragility fractures, to guide decisions regarding treatment, and to monitor responses to therapy. Skeletal assessments have been recommended for children with recurrent fractures, bone pain, bone deformities, or "osteopenia" (a term describing the appearance of "washed out" bones) on standard radiographs or to monitor therapy.[8,11,12] Details about the number of fractures and impacts causing them should guide the decision of whether bone

densitometry is indicated. Most concerning are low-impact fractures occurring from a standing height or less. Specific recommendations have been proposed for monitoring bone health in cystic fibrosis[13] and childhood cancer.[14] For example, a baseline DXA is recommended by 18 years of age or 2 years after the end of chemotherapy (for cancer survivors) but earlier in patients with more severe disease, low body weight, chronic glucocorticoid therapy, delayed puberty, gonadal failure, or a history of fracture. Another clinical scenario in which a DXA assessment is warranted is in female adolescents with nutritional concerns (eg, related to an eating disorder and/or excessive exercise), with scans recommended after 6 or more months of amenorrhea.

The most rigorous and comprehensive recommendations related to bone densitometry were developed by the PDC after extensive analysis of all relevant literature.[8] The PDC guidelines identify a list of the primary and secondary disorders that have been associated with low bone mass and increased fracture risk (Table 1). PDC guidelines recommend that the initial densitometry examination be performed when the patient may benefit from intervention and when the results of densitometry would influence management.[8] These parameters provide general guidance for the pediatrician and may help to secure payment for densitometry from insurance providers.

Beyond these guidelines, the decision to order bone densitometry in an individual patient requires clinical judgment. The risk of bone fragility is influenced by the age of onset and severity of any underlying disorder, associated risk factors such as poor nutrition or inactivity, and exposure to irradiation or to potentially bone-toxic drugs (eg, glucocorticoids, methotrexate, or anticonvulsants). A family history

TABLE 1 Diseases or Therapies That May Affect the Skeleton

Primary bone disorders
   o Idiopathic juvenile osteoporosis
   o Osteogenesis imperfecta
Potential secondary bone diseases
   o Chronic inflammatory disorders
      - Inflammatory bowel disease
      - Juvenile idiopathic arthritis
      - Celiac disease
      - Cystic fibrosis
   o Chronic immobilization
      - Cerebral palsy
      - Myopathic disease
      - Epidermolysis bullosa
   o Endocrine disturbance
      - Turner syndrome
      - Anorexia nervosa
      - Type 1 diabetes
   o Cancer and therapies with adverse effects on bone health
      - Acute lymphoblastic leukemia
      - Chemotherapy for childhood cancer
      - Transplantation (nonrenal)
   o Hematologic disorders
      - Thalassemia
      - Sickle cell disease
   o Genetic disorders
      - Ehlers Danlos syndrome
      - Galactosemia
      - Marfan syndrome

Adapted from Bishop et al.[15] These are among conditions for which consideration of DXA screening and other diagnostic testing for bone health is warranted.

of bone fragility is relevant, because an estimated 60% to 80% of the variability in bone mass between individuals is determined by genetic factors.[6] This history is best assessed by asking about recurrent fractures or hip fractures in family members. The decision to evaluate an otherwise healthy child with a history of fractures will depend on the number of broken bones and the intensity of the trauma causing the injury. Low-trauma fractures are defined as those occurring from a standing height or less. A final consideration before ordering DXA scans should be how the results will influence patient management. For example, it may not be helpful to document that BMD is low for age in a child with cerebral palsy if the child has not had a fracture, because low BMD alone is not considered an indication for bisphosphonate therapy.[8] Finally, it is important to consider whether the patient can

remain still for the DXA without sedation.

ORDERING DXA FOR CHILDREN AND ADOLESCENTS

The preferred skeletal sites for DXA measurements in children are lumbar spine (L1–4) and total body, not including the head.[10] The cranium should be excluded from the total body scan analysis, because the head constitutes a large portion of the total body bone mass but changes little with growth, activity, or disease; inclusion of the skull potentially masks gains or losses at other skeletal sites.[16] For children younger than 5 years old, the spine bone mineral content (BMC) and BMD can be measured; whole-body measurements are feasible only for those aged 3 years or older. DXA measurements of the hip region (total hip or femoral neck) are not as reliable in younger patients (<13 years) because of difficulties in

identifying the bony landmarks for this region of interest.

Scans of alternative regions of interest are recommended in special cases. DXA assessments of the lateral distal femur can be valuable in children with immobilization disorders and in those with contractures who cannot be positioned properly for spine or whole-body studies.[17] The distal radius can be measured in patients who exceed the weight limit for the DXA table or those who cannot transfer onto the table because of a mobilization disorder. Scanning of these alternate skeletal sites also may be necessary in patients with metal hardware (eg, rodding for scoliosis) in the standard regions of interest.

A vertebral fracture that occurs without major trauma is an important indication of abnormal bone fragility.[8] Because these fractures can be asymptomatic, some type of imaging is needed to rule out vertebral fractures in patients at high risk, such as those receiving long-term glucocorticoid therapy. In the past, a lateral thoracolumbar radiograph has been used to assess for loss of vertebral height.[18] Alternatively, vertebral fracture analysis (VFA) by DXA has been used with far less radiation than conventional radiography. Studies using older software found that DXA VFA had lower diagnostic accuracy compared with lateral spine radiography in children.[19] Newer VFA software may provide sufficient image quality to screen for spine fractures with the use of DXA.[20]

INTERPRETATION OF DXA RESULTS

Bone mass, as measured by DXA, is reported as BMC (g) or areal BMD (g/cm^2). These values are compared with reference values from healthy youth of similar age, sex, and race/ethnicity to calculate a z score, the number of SDs from the expected mean. Abundant pediatric reference data are now available for children and teenagers but not for infants.[10] It is essential to select norms collected by using equipment from the same manufacturer as that used for the patient because of systematic differences in software.[10] Peak bone mass is achieved in the second or third decade, depending on the skeletal site.[21] Therefore, T-scores (which compare the patient's BMD with that of a healthy young adult) should not be used before 20 years of age. Unfortunately, some older software packages from DXA manufacturers automatically generate a T-score, even in younger subjects. The ordering physician must be careful to not use T-scores when interpreting DXA results.

The appropriate interpretation of DXA results may require more than the calculation of z scores. Children with chronic illness often have delayed growth and pubertal development, factors that contribute to a low bone mass for age or sex. BMD, as measured by DXA, corrects bone mineral for the area (height and width) but not for the volume (height, width, and thickness) of bone. For this reason, if 2 individuals with identical "true" volumetric bone density are compared, the shorter person will have a lower BMD than the taller one.[9,22] Similarly, a child with delayed puberty will not have had the gains in bone size, geometry, and density that occur with sex steroid exposure. Controversy persists about the optimal method to adjust for variations in bone size, body composition, and maturity as well as the criteria by which the "best method" is defined; ideally, the adjustment method would prove to be a stronger predictor of fracture.[22]

The PDC guidelines recommend that BMD in children with delayed growth or puberty be adjusted for height or height age or compared with reference data with age-, sex-, and height-specific z scores.[10] DXA

reference data corrected for all these variables have been published.[23]

The terms "osteopenia" and "osteoporosis" are used in older adults to describe lesser or greater deficits in bone mass. These terms should not be used to describe densitometry findings in pediatric patients. Instead, a BMC or BMD z score that is >2 SDs below expected (< –2.0) is referred to as "low for age."[10] The following criteria for osteoporosis in a pediatric patient were agreed on in the 2013 PDC guidelines[8]:

- one or more vertebral fractures occurring in the absence of local disease or high-energy trauma (measuring BMD can add to the assessment of these patients but is not required as a diagnostic criterion); or

- low bone density (BMC or areal BMD z scores < –2.0) and a significant fracture history (2 or more long bone fractures before 10 years of age or 3 or more long bone fractures before 19 years of age).

Last, it is important to recognize that there are certain diseases in pediatrics (eg, end-stage renal disease and spinal vertebral fractures) in which DXA measures do not accurately reflect fracture risk or bone health.[10]

INTERPRETING LONGITUDINAL DATA

Repeat DXA studies are performed to monitor the skeletal response to ongoing illness, to recovery from illness, or to bone-active therapies. Repeat measurements must be made on densitometry equipment from the same manufacturer with the use of the same software to avoid variability attributable to software programs alone. For a change in BMD to be technically meaningful, it must exceed the variability that is observed when DXA measurements are repeated in the same individual. The "least significant change" refers

to the smallest percentage difference in measurements that exceeds the variability or "noise" from repeated measurements.[24] In densitometry centers that are able to perform a precision study, a least significant change of 3% or less usually can be achieved.[24] However, some hospital radiation safety committees prohibit DXA centers from carrying out these protocols. It should also be recognized that interval growth changes and accompanying increases in bone size make it more difficult to differentiate true increases in density from changes in areal BMD that are related to growth. Therefore, careful interpretation by an expert in pediatric densitometry is needed.

Longitudinal changes in bone densitometry must also take into account interval changes in growth and maturity. To assess whether observed gains in bone mass and size are appropriate for age and pubertal stage requires thoughtful assessment of z scores, as described previously. The recommended interval between repeat densitometry studies will depend on the progression of disease or the type of intervention being used. The minimal interval between scans generally is 6 months,[10] but a year often is more appropriate in clinical practice to allow for the detection of meaningful changes.

ABILITY OF BONE DENSITOMETRY TO PREDICT FRACTURES

Low BMD is a sufficiently powerful predictor of fracture in older adults that it has been used as a diagnostic criterion for "osteoporosis" in older individuals.[25] Reduced BMD also is associated with increased fracture risk in children and teenagers, but the data are not sufficient to establish the diagnosis of osteoporosis on the basis of bone densitometry criteria alone.[10,26] In studies in otherwise healthy youth, children with a history of fracture have been shown to have reduced spine or whole-body bone mass or smaller bone area for height.[4,26] One study showed diminished bone density (by DXA) and bone strength (by HR-pQCT) in women and men who sustained a mild trauma distal forearm fracture during childhood.[27]

Less is known about the relationship between low bone mass and fracture risk in children with chronic illness, because studies in these patient populations have been limited to smaller cohorts with varying diagnoses and risk factors for poor bone health. The most common site of fractures in these children may not be the forearm; lower extremity fractures are common in immobilized children,[28,29] and spine fractures are more common in young patients with childhood leukemia, osteogenesis imperfecta, or exposure to glucocorticoids.[30,31]

Clinical variables have been shown to influence the risk of fractures in older adults independent of their bone mass by densitometry. Age, weight, alcohol or smoking history, glucocorticoid use, and a history of previous fracture are used to calculate the absolute fracture risk.[25] The contribution of these or other clinical variables to fracture risk in children has not been established. However, bone densitometry by DXA is only part of a comprehensive skeletal health screening that includes review of nutrition, physical activity, pubertal stage, disease severity, patient and family fracture history, and medication exposure. A child with low bone mass for age or one with a significant fracture history would likely benefit from evaluation by a provider with expertise in bone (eg, a pediatric endocrinologist, nephrologist, geneticist, neurologist, or rheumatologist).[1,6,26,32]

RISKS AND COSTS OF DENSITOMETRY

Exposure to the very low doses of ionizing radiation with DXA poses no known health risk. The estimated

5 to 6 μSv of radiation exposure from a spine and whole-body DXA scan is far less than the 80 μSv accumulated during a round-trip transatlantic flight.[33] More concerning is the potential risk of misdiagnosis if DXA data are not interpreted by skilled professionals at pediatric densitometry centers. An important study revealed errors in 88% of the scans from children referred for an osteoporosis intervention study; 62% of the errors involved a misdiagnosis of osteoporosis on the basis of inappropriate use of a T-score.[34] Errors in interpreting DXA results generate considerable parental concern and can result in costly and unnecessary use of pharmacologic agents and restrictions on physical activity.

THERAPY FOR CHILDHOOD SKELETAL FRAGILITY

Treatment options for children with low bone mass and fractures are more limited than in adults, underscoring the importance of accurate skeletal assessments.[35] General measures to address skeletal risk factors are safe and appropriate first steps for all patients. All strategies to optimize bone health should be considered.[36] Calcium intake should meet current recommended daily intake of 500 mg for children 1 to 3 years of age, 800 mg for children 4 to 8 years of age, and 1300 mg for children and adolescents 9 to 18 years of age.[7,36,37] Routine screening of vitamin D levels is not indicated in healthy youth. However, the adequacy of total body vitamin D stores should be assessed in youth at risk of bone fragility by measuring by measuring serum concentrations of 25-hydroxyvitamin D. Concentrations of at least 20 ng/mL (50 nmol/L) have been recommended for healthy children, but some experts aim for a serum 25-hydroxyvitamin D concentration >30 ng/mL in populations at increased risk of fracture.[7,36] Weight-bearing activity should be encouraged, and even short periods of high-intensity

exercise (eg, jumping 10 minutes/ day, 3 times/week) have produced measurable gains in bone mass.[38] The childhood and teenage years appear to be of particular importance for bone accretion. The Iowa Bone Development Study (a prospective cohort study) showed 10% to 16% greater hip BMC and 8% greater hip areal BMD in participants who accumulated the greatest amount of activity from childhood through adolescence (12-year follow-up).[39] For patients with limited mobility, reducing immobility through physical therapy[40] or the use of vibrating platforms can be helpful.[29,41] Reducing inflammation, undernutrition, or hormone imbalances also is necessary. In children with inflammatory bowel disease, 1 study showed that a reduction in inflammation through the use of anti–tumor necrosis factor α therapy led to appreciable differences in bone structure and density.[42]

If general measures fail to prevent further bone loss and fracture, pharmacologic therapy may be considered. None of the drugs used to treat bone fragility in the elderly have yet been approved by the Food and Drug Administration for pediatric use.[35,43] Nevertheless, therapy with bisphosphonates is considered reasonable for children with moderate to severe osteogenesis imperfecta (2 or more fractures in a year or vertebral compression fractures).[44] For secondary osteoporosis attributable to chronic disease, bisphosphonates may be used on a compassionate basis to treat low-trauma fractures of the spine or extremities.[45] When pharmacologic therapy is considered, referral to a specialist with expertise in pediatric bone disorders is advised.

SUMMARY

DXA has been established as a valuable tool as part of a comprehensive skeletal assessment in children and teenagers. Normative data are accumulating for the use of this tool in infants, but they have not yet been fully integrated into clinical practice.[46] Acquiring and interpreting densitometry data in younger patients remain challenging and should be performed in consultation with experts. Panels of pediatric experts have set standards for when and how to perform DXAs on the basis of the best-available data; experts can be located through the International Society for Clinical Densitometry (www.iscd.org).[8,10] Ongoing research will serve to refine the best modalities for assessing bone strength in children and to determine the key clinical variables that influence fracture risk independent of bone.

LEAD AUTHORS

Laura K. Bachrach, MD
Catherine M. Gordon, MD, MSc

SECTION ON ENDOCRINOLOGY EXECUTIVE COMMITTEE, 2015–2016

Irene N. Sills, MD, Chairperson
Jane L. Lynch, MD, Chairperson-Elect
Samuel J. Casella, MD, MSc
Linda A. DiMeglio, MD, MPH
Jose L. Gonzalez, MD, JD, MSEd
Kupper Wintergerst, MD
Paul B. Kaplowitz, MD, PhD, Immediate Past Chairperson

STAFF

Laura N. Laskosz, MPH

ABBREVIATIONS

BMC: bone mineral content
BMD: bone mineral density
DXA: dual-energy radiograph absorptiometry
HR-pQCT: high-resolution peripheral quantitative computed tomography
PDC: Pediatric Position Development Conference
pQCT: peripheral quantitative computed tomography
QCT: quantitative computed tomography
VFA: vertebral fracture analysis

REFERENCES

1. Boyce AM, Gafni RI. Approach to the child with fractures. *J Clin Endocrinol Metab.* 2011;96(7):1943–1952

2. Cooper C, Dennison EM, Leufkens HG, Bishop N, van Staa TP. Epidemiology of childhood fractures in Britain: a study using the general practice research database. *J Bone Miner Res.* 2004;19(12):1976–1981

3. Goulding A, Grant AM, Williams SM. Bone and body composition of children and adolescents with repeated forearm fractures. *J Bone Miner Res.* 2005;20(12):2090–2096

4. Clark EM, Ness AR, Bishop NJ, Tobias JH. Association between bone mass and fractures in children: a prospective cohort study. *J Bone Miner Res.* 2006;21(9):1489–1495

5. Khosla S, Melton LJ III, Dekutoski MB, Achenbach SJ, Oberg AL, Riggs BL. Incidence of childhood distal forearm fractures over 30 years: a population-based study. *JAMA.* 2003;290(11):1479–1485

6. Rizzoli R, Bianchi ML, Garabédian M, McKay HA, Moreno LA. Maximizing bone mineral mass gain during growth for the prevention of fractures in the adolescents and the elderly. *Bone.* 2010;46(2):294–305

7. Simoneau T, Gordon CM. Vitamin D: recent recommendations and discoveries. *Adolesc Med State Art Rev.* 2014;25(2):239–250

8. Gordon CM, Leonard MB, Zemel BS; International Society for Clinical Densitometry. 2013 Pediatric Position Development Conference: executive summary and reflections. *J Clin Densitom.* 2014;17(2):219–224

9. Specker BL, Schoenau E. Quantitative bone analysis in children: current methods and recommendations. *J Pediatr.* 2005;146(6):726–731

10. Crabtree NJ, Arabi A, Bachrach LK, et al; International Society for Clinical Densitometry. Dual-energy X-ray absorptiometry interpretation and reporting in children and adolescents: the revised 2013 ISCD Pediatric Official Positions. *J Clin Densitom.* 2014;17(2):225–242

11. Fewtrell MS; British Paediatric and Adolescent Bone Group. Bone densitometry in children assessed by dual x ray absorptiometry: uses and pitfalls. *Arch Dis Child.* 2003;88(9):795–798

12. Adams J, Shaw N, eds. *A Practical Guide to Bone Densitometry in Children.* Camerton,Bath, United Kingdom: National Osteoporosis Society; 2004

13. Aris RM, Merkel PA, Bachrach LK, et al. Guide to bone health and disease in cystic fibrosis. *J Clin Endocrinol Metab.* 2005;90(3):1888–1896

14. Wasilewski-Masker K, Kaste SC, Hudson MM, Esiashvili N, Mattano LA, Meacham LR. Bone mineral density deficits in survivors of childhood cancer: long-term follow-up guidelines and review of the literature. *Pediatrics.* 2008;121(3). Available at: www.pediatrics.org/cgi/content/full/121/3/e705

15. Bishop N, Braillon P, Burnham J, et al. Dual-energy X-ray aborptiometry assessment in children and adolescents with diseases that may affect the skeleton: the 2007 ISCD pediatric official positions. *J Clin Densitom.* 2008;11(1):29–42

16. Taylor A, Konrad PT, Norman ME, Harcke HT. Total body bone mineral density in young children: influence of head bone mineral density. *J Bone Miner Res.* 1997;12(4):652–655

17. Zemel BS, Stallings VA, Leonard MB, et al. Revised pediatric reference data for the lateral distal femur measured by Hologic Discovery/Delphi dual-energy X-ray absorptiometry. *J Clin Densitom.* 2009;12(2):207–218

18. Genant HK, Wu CY, van Kuijk C, Nevitt MC. Vertebral fracture assessment using a semiquantitative technique. *J Bone Miner Res.* 1993;8(9):1137–1148

19. Mäyränpää MK, Helenius I, Valta H, Mäyränpää MI, Toiviainen-Salo S, Mäkitie O. Bone densitometry in the diagnosis of vertebral fractures in children: accuracy of vertebral fracture assessment. *Bone.* 2007;41(3):353–359

20. Divasta AD, Feldman HA, Gordon CM. Vertebral fracture assessment in adolescents and young women with anorexia nervosa: a case series. *J Clin Densitom.* 2014;17(1):207–211

21. Baxter-Jones AD, Faulkner RA, Forwood MR, Mirwald RL, Bailey DA. Bone mineral accrual from 8 to 30 years of age: an estimation of peak bone mass. *J Bone Miner Res.* 2011;26(8):1729–1739

22. Bachrach LK. Osteoporosis in children: still a diagnostic challenge. *J Clin Endocrinol Metab.* 2007;92(6):2030–2032

23. Zemel BS, Leonard MB, Kelly A, et al. Height adjustment in assessing dual energy X-ray absorptiometry measurements of bone mass and density in children. *J Clin Endocrinol Metab.* 2010;95(3):1265–1273

24. Shepherd JA, Wang L, Fan B, et al. Optimal monitoring time interval between DXA measures in children. *J Bone Miner Res.* 2011;26(11):2745–2752

25. Kanis JA, Oden A, Johnell O, et al. The use of clinical risk factors enhances the performance of BMD in the prediction of hip and osteoporotic fractures in men and women. *Osteoporos Int.* 2007;18(8):1033–1046

26. Bishop N, Arundel P, Clark E, et al; International Society of Clinical Densitometry. Fracture prediction and the definition of osteoporosis in children and adolescents: the ISCD 2013 pediatric official positions. *J Clin Densitom.* 2014;17(2):275–280

27. Farr JN, Khosla S, Achenbach SJ, et al. Diminished bone strength is observed in adult women and men who sustained a mild trauma distal forearm fracture during childhood. *J Bone Miner Res.* 2014;29(10):2193–2202

28. Henderson RC, Lark RK, Gurka MJ, et al. Bone density and metabolism in children and adolescents with moderate to severe cerebral palsy. *Pediatrics.* 2002;110(1 pt 1):e5

29. Mughal MZ. Fractures in children with cerebral palsy. *Curr Osteoporos Rep.* 2014;12(3):313–318

30. Halton J, Gaboury I, Grant R, et al; Canadian STOPP Consortium. Advanced vertebral fracture among newly diagnosed children with acute lymphoblastic leukemia: results of the Canadian Steroid-Associated Osteoporosis in the Pediatric Population (STOPP) research program. *J Bone Miner Res.* 2009;24(7):1326–1334

31. Cummings EA, Ma J, Fernandez CV, et al; Canadian STOPP Consortium (National Pediatric Bone Health Working Group). Incident vertebral fractures in children with leukemia during the four years following diagnosis. *J Clin Endocrinol Metab.* 2015;100(9):3408–3417

32. Ma NS, Gordon CM. Pediatric osteoporosis: where are we now? *J Pediatr.* 2012;161(6):983–990

33. Lewis MK, Blake GM, Fogelman I. Patient dose in dual X-ray absorptiometry. *Osteoporos Int.* 1994;4(1):11–15

34. Gafni RI, Baron J. Overdiagnosis of osteoporosis in children due to misinterpretation of dual-energy X-ray absorptiometry (DEXA). *J Pediatr.* 2004;144(2):253–257

35. Bachrach LK. Diagnosis and treatment of pediatric osteoporosis. *Curr Opin Endocrinol Diabetes Obes.* 2014;21(6):454–460

36. Golden NH, Abrams SA; Committee on Nutrition. Optimizing bone health in children and adolescents. *Pediatrics.* 2014;134(4):e1229–e1243

37. American Academy of Pediatrics. Dietary Reference Intakes for calcium and vitamin D [statement of endorsement]. *Pediatrics.* 2012;130(5). Available at: www.pediatrics.org/cgi/content/full/130/5/e1424

38. Tan VPS, Macdonald HM, Kim S, et al. Influence of physical activity on bone strength in children and adolescents: a systematic review and narrative synthesis. *J Bone Miner Res.* 2014;29(10):2161–2181

39. Janz KF, Letuchy EM, Burns TL, Eichenberger Gilmore JM, Torner JC, Levy SM. Objectively measured physical activity trajectories predict adolescent bone strength: Iowa Bone Development Study. *Br J Sports Med.* 2014;48(13):1032–1036

40. Chad KE, Bailey DA, McKay HA, Zello GA, Snyder RE. The effect of a weight-bearing physical activity program on bone mineral content and estimated volumetric density in children with spastic cerebral palsy. *J Pediatr.* 1999;135(1):115–117

41. Ward K, Alsop C, Caulton J, Rubin C, Adams J, Mughal Z. Low magnitude mechanical loading is osteogenic in children with disabling conditions. *J Bone Miner Res.* 2004;19(3):360–369

42. Griffin LM, Thayu M, Baldassano RN, et al. Improvements in bone density and structure during anti-TNF-α therapy in pediatric Crohn's disease. *J Clin Endocrinol Metab.* 2015;100(7):2630–2639

43. Bachrach LK, Ward LM. Bisphophonate use in childhood osteoporosis. *J Clin Endocrinol Metab.* 2009;94(2):400–409

44. Rauch F, Glorieux FH. Clinical review 1: bisphosphonate treatment in osteogenesis imperfecta: which drug, for whom, for how long? *Ann Med.* 2005;37(4):295–302

45. Ward L, Tricco AC, Phuong P, et al. Bisphosphonate therapy for children and adolescents with secondary osteoporosis [review]. *Cochrane Database Syst Rev.* 2007;4:CD005324

46. Kalkwarf HJ, Abrams SA, DiMeglio LA, Koo WW, Specker BL, Weiler H; International Society for Clinial Densitometry. Bone densitometry in infants and young children: the 2013 ISCD pediatric official positions. *J Clin Densitom.* 2014;17(2):243–257

Children and Adolescents and Digital Media

. . . .

- *Technical Report*

TECHNICAL REPORT

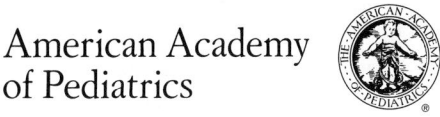

Children and Adolescents and Digital Media

Yolanda (Linda) Reid Chassiakos, MD, FAAP, Jenny Radesky, MD, FAAP, Dimitri Christakis, MD, FAAP, Megan A. Moreno, MD, MSEd, MPH, FAAP, Corinn Cross, MD, FAAP, COUNCIL ON COMMUNICATIONS AND MEDIA

abstract

Today's children and adolescents are immersed in both traditional and new forms of digital media. Research on traditional media, such as television, has identified health concerns and negative outcomes that correlate with the duration and content of viewing. Over the past decade, the use of digital media, including interactive and social media, has grown, and research evidence suggests that these newer media offer both benefits and risks to the health of children and teenagers. Evidence-based benefits identified from the use of digital and social media include early learning, exposure to new ideas and knowledge, increased opportunities for social contact and support, and new opportunities to access health promotion messages and information. Risks of such media include negative health effects on sleep, attention, and learning; a higher incidence of obesity and depression; exposure to inaccurate, inappropriate, or unsafe content and contacts; and compromised privacy and confidentiality. This technical report reviews the literature regarding these opportunities and risks, framed around clinical questions, for children from birth to adulthood. To promote health and wellness in children and adolescents, it is important to maintain adequate physical activity, healthy nutrition, good sleep hygiene, and a nurturing social environment. A healthy Family Media Use Plan (www.healthychildren.org/MediaUsePlan) that is individualized for a specific child, teenager, or family can identify an appropriate balance between screen time/online time and other activities, set boundaries for accessing content, guide displays of personal information, encourage age-appropriate critical thinking and digital literacy, and support open family communication and implementation of consistent rules about media use.

INTRODUCTION

What Are the Differences Between Traditional Media and New Digital or Social Media?

Today's generation of children and adolescents are surrounded by and immersed in a digital environment. Traditional media, such as television

Technical reports from the American Academy of Pediatrics benefit from expertise and resources of liaisons and internal (AAP) and external reviewers. However, technical reports from the American Academy of Pediatrics may not reflect the views of the liaisons or the organizations or government agencies that they represent.

The guidance in this report does not indicate an exclusive course of treatment or serve as a standard of medical care. Variations, taking into account individual circumstances, may be appropriate.

All technical reports from the American Academy of Pediatrics automatically expire 5 years after publication unless reaffirmed, revised, or retired at or before that time.

DOI: 10.1542/peds.2016-2593

PEDIATRICS (ISSN Numbers: Print, 0031-4005; Online, 1098-4275).

Copyright © 2016 by the American Academy of Pediatrics

FINANCIAL DISCLOSURE: The authors have indicated they do not have a financial relationship relevant to this article to disclose.

FUNDING: No external funding.

POTENTIAL CONFLICT OF INTEREST: The authors have indicated they have no potential conflicts of interest to disclose.

To cite: Reid Chassiakos Y, Radesky J, Christakis D, et al., AAP COUNCIL ON COMMUNICATIONS AND MEDIA. Children and Adolescents and Digital Media. *Pediatrics.* 2016;138(5): e20162593

(TV), radio, and periodicals, have been supplemented by new digital technologies that promote interactive and social engagement and allow children and teenagers instant access to entertainment, information, and knowledge; social contact; and marketing. Traditional media, also referred to as broadcast media, typically were created externally by an established production source, such as a film studio, TV network, or editorial staff and were provided either to individuals or to a broader audience for passive viewing or reading. In contrast, newer digital media, which include social and interactive media, are a form of media in which users can both consume and actively create content. Examples include applications (apps), multiplayer video games, YouTube videos, or video blogs (vlogs). For children and young adults today, this evolving integration of passively viewed and interactive media is seamless and natural; the distinctions and boundaries between traditional/broadcast and interactive/social media have become blurred or imperceptible.

Digital media allow information sharing across a variety of media formats, including text, photographs, video, and audio. Today's video games, for example, often represent a merging of both traditional and social media, as users can virtually "inhabit" impressively produced worlds and interact with other users in remote locations. Video game participants can even work collaboratively to cocreate virtual worlds. Thus, digital media can provide an engaging experience in which the media experiences of children and teenagers become highly personalized.

MEDIA USE ESTIMATES

How Are Media Usage Patterns Changing in Young Children?

The evolution of media from traditional to newer forms of digital media in the past decade has resulted in changes in the patterns of media use. For example, in 1970, children began to regularly watch TV at 4 years of age, whereas today, children begin interacting with digital media at 4 *months* of age.

As new media platforms and social media have been incorporated into children's media diets, hours spent in TV viewing have slowly decreased over the past 2 decades. Loprinzi and Davis[1] examined trends in parent-reported TV viewing among preschoolers 2 to 5 years of age (n = 5724) and children 6 to 11 years of age (n = 7104) between 2001 and 2012 using data from the National Health and Nutrition Examination Survey (NHANES), showing significant decreases in mean TV viewing over time, primarily for preschoolers and, to a lesser extent, for school-aged children. Non-Hispanic white boys demonstrated the largest decrease in mean viewing of 29%, from 2.24 hours of TV per day down to 1.59 hours of TV per day. Despite these decreases, the majority of parents still reported that their children watched TV for 2 or more hours per day.

It is unclear whether these decreases are in part the result of parents heeding expert recommendations to limit screen time (evidence would suggest not)[2] or whether they represent a displacement of TV viewing by the use of novel platforms. In young children, use of mobile devices, such as smartphones and tablet computers, has risen dramatically since the Kaiser Family Foundation first began surveying parents of 0- to 8-year-olds about their technology use.[3] For example, in 2011, 52% of children 0 to 8 years of age had access to a mobile device (although only 38% had ever used one). By 2013, this access had increased to 75% of 0- to 8-year-olds.[4] Although these national surveys continued to demonstrate a digital divide on the basis of economic status, with less access to mobile technology and the Internet in lower-income families, a smaller study in 2015 called this disparity into question by showing that almost all (96.6%) 0- to 4-year-olds recruited from a low-income pediatric clinic had used mobile devices, and 75% owned their own device.[5] This study also showed that most 2-year-olds used mobile devices on a daily basis and that most of the 1-year-olds assessed (92.2%) had already used a mobile device. Although a digital divide likely still exists in terms of access to quality content and reliable Wi-Fi, it is now clear that most young children seen by a pediatric health care provider will have used or have been exposed to mobile technology.

Exactly what young children are doing on mobile technology has not been studied in great detail, because mobile device usage is relatively recent and methodologically difficult to assess. By parent report, most children in the Kabali et al study[5] watched YouTube or Netflix primarily, and smaller proportions watched educational programs and played early-learning apps (eg, alphabet and counting apps). A large minority also played games or watched cartoons. Common Sense Media's Zero to Eight survey has found disparities in the use of educational media on mobile devices, with 54% of children from higher-income families often or sometimes using educational content on mobile devices but only 28% of children from lower-income families doing so.[4] Thus, younger children and those from lower-income families are more likely to use mobile devices for entertainment purposes.

How Are Media Being Used in Older Children and Teens Today? Which Modes of Use Are Most Popular?

Studies show that social media use patterns and rates among older children and adolescents have continued to grow over the past decade, aided in part by the recent rise in mobile phone use among children and teenagers. At present, approximately three-quarters of teenagers own a smartphone, 24% of adolescents describe themselves as "constantly connected" to the Internet[6] and 50% report feeling "addicted" to their phones.[7] Mobile apps provide a breadth of specific functions, such as gaming, photo and video sharing, and global positioning system monitoring. Social media sites and their associated mobile apps provide a platform for users to create an online identity, communicate with others, and build a social network. Among the myriad accessible social networking sites, Facebook remains the most popular, with 71% of 13- to 17-year-olds surveyed by the Pew Research Center in 2014 and 2015 reporting using this site/app.[6] However, adolescents today do not typically dedicate themselves to just 1 site; most teenagers maintain a "social media portfolio" of several selected sites including, as indicated by rates of use in the Pew survey, Instagram (52%), Snapchat (41%), Twitter (33%), Google+ (33%), Vine (24%), Tumblr (14%), and other social media (11%).[6]

As communication moves from face-to-face and voice-only phone conversations to more screen-to-screen interactions via apps, such as FaceTime or Skype, daily communication is becoming intertwined with screen time. Texting, using a smartphone keyboard to send a written message or a visual symbol (emoji) to another smartphone, also has become a prominent means of communication for teenagers.

Lines are also becoming blurred between media use for communication versus for entertainment. With the ability

to message your opponent while engaging in a remote video game or tweet while watching a TV show, viewers and gamers often link their entertainment to social media. Modes of communication have become more fluid, with conversations jumping back and forth between text messages to social media sites. Text messages also may include links to media, such as personal videos, YouTube videos, and links to Web sites and social networking sites.

Pew data from 2012 suggest that teenagers between 14 and 17 years of age sent a median of 100 texts a day. With all likelihood, this number will continue to increase as new data become available. Texting no longer is limited to cellular phone systems but can be facilitated by messaging apps, such as Kik or WhatsApp. Pew data from 2015 show that these apps are most popular with Latino (46%) and African-American (47%) teenagers, compared with white teenagers (24%).[6]

Video games also remain very popular among families; it is estimated that 4 out of 5 households own a device used to play video games, and approximately half of US homes own a dedicated game console.[8] Video games also are available via apps on mobile devices. Additionally, apps that have a practical function are also being marketed with a gaming perspective; this approach is known as "gamification."

It is common for adolescents today to engage in more than 1 form of media at the same time, a practice referred to as media multitasking. This multitasking may include watching TV and using a computer[9] or being online and engaging in more than 1 activity. In one study of older adolescents, approximately 50% of the time students were online, they were engaged in more than 1 activity.[10]

GAMIFICATION AND ADVERTISING

What Is Gamification? What Is the Impact of Gamification on Media Use by Children?

Gamification applies gaming elements to a real-world activity in a seamless, user-friendly, and attractive way. Commercial video games have incorporated cutting-edge graphics, behavioral reinforcers (ie, for reaching certain levels of play), and exciting stories, which have been delivered through stationary personal computers, dedicated gaming consoles, or multiplayer networks. One key difference today is the portability achieved via smartphones, mobile Wi-Fi, and broad social networks, which has changed how and where games can be played and how gaming functions can be applied. These portable "games" can now be integrated into daily life by functioning as sources for information and guidance and by providing motivation to achieve academic and wellness goals. For example, the Nike+ app tracks exercisers' routes, pace, steps, distance, and time and challenges runners to compete with friends and improve their performance. Such design also serves to reinforce behavior (both health behaviors and for using the app), resulting in more engagement with both.[11]

How Have Mobile and Social Media Changed the Ability of Advertisers to Reach Children and Teenagers?

Newer media have provided expanding opportunities for marketers and advertisers to adapt their messages to reach millions of children and teenagers.[12] These newer forms of media may broaden the types of products and behaviors to which children and adolescents are exposed. For example, although restrictions may exist to limit exposure to advertisements for alcohol in traditional media, research suggests that the major alcohol brands maintain a strong presence on Facebook, Twitter, and YouTube.[13,14] From a marketing perspective, social media are consumer focused, allowing interaction and input that can build relationships.[15] Social media also allow targeted ads that reflect content that users have posted on their own pages. In one study, researchers found that placing content related to exercise or nutrition as a status update on Facebook led to advertisements for sports gear and diets as well as junk food.[15] Thus, social media ads can directly address individuals or groups who would be interested and responsive. Social media ads may also be interactive and are more affordable to create and disseminate. However, this ability for marketers to reach children through social media is understudied.

Marketing to parents of young children also is common, because advertisers know that many parents fear that their children may fall behind in the skilled use of technology without early exposure to it.[16] In reality, parents can be reassured that their children will learn to use digital media quickly when they are introduced at home or in school.

BENEFITS AND OPPORTUNITIES OF MEDIA USE

Fortunately, new media use is not without its benefits, but these benefits largely depend on a child's age and developmental stage, a child's characteristics, how the media are used (eg, with a parent or without), and the media content and design.

Early Childhood

At What Age Can Infants and Toddlers Learn From Screens?

Evidence continues to show limited educational benefits of media for children younger than 2 years. Earlier American Academy of Pediatrics (AAP) recommendations to discourage media exposure for children younger than 2 years were based on research on TV and videos, which showed that in-person interactions with parents are much more effective than video for learning of new verbal or nonverbal problem-solving skills.[17] This research showed that infants and toddlers experience what was referred to as the "video deficit:" difficulty learning from 2-dimensional video representations at younger than 30 months of age. The video deficit is thought to be attributable to infants' and young toddlers' lack of symbolic thinking, immature attentional controls, and the memory flexibility required to effectively transfer knowledge from a 2-dimensional platform to a 3-dimensional world.[18] Before 2 years of age, children are still developing cognitive, language, sensorimotor, and social-emotional skills, which require hands-on exploration and social interaction with trusted caregivers for successful maturation.

Therefore, adult interaction remains crucial for toddlers to learn effectively from digital media. For example, from 12 to 24 months of age, toddlers can begin to learn novel words from commercially available "word learning" videos, but only if their parents watch with them and reteach the words, essentially using the videos as a learning scaffold to build the language skills.[19,20] In one longitudinal study of low-income families, 14-month-olds whose mothers had talked with them during educational TV programming since infancy showed more advanced language development than infants whose mothers did not talk with them during media use (although this finding also may have reflected how much mothers spoke to children in general).[21] The few experimental studies showing independent learning of words from videos at this age have been limited by their low ecologic validity[22] or have shown that toddlers lose the knowledge learned over time without repetition.[23]

More recent research has shown that, under particular conditions, children between 15 and 24 months of age can learn from repeated viewing of video demonstrations without adult help. Dayanim and Namy showed that 15-month-olds could learn the meaning of sign language symbols after 3 weeks of watching a commercially available video 4 times per week.[24] However, children in a comparison study group whose parents used a book of sign language symbols to teach the content retained more knowledge about the symbols' meanings for a longer period of time.

Building parasocial relationships with TV or video characters (ie, the perceived relationship that audience members develop with characters who speak to them, such as Elmo or Dora) also has been shown to improve toddlers' learning. Calvert et al[25] showed that, after 3 months of playing with a personalized interactive toy, 21-month-olds could learn how to stack cups from a video demonstration by the same character, suggesting that building an emotional bond with an on-screen character improves learning potential. However, a primary limitation of such experimental studies is that they do not examine how repeated media use displaces other activities, and they do not examine longer-term outcomes. For example, in the study by Calvert and colleagues,[25] children randomly assigned to the group that did not receive the interactive toy for 3 months actually scored better in terms of language development at 21 months of age.

Are Touchscreens More Educational?

Pedagogic theory has long emphasized that interaction improves learning. This understanding has been the motivation for recommending coviewing of media, along with evidence that parent interaction increases young children's engagement with media and understanding of content.[26] The interactivity of new media via touchscreens allows apps to "know" whether a child is responding accurately and tailor responses, reinforcement, and next steps to the child's input. Theoretically, this may increase educational potential by providing scaffolding to build skills at the child's edge of competence.

Empirical evidence regarding interactive media use in infants and toddlers is sparse. At 24 months of age, a child can learn words from live video-chatting with a responsive adult[27] or from carefully designed, interactive screen interfaces that prompt the child to tap on relevant learning items.[28] Starting at 15 months of age, toddlers can learn novel words from touchscreens in laboratory-based studies (with specially designed, not commercial, apps) but have trouble transferring this knowledge to the 3-dimensional world,[29] particularly if they regularly use touchscreen platforms to view entertainment media.

Is Skyping Appropriate for Infants and Toddlers?

Many parents now use video-chat (eg, Skype, Facetime) as an interactive media form that facilitates social connection with distant relatives. New evidence shows that infants and toddlers regularly engage in video-chatting,[30] but the same principles regarding need for parental support would apply in order for infants and toddlers to understand what they are seeing. Because video-chat episodes usually are brief,[30] promote social connection, and involve support from adults, this practice should not be discouraged in infants and toddlers.

What Is the Best Approach to Selecting Quality Content for Young Children?

High-quality TV programs (eg, Public Broadcasting Service [PBS]

programs, such as *Sesame Street* and *Mister Rogers' Neighborhood*) can demonstrably improve cognitive, linguistic, and social outcomes for children 3 to 5 years of age. Although there have been few large community-based, randomized trials, many observational studies and some small experimental ones have demonstrated that preschoolers can learn literacy, numeracy, and prosocial skills from high-quality TV programs.[31,32] In addition, Sesame Workshop and other child content creators have been responding to current child health and developmental needs (eg, obesity, resilience) by crafting programming aimed at teaching parents and children relevant knowledge and skills.

Choosing PBS content has been found to be protective of poor executive function outcomes observed in children who start consuming media in early infancy.[33] Preschoolers randomly assigned to change from inappropriate or violent content to high-quality prosocial programming were found to have significant improvements in their externalizing and internalizing behavior,[32] which also speaks to the importance of content. For families who find it difficult to modify the overall amount of media use in their homes, changing to high-quality content may be a more actionable alternative; to make these changes, pediatric providers can direct them toward curation services, such as Common Sense Media, for reviews of videos, apps, TV shows, and movies.

Are "Educational" Apps and e-Books Really Educational?

As content from PBS high-quality programs is translated into apps and game formats (eg, *Martha Speaks*, *Big Bird's Words*, and *Cookie Monster's Challenge* apps), educational benefits have been shown in preschoolers.[34] Unfortunately, very few of the commercially available apps found

in the educational section of app stores have evidence-based design input with demonstrated learning effectiveness. In fact, recent reviews of hundreds of toddler/preschooler apps labeled as educational have demonstrated that most apps show low educational potential, target only rote academic skills (eg, ABCs, colors), are not based on established curricula, and include almost no input from developmental specialists or educators.[35,36] An additional concern is that the formal features (ie, bells and whistles) that are designed to engage the child in an interactive experience may actually decrease the child's comprehension or distract from social interaction between caregivers and children during use, as has been shown for e-books,[37] which is important, because active parent involvement in both digital play and book reading improves children's learning from the experience.[38,39]

One reason that children may be less socially engaged during digital play is that gaming design involves behavioral reinforcement meant to achieve a maximum duration of engagement, which may explain why interrupting children's digital play leads to tantrums, particularly when games or videos are set on autoadvance.[40] To address these concerns, academic and industry leaders have recently recommended creating digital products for children that are appropriately engaging, but not distracting; that are designed to be used by a dual audience (ie, both parent and child) to facilitate family participation in media use and modeling of more effective social and learning interactions[35,41]; and that have automatic "stops" as the default design to encourage children and caregivers to pause the game use and turn to the 3-dimensional world.[40]

One recent app, for example, demonstrates such an adult–child dyad-centered design. Bedtime Math creates a platform and a structure for parents and children to read stories and answer math problems together on a nightly basis. It is one of the few apps that has been tested in a randomized controlled community-based trial and shown benefits.[42] Embedding, indeed requiring, social interactivity for functionality may hold great promise for even younger children as well. However, recent population-based surveys suggest that joint media engagement[43] (and designs to facilitate it)[35] is not as common as individual use.

School-Aged Children and Teenagers

How Can Media Use in Older Children and Teenagers Increase Collaboration and Tolerance?

Research studies as well as anecdotal reports have suggested benefits of media use for today's children and adolescents, such as communication and engagement.[44] Additional benefits include exposure to new ideas and immersive learning experiences. Many social media platforms provide tools that students can use to touch base with and collaborate with others on projects. Communicating across distance is made easier by social media; these communications may include connecting via video-chatting with family or friends who are separated geographically. Traditional and social media can also raise awareness of current events and issues, and social media can provide tools to promote community participation and civic engagement.

A study by Kidd and Castano[45] indicated that reading literary fiction improves empathy in children. Although books are a traditional form of media, the study indicates that exposure to character-focused media can break stereotypes and help children understand people from whom they differ. Internet usage/digital media consumption is positioned to have a similar impact, which is important to help children learn about, understand, and empathize with marginalized groups.

How Can Social Media Be Used To Promote Improved Health?

Health benefits of social media may include enhanced access to valuable support networks. These networks may be particularly helpful for patients with ongoing illnesses, conditions, or disabilities[46] as well as for those identifying as lesbian, gay, bisexual, transgender, questioning, or intersex (LGBTQI) seeking helpful information or a welcoming community. Recent literature indicates that transgender teenagers who feel supported by their families have lower rates of depression and anxiety.[47] Connections with a supportive online community (eg, the "It Gets Better" project) may be beneficial to teenagers who identify as LGBTQI, but most such programs have not been studied to determine effects and outcomes.

Research also supports the use of social media to foster social inclusion or peer-to-peer connection among patients who might otherwise feel excluded, for example, patients with obesity[48] or mental illness.[13] Individuals with mental illness report greater social connectedness and feelings of group belonging when using social media in this manner, because they foster the ability to share personal stories and strategies for coping with challenges.[14] The advantages of these connections include avoiding feared stigma, enhancing social networks, learning about resources from peers online, and gaining information and insight. However, risks of such interactions can include exposure to misinformation, negativity or hostility in communications, delays in seeking out traditional resources, and unhealthy influences.

Young adults describe the benefits of seeking health information online and through social media and recognize these channels as useful supplementary sources of information to health care visits.[15]

Social media may be used to enhance health and wellness and promote healthier behaviors, such as smoking cessation and balanced nutrition.[44] However, there are a myriad of easily accessible Web sites and social networks that facilitate and even promote unhealthy behaviors, such as disordered eating. "Pro-ana" (anorexia nervosa) and "pro-mia (bulimia)" sites, for example, are forums in which peers actively support restricted eating or purging and frequently offer life-threatening suggestions and advice.[49]

Do Screen Time Limits Apply for Children With Disabilities Who Use Mobile Devices To Communicate?

An important benefit from new media has been the development and use of technology-aided interventions in children and adolescents with disabilities, particularly through the expanding use of assistive and interactive digital media to learn and to communicate in youth with autism spectrum disorder (ASD),[50] physical disabilities, speech impairment, and intellectual disability to learn and communicate.[51] However, because teenagers with ASD have higher rates of problematic media use,[52,53] limits still should be placed on entertainment media use, such as watching videos or playing gaming apps, which can represent a restricted interest in children with ASD.

HEALTH AND DEVELOPMENTAL RISKS OF MEDIA USE

What Are the Developmental and Behavioral Risks in Early Childhood?

Population-based studies continue to show associations between excessive TV viewing in early childhood and cognitive,[54–56] language,[57,58] and social/emotional delays.[59–62] Possible mechanisms for these outcomes include the effects of viewing inappropriate, adult-oriented content[54] (as well as some inappropriate child-directed content),[58] a decrease in parent–child interaction when the TV is on,[63] and poorer family functioning in households with high media use.[60]

An earlier age of media use onset, greater cumulative hours of media use, and content that is not of high quality all are significant independent predictors of poor executive functioning (impulse control, self-regulation, mental flexibility)[33] as well as "theory of mind" deficits (ie, the ability to understand others' thoughts and feelings) in preschoolers.[64] Media multitasking, once thought to be a pastime only of only adolescents, now is observed even in children younger than 4 years.[13] The orienting response to novel stimuli is very strong in young children, so their attention is drawn to the engaging and quickly changing features of digital media, such as animation, sounds, and highlighted features they can tap and swipe.[65] These features, however, may decrease young children's comprehension.[66] It is unknown whether rapid shifts in attention to and from digital stimuli may have long-term effects on children's attention span or information processing.

Because strong associations between violent media content and child aggressive behavior have been clearly documented,[67] parents should continue to monitor the content of their children's media. Today, more children own and use mobile devices independently,[13] making monitoring and regulation much more difficult.[16,68] More research is needed on how parents can best supervise and guide their children's media use.

Are Certain Children or Families More Susceptible to These Risks?

TV has been used as an "electronic babysitter" for decades, but recent evidence suggests that excessive media use is more likely in infants and toddlers with a "difficult"

temperament[69,70] or self-regulation problems.[71] Toddlers with social-emotional delays are more likely to be given a mobile device to calm them down,[72] especially if their parents are facing parenting control challenges. However, it is not clear whether more "difficult" infants and toddlers have more positive or negative outcomes over time when exposed to longer media duration, which likely depends on content quality and other contextual factors. For example, Linebarger et al[73] found that the quality of parenting can modify associations between media use and child development: inappropriate content and inconsistent parenting had cumulative negative effects on low-income preschoolers' executive function, and warm parenting and educational content interacted to produce additive benefits.

Is Media Use Linked to Obesity?

High levels of media use are linked to obesity and cardiovascular risk[74] throughout the life course, but these associations are observed starting in early childhood. For example, heavy media use during preschool years is associated with small but significant increases in BMI,[75] which sets the stage for greater weight gain later in childhood. The association between using ≥2 hours of media per day and obesity persists even after adjusting for children's psychosocial risk factors or behavioral problems.[76] Research in preschoolers often uses a 2-hour cutoff to define excessive media use, but a recent study of 2-year-olds found that BMI increased for **every hour per week** of media consumed.[77] Moreover, media use behaviors may explain some of the obesity risk disparities among young black and Hispanic children.[78] None of these studies examined mobile media specifically, which may be more easily used during meals and, therefore, distract children from satiety cues.[79]

Studies of older children and teenagers show clear correlations between increases in hours of TV viewing and higher risk of obesity.[80] In a 1996 study of 5- to 10-year-olds, the odds of being overweight were 4.6 times greater for youth watching more than 5 hours of TV per day compared with those watching 0 to 2 hours.[81] This study greatly influenced the AAP recommendations for 2 hours or less of sedentary screen time daily for children 2 through 18 years of age. However, a more recent study in the Netherlands of children 4 through 13 years of age found that watching TV **over 1.5 hours per day** was a significant risk factor for obesity. In this study, however, an association between TV and obesity was only found for children 4 through 9 years of age.[82] A large international study with almost 300 000 children and adolescents found that watching **between 1 and 3 hours of TV a day** led to a 10% to 27% increase in risk of obesity.[83] These more recent studies suggest that setting limits of TV viewing to between **1 and 1.5 hours a day** may be more effective to prevent obesity than the 2 hours per day standard presented in earlier AAP recommendations.

Additional studies have identified relevant factors around TV viewing beyond solely the number of hours for families to use in developing household rules. Another recent study found that the association between TV viewing and obesity risk was only significant for children who were already at the higher end of the BMI distribution.[84] A large study using a national dataset of children reported that it was not just the hours of TV viewing that predicted obesity, but the combination of low physical activity and high sedentary TV viewing that was most contributory to obesity risk.[85] A 2008 study directly examined the AAP recommendations for 2 hours a day or less of sedentary media consumption and found that **boys who exceeded 2 hours a day of sedentary media use** were 1.7 times more likely to be overweight compared with those who had 2 hours a day or less of sedentary media use. The results for girls were much less impressive, in that girls with over 2 hours a day of sedentary media use were only 1.2 times more likely to be overweight compared with girls who had 2 hours or less of media use time.[86]

The association between TV viewing and obesity previously attributed to food advertising[87] may now be decreased, because children watch more videos from streaming services (eg, Netflix, Hulu), which do not contain advertisements, but this has yet to be studied.

Another area of obesity risk is the presence of a TV in the bedroom. A 2007 study found that having a TV in the bedroom was an independent risk factor for obesity. A more recent study found that the combination of a TV in the bedroom and greater use of screen time had the strongest association with obesity.[88]

Fortunately, studies also suggest that making efforts to reduce children's sedentary media use can have positive health effects. An intervention study focused on third and fourth graders worked with the participants to reduce time spent watching TV and playing video games. The study demonstrated that children in the intervention group reported reduced TV viewing and meals in front of the TV and had reduced BMIs, illustrating that interventions to reduce sedentary media use can positively impact health behaviors as well as BMI.[89]

How Does Media Use Affect Sleep?

There is a growing body of evidence that suggests that media use negatively affects sleep.[90] Increased duration of media exposure and the presence of a TV, computer, or

mobile device in the bedroom in early childhood have been associated with fewer minutes of sleep per night, especially among children of racial/ethnic minority groups.[91] Later bedtimes after evening media use and violent content in the media also may be contributing factors,[92] and suppression of endogenous melatonin by blue light emitted from screens is another possible cause.[93] Associations between media and sleep are seen in infants as well; 6- to 12-month-olds who were exposed to screen media in the evening hours showed significantly shorter night-time sleep duration than those who had no evening screen exposure.[94]

Studies of older children and teenagers have found that participants with higher social media use[95] or who sleep with mobile devices in their room[96,97] were at greater risk for sleep disturbances. One study of adults found that taking a phone into the bedroom led to longer sleep latency, worse sleep quality, more sleep disturbance, and more daytime dysfunction.[98] This study illustrates the multiple mechanisms by which media use around bedtime, or during bedtime, can disrupt sleep and affect daytime function.

Bruni et al[90] studied the use of technology on sleep quality in adolescents and preadolescents. Adolescents' bad sleep quality was associated consistently with greater mobile phone use and the number of devices in the bedroom, and in preadolescents, bad sleep quality was associated with greater Internet use and later media turn-off time. The authors concluded that evening circadian preference, mobile phone and Internet use, the number of other activities engaged in after 9:00 PM, later media turning-off time, and the number of devices in the bedroom have different, but significant, negative influences on sleep quality in preadolescents and adolescents.[90] Similarly, Lemola et al[99] reported

associations between electronic media use in bed before sleep, sleep difficulties, and symptoms of depression in teenagers.

Daytime screen use may also affect sleep. According to a Norwegian study, daytime and bedtime use of electronic devices *both* affected sleep measures, with an increased risk of short sleep duration, long sleep onset latency, and increased sleep deficiency. A dose–response relationship emerged between sleep duration and use of electronic devices.[100] Ensuring that children and teenagers obtain the necessary hours of healthy sleep is an important goal of a Family Media Use Plan (www.healthychildren.org/MediaUsePlan).

What Are the Risks of Social Media Use In School-Aged Children and Teenagers?

The links between media and health behaviors among adolescents have been backed by decades of evidence in traditional media.[101-104] Studies have shown that exposure to alcohol or tobacco use or risky sexual behaviors in TV or movies is associated with initiation of these behaviors,[101,102,105,106] leading some to describe TV as a "superpeer."[107] A growing body of evidence suggests that these influences also are strong in digital and social media. Several studies have illustrated that adolescents' displays on social media frequently include portrayal of risky health behaviors, such as illegal alcohol use or overuse, illicit substance use, high-risk sexual behaviors, and harmful behaviors, such as self-injury and disordered eating.[108-112] A growing body of evidence suggests that peer viewers of this content are influenced to see these behaviors as normative and desirable.[113-115] Social media combine the power of interpersonal persuasion with the reach of mass media. Fogg described this mass interpersonal persuasion as "the most significant advance in persuasion since radio was invented in the 1890s."[116]

Although restrictions exist to protect youth and children from exposure to alcohol, tobacco, and marijuana advertisements on traditional media platforms, such as TV, there is concern about the extent to which youth are exposed to promotion of these substances on social media Web sites from marketers or peers. For example, research from both the United States and the United Kingdom indicate that the major alcohol brands maintain a strong advertising presence on Facebook, Twitter, and YouTube.[13,14] Targeted advertising via social media may have a significant effect on adolescent behavior.

How Does Media Use in School-Aged Children and Teenagers Relate to Mental Health?

Research studies have identified both benefits and concerns regarding mental health and media use. In one longitudinal panel survey, 396 white and black preadolescent boys and girls were assessed to determine the long-term effects of TV consumption on global self-esteem. TV exposure was found to be significantly related to self-esteem, but whether it increased or decreased self-esteem was influenced by demographic factors. Greater exposure resulted in a decrease in self-esteem for both white and black girls and for black boys but resulted in an increase in self-esteem for white boys.[117] Analyzing these results, the authors postulate that the majority of the TV content served to reinforce both gender-role and racial stereotypes, which tended to be positive for white boys but not the other groups. The authors suggested that the black children and white girls could be internalizing the "social norms" portrayed and using these messages as a basis for self-evaluation, negatively affecting their self-esteem. There is also an opportunity cost when more TV viewing displaces real-life experiences that might build self-esteem.

The interactive and selective components of social media may offset some of these traditional media drawbacks, because social media use in moderation can enhance social support and connection. However, use in moderation and the specific way in which social media are used may be the key. Previous research has suggested a U-shaped relationship between Internet use and depression, with increased risks for depression at both the high and low ends of Internet use.[118,119] A recent study examined social media use and depression and found a positive association.[120] Older adolescents who used social media passively by solely viewing content reported declines in well-being and life satisfaction, whereas those who used social media actively by interacting with others and posting content did not experience these declines.[121] Another study found that teenagers who used Instagram to follow strangers and engage in social comparisons had higher depression symptoms, but others who followed friends and engaged in less social comparison had fewer depression symptoms.[122] These studies illustrate that, beyond the number of hours spent on social media, a key factor is how an individual uses social media.

Do Children and Adolescents Understand the Privacy Risks Associated With Social Media Use?

An important issue across all social media and interactive apps is privacy, because content that a child or adolescent chooses to post on any site or app becomes public in some way. Removal of such content may be difficult or impossible. Previous work suggests that adolescents vary in their understanding of privacy practices, and even among those who do know how to set privacy settings, many choose not to do so.[123–125]

Despite efforts by some social media sites to protect privacy or even to delete content after it is viewed, privacy violations and content sharing are always possible.[126,127] This risk illustrates the need for continued discussion about media and privacy with children and teenagers with parents, caregivers, teachers, and other responsible adults. These discussions should be included in schools through their digital citizenship programs and in pediatric well-child examinations with parents and teenagers. Pediatricians can introduce and work with families to develop a Family Media Use Plan (see the AAP guide to making a plan at www.healthychildren.org/MediaUsePlan) that can mitigate or avoid such risks.

Is Cyberbullying Different From Traditional Bullying?

Cyberbullying is commonly defined as "an aggressive, intentional act or behavior that is carried out by a group or an individual, using electronic forms of contact, repeatedly and over time against a victim who cannot easily defend him or herself."[128] Unfortunately, there are many online platforms in which bullying may take place, including E-mail, blogs, social networking Web sites/apps, online games, and text messaging. There is clear overlap between cyberbullying and traditional bullying,[129] but several features of online bullying present new challenges. These challenges include that perpetrators can bully at any time of day and can be anonymous, the rapidity with which information can spread online,[130] and the fluidity with which bully and target roles can switch in the online world. Estimates of the number of youth who experience cyberbullying vary, ranging from 10% to 40%, depending on the age group and how cyberbullying is defined.

Cyberbullying shares many similarities and a few key differences with traditional bullying. For example, victims of cyberbullying often do not know who the bully is or why they are being targeted, the hurtful actions of a cyberbully can reach a child or teenager anytime he or she uses a smartphone or computer (so there is no safe haven of home), and the bullying messages can also spread virally through the Internet to many other people at school or in the community, making this type of bullying potentially very embarrassing and lasting.

Descriptive research has shown that vulnerable populations exist and are more likely to be targeted for bullying. Youths identifying as LGBTQI are more likely to be victimized in bullying dynamics and are at risk online as well.[131] Children and adolescents with ASD are a population particularly vulnerable to bullying (https://www. autismspeaks.org/family-services/ bullying) and could easily be a target for cyberbullying. The 2016 National Academies of Sciences, Engineering, and Medicine report, "Preventing Bullying Through Science, Policy, and Practice,"[132] addressed the concept of populations vulnerable to bullying to propose that there is a need for research that moves beyond descriptive studies and labeling of youth as vulnerable and considers processes that can explain why individuals may have differences in their bullying experiences and consequences depending on their context.

Previous studies have examined the negative effects that cyberbullying can have on both bullies and victims. Victims are more likely to report lower grades and other academic problems as a result of the experience. Similar to traditional bullying, cyberbullying can lead to short- and long-term[133,134] negative social, academic, and health[134–137] consequences for both the perpetrator and target. Both bullies and victims often report higher

levels of depression and lower self-esteem. Victims were at higher risk of both suicidal ideation and suicide attempts.

Fortunately, newer studies suggest that interventions targeting bullying also may reduce cyberbullying.[138] Moreno states: "Parents can play a role in preventing cyberbullying by educating their children about appropriate online behaviors. Parents should have discussions early and often about their child's friendships and relationships to develop and maintain open communication about these topics."[139] The Centers for Disease Control and Prevention panel reviewing effective prevention strategies recommends media literacy education as a "promising approach," along with collaborative strategies among teenagers, parents, and schools that encourage victims to report cyberbullying and seek adult support.[140]

What Is Sexting and How Can the Risks of Sexting Be Avoided or Addressed?

Sexting is a serious issue in adolescence. Sexting is commonly defined as the electronic transmission of nude or seminude images as well as sexually explicit text messages.[111] It is estimated that approximately 12% of youth 10 to 19 years of age have ever sent a sexual photo to someone else[112]; sadly, many youth who have participated in sexting report having felt pressured into sending a sext. When dealing with youth and sexting, adults, authorities, and schools need to be aware that the situation may be more complicated.

Spencer et al[141] examined sexting and youth in an urban population; 55 youth presenting for care at the Teen Health Center at Children's Hospital Los Angeles were surveyed to evaluate prevalence and sexting behaviors, such as forwarding sexts, reasons for sending sexts, and youths' concerns regarding sexting. Of those

surveyed, 48.5% of girls and 63.6% of boys had sent a sext, and 70% of girls and 82% of boys had received a sext. The authors report that girls expressed significantly more concern than boys about how sexting could affect their reputation, including getting caught by an adult with a sext and how others would think of them. Fortunately, 52% of respondents said they would be comfortable talking with their doctor about sexting. Pediatricians may, therefore, find their teen patients receptive to a conversation about sexting and its implications and risks.

Ybarra and Mitchell, in their article, "'Sexting' and its relation to sexual activity and sexual risk behavior in a national survey of adolescents,"[142] suggest that sexting is related to behaviors indicative of psychosocial challenge and risky sexual behavior for some youth. Significant findings include a higher frequency of sexting among females and lesbian, gay, and bisexual youth. Additionally, a greater number of past-year sex partners and a greater odds of depression and substance abuse were found among teenagers who sext.

Findings related to lesbian, gay, and bisexual populations are consistent with previous studies on sexting; of note, transgender youth were not included. Earlier research had demonstrated a significant association between sexting and risky sexual behaviors in lesbian, gay, bisexual, and transgender youth.[142]

Ybarra and Mitchell's study[142] found that sexting was indicative of sexual activity and risky sexual behaviors, and further research may identify predictive outcomes of sexting. One study suggests that sexting may precede sexual intercourse.[142] The predictive value of a sexting history may inform sex education and HEEADSSS (home, education & employment, eating, activities, drugs, sexuality, suicide/depression, and safety) assessments. Moreover, discussions between pediatricians and teenagers about sexting may indicate risky sexual behaviors and a number of psychosocial issues, such as depression, anxiety, and low self-esteem, that may be further addressed.

Temple et al[143] examined whether adolescents who report sexting exhibited more psychosocial health problems than their nonsexting counterparts. The authors reported that teen sexting was significantly associated with symptoms of depression, impulsivity, and substance use. When adjusted for previous sexual behavior, age, gender, race/ethnicity, and parent education, however, sexting was only related to impulsivity and substance use. The authors concluded that "while teen sexting appears to correlate with impulsive and high-risk behaviors (substance use), we did not find sexting to be a marker of mental health."[143]

Sexting is a behavior that will likely continue and expand with technologic advances that make photography and communication more accessible. Active debate continues regarding the ethical and legal components of sexting, especially among underage youth. Concerns include the identification of sexts as pornography or sexual misconduct. Even consensual, noncoercive sexting may result in criminal prosecution that may lead to long-term legal consequences.

Addressing risky sexual behaviors and psychological symptoms associated with sexting through education and guidance should help to promote wellness and responsibility within adolescent populations. Further research evaluating sexting among gender minority populations (eg, transgender adolescents) also will be valuable in understanding and discouraging the behavior

and providing safer and less risky alternatives for social connections.

CHILD PORNOGRAPHY AND CHILD ABUSE

How Has Social Media Changed the Landscape of Child Pornography and Child Abuse?

Unfortunately, the Internet has also created opportunities for the exploitation of children by sex offenders. Online predators can gain access to children and teenagers through social networking, chat rooms, E-mail, and online games. Cases of child trafficking, cybergrooming, and sexual abuse for private and commercial purposes have increased with the help of the anonymous cyberspace environment. For example, online grooming leads to establishment of a trusting relationship, often with the perpetrator misrepresenting himself as another child or teenager. This developing online relationship may lead to sexting or to convincing the child to meet the perpetrator in person. Children may be deceived, tricked, or coerced into engaging in sexual acts for the production of child sexual abuse materials (child pornography), which then can circulate online for years to come. Child sexual abuse images often involve young and very young children. Of 43 597 children assessed in sexual abuse images and videos, 49.6% appeared to have a sexual maturity rating of 1, and 28.7% appeared to have a sexual maturity rating of 2.[144] Besides the adverse effects associated with child sexual abuse,[145,146] victims who have had online sexual images (pornography and sexting) posted may experience significant anxiety and stress related to knowledge that the abuse images may be downloaded and viewed by millions of people for an indefinite period of time. Thus, the exploitation continues for months and years after the images were obtained.[144]

Online child sexual exploitation also may involve recruitment and advertisement of children for prostitution and other forms of exploitation.[147] The Internet may be used by human traffickers to facilitate movement of victims and to manage a criminal network.[148]

Internet-initiated sex crimes involving offenders who meet and groom children online tend to involve adolescents rather than very young children: 99% of victims in one study were 13 to 17 years old, and 48% were 13 to 14 years old. Many of these crimes involve face-to-face sexual contact, which the victim perceives as "consensual." Sexual relationships in early adolescence are associated with an increased risk of social, academic, and behavioral adverse outcomes.[149,150]

Research has shown that parents underestimate the likelihood that their child might engage in online conversation with people they do not know. Therefore, it is critical that parents promote online safety with their children from an early age, monitor children's Internet use, and use tools, such as parental control software, to maintain awareness of their child's online activities.[151] Pediatricians should consider asking appropriate questions to explore this possibility and to educate youth about protecting themselves from exploitation. All health care professionals should report any suspicions of sexual abuse/exploitation as per child abuse reporting laws.

USE OF MEDIA BY PARENTS AND CAREGIVERS

What Effect Does Parent Media Use Have on Young and School-Aged Children and Teenagers?

Parents and caregivers play an important role in modeling optimal behaviors for their children in general, including when it comes to the consumption and use of media. The growth of digital and social media, particularly in the last 5 years, has seen dramatic increases in adults' use of social media as well as use by children and teenagers; more than 70% of adults now use social media[152] and 27% report feeling "addicted" to their mobile devices.[7] Social media can provide positive social experiences for adults, such as opportunities for parents to connect with their child in a college dorm via video-chatting services. Such services also can promote social and emotional connection among distant relatives or deployed parents and children. However, some parents can, themselves, overuse digital media. For example, research has shown that parents' own TV viewing distracts from parent–child interactions[153] and children's play.[154] Children younger than 2 years are more likely to be exposed to and watch inappropriate "background" media (eg, TV) than older children.[155] Heavy parent use of mobile devices is associated with fewer verbal and nonverbal interactions between parents and children[156] and may be associated with more parent–child conflict.[157]

Because parent media use is a strong predictor of child media habits,[158] reducing parental TV viewing, including "background" TV, and enhancing parent–child interactions may be an important area of behavior change that pediatricians can help to facilitate. Because parent–child interactions during family routines are an important opportunity for emotional connection, have been shown to be protective of child health outcomes, such as asthma and high-risk behavior,[159] and are the primary driver of early childhood development of language, cognition, social skills, and emotion regulation, it is important to preserve them. Parents often report feeling that technology speeds up their lives and work demands[160] and that it is difficult to multitask between technology and childrearing, so pediatric providers can support their efforts to create boundaries and "unplugged" zones in their households.

THE FAMILY MEDIA USE PLAN

- How can pediatric health care providers help families use media in healthy ways?

- What is the AAP Family Media Use Plan?

Pediatricians and other pediatric health care professionals can be helpful resources for families seeking specific advice about how to develop and individualize family rules and guidelines to meet their distinct needs. Unfortunately, only 16% of pediatricians ask families about their media use. In addition, only 29% of parents report relying on their pediatrician for advice about broadcast and social media, although those who do tend to follow AAP recommendations.[161]

When discussing media use with families, pediatric health care providers can print out and help families begin completing the AAP Family Media Use Plan (www.healthychildren.org/MediaUsePlan). Providers can discuss with parents and developmentally ready children how each of the media-specific behaviors and health concerns can be addressed through practical, family-centered approaches. The Family Media Use Plan can act as a teaching tool through which pediatricians can provide information about the benefits and health risks of both traditional and new media. The potential risks of interactive media, such as reduced physical activity, inadequate sleep, and unhealthy influences like cyberbullying and weight bias, are important to discuss with families as well.

The plan also can be a tool through which the pediatrician can explore and understand each family's values and health goals—for example, how good nutrition, an active lifestyle, good sleep hygiene, parent–child emotional connection, and creative play fit into the family's typical day—and identify areas in which good health and wellness can be enhanced. Pediatricians can suggest ways in which media can be used to connect, learn, and create instead of simply consume.

These discussions can also allow pediatric health care providers to consider screening for problematic Internet use and Internet gaming disorder using validated tools, such as the Internet Gaming Disorder scale (https://www.researchgate.net/publication/270652917_The_Internet_Gaming_Disorder_Scale) and the Problematic and Risky Internet Use Screening Scale (http://mediad.publicbroadcasting.net/p/kplu/files/201502/PRIUSS_scale_and_guidelines.pdf).

If challenges in implementing a media use plan are anticipated, pediatric health care providers can consider introducing motivational interviewing or engaging in problem solving with parents and children about possible solutions. The pediatrician has an opportunity to discuss specific tools to address identified family needs and concerns, including social services and community resources, if needed. Finally, the pediatrician may be able to provide families with referrals to educational and informational resources, such as vetted Web sites (eg, www.HealthyChildren.org).

CONCLUSIONS

New digital and social media facilitate and promote social interactions as well as participation and engagement that involve both viewing and creating content. The effects of media use, however, are multifactorial and depend on the type of media, the type of use, the amount and extent of use, and the characteristics of the individual child or adolescent using the media. Children today are growing up in an era of highly personalized media use experiences; therefore, parents should be encouraged to develop personalized Family Media Use Plans for their families that attend to each child's age, health, temperament, and developmental stage and ensure that each child can practice and benefit from the essentials for healthy growth and development, such as a healthy diet, good sleep hygiene, adequate physical activity, and positive social interactions.

Parents should recognize and understand their own roles in modeling appropriate media use and balance between media time and other activities. Pediatricians can help families identify and adopt a healthy Family Media Use Plan, minimize unhealthy habits and behaviors, and recognize and address issues that occur related to the use of traditional and new media that can negatively affect health, wellness, social and personal development, and academic performance and success.

LEAD AUTHORS

Yolanda (Linda) Reid Chassiakos, MD, FAAP
Jenny Radesky, MD, FAAP
Dimitri Christakis, MD, FAAP
Megan A. Moreno, MD, MSEd, MPH, FAAP
Corinn Cross, MD, FAAP

COUNCIL ON COMMUNICATIONS AND MEDIA EXECUTIVE COMMITTEE, 2016–2017

David Hill, MD, FAAP, Chairperson
Nusheen Ameenuddin, MD, MPH, FAAP
Yolanda (Linda) Reid Chassiakos, MD, FAAP
Corinn Cross, MD, FAAP
Jenny Radesky, MD, FAAP
Jeffrey Hutchinson, MD, FAAP
Rhea Boyd, MD, FAAP
Robert Mendelson, MD, FAAP
Megan A. Moreno, MD, MSEd, MPH, FAAP
Justin Smith, MD, FAAP
Wendy Sue Swanson, MD, MBE, FAAP

LIAISONS

Kris Kaliebe, MD – *American Academy of Child and Adolescent Psychiatry*
Jennifer Pomeranz, JD, MPH – *American Public Health Association*
Brian Wilcox, PhD – *American Psychological Association*

STAFF

Thomas McPheron

ABBREVIATIONS

AAP: American Academy of Pediatrics
app: application
ASD: autism spectrum disorder
LGBTQI: lesbian, gay, bisexual, transgender, questioning, or intersex
PBS: Public Broadcasting Service
TV: television

REFERENCES

1. Loprinzi PD, Davis RE. Secular trends in parent-reported television viewing among children in the United States, 2001-2012. *Child Care Health Dev.* 2016;42(2):288–291

2. Screening out screen time: parents limit media use for young children. *C.S. Mott Children's Hospital National Poll on Children's Health.* 2014;21(1):1–2. Available at: www.mottnpch.org/reports-surveys/screening-out-screen-time-parents-limit-media-use-young-children. Accessed May 16, 2016

3. Rideout V. *Zero to Eight: Children's Media Use in America.* San Francisco, CA: Common Sense Media; 2011

4. Rideout V. *Zero to Eight: Children's Media Use in America.* San Francisco, CA: Common Sense Media; 2013

5. Kabali HK, Irigoyen MM, Nunez-Davis R, et al. Exposure and use of mobile media devices by young children. *Pediatrics.* 2015;136(6):1044–1050

6. Lenhart A. *Teens, Social Media & Technology Overview 2015.* Washington, DC: Pew Internet and American Life Project; 2015

7. Felt LJ, Robb MB. *Technology Addiction: Concern, Controversy, and Finding a Balance.* San Francisco, CA: Common Sense Media; 2016, Available at https://www.commonsensemedia.org/research/technology-addiction-concern-controversy-and-finding-balance. Accessed May 16, 2016

8. Entertainment Software Association. *2015 Sales, Demographic, and Usage Data. Essential Facts About the Computer and Video Game Industry.* Washington, DC: Entertainment Software Association; 2015

9. Brasel SA, Gips J. Media multitasking behavior: concurrent television and computer usage. *Cyberpsychol Behav Soc Netw.* 2011;14(9):527–534

10. Moreno MA, Jelenchick L, Koff R, Eickhoff JE, Diermyer C, Christakis DA. Internet use and multitasking among older adolescents: an experience sampling approach. *Comput Human Behav.* 2012;28(4):1097–1102

11. Kim B. The popularity of gamification in the mobile and social era. *Libr Technol Rep.* 2015;51(2):5–9

12. Blakeman R. *Nontraditional Media in Marketing and Advertising.* Thousand Oaks, CA: Sage Publications; 2014

13. Winpenny EM, Marteau TM, Nolte E. Exposure of children and adolescents to alcohol marketing on social media websites. *Alcohol Alcohol.* 2014;49(2):154–159

14. Jernigan DH, Rushman AE. Measuring youth exposure to alcohol marketing on social networking sites: challenges and prospects. *J Public Health Policy.* 2014;35(1):91–104

15. Villiard H, Moreno MA. Fitness on facebook: advertisements generated in response to profile content. *Cyberpsychol Behav Soc Netw.* 2012;15(10):564–568

16. Radesky JS, Eisenberg S, Kistin CJ, et al. Overstimulated consumers or next-generation learners? Parent tensions about child mobile technology use. *Ann Fam Med.* 2016, In press

17. Brown A; Council on Communications and Media. Media use by children younger than 2 years. *Pediatrics.* 2011;128(5):1040–1045

18. Barr R. Memory constraints on infant learning from picture books, television, and touchscreens. *Child Dev Perspect.* 2013;7(4):205–210

19. DeLoache JS, Chiong C, Sherman K, et al. Do babies learn from baby media? *Psychol Sci.* 2010;21(11):1570–1574

20. Richert RA, Robb MB, Fender JG, Wartella E. Word learning from baby videos. *Arch Pediatr Adolesc Med.* 2010;164(5):432–437

21. Mendelsohn AL, Brockmeyer CA, Dreyer BP, Fierman AH, Berkule-Silberman SB, Tomopoulos S. Do verbal interactions with infants during electronic media exposure mitigate adverse impacts on their language development as toddlers? *Infant Child Dev.* 2010;19(6):577–593

22. Vandewater EA, Barr RF, Park SE, Lee S. A US Study of transfer of learning from video to books in toddlers. *J Child Media.* 2010;4(4):451–467

23. Brito N, Barr R, McIntyre P, Simcock G. Long-term transfer of learning from books and video during toddlerhood. *J Exp Child Psychol.* 2012;111(1):108–119

24. Dayanim S, Namy LL. Infants learn baby signs from video. *Child Dev.* 2015;86(3):800–811

25. Calvert SL, Richards MN, Kent CC. Personalized interactive characters for toddlers' learning of seriation from a video presentation. *J Appl Dec Psychol.* 2014;35(3):148–155

26. Fidler AE, Zack E, Barr R. Television viewing patterns in 6-to 18-month-olds: the role of caregiver–infant interactional quality. *Infancy.* 2010;15(2):176–196

27. Roseberry S, Hirsh-Pasek K, Golinkoff RM. Skype me! Socially contingent interactions help toddlers learn language. *Child Dev.* 2014;85(3):956–970

28. Kirkorian HL, Choi K, Pempek TA. Toddlers' word learning from contingent and noncontingent video on touch screens. *Child Dev.* 2016;87(2):405–413

29. Zack E, Gerhardstein P, Meltzoff AN, Barr R. 15-month-olds' transfer of learning between touch screen and real-world displays: language cues and cognitive loads. *Scand J Psychol.* 2013;54(1):20–25

30. McClure ER, Chentsova-Dutton YE, Barr RF, Holochwost SJ, Parrott WG.
"Facetime doesn't count": video chat as an exception to media restrictions for infants and toddlers. *Int J Child-Computer Interact.* 2015;6:1–6

31. Anderson DR, Huston AC, Schmitt KL, Linebarger DL, Wright JC. Early childhood television viewing and adolescent behavior: the recontact study. *Monogr Soc Res Child Dev.* 2001;66(1):I–VIII, 1–147

32. Christakis DA, Garrison MM, Herrenkohl T, et al. Modifying media content for preschool children: a randomized controlled trial. *Pediatrics.* 2013;131(3):431–438

33. Nathanson AI, Aladé F, Sharp ML, Rasmussen EE, Christy K. The relation between television exposure and executive function among preschoolers. *Dev Psychol.* 2014;50(5):1497–1506

34. Chiong C, Shuler C. *Learning: is there an app for that? Investigations of young children's usage and learning with mobile devices and apps.* New York, NY: The Joan Ganz Cooney Center at Sesame Workshop; 2010, Available at http://www-tc.pbskids.org/read/files/cooney_learning_apps.pdf. Accessed May 9, 2016

35. Vaala S, Ly A, Levine M. *Getting a Read on the App Stores: A Market Scan and Analysis of Children's Literacy Apps.* New York: The Joan Ganz Cooney Center at Sesame Workshop; 2015. Available at www.joanganzcooneycenter.org/wp-content/uploads/2015/12/jgcc_gettingaread.pdf. Accessed May 9, 2016

36. Guernsey L, Levine MH. *Tap Click Read: Growing Readers in a World of Screens.* San Francisco, CA: Jossey-Bass; 2015

37. Bus AG, Takacs ZK, Kegel CA. Affordances and limitations of electronic storybooks for young children's emergent literacy. *Dev Rev.* 2015;35:79–97

38. Lauricella AR, Barr R, Calvert SL. Parent–child interactions during traditional and computer storybook reading for children's comprehension: implications for electronic storybook design. *Int J Child-Computer Interact.* 2014;2(1):17–25
39. Strouse GA, O'Doherty K, Troseth GL. Effective coviewing: Preschoolers' learning from video after a dialogic questioning intervention. *Dev Psychol.* 2013;49(12):2368–2382

40. Hiniker A, Suh H, Cao S, Kientz JA. Screen time tantrums: how families manage screen media experiences for toddlers and preschoolers. In: *CHI'16. Proceedings of the 2016 CHI Conference on Human Factors in Computing Systems;* May 7–12, 2016; New York, NY. 648–660. Available at: http://dl.acm.org/citation.cfm?doid=2858036.2858278. Accessed May 9, 2016

41. Hirsh-Pasek K, Zosh JM, Golinkoff RM, Gray JH, Robb MB, Kaufman J. Putting education in "educational" apps: lessons from the science of learning. *Psychol Sci Public Interest.* 2015;16(1):3–34

42. Berkowitz T, Schaeffer MW, Maloney EA, et al. Math at home adds up to achievement in school. *Science.* 2015;350(6257):196–198

43. Wartella E. *Parenting in the Age of Digital Technology.* Chicago, IL: Northwestern University Press; 2013

44. Moreno MA, Gannon KE. Social media and health. In: Rosen D, Joffe A, eds. AM STARs Adolescent Medicine: State of the Art Reviews. Young Adult Health. 2013;24(3):538–552

45. Kidd DC, Castano E. Reading literary fiction improves theory of mind. *Science.* 2013;342(6156):377–380

46. Naslund JA, Aschbrenner KA, Marsch LA, Bartels SJ. The future of mental health care: peer-to-peer support and social media. *Epidemiol Psychiatr Sci.* 2016;25(2):113–122

47. Olson KR, Durwood L, DeMeules M, McLaughlin KA. Mental health of transgender children who are supported in their identities. *Pediatrics.* 2016;137(3). Available at: http://pediatrics.aappublications.org/content/137/3/e20153223.

48. Dickins M, Browning C, Feldman S, Thomas S. Social inclusion and the Fatosphere: the role of an online weblogging community in fostering social inclusion. *Sociol Health Illn.* 2016;38(5):797–811

49. Social Issues Research Centre. Totally in control: the rise of pro-ana/pro-mia websites. Available at: www.sirc.org/articles/totally_in_control2.shtml. Accessed May 9, 2016

50. Odom SL, Thompson JL, Hedges S, et al. Technology-aided interventions and instruction for adolescents with autism spectrum disorder. *J Autism Dev Disord.* 2015;45(12):3805–3819

51. Desch LW, Gaebler-Spira D; Council on Children With Disabilities. Prescribing assistive-technology systems: focus on children with impaired communication. *Pediatrics.* 2008;121(6):1271–1280

52. Mazurek MO, Wenstrup C. Television, video game and social media use among children with ASD and typically developing siblings. *J Autism Dev Disord.* 2013;43(6):1258–1271

53. Mazurek MO, Shattuck PT, Wagner M, Cooper BP. Prevalence and correlates of screen-based media use among youths with autism spectrum disorders. *J Autism Dev Disord.* 2012;42(8):1757–1767

54. Tomopoulos S, Dreyer BP, Berkule S, Fierman AH, Brockmeyer C, Mendelsohn AL. Infant media exposure and toddler development. *Arch Pediatr Adolesc Med.* 2010;164(12):1105–1111

55. Schmidt ME, Rich M, Rifas-Shiman SL, Oken E, Taveras EM. Television viewing in infancy and child cognition at 3 years of age in a US cohort. *Pediatrics.* 2009;123(3). Available at: http://pediatrics.aappublications.org/content/123/3/e370

56. Lin LY, Cherng RJ, Chen YJ, Chen YJ, Yang HM. Effects of television exposure on developmental skills among young children. *Infant Behav Dev.* 2015;38:20–26

57. Zimmerman FJ, Christakis DA, Meltzoff AN. Associations between media viewing and language development in children under age 2 years. *J Pediatr.* 2007;151(4):364–368

58. Duch H, Fisher EM, Ensari I, et al. Association of screen time use and language development in Hispanic toddlers: a cross-sectional and longitudinal study. *Clin Pediatr (Phila).* 2013;52(9):857–865

59. Tomopoulos S, Dreyer BP, Valdez P, et al. Media content and externalizing behaviors in Latino toddlers. *Ambul Pediatr.* 2007;7(3):232–238

60. Hinkley T, Verbestel V, Ahrens W, et al; IDEFICS Consortium. Early childhood electronic media use as a predictor of poorer well-being: a prospective cohort study. *JAMA Pediatr.* 2014;168(5):485–492

61. Pagani LS, Fitzpatrick C, Barnett TA, Dubow E. Prospective associations between early childhood television exposure and academic, psychosocial, and physical well-being by middle childhood. *Arch Pediatr Adolesc Med.* 2010;164(5):425–431

62. Conners-Burrow NA, McKelvey LM, Fussell JJ. Social outcomes associated with media viewing habits of low-income preschool children. *Early Educ Dev.* 2011;22(2):256–273

63. Christakis DA, Gilkerson J, Richards JA, et al. Audible television and decreased adult words, infant vocalizations, and conversational turns: a population-based study. *Arch Pediatr Adolesc Med.* 2009;163(6):554–558

64. Nathanson AI, Sharp ML, Alade F, Rasmussen EE, Christy K. The relation between television exposure and theory of mind among preschoolers. *Dev Psychol.* 2014;50(5):1497–1506

65. Rothbart MK, Posner MI. The developing brain in a multitasking world. *Dev Rev.* 2015;35(35):42–63

66. Goodrich SA, Pempek TA, Calvert SL. Formal production features of infant and toddler DVDs. *Arch Pediatr Adolesc Med.* 2009;163(12):1151–1156

67. American Academy of Pediatrics, Council on Communications and Media. Virtual violence statement. *Pediatrics.* 2016;138(1). Available at: http://pediatrics.aappublications.org/content/early/2016/07/14/peds.2016-1298.

68. Hiniker A, Schoenebeck SY, Kientz JA. Not at the dinner table: parents' and children's perspectives on family technology rules. In: *CSCW '16: Proceedings of the 19th ACM Conference on Computer-Supported Cooperative Work & Social Computing;* February 27–March 2, 2016; New York,

NY. 1376–1389., Available at http://dl.acm.org/citation.cfm?doid=2818048.2819940. Accessed May 9, 2016

69. Thompson AL, Adair LS, Bentley ME. Maternal characteristics and perception of temperament associated with infant TV exposure. *Pediatrics.* 2013;131(2). Available at: http://pediatrics.aappublications.org/content/131/2/e390

70. Sugawara M, Matsumoto S, Murohashi H, Sakai A, Isshiki N. Trajectories of early television contact in Japan: relationship with preschoolers' externalizing problems. *J Child Media.* 2015;9(4):453–471

71. Radesky JS, Silverstein M, Zuckerman B, Christakis DA. Infant self-regulation and early childhood media exposure. *Pediatrics.* 2014;133(5). Available at: http://pediatrics.aappublications.org/content/133/5/e1172

72. Radesky JS, Peacock-Chambers E, Zuckerman B, Silverstein M. Use of mobile technology to calm upset children: associations with social-emotional development. *JAMA Pediatr.* 2016;170(4):397–399

73. Linebarger DL, Barr R, Lapierre MA, Piotrowski JT. Associations between parenting, media use, cumulative risk, and children's executive functioning. *J Dev Behav Pediatr.* 2014;35(6):367–377

74. Bel-Serrat S, Mouratidou T, Santaliestra-Pasías AM, et al; IDEFICS consortium. Clustering of multiple lifestyle behaviours and its association to cardiovascular risk factors in children: the IDEFICS study. *Eur J Clin Nutr.* 2013;67(8):848–854

75. Cox R, Skouteris H, Rutherford L, Fuller-Tyszkiewicz M, Dell' Aquila D, Hardy LL. Television viewing, television content, food intake, physical activity and body mass index: a cross-sectional study of preschool children aged 2-6 years. *Health Promot J Austr.* 2012;23(1):58–62

76. Suglia SF, Duarte CS, Chambers EC, Boynton-Jarrett R. Social and behavioral risk factors for obesity in early childhood. *J Dev Behav Pediatr.* 2013;34(8):549–556

77. Wen LM, Baur LA, Rissel C, Xu H, Simpson JM. Correlates of body mass

index and overweight and obesity of children aged 2 years: findings from the healthy beginnings trial. *Obesity (Silver Spring)*. 2014;22(7):1723–1730

78. Taveras EM, Gillman MW, Kleinman KP, Rich-Edwards JW, Rifas-Shiman SL. Reducing racial/ethnic disparities in childhood obesity: the role of early life risk factors. *JAMA Pediatr*. 2013;167(8):731–738

79. Bellissimo N, Pencharz PB, Thomas SG, Anderson GH. Effect of television viewing at mealtime on food intake after a glucose preload in boys. *Pediatr Res*. 2007;61(6):745–749

80. Proctor MH, Moore LL, Gao D, et al. Television viewing and change in body fat from preschool to early adolescence: The Framingham Children's Study. *Int J Obes Relat Metab Disord*. 2003;27(7):827–833

81. Gortmaker SL, Must A, Sobol AM, Peterson K, Colditz GA, Dietz WH. Television viewing as a cause of increasing obesity among children in the United States, 1986-1990. *Arch Pediatr Adolesc Med*. 1996;150(4):356–362

82. de Jong E, Visscher TL HiraSing RA, Heymans MW, Seidell JC, Renders CM. Association between TV viewing, computer use and overweight, determinants and competing activities of screen time in 4- to 13-year-old children. *Int J Obes*. 2013;37(1):47–53

83. Braithwaite I, Stewart AW, Hancox RJ, Beasley R, Murphy R, Mitchell EA; ISAAC Phase Three Study Group. The worldwide association between television viewing and obesity in children and adolescents: cross sectional study. *PLoS One*. 2013;8(9):e74263

84. Mitchell JA, Rodriguez D, Schmitz KH, Audrain-McGovern J. Greater screen time is associated with adolescent obesity: a longitudinal study of the BMI distribution from Ages 14 to 18. *Obesity (Silver Spring)*. 2013;21(3):572–575

85. Sisson SB, Broyles ST, Baker BL, Katzmarzyk PT. Screen time, physical activity, and overweight in U.S. youth: national survey of children's health 2003. *J Adolesc Health*. 2010;47(3):309–311

86. Laurson KR, Eisenmann JC, Welk GJ, Wickel EE, Gentile DA, Walsh DA. Combined influence of physical activity and screen time recommendations on childhood overweight. *J Pediatr*. 2008;153(2):209–214

87. Zimmerman FJ, Bell JF. Associations of television content type and obesity in children. *Am J Public Health*. 2010;100(2):334–340

88. Wethington H, Pan L, Sherry B. The association of screen time, television in the bedroom, and obesity among school-aged youth: 2007 National Survey of Children's Health. *J Sch Health*. 2013;83(8):573–581

89. Robinson TN. Reducing children's television viewing to prevent obesity: a randomized controlled trial. *JAMA*. 1999;282(16):1561–1567

90. Bruni O, Sette S, Fontanesi L, Baiocco R, Laghi F, Baumgartner E. Technology use and sleep quality in preadolescence and adolescence. *J Clin Sleep Med*. 2015;11(12):1433–1441

91. Cespedes EM, Gillman MW, Kleinman K, Rifas-Shiman SL, Redline S, Taveras EM. Television viewing, bedroom television, and sleep duration from infancy to mid-childhood. *Pediatrics*. 2014;133(5). Available at: http://pediatrics.aappublications.org/content/133/5/e1163

92. Garrison MM, Christakis DA. The impact of a healthy media use intervention on sleep in preschool children. *Pediatrics*. 2012;130(3):492–499

93. Salti R, Tarquini R, Stagi S, et al. Age-dependent association of exposure to television screen with children's urinary melatonin excretion? *Neuroendocrinol Lett*. 2006;27(1-2):73–80

94. Vijakkhana N, Wilaisakditipakorn T, Ruedeekhajorn K, Pruksananonda C, Chonchaiya W. Evening media exposure reduces night-time sleep. *Acta Paediatr*. 2015;104(3):306–312

95. Levenson JC, Shensa A, Sidani JE, Colditz JB, Primack BA. The association between social media use and sleep disturbance among young adults. *Prev Med*. 2016;85:36–41

96. Buxton OM, Chang AM, Spilsbury JC, Bos T, Emsellem H, Knutson KL. Sleep in the modern family: protective family routines for child and adolescent sleep. *Sleep Health*. 2015;1(1):15–27

97. Arora T, Broglia E, Thomas GN, Taheri S. Associations between specific technologies and adolescent sleep quantity, sleep quality, and parasomnias. *Sleep Med*. 2014;15(2):240–247

98. Exelmans L, Van den Bulck J. Bedtime mobile phone use and sleep in adults. *Soc Sci Med*. 2016;148:93–101

99. Lemola S, Perkinson-Gloor N, Brand S, Dewald-Kaufmann JF, Grob A. Adolescents' electronic media use at night, sleep disturbance, and depressive symptoms in the smartphone age. *J Youth Adolesc*. 2015;44(2):405–418

100. Hysing M, Pallesen S, Stormark KM, Jakobsen R, Lundervold AJ, Sivertsen B. Sleep and use of electronic devices in adolescence: results from a large population-based study. *BMJ Open*. 2015;5(1):e006748

101. Gidwani PP, Sobol A, DeJong W, Perrin JM, Gortmaker SL. Television viewing and initiation of smoking among youth. *Pediatrics*. 2002;110(3):505–508

102. Dalton MA, Beach ML, Adachi-Mejia AM, et al. Early exposure to movie smoking predicts established smoking by older teens and young adults. *Pediatrics*. 2009;123(4). Available at: http://pediatrics.aappublications.org/content/123/4/e551

103. Dalton MA, Sargent JD, Beach ML, et al. Effect of viewing smoking in movies on adolescent smoking initiation: a cohort study. *Lancet*. 2003;362(9380):281–285

104. Titus-Ernstoff L, Dalton MA, Adachi-Mejia AM, Longacre MR, Beach ML. Longitudinal study of viewing smoking in movies and initiation of smoking by children. *Pediatrics*. 2008;121(1):15–21

105. Robinson TN, Chen HL, Killen JD. Television and music video exposure and risk of adolescent alcohol use. *Pediatrics*. 1998;102(5):E54

106. Klein JD, Brown JD, Childers KW, Oliveri J, Porter C, Dykers C. Adolescents' risky behavior and mass media use. *Pediatrics*. 1993;92(1):24–31

107. Strasburger VC, Wilson BJ, Jordan A. *Children, adolescents and the media*. Thousand Oaks, CA: Sage Publications; 2008

108. Hinduja S, Patchin JW. Personal information of adolescents on the Internet: A quantitative content analysis of MySpace. *J Adolesc*. 2008;31(1):125–146

109. Moreno MA, Parks MR, Zimmerman FJ, Brito TE, Christakis DA. Display of health risk behaviors on MySpace by adolescents: prevalence and associations. *Arch Pediatr Adolesc Med*. 2009;163(1):27–34

110. Moreno MA, Parks M, Richardson LP. What are adolescents showing the world about their health risk behaviors on MySpace? *MedGenMed*. 2007;9(4):9

111. McGee JB, Begg M. What medical educators need to know about "Web 2.0". *Med Teach*. 2008;30(2):164–169

112. Moreno MA, Ton A, Selkie E, Evans Y. Secret Society 123: understanding the language of self-harm on Instagram. *J Adolesc Health*. 2016;58(1):78–84

113. Moreno MA, Briner LR, Williams A, Walker L, Christakis DA. Real use or "real cool": adolescents speak out about displayed alcohol references on social networking websites. *J Adolesc Health*. 2009;45(4):420–422

114. Moreno MA, Kota R, Schoohs S, Whitehill JM. The Facebook influence model: a concept mapping approach. *Cyberpsychol Behav Soc Netw*. 2013;16(7):504–511

115. Litt DM, Stock ML. Adolescent alcohol-related risk cognitions: the roles of social norms and social networking sites. *Psychol Addict Behav*. 2011;25(4):708–713

116. Fogg BJ. Mass interpersonal persuasion: an early view of a new phenomenon. In: Oinas-Kukkonen H, Hasle P, Harjumaa M, Segerståhl K, Øhrstrøm P, eds. *Persuasive Technology, Third International Conference, PERSUASIVE 2008, Oulu, Finland, June 4–6, 2008, Proceedings*. Berlin, Germany: Springer-Verlag Berlin Heidelberg; 2008:23–34

117. Martins N, Harrison K. Racial and gender differences in the relationship between children's television use and self-esteem a longitudinal panel study communication research. *Communic Res*. 2012;39(3):338–357

118. Bélanger RE, Akre C, Berchtold A, Michaud PA. A U-shaped association between intensity of Internet use and adolescent health. *Pediatrics*. 2011;127(2). Available at: http://pediatrics.aappublications.org/content/127/2/e330

119. Moreno MA, Jelenchick L, Koff RN, Eickhoff J. Depression and internet use among older adolescents: an experience sampling approach. *Psychology (Irvine)*. 2012;3(9A):743–748

120. Lin LY, Sidani JE, Shensa A, et al. Association between social media use and depression among U.S. young adults. *Depress Anxiety*. 2016;33(4):323–331

121. Kross E, Verduyn P, Demiralp E, et al. Facebook use predicts declines in subjective well-being in young adults. *PLoS One*. 2013;8(8):e69841

122. Lup K, Trub L, Rosenthal L. Instagram #instasad?: exploring associations among instagram use, depressive symptoms, negative social comparison, and strangers followed. *Cyberpsychol Behav Soc Netw*. 2015;18(5):247–252

123. Boyd D, Marwick AE. Social privacy in networked publics: teens' attitudes, practices, and strategies. In: *A Decade in Internet Time: Symposium on the Dynamics of the Internet and Society*, September 21–24, 2011; Oxford, U.K.:1-29

124. Madden M, Lenhart A, Cortesi S, et al. *Teens, Social Media, and Privacy*. Washington, DC: Pew Research Center; 2013

125. Moreno MA, Kelleher E, Ameenuddin N, Rastogi S. Young adult females' views regarding online privacy protection at two time points. *J Adolesc Health*. 2014;55(3):347–351

126. Hoadley CM, Xu H, Lee JJ, Rosson MB. Privacy as information access and illusory control: the case of the Facebook News Feed privacy outcry. *Electron Commer Res Appl*. 2010;9(1):50–60

127. Tsukayama H. Facebook draws fire from privacy advocates over ad changes. *The Washington Post*. June 12, 2014. Available at: https://www.washingtonpost.com/news/the-switch/wp/2014/06/12/privacy-experts-say-facebook-changes-open-up-unprecedented-data-collection/. Accessed May 9, 2016

128. Smith PK, Mahdavi J, Carvalho M, Fisher S, Russell S, Tippett N. Cyberbullying: its nature and impact in secondary school pupils. *J Child Psychol Psychiatry*. 2008;49(4):376–385

129. Waasdorp TE, Bradshaw CP. The overlap between cyberbullying and traditional bullying. *J Adolesc Health*. 2015;56(5):483–488

130. Raskauskas J, Stoltz AD. Involvement in traditional and electronic bullying among adolescents. *Dev Psychol*. 2007;43(3):564–575

131. Schneider SK, O'Donnell L, Stueve A, Coulter RW. Cyberbullying, school bullying, and psychological distress: a regional census of high school students. *Am J Public Health*. 2012;102(1):171–177

132. Rivara F, Le Menestrel S, eds. *Preventing Bullying Through Science, Policy, and Practice*. Washington, DC: National Academies of Sciences, Engineering, and Medicine; 2016, Available at www.nap.edu/catalog/23482/preventing-bullying-through-science-policy-and-practice. Accessed May 9, 2016

133. McDougall P, Vaillancourt T. Long-term adult outcomes of peer victimization in childhood and adolescence: Pathways to adjustment and maladjustment. *Am Psychol*. 2015;70(4):300–310

134. Vaillancourt T, Brittain HL, McDougall P, Duku E. Longitudinal links between childhood peer victimization, internalizing and externalizing problems, and academic functioning: developmental cascades. *J Abnorm Child Psychol*. 2013;41(8):1203–1215

135. Vaillancourt T, Duku E, Decatanzaro D, Macmillan H, Muir C, Schmidt LA. Variation in hypothalamic-pituitary-adrenal axis activity among bullied and non-bullied children. *Aggress Behav*. 2008;34(3):294–305

136. Vaillancourt T, Duku E, Becker S, et al. Peer victimization, depressive

symptoms, and high salivary cortisol predict poorer memory in children. *Brain Cogn.* 2011;77(2):191–199

137. Selkie E, Kota R, Moreno M. Relationship between cyberbullying experiences and depressive symptoms in female college students. *J Adolesc Health.* 2014;54(2):S28

138. Del Rey R, Casas JA, Ortega R. Impact of the ConRed program on different cyberbulling roles. *Aggress Behav.* 2016;42(2):123–135

139. Moreno MA. Cyberbullying. *JAMA Pediatr.* 2014;168(5):500

140. David-Ferdon C, Hertz MF. *Electronic Media and Youth Violence: A CDC Issue Brief for Researchers.* Atlanta, GA: Centers for Disease Control and Prevention; 2009

141. Spencer J, Olson J, Schrager S, Tanaka D, Belzer M. Sexting and adolescents: a descriptive study of sexting and youth in an urban population. *J Adolesc Health.* 2015;56(2 Suppl 1):S22

142. Ybarra ML, Mitchell KJ. "Sexting" and its relation to sexual activity and sexual risk behavior in a national survey of adolescents. *J Adolesc Health.* 2014;55(6):757–764

143. Temple JR, Le VD, van den Berg P, Ling Y, Paul JA, Temple BW. Brief report: Teen sexting and psychosocial health. *J Adolesc.* 2014;37(1):33–36

144. Stanley J. Child abuse and the Internet. *National Child Protection Clearinghouse Series.* 2001;15:1–18

145. Kendall-Tackett KA, Williams LM, Finkelhor D. Impact of sexual abuse on children: a review and synthesis of recent empirical studies. *Psychol Bull.* 1993;113(1):164–180

146. Irish L, Kobayashi I, Delahanty DL. Long-term physical health consequences of childhood sexual abuse: a meta-analytic review. *J Pediatr Psychol.* 2010;35(5):450–461

147. Aiken M, Moran M, Berry M. Child abuse material and the Internet: cyberpsychology of online child related sex offending. Paper presented at the *29th Meeting of the INTERPOL Specialist Group on Crimes Against Children*; Lyons, France; September 5–7, 2011

148. Mitchell KJ, Wolak J, Finkelhor D. Are blogs putting youth at risk for online sexual solicitation or harassment? *Child Abuse Negl.* 2008;32(2):277–294

149. Halpern CT, Kaestle CE, Hallfors DD. Perceived physical maturity, age of romantic partner, and adolescent risk behavior. *Prev Sci.* 2007;8(1):1–10

150. Neemann J, Hubbard J, Masten AS. The changing importance of romantic relationship involvement to competence from late childhood to late adolescence. *Dev Psychopathol.* 1995;7(4):727–750

151. Steel CM. Child pornography in peer-to-peer networks. *Child Abuse Negl.* 2009;33(8):560–568

152. Brenner J, Smith A. *72% of Online Adults are Social Networking Site Users.* Washington, DC: Pew Internet American Life Project; 2013

153. Kirkorian HL, Pempek TA, Murphy LA, Schmidt ME, Anderson DR. The impact of background television on parent-child interaction. *Child Dev.* 2009;80(5):1350–1359

154. Schmidt ME, Pempek TA, Kirkorian HL, Lund AF, Anderson DR. The effects of background television on the toy play behavior of very young children. *Child Dev.* 2008;79(4):1137–1151

155. Tomopoulos S, Cates CB, Dreyer BP, Fierman AH, Berkule SB, Mendelsohn AL. Children under the age of two are more likely to watch inappropriate background media than older children. *Acta Paediatr.* 2014;103(5):546–552

156. Radesky J, Miller AL, Rosenblum KL, Appugliese D, Kaciroti N, Lumeng JC. Maternal mobile device use during a structured parent-child interaction task. *Acad Pediatr.* 2015;15(2):238–244

157. Radesky JS, Kistin CJ, Zuckerman B, et al. Patterns of mobile device use by caregivers and children during meals in fast food restaurants. *Pediatrics.* 2014;133(4). Available at: http://pediatrics.aappublications.org/content/133/4/e843

158. Jago R, Stamatakis E, Gama A, et al. Parent and child screen-viewing time and home media environment. *Am J Prev Med.* 2012;43(2):150–158

159. Fiese BH, Winter MA, Botti JC. The ABCs of family mealtimes: observational lessons for promoting healthy outcomes for children with persistent asthma. *Child Dev.* 2011;82(1):133–145

160. Chesley N. Information and communication technology use, work intensification, and employee strain and distress. *Work Employ Soc.* 2014;28(4):589–610

161. Schmidt ME, Haines J, O'Brien A, et al. Systematic review of effective strategies for reducing screen time among young children. *Obesity (Silver Spring).* 2012;20(7):1338–1354

Codeine: Time to Say "No"

• •

• *Clinical Report*

CLINICAL REPORT Guidance for the Clinician in Rendering Pediatric Care

American Academy
of Pediatrics

DEDICATED TO THE HEALTH OF ALL CHILDREN™

Codeine: Time to Say "No"

Joseph D. Tobias, MD, Thomas P. Green, MD, Charles J. Coté, MD, SECTION ON
ANESTHESIOLOGY AND PAIN MEDICINE, COMMITTEE ON DRUGS

abstract

Codeine has been prescribed to pediatric patients for many decades as
both an analgesic and an antitussive agent. Codeine is a prodrug with little
inherent pharmacologic activity and must be metabolized in the liver into
morphine, which is responsible for codeine's analgesic effects. However,
there is substantial genetic variability in the activity of the responsible
hepatic enzyme, *CYP2D6*, and, as a consequence, individual patient response
to codeine varies from no effect to high sensitivity. Drug surveillance has
documented the occurrence of unanticipated respiratory depression and
death after receiving codeine in children, many of whom have been shown
to be ultrarapid metabolizers. Patients with documented or suspected
obstructive sleep apnea appear to be at particular risk because of opioid
sensitivity, compounding the danger among rapid metabolizers in this
group. Recently, various organizations and regulatory bodies, including the
World Health Organization, the US Food and Drug Administration, and the
European Medicines Agency, have promulgated stern warnings regarding
the occurrence of adverse effects of codeine in children. These and other
groups have or are considering a declaration of a contraindication for
the use of codeine for children as either an analgesic or an antitussive.
Additional clinical research must extend the understanding of the risks and
benefits of both opioid and nonopioid alternatives for orally administered,
effective agents for acute and chronic pain.

DOI: 10.1542/peds.2016-2396

PEDIATRICS (ISSN Numbers: Print, 0031-4005; Online, 1098-4275).

Copyright © 2016 by the American Academy of Pediatrics

FINANCIAL DISCLOSURE: The authors have indicated they do
not have a financial relationship relevant to this article to
disclose.

FUNDING: No external funding.

POTENTIAL CONFLICT OF INTEREST: The authors have
indicated they have no potential conflicts of interest to
disclose.

To cite: Tobias JD, Green TP, Coté CJ, AAP SECTION ON
ANESTHESIOLOGY AND PAIN MEDICINE, AAP COMMITTEE ON
DRUGS. Codeine: Time To Say "No". *Pediatrics*. 2016;138(4):
e20162396

INTRODUCTION

Effective pain management for pediatric patients remains problematic,
with studies showing that significant improvements and alterations
in practice may be needed to provide safe and adequate analgesia.[1-3]
These issues are further complicated by the limited number of child-
appropriate pain formulations and medications, parental perceptions
about the need for such analgesics, and differences in metabolism and
oral bioavailability between children and adults.[1,4] Similarly, there are
few evidence-based therapies for children with cough.[5] The purpose of
this clinical report is to present up-to-date information regarding risks
related to pharmacogenetic variations in codeine metabolism and to

outline the therapeutic and safety implications in the treatment of pain or cough in children.

BACKGROUND

Codeine (3-methylmorphine) is a naturally occurring methylated morphine that has seen widespread clinical use for >50 years as an analgesic and an antitussive agent. Historically, codeine was considered an optimal oral analgesic for the outpatient treatment of acute pain of various etiologies in children, partly because of the perception that it was a safe opioid analgesic with a wide therapeutic index and a limited risk of respiratory depression.[6] It was the primary agent used for outpatient analgesia after adenotonsillectomy in children and was recommended as a step 2 medication in the World Health Organization Pain Ladder for the treatment of moderate pain.[7] However, codeine itself has no analgesic effect; it is a prodrug that must be metabolized to morphine to be effective. Furthermore, increased understanding of pharmacogenetics and ongoing safety investigations have shown a large variation in the conversion of codeine to morphine. This genetics-based interpatient variation produces considerable variability in the therapeutic response to recommended codeine dosing, ranging from a lack of effect because of low morphine levels to fatalities related to excessive morphine levels.[8]

Despite these concerns and the potential hazards, codeine continues to be widely available from many pharmacies and inpatient hospital formularies for use in outpatient pediatric settings and is commonly prescribed to pediatric patients.[9,10] One study from 2011 reported that, among dispensed prescriptions for selected opioids, codeine was prescribed to >800 000 patients younger than 11 years, more than any other opioid in the study.[11]

During the years 2007–2011, otolaryngologists were the most frequent prescribers of codeine/ acetaminophen liquid formulations (19.6%), followed by dentists (13.3%), pediatricians (12.7%), and general practice/family physicians (10.1%).[11] Two other studies reported the use of opioids in pediatric emergency departments in the period 2001–2010. In 1 study, the frequency of codeine administration in emergency departments both for pain associated with injury and for cough remained unchanged during this period.[9] The other longitudinal study covering the same time period showed that overall codeine use remained constant in adolescents but has decreased in younger age groups.[12]

In the last 5 years, various organizations and regulatory bodies have promulgated warnings regarding adverse responses associated with codeine, as follows:

1. March 2011: The World Health Organization deleted codeine from its list of essential medications for children because of concerns that its "efficacy and safety were questionable in an unpredictable portion of the paediatric population."[13]

2. August 2012: The US Food and Drug Administration (FDA) issued a safety alert regarding the use of codeine in children after tonsillectomy, adenoidectomy, or adenotonsillectomy.[14]

3. February 2013: An update from the FDA added a "black box warning" to the drug label of codeine and codeine-containing preparations. The warning advises health care professionals "to prescribe an alternative analgesic [to codeine] for postoperative pain control in children undergoing tonsillectomy and/or adenoidectomy." A contraindication was added to restrict codeine use in such

patients. The "Warnings/ Precautions," "Pediatric Use," and "Patient Counseling Information" sections of the label were also updated.[15]

4. June 2013: The European Medicines Agency issued a report recommending the restriction of codeine for the treatment of pain to children older than 12 years as well as a contraindication to its use in children younger than 18 years undergoing tonsillectomy and/or adenoidectomy. In addition, it recommended against codeine use in breastfeeding women.[16]

5. June 2013: Health Canada announced that it had reviewed the safety of prescription pain and cough medications containing codeine and recommended against their use in children younger than 12 years.[17]

6. March 2015: The European Medicines Agency completed a review of the use of codeine for cough and cold and recommended against its use in children younger than 12 years as well as children and adolescents between 12 and 18 years who have problems with breathing.[18]

GENETIC VARIABILITY IN CODEINE METABOLISM

Codeine is a prodrug that has limited affinity for the μ-opioid receptor and no analgesic effects. After an oral dose, the majority of codeine undergoes hepatic glucuronidation or N-demethylation to inactive metabolites. The analgesic properties result from hepatic metabolism and conversion of the parent compound (codeine) to morphine and the active metabolite morphine-6-glucuronide. The conversion from codeine to morphine is regulated by the cytochrome P450 2D6 (CYP2D6) enzyme system.[19,20]

The activity of *CYP2D6* varies significantly as a function of genetic polymorphisms. More than 70 different alleles have been identified, with individuals inheriting 1 allele from each parent. The level of enzyme activity from each allele has been broadly classified according to the following scheme: normal function = 1, reduced function = 0.5, and no function = 0. The enzyme activity for an individual is the sum of activity from each parent's allele. On the basis of these additive scores, individuals can be classified as extensive (score of 1–2), intermediate (0.5), or poor (0) metabolizers. It has also been increasingly recognized that some individuals may have significantly more activity related to gene duplication.

The prevalence of the different levels of activity varies among ethnic backgrounds, with poor metabolizers overrepresented in people of northern European Caucasian descent. Poor metabolizers initially received the greatest attention because of codeine's lack of efficacy in such patients.[21–23] As our understanding of the influence of genetic variations on pharmacokinetics has improved, attention has become more focused on individuals who are ultrarapid metabolizers secondary to gene duplications. This latter group has ≥2 copies of the *CYP2D6* gene, which can result in an enzyme activity score ≥3, indicating a very high level of enzyme activity. The result in these patients is the production of large amounts of morphine that can cause respiratory depression or apnea, even after normal therapeutic doses of oral codeine.[19,23,24] The frequency of the ultrarapid metabolizer genotype has been estimated at ~29% of patients of African/Ethiopian heritage, ~21% of those from Saudi Arabia and other Middle Eastern countries, and ~3.4% to 6.5% of African-American and white persons.[19,20,23,24]

Intermediate metabolism tends to be more common in Asians than in whites,[25] but poor metabolism is less common.[26]

REPORTS OF ADVERSE EFFECTS

The evidence linking the use of codeine with life-threatening or fatal respiratory depression is based on a series of case reports that have appeared in the literature regularly since 2004.[27–34] The publication of these reports initiated an evaluation by the FDA, which included a review of the literature as well as reports submitted to the FDA Adverse Event Reporting System from 1969 through May 2012.[35] The search revealed 13 cases of pediatric deaths (*n* = 10) or respiratory depression (*n* = 3) attributed to the therapeutic use of codeine, 7 of which had been published in the medical literature. The age range was slightly wider than the initial reports (21 months to 9 years of age). The majority occurred during the postoperative period after adenoidectomy or adenotonsillectomy with the recommended codeine dose and dosing interval. However, 1 clinical study proposed that repeated episodes of hypoxemia result in altered μ-opioid receptors and greater analgesic potency of opioids in this setting.[36]

Three additional pediatric deaths related to codeine were reported in 2013.[37] These included a 10-year-old child who had undergone orthopedic surgery, a 4-year-old treated after tonsillectomy, and a third child who received codeine as a cough suppressant, albeit in a higher dose than was prescribed.

Most recently, a review by the FDA of the Adverse Event Reporting System data from 1965 to 2015 in children who had used codeine or any codeine-containing products revealed a total of 64 cases of severe respiratory depression and 24 codeine-related deaths, 21 of which were in children younger than 12 years.[38]

USE OF CODEINE AND ITS ALTERNATIVES FOR ANALGESIA

Even before these reports of adverse events, many physicians had concerns regarding the efficacy of codeine, mostly related to its lack of effect in a significant proportion of the population (poor metabolizers). Although *CYP2D6* genotyping that could identify patients at higher risk is available (although currently expensive), patients with normal metabolism are also at theoretical risk of high morphine levels. Therefore, further investigation is required to determine the value of such testing, which will depend on the population in whom it is applied. As such, physicians are faced with considering alternative analgesic agents to use when oral administration is needed postoperatively or in the outpatient setting.

In the United States, many physicians have switched to prescribing oxycodone for analgesia. Oxycodone is a semisynthetic opioid that is an active analgesic, not a prodrug like codeine. Metabolism is via N-demethylation by the *CYP3A4* enzyme system to inactive metabolites. A minor percentage of oxycodone is metabolized by the *CYP2D6* enzyme system to the active metabolite noroxymorphone, so ultrarapid metabolizers may be at some risk of opiate toxicity. Oxycodone is available in a liquid formulation both alone and in combination with acetaminophen. However, data are currently insufficient to unequivocally endorse the widespread use of oxycodone in infants and children. One study has shown considerable variability in absorption and oral bioavailability in children.[39] Another recent preliminary pharmacokinetic study in children younger than 6 years showed significant differences in onset of absorption and peak levels of oxycodone and plasma concentrations of noroxymorphone on the basis of *CYP2D6* genotypes.[40]

Hydrocodone is also a potential alternative for analgesia, but *CYP2D6* is responsible for the conversion of hydrocodone to an active metabolite, hydromorphone. Ultrarapid metabolizers may have up to an eightfold greater plasma concentration of hydromorphone, whereas poor metabolizers receive minimal analgesia.[41]

Given the problems with codeine and potential concerns with the other available agents, the use of an oral morphine elixir has been suggested by some as an alternative.[20,42] However, although there is extensive experience with intravenous morphine in children, there is little clinical experience and very limited comparative clinical data on safety and efficacy available for the oral formulation.

Additional options for pain relief include less familiar and less commonly used medications, such as tramadol. Tramadol has a longer half-life (6–7 hours) than other oral agents as well as an active metabolite with a half-life of 10 to 11 hours. Unlike other weak opioids, it has a unique dual mechanism of action, including agonism at the μ-opioid receptor, and inhibits reuptake of neurotransmitters (norepinephrine and serotonin) within the central nervous system. Primary metabolism occurs through hepatic N-demethylation by the cytochrome *CYP3A4* enzyme system to an inactive metabolite. A smaller percentage is metabolized by o-demethylation (*CYP2D6* enzyme) to the active metabolite desmethyltramadol. Although preliminary studies in the pediatric population have shown effective analgesia,[43–46] there are reasons to be concerned about potential problems with tramadol that are similar to those encountered

with codeine. Although tramadol is not dependent on metabolism for its analgesic effect, it is partially dependent on the *CYP2D6* enzyme system for metabolism, which could lead to drug accumulation in poor metabolizers.[47] In addition, the o-demethylated (*CYP2D6*-dependent) metabolite has a much higher affinity for the μ-opioid receptor, and a case report of administration of tramadol to a child with ultrarapid metabolism and subsequent respiratory depression was recently published.[48] Furthermore, many other drugs, including selective serotonin reuptake inhibitors, tricyclic antidepressants, and some antiepileptic drugs, inhibit the metabolism of tramadol, leading to undesirable tramadol accumulation. As such, further investigation must be conducted before the widespread use of tramadol in children for pain relief.

A similar agent, tapentadol, is a centrally acting analgesic with a dual mode of action as an agonist at the μ-opioid receptor and as a norepinephrine reuptake inhibitor within the central nervous system. In contradistinction to tramadol, it has only weak effects on the reuptake of serotonin and is a significantly more potent opioid agonist. It has no active metabolites. It was approved by the FDA in 2011 for use in adults; to date, there are no data regarding its use in the pediatric population. There is 1 report from a poison control center review of 124 unintended exposures, one of which resulted in coma and respiratory depression in a 9-month-old child.[49]

Concerns regarding opioids in children with sleep-disordered breathing have led to a reevaluation of postoperative nonopioid analgesics, such as acetaminophen and nonsteroidal antiinflammatory drugs (NSAIDs), such as ibuprofen, for children with mild to moderate pain.[50–54] In addition, there are intravenous formulations of

acetaminophen and an NSAID (ketorolac).[55,56] Although previously thought to potentially increase the incidence of postoperative bleeding, some evidence suggests that NSAIDs can be incorporated into the postoperative regimen without adversely affecting the postoperative course in most children without underlying bleeding diatheses.[53,54] The effective use of these nonopioid agents may significantly reduce or, in some cases, eliminate the need for opioids. Further studies of other nonopioid analgesics, including dextromethorphan and dexmedetomidine, are also needed.

It is clear that one of the keys to improving analgesia and reducing opioid-related adverse effects is both provider and parental education regarding the effective use of nonopioid analgesics.[1,57] The answer may not lie in using more medication or different medications but merely using more effectively other options that are currently available.

USE OF CODEINE AS AN ANTITUSSIVE AGENT IN CHILDREN

Codeine is also prescribed as an antitussive agent and is still available in over-the-counter cough and cold formulations without a prescription from outpatient pharmacies in 28 US states and the District of Columbia.[38] However, neither the value of suppressing cough nor the effectiveness of codeine in children with acute illnesses has been shown,[58–60] and the risks of codeine administration described previously also apply to children receiving this agent as an antitussive agent. In April 2015, the European Medicines Agency announced that codeine must not be used to treat cough and cold in children younger than 12 years[18] and further cautioned that codeine is not recommended in children and adolescents between 12 and 18 years of age with compromised respiratory function, including those with asthma and other chronic breathing problems. On July 1, 2015, the FDA issued a drug safety communication stating that it is investigating the possible risks of using codeine-containing medicines to treat coughs and colds in children younger than 18 years because of the potential for serious adverse effects, including slowed or difficult breathing.[61] An FDA advisory panel met in December 2015[38] and, by an overwhelming majority vote, recommended that the use of codeine in the treatment of cough in all children up to 18 years of age should be contraindicated. Final agency action on this recommendation is pending at this time. Alternative therapies for cough have recently been reviewed.[62]

SUMMARY

Published reports and clinical evidence have shown the potential dangers of codeine as an analgesic or as an antitussive. Although these concerns have been emphasized by the FDA, the European Medicines Agency, Health Canada, and the American Academy of Pediatrics, regular codeine administration to children continues.[9,10,63] The life-threatening events and deaths in these reports share a number of common features in that the majority of the children (1) were relatively young, (2) were placed on a postoperative pain regimen of scheduled acetaminophen and codeine, and (3) had undergone adenotonsillectomy for sleep-disordered breathing. However, physicians cannot assume that such problems will occur only after adenotonsillectomy. Given the increasing prevalence of obesity in the United States, it is likely that some patients presenting for nonotolaryngologic procedures may have undiagnosed sleep-disordered breathing and may also be at risk if they require extended postoperative analgesia.

Additional measures are needed to prevent future problems with the use of codeine in the pediatric population. Improved education of parents and more formal restrictions regarding its use in children, regardless of age, are necessary. The evolving information about the genetic variability in drug metabolism will yield important insights to guide physicians in the safe and effective treatment of their patients. Additional clinical research must extend the understanding of the risks and benefits of both opioid and nonopioid alternatives for orally administered, effective agents for acute pain.

LEAD AUTHORS

Joseph D. Tobias, MD, FAAP
Thomas P. Green, MD, FAAP
Charles J. Coté, MD, FAAP

SECTION ON ANESTHESIOLOGY AND PAIN MEDICINE EXECUTIVE COMMITTEE, 2014–2015

Joseph D. Tobias, MD, FAAP
Rita Agarwal, MD, FAAP
Corrie T.M. Anderson, MD, FAAP
Courtney Alan Hardy, MD, FAAP
Anita Honkanen, MD, FAAP
Mohamed A. Rehman, MD, FAAP

LIAISONS

Carolyn Bannister, MD
Randall Flick, MD
Constance S. Houck, MD
Carolyn Bannister

STAFF

Jennifer Riefe

COMMITTEE ON DRUGS, 2014–2015

Kathleen Neville, MD, MS, FAAP, Chairperson
Thomas P. Green, MD, FAAP
Constance S. Houck, MD, FAAP
Bridgette Jones, MD, MSc, FAAP
Ian M. Paul, MD, MSc, FAAP
Janice E. Sullivan, MD, FAAP
John N. Van Den Anker, MD, PhD, FAAP

LIAISONS

John J. Alexander, MD, FAAP – *Food and Drug Administration*
R. Phillip Heine, MD – *American College of Obstetricians and Gynecologists*
Janet D. Cragan, MD, MPH, FAAP – *Centers for Disease Control and Prevention*

Michael J. Rieder, MD, FAAP – *Canadian Paediatric Society*
Adelaide S. Robb, MD – *American Academy of Child and Adolescent Psychiatry*
Hari Cheryl Sachs, MD, FAAP – *Food and Drug Administration*
Anne Zajicek, MD, PharmD, FAAP – *National Institutes of Health*

STAFF

Raymond J. Koteras, MHA

ABBREVIATIONS

FDA: Food and Drug Administration
NSAID: nonsteroidal antiinflammatory drug

REFERENCES

1. Fortier MA, MacLaren JE, Martin SR, Perret-Karimi D, Kain ZN. Pediatric pain after ambulatory surgery: where's the medication? *Pediatrics.* 2009;124(4):e588–e595

2. Shum S, Lim J, Page T, et al. An audit of pain management following pediatric day surgery at British Columbia Children's Hospital. *Pain Res Manag.* 2012;17(5):328–334

3. Stewart DW, Ragg PG, Sheppard S, Chalkiadis GA. The severity and duration of postoperative pain and analgesia requirements in children after tonsillectomy, orchidopexy, or inguinal hernia repair. *Paediatr Anaesth.* 2012;22(2):136–143

4. Rony RY, Fortier MA, Chorney JM, Perret D, Kain ZN. Parental postoperative pain management: attitudes, assessment, and management. *Pediatrics.* 2010;125(6):e1372–e1378

5. Paul IM. Therapeutic options for acute cough due to upper respiratory infections in children. *Lung.* 2012;190(1):41–44

6. Ewah BN, Robb PJ, Raw M. Postoperative pain, nausea and vomiting following paediatric day-case tonsillectomy. *Anaesthesia.* 2006;61(2):116–122

7. Tremlett M, Anderson BJ, Wolf A. Pro-con debate: is codeine a drug that still

has a useful role in pediatric practice? *Paediatr Anaesth.* 2010;20(2):183–194

8. Madadi P, Koren G. Pharmacogenetic insights into codeine analgesia: implications to pediatric codeine use. *Pharmacogenomics.* 2008;9(9):1267–1284

9. Kaiser SV, Asteria-Penaloza R, Vittinghoff E, Rosenbluth G, Cabana MD, Bardach NS. National patterns of codeine prescriptions for children in the emergency department. *Pediatrics.* 2014;133(5):e1139–e1147

10. Cartabuke RS, Tobias JD, Taghon T, Rice J. Current practices regarding codeine administration among pediatricians and pediatric subspecialists. *Clin Pediatr (Phila).* 2014;53(1):26–30

11. Racoosin JA. Death and respiratory arrest related to ultra-rapid metabolism of codeine to morphine. Available at: www.fda.gov/downloads/AdvisoryCommittees/CommitteesMeetingMaterials/PediatricAdvisoryCommittee/UCM343601.pdf. Accessed January 6, 2016

12. Mazer-Amirshahi M, Mullins PM, Rasooly IR, van den Anker J, Pines JM. Trends in prescription opioid use in pediatric emergency department patients. *Pediatr Emerg Care.* 2014;30(4):230–235

13. World Health Organization. Unedited report of the 18th Expert Committee on the Selection and Use of Essential Medicines. Geneva, Switzerland: World Health Organization; 2011. Available at: www.who.int/selection_medicines/Complete_UNEDITED_TRS_18th.pdf. Accessed February 1, 2016

14. US Food and Drug Administration. Drug safety communication. Codeine use in certain children after tonsillectomy and or adenoidectomy may lead to rare but life threatening adverse events or death. Rockville, MD: US Food and Drug Administration; 2012. Available at: www.fda.gov/Drugs/Drugsafety/ucm313631.htm. Accessed February 23, 2016

15. US Food and Drug Administration. Drug safety communication. Safety review update of codeine use in children: a new boxed warning and contraindication on use after tonsillectomy and or adenoidectomy.

Rockville, MD: US Food and Drug Administration; 2013. Available at: www.fda.gov/Drugs/Drugsafety/ucm339112.htm. Accessed February 23, 2016

16. European Medicines Agency. Codeine-containing medicines. 2013. Available at: www.ema.europa.eu/ema/index.jsp?curl=pages/medicines/human/referrals/Codeinecontaining_medicines/human_referral_prac_000008.jsp&mid=WC0b01ac05805c516f. Accessed February 23, 2016

17. Health Canada. Health Canada's review recommends codeine only be used in patients aged 12 and over. Ottawa, Canada: Health Canada; 2013. Available at: www.healthycanadians.gc.ca/recall-alert-rappel-avis/hcsc/2013/33915aeng.php. Accessed February 23, 2016

18. European Medicines Agency. Codeine not to be used in children below 12 years for cough and cold. London, United Kingdom: European Medicines Agency; 2015. Available at: www.ema.europa.eu/ema/index.jsp?curl=pages/medicines/human/referrals/Codeine_containing_medicinal_products_for_the_treatment_of_cough_and_cold_in_paediatric_patients/human_referral_prac_000039.jsp&mid=WC0b01ac05805c516f. Accessed February 23, 2016

19. Cascorbi I. Pharmacogenetics of cytochrome p4502D6: genetic background and clinical implication. *Eur J Clin Invest.* 2003;33(suppl 2):17–22

20. Tremlett MR. Wither codeine? *Paediatr Anaesth.* 2013;23(8):677–683

21. May DG. Genetic differences in drug disposition. *J Clin Pharmacol.* 1994;34(9):881–897

22. Poulsen L, Riishede L, Brøsen K, Clemensen S, Sindrup SH. Codeine in post-operative pain: study of the influence of sparteine phenotype and serum concentrations of morphine and morphine-6-glucuronide. *Eur J Clin Pharmacol.* 1998;54(6):451–454

23. VanderVaart S, Berger H, Sistonen J, et al. CYP2D6 polymorphisms and codeine analgesia in postpartum pain management: a pilot study. *Ther Drug Monit.* 2011;33(4):425–432

24. de Leon J, Dinsmore L, Wedlund P. Adverse drug reactions to oxycodone and hydrocodone in CYP2D6 ultrarapid metabolizers. *J Clin Psychopharmacol.* 2003;23(4):420–421

25. Dean L. Codeine therapy and the CYP2D6 genotype. *Med Genet Summ* [online]. September 20, 2012. Available at: www.ncbi.nlm.nih.gov/books/NBK100662/. Accessed January 6, 2016

26. Sohn DR, Shin SG, Park CW, Kusaka M, Chiba K, Ishizaki T. Metoprolol oxidation polymorphism in a Korean population: comparison with native Japanese and Chinese populations. *Br J Clin Pharmacol.* 1991;32(4):504–507

27. Koren G, Cairns J, Chitayat D, Gaedigk A, Leeder SJ. Pharmacogenetics of morphine poisoning in a breastfed neonate of a codeine-prescribed mother. *Lancet.* 2006;368(9536):704

28. Gasche Y, Daali Y, Fathi M, et al. Codeine intoxication associated with ultrarapid CYP2D6 metabolism. *N Engl J Med.* 2004;351(27):2827–2831

29. Madadi P, Koren G, Cairns J, et al. Safety of codeine during breast feeding: fatal morphine poisoning in the breastfed neonate of a mother prescribed codeine. *Can Fam Physician.* 2007;53(1):33–35

30. Ferner RE. Did the drug cause death? Codeine and breastfeeding. *Lancet.* 2008;372(9639):606–608

31. Voronov P, Przybylo HJ, Jagannathan N. Apnea in a child after oral codeine: a genetic variant—an ultra-rapid metabolizer. *Paediatr Anaesth.* 2007;17(7):684–687

32. Ciszkowski C, Madadi P, Phillips MS, Lauwers AE, Koren G. Codeine, ultrarapid-metabolism genotype, and postoperative death. *N Engl J Med.* 2009;361(8):827–828

33. Kelly LE, Rieder M, van den Anker J, et al. More codeine fatalities after tonsillectomy in North American children. *Pediatrics.* 2012;129(5):e1343–e1347

34. Lynn AM, Nespeca MK, Opheim KE, Slattery JT. Respiratory effects of intravenous morphine infusions in neonates, infants, and children after cardiac surgery. *Anesth Analg.* 1993;77(4):695–701

35. Racoosin JA, Roberson DW, Pacanowski MA, Nielsen DR. New evidence about an old drug—risk with codeine after adenotonsillectomy. *N Engl J Med.* 2013;368(23):2155–2157

36. Brown KA, Laferrière A, Lakheeram I, Moss IR. Recurrent hypoxemia in children is associated with increased analgesic sensitivity to opiates. *Anesthesiology.* 2006;105(4):665–669

37. Friedrichsdorf SJ, Nugent AP, Strobl AQ. Codeine-associated pediatric deaths despite using recommended dosing guidelines: three case reports. *J Opioid Manag.* 2013;9(2):151–155

38. Seymour S. Briefing document, Joint Pulmonary-Allergy Drugs and Drug Safety and Risk Management Advisory Committee Meeting; December 10, 2015. Available at: www.fda.gov/AdvisoryCommittee s/CommitteesMeetingMaterials/ Drugs/Pulmonary-AllergyDrugsAdvis oryCommittee/ucm433815.htm. Accessed February 23, 2016

39. Kokki H, Rasanen I, Reinikainen M, Suhonen P, Vanamo K, Ojanperä I. Pharmacokinetics of oxycodone after intravenous, buccal, intramuscular and gastric administration in children. *Clin Pharmacokinet.* 2004;43(9):613–622

40. Sriswasdi P, Dube C, Perieira L, et al. Population Pharmacokinectics and Pharmacogenomics of Oral Oxycodone in Pediatric Surgical Patients. In: Proceedings from the Annual American Society of Anesthesiologist Meeting; October 24-28, 2015; San Diego, CA. Abstract 3200.

41. Stauble ME, Moore AW, Langman LJ, et al. Hydrocodone in postoperative personalized pain management: pro-drug or drug?. *Clin Chim Acta.* 2014;429:26–29

42. Anderson BJ. Is it farewell to codeine? *Arch Dis Child.* 2013;98(12):986–988

43. Payne KA, Roelofse JA, Shipton EA. Pharmacokinetics of oral tramadol drops for postoperative pain relief in children aged 4 to 7 years—a pilot study. *Anesth Prog.* 2002;49(4):109–112

44. Rose JB, Finkel JC, Arquedas-Mohs A, Himelstein BP, Schreiner M, Medve RA. Oral tramadol for the treatment of pain of 7-30 days' duration in children. *Anesth Analg.* 2003;96(1):78–81

45. Finkel JC, Rose JB, Schmitz ML, et al. An evaluation of the efficacy and tolerability of oral tramadol hydrochloride tablets for the treatment of postsurgical pain in children. *Anesth Analg.* 2002;94(6):1469–1473

46. Tobias JD. Tramadol for postoperative analgesia in adolescents following orthopedic surgery in a third world country. *Am J Pain Manage.* 1996;6:51–53

47. Xu J, Zhang XC, Lv XQ, et al. Effect of the cytochrome P450 2D6*10 genotype on the pharmacokinetics of tramadol in post-operative patients. *Pharmazie.* 2014;69(2):138–141

48. Orliaguet G, Hamza J, Couloigner V, et al. A case of respiratory depression in a child with ultrarapid CYP2D6 metabolism after tramadol. *Pediatrics.* 2015;135(3):e753–e755

49. Borys D, Stanton M, Gummin D, Drott T. Tapentadol toxicity in children. *Pediatrics.* 2015;135(2):e392–e396

50. Mattos JL, Robison JG, Greenberg J, Yellon RF. Acetaminophen plus ibuprofen versus opioids for treatment of post-tonsillectomy pain in children. *Int J Pediatr Otorhinolaryngol.* 2014;78(10):1671–1676

51. Merry AF, Edwards KE, Ahmad Z, Barber C, Mahadevan M, Frampton C. Randomized comparison between the combination of acetaminophen and ibuprofen and each constituent alone for analgesia following tonsillectomy in children. *Can J Anaesth.* 2013;60(12):1180–1189

52. Kelly LE, Sommer DD, Ramakrishna J, et al. Morphine or ibuprofen for post-tonsillectomy analgesia: a randomized trial. *Pediatrics.* 2015;135(2):307–313

53. Bedwell JR, Pierce M, Levy M, Shah RK. Ibuprofen with acetaminophen for postoperative pain control following tonsillectomy does not increase emergency department utilization. *Otolaryngol Head Neck Surg.* 2014;151(6):963–966

54. Yaman H, Belada A, Yilmaz S. The effect of ibuprofen on postoperative hemorrhage following tonsillectomy in children. *Eur Arch Otorhinolaryngol.* 2011;268(4):615–617

55. Sucato DJ, Lovejoy JF, Agrawal S, Elerson E, Nelson T, McClung A. Postoperative ketorolac does not predispose to pseudoarthrosis following posterior spinal fusion and instrumentation for adolescent idiopathic scoliosis. *Spine.* 2008;33(10):1119–1124

56. Sinatra RS, Jahr JS, Reynolds LW, Viscusi ER, Groudine SB, Payen-Champenois C. Efficacy and safety of single and repeated administration of 1 gram intravenous acetaminophen injection (paracetamol) for pain management after major orthopedic surgery. *Anesthesiology.* 2005;102(4):822–831

57. Jenkins BN, Fortier MA. Developmental and cultural perspectives on children's postoperative pain management at home. *Pain Manag.* 2014;4(6):407–412

58. American Academy of Pediatrics Committee on Drugs. Use of codeine- and dextromethorphan-containing cough remedies in children. *Pediatrics.* 1997;99(6):918–920

59. Smith SM, Schroeder K, Fahey T. Over-the-counter (OTC) medications for acute cough in children and adults in ambulatory settings. *Cochrane Database Syst Rev.* 2008;4:CD001831

60. Goldman RD. Codeine for acute cough in children. *Can Fam Physician.* 2010;56(12):1293–1294

61. Drug Safety Communication. FDA evaluating the potential risks of using codeine cough-and-cold medicines in children. Rockville, MD: US Food and Drug Administration; July 1, 2015. Available at: www.fda.gov/Drugs/ DrugSafety/ucm453125.htm. Accessed February 23, 2016

62. Lowry JA, Leeder JS. Over-the-counter medications: update on cough and cold preparations. *Pediatr Rev.* 2015;36(7):286–297, quiz 298

63. Woolf AD, Greco C. Why can't we retire codeine? *Pediatrics.* 2014;133(5). Available at: www.pediatrics.org/cgi/ content/full/133/5/e1354

Contraception for HIV-Infected Adolescents

• *Clinical Report*

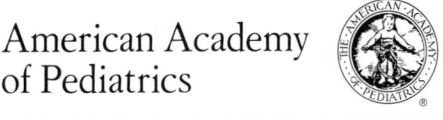

CLINICAL REPORT   Guidance for the Clinician in Rendering Pediatric Care

Contraception for HIV-Infected Adolescents

Athena P. Kourtis, MD, PhD, MPH, FAAP, Ayesha Mirza, MD, FAAP, COMMITTEE ON PEDIATRIC AIDS

abstract

Access to high-quality reproductive health care is important for adolescents and young adults with HIV infection to prevent unintended pregnancies, sexually transmitted infections, and secondary transmission of HIV to partners and children. As perinatally HIV-infected children mature into adolescence and adulthood and new HIV infections among adolescents and young adults continue to occur in the United States, medical providers taking care of such individuals often face issues related to sexual and reproductive health. Challenges including drug interactions between several hormonal methods and antiretroviral agents make decisions regarding contraceptive options more complex for these adolescents. Dual protection, defined as the use of an effective contraceptive along with condoms, should be central to ongoing discussions with HIV-infected young women and couples wishing to avoid pregnancy. Last, reproductive health discussions need to be integrated with discussions on HIV care, because a reduction in plasma HIV viral load below the level of detection (an "undetectable viral load") is essential for the individual's health as well as for a reduction in HIV transmission to partners and children.

DOI: 10.1542/peds.2016-1892

PEDIATRICS (ISSN Numbers: Print, 0031-4005; Online, 1098-4275).

Copyright © 2016 by the American Academy of Pediatrics

FINANCIAL DISCLOSURE: The authors have indicated they do not have a financial relationship relevant to this article to disclose.

FUNDING: No external funding.

POTENTIAL CONFLICT OF INTEREST: The authors have indicated they have no potential conflicts of interest to disclose.

To cite: Kourtis AP, Mirza A, AAP COMMITTEE ON PEDIATRIC AIDS. Contraception for HIV-Infected Adolescents. *Pediatrics.* 2016;138(3):e20161892

INTRODUCTION

The American Academy of Pediatrics (AAP) recommends that pediatricians develop a working knowledge of existing contraceptive methods for adolescents and has recently published a clinical report to address this issue.[1] Because the evidence base for contraception for HIV-infected adolescents has recently expanded, the goal of this clinical report is to provide a description and rationale for best practices in counseling and administering contraception for adolescents with HIV infection.

HIV type 1–infected adolescents represent an important subgroup within the adolescent population. The availability of combination antiretroviral therapy (cART) in the United States has led to increasing numbers of children who acquired HIV infection through mother-to-child transmission who survive into adolescence and young adulthood. In addition, there is also a growing population of horizontally HIV-infected youth. Reproductive health education for pediatric patients as well as their health care providers represents an important and unmet need in this vulnerable population. Pediatricians providing care for adolescents with HIV infection can help them make informed choices by addressing their contraceptive needs. The AAP recently published a clinical report and accompanying technical report entitled "Contraception for Adolescents."[1] The American College of Obstetricians and Gynecologists has also issued an opinion statement acknowledging that adolescents who are HIV infected should receive sexual and reproductive health counseling and care.[2] The intent of this clinical report is to address specific considerations and guidance related to contraceptive options available for HIV-infected adolescents.

HIV-INFECTED ADOLESCENTS IN THE UNITED STATES

At the end of 2012, there were an estimated 10 832 people in the United States and 6 dependent areas (American Samoa, Guam, the Northern Mariana Islands, Puerto Rico, the Republic of Palau, and the US Virgin Islands) living with perinatally acquired HIV infection.[3] In 2010, young people aged 13 to 24 years represented 17% of the US population but accounted for an estimated 26% of all new (47 500) HIV infections.[4] This number represented the second largest percentage of new infections in 2010 (the largest group being among those aged 25–34 years [31%]).[5]

Although the majority of new HIV infections among youth occur among gay and bisexual males, female youth in the United States continue to remain vulnerable, with certain ethnic groups at higher risk than others. In 2010, black youth accounted for an estimated

57% of all new HIV infections in youth in the United States, followed by Hispanic/Latino (20%) and white (20%) youth (both male and female).[6] Available data show that a majority of individuals 15 to 24 years of age in the United States do not perceive that they are at risk of acquiring HIV infection and thus are unlikely to take measures to prevent themselves from contracting HIV. Data also show that more than 60% of HIV-infected youth in the United States do not know that they are infected.[7]

As they age, HIV-infected adolescents are more likely to engage in sexual activity, similar to uninfected youth populations.[8] According to the 2013 Youth Risk Behavior Surveillance conducted by the Centers for Disease Control and Prevention (CDC) among students nationwide in grades 9 through 12, 48.6% of students reported ever having sexual intercourse, with 34% nationwide reporting sexual activity within the 3 months before the survey and 5.6% of students nationwide reporting having had sexual intercourse before the age of 13 years.[9] Among currently sexually active students, 13.7% reported that neither they nor their partner had used any method to prevent pregnancy during the last sexual intercourse.[9] HIV-infected youth can likewise engage in high-risk sexual behaviors, and high rates of unintended pregnancy have been documented in that group.[8,10,11] These statistics underscore the importance of reproductive counseling in HIV-infected youth.

Approximately 280 000 HIV-infected women and an estimated 140 000 serodiscordant couples live in the United States, many of whom desire children.[12] Data from a multisite US-based cross-sectional study indicate that there is limited discussion of preconception issues between HIV care providers and their patients.[12,13] When such discussions

do occur, the majority are initiated by patients. Other studies also support this finding.[14,15] The routine provision of preconception care and counseling for these individuals is a critical need and represents an ongoing challenge. Available data support the fact that unintended pregnancies in this population continue to occur.[11] The estimated number of women with HIV giving birth in the United States increased from 6075 to 6422 births in 2000 to 8650 to 8900 in 2006[16] (a 30% increase). Access to medical care and discussion of fertility intentions may aid in decreasing the risk of an unplanned pregnancy in this population.[12]

REPRODUCTIVE HEALTH ISSUES SPECIFIC TO HIV-INFECTED ADOLESCENTS

Multiple demographic, psychological, sexual, medical, and relationship-based factors play a role in the reproductive decision-making of HIV-infected adolescents and young adults.[12-15] Data suggest that discussions with HIV-infected adolescents about reproductive health led by clinical care providers may not focus as much on family planning but rather on the prevention of sexually transmitted infections (STIs).[17,18] Discussions about pregnancy prevention may have insufficient content related to pregnancy planning in youth as well as in older women.[19] These findings may reflect general discomfort among pediatric health care providers when addressing issues related to sexuality in adolescent patients and concern for potential drug interactions between certain antiretroviral drugs and hormonal contraception.

The physician-patient relationship also affects reproductive decision-making. Adolescents with chronic medical conditions are faced with many challenges as they transition from pediatric to adult care, including the loss of a long-standing physician-patient relationship.[20,21] The medical home may represent the only stable environment some of these adolescents have ever known.[22] Once the transition in care from a pediatric to an adult provider occurs, perinatally HIV-infected adolescents, in particular, may have difficulty expressing their medical needs, particularly those related to sexual and reproductive health. In addition, both perinatally and horizontally HIV-infected youth may experience neurocognitive deficits.[23,24] This situation can not only make the transition more difficult but also may present ongoing challenges for both retention in care and adherence to life-saving cART. Impairment in cognitive ability and reasoning may also present a major barrier to complicated discussions about reproductive health and contraceptive counseling.

The integration of family planning services within HIV treatment, care, and prevention programs has resulted in an increase in contraceptive use.[25-27] The integration of services is an as-yet underutilized strategy that holds promise, particularly because multiple appointments with different providers pose another barrier to receiving appropriate care. Providers report systemic barriers to providing sexual and reproductive health education, such as overbooked clinics and large patient loads, which limit the length of one-on-one time with patients. In some cases, lack of adequate training on how to effectively provide sexual and reproductive health education and discuss these topics with minors presents an additional barrier.[18] The use of reproductive life planning tools, such as those available on the CDC Web site, may aid providers as they approach these topics with their adolescent patients.[28]

CONFIDENTIALITY AND CONSENT: STATE LAWS

Laws in all 50 states and the District of Columbia allow minors to consent to testing and treatment of STIs. Some states allow, but do not require, a physician to inform a minor's parents that he or she is seeking or receiving STI services when the physician deems it in the minor's best interests. Iowa is the only state that requires that parents be notified if their child tests positive for HIV infection. Laws in 26 states and the District of Columbia explicitly give minors the authority to consent to contraceptive services. Twenty states allow only certain categories of minors to consent to contraceptive services, and 4 states have no relevant policy or case law.[29,30] Improved access to contraceptive health care with fewer restrictions to family planning reduces unplanned pregnancies and teen births. For example, states with policies that expand access to family planning services for adolescents have been associated with lower teen birth rates, at least for some teenagers.[31]

Familiarity with national and state laws regarding contraceptive treatment of minors is important to provide quality health care to adolescents. Maintaining confidentiality within the limitations permitted by law is paramount to patient trust and the likelihood that an adolescent will return for appropriate guidance and care. Confidentiality is particularly important when sexual behaviors are discussed and may be a major factor in adolescents' decisions to disclose such behaviors to their health care providers and, in turn, use appropriate health services. Because adolescents are often covered by their parents' health insurance, unintended disclosure of health services to parents may further complicate confidentiality. It is important to explain to adolescents when prescribing contraceptive

agents that there is a potential for unintended disclosure to parents through health plan communications. The AAP recommends that pediatricians put sexuality education into a lifelong perspective and actively encourage parents to discuss sexuality and contraception consistent with the family's attitudes, values, beliefs, and circumstances beginning early in the child's life.[32]

Physicians who provide care for adolescent minors have an ethical duty to promote autonomy and advocate for patients to be involved in medical decision-making that affects their care, including reproductive health. However, they also have a responsibility to recognize when the decision-making capacity of the individual minor may compromise such decisions and when decisions are not in the best interest of the patient. Recognizing that situations vary, physicians generally should encourage parental involvement and should try to correct misconceptions that the minor may have about the consequences of parental involvement. The Society for Adolescent Health and Medicine recommends that physicians promote effective communication between adolescents and their parents,[33] a position that is endorsed by the AAP and the American Medical Association.[32,34]

METHODS OF CONTRACEPTION

Several resources provide indications and specific practice recommendations for the use of particular contraceptive options in HIV-infected females.[1,2,35] Detailed guidance about the use of various contraceptive methods in women with medical conditions, including HIV infection, is found in the US Medical Eligibility Criteria for Contraceptive Use.[35] Even though HIV infection alone does not preclude the use of any hormonal contraceptive method,[35] medical conditions and medications used in HIV-infected adolescents may influence contraceptive choices.

This report is based on the AAP technical report on contraception for adolescents[1] but focuses on the appropriateness and considerations of each contraceptive method for HIV-infected adolescents. As in the previous report, contraceptive methods are presented in general order of effectiveness, starting with the most effective reversible methods, the long-acting reversible contraceptive (LARC) methods (contraceptive implants and intrauterine devices [IUDs]). LARC methods usually are ideal contraceptive methods for the adolescent population, because they are user-independent options that eliminate the need for regular adherence for effectiveness. In addition, many HIV-infected adolescents are challenged by daily adherence to cART, so adding an additional medication to which they need to adhere may be undesirable. Hormonal contraceptive methods do not protect against STIs; a barrier method, such as a condom, is recommended for concurrent protection against STIs. Dual method use—the use of a condom in conjunction with a highly effective contraceptive method—should be encouraged for adolescents,[1] because the former can prevent transmission of HIV and other STIs to sexual partners. Recommending dual protection use should be a central component of reproductive health counseling for HIV-infected adolescents.

Progestin Implants

Implants are a highly effective user- and coitus-independent contraceptive method.[1] The progestin implant Nexplanon (Merck, Whitehouse Station, NJ) consists of a single rod containing etonogestrel, the active metabolite of the progestin desogestrel. Implants have a failure rate of less than 1%, a Food and Drug Administration–approved duration of action of 3 years, and very low complication rates.[36] In addition, there is evidence that the effectiveness of the implant is unchanged at 4 years of use.[37] Studies in adolescents have shown that progestin implants are more effective than shorter-acting methods in preventing unintended pregnancy,[38] primarily because they have very low adherence requirements and their typical-use effectiveness approximates perfect-use effectiveness. Changes in menstrual bleeding patterns are the most common side effect and the principal reason for method discontinuation.[39] Data are scant on the effect of progestin implants on bone mineral density.[40,41]

The efficacy of progestin implants may be impaired by hepatic enzyme–inducing drugs that act on the cytochrome P450 pathway. Implants, in particular, are potentially more vulnerable to the effect of these inducers than other progestin methods, such as injectable contraceptives, because hormonal levels are closer to the lowest therapeutic blood concentration needed for contraceptive efficacy. Emerging evidence indicates reduced levonorgestrel concentrations in women who use levonorgestrel implants and receive efavirenz-containing antiretroviral therapy; contraceptive failures have been described in such women.[42–47] It should be noted that levonorgestrel implants are not available in the United States but are available in several other parts of the world. Several case reports and a pharmacokinetics study also suggest that efavirenz[48] may decrease the efficacy of etonogestrel implants (eg, Nexplanon), although additional data are needed.[47,49] Failure of the etonogestrel implant was reported in 2 patients receiving efavirenz-based therapy.[50] Prospectively collected data are not yet available to accurately quantify the interaction of efavirenz with progestin implants, to note the time of contraceptive failure, and to comparatively evaluate against other contraceptive options for HIV-infected women. Data on adolescents specifically are not available. Initial concerns about a possible pharmacokinetic interaction of levonorgestrel with nevirapine have not been confirmed by subsequent studies.[45] The National Institutes of Health (NIH) guidance is to use an alternative or additional contraceptive method when efavirenz, nevirapine, or most protease inhibitors (PIs) are administered to HIV-infected individuals.[51,52] The CDC and the World Health Organization (WHO) state that the benefits of using progestin implants outweigh any risks with concomitant administration of an antiretroviral agent in HIV-infected women.[35,53]

Intrauterine Devices

IUDs are another type of LARC. Four IUDs currently are approved in the United States: a copper-containing IUD (copper T380-A; ParaGard; Teva North America, North Wales, PA) and 3 levonorgestrel-releasing IUDs (52 mg levonorgestrel; Mirena; Berlax, Montville, NJ; 52 mg levonorgestrel; Liletta; Actavis, San Francisco, CA; and 13.5 mg levonorgestrel; Skyla; Bayer HealthCare Pharmaceuticals, Wayne, NJ). They are appropriate for adolescents and are generally safe and effective methods of contraception with a failure rate of less than 1%.[54,55] The 13.5-mg levonorgestrel IUD is approved for 3 years,[56] and the 52-mg levonorgestrel IUD, depending on formulation, is approved for 3 years (Liletta) or 5 years (Mirena), although data for Mirena suggest that it remains effective for up to 7 years.[57] The copper IUD is approved for 10 years, but data support its use for 12 years.[58] Women will continue to have regular menstrual cycles with the copper IUD; however, these cycles may be heavier with more cramping initially. With the levonorgestrel IUD, menses will become more irregular; however, overall bleeding will be less, with many women experiencing amenorrhea. Individuals with painful menses may have significant improvement of their symptoms with the levonorgestrel IUD.[54]

Despite earlier concerns, IUDs are now considered safe for nulliparous adolescents,[1] because they do not cause tubal infertility in nulliparous women.[35,59] There is a small risk of pelvic infection after insertion, but this increased risk does not extend beyond the first 21 days after insertion.[60,61] Although an ongoing active STI or other pelvic infection is a contraindication to IUD placement, an IUD may be inserted in an asymptomatic adolescent at high risk of an STI with screening on the day of insertion. The treatment of any new STI can be subsequently provided without IUD removal.[1,62] A recent systematic review found an overall low incidence of pelvic inflammatory disease among women with HIV who use IUDs and no differences in infectious complications when comparing IUD complication rates by HIV disease stage; however, the evidence was limited and of fair to poor quality.[63]

HIV infection is not a contraindication to IUD use. The use of an IUD in the context of HIV infection is classified according to CDC US medical eligibility criteria for contraceptive use as category 2, meaning that HIV is a condition for which the advantages of using the IUD generally outweigh theoretical or proven risks.[1,35] However, the use of an IUD by an individual with advanced HIV disease is classified as category 3, meaning that risks generally outweigh benefits, including the theoretical risk of infection with IUD insertion. Therefore, such women should use an alternative

contraceptive method other than an IUD until their immunologic and clinical status improves with cART. For women with an IUD already in place who progress to advanced HIV disease, the IUD can remain in place. However, these women may be at increased risk of pelvic infection.[35,53]

IUD use did not adversely affect HIV disease progression when compared with hormonal contraceptive use and was not associated with increased risk of HIV transmission to partners.[35] Several small studies have found that levonorgestrel IUDs were not associated with increased genital shedding of HIV.[64,65] Limited data also suggest that the efficacy of the levonorgestrel IUD is unlikely to be affected by antiretroviral therapy.[64,66] Furthermore, evidence suggests that there is no higher risk of overall or infectious complications in HIV-infected compared with uninfected women.[65,67,68]

Progestin-Only Injectable Contraception

Depot medroxyprogesterone acetate (DMPA), known by the brand name Depo-Provera (Pfizer, New York, NY), is progestin given as a single injection approximately every 13 weeks (up to 15 weeks) with the use of a dose of either 150 mg delivered intramuscularly or 104 mg delivered subcutaneously.[1] This contraceptive method is highly effective at preventing pregnancy, with a 1-year probability of pregnancy of approximately 6% for typical use and 0.2% with perfect use.[1] Similar to the LARC methods, DMPA can be administered to those with contraindications to estrogens and is convenient for many adolescents; however, it requires injections approximately every 13 weeks. Its main side effects are weight gain, a delayed return to fertility, menstrual bleeding irregularities, and bone mineral loss, which is largely reversible after DMPA discontinuation.[1,69,70]

Patients receiving DMPA injections should be counseled about age-appropriate recommendations for supplementation with calcium and vitamin D and regular weight-bearing exercise as well as avoidance of smoking and alcohol to maintain skeletal health.[1] Some providers obtain dual-energy radiograph absorptiometry scans in adolescent patients at baseline when they begin DMPA injections. However, there is no evidence to recommend this practice; moreover, initial bone mineral density losses stabilize by 5 years, with return to pre-use levels on discontinuation of progestin injections.[55] Given the uncertainty surrounding the interaction between progestin-only injectables (particularly DMPA) and the risk of HIV transmission to male partners,[35,53,67,71] as will be discussed later, women with HIV infection need to be informed that progestin-only injectables may or may not increase their risk of HIV transmission to partners. There is insufficient evidence to confirm any risk of disease progression[72]; however, further research is warranted. Women and couples at high risk of HIV who are considering progestin-only injectables should also be informed about and have access to HIV-preventive measures, including male and female condoms.[53] Levels of DMPA do not appear to be reduced by the use of antiretroviral agents (including efavirenz, zidovudine, lamivudine, nevirapine, and nelfinavir)[73–75]; indeed, this agent is largely free of antiretroviral interactions and can be administered with all classes of antiretroviral agents. Although both HIV disease and the antiretroviral agen tenofovir disoproxil fumarate can cause decreases in bone mineral density,[76] the effects of concomitant use of DMPA and tenofovir disoproxil fumarate on adolescent bone health are not known.

Combined Oral Contraceptives

Combined oral contraceptives (COCs) contain an estrogen and a progestin and are available by prescription. They are the most commonly used method of hormonal contraception among adolescents in the United States[1] and are the prototype of other combined methods of birth control, such as the vaginal ring and transdermal patch, which have similar efficacy and clinical profiles. In almost every pill, the estrogen component is ethinyl estradiol in varying amounts, with the "low dose" pill (30–35 μg) being the first line for adolescents.[1] Their typical-use failure rates are 9% in adults and may be higher in adolescents,[1,77] because they depend on user adherence. Approaches to increase adherence include support from a family member, friend, or partner or cell phone alarms[1] and should include instructions if 1 or more pills are missed. As with all estrogen-containing contraceptive methods, COCs have some contraindications[1,35]; however, most of these are uncommon in the adolescent. Interactions with several classes of medications, including some antiretroviral agents,[1,35,51,52] are one of the main factors limiting the use of COCs in HIV-infected women. Such interactions lead mainly to a decrease in contraceptive hormonal levels, potentially leading to decreased contraceptive effectiveness, and will be summarized in a later section. A decrease in contraceptive effectiveness of COCs is observed particularly with concurrent administration of a ritonavir-boosted PI; an alternative or additional contraceptive method should be considered when any boosted PI regimen is used. Because nevirapine and efavirenz induce the metabolism of COCs and reduce hormonal levels, an alternative or additional contraceptive method should also be considered in women who are taking these antiretroviral agents;

however, other nonnucleoside reverse transcriptase inhibitors (NNRTIs), such as etravirine and rilpivirine, do not seem to cause the same reduction.[38]

COCs do not have any significant interactions with nucleoside reverse transcriptase inhibitors, integrase inhibitors such as raltegravir and dolutegravir, entry inhibitors such as maraviroc, or fusion inhibitors such as enfuvirtide. Preliminary data suggest that elvitegravir/cobicistat may alter hormonal concentrations; the clinical significance of this finding is not fully known, but COCs with greater than 30 μg ethinyl estradiol or alternative contraceptives may need to be considered.[51]

Most of the available evidence has found no statistically significant association between the use of COCs and HIV acquisition, HIV transmission to partners, or HIV disease progression; however, the quality of the available evidence is generally considered low.[53,72,78,79]

Contraceptive Vaginal Ring, Transdermal Contraceptive Patch

These methods have efficacy, benefits, side effects, and drug interactions comparable to other combined hormonal methods but represent simpler regimens. Despite the simplified regimen afforded by these methods (weekly for the patch and monthly for the vaginal ring), studies suggest variable rates of acceptability and low long-term continuation rates among adolescents.[78,80,81] For HIV-infected adolescents, drug interaction considerations are similar to those of COCs mentioned previously.[35,52] As with other hormonal methods, a condom should always be used concurrently for STI/HIV protection.

Progestin-Only Pills

Progestin-only pills are not typically recommended as a first-choice method in adolescents, because they require particular timing of pill

administration relative to coitus.[1] In addition, they are less effective than other progestin-only methods, including the progestin-containing IUD, implant, and injectables.[1] There is currently no available information regarding the risk of HIV acquisition or transmission to partners with the use of progestin-only pills. On the basis of limited data, progestin levels with progestin-only pills do not appear to be reduced by some PIs,[82] but contraceptive efficacy data are not available. Data on hormonal levels when progestin-only pills are used with other antiretroviral agents, such as efavirenz or nevirapine, are not available.[47] Recommendations for use with antiretroviral drugs are generally the same as those for COCs discussed previously.[35,51]

Male Condoms

Male condoms are the preferred method of barrier contraception because of their demonstrated ability to decrease the transmission of STIs, including HIV.[1,79] In addition, they are the most common contraceptive method used by adolescents.[83] They need to be used correctly and consistently with each act of sexual intercourse; therefore, their typical-use failure rate is 18% for all users and can be higher among adolescents, in contrast to a perfect-use failure rate of 2%.[84] Latex condoms should only be used with water-based lubricants[85]; natural membrane condoms do not provide adequate STI protection.[79] The high typical-use failure rate for pregnancy prevention, but added protection from STIs, has led to the recommendation for dual contraception with a condom plus a highly effective hormonal or other long-acting contraceptive method.[79] More information on condoms can be found in the AAP policy statement on condom use by adolescents.[79] HIV-infected adolescents should always use a condom to prevent HIV transmission to partners.

Emergency Contraception

Several products are available for emergency contraception in the United States, including a progestin-only dedicated emergency contraception product (levonorgestrel-based pill), high-dose combined estrogen-progestin pills, ulipristal acetate (a progesterone receptor modulator), and the copper IUD.[1] All of these methods can prevent pregnancy when initiated up to 5 days after an act of unprotected sexual intercourse but are more effective the earlier they are used. More information on emergency contraception can be found in the AAP policy statement on emergency contraception.[86] Plan B One-Step (levonorgestrel) is approved by the Food and Drug Administration as a nonprescription product for all women of childbearing potential,[87] and generic versions are approved as nonprescription products for adolescent females and women aged ≥17 years, even though proof of age is not required for purchase.[1] Counseling and advance provision of emergency contraception should be a part of anticipatory guidance for adolescents.[1] Recommendations are not different for HIV-infected adolescents; however, drug interactions with antiretroviral agents may need to be considered. Limited evidence suggests that levonorgestrel levels are significantly reduced among women using levonorgestrel emergency contraception who are receiving efavirenz, but no efficacy data are available.[44] Data for interactions of other types of emergency contraception and other antiretroviral agents are not available.[47] However, ulipristal acetate is predominantly metabolized by CYP3A4, so interactions can be expected.[51,52] The efficacy of the copper IUD is not affected by antiretroviral agents.

Spermicides, Diaphragm, Cervical Cap

HIV infection is a contraindication to the use of spermicides, because there is an increased risk of genital lesions and resulting viral shedding and transmission of HIV associated with nonoxynol-9.[35,88] Diaphragms and cervical caps are contraindicated in HIV-infected individuals for similar reasons, mainly because of concerns about the spermicide.[89]

Fertility Awareness and Other Periodic Abstinence Methods

Although strict abstinence is obviously an effective means of birth control, it is not a realistic option for adolescents after their sexual debut. Fertility awareness and other periodic abstinence methods are not recommended for adolescents, because they have high failure rates.[1] A condom should always be used by HIV-infected adolescents to prevent the transmission of HIV infection to partners.

Withdrawal

This method has a high contraceptive failure rate,[1] and it provides no STI/HIV protection; therefore, it is not recommended as a contraceptive method.

HORMONAL CONTRACEPTION AND HIV RISK

Concerns have been raised about the effects of hormonal contraception on the risk of HIV acquisition, the risk of HIV transmission from female to male partners, and HIV disease progression. Some observational studies have documented an increased risk of HIV acquisition, transmission, and disease progression associated with changes in the genital tract during contraceptive use.[90–94] Most relevant to this clinical report are the possible associations of hormonal contraception with the risk of HIV transmission to partners and with

HIV disease progression. A secondary analysis from 2 longitudinal studies of HIV incidence that followed serodiscordant couples in Africa reported that DMPA use increased the risk of HIV transmission from infected women to their male partners.[95] Among serodiscordant couples in which the HIV-negative partner was male, the rates of HIV transmission were 2.61 per 100 person-years when women used hormonal contraception and 1.51 per 100 person-years when women did not use hormonal contraception (P = .02). This study was subject to confounding, because it was not designed to examine HIV risk with hormonal contraception and only a small proportion of women used hormonal contraceptives (11% of total person-years of follow-up). In addition, these women were not receiving antiretroviral therapy. Indirect evidence on the risk of HIV transmission from female to male partners from 11 studies that assessed genital HIV shedding is mixed.[96] Studies have reported an association between hormonal contraceptive use and increased frequency of shedding of HIV DNA, but not RNA, in the genital tract,[94,97–99] although this finding has not been consistently documented in all studies.[93,96] Most studies were cross-sectional, had small sample sizes, and evaluated different markers of transmissibility (HIV DNA versus RNA). Their results are thus difficult to compare or generalize.

Evidence on the effects of hormonal contraception on HIV disease progression was reviewed.[72] Ten cohort studies consistently found no association with hormonal contraceptive use and HIV disease progression compared with nonuse of hormonal contraceptives. One randomized controlled trial found that hormonal contraceptive use was associated with an increased risk of HIV disease progression compared with copper IUD use, but this study had important methodologic shortcomings.[72] Thus, the preponderance of evidence suggests that HIV-infected women can use hormonal contraceptive methods without concerns for HIV disease progression.[72]

A recent WHO[100] consultation concluded that there was, as yet, insufficient evidence to support a change in current guidelines on the use of hormonal contraceptives for women living with HIV or those at high risk of HIV infection.[100] The CDC supports this guidance and has added clarification that strongly encourages condom use and other measures to prevent HIV infection for at-risk women.[35] The WHO encouraged further investigation of the relationship of hormonal contraception and HIV risk. Because most of the available information on HIV risk derives from studies on women who used DMPA or COCs, very limited or no information is currently available on HIV risk related to other hormonal methods, such as progestin implants or progestin-releasing IUDs.

INTERACTIONS OF HORMONAL CONTRACEPTION AND ANTIRETROVIRAL DRUGS

Hormonal contraceptives are primarily metabolized in the liver by the cytochrome P450 system. Antiretroviral agents have varying effects on this metabolic pathway; this is the main biological reason for the interaction between the 2 drug categories, although other metabolic pathways are sometimes involved. Special consideration is necessary for women who use some hormonal methods (ie, combined hormonal contraceptive methods, progestin-only pills, emergency contraceptive pills, or etonogestrel implants) with certain antiretroviral regimens (particularly those containing efavirenz and ritonavir-boosted PIs).[53] In addition, because

efavirenz use may be associated with neural tube defects after early fetal exposure, women receiving efavirenz should avoid becoming pregnant, and treatment with efavirenz should be avoided during the first 8 weeks of pregnancy whenever possible.[51]

Data on drug interactions between antiretroviral therapy and hormonal contraceptives come primarily from drug-label pharmacokinetics and limited clinical studies, and the clinical implications of observed alterations in hormonal or antiretroviral levels are not always known. In addition, the magnitude of change in drug levels that may reduce contraceptive efficacy or increase adverse effects is not completely known; therefore, the quality of evidence is deemed low.[35,100] Up-to-date information regarding drug interactions with antiretroviral agents can be found within the regularly updated CDC, WHO, and NIH guidelines[35,51–53] Because definitive, high-quality studies on pregnancy rates among women taking hormonal contraceptives and receiving antiretroviral therapy do not exist, dosing recommendations are based on expert opinion.[51] The recommendations referred to in this clinical report are based on the consensus of the NIH expert panel[51] and may be slightly different from those of other sources, including the CDC and the WHO.

A summary of the available evidence on interactions with hormonal contraceptives by antiretroviral class is presented in Table 1. Interactions with hormonal contraceptives may differ among individual antiretroviral agents in each class. In general, nucleoside reverse transcriptase inhibitors and entry inhibitors do not appear to have significant interactions with hormonal contraceptive methods.[51,53,101] With regard to NNRTIs, 3 clinical studies, including 1 large study, found that the use of nevirapine-containing cART did not increase ovulation or

pregnancy rates in women taking COCs.[102–105] For efavirenz-containing cART, a pharmacokinetic study showed consistently significant decreases in contraceptive hormone levels in women taking COCs, and a small clinical study showed higher ovulation rates in women taking efavirenz-containing cART and COCs.[44,102,106] The newer NNRTIs, etravirine and rilpivirine, do not interact with COCs.[101,107] On the basis of primarily pharmacokinetic data, the efficacy of DMPA is likely not affected by NNRTIs. Efavirenz, but likely not nevirapine, decreases levonorgestrel levels and may decrease contraceptive efficacy in women using levonorgestrel implants[45] or levonorgestrel for emergency contraception[52]; data on interactions of efavirenz with etonogestrel implants are even more scarce.

As mentioned earlier, pharmacokinetic data suggest decreases in COC hormone levels with ritonavir-boosted PIs. For women using ritonavir-boosted PIs who are taking combination hormonal contraceptives (COC pills, patches, or rings) or progestin-only pills, the use of an alternative or additional method of contraception is recommended.[35,51,52] Atazanavir increases ethinyl estradiol concentrations by 50% or more, so with unboosted atazanavir, COCs with concentrations of ethinyl estradiol less than 30 µg are needed.[35,51,52] On the basis of primarily pharmacokinetic data, the effectiveness of DMPA is likely not affected by PIs.[53] The concomitant use of hormonal contraceptives and preexposure prophylaxis regimens has been evaluated in only a few studies; preexposure prophylaxis was shown to be efficacious in women using DMPA and in their partners.[108] Similarly, concomitant oral tenofovir/emtricitabine use was not associated with changes in plasma levonorgestrel concentrations

TABLE 1 Interactions of Hormonal Contraceptives With Antiretroviral Drugs by Drug Class

Antiretroviral Class[a]	Hormonal Contraceptive Type					
	Progestin Implants	Levonorgestrel IUD[b]	Progestin Injectables (DMPA)	Combined Hormonal Methods and Progestin-Only Pills	Emergency Contraception
NRTIs	No known interactions	No known interactions	No known interactions	No known interactions	No known interactions
NNRTIs	Potential interaction with efavirenz may limit its contraceptive efficacy; more data are needed	No known interactions	No known interactions	Interactions with efavirenz may decrease hormonal contraceptive levels and contraceptive efficacy; alternative or additional contraceptive methods are recommended	Interactions of levonorgestrel emergency contraception with efavirenz may limit efficacy; possible interactions of ulipristal with NNRTIs; no clinical data
PIs	Potential interaction, very limited clinical data	No known interactions	No known interactions	Interactions with most ritonavir-boosted PIs may decrease hormone contraceptive levels and contraceptive efficacy; alternative or additional contraceptive methods are recommended	Possible interaction of ulipristal with elvitegravir/cobicistat; no clinical data
Integrase inhibitors	No known interactions	No known interactions	No known interactions	Possible interaction with elvitegravir/cobicistat	Possible interaction of ulipristal with elvitegravir/cobicistat
Entry/fusion inhibitors	No known interactions	No known interactions	No known interactions	No known interactions	No known interactions

The concurrent use of male condoms for protection against STIs, for additional protection against unintended pregnancy, and for prevention of transmission of HIV infection to partners is always recommended for HIV-infected women. NRTI, nucleoside reverse transcriptase inhibitor.

[a] NRTIs include abacavir, tenofovir, zidovudine, lamivudine, didanosine, emtricitabine, and stavudine; NNRTIs include efavirenz, etravirine, nevirapine, and rilpivirine; PIs include ritonavir-boosted atazanavir, darunavir, fosamprenavir, lopinavir, saquinavir and tipranavir; unboosted atazanavir, fosamprenavir, indinavir, nelfinavir; integrase inhibitors include raltegravir, dolutegravir, and elvitegravir/cobicistat; entry/fusion inhibitors include maraviroc, vicriviroc, and enfuvirtide.

[b] An alternative contraceptive method is recommended for women with severe/advanced clinical HIV disease, until improvement with antiretroviral therapy. If a woman with an IUD develops severe clinical disease, the IUD does not need to be removed, but careful monitoring for pelvic infection is recommended.

among women using a levonorgestrel implant in the first year of use.[109]

The efficacy of cART does not appear to be affected by the use of hormonal contraceptive methods on the basis of limited clinical data.[66,110-114] Very few data are available on whether hormonal contraceptive methods and cART taken together lead to worsening of side effects of contraceptives or increased antiretroviral toxicity. Pharmacokinetic data suggest that COCs, DMPA, and progestin implants are unlikely to have an effect on cART toxicity.[90] Complete information on all contraceptive methods and possible interactions with antiretroviral agents can be found in the CDC-issued Medical Eligibility Criteria for Contraceptive Use[35] and the regularly updated NIH guidance.[51]

CONCLUSIONS

The use of effective contraception is necessary in sexually active HIV-infected adolescents, because it prevents unintended pregnancy, promotes family planning, and prevents mother-to-child transmission of HIV. The promotion of these methods, in conjunction with education regarding dual protection use, is important. However, several of the antiretroviral drugs used in currently recommended regimens for adults and adolescents in the United States[52] have interactions with some hormonal contraceptives, which may limit their efficacy. The evidence on pharmacologic interactions and their clinical significance is still emerging. Interactions of LARCs with antiretroviral agents are particularly important to determine, because LARCs are the most effective contraceptive methods. The effect of hormonal contraceptives on local cervicovaginal concentrations of antiretroviral drugs administered topically or systemically will also need to be studied.[110] There is a need for the development of long-acting, safe, multipurpose prevention technologies that address multiple sexual and reproductive health needs of adolescents and young adults as well as decreased user adherence requirements.[115] Such proof-of-concept technologies might include genitally applied products that can afford antiviral and contraceptive activity and have longer duration of action.[110]

Comprehensive reproductive health counseling and care is an important aspect of care for HIV-infected adolescent females. This care includes the capacity to provide appropriate contraceptive guidance, delivery, and monitoring. Encouraging abstinence,[116] delay of sexual initiation, correct and consistent condom use, and adherence to the antiretroviral regimen are important strategies to improve adolescents' health, prevent unintended pregnancies, and prevent HIV transmission to partners. Clinics and physician practices providing primary care for HIV-infected female adolescents need to include comprehensive reproductive health counseling and care and have the capability to provide appropriate contraceptive guidance, delivery, and monitoring. Addressing adolescent reproductive health issues in the medical home and during routine visits, where family planning services are integrated into care, along with antiretroviral therapy adherence and risk-reduction counseling, may be one of the best ways to address the sexual and reproductive health needs of HIV-infected adolescents.

ACKNOWLEDGMENT

We thank Dr Lisa Haddad for her helpful comments on the manuscript.

LEAD AUTHORS

Athena P. Kourtis, MD, PhD, MPH, FAAP
Ayesha Mirza, MD, FAAP

ABBREVIATIONS

AAP: American Academy of Pediatrics
cART: combination antiretroviral therapy
CDC: Centers for Disease Control and Prevention
COC: combined oral contraceptive
DMPA: depot medroxyprogesterone acetate
IUD: intrauterine device
LARC: long-acting reversible contraceptive
NIH: National Institutes of Health
NNRTI: nonnucleoside reverse transcriptase inhibitor
PI: protease inhibitor
STI: sexually transmitted infection
WHO: World Health Organization

REFERENCES

1. Ott MA, Sucato GS; Committee on Adolescence. Contraception for adolescents. Pediatrics. 2014;134(4). Available at: www.pediatrics.org/cgi/content/full/134/4/e1257

2. American College of Obstetricians and Gynecologists; Women's Health Care Physicians. Committee Opinion No. 572: reproductive health care for adolescents with human immunodeficiency virus. Obstet Gynecol. 2013;122(3):721–726

3. Centers for Disease Control and Prevention. HIV Surveillance Report. February 2015. Available at: www.cdc.gov/hiv/library/reports/surveillance/. Accessed January 4, 2016

4. Centers for Disease Control and Prevention. Estimated HIV incidence in the United States, 2007–2010. HIV Surveillance Supplemental Report. 2012;17(4). Available at: www.cdc.gov/hiv/pdf/statistics_hssr_vol_17_no_4.pdf. Accessed January 4, 2016

5. Centers for Disease Control and Prevention. New HIV infections in the United States. Available at: www.cdc.gov/nchhstp/newsroom//docs/2012/HIV-Infections-2007-2010.pdf. Accessed January 4, 2016

6. Centers for Disease Control and Prevention. HIV among Youth. Available at: www.cdc.gov/hiv/risk/age/youth/index.html?s_cid=tw_std0141316. Accessed January 4, 2016

7. Centers for Disease Control and Prevention. Vital signs: HIV infection, testing, and risk behaviors among youths—United States. MMWR Morb Mortal Wkly Rep. 2012;61(47):971–976

8. Mellins CA, Tassiopoulos K, Malee K, et al; Pediatric HIV/AIDS Cohort Study. Behavioral health risks in perinatally HIV-exposed youth: co-occurrence of sexual and drug use behavior, mental health problems, and nonadherence to antiretroviral treatment. AIDS Patient Care STDS. 2011;25(7):413–422

9. Kann L, Kinchen S, Shanklin SL, et al; Centers for Disease Control and Prevention. Youth risk behavior surveillance—United States, 2013. MMWR Suppl. 2014;63(4):1–168. Available at: www.cdc.gov/mmwr/pdf/ss/ss6304.pdf. Accessed January 4, 2016

10. Elkington KS, Bauermeister JA, Santamaria EK, Dolezal C, Mellins CA. Substance use and the development of sexual risk behaviors in youth perinatally exposed to HIV. J Pediatr Psychol. 2015;40(4):442–454

11. Sutton MY, Patel R, Frazier EL. Unplanned pregnancies among

HIV-infected women in care-United States. *J Acquir Immune Defic Syndr.* 2014;65(3):350–358

12. Rahangdale L, Stewart A, Stewart RD, et al; HOPES (HIV and OB Pregnancy Education Study). Pregnancy intentions among women living with HIV in the United States. *J Acquir Immune Defic Syndr.* 2014;65(3):306–311

13. Centers for Disease Control and Prevention. HIV among pregnant women, infants, and children. Available at: www.cdc.gov/hiv/risk/gender/pregnantwomen/facts/index.html. Accessed January 4, 2016

14. Finocchario-Kessler S, Bastos FI, Malta M, et al; Rio Collaborative Group. Discussing childbearing with HIV-infected women of reproductive age in clinical care: a comparison of Brazil and the US. *AIDS Behav.* 2012;16(1):99–107

15. Steiner RJ, Finocchario-Kessler S, Dariotis JK. Engaging HIV care providers in conversations with their reproductive-age patients about fertility desires and intentions: a historical review of the HIV epidemic in the United States. *Am J Public Health.* 2013;103(8):1357–1366

16. Whitmore SK, Zhang X, Taylor AW, Blair JM. Estimated number of infants born to HIV-infected women in the United States and five dependent areas, 2006. *J Acquir Immune Defic Syndr.* 2011;57(3):218–222

17. Fair C, Wiener L, Zadeh S, et al. Reproductive health decision-making in perinatally HIV-infected adolescents and young adults. *Matern Child Health J.* 2013;17(5):797–808

18. Albright JN, Fair CD. Providers caring for adolescents with perinatally-acquired HIV: current practices and barriers to communication about sexual and reproductive health. *AIDS Patient Care STDS.* 2014;28(11):587–593

19. Finocchario-Kessler S, Dariotis JK, Sweat MD, et al. Do HIV-infected women want to discuss reproductive plans with providers, and are those conversations occurring? *AIDS Patient Care STDS.* 2010;24(5):317–323

20. Committee on Pediatric Aids. Transitioning HIV-infected youth into adult health care. *Pediatrics.* 2013;132(1):192–197

21. Cooley WC, Sagerman PJ; American Academy of Pediatrics; American Academy of Family Physicians; American College of Physicians; Transitions Clinical Report Authoring Group. Supporting the health care transition from adolescence to adulthood in the medical home. *Pediatrics.* 2011;128(1):182–200

22. Fair CD, Sullivan K, Dizney R, Stackpole A. "It's like losing a part of my family": transition expectations of adolescents living with perinatally acquired HIV and their guardians. *AIDS Patient Care STDS.* 2012;26(7):423–429

23. Nichols SL, Bethel J, Garvie PA, et al. Neurocognitive functioning in antiretroviral therapy-naïve youth with behaviorally acquired human immunodeficiency virus. *J Adolesc Health.* 2013;53(6):763–771

24. Mellins CA, Malee KM. Understanding the mental health of youth living with perinatal HIV infection: lessons learned and current challenges. *J Int AIDS Soc.* 2013;16:18593

25. Baumgartner JN, Green M, Weaver MA, et al. Integrating family planning services into HIV care and treatment clinics in Tanzania: evaluation of a facilitated referral model. *Health Policy Plan.* 2014;29(5):570–579

26. Berer M. HIV/AIDS, sexual and reproductive health: intersections and implications for national programmes. *Health Policy Plan.* 2004;19(suppl 1):i62–i70

27. Tao AR, Onono M, Baum S, et al. Providers' perspectives on male involvement in family planning in the context of a cluster-randomized controlled trial evaluating integrating family planning into HIV care in Nyanza Province, Kenya. *AIDS Care.* 2015;27(1):31–37

28. Centers for Disease Control and Prevention. Preconception health and health care: my reproductive life plan. Available at: www.cdc.gov/preconception/documents/reproductivelifeplan-worksheet.pdf. Accessed January 4, 2016

29. Guttmacher Institute. State policies in brief: an overview of Minors' Consent Law. Available at: www.guttmacher.org/statecenter/spibs/spib_OMCL.pdf. Accessed January 4, 2016

30. Guttmacher Institute. State policies in brief: minors' access to STI services. Available at: www.guttmacher.org/statecenter/spibs/spib_MASS.pdf. Accessed January 4, 2016

31. Beltz MA, Sacks VH, Moore KA, Terzian M. State policy and teen childbearing: a review of research studies. *J Adolesc Health.* 2015;56(2):130–138

32. Committee on Adolescent Health; Committee on Psychosocial Aspects of Child and Family Health. Sexuality education for children and adolescents. *Pediatrics.* 2001;108(2):498–502. Reaffirmed October 2004

33. Ford C, English A, Sigman G. Confidential health care for adolescents: position paper for the Society for Adolescent Medicine. *J Adolesc Health.* 2004;35(2):160–167

34. American Medical Association. The AMA code of medical ethics' opinion on confidential services for children and adolescents. *AMA J Ethics.* 2012;14:778–779. Available at: http://journalofethics.ama-assn.org/2012/10/coet1-1210.html. Accessed January 4, 2016

35. Centers for Disease Control and Prevention. U.S. medical eligibility criteria for contraceptive use, 2010. *MMWR Recomm Rep.* 2010;59(RR-4):1–86

36. Raymond GE. Contraceptive implants. In: Hatcher RA, Trussell J, Nelson AL, Cates W Jr, Kowal D, Policar MS, eds. *Contraceptive Technology.* 20th revised ed. Atlanta, GA: Ardent Media, Inc; 2011:193–203

37. McNicholas C, Maddipati R, Zhao Q, Swor E, Peipert JF. Use of the etonogestrel implant and levonorgestrel intrauterine device beyond the U.S. Food and Drug Administration-approved duration. *Obstet Gynecol.* 2015;125(3):599–604

38. Lewis LN, Doherty DA, Hickey M, Skinner SR. Implanon as a contraceptive choice for teenage mothers: a comparison of contraceptive choices, acceptability

and repeat pregnancy. *Contraception.* 2010;81(5):421–426

39. Darney P, Patel A, Rosen K, Shapiro LS, Kaunitz AM. Safety and efficacy of a single-rod etonogestrel implant (Implanon): results from 11 international clinical trials. *Fertil Steril.* 2009;91(5):1646–1653

40. Beerthuizen R, van Beek A, Massai R, Mäkäräinen L, Hout J, Bennink HC. Bone mineral density during long-term use of the progestagen contraceptive implant Implanon compared to a non-hormonal method of contraception. *Hum Reprod.* 2000;15(1):118–122

41. Pongsatha S, Ekmahachai M, Suntornlimsiri N, Morakote N, Chaovisitsaree S. Bone mineral density in women using the subdermal contraceptive implant Implanon for at least 2 years. *Int J Gynaecol Obstet.* 2010;109(3):223–225

42. Perry SH, Swamy P, Preidis GA, Mwanyumba A, Motsa N, Sarero HN. Implementing the Jadelle implant for women living with HIV in a resource-limited setting: concerns for drug interactions leading to unintended pregnancies. *AIDS.* 2014;28(5):791–793

43. Tseng A, Hills-Nieminen C. Drug interactions between antiretrovirals and hormonal contraceptives. *Expert Opin Drug Metab Toxicol.* 2013;9(5):559–572

44. Carten ML, Kiser JJ, Kwara A, Mawhinney S, Cu-Uvin S. Pharmacokinetic interactions between the hormonal emergency contraception, levonorgestrel (Plan B), and efavirenz. *Infect Dis Obstet Gynecol.* 2012;2012:137192

45. Scarsi K, Lamorde M, Darin K, et al. Efavirenz- but not nevirapine-based antiretroviral therapy decreases exposure to the levonorgestrel released from a sub-dermal contraceptive implant. *J Int AIDS Soc.* 2014;17(4 suppl 3):19484

46. Scarsi KNS, Byakika-Kibwika P. Levonorgestrel implant + EFV-based ART: unintended pregnancies and associated PK data. In: A report from the Conference on Retroviruses and Opportunistic Infections; February 23-26, 2015; Seattle, WA. Abstract 85LB

47. US Agency for International Development. Drug interactions between hormonal contraceptive methods and anti-retroviral medications used to treat HIV. Technical Issue Brief; October 2014:1–4. Available at: www.cdc.gov/globalaids/resources/pmtct-care/docs/hc_art-brief_final.pdf. Accessed January 4, 2016

48. Vieira CS, Bahamondes MV, de Souza RM, et al. Effect of antiretroviral therapy including lopinavir/ritonavir or efavirenz on etonogestrel-releasing implant pharmacokinetics in HIV-positive women. *J Acquir Immune Defic Syndr.* 2014;66(4):378–385

49. Kreitchmann R, Innocente AP, Preussler GM. Safety and efficacy of contraceptive implants for HIV-infected women in Porto Alegre, Brazil. *Int J Gynaecol Obstet.* 2012;117(1):81–82

50. Leticee N, Viard JP, Yamgnane A, Karmochkine M, Benachi A. Contraceptive failure of etonogestrel implant in patients treated with antiretrovirals including efavirenz. *Contraception.* 2012;85(4):425–427

51. National Institutes of Health. Recommendations for use of antiretroviral drugs in pregnant HIV-1-infected women for maternal health and interventions to reduce perinatal HIV transmission in the United States. Available at: https://aidsinfo.nih.gov/guidelines/html/3/perinatal-guidelines/0. Accessed January 4, 2016

52. National Institutes of Health. Guidelines for the use of antiretroviral agents in HIV-1-infected adults and adolescents. Available at: https://aidsinfo.nih.gov/contentfiles/lvguidelines/adultandadolescentgl.pdf. Accessed January 4, 2016

53. World Health Organization. Medical eligibility criteria for contraceptive use. 5th ed. Executive summary. Geneva, Switzerland: World Health Organization; 2015. Available at: www.who.int/reproductivehealth/publications/family_planning/Ex-Summ-MEC-5/en/. Accessed January 4, 2016

54. Deans G, Schwarz EB. Intrauterine contraceptives (IUCs). In: Hatcher RA, Trussell J, Nelson AL, Cates W Jr, Kowal D, Policar MS, eds. *Contraceptive Technology.* 20th revised ed. Atlanta, GA: Ardent Media, Inc; 2011:147–182

55. Centers for Disease Control and Prevention. U.S. selected practice recommendations for contraceptive use, 2013: adapted from the World Health Organization selected practice recommendations for contraceptive use, 2nd edition. *MMWR Recomm Rep.* 2013;62(RR-5):1–46. Available at: www.cdc.gov/mmwr/preview/mmwrhtml/rr6205a1.htm. Accessed January 4, 2016

56. Bayer HealthCare Pharmaceuticals. Skyla [package insert]. 2013. Available at: http://labeling.bayerhealthcare.com/html/products/pi/Skyla_PI.pdf. Accessed January 4, 2016

57. Bayer HaelthCare Pharmaceuticals Inc. Mirena [package insert]. 2014. Available at: http://labeling.bayerhealthcare.com/html/products/pi/Mirena_PI.pdf. Accessed January 4, 2016

58. Teva Women's Health I. ParaGuard T 380A [package insert]. 2013. Available at: www.paragard.com/Pdf/ParaGard-PI.pdf. Accessed January 4, 2016

59. Hubacher D, Lara-Ricalde R, Taylor DJ, Guerra-Infante F, Guzmán-Rodríguez R. Use of copper intrauterine devices and the risk of tubal infertility among nulligravid women. *N Engl J Med.* 2001;345(8):561–567

60. Mohllajee AP, Curtis KM, Peterson HB. Does insertion and use of an intrauterine device increase the risk of pelvic inflammatory disease among women with sexually transmitted infection? A systematic review. *Contraception.* 2006;73(2):145–153

61. Farley TM, Rosenberg MJ, Rowe PJ, Chen JH, Meirik O. Intrauterine devices and pelvic inflammatory disease: an international perspective. *Lancet.* 1992;339(8796):785–788

62. Tepper NK, Marchbanks PA, Curtis KMUS. U.S. selected practice recommendations for contraceptive use, 2013. *J Womens Health (Larchmt).* 2014;23(2):108–111

63. Tepper NK, Curtis KM, Nanda K, Jamieson DJ. Safety of intrauterine devices among women with HIV: a systematic review [published online ahead of print June 22,

2016]. *Contraception*.10.1016/j.
contraception.2016.06.011

64. Heikinheimo O, Lehtovirta P, Suni
J, Paavonen J. The levonorgestrel-
releasing intrauterine system (LNG-
IUS) in HIV-infected women—effects
on bleeding patterns, ovarian function
and genital shedding of HIV. *Hum
Reprod*. 2006;21(11):2857–2861

65. Lehtovirta P, Paavonen J, Heikinheimo
O. Experience with the levonorgestrel-
releasing intrauterine system among
HIV-infected women. *Contraception*.
2007;75(1):37–39

66. Heikinheimo O, Lehtovirta P, Aho
I, Ristola M, Paavonen J. The
levonorgestrel-releasing intrauterine
system in human immunodeficiency
virus-infected women: a 5-year
follow-up study. *Am J Obstet Gynecol*.
2011;204(2):126.e1–126.e4

67. Morrison CS, Chen PL, Kwok C, et
al. Hormonal contraception and the
risk of HIV acquisition: an individual
participant data meta-analysis. *PLoS
Med*. 2015;12(1):e1001778

68. Stringer EM, Kaseba C, Levy J,
et al. A randomized trial of the
intrauterine contraceptive device vs
hormonal contraception in women
who are infected with the human
immunodeficiency virus. *Am J Obstet
Gynecol*. 2007;197(2):144.e1–144.e8

69. Pfizer. Depo-provera CI [package
insert]. 2010. Available at: www.
accessdata.fda.gov/drugsatfda_
docs/label/2010/020246s036lbl.pdf.
Accessed January 4, 2016

70. Beksinska ME, Kleinschmidt I, Smit
JA, Farley TM, Rees HV. Bone mineral
density in young women aged 19-24
after 4-5 years of exclusive and mixed
use of hormonal contraception.
Contraception. 2009;80(2):128–132

71. Polis CB, Phillips SJ, Curtis KM, et al.
Hormonal contraceptive methods and
risk of HIV acquisition in women: a
systematic review of epidemiological
evidence. *Contraception*.
2014;90(4):360–390

72. Phillips SJ, Curtis KM, Polis CB. Effect
of hormonal contraceptive methods on
HIV disease progression: a systematic
review. *AIDS*. 2013;27(5):787–794

73. Nanda K, Amaral E, Hays M, Viscola
MA, Mehta N, Bahamondes L.

Pharmacokinetic interactions
between depot medroxyprogesterone
acetate and combination
antiretroviral therapy. *Fertil Steril*.
2008;90(4):965–971

74. Cohn SE, Park JG, Watts DH, et al;
ACTG A5093 Protocol Team. Depo-
medroxyprogesterone in women
on antiretroviral therapy: effective
contraception and lack of clinically
significant interactions. *Clin
Pharmacol Ther*. 2007;81(2):222–227

75. Watts DH, Park JG, Cohn SE, et al.
Safety and tolerability of depot
medroxyprogesterone acetate among
HIV-infected women on antiretroviral
therapy: ACTG A5093. *Contraception*.
2008;77(2):84–90

76. Puthanakit T, Siberry GK. Bone health
in children and adolescents with
perinatal HIV infection. *J Int AIDS Soc*.
2013;16:18575

77. Nelson AL. Combined oral
contraceptives. In: Hatcher RA,
Trussell J, Nelson AL, Cates W Jr, Kowal
D, Policar MS, eds. *Contraceptive
Technology*. 20th revised ed. Atlanta,
GA: Ardent Media, Inc; 2011:249–319

78. Stewart FH, Brown BA, Raine TR,
Weitz TA, Harper CC. Adolescent and
young women's experience with the
vaginal ring and oral contraceptive
pills. *J Pediatr Adolesc Gynecol*.
2007;20(6):345–351

79. Committee on Adolescence. Condom
use by adolescents. *Pediatrics*.
2013;132(5):973–981

80. Gilliam ML, Neustadt A, Kozloski M,
Mistretta S, Tilmon S, Godfrey E.
Adherence and acceptability of the
contraceptive ring compared with the
pill among students: a randomized
controlled trial. *Obstet Gynecol*.
2010;115(3):503–510

81. Bakhru A, Stanwood N. Performance
of contraceptive patch compared
with oral contraceptive pill in a
high-risk population. *Obstet Gynecol*.
2006;108(2):378–386

82. Atrio J, Stanczyk FZ, Neely M, Cherala
G, Kovacs A, Mishell DR Jr. Effect
of protease inhibitors on steady-
state pharmacokinetics of oral
norethindrone contraception in HIV-
infected women. *J Acquir Immune
Defic Syndr*. 2014;65(1):72–77

83. Martinez G, Copen CE, Abma JC.
Teenagers in the United States:
sexual activity, contraceptive use,
and childbearing, 2006-2010 national
survey of family growth. *Vital Health
Stat 23*. 2011;(6):1–35

84. Warner L, Steiner MJ. Male condoms.
In: Hatcher RA, Trussell J, Nelson AL,
Cates W Jr, Kowal D, Policar MS, eds.
Contraceptive Technology. 20th revised
ed. Atlanta, GA: Ardent Media, Inc;
2011:371–382

85. Centers for Disease Control and
Prevention. Condom fact sheet
in brief. Available at: www.cdc.
gov/condomeffectiveness/docs/
condomfactsheetinbrief.pdf. Accessed
January 4, 2016

86. Committee on Adolescence.
Emergency contraception. *Pediatrics*.
2012;130(6):1174–1182

87. US Food and Drug Administration. FDA
approves Plan B One-Step emergency
contraceptive for use without a
prescription for all women of childbearing potential [news release].
Silver Spring, MD: US Food and
Drug Administration; June 20, 2013.
Available at: www.fda.gov/NewsEvents/
Newsroom/PressAnnouncements/
ucm358082.htm. Accessed January 4,
2016

88. Wilkinson D, Tholandi M, Ramjee G,
Rutherford GW. Nonoxynol-9 spermicide
for prevention of vaginally acquired
HIV and other sexually transmitted
infections: systematic review and
meta-analysis of randomised
controlled trials including more
than 5000 women. *Lancet Infect Dis*.
2002;2(10):613–617

89. Cates W Jr. Vaginal barriers and
spermicides. In: Hatcher RA, Trussell J,
Nelson AL, Cates W Jr, Kowal D, Policar
MS, eds. *Contraceptive Technology*.
20th revised ed. Atlanta, GA: Ardent
Media, Inc; 2011:391–405

90. US Agency for International
Development. *Hormonal
Contracception and HIV* [technical
brief]. Washington, DC: US Agency for
International Development; 2013

91. Baeten JM, Lavreys L, Overbaugh J. The
influence of hormonal contraceptive
use on HIV-1 transmission and
disease progression. *Clin Infect Dis*.
2007;45(3):360–369

92. Blish CA, Baeten JM. Hormonal contraception and HIV-1 transmission. *Am J Reprod Immunol.* 2011;65(3):302–307

93. Roccio M, Gardella B, Maserati R, Zara F, Iacobone D, Spinillo A. Low-dose combined oral contraceptive and cervicovaginal shedding of human immunodeficiency virus. *Contraception.* 2011;83(6):564–570

94. Mostad SB, Overbaugh J, DeVange DM, et al. Hormonal contraception, vitamin A deficiency, and other risk factors for shedding of HIV-1 infected cells from the cervix and vagina. *Lancet.* 1997;350(9082):922–927

95. Heffron R, Donnell D, Rees H, et al; Partners in Prevention HSV/HIV Transmission Study Team. Use of hormonal contraceptives and risk of HIV-1 transmission: a prospective cohort study. *Lancet Infect Dis.* 2012;12(1):19–26

96. Polis CB, Phillips SJ, Curtis KM. Hormonal contraceptive use and female-to-male HIV transmission: a systematic review of the epidemiologic evidence. *AIDS.* 2013;27(4):493–505

97. Clemetson DB, Moss GB, Willerford DM, et al. Detection of HIV DNA in cervical and vaginal secretions: prevalence and correlates among women in Nairobi, Kenya. *JAMA.* 1993;269(22):2860–2864

98. Kovacs A, Wasserman SS, Burns D, et al; DATRI Study Group; WIHS Study Group. Determinants of HIV-1 shedding in the genital tract of women. *Lancet.* 2001;358(9293):1593–1601

99. Wang CC, McClelland RS, Overbaugh J, et al. The effect of hormonal contraception on genital tract shedding of HIV-1. *AIDS.* 2004;18(2):205–209

100. World Health Organization. Hormonal contraceptive methods for women at high risk of HIV and living with HIV. 2014 Guidance statement. Geneva, Switzerland: World Health Organization; 2014. Available at: http://apps.who.int/iris/bitstream/10665/128537/1/WHO_ RHR_14.24_eng.pdf?ua=1. Accessed January 4, 2016

101. Crauwels HM, van Heeswijk RP, Buelens A, Stevens M, Hoetelmans RM. Lack of an effect of rilpivirine on the pharmacokinetics of ethinylestradiol and norethindrone in healthy volunteers. *Int J Clin Pharmacol Ther.* 2014;52(2):118–128

102. Landolt NK, Phanuphak N, Ubolyam S, et al. Efavirenz, in contrast to nevirapine, is associated with unfavorable progesterone and antiretroviral levels when coadministered with combined oral contraceptives. *J Acquir Immune Defic Syndr.* 2013;62(5):534–539

103. Mildvan D, Yarrish R, Marshak A, et al. Pharmacokinetic interaction between nevirapine and ethinyl estradiol/norethindrone when administered concurrently to HIV-infected women. *J Acquir Immune Defic Syndr.* 2002;29(5):471–477

104. Nanda K, Delany-Moretlwe S, Dubé K, et al. Nevirapine-based antiretroviral therapy does not reduce oral contraceptive effectiveness. *AIDS.* 2013;27(suppl 1):S17–S25

105. Stuart GS, Moses A, Corbett A, et al. Combined oral contraceptives and antiretroviral PK/PD in Malawian women: pharmacokinetics and pharmacodynamics of a combined oral contraceptive and a generic combined formulation antiretroviral in Malawi. *J Acquir Immune Defic Syndr.* 2011;58(2):e40–e43

106. Sevinsky H, Eley T, Persson A, et al. The effect of efavirenz on the pharmacokinetics of an oral contraceptive containing ethinyl estradiol and norgestimate in healthy HIV-negative women. *Antivir Ther.* 2011;16(2):149–156

107. Schöller-Gyüre M, Kakuda TN, Woodfall B, et al. Effect of steady-state etravirine on the pharmacokinetics and pharmacodynamics of ethinylestradiol and norethindrone. *Contraception.* 2009;80(1):44–52

108. Heffron R, Mugo N, Were E, et al; Partners PrEP Study Team. Preexposure prophylaxis is efficacious for HIV-1 prevention among women using depot medroxyprogesterone acetate for contraception. *AIDS.* 2014;28(18):2771–2776

109. Todd CS, Deese J, Wang M, et al; FEM-PrEP Study Group. Sino-implant (II)® continuation and effect of concomitant tenofovir disoproxil fumarate-emtricitabine use on plasma levonorgestrel concentrations among women in Bondo, Kenya. *Contraception.* 2015;91(3):248–252

110. Thurman AR, Anderson S, Doncel GF. Effects of hormonal contraception on antiretroviral drug metabolism, pharmacokinetics and pharmacodynamics. *Am J Reprod Immunol.* 2014;71(6):523–530

111. Polis CB, Nakigozi G, Ssempijja V, et al. Effect of injectable contraceptive use on response to antiretroviral therapy among women in Rakai, Uganda. *Contraception.* 2012;86(6):725–730

112. Chu JH, Gange SJ, Anastos K, et al. Hormonal contraceptive use and the effectiveness of highly active antiretroviral therapy. *Am J Epidemiol.* 2005;161(9):881–890

113. Hubacher D, Liku J, Kiarie J, et al. Effect of concurrent use of anti-retroviral therapy and levonorgestrel sub-dermal implant for contraception on CD4 counts: a prospective cohort study in Kenya. *J Int AIDS Soc.* 2013;16:18448

114. Johnson D, Kempf MC, Wilson CM, Shrestha S. Hormonal contraceptive use and response to antiretroviral therapy among adolescent females. *HIV and AIDS Review.* 2011;10(3):65–69

115. Friend DR, Clark JT, Kiser PF, Clark MR. Multipurpose prevention technologies: products in development. *Antiviral Res.* 2013;100(suppl):S39–S47

116. Underhill K, Montgomery P, Operario D. Abstinence-plus programs for HIV infection prevention in high-income countries. *Cochrane Database Syst Rev.* 2008;1:CD007006

Countering Vaccine Hesitancy

- *Clinical Report*

CLINICAL REPORT   Guidance for the Clinician in Rendering Pediatric Care

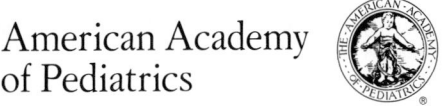

American Academy
of Pediatrics

DEDICATED TO THE HEALTH OF ALL CHILDREN™

Countering Vaccine Hesitancy

Kathryn M. Edwards, MD, Jesse M. Hackell, MD, THE COMMITTEE ON INFECTIOUS DISEASES, THE COMMITTEE ON PRACTICE AND AMBULATORY MEDICINE

Immunizations have led to a significant decrease in rates of vaccine-preventable diseases and have made a significant impact on the health of children. However, some parents express concerns about vaccine safety and the necessity of vaccines. The concerns of parents range from hesitancy about some immunizations to refusal of all vaccines. This clinical report provides information about addressing parental concerns about vaccination.

abstract

Clinical reports from the American Academy of Pediatrics benefit from expertise and resources of liaisons and internal (AAP) and external reviewers. However, clinical reports from the American Academy of Pediatrics may not reflect the views of the liaisons or the organizations or government agencies that they represent.

The guidance in this report does not indicate an exclusive course of treatment or serve as a standard of medical care. Variations, taking into account individual circumstances, may be appropriate.

All clinical reports from the American Academy of Pediatrics automatically expire 5 years after publication unless reaffirmed, revised, or retired at or before that time.

DOI: 10.1542/peds.2016-2146

PEDIATRICS (ISSN Numbers: Print, 0031-4005; Online, 1098-4275).

Copyright © 2016 by the American Academy of Pediatrics

FINANCIAL DISCLOSURE: Dr Hackell has indicated that a family member has stock or equity in Pfizer and GlaxoSmithKline.

FUNDING: No external funding.

POTENTIAL CONFLICT OF INTEREST: The authors have indicated they have no potential conflicts of interest to disclose.

To cite: Edwards KM, Hackell JM, AAP THE COMMITTEE ON INFECTIOUS DISEASES, THE COMMITTEE ON PRACTICE AND AMBULATORY MEDICINE. Countering Vaccine Hesitancy. *Pediatrics.* 2016;138(3):e20162146

INTRODUCTION

Immunizations have had an enormous impact on the health of children, and the prevention of disease by vaccination is one of the single greatest public health achievements of the last century. However, over the past decade acceptance of vaccines has been challenged by individuals and groups who question their benefit.[1] Increasing numbers of people are requesting alternative vaccination schedules[2,3] or postponing or declining vaccination.[4] In a national telephone survey of 1500 parents of children 6 to 23 months of age conducted in 2010 with a response rate of 46%, approximately 3% of respondents had refused all vaccines and 19.4% had refused or delayed at least 1 of the recommended childhood vaccines.[5] A study conducted in a metropolitan area of Oregon reported that rates of alternative immunization schedule usage have increased nearly fourfold in recent years,[3] and in some parts of the country the use of "personal belief exemptions" from vaccinations has grown to rates in excess of 5% of the school-aged population.[6]

The Periodic Survey of Fellows (PS#66) conducted by the American Academy of Pediatrics (AAP) in 2006 revealed that 75% of pediatricians surveyed had encountered parents who refused a vaccine,[7] and a follow-up survey in 2013 (PS#84) revealed that this figure had increased to 87% of pediatricians.[8] According to the survey, pediatricians stated that the proportion of parents who refused 1 or more vaccines increased from 9.1% to 16.7% during the 7-year interval between surveys.[7,8] Physicians stated that the most common reasons parents refused vaccines were that they believed that vaccines are unnecessary (which showed an increase over the 7-year span) and that they had concerns

TABLE 1 Categorization of Parental Attitudes Toward Vaccines[12,14]

Immunization advocate	Parents agree that vaccines are necessary and safe. Parents have a strong relationship with their health care provider.
Go along to get along	Parents do not question vaccines, would like to vaccinate their children, but may lack a detailed knowledge of vaccines.
Cautious acceptor	Parents may have minor concerns about vaccines but ultimately vaccinate their children.
Fence-sitter	Parents have significant concerns about vaccines and tend to be knowledgeable about vaccines. Parents may vaccinate their child or may refuse or delay vaccines. Parents may have significant concerns about vaccines and may have a neutral relationship with their health care provider.
Refuser	Parents refuse all vaccines for their child. Their reasons for refusal may include distrust in the medical system, safety concerns, and religious beliefs.

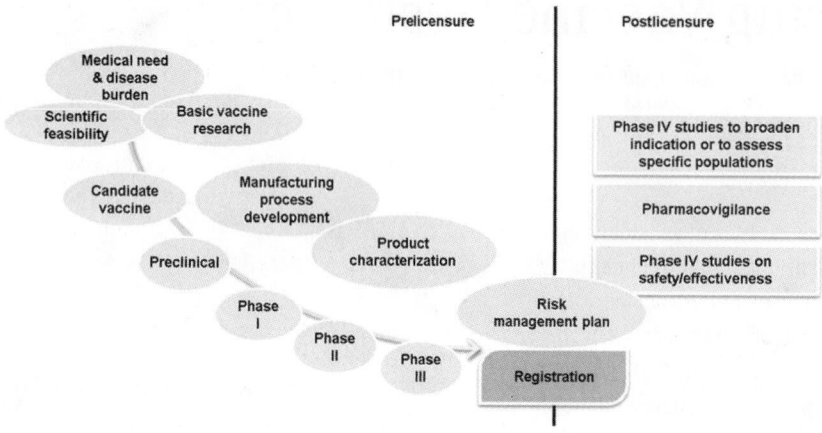

FIGURE 1
Vaccine pipeline: prelicensure and postlicensure vaccine development activities. From Hardt K, Schmidt-Ott R, Glismann S, Adegbola RA, Meurice F. Sustaining vaccine confidence in the 21st century. *Vaccines.* 2013;1(3):204–224. Copyright © 2013 by the authors; licensee MDPI, Basel, Switzerland. Reproduced under the terms and conditions of the Creative Commons Attribution license (http://creativecommons.org/licenses/by/3.0/).

about autism (which declined between survey years). In both 2006 and 2013, pediatricians reported that they were able to convince approximately 30% of parents to vaccinate their children when they initially refused. Another observational study found that when physicians continued to engage parents, up to 47% of parents ultimately accepted vaccines after initially refusing them.[9] Although the majority of parents accept vaccines, the increasing frequency of refusal and the requests for alternative vaccine schedules indicate that there are still significant barriers to overcome.[10]

TERMINOLOGY

The term *vaccine hesitancy* has emerged to depolarize the "pro" versus "anti" vaccination alignment and to express the spectrum

of parental attitudes toward vaccines.[1] Vaccine hesitancy has been characterized recently by a committee at the World Health Organization as "a behavior, influenced by a number of factors including issues of confidence (do not trust a vaccine or a provider), complacency (do not perceive a need for a vaccine or do not value the vaccine), and convenience (access)."[11] Vaccine-hesitant individuals are a heterogeneous group who hold varying degrees of indecision about specific vaccines or about vaccinations in general. Vaccine-hesitant individuals may accept all vaccines but remain concerned about them, they may refuse or delay some vaccines but accept others, or they may refuse all vaccines. The latter group refusing all vaccines is estimated at approximately 3% of parents, although the prevalence may vary geographically.[4,12,13]

The concept that parental vaccine hesitancy is a spectrum has been confirmed in several studies[4,14,15] and was well described in a recent review by Leask et al[12] (Table 1). Some parents who totally refuse vaccines may be fixed and unswayable in their beliefs and may not respond to the pediatrician attempting to change their views. The AAP recommends that pediatricians continue to engage with vaccine-hesitant parents, provide other health care services to their children, and attempt to modify their opposition to vaccines.[16–18] Fortunately, most vaccine-hesitant parents are responsive to vaccine information, consider vaccinating their children, and are not opposed to all vaccines. Responding to vaccine-hesitant parents is the focus of this clinical report.

VACCINES ARE TESTED THOROUGHLY

Vaccine development is a long and arduous process, often lasting many years and involving a combination of public and private partnerships. The current system for developing, testing, and regulating vaccines requires that the vaccines demonstrate both safety and efficacy before licensure and that long-term safety is monitored (http://www.historyofvaccines.org/content/articles/vaccine-development-testing-and-regulation; Fig 1). The first step in vaccine discovery involves the identification of a need for a vaccine and an understanding of the mechanism of protective immunity against that disease.

If the vaccine appears promising in preclinical studies, the vaccine sponsor submits an application for an Investigational New Drug to the US Food and Drug Administration (FDA). Law requires that the sponsor describe the manufacturing and testing processes, summarize the laboratory reports, and describe the proposed studies to evaluate the vaccine. As with therapeutic drugs, vaccine evaluation includes phase I through phase III testing. Phase I trials are intended to assess the safety of the candidate vaccine and to determine the type and extent of immune response that the vaccine provokes.

Phase II testing involves several hundred volunteers, some of whom belong to groups at risk for acquiring the disease. These trials generally are randomized and controlled and usually include a placebo group or a standard licensed vaccine when a new vaccine for that disease is being tested.

Phase III vaccine trials are designed to determine whether the vaccine will prevent the disease in question and to assess the vaccine's safety when administered to a large number of subjects. These studies often involve thousands or tens of thousands of participants, depending on the incidence of disease and the rates of adverse events to be detected. If these studies show the vaccine to be effective and safe, it is then licensed.

VACCINE SAFETY IS ACTIVELY MONITORED AFTER LICENSURE

Once vaccines are licensed, a number of processes are in place to ensure that the safety of vaccines is monitored. In 1990, the Centers for Disease Control and Prevention (CDC) and FDA established the Vaccine Adverse Events Reporting System (VAERS), a voluntary passive reporting system that serves as a signal detection system for adverse events associated with vaccines (http://vaers.hhs.gov/index). Anyone who suspects an association between a vaccination and an adverse event can report the event to VAERS. The CDC and the FDA then investigate the event.[19] VAERS has successfully identified several adverse events related to vaccination in the past, such as intussusception after administration of the RotaShield (Wyeth Laboratories Inc, Marietta, PA) rotavirus vaccine, which was identified in 1999, leading to the ultimate withdrawal of that vaccine from the market.[20]

In 1990, the CDC also established the Vaccine Safety Datalink (VSD) to monitor vaccine safety. The VSD is composed of a number of large health provider groups with linked databases with comprehensive information about vaccines administered and health care encounters.[21] Because the VSD involves millions of individuals, it can be used to detect rare events and was used to study the possible, but subsequently disproven, association between Guillain–Barré syndrome and meningococcal vaccination.[22] Another parallel system to the VSD is the Post-Licensure Rapid Immunization Safety Monitoring system.[23] This system uses health insurance claims data from 107 million individuals to actively monitor vaccine safety. In addition, the CDC has also established the Clinical Immunization Safety Assessment Project, a group of academic health care centers, to address specific questions about vaccine safety from individual health care providers (http://www.cdc.gov/vaccinesafety/activities/cisa.html).[24]

In summary, vaccines are comprehensively evaluated before their licensure. They are developed and tested in large numbers of subjects, regulated by the FDA, and carefully monitored after licensure through a comprehensive safety surveillance system funded by the CDC and the FDA. In rare instances in which safety concerns are identified, regulatory or other actions to safeguard public health are taken.

HISTORICAL VACCINE OPPOSITION

Before discussing the recent increase in vaccine hesitancy, it is valuable to recall that opposition to vaccination is not a new occurrence. In the early 1800s in Europe, Jenner promoted vaccination against smallpox by using material obtained from cowpox lesions.[25] However, over the next several decades, increasing rates of opposition to smallpox vaccination were seen in the United Kingdom, requiring vaccination to be mandated by law.[25] Similar obstacles to universal smallpox vaccination were also encountered in the United States. In the 1850s, a number of parents and physicians challenged mandatory smallpox vaccination, and in 1905 in the case *Jacobson v Massachusetts,* the US Supreme Court supported the rights of states to pass laws mandating smallpox vaccine.[6] However, although vaccine hesitancy is not a new phenomenon, it may have a greater effect on public health today. With the ease of global travel, vaccine-preventable diseases are spread more quickly and may unexpectedly appear in areas where health care professionals are unfamiliar with their clinical presentation.

CURRENT VACCINE EXEMPTIONS

Herd immunity is a fundamental concept that contributes to the success of many vaccination programs. Control of many vaccine-preventable diseases is contingent on a significant proportion of the population in a community being immune.[26] Depending on the disease, the percentage of individuals required to achieve herd immunity in a community ranges from 30% to 95%.[27] Traditionally, immunization rates have been maintained in the United States through mandatory vaccination requirements for entry into and advancement through licensed child care centers and schools. However, recent years have seen a marked increase in the availability and use of "philosophical" or "personal belief" exemptions from vaccination. Over the period from 2005 through 2011, Omer et al[28] reported that the unadjusted rates for nonmedical exemptions in states that allowed for philosophical exemptions were 2.5 times higher than in states that allowed only religious exemptions. In Arkansas, rates of overall exemptions increased an average of 23% per year once philosophical exemptions were allowed.[29] Studies have demonstrated that parents who refuse vaccines are more likely to be white and more highly educated than those who do not.[4,6,30,31] In addition, the prevalence of vaccine-hesitant parents seems to vary geographically.[6,32] It is unclear whether requiring a mandatory physician visit or educational module for parents who apply for vaccine exemption in states with philosophical exemptions is effective in reducing refusals.[32]

Children who are philosophically exempted from vaccination not only are at greater risk of developing vaccine-preventable disease but also put vaccinated children and medically exempt children who live in the same area at risk.[33-35] Vaccine-preventable diseases occurring in vaccinated children may result from waning immunity after immunization or may be attributable to an ineffective immune response to vaccine initially. In January 2015, a measles outbreak occurred in California, where an estimated 3.1% of kindergartners had a nonmedical exemption from receiving the measles–mumps–rubella (MMR) vaccine.[36] The majority of cases occurred in children who either had

not received measles vaccine (45%) or had unknown vaccination status (38%).[37] Of the cases in unvaccinated children, 43% of parents cited philosophical or religious objects to vaccine. An additional 40% of unvaccinated children could not receive the vaccine because they were too young. This outbreak, which spread to multiple states, has sparked intense debate about vaccine exemptions and the government's role in limiting nonmedical exemptions. Whether the 2015 outbreak and legislation resulting from this outbreak will have a long-lasting effect on public policy and parental choices is not clear at this time. For these reasons, we believe the better approach is to work to eliminate all nonmedical exemptions for childhood vaccines, a position that is shared by the American Medical Association and the Infectious Diseases Society of America and is currently the basis of a policy statement being developed by the AAP. There has also been greater recognition among pediatricians that delayed or incomplete vaccination schedules are probably responsible, at least in part, for the spread of measles in that outbreak.[38-40] As a result, more pediatricians are becoming concerned about the risk unimmunized children pose to other children in their practices, both immunized children and those too young or otherwise unable to be immunized. Some are electing to dismiss families who refuse vaccines from their practices.[7] The ethical considerations of patient dismissal are complex and are discussed in a subsequent section of this statement as well as in a comprehensive review by Diekema.[41]

FACTORS INVOLVED IN VACCINE ACCEPTANCE

The evolution of vaccine confidence over the course of vaccine introduction is summarized in a figure that first appeared in a

1994 article by Chen et al[19] (Fig 2), which succinctly outlines many of the pivotal factors that must be considered when discussing vaccine hesitancy. As shown in Fig 2, disease incidence is highest before the development and implementation of a vaccine program. At this time, the public generally is eager to accept a new vaccine, particularly if the morbidity and mortality associated with the disease are considerable. Then, after the vaccine is developed and proven efficacious, individuals are eager to be vaccinated, and coverage increases, with subsequent declines in disease incidence ("increasing coverage" phase). However, as vaccine uptake peaks, the disease incidence declines, and the total number of adverse events after vaccination increases. Whether the adverse events were causally related or only temporally associated with vaccine administration can be difficult to determine, but these adverse events may lead to loss of confidence in the vaccine as the public perceives the risk of vaccination to outweigh the risk of disease ("loss of confidence" phase). This, in turn, may increase vaccine refusal and ultimately lead to disease resurgence. Then, after disease resurgence or an outbreak, as the public again appreciates the increasing burden of disease, vaccine acceptance is restored and vaccination rates increase ("resumption of confidence" phase). Unfortunately, a recent study during an outbreak of pertussis in the state of Washington suggested that, despite an increase in pertussis cases, parents did not have a "resumption in vaccine confidence" and did not increase pertussis vaccine uptake.[42] In the rare incidents in which disease is eradicated by vaccine, as occurred with smallpox, vaccination can stop ("eradication" phase). This conceptual framework is more applicable to diseases for which the time between exposure and infection is short, such as measles, pertussis, or polio, and less relevant to, for example, vaccines against human papillomavirus (HPV), for which the benefits of immunization in preventing cancer may take years or decades to become apparent. Figure 2 clearly highlights the delicate balance between perceived risk and benefit for each vaccine and how this balance is linked integrally to vaccine acceptance.

PARENTS' VARIED CONCERNS ABOUT VACCINES SHOULD BE ADDRESSED

A number of studies have attempted to define the reasons why parents are vaccine hesitant, and these factors are summarized in Table 2.[1,4,5,15,43–45] In 1 study, 44% of parents reported concern over pain associated with receiving multiple injections during a single visit, 34% expressed unease about receiving too many vaccines at a single visit, 26% worried about the development of autism or other potential learning difficulties after receiving vaccines, 13.5% expressed concern that vaccines could lead to chronic illnesses, and 13.2% stated that vaccines were not tested enough for safety before their use.[45] Concerns about vaccine safety and questions about the necessity of vaccines are often cited as reasons for vaccine refusal.[43,46–48] One survey found that parents who decide to not vaccinate their children have a greater distrust of health care professionals and the government and are more likely to use complementary and alternative medicine, compared with parents who vaccinate their children.[47] Freed et al[43] also conducted an online survey of several thousand parents to identify vaccine concerns. Most of the surveyed parents agreed that vaccines protected their children from diseases; however, more than half expressed concerns regarding serious adverse effects of vaccines. Overall, 11.5% of parents in that study had refused at least 1 recommended vaccine, and the fear

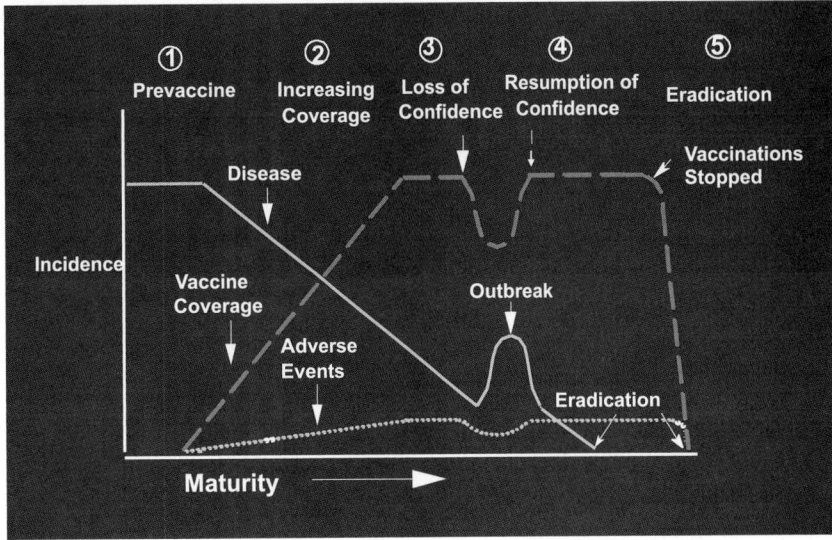

FIGURE 2

Evolution of a vaccine program. Reproduced with permission. Chen RT, Orenstein WA. Epidemiologic methods in immunization programs. *Epidemiol Rev.* 1996;18(2):102. Copyright © 1996 by the Oxford University Press.

TABLE 2 Parental Concerns About Vaccines

Vaccine safety
    Too many vaccines
    Development of autism
    Vaccine additives (thimerosal, aluminum)
    Overload the immune system
    Serious adverse reactions
    Potential for long-term adverse events
    Inadequate research performed before licensure
    May cause pain to the child
    May make the child sick
Necessity of vaccines
    Disease is more "natural" than vaccine
    Parents do not believe diseases being prevented are serious
    Vaccine-preventable diseases have disappeared
    Not all vaccines are needed
    Vaccines do not work
Freedom of choice
    Parents have the right to choose whether to immunize their child
    Parents know what's best for their child
    Believe that the risks outweigh the benefits of vaccine
    Do not trust organized medicine, public health
    Do not trust government health authorities
    Do not trust pharmaceutical companies
    Ethical, moral, or religious reasons

that vaccines could cause autism was often cited as a reason for refusal.[43]

Parental concerns must be addressed, and concerns will vary among parents. For example, vaccine safety and triggering early sexual activity are often cited as parental concerns about the HPV vaccine.[49] Reassuring parents that the vaccine is safe and

that there is no evidence that HPV vaccine increases sexual activity may dispel their concerns.[50] Some parents are concerned primarily about the pain associated with immunizations. Strategies to reduce pain include administering vaccines quickly without aspirating, holding the child upright, administering the most painful vaccine last, and

TABLE 3 Number of Immunogenic Proteins and Polysaccharides Contained in Vaccines Over the Past 100 Years

1890		1960		1980		2000	
Vaccine	Proteins	Vaccine	Proteins	Vaccine	Proteins	Vaccine	Proteins and Polysaccharides
Smallpox	~200	Smallpox	~200	Diphtheria	1	Diphtheria	1
Total	~200	Diphtheria	1	Tetanus	1	Tetanus	1
		Tetanus	1	WC-pertussis	~3000	AC-pertussis	2–5
		WC-pertussis	~3000	Polio	15	Polio	15
		Polio	15	Measles	10	Measles	10
		Total	~3217	Mumps	9	Mumps	9
				Rubella	5	Rubella	5
				Total	~3041	Hib	2
						Varicella	69
						Pneumococcus	8
						Hepatitis B	1
						Total	123–126

Adapted from Offit et al.[52]

AC-pertussis, acellular pertussis vaccine; WC-pertussis, whole cell pertussis vaccine.

providing tactile stimulation.[51] Breastfeeding, feeding sweet-tasting solutions, and topical anesthetics are other tools that can be used before vaccine administration to decrease pain. Distraction strategies, including pinwheels, deep breathing exercises, and toys, can be used in older children to decrease anxiety and pain. Although rigorously controlled studies of these techniques have not been performed, studies of other painful procedures lend support to their use in vaccination.[51,52]

Providers should address specific parental questions about the production and composition of the vaccines by directly providing the information requested. For example, for concerns about the presence of mercury (thimerosal) in vaccines, parents can be reassured that currently, none of the single-dose vaccine preparations given to infants contain any mercury. The opposition to the presence of aluminum as an adjuvant in some vaccines can be addressed by providing evidence for both the necessity of the aluminum for a vigorous immune response and the lack of evidence for its toxicity. The religious argument that vaccines contain cells derived from aborted human fetuses can be answered in statements from major religious denominations either acknowledging that the vaccines do not contain such cells or that the earlier use of fetal

cell lines in vaccine production does not prohibit the use of these vaccines many years after the fetal cells were obtained.[53]

A specific response to the parental concern of "too many vaccines" and the potential for "overwhelming the immune system" was provided by Offit et al.[54] As shown in Table 3, the number of immunogenic proteins and polysaccharides contained in currently licensed vaccines is significantly smaller than the number of antigens contained in earlier vaccines and in naturally circulating organisms that infected children before universal vaccination. Sharing a copy of Table 3 could provide the necessary reassurance to parents who have concerns regarding "too many vaccines."

COUNTERING VACCINE HESITANCY CAN BE CHALLENGING

Even the use of targeted discussion strategies may not be adequate to counter vaccine hesitancy. A recent study reported by Nyhan et al[55] recruited a nationally representative sample of parents through random digit dialing and address-based sampling and randomly assigned them to 1 of 5 groups: providing textual information explaining the lack of evidence that MMR vaccine causes autism, supplying textual information about the dangers of

the diseases prevented by MMR vaccine, showing visual images of children who have diseases prevented by MMR vaccine, providing a dramatic audio narrative about an infant who almost died of measles, and no intervention. None of the interventions increased parental intent to vaccinate a future child. Thus, the authors concluded that current public health communications about vaccines may not be effective, and for some vaccine-hesitant parents, they may actually increase misperceptions and reduce vaccination intention. However, a limitation of this study was that it was Web based and did not examine the effect of direct one-to-one personal communication between the pediatrician and the parent.

Providing vaccine information is time consuming. Kempe et al[56] found that 53% of physicians spend 10 to 19 minutes discussing vaccines with concerned parents, and 8% of physicians spend 20 minutes or more with these parents. They also reported that pediatricians experienced decreased job satisfaction because of time spent with parents with significant vaccine concerns. Physicians have several options to deal with this problem, ranging from scheduling longer well-care visits, with some loss of overall efficiency; simply not having the discussion and acceding to a parent's request to defer, delay, or skip a vaccination; or dismissing such families from their practice. Permitting alternative vaccine schedules reduces vaccine timeliness and complicates an already complex vaccine schedule.[57] A study by Robison et al[3] demonstrated that children whose parents chose to limit vaccinations had more total visits for immunizations and by both 9 and 19 months of age were substantially less likely to be caught up on their immunization series. The additional time and costs associated with longer and more frequent well-child and immunization visits for parents with vaccine concerns are substantial, and by decreasing the efficiency of primary care providers, they may have a significant effect on access to health care services for all children.

PEDIATRICIANS PLAY AN IMPORTANT ROLE

With all the challenges acknowledged, the single most important factor in getting parents to accept vaccines remains the one-on-one contact with an informed, caring, and concerned pediatrician.[58] In a study reported in *Pediatrics,* parents of more than 7000 children 19 to 35 months of age were surveyed to determine whether they believed vaccines were safe and what influence their primary care providers had on their decisions to vaccinate.[45] Nearly 80% of parents stated that their decision to vaccinate was positively influenced by their primary care provider. The study concluded, "Health care providers have a positive influence on parents to vaccinate their children, including parents who believe that vaccinations are unsafe. Physicians, nurses, and other health care professionals should increase their efforts to build honest and respectful relationships with parents, especially when parents express concerns about vaccine safety or have misconceptions about the benefits and risks of vaccinations." In

another study, Smith et al[59] clearly demonstrated that parents whose children were vaccinated listed their pediatrician as a strong influence on their decision to vaccinate. A well-informed pediatrician who effectively addresses parental concerns and strongly supports the benefits of vaccination has enormous influence on parental vaccine acceptance.

ATTENTIVENESS TO PARENTS' CONCERNS IS IMPORTANT WHILE CORRECTING MISCONCEPTIONS

After acknowledging the varied concerns of vaccine-hesitant parents, the pediatrician needs to communicate with the parents about the development and safety testing of vaccines, the reasons for immunizing, and the risks of not doing so. An important aspect of communication with vaccine-hesitant parents is to clearly articulate the message that vaccines are safe and effective, and serious disease can occur if your child and family are not immunized. The safety of the currently recommended vaccines administered according to their established schedules was strongly affirmed by the Institute of Medicine in 2013.[60] A recent report commissioned by the Agency for Healthcare Research and Quality, on behalf of the National Vaccine Program Office, and an accompanying editorial also affirmed the safety of vaccines recommended for routine immunization of children.[61,62] It is important to present this safety information in a nonconfrontational dialogue with the parents while listening to and acknowledging their concerns. Misconceptions should be corrected, because both parents and pediatricians are in agreement in wanting the best for the children's health and well-being.[63]

THE CURRENT VACCINE SCHEDULE IS THE ONLY RECOMMENDED SCHEDULE

It is extremely important that the pediatrician remain up to date on

the current recommended vaccine schedule and support it as the only evidence-based schedule that has been tested and approved by multiple authoritative experts for safety and efficacy.[60] No alternative vaccine schedules have been evaluated and found to provide better safety or efficacy than the recommended schedule, supported by the Advisory Committee on Immunization Practices of the CDC and the Committee on Infectious Diseases of the AAP (the committee that produces the *Red Book*). Pediatricians who routinely recommend limiting the numbers of vaccines administered at a single visit such that vaccines are administered late are providing care that deviates from the standard evidence-based schedule recommended by these bodies. Situational deviation from these recommendations may be considered a last resort if, after reasonable attempts to convince hesitant parents, it is the only way to achieve the ultimate goal of immunizing a child. All who provide vaccines must be capable of articulating the safety and efficacy of the standard schedule and refrain from suggesting that delaying or deferring vaccines may be safer or more effective, because there is no evidence to support this viewpoint.

Pediatricians should not overestimate parental vaccine hesitancy or mistake a simple lack of knowledge for hesitancy or opposition.[64] Opel et al[9] reported that only 55% of practitioners routinely provide parents with the rationale for why vaccines are administered and their potential adverse effects. They reported that nearly half of parents who were initially vaccine hesitant ultimately accepted vaccines after practitioners provided a rationale for vaccine administration. Parental education can be provided through Vaccine Information Statements (VISs) given to parents before vaccine administration, through an online review of the VIS before the routine immunization visit, or through referral to authoritative Web sites, such as that of the CDC (http://www.cdc.gov/vaccines/vpd-vac/default.htm). One study reported that the majority of mothers preferred receiving vaccine information before the initial immunization visit.[65] The provision of a VIS is required at each immunization encounter for each vaccine, and counseling about vaccine-preventable diseases and vaccine adverse effects is required to correctly bill for vaccine administration. If parents refuse vaccination, a vaccine refusal waiver, used by many pediatricians in the event of deviations from the recommended vaccine schedule, can be obtained from the AAP Web site (https://www.aap.org/en-us/advocacy-and-policy/aap-health-initiatives/immunization/Pages/refusal-to-vaccinate.aspx), and parents may be asked to sign it.

PRESUMPTIVE DELIVERY STRATEGY

Another effective communication approach is the presumptive delivery strategy. Opel et al[9] demonstrated that the majority of parents accepted the provider's vaccine recommendations when they were presented as required immunizations to maintain optimal disease prevention. This approach may not work well with some parents, however, and pediatricians may use it selectively based on their experience. In addition, pediatricians who began practicing medicine before the introduction of many of today's routinely recommended vaccines have first-hand knowledge of these preventable diseases and often use that experience to effectively communicate the need for vaccines and the rationale for their administration according to established recommendations. One study conducted among 542 primary care providers in the United States

demonstrated that recent graduates were less likely to believe that vaccines were safe and efficacious than their older colleagues[66]; whether this is attributable to lack of first-hand experience with vaccine-preventable diseases or lack of comprehensive vaccine education is unclear. Educational efforts during residency training programs should provide trainees with a comprehensive understanding of the effect of vaccines on disease burden and the knowledge to evaluate the safety of vaccines as well as effective communication strategies. Only 48.5% of 303 US pediatric residents surveyed reported training in communication strategies for vaccine-hesitant patients during residency, and nearly 80% requested more education about the adverse effects of vaccines.[67] One study found that a brief single educational intervention may not be sufficient to provide physicians with the skills to counteract vaccine hesitancy and suggested that more research is needed to determine the most effective educational interventions.[68]

PERSONALIZING THE MESSAGE THAT VACCINES ARE SAFE AND EFFECTIVE CAN BE POWERFUL

The presentation of basic medical information may not be sufficient to reassure parents about the safety and necessity of vaccines. Developing a trusting relationship with parents is key to influencing parental decision-making around vaccines.[69] Parents often are more likely to be persuaded by stories and anecdotes about the successes of vaccines. Personal examples of children who were sick with vaccine-preventable illnesses can be much more effective than simply reading the numbers of children infected with a disease each year in the VIS. The Web site www.immunize.org/reports is an excellent source of such cases. A recent study by Kempe et al[56] demonstrated that physicians reported the greatest

success convincing skeptical parents using messages that relied on their personal choices and experiences. Physicians relating that they have immunized all of their children, their grandchildren, or themselves provide a compelling message that they are confident in the safety of the vaccines.

Other techniques, such as the use of parent-centered motivational interviewing, have been suggested as an effective way to personalize communication. Having parents verbalize their questions and concerns, followed by a focused response to their concerns, may be an effective communication strategy. However, the effect of motivational interviewing and other communication techniques requires careful assessment. It is encouraging that both AAP Periodic Surveys of Fellows from 2006 and 2013 indicated that one-third of parents who initially refused ≥1 vaccines ultimately changed their minds and gave permission for vaccination. Although these conversations may be difficult and frustrating, they clearly represent time well spent. A summary of points that may be useful in these conversations is found in Table 4.

DISMISSAL OF PATIENTS WHO REFUSE VACCINATION

Some families still will not be persuaded to vaccinate.[56] After multiple attempts to convince families to vaccinate have failed, some pediatricians have chosen to dismiss families as a last resort.[7,8,70] Arguments have been made that these families should not be dismissed on the basis of public health principles, because nonvaccinating families might cluster in certain practices, making them the focal point for outbreaks.[71] Ethical arguments against dismissal have also been made.[41,72,73] In addition, there are dilemmas for the many pediatricians who continue to care for these families, including potentially exposing other patients to vaccine-preventable diseases from those who are unimmunized. Finally, many pediatricians may feel obligated to continue to care for children in families who refuse immunizations.

There are no published data regarding the eventual outcome of strict "vaccinate or be dismissed" policies on the eventual acceptance of vaccines, and additional studies are needed. However, there is anecdotal evidence that when pediatricians give parents the choice between immunizing their child or being dismissed, some parents accept vaccination, even when other efforts at persuasion have failed.

It should be noted that the same legal and ethical constraints exist to dismissal for any permissible reason, including failure to vaccinate. Dismissal must be conducted in a manner consistent with applicable state laws prohibiting abandonment of patients. Although these laws vary from state to state, official notification of the parents or legal guardian is required, along with the provision of information for finding a new physician. Furthermore, the dismissing physician is obligated to continue current treatment and provide emergency care for a reasonable period of time, usually 30 days.[74,75]

Certain practice settings may also limit the ability to dismiss a patient. Employees of hospitals and large health care organizations are often unable to dismiss patients by official organizational policy. In areas of the country where there may be limited access to pediatric care, the pediatrician should carefully evaluate the availability of other qualified providers for the family. If there are no other qualified physicians in the area, the pediatrician is faced with the problem of leaving a family without adequate health care. In

TABLE 4 Communication Highlights

Vaccines are safe and effective, and serious disease can occur if your child and family are not immunized.
Vaccine-hesitant individuals are a heterogeneous group, and their individual concerns should be respected and addressed.
Vaccine are tested thoroughly before licensure, and vaccine safety assessment networks exist to monitor vaccine safety after licensure.
Nonmedical vaccine exemptions increase rates of unvaccinated children.
Unvaccinated children put vaccinated children and medically exempt children who live in that same area at risk.
Pediatricians and other health care providers play a major role in educating parents about the safety and effectiveness of vaccines. Strong provider commitment to vaccination can influence hesitant or resistant parents.
Personalizing vaccine acceptance is often an effective approach.
The majority of parents accepted the provider's vaccine recommendations when they were presented as required immunizations to maintain optimal disease prevention.
The current vaccine schedule is the only one recommended by the CDC and the AAP. Alternative schedules have not been evaluated.

these situations, the pediatrician should continue to provide care to the patient and family.

The decision to dismiss a family who continues to refuse immunization is not one that should be made lightly, nor should it be made without considering and respecting the reasons for the parents' point of view.[44] Nevertheless, the individual pediatrician may consider dismissal of families who refuse vaccination as an acceptable option. In all practice settings, consistency, transparency, and openness regarding the practice's policy on vaccines is important.

CONCLUSIONS

Vaccine discussions continue to occupy the media and Internet, and every parent of a child for whom vaccination is recommended is exposed to these messages on a regular basis. Data have shown that participation in social media reinforces one's beliefs about vaccination, no matter what those beliefs are.[76] The pediatrician is often the only medically trained person available to discuss vaccine matters with parents, and it is incumbent on him or her to provide scientifically based and balanced information when these questions are asked. Table 5 provides a summary of some

of the available resources to aid the pediatrician.

The pediatrician should also appreciate that vaccine-hesitant parents are a heterogeneous group and that specific parental vaccine concerns should be individually identified and addressed. Although many techniques for working with vaccine-hesitant parents have been suggested, scant data are available to determine the efficacy of these methods.[77] Additional research on communication techniques is needed. The clear message parents should hear is that vaccines are safe and effective, and serious disease can occur if your child and family are not immunized. Pediatricians should keep in mind that many, if not most, vaccine-hesitant parents are not opposed to vaccinating their children; rather, they are seeking guidance about the issues involved, beginning with the complexity of the schedule and the number of vaccines proposed. Parents may be unsure of the need for vaccines, because most have never experienced the diseases vaccines are designed to prevent, and they have concerns about possible adverse effects of these vaccines.

Pediatricians facing concerned parents on a regular basis should be prepared to discuss the science behind the current vaccine schedule and the extensive testing of each

TABLE 5 Vaccine Resources

Tools

    AAP refusal to vaccinate form: https://www.aap.org/en-us/Documents/immunization_refusaltovaccinate.pdf

    Risk communication videos: https://www.aap.org/en-us/advocacy-and-policy/aap-health-initiatives/immunization/Pages/vaccine-hesitant-parents.aspx#Video

    Navigating Vaccine Hesitancy: https://www.aap.org/en-us/Documents/immunization_hesitancy.pdf (will be available soon)

Education

    Pedialink modules: https://pedialink.aap.org/visitor

        Adolescent Immunizations: Strongly Recommending the HPV Vaccine: http://shop.aap.org/Adolescent-Immunizations-Strongly-Recommending-the-HPV-Vaccine

        Challenging Cases: Vaccine Hesitancy: http://bit.ly/cc-vaccinehesitancy. This module is the educational component of the clinical report.

    AAP Immunization Web site: https://www.aap.org/en-us/advocacy-and-policy/aap-health-initiatives/immunization/Pages/default.aspx

    (The following are some of the specific pages within the above site)

        Parental Refusal Resource Page: https://www.aap.org/en-us/advocacy-and-policy/aap-health-initiatives/immunization/Pages/refusal-to-vaccinate.aspx

        Vaccine-Hesitant Parents: https://www.aap.org/en-us/advocacy-and-policy/aap-health-initiatives/immunization/Pages/vaccine-hesitant-parents.aspx

        Information for families: https://www.healthychildren.org/english/safety-prevention/immunizations/pages/default.aspx

        Common Parental Concerns: https://www.aap.org/en-us/advocacy-and-policy/aap-health-initiatives/immunization/Pages/Common-Parental-Concerns.aspx

    HealthyChildren.org (for parents): http://www.healthychildren.org/English/safety-prevention/Pages/default.aspx (same as above)

    CDC/AAP Provider Resources for Vaccine Conversations With Parents: http://www.cdc.gov/vaccines/hcp/patient-ed/conversations/index.html

    Immunization Action Coalition: http://www.immunize.org/

    Children's Hospital of Philadelphia: http://www.chop.edu/service/vaccine-education-center/home.html

    National Foundation for Infectious Diseases: http://www.nfid.org/

    Families Fighting flu: www.familiesfightingflu.org

    Vaccine Resource library: www.path.org/vaccineresources

    Every Child by Two: www.ecbt.org

    Parents of Kids With Infectious Diseases: www.pkids.org

Policy

    Responding to Parental Refusals of Immunization of Children: http://pediatrics.aappublications.org/content/115/5/1428.full

    Medical Versus Nonmedical Immunization Exemptions for Child Care and School Attendance: http://www.pediatrics.org/cgi/doi/10.1542/peds.2016.2146

    2016 Immunization Schedules: http://www2.aap.org/immunization/IZSchedule.html

    COID Policy Collection page: http://pediatrics.aappublications.org/cgi/collection/committee_on_infectious_diseases

    Red Book

        Discussing Vaccines With Patients and Parents

            Discussing Vaccines With Patients and Parents (pp. 7–9)

            Addressing Parents' Questions About Vaccine Safety and Effectiveness (p. 9)

            Common Misconceptions About Immunizations and the Institute of Medicine Findings (pp. 10–11)

            Resources for Optimizing Communications With Parents About Vaccines (p. 12)

            Parental Refusal of Immunizations (pp. 12–13)

    Assessing the State of Vaccine Confidence in the United States: Recommendations From the National Vaccine Advisory Committee: http://www.hhs.gov/sites/default/files/nvpo/nvac/reports/nvac-vaccine-confidence-public-health-report-2015.pdf

Journal articles

    Childhood Immunization: When Physicians and Parents Disagree: http://pediatrics.aappublications.org/content/128/Supplement_4/S167.full

    Safety of Vaccines Used for Routine Immunization of US Children: A Systematic Review: http://pediatrics.aappublications.org/content/early/2014/06/26/peds.2014-1079.full.pdf+html

    Commentary in *Pediatrics*: Vaccines: Can Transparency Increase Confidence and Reduce Hesitancy? http://pediatrics.aappublications.org/content/early/2014/06/26/peds.2014-1494.full.pdf+html

    Children whose parents refused vitamin K at birth are 14.6 times more likely to be unimmunized by age 15 mo. This provides an opportunity to identify a subset of likely vaccine-hesitant parents at birth and engage them with targeted information.

        News release: http://www.aap.org/en-us/about-the-aap/aap-press-room/Pages/Parents-Who-Refuse-Vitamin-K-for-Newborn-Also-More-Likely-to-Refuse-Vaccines.aspx

        Study: http://pediatrics.aappublications.org/content/early/2014/08/12/peds.2014-1092

    A survey found that parents who were informed about the MMR vaccine's direct benefits to their child, rather than the vaccine's benefits to society as a whole, were more likely to immunize.

        News release: http://www.aap.org/en-us/about-the-aap/aap-press-room/Pages/Emphasizing-MMR-Vaccine%27s-Benefits-for-Children-Increases-Parents%27-Intent-to-Immunize.aspx

        Study: http://pediatrics.aappublications.org/content/early/2014/08/12/peds.2013-4077

        MedScape story: http://www.medscape.com/viewarticle/830062?src=rss

    A pertussis epidemic in Washington State did not increase parents' intent to vaccinate their children.

        Study: http://pediatrics.aappublications.org/content/early/2014/08/12/peds.2013-3637.full.pdf+html

        Commentary: http://pediatrics.aappublications.org/content/early/2014/08/12/peds.2014-1883.full.pdf+html

        HealthDay story: http://health.usnews.com/health-news/articles/2014/08/18/doctors-id-new-ways-to-get-more-kids-vaccinated

Research

    Periodic Survey #66 (2006): Vaccine Refusals: http://www.aap.org/en-us/professional-resources/Research/Pages/PS66_Executive_Summary_PediatriciansAttitudesandPracticesSurroundingtheDeliveryofImmunizationsPart2.aspx

    Periodic Survey #84(2013) Vaccine Delays/Refusals and Risk–Benefit Information Abstracts

        Vaccine Refusals and Requests for Alternate Vaccine Schedules (AVS): National Surveys of Pediatricians Pediatric Academic Societies (PAS) May 2014

TABLE 5 Continued

Images

Red Book Online Visual Library: http://aapredbook.aappublications.org/site/visual

Photos, videos, and family stories regarding vaccine-preventable diseases: http://www2.aap.org/immunization/illnesses/illnesses.html

---

vaccine before and after licensure, remind the parents of the severity of the diseases being prevented, address the questions that are causing parental concerns and, most importantly, emphasize that infants and children are the ones at greatest risk of disease. The on-time administration of vaccines is the most effective way to prevent what have in the past been severe and often fatal childhood illnesses. Delaying any vaccine past the recommended administration date greatly increases the period of time that a child remains susceptible to disease and also exposes even vaccinated children to additional risk.[35,78]

Countering vaccine hesitancy can best be accomplished in the course of clinical practice through open communication and discussion between the pediatrician and the parents. Because most parents agree to vaccinate their children, this dialogue, which can be started as early as the prenatal interview visit[79] if possible, should be an ongoing process. Continued research is needed on the best methods to communicate the safety and effectiveness of vaccines. Providing vaccine-related information before the first immunization visit may permit parents to clearly formulate their concerns so that they can be fully addressed by the pediatrician. Most parents need and want education about the best way to provide care for their children, including vaccinations. Dealing with vaccine hesitancy is a wonderful opportunity to continue to provide this information and education to families.

LEAD AUTHORS

Kathryn M. Edwards, MD, FAAP

Jesse M. Hackell, MD, FAAP

COMMITTEE ON INFECTIOUS DISEASES, 2015–2016

Carrie L. Byington, MD, FAAP, Chairperson

Yvonne A. Maldonado, MD, FAAP, Vice Chairperson

Elizabeth D. Barnett MD, FAAP

H. Dele Davies, MD, MS, MHCM, FAAP

Kathryn M. Edwards, MD, FAAP

Ruth Lynfield, MD, FAAP

Flor M. Munoz, MD, FAAP

Dawn Nolt, MD, MPH

Ann-Christine Nyquist, MD, MSPH, FAAP

Mobeen H. Rathore, MD, FAAP

Mark H. Sawyer, MD, FAAP

William J. Steinbach, MD, FAAP

Tina Q. Tan, MD, FAAP

Theoklis E. Zaoutis, MD, MSCE, FAAP

FORMER COMMITTEE MEMBERS

Dennis L. Murray, MD, FAAP

Gordon E. Schutze, MD, FAAP

Rodney E. Willoughby Jr, MD, FAAP

EX OFFICIO

Henry H. Bernstein, DO, MHCM, FAAP – Red Book Online Associate Editor

Michael T. Brady, MD, FAAP, Red Book Associate Editor

Mary Anne Jackson, MD, FAAP, Red Book Associate Editor

David W. Kimberlin, MD, FAAP – Red Book Editor

Sarah S. Long, MD, FAAP – Red Book Associate Editor

H. Cody Meissner, MD, FAAP – Visual Red Book Associate Editor

CONTRIBUTOR

Annabelle de St Maurice, MD, FAAP – Vanderbilt University

LIAISONS

Douglas Campos-Outcalt, MD, MPA – American Academy of Family Physicians

Amanda C. Cohn, MD, FAAP – Centers for Disease Control and Prevention

Jamie Deseda-Tous, MD – Sociedad Latinoamericana de Infectologia Pediatrica (SLIPE)

Karen M. Farizo, MD – US Food and Drug Administration

Marc Fischer, MD, FAAP – Centers for Disease Control and Prevention

Bruce G. Gellin, MD, MPH – National Vaccine Program Office

Richard L. Gorman, MD, FAAP – National Institutes of Health

Natasha Halasa, MD, MPH, FAAP – Pediatric Infectious Diseases Society

Joan L. Robinson, MD – Canadian Paediatric Society

Geoffrey R. Simon, MD, FAAP – Committee on Practice Ambulatory Medicine

Jeffrey R. Starke, MD, FAAP – American Thoracic Society

STAFF

Jennifer M. Frantz, MPH

COMMITTEE ON PRACTICE AND AMBULATORY CARE, 2015–2016

Geoffrey R. Simon, MD, FAAP – Chair

Cynthia N. Baker, MD, FAAP

Graham A. Barden III, MD, FAAP

Oscar "Skip" W. Brown III, MD, FAAP

Jesse M. Hackell, MD, FAAP

Amy P. Hardin, MD, FAAP

Kelley E. Meade, MD, FAAP

Scot B. Moore, MD, FAAP

Julia E. Richerson, MD, FAAP

STAFF

Elizabeth Sobczyk, MPH, MSW

The AAP acknowledges the significant contributions of Annabelle de St Maurice MD, FAAP – Vanderbilt University.

ABBREVIATIONS

AAP: American Academy of Pediatrics

CDC: Centers for Disease Control and Prevention

FDA: US Food and Drug Administration

HPV: human papillomavirus

MMR: measles–mumps–rubella

VAERS: Vaccine Adverse Events Reporting System

VIS: Vaccine Information Statement

VSD: Vaccine Safety Datalink

REFERENCES

1. Larson HJ, Jarrett C, Eckersberger E, Smith DM, Paterson P. Understanding vaccine hesitancy around vaccines and vaccination from a global perspective: a systematic review of published literature, 2007–2012. Vaccine. 2014;32(19):2150–2159

2. Dempsey AF, Schaffer S, Singer D, Butchart A, Davis M, Freed GL. Alternative vaccination schedule preferences among parents of young children. *Pediatrics*. 2011;128(5):848–856

3. Robison SG, Groom H, Young C. Frequency of alternative immunization schedule use in a metropolitan area. *Pediatrics*. 2012;130(1):32–38

4. Gust DA, Darling N, Kennedy A, Schwartz B. Parents with doubts about vaccines: which vaccines and reasons why. *Pediatrics*. 2008;122(4):718–725

5. McCauley MM, Kennedy A, Basket M, Sheedy K. Exploring the choice to refuse or delay vaccines: a national survey of parents of 6- through 23-month-olds. *Acad Pediatr*. 2012;12(5):375–383

6. Omer SB, Salmon DA, Orenstein WA, deHart MP, Halsey N. Vaccine refusal, mandatory immunization, and the risks of vaccine-preventable diseases. *N Engl J Med*. 2009;360(19):1981–1988

7. American Academy of Pediatrics; Committee on Community Health Services. Periodic Survey #66: Pediatricians' Attitudes and Practices Surrounding the Delivery of Immunizations. 2006. Available at: https://www.aap.org/en-us/professional-resources/Research/Pages/PS66_Executive_Summary_PediatriciansAttitudesandPracticesSurroundingtheDeliveryofImmunizationsPart2.aspx?nfstatus=401&nftoken=00000000-0000-0000-0000-000000000000&nfstatusdescription=ERROR:+No+local+token. Accessed July 25, 2016

8. Hough-Telford C, Kimberlin DW, Aban I, et al. Vaccine delays, refusals, and patient dismissals: a survey of pediatricians. *Pediatrics*. 2016;138(3):e20162127

9. Opel DJ, Heritage J, Taylor JA, et al. The architecture of provider–parent vaccine discussions at health supervision visits. *Pediatrics*. 2013;132(6):1037–1046

10. Kempe A, O'Leary ST, Kennedy A, et al. Physician response to parental requests to spread out the recommended vaccine schedule. *Pediatrics*. 2015;135(4):666–677

11. World Health Organization. Immunization, Vaccines and Biologicals. SAGE Working Group Dealing With Vaccine Hesitancy. 2012. Available at: www.who.int/immunization/sage/sage_wg_vaccine_hesitancy_apr12/en/. Accessed October 6, 2014

12. Leask J, Kinnersley P, Jackson C, Cheater F, Bedford H, Rowles G. Communicating with parents about vaccination: a framework for health professionals. *BMC Pediatr*. 2012;12:154

13. Kahan DM. Vaccine Risk Perceptions and Ad Hoc Risk Communication: An Empirical Assessment. CCP Risk Perception Studies Report No. 17 Yale Law & Economics Research Paper No. 491. Available at: http://papers.ssrn.com/sol3/papers.cfm?abstract_id=2386034. Accessed July 25, 2016

14. Gust D, Brown C, Sheedy K, Hibbs B, Weaver D, Nowak G. Immunization attitudes and beliefs among parents: beyond a dichotomous perspective. *Am J Health Behav*. 2005;29(1):81–92

15. Smith PJ, Humiston SG, Marcuse EK, et al. Parental delay or refusal of vaccine doses, childhood vaccination coverage at 24 months of age, and the Health Belief Model. *Public Health Rep*. 2011;126(suppl 2):135–146

16. Diekema DS; American Academy of Pediatrics Committee on Bioethics. Responding to parental refusals of immunization of children. *Pediatrics*. 2005;115(5):1428–1431

17. Reaffirmation: responding to parents who refuse immunization for their children. *Pediatrics*. 2013;131(5). Available at: www.pediatrics.org/cgi/content/full/131/5/e1696

18. Diekema DS. Improving childhood vaccination rates. *N Engl J Med*. 2012;366(5):391–393

19. Chen RT, Rastogi SC, Mullen JR, et al. The Vaccine Adverse Event Reporting System (VAERS). *Vaccine*. 1994;12(6):542–550

20. Iskander JK, Miller ER, Chen RT. The role of the Vaccine Adverse Event Reporting system (VAERS) in monitoring vaccine safety. *Pediatr Ann*. 2004;33(9):599–606

21. McNeil MM, Gee J, Weintraub ES, et al. The Vaccine Safety Datalink: successes and challenges monitoring vaccine safety. *Vaccine*. 2014;32(42):5390–5398

22. Centers for Disease Control and Prevention (CDC). Update: Guillain–Barré syndrome among recipients of Menactra meningococcal conjugate vaccine--United States, October 2005–February 2006. *MMWR Morb Mortal Wkly Rep*. 2006;55(13):364–366

23. Baker MA, Nguyen M, Cole DV, Lee GM, Lieu TA. Post-licensure Rapid Immunization Safety Monitoring program (PRISM) data characterization. *Vaccine*. 2013;31(suppl 10):K98–K112

24. Williams SE, Klein NP, Halsey N, et al. Overview of the clinical consult case review of adverse events following immunization: Clinical Immunization Safety Assessment (CISA) network 2004–2009. *Vaccine*. 2011;29(40):6920–6927

25. Wolfe RM, Sharp LK. Anti-vaccinationists past and present. *BMJ*. 2002;325(7361):430–432

26. May T, Silverman RD. "Clustering of exemptions" as a collective action threat to herd immunity. *Vaccine*. 2003;21(11–12):1048–1051

27. Fine PEM, Mulholland K. Community immunity. In: Plotkin SA, Orenstein WA, Offit PA, eds. *Vaccine*, 6th ed. Philadelphia, PA: Saunders; 2013:1395–1412

28. Omer SB, Richards JL, Ward M, Bednarczyk RA. Vaccination policies and rates of exemption from immunization, 2005–2011. *N Engl J Med*. 2012;367(12):1170–1171

29. Safi H, Wheeler JG, Reeve GR, et al. Vaccine policy and Arkansas childhood immunization exemptions: a multi-year review. *Am J Prev Med*. 2012;42(6):602–605

30. Smith PJ, Chu SY, Barker LE. Children who have received no vaccines: who are they and where do they live? *Pediatrics*. 2004;114(1):187–195

31. Wei F, Mullooly JP, Goodman M, et al. Identification and characteristics of vaccine refusers. *BMC Pediatr*. 2009;9:18

32. Wang E, Clymer J, Davis-Hayes C, Buttenheim A. Nonmedical

exemptions from school immunization requirements: a systematic review. *Am J Public Health.* 2014;104(11):e62–e84

33. Feikin DR, Lezotte DC, Hamman RF, Salmon DA, Chen RT, Hoffman RE. Individual and community risks of measles and pertussis associated with personal exemptions to immunization. *JAMA.* 2000;284(24):3145–3150

34. Carrel M, Bitterman P. Personal belief exemptions to vaccination in California: a spatial analysis. *Pediatrics.* 2015;136(1):80–88

35. Phadke VKBR, Bednarczyk RA, Salmon DA, Omer SB. Association between vaccine refusal and vaccine-preventable diseases in the United States: a review of measles and pertussis. *JAMA.* 2016;315(11):1149–1158

36. Seither R, Masalovich S, Knighton CL, Mellerson J, Singleton JA, Greby SM; Centers for Disease Control and Prevention (CDC). Vaccination coverage among children in kindergarten: United States, 2013–14 school year. *MMWR Morb Mortal Wkly Rep.* 2014;63(41):913–920

37. Clemmons NS, Gastanaduy PA, Fiebelkorn AP, Redd SB, Wallace GS; Centers for Disease Control and Prevention (CDC). Measles: United States, January 4–April 2, 2015. *MMWR Morb Mortal Wkly Rep.* 2015;64(14):373–376

38. Wightman A, Opel DJ, Marcuse EK, Taylor JA. Washington State pediatricians' attitudes toward alternative childhood immunization schedules. *Pediatrics.* 2011;128(6):1094–1099

39. Yang YT, Silverman RD. Legislative prescriptions for controlling nonmedical vaccine exemptions. *JAMA.* 2015;313(3):247–248

40. Gostin LO. Law, ethics, and public health in the vaccination debates: politics of the measles outbreak. *JAMA.* 2015;313(11):1099–1100

41. Diekema DS. Provider dismissal of vaccine-hesitant families: misguided policy that fails to benefit children. *Hum Vaccin Immunother.* 2013;9(12):2661–2662

42. Wolf ER, Rowhani-Rahbar A, Opel DJ. The impact of epidemics of vaccine-preventable disease on vaccine uptake: lessons from the 2011–2012 US pertussis epidemic. *Expert Rev Vaccines.* 2015;14(7):923–933

43. Freed GL, Clark SJ, Butchart AT, Singer DC, Davis MM. Parental vaccine safety concerns in 2009. *Pediatrics.* 2010;125(4):654–659

44. Dube E, Vivion M, Sauvageau C, Gagneur A, Gagnon R, Guay M. "Nature does things well, why should we interfere?": vaccine hesitancy among mothers. *Qual Health Res.* 2015;26(3):411–425

45. Kennedy A, Basket M, Sheedy K. Vaccine attitudes, concerns, and information sources reported by parents of young children: results from the 2009 HealthStyles survey. *Pediatrics.* 2011;127(suppl 1):S92–S99

46. Kennedy AM, Brown CJ, Gust DA. Vaccine beliefs of parents who oppose compulsory vaccination. *Public Health Rep.* 2005;120(3):252–258

47. Salmon DA, Moulton LH, Omer SB, DeHart MP, Stokley S, Halsey NA. Factors associated with refusal of childhood vaccines among parents of school-aged children: a case–control study. *Arch Pediatr Adolesc Med.* 2005;159(5):470–476

48. Wenger OK, McManus MD, Bower JR, Langkamp DL. Underimmunization in Ohio's Amish: parental fears are a greater obstacle than access to care. *Pediatrics.* 2011;128(1):79–85

49. Darden PM, Thompson DM, Roberts JR, et al. Reasons for not vaccinating adolescents: National Immunization Survey of Teens, 2008–2010. *Pediatrics.* 2013;131(4):645–651

50. Bednarczyk RA, Davis R, Ault K, Orenstein W, Omer SB. Sexual activity–related outcomes after human papillomavirus vaccination of 11- to 12-year-olds. *Pediatrics.* 2012;130(5):798–805

51. Taddio A, Appleton M, Bortolussi R, et al Reducing the pain of childhood vaccination: an evidence-based clinical practice guideline (summary). *CMAJ.* 2010;182(18):1989–1995

52. Reis EC, Roth EK, Syphan JL, Tarbell SE, Holubkov R. Effective pain reduction for multiple immunization injections in young infants. *Arch Pediatr Adolesc Med.* 2003;157(11):1115–1120

53. Grabenstein JD. What the world's religions teach, applied to vaccines and immune globulins. *Vaccine.* 2013;31(16):2011–2023

54. Offit PA, Quarles J, Gerber MA, et al. Addressing parents' concerns: do multiple vaccines overwhelm or weaken the infant's immune system? *Pediatrics.* 2002;109(1):124–129

55. Nyhan B, Reifler J, Richey S, Freed GL. Effective messages in vaccine promotion: a randomized trial. *Pediatrics.* 2014;133(4). Available at: www.pediatrics.org/cgi/content/full/133/4/e835

56. Kempe A, Daley MF, McCauley MM, et al. Prevalence of parental concerns about childhood vaccines: the experience of primary care physicians. *Am J Prev Med.* 2011;40(5):548–555

57. Offit PA, Moser CA. The problem with Dr Bob's alternative vaccine schedule. *Pediatrics.* 2009;123(1). Available at: www.pediatrics.org/cgi/content/full/123/1/e164

58. Taylor JA, Darden PM, Slora E, Hasemeier CM, Asmussen L, Wasserman R. The influence of provider behavior, parental characteristics, and a public policy initiative on the immunization status of children followed by private pediatricians: a study from Pediatric Research in Office Settings. *Pediatrics.* 1997;99(2):209–215

59. Smith PJ, Kennedy AM, Wooten K, Gust DA, Pickering LK. Association between health care providers' influence on parents who have concerns about vaccine safety and vaccination coverage. *Pediatrics.* 2006;118(5). Available at: www.pediatrics.org/cgi/content/full/118/5/e1287

60. The Childhood Immunization Schedule and Safety. *Stakeholder Concerns, Scientific Evidence and Future Studies.* Washington, DC: Institute of Medicine of the National Academies; 2013

61. Maglione MA, Das L, Raaen L, et al. Safety of vaccines used for routine immunization of U.S. children: a systematic review. *Pediatrics.* 2014;134(2):325–337

62. Byington CL. Vaccines: can transparency increase confidence and reduce hesitancy? *Pediatrics.* 2014;134(2):377–379

63. Healy CM, Pickering LK. How to communicate with vaccine-hesitant parents. *Pediatrics*. 2011;127(suppl 1):S127–S133

64. Healy CM, Montesinos DP, Middleman AB. Parent and provider perspectives on immunization: are providers overestimating parental concerns? *Vaccine*. 2014;32(5):579–584

65. Vannice KS, Salmon DA, Shui I, et al. Attitudes and beliefs of parents concerned about vaccines: impact of timing of immunization information. *Pediatrics*. 2011;127(suppl 1):S120–S126

66. Mergler MJ, Omer SB, Pan WK, et al. Are recent medical graduates more skeptical of vaccines? *Vaccines (Basel)*. 2013;1(2):154–166

67. Williams SE, Swan R. Formal training in vaccine safety to address parental concerns not routinely conducted in US pediatric residency programs. *Vaccine*. 2014;32(26):3175–3178

68. Henrikson NB, Opel DJ, Grothaus L, et al. Physician communication training and parental vaccine hesitancy: a randomized trial. *Pediatrics*. 2015;136(1):70–79

69. Benin AL, Wisler-Scher DJ, Colson E, Shapiro ED, Holmboe ES. Qualitative analysis of mothers' decision-making about vaccines for infants: the importance of trust. *Pediatrics*. 2006;117(5):1532–1541

70. Block SL. The pediatrician's dilemma: refusing the refusers of infant vaccines. *J Law Med Ethics*. 2015;43(3):648–653

71. Halperin B, Melnychuk R, Downie J, Macdonald N. When is it permissible to dismiss a family who refuses vaccines? Legal, ethical and public health perspectives. *Paediatr Child Health*. 2007;12(10):843–845

72. Chervenak FA, McCullough LB, Brent RL. Professional responsibility and early childhood vaccination. *J Pediatr*. 2016;169(2):305–309

73. Diekema DS. Physician dismissal of families who refuse vaccination: an ethical assessment. *J Law Med Ethics*. 2015;43(3):654–660

74. Lippman H, Davenport J. Patient dismissal: the right way to do it. *J Fam Pract*. 2011;60(3):135–140

75. American Academy of Pediatrics. *Medicolegal Issues in Pediatrics*. 7th ed. Elk Grove Village, IL: American Academy of Pediatrics; 2012:58–59

76. Salathé M, Khandelwal S. Assessing vaccination sentiments with online social media: implications for infectious disease dynamics and control. *PLOS Comput Biol*. 2011;7(10):e1002199

77. Sadaf A, Richards JL, Glanz J, Salmon DA, Omer SB. A systematic review of interventions for reducing parental vaccine refusal and vaccine hesitancy. *Vaccine*. 2013;31(40):4293–4304

78. Luman ET, Barker LE, Shaw KM, McCauley MM, Buehler JW, Pickering LK. Timeliness of childhood vaccinations in the United States: days undervaccinated and number of vaccines delayed. *JAMA*. 2005;293(10):1204–1211

79. Cohen GJ; Committee on Psychosocial Aspects of Child and Family Health. The prenatal visit. *Pediatrics*. 2009;124(4):1227–1232

Disclosure of Adverse Events in Pediatrics

· ·

- *Policy Statement*

629

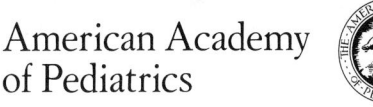

POLICY STATEMENT Organizational Principles to Guide and Define the Child Health
Care System and/or Improve the Health of all Children

DEDICATED TO THE HEALTH OF ALL CHILDREN™

Disclosure of Adverse Events in Pediatrics

COMMITTEE ON MEDICAL LIABILITY AND RISK MANAGEMENT, COUNCIL ON QUALITY IMPROVEMENT AND PATIENT SAFETY

abstract

Despite increasing attention to issues of patient safety, preventable adverse events (AEs) continue to occur, causing direct and consequential injuries to patients, families, and health care providers. Pediatricians generally agree that there is an ethical obligation to inform patients and families about preventable AEs and medical errors. Nonetheless, barriers, such as fear of liability, interfere with disclosure regarding preventable AEs. Changes to the legal system, improved communications skills, and carefully developed disclosure policies and programs can improve the quality and frequency of appropriate AE disclosure communications.

INTRODUCTION

Patient safety has been characterized as 1 of the 6 domains of health care quality by the Institute of Medicine (IOM),[1] which attributed 44 000 to 98 000 inpatient deaths annually to medical errors (MEs) in the United States.[2] The American Academy of Pediatrics has called attention to the importance of pediatric patient safety since 2001[3] and recommended improved identification and reporting of MEs and adverse events (AEs) to improve the culture of safety in pediatric care.[4]

The IOM defines "patient safety" as the prevention of patient harm and freedom from accidental injury in the health care setting.[5] An AE occurs when patient harm is caused by medical care.[2] A ME is an act of commission or omission that unreasonably increases risk of an undesirable patient outcome. AEs may be determined to be preventable (when patient harm is related to a ME) or nonpreventable (when patient harm occurs in the absence of ME). An ME that causes patient harm becomes a preventable AE. An ME that has the potential to cause patient harm but does not do so is referred to as a potential AE or near miss. These concepts and their relationships are illustrated in Fig 1.

The magnitude of harm to patients from AEs can be estimated but has not been quantified reliably. One investigation reported 12.91 AEs per 1000 hospital discharges among patients from birth through 15 years of age,

Policy statements from the American Academy of Pediatrics benefit from expertise and resources of liaisons and internal (AAP) and external reviewers. However, policy statements from the American Academy of Pediatrics may not reflect the views of the liaisons or the organizations or government agencies that they represent.

The guidance in this statement does not indicate an exclusive course of treatment or serve as a standard of medical care. Variations, taking into account individual circumstances, may be appropriate.

All policy statements from the American Academy of Pediatrics automatically expire 5 years after publication unless reaffirmed, revised, or retired at or before that time.

DOI: 10.1542/peds.2016-3215

Accepted for publication Sep 26, 2016

PEDIATRICS (ISSN Numbers: Print, 0031-4005; Online, 1098-4275).

Copyright © 2016 by the American Academy of Pediatrics

FINANCIAL DISCLOSURE: The authors have indicated they do not have a financial relationship relevant to this article to disclose.

FUNDING: No external funding.

POTENTIAL CONFLICT OF INTEREST: The authors have indicated they have no potential conflicts of interest to disclose.

To cite: AAP COMMITTEE ON MEDICAL LIABILITY AND RISK MANAGEMENT and AAP COUNCIL ON QUALITY IMPROVEMENT AND PATIENT SAFETY. Disclosure of Adverse Events in Pediatrics. Pediatrics. 2016;138(6):e20163215

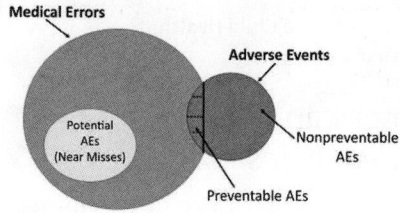

FIGURE 1
AEs and MEs.

with "negligence" identified in 28% of events.[6] In a study of 3700 pediatric hospitalizations, 1% of patients experienced AEs, and 60% of these were determined to be preventable.[7] Among Canadian inpatient pediatric AEs, the overall rate was 9.2%, and those related to surgery were most frequent.[8] Almost half of the AEs in this study were determined to be preventable. A prospective study at 6 pediatric practices found that 3% of patients had preventable adverse drug events.[9] There have been wide variations in estimates of the incidence of AEs in the pediatric inpatient setting and even more uncertainty about the rates of MEs and AEs in the outpatient setting, where most pediatric care occurs.[4,10] What is clear is that pediatric AEs are frequent occurrences, with significant patient morbidity and mortality. The economic cost of AEs was estimated at between $393 and $958 billion in 2006, at which time these amounts were equal to 18% to 45% of total US health care spending.[11] Specific costs for the subset of cases involving children have not been quantified.

AEs not only affect patients and their families but also may have devastating effects on health care providers, who may suffer emotional consequences both from preventable AEs and from subsequent malpractice litigation.[12] Affected clinicians may feel guilt, shame, and isolation, and these feelings may be exacerbated by negative reactions from their colleagues.[13-16] Anticipated or actual punitive consequences can add additional emotional and financial burdens on providers.[17]

The concepts of reporting and disclosure of AEs should be distinguished. "Reporting" refers to the exchange of information among providers and regulators. Reporting systems may be internal to health care organizations or may be required by licensing boards and governmental agencies. These systems may be voluntary or mandatory, and some organizations may use automated AE reporting (eg, bar-code systems and computerized provider order entry). Although in the past, many AE reporting systems focused on punitive consequences, such an approach has been found to deter further reporting. Thus, the current trend has been to reward the reporting of AEs with positive feedback and to use existing reports to develop systematic remedies to promote a safer patient care environment. "Disclosure," in contrast, is communication directed from health care personnel to the affected patient and/or family about an AE. Disclosure is a description of what is known and does not include speculation about causation or individuals' motivations or assumptions about judgment or fault.

The IOM noted that most MEs are attributable to flaws in systems rather than individuals and called for a "dramatic improvement in the reliability and safety" of the health care process.[2] For this improvement to occur, AEs must first be identified and given attention to understand their preventable causes and to allow for systematic safety improvements. Disclosure and open communication with patients and their families after an AE may provide benefit to the patient and to the health care provider, reduce consequential harms, allow for better follow-up, and promote a safety culture. Additionally, patients and caregivers most often desire complete disclosure of AEs and may be less likely to pursue litigation against their health care providers

if complete disclosure is done.[18] Conversely, lack of communication may make patients feel worse and may erode the sense of trust in their caregivers that is key to healing and to optimal health care.[18] The health care provider's self-perception and self-confidence may deteriorate when health care outcomes are poor.[15,16] Full and open communication may alleviate the provider's feelings of anxiety, disgrace, and guilt.[19] However, those feelings may also persist and may even be an obstacle to full disclosure. Pediatric clinicians and institutions should be alert to the involved provider becoming a "second victim" of an ME.[17]

ETHICAL CONSIDERATIONS IN DISCLOSURE

In addition to the quality-control and systems-improvement benefits of disclosure, physicians broadly acknowledge that disclosure of AEs is an ethical obligation.[20-23] Although there is evidence that they often do not "practice what they preach,"[13,18,24-27] physicians and medical trainees, in particular, agree that physicians have an ethical obligation to their patients to disclose preventable AEs.[21,26-28] In an anonymous survey among pediatric residents and attending pediatricians, pediatricians in private practice were less likely to report errors than other attending pediatricians (72% vs 92%; P < .001).[25] Most agreed that disclosing a serious error would be difficult (overall, 88%; attending pediatricians, 86%; residents, 96%; P = .005). More residents than attending pediatricians had received education about how to disclose errors (57% vs 29%; P < .001).

BARRIERS TO DISCLOSURE

Despite the compelling benefits and ethical imperatives for AE disclosure, many physicians nevertheless continue to have difficulty completing the task of informing patients and their families about AEs and MEs.[13,21,25,29] Several barriers can create obstacles to disclosure, including perceived legal risks and the cautionary advice of legal counsel, concerns that disclosure might harm patients, a lack of confidence in disclosure skills, and a fear of embarrassment.[14,25,30–32] Language and cultural differences may also interfere with meaningful communication about AEs.[14] Among these barriers, perceived legal risks and legal advice cautioning against disclosure may be the most significant.[27,32]

LEGAL RISKS ASSOCIATED WITH DISCLOSURE AND APOLOGY

Historically, lawyers advised their physician-clients not to disclose MEs and did so with sound legal justification.[33–36] In the US legal system, previous statements by an observer of an event generally are not permitted to be introduced in court as evidence about that event.[37] In other words, a courtroom witness can testify about what he knows from his own observation but not about what someone else told him about the event. This "hearsay rule" presumes that bringing a witness into the courtroom to discuss what he actually knows from firsthand experience is more informative and more reliable than having someone else recount what another observer, on some previous occasion, said that she had seen.[37] However, the law recognizes the possibility that a witness might be less likely to fully and truthfully describe his observations when that witness has become the defendant in the lawsuit. Moreover, that defendant-witness might recant truthful statements that he might have previously made about the event. Therefore, a well-established exception to the hearsay rule permits previous, self-incriminating statements by defendants to be admitted into evidence, even though those

statements are hearsay.[38] This "admission of a party-opponent" exception has been used by plaintiffs in numerous cases to quote a defendant-physician's earlier admission of fault to help prove that the physician-defendant committed malpractice.[36]

The concept of "apology" generates similar legal concerns but may be even more problematic because of variations in definition. "Apology" is defined by *Webster's Dictionary* as "a statement that you are sorry about something" or "an expression of regret for having done or said something wrong."[39] This definition does not include any acknowledgment of fault. Alternatively, "apology" may be defined as "an admission of error or discourtesy accompanied by an expression of regret." This lack of clarity in what it means "to apologize" can result in plaintiffs asserting in court that a physician-defendant "admitted" to fault, when the physician-defendant had no intention of admitting fault in the course of the apology.[40]

Some lawmakers have attempted to encourage physician disclosure and apology by reducing this legal risk through legislative changes to the hearsay rule exceptions.[30,33,41] Many state legislatures have attempted to encourage disclosures and apologies by adopting "apology laws," intended to encourage physician-patient communications about AEs by limiting, or even completely excluding, plaintiffs' ability to use such communications as evidence against the physician in later litigation.[30,41] "Sympathy-only" apology laws bar the use of physician expressions of sympathy by plaintiffs at trial to prove negligence but do permit plaintiffs to use physician statements that expressly admitted fault.[30] On the other hand, "admission of fault" apology laws prevent plaintiffs from using virtually any previous physician disclosures to the

patient and family, even when the physician admitted responsibility for an ME or other improper care, to prove negligence at trial.[30],*

The effects of these apology laws in reducing liability risks remain unclear. Nevertheless, there is some evidence that they may be effective in reducing liability risks. For example, in *Deitsch v INOVA Health Care Services*, the plaintiff alleged that the defendant cardiologist was negligent in failing to personally evaluate a tachycardic patient in the emergency department.[42] The cardiologist subsequently met with the family in the ICU and reportedly stated, "I am sorry I wasn't there."[42] The Circuit Court of Virginia prohibited the plaintiffs from using this statement at trial, declaring that this "expression of sympathy and benevolence" was precisely the type of communication that the Virginia apology law was enacted to protect.[42] Similarly, in *Airasian v Shaak*, the Georgia Court of Appeals prohibited the plaintiffs from using as evidence the defendant surgeon's postoperative statement to the patient's wife that "this [need for a second, emergency surgery] was my fault."[43]

The *Deitsch* and *Airasian* cases demonstrate how apology laws can protect physician disclosures about AEs, thus encouraging other physicians to communicate with patients and potentially preserving physician-patient relationships, improving patient and family satisfaction, and helping to identify systems weaknesses leading to AEs. However, some apology laws, particularly sympathy-only apology laws, may not provide protection and reassurance sufficient to encourage disclosure.[33,36] Mastroianni et al opined that "sympathy-only" apology laws have a fatal structural weakness in that they do not protect the key

---

*For information on current state apology laws, please contact the AAP Division of State Government Affairs at 800/433-9016, extension 7799, or at stgov@aap.org.

information that patients want communicated to them after an AE.[33] These authors observed that patients (and families) want full and clear explanations and accountability for adverse outcomes. Mere expressions of sympathy, in the absence of full disclosure and accountability, may be unsatisfactory to patients and may fail to bring about systems improvements that might prevent future adverse outcomes.[13]

There is evidence that disclosure, even in the absence of protective apology laws, may reduce liability risks and litigation costs.[44,45] Nevertheless, some researchers have suggested a theoretical risk that the sheer volume of patients who could be put on notice of MEs by full disclosure policies might result in a greater volume of lawsuits.[46]

FACILITATING BETTER DISCLOSURE

In the event of a preventable AE, the pediatrician's first responsibility is to attend to the immediate medical needs of the patient. Thereafter, improved physician-patient communication may contribute to enhanced patient satisfaction, better ongoing medical care for the patient, and prevention of future AEs. Moreover, full disclosure about such events is ethically indicated. Therefore, pediatricians should endeavor to provide appropriate disclosure when their patients experience preventable AEs. Pediatricians can help facilitate such disclosures in at least 2 ways: developing and implementing disclosure policies and procedures for their own practices, and supporting public policies that facilitate disclosure.

Unfortunately, preventable AEs are often the result of a cascade of errors rather than a single mistake.[47] Gaining a clear understanding of whether an ME occurred, how it occurred, and whether and how it affected a patient may be a

difficult and complex process. Hasty confessions have the potential to generate legally admissible admissions of fault, even if the confession later turns out to have been erroneous. To reduce the risks of inaccurate or premature admissions of fault, practices and hospitals may choose to establish disclosure policies that govern how preventable AEs are investigated and how the findings of such investigations are communicated to patients and families.

Pediatricians can prepare for future AEs by developing disclosure policies and procedures. Disclosure plans will help pediatricians determine in advance what types of information that they will communicate with patients and families when AEs occur. Pediatricians can be ready to appropriately express their sympathy about adverse outcomes and to declare their willingness and intention to investigate the cause(s) of the AE, to take measures (when appropriate) to prevent similar events in the future, and to provide ongoing necessary medical care and support to the affected patient and family. Pediatricians can also be prepared to take appropriate steps to protect themselves from unnecessary and inappropriate medical liability, by having a plan in place to notify medical malpractice insurance carriers and to consult with legal counsel.

EDUCATION ON DISCLOSURE OF PREVENTABLE AES

Education regarding practical disclosure skills and patient safety can be valuable to pediatric trainees and clinicians at all levels of experience. Simulation technology has been successfully used as one technique to assist in this learning.[48] Several other approaches to resident patient safety curricula have been reported.[49]

CONCLUSIONS

There is little doubt that patients, families, and physicians are better served when full and honest communications can take place after AEs. The American Academy of Pediatrics and its members can help to promote such communications by becoming informed about, and encouraging, state apology laws and other public policies that support disclosure.

RECOMMENDATIONS

1. Pediatric health care providers and institutions should develop and implement their own policies and procedures for identifying and disclosing AEs to patients and families in an honest and empathetic manner as part of a nonpunitive culture of ME reporting.

2. Pediatric institutions and practices should develop policies and procedures to provide emotional support for clinicians involved in AEs.

3. Pediatric medical educators should develop and implement educational programs regarding identification and prevention of MEs and communication about AEs with patients and their families as part of a comprehensive patient safety curriculum.

4. Additional research is needed on the consequences of various approaches to disclosure as well as of the effectiveness of disclosure education.

5. State legislators and other governmental and regulatory bodies are encouraged to continue developing apology laws and other mechanisms to reduce liability risks associated with disclosure.

LEAD AUTHORS

William M. McDonnell, MD, JD, FAAP

Daniel R. Neuspiel, MD, MPH, FAAP

ABBREVIATIONS

AE: adverse event
IOM: Institute of Medicine
ME: medical error

REFERENCES

1. Institute of Medicine, Committee on Quality of Health Care in America. *Crossing the Quality Chasm: A New Health System for the 21st Century.* Washington, DC: National Academy Press; 2001

2. Kohn LT, Corrigan JM, Donaldson MS, eds. *To Err Is Human: Building a Safer Health System.* Washington, DC: National Academy Press; 2000

3. Lannon CM, Coven BJ, Lane France F, et al; National Initiative for Children's Health Care Quality Project Advisory Committee. Principles of patient safety in pediatrics. *Pediatrics.* 2001;107(6):1473–1475

4. Miller MR, Takata G, Stucky ER, Neuspiel DR; Steering Committee on Quality Improvement and Management and Committee on Hospital Care. Policy statement—principles of pediatric patient safety: reducing harm due to medical care. *Pediatrics.* 2011;127(6):1199–1210

5. Aspden P, Corrigan J, Wolcott J, et al, eds; Institute of Medicine, Committee on Data Standards for Patient Safety. *Patient Safety: Achieving a New Standard for Care.* Washington, DC: National Academies Press; 2004

6. Leape LL, Brennan TA, Laird N, et al. The nature of adverse events in hospitalized patients. Results of the Harvard Medical Practice Study II. *N Engl J Med.* 1991;324(6):377–384

7. Woods D, Thomas E, Holl J, Altman S, Brennan T. Adverse events and preventable adverse events in children. *Pediatrics.* 2005;115(1):155–160

8. Matlow AG, Baker GR, Flintoft V, et al. Adverse events among children in Canadian hospitals: the Canadian Paediatric Adverse Events Study. *CMAJ.* 2012;184(13):E709–E718

9. Kaushal R, Goldmann DA, Keohane CA, et al. Adverse drug events in pediatric outpatients. *Ambul Pediatr.* 2007;7(5):383–389

10. Neuspiel DR, Stubbs EH. Patient safety in ambulatory care. *Pediatr Clin North Am.* 2012;59(6):1341–1354

11. Goodman JC, Villarreal P, Jones B. The social cost of adverse medical events, and what we can do about it. *Health Aff (Millwood).* 2011;30(4):590–595

12. Wu AW. Medical error: the second victim. The doctor who makes the mistake needs help too. *BMJ.* 2000;320(7237):726–727

13. Gallagher TH, Waterman AD, Ebers AG, Fraser VJ, Levinson W. Patients' and physicians' attitudes regarding the disclosure of medical errors. *JAMA.* 2003;289(8):1001–1007

14. Berlinger N, Wu AW. Subtracting insult from injury: addressing cultural expectations in the disclosure of medical error. *J Med Ethics.* 2005;31(2):106–108

15. Abd Elwahab S, Doherty E. What about doctors? The impact of medical errors. *Surgeon.* 2014;12(6):297–300

16. Waterman AD, Garbutt J, Hazel E, et al. The emotional impact of medical errors on practicing physicians in the United States and Canada. *Jt Comm J Qual Patient Saf.* 2007;33(8):467–476

17. Marmon LM, Heiss K. Improving surgeon wellness: the second victim syndrome and quality of care. *Semin Pediatr Surg.* 2015;24(6):315–318

18. Helmchen LA, Richards MR, McDonald TB. How does routine disclosure of medical error affect patients' propensity to sue and their assessment of provider quality? Evidence from survey data. *Med Care.* 2010;48(11):955–961

19. Bell SK, Mann KJ, Truog R, Lantos JD. Should we tell parents when we've made an error? *Pediatrics.* 2015;135(1):159–163

20. Bernstein M, Brown B. Doctors' duty to disclose error: a deontological or Kantian ethical analysis. *Can J Neurol Sci.* 2004;31(2):169–174

21. Gallagher TH, Waterman AD, Garbutt JM, et al. US and Canadian physicians' attitudes and experiences regarding disclosing errors to patients. *Arch Intern Med.* 2006;166(15):1605–1611

22. Stokes SL, Wu AW, Pronovost PJ. Ethical and practical aspects of disclosing adverse events in the emergency department. *Emerg Med Clin North Am.* 2006;24(3):703–714

23. Waite M. To tell the truth: the ethical and legal implications of disclosure of medical error. *Health Law J.* 2005;13:1–33

24. Blendon RJ, DesRoches CM, Brodie M, et al. Views of practicing physicians and the public on medical errors. *N Engl J Med.* 2002;347(24):1933–1940

25. Garbutt J, Brownstein DR, Klein EJ, et al. Reporting and disclosing medical errors: pediatricians' attitudes and behaviors. *Arch Pediatr Adolesc Med.* 2007;161(2):179–185

26. Cole AP, Block L, Wu AW. On higher ground: ethical reasoning and its relationship with error disclosure. *BMJ Qual Saf.* 2013;22(7):580–585

27. Varjavand N, Bachegowda LS, Gracely E, Novack DH. Changes in intern attitudes toward medical error and disclosure. *Med Educ.* 2012;46(7):668–677

28. Parker M. A fair dinkum duty of open disclosure following medical error. *J Law Med*. 2012;20(1):35–43

29. Gallagher TH, Studdert D, Levinson W. Disclosing harmful medical errors to patients. *N Engl J Med*. 2007;356(26):2713–2719

30. McDonnell WM, Guenther E. Narrative review: do state laws make it easier to say "I'm sorry?" *Ann Intern Med*. 2008;149(11):811–816

31. Gallagher THA. A 62-year-old woman with skin cancer who experienced wrong-site surgery: review of medical error. *JAMA*. 2009;302(6):669–677

32. Lamb RM, Studdert DM, Bohmer RMJ, Berwick DM, Brennan TA. Hospital disclosure practices: results of a national survey. *Health Aff (Millwood)*. 2003;22(2):73–83

33. Mastroianni AC, Mello MM, Sommer S, Hardy M, Gallagher TH. The flaws in state "apology" and "disclosure" laws dilute their intended impact on malpractice suits. *Health Aff (Millwood)*. 2010;29(9):1611–1619

34. Hyman DA. When and why lawyers are the problem. *Depaul L Rev*. 2008;57(2):267–280

35. Tabler N. Should physicians apologize for medical errors? *Health Lawyer*. 2007;19:23–30

36. Raper SE. No role for apology: remedial work and the problem of medical injury. *Yale J Health Policy Law Ethics*. 2011;11(2):267–330

37. Broun KS, Dix GE, Imwinkelried DJ, et al. The hearsay rule and its exceptions: the hearsay rule. In: Broun KS, Dix GE, Imwinkelried DJ, et al, eds. *McCormick on Evidence*. 7th ed. Eagan, MN: Thomson Reuters; 2013:175–257

38. Broun KS, Dix GE, Imwinkelried DJ, et al. The hearsay rule and its exceptions: admissions of a party-opponent. In: Broun KS, Dix GE, Imwinkelried DJ, et al, eds. *McCormick on Evidence*. 7th ed. Eagan, MN: Thomson Reuters; 2013:259–350

39. *Merriam-Webster Dictionary*. Available at: www.merriam-webster.com/dictionary/apology. Accessed May 24, 2016

40. *Johnson v Randall Smith*, 989 NE2d 35 (Ohio 2013)

41. Clinton HR, Obama B. Making patient safety the centerpiece of medical liability reform. *N Engl J Med*. 2006;354(21):2205–2208

42. *Deitsch v INOVA Health Care Services*, 2005 WL 4876742, No. 223119 (Va Cir Ct 2005)

43. *Airasian v Shaak*, 289 Ga App 540, 657 S.E.2d 600 (2008)

44. Kachalia A, Kaufman SR, Boothman R, et al. Liability claims and costs before and after implementation of a medical error disclosure program. *Ann Intern Med*. 2010;153(4):213–221

45. Wu AW, Huang IC, Stokes S, Pronovost PJ. Disclosing medical errors to patients: it's not what you say, it's what they hear. *J Gen Intern Med*. 2009;24(9):1012–1017

46. Studdert DM, Mello MM, Gawande AA, Brennan TA, Wang YC. Disclosure of medical injury to patients: an improbable risk management strategy. *Health Aff (Millwood)*. 2007;26(1):215–226

47. Reason J. Human error: models and management. *BMJ*. 2000;320(7237):768–770

48. Matos FM, Raemer DB. Mixed-realism simulation of adverse event disclosure: an educational methodology and assessment instrument. *Simul Healthc*. 2013;8(2):84–90

49. Neuspiel DR, Hyman D, Lane M. Quality improvement and patient safety in the pediatric ambulatory setting: current knowledge and implications for residency training. *Pediatr Clin North Am*. 2009;56(4):935–951

Establishing a Standard Protocol for the Voiding Cystourethrography

- *Clinical Report*

CLINICAL REPORT Guidance for the Clinician in Rendering Pediatric Care

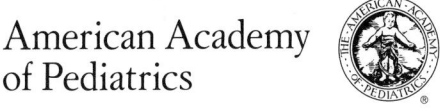

American Academy
of Pediatrics

DEDICATED TO THE HEALTH OF ALL CHILDREN™

Establishing a Standard Protocol for the Voiding Cystourethrography

Dominic Frimberger, MD, Maria-Gisela Mercado-Deane, MD, FAAP, SECTION ON UROLOGY, SECTION ON RADIOLOGY

abstract

The voiding cystourethrogram (VCUG) is a frequently performed test to diagnose a variety of urologic conditions, such as vesicoureteral reflux. The test results determine whether continued observation or an interventional procedure is indicated. VCUGs are ordered by many specialists and primary care providers, including pediatricians, family practitioners, nephrologists, hospitalists, emergency department physicians, and urologists. Current protocols for performing and interpreting a VCUG are based on the International Reflux Study in 1985. However, more recent information provided by many national and international institutions suggests a need to refine those recommendations. The lead author of the 1985 study, R.L. Lebowitz, agreed to and participated in the current protocol. In addition, a recent survey directed to the chairpersons of pediatric radiology of 65 children's hospitals throughout the United States and Canada showed that VCUG protocols vary substantially. Recent guidelines from the American Academy of Pediatrics (AAP) recommend a VCUG for children between 2 and 24 months of age with urinary tract infections but did not specify how this test should be performed. To improve patient safety and to standardize the data obtained when a VCUG is performed, the AAP Section on Radiology and the AAP Section on Urology initiated the current VCUG protocol to create a consensus on how to perform this test.

DOI: 10.1542/peds.2016-2590

PEDIATRICS (ISSN Numbers: Print, 0031-4005; Online, 1098-4275).

FINANCIAL DISCLOSURE: The authors have indicated they do not have a financial relationship relevant to this article to disclose.

FUNDING: No external funding.

POTENTIAL CONFLICT OF INTEREST: The authors have indicated they have no potential conflicts of interest to disclose.

To cite: Frimberger D, Mercado-Deane MG, AAP SECTION ON UROLOGY, AAP SECTION ON RADIOLOGY. Establishing a Standard Protocol for the Voiding Cystourethrography. Pediatrics. 2016;138(5):e20162590

INTRODUCTION

The voiding cystourethrogram (VCUG) and the nuclear cystogram are the accepted tests in national and international institutions to diagnose vesicoureteral reflux (VUR). The VCUG aims to image the urinary tract, including the urethra, bladder, ureters, and kidneys, during bladder filling and emptying. The VCUG has many components that can be individually reviewed on the basis of evidence, but no evidence-based protocol for the VCUG per se is available. The International Reflux Study in 1985[1] is the only published protocol. However, a recent survey directed to the chairpersons of pediatric radiology of 65 children's hospitals in the United States and Canada showed that VCUG protocols vary substantially.[2] The use of different VCUG protocols raises concerns about patient safety and does not allow valid comparison of data and outcomes between individuals and institutions. Unlike the VCUG, most imaging studies are performed by using protocols that have national and often international consensus that allow the comparison of results across centers and achieve a uniform level of patient safety. Recent guidelines from the American Academy of Pediatrics (AAP) recommend a VCUG for children between 2 and 24 months of age with a urinary tract infection but did not specify how this test should be performed.[3] Ward et al[4] compared the radiation exposure and effective dose in children undergoing VCUG. They found an 8 times reduced radiation exposure when using grid-controlled, variable-rate pulsed fluoroscopy versus conventional continuous fluoroscopy. To strike the balance between obtaining high-quality images and minimizing radiation exposure, radiology departments should observe the "as low as (is) reasonably achievable" (ALARA) and Image Gently guidelines. Image Gently is an initiative of the Alliance for Radiation Safety in Pediatric Imaging. Both promote radiation protection for the patient and radiologic personnel.[5,6]

Differences in individual test parameters can have a significant effect on the outcome of the test and have the potential to influence management protocols for individual patients. In a study in 183 patients after minimally invasive ureteral injection therapy, 60% of patients with a postoperative positive VCUG result did not show VUR until the bladder was filled over the age-adjusted bladder capacity.[7] If an alternative protocol had been used that filled the bladder just to the age-adjusted capacity, those patients would have had a negative study result, and their surgery would have been considered successful. Therefore, the postoperative success rates would be a function not only of the surgical

technique and skill of the surgeon but also of the specific VCUG imaging technique.

Many components of the VCUG are universally accepted and performed equally throughout different institutions. Little discussion exists regarding the necessity to empty the bladder before the test and to use a small nonballoon catheter for filling. The use of more than 1 bladder filling is a common standard, because several groups showed that cyclic filling increases the reliability to detect VUR.[8,9] It is also well established that several voiding cycles may be necessary to detect the presence of an ectopic, refluxing ureter.[10] The documented relationship between bladder volume at the onset of VUR and outcome causes many pediatric urologists to ask their radiology departments to note the bladder volume when VUR first occurs. Bladder volume when VUR first occurs is important, because previous studies have shown that VUR occurring at lower bladder volumes and pressure has a tendency to resolve spontaneously less often, independent of grade.[11] In addition, Alexander et al[8] verified that bladder volume at the onset of VUR is an independent risk factor for breakthrough febrile urinary tract infection.

The VCUG can be a traumatizing test for patients and parents alike. Sedation can be used as long as the effects do not alter the voiding phase and therefore the outcome of the test. However, patient and parent education, along with providing a comfortable environment with well-trained staff and the addition of child life specialists when available, is of great importance to minimize stress.[12,13]

The multitude of data on the effect of the VCUG technique on test outcome has caused many departments to adapt similar parameters of the VCUG in their protocols, such as the practice guidelines of the American College of Radiology.[14] However, other components of the VCUG are controversial, such as the use of

sedation or immobilization. These controversies lead to different protocols among institutions, making it problematic to compare outcomes even when the details of the technique are reported.

Standard evidence-based protocols in medicine are important to minimize patient risk and to improve the validity of comparing data and outcomes between individuals and institutions. Great efforts were made to ensure that the renal scan protocol used in the Randomized Intervention for Children with VesicoUreteral Reflux (RIVUR) Study was uniform across the participating centers.[15] However, the very test that evaluated the presence and grade of VUR was not standardized. To improve our understanding of VUR, a standardized protocol of how to perform the diagnostic VCUG study is necessary.

Because the VCUG is ordered by many different pediatric specialties and the test results are used to determine treatment of the individual patient, this statement disseminates the current protocol to reach the broad community of pediatric health care providers. Medical circumstances can make it necessary to alter the protocol to accommodate a patient's specific needs; in those cases, the reasons should be documented and the changes noted in the report.

VCUG TEMPLATE

Patient Name; Date of Birth; Medications; Medical Record Number

Date of Study

Reason for Examination: Information Provided by Ordering Physician

Comparison: Previous Studies

Technique

Informed consent is obtained and documented in the patient's record.

1. Observe ALARA and Image Gently principles (see ALARA/Image Gently Principles).[5,6]

2. Observe recommendations for possible sedation (see Sedation).

3. Observe recommendations for possible immobilization (see Immobilization).

4. Toilet trained: allow patient to void in private bathroom immediately before the study.

5. After voiding and for non–toilet-trained individuals: insert a small age-appropriate (3.5–8 French) nonballoon catheter with the use of sterile technique (see Sterile Catheterization).

6. Measure postvoid residual (PVR) urine in milliliters.

7. Obtain a single anterior-posterior (AP) scout image covering the kidneys, ureters, and bladder (KUB).

8. Retrograde fill the bladder (see Bladder Filling) with radiographic contrast (see Contrast) at body temperature.

9. During filling, obtain multiple spot images in AP, right and left oblique, and lateral positions (see Spot Images).

10. Fill bladder until voiding occurs and stop contrast flow (see Bladder Filling).

11. Obtain voiding images of the urethra (see Spot Images).

12. Refill bladder until voiding occurs (see Cyclic Voiding, Bladder Filling).

13. Obtain voiding and postvoid images of the kidneys and bladder (see Spot Images).

14. Record maximum amount of contrast instilled.

Findings

Scout Image

1. Osseous structures, especially symphysis and spine and surrounding soft tissues

2. Any other abnormalities

3. Bowel gas pattern and amount of stool in various portions of the colon to assess for constipation

Bladder

1. Shape and contour

2. Filling defects, trabeculations, or other abnormalities

3. Maximum bladder capacity (at time of first void if cyclic study)

4. Estimate of PVR volume (mild, moderate, or large)

5. Note position and appearance of the bladder neck

VUR

1. Record onset of VUR for each side: (a) approximate bladder volume at which reflux occurred and (b) onset of reflux during filling or voiding.

2. Grade VUR according to the International Reflux Study (see VUR Grading).

3. Comment on the insertion site and anatomy of the ureter(s): (a) normal versus ectopic, (b) single versus duplicated or bifid system, and (c) insertion near or in a diverticulum.

4. Assess drainage of VUR after void. In some patients with VUR, recatheterization may be necessary to assess drainage of the refluxed material, especially in non–toilet-trained children.

Voiding

1. Record bladder volume at onset of voiding.

2. Note appearance of bladder neck as child voids.

3. Estimate bladder volume residual (mild, moderate, or large).

Urethra

1. Record urethral abnormalities including dilatation, valves, strictures, and the appearance in the region of the external sphincter.

2. Record reflux into ejaculatory ducts.

Impression

Summarize findings.

DEFINITION OF PARAMETERS

ALARA and Image Gently Principles

As defined in Title 10, Section 20.1003, of the Code of Federal Regulations (10 CFR 20.1003), ALARA is an acronym for "as low as (is) reasonably achievable," which means making every reasonable effort to maintain exposures to ionizing radiation as far below the dose limits as is practical, consistent with the purpose for which the licensed activity is undertaken, taking into account the state of technology, the economics of improvements in relation to the state of technology, the economics of improvements in relation to benefits to the public health and safety, and other societal and socioeconomic considerations, and in relation to the utilization of nuclear energy and licensed materials in the public interest (US Nuclear Regulatory Commission; last updated December 10, 2012).

The Image Gently Campaign is an initiative of the Alliance for Radiation Safety in Pediatric Imaging. The campaign goal is to change practice by increasing awareness of the opportunities to promote radiation protection in the imaging of children (www.pedrad.org/associations/5364/ig and http://www.imagegently.org/Portals/6/Radiologists/Background4radiologists.pdf).

Sedation

1. Child and family education, preparation, and support during the examination are important for the success of the study (use a certified child life specialist if available).[13]

2. Encourage supportive family members to be present in the fluoroscopic suite.

3. The use of sedation is acceptable in certain situations when all less intrusive methods fail to achieve a relaxed atmosphere for the child and/or family.

4. Because voiding is an integral part of the VCUG, if sedation is used, it should not interfere with voiding.

5. The specific sedation used (oral, intravenous, or inhalation) is at the discretion of the physician and the institution's guidelines. When sedation is used, it should follow the guidelines for preparation, monitoring, and recovery as set forth by the AAP.[16]

6. Because sedation may alter results, its use should be noted in reports, presentations, and manuscripts.

Immobilization

High-quality images with observation of the ALARA and Image Gently principles are required. Restraining devices usually are not necessary but can be used in certain situations.

Contrast Material

Commonly used contrast materials include the following: iothalamate meglumine (Cysto-Conray 17%; Mallinckrodt Pharmaceuticals, manufactured by Liebel-Flarsheim Company LLC, Raleigh, NC) and full-strength diatrizoate meglumine (Cystografin; Bracco Diagnostics, Monroe Township, NJ). The type of contrast should be identified in the report.

Sterile Catheterization

Strict adherence to the principles of medical and surgical asepsis should be followed:

1. Wash hands, clean perimeatal region with antiseptic solution and provide a sterile field.

2. Wash hands, reapply sterile gloves, then insert catheter.

3. Appropriate use of lidocaine or other anesthetic gel has been shown to reduce discomfort but requires adequate contact time to be effective. In boys, lidocaine gel is instilled into the urethra. Lidocaine gel on a gauze pad can be applied to the interlabial area in girls, followed by instillation of gel into the urethra.[17]

4. Placement of the catheter is facilitated by clear identification of the urethral meatus, and exposure is often facilitated by an assistant for girls.

5. Collect urine in a sterile container and record PVR.

6. Send urine for analysis and culture as indicated.

Radiology departments can make specific arrangements to send a urine specimen for analysis and culture if requested by the ordering physician.

Spot Images

Images must be of high quality and should be taken in accordance with the ALARA and Image Gently principles. The usual number of images is KUB + 12 images. Images should be saved from the fluoroscopic imaging rather than obtained by separate reexposures to reduce radiation. If there is pathology, additional images can be obtained to show the abnormality.

Recommended images for the different VCUG phases are as follows:

First fill:

1. AP early first fill
2. AP late first fill
3. At late first fill: AP right anterior oblique, AP left anterior oblique, lateral spine included

Second fill:

AP right anterior oblique and AP left anterior oblique

Voiding Phase

1. AP bladder when voiding occurs:
   d. Females: AP urethra (2–4 images)
   e. Males: lateral to oblique, entire urethra during voiding from the bladder neck to the tip of the penis (2–4 images)

Postvoid

Single KUB, including bladder, ureters, and kidneys.

Bladder Filling

1. Fill bladder with gravity at 100 cm above the examination table.

2. If filling pump is used, infuse at 10% of expected bladder capacity per minute.

3. Estimated bladder capacity as follows[18,19]:
   a. For patients <2 years of age: weight (kg) × 7
   b. For patients >2 to 14 years of age:
      i. In ounces: age in years + 1
      ii. In milliliters: (age in years × 30) + 30
   c. For patients >14 years of age: 500 mL

4. Record infused volume[20]:
   a. Standard: record volume:
      i. At onset of VUR
      ii. Maximum volume infused at time of void
      iii. PVR estimate (mild, moderate, or large)
   b. Additional recommendation for complex cases:
      i. Volume when child is uncomfortable
      ii. Volume when voiding with strong stream

5. Fill bladder until voiding occurs. If bladder filling reaches >2 times bladder capacity and no voiding takes place, consider subsequent

evaluation of patient with videourodynamic study.

Cyclic VCUG

At least 2 voiding cycles are recommended to identify a potential ectopic ureter or intermittent VUR.[21]

1. Child can void around the catheter for the first void.

2. Refill bladder and remove catheter for second void.

3. If an ectopic ureter and VUR is identified on first void and good urethral images are obtained, there may be no need for a second cycle.

VUR Grading

Grade I: ureter only

Grade II: ureter, pelvis, and calyces; no dilatation; normal calyceal fornices

Grade III: mild or moderate dilatation and/or tortuosity of the ureter and mild or moderate dilatation of the renal pelvis; no or only slight blunting of the fornices

Grade IV: moderate dilatation and/ or tortuosity of the ureter and moderate dilatation of the renal pelvis and calyces; blunting of the sharp angle of the fornices but maintenance of the papillary impressions in the majority of calyces

Grade V: gross dilatation and tortuosity of the ureter; severe dilatation of the renal pelvis and calyces; the papillary impressions are no longer visible in the majority of calyces

ACKNOWLEDGMENTS

The current clinical report is the work of the VCUG consensus team, working together closely in collecting and analyzing the available data. The authors thank the members of the team who contributed to the development and writing of this report: Dr Christopher S. Cooper, MD, FAAP, Dr Stuart B. Bauer, MD, FAAP, Dr Mark P. Cain, MD, FAAP, Dr Saul P. Greenfield, MD, FAAP, Dr Andrew J. Kirsch, MD, and Dr Faridali Ramji, MD. The authors also express their sincere gratitude to Ms Kathleen Ozmeral for her help in developing this report.

LEAD AUTHORS

Dominic Frimberger, MD
Maria-Gisela Mercado-Deane, MD, FAAP

SECTION ON UROLOGY EXECUTIVE COMMITTEE, 2014–2015

Patrick H. McKenna, MD, FAAP, Chairperson
J. Christopher Austin, MD, FAAP
Paul F. Austin, MD, FAAP
Christopher S. Cooper, MD, FAAP
Saul P. Greenfield, MD, FAAP
C.D. Anthony Herndon, MD, FAAP
Thomas F. Kolon, MD, FAAP
Andrew E. MacNeily, MD, FAAP
John M. Park, MD, FAAP
Julian H. Wan, MD, FAAP, Immediate Past Chairperson

SECTION ON RADIOLOGY EXECUTIVE COMMITTEE, 2014–2015

Maria-Gisela Mercado-Deane, MD, FAAP, Chairperson
Aparna Annam, DO, FAAP
Dorothy Bulas, MD, FAAP
John Cassese, MD, FAAP
Sarah Milla, MD, FAAP
F. Glen Seidel, MD, FAAP
Christopher Cassady, MD, FAAP, Immediate Past Chairperson

STAFF

Kathleen Kuk Ozmeral

ABBREVIATIONS

AAP: American Academy of Pediatrics
ALARA: as low as (is) reasonably achievable
AP: anterior-posterior
KUB: kidneys, ureters, and bladder
PVR: postvoid residual
VCUG: voiding cystourethrogram
VUR: vesicoureteral reflux

REFERENCES

1. Lebowitz RL, Olbing H, Parkkulainen KV, Smellie JM, Tamminen-Möbius TE; International Reflux Study in Children. International system of radiographic grading of vesicoureteric reflux. *Pediatr Radiol.* 1985;15(2):105–109

2. Palmer BW, Ramji FG, Snyder CT, Hemphill M, Kropp BP, Frimberger D. Voiding cystourethrogram—are our protocols the same? *J Urol.* 2011;186(4 suppl):1668–1671

3. Roberts KB; Subcommittee on Urinary Tract Infection; Steering Committee on Quality Improvement and Management. Urinary tract infection: clinical practice guideline for the diagnosis and management of the initial UTI in febrile infants and children 2 to 24 months. *Pediatrics.* 2011;128(3):595–610

4. Ward VL, Strauss KJ, Barnewolt CE, et al. Pediatric radiation exposure and effective dose reduction during voiding cystourethrography. *Radiology.* 2008;249(3):1002–1009

5. ALARA: as defined in title 10, section 20.1003, of the Code of Federal Regulations (10 CFR 20.1003). US Nuclear Regulatory Commission; last updated December 10, 2012. Available at: http://www.nrc.gov/reading-rm/basic-ref/glossary/alara.html. Accessed September 8, 2016

6. Alliance for Pediatric Radiation in Imaging. Image Gently. Available at: www.imagegently.org. Accessed January 25, 2016

7. Palmer BW, Frimberger D. Clinical and radiographic success after dextranomer/hyaluronic acid copolymer injection for the treatment of vesicoureteral reflux. Presented at: South Central Section of the American Urological Association; San Antonio, TX; September 14–17, 2011. Abstract 48

8. Alexander SE, Arlen AM, Storm DW, Kieran K, Cooper CS. Bladder volume at onset of vesicoureteral reflux is an independent risk factor for breakthrough febrile urinary tract infection. *J Urol.* 2015;193(4):1342–1346

9. Papadopoulou F, Efremidis SC, Oiconomou A, et al. Cyclic voiding cystourethrography: is vesicoureteral

reflux missed with standard voiding cystourethrography? [published correction appears in *Eur Radiol.* 2002;12(1):260]. *Eur Radiol.* 2002;12(3):666–670

10. Polito C, Moggio G, La Manna A, Cioce F, Cappabianca S, Di Toro R. Cyclic voiding cystourethrography in the diagnosis of occult vesicoureteric reflux. *Pediatr Nephrol.* 2000;14(1):39–41

11. McMillan ZM, Austin JC, Knudson MJ, Hawtrey CE, Cooper CS. Bladder volume at onset of reflux on initial cystogram predicts spontaneous resolution. *J Urol.* 2006;176(4 pt 2):1838–1841

12. Stokland E, Andréasson S, Jacobsson B, Jodal U, Ljung B. Sedation with midazolam for voiding cystourethrography in children: a randomised double-blind study. *Pediatr Radiol.* 2003;33(4):247–249

13. Salmon K, McGuigan F, Pereira JK. Brief report: optimizing children's memory and management of an invasive medical procedure: the influence of procedural narration and distraction. *J Pediatr Psychol.* 2006;31(5):522–527

14. American College of Radiology; Society for Pediatric Radiology. ACR–SPR Practice Parameter for the Performance of Voiding Cystourethrography in Children. Reston, VA: American College of Radiology and the Society for Pediatric Radiology; revised 2014 (Resolution 13). Available at: www.acr.org/~/media/ACR/Documents/PGTS/guidelines/Voiding_Cystourethrography.pdf. Accessed January 25, 2016

15. Hoberman A, Greenfield SP, Mattoo TK, et al; RIVUR Trial Investigators. Antimicrobial prophylaxis for children with vesicoureteral reflux. *N Engl J Med.* 2014;370(25):2367–2376

16. Coté CJ, Wilson S; American Academy of Pediatrics; American Academy of Pediatric Dentistry. Guidelines for monitoring and management of pediatric patients before, during, and after sedation for diagnostic and therapeutic procedures: update 2016. *Pediatrics.* 2016;138(1):e20161212

17. Gerard LL, Cooper CS, Duethman KS, Gordley BM, Kleiber CM. Effectiveness of lidocaine lubricant for discomfort during pediatric urethral catheterization. *J Urol.* 2003;170(2 pt 1):564–567

18. Fairhurst JJ, Rubin CM, Hyde I, Freeman NV, Williams JD. Bladder capacity in infants. *J Pediatr Surg.* 1991;26(1):55–57

19. Hjälmås K. Urodynamics in normal infants and children. *Scand J Urol Nephrol Suppl.* 1988;114:20–27

20. Cooper CS, Madsen MT, Austin JC, Hawtrey CE, Gerard LL, Graham MM. Bladder pressure at the onset of vesicoureteral reflux determined by nuclear cystometrogram. *J Urol.* 2003;170(4 pt 2):1537–1540; discussion: 1540

21. Jequier S, Jequier JC. Reliability of voiding cystourethrography to detect reflux. *AJR Am J Roentgenol.* 1989;153(4):807–810

Evaluation and Management of Children and Adolescents With Acute Mental Health or Behavioral Problems. Part I: Common Clinical Challenges of Patients With Mental Health and/or Behavioral Emergencies

• •

- *Clinical Report*

CLINICAL REPORT Guidance for the Clinician in Rendering Pediatric Care

American Academy
of Pediatrics

DEDICATED TO THE HEALTH OF ALL CHILDREN™

Evaluation and Management of Children and Adolescents With Acute Mental Health or Behavioral Problems. Part I: Common Clinical Challenges of Patients With Mental Health and/or Behavioral Emergencies

Thomas H. Chun, MD, MPH, FAAP, Sharon E. Mace, MD, FAAP, FACEP, Emily R. Katz, MD, FAAP, AMERICAN ACADEMY OF PEDIATRICS, COMMITTEE ON PEDIATRIC EMERGENCY MEDICINE, AND AMERICAN COLLEGE OF EMERGENCY PHYSICIANS, PEDIATRIC EMERGENCY MEDICINE COMMITTEE

INTRODUCTION

Mental health problems are among the leading contributors to the global burden of disease.[1] Unfortunately, pediatric populations are not spared of mental health problems. In the United States, 21% to 23% of children and adolescents have a diagnosable mental health or substance use disorder.[2,3] Among patients of emergency departments (EDs), 70% screen positive for at least 1 mental health disorder,[4] 23% meet criteria for 2 or more mental health concerns,[5] 45% have a mental health problem resulting in impaired psychosocial functioning,[5] and 10% of adolescents endorse significant levels of psychiatric distress at the time of their ED visit.[6] In pediatric primary care settings, the reported prevalence of mental health and behavioral disorders is between 12% to 22% of children and adolescents.[7]

Although the American Academy of Pediatrics (AAP) has published a policy statement on mental health competencies and a Mental Health Toolkit for pediatric primary care providers, no such guidelines or resources exist for clinicians who care for pediatric mental health emergencies.[8,9] This clinical report supports the 2006 joint policy statement of the AAP and American College of Emergency Physicians (ACEP) on pediatric mental health emergencies, with the goal of addressing the knowledge gaps in this area.[10,11] The report is written primarily from the perspective of ED clinicians, but it is intended for all clinicians who care for children and adolescents with acute mental health and behavioral problems.

Recent epidemiologic studies of mental health visits have revealed a rapid burgeoning of both ED and primary care visits.[12–20] An especially problematic trend is the increase in "boarding" of psychiatric patients in

DOI: 10.1542/peds.2016-1570

PEDIATRICS (ISSN Numbers: Print, 0031-4005; Online, 1098-4275).

FINANCIAL DISCLOSURE: The authors have indicated they do not have a financial relationship relevant to this article to disclose.

FUNDING: No external funding.

POTENTIAL CONFLICT OF INTEREST: The authors have indicated they have no potential conflicts of interest to disclose.

To cite: Chun TH, Mace SE, AAP FACEP, Katz ER. Evaluation and Management of Children and Adolescents With Acute Mental Health or Behavioral Problems. Part I: Common Clinical Challenges of Patients With Mental Health and/or Behavioral Emergencies. Pediatrics. 2016;138(3):e20161570

the ED and inpatient pediatric beds (ie, extended stays lasting days or even weeks). Although investigation of boarding practices is still in its infancy, the ACEP[21] and the American Medical Association[22] have both expressed concern about it, because it significantly taxes the functioning and efficiency of both the ED and hospital, and mental health services may not be available in the ED.[23-26]

In addition, compared with other pediatric care settings, ED patients are known to be at higher risk of mental health disorders, including depression,[27,28] anxiety,[29] posttraumatic stress disorder,[30] and substance abuse.[31] These mental health conditions may be unrecognized not only by treating clinicians but also by the child/adolescent and his or her parents.[32-36] A similar phenomenon has been described with suicidal patients. Individuals who have committed suicide frequently visited a health care provider in the months preceding their death.[37,38] Although a minority of suicidal patients present with some form of self-harm, many have vague somatic complaints (eg, headache, gastrointestinal tract distress, back pain, concern for a sexually transmitted infection) masking their underlying mental health condition.[34–36]

Despite studies demonstrating moderate agreement between emergency physicians and psychiatrists in the assessment and management of patients with mental health problems,[39,40] ED clinicians frequently cite lack of training and confidence in their abilities as barriers to caring for patients with mental health emergencies.[41–44] Another study of emergency medicine and pediatric emergency medicine training programs found that formal training in psychiatric problems is not required nor offered by most programs.[45] Pediatric primary care providers report similar barriers to caring for their patients with mental health problems.[46,47]

Part I of this clinical report focuses on the issues relevant to patients presenting to the ED with a mental health chief complaint and covers the following topics:

- Medical clearance of pediatric psychiatric patients

- Suicidal ideation and suicide attempts

- Involuntary hospitalization

- Restraint of the agitated patient

  o Verbal restraint

  o Chemical restraint

  o Physical restraint

- Coordination with the medical home

Part II discusses challenging patients with primarily medical or indeterminate presentations, in which the contribution of an underlying mental health condition may be unclear or a complicating factor, including:

- Somatic symptom and related disorders

- Adverse effects to psychiatric medications

  o Antipsychotic adverse effects

  o Neuroleptic malignant syndrome

  o Serotonin syndrome

- Children with special needs in the ED (autism spectrum and developmental disorders)

- Mental health screening in the ED

An executive summary of this clinical report can be found at www.pediatrics.org/cgi/doi/10.1542/peds.2016-1571.

MEDICAL CLEARANCE OF PEDIATRIC PSYCHIATRIC PATIENTS

Background

Medical clearance can be defined as the process of excluding acute medical illnesses or injuries in patients presenting with psychiatric complaints. Concern that medical illness may be the underlying cause of a psychiatric problem has led some to suggest "that emergency patients with psychiatric complaints receive a full medical evaluation."[48] Medical clearance originates from the perspective that an ED evaluation of a psychiatric patient may be the only opportunity to diagnose underlying illnesses or injuries that could result in morbidity or mortality because resources for diagnosing and treating medical conditions may not be readily available in some psychiatric facilities. In addition, many psychiatric complaints and disorders can be exacerbated or precipitated by medical illness,[49] and some psychiatric patients may have unmet medical needs.[50-52]

Medical Diseases in ED Psychiatric Patients

Previous studies of medical conditions in ED psychiatric patients have been almost exclusively conducted with adults and have had highly variable findings. Past reports have found underlying medical problems in 19% to 63% of ED psychiatric patients.[53-55] Studies of adults admitted to psychiatric units after an ED medical evaluation have had similarly disparate results. Some have reported missed medical conditions in up to half of patients,[53,56] including diabetes, uremic and hepatic encephalopathy, pneumonia, urinary tract infections, and sepsis,[57] but another found that only 4% (12 of 298) needed treatment of a medical condition within 24 hours of admission to the psychiatric unit.[58] To address these concerns, some have suggested a standardized evaluation and documentation of the ED medical evaluation.[59] Major limitations of these studies are that they are from older literature, and they did not include children. More recent adult and pediatric studies, discussed later, suggest that significant rates of medical morbidity in psychiatric patients may be less likely.

Some authors argue that it is not possible to rule out all potential medical etiologies for psychiatric symptoms and believe that the role of the ED evaluation is to determine whether the patient is "medically stable" rather than "medically cleared."[60] Although the concept of "medical stability," which can be defined as the lack of medical conditions requiring acute evaluation and/or treatment, is gaining traction, for the purposes of this discussion, the term "medical clearance" will be used. A growing body of adult and pediatric studies suggest that an ED patient's history, physical examination, and vital signs provide important data for determining the appropriate medical evaluation for a psychiatric patient. These findings support the 2006 ACEP policy statement, which recommends "focused medical assessment" for ED psychiatric patients, in which laboratory testing is obtained on the basis of history and physical examination rather than a predetermined battery of tests for all patients with psychiatric complaints.[61] When ED resource utilization and the cost of medical screening evaluations for pediatric psychiatric patients are considered, additional questions are raised about such evaluations and whether the ED is the optimal site for them.[62,63]

The Goals of Medical Clearance

Medical clearance of psychiatric patients focuses on determining whether the patient's behavioral or psychiatric signs and symptoms are caused or exacerbated by an underlying medical condition and whether there are medical conditions that would benefit from acute treatment in the ED. Given the vast number of medical illnesses that can masquerade as a behavioral problem or psychiatric disorder,

a comprehensive list of such conditions is beyond the scope of this article. Table 1 focuses on medical conditions that can be evaluated within the context and time frame of an ED visit. Examples of medical conditions requiring ED treatment includes suturing, wound or injury care, and treatment of an overdose. In addition, some psychiatric patients may have comorbidities that are not contributing to their behavioral or psychiatric complaints but would benefit from ED care, such as asthma or diabetes.[58]

Key elements for detecting underlying medical condition(s) include careful assessment of abnormal vital signs, a complete history and physical examination, with particular attention to the neurologic, cardiac, and respiratory systems.[64] Various screening tools have been developed to assist in the medical clearance of psychiatric patients in the ED,[60,65] although these authors also stress the importance of an adequate history and physical examination and do not mandate laboratory or other investigations.[65] After medical clearance has been performed, the AAP and ACEP support the development of transport protocols to definitive psychiatric treatment facilities for EDs that transfer patients with mental health care needs.[10,11]

Diagnostic Laboratory Testing and Medical Clearance

In 1 study of emergency physicians, "routine testing" was performed in 35% of respondents, with 16% of the testing performed because it was ED protocol and 84% of the testing performed at request of the mental health service. Of those with protocol testing, the most frequently ordered tests were urine toxicology screen (86%), serum alcohol (85%), complete blood cell count (56%), electrolytes (56%), blood urea nitrogen (45%), creatinine (40%), serum toxicology screen (31%), and

electrocardiogram (18%).[66] Other commonly obtained laboratory evaluations for medical clearance include testing for pregnancy and sexually transmitted infections.

Recently, the utility of routine medical screening tests has been questioned. In contrast to the older literature, more contemporary studies are finding much lower rates of unsuspected, clinically emergent, or urgent laboratory abnormalities. Two studies of adult ED patients with psychiatric complaints found low rates of clinically significant abnormalities on routine laboratory testing,[55,67] the majority (94%) of which were clinically suspected on the basis of the patient's history and physical examination.[55] Similar results have been reported in admitted adult psychiatric patients after an ED evaluation. One study of 250 psychiatric inpatients found a mean of 27.7 tests were ordered per patient, with only 4% (11 of 250) having "important" medical problems discovered and less than 1 test in 50 resulting in any clinically useful information.[10] Another study identified only 1 patient of 519 (0.2%) with an abnormal laboratory test result that would have changed ED management or patient disposition.[68]

Similar results have emerged for ED pediatric psychiatric patients. Several studies have found little to no utility for routine urine drug testing. Shihabuddin et al evaluated such testing in 547 patients presenting with a psychiatric complaint. A positive result was found in 20.8% of patients, half of which were suspected on the basis of the patients' reported substance use history. Urine drug testing resulted in no changes in patient management, and all were medically cleared.[69] Fortu et al examined 652 (385 routine and 267 medically indicated) urine toxicology screens.[70] For the routine toxicology screens, only 5% were positive, and there were no changes

TABLE 1 Medical Disorders That Can Present as a Psychiatric Disorder or Behavioral Problem[a]

Neurologic (CNS) Diseases
  Stroke/transient ischemic attacks
  Hemorrhage: intracerebral, subdural, subarachnoid, epidural
  CNS vascular: aneurysms, venous thrombosis, ischemia, vertebrobasilar insufficiency
  CNS malignancy/tumors
  CNS trauma: primary injury, secondary injury or sequelae of head trauma
  CNS infections: meningitis, encephalitis, abscess (brain, epidural, spinal), HIV, syphilis
  Congenital malformations
  Hydrocephalus
  Seizures
  Headaches including migraines
  Neurodegenerative disorders: multiple sclerosis, Huntington chorea
  Tuberous sclerosis
  Delirium ("ICU psychosis")
Metabolic, Endocrine, and Electrolyte Disturbances
  Hyponatremia
  Hypocalcemia
  Hypoglycemia
  Hyperglycemia
  Ketoacidosis
  Uremia
  Hyperammonemia
  Inborn errors of metabolism: lipid storage diseases, Gaucher disease, Niemann-Pick disease
  Thyroid disease: hyperthyroidism, thyroid storm, hypothyroidism
  Adrenal disease: Addison disease, Cushing disease
  Pituitary: hypopituitarism
  Parathyroid disease: hypoparathyroidism, hyperparathyroidism
  Pheochromocytoma
Respiratory
  Hypoxia
  Hypercarbia/hypercapnia
  Respiratory failure
Medications
  Drug withdrawal: alcohol, amphetamines, barbiturates, benzodiazepines, cocaine, psychiatric
    medications
  Drug overdose:
    Drugs of abuse: phencyclidine, heroin, cocaine, marijuana, MDMA (3,4-methylenedioxy-
      methamphetamine), LSD (lysergic acid diethylamide), alcohol, amphetamines, "bath salts"
    Prescription drugs: steroids, birth control, antihypertensives, statins, anticonvulsants,
      barbiturates, benzodiazepines, opioids, anticholinergics, antibiotics, antifungal agents, antiviral
      agents, asthmatic medications, muscle relaxants, gastrointestinal tract drugs, anesthetics,
      anticholinergics, cardiac medications (such as digoxin), decongestants, antiarrhythmics,
      immunosuppressives
    Drugs for psychiatric patients: antidepressants, antipsychotics, lithium
Hematologic/Oncologic
  Malignancies
  Tumors
  Paraneoplastic syndromes
Inflammatory/Rheumatologic
  Sarcoidosis
  Systemic lupus erythematosus
Toxins
  Carbon monoxide
  Lead poisoning
  Organophosphates
  Volatile substances
Other
  Fever
  Child maltreatment

[a] This is not an exhaustive inclusive list but one that provides examples of the many diseases/conditions and drugs/medications that can masquerade as a psychiatric/behavioral disorder.

in management and no significant differences in disposition between those with positive and negative toxicology screens. Tenenbein reviewed 3 retrospective case studies of urine drug testing in children and concluded, "The emergency drug screen is unlikely to impact significantly upon the management of the patient in the emergency department."[71]

Santiago et al prospectively studied 208 children and adolescents presenting to the ED with psychiatric conditions.[62] Half of the patients underwent medical testing, 26% (55 patients) were medically indicated (ie, because of clinical suspicions based on the elicited history and physical examination), and 24% (54 patients) were obtained at the request of the mental health consultant. Only 3 patients had laboratory abnormalities that required further medical intervention, all of which were suspected on the basis of patient's presenting history and physical examination. Among patients for whom "routine testing" was performed, 9% (5 patients) had unsuspected abnormalities, none of which altered ED patient management.

Two recent studies of ED pediatric psychiatric patients have raised similar questions about the utility of routine medical testing and of "medical clearance" evaluations. Donofrio et al investigated the utility of extensive laboratory testing of these patients.[72] Of 1082 eligible patients, more than 68% had multiple laboratory testing, including urine toxicology, urinalysis, and blood tests for complete blood cell count, electrolytes, hepatic transferases, thyroid stimulating hormone, and syphilis. Of these tested patients, only 7 had a laboratory abnormality that resulted in a disposition change. Not only was the number of disposition changing laboratory abnormalities low, only 1 of these abnormalities was not suspected from the patient's history and physical examination. Santillanes et al studied all patients referred to their ED for medical screening clearance by a mobile psychiatric crisis team.[63] All patients had been placed on an involuntary psychiatric hold. Among 789 patients, 9.1% met criteria for a medical screening examination (ie, altered mental status, ingestion, hanging, traumatic injury, sexual assault, or medical complaints), and only 1.2% (9 patients) were admitted for medical reasons. Of these 9 patients, only 2 did not meet criteria for a medical screening evaluation, although both patients' conditions (possible disorientation and urinary tract infection in an HIV-positive patient) were suspected on the basis of a basic history and physical examination.

Diagnostic Radiology Testing and Medical Clearance

All studies of radiographic evaluation of psychiatric patients have been conducted with adults. Although central nervous system (CNS) abnormalities such as oligodendroglioma, glioblastoma, meningioma, intracerebral cysts, and hydrocephalus can present with primarily psychiatric symptoms,[73] other studies have found low rates of clinically significant findings on computed tomography (CT) scan. In 1 study of 127 young military recruits with new-onset psychosis, none had clinically significant findings on brain CT scans.[74] In another analysis of new-onset acute psychosis in patients admitted to a psychiatric unit, only 1.2% had clinically significant findings.[75] A larger study of 397 patients with a psychiatric presentation and no focal neurologic findings detected specific abnormalities in 5%, all of which had no relevance to the patient's condition. The pretest probability of a space occupying lesion or any relevant abnormality was no greater than finding one

in the general population.[76] These findings have led some authors to question the utility of routine brain CT scans.[64] Given the concerns about the long-term effects of radiation exposure on pediatric patients,[77–79] the utility of routine brain CT in children and adolescents is, at best, unclear.

Summary

The current body of literature supports focused medical assessments for ED psychiatric patients, in which laboratory and radiographic testing is obtained on the basis of a patient's history and physical examination. Routine diagnostic testing generally is low yield, costly, and unlikely to be of value or affect the disposition or management of ED psychiatric patients. When patients are clinically stable (ie, alert, cooperative, normal vital signs, with noncontributory history and physical examination and psychiatric symptoms), the ACEP states that routine laboratory testing need not be performed as part of the ED assessment.[61] If a discrepancy occurs between the ED and psychiatry clinicians regarding the appropriate ED medical evaluation of a psychiatric patient, direct communication between the ED and psychiatry attending physicians may be helpful. For patients with concerning findings on history and/or physical examination (eg, altered mental status or unexplained vital signs abnormalities) or with new-onset or acute changes in psychiatric symptoms, a careful evaluation for possible underlying medical conditions may be important.

SUICIDAL IDEATION AND SUICIDE ATTEMPTS

For an extended discussion on the assessment and management of suicidal adolescents, please refer to the AAP clinical report on suicide.[80]

Epidemiology and Risk Factors

Suicide is the third leading cause of death among people 10 to 24 years of age, accounting for more than 4000 deaths per year.[81] Although only a small percentage of suicide attempts lead to medical attention,[82] they nonetheless account for a significant number of ED visits.[83] Suicidal ideation in the absence of a suicide attempt is also a common chief complaint in pediatric EDs.

Approximately 16% of teenagers report having seriously considered suicide in the past year, 12.8% report having planned a suicide attempt, and 7.8% report having attempted suicide in the past year. Females are more likely to consider and attempt suicide, but males are more than 5 times more likely to die by suicide. The higher fatality rate among males is primarily accounted for by their use of more lethal means: males are more likely to attempt suicide via firearms and hanging, whereas females are more likely to attempt via overdose.[82]

American Indian/Alaska Native males have the highest suicide rates among ethnic groups. Non-Hispanic white males are also at increased risk.[81] Adolescents who have previous suicide attempts,[84] impulsivity, a mood or disruptive behavior disorder,[85] recent psychiatric hospitalization,[86,87] substance abuse,[88] a family history of suicide,[89] or a history of sexual or physical abuse[90]; are homeless/runaway[91]; or who identify as lesbian, gay, bisexual, or transgender[92] are also at higher risk for attempting and/or completing suicide. Suicide and suicide attempts are often precipitated by significant psychosocial stressors. These can include family conflict, the breakup of a romantic relationship, bullying, academic difficulties, or disciplinary actions/legal troubles. Younger patients tend to be triggered more often by family conflict, whereas older adolescents are more likely to cite peer or romantic conflicts as a precipitant.[93]

Evaluation

For patients reporting current or recent suicidal ideation and those who present after clear or suspected intentional self-injury, best practices include an evaluation by a clinician experienced in evaluating pediatric mental health conditions. Whenever concern for suicidal ideation or attempt is present, having the patient undergo a personal and belongings search, change into hospital attire, and be placed in as safe a setting as possible (eg, a room without easy access to medical equipment) with close staff supervision may be important.

Interviewing patients and caregivers both together and separately may be beneficial. Obtaining collateral information from caregivers or other individuals who may have knowledge about the patient's state of mind or the details of the event in question often has significant clinical utility, as patients frequently minimize the severity of their symptoms or the intention behind their acts. When interviewing adolescents alone, a discussion about the limits of patient confidentiality may facilitate an open and honest conversation. If there are significant concerns that the patient may be at high risk of harm to himself or herself or others (see "Determination of Level of Care"), the physician may decide to break doctor-patient confidentiality.

A thorough medical examination with careful evaluation for signs of self-injury or toxidromes and a mental status examination may be helpful. The mental status examination typically includes assessment of the patient's appearance, behavior, thought process, thought content (including presence or absence of hallucinations or delusions), mood and affect, and insight and judgment. An evaluation for delirium may also be indicated. When suspicion of delirium is high, a number of screening tools (eg, the Folstein Mini-Mental Status Examination)[94] may be useful.

Determination of Level of Care

No validated criteria exist for assessing level of risk for subsequent suicide or determining level of care. However, most experts agree that patients who continue to endorse a desire to die, remain agitated or severely hopeless, cannot engage in a discussion around safety planning, do not have an adequate support system, cannot be adequately monitored or receive follow-up care, or had a high-lethality suicide attempt or an attempt with clear expectation of death may be at high risk of suicide, and consideration should be given to admission to an inpatient psychiatric facility once medically cleared.[80] Additional risk factors, such as gender, comorbid substance abuse, and high levels of anger or impulsivity, may also be considered.

Patients who do not meet criteria for inpatient psychiatric hospitalization may be candidates for outpatient mental health treatment and intervention. Where available, partial hospital programs, intensive outpatient services, or in-home treatment/crisis stabilization interventions may be considered, especially when ED clinicians believe that a patient may benefit from more intensive or urgent treatment. Experts suggest that even patients who are deemed to be at relatively low risk of future suicidal or self-injurious acts benefit from outpatient follow-up. Whenever possible, a follow-up appointment with the medical home provider and an outpatient mental health clinician may be helpful. When outpatient mental health services are not readily accessible or wait times for intake appointments are considerable, the medical home providers can play an important bridging role. These providers may also continue to work with patients and families to promote engagement in and adherence to mental health treatment. Consensus expert opinion suggests direct contact with these outpatient providers, either by the mental health consultant or the ED clinician, documentation of this contact, and documentation of the discharge treatment plan.[95,96]

Discharge Planning

Some patients evaluated in the ED for suicidal ideation or a suicide attempt struggle to obtain follow-up care.[97,98] The ED visit may, therefore, be a valuable link in obtaining care for these patients. ED physicians may stress the importance of follow-up to both the patient and the family and attempt to identify and address barriers to subsequent treatment. Counseling and educating families about suicide risk and treatment may be beneficial. The greatest risk of reattempting suicide is in the months after an initial attempt. In addition, given that counseling takes time to work, emphasizing the importance of consistent follow-up may help patients and families.[99-101]

Although having a patient sign a no-suicide contract has not been shown to prevent subsequent suicides,[95] a safety-planning discussion is still an important element of ED care. A safety plan typically includes steps such as identification of (1) warning signs and potential triggers for recurrence of suicidal ideation; (2) coping strategies the patient may use if suicidal ideation returns; (3) healthy activities that could provide distraction or suppression of suicidal thoughts; (4) responsible social supports to which the patient could turn if suicidal urges recur; (5) contact information for professional supports, including instructions on how and when to reaccess emergency services; and (6) means restriction.[102]

Studies suggest that means restriction counseling may be a key component of discharge planning discussions. A large percentage of suicide attempts are impulsive. One study of patients 13 to 34 years of age who had near-lethal suicide attempts found that 24% of patients went from deciding to attempt suicide to implementing their plan within 0 to 5 minutes, 24% took 5 to 19 minutes, and 23% took 20 minutes to 1 hour.[103] Several studies have demonstrated that patients usually misjudge the lethality of their suicide attempts.[104–106] There is also a wide variation in the case-fatality rates of common methods of suicide attempt, ranging from 85% for gunshot wounds to 2% for ingestions and 1% for cutting.[107] It follows that interventions that decrease access to more lethal means and/or increase the amount of time and effort it takes for someone to carry out their suicidal plan and, as a result, increase the amount of time they have to reconsider or for someone to intervene may have a positive effect.

It may be helpful to ask and counsel patients and families about restricting access to potentially lethal means, including access to such means in the homes of friends or family. Means restriction counseling includes suggestions for securing knives, locking up medicines, and removing firearms. It is important to note that parents often underestimate their children's abilities to locate and access firearms and that simply having a gun in the home has been shown to double the risk of youth suicide.[108,109] Families who are reluctant to permanently remove firearms from the home may be open to temporarily relocating them (eg, for safe keeping with a relative, friend, or local law enforcement) until the child is in a better emotional state. If families insist on keeping firearms in the home, counseling them on how to store them as safely as possible (eg,

by locking all firearms unloaded in a specialized or tamper-proof safe, separately locking or temporarily removing ammunition, and restricting access to keys or lock combinations) may be helpful. Given the high rates of drug and alcohol intoxication among individuals who attempt and complete suicide, physicians may also want to suggest alcohol access restriction and, where indicated, referral for substance abuse counseling and treatment.

INVOLUNTARY HOSPITALIZATION

Under certain circumstances, physicians may insist on admission to a psychiatric inpatient unit over the objections of patients and/or their guardians. This type of admission is often referred to as a "psychiatric hold." Every state has laws governing involuntary admission for inpatient psychiatric hospitalization. Specific details of such laws vary from state to state, as do laws regarding confidentiality and an adolescent's right to seek mental health or substance abuse treatment without parental consent. As such, ED clinicians may benefit from familiarizing themselves with the relevant laws, statutes, and involuntary commitment procedures in the states in which they practice. In general, physicians are able to admit a patient against his or her will for a brief period of time, typically up to 72 hours, but ranging from 1 to 30 days. After that initial period, the psychiatric facility works to obtain a court order for civil commitment for ongoing treatment, if the patient and/or his or her guardian still object to the hospitalization. Criteria for involuntary hospitalization typically include the patient having a mental disorder and being at immediate risk of harm to self or others. Some states also allow for involuntary hospitalization if the patient is "gravely disabled." The criteria for being gravely disabled may include

the inability to meet basic physical needs including nourishment, shelter, safety, and/or basic medical care.[110] State laws differ over whether and, if so, at what age, assent for psychiatric admission must be obtained from minors. For more information on related state laws, contact the AAP Division of State Government Affairs at stgov@aap.org.

RESTRAINT OF THE AGITATED PATIENT

Restraint typically refers to methods of restricting an individual's freedom of movement, physical activity, or normal access to his or her body because of concerns about the person harming himself or herself or others. Some experts believe that interventions to help control a person's activity and behavior span a wide gamut, including verbal and behavioral strategies and favor the term "de-escalation interventions." Restraints may be used for either "medical" or "psychiatric" patients[111] and have been subdivided into verbal, chemical, and physical restraints. Chemical restraint, sometimes called "rapid tranquilization," is the use of pharmacologic means for the acute management of an agitated patient.[112]

Four guiding principles for working with agitated patients are as follows: (1) maximizing the safety of the patient and treating staff; (2) assisting the patient in managing his or her emotions and maintaining or regaining control of his or her behavior; (3) using the least restrictive, age-appropriate methods of restraint possible; and (4) minimizing coercive interventions that may exacerbate agitation.[113]

Verbal Restraint

The general principles of verbal restraint can be found across a wide variety of disciplines, including various psychotherapeutic approaches (eg, anger management, stress reduction), linguistic science, law enforcement, martial arts, and nursing.[113–116] Although consensus is that verbal restraint is preferable to chemical or physical restraint,[117] reviews of the literature find primarily case studies, with a paucity of rigorous studies of verbal restraint, and little on specific strategies or efficacy.[113,118] For example, although a study by Jonikas et al found a decrease in restraint use, it was not clear whether the decrease was attributable to staff training in de-escalation techniques or to crisis intervention training, which occurred at the same time.[119] Other protocols emphasize the importance of prevention in behavior management protocols.[115,120]

Detailed in Table 2 are Fishkind's "Ten Commandments of De-escalation," which incorporate practical, commonly used verbal restraint strategies.[112–114,121–123] Other strategies that may improve the chances of successful de-escalation include a calming physical environment with decreased sensory stimulation, rooms that have been "safety-proofed" (ie, removal or securing of objects that could be used as weapons) or close monitoring if this is not possible,[113] modifying or eliminating triggers of agitation (eg, an argumentative acquaintance, friend, or family or staff member, a long ED wait time),[117,124,125] and staff training in behavioral emergencies.[126,127] A child life specialist may also be an excellent resource to help calm an agitated child. To minimize risk to themselves, health care providers may take precautions, such as removing neck ties, stethoscopes, or securing long hair.

Chemical Restraint

All controlled trials of medications for acute agitation in the ED or inpatient psychiatric setting have been conducted with adults. In the literature, different terms have been used to describe the use of medications to treat agitation, violent or aggressive behavior, or excessive psychomotor activity (eg, psychosis or mania), including pharmacologic or chemical restraint[128] and rapid tranquilization.[112] The 3 most commonly used classes of drugs for this purpose are the typical antipsychotics, atypical antipsychotics, and benzodiazepines.[124,125,129]

Antipsychotics

Antipsychotics exert their effect primarily as CNS dopamine receptor antagonists.[130,131] "Low-potency" agents (eg, chlorpromazine and thioridazine) are more sedating, with fewer extrapyramidal symptoms than "high-potency" agents (eg, haloperidol and droperidol), which are less sedating but more likely to cause extrapyramidal symptoms.[132] The second-generation "atypical" antipsychotics are both serotonin-dopamine receptor antagonists.[130] Some consider aripiprazole the first "third-generation" antipsychotic, because it has partial dopamine receptor agonist activity, distinguishing it from other antipsychotics.[130,132,133] Antipsychotics also have varying ability to block other CNS neurotransmitters, which, combined with their disparate affinity for the postsynaptic D_2 receptors, account for the side effect profiles of each medication, which are discussed in greater detail below and in part II of this clinical report.[130,132]

Benzodiazepines

Benzodiazepines exert their CNS depressant effect by binding to presynaptic γ-aminobutyric acid (GABA) receptors. GABA, the primary CNS inhibitory neurotransmitter, decreases neuronal excitability. Benzodiazepines that have been commonly used to treat agitation are lorazepam, midazolam, and diazepam. Some experts prefer lorazepam for the management of acute agitation because it has fast onset of action, rapid and complete absorption, and no active metabolites. Midazolam may have a more rapid onset of action, but it also has a shorter duration of action. Diazepam has a longer half-life and erratic absorption when given intramuscularly (IM).[134,135]

Less Commonly Used Drugs

Other drugs also used for management of the agitated patient include the antihistamines diphenhydramine, and hydroxyzine and the α-adrenergic agent clonidine.[117,134,136,137] Diphenhydramine and hydroxyzine have sedative effects and are commonly used as nighttime sleep aids for insomnia. Clonidine is a presynaptic $α_2$-agonist, often used off-label for attention-deficit/hyperactivity disorder and opiate withdrawal. Doses are typically given at night because a significant effect of the medication is somnolence. Although there have been some controlled trials of diphenhydramine as a sedative,[138,139] clonidine has been less well studied.[140]

Drug Selection for Chemical Restraint

Drug selection for chemical restraint will depend largely on the specific details of the clinical scenario (Table 3) and collaboration among ED, psychiatric, and pharmacy colleagues. The combination of a benzodiazepine and an antipsychotic is a regimen frequently suggested by experts for acutely agitated patients, including children and adolescents[124,134,141–147] (Table 4). The route of administration, orally or IM, will depend on the patient's condition. The choice of medication(s) also depend(s) on the patient's current medications. If a patient is already on an antipsychotic, an additional or increased dose of that medication may be preferred.[61,145,147]

TABLE 2 Verbal Restraint Strategies

	Guiding Principle	Strategies, Suggestions, and Examples
1. Respect personal space	• Physical environment can make a patient feel threatened and/or vulnerable	• Two arms' length distance from patient • Unobstructed path out of room for both patient and ED staff
2. Minimize provocative behavior	• Posture and behavior can make a patient feel threatened and/or vulnerable • Concealed hands might imply a hidden weapon	• Calm demeanor and facial expressions • Visible, unclenched hands • Minimize defensive and/or confrontational body language, eg, hands on hips, arms crossed, aggressive posture, directly facing patient (instead, stand at an angle to the patient)
3. Establish verbal contact	• Multiple messages and "messengers" may confuse and agitate the patient	• Ideally, designate 1 or limited staff members to interact with the patient • Introduce self and staff to patient • Orient patient to ED and what to expect • Reassure patient that you will help him or her
4. Be concise	• Agitated patients may be impaired in verbally processing information • Repeating the message may be helpful	• Simple language, concise sentences • May be helpful to frequently repeat/reinforce message • Allow the patient adequate time to process information and respond
5. Identify patient's goals and expectations	• Use body language and verbal acknowledgment to convey	• "I'd like to know what you hoped or expected would happen here." • "What helps you at times like this?" • "Even if I can't provide it, I'd like to know so we can work on it."
6. Use active listening	• Convey to the patient that what he or she said is heard, understood, and valued	• "Tell me if I have this right …" • "What I heard is that …"
7. Agree <u>OR</u> agree to disagree	• Builds empathy for patient's situation • Minimize arguing	• (Agree) "What you're (specific example) going through/experiencing is difficult." • (Agree) "I think everyone would want (the same as you)." • (Agree) "That (what patient is complaining about) would upset other people too." • (Agree to disagree) "People have a lot of different views on (the focus of disagreement)."
8. Clear limits and expectations	• Reasonable and respectful limit setting • Set expectations of mutual respect and dignity, as well as consequences of unacceptable behaviors • Minimize "bargaining" • Coach patient on how to maintain control	• "We're here to help, but it's also important that we're safe with each other and respect each other." • "Safety comes first. If you're having a hard time staying safe or controlling your behavior, we will … (clear, nonpunitive consequence)." • "It'll help me if you (sit, calm yourself, etc). I can better understand you if you calmly tell me your concerns."
9. Offer choices and optimism	• Realistic choice helps empower the patient, regain control of himself/herself, and feel like a partner in the process • Link patient's goals to his or her action • Minimize deception and/or bargaining	• "Instead of (violence/agitation), what else could you do? Would (offer choice) help?" • Acts of kindness (eg, food, blanket, magazine, access to a phone or family member) may help • "You'd like (desired outcome). How can we work together to accomplish (their goal)?"
10. Debrief patient and staff	• If an involuntary intervention is indicated, debriefing may help restore working relationship with the patient and help staff plan for possible future interventions	• Explain why the intervention was necessary • Ask patient to explain his or her perspective • Review options/alternative strategies if the situation arises again

TABLE 3 Acute Agitation Medication Considerations

Suspected Etiology of Agitation	Symptom Severity	
	Mild/Moderate	Severe
Medical/intoxication	Benzodiazepine	Benzodiazepine first, consider adding antipsychotic
Psychiatric	Benzodiazepine or antipsychotic	Antipsychotic
Unknown	Dose of benzodiazepine or antipsychotic; consider a dose of the other medication if the first dose is not effective	

In situations in which the cause of agitation is unclear, many clinicians prefer a stepwise rather than combination approach, administering either a benzodiazepine or first-generation antipsychotic. When treating an agitated patient with a known psychiatric disorder, either a first- or second-generation antipsychotic is generally preferred.

TABLE 4 Medications for the Acutely Agitated Pediatric Patient[a]

Drug: How Supplied	Dose: Route of Administration	Time: Course/Onset Peak/Duration	Side Effects	Advantages	Comments
Benzodiazepines	See individual drugs	See individual drugs	• Sedation	• No EPS	• Contraindicated for intoxication due to other GABAergic drugs (eg, barbiturates, benzodiazepine abuse) • Use with caution in patients with respiratory compromise
			• Respiratory depression	• Preferred agent for many intoxications (eg, cocaine can cause seizures), withdrawal (eg, alcohol)	• Pregnancy class D
			• Hypotension • Paradoxical disinhibition (especially younger children and those with developmental disabilities)		
Lorazepam PO, IM, IV	0.05–0.1 mg/kg PO/IM/IV Usual dose: Adult: 2 mg PO/IM May repeat every 30–60 min	Onset: 5–10 min IV 15 min IM 20–30 min PO Peak: 30 min IV 1 h IM 2 h PO Duration: 2 h IV 6–8 h PO/IM			• Most commonly used drug for acute pediatric agitation
Midazolam PO, IM, IV	0.1 mg/kg PO/IM/IV Usual dose: Adult: 2 mg/PO/IM May repeat every 30–60 min	Onset: 5–10 min IV 10–15 min IM 20 min PO Peak: 5–15 min IV 15–30 min IM 1 h PO Duration: 3–4 h			
Antipsychotics First-generation, "typical antipsychotics"[b]			• Prolonged QT_c • Torsades de pointes • Dysrhythmias • Hypotension • Dystonia/EPS[c] • NMS		• Pregnancy class C
Haloperidol PO, IM	0.025–0.075 mg/kg IM/PO	Onset:		• Most commonly used drug in adults for acute agitation	• Lowers seizure threshold in animals

TABLE 4 Continued

Drug: How Supplied	Dose: Route of Administration	Time: Course/Onset Peak/ Duration	Side Effects	Advantages	Comments
	Usual dose:	20–30 min IM		• Second most commonly used drug in pediatric patients • Low addiction potential • High therapeutic index • Lack of tolerance	
	Child: 0.5–2 mg Adolescent: 2–5 mg Adult: 5–10 mg	45–60 min PO Peak: 60 min IM 3 h PO			
	May repeat IM every 20–30 min, PO every 60 min Usual total dose for tranquilization: 10–20 mg (adults)	Duration: 4–8 h			
Second-generation, "atypical antipsychotics"			• Same as first-generation drugs	• May be better tolerated and may cause fewer EPS than first-generation drugs • May have higher risk of dystonia, especially with higher doses and in male and/or young patients	• Pregnancy class C
			• Hyperglycemia		
			• Hyperprolactinemia		
Risperidone PO (liquid, tablet, ODT), IM	0.025–0.050 mg/kg PO/IM Usual dose: Child: 0.25–0.50 mg Adolescent: 0.5–1 mg May repeat PO every 60 min	Onset: 30–60 min PO Peak: 1–2 h PO			
Olanzepine PO (tablet, ODT) IM	0.1 mg/kg PO/IM	Onset:	• Postinjection delirium/sedation		• FDA investigating 2 unexplained deaths 3–4 d after appropriate IM dose • Consider monitoring for at least 3 h after IM injection
	Usual dose:	10–20 min IM			
	Child: 2.5 mg Adolescent: 5–10 mg Adult: 10 mg Maximum: 30 mg daily	20–30 min PO Peak: 15–45 min IM 6 h PO			
	May repeat IM every 20–30 min, PO every 30–45 min	Duration: 24 h			
Ziprasidone PO, IM	Usual dose: Younger adolescent (12–16 y): 10 mg Older adolescent (>16 y): 10–20 mg Maximum: 40 mg daily May repeat every 2 h	Onset: 60 min IM 4–5 h PO Peak: IM ≤60 min PO 6–8 h PO			
Combinations[d] Antipsychotic (typical) + benzodiazepine	Haloperidol + lorazepam or midazolam				

TABLE 4 Continued

Drug: How Supplied	Dose: Route of Administration	Time: Course/Onset Peak/Duration	Side Effects	Advantages	Comments
Antipsychotic (typical) + antihistamine	Haloperidol + diphenhydramine				
Antipsychotic (atypical) + benzodiazepine	Risperidone + lorazepam or midazolam				
Antipsychotic (atypical) + antihistamine	Risperidone + diphenhydramine				

Side effects for all drugs in the class are given in the row for the drug class. Side effects for a specific drug in the class are given in the row for the drug class. Pregnancy class is based on limited data, but according to Lexicomp (http://www.wolterskluwercdi.com/lexicomp-online/community-pharmacy/), the benzodiazepines are class D and the first- and second-generation antipsychotics listed in the table are class C (last accessed December 2, 2013). EPS, extrapyramidal symptom; FDA, US Food and Drug Administration; IV, intravenous; NMS, neuroleptic malignant syndrome; ODT, oral disintegrating tablet; PO, oral administration.

a This table provides suggestions for some of the most commonly used drugs for management of the agitated pediatric patient. Child (prepubertal) ages 6–12 y; adolescent 13 y or older. Adult doses have been used in adolescents with high BMI.[125] [129,135,143,148,149]

b Chlorpromazine, a phenothiazine that can be used to treat nausea/vomiting and intractable hiccups, has also been used with agitated patients[118,126,150] but has many of the same adverse effects as the other drugs (extrapyramidal/dystonic symptoms, neuroleptic malignant syndrome) as well as anticholinergic side effects and a decrease in the seizure threshold, without having any major advantages over the other drugs.

c EPSs include dystonia and akathisia, which may be treated with diphenhydramine (1.0 mg/kg/dose IV or PO, maximum 50 mg, usual dose in adults is 25 mg or 50 mg) and/or benztropine (1–2 mg in adults).

d Studies of the coadministration of these drugs have been reported. There may be research with other combinations studied in the future. Combinations of a butyrophenone (eg, haloperidol) and a benzodiazepine (eg, lorazepam) may be given together for an additive effect and may be administered in the same syringe. Data in some adult studies suggest that coadministration of a butyrophenone with a benzodiazepine may be more effective than either medication alone.

In other clinical situations, benzodiazepines alone may be the drug of choice. A common scenario is when the agitation is attributable to drug withdrawal or drug intoxication, especially drugs that decrease seizure threshold (eg, cocaine).[117,123,143,145,151] Because of their anticholinergic properties, antipsychotics may worsen the condition of patients who present with intoxication from drugs with anticholinergic properties (eg, hallucinogens) or with an anticholinergic delirium.[123,124,143]

Adverse Effects of and Clinical Monitoring During Chemical Restraint

Monitoring of patients who have received chemical restraint is similar to patients under physical restraint, which are discussed in detail in the subsequent section on physical restraint.[152–154] Medications used for chemical restraint may result in myriad adverse effects that benefit from close medical monitoring, including respiratory depression; hypotension; paradoxical behavioral disinhibition from benzodiazepines, especially in younger children and those with developmental disabilities[134,148,155]; dystonic reactions; orthostatic hypotension; sinus tachycardia; and other dysrhythmias attributable to antipsychotics.[61,130,132–134,149] Given these concerns, monitoring patients who receive antipsychotics may include close clinical observation, cardiorespiratory monitoring, pulse oximetry,[156] and/or an electrocardiogram, when and if the patient will tolerate them.

The most feared cardiac adverse effect of antipsychotics is a quinidine-like QT_c prolongation, resulting in dysrhythmias such as torsades de pointes. QT_c prolongation has been noted to occur with therapeutic dosing of antipsychotics and is possible with any antipsychotic medication. Potential risk factors for QT_c prolongation and dysrhythmia include coadministration with

TABLE 5 QT-Interval-Prolonging Medications in Pediatrics

Antiemetics	Cardiac	Antidepressants
• Ondansetron	• Adenosine	• Fluoxetine
• Dolasetron	• Dopamine	• Sertraline
Macrolides	• Epinephrine	• Paroxetine
• Azithromycin	• Dobutamine	• Venlafaxine
• Clarithromycin	• Quinidine	• Amitriptyline
• Erythromycin	• Procainamide	• Desipramine
Fluoroquinolones	• Flecainide	• Imipramine
• Ciprofloxacin	• Amiodarone	Mood-stabilizing agents
• Levofloxacin	• Bretylium	• Lithium
• Moxifloxacin	• Nicardipine	Antipsychotics
Other Antibiotics	• Sotalol	• Please see Table 4 at www. pediatrics.org/cgi/doi/10.1542/ peds.2016-1573
• Amantadine	Antihistamines	Other medications
• Trimethoprim-sulfamethoxazole	• Diphenhydramine	• Cisapride
Antimalarials	• Hydroxyzine	• Octreotide
• Quinine	• Loratadine	• Pentamidine
• Chloroquine	• Astemizole	• Tacrolimus
Neurologic	• Terfenadine	• Vasopressin
• fos-Phenytoin	Respiratory tract	
• Sumatriptan	• Albuterol	
• Zolmitriptan	• Terbutaline	
• Chloral hydrate	• Phenylephrine	
	• Pseudoephedrine	

This is an incomplete list of QT-interval-prolonging medications, limited to those that are commonly used in pediatrics. For a more comprehensive list, please refer to the cited references Haddad et al, Olsen et al, and Yap et al.[159–161]

other drugs that prolong the QT_c; administration of high doses of haloperidol[157,158]; and underlying medical illness (eg, electrolyte abnormalities, hepatic or renal impairment, heart failure, elderly, congenital long QT syndromes). Among the typical and atypical antipsychotics, thioridazine and ziprasidone, respectively, are associated with the greatest degrees of QTc prolongation.[130,134,145,159] Many other commonly used pediatric medications may prolong the QT_c, including antiemetics (eg, ondansetron), antibiotics such as macrolides, fluoroquinolones, and antifungal agents (eg, ketoconazole), antiarrhythmics, and other psychiatric medications (Table 5).[160–162] US Food and Drug Administration "black box" warnings have been issued for both droperidol and thioridazine because of this risk, although the actual clinical risk of and dangers from antipsychotic-induced cardiac dysrhythmias is unclear and is being vigorously debated.[61,134,149,163–168] However, since the black box

warning, the use of droperidol has declined exponentially.[114,117,125,157]

Acute dystonia usually presents as involuntary motor tics or spasms usually involving the face, neck, back, and limb muscles and may occur after antipsychotic administration. Oculogyric crisis is a specific form of acute dystonia, characterized by continuous rotatory eye movements. A rare, life-threatening form of dystonia is laryngeal dystonia, which presents as a choking sensation, difficulty breathing, or stridor. Acute dystonia is commonly treated with diphenhydramine or benztropine administered intravenously or IM. Additional doses of these medications may be indicated, given that their half-life is shorter than antipsychotics.

Among the less commonly used chemical restraint medications, antihistamines, such as diphenhydramine and hydroxyzine, can cause anticholinergic adverse effects including dry mouth, dry skin, urinary retention, constipation, flushing, dizziness,

mydriasis, delirium, and conduction abnormalities. Clonidine can result in hypotension and sedation.[136,137]

Physical Restraint

Physical restraint involves the use of mechanical restrictive devices to limit physical activity. Some differentiate physical restraint from "therapeutic holding," a method in which health care providers or caregivers hold the individual to contain the agitated behavior. Therapeutic holding is most often used in patients of younger ages as a method to help patients regain control of their behavior.[169] In 1 study, restraint was achieved with a mean of 3.5 people per patient, with patients held for an average of 21 minutes.[170] Another technique is seclusion, which refers to the placement of an individual in isolation in an enclosed space.[171]

The prevalence of the use of physical restraints among ED adult psychiatric patients varies widely, ranging from 8% to 59%.[172-177] There are much fewer data on the use of restraint among pediatric patients.[62,144]

Complications of Physical Restraints

Over the past 2 decades, there has been increasing concern regarding adverse events, including deaths, associated with the use of physical restraints in psychiatric facilities.[111] The New York State Commission on Quality of Care in 1994 reported 111 deaths over a 10-year period in New York facilities that were linked to the use of physical restraints.[178] Four years later, the *Hartford Courant* detailed 142 mortalities nationwide attributed to physical restraint use, with children disproportionately represented among the deaths.[179] Among child and adolescent psychiatric facilities, between 1993 and 2003, 45 deaths were ascribed to the use of restraints.[180]

There is also significant morbidity associated with the use of physical restraints. The most common complication is skin breakdown at the site of the restraint, with the possibility of neurovascular damage also occurring.[123] Rhabdomyolysis may occur, especially in patients who continue to struggle, which can lead to kidney failure. Other reported complications include accidental strangulation from vest restraints, brachial plexus injuries, electrolyte abnormalities, hyperthermia, deep vein thrombosis, pulmonary injury/diseases, and asphyxia.[171]

Physical Restraint Policies and Regulations

Because of increasing awareness of the potential complications and dangers of physical restraint, federal agencies and hospital accreditation organizations have developed formal regulations regarding physical restraint. In 2006, the Centers for Medicare and Medicaid Services published its most recent guidelines on patients' rights regarding the use of restraints and seclusion.[152] The US General Accounting Office and The Joint Commission (formerly, The Joint Commission for the Accreditation of Health Care Organizations) have published similar policies and regulations.[153,181] Medical professional organizations, including the AAP,[182] the ACEP,[183] the American Academy of Child and Adolescent Psychiatry,[115] and the American Medical Association,[184] all have policies supporting these regulations, the principles of the humane and least restrictive possible use of restraint, and the need for further research in this area.

The use of restraints remains controversial. Although restraints can be a component of patient treatment in certain situations,[61,182,185] the use of restraints and seclusion has been questioned by some. According to the National Association of State Mental Health Program Directors, "Seclusion and restraint should be considered a security measure, not a form of

'medical treatment' that should only be used as 'last resort measure.'"[186] Adding to the complexity of this issue, it is important to keep in mind the potential liability for failure to restrain a patient who loses control and injures someone and/or destroys property, which may be greater than the liability for appropriately restraining an aggressive/violent patient.[114]

Indications for the Use of Physical Restraints

There are specific indications for the use of restraints: when the patient is an acute danger to harm himself/herself or others,[111,123,124,176,187] to prevent significant disruption of the treatment plan including considerable disruption of property, and when other less restrictive measures have failed or are not possible options.[61,129,182,185] It is unethical to use restraints for convenience or punishment and when prohibited by law or regulation or by untrained personnel.[185]

Techniques for Application of Physical Restraints

If other less restrictive measures have failed, nursing staff may initiate restraint use in extenuating circumstances, with a physician or other licensed independent practitioner performing a face-to-face evaluation and reviewing and approving the order within 1 hour.[123] Sometimes, the mere show of force by a cohort of trained professionals may induce the agitated/violent individual to deescalate, rendering restraint unnecessary. When possible, 5 or more individuals may be included in the application of physical restraints. One person supports the head, and 4 other individuals secure each limb. Experts suggest applying restraints securely to each extremity, then to the bed frame rather than the side rails. Maximizing patient safety includes allowing the patient's head to rotate freely, elevating the head of the bed, if possible, to decrease the risk of

aspiration. If a female patient is being restrained, having at least 1 female on the restraint team may be helpful. In some cases, a "sandwiching" technique between 2 mattresses has been used, with careful monitoring for risk for asphyxia.[122]

Although definitive studies evaluating the best and safest restraint practices are lacking, experts suggest the use of age-appropriate or leather restraints. Restraints made of softer, makeshift, or other materials may be less effective and more likely to result in patient injury. After their review of deaths of patients who were being physically restrained, The Joint Commission made the following suggestions[188]:

- Proper staff training on alternatives to and proper application of physical restraints

- Continuous monitoring of restrained patients

- Supine positioning, with

  o the head of the bed elevated, and

  o free cervical range of motion, to decrease aspiration risk

- Prone positioning may be used if other measures have failed or are not possible. Deaths have been associated with its use. If used, helpful strategies include the following:

  o monitoring for airway obstruction,

  o minimizing or eliminating pressure on the neck and back, and

  o discontinuing as soon as possible

- Minimize covering of the patient's face or head

- Minimize the use of high vests, waist restraints, and beds with unprotected, split side rails

- Remove smoking materials from the patient

- Minimize restraint of medically compromised or unstable patients

- In cases of agitation because of suspected illicit stimulant use, chemical restraint may be preferable, as a rapid increase in serum potassium secondary to rhabdomyolysis may result in cardiac arrest.

The Joint Commission guidelines also include a schedule for the evaluation of the need for and ordering of restraints, as well as patient monitoring and assistance, by a licensed independent practitioner (licensed independent practitioner; eg, physician, nurse practitioner, physician assistant) and the staff members who apply or monitor the restrained patient (Table 6).[153]

Techniques for Removal of Restraints

Before removal of restraints, it may be helpful to inform the patient of what behavior is expected to minimize the chance that restraints will be reapplied. The same number of staff members that was used to apply the restraints may be present when the restraints are removed. A common strategy is removing 1 restraint at a time, usually starting with 1 lower extremity, next the other leg, then 1 of the upper extremities, and then the other arm, to monitor the patient's response. If the patient becomes violent or disruptive, then the limb restraint(s) may be reapplied; if the patient is cooperative, the restraint removal process may continue.

COORDINATION WITH THE MEDICAL HOME

Experts strongly endorse the benefits of a "medical home"—patient-centered care that is coordinated and integrated by the patient's personal physician, especially for high-risk and/or high-utilization patients.[189,190] The AAP also supports the integration of mental health treatment within the medical home so that youth can "benefit from the strength and skills of the primary care clinician in establishing rapport with the child and family, using the primary care clinicians' unique

TABLE 6 The Joint Commission Requirements for Evaluating and Ordering Restraint

	Age		
	<9 y	9–17 y	>18 y
LIP in-person evaluation to order restraint	Within 1 h of placement of restraints	Within 1 h of placement of restraints	Within 1 h of placement of restraints
Renew restraint order by qualified staff	Every 1 h	Every 2 h	Every 4 h
LIP in-person evaluation to renew restraint order	Every 4 h	Every 4 h	Every 8 h
Assessments every 15 min (all ages)	• Vital signs • Signs of injury due to restraint or seclusion • Nutrition/hydration • Extremities circulation and range of motion • Hygiene and elimination (bowel/bladder) • Physical and psychological status/comfort • Readiness to discontinue restraint		

LIP, licensed independent practitioner.

opportunities to engage children and families in mental health care without stigma."[191] Unfortunately, nearly half of adolescents lack a medical home, with those with mental health problems being even less likely to have the benefit of a medical home.[192] Whenever possible, best practices include consulting primary care pediatricians regarding level-of-care determination, follow-up planning, and referrals. When referral to an outpatient mental health specialist is indicated, providers who are either colocated within or have established collaborations with the medical home may be strongly considered. The medical home provider can follow up with the family to help facilitate and encourage adequate aftercare. In circumstances when a referral to a mental health specialist or higher level of psychiatric care is either not indicated or unavailable, encouraging patients to seek follow-up treatment through their medical home may be beneficial.

There are likely additional health benefits to involving a child's medical home in the aftercare plan. Although data in children are limited, there is a body of data demonstrating that access to primary care may be problematic and morbidity and

mortality are increased in adults with psychiatric illness. In fact, studies suggest that the life expectancy of adults with severe psychiatric illness is between 13 and 35 years lower than their peers without psychiatric illness.[193] Pediatric studies have demonstrated increased rates of obesity and worse self-reported health in adolescents with mental illness.[194] Youth with attention-deficit/hyperactivity disorder and developmental disabilities, such as autism spectrum disorders, have been found to have elevated rates of medical conditions including asthma, frequent ear infections, severe headaches or migraines, and seizures. They also have increased utilization of specialists and higher unmet health needs, including delays in care and inability to afford prescriptions.[150] Therefore, emergency physicians may have a significant effect on children presenting with mental health concerns by referring and encouraging them to participate in coordinated care through a suitable medical home.

LEAD AUTHORS

Thomas H. Chun, MD, MPH, FAAP
Sharon E. Mace, MD, FAAP, FACEP
Emily R. Katz, MD, FAAP

ABBREVIATIONS

AAP: American Academy of Pediatrics
ACEP: American College of Emergency Physicians
CNS: central nervous system
CT: computed tomography
ED: emergency department
GABA: γ-aminobutyric acid
IM: intramuscularly

REFERENCES

1. World Health Organization. *The Global Burden of Disease: 2004 Update.* Geneva, Switzerland: World Health Organization Press; 2008

2. Merikangas KR, He JP, Burstein M, et al. Lifetime prevalence of mental disorders in U.S. adolescents: results from the National Comorbidity Survey Replication—Adolescent Supplement (NCS-A). *J Am Acad Child Adolesc Psychiatry.* 2010;49(10):980–989

3. National Institute of Mental Health, Substance Abuse and Mental Health Services Administration, Department of Health and Human Services. *Mental Health: A Report of the Surgeon General. Executive Summary.* Rockville, MD: US Department of Health and Human Services; 1999

4. Grupp-Phelan J, Delgado SV, Kelleher KJ. Failure of psychiatric referrals from the pediatric emergency department. *BMC Emerg Med.* 2007;7:12

5. Grupp-Phelan J, Wade TJ, Pickup T, et al. Mental health problems in children and caregivers in the emergency department setting. *J Dev Behav Pediatr.* 2007;28(1):16–21

6. Fein JA, Pailler ME, Barg FK, et al. Feasibility and effects of a Web-based adolescent psychiatric assessment administered by clinical staff in the pediatric emergency department. *Arch Pediatr Adolesc Med.* 2010;164(12):1112–1117

7. Sheldrick RC, Merchant S, Perrin EC. Identification of developmental-behavioral problems in primary care: a systematic review. *Pediatrics.* 2011;128(2):356–363

8. Committee on Psychosocial Aspects of Child and Family Health and Task Force on Mental Health. Policy statement—The future of pediatrics: mental health competencies for pediatric primary care. *Pediatrics.* 2009;124(1):410–421

9. Foy JM, Kelleher KJ, Laraque D; American Academy of Pediatrics Task Force on Mental Health. Enhancing pediatric mental health care: strategies for preparing a primary care practice. *Pediatrics.* 2010;125(suppl 3):S87–S108

10. Dolan MA, Mace SE; American Academy of Pediatrics, Committee on Pediatric Emergency Medicine; American College of Emergency Physicians and Pediatric Emergency Medicine Committee. Pediatric mental health emergencies in the emergency medical services system. *Pediatrics.* 2006;118(4):1764–1767

11. American College of Emergency Physicians, Pediatric Emergency Medicine Committee. American Academy of Pediatrics, Committee on Pediatric Emergency Medicine. Pediatric mental health emergencies in the emergency medical services system. *Ann Emerg Med.* 2006;48(4):484–486

12. Sills MR, Bland SD. Summary statistics for pediatric psychiatric visits to US emergency departments, 1993–1999. *Pediatrics.* 2002;110(4). Available at: www.pediatrics.org/cgi/content/full/110/4/e40

13. Goldstein AB, Silverman MA, Phillips S, Lichenstein R. Mental health visits in a pediatric emergency department and their relationship to the school calendar. *Pediatr Emerg Care.* 2005;21(10):653–657

14. Larkin GL, Claassen CA, Emond JA, Pelletier AJ, Camargo CA. Trends in U.S. emergency department visits for mental health conditions, 1992 to 2001. *Psychiatr Serv.* 2005;56(6):671–677

15. Grupp-Phelan J, Harman JS, Kelleher KJ. Trends in mental health and chronic condition visits by children presenting for care at U.S. emergency departments. *Public Health Rep.* 2007;122(1):55–61

16. Mahajan P, Alpern ER, Grupp-Phelan J, et al; Pediatric Emergency Care Applied Research Network (PECARN). Epidemiology of psychiatric-related visits to emergency departments in a multicenter collaborative research pediatric network. *Pediatr Emerg Care.* 2009;25(11):715–720

17. Newton AS, Ali S, Johnson DW, et al. A 4-year review of pediatric mental health emergencies in Alberta. *CJEM.* 2009;11(5):447–454

18. Pittsenbarger ZE, Mannix R. Trends in pediatric visits to the emergency department for psychiatric illnesses. *Acad Emerg Med.* 2014;21(1):25–30

19. Anderson LE, Chen ML, Perrin JM, Van Cleave J. Outpatient visits and medication prescribing for us children with mental health conditions. *Pediatrics.* 2015;136(5). Available at: www.pediatrics.org/cgi/content/full/136/5/e1178

20. Olfson M, Blanco C, Wang S, Laje G, Correll CU. National trends in the mental health care of children, adolescents, and adults by office-based physicians. *JAMA Psychiatry.* 2014;71(1):81–90

21. American College of Emergency Physicians. *ACEP Psychiatric and Substance Abuse Survey 2008.* Irving, TX: American College of Emergency Physicians; 2008

22. American Medical Association. *Report of the Council on Medical Service: Access to Psychiatric Beds and Impact on Emergency Medicine.* Chicago, IL: American Medical Association; 2007

23. Claudius I, Donofrio JJ, Lam CN, Santillanes G. Impact of boarding pediatric psychiatric patients on a medical ward. *Hosp Pediatr.* 2014;4(3):125–132

24. Kutscher B. Bedding, not boarding. Psychiatric patients boarded in hospital EDs create crisis for patient care and hospital finances. *Mod Healthc.* 2013;43(46):15–17

25. Nicks BA, Manthey DM. The impact of psychiatric patient boarding in emergency departments. *Emerg Med Int.* 2012;2012:360308

26. Wharff EA, Ginnis KB, Ross AM, Blood EA. Predictors of psychiatric boarding in the pediatric emergency department: implications for emergency care. *Pediatr Emerg Care.* 2011;27(6):483–489

27. Biros MH, Hick K, Cen YY, et al. Occult depressive symptoms in adolescent emergency department patients. *Arch Pediatr Adolesc Med.* 2008;162(8):769–773

28. Scott EG, Luxmore B, Alexander H, Fenn RL, Christopher NC. Screening for adolescent depression in a pediatric emergency department. *Acad Emerg Med.* 2006;13(5):537–542

29. Ramsawh HJ, Chavira DA, Kanegaye JT, Ancoli-Israel S, Madati PJ, Stein MB. Screening for adolescent anxiety disorders in a pediatric emergency department. *Pediatr Emerg Care.* 2012;28(10):1041–1047

30. Winston FK, Kassam-Adams N, Garcia-España F, Ittenbach R, Cnaan A. Screening for risk of persistent posttraumatic stress in injured children and their parents. *JAMA.* 2003;290(5):643–649

31. Rhodes KV, Gordon JA, Lowe RA; Society for Academic Emergency Medicine Public Health and Education Task Force Preventive Services Work Group. Preventive care in the emergency department, Part I: Clinical preventive services—are they relevant to emergency medicine? Society for Academic Emergency Medicine Public Health and Education Task Force Preventive Services Work Group. *Acad Emerg Med.* 2000;7(9):1036–1041

32. Downey LV, Zun LS, Burke T. Undiagnosed mental illness in the emergency department. *J Emerg Med.* 2012;43(5):876–882

33. Pan YJ, Lee MB, Chiang HC, Liao SC. The recognition of diagnosable psychiatric disorders in suicide cases' last medical contacts. *Gen Hosp Psychiatry.* 2009;31(2):181–184

34. Porter SC, Fein JA, Ginsburg KR. Depression screening in adolescents with somatic complaints presenting to the emergency department. *Ann Emerg Med.* 1997;29(1):141–145

35. Slap GB, Vorters DF, Chaudhuri S, Centor RM. Risk factors for attempted suicide during adolescence. *Pediatrics.* 1989;84(5):762–772

36. Slap GB, Vorters DF, Khalid N, Margulies SR, Forke CM. Adolescent suicide attempters: do physicians recognize them? *J Adolesc Health.* 1992;13(4):286–292

37. Luoma JB, Martin CE, Pearson JL. Contact with mental health and primary care providers before suicide: a review of the evidence. *Am J Psychiatry.* 2002;159(6):909–916

38. Gairin I, House A, Owens D. Attendance at the accident and emergency department in the year before suicide: retrospective study. *Br J Psychiatry.* 2003;183:28–33

39. Garbrick L, Levitt MA, Barrett M, Graham L. Agreement between emergency physicians and psychiatrists regarding admission decisions. *Acad Emerg Med.* 1996;3(11):1027–1030

40. Tse SK, Wong TW, Lau CC, Yeung WS, Tang WN. How good are accident and emergency doctors in the evaluation of psychiatric patients? *Eur J Emerg Med.* 1999;6(4):297–300

41. Cronholm PF, Barg FK, Pailler ME, Wintersteen MB, Diamond GS, Fein JA. Adolescent depression: views of health care providers in a pediatric emergency department. *Pediatr Emerg Care*. 2010;26(2):111–117

42. Habis A, Tall L, Smith J, Guenther E. Pediatric emergency medicine physicians' current practices and beliefs regarding mental health screening. *Pediatr Emerg Care*. 2007;23(6):387–393

43. Hoyle JD Jr, White LJ; Emergency Medical Services for Children. Health Resources Services Administration. Maternal and Child Health Bureau. National Association of EMS Physicians. Treatment of pediatric and adolescent mental health emergencies in the United States: current practices, models, barriers, and potential solutions. *Prehosp Emerg Care*. 2003;7(1):66–73

44. Hoyle JD Jr, White LJ. Pediatric mental health emergencies: summary of a multidisciplinary panel. *Prehosp Emerg Care*. 2003;7(1):60–65

45. Santucci KA, Sather J, Baker MD. Emergency medicine training programs' educational requirements in the management of psychiatric emergencies: current perspective. *Pediatr Emerg Care*. 2003;19(3):154–156

46. Horwitz SM, Storfer-Isser A, Kerker BD, et al. Barriers to the identification and management of psychosocial problems: changes from 2004 to 2013. *Acad Pediatr*. 2015;15(6):613–620

47. Al-Osaimi FD, Al-Haidar FA. Assessment of pediatricians' need for training in child psychiatry. *J Family Community Med*. 2008;15(2):71–75

48. Riba M, Hale M. Medical clearance: fact or fiction in the hospital emergency room. *Psychosomatics*. 1990;31(4):400–404

49. Glauser JG. Functional versus organic illness: identifying medical illness in patients with psychiatric symptoms. *Crit Decis Emerg Med*. 2005;19(6):12–21

50. Newcomer JW. Metabolic considerations in the use of antipsychotic medications: a review of recent evidence. *J Clin Psychiatry*. 2007;68(suppl 1):20–27

51. Allen MH, Currier GW. Medical assessment in the psychiatric emergency service. *New Dir Ment Health Serv*. 1999;82(82):21–28

52. Krummel S, Kathol RG. What you should know about physical evaluations in psychiatric patients. Results of a survey. *Gen Hosp Psychiatry*. 1987;9(4):275–279

53. Hall RC, Gardner ER, Stickney SK, LeCann AF, Popkin MK. Physical illness manifesting as psychiatric disease. II. Analysis of a state hospital inpatient population. *Arch Gen Psychiatry*. 1980;37(9):989–995

54. Henneman PL, Mendoza R, Lewis RJ. Prospective evaluation of emergency department medical clearance. *Ann Emerg Med*. 1994;24(4):672–677

55. Olshaker JS, Browne B, Jerrard DA, Prendergast H, Stair TO. Medical clearance and screening of psychiatric patients in the emergency department. *Acad Emerg Med*. 1997;4(2):124–128

56. Herridge CF. Physical disorders in psychiatric illness. A study of 209 consecutive admissions. *Lancet*. 1960;2(7157):949–951

57. Worster A, Elliott L, Bose TJ, Chemeris E. Reliability of vital signs measured at triage. *Eur J Emerg Med*. 2003;10(2):108–110

58. Tintinalli JE, Peacock FW IV, Wright MA. Emergency medical evaluation of psychiatric patients. *Ann Emerg Med*. 1994;23(4):859–862

59. Pinto T, Poynter B, Durbin J. Medical clearance in the psychiatric emergency setting: a call for more standardization. *Healthc Q*. 2010;13(2):77–82

60. Zun LS. Evidence-based evaluation of psychiatric patients. *J Emerg Med*. 2005;28(1):35–39

61. Lukens TW, Wolf SJ, Edlow JA, et al; American College of Emergency Physicians Clinical Policies Subcommittee (Writing Committee) on Critical Issues in the Diagnosis and Management of the Adult Psychiatric Patient in the Emergency Department. Clinical policy: critical issues in the diagnosis and management of the adult psychiatric patient in the emergency department. *Ann Emerg Med*. 2006;47(1):79–99

62. Santiago LI, Tunik MG, Foltin GL, Mojica MA. Children requiring psychiatric consultation in the pediatric emergency department: epidemiology, resource utilization, and complications. *Pediatr Emerg Care*. 2006;22(2):85–89

63. Santillanes G, Donofrio JJ, Lam CN, Claudius I. Is medical clearance necessary for pediatric psychiatric patients? *J Emerg Med*. 2014;46(6):800–807

64. Glauser J, Marshall M. Medical clearance of psychiatric patients. *Emerg Med Rep*. 2011;32(23):273–283

65. Shah SJ, Fiorito M, McNamara RM. A screening tool to medically clear psychiatric patients in the emergency department. *J Emerg Med*. 2012;43(5):871–875

66. Broderick KB, Lerner EB, McCourt JD, Fraser E, Salerno K. Emergency physician practices and requirements regarding the medical screening examination of psychiatric patients. *Acad Emerg Med*. 2002;9(1):88–92

67. Korn CS, Currier GW, Henderson SO. "Medical clearance" of psychiatric patients without medical complaints in the emergency department. *J Emerg Med*. 2000;18(2):173–176

68. Janiak BD, Atteberry S. Medical clearance of the psychiatric patient in the emergency department. *J Emerg Med*. 2012;43(5):866–870

69. Shihabuddin BS, Hack CM, Sivitz AB. Role of urine drug screening in the medical clearance of pediatric psychiatric patients: is there one? *Pediatr Emerg Care*. 2013;29(8):903–906

70. Fortu JM, Kim IK, Cooper A, Condra C, Lorenz DJ, Pierce MC. Psychiatric patients in the pediatric emergency department undergoing routine urine toxicology screens for medical clearance: results and use. *Pediatr Emerg Care*. 2009;25(6):387–392

71. Tenenbein M. Do you really need that emergency drug screen? *Clin Toxicol (Phila)*. 2009;47(4):286–291

72. Donofrio JJ, Santillanes G, McCammack BD, et al. Clinical utility of screening laboratory tests in pediatric psychiatric patients presenting to the

emergency department for medical clearance. *Ann Emerg Med.* 2013

73. Bunevicius A, Deltuva VP, Deltuviene D, Tamasauskas A, Bunevicius R. Brain lesions manifesting as psychiatric disorders: eight cases. *CNS Spectr.* 2008;13(11):950–958

74. Bain BK. CT scans of first-break psychotic patients in good general health. *Psychiatr Serv.* 1998;49(2):234–235

75. Gewirtz G, Squires-Wheeler E, Sharif Z, Honer WG. Results of computerised tomography during first admission for psychosis. *Br J Psychiatry.* 1994;164(6):789–795

76. Agzarian MJ, Chryssidis S, Davies RP, Pozza CH. Use of routine computed tomography brain scanning of psychiatry patients. *Australas Radiol.* 2006;50(1):27–28

77. Brody AS, Frush DP, Huda W, Brent RL; American Academy of Pediatrics Section on Radiology. Radiation risk to children from computed tomography. *Pediatrics.* 2007;120(3):677–682

78. Newman B, Callahan MJ. ALARA (as low as reasonably achievable) CT 2011--executive summary. *Pediatr Radiol.* 2011;41(Suppl 2):453–455

79. Mathews JD, Forsythe AV, Brady Z, et al. Cancer risk in 680,000 people exposed to computed tomography scans in childhood or adolescence: data linkage study of 11 million Australians. *BMJ.* 2013;346:f2360

80. Shain BN; American Academy of Pediatrics Committee on Adolescence. Suicide and suicide attempts in adolescents. *Pediatrics.* 2016;138(1):e20161420

81. Centers for Disease Conrol and Prevention. Leading Causes of Death 1999–2010. Web-Based Injury Statistics Query and Reporting System (WISQARS) [database]. Available at: https://www.cdc.gov/injury/wisqars/. Accessed April 14, 2012

82. Eaton DK, Kann L, Kinchen S, et al; Centers for Disease Control and Prevention (CDC). Youth risk behavior surveillance—United States, 2011. *MMWR Surveill Summ.* 2012;61(4):1–162

83. Ting SA, Sullivan AF, Boudreaux ED, Miller I, Camargo CA Jr. Trends in US emergency department visits for attempted suicide and self-inflicted injury, 1993–2008. *Gen Hosp Psychiatry.* 2012;34(5):557–565

84. Shaffer D, Craft L. Methods of adolescent suicide prevention. *J Clin Psychiatry.* 1999;60(suppl 2):70–74, discussion 75–76, 113–116

85. Foley DL, Goldston DB, Costello EJ, Angold A. Proximal psychiatric risk factors for suicidality in youth: the Great Smoky Mountains Study. *Arch Gen Psychiatry.* 2006;63(9):1017–1024

86. Lewinsohn PM, Rohde P, Seeley JR. Psychosocial risk factors for future adolescent suicide attempts. *J Consult Clin Psychol.* 1994;62(2):297–305

87. Shaffer D, Gould MS, Fisher P, et al. Psychiatric diagnosis in child and adolescent suicide. *Arch Gen Psychiatry.* 1996;53(4):339–348

88. Esposito-Smythers C, Spirito A. Adolescent substance use and suicidal behavior: a review with implications for treatment research. *Alcohol Clin Exp Res.* 2004;28(suppl 5):77S–88S

89. McKeown RE, Garrison CZ, Cuffe SP, Waller JL, Jackson KL, Addy CL. Incidence and predictors of suicidal behaviors in a longitudinal sample of young adolescents. *J Am Acad Child Adolesc Psychiatry.* 1998;37(6):612–619

90. Brown J, Cohen P, Johnson JG, Smailes EM. Childhood abuse and neglect: specificity of effects on adolescent and young adult depression and suicidality. *J Am Acad Child Adolesc Psychiatry.* 1999;38(12):1490–1496

91. Smart RG, Walsh GW. Predictors of depression in street youth. *Adolescence.* 1993;28(109):41–53

92. McDaniel JS, Purcell D, D'Augelli AR. The relationship between sexual orientation and risk for suicide: research findings and future directions for research and prevention. *Suicide Life Threat Behav.* 2001;31(Suppl):84–105

93. Olverholser J. Predisposing factors in suicide attempts: life stressors. In: Spirito A, Overholser JC, eds. *Evaluating and Treating Adolescent Suicide Attempters: From Research to Practice.* New York, NY: Academic Press; 2002:42–54

94. Folstein MF, Folstein SE, McHugh PR. "Mini-Mental State." A practical method for grading the cognitive state of patients for the clinician. *J Psychiatr Res.* 1975;12(3):189–198

95. American Academy of Child and Adolescent Psychiatry. Practice parameter for the assessment and treatment of children and adolescents with suicidal behavior. *J Am Acad Child Adolesc Psychiatry.* 2001;40(suppl 7):24S–51S

96. Fontanella CA, Bridge JA, Campo JV. Psychotropic medication changes, polypharmacy, and the risk of early readmission in suicidal adolescent inpatients. *Ann Pharmacother.* 2009;43(12):1939–1947

97. Spirito A, Lewander WJ, Levy S, Kurkjian J, Fritz G. Emergency department assessment of adolescent suicide attempters: factors related to short-term follow-up outcome. *Pediatr Emerg Care.* 1994;10(1):6–12

98. Trautman PD, Stewart N, Morishima A. Are adolescent suicide attempters noncompliant with outpatient care? *J Am Acad Child Adolesc Psychiatry.* 1993;32(1):89–94

99. Prinstein MJ, Nock MK, Simon V, Aikins JW, Cheah CS, Spirito A. Longitudinal trajectories and predictors of adolescent suicidal ideation and attempts following inpatient hospitalization. *J Consult Clin Psychol.* 2008;76(1):92–103

100. Spirito A, Plummer B, Gispert M, et al. Adolescent suicide attempts: outcomes at follow-up. *Am J Orthopsychiatry.* 1992;62(3):464–468

101. Yen S, Weinstock LM, Andover MS, Sheets ES, Selby EA, Spirito A. Prospective predictors of adolescent suicidality: 6-month post-hospitalization follow-up. *Psychol Med.* 2013;43(5):983–993

102. Sher L, LaBode V. Teaching health care professionals about suicide safety planning. *Psychiatr Danub.* 2011;23(4):396–397

103. Simon OR, Swann AC, Powell KE, Potter LB, Kresnow MJ, O'Carroll PW. Characteristics of impulsive suicide attempts and attempters. *Suicide Life Threat Behav.* 2001;32(suppl 1):49–59

104. Brown GK, Henriques GR, Sosdjan D, Beck AT. Suicide intent and accurate expectations of lethality: predictors of medical lethality of suicide attempts. *J Consult Clin Psychol.* 2004;72(6):1170–1174

105. Swahn MH, Potter LB. Factors associated with the medical severity of suicide attempts in youths and young adults. *Suicide Life Threat Behav.* 2001;32(suppl 1):21–29

106. Plutchik R, van Praag HM, Picard S, Conte HR, Korn M. Is there a relation between the seriousness of suicidal intent and the lethality of the suicide attempt? *Psychiatry Res.* 1989;27(1):71–79

107. Vyrostek SB, Annest JL, Ryan GW. Surveillance for fatal and nonfatal injuries—United States, 2001. *MMWR Surveill Summ.* 2004;53(7):1–57

108. Baxley F, Miller M. Parental misperceptions about children and firearms. *Arch Pediatr Adolesc Med.* 2006;160(5):542–547

109. Brent DA, Perper JA, Allman CJ, Moritz GM, Wartella ME, Zelenak JP. The presence and accessibility of firearms in the homes of adolescent suicides. A case-control study. *JAMA.* 1991;266(21):2989–2995

110. Treatment Advocacy Center. State Standards Charts for Assisted Treatment. Civil Commitment Criteria and Initiation Procedures by State. Available at: www.treatmentadvocacy center.org/storage/documents/State_ Standards_Charts_for_Assisted_ Treatment_-_Civil_Commitment_ Criteria_and_Initiation_Procedures. pdf. Accessed July 9, 2015

111. Glezer A, Brendel RW. Beyond emergencies: the use of physical restraints in medical and psychiatric settings. *Harv Rev Psychiatry.* 2010;18(6):353–358

112. Hockberger RS. Richards J. Thought disorders. In: Marx JA, Hockberger R, Walls RM, eds. *Rosen's Emergency Medicine: Concepts and Clinical Practice.* Philadelphia, PA: Saunders; 2014:1460–1465

113. Richmond JS, Berlin JS, Fishkind AB, et al. Verbal de-escalation of the agitated patient: consensus statement of the American Association for Emergency Psychiatry Project BETA De-escalation Workgroup. *West J Emerg Med.* 2012;13(1):17–25

114. Heiner JD, Moore GP. The combative patient. In: Marx JA, Hockberger R, Walls RM, eds. *Rosen's Emergency Medicine: Concepts and Clinical Practice.* Philadelphia, PA: Saunders; 2014:2414–2421

115. Masters KJ, Bellonci C, Bernet W, et al; American Academy of Child and Adolescent Psychiatry. Practice parameter for the prevention and management of aggressive behavior in child and adolescent psychiatric institutions, with special reference to seclusion and restraint. *J Am Acad Child Adolesc Psychiatry.* 2002;41(suppl 2):4S–25S

116. Stevenson S. Heading off violence with verbal de-escalation. *J Psychosoc Nurs Ment Health Serv.* 1991;29(9):6–10

117. Adimando AJ, Poncin YB, Baum CR. Pharmacological management of the agitated pediatric patient. *Pediatr Emerg Care.* 2010;26(11):856–860, quiz 861–863

118. Delaney KR. Evidence base for practice: reduction of restraint and seclusion use during child and adolescent psychiatric inpatient treatment. *Worldviews Evid Based Nurs.* 2006;3(1):19–30

119. Jonikas JA, Cook JA, Rosen C, Laris A, Kim JB. A program to reduce use of physical restraint in psychiatric inpatient facilities. *Psychiatr Serv.* 2004;55(7):818–820

120. dosReis S, Barnett S, Love RC, Riddle MA; Maryland Youth Practice Improvement Committee. A guide for managing acute aggressive behavior of youths in residential and inpatient treatment facilities. *Psychiatr Serv.* 2003;54(10):1357–1363

121. Fishkind A. Calming agitation with words, not drugs: 10 commandments for safety. *Curr Psychiatr.* 2002;1(4):32–39

122. Larkin GL, Beautrais AL. Behavioral disorders: emergency assessment. In: Tintinalli JE, Stapczynski S, Ma OJ, Cline DM, Cydulka RK, Meck_lereds GD, eds. *Tintinalli's Emergency Medicine: A Comprehensive Study Guide.* New York, NY: McGraw-Hill Education; 2011:1939–1946

123. Rossi J, Swan MC, Isaacs ED. The violent or agitated patient. *Emerg Med Clin North Am.* 2010;28(1):235–256, x

124. Marder SR. A review of agitation in mental illness: treatment guidelines and current therapies. *J Clin Psychiatry.* 2006;67(suppl 10):13–21

125. Mace SE. Behavioral and psychiatric disorders in children and infants. In: Tintinalli JE, Stapczynski S, Ma OJ, Cline DM, Cydulka RK, Meck_lereds GD, eds. *Tintinalli's Emergency Medicine: A Comprehensive Study Guide.* New York, NY: McGraw-Hill Education; 2011:967–971

126. Allen MH, Forster P, Zealberg J, Currier G; American Psychiatric Association, Task Force on Psychiatric Emergency Services. *Report and Recommendations Regarding Psychiatric Emergency and Crisis Services: A Review and Model Program Descriptions.* Bloomfield, CT: American Association for Emergency Psychiatry; 2002

127. Cowin L, Davies R, Estall G, Berlin T, Fitzgerald M, Hoot S. De-escalating aggression and violence in the mental health setting. *Int J Ment Health Nurs.* 2003;12(1):64–73

128. Tan D. Medications for psychiatric emergencies. In: Khouzam HR, Tan DT, Gill TS, eds. *Handbook of Emergency Psychiatry.* Philadelphia, PA: Mosby-Elsevier; 2007:22–31

129. Downes MA, Healy P, Page CB, Bryant JL, Isbister GK. Structured team approach to the agitated patient in the emergency department. *Emerg Med Australas.* 2009;21(3):196–202

130. Miyamoto S, Lieberman JA, Fleischacker WW, Marder SR. Antipsychotic drugs. In: Tasman A, Kay J, Lieberman A, First MB, Maj M, eds. *Psychiatry.* 3rd ed. West Sussex, England: John Wiley & Sons; 2008:2161–2201

131. Smith T, Horwath E, Cournos F. Schizophrenia and other psychotic disorders. In: Cutler JL, Marcus E, eds. *Psychiatry.* New York, NY: Oxford University Press; 2010:101–131

132. Levine M, LoVecchio F. Antipsychotics. In: Tintinalli JE, Stapczynski S, Ma OJ, Cline DM, Cydulka RK, Meck_lereds GD,

eds. *Tintinalli's Emergency Medicine: A Comprehensive Study Guide.* New York, NY: McGraw-Hill Education; 2011:1207–1211

133. Minns AB, Clark RF. Toxicology and overdose of atypical antipsychotics. *J Emerg Med.* 2012;43(5):906–913

134. Sonnier L, Barzman D. Pharmacologic management of acutely agitated pediatric patients. *Paediatr Drugs.* 2011;13(1):1–10

135. Nobay F, Simon BC, Levitt MA, Dresden GM. A prospective, double-blind, randomized trial of midazolam versus haloperidol versus lorazepam in the chemical restraint of violent and severely agitated patients. *Acad Emerg Med.* 2004;11(7):744–749

136. May DE, Kratochvil CJ. Attention-deficit hyperactivity disorder: recent advances in paediatric pharmacotherapy. *Drugs.* 2010;70(1):15–40

137. Yoon EY, Cohn L, Rocchini A, Kershaw D, Clark SJ. Clonidine utilization trends for Medicaid children. *Clin Pediatr (Phila).* 2012;51(10):950–955

138. Cengiz M, Baysal Z, Ganidagli S. Oral sedation with midazolam and diphenhydramine compared with midazolam alone in children undergoing magnetic resonance imaging. *Paediatr Anaesth.* 2006;16(6):621–626

139. Roach CL, Husain N, Zabinsky J, Welch E, Garg R. Moderate sedation for echocardiography of preschoolers. *Pediatr Cardiol.* 2010;31(4):469–473

140. Lustig SL, Botelho C, Lynch L, Nelson SV, Eichelberger WJ, Vaughan BL. Implementing a randomized clinical trial on a pediatric psychiatric inpatient unit at a children's hospital: the case of clonidine for post-traumatic stress. *Gen Hosp Psychiatry.* 2002;24(6):422–429

141. Battaglia J, Moss S, Rush J, et al. Haloperidol, lorazepam, or both for psychotic agitation? A multicenter, prospective, double-blind, emergency department study. *Am J Emerg Med.* 1997;15(4):335–340

142. Chan EW, Taylor DM, Knott JC, Phillips GA, Castle DJ, Kong DC. Intravenous droperidol or olanzapine as an adjunct to midazolam for the acutely agitated

patient: a multicenter, randomized, double-blind, placebo-controlled clinical trial. *Ann Emerg Med.* 2013;61(1):72–81

143. Allen MH. Managing the agitated psychotic patient: a reappraisal of the evidence. *J Clin Psychiatry.* 2000;61(suppl 14):11–20

144. Dorfman DH, Mehta SD. Restraint use for psychiatric patients in the pediatric emergency department. *Pediatr Emerg Care.* 2006;22(1):7–12

145. Isaacs E. The violent patient. In: Marx JA, Hockberger R, Walls RM, eds. *Rosen's Emergency Medicine: Concepts and Clinical Practice.* Philadelphia, PA: Saunders; 2014:1460–1465

146. Bieniek SA, Ownby RL, Penalver A, Dominguez RA. A double-blind study of lorazepam versus the combination of haloperidol and lorazepam in managing agitation. *Pharmacotherapy.* 1998;18(1):57–62

147. Currier GW, Medori R. Orally versus intramuscularly administered antipsychotic drugs in psychiatric emergencies. *J Psychiatr Pract.* 2006;12(1):30–40

148. Garris S, Hughes C. Management of acute agitation. In: Tintinalli JE, Stapczynski S, Ma OJ, Cline DM, Cydulka RK, Mecklereds GD, eds. *Tintinalli's Emergency Medicine: A Comprehensive Study Guide.* New York, NY: McGraw-Hill Education; 2011

149. Whittler MA, Lavonas EJ. Antipsychotics. In: Marx JA, Hockberger RS, Walls RM, et al, eds. *Rosen's Emergency Medicine: Concepts and Clinical Practice.* Philadelphia, PA: Saunders; 2014:2042–2046

150. Schieve LA, Gonzalez V, Boulet SL, et al. Concurrent medical conditions and health care use and needs among children with learning and behavioral developmental disabilities, National Health Interview Survey, 2006–2010. *Res Dev Disabil.* 2012;33(2):467–476

151. Sorrentino A. Chemical restraints for the agitated, violent, or psychotic pediatric patient in the emergency department: controversies and recommendations. *Curr Opin Pediatr.* 2004;16(2):201–205

152. Centers for Medicare & Medicaid Services (CMS), DHHS. Medicare and Medicaid programs; hospital conditions of participation: patients' rights. Final rule. *Fed Regist.* 2006;71(236):71377–71428

153. The Joint Commission. *Standards on Restraint and Seclusion.* Oakbrook Terrace, IL: The Joint Commission; 2009

154. Health Care Finance Administration. Medicare and Medicaid Programs; Hospital Conditions of Participation: Patients' Rights; Interim Final Rule. *Fed Regist.* 1999;64(127):36088–36089

155. Baren JM, Mace SE, Hendry PL, Dietrich AM, Goldman RD, Warden CR. Children's mental health emergencies—part 2: emergency department evaluation and treatment of children with mental health disorders. *Pediatr Emerg Care.* 2008;24(7):485–498

156. Masters KJ. Pulse oximetry use during physical and mechanical restraints. *J Emerg Med.* 2007;33(3):289–291

157. Walters H, Killius K. *Guidelines for the Acute Psychotropic Medication Management of Agitation in Children and Adolescents.* Boston, MA: Boston Medical Center Emergency Department Policy and Procedure Guidelines; 2012

158. Meyer-Massetti C, Cheng CM, Sharpe BA, Meier CR, Guglielmo BJ. The FDA extended warning for intravenous haloperidol and torsades de pointes: how should institutions respond? *J Hosp Med.* 2010;5(4):E8–E16

159. Haddad PM, Anderson IM. Antipsychotic-related QTc prolongation, torsade de pointes and sudden death. *Drugs.* 2002;62(11):1649–1671

160. Olsen KM. Pharmacologic agents associated with QT interval prolongation. *J Fam Pract.* 2005;(suppl):S8–S14

161. Yap YG, Camm AJ. Drug induced QT prolongation and torsades de pointes. *Heart.* 2003;89(11):1363–1372

162. Labellarte MJ, Crosson JE, Riddle MA. The relevance of prolonged QTc measurement to pediatric psychopharmacology. *J Am Acad Child Adolesc Psychiatry.* 2003;42(6):642–650

163. Bailey P, Norton R, Karan S. The FDA droperidol warning: is it justified? *Anesthesiology.* 2002;97(1):288–289

164. Chase PB, Biros MH. A retrospective review of the use and safety of droperidol in a large, high-risk, inner-city emergency department patient population. *Acad Emerg Med.* 2002;9(12):1402–1410

165. Dershwitz M. Droperidol: should the black box be light gray? *J Clin Anesth.* 2002;14(8):598–603

166. Gan TJ, White PF, Scuderi PE, Watcha MF, Kovac A. FDA "black box" warning regarding use of droperidol for postoperative nausea and vomiting: is it justified? *Anesthesiology.* 2002;97(1):287

167. Hilt RJ, Woodward TA. Agitation treatment for pediatric emergency patients. *J Am Acad Child Adolesc Psychiatry.* 2008;47(2):132–138

168. Horowitz BZ, Bizovi K, Moreno R. Droperidol—behind the black box warning. *Acad Emerg Med.* 2002;9(6):615–618

169. Baren JM, Mace SE, Hendry PL, Dietrich AM, Grupp-Phelan J, Mullin J. Children's mental health emergencies—part 1: challenges in care: definition of the problem, barriers to care, screening, advocacy, and resources. *Pediatr Emerg Care.* 2008;24(6):399–408

170. Miller D, Walker MC, Friedman D. Use of a holding technique to control the violent behavior of seriously disturbed adolescents. *Hosp Community Psychiatry.* 1989;40(5):520–524

171. Di Lorenzo R, Baraldi S, Ferrara M, Mimmi S, Rigatelli M. Physical restraints in an Italian psychiatric ward: clinical reasons and staff organization problems. *Perspect Psychiatr Care.* 2012;48(2):95–107

172. Allen MH, Currier GW. Use of restraints and pharmacotherapy in academic psychiatric emergency services. *Gen Hosp Psychiatry.* 2004;26(1):42–49

173. Beck JC, White KA, Gage B. Emergency psychiatric assessment of violence. *Am J Psychiatry.* 1991;148(11):1562–1565

174. Bell CC, Palmer JM. Security procedures in a psychiatric emergency service. *J Natl Med Assoc.* 1981;73(9):835–842

175. Currier GW, Allen MH. Emergency psychiatry: physical and chemical restraint in the psychiatric emergency service. *Psychiatr Serv.* 2000;51(6):717–719

176. Currier GW, Walsh P, Lawrence D. Physical restraints in the emergency department and attendance at subsequent outpatient psychiatric treatment. *J Psychiatr Pract.* 2011;17(6):387–393

177. Lavoie FW. Consent, involuntary treatment, and the use of force in an urban emergency department. *Ann Emerg Med.* 1992;21(1):25–32

178. Sundram CJ, Stack EW, Benjamin WP. *Restraint and Seclusion Practices in New York State Psychiatric Facilities.* Albany, NY: New York State Commission on Quality of Care for the Mentally Disabled; 1994

179. Weiss EM, Altamira D, Blinded DF, et al. Deadly restraint: a Hartford Courant investigative report. *Hartford Courant.* October 11-15, 1998:A10

180. Nunno MA, Holden MJ, Tollar A. Learning from tragedy: a survey of child and adolescent restraint fatalities. *Child Abuse Negl.* 2006;30(12):1333–1342

181. US General Accounting Office. *Report to Congressional Requestors: Mental Health: Improper Restraint or Seclusion Places People at Risk. US Department of Health and Human Services.* Washington, DC: US General Accounting Office; 1999

182. American Academy of Pediatrics Committee on Pediatric Emergency Medicine. The use of physical restraint interventions for children and adolescents in the acute care setting. *Pediatrics.* 1997;99(3):497–498

183. American College of Emergency Physicians. Emergency physicians' patient care responsibilities outside the emergency department. *Ann Emerg Med.* 2006;47(3):304

184. Brown RL, Genel M, Riggs JA; American Medical Association, Council on Scientific Affairs. Use of seclusion and restraint in children and adolescents. Council on Scientific Affairs, American Medical Association. *Arch Pediatr Adolesc Med.* 2000;154(7):653–656

185. American Psychiatric Association, Task Force on the Psychiatric Uses of Seclusion and Restraint. *Seclusion and Restraint: The Psychiatric Uses (Task Force Report 22).* Washington, DC: American Psychiatric Association; 1985

186. Medical Directors Council of the National Association of State Mental Health Program Directors. *Reducing the Use of Seclusion and Restraints: Findings, Strategies and Recommendations.* Alexandria, VA: National Association of State Mental Health Program Directors; 1999

187. Fisher WA. Restraint and seclusion: a review of the literature. *Am J Psychiatry.* 1994;151(11):1584–1591

188. The Joint Commission. Preventing Restraint Deaths. In: *Sentinel Event Alert.* Oakbrook Terrace, IL: The Joint Commission; 1998:2

189. Higgins S, Chawla R, Colombo C, Snyder R, Nigam S. Medical homes and cost and utilization among high-risk patients. *Am J Manag Care.* 2014;20(3):e61–e71

190. Schwenk TL. The patient-centered medical home: one size does not fit all. *JAMA.* 2014;311(8):802–803

191. American Academy of Child and Adolescent Psychiatry Committee on Health Care Access and Economics Task Force on Mental Health. Improving mental health services in primary care: reducing administrative and financial barriers to access and collaboration. *Pediatrics.* 2009;123(4):1248–1251

192. Adams SH, Newacheck PW, Park MJ, Brindis CD, Irwin CE Jr. Medical home for adolescents: low attainment rates for those with mental health problems and other vulnerable groups. *Acad Pediatr.* 2013;13(2):113–121

193. DE Hert M, Correll CU, Bobes J, et al. Physical illness in patients with severe mental disorders. I. Prevalence, impact of medications and disparities in health care. *World Psychiatry.* 2011;10(1):52–77

194. Burnett-Zeigler I, Walton MA, Ilgen M, et al. Prevalence and correlates of mental health problems and treatment among adolescents seen in primary care. *J Adolesc Health.* 2012;50(6):559–564

Evaluation and Management of Children and Adolescents With Acute Mental Health or Behavioral Problems. Part I: Common Clinical Challenges of Patients With Mental Health and/or Behavioral Emergencies— Executive Summary

- *Clinical Report*

CLINICAL REPORT Guidance for the Clinician in Rendering Pediatric Care

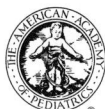

American Academy
of Pediatrics

DEDICATED TO THE HEALTH OF ALL CHILDREN™

Executive Summary: Evaluation and Management of Children and Adolescents With Acute Mental Health or Behavioral Problems. Part I: Common Clinical Challenges of Patients With Mental Health and/or Behavioral Emergencies

Thomas H. Chun, MD, MPH, FAAP, Sharon E. Mace, MD, FAAP, FACEP, Emily R. Katz, MD, FAAP,
AMERICAN ACADEMY OF PEDIATRICS, COMMITTEE ON PEDIATRIC EMERGENCY MEDICINE, AMERICAN
COLLEGE OF EMERGENCY PHYSICIANS, PEDIATRIC EMERGENCY MEDICINE COMMITTEE

EXECUTIVE SUMMARY

The number of children and adolescents seen in emergency departments (EDs) and primary care settings for mental health problems has skyrocketed in recent years, with up to 23% of patients in both settings having diagnosable mental health conditions.[1-4] Even when a mental health problem is not the focus of an ED or primary care visit, mental health conditions, both known and occult, may challenge the treating clinician and complicate the patient's care.[4]

Although the American Academy of Pediatrics has published a policy statement on mental health competencies and a Mental Health Toolkit for pediatric primary care providers, no such guidelines or resources exist for clinicians who care for pediatric mental health emergencies.[5,6] Many ED and primary care physicians report a paucity of training and lack of confidence in caring for pediatric psychiatry patients. The 2 clinical reports (www.pediatrics.org/cgi/doi/10.1542/peds.2016-1570 and www.pediatrics.org/cgi/doi/10.1542/peds.2016-1573) support the 2006 joint policy statement of the American Academy of Pediatrics and the American College of Emergency Physicians on pediatric mental health emergencies,[7] with the goal of addressing the knowledge gaps in this area. Although written primarily from the perspective of ED clinicians, they are intended for all clinicians who care for children and adolescents with acute mental health and behavioral problems.

The clinical reports are organized around the common clinical challenges pediatric caregivers face, both when a child or adolescent presents with a psychiatric chief complaint or emergency (part I) and also when a mental

This document is copyrighted and is property of the American Academy of Pediatrics and its Board of Directors. All authors have filed conflict of interest statements with the American Academy of Pediatrics. Any conflicts have been resolved through a process approved by the Board of Directors. The American Academy of Pediatrics has neither solicited nor accepted any commercial involvement in the development of the content of this publication.

Clinical reports from the American Academy of Pediatrics benefit from expertise and resources of liaisons and internal (AAP) and external reviewers. However, clinical reports from the American Academy of Pediatrics may not reflect the views of the liaisons or the organizations or government agencies that they represent.

The guidance in this report does not indicate an exclusive course of treatment or serve as a standard of medical care. Variations, taking into account individual circumstances, may be appropriate.

All clinical reports from the American Academy of Pediatrics automatically expire 5 years after publication unless reaffirmed, revised, or retired at or before that time.

DOI: 10.1542/peds.2016-1571

PEDIATRICS (ISSN Numbers: Print, 0031-4005; Online, 1098-4275).

To cite: Chun TH, Mace SE, Katz ER, AMERICAN ACADEMY OF PEDIATRICS. Executive Summary: Evaluation and Management of Children and Adolescents With Acute Mental Health or Behavioral Problems. Part I: Common Clinical Challenges of Patients With Mental Health and/or Behavioral Emergencies. *Pediatrics.* 2016;138(3):e20161571

health condition may be an unclear or complicating factor in a non–mental health clinical presentation (part II). Part II of the clinical reports (www.pediatrics.org/cgi/doi/10.1542/peds.2016-1573) includes discussions of somatic symptom and related disorders, adverse effects of psychiatric medications including neuroleptic malignant syndrome and serotonin syndrome, caring for children with special needs such as autism and developmental disorders, and mental health screening. This executive summary is an overview of part I of the clinical reports. The full text of the below topics can be accessed online at (www.pediatrics.org/cgi/doi/10.1542/peds.2016-1570). Key considerations are shown in the following sections.

1. ED Medical Clearance of Pediatric Psychiatric Patients

- Definition

  1. Medical clearance is the process of excluding potential medical conditions causing or exacerbating the patient's psychiatric symptoms as well as evaluating the patient for medical diseases or injuries for which acute diagnostic or therapeutic interventions in the ED may be indicated.[8,9]

  2. Some favor the term "medically stable," because the goal of the ED visit is not to exclude all possible medical etiologies but rather to rule out acute medical conditions.[10]

  3. For patients with unexplained vital sign abnormalities, a concerning history, or physical examination findings or with new onset or acute changes in their neurologic or psychiatric symptoms, a careful evaluation for potential underlying medical conditions may be important.[11]

- Laboratory Testing

  1. Despite the large number of medical conditions (see

Table 1 at [www.pediatrics.org/cgi/doi/10.1542/peds.2016-1570]) that can present with mental health symptoms, there is a growing body of both pediatric and adult literature that casts doubt on the utility of routinely obtaining laboratory or radiologic testing for these patients.[12-19] This literature supports the position of the American College of Emergency Physicians for focused medical assessments and judicious testing of these ED patients.[11]

  2. Mental health consultants often request pregnancy (females), toxicology, and sexually transmitted infection testing for adolescent patients. Whether to obtain these or other medical tests or evaluations can usually be decided with a direct conversation between the ED and mental health clinicians.

2. Suicidal Ideation and Suicide Attempts

- Epidemiology

  1. Suicide is one of the leading causes of death in adolescents,[20] and suicide attempts are one of the most common ED mental health presentations.[21,22] Epidemiologic studies in teenagers have found that 16% reported seriously considering suicide and 7.8% have attempted suicide in the past year.[23]

  2. More females consider and attempt suicide, although males are far more likely to die of suicide because of their frequent use of more lethal means (eg, firearms, hanging).[23] Native Americans have the highest suicide rates among ethnic groups.[21]

- Risk factors: previous suicide attempt(s); mood (eg, depression, bipolar disorder, mood swings,

irritable mood, etc), impulsivity, or disruptive behavior disorders; substance abuse; recent psychiatric hospitalization; family history of suicide; interpersonal violence (eg, physical or sexual abuse, bullying, antisocial behavior); homelessness or runaway behavior; self-identification as lesbian, gay, bisexual, or transgender; hopelessness; history of aggressive or impulsive behavior; cultural/religious beliefs; recent loss or stress (eg, relational, social, work, financial, etc) of the patient or family; physical illness; recent high-profile suicides; access to lethal methods; social isolation; and barriers or unwillingness to seek mental health care.[24-29]

- Assessment

  1. Suicidal ideation and attempts are often precipitated by psychosocial stressors.[29] As such, evaluating the pediatric patient for suicide risk includes inquiring about his or her current psychosocial situation, interviewing both the patient and his or her caregivers (eg, family members, school or mental health personnel), and assessing for the aforementioned suicide risk factors.

  2. The ED management of patients with suicidal ideation and attempts includes an evaluation of their current mental health state. Children and adolescents frequently misjudge the lethality of their actions. A potential pitfall is to equate the lethality of a suicide attempt with the patient's suicide intent. A patient whose suicide attempt had low medical lethality may, in fact, have a significant wish to harm himself or herself or to die.[30-32]

  3. The ED workup of patients presenting for suicidal ideation or attempt includes evaluation for signs of self-injury (which

can be concealed under clothing) or occult toxidromes as well as questions about suicidal intent, suicide plans, and other self-injurious behaviors.

- Disposition: The decision for inpatient versus outpatient management depends on many factors, including a careful assessment of suicide risk, and may include consultation with a mental health clinician. Outpatient management may be considered for low-risk patients (those with a low risk of future self-harm, adequate supervision, mental health follow-up, and safety planning; eg, the patient can identify his or her warning signs or triggers for recurrent suicidal ideation and have appropriate coping strategies if he or she becomes suicidal again, such as healthy activities and social support, and means restrictions, that is, limiting access to mechanisms for self-harm, such as firearms, other weapons, medications, etc).[33] "Contracting for safety"/suicide prevention agreements are controversial and remain unproven.[34]

- Involuntary hospitalization: Under certain circumstances, physicians may insist on admission to a psychiatric unit over the objections of patients and/or their parents/guardians, when clinically indicated. Every state has laws governing involuntary admission for inpatient psychiatric hospitalization. These laws vary from state to state, as do laws regarding confidentiality and an adolescent's right to seek mental health or substance abuse treatment without parental consent. As such, it may be beneficial for ED clinicians to familiarize themselves with their state's relevant laws, statutes, and involuntary commitment procedures. For more information on related state laws, contact the American Academy of Pediatrics' Division of State Government Affairs at stgov@aap.org.

3. Restraint of the Agitated Patient

- Agitated behavior is the final common pathway for a wide number of medical and psychiatric conditions and, in some cases, a combination of the two. Determining the underlying cause of the agitation often guides treatment choices.

- The 4 guiding principles of working with agitated patients are as follows[35]:

  1. prioritizing the safety of the patient and the treating staff;

  2. assisting the patient in managing his or her emotions and regaining control of his or her behavior;

  3. utilizing age-appropriate and the least-restrictive methods possible; and

  4. recognizing that coercive interventions may exacerbate the agitation.

- Monitoring and evaluation of restrained patients (see Table 6 at [www.pediatrics.org/cgi/doi/10.1542/peds.2016-1570]) may include the following[36–38]:

  1. in-person evaluation by a licensed independent practitioner within 1 hour of placement of restraints;

  2. review and renewal of restraint orders on a frequent basis (1–8 hours, depending the patient's age); and

  3. frequent assessment of vital signs, injury attributable to restraint, nutrition and hydration status, peripheral circulation, hygiene and elimination status, physical and psychological status, and readiness to discontinue restraint.

- Verbal restraint/de-escalation

  1. A calming (eg, quiet room, soft/decreased lighting, elimination of triggers of agitation) and safe (eg, removal or securing of objects that can be used as weapons, padded walls) physical environment may help de-escalate a patient.[35,39,40]

  2. Common verbal restraint (see Table 2 at [www.pediatrics.org/cgi/doi/10.1542/peds.2016-1570]) strategies include the following[41]:

     a. respecting personal space;

     b. minimizing behavior and/or interventions the patient may find provocative;

     c. using clear, concise language and expectations;

     d. active listening, especially regarding the patient's goals; and

     e. offering clear, realistic choices without "bargaining."

- Chemical restraint

  1. The most commonly used medications for agitation are antihistamines, benzodiazepines, and antipsychotics.[42,43]

  2. Choice of medication(s) usually depends on many factors, including the severity and underlying cause of the agitated behavior; collaboration between ED, psychiatric, and pharmacy colleagues; and which medication(s), if any, the patient is currently taking (see Tables 3 and 4 at [www.pediatrics.org/cgi/doi/10.1542/peds.2016-1570]).[42,43]

     a. Diphenhydramine may be used for mild agitation.

     b. Benzodiazepines are common first-line drugs for medical causes of agitation.

     c. Either benzodiazepines or antipsychotics may be used

for psychiatric causes of agitation.

d. Some experts favor a combination of an antipsychotic with either a benzodiazepine or an antihistamine for severe agitation.[43,44]

3. Monitoring and precautions

a. For patients receiving chemical restraint, consider the same monitoring and reassessment precautions as for physical restraint.[37,38]

b. Antipsychotics may cause QT_c prolongation and dysrhythmias, especially in patients with underlying cardiac conditions and/or who are taking other QT_c-prolonging medication.[45–47] Many medications commonly used in pediatrics (see Table 5 at [www.pediatrics.org/cgi/doi/10.1542/peds.2016-1570]) can affect QT_c duration. If there are significant concerns for dysrhythmia, cardiac monitoring may be considered for patients receiving antipsychotics.

c. Antipsychotics can exacerbate symptoms in patients with anticholinergic or sympathomimetic toxidromes or delirium.

- Physical restraint

1. Physical restraints have resulted in the death of psychiatric patients and have disproportionately affected children.[48,49]

2. Federal, regulatory, and accreditation agencies all have guidelines and regulations regarding physical restraint.[37,38]

3. Guidelines for when physical restraint may be indicated include the following[11,50–54]:

a. an imminent risk of harm to self or others;

b. significant risk of disrupting treatment; and

c. less restrictive means have failed.

4. For the application of restraints, when possible:

a. apply restraints with ≥ 5 providers, one for each extremity and one for the patient's head;

b. use leather or other age-appropriate restraints; and

c. secure restraints to the bed frame.

5. To maximize safety during physical restraint, experts suggest, when possible[38]:

a. staff training of alternatives to and proper application of restraints;

b. continuous patient monitoring;

c. utilize the supine position, with free cervical range of motion and elevation of the head of the bed, to reduce aspiration risk;

d. utilize the prone position only if other measures have failed or are not possible; if the prone position is used, monitoring for airway obstruction and excessive pressure on the back and neck of the patient may be helpful, because death has been associated with these factors and prone restraint; experts suggest discontinuing prone positioning as soon as possible[38];

e. minimize covering of the patient's face or head, to reduce aspiration risk;

f. minimize use of high vests, waist restraints, or beds with unprotected side rails to

reduce the risk of respiratory compromise and falls;

g. minimize restraint of medically compromised or unstable patients; and

h. in cases of agitation attributable to suspected illicit stimulant use, chemical restraint may be preferable, because a rapid increase in serum potassium secondary to rhabdomyolysis may result in cardiac arrest.

4. Coordination With the Medical Home

- Coordinating mental health care with the medical home (ie, patient-centered care, coordinated and integrated by the patient's personal physician) offers several benefits.[55,56]

1. Coordinating with the medical home decreases redundant care for high-risk or high-utilization patients.

2. The medical home may be a unique opportunity to address mental health care without stigma.[55]

3. For patients without a medical home, identifying and promptly referring them to a personal physician may be beneficial.

4. Children and adolescents with mental health problems and those taking psychiatric medications are at increased risk of medical problems, including asthma, ear infections, headaches or migraines, seizures, and obesity/metabolic syndrome.

LEAD AUTHORS

Thomas H. Chun, MD, MPH, FAAP
Sharon E. Mace, MD, FAAP, FACEP
Emily R. Katz, MD, FAAP

AMERICAN ACADEMY OF PEDIATRICS, COMMITTEE ON PEDIATRIC EMERGENCY MEDICINE, 2015-2016

Joan E. Shook, MD, MBA, FAAP, Chairperson
James M. Callahan, MD, FAAP
Thomas H. Chun, MD, MPH, FAAP
Gregory P. Conners, MD, MPH, MBA, FAAP
Edward E. Conway Jr, MD, MS, FAAP
Nanette C. Dudley, MD, FAAP
Toni K. Gross, MD, MPH, FAAP
Natalie E. Lane, MD, FAAP
Charles G. Macias, MD, MPH, FAAP
Nathan L. Timm, MD, FAAP

LIAISONS

Kim Bullock, MD — *American Academy of Family Physicians*
Elizabeth Edgerton, MD, MPH, FAAP — *Maternal and Child Health Bureau*
Tamar Magarik Haro — *AAP Department of Federal Affairs*
Madeline Joseph, MD, FACEP, FAAP — *American College of Emergency Physicians*
Angela Mickalide, PhD, MCHES — *EMSC National Resource Center*
Brian R. Moore, MD, FAAP — *National Association of EMS Physicians*
Katherine E. Remick, MD, FAAP — *National Association of Emergency Medical Technicians*
Sally K. Snow, RN, BSN, CPEN, FAEN — *Emergency Nurses Association*
David W. Tuggle, MD, FAAP — *American College of Surgeons*
Cynthia Wright-Johnson, MSN, RNC — *National Association of State EMS Officials*

FORMER MEMBERS AND LIAISONS, 2013-2015

Alice D. Ackerman, MD, MBA, FAAP
Lee Benjamin, MD, FACEP, FAAP - *American College of Physicians*
Susan M. Fuchs, MD, FAAP
Marc H. Gorelick, MD, MSCE, FAAP
Paul Sirbaugh, DO, MBA, FAAP - *National Association of Emergency Medical Technicians*
Joseph L. Wright, MD, MPH, FAAP

STAFF

Sue Tellez

AMERICAN COLLEGE OF EMERGENCY PHYSICIANS, PEDIATRIC EMERGENCY MEDICINE COMMITTEE, 2013–2014

Lee S. Benjamin, MD, FACEP, Chairperson
Isabel A. Barata, MD, FACEP, FAAP
Kiyetta Alade, MD
Joseph Arms, MD
Jahn T. Avarello, MD, FACEP
Steven Baldwin, MD
Kathleen Brown, MD, FACEP
Richard M. Cantor, MD, FACEP
Ariel Cohen, MD
Ann Marie Dietrich, MD, FACEP
Paul J. Eakin, MD
Marianne Gausche-Hill, MD, FACEP, FAAP
Michael Gerardi, MD, FACEP, FAAP
Charles J. Graham, MD, FACEP
Doug K. Holtzman, MD, FACEP
Jeffrey Hom, MD, FACEP
Paul Ishimine, MD, FACEP
Hasmig Jinivizian, MD
Madeline Joseph, MD, FACEP

Sanjay Mehta, MD, Med, FACEP
Aderonke Ojo, MD, MBBS
Audrey Z. Paul, MD, PhD
Denis R. Pauze, MD, FACEP
Nadia M. Pearson, DO
Brett Rosen, MD
W. Scott Russell, MD, FACEP
Mohsen Saidinejad, MD
Harold A. Sloas, DO
Gerald R. Schwartz, MD, FACEP
Orel Swenson, MD
Jonathan H. Valente, MD, FACEP
Muhammad Waseem, MD, MS
Paula J. Whiteman, MD, FACEP
Dale Woolridge, MD, PhD, FACEP

FORMER COMMITTEE MEMBERS

Carrie DeMoor, MD
James M. Dy, MD
Sean Fox, MD
Robert J. Hoffman, MD, FACEP
Mark Hostetler, MD, FACEP
David Markenson, MD, MBA, FACEP
Annalise Sorrentino, MD, FACEP
Michael Witt, MD, MPH, FACEP

STAFF

Dan Sullivan

Stephanie Wauson

ABBREVIATION

ED: emergency department

FINANCIAL DISCLOSURE: The authors have indicated they do not have a financial relationship relevant to this article to disclose.

FUNDING: No external funding.

POTENTIAL CONFLICT OF INTEREST: The authors have indicated they have no potential conflicts of interest to disclose.

REFERENCES

1. Mahajan P, Alpern ER, Grupp-Phelan J, et al; Pediatric Emergency Care Applied Research Network (PECARN). Epidemiology of psychiatric-related visits to emergency departments in a multicenter collaborative research pediatric network. *Pediatr Emerg Care.* 2009;25(11):715–720

2. Pittsenbarger ZE, Mannix R. Trends in pediatric visits to the emergency department for psychiatric illnesses. *Acad Emerg Med.* 2014;21(1):25–30

3. Sheldrick RC, Merchant S, Perrin EC. Identification of developmental-behavioral problems in primary care: a systematic review. *Pediatrics.* 2011;128(2):356–363

4. Grupp-Phelan J, Wade TJ, Pickup T, et al. Mental health problems in children and caregivers in the emergency department setting. *J Dev Behav Pediatr.* 2007;28(1):16–21

5. Committee on Psychosocial Aspects of Child and Family Health; Task Force on Mental Health. The future of pediatrics: mental health competencies for pediatric primary care [policy statement]. *Pediatrics.* 2009;124(1):410–421

6. Foy JM, Kelleher KJ, Laraque D; American Academy of Pediatrics Task Force on Mental Health. Enhancing pediatric mental health care: strategies for preparing a

primary care practice. *Pediatrics.* 2010;125(suppl 3):S87–S108

7. Dolan MA, Mace SE; American Academy of Pediatrics, Committee on Pediatric Emergency Medicine; American College of Emergency Physicians and Pediatric Emergency Medicine Committee. Pediatric mental health emergencies in the emergency medical services system. *Pediatrics.* 2006;118(4):1764–1767

8. Glauser J, Marshall M. Medical clearance of psychiatric patients. *Emerg Med Rep.* 2011;32(23):273–286

9. Riba M, Hale M. Medical clearance: fact or fiction in the hospital

emergency room. *Psychosomatics.* 1990;31(4):400–404

10. Zun LS. Evidence-based evaluation of psychiatric patients. *J Emerg Med.* 2005;28(1):35–39

11. Lukens TW, Wolf SJ, Edlow JA, et al; American College of Emergency Physicians Clinical Policies Subcommittee (Writing Committee) on Critical Issues in the Diagnosis and Management of the Adult Psychiatric Patient in the Emergency Department. Clinical policy: critical issues in the diagnosis and management of the adult psychiatric patient in the emergency department. *Ann Emerg Med.* 2006;47(1):79–99

12. Agzarian MJ, Chryssidis S, Davies RP, Pozza CH. Use of routine computed tomography brain scanning of psychiatry patients. *Australas Radiol.* 2006;50(1):27–28

13. Donofrio JJ, Santillanes G, McCammack BD, et al. Clinical utility of screening laboratory tests in pediatric psychiatric patients presenting to the emergency department for medical clearance. *Ann Emerg Med.* 2014;63(6):666–75.e3

14. Fortu JM, Kim IK, Cooper A, Condra C, Lorenz DJ, Pierce MC. Psychiatric patients in the pediatric emergency department undergoing routine urine toxicology screens for medical clearance: results and use. *Pediatr Emerg Care.* 2009;25(6):387–392

15. Janiak BD, Atteberry S. Medical clearance of the psychiatric patient in the emergency department. *J Emerg Med.* 2012;43(5):866–870

16. Santiago LI, Tunik MG, Foltin GL, Mojica MA. Children requiring psychiatric consultation in the pediatric emergency department: epidemiology, resource utilization, and complications. *Pediatr Emerg Care.* 2006;22(2):85–89

17. Santillanes G, Donofrio JJ, Lam CN, Claudius I. Is medical clearance necessary for pediatric psychiatric patients? *J Emerg Med.* 2014;46(6):800–807

18. Shihabuddin BS, Hack CM, Sivitz AB. Role of urine drug screening in the medical clearance of pediatric psychiatric patients: is there one? *Pediatr Emerg Care.* 2013;29(8):903–906

19. Tenenbein M. Do you really need that emergency drug screen? *Clin Toxicol (Phila).* 2009;47(4):286–291

20. Shain BN; American Academy of Pediatrics, Committee on Adolescence. Suicide and suicide attempts in adolescents. *Pediatrics.* 2016;138(1):e20161420

21. Centers for Disease Control and Prevention, National Center for Injury Prevention and Control. Web-based Injury Statistics Query and Reporting System (WISQARS) [database]. Available at: www.cdc.gov/injury/wisqars/. Accessed July 7, 2015

22. Ting SA, Sullivan AF, Boudreaux ED, Miller I, Camargo CA Jr. Trends in US emergency department visits for attempted suicide and self-inflicted injury, 1993-2008. *Gen Hosp Psychiatry.* 2012;34(5):557–565

23. Eaton DK, Kann L, Kinchen S, et al; Centers for Disease Control and Prevention. Youth risk behavior surveillance—United States, 2011. *MMWR Surveill Summ.* 2012;61(4 SS-4):1–162

24. Brown J, Cohen P, Johnson JG, Smailes EM. Childhood abuse and neglect: specificity of effects on adolescent and young adult depression and suicidality. *J Am Acad Child Adolesc Psychiatry.* 1999;38(12):1490–1496

25. Esposito-Smythers C, Spirito A. Adolescent substance use and suicidal behavior: a review with implications for treatment research. *Alcohol Clin Exp Res.* 2004;28(5 suppl):77S–88S

26. Foley DL, Goldston DB, Costello EJ, Angold A. Proximal psychiatric risk factors for suicidality in youth: the Great Smoky Mountains Study. *Arch Gen Psychiatry.* 2006;63(9):1017–1024

27. McDaniel JS, Purcell D, D'Augelli AR. The relationship between sexual orientation and risk for suicide: research findings and future directions for research and prevention. *Suicide Life Threat Behav.* 2001;31(suppl):84–105

28. McKeown RE, Garrison CZ, Cuffe SP, Waller JL, Jackson KL, Addy CL. Incidence and predictors of suicidal behaviors in a longitudinal sample of young adolescents. *J Am Acad Child Adolesc Psychiatry.* 1998;37(6):612–619

29. Overholser J. Predisposing factors in suicide attempts: life stressors. In: Spirito A, Overholser JC, Overholser J, eds. *Evaluating and Treating Adolescent Suicide Attempters: From Research to Practice.* New York, NY: Academic Press; 2002:42–54

30. Brown GK, Henriques GR, Sosdjan D, Beck AT. Suicide intent and accurate expectations of lethality: predictors of medical lethality of suicide attempts. *J Consult Clin Psychol.* 2004;72(6):1170–1174

31. Plutchik R, van Praag HM, Picard S, Conte HR, Korn M. Is there a relation between the seriousness of suicidal intent and the lethality of the suicide attempt? *Psychiatry Res.* 1989;27(1):71–79

32. Swahn MH, Potter LB. Factors associated with the medical severity of suicide attempts in youths and young adults. *Suicide Life Threat Behav.* 2001;32(1 suppl):21–29

33. Sher L, LaBode V. Teaching health care professionals about suicide safety planning. *Psychiatr Danub.* 2011;23(4):396–397

34. American Academy of Child and Adolescent Psychiatry. Practice parameter for the assessment and treatment of children and adolescents with suicidal behavior. *J Am Acad Child Adolesc Psychiatry.* 2001;40(7 suppl):24S–51S

35. Richmond JS, Berlin JS, Fishkind AB, et al. Verbal de-escalation of the agitated patient: consensus statement of the American Association for Emergency Psychiatry Project BETA De-escalation Workgroup. *West J Emerg Med.* 2012;13(1):17–25

36. Health and Human Services Division, US General Accounting Office, ed. Report to Congressional Requestors: Mental Health: Improper Restraint or Seclusion Places People at Risk. Washington, DC: US General Accounting Office; 1999

37. Centers for Medicare and Medicaid Services; Department of Health and Human Services. Medicare and Medicaid programs; hospital conditions of participation: patients' rights. Final rule. *Fed Regist.* 2006;71(236):71377–71428

38. The Joint Commission. *Standards on Restraint and Seclusion.* Oakbrook Terrace, IL: The Joint Commission; 2009

39. Cowin L, Davies R, Estall G, Berlin T, Fitzgerald M, Hoot S. De-escalating aggression and violence in the mental health setting. *Int J Ment Health Nurs.* 2003;12(1):64–73

40. American Psychiatric Association, Task Force on the Psychiatric Use of Seclusion and Restraint. *Seclusion and Restraint: The Psychiatric Uses.* Washington, DC: American Psychiatric Association; 1985. Task Force Report 22.

41. Fishkind A. Calming agitation with words, not drugs: 10 commandments for safety. *Curr Psychiatr.* 2002;1(4):32–39

42. Adimando AJ, Poncin YB, Baum CR. Pharmacological management of the agitated pediatric patient. *Pediatr Emerg Care.* 2010;26(11):856–860; quiz: 861–863

43. Sonnier L, Barzman D. Pharmacologic management of acutely agitated pediatric patients. *Paediatr Drugs.* 2011;13(1):1–10

44. Marder SR. A review of agitation in mental illness: treatment guidelines and current therapies. *J Clin Psychiatry.* 2006;67(suppl 10):13–21

45. Labellarte MJ, Crosson JE, Riddle MA. The relevance of prolonged QTc measurement to pediatric psychopharmacology. *J Am Acad Child Adolesc Psychiatry.* 2003;42(6):642–650

46. Olsen KM. Pharmacologic agents associated with QT interval prolongation. *J Fam Pract.* 2005;(suppl):S8–S14

47. Yap YG, Camm AJ. Drug induced QT prolongation and torsades de pointes. *Heart.* 2003;89(11):1363–1372

48. Nunno MA, Holden MJ, Tollar A. Learning from tragedy: a survey of child and adolescent restraint fatalities. *Child Abuse Negl.* 2006;30(12):1333–1342

49. Weiss EM, Altamira D, Blinded DF, et al. Deadly restraint: a Hartford Courant investigative report. *Hartford Courant.* October 11–15, 1998:A10

50. American Academy of Pediatrics Committee on Pediatric Emergency Medicine. The use of physical restraint interventions for children and adolescents in the acute care setting. *Pediatrics.* 1997;99(3):497–498

51. Currier GW, Walsh P, Lawrence D. Physical restraints in the emergency department and attendance at subsequent outpatient psychiatric treatment. *J Psychiatr Pract.* 2011;17(6):387–393

52. Downes MA, Healy P, Page CB, Bryant JL, Isbister GK. Structured team approach to the agitated patient in the emergency department. *Emerg Med Australas.* 2009;21(3):196–202

53. Glezer A, Brendel RW. Beyond emergencies: the use of physical restraints in medical and psychiatric settings. *Harv Rev Psychiatry.* 2010;18(6):353–358

54. Rossi J, Swan MC, Isaacs ED. The violent or agitated patient. *Emerg Med Clin North Am.* 2010;28(1):235–256

55. American Academy of Child and Adolescent Psychiatry Committee on Health Care Access and Economics Task Force on Mental Health. Improving mental health services in primary care: reducing administrative and financial barriers to access and collaboration. *Pediatrics.* 2009;123(4):1248–1251

56. Schwenk TL. The patient-centered medical home: one size does not fit all. *JAMA.* 2014;311(8):802–803

Evaluation and Management of Children With Acute Mental Health or Behavioral Problems. Part II: Recognition of Clinically Challenging Mental Health Related Conditions Presenting With Medical or Uncertain Symptoms

• •

• *Clinical Report*

CLINICAL REPORT   Guidance for the Clinician in Rendering Pediatric Care

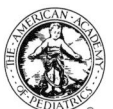

American Academy
of Pediatrics

DEDICATED TO THE HEALTH OF ALL CHILDREN™

Evaluation and Management of Children With Acute Mental Health or Behavioral Problems. Part II: Recognition of Clinically Challenging Mental Health Related Conditions Presenting With Medical or Uncertain Symptoms

Thomas H. Chun, MD, MPH, FAAP, Sharon E. Mace, MD, FAAP, FACEP, Emily R. Katz, MD, FAAP,
AMERICAN ACADEMY OF PEDIATRICS Committee on Pediatric Emergency Medicine, AMERICAN
COLLEGE OF EMERGENCY PHYSICIANS Pediatric Emergency Medicine Committee

INTRODUCTION

Part I of this clinical report (http://www.pediatrics.org/cgi/doi/10.1542/peds.2016-1570) discusses the common clinical issues that may be encountered in caring for children and adolescents presenting to the emergency department (ED) or primary care setting with a mental health condition or emergency and includes the following:

- Medical clearance of pediatric psychiatric patients

- Suicidal ideation and suicide attempts

- Involuntary hospitalization

- Restraint of the agitated patient

  o Verbal restraint

  o Chemical restraint

  o Physical restraint

- Coordination with the medical home

Part II discusses the challenges a pediatric clinician may face when evaluating patients with a mental health condition, which may be contributing to or a complicating factor for a medical or indeterminate clinical presentation. Topics covered include the following:

- Somatic symptom and related disorders

- Adverse effects of psychiatric medications

DOI: 10.1542/peds.2016-1573

PEDIATRICS (ISSN Numbers: Print, 0031-4005; Online, 1098-4275).

To cite: Chun TH, Mace SE, Katz ER, AAP AMERICAN ACADEMY OF PEDIATRICS Committee on Pediatric Emergency Medicine. Evaluation and Management of Children With Acute Mental Health or Behavioral Problems. Part II: Recognition of Clinically Challenging Mental Health Related Conditions Presenting With Medical or Uncertain Symptoms. *Pediatrics.* 2016;138(3):e20161573

TABLE 1 Common Symptoms of Somatic Symptom and Related Disorders[14]

Pseudoneurologic	Gastrointestinal symptoms
Amnesia	Abdominal pain
Difficulty with swallowing or voice	Nausea
Vision or hearing impairment	Vomiting
Syncope	Bloating
Seizure	Diarrhea
Paralysis or paresis	Multiple food intolerances
Pain symptoms	Cardiopulmonary symptoms
Headache	Chest pain
Back pain	Dyspnea
Extremity pain	Palpitations
Dysuria	Dizziness

o Antipsychotic adverse effects

o Neuroleptic malignant syndrome

o Serotonin syndrome

- Children with special needs (autism spectrum disorders [ASDs] and developmental disorders [DDs])

- Mental health screening

The report is written primarily from the perspective of ED clinicians, but it is intended for all clinicians who care for children and adolescents with acute mental health and behavioral problems. An executive summary of this clinical report can be found at http://www.pediatrics.org/cgi/doi/10.1542/peds.2016-1574.

SOMATIC SYMPTOM AND RELATED DISORDERS

Overview

The *Diagnostic and Statistical Manual of Mental Disorders, Fifth Edition* recognizes 7 distinct somatic symptom and related disorders, including somatic symptom disorder, illness anxiety disorder, conversion disorder (functional neurologic symptom disorder), psychological factors affecting other medical conditions, factitious disorder, other specified somatic symptom and related disorder, and unspecified somatic symptom and related disorder.[1] Each disorder has specific diagnostic criteria, which apply to both adults and children and which are not adjusted for children. All these disorders

refer to an individual's subjective experience of physical symptoms. These diagnoses can also be applied to situations in which the level of distress or disability is thought to be disproportionate to what is typically associated with the physical findings. For example, when a medical condition is present, if the physical problems do not fully explain the reported symptoms or severity, a somatic symptom and related disorder may apply.[2]

Additional criteria for somatic symptom disorders include the requirement that the complaints or fixations are not associated with material gain, nor are they intentionally produced.[3] Symptoms that are intentionally created are classified as factitious disorders; those that result in material gain are categorized as malingering. Lastly, the symptoms result in significant impairment in psychosocial functioning (eg, relationships with family or friends, academic or occupational difficulties).[1]

Epidemiologic studies have found that somatic symptom and related disorders are both common and a significant contributor to health care usage and costs. In adult primary care populations, between 10% and 15% of patients have a diagnosis of 1 of these disorders.[4] Among children and adolescents, recurrent abdominal pain and headaches account for 5% and between 20% and 55% of pediatric office visits, respectively; 10% of adolescents report frequent

headaches, chest pain, nausea, and fatigue.[5] Patients with somatic symptom and related disorders use all types of medical services (eg, primary, specialty, ED, and mental health care) more frequently,[4,6–8] are more likely to "doctor shop,"[4] and in 2005, were estimated to have incrementally added $265 billion to the cost of health care in the United States.[9]

Clinical Features and Studies of Pediatric Somatic Symptom and Related Disorders

The clinical presentations of somatic symptom and related disorders are myriad, most often involving neurologic, pain, autonomic, or gastrointestinal tract symptoms (Table 1). Children and adolescents often report such symptoms[10,11] and often have multiple visits for these symptoms in primary care and other settings.[3,5,12,13] Vague, poorly described complaints, recent or current stressful events, symptoms that fluctuate with activity or stress, and lack of physical findings and laboratory abnormalities are common.[3]

Symptoms of pediatric somatic symptom and related disorders often do not meet strict *Diagnostic and Statistical Manual of Mental Disorders, Fifth Edition* diagnostic criteria and defy categorization. Other difficulties in caring for patients with these disorders in the ED are that few patients will have received a formal diagnosis, and ED clinicians rarely have access to sufficient clinical information to confirm the diagnosis.[15–17] In addition, the diagnosis of a "psychosomatic" illness can be stigmatizing to patients and families, resulting in them feeling unheard, disrespected, and defensive about their symptoms.[5] For these and other reasons, some prefer the term "medically unexplained symptoms".[2,6,18,19]

Several studies, including 1 performed jointly in the Pediatric

Research in Office Settings and Ambulatory Sentinel Practice Network collaboratives, have identified demographic and risk factors associated with pediatric somatic symptom and related disorders.[2,8,20,21] Patients who are adolescents, female, from minority ethnicities, from nonintact families, or from urban dwellings; who have past histories of psychological trauma; whose parents have lower education levels; and who have other family members with somatic symptom and related disorders are more likely to present with unexplained medical symptoms. Such patients are also at much higher risk of comorbid psychiatric problems.[8]

Other studies have approached this topic by investigating the prevalence of and relationships between psychiatric conditions in patients with unexplained medical symptoms. Emiroğlu et al[22] studied 31 patients referred to a pediatric neurology clinic for headache, vertigo, and syncope. When comprehensive testing did not reveal an identifiable medical cause for their symptoms, the patients were interviewed by a child psychiatrist. A large majority (93.5%) were found to have a diagnosable disorder according to *Diagnostic and Statistical Manual of Mental Disorders, Fourth Edition* criteria, the most common being mood and somatic symptom and related disorders. Other pediatric headache studies have found similar results.[23,24] Guidetti et al[25] followed patients for 8 years after referral to a pediatric neurology headache clinic. At follow-up, persistence or worsening of headaches was highly associated with the presence of comorbid psychiatric conditions, and resolution of headaches strongly correlated with the absence of mental health conditions. In this study, the most common mental health conditions were anxiety disorders and depression.

Other studies in other settings echo these findings. In a pediatric cardiology clinic study, Tunaoglu et al[26] reported a prevalence of 74% for psychiatric disorders, primarily depression, anxiety, and somatic symptom and related disorders, in patients referred for chest pain with normal medical workups. Campo et al[27] recruited patients from a pediatric primary care office. Using standardized psychiatric interviews, they found that patients with recurrent abdominal pain were significantly more likely to be diagnosed with anxiety (79%) and depressive disorders (43%) than controls. In a study from a pediatric rheumatology clinic, Kashikar-Zuck et al[28] also conducted standardized psychiatric interviews among patients with juvenile fibromyalgia. A high prevalence of current and lifetime anxiety and mood disorders was detected in this population.

Somatic Symptom and Related Disorders and the ED

Somatic symptom and related disorders are a particularly vexing problem in the ED because of the potential harm to patients that may result from diagnostic uncertainty. It is understandable that a patient with 1 of these disorders might undergo extensive, invasive testing such as a lumbar puncture, be exposed to radiographic studies with ionizing radiation, or be given potent medications to treat their symptoms, which in turn could result in significant respiratory, cardiac, central nervous system (CNS), or hematologic adverse effects, potentially necessitating additional medications or procedures such as endotracheal intubation and mechanical ventilation to treat these adverse effects.

Psychogenic nonepileptic seizures (PNES, previously called "pseudoseizures") in pediatric ED patients are an illustrative example of this conundrum. In their review

of identified PNES patients (the authors recognize that PNES is often unrecognized and underdiagnosed in the ED), Selbst and Clancy[29] found that all had multiple previous ED visits, 8 of 10 patients had been prescribed anticonvulsants in the past, 6 received anticonvulsants either in the ED or before arrival in the ED by prehospital personnel, all but 1 had invasive procedures and testing, and 8 were admitted to the hospital. Other studies have found similar rates of extensive medical testing in children with PNES.[30] Accurate diagnosis and appropriate referrals for these patients may be important, as Wyllie et al[31] found that on follow-up, 72% of patients' PNES had resolved after psychiatric treatment. A particularly challenging problem when treating potential PNES in the ED is that some of these patients will have both a true seizure disorder and PNES, making airway management and the decision to give anticonvulsants for apparent seizure activity difficult and complex for ED physicians.

Several studies have investigated the impact of somatic symptom and related disorders on emergency department patients. Knockaert et al[32] prospectively enrolled 578 adult patients presenting to a Belgian ED with chest pain. Although the majority of these patients were found to have a cardiac or pulmonary disease as the etiology of their chest pain, the authors classified "somatization disorder" as the third leading cause (9.2%) of these ED visits. Another interesting finding from this study was that somatization disorder was more common among patients who were self-referred to the ED and those brought by ambulance. Although formal psychiatric evaluation was not performed on all patients, and classification as somatization disorder was based on the available clinical information and the final discharge diagnoses, the authors believe that their methods underestimated the true prevalence. Other studies have found a higher prevalence of mental health disorders among adult ED patients with chest pain.[17]

Lipsitz et al[33] studied 32 pediatric ED patients who presented with chest pain and for whom no medical cause was found. Using a semistructured *Diagnostic and Statistical Manual of Mental Disorders, Fourth Edition* interview to detect anxiety disorders, they found that 81% met diagnostic criteria for an anxiety disorder, with 28% meeting full criteria for panic disorder. Other pain symptoms such as headaches, abdominal pain, and back pain were common in these children, as were impaired quality of life and multiple domains of daily functioning. In a secondary analysis of a larger study on maternal and pediatric mental health problems, Dang et al[34] explored the relationship between mothers' somatic symptoms and subsequent pediatric ED use for their child. Maternal somatic symptoms were assessed with the Patient Health Questionnaire 15, a validated measure for inquiring about common somatic problems in outpatient settings. After covariates were adjusted for, mothers with high somatic symptom scores reported higher rates of depression symptoms, difficulty caring for themselves and their child, and a greater use of the ED for their child (odds ratio, 1.8; 95% confidence interval [CI], 0.99–3.38; P = .055).

Although there are no known studies of interventions for pediatric ED patients, Abbass et al[35] performed an intriguing prospective study of adult ED patients with suspected somatic symptom and related disorders. If the treating ED physician made a provisional diagnosis of somatization after completing the medical evaluation of the patient, a referral was made for an outpatient mental health evaluation and intensive, short-term psychotherapy.

The mental health evaluation and treatment typically took place a few weeks after the ED visit, with patients receiving a mean of 3.8 psychotherapy sessions (range: 1–25 sessions). After the psychotherapy intervention, at 1-year follow-up, they found a mean reduction of 3.2 ED (69%) visits per patient (SD, 6.4; 95% CI, 1.3–5.0; P < .001), compared with the year before the index ED visit. In addition, at follow-up patients reported significant improvement in their somatic symptoms and high satisfaction with the psychotherapeutic referral and intervention. Although this was not a randomized controlled trial, patients who were referred to psychotherapy but did not attend treatment did not show any changes in their ED use at 1 year follow-up.

Treatment Strategies

Medically unexplained symptoms are extremely frustrating for patients, families, and medical providers. Parents and children often think that they are not being listened to and that physicians have misdiagnosed the problem, or potential causes of the symptoms have not been adequately evaluated.[2,10] These feelings can be intense and may be rooted in a fear that a medical illness is being missed, frustration over the lack of success in resolving the symptoms, the stigma of being labeled or perceived as "psychosomatic," or difficulty in acknowledging that psychological and physical symptoms may be related.[18]

Prognosis often is unpredictable. In some cases, the episode can be brief and resolve. In other cases, the course is chronic and difficult to treat. The chronicity of the symptoms and previous response to treatment may be informative about the likely treatment course. Most experts agree that an empathetic, consistent, multidisciplinary, long-term treatment plan is helpful for chronic

cases.[2,5,10,18] This may include various psychotherapies (eg, cognitive–behavioral, rehabilitative, operant interventions, self-management strategies, and family or group therapy), consistent communication between all treating providers, and comprehensive treatment of comorbid psychiatric conditions.[2]

Although these treatment modalities are not practical or possible for the ED setting, there are some strategies that are applicable and may be helpful. Experts suggest the following[2,5,18]:

- *Provide reassurance*: First and foremost, it is important to convey to the patient and family that the patient's symptoms are being heard and taken seriously. Taking time to obtain a detailed history and comprehensive physical examination can help accomplish this goal. Some children and families may be reassured by the knowledge that their symptoms are not life or limb threatening. In addition, eliciting and addressing the child's and family's anxiety and fears about the patient's symptoms may be both clinically illuminating for the ED provider and comforting to the patient and family. It may also be important to reaffirm that their ED and outpatient providers are working and will continue to work with them to continue to evaluate and treat their symptoms.

- *Communicate*: Strategies to improve communication include emphasizing collaboration between the patient, family, and all caregivers; identifying common goals and outcomes; and introducing the idea of working on improving functioning in addition to working toward symptom resolution. In addition, educating the patient and family about the limitations of the ED setting, as well as the benefits of other settings for evaluation and treatment, may be helpful. Lastly, exploring the patient and family's openness to the possibility that the symptoms may be psychologically related may be an important first step. Determining and using terms such as stress, temperament, anxiety, "nerves," and other terms that are acceptable to the patient and family may assist in this goal.

- *Coordinate care*: Contacting and communicating with all involved care providers may be time consuming but is important in implementing a cohesive, comprehensive evaluation and treatment plan and may have the added benefit of providing reassurance to the patient and family as well as decreasing frustration and improving satisfaction.

ADVERSE EFFECTS OF PSYCHIATRIC MEDICATIONS

The use of all psychotropic medications in pediatric populations over the last 2 decades has markedly increased.[36,37] Antipsychotic use, in particular, has shown large increases.[38] Especially notable is their burgeoning off-label use,[39-41] including in preschool-aged children.[42-44] Given the frequency and multiple medication regimens with which psychotropic agents are being prescribed,[36] ED clinicians are likely to encounter children and adolescents taking 1 or many of these medications. This section focuses on the clinical problems and diagnostic and treatment dilemmas one may encounter in the ED when caring for pediatric patients on antipsychotics and antidepressants.

An additional important consideration for ED clinicians is that many commonly used medications not typically thought of as psychotropic agents have dopaminergic and serotonergic properties similar to those of antipsychotics and antidepressants. For example, drugs used as antiemetics and for

TABLE 2 Antipsychotic Adverse Symptoms

Neurotransmitter	Symptoms	Antipsychotics Commonly Associated With Symptom
Dopamine		
Nigrostriatal tract	Extrapyramidal symptoms (eg, dystonia, dyskinesia, akathisia, Parkinsonism)	High-potency "typical" antipsychotics (haloperidol)
Tuberoinfundibular tract	Hyperprolactinemia	All "typical" antipsychotics, risperidone
Preoptic tract	Hypothermia	Rare, possibly more common with atypical antipsychotics
Acetylcholine (muscarinic)	Sinus tachycardia, dry mucous membranes, mydriasis, urinary retention	Low-potency "typical" antipsychotics (chlorpromazine)
α-Adrenergic	Orthostatic hypotension, reflex tachycardia	Atypical antipsychotics
Histamine	Sedation	"Typical" antipsychotics
Mechanism unknown		
Potential etiology: Pancreatic versus CNS adrenergic α_1, α_2, dopamine D_2, muscarinic, histamine H_1, serotonin$_1$, serotonin$_2$, or serotonin$_6$	Wt gain, obesity, hyperlipidemia, metabolic syndrome, impaired glucose tolerance, hyperglycemia, type 2 diabetes	Atypical antipsychotics Highest risk: clozapine, olanzapine Lower risk: quetiapine, risperidone Lowest risk: ziprasidone, aripiprazole

migraines (ie, prochlorperazine, metoclopramide, promethazine, and trimethobenzamide) are phenothiazines, the same type of medications as first-generation, "typical" antipsychotics. Droperidol, which has been used as an antiemetic and for agitation, is a butyrophenone, the same class as the antipsychotic haloperidol.[45] The number and scope of medications with serotonergic effects are surprising and are detailed in this section. Either alone or in combination with psychotropic serotonergic drugs, these medications can result in serotonin toxicity. Given how frequently these medications are used in clinical practice, familiarizing oneself with them and their potential adverse effects may be beneficial to ED clinicians.

Antipsychotic Adverse Effects

Antipsychotics are prescribed for various childhood disorders, including oppositional–defiant disorder, conduct disorder, attention-deficit/hyperactivity disorder, and ASDs.[46-49] These medications have

also been used as antiemetics and antipruritics and to treat headaches, hiccups, and various neurologic disorders such as Parkinson disease, hemiballismus, ballismus, Tourette syndrome, and Huntington chorea.[50,51]

The common adverse effects of antipsychotics can be conceptualized and organized around the CNS neurotransmitters on which they act.[45,50-54] Table 2 lists the common adverse effects of antipsychotics and the medications with which they are most commonly associated.

It is important to note that antipsychotics have other clinically significant effects, including "black box" warnings from the US Food and Drug Administration (FDA) for thioridazine and droperidol because of their potential to cause dysrhythmias. Almost all antipsychotics cause some degree of QT_c prolongation because of a quinidinelike effect. For most of the medications, however, the degree of QT_c prolongation is small, which has given rise to a debate about the actual risk of dysrhythmias and torsades de pointes with antipsychotics administered in their usual doses and routes of administration.[45,47,48,55-60] Of note, intravenous (IV) haloperidol has been studied[61] but carries an FDA non–black box warning because of deaths associated with high doses and IV administration.[62] Therefore, experts suggest that intramuscular dosing of antipsychotics in the ED is the parental preferred route of administration. Table 3 details the factors that are thought to increase the risk of QT_c prolongation and sudden death.[48,51,63,64] Table 4 lists the degree of QT_c prolongation for common antipsychotics.[65]

Cardiac: Black Box Warning

Both thioridazine and droperidol have been issued FDA black box warnings for a potential association with prolonged QT interval, torsades de pointes, and sudden death. Since then, several studies have disputed this risk with droperidol.[55-60] A large retrospective review of 2468 patients given droperidol in the ED found that no cardiovascular event occurred that did not have an alternative explanation, and only 6 serious adverse events occurred, with 1 cardiac arrest in a patient with a normal QT interval out of 2468 patients (0.2% = 6/2468).[56] A pediatric study also suggested the safety and efficacy of droperidol when used to treat agitation, nausea and vomiting, headache, and pain.[66] Thus, "although droperidol can be associated with prolongation of the QT interval, there is not convincing evidence that the drug causes severe cardiac events."[60] Despite these and other studies, since the black box warning was issued, use of droperidol has declined exponentially.[67,68]

Neurologic

·Acute extrapyramidal syndromes associated with antipsychotic medications include acute dystonia, akathisia, and a Parkinsonian syndrome. Acute dystonia is characterized by involuntary motor

TABLE 3 Risk Factors for QT_c Prolongation or Dysrhythmias With Antipsychotic Use

Coadministration with other QT_c-prolonging medications
IV administration or high doses
Medically ill patients
Electrolyte abnormalities
Hepatic, renal, or cardiac impairment
Congenital long QT syndromes

tics or spasms usually involving the face, the extraocular muscles (oculogyric crisis), and the neck, back, and limb muscles and tends to occur after the first few doses of medication or after an increase in dosage. Laryngeal dystonia is a rare, potentially life-threatening adverse event that presents as a choking sensation, difficulty breathing, or stridor.[45,48]

Akathisia is a subjective feeling of restlessness, which generally occurs within the first few days of antipsychotic medication administration. Akathisia is found in up to 25% of patients[51] and has also been reported in patients receiving a single, standard dose (10 mg) of prochlorperazine. Both acute dystonia and acute akathisia tend to occur early in the course of treatment (ie, days to weeks after beginning an antipsychotic) and are easily reversed. To minimize these adverse effects, some advocate coadministering 25 to 50 mg of diphenhydramine or 1 to 2 mg of benztropine when giving an antipsychotic.[69] Others prefer to treat with anticholinergic agents (ie, diphenhydramine or benztropine) only if acute symptoms occur, followed by 2 days of oral therapy, given the prolonged half-life of antipsychotics.

The delayed-onset neurologic syndromes are Parkinsonism and tardive dyskinesia. The hallmarks of Parkinsonism are shuffling gait, cogwheel muscle rigidity, mask facies, bradykinesia or akinesia, pill-rolling tremors, and cognitive impairment. These symptoms are found in up to 13% of patients and

TABLE 4 QT_c Prolongation Associated With Antipsychotics

Medication	Mean QT_c Prolongation, ms
Thioridazine	25–30
Ziprasidone	5–22
Pimozide	13
Clozapine	8–10
Haloperidol	7
Quetiapine	6
Risperidone	0–5
Olanzapine	2
Aripiprazole	0

generally occur weeks to months after the patient starts antipsychotic therapy.[51] Drug-induced Parkinsonism syndrome is often treated by adding an anticholinergic agent, adding a dopaminergic agonist (eg, amantadine), or decreasing the dosage of a typical antipsychotic or switching to an atypical antipsychotic. Considering the diagnosis of drug-induced Parkinsonism may be important, because early diagnosis and rapid withdrawal of the antipsychotic drug may improve the possibility of complete recovery.[50] Tardive dyskinesia is characterized by rapid involuntary facial movements (eg, blinking, grimacing, chewing, or tongue movements) and extremity or truncal movements. Respiratory dyskinesia is often undiagnosed, can lead to recurrent aspiration pneumonia, and includes orofacial dyskinesia, dysphonia, dyspnea, and respiratory alkalosis.[45] Tardive dyskinesia occurs in 5% of young patients per year and is more common with older, "typical" antipsychotics.[50]

Although antipsychotic medications have been noted to lower the seizure threshold in a dose-dependent manner, antipsychotic medication–induced seizures are rare (usually <1%) when therapeutic doses are used, except for clozapine, which has a 5% incidence of seizures at high dosages.[45,51]

Metabolic

Adverse effects, such as weight gain, hyperglycemia, and

hyperlipidemia, are common, especially with second-generation, "atypical" antipsychotics.[45,50,51,70] Antipsychotics vary in their metabolic adverse effects, with the highest risk associated with clozapine and olanzapine, an intermediate risk with quetiapine, risperidone, and chlorpromazine, and the lowest risk with haloperidol, ziprasidone, and aripiprazole.[53]

Other

Agranulocytosis is a potential adverse effect of the atypical antipsychotic drug clozapine. Patients on clozapine regularly have complete blood cell counts performed, usually weekly or monthly, to monitor for this adverse effect. Other adverse effects of various atypical antipsychotics include somnolence, anxiety, agitation, oral hypoesthesia, headache, nausea, vomiting, insomnia, and tremor.[51]

Neuroleptic Malignant Syndrome

Neuroleptic malignant syndrome (NMS) is a potentially lethal syndrome consisting of the tetrad of mental status changes, fever, hypertonicity or rigidity, and autonomic dysfunction. It is presumed to be attributable to a lack of dopaminergic activity in the CNS, although hyperactivity of the sympathetic nervous system may also be involved. The deficiency of central dopaminergic activity can be attributable to dopamine antagonists or dopamine receptor blockade, dysfunction of the dopamine receptors, or withdrawal of dopamine agonists.[50,71,72]

With the increasing use of antipsychotic medications in the pediatric population, clinicians caring for children and adolescents may encounter this syndrome.[73] Given that NMS can be difficult to recognize and attenuated or incomplete presentations are possible, NMS is challenging to diagnose.[71,74] The incidence of NMS has been difficult

to determine, with estimates ranging from 0.02% to 3%.[45,71,75] Fortunately, mortality from NMS has decreased from 76% in the 1960s to <10% to 15% more recently.[72,76-78] Experts suggest considering NMS in the differential diagnosis of patients presenting with fever and altered mental status who are taking or may have taken an antipsychotic.[74]

NMS affects patients of all ages, with an apparent predominance in young adults and male patients (2:1).[73,79-81] It is unclear whether these are truly risk factors or reflect the patient population with the greatest use of antipsychotic medications.[75] Coadministration of psychotropic agents seems to be an especially high risk factor for precipitating NMS; in 1 study, more than half of people with reported NMS cases were taking concomitant psychotropic agents.[77] Other risk factors include dehydration, physical exhaustion, preexisting organic brain disease, and the use of long-acting depot antipsychotics. Neither duration of exposure to the drug nor toxic overdoses of antipsychotics appear to be associated with NMS. In addition, reintroducing the original precipitating drug may not lead to a reoccurrence of NMS, although patients with a history of NMS are at increased risk of recurrence.[76,77] The onset of NMS generally occurs within 7 days of starting or increasing antipsychotics and may last for 5 to 10 days even after the initiating agent is stopped. With depot forms of antipsychotics, however, onset of NMS symptoms may be more insidious and may last longer, up to 15 to 30 days.[71,76,82]

It was initially thought that newer atypical antipsychotics, which have both serotonin and dopamine-blocking properties, would not cause NMS because of their lower activity at dopamine receptors and their greater antiserotoninergic activity. This has not turned out to

be the case. Both second-generation atypical antipsychotics and the third-generation aripiprazole, which has partial dopamine agonist activity, have all been implicated in causing NMS.[76,79,83-87]

Despite its name, NMS can also be triggered by the administration or withdrawal of other, nonantipsychotic medications. Administration of tricyclic antidepressants, selective serotonin reuptake inhibitors (SSRIs), and lithium have been associated with NMS.[75] NMS also has been associated with the abrupt withdrawal of medications (eg, dopaminergic drugs used to treat Parkinson disease, such as levodopa, as well as baclofen, amantadine, some antipsychotics, and some antidepressants).[74] Lastly, the introduction to this section enumerates some of the medications commonly thought to be antiemetics or antimigraine therapies. They are, in fact, phenothiazines (ie, the same class of medications as first-generation, typical antipsychotics), but because of the clinical conditions for which they are used, they may not be suspected for being at risk for triggering NMS.

Pathophysiology

The cause of NMS is postulated to be a lack of dopaminergic activity in the CNS, principally affecting the D_2 receptors. Dopamine D_2 receptor antagonism leads to the manifestations of the NMS. Blockade of D_2 receptors in the hypothalamus produces an increased set point and loss of heat-dissipating mechanisms. Antagonism of the D_2 receptors in the nigrostriatal pathways and spinal cord via extrapyramidal pathways produces muscle rigidity and tremor. In the periphery, the increased release of calcium from the sarcoplasmic reticulum causes increased contractility, leading to muscle rigidity, increased heat production (with worsening of hyperthermia), and muscle cell

TABLE 5 Differential Diagnosis of NMS[72,89]

Toxicologic	Psychiatric
Serotonin syndrome	Delirium
Anticholinergic poisoning	Lethal catatonia
Sympathomimetics	Factitious fever
Malignant hyperthermia	Munchausen syndrome
Monoamine oxidase inhibitor	CNS
Monoamine oxidase inhibitor interaction with drugs	Intracranial tumors
or foods	
Central anticholinergic syndrome	Vasculitis
Lithium	Stroke
Phencyclidine	Seizure
Infectious disease	Other
Encephalitis	Heatstroke
Meningitis	Rheumatologic (eg, systemic lupus
	erythematosus, lupus cerebritis)
Tetanus	Malignancies
Endocrine	HIV/AIDS
Pheochromocytoma	Porphyria
Thyroid disease	Familial Mediterranean fever
Adrenal disease	

breakdown with elevated creatine kinase and rhabdomyolysis. In addition, D_2 receptor antagonism by eliminating tonic inhibition of the sympathetic nervous system leads to sympathoadrenal hyperactivity and autonomic instability.[72,75]

Clinical Presentation

The hallmarks of NMS are hyperthermia, altered mental status, muscle rigidity, and autonomic instability. Manifestations of autonomic dysfunction, which may occur before other symptoms, include fever up to 41°C or higher, tachycardia, blood pressure instability, diaphoresis, pallor, cardiac dysrhythmia, diaphoresis, sialorrhea, and dysphagia.[71,88]

The most common neurologic finding is lead pipe rigidity, although akinesia, dyskinesia, or waxy flexibility may be present.[45,77] The alteration in mental status often takes the form of delirium but varies from alert mutism to agitation to stupor to coma.[50,76] Motor abnormalities may include rigidity, akinesia, intermittent tremors, and involuntary movements. Other less common neurologic or neuromuscular signs include a positive Babinski, chorea, seizures, opisthotonos, trismus, and oculogyric crisis.[76,86]

Complications include renal failure from rhabdomyolysis, thromboemboli, dysrhythmias, cardiovascular collapse, and respiratory failure from aspiration pneumonia or tachypneic hypoventilation caused by diminished chest wall compliance from muscle rigidity, which may result in endotracheal intubation and ventilatory support.[50,71]

Diagnosis

Because there are no pathognomonic clinical or laboratory criteria, NMS is a clinical diagnosis. The differential diagnosis for NMS is broad and is outlined in Table 5. An important component of the diagnosis is a history of antipsychotic use or withdrawal of a dopaminergic agent.[45,86] Numerous diagnostic criteria have been proposed, which have included the classic clinical symptoms and other supplemental criteria.[1,79,81,88] Additional proposed criteria include elevated creatine kinase,[81] leukocytosis, incontinence, dysphagia, mutism, and metabolic acidosis.[1,79,81]

Recently, a Delphi panel of international NMS experts convened to discuss NMS diagnostic criteria.[90] Although its purpose was not to create a new set of criteria, the

results reflect consensus on the relative importance of individual clinical and diagnostic features for making a diagnosis of NMS. On a 100-point scoring system (ie, the total number of points sum up to 100), each clinical feature of NMS was assigned a number of "priority points." The point system is not meant to be used as a method for making the diagnosis of NMS; that is, there is no threshold number of points that indicate the presence or absence of NMS. Rather, it is meant to help clinicians determine which features of NMS are more important in making the diagnosis. The greater the number of points assigned, the greater the significance of the feature in making the diagnosis of NMS. The Delphi panel made the following assignments: exposure to dopamine antagonist or withdrawal of dopamine agonist within 3 days (20 points), hyperthermia (>100.4°F oral on ≥2 occasions [18 points]), rigidity (17 points), mental status alteration (13 points), creatine kinase elevation (≥4 times upper limit of normal [10 points]), sympathetic nervous system lability (10 points), hypermetabolism (5 points), and negative workup for infectious, toxic, metabolic, or neurologic causes (7 points). Sympathetic nervous system lability was defined as 2 or more of the following: elevated (systolic or diastolic ≥25% of baseline) or fluctuations (≥20 mm Hg diastolic or ≥25 mm Hg systolic change within 24 hours) in blood pressure, diaphoresis, or urinary incontinence. Hypermetabolism was defined as a heart rate increase ≥25% above baseline and respiratory rate ≥50% above baseline.

Leukocytosis, generally in the range of 15 000 to 30 000 cells per cubic millimeter, and electrolyte findings consistent with dehydration may be present. The etiology of elevated alkaline phosphatase, lactic dehydrogenase, and transaminases indicating impaired liver function is unknown but may be secondary to acute fatty liver changes from the hyperpyrexia. An elevated serum aldolase and creatine kinase, often greater than 16 000 IU/L, may be attributable to severe, sustained muscle contractions. The elevated creatine kinase may lead to rhabdomyolysis, acute myoglobinuria, and renal failure. A nonspecific common finding is the presence of a low serum iron concentration in patients with NMS.[77,86,91] If a lumbar puncture is performed, the cerebrospinal fluid results may be normal or have nonspecific findings. Findings on an EEG, if obtained, are variable. The EEG results may be normal or demonstrate findings of a nonspecific encephalopathy, such as diffuse slowing.[71,76] There are no specific findings on postmortem histopathology of the brain.[71]

Differentiating NMS from serotonin syndrome and other toxidromes can be challenging. Clinical features that may help are detailed in Table 7 and the section on serotonin syndrome.

Treatment

Management of NMS involves primarily supportive care and removal of the initiating agent. If NMS is triggered by the abrupt withdrawal of an anti-Parkinsonism drug, reintroduction of the drug may be considered.[72] Cardiorespiratory compromise may be managed with standard, supportive measures. Dehydration or elevated creatine kinase and rhabdomyolysis may be treated with IV fluids. If renal failure occurs, hemodialysis may be necessary (however, dialysis does not remove antipsychotics that are protein bound). For agitation, experts suggest benzodiazepines as the first-line agent. Fever can be treated with external cooling measures, such as cooling blankets.[72,75]

Suggestions for NMS treatment are based on case reports and clinical experience, not rigorous clinical trials, limiting the strength of the evidence base. The most frequently administered drugs have been dantrolene, bromocriptine, and amantadine. Dantrolene decreases muscle rigidity, and thermogenesis caused by the tonic contraction of muscles. It blocks the release of calcium from smooth muscle cells' sarcoplasmic reticulum, uncoupling actin and myosin chains, resulting in muscle relaxation. Commonly used dosages in NMS are 1 mg/kg by IV push followed by 0.25 to 0.75 mg/kg every 6 hours. The drug may be continued until symptoms resolve or a maximum of 10 mg/kg is reached.[72,77]

The utility of CNS dopaminergic agents is unclear and controversial. Therefore, consultation with a toxicologist or poison control center may be helpful. Bromocriptine is a centrally acting dopamine agonist. Experts suggest an initial dosage of 1.25 to 2.5 mg twice a day, which may be increased to 10 mg 3 times a day. Muscle rigidity usually responds quickly to bromocriptine, but fever, blood pressure, and creatine kinase levels may take several days to normalize. Amantadine has dopaminergic and anticholinergic effects. A common starting dosage is 100 mg orally, with a maximum dosage of 200 mg twice a day.[72,77,86] Benzodiazepines are often used for agitation and rigidity. Electroconvulsive therapy has been used in some pharmacotherapy-resistant cases.[72,77]

ED clinicians may not have seen or treated many cases of NMS. Potential resources for caring for these patients include toxicologists, a poison control center, and the NMS Information Service, which can be accessed through its Web site (http://www.nmsis.org/index.asp). Staffed by NMS experts, the NMS Information Service provides information, education, and phone consultation regarding the diagnosis and treatment of NMS.

Serotonin Syndrome

Serotonin syndrome occurs in all ages, from infants and children to older adults. It has even been reported in newborn infants as a result of in utero exposure.[92] The incidence of and mortality from serotonin syndrome have been increasing and may escalate in the future[93,94] because of the growing number and use of proserotonergic medications, such as SSRIs, other classes of psychiatric medications (eg, other antidepressants and anxiolytics), antibiotics, opiate analgesics, antiemetics, anticonvulsants, antimigraine drugs, anti-Parkinsonism drugs, muscle relaxants, and weight-reduction or bariatric medications (Table 6). In addition to prescription medications, a wide variety of over-the-counter medications, herbal and dietary supplements, and drugs of abuse have all been associated with serotonin syndrome.[95]

Serotonin syndrome occurs in approximately 16% to 18% of patients who overdose with an SSRI.[93] The true incidence of serotonin syndrome is difficult to estimate, given that many instances are probably undiagnosed or misdiagnosed.[96,97] Variable clinical manifestations (eg, lack of the classic triad of symptoms), wide spectrum of disease from mild to life-threatening, symptoms that are easily misattributed to the patient's underlying mental condition (eg, anxiety and akathisia), lack of awareness of the disorder, and the vast number of medications, other agents, and combinations of medicines or agents that can cause serotonin syndrome all may contribute to missed diagnoses.[93,97,98]

Pathophysiology

In the CNS, serotonin (5-hydroxytryptamine) regulates temperature, attention, and behavior. Peripherally, serotonin

TABLE 6 Medications and Other Agents Associated With Serotonin Syndrome

Psychiatric drugs
    Antianxiety drugs: direct serotonin antagonists
        Buspirone
    Antimanic drugs: increased postsynaptic receptor sensitivity
        Lithium
        Antidepressants
    Antidepressants: tricyclic antidepressants
        Amitriptyline
        Clomipramine
        Nortriptyline
    Antidepressants: monoamine oxidase inhibitors
        Phenelzine
    Antidepressants: SSRIs
        Citalopram
        Fluoxetine
        Paroxetine
        Sertraline
    Antidepressants: $5HT_{2A}$ receptor blockers
        Nefazodone
        Trazodone
    Antidepressants: serotonin-norepinephrine reuptake inhibitors
        Venlafaxine
        Duloxetine
Nonpsychiatric drugs
    Skeletal muscle relaxants
        Cyclobenzaprine
    Opioid analgesics
        Fentanyl
        Meperidine
        Oxycodone
        Pentazocine
        Tramadol
        Hydrocodone
    Antibiotics
        Linezolid
    Antiretroviral (protease inhibitor)
        Ritonavir
    Anticonvulsants
        Carbamazepine
        Valproic acid
    Antiemetics
        Metoclopramide (Reglan)
        $5HT_3$ receptor antagonists
        Ondansetron
    Antimigraine drugs
        Ergot alkaloids: ergotamines
        Triptans (5 HT_{1B} and $5HT_{1B}$ receptor agonists; eg, sumatriptan)
        Antiparkinsonian drugs
        Carbidopa/levodopa
    Bariatric medications (weight reduction)
        Sibutramine
Over-the-counter medications
    Dextromethorphan (cough suppressants and cold remedies)
Drugs of abuse
    3,4–Methylenedioxymethamphetamine (Ecstasy)
    Cocaine
    Lysergic acid diethylamide
    Methamphetamine
Herbals
    Hypericum perforatum (St John's wort)
Dietary supplements
    Panax ginseng (ginseng)
    L-tryptophan
    5-hydroxytryptophan

This is not an all-inclusive list but gives an overview of the wide range of agents that can trigger the serotonin syndrome. Drugs are listed by their therapeutic category. This list is not intended to endorse any given drug or product.

modulates gastrointestinal tract motility, vasoconstriction, bronchoconstriction, and platelet aggregation. Seven families of serotonin receptors have been identified, with serotonin syndrome resulting from excess CNS serotonin,[98,99] primarily caused by overstimulation of serotonin$_{2A}$ receptors.[100,101]

Excessive serotonin activity may result from myriad mechanisms, including increased release of serotonin (eg, cocaine, amphetamines), increased production of serotonin (eg, L-tryptophan in stimulant products), inhibiting reuptake of synaptic serotonin (eg, tricyclic antidepressants, SSRIs), decreased neuronal metabolism of serotonin via inhibition of monoamine oxidase inhibitors, direct stimulation of serotonin receptors (eg, lysergic acid diethylamide, migraine drugs such as sumatriptan, buspirone), and increased postsynaptic receptor responsivity (eg, lithium).[93,95]

A single dose of a single proserotonergic agent may precipitate serotonin syndrome. However, many cases occur after exposure to 2 or more drugs that increase the serotonin activity. Examples of combinations of proserotonergic medications causing serotonin syndrome include reports of SSRIs and fentanyl (given during procedural sedation),[102] erythromycin,[96] and St John's wort (an over-the-counter herbal supplement).[95] In addition, serotonin syndrome has also been reported in a patient withdrawing from a serotonergic agent.[100]

Clinical Presentation

The clinical triad of the serotonin syndrome consists of mental status changes, autonomic hyperactivity, and neuromuscular abnormalities. One of the greatest challenges of this diagnosis is its extremely variable presentation. Many patients do not exhibit all these clinical characteristics.[103] Some patients will have severe symptoms, such as high fever (up to 41.1°C), severe hypertension, and tachycardia that may deteriorate into hypotension, shock, agitated delirium, muscular rigidity, and hypertonicity. Mild cases may range from tremor and diarrhea to tachycardia and hypertension but no fever. Symptom onset is generally rapid, often within minutes of exposure to the precipitating agent, with most patients presenting within 6 to 24 hours.[100]

Agitated delirium is the most common form of mental status change, although this too has a wide spectrum of severity, including mild agitation, hypervigilance, slightly pressured speech, and easy startle. Diaphoresis, shivering, mydriasis, increased bowel sounds, and diarrhea are common signs of autonomic dysfunction.[95,100] Myoclonus is the most common neuromuscular finding,[98] but other abnormalities are possible, including muscular rigidity, hypertonicity (which may in turn contribute to hyperthermia), hyperreflexia and clonus (which are more pronounced in the lower than the upper extremities), horizontal ocular clonus, tremor, and akathisia. In some cases, muscle hypertonicity may be so severe that it overpowers and obscures tremor and hyperreflexia.

Significant morbidity and mortality are associated with serotonin syndrome. Severe cases are characterized by rhabdomyolysis with an elevated creatine kinase, metabolic acidosis, elevated serum aminotransferase, renal failure with an elevated serum creatinine, seizures, and disseminated intravascular coagulopathy. Approximately one-quarter of patients are treated with intubation, mechanical ventilation, and admission to an ICU. The mortality rate is approximately 11%, with the most common cause of death being inadequate management of hyperthermia.[98]

Diagnosis

The differential diagnosis of serotonin syndrome includes other disorders precipitated by medications or drug toxicity reactions (eg, NMS and malignant hyperthermia, anticholinergic syndrome, and withdrawal syndromes including delirium tremens); CNS disorders spanning infection (meningitis, encephalitis), tumors, and seizures; and psychiatric disorders such as acute catatonia.

Differentiating between serotonin syndrome and other medication-induced syndromes can be challenging and may be important, given that treatment may differ depending on the underlying etiology. Table 7 details both the similar and differentiating features of these syndromes. The most common clinical finding of serotonin syndrome is myoclonus, which occurs in slightly more than half (57%) of cases.[98] Some experts believe that clonus and hyperreflexia are "highly diagnostic for the serotonin syndrome and their occurrence in the setting of serotonergic drug use establishes the diagnosis."[100]

As with NMS, there are no pathognomonic laboratory or radiographic findings of serotonin syndrome. Testing may be obtained on the basis of clinical suspicion and may include a complete blood cell count, electrolytes, serum urea nitrogen, creatinine, arterial blood gas (checking respiratory status and for metabolic acidosis), hepatic transaminases, creatine kinase, urinalysis, toxicology screens, coagulation studies, electrocardiography, EEG, and brain imaging studies.

Clinical diagnostic criteria for serotonin syndrome have been proposed.[104,105] Hunter criteria[104] have a higher sensitivity (84% vs 75%) and specificity (97% vs 96%) than Sternbach criteria.[105] In addition, the use of the Sternbach criteria may exclude mild, early, or subacute serotonin syndrome. Others prefer modified Dunkley criteria.[100,104] According to the modified Dunkley criteria, the diagnosis can be made if the patient has taken a serotonergic drug within the last 5 weeks and has any of the following: tremor and hyperreflexia; spontaneous clonus; muscle rigidity, temperature >38°C, and either ocular clonus or inducible clonus; ocular clonus and either agitation or diaphoresis; or inducible clonus and either agitation or diaphoresis.[100] Other variations of these diagnostic criteria have been proposed. They all include a serotonergic drug having been started or the dosage increased and other possible etiologies (eg, NMS, substance abuse, withdrawal, infection, other toxidromes) having been ruled out, plus the presence of specific signs and symptoms.[95,106,107]

Treatment

Treatment often involves discontinuing the precipitating agent and providing supportive care. Supportive care may include treatment of agitation (eg, benzodiazepines), amelioration of hyperthermia, and management of the autonomic instability (eg, IV fluids and other agents to address abnormal vital signs). In addition, for those with severe serotonin syndrome (eg, temperature >41.1°C), emergency sedation, neuromuscular paralysis, and intubation may be considered. Physical restraints may be detrimental, because they may exacerbate isometric contractions, thereby worsening hyperthermia and lactic acidosis and increasing mortality.[98]

In severe cases, serotonin$_{2A}$ antagonists may be considered, with cyproheptadine being most commonly used. The adult dosage of

TABLE 7 Differentiation of the Drug Toxicity Syndromes

	Serotonin Syndrome	NMS	Malignant Hyperthermia	Anticholinergic Poisoning
Etiology	Excessive serotonin	Decreased dopamine	Calcium release from sarcoplasmic reticulum	Inhibit acetylcholine binding to muscarinic receptors
Precipitant	Proserotonergic drugs	Dopamine antagonist or withdrawal of dopaminergic drug	Inhalational anesthetic with or without succinylcholine	Anticholinergic drugs or antimuscarinic drugs
History	Nonidiosyncratic, add new drug, ↑ dosage of drug, or add second drug	Idiosyncratic, exposure to dopamine antagonist drug or withdrawal from dopaminergic drug	Inherited (+ family history) or new genetic mutation	Anticholinergic drug exposure antihistamines, tricyclic antidepressants, sleep aids, cold preparations, diphenhydramine, atropine
Onset	Minutes to hours Usual: 6–24 h	Days Usual: 1–7 d	Hours Usual: <12 h	Minutes to hours Usual: 0.5–24 h
Vital signs				
Temperature	Elevated (≤41.1°C)	Elevated (≤41.1°C)	Elevated (≤46°C)	Mild elevation (<38.8°C)
Heart rate	Tachycardia	Tachycardia	Tachycardia	Tachycardia
Respirations	Tachypnea	Tachypnea	Tachypnea	Tachypnea
Blood pressure	Hypertension (may deteriorate to hypotension)	Hypertension	Hypertension	Hypertension (mild)
Mental status	Agitated delirium	Variable: alert, mutism, stupor, coma	Agitation	Agitated delirium
Neuromuscular abnormalities				
Muscle tone	Increased, lower extremities greater than upper extremities	"Lead pipe" rigidity	Rigor mortis–like rigidity (masseters or generalized)	Normal
Muscle reflexes	Hyperreflexic, clonus; may be masked by hypertonicity	Slowed, bradyreflexic	Hyporeflexic	Normal
Physical examination				
Skin	Diaphoretic	Diaphoretic	Diaphoretic, mottled	Hot, dry, erythema[a]
Pupils	Mydriasis	Normal	Normal	Mydriasis
Mucous membranes	Sialorrhea	Sialorrhea	Normal	Dry[a]
Gastrointestinal motility	Hyperactive bowel sounds, may have diarrhea	Normal or hypoactive bowel sounds	Hypoactive bowel sounds	Hypoactive or absent bowel sounds
Treatment considerations				
General	Discontinue precipitant drug, supportive care, benzodiazepine for agitation			
Specific	If severe: serotonin$_{2A}$ antagonists (eg, cyproheptadine)	If severe: smooth muscle relaxant (eg, dantrolene), dopamine agonists (eg, bromocriptine, amantadine)	If severe: dantrolene	Sodium bicarbonate for prolonged QRS or dysrhythmias, treat hyperthermia, physostigmine

All of these drug toxicity syndromes can present with altered mental status, autonomic dysfunction, and neuromuscular abnormalities as manifested by abnormal vital signs including fever, hypertension, and tachycardia. Treatment in all 4 syndromes may include removing the precipitating agent and providing supportive care. Other specific therapy may differ depending on the disorder. Not all patients will have all the classic signs and symptoms. For example, a patient with mild serotonin syndrome may be afebrile but have tachycardia and hypertension. Typical findings are listed in this table.

[a] Anticholinergic syndrome described as "Red as a beet, dry as a bone, hot as a hare, blind as a bat, mad as a hatter, full as a flask."

cyproheptadine is usually 12 to 24 mg over 24 hours, typically starting with 12 mg, followed by 2 mg every 2 hours for continuing symptoms, and a maintenance dose of 8 mg every 6 hours, given orally. There is no parenteral form, but tablets have been crushed and administered via a nasogastric tube. The pediatric dosage is usually 0.25 mg/kg per day, divided into 2 or 3 doses daily, up to a maximum of 12 mg. Chlorpromazine, an antagonist of serotonin$_{2A}$ receptors as well, is available in a parenteral form but has the disadvantage that it can cause hypotension and may increase muscle rigidity, decrease the seizure threshold, and worsen NMS.[98] Both drugs may be effective,[108] but cyproheptadine is preferred by most experts.[99,100]

Low dosages of direct-acting sympathomimetic amines (eg, phenylephrine, norepinephrine, and epinephrine) or short-acting drugs such as esmolol or nitroprusside have been used to manage fluctuating blood pressure and heart rate. Use of indirect agents (eg, dopamine) may not be efficacious, because the mechanism of action of these drugs includes intracellular metabolism via catecholamine-O-methyl transferase to metabolize the dopamine to epinephrine and norepinephrine, which may result in overshooting the desired effect.

Management of hyperthermia often involves terminating the extreme muscle activity. In addition to treating agitation, benzodiazepines may be useful in controlling muscular activity in moderate cases. In severe cases, paralysis with nondepolarizing drugs (eg, vecuronium or rocuronium) and intubation may be considered. Some experts suggest that succinylcholine may be risky with these patients, secondary to hyperkalemia and rhabdomyolysis, which may be present and ultimately result in dysrhythmias. Because the fever of NMS is secondary to muscular hyperactivity and not effects on the hypothalamic thermoregulation set point, antipyretics typically are not efficacious.[96,99,108]

Patients with serotonin syndrome can deteriorate rapidly; therefore, close observation and preparation for rapid intervention may be considered. In milder cases, evaluation, observation, and discharge with close, additional outpatient management may be considered. As mentioned previously, discussing these patients' care with a toxicologist or poison control center may be helpful.

CHILDREN WITH SPECIAL NEEDS

Autism Spectrum and Developmental Disorders

In recent years, there has been a sharp increase in the incidence of ASDs and DDs,[109] with corresponding interest and growth in treatment strategies. Investigated therapeutic modalities include psychobehavioral therapies,[110-115] psychopharmacology,[116-118] occupational and language therapies,[119-121] and complementary and alternative medicines.[122] Unfortunately, many studies have had methodologic limitations (eg, small sample sizes, variability in study populations, methods or interventions used, and outcomes measures) and are not applicable to the medical setting.[123-125] Three evidence-based reviews of this topic conclude that there is adequate evidence for only a limited number of therapies (eg, pharmacotherapy), although several other strategies show promise (eg, early and intensive behavioral therapy, social skills training, and visual communication systems).[125-128] Given these limitations, the strategies discussed below are based primarily on expert, consensus opinion.

ASD-DD–Sensitive Care Resources

A wide range of ED health professionals can champion, organize, design, and coordinate ASD-sensitive ED care, including physicians, nurses, nursing assistants, nurse practitioners and physician assistants, social workers, and child life specialists. Non-ED professionals who may be helpful include developmental–behavioral pediatricians, child psychologists and psychiatrists, special education teachers, speech–language therapists, and occupational therapists.

Often, the most important ASD-DD "experts" to consult are the child's parents. Parents of children with ASDs or DDs know what strategies work with their children (eg, which words, actions, or stimuli calm and help their child and which have the opposite effect). Parents can also be "interpreters" for ED clinicians, deciphering the significance of their child's actions and behaviors and facilitating communication with their child. Spending some time asking parents about their child is likely to be a productive, efficient method for tailoring effective ED care for these patients.

Strategies for ASD-DD–Sensitive ED Care

Typical strategies for caring for children with ASD-DD are listed in Table 8.[128] Children with ASD-DD are often hypersensitive to environmental stimuli (eg, light, sound, and activity). Simple solutions include using a quiet office or counseling room (if available) instead of a loud, stimulating examination room. If this type of patient space is not available, an alternative solution may be to use a quiet examination room, away from the busy, noisy areas of the ED, with dimmed lighting (eg, turning off some lights or using a single lamp).

Studies have demonstrated that visual communication systems (VCSs) can improve communication with children with language disabilities.[129-132] VCS products are the most commonly used communication adjuncts and are widely available. There are numerous commercial or free and print and electronic products (eg, Web sites, "apps," devices). A visual schedule (Fig 1) exemplifies how a VCS can be used to prepare a child with ASD-DD for an upcoming event or activity. Visual schedules help children organize themselves, understand what will happen next, highlight or introduce activities that are unfamiliar to them, and create smoother transitions, all of which may decrease children's anxiety.

If a child has his or her own personal VCS, it may be advantageous to use

TABLE 8 Nonpharmacologic Strategies for Caring for Children With ASD-DD

Environmental modification (light, noise, other stimuli)
Visual communication systems
Transition planning
Occupational or physical therapy techniques

Triage Schedule

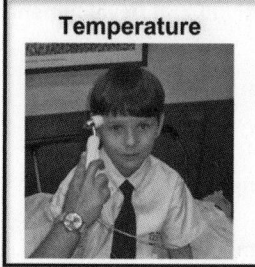
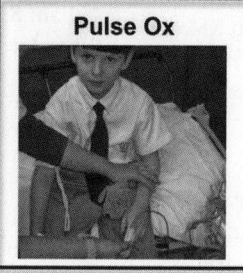
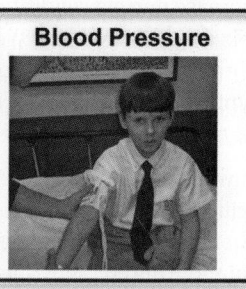

FIGURE 1
Digital photograph visual schedule. Photo credit: Thomas H. Chun, MD, MPH, FAAP.

Triage Schedule

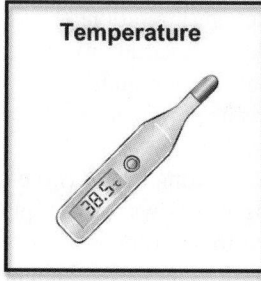
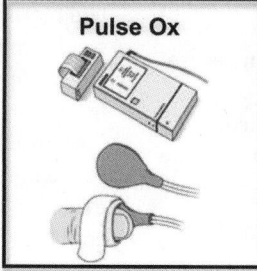
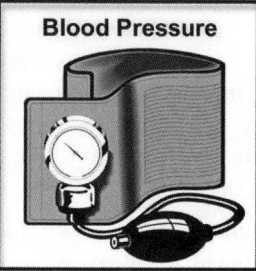

FIGURE 2
Clip art visual schedule.

the VCS, because the child will be familiar with pictures. A potential disadvantage of a personal VCS is that the set of images may not have the necessary medical pictures. A simple and inexpensive solution to this problem is to create a custom set of images of the ED setting. This can easily be done with clip art or digital photography images, which are then printed and laminated. If digital photography is used, taking pictures of the ED staff, equipment, and commonly performed procedures is a simple method for creating a customized VCS for your setting (Fig 2).

Transitions are often problematic for children with ASD-DD, including changing from 1 activity to the next, moving from 1 setting to another (especially new settings), and breaks or deviations from their usual routines. For these reasons, a medical visit may be upsetting or unsettling to these children. Fortunately, many parents are familiar with anticipating and planning for these types of transitions. For example, these parents talk to their children before a new experience, describe what will happen and the sequence of events, and explain what might be upsetting to the children and how they will handle these stressful situations. Preparing children with ASD-DD for a medical visit ideally begins before or while en route to the visit and is an ongoing process once they arrive.

Anticipating and building breaks in a schedule may be helpful. Many children with ASD-DD are able to remain on task for only short periods of time. Regular, brief breaks in the schedule may be helpful to these children. As time consuming as it may be, in the total calculus of planning

the ED visit this may still be a time-neutral strategy relative to the time consumed by unsuccessful strategies. At the least, this strategy is likely to be more satisfactory to children, their parents, and ED clinicians.

Desensitization strategies that are used with all children (eg, gradually approaching and engaging with children, bending down to interact at children's level, allowing children to play with medical instruments or to use them on you or their parent first, distracting them with a toy or game, and having children held or comforted by parents while they are examined) also may help with children with ASD-DD. For some, however, the same strategies may benefit from significant augmentation, literally breaking each step down into several incremental, smaller steps. It may take several visits and interactions and multiple attempts before children will allow you to approach and examine them.

Other children with ASD-DD are very sensitive about their personal space. Starting at the periphery (ie, toes and fingers) and slowly moving centrally may help relax children and facilitate the examination. These types of desensitization strategies have been successfully used for phlebotomy attempts in children with ASD-DD.[133]

Many children with ASD-DD find value in occupational therapy (OT). OT techniques that are directly applicable to medical settings involve sensory integration and tasks that can be used as distraction techniques. Children with ASD-DD have variable responses to touch, with some finding it soothing and others becoming distressed by touch. Some find "deep pressure" (ie, the feeling of weight on their bodies) relaxing, but others respond to light touch. Devices such as weighted blankets or shawls for deep pressure and gentle massaging devices for light touch frequently are used. These products can be purchased through OT supply vendors, but simple substitutes can be found easily in medical settings. For example, a radiology lead vest or apron is an easy facsimile of a weighted blanket. Gently stroking the child with gauze or cast underpadding provides an excellent light touch massage.

Distraction may be a useful adjunct in children with ASD-DD. Occupying a child's hands or body with "fidget toys" is a typical strategy. OT devices (eg, grip strengthening and manual dexterity devices, devices to improve balance) also may serve this function. With appropriate supervision, simple substitutes for these devices are also easily made (eg, a loosely wound roll of gauze or cast underpadding can be a substitute for a squeeze toy). Rocking in a rocking chair or nylon folding sports stadium seat also can calm children (Fig 3).

Psychopharmacology and ASD-DD

There are no rigorous evidence-based guidelines regarding psychotropic medications for children with ASD-DD. Although there is strong evidence for the use of psychotropic medications in ASD-DD,[116,117,125] there are no controlled trials of these medications for acute agitation or sedation. Currently, there are no known contraindications to using common sedating medications for children with ASD-DD, although some experts believe that atypical medication responses may be more common (eg, idiosyncratic, disinhibition, or paradoxical reactions). Inquiring about the previous reaction to medications often is helpful, as may be beginning with lower medication dosages to observe and determine the child's response to the medication.[134]

MENTAL HEALTH SCREENING

For a discussion of mental health screening strategies in primary care settings, please refer to the American

Academy of Pediatrics clinical report on screening for behavioral and emotional problems.[135]

The Advantages of the ED Setting

The ED may be an ideal setting for screening and identifying high-risk, difficult-to-reach pediatric populations with mental health problems. Many teenagers either do not have a primary care provider or face significant barriers to accessing such health care. For these adolescents, the ED often is their main or only source of medical care.[136,137] Other high-risk groups for mental health and substance use problems are homeless adolescents and school dropouts,[138–143] both of whom disproportionately seek medical care in the ED.

Finally, male adolescents may preferentially seek care in EDs because they are less likely to participate in primary or mental health care.[144,145]

Feasibility and Acceptability of ED Mental Health Screening

Several rapid, efficient, and accurate ED mental health screening tools have been developed and show promising results. As few as 2 screening questions have been found to be helpful in detecting depression in both adult and pediatric ED settings as well as problematic adolescent alcohol use.[146–148] A 4-question adolescent suicide screen has been shown to have good sensitivity, specificity, and predictive value across a range of teenagers seeking care in the ED and can be accurately administered by non–mental health professionals.[149–151] Similarly, an 8-question screen was shown to have excellent predictive characteristics for detecting posttraumatic stress symptoms in children who sustained traffic-related injuries.[152]

Given the clinical and time pressures of the ED setting, it is important that mental health screening be

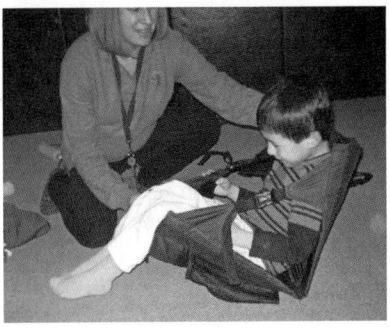

FIGURE 3
Example of rocking in a sports chair. Photo credit: Thomas H. Chun, MD, MPH, FAAP.

acceptable to adolescents, their parents, and ED clinicians. Numerous studies have shown the acceptability of such screening. Teenagers and parents both report favorable attitudes toward mental health screening during an ED visit.[153,154] In this study, suicide and drug and alcohol screening rated as more important than other mental health problems. Female adolescents and their parents, more than male adolescents, expressed positive views on screening. In another study, both teenagers and their caregivers perceived ED depression screening as a sign of caring and concern for the adolescent.[155] Suicide screening has been found to be acceptable to 60% to 66% of patients and parents, with 96% of participants agreeing that suicide screening is appropriate in the ED.[149,150,156]

What do ED clinicians think about mental health screening in the ED? Is such screening acceptable to them? Perceived and real barriers to such screening exist, including lack of training, time constraints, and increasing ED patients' length of stay. Williams et al[154] investigated this question and found that 99% of physicians and 97% of nurses stated that a brief, validated screening tool did not interfere with patient care. In addition, research staff endorsed "no difficulty" in administering the screen to 73% of participants. Lastly, a significant and important finding of the study by Horowitz et al[149] was that real-time evaluation of positive suicide screens did not increase ED patients' length of stay.

ED Mental Health Screens

Many mental health screening tools have been developed or tested in the ED setting. Although not validated in general ED populations, they have the potential to increase ED mental health screening. One example is an abbreviated version of the Home, Education/School, Activities, Drugs, Depression, Sexuality, Suicide, Safety (HEADDSSS) mnemonic for adolescent psychosocial assessment, which was adapted for and tested in an ED.[157] The Home, Education, Activities and Peers, Drugs and Alcohol, Suicidality, Emotions and Behaviors, Discharge Resources (HEADS-ED) was found to be reliable and accurate, with good concurrent and predictive validity for future psychiatric evaluation and hospitalization.[158]

Horowitz et al[149,151,159] have performed several studies on ED suicide screening, most recently by using multiple logistic regression modeling to determine which suicide screening questions best screen for and identify occult suicidal youth.[150] A 4-question model was found to optimize sensitivity (97%; 95% CI, 91%–99%), specificity (88%; 95% CI, 84%–91%), and negative predictive value (99%, 95% CI, 98%–99%) for ED patients presenting with both psychiatric and nonpsychiatric conditions. The 4 domains of suicidal ideation are current suicidal ideation, past suicide attempts, current wish to die, and current thoughts of being better off dead. Given the prevalence of suicidal ideation and attempts and the morbidity and mortality associated with attempts, screening patients with unclear or high risk of suicide (eg, those presenting with ingestions, acute intoxication, single-car motor vehicle crashes, and significant falls) also may be important.

Both depression and alcohol abuse may be screened for with 2 questions. Rutman et al[147] found that the 2 questions "During the past month, have you often been bothered by feeling down, depressed, or hopeless?" and "During the past month, have you often been bothered by little interest or pleasure in doing things?" were 78% sensitive (95% CI, 73%–84%) and 82% specific (95% CI, 77%–87%) for adolescent depression. These 2 questions have similar screening properties in adult ED patients as well.[146] Both Newton et al and the National Institute of Alcohol Abuse and Alcoholism (NIAAA) have developed 2-question screens for problematic teenage alcohol use.[148,160] Newton et al also believe that a single question may efficiently screen for marijuana use. They used the following questions: "In the past year, have you sometimes been under the influence of alcohol in situations where you could have caused an accident or gotten hurt?", "Have there often been times when you have a lot more to drink than you intended to have?", and "In the past year, how often have your used cannabis: 0 to 1 time, or greater than 2 times?" Teenagers who answer "yes" to 1 alcohol question or to the marijuana question have an eightfold and sevenfold increased risk of having a substance use disorder, respectively. The 2 NIAAA questions vary according to the patient's age and explore the patient's and their friends' experience with alcohol. The NIAAA currently is investigating the reliability as well as the concurrent, convergent, discriminant, and predictive validity of this screen.[161]

Computerized screening may add advantages and efficiency to ED mental health screening. They can be administered with little ED clinician time or effort and have been used successfully in both pediatric and general ED settings for general health and mental health screening, alcohol use,[162-164] interpersonal and intimate partner violence,[165,166] weapons,[167] injury prevention,[168] and HIV risk behaviors.[169] Adolescents not only rated these screens as highly acceptable but also may prefer such health interventions.[170-172] Fein and Pailler[140,173] have developed and implemented an electronic tool for universal screening of ED adolescent physical and mental health risks. The screen was presented to patients by a nurse or medical technician. After the screen was scored, the adolescent's results were printed out and reviewed by the treating physicians. This method resulted in a 68% increase in identification of psychiatric illnesses and subsequently a 47% increase in mental health assessments.

LEAD AUTHORS

Thomas H. Chun, MD, MPH, FAAP
Sharon E. Mace, MD, FAAP, FACEP
Emily R. Katz, MD, FAAP

AMERICAN ACADEMY OF PEDIATRICS COMMITTEE ON PEDIATRIC EMERGENCY MEDICINE, 2014–2015

Joan E. Shook, MD, MBA, FAAP, Chairperson
James M. Callahan, MD, FAAP
Thomas H. Chun, MD, MPH, FAAP
Gregory P. Conners, MD, MPH, MBA, FAAP
Edward E. Conway Jr, MD, MS, FAAP
Nanette C. Dudley, MD, FAAP
Toni K. Gross, MD, MPH, FAAP
Natalie E. Lane, MD, FAAP
Charles G. Macias, MD, MPH, FAAP
Nathan L. Timm, MD, FAAP

LIAISONS

Kim Bullock, MD – *American Academy of Family Physicians*
Elizabeth Edgerton, MD, MPH, FAAP – *Maternal and Child Health Bureau*
Tamar Magarik Haro – *AAP Department of Federal Affairs*
Madeline Joseph, MD, FACEP, FAAP – *American College of Emergency Physicians*
Angela Mickalide, PhD, MCHES – *EMSC National Resource Center*
Brian R. Moore, MD, FAAP – *National Association of EMS Physicians*
Katherine E. Remick, MD, FAAP – *National Association of Emergency Medical Technicians*
Sally K. Snow, RN, BSN, CPEN, FAEN – *Emergency Nurses Association*
David W. Tuggle, MD, FAAP – *American College of Surgeons*

> **ABBREVIATIONS**
>
> ASD: autism spectrum disorder
> CI: confidence interval
> CNS: central nervous system
> DD: developmental disorder
> ED: emergency department
> FDA: US Food and Drug Administration
> IV: intravenous
> NIAAA: National Institute of Alcohol Abuse and Alcoholism
> NMS: neuroleptic malignant syndrome
> OT: occupational therapy
> PNES: psychogenic nonepileptic seizures
> SSRI: selective serotonin reuptake inhibitor
> VCS: visual communication system

REFERENCES

1. American Psychiatric Association. *Diagnostic and Statistical Manual of Mental Disorders.* 5th ed (DSM-5). Washington, DC: American Psychiatric Association Press; 2013

2. Dell ML, Campo JV. Somatoform disorders in children and adolescents. *Psychiatr Clin North Am.* 2011;34(3):643–660

3. Sater N, Constantino JN. Pediatric emergencies in children with psychiatric conditions. *Pediatr Emerg Care.* 1998;14(1):42–50

4. Barsky AJ, Orav EJ, Bates DW. Distinctive patterns of medical care utilization in patients who somatize. *Med Care.* 2006;44(9):803–811

5. Silber TJ. Somatization disorders: diagnosis, treatment, and prognosis. *Pediatr Rev.* 2011;32(2):56–63, quiz 63–64

6. Reid S, Wessely S, Crayford T, Hotopf M. Medically unexplained symptoms in frequent attenders of secondary health care: retrospective cohort study. *BMJ.* 2001;322(7289):767

7. Livingston R, Witt A, Smith GR. Families who somatize. *J Dev Behav Pediatr.* 1995;16(1):42–46

8. Campo JV, Jansen-McWilliams L, Comer DM, Kelleher KJ. Somatization in pediatric primary care: association with psychopathology, functional impairment, and use of services. *J Am Acad Child Adolesc Psychiatry.* 1999;38(9):1093–1101

9. Barsky AJ, Orav EJ, Bates DW. Somatization increases medical utilization and costs independent of psychiatric and medical comorbidity. *Arch Gen Psychiatry.* 2005;62(8):903–910

10. Campo JV, Fritsch SL. Somatization in children and adolescents. *J Am Acad Child Adolesc Psychiatry.* 1994;33(9):1223–1235

11. Garralda ME. Somatisation in children. *J Child Psychol Psychiatry.* 1996;37(1):13–33

12. Garralda ME, Bailey D. Children with psychiatric disorders in primary care. *J Child Psychol Psychiatry.* 1986;27(5):611–624

13. Garralda ME, Bailey D. Psychosomatic aspects of children's consultations in primary care. *Eur Arch Psychiatry Neurol Sci.* 1987;236(5):319–322

14. Schecker N. Childhood conversion reactions in the emergency department: Part II--general and specific features. *Pediatr Emerg Care.* 1990;6(1):46–51

15. Lee J, Dade LA. The buck stops where? What is the role of the emergency physician in managing panic disorder in chest pain patients? *CJEM.* 2003;5(4):237–238

16. Pollard CA, Lewis LM. Managing panic attacks in emergency patients. *J Emerg Med.* 1989;7(5):547–552

17. Fleet RP, Dupuis G, Marchand A, Burelle D, Arsenault A, Beitman BD. Panic disorder in emergency department chest pain patients: prevalence, comorbidity, suicidal ideation, and physician recognition. *Am J Med.* 1996;101(4):371–380

18. Garralda ME. Unexplained physical complaints. *Pediatr Clin North Am.* 2011;58(4):803–813, ix

19. Stephenson DT, Price JR. Medically unexplained physical symptoms in emergency medicine. *Emerg Med J.* 2006;23(8):595–600

20. Alfvén G. The covariation of common psychosomatic symptoms among children from socio-economically differing residential areas. An epidemiological study. *Acta Paediatr.* 1993;82(5):484–487

21. Haugland S, Wold B, Stevenson J, Aaroe LE, Woynarowska B. Subjective health complaints in adolescence. A cross-national comparison of prevalence and dimensionality. *Eur J Public Health.* 2001;11(1):4–10

22. Emiroğlu FN, Kurul S, Akay A, Miral S, Dirik E. Assessment of child neurology outpatients with headache, dizziness, and fainting. *J Child Neurol.* 2004;19(5):332–336

23. Egger HL, Angold A, Costello EJ. Headaches and psychopathology in children and adolescents. *J Am Acad Child Adolesc Psychiatry.* 1998;37(9):951–958

24. Galli F, Patron L, Russo PM, Bruni O, Ferini-Strambi L, Guidetti V. Chronic daily headache in childhood and adolescence: clinical aspects and a 4-year follow-up [published correction appears in *Cephalalgia.* 2004;24(11):1011]. *Cephalalgia.* 2004;24(10):850–858

25. Guidetti V, Galli F, Fabrizi P, et al. Headache and psychiatric comorbidity: clinical aspects and outcome in an 8-year follow-up study. *Cephalalgia.* 1998;18(7):455–462

26. Tunaoglu FS, Olguntürk R, Akcabay S, Oguz D, Gücüyener K, Demirsoy S. Chest pain in children referred to a cardiology clinic. *Pediatr Cardiol.* 1995;16(2):69–72

27. Campo JV, Bridge J, Ehmann M, et al. Recurrent abdominal pain, anxiety, and depression in primary care. *Pediatrics.* 2004;113(4):817–824

28. Kashikar-Zuck S, Parkins IS, Graham TB, et al. Anxiety, mood, and behavioral disorders among pediatric patients with juvenile fibromyalgia syndrome. *Clin J Pain.* 2008;24(7):620–626

29. Selbst SM, Clancy R. Pseudoseizures in the pediatric emergency department. *Pediatr Emerg Care.* 1996;12(3):185–188

30. Bhatia MS, Sapra S. Pseudoseizures in children: a profile of 50 cases. *Clin Pediatr (Phila).* 2005;44(7):617–621

31. Wyllie E, Glazer JP, Benbadis S, Kotagal P, Wolgamuth B. Psychiatric features of children and adolescents with pseudoseizures. *Arch Pediatr Adolesc Med.* 1999;153(3):244–248

32. Knockaert DC, Buntinx F, Stoens N, Bruyninckx R, Delooz H. Chest pain in the emergency department: the broad spectrum of causes. *Eur J Emerg Med.* 2002;9(1):25–30

33. Lipsitz JD, Gur M, Sonnet FM, et al. Psychopathology and disability in children with unexplained chest pain presenting to the pediatric emergency department. *Pediatr Emerg Care.* 2010;26(11):830–836

34. Dang AT, Ho M, Kroenke K, Grupp-Phelan J. Maternal somatic symptoms, psychosocial correlates, and subsequent pediatric emergency department use. *Pediatr Emerg Care.* 2013;29(2):170–174

35. Abbass A, Campbell S, Magee K, Tarzwell R. Intensive short-term dynamic psychotherapy to reduce rates of emergency department return visits for patients with medically unexplained symptoms: preliminary evidence from a pre–post intervention study. *CJEM.* 2009;11(6):529–534

36. Comer JS, Olfson M, Mojtabai R. National trends in child and adolescent psychotropic polypharmacy in office-based practice, 1996–2007. *J Am Acad Child Adolesc Psychiatry.* 2010;49(10):1001–1010

37. Olfson M, Blanco C, Wang S, Laje G, Correll CU. National trends in the mental health care of children, adolescents, and adults by office-based physicians. *JAMA Psychiatry.* 2014;71(1):81–90

38. Pringsheim T, Lam D, Patten SB. The pharmacoepidemiology of antipsychotic medications for Canadian children and adolescents: 2005–2009. *J Child Adolesc Psychopharmacol.* 2011;21(6):537–543

39. Alexander GC, Gallagher SA, Mascola A, Moloney RM, Stafford RS. Increasing off-label use of antipsychotic medications in the United States, 1995–2008. *Pharmacoepidemiol Drug Saf.* 2011;20(2):177–184

40. Matone M, Localio R, Huang YS, dosReis S, Feudtner C, Rubin D. The relationship between mental health diagnosis and treatment with second-generation antipsychotics over time: a national study of US Medicaid-enrolled children. *Health Serv Res.* 2012;47(5):1836–1860

41. Pathak P, West D, Martin BC, Helm ME, Henderson C. Evidence-based use of second-generation antipsychotics in a state Medicaid pediatric population, 2001–2005. *Psychiatr Serv.* 2010;61(2):123–129

42. Harrison JN, Cluxton-Keller F, Gross D. Antipsychotic medication prescribing trends in children and adolescents. *J Pediatr Health Care.* 2012;26(2):139–145

43. Cooper WO, Arbogast PG, Ding H, Hickson GB, Fuchs DC, Ray WA. Trends in prescribing of antipsychotic medications for US children. *Ambul Pediatr.* 2006;6(2):79–83

44. Olfson M, Crystal S, Huang C, Gerhard T. Trends in antipsychotic drug use by very young, privately insured children.

J Am Acad Child Adolesc Psychiatry. 2010;49(1):13–23

45. Whittler MA, Lavonas EJ. Antipsychotics. In: Marx JA, Hockberger R, Walls RM, eds. *Rosen's Emergency Medicine: Concepts and Clinical Practice.* Philadelphia, PA: Saunders; 2014:2042–2046

46. Amaral DG, Rubenstein JLR, Rogers SJ. Neuroscience of autism. In: Tasman A, Kay J, Lieberman A, First MB, Maj M, eds. *Psychiatry.* 3rd ed. West Sussex, England: John Wiley & Sons; 2008:386–392

47. Hilt RJ, Woodward TA. Agitation treatment for pediatric emergency patients. *J Am Acad Child Adolesc Psychiatry.* 2008;47(2):132–138

48. Sonnier L, Barzman D. Pharmacologic management of acutely agitated pediatric patients. *Paediatr Drugs.* 2011;13(1):1–10

49. Newcorn JH, Ivanov I, Sharma V. Childhood disorders: attention-deficit and disruptive behavior disorders. In: Tasman A, Kay J, Lieberman A, First MB, Maj M, eds. *Psychiatry.* 3rd ed. West Sussex, England: John Wiley & Sons; 2008:816–831

50. Levine M, LoVecchio F. Antipsychotics. In: Tintinalli JE, Stapczynski S, Ma OJ, Cline DM, Cydulka RK, Mecklereds GD, eds. *Tintinalli's Emergency Medicine: A Comprehensive Study Guide.* New York, NY: McGraw-Hill Education; 2011:1207–1211

51. Miyamoto S, Merrill DB, Lieberman JA, Fleischacker WW, Marder SR. Antipsychotic drugs. In: Tasman A, Kay J, Lieberman A, First MB, Maj M, eds. *Psychiatry.* 3rd ed. West Sussex, England: John Wiley & Sons; 2008:2161–2201

52. Guenette MD, Giacca A, Hahn M, et al. Atypical antipsychotics and effects of adrenergic and serotonergic receptor binding on insulin secretion in-vivo: an animal model. *Schizophr Res.* 2013;146(1–3):162–169

53. Reynolds GP, Kirk SL. Metabolic side effects of antipsychotic drug treatment: pharmacological mechanisms. *Pharmacol Ther.* 2010;125(1):169–179

54. Starrenburg FC, Bogers JP. How can antipsychotics cause diabetes mellitus? Insights based on receptor-binding profiles, humoral factors and transporter proteins. *Eur Psychiatry.* 2009;24(3):164–170

55. Bailey P, Norton R, Karan S. The FDA droperidol warning: is it justified? *Anesthesiology.* 2002;97(1):288–289

56. Chase PB, Biros MH. A retrospective review of the use and safety of droperidol in a large, high-risk, inner-city emergency department patient population. *Acad Emerg Med.* 2002;9(12):1402–1410

57. Dershwitz M. Droperidol: should the black box be light gray? *J Clin Anesth.* 2002;14(8):598–603

58. Gan TJ, White PF, Scuderi PE, Watcha MF, Kovac A. FDA "black box" warning regarding use of droperidol for postoperative nausea and vomiting: is it justified? *Anesthesiology.* 2002;97(1):287

59. Horowitz BZ, Bizovi K, Moreno R. Droperidol: behind the black box warning. *Acad Emerg Med.* 2002;9(6):615–618

60. Lukens TW, Wolf SJ, Edlow JA, et al; American College of Emergency Physicians Clinical Policies Subcommittee (Writing Committee) on Critical Issues in the Diagnosis and Management of the Adult Psychiatric Patient in the Emergency Department. Clinical policy: critical issues in the diagnosis and management of the adult psychiatric patient in the emergency department. *Ann Emerg Med.* 2006;47(1):79–99

61. Walters H, Killius K. *Guidelines for the Acute Psychotropic Medication Management of Agitation in Children and Adolescents.* Boston, MA: Boston Medical Center Emergency Department Policy and Procedure Guidelines; 2012

62. Meyer-Massetti C, Cheng CM, Sharpe BA, Meier CR, Guglielmo BJ. The FDA extended warning for intravenous haloperidol and torsades de pointes: how should institutions respond? *J Hosp Med.* 2010;5(4):E8–E16

63. Haddad PM, Anderson IM. Antipsychotic-related QTc prolongation, torsade de pointes and sudden death. *Drugs.* 2002;62(11):1649–1671

64. Isaacs E. The violent patient. In: Marx JA, Hockberger R, Walls RM, eds. *Rosen's Emergency Medicine: Concepts and Clinical Practice.* Philadelphia, PA: Saunders; 2014:1460–1465

65. Gören JL, Dinh TA. Psychotropics and sudden cardiac death. *R I Med J (2013).* 2013;96(3):38–41

66. Szwak K, Sacchetti A. Droperidol use in pediatric emergency department patients. *Pediatr Emerg Care.* 2010;26(4):248–250

67. Baren JM, Mace SE, Hendry PL, Dietrich AM, Goldman RD, Warden CR. Children's mental health emergencies--part 2: emergency department evaluation and treatment of children with mental health disorders [published correction appears in *Pediatr Emerg Care.* 2008;24(11):748]. *Pediatr Emerg Care.* 2008;24(7):485–498

68. Hockberger R, Walls R. Thought disorders. In: Marx JA, Hockberger R, Walls RM, eds. *Rosen's Emergency Medicine: Concepts and Clinical Practice.* Philadelphia, PA: Saunders; 2014:1430–1436

69. Pringsheim T, Doja A, Belanger S, Patten S; Canadian Alliance for Monitoring Effectiveness and Safety of Antipsychotics in Children (CAMESA) guideline group. Treatment recommendations for extrapyramidal side effects associated with second-generation antipsychotic use in children and youth. *Paediatr Child Health.* 2011;16(9):590–598

70. Minns AB, Clark RF. Toxicology and overdose of atypical antipsychotics. *J Emerg Med.* 2012;43(5):906–913

71. Guzé BH, Baxter LR Jr. Current concepts. Neuroleptic malignant syndrome. *N Engl J Med.* 1985;313(3):163–166

72. Meeks TW, Jeste DV. Medication-induced movement disorders. In: Tasman A, Kay J, Lieberman A, First MB, Maj M, eds. *Psychiatry.* 3rd ed. West Sussex, England: John Wiley & Sons; 2008:2142

73. Silva RR, Munoz DM, Alpert M, Perlmutter IR, Diaz J. Neuroleptic malignant syndrome in children and adolescents. *J Am Acad Child Adolesc Psychiatry.* 1999;38(2):187–194

74. Young MC, Miller AD, Clark RF. Antipsychotic agents. In: Wolfson AB, Hendey GW, Ling LJ, Rosen CL, Schaider

JJ, Sharieff GQ, eds. *Harwood-Nuss Clinical Practice of Emergency Medicine*. Philadelphia, PA: Wolters-Kluwer/Lippincott Williams & Wilkins; 2010:1493–1497

75. Margetić B, Aukst-Margetić B. Neuroleptic malignant syndrome and its controversies. *Pharmacoepidemiol Drug Saf*. 2010;19(5):429–435

76. Jacobson JL. Neuroleptic malignant syndrome. In: Jacobson JL, ed. *Psychiatric Secrets*. Philadelphia, PA: Hanley & Belfus; 2000:447–451

77. Perry PJ, Wilborn CA. Serotonin syndrome vs neuroleptic malignant syndrome: a contrast of causes, diagnoses, and management. *Ann Clin Psychiatry*. 2012;24(2):155–162

78. Shalev A, Hermesh H, Munitz H. Mortality from neuroleptic malignant syndrome. *J Clin Psychiatry*. 1989;50(1):18–25

79. Caroff SN, Mann SC. Neuroleptic malignant syndrome. *Med Clin North Am*. 1993;77(1):185–202

80. Chung T, Smith GT, Donovan JE, et al. Drinking frequency as a brief screen for adolescent alcohol problems. *Pediatrics*. 2012;129(2):205–212

81. Levenson JL. Neuroleptic malignant syndrome. *Am J Psychiatry*. 1985;142(10):1137–1145

82. Agar L. Recognizing neuroleptic malignant syndrome in the emergency department: a case study. *Perspect Psychiatr Care*. 2010;46(2):143–151

83. Bajjoka I, Patel T, O'Sullivan T. Risperidone-induced neuroleptic malignant syndrome. *Ann Emerg Med*. 1997;30(5):698–700

84. Kogoj A, Velikonja I. Olanzapine induced neuroleptic malignant syndrome: a case review. *Hum Psychopharmacol*. 2003;18(4):301–309

85. Trollor JN, Chen X, Chitty K, Sachdev PS. Comparison of neuroleptic malignant syndrome induced by first- and second-generation antipsychotics. *Br J Psychiatry*. 2012;201(1):52–56

86. Wijdicks EFM. Neuroleptic malignant syndrome. In: Aminoff MJ, ed. *UpToDate*. Updated May 30, 2014. Available at: www.uptodate.com/contents/neuroleptic-malignant-syndrome. Accessed July 7, 2015

87. Hammerman S, Lam C, Caroff SN. Neuroleptic malignant syndrome and aripiprazole. *J Am Acad Child Adolesc Psychiatry*. 2006;45(6):639–641

88. Martel ML, Biros MH. Psychotropic medications and rapid tranquilization. In: Tintinalli JE, Stapczynski S, Ma OJ, Cline DM, Cydulka RK, Mecklereds GD, eds. *Tintinalli's Emergency Medicine: A Comprehensive Study Guide*. New York, NY: McGraw-Hill Education; 2011:1952–1955

89. Hatfield-Keller E, Thomas HA. Fever. In: Wolfson AB, Hendey GW, Ling LJ, Rosen CL, Schaider JJ, Sharieff GQ, eds. *Harwood-Nuss Clinical Practice of Emergency Medicine*. Philadelphia, PA: Wolters-Kluwer/Lippincott Williams & Wilkins; 2010:99–101

90. Gurrera RJ, Caroff SN, Cohen A, et al. An international consensus study of neuroleptic malignant syndrome diagnostic criteria using the Delphi method. *J Clin Psychiatry*. 2011;72(9):1222–1228

91. Anglin RE, Rosebush PI, Mazurek MF. Neuroleptic malignant syndrome: a neuroimmunologic hypothesis. *CMAJ*. 2010;182(18):E834–E838

92. Isbister GK, Dawson A, Whyte IM, Prior FH, Clancy C, Smith AJ. Neonatal paroxetine withdrawal syndrome or actually serotonin syndrome? *Arch Dis Child Fetal Neonatal Ed*. 2001;85(2):F147–F148

93. Kant S, Liebelt E. Recognizing serotonin toxicity in the pediatric emergency department. *Pediatr Emerg Care*. 2012;28(8):817–821, quiz 822–824

94. Spirko BA, Wiley JF II. Serotonin syndrome: a new pediatric intoxication. *Pediatr Emerg Care*. 1999;15(6):440–443

95. Birmes P, Coppin D, Schmitt L, Lauque D. Serotonin syndrome: a brief review. *CMAJ*. 2003;168(11):1439–1442

96. Ables AZ, Nagubilli R. Prevention, recognition, and management of serotonin syndrome. *Am Fam Physician*. 2010;81(9):1139–1142

97. Christensen RC. Identifying serotonin syndrome in the emergency department. *Am J Emerg Med*. 2005;23(3):406–408

98. Mills KC, Bora KM. Atypical antidepressants, serotonin reuptake

inhibitors, and serotonin syndrome. In: Tintinalli JE, Stapczynski S, Ma OJ, Cline DM, Cydulka RK, Mecklereds GD, eds. *Tintinalli's Emergency Medicine: A Comprehensive Study Guide*. New York, NY: McGraw-Hill Education; 2011:1198–1203

99. Isbister GK, Buckley NA, Whyte IM. Serotonin toxicity: a practical approach to diagnosis and treatment. *Med J Aust*. 2007;187(6):361–365

100. Boyer EW, Shannon M. The serotonin syndrome. *N Engl J Med*. 2005;352(11):1112–1120

101. Isbister GK, Buckley NA. The pathophysiology of serotonin toxicity in animals and humans: implications for diagnosis and treatment. *Clin Neuropharmacol*. 2005;28(5):205–214

102. Kirschner R, Donovan JW. Serotonin syndrome precipitated by fentanyl during procedural sedation. *J Emerg Med*. 2010;38(4):477–480

103. Barthold CL, Graudins A. Serotonin re-uptake inhibitors and the serotonin syndrome. In: Wolfson AB, Hendey GW, Ling LJ, Rosen CL, Schaider JJ, Sharieff GQ, eds. *Harwood-Nuss Clinical Practice of Emergency Medicine*. Philadelphia, PA: Wolters-Kluwer/Lippincott Williams & Wilkins; 2010:1510–1513

104. Dunkley EJ, Isbister GK, Sibbritt D, Dawson AH, Whyte IM. The Hunter Serotonin Toxicity Criteria: simple and accurate diagnostic decision rules for serotonin toxicity. *QJM*. 2003;96(9):635–642

105. Sternbach H. The serotonin syndrome. *Am J Psychiatry*. 1991;148(6):705–713

106. Boland RJ, Keller MB. Antidepressants. In: Tasman A, Kay J, Lieberman A, First MB, Maj M, eds. *Psychiatry*. 3rd ed. West Sussex, England: John Wiley & Sons; 2008:2142

107. Radomski JW, Dursun SM, Reveley MA, Kutcher SP. An exploratory approach to the serotonin syndrome: an update of clinical phenomenology and revised diagnostic criteria. *Med Hypotheses*. 2000;55(3):218–224

108. Gillman PK. The serotonin syndrome and its treatment. *J Psychopharmacol*. 1999;13(1):100–109

109. Autism and Developmental Disabilities Monitoring Network Surveillance Year

2008 Principal Investigators; Centers for Disease Control and Prevention. Prevalence of autism spectrum disorders: Autism and Developmental Disabilities Monitoring Network, 14 sites, United States, 2008. *MMWR Surveill Summ.* 2012;61(3):1–19

110. Foxx RM. Applied behavior analysis treatment of autism: the state of the art. *Child Adolesc Psychiatr Clin N Am.* 2008;17(4):821–834, ix

111. Hodgetts S, Hodgetts W. Somatosensory stimulation interventions for children with autism: literature review and clinical considerations. *Can J Occup Ther.* 2007;74(5):393–400

112. Karkhaneh M, Clark B, Ospina MB, Seida JC, Smith V, Hartling L. Social Stories to improve social skills in children with autism spectrum disorder: a systematic review. *Autism.* 2010;14(6):641–662

113. LeBlanc LA, Gillis JM. Behavioral interventions for children with autism spectrum disorders. *Pediatr Clin North Am.* 2012;59(1):147–164, xi–xii

114. Meindl JN, Cannella-Malone HI. Initiating and responding to joint attention bids in children with autism: a review of the literature. *Res Dev Disabil.* 2011;32(5):1441–1454

115. Virués-Ortega J. Applied behavior analytic intervention for autism in early childhood: meta-analysis, meta-regression and dose–response meta-analysis of multiple outcomes. *Clin Psychol Rev.* 2010;30(4):387–399

116. McPheeters ML, Warren Z, Sathe N, et al. A systematic review of medical treatments for children with autism spectrum disorders. *Pediatrics.* 2011;127(5). Available at: www.pediatrics.org/cgi/content/full/127/5/e1312

117. Siegel M, Beaulieu AA. Psychotropic medications in children with autism spectrum disorders: a systematic review and synthesis for evidence-based practice. *J Autism Dev Disord.* 2012;42(8):1592–1605

118. Sung M, Fung DS, Cai Y, Ooi YP. Pharmacological management in children and adolescents with pervasive developmental disorder. *Aust N Z J Psychiatry.* 2010;44(5):410–428

119. Case-Smith J, Arbesman M. Evidence-based review of interventions for autism used in or of relevance to occupational therapy. *Am J Occup Ther.* 2008;62(4):416–429

120. Oriel KN, George CL, Peckus R, Semon A. The effects of aerobic exercise on academic engagement in young children with autism spectrum disorder. *Pediatr Phys Ther.* 2011;23(2):187–193

121. Polatajko HJ, Cantin N. Exploring the effectiveness of occupational therapy interventions, other than the sensory integration approach, with children and adolescents experiencing difficulty processing and integrating sensory information. *Am J Occup Ther.* 2010;64(3):415–429

122. Rossignol DA. Novel and emerging treatments for autism spectrum disorders: a systematic review. *Ann Clin Psychiatry.* 2009;21(4):213–236

123. Mesibov GB, Shea V. Evidence-based practices and autism. *Autism.* 2011;15(1):114–133

124. Reichow B, Volkmar FR, Cicchetti DV. Development of the evaluative method for evaluating and determining evidence-based practices in autism. *J Autism Dev Disord.* 2008;38(7):1311–1319

125. Warren Z, Veenstra-VanderWeele J, Stone W, et al. *Therapies for Children With Autism Spectrum Disorders.* Comparative Effectiveness Review no. 26. (Prepared by the Vanderbilt Evidence-Based Practice Center under contract no. 290-02-HHSA-290-2007-10065-I.) AHRQ publication no. 11-EHC029-EF. Rockville, MD: Agency for Healthcare Research and Quality; 2011

126. Maglione MA, Gans D, Das L, Timbie J, Kasari C; Technical Expert Panel; HRSA Autism Intervention Research–Behavioral (AIR-B) Network. Nonmedical interventions for children with ASD: recommended guidelines and further research needs. *Pediatrics.* 2012;130(suppl 2):S169–S178

127. Wong C, Odom SL, Hume K, et al. *Evidence Based Practices for Children, Youth, and Young Adults With Autism Spectrum Disorder.* Chapel Hill, NC: University of North Carolina; 2013

128. Chun TH, Berrios-Candelaria R. Caring for children with autism in emergencies: What can we learn from . . . Broadway? *Contemp Pediatr.* 2012;29(9):56–65

129. Ganz JB, Davis JL, Lund EM, Goodwyn FD, Simpson RL. Meta-analysis of PECS with individuals with ASD: investigation of targeted versus non-targeted outcomes, participant characteristics, and implementation phase. *Res Dev Disabil.* 2012;33(2):406–418

130. Gordon K, Pasco G, McElduff F, Wade A, Howlin P, Charman T. A communication-based intervention for nonverbal children with autism: what changes? Who benefits? *J Consult Clin Psychol.* 2011;79(4):447–457

131. Howlin P, Gordon RK, Pasco G, Wade A, Charman T. The effectiveness of Picture Exchange Communication System (PECS) training for teachers of children with autism: a pragmatic, group randomised controlled trial. *J Child Psychol Psychiatry.* 2007;48(5):473–481

132. Yoder PJ, Lieberman RG. Brief report: randomized test of the efficacy of picture exchange communication system on highly generalized picture exchanges in children with ASD. *J Autism Dev Disord.* 2010;40(5):629–632

133. Autism Treatment Network. Blood draw tool kit (for parents and medical providers). Available at: www.autismspeaks.org/science/resources-programs/autism-treatment-network/tools-you-can-use/blood-draw-toolkits. Accessed July 5, 2015

134. Sullivan M. Autism demands attention in the emergency department. *ACEP News.* April 17, 2012

135. Weitzman C, Wegner L; Section on Developmental and Behavioral Pediatrics; Committee on Psychosocial Aspects of Child and Family Health; Council on Early Childhood; Society for Developmental and Behavioral Pediatrics; American Academy of Pediatrics. Promoting optimal development: screening for behavioral and emotional problems. *Pediatrics.* 2015;135(2):384–395

136. Oster A, Bindman AB. Emergency department visits for ambulatory care sensitive conditions: insights

into preventable hospitalizations. *Med Care*. 2003;41(2):198–207

137. Wilson KM, Klein JD. Adolescents who use the emergency department as their usual source of care. *Arch Pediatr Adolesc Med*. 2000;154(4):361–365

138. Klein JD, Woods AH, Wilson KM, Prospero M, Greene J, Ringwalt C. Homeless and runaway youths' access to health care. *J Adolesc Health*. 2000;27(5):331–339

139. Chen CM, Yi HY, Faden VB. *Trends in Underage Drinking in the United States, 1991–2009. National Institute on Alcohol Abuse and Alcoholism. Surveillance Report #91.* Bethesda, MD: US Department of Health and Human Services; 2011

140. Fein JA, Pailler ME, Barg FK, et al. Feasibility and effects of a Web-based adolescent psychiatric assessment administered by clinical staff in the pediatric emergency department. *Arch Pediatr Adolesc Med*. 2010;164(12):1112–1117

141. Grupp-Phelan J, Delgado SV, Kelleher KJ. Failure of psychiatric referrals from the pediatric emergency department. *BMC Emerg Med*. 2007;7:12

142. Grupp-Phelan J, Wade TJ, Pickup T, et al. Mental health problems in children and caregivers in the emergency department setting. *J Dev Behav Pediatr*. 2007;28(1):16–21

143. Monti PM, Colby SM, Barnett NP, et al. Brief intervention for harm reduction with alcohol-positive older adolescents in a hospital emergency department. *J Consult Clin Psychol*. 1999;67(6):989–994

144. Marcell AV, Klein JD, Fischer I, Allan MJ, Kokotailo PK. Male adolescent use of health care services: where are the boys? *J Adolesc Health*. 2002;30(1):35–43

145. Chandra A, Minkovitz CS. Stigma starts early: gender differences in teen willingness to use mental health services. *J Adolesc Health*. 2006;38(6):754.e1–754.e8

146. Haughey MT, Calderon Y, Torres S, Nazario S, Bijur P. Identification of depression in an inner-city population using a simple screen. *Acad Emerg Med*. 2005;12(12):1221–1226

147. Rutman MS, Shenassa E, Becker BM. Brief screening for adolescent depressive symptoms in the emergency department. *Acad Emerg Med*. 2008;15(1):17–22

148. Newton AS, Gokiert R, Mabood N, et al. Instruments to detect alcohol and other drug misuse in the emergency department: a systematic review. *Pediatrics*. 2011;128(1). Available at: www.pediatrics.org/cgi/content/full/128/1/e180

149. Horowitz L, Ballard E, Teach SJ, et al. Feasibility of screening patients with nonpsychiatric complaints for suicide risk in a pediatric emergency department: a good time to talk? *Pediatr Emerg Care*. 2010;26(11):787–792

150. Horowitz LM, Bridge JA, Teach SJ, et al. Ask Suicide-Screening Questions (ASQ): a brief instrument for the pediatric emergency department. *Arch Pediatr Adolesc Med*. 2012;166(12):1170–1176

151. Horowitz LM, Wang PS, Koocher GP, et al. Detecting suicide risk in a pediatric emergency department: development of a brief screening tool. *Pediatrics*. 2001;107(5):1133–1137

152. Winston FK, Kassam-Adams N, Garcia-España F, Ittenbach R, Cnaan A. Screening for risk of persistent posttraumatic stress in injured children and their parents. *JAMA*. 2003;290(5):643–649

153. O'Mara RM, Hill RM, Cunningham RM, King CA. Adolescent and parent attitudes toward screening for suicide risk and mental health problems in the pediatric emergency department. *Pediatr Emerg Care*. 2012;28(7):626–632

154. Williams JR, Ho ML, Grupp-Phelan J. The acceptability of mental health screening in a pediatric emergency department. *Pediatr Emerg Care*. 2011;27(7):611–615

155. Pailler ME, Cronholm PF, Barg FK, Wintersteen MB, Diamond GS, Fein JA. Patients' and caregivers' beliefs about depression screening and referral in the emergency department. *Pediatr Emerg Care*. 2009;25(11):721–727

156. King CA, O'Mara RM, Hayward CN, Cunningham RM. Adolescent suicide risk screening in the emergency department. *Acad Emerg Med*. 2009;16(11):1234–1241

157. Goldenring JM, Rosen DS. Getting into adolescent heads: an essential update. *Contemp Pediatr*. 2004;21(1):64–90

158. Cappelli M, Gray C, Zemek R, et al. The HEADS-ED: a rapid mental health screening tool for pediatric patients in the emergency department. *Pediatrics*. 2012;130(2). Available at: www.pediatrics.org/cgi/content/full/130/2/e321

159. Horowitz LM, Ballard ED, Pao M. Suicide screening in schools, primary care and emergency departments. *Curr Opin Pediatr*. 2009;21(5):620–627

160. National Institute of Alcohol Abuse and Alcoholism. *Alcohol Screening and Brief Intervention for Youth: A Practitioner's Guide*. Bethesda, MD: National Institutes of Health; 2011

161. National Institute of Alcohol Abuse and Alcoholism. Evaluation of NIAAA's Alcohol Screening Guide for Children and Adolescents. Bethesda, MD: National Institute of Alcohol Abuse and Alcoholism; 2011. Available at: http://grants.nih.gov/grants/guide/rfa-files/RFA-AA-12-008.html. Accessed July 5, 2015

162. Maio RF, Shope JT, Blow FC, et al. A randomized controlled trial of an emergency department-based interactive computer program to prevent alcohol misuse among injured adolescents. *Ann Emerg Med*. 2005;45(4):420–429

163. Suffoletto B, Callaway C, Kristan J, Kraemer K, Clark DB. Text-message–based drinking assessments and brief interventions for young adults discharged from the emergency department. *Alcohol Clin Exp Res*. 2012;36(3):552–560

164. Walton MA, Chermack ST, Shope JT, et al. Effects of a brief intervention for reducing violence and alcohol misuse among adolescents: a randomized controlled trial. *JAMA*. 2010;304(5):527–535

165. Walton MA, Cunningham RM, Goldstein AL, et al. Rates and correlates of violent behaviors among adolescents treated in an urban emergency department. *J Adolesc Health*. 2009;45(1):77–83

166. Whiteside LK, Walton MA, Stanley R, et al. Dating aggression and risk behaviors among teenage girls seeking gynecologic care. *Acad Emerg Med.* 2009;16(7):632–638

167. Cunningham RM, Resko SM, Harrison SR, et al. Screening adolescents in the emergency department for weapon carriage. *Acad Emerg Med.* 2010;17(2):168–176

168. Gielen AC, McKenzie LB, McDonald EM, et al. Using a computer kiosk to promote child safety: results of a randomized, controlled trial in an urban pediatric emergency department. *Pediatrics.* 2007;120(2):330–339

169. Choo EK, Ranney ML, Aggarwal N, Boudreaux ED. A systematic review of emergency department technology-based behavioral health interventions. *Acad Emerg Med.* 2012;19(3):318–328

170. Heron KE, Smyth JM. Ecological momentary interventions: incorporating mobile technology into psychosocial and health behaviour treatments. *Br J Health Psychol.* 2010;15(pt 1):1–39

171. Kit Delgado M, Ginde AA, Pallin DJ, Camargo CA Jr. Multicenter study of preferences for health education in the emergency department population. *Acad Emerg Med.* 2010;17(6):652–658

172. Ranney ML, Choo EK, Wang Y, Baum A, Clark MA, Mello MJ. Emergency department patients' preferences for technology-based behavioral interventions. *Ann Emerg Med.* 2012;60(2):218–27.e48

173. Pailler ME, Fein JA. Computerized behavioral health screening in the emergency department. *Pediatr Ann.* 2009;38(3):156–160

Evaluation and Management of Children With Acute Mental Health or Behavioral Problems. Part II: Recognition of Clinically Challenging Mental Health Related Conditions Presenting With Medical or Uncertain Symptoms—Executive Summary

- *Clinical Report*

CLINICAL REPORT   Guidance for the Clinician in Rendering Pediatric Care

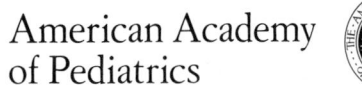
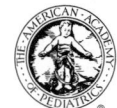

American Academy
of Pediatrics

DEDICATED TO THE HEALTH OF ALL CHILDREN™

Executive Summary: Evaluation and Management of Children With Acute Mental Health or Behavioral Problems. Part II: Recognition of Clinically Challenging Mental Health Related Conditions Presenting With Medical or Uncertain Symptoms

Thomas H. Chun, MD, MPH, FAAP, Sharon E. Mace, MD, FAAP, FACEP, Emily R. Katz, MD, FAAP, AMERICAN ACADEMY OF PEDIATRICS, COMMITTEE ON PEDIATRIC EMERGENCY MEDICINE, AMERICAN COLLEGE OF EMERGENCY PHYSICIANS, PEDIATRIC EMERGENCY MEDICINE COMMITTEE

EXECUTIVE SUMMARY

The number of children and adolescents seen in emergency departments (EDs) and primary care settings for mental health problems has skyrocketed in recent years, with up to 23% of patients in both settings having diagnosable mental health conditions.[1-4] Even when a mental health problem is not the focus of an ED or primary care visit, mental health conditions, both known and occult, may challenge the treating clinician and complicate the patient's care.[4]

Although the American Academy of Pediatrics (AAP) has published a policy statement on mental health competencies and a Mental Health Toolkit for pediatric primary care providers, no such guidelines or resources exist for clinicians who care for pediatric mental health emergencies.[5,6] Many ED and primary care physicians report paucity of training and lack of confidence in caring for pediatric psychiatry patients. The 2 clinical reports support the 2006 joint policy statement of the AAP and the American College of Emergency Physicians on pediatric mental health emergencies, [7] with the goal of addressing the knowledge gaps in this area. Although written primarily from the perspective of ED clinicians, it is intended for all clinicians who care for children and adolescents with acute mental health and behavioral problems. They are organized around the common clinical challenges pediatric caregivers face, both when a child or adolescent presents with a psychiatric chief complaint or emergency (part I) and when a mental health condition may be an unclear or complicating factor in a non–mental health ED presentation (part II). Part I of the clinical reports

DOI: 10.1542/peds.2016-1574

Accepted for publication May 12, 2016

PEDIATRICS (ISSN Numbers: Print, 0031-4005; Online, 1098-4275).

To cite: Chun TH, Mace SE, AAP FACEP, Katz ER. Executive Summary: Evaluation and Management of Children With Acute Mental Health or Behavioral Problems. Part II: Recognition of Clinically Challenging Mental Health Related Conditions Presenting With Medical or Uncertain Symptoms. *Pediatrics.* 2016;138(2):e20161574 includes discussions of Medical Clearance of Pediatric Psychiatric Patients, Suicide and Suicidal Ideation, Restraint of the Agitated Patient Including Verbal, Chemical, and Physical Restraint, and Coordination of Care With the Medical Home, and it can be accessed online at www.pediatrics.org/cgi/doi/10.1542/peds.2016-1570. This executive summary is an overview of part II of the clinical reports. Full text of the following topics can be accessed online at www.pediatrics.org/cgi/doi/10.1542/peds.2016-1573.

Key considerations include the following:

Somatic Symptom and Related Disorders

- Somatic symptom and related disorders encompass conditions in which physical symptoms are not intentionally produced or associated with material gain.[8] These disorders are common and are significant contributors to health care usage and costs, because they cause significant functional impairment.[9–11]

- Symptoms of pediatric somatic symptom and related disorders often do not meet strict diagnostic criteria and defy categorization.[12,13] Clinical presentations are myriad, most often involving neurologic, pain, autonomic, or gastrointestinal tract symptoms.[14,15] Patients often have vague, poorly described complaints, recent or current stressful events, and symptoms that fluctuate with activity or stress and often have multiple medical visits for these symptoms.[16]

- *Risk factors:* Studies have found higher rates of somatic symptom and related disorders in patients who are adolescent, female, or of minority ethnicities; patients who live in urban areas; patients from nonintact families; patients whose parents have lower education level; patients whose family members

have somatic symptom and related disorders; and patients who have histories of psychological trauma. Comorbid depression and anxiety disorders are common.[8,17]

- *Somatic symptom and related disorders and the ED:* Caring for such patients in the ED can be particularly vexing, because few patients will have received a formal diagnosis, and ED clinicians often do not have access to sufficient clinical information to confirm the diagnosis.[12,13] In addition, diagnosing a "psychosomatic" illness may be stigmatizing to patients and families and may result in them feeling unheard, disrespected, and defensive about their symptoms.[18] Because of diagnostic uncertainty, patients with somatic symptom and related disorders are at risk for extensive, invasive, or potentially harmful testing and interventions in the ED.[19,20]

- *ED management strategies*[8,18,21]: ED clinicians may consider doing the following:

    i. Reassure the patient and family that the patient's symptoms are being heard and taken seriously and that testing and treatment that are medically indicated will be performed.

    ii. Emphasize collaboration between the patient, family, and all caregivers; make referrals as needed; and identify common goals and outcomes. Educating the patient and family about the limitations of the ED setting and what are alternative settings for evaluation and treatment may be beneficial.

    iii. Introduce the concept of working on improving functioning while also working on symptom resolution.

    iv. Coordinate the patient's care with the medical home and other involved care providers to help the ED clinician avoid unnecessary testing or intervention and reassure the patient and family.

Adverse Effects of Psychiatric Medications

- In recent years, the use of medications for mental health conditions, especially antipsychotics, is burgeoning among children and adolescents.[22–25]

- Many medications commonly used as antiemetics or for migraines (eg, prochlorperazine, metoclopramide, and promethazine) are phenothiazines, the same class of medications as first-generation "typical" antipsychotics.[26] In addition, other medications commonly used in pediatrics have serotonergic properties. Therefore, a working knowledge of the adverse effects of these medications may be helpful to ED clinicians.

- Antipsychotics:

    i. Although antipsychotics exert their effect primarily through the brain's dopaminergic system, they also affect numerous other neurotransmitter systems. Table 2 in the clinical report (see Table 2 at www.pediatrics.org/cgi/doi/10.1542/peds.2016-1573) lists the common adverse effects, which neurotransmitter system is involved, and which adverse effects are most commonly seen with which antipsychotics.

    ii. *QT_c prolongation:* Almost all antipsychotics cause some degree of QT_c prolongation because of a quinidinelike effect (see Table 4 at www.

pediatrics.org/cgi/doi/10. 1542/peds.2016-1573). Risk factors (see Table 3 at www.pediatrics.org/cgi/ doi/10.1542/peds.2016- 1573) for QT_c prolongation and sudden death include coadministration of other QT_c-prolonging medications (see Table 5 at www. pediatrics.org/cgi/doi/10. 1542/peds.2016-1570); intravenous administration or high dosage; medically ill patients; electrolyte abnormalities; hepatic, renal, or cardiac impairment; and congenital long QT syndromes.[27–29]

iii. *Black box warning:* Because of this risk, thioridazine and, more controversially, droperidol carry Food and Drug Administration "black box" warnings.

iv. *Extrapyramidal symptoms:* Dystonia, akathisia, Parkinsonism, and tardive dyskinesia are typical extrapyramidal symptoms. Acute dystonic reactions, the most commonly encountered extrapyramidal symptoms, often respond to diphenhydramine or benztropine. Laryngeal dystonia is rare but potentially life threatening.[26,28]

v. *Metabolic syndrome:* Hyperglycemia, hyperlipidemia, and obesity are often associated with atypical antipsychotic use, with variable severity between medications (see Table 2 at www.pediatrics. org/cgi/doi/10.1542/peds. 2016-1573).[30]

vi. *Agranulocytosis:* This rare adverse effect is most commonly associated with clozapine and less

commonly with risperidone and olanzapine.[31]

vii. *Neuroleptic malignant syndrome (NMS):* NMS is a potentially lethal condition consisting of the tetrad of mental status changes, fever, muscular hypertonicity or rigidity, and autonomic dysfunction caused by central dopamine deficiency and can occur with any antipsychotic.[32,33]

1. NMS occurs idiosyncratically but is most common within 7 days of starting or increasing antipsychotic doses and later (15–30 days) if depot medications have been used.[32,34]

2. In addition to the classic tetrad, symptoms can include tachycardia, blood pressure instability, diaphoresis, pallor, cardiac dysrhythmia, diaphoresis, sialorrhea, dysphagia, rhabdomyolysis, renal failure, thromboembolic events, hypoventilation, and respiratory failure.[32,35]

3. NMS is a clinical diagnosis, because there are no pathognomonic clinical or laboratory criteria. Leukocytosis and elevated serum creatine phosphokinase and aldose are commonly observed.[36]

4. Treatment may include supportive measures, such as removal of the initiating agent, and when indicated may also include intravenous fluids for dehydration and rhabdomyolysis, benzodiazepines for agitation, external cooling measures, and cardiorespiratory support. The smooth muscle relaxant dantrolene may be used to

directly treat the abnormal muscle contractions of NMS.[37,38] The utility of central nervous system dopaminergic agents, such as bromocriptine and amantadine, is less clear and controversial.

5. Potential resources for caring for patients with NMS include toxicologists, a poison control center, and the NMS Information Service, which can be accessed through its Web site (http://www.nmsis. org/index.asp).[37,38]

• Serotonin syndrome:

i. Given the large number of non–mental health medications with serotonergic properties (see Table 6 at www.pediatrics. org/cgi/doi/10.1542/peds. 2016-1573) in addition to antidepressants and some antipsychotics, it is not surprising that the incidence of serotonin syndrome is increasing. It can occur in cases of overdose but also in the course of standard use.[39,40] The classic clinical triad consists of mental status changes, autonomic hyperactivity, and neuromuscular abnormalities, although many patients do not exhibit all these clinical characteristics. Given the wide variability in the severity of symptoms and the lack of pathognomonic clinical and laboratory findings, diagnosing serotonin syndrome can be particularly challenging.[40,41]

ii. *Signs and symptoms:* Agitated delirium is the most common form of mental status change, although it also has a wide spectrum of severity, including mild agitation, hypervigilance, slightly pressured speech, and easy startle. Diaphoresis, shivering, mydriasis, increased bowel sounds, and diarrhea are common signs of autonomic dysfunction. Myoclonus is the most common neuromuscular finding, but other abnormalities are possible, including, muscular rigidity, hypertonicity, hyperreflexia, clonus, horizontal ocular clonus, tremor, akathisia, and seizures.[39,42] Laboratory findings can include elevated CPK and hepatic transaminases, metabolic acidosis, renal failure, and disseminated intravascular coagulopathy.

iii. *Diagnosis:* Differentiating serotonin syndrome from other medication-induced syndromes can be challenging. Table 7 in the clinical report (www. pediatrics.org/cgi/doi/10. 1542/peds.2016-1573) details both the similar and differentiating features of these syndromes. In addition to the aforementioned laboratory abnormalities, other diagnostic testing may include a complete blood cell count, serum electrolytes, arterial blood gas, urinalysis, toxicology screens, electrocardiogram, electroencephalogram, and brain imaging studies.

iv. *Treatment:* Similar to NMS, treatment of serotonin syndrome most often includes supportive measures. For severe cases, centrally acting serotonin agents may be considered, including cyproheptadine

and chlorpromazine. Some experts prefer cyproheptadine, because chlorpromazine may cause hypotension and increase muscle rigidity, decrease seizure threshold, and worsen NMS (eg, in diagnostically challenging cases when the diagnosis is unclear and the patient has NMS, not serotonin syndrome).[42,43] Toxicologists, poison control centers, and the NMS Information Service, as mentioned previously in the NMS section, may be helpful resources in caring for these patients. Evaluation and observation in the ED and additional outpatient management may be considered in mild cases.

Children With Special Needs: Caring for Patients With Autism Spectrum Disorders and Developmental Disorders

- In recent years, there has been a sharp increase in the incidence of autism spectrum disorders, with corresponding interest and growth in treatment strategies. Most studies have methodological or generalizability limitations. Therefore, the following strategies are based primarily on expert, consensus opinion.

- *Resources:* Often, the most important autism spectrum disorder or developmental delay (ASD-DD) "expert" to consult is the child's parent. Parents of children with ASD-DD often know what strategies work with their child (eg, which words, actions, stimuli, calm and help their child) and which have the opposite effect. They can also be an "interpreter" for ED clinicians, deciphering the significance of their child's actions and behaviors and facilitating communication with their child. Spending some time asking the parents about their child can be

a very productive, efficient method for tailoring effective ED care for patients with ASD-DD. A wide range of ED professionals can assist with or champion ASD-DD–sensitive care, including physicians, nurses, nursing assistants, nurse practitioners or physician assistants, social workers, and child life specialists. Non-ED resources that may be helpful include developmental–behavioral pediatricians, child psychologist and psychiatrists, special education teachers, speech–language therapists, and occupational therapists.

- *Strategies:* A variety of environmental modifications, communication adjuncts, and distraction techniques may assist in caring for children with ASD-DD (see Table 8 at www. pediatrics.org/cgi/doi/10. 1542/peds.2016-1573). A quiet, darkened room may be soothing to a child with an ASD-DD. These children often communicate with a visual communication system (VCS).[44] If they do not have their usual VCS, a wide variety of free and commercial products are available. Digital photography is an alternative, inexpensive method of creating a custom VCS for the ED. Transition planning and desensitization strategies may help children with ASD-DD acclimate to the ED and the care they will receive. Distraction techniques that may be useful include physical activity, electronic games, and tactile stimulation.

- *Medications:* There are no rigorous, evidence-based recommendations for which medications to use for children with ASD-DD. Although there are no known contraindications, other than the patient's past response to medications, atypical, idiosyncratic responses to medications may be common with these patients. Consultation with an ASD-DD expert before starting medication may be helpful. Many suggest starting with lower medication dosages and closely monitoring the patient's response.[45]

Mental Health Screening

- *Advantages of the ED:* Many children and adolescents who visit EDs are at high risk of mental health problems that may not be addressed in other settings.[46,47] For example, they may not attend school or have a medical home, effectively making the ED the sole safety net for these patients.[48,49]

- *Feasibility and acceptability of ED mental health screening:* Many rapid and efficient mental health screening tools have been tested in the ED, including for depression, suicide, anxiety, and posttraumatic stress.[50–53] Studies have found these screening tools to have high feasibility (eg, they can be completed in a few seconds to a few minutes) and acceptability by patients, their families, and ED clinicians.[54–58] Electronic screening tools have been developed, are being tested, and may be advantageous to the ED setting.[59–61]

LEAD AUTHORS

Thomas H. Chun, MD, MPH, FAAP
Sharon E. Mace, MD, FAAP, FACEP
Emily R. Katz, MD, FAAP

AMERICAN ACADEMY OF PEDIATRICS, COMMITTEE ON PEDIATRIC EMERGENCY MEDICINE, 2015-2016

Joan E. Shook, MD, MBA, FAAP, Chairperson
James M. Callahan, MD, FAAP
Thomas H. Chun, MD, MPH, FAAP
Gregory P. Conners, MD, MPH, MBA, FAAP
Edward E. Conway Jr, MD, MS, FAAP
Nanette C. Dudley, MD, FAAP

Toni K. Gross, MD, MPH, FAAP
Natalie E. Lane, MD, FAAP
Charles G. Macias, MD, MPH, FAAP
Nathan L. Timm, MD, FAAP

LIAISONS

Kim Bullock, MD — *American Academy of Family Physicians*
Elizabeth Edgerton, MD, MPH, FAAP — *Maternal and Child Health Bureau*
Brian R. Moore, MD, FAAP — *National Association of EMS Physicians*
Tamar Magarik Haro — *AAP Department of Federal Affairs*
Madeline Joseph, MD, FACEP, FAAP — *American College of Emergency Physicians*
Angela Mickalide, PhD, MCHES — EMSC National Resource Center
Katherine E. Remick, MD, FAAP — National Association of Emergency Medical Technicians
Sally K. Snow, RN, BSN, CPEN, FAEN — Emergency Nurses Association
David W. Tuggle, MD, FAAP — American College of Surgeons
Cynthia Wright-Johnson, MSN, RNC — National Association of State EMS Officials

FORMER MEMBERS AND LIAISONS, 2013-2015

Alice D. Ackerman, MD, MBA, FAAP
Lee Benjamin, MD, FACEP, FAAP - *American College of Physicians*
Susan M. Fuchs, MD, FAAP
Marc H. Gorelick, MD, MSCE, FAAP
Paul Sirbaugh, DO, MBA, FAAP - *National Association of Emergency Medical Technicians*
Joseph L. Wright, MD, MPH, FAAP

STAFF

Sue Tellez

AMERICAN COLLEGE OF EMERGENCY PHYSICIANS, PEDIATRIC EMERGENCY MEDICINE COMMITTEE, 2013–2014

Lee S. Benjamin, MD, FACEP, Chairperson
Isabel A. Barata, MD, FACEP, FAAP
Kiyetta Alade, MD
Joseph Arms, MD
Jahn T. Avarello, MD, FACEP
Steven Baldwin, MD
Kathleen Brown, MD, FACEP
Richard M. Cantor, MD, FACEP
Ariel Cohen, MD
Ann Marie Dietrich, MD, FACEP
Paul J. Eakin, MD

Marianne Gausche-Hill, MD, FACEP, FAAP
Michael Gerardi, MD, FACEP, FAAP
Charles J. Graham, MD, FACEP
Doug K. Holtzman, MD, FACEP
Jeffrey Hom, MD, FACEP
Paul Ishimine, MD, FACEP
Hasmig Jinivizian, MD
Madeline Joseph, MD, FACEP
Sanjay Mehta, MD, MEd, FACEP
Aderonke Ojo, MD, MBBS
Audrey Z. Paul, MD, PhD
Denis R. Pauze, MD, FACEP
Nadia M. Pearson, DO
Brett Rosen, MD
W. Scott Russell, MD, FACEP
Mohsen Saidinejad, MD
Harold A. Sloas, DO
Gerald R. Schwartz, MD, FACEP
Orel Swenson, MD
Jonathan H. Valente, MD, FACEP
Muhammad Waseem, MD, MS
Paula J. Whiteman, MD, FACEP
Dale Woolridge, MD, PhD, FACEP

FORMER COMMITTEE MEMBERS

Carrie DeMoor, MD
James M. Dy, MD
Sean Fox, MD
Robert J. Hoffman, MD, FACEP
Mark Hostetler, MD, FACEP
David Markenson, MD, MBA, FACEP
Annalise Sorrentino, MD, FACEP
Michael Witt, MD, MPH, FACEP

STAFF

Dan Sullivan
Stephanie Wauson

ABBREVIATIONS

AAP: American Academy of Pediatrics
ASD-DD: autism spectrum disorder or developmental delay
ED: emergency department
NMS: neuroleptic malignant syndrome
VCS: visual communication system

FINANCIAL DISCLOSURE: The authors have indicated they do not have a financial relationship relevant to this article to disclose.

FUNDING: No external funding.

POTENTIAL CONFLICT OF INTEREST: The authors have indicated they have no potential conflicts of interest to disclose.

REFERENCES

1. Mahajan P, Alpern ER, Grupp-Phelan J, et al; Pediatric Emergency Care Applied Research Network (PECARN). Epidemiology of psychiatric-related visits to emergency departments in a multicenter collaborative research pediatric network. *Pediatr Emerg Care.* 2009;25(11):715–720

2. Pittsenbarger ZE, Mannix R. Trends in pediatric visits to the emergency department for psychiatric illnesses. *Acad Emerg Med.* 2014;21(1):25–30

3. Sheldrick RC, Merchant S, Perrin EC. Identification of developmental–behavioral problems in primary care: a systematic review. *Pediatrics.* 2011;128(2):356–363

4. Grupp-Phelan J, Wade TJ, Pickup T, et al. Mental health problems in children and caregivers in the emergency department setting. *J Dev Behav Pediatr.* 2007;28(1):16–21

5. Committee on Psychosocial Aspects of Child and Family Health and Task Force on Mental Health. Policy statement--The future of pediatrics: mental health competencies for pediatric primary care. *Pediatrics.* 2009;124(1):410–421

6. Foy JM, Kelleher KJ, Laraque D; American Academy of Pediatrics Task Force on Mental Health. Enhancing pediatric mental health care: strategies for preparing a primary care practice. *Pediatrics.* 2010;125(suppl 3):S87–S108

7. Dolan MA, Mace SE; American Academy of Pediatrics, Committee on Pediatric Emergency Medicine; American College of Emergency Physicians and Pediatric Emergency Medicine Committee. Pediatric mental health emergencies in the emergency medical services system. *Pediatrics.* 2006;118(4):1764–1767

8. Dell ML, Campo JV. Somatoform disorders in children and adolescents. *Psychiatr Clin North Am.* 2011;34(3):643–660

9. Barsky AJ, Orav EJ, Bates DW. Somatization increases medical utilization and costs independent of psychiatric and medical comorbidity. *Arch Gen Psychiatry.* 2005;62(8):903–910

10. Campo JV, Jansen-McWilliams L, Comer DM, Kelleher KJ. Somatization in pediatric primary care: association with psychopathology, functional impairment, and use of services. *J Am Acad Child Adolesc Psychiatry.* 1999;38(9):1093–1101

11. Reid S, Wessely S, Crayford T, Hotopf M. Medically unexplained symptoms in frequent attenders of secondary health care: retrospective cohort study. *BMJ.* 2001;322(7289):767

12. Fleet RP, Dupuis G, Marchand A, Burelle D, Arsenault A, Beitman BD. Panic disorder in emergency department chest pain patients: prevalence, comorbidity, suicidal ideation, and physician recognition. *Am J Med.* 1996;101(4):371–380

13. Pollard CA, Lewis LM. Managing panic attacks in emergency patients. *J Emerg Med.* 1989;7(5):547–552

14. Campo JV, Fritsch SL. Somatization in children and adolescents. *J Am Acad Child Adolesc Psychiatry.* 1994;33(9):1223–1235

15. Garralda ME. Somatisation in children. *J Child Psychol Psychiatry.* 1996;37(1):13–33

16. Sater N, Constantino JN. Pediatric emergencies in children with psychiatric conditions. *Pediatr Emerg Care.* 1998;14(1):42–50

17. Haugland S, Wold B, Stevenson J, Aaroe LE, Woynarowska B. Subjective health complaints in adolescence. A cross-national comparison of prevalence and dimensionality. *Eur J Public Health.* 2001;11(1):4–10

18. Silber TJ. Somatization disorders: diagnosis, treatment, and prognosis. *Pediatr Rev.* 2011;32(2):56–63, quiz 63–64

19. Bhatia MS, Sapra S. Pseudoseizures in children: a profile of 50 cases. *Clin Pediatr (Phila).* 2005;44(7):617–621

20. Selbst SM, Clancy R. Pseudoseizures in the pediatric emergency department. *Pediatr Emerg Care.* 1996;12(3):185–188

21. Garralda ME. Unexplained physical complaints. *Pediatr Clin North Am.* 2011;58(4):803–813, ix

22. Alexander GC, Gallagher SA, Mascola A, Moloney RM, Stafford RS. Increasing off-label use of antipsychotic medications in the United States, 1995–2008. *Pharmacoepidemiol Drug Saf.* 2011;20(2):177–184

23. Harrison JN, Cluxton-Keller F, Gross D. Antipsychotic medication prescribing trends in children and adolescents. *J Pediatr Health Care.* 2012;26(2):139–145

24. Matone M, Localio R, Huang YS, dosReis S, Feudtner C, Rubin D. The relationship between mental health diagnosis and treatment with second-generation antipsychotics over time: a national study of US Medicaid-enrolled children. *Health Serv Res.* 2012;47(5):1836–1860

25. Pringsheim T, Doja A, Belanger S, Patten S; Canadian Alliance for Monitoring Effectiveness and Safety of Antipsychotics in Children (CAMESA) guideline group. Treatment recommendations for extrapyramidal side effects associated with second-generation antipsychotic use in children and youth. *Paediatr Child Health.* 2011;16(9):590–598

26. Whittler MA, Lavonas EJ. Antipsychotics. In: Marx JA, Hockberger RS, Walls RM, et al, eds. *Rosen's Emergency Medicine: Concepts and Clinical Practice.* Philadelphia, PA: Saunders; 2014:2042–2046

27. Lukens TW, Wolf SJ, Edlow JA, et al; American College of Emergency Physicians Clinical Policies Subcommittee (Writing Committee) on Critical Issues in the Diagnosis and Management of the Adult Psychiatric Patient in the Emergency Department. Clinical policy: critical issues in the diagnosis and management of the adult psychiatric patient in the emergency department. *Ann Emerg Med.* 2006;47(1):79–99

28. Sonnier L, Barzman D. Pharmacologic management of acutely agitated pediatric patients. *Paediatr Drugs.* 2011;13(1):1–10

29. Hilt RJ, Woodward TA. Agitation treatment for pediatric emergency patients. *J Am Acad Child Adolesc Psychiatry.* 2008;47(2):132–138

30. Reynolds GP, Kirk SL. Metabolic side effects of antipsychotic drug treatment: pharmacological mechanisms. *Pharmacol Ther.* 2010;125(1):169–179

31. Miyamoto S, Lieberman JA, Fleischacker WW, Marder SR. Antipsychotic drugs. In: Tasman A, Kay J, Lieberman A, First MB, Maj M, eds. *Psychiatry*. 3rd ed. West Sussex, England: John Wiley & Sons; 2008:2161–2201

32. Guzé BH, Baxter LR Jr. Current concepts. Neuroleptic malignant syndrome. *N Engl J Med*. 1985;313(3):163–166

33. Levine M, LoVecchio F. Antipsychotics. In: Tintinalli JE, Stapczynski S, Ma OJ, Cline DM, Cydulka RK, Mecklereds GD, eds. *Tintinalli's Emergency Medicine: A Comprehensive Study Guide*. New York, NY: McGraw-Hill Education; 2011:1207–1211

34. Agar L. Recognizing neuroleptic malignant syndrome in the emergency department: a case study. *Perspect Psychiatr Care*. 2010;46(2):143–151

35. Martel ML, Biros MH. Psychotropic medications and rapid tranquilization. In: Tintinalli JE, Stapczynski S, Ma OJ, Cline DM, Cydulka RK, Mecklereds GD, eds. *Tintinalli's Emergency Medicine: A Comprehensive Study Guide*. New York, NY: McGraw-Hill Education; 2011:1952–1955

36. Wijdicks EFM. Neuroleptic malignant syndrome. In: Aminoff MJ, ed. *UpToDate*. Updated May 30, 2014. Available at: www.uptodate.com/contents/neuroleptic-malignant-syndrome. Accessed July 7, 2015

37. Meeks TW, Jeste DV. Medication-induced movement disorders. In: Tasman A, Kay J, Lieberman A, First MB, Maj M, eds. *Psychiatry*. 3rd ed. West Sussex, England: John Wiley & Sons; 2008:2142

38. Perry PJ, Wilborn CA. Serotonin syndrome vs neuroleptic malignant syndrome: a contrast of causes, diagnoses, and management. *Ann Clin Psychiatry*. 2012;24(2):155–162

39. Birmes P, Coppin D, Schmitt L, Lauque D. Serotonin syndrome: a brief review. *CMAJ*. 2003;168(11):1439–1442

40. Kant S, Liebelt E. Recognizing serotonin toxicity in the pediatric emergency department. *Pediatr Emerg Care*. 2012;28(8):817–821, quiz 822–824

41. Christensen RC. Identifying serotonin syndrome in the emergency department. *Am J Emerg Med*. 2005;23(3):406–408

42. Boyer EW, Shannon M. The serotonin syndrome. *N Engl J Med*. 2005;352(11):1112–1120

43. Isbister GK, Buckley NA, Whyte IM. Serotonin toxicity: a practical approach to diagnosis and treatment. *Med J Aust*. 2007;187(6):361–365

44. Ganz JB, Davis JL, Lund EM, Goodwyn FD, Simpson RL. Meta-analysis of PECS with individuals with ASD: investigation of targeted versus non-targeted outcomes, participant characteristics, and implementation phase. *Res Dev Disabil*. 2012;33(2):406–418

45. Sullivan M. Autism demands attention in the emergency department. *ACEP News*. April 17, 2012

46. Oster A, Bindman AB. Emergency department visits for ambulatory care sensitive conditions: insights into preventable hospitalizations. *Med Care*. 2003;41(2):198–207

47. Wilson KM, Klein JD. Adolescents who use the emergency department as their usual source of care. *Arch Pediatr Adolesc Med*. 2000;154(4):361–365

48. Klein JD, Woods AH, Wilson KM, Prospero M, Greene J, Ringwalt C. Homeless and runaway youths' access to health care. *J Adolesc Health*. 2000;27(5):331–339

49. Marcell AV, Klein JD, Fischer I, Allan MJ, Kokotailo PK. Male adolescent use of health care services: where are the boys? *J Adolesc Health*. 2002;30(1):35–43

50. Haughey MT, Calderon Y, Torres S, Nazario S, Bijur P. Identification of depression in an inner-city population using a simple screen. *Acad Emerg Med*. 2005;12(12):1221–1226

51. Horowitz LM, Bridge JA, Teach SJ, et al. Ask Suicide-Screening Questions (ASQ): a brief instrument for the pediatric emergency department. *Arch Pediatr Adolesc Med*. 2012;166(12):1170–1176

52. Newton AS, Gokiert R, Mabood N, et al. Instruments to detect alcohol and other drug misuse in the emergency department: a systematic review. *Pediatrics*. 2011;128(1). Available at: www.pediatrics.org/cgi/content/full/128/1/e180

53. Winston FK, Kassam-Adams N, Garcia-España F, Ittenbach R, Cnaan A. Screening for risk of persistent posttraumatic stress in injured children and their parents. *JAMA*. 2003;290(5):643–649

54. Horowitz L, Ballard E, Teach SJ, et al. Feasibility of screening patients with nonpsychiatric complaints for suicide risk in a pediatric emergency department: a good time to talk? *Pediatr Emerg Care*. 2010;26(11):787–792

55. King CA, O'Mara RM, Hayward CN, Cunningham RM. Adolescent suicide risk screening in the emergency department. *Acad Emerg Med*. 2009;16(11):1234–1241

56. O'Mara RM, Hill RM, Cunningham RM, King CA. Adolescent and parent attitudes toward screening for suicide risk and mental health problems in the pediatric emergency department. *Pediatr Emerg Care*. 2012;28(7):626–632

57. Pailler ME, Cronholm PF, Barg FK, Wintersteen MB, Diamond GS, Fein JA. Patients' and caregivers' beliefs about depression screening and referral in the emergency department. *Pediatr Emerg Care*. 2009;25(11):721–727

58. Williams JR, Ho ML, Grupp-Phelan J. The acceptability of mental health screening in a pediatric emergency department. *Pediatr Emerg Care*. 2011;27(7):611–615

59. Kit Delgado M, Ginde AA, Pallin DJ, Camargo CA Jr. Multicenter study of preferences for health education in the emergency department population. *Acad Emerg Med*. 2010;17(6):652–658

60. Pailler ME, Fein JA. Computerized behavioral health screening in the emergency department. *Pediatr Ann*. 2009;38(3):156–160

61. Ranney ML, Choo EK, Wang Y, Baum A, Clark MA, Mello MJ. Emergency department patients' preferences for technology-based behavioral interventions. *Ann Emerg Med*. 2012;60(2):218–27.e48

Evaluation and Referral for Developmental Dysplasia of the Hip in Infants

- *Clinical Report*

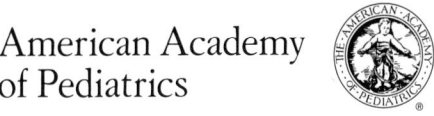

CLINICAL REPORT   Guidance for the Clinician in Rendering Pediatric Care

American Academy
of Pediatrics

DEDICATED TO THE HEALTH OF ALL CHILDREN™

Evaluation and Referral for Developmental Dysplasia of the Hip in Infants

Brian A. Shaw, MD, FAAOS, FAAP, Lee S. Segal, MD, FAAOS, FAAP, SECTION ON ORTHOPAEDICS

abstract

Developmental dysplasia of the hip (DDH) encompasses a wide spectrum of clinical severity, from mild developmental abnormalities to frank dislocation. Clinical hip instability occurs in 1% to 2% of full-term infants, and up to 15% have hip instability or hip immaturity detectable by imaging studies. Hip dysplasia is the most common cause of hip arthritis in women younger than 40 years and accounts for 5% to 10% of all total hip replacements in the United States. Newborn and periodic screening have been practiced for decades, because DDH is clinically silent during the first year of life, can be treated more effectively if detected early, and can have severe consequences if left untreated. However, screening programs and techniques are not uniform, and there is little evidence-based literature to support current practice, leading to controversy. Recent literature shows that many mild forms of DDH resolve without treatment, and there is a lack of agreement on ultrasonographic diagnostic criteria for DDH as a disease versus developmental variations. The American Academy of Pediatrics has not published any policy statements on DDH since its 2000 clinical practice guideline and accompanying technical report. Developments since then include a controversial US Preventive Services Task Force "inconclusive" determination regarding usefulness of DDH screening, several prospective studies supporting observation over treatment of minor ultrasonographic hip variations, and a recent evidence-based clinical practice guideline from the American Academy of Orthopaedic Surgeons on the detection and management of DDH in infants 0 to 6 months of age. The purpose of this clinical report was to provide literature-based updated direction for the clinician in screening and referral for DDH, with the primary goal of preventing and/or detecting a dislocated hip by 6 to 12 months of age in an otherwise healthy child, understanding that no screening program has eliminated late development or presentation of a dislocated hip and that the diagnosis and treatment of milder forms of hip dysplasia remain controversial.

DOI: 10.1542/peds.2016-3107

PEDIATRICS (ISSN Numbers: Print, 0031-4005; Online, 1098-4275).

FINANCIAL DISCLOSURE: The authors have indicated they do not have a financial relationship relevant to this article to disclose.

FUNDED: No external funding.

POTENTIAL CONFLICT OF INTEREST: The authors have indicated they have no potential conflicts of interest to disclose.

To cite: Shaw BA, Segal LS, AAP SECTION ON ORTHOPAEDICS. Evaluation and Referral for Developmental Dysplasia of the Hip in Infants. *Pediatrics.* 2016;138(6):e20163107

INTRODUCTION

Early diagnosis and treatment of developmental dysplasia of the hip (DDH) is important to provide the best possible clinical outcome. DDH encompasses a spectrum of physical and imaging findings, from mild instability and developmental variations to frank dislocation. DDH is asymptomatic during infancy and early childhood, and, therefore, screening of otherwise healthy infants is performed to detect this uncommon condition. Traditional methods of screening have included the newborn and periodic physical examination and selected use of radiographic imaging. The American Academy of Pediatrics (AAP) promotes screening as a primary care function. However, screening techniques and definitions of clinically important clinical findings are controversial, and despite abundant literature on the topic, quality evidence-based literature is lacking.

The AAP last published a clinical practice guideline on DDH in 2000 titled "Early Detection of Developmental Dysplasia of the Hip."[1] The purpose of this clinical report is to provide the pediatrician with updated information for DDH screening, surveillance, and referral based on recent literature, expert opinion, policies, and position statements of the AAP and the Pediatric Orthopaedic Society of North America (POSNA), and the 2014 clinical practice guideline of the American Academy of Orthopaedic Surgeons (AAOS).[1–3]

DEFINITIONS

A contributing factor to the DDH screening debate is lack of a uniform definition of DDH. DDH encompasses a spectrum of pathologic hip disorders in which hips are unstable, subluxated, or dislocated and/ or have malformed acetabula.[1] However, imaging advancements, primarily ultrasonography, have created uncertainty regarding whether minor degrees of anatomic and physiologic variability are clinically significant or even abnormal, particularly in the first few months of life.

Normal development of the femoral head and acetabulum is codependent; the head must be stable in the hip socket for both to form spherically and concentrically. If the head is loose in the acetabulum, or if either component is deficient, the entire hip joint is at risk for developing incongruence and lack of sphericity. Most authorities refer to looseness as instability or subluxation and the actual physical deformity of the femoral head and/or acetabulum as dysplasia, but some consider hip instability itself to be dysplasia. Further, subluxation can be static (in which the femoral head is relatively uncovered without stress) or dynamic (the hip partly comes out of the socket with stress). The Ortolani maneuver, in which a subluxated or dislocated femoral head is reduced into the acetabulum with gentle hip abduction by the examiner, is the most important clinical test for detecting newborn dysplasia. In contrast, the Barlow maneuver, in which a reduced femoral head is gently adducted until it becomes subluxated or dislocated, is a test of laxity or instability and has less clinical significance than the Ortolani maneuver. In a practical sense, both maneuvers are performed seamlessly in the clinical assessment of an infant's hip. Mild instability and morphologic differences at birth are considered by some to be pathologic and by others to be normal developmental variants.

In summary, there is lack of universal agreement on what measurable parameters at what age constitute developmental variation versus actual disease. Despite these differences in definition, there is universal expert agreement that a hip will fare poorly if it is unstable and morphologically abnormal by 2 to 3 years of age. It is the opinion of the AAP that DDH fulfills most screening criteria outlined by Wilson and Jungner[4] and that screening efforts are worthwhile to prevent a subluxated or dislocated hip by 6 to 12 months of age.

> The Ortolani maneuver, in which a subluxated or dislocated femoral head is reduced into the acetabulum with gentle hip abduction by the examiner, is the most important clinical test for detecting newborn hip dysplasia.

INCIDENCE, RISK FACTORS, AND NATURAL HISTORY

Incidence

The incidence of developmental dislocation of the hip is approximately 1 in 1000 live births. The incidence of the entire spectrum of DDH is undoubtedly higher but not truly known because of the lack of a universal definition. Rosendahl et al[5] noted a prevalence of dysplastic but stable hips of 1.3% in the general population. A study from the United Kingdom reported a 2% prevalence of DDH in girls born in the breech position.[6]

Risk Factors

Important risk factors for DDH include breech position, female sex, incorrect lower-extremity swaddling, and positive family history. These risk factors are thought to be additive. Other suggested findings, such as being the first born or having torticollis, foot abnormalities, or oligohydramnios, have not been proven to increase the risk of "nonsyndromic" DDH.[3,7]

Breech presentation may be the most important single risk factor, with DDH reported in 2% to 27% of boys and girls presenting in the breech position.[6,8,9] Frank breech presentation in a girl (sacral presentation with hips flexed and knees extended) appears to have the highest risk.[1] Most evidence supports the breech position toward the end of pregnancy rather than breech delivery that contributes to DDH. There is no clear demarcation of timing of this risk; in other words, the point during pregnancy when the DDH risk is normalized by spontaneous or external version from breech to vertex position. Mode of delivery (cesarean) may decrease the risk of DDH with breech positioning.[10-12] A recent study suggested that breech-associated DDH is a milder form than DDH that is not associated with breech presentation, with more rapid spontaneous normalization.[13]

Genetics may contribute more to the risk of DDH than previously considered "packaging effects." If a monozygotic twin has DDH, the risk to the other twin is approximately 40%, and the risk to a dizygotic twin is 3%.[14,15] Recent research has confirmed that the familial relative risk of DDH is high, with first-degree relatives having 12 times the risk of DDH over controls.[16-18] The left hip is more likely to be dysplastic than the right, which may be because of the more common in utero left occiput anterior position in nonbreech infants.[1] The AAOS clinical practice guideline considers breech presentation and family history to be the 2 most important risk factors in DDH screening.[3]

A lesser-known but important risk factor is the practice of swaddling, which has been gaining popularity in recent years for its noted benefits of enhancing better sleep patterns and duration and minimizing hypothermia. However, these benefits are countered by the apparent increased rates of DDH observed in several ethnic groups, such as Navajo Indian and Japanese populations, that have practiced traditional swaddling techniques.

Traditional swaddling maintains the hips in an extended and adducted position, which increases the risk of DDH. However, the concept of "safe swaddling," which allows for hip flexion and abduction and knee flexion, has been shown to lessen the risk of DDH (http://hipdysplasia.org/developmental-dysplasia-of-the-hip/hip-healthy-swaddling/). Parents can be taught the principles of safe infant sleep, including supine position in the infant's own crib and not the parent's bed, with no pillows, bumpers, or loose blankets.[19-24] The POSNA, International Hip Dysplasia Institute, AAOS, United States Bone and Joint Initiative, and Shriners Hospitals for Children have published a joint statement regarding the importance of safe swaddling in preventing DDH.[25]

In general, risk factors are poor predictors of DDH. Female sex, alone without other known risk factors, accounts for 75% of DDH. This emphasizes the importance of a careful physical examination of all infants in detecting DDH.[6] A recent survey showed poor consensus on risk factors for DDH from a group of experts.[26]

> In general, risk factors are poor predictors of DDH. Female sex, alone without other known risk factors, accounts for 75% of DDH.

Natural History

Clinical and imaging studies show that the natural history of mild dysplasia and instability noted in the first few weeks of life is typically benign. Barlow-positive (subluxatable and dislocatable) hips resolve spontaneously, and Barlow himself noted that the mild dysplasia in all 250 newborn infants with positive test results in his original study resolved spontaneously.[27-32]

Conversely, the natural history of a child with hip dysplasia at the more

severe end of the disease spectrum (subluxation or dislocation) by walking age is less satisfactory than children treated successfully at a younger age. Without treatment, these children will likely develop a limp, limb length discrepancy, and limited hip abduction. This may result in premature degenerative arthritis in the hip, knee, and low back. The burden of disability is high, because most affected people become symptomatic in their teens and early adult years, and most require complex hip salvage procedures and/or replacement at an early age.

SCREENING AND DIAGNOSIS

The 2000 AAP clinical practice guideline recommended that all newborn infants be screened for DDH by physical examination, with follow-up at scheduled well-infant periodic examinations. The POSNA, the Canadian Task Force on DDH, and the AAOS have also advocated newborn and periodic screening. A 2006 report by the US Preventive Services Task Force (USPSTF) resulted in controversy regarding DDH screening. By using a data-driven model and a strong emphasis on the concept on predictors of poor health, the USPSTF report gave an "I" recommendation, meaning that the evidence was insufficient to recommend routine screening for DDH in infants as a means to prevent adverse outcomes.[1-3,33-35] However, on the basis of the body of evidence when evaluated from the perspective of a clinical practice model, the AAP advocates for DDH screening.

In its report, the USPSTF noted that avascular necrosis (AVN) is the most common (up to 60%) and severe potential harm of both surgical and nonsurgical interventions.[33] Williams et al[36] reported the risk of AVN to be less than 1% with screening, early detection, and the use of the Pavlik harness. In a long-term follow-up study of a randomized controlled trial from Norway, the authors reported no cases of AVN and no increased risk of harm with increased treatment.[37] The USPSTF also raised concerns about the psychological consequences or stresses with early diagnosis and intervention. Gardner et al[38] found that the use of hip ultrasonography allowed for reduction of treatment rates without adverse clinical or psychological outcomes. Thus, the concerns of AVN and psychological distress or potential predictors of poor health have not been supported in literature not referenced in the USPSTF report.

In 2 well-designed, randomized controlled trial studies from Norway, the prevalence of late DDH presentation was reduced from 2.6 to 3.0 per 1000 to 0.7 to 1.3 per 1000 by using either selective or universal hip ultrasonographic screening. Neither study reached statistical significance because of the inadequate sample size on the basis of prestudy rates of late-presentation DDH. Despite this, both centers have introduced selective hip ultrasonography as part of their routine newborn screening.[39,40] Clarke et al[32] also demonstrated a decrease in late DDH presentation from 1.28 per 1000 to 0.74 per 1000 by using selective hip ultrasonography in a prospective cohort of patients over a 20-year period.

The term "surveillance" may be useful nomenclature to consider in place of screening, because, by definition, it means the close monitoring of someone or something to prevent an adverse outcome. The term surveillance reinforces the concept of periodic physical examinations as part of well-child care visits until 6 to 9 months of age and the use of selective hip ultrasonography as an adjunct imaging tool or an anteroposterior radiograph of the pelvis after 4 months of age for infants with identified risk factors.[3,5,32,41]

Wilson and Jungner[4] outlined 10 principles or criteria to consider

when determining the utility of screening for a disease. The AAP believes DDH fulfills most of these screening criteria (Table 1), except for an understanding of the natural history of hip dysplasia and an agreed-on policy of whom to treat. The 2006 USPSTF report and the AAOS clinical practice guideline provide a platform to drive future research in these 2 areas. Screening for DDH is important, because the condition is initially occult, easier to treat when identified early, and more likely to cause long-term disability if detected late. A reasonable goal for screening is to prevent the late presentation of DDH after 6 months of age.

Physical Examination

The physical examination is by far the most important component of a DDH screening program, with imaging by radiography and/or ultrasonography playing a secondary role. It remains the "cornerstone" of screening and/or surveillance for DDH, and the available evidence supports that primary care physicians serially examine infants previously screened with normal hip examinations on subsequent visits up to 6 to 9 months of age.[3,41-44] Once a child is walking, a dislocated hip may manifest as an abnormal gait.

The 2000 AAP clinical practice guideline gave a detailed description of the examination, including observing for limb length discrepancy, asymmetric thigh or gluteal folds, and limited or asymmetric abduction, as well as performing Barlow and Ortolani tests.[1] It is essential to perform these manual tests gently. By ~3 months of age, a dislocated hip becomes fixed, limiting the usefulness and sensitivity of the Barlow and Ortolani tests. By this age, restricted, asymmetric hip abduction of the involved hip becomes the most important finding (see video available at http://www.

TABLE 1 World Health Organization Criteria for Screening for Health Problems

1.	The condition should be an important health problem
2.	There should be a treatment of the condition
3.	Facilities for the diagnosis and treatment should be available
4.	There should be a latent stage of the disease
5.	There should be a suitable test or examination for the condition
6.	The test should be acceptable to the population
7.	The natural history of the disease should be adequately understood
8.	There should be an agreed-on policy on whom to treat
9.	The total cost of finding a case should be economically balanced in relation to medical expenditures as a whole
10.	Case finding should be a continuous process

aap.org/sections/ortho). Diagnosing bilateral DDH in the older infant can be difficult because of symmetry of limited abduction.

Although ingrained in the literature, the significance and safety of the Barlow test is questioned. Barlow stated in his original description that the test is for laxity of the hip joint rather than for an existing dislocation. The Barlow test has no proven predictive value for future hip dislocation. If performed frequently or forcefully, it is possible that the maneuver itself could create instability.[45,46] The AAP recommends, if the Barlow test is performed, that it be done by gently adducting the hip while palpating for the head falling out the back of the acetabulum and that no posterior-directed force be applied. One can think of the Barlow and Ortolani tests as a continuous smooth gentle maneuver starting with the hip flexed and adducted, with gentle anterior pressure on the trochanter while the hip is abducted to feel whether the hip is locating into the socket, followed by gently adducting the hip and relieving the anterior pressure on the trochanter while sensing whether the hip slips out the back. The examiner should not attempt to forcefully dislocate the femoral head (see video available at http://www.aap.org/sections/ortho).

"Hip clicks" without the sensation of instability are clinically insignificant.[47] Whereas the Ortolani sign represents the palpable sensation of the femoral head moving into the acetabulum over the hypertrophied rim of the acetabular cartilage (termed neolimbus), isolated high-pitched clicks represent the movement of myofascial tissues over the trochanter, knee, or other bony prominences and are not a sign of hip dysplasia or instability.

Radiography

Plain radiography becomes most useful by 4 to 6 months of age, when the femoral head secondary center of ossification forms.[48] Limited evidence supports obtaining a properly positioned anteroposterior radiograph of the pelvis.[3] If the pelvis is rotated or if a gonadal shield obscures the hip joint, then the radiograph should be repeated. Hip asymmetry, subluxation, and dislocation can be detected on radiographs when dysplasia is present. There is debate about whether early minor radiographic variability (such as increased acetabular index) constitutes actual disease.[31] Radiography is traditionally indicated for diagnosis of the infant with risk factors or an abnormal examination after 4 months of age.[1,2,8,49]

Ultrasonography

Ultrasonography can provide detailed static and dynamic imaging of the hip before femoral head ossification. The American Institute of Ultrasound in Medicine and the American College of Radiology published a joint guideline for the standardized performance of the infantile hip ultrasonographic examination.[50] Static ultrasonography shows coverage of the femoral head by the cartilaginous acetabulum (α angle) at rest, and dynamic ultrasonography demonstrates a real-time image of the Barlow and Ortolani tests.

Ultrasonographic imaging can be universal for all infants or selective for those at risk for having DDH. Universal newborn ultrasonographic screening is not recommended in North America because of the expense, inconvenience, inconsistency, subjectivity, and high false-positive rates, given an overall population disease prevalence of 1% to 2%.[3] Rather, selective ultrasonographic screening is recommended either to clarify suspicious findings on physical examination after 3 to 4 weeks of age or to detect clinically silent DDH in the high-risk infant from 6 weeks to 4 to 6 months of age.[1,2,35,50] Two prospective randomized clinical trials from Norway support selective ultrasonographic imaging when used in conjunction with high-quality clinical screening.[39,40]

Roposch and colleagues[51,52] contend that experts cannot reach a consensus on what is normal, abnormal, developmental variation, or simply uncertain regarding much ultrasonographic imaging, thereby confounding referral and treatment recommendations. Several studies have demonstrated that mild ultrasonographic abnormalities usually resolve spontaneously, fueling the controversy over what imaging findings constitute actual disease requiring treatment.[5,30,51,53–56]

The concept of surveillance for DDH emphasizes the importance of repeated physical examinations and the adjunct use of selective hip ultrasonography after 6 weeks of age or an anteroposterior radiograph of the pelvis after 4 months of age for infants with questionable or abnormal findings on physical examination or with identified risk factors. Ultrasonography is not necessary for a frankly dislocated hip (Ortolani positive) but may be desired by the treating physician. Physiologic joint capsular laxity and immature acetabular development before 6 weeks of age may limit the accuracy of hip ultrasonography interpretations.[39,40] There is no consensus on exact timing of and indications for ultrasonography among expert groups.[26,57] However, ultrasonographic imaging does have a management role in infants younger than 6 weeks undergoing abduction brace treatment of unstable hips identified on physical examination.[3]

REFERRAL, ADJUNCTIVE IMAGING, AND TREATMENT

Referral

Early detection and referral of infants with DDH allows appropriate intervention with bracing or casting, which may prevent the need for reconstructive surgery. Primary indications for referral include an unstable (positive Ortolani test result) or dislocated hip on clinical examination. Because most infants with a positive Barlow test result at either the newborn or 2-week examination stabilize on their own, these infants should have sequential follow-up examinations as part of the concept of surveillance. This recommendation differs from the 2000 AAP clinical practice guideline.[1] Any child with limited hip abduction or asymmetric hip abduction after the neonatal period (4 weeks) should be referred. Relative indications for referral include infants with risk factors for DDH, a questionable examination, and pediatrician or parental concern.[1]

Adjunctive Imaging

Recommendations for the evaluation and management of infants with risk factors for DDH but with normal findings on physical examination continue to evolve. The 2000 AAP clinical practice guideline recommended hip ultrasonography at 6 weeks of age or radiography of the pelvis and hips at 4 months of age in girls with a positive family history of DDH or breech presentation. The AAP clinical practice guideline also stated that hip ultrasonographic examinations remain an option for all infants born breech.[1] The recent AAOS report found that moderate evidence supports an imaging study before 6 months of age in infants with breech presentation, family history, and/or history of clinical instability.[3,58–60]

> Consider imaging before 6 months of age for male or female infants with normal findings on physical examination and the following risk factors:
>
> 1. Breech presentation in third trimester (regardless of cesarean or vaginal delivery)
> 2. Positive family history
> 3. History of previous clinical instability
> 4. Parental concern
> 5. History of improper swaddling
> 6. Suspicious or inconclusive physical examination

Refinement in the term "breech presentation" as a risk factor for DDH is needed to determine whether selective hip ultrasonography at 6 weeks or radiography before 6 months of age is needed for an infant with a normal clinical hip examination. More specific variables, such as mode of delivery, type of breech position, or breech position at any time during the pregnancy or in the third trimester, have received little attention to date. The AAOS clinical practice guideline reported 6 studies addressing breech presentation, but all were considered low-strength evidence.[3] Thus, the literature is not adequate enough to allow specific guidance. The risk is thought to be greater for frank breech (hips flexed, knees extended) in the last trimester.[1]

Lacking expert consensus of risk factors for DDH,[26] the questions of whether to obtain additional imaging studies with a normal clinical hip examination is ultimately best left to one's professional judgment. One must consider, however, that the overall probability of a clinically stable hip to later dislocate is very low.

Because of the variability in performance and interpretation of the hip ultrasonographic examination and varying thresholds for treatment, the requesting physician might consider developing a regional protocol in conjunction with a consulting pediatric orthopedist and pediatric radiologist. Specific criteria for imaging and referral based on local resources can promote consistency in evaluation and treatment of suspected DDH. Realistically, many families may not have ready access to quality infant hip ultrasonography, and this may determine the choice of obtaining a pelvic radiograph instead of an ultrasound.[61]

Treatment

Recommendations for treatment are based on the clinical hip examination and the presence or absence of imaging abnormalities. Infants with a stable clinical hip examination but with abnormalities noted on ultrasonography can be observed without a brace.[3,56]

The initiation of abduction brace treatment, either immediate or delayed, for clinically unstable hips is supported by several studies.[3,62–64] In a randomized clinical trial, Gardiner and Dunn[62] found no difference in hip ultrasonography findings or clinical outcome for infants with dislocatable hips treated with either immediate or delayed abduction bracing at 6- and 12-month follow-up. The infants in the delayed group (2 weeks) were treated with abduction bracing if hip instability persisted or the hip

ultrasonographic abnormalities did not improve.[62]

RISKS OF TREATMENT

Treatment of clinically unstable hips usually consists of bracing when discovered in early infancy and closed reduction with adductor tenotomy and spica cast immobilization when noted later. After 18 months of age, open surgery is generally recommended.

As previously noted, the 2006 USPSTF report noted a high rate of AVN, up to 60% with both surgical and nonsurgical intervention.[33] Other studies have reported much lower rates of AVN.[36,37] One prospective study reported a zero prevalence of AVN by 6 years of age in mildly dysplastic hips treated with bracing.[30]

However, abduction brace treatment is not innocuous. The potential risks include AVN, temporary femoral nerve palsy, and obturator (inferior) hip dislocation.[65–67] One study demonstrated a 7% to 14% risk of complications after treatment in a Pavlik harness. The risk was greater in hips that did not reduce in the brace.[33] Precautions such as avoiding forced abduction in the harness, stopping treatment after 3 weeks if the hip does not reduce, and proper strap placement with weekly monitoring is important to minimize the risks associated with brace treatment.[68,69] Double diapering is a probably harmless but ineffective treatment of true DDH.

What remains controversial is whether the selective use of ultrasonography reduces or increases treatment. A randomized controlled study from the United Kingdom showed that approximately half of all positive physical examination findings were falsely positive (ie, normal ultrasonography results) and that the use of ultrasonography in clinically suspect hips actually reduced DDH treatment.[60] However, in the United States and Canada,[21] the reverse appears to be true. In the current medicolegal climate that encourages a defensive approach, liberal use of ultrasonography in the United States and Canada has clearly fostered overdiagnosis and overtreatment of DDH, despite best-available literature supporting observation of mild dysplasia.[33–35,70]

MEDICOLEGAL RISK TO THE PEDIATRICIAN

Undetected or late-developing DDH is a liability concern for the pediatrician, generating anxiety and a desire for guidance in best screening methodology.[71] Unfortunately, this fear may also provoke overdiagnosis and overtreatment. "Late-presenting" DDH is a more accurate term than "missed" to use when DDH is first diagnosed in a walking-aged child who had appropriate clinical examinations during infancy.[72,73]

Although there is no universally recognized DDH screening standard, the AAP endorses the concept of surveillance or periodic physical examinations until walking age, with selective use of either hip ultrasonography or radiography, depending on age. The AAP cautions against overreliance on ultrasonography as a diagnostic test and encourages its use as an adjunctive secondary screen and an aid to treatment of established DDH. Notably, no screening program has been shown to completely eliminate the risk of a late-presenting dislocated hip.[69]

The electronic health record can be used to provide a template, reminder, and documentation tool for the periodic examination. It also can be useful in the transition and comanagement of children with suspected DDH by providing effective information transfer between consultants and primary care physicians and ensuring follow-up. Accurate documented communication between providers is important to provide continuity of care for this condition, and it is also important to explain to the parent(s) and document those instances when observation is used as a planned strategy so it is less likely to be misinterpreted as negligence.

BEST PRACTICES AND STATE OF THE ART

1. The AAP, POSNA, AAOS, and Canadian DDH Task Force recommend newborn and periodic surveillance physical examinations for DDH to include detection of limb length discrepancy, examination for asymmetric thigh or buttock (gluteal) creases, performing the Ortolani test for stability (performed gently and which is usually negative after 3 months of age), and observing for limited abduction (generally positive after 3 months of age). Use of electronic health records can be considered to prompt and record the results of periodic hip examinations. The AAP recommends against universal ultrasonographic screening.

2. Selective hip ultrasonography can be considered between the ages of 6 weeks and 6 months for "high-risk" infants without positive physical findings. High risk is a relative and controversial term, but considerations include male or female breech presentation, a positive family history, parental concern, suspicious but inconclusive periodic examination, history of a previous positive instability physical examination, and history of tight lower-extremity swaddling. Because most DDH occurs in children without risk factors, physical examination remains the primary screening tool.

3. It is important that infantile hip ultrasonography be performed and interpreted per American Institute of Ultrasound in Medicine and the American College of Radiology guidelines by experienced, trained examiners. Developing local criteria for screening imaging and referral based on best resources may promote more uniform and cost-effective treatment. Regional variability of ultrasonographic imaging quality can lead to under- or overtreatment.

4. Most minor hip anomalies observed on ultrasonography at 6 weeks to 4 months of age will resolve spontaneously. These include minor variations in α and β angles and subluxation ("uncoverage") with stress maneuvers. Current levels of evidence do not support recommendations for treatment versus observation in any specific case of minor ultrasonographic variation. Care is, therefore, individualized through a process of shared decision-making in this setting of inadequate information.

5. Radiography (anteroposterior and frog pelvis views) can be considered after 4 months of age for the high-risk infant without physical findings or any child with positive clinical findings. Age 4 to 6 months is a watershed during which either imaging modality may be used; radiography is more readily available, has a lower rate of false-positive results, and is less expensive than ultrasonography but involves a very low dose of radiation.

6. A referral to an orthopedist for DDH does not require

ultrasonography or radiography. The primary indication for referral includes an unstable (positive Ortolani test result) or dislocated hip on clinical examination. Any child with limited hip abduction or asymmetric hip abduction after the neonatal period (4 weeks of age) should be referred for evaluation. Relative indications for referral include infants with risk factors for DDH, a questionable examination, and pediatrician or parental concern.

7. Evidence strongly supports screening for and treatment of hip dislocation (positive Ortolani test result) and initially observing milder early forms of dysplasia and instability (positive Barlow test result). Depending on local custom, either the pediatrician or the orthopedist can observe mild forms by periodic examination and possible follow-up imaging, but actual treatment should be performed by an orthopedist.

8. A reasonable goal for the primary care physician should be to diagnose hip subluxation or dislocation by 6 months of age by using the periodic physical examination. Selective ultrasonography or radiography may be used in consultation with a pediatric radiologist and/or orthopedist. No screening program has been shown to completely eliminate the risk of a late presentation of DDH. There is no high-level evidence that milder forms of dysplasia can be prevented by screening and early treatment.

9. Tight swaddling of the lower extremities with the hips adducted and extended should be avoided. The concept of "safe" swaddling, which

does not restrict hip motion, minimizes the risk of DDH.

10. Treatment of neonatal DDH is not an emergency, and in-hospital initiation of bracing is not required. Orthopaedic consultation can be safely obtained within several weeks of discharge for an infant with a positive Ortolani test result. Infants with a positive Barlow test results should be reexamined and referred to an orthopedist if they continue to show clinical instability.

ACKNOWLEDGMENTS

The authors thank Charles Price, MD, FAAP, Ellen Raney, MD, FAAP, Joshua Abzug, MD, FAAP, and William Hennrikus, MD, FAAP, for their valuable contributions to this report.

LEAD AUTHORS

Brian A. Shaw, MD, FAAOS, FAAP
Lee S. Segal, MD, FAAP

SECTION ON ORTHOPAEDICS EXECUTIVE COMMITTEE, 2014–2015

Norman Y. Otsuka, MD, FAAP, Chairperson
Richard M. Schwend, MD, FAAP, Immediate Past Chairperson
Theodore John Ganley, MD, FAAP
Martin Joseph Herman, MD, FAAP
Joshua E. Hyman, MD, FAAP
Brian A. Shaw, MD, FAAOS, FAAP
Brian G. Smith, MD, FAAP

STAFF

Niccole Alexander, MPP

ABBREVIATIONS

AAOS: American Academy of Orthopaedic Surgeons
AAP: American Academy of Pediatrics
AVN: avascular necrosis
DDH: developmental dysplasia of the hip
POSNA: Pediatric Orthopaedic Society of North America
USPSTF: US Preventive Services Task Force

REFERENCES

1. American Academy of Pediatrics. Clinical practice guideline: early detection of developmental dysplasia of the hip. Committee on Quality Improvement, Subcommittee on Developmental Dysplasia of the Hip. *Pediatrics*. 2000;105(4 pt 1):896–905

2. Schwend RM, Schoenecker P, Richards BS, Flynn JM, Vitale M; Pediatric Orthopaedic Society of North America. Screening the newborn for developmental dysplasia of the hip: now what do we do? *J Pediatr Orthop*. 2007;27(6):607–610

3. American Academy of Orthopaedic Surgeons. *Detection and Nonoperative Management of Pediatric Developmental Dysplasia of the Hip in Infants Up to Six Months of Age. Evidence-Based Clinical Practice Guideline*. Rosemont, IL: American Academy of Orthopaedic Surgeons; 2014

4. Wilson JMG, Jungner G. *Principles and Practice of Screening for Disease*. Geneva, Switzerland: World Health Organization; 1968

5. Rosendahl K, Dezateux C, Fosse KR, et al. Immediate treatment versus sonographic surveillance for mild hip dysplasia in newborns. *Pediatrics*. 2010;125(1). Available at: www.pediatrics.org/cgi/content/full/125/1/e9

6. Bache CE, Clegg J, Herron M. Risk factors for developmental dysplasia of the hip: ultrasonographic findings in the neonatal period. *J Pediatr Orthop B*. 2002;11(3):212–218

7. Barr LV, Rehm A. Should all twins and multiple births undergo ultrasound examination for developmental dysplasia of the hip? A retrospective study of 990 multiple births. *Bone Joint J*. 2013;95-B(1):132–134

8. Imrie M, Scott V, Stearns P, Bastrom T, Mubarak SJ. Is ultrasound screening for DDH in babies born breech sufficient? *J Child Orthop*. 2010;4(1):3–8

9. Suzuki S, Yamamuro T. Avascular necrosis in patients treated with the Pavlik harness for congenital dislocation of the hip. *J Bone Joint Surg Am*. 1990;72(7):1048–1055

10. Fox AE, Paton RW. The relationship between mode of delivery and

developmental dysplasia of the hip in breech infants: a four-year prospective cohort study. *J Bone Joint Surg Br.* 2010;92(12):1695–1699

11. Lowry CA, Donoghue VB, O'Herlihy C, Murphy JF. Elective Caesarean section is associated with a reduction in developmental dysplasia of the hip in term breech infants. *J Bone Joint Surg Br.* 2005;87(7):984–985

12. Panagiotopoulou N, Bitar K, Hart WJ. The association between mode of delivery and developmental dysplasia of the hip in breech infants: a systematic review of 9 cohort studies. *Acta Orthop Belg.* 2012;78(6):697–702

13. Sarkissian EJ, Sankar WN, Baldwin K, Flynn JM. Is there a predilection for breech infants to demonstrate spontaneous stabilization of DDH instability? *J Pediatr Orthop.* 2014;34(5):509–513

14. Dodinval P. Hérédité de la maladie luxante de la hanche (MLH) [Heredity in congenital dislocation of the hip]. *Acta Orthop Belg.* 1990;56(1 pt A):7–11

15. Tönnis D. Inheritance. In: Tönnis D, ed. *Congenital Dysplasia and Dislocation of the Hip in Children and Adults.* Berlin, Germany: Springer-Verlag; 1984:61–62

16. Stevenson DA, Mineau G, Kerber RA, Viskochil DH, Schaefer C, Roach JW. Familial predisposition to developmental dysplasia of the hip. *J Pediatr Orthop.* 2009;29(5):463–466

17. Schiffern AN, Stevenson DA, Carroll KL, et al. Total hip arthroplasty, hip osteoarthritis, total knee arthroplasty, and knee osteoarthritis in patients with developmental dysplasia of the hip and their family members: a kinship analysis report. *J Pediatr Orthop.* 2012;32(6):609–612

18. Carroll KL, Schiffern AN, Murray KA, et al. The occurrence of occult acetabular dysplasia in relatives of individuals with developmental dysplasia of the hip. *J Pediatr Orthop.* 2016;36(1):96–100

19. Mahan ST, Kasser JR. Does swaddling influence developmental dysplasia of the hip? *Pediatrics.* 2008;121(1):177–178

20. van Sleuwen BE, Engelberts AC, Boere-Boonekamp MM, Kuis W, Schulpen TW, L'Hoir MP. Swaddling: a systematic review. *Pediatrics.* 2007;120(4). Available at: www.pediatrics.org/cgi/content/full/120/4/e1097

21. Wang E, Liu T, Li J, et al. Does swaddling influence developmental dysplasia of the hip? An experimental study of the traditional straight-leg swaddling model in neonatal rats. *J Bone Joint Surg Am.* 2012;94(12):1071–1077

22. Gerard CM, Harris KA, Thach BT. Physiologic studies on swaddling: an ancient child care practice, which may promote the supine position for infant sleep. *J Pediatr.* 2002;141(3):398–403

23. Oden RP, Powell C, Sims A, Weisman J, Joyner BL, Moon RY. Swaddling: will it get babies onto their backs for sleep? *Clin Pediatr (Phila).* 2012;51(3):254–259

24. Canillas F, Delgado-Martos MJ, Martos-Rodriguez A, Quintana-Villamandos B, Delgado-Baeza E. Contribution to the initial pathodynamics of hip luxation in young rats. *J Pediatr Orthop.* 2012;32(6):613–620

25. Pediatric Orthopaedic Society of North America, International Hip Dysplasia Institute, American Academy of Orthopaedic Surgeons, United States Bone and Joint Initiative, Shriners Hospitals for Children. Position Statement: Swaddling and Developmental Hip Dysplasia. Rosemont, IL: Pediatric Orthopaedic Society of North America; 2015. Available at: www.aaos.org/uploadedFiles/PreProduction/About/Opinion_Statements/position/1186%20Swaddling%20and%20Developmental%20Hip%20Dysplasia%281%29.pdf. Accessed January 12, 2016

26. Roposch A, Liu LQ, Protopapa E. Variations in the use of diagnostic criteria for developmental dysplasia of the hip. *Clin Orthop Relat Res.* 2013;471(6):1946–1954

27. Barlow TG. Early diagnosis and treatment of congenital dislocation of the hip. *J Bone Joint Surg Br.* 1962;44B(2):292–301

28. Barlow TG. Congenital dislocation of the hip in the newborn. *Proc R Soc Med.* 1966;59(11 part 1):1103–1106

29. Barlow TG. Neonatal hip dysplasia—treatment, results and complications. *Proc R Soc Med.* 1975;68(8):475

30. Brurås KR, Aukland SM, Markestad T, Sera F, Dezateux C, Rosendahl K. Newborns with sonographically dysplastic and potentially unstable hips: 6-year follow-up of an RCT. *Pediatrics.* 2011;127(3). Available at: www.pediatrics.org/cgi/content/full/127/3/e661

31. Mladenov K, Dora C, Wicart P, Seringe R. Natural history of hips with borderline acetabular index and acetabular dysplasia in infants. *J Pediatr Orthop.* 2002;22(5):607–612

32. Clarke NM, Reading IC, Corbin C, Taylor CC, Bochmann T. Twenty years' experience of selective secondary ultrasound screening for congenital dislocation of the hip. *Arch Dis Child.* 2012;97(5):423–429

33. Shipman SA, Helfand M, Moyer VA, Yawn BP. Screening for developmental dysplasia of the hip: a systematic literature review for the US Preventive Services Task Force. *Pediatrics.* 2006;117(3). Available at: www.pediatrics.org/cgi/content/full/117/3/e557

34. US Preventive Services Task Force. Screening for developmental dysplasia of the hip: recommendation statement. *Pediatrics.* 2006;117(3):898–902

35. Patel H; Canadian Task Force on Preventive Health Care. Preventive health care, 2001 update: screening and management of developmental dysplasia of the hip in newborns. *CMAJ.* 2001;164(12):1669–1677

36. Williams PR, Jones DA, Bishay M. Avascular necrosis and the Aberdeen splint in developmental dysplasia of the hip. *J Bone Joint Surg Br.* 1999;81(6):1023–1028

37. Laborie LB, Engesæter IØ, Lehmann TG, Eastwood DM, Engesæter LB, Rosendahl K. Screening strategies for hip dysplasia: long-term outcome of a randomized controlled trial. *Pediatrics.* 2013;132(3):492–501

38. Gardner F, Dezateaux C, Elbourne D, Gray A, King A, Quinn A; Collaborative Hip Trial Group. The hip trial: psychological consequences for mothers of using ultrasound to manage infants with developmental hip dysplasia. *Arch Dis Child Fetal Neonatal Ed.* 2005;90(1):F17–F24

39. Rosendahl K, Markestad T, Lie RT. Ultrasound screening for developmental dysplasia of the hip in the neonate: the effect on treatment rate and prevalence of late cases. *Pediatrics.* 1994;94(1):47–52

40. Holen KJ, Tegnander A, Bredland T, et al. Universal or selective screening of the neonatal hip using ultrasound? A prospective, randomised trial of 15,529 newborn infants. *J Bone Joint Surg Br.* 2002;84(6):886–890

41. Hagans JF, Shaw JS, Duncan P, eds. *Bright Futures: Guidelines for Health Supervision of Infants, Children, and Adolescents, Third Edition. Pocket Guide.* Elk Grove Village, IL: American Academy of Pediatrics; 2008

42. Catterall A. The early diagnosis of congenital dislocation of the hip. *J Bone Joint Surg Br.* 1994;76(4):515–516

43. Wirth T, Stratmann L, Hinrichs F. Evolution of late presenting developmental dysplasia of the hip and associated surgical procedures after 14 years of neonatal ultrasound screening. *J Bone Joint Surg Br.* 2004;86(4):585–589

44. Myles JW. Secondary screening for congenital displacement of the hip. *J Bone Joint Surg Br.* 1990;72(2):326–327

45. Moore FH. Examining infants' hips—can it do harm? *J Bone Joint Surg Br.* 1989;71(1):4–5

46. Jones DA. Neonatal hip stability and the Barlow test. A study in stillborn babies. *J Bone Joint Surg Br.* 1991;73(2):216–218

47. Bond CD, Hennrikus WL, DellaMaggiore ED. Prospective evaluation of newborn soft-tissue hip "clicks" with ultrasound. *J Pediatr Orthop.* 1997;17(2):199–201

48. Scoles PV, Boyd A, Jones PK. Roentgenographic parameters of the normal infant hip. *J Pediatr Orthop.* 1987;7(6):656–663

49. Karmazyn BK, Gunderman RB, Coley BD, et al; American College of Radiology. ACR Appropriateness Criteria on developmental dysplasia of the hip—child. *J Am Coll Radiol.* 2009;6(8):551–557

50. American Institute of Ultrasound in Medicine; American College of Radiology. AIUM practice guideline for the performance of an ultrasound examination for detection and assessment of developmental dysplasia of the hip. *J Ultrasound Med.* 2009;28(1):114–119

51. Roposch A, Wright JG. Increased diagnostic information and understanding disease: uncertainty in the diagnosis of developmental hip dysplasia. *Radiology.* 2007;242(2):355–359

52. Roposch A, Moreau NM, Uleryk E, Doria AS. Developmental dysplasia of the hip: quality of reporting of diagnostic accuracy for US. *Radiology.* 2006;241(3):854–860

53. Burger BJ, Burger JD, Bos CF, Obermann WR, Rozing PM, Vandenbroucke JP. Neonatal screening and staggered early treatment for congenital dislocation or dysplasia of the hip. *Lancet.* 1990;336(8730):1549–1553

54. Dunn PM, Evans RE, Thearle MJ, Griffiths HE, Witherow PJ. Congenital dislocation of the hip: early and late diagnosis and management compared. *Arch Dis Child.* 1985;60(5):407–414

55. Sampath JS, Deakin S, Paton RW. Splintage in developmental dysplasia of the hip: how low can we go? *J Pediatr Orthop.* 2003;23(3):352–355

56. Wood MK, Conboy V, Benson MK. Does early treatment by abduction splintage improve the development of dysplastic but stable neonatal hips? *J Pediatr Orthop.* 2000;20(3):302–305

57. Shorter D, Hong T, Osborn DA. Screening programmes for developmental dysplasia of the hip in newborn infants. *Cochrane Database Syst Rev.* 2011;(9):CD004595

58. Paton RW, Srinivasan MS, Shah B, Hollis S. Ultrasound screening for hips at risk in developmental dysplasia. Is it worth it? *J Bone Joint Surg Br.* 1999;81(2):255–258

59. Paton RW, Hinduja K, Thomas CD. The significance of at-risk factors in ultrasound surveillance of developmental dysplasia of the hip. A ten-year prospective study. *J Bone Joint Surg Br.* 2005;87(9):1264–1266

60. Elbourne D, Dezateux C, Arthur R, et al; UK Collaborative Hip Trial Group. Ultrasonography in the diagnosis and management of developmental hip dysplasia (UK Hip Trial): clinical and economic results of a multicentre randomised controlled trial. *Lancet.* 2002;360(9350):2009–2017

61. Pacana MJ, Hennrikus WL, Slough J, Curtin W. Ultrasound examination for infants born breech by elective cesarean section with a normal hip exam for instability [published online ahead of print October 21, 2015]. *J Pediatr Orthop.* Doi:10.1097/BPO.0000000000000668

62. Gardiner HM, Dunn PM. Controlled trial of immediate splinting versus ultrasonographic surveillance in congenitally dislocatable hips. *Lancet.* 1990;336(8730):1553–1556

63. Paton RW, Hopgood PJ, Eccles K. Instability of the neonatal hip: the role of early or late splintage. *Int Orthop.* 2004;28(5):270–273

64. Lorente Moltó FJ, Gregori AM, Casas LM, Perales VM. Three-year prospective study of developmental dysplasia of the hip at birth: should all dislocated or dislocatable hips be treated? *J Pediatr Orthop.* 2002;22(5):613–621

65. Suzuki S, Kashiwagi N, Kasahara Y, Seto Y, Futami T. Avascular necrosis and the Pavlik harness. The incidence of avascular necrosis in three types of congenital dislocation of the hip as classified by ultrasound. *J Bone Joint Surg Br.* 1996;78(4):631–635

66. Murnaghan ML, Browne RH, Sucato DJ, Birch J. Femoral nerve palsy in Pavlik harness treatment for developmental dysplasia of the hip. *J Bone Joint Surg Am.* 2011;93(5):493–499

67. Rombouts JJ, Kaelin A. Inferior (obturator) dislocation of the hip in neonates. A complication of treatment by the Pavlik harness. *J Bone Joint Surg Br.* 1992;74(5):708–710

68. Mubarak S, Garfin S, Vance R, McKinnon B, Sutherland D. Pitfalls in the use of the Pavlik harness for treatment of congenital dysplasia, subluxation, and dislocation of the hip. *J Bone Joint Surg Am.* 1981;63(8):1239–1248

69. Kitoh H, Kawasumi M, Ishiguro N. Predictive factors for unsuccessful treatment of developmental dysplasia of the hip by the Pavlik harness. *J Pediatr Orthop.* 2009;29(6):552–557

70. Sucato DJ, Johnston CE II, Birch JG, Herring JA, Mack P. Outcome of ultrasonographic hip abnormalities in clinically stable hips. *J Pediatr Orthop.* 1999;19(6):754–759

71. McAbee GN, Donn SM, Mendelson RA, McDonnell WM, Gonzalez JL, Ake JK. Medical diagnoses commonly associated with pediatric malpractice lawsuits in the United States. *Pediatrics.* 2008;122(6). Available at: www.pediatrics.org/cgi/content/full/122/6/e1282

72. Davies SJ, Walker G. Problems in the early recognition of hip dysplasia. *J Bone Joint Surg Br.* 1984;66(4):479–484

73. Ilfeld FW, Westin GW, Makin M. Missed or developmental dislocation of the hip. *Clin Orthop Relat Res.* 1986;(203):276–281

Families Affected by Parental Substance Use

- *Clinical Report*

CLINICAL REPORT Guidance for the Clinician in Rendering Pediatric Care

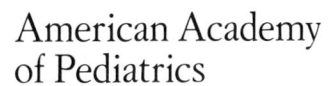

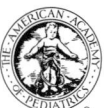

DEDICATED TO THE HEALTH OF ALL CHILDREN™

Families Affected by Parental Substance Use

Vincent C. Smith, MD, MPH, FAAP, Celeste R. Wilson, MD, FAAP, COMMITTEE ON SUBSTANCE USE AND PREVENTION

abstract

Children whose parents or caregivers use drugs or alcohol are at increased risk of short- and long-term sequelae ranging from medical problems to psychosocial and behavioral challenges. In the course of providing health care services to children, pediatricians are likely to encounter families affected by parental substance use and are in a unique position to intervene. Therefore, pediatricians need to know how to assess a child's risk in the context of a parent's substance use. The purposes of this clinical report are to review some of the short-term effects of maternal substance use during pregnancy and long-term implications of fetal exposure; describe typical medical, psychiatric, and behavioral symptoms of children and adolescents in families affected by substance use; and suggest proficiencies for pediatricians involved in the care of children and adolescents of families affected by substance use, including screening families, mandated reporting requirements, and directing families to community, regional, and state resources that can address needs and problems.

Clinical reports from the American Academy of Pediatrics benefit from expertise and resources of liaisons and internal (AAP) and external reviewers. However, clinical reports from the American Academy of Pediatrics may not reflect the views of the liaisons or the organizations or government agencies that they represent.

The guidance in this report does not indicate an exclusive course of treatment or serve as a standard of medical care. Variations, taking into account individual circumstances, may be appropriate.

All clinical reports from the American Academy of Pediatrics automatically expire 5 years after publication unless reaffirmed, revised, or retired at or before that time.

DOI: 10.1542/peds.2016-1575

PEDIATRICS (ISSN Numbers: Print, 0031-4005; Online, 1098-4275).

Copyright © 2016 by the American Academy of Pediatrics

FINANCIAL DISCLOSURE: The authors have indicated they have no financial relationships relevant to this article to disclose.

FUNDING: No external funding.

POTENTIAL CONFLICT OF INTEREST: The authors have indicated they have no potential conflicts of interest to disclose.

To cite: Smith VC, Wilson CR, AAP COMMITTEE ON SUBSTANCE USE AND PREVENTION. Families Affected by Parental Substance Use. *Pediatrics.* 2016;138(2):e20161575

INTRODUCTION

In the course of providing health care services to children, pediatricians often encounter families affected by substance use, distribution, manufacturing, or cultivation that ultimately places parents and their children at risk. Substance use can include illicit substances such as marijuana, heroin, cocaine, and methamphetamine (eg, crystal meth), as well as misuse of alcohol and prescription medications. As defined by the National Alliance for Drug Endangered Children, drug-endangered children are those who are at risk for suffering physical or emotional harm as a result of their caregiver's substance use, possession, manufacturing, cultivation, or distribution.[1,2] Children also may be endangered when parents' substance use interferes with their ability to raise their children and provide a safe, nurturing environment.[1] Parents' substance use may affect their ability to consistently prioritize the child's basic physical and emotional needs over their own need for substances. Cigarette smoking often accompanies substance use and can pose additional hazards to children (www2.aap.org/richmondcenter). Furthermore, the home environment may be unsanitary or unsafe, particularly if illegal or legal drugs, chemicals, or paraphernalia are accessible or if drugs are being cultivated or manufactured in the home. Such conditions can lead to poor child health and developmental outcomes or child maltreatment and even child death.

Children exposed to a parent's substance use commonly experience educational delays and inadequate medical and dental care.[3] Almost a quarter of children of mothers with identified substance use disorders (SUDs) do not receive routine child health maintenance services in their first 2 years of life.[3] Children of parents with SUDs are also at greater risk of later mental health and behavioral problems, including SUDs.[4,5] Pediatricians have an opportunity to help break multigenerational cycles of child abuse and neglect and substance use by being informed about the effects of parental substance use on children, intervening when necessary, and collaborating with the family, other health care providers, and appropriate government agencies to address the issues involved.

Pediatricians are in a unique position to identify and assess a child's risk in the context of a parent's SUD and intervene to protect the child. Research has shown that a majority of parents are accepting of their child's pediatrician asking them about their own substance use.[6] Pediatricians can include questions about the extent of family substance use as part of the routine family assessment during health supervision visits or when clinically indicated.[7] Given the risks to health and development, children in families with known or suspected parental SUDs may warrant more frequent appointments with their pediatrician for close medical follow-up or

developmental evaluation. For example, children may have their ears examined for chronic otitis media because of greater exposure to smoke or large breathable particulates in their homes or for more frequent developmental assessments, given risks of emotional and behavioral disorders, delays in expressive language, and mental illness.

Pediatricians who help identify substance use problems in a child's family members are not expected to solve, manage, or treat these problems; rather, they can assist families by working in partnership with other professionals to provide access to state, regional, and local resources available to families. Being familiar with effective harm reduction strategies and being prepared to inform public debate on how to use evidence-based strategies to protect and advocate for children whose parents have SUDs are important roles that the pediatrician can assume. In addition, medical professionals are mandatory reporters of suspected child maltreatment and may be the only professionals who have the opportunity to recognize that a child, especially one of preschool age, has been abused or neglected.

The purposes of this clinical report are to review some of the short-term effects of maternal substance use during pregnancy and long-term implications of fetal exposure; describe typical medical, psychiatric, and behavioral symptoms of children and adolescents in families affected by substance use; and suggest proficiencies for pediatricians involved in the care of children and adolescents of families affected by substance use, including screening families, mandated reporting requirements, and directing families to community, regional, or state resources that can address needs and problems. Throughout this report, the term parent is used, but

the discussion could apply to any primary adult who cares for a child, including guardians, grandparents, and foster parents.

EPIDEMIOLOGY OF SUBSTANCE USE IN THE UNITED STATES

A 2013 national government survey on drug use and health reported that more than 9.4% of the US population 12 years and older uses psychoactive substances.[8] In 2013, an estimated 24.6 million Americans 12 years or older had used an illicit substance in the 30 days before the survey.[8] The total annual societal cost of substance use in terms of lost goods, lost productivity, treatment, and medical services in the United States is estimated to be $510.8 billion.[9] This estimate includes costs related to alcohol and drug treatment and prevention services; substance use–related medical condition management and sequelae; lost earnings attributable to premature death, substance use–related illness, and loss of employment; goods and services associated with substance use–related crime, criminal justice, motor vehicle crashes, property damage, and fires; and police, fire department, adjudication, and sanctioning expenses.[9]

Exposure to substances begins prenatally for many infants. Specifically, a study by Patrick et al[10] of a nationally representative sample of infants demonstrated that in 2012, approximately 22 000 infants were diagnosed with neonatal abstinence syndrome. Neonatal abstinence syndrome includes a combination of physiologic and neurobehavioral signs that include such things as sweating, irritability, increased muscle tone and activity, feeding problems, diarrhea, and seizures and is the result of prenatal exposure to opioids followed by withdrawal at birth.[11] This problem persists, as evidenced by a recent study that showed among 112 029 pregnant women, 31 354 (28.0%) were prescribed at least 1 opioid pain reliever during pregnancy.[12]

It is estimated that 1 in 5 children grows up in a home in which someone uses drugs or misuses alcohol.[7] The exact number of children living with adults with SUDs is unknown[13]; however, an estimated 8.3 million children younger than 18 years (12%) were residing with at least 1 substance-dependent or substance-using parent between 2002 and 2007.[14]

IMPLICATIONS OF FETAL EXPOSURE SECONDARY TO MATERNAL SUBSTANCE USE

Detailed discussions of short- and long-term effects of prenatal substance use on the exposed fetus are available elsewhere.[11,15–17] A brief description follows (Table 1).

Short-term Medical Effects of Fetal Exposure

The detrimental effects of fetal exposure to alcohol are well documented.[11,15,17] Fetal alcohol spectrum disorders, fetal alcohol effects, prenatal complications (eg, prematurity, low birth weight), and prolonged postnatal hospitalization all are associated with alcohol use during the prenatal period, but a full review is beyond the scope of this report.

Because there is passive diffusion across the placenta of substances smaller than 500 dalton (d), most illicit and some other substances used by a pregnant woman will directly affect the fetus (eg, methamphetamine = 149 d, buprenorphine = 467 d, tetrahydrocannabinol [THC] = 314 d).[18] Exposure to substances during the first trimester can affect the structure of the developing fetal brain, and exposure during the second and third trimesters may affect brain function.[18] Marijuana crosses the placenta, and its psychoactive

TABLE 1 Short- and Long-term Effects of Fetal Substance Exposure

Effect	Alcohol	Marijuana	Opiates	Cocaine	Methamphetamine
Short-term effects or birth outcome					
Fetal growth	+++	+/−	+	+	+
Anomalies	+++	−	−	−	−
Withdrawal	−	−	+++	-	Unknown
Neurobehavior	+	+	+	+	−
Long-term effects					
Growth	+++	−	−	+/−	Unknown
Behavior	+++	+	+	+	Unknown
Cognition	+++	+	+/−	+	Unknown
Language	+	-	Unknown	+	Unknown
Achievement	+++	+	Unknown	+/−	Unknown

Adapted with permission from Behnke et al (2013).[11] +++, strong effect; +, effect; +/−, no consensus about effect; −, no known effect.

constituents are fat soluble and can bind to cannabinoid receptors in the fetal brain.[19] Newborn infants can have small-for-gestational-age head circumference after prenatal exposure to cannabis.[19] Fetal exposure to cannabis has been associated with subtle neurobehavioral disturbances (ie, exaggerated and prolonged startle reflexes and increased hand–mouth behavior), high-pitched cries, and sleep cycle disturbances with electroencephalographic changes in the newborn period.[11,19] Repeated fetal exposure to cannabis disrupts endocannabinoid signaling, particularly the temporal dynamics of the CB1 cannabinoid receptor, and alters fetal cortical circuitry development.[16] Interference with the endocannabinoid system disrupts normal neurobiological development, particularly of neurotransmitter maturation and neuronal survival.[19]

Effects of fetal cocaine and opioid exposure may appear during the newborn period as any of the following symptoms of withdrawal: irritability, poor and irregular feeding patterns, frequent crying, tremulousness, increased respiratory and heart rates, hypertonia, an exaggerated startle response, vomiting, frantic sucking, and difficulty being consoled.[6,11] Prenatal cocaine exposure can have effects on neurobehavior, which may manifest clinically as lability of state, decreased behavioral

and autonomic regulation, and poor alertness and orientation.[11] Prenatal cocaine exposure also may hinder fetal growth.[11] Similarly, prenatal methamphetamine exposure can inhibit fetal growth and alter neurobehavior (ie, poor movement quality, decreased arousal, and increased stress).[11] Prenatal buprenorphine exposure causes fewer withdrawal symptoms and, similar to methadone, has a longer duration of action than other opioids.[20]

Long-term Medical Effects of Fetal Exposure

Children with prenatal drug exposure are more likely to develop disruptive behavioral disorders such as oppositional defiant disorder; impaired intellectual and academic achievement; and cognitive problems, such as delayed language development, poor memory, and the inability to learn from mistakes.[2,6] Children who were exposed to drugs prenatally also have a higher risk of developing an SUD.[2,6] Prenatal drug exposure is associated with increased rates of anxiety and mood disorders, lower self-esteem, and perceived lack of control over their environment.[6]

Fetal alcohol exposure continues to affect growth, cognition, behavior, language, and achievement throughout life.[11,17] Children exposed in utero to cannabis may have a small-for-age head circumference well into their teenage years and permanent neurobehavioral, cognitive, and intellectual deficits that vary depending on the timing and degree of in utero exposure.[16,19] Specifically, heavy use (defined as more than 1 joint, or approximately 10 mg of THC, per day) during the first trimester has been associated with lower verbal reasoning skills in the child, whereas second trimester use was associated with impairments of the child's composite short-term memory.[19] Children exposed prenatally to heavy amounts of cannabis often struggle with tasks requiring visual memory, analysis, and integration; acquire language skills slowly; show increased levels of aggression; and display poor attention span.[19]

Mothers who have heroin addiction or are receiving medication-assisted treatment with methadone may have infants who exhibit increased activity as well as poorer coordination during childhood than children of similar age without prenatal opioid exposure.[4] Children with prenatal heroin exposure have more behavioral problems (including hyperactivity, brief attention span, sleep disturbance, and temper outbursts) at 12 to 24 months of age; language delay at 24 to 32 months of age; and, overall, more difficulties learning when compared with their age-matched peers.[4] Similarly, children of mothers treated prenatally with methadone maintenance are more impulsive, immature, and irresponsible than their unexposed peers and also perform poorly on intelligence tests at 3 to 7 years of age.[4] Information about the long-term developmental outcomes of prenatal buprenorphine exposure is limited, and many of the reports have conflicting findings.[20] Several studies have found that children with fetal exposure to prescribed buprenorphine score lower on Bayley cognitive and language scales compared with children who were not exposed

TABLE 2 General Warning Signs for Child Abuse

Frequent injuries, bruising, welts, or burns that cannot be sufficiently explained (eg, cigarette burns, bruises on the face, lips, and mouth or on several surface planes at the same time).
Withdrawn, fearful, or extreme behavior.
Clusters of bruises, welts, or burns, indicating repeated contact with a hand or instrument.
Injuries appear to have a pattern (eg, straight lines or circles) such as marks from a hand, belt, or electric cord.
Any bruise without a plausible explanation in an infant who is not yet cruising is suspicious for abuse.
Unusual injuries on children where children do not usually get injured (eg, the torso, back, neck, buttocks, or thighs).
Is always watchful and "on alert," as if waiting for something bad to happen.
Shies away from touch, flinches at sudden movements, or seems afraid to go home.

Adapted from www.mass.gov/eohhs/gov/departments/dcf/child-abuse-neglect/warning-signs.html. The list presents some general warning signs but is not comprehensive. The criteria for abuse and neglect may vary by region or state. Pediatricians should check their state and local laws for more detailed information.

prenatally.[20] There is also some evidence of decreased myelination and disrupted striatal cholinergic activity in children of women who received buprenorphine during pregnancy.[20] Prenatal exposure to cocaine may result in behavior, cognition, and language deficits in children.[11] Children who were exposed to crystal methamphetamine prenatally may have developmental delays in communication, personal and social skills, fine and gross motor skills, and problem-solving skills as well as aggressive or withdrawn behaviors.[21]

PSYCHOSOCIAL IMPACT OF LIVING IN A FAMILY AFFECTED BY PARENTAL SUBSTANCE USE

Parental substance use is associated with myriad family and social problems.[22-27] Whether secondary to inconsistency in parenting, disruption or lack of healthy family routines and rituals, or parental conflict and stress, children of substance-using parents typically are denied the security that is associated with structure and stability provided by appropriate parenting. The parent's SUD and the violent and erratic behavior that may be associated place the child at higher risk of being abused or neglected (Tables 2 and 3).[21,28-31] Children whose parents use substances and misuse alcohol are 3 times as likely to be physically,

emotionally, or sexually abused and 4 times as likely to be emotionally or physically neglected.[21,32] Higher rates of neglect have been noted in rural populations.[33] The neonatal period, when infants are the most vulnerable, is the period of highest risk of harm.[32] Parenting impairment varies to different degrees depending on which substances parents use.[34] Mandatory involvement of child protective services helps ensure a child's safety but may result in the child being placed in an alternate living situation with a relative (ie, kinship care) or unrelated caregiver.[35] Nonetheless, transition into foster care may be necessary to protect a child's physical safety.

The home environment may lack appropriate childproofing safety measures because of transience of housing and parents being distracted by substance use or alcohol misuse. The use of open flames or lighters for the consumption or production of drugs may increase the dangers of accidental burns, fires, and explosions where children live. Children are at increased risk of acquiring infectious diseases because of exposure to needles and drug paraphernalia.[21] Because of the significant cost of illicit substance use, household funds may be more limited, and parents with an SUD may struggle to meet their household financial demands.[3] Homes used to produce crystal methamphetamine may be unsafe and uninhabitable because of the presence of toxic ingredients and byproducts, including mercury, lead, and other large breathable particulates that settle close to the floor.[21] Home production of butane-extracted cannabis may lead to explosions or house fires. Children living in these chaotic home environments may be at risk for having contact with people in their house using or buying drugs; witnessing criminal behavior and interacting with criminals; ingesting or inhaling drugs or chemicals; being exposed to deplorable living conditions, including human waste, vermin, insects, clutter, garbage, and filth; and being subjected to sexual abuse and trafficking.

Because of potential for abuse, neglect, and a hazardous home environment, children whose parents have SUDs tend to come to the attention of child welfare agencies at a younger age than other children and are more likely than other children to be placed and remain in foster care.[36] Many families receiving child welfare services are affected by parental substance use.[37–39] The US Department of Health and Human Services concluded that parental substance abuse is a contributing factor for one-third to two-thirds of children being involved with the child welfare system.[37] This estimate is based on very old data, and as noted by a recent review, parental SUD prevalence rates based on these older data may no longer be representative of current trends, but more current data are lacking.[38]

Despite early maternal intentions and supportive interventions, 27% of children born to women with significant SUDs needed the involvement of child protective services during the preschool years.[40] An estimated 20% of substantiated cases of child abuse or neglect were associated with an SUD in the caregiver, and nearly 10% involved a caregiver with an alcohol use disorder.[41]

Although the link between child abuse and neglect and substance use is well

TABLE 3 General Warning Signs for Child Neglect

Lack of medical or dental care
Lack of personal care or hygiene (eg, unbathed, matted and unwashed hair, lice or scabies, or noticeable body odor)
Clothes are ill-fitting, filthy, or inappropriate for the weather
Missing key pieces of clothing (eg, underwear, socks, shoes)
Poor school attendance or frequent tardiness
Lack of supervision (eg, young children left unattended or with other children too young to protect or care for them or being left alone or allowed to play in unsafe situations and environments)
Lack of proper nutrition
Lack of adequate shelter
Lack of primary medical care, dental care, or immunizations as well as untreated illnesses or injuries
Self-destructive feelings or behavior

Adapted from www.mass.gov/eohhs/gov/departments/dcf/child-abuse-neglect/warning-signs.html. The list presents some general warning signs but is not comprehensive. The criteria for abuse and neglect may vary by region or state. Pediatricians should check their state and local laws for more detailed information.

documented, it is not necessarily a direct causal relationship, because a significant portion of adults with SUDs also have concurrent mental illness, including anxiety, depression, and posttraumatic stress disorder.[32] Parents with SUDs often experience financial instability, food and housing insecurity, a chaotic living environment, inconsistent employment, domestic violence, social stigma or isolation, incarceration, and stress.[3,32] Parental substance use has been linked with negative parental behaviors that include lower levels of parental involvement, limited or absent parental monitoring, ineffective control of children's behaviors, and poor discipline skills including use of coercive control, harsh discipline, and failure to follow through.[42] Collectively, these factors all contribute to substance use and child mistreatment. Any single factor, such as prenatal substance exposure, may be less salient to the overall developmental outcome of these children than the cumulative effects of exposure in the context of multiple home environmental and circumstance risks.

MEDICAL, PSYCHIATRIC, AND BEHAVIORAL SYMPTOMS OF CHILDREN AND ADOLESCENTS IN FAMILIES AFFECTED BY PARENTAL SUBSTANCE USE

Children and adolescents of parents with SUDs are at greater

risk of having problems ranging from serious medical conditions to psychobehavioral difficulties. Compared with their peers whose parents do not have SUDs, they are twice as likely to sustain serious injuries, increasing the risks of missed time from school, hospitalization, or surgical treatment.[43–47] A recent study found that 23% of children whose mothers were substance users were not engaged with routine child health services at any point during the first 2 years of life.[3] Mothers of drug-exposed newborn infants may be ill equipped to cope with their infants' health care needs.[6] Youth whose parents have SUDs are more likely to be neglected, and chronic neglect has more long-term implications for a child's mental health and development than do abuse and other forms of maltreatment.[48]

Mental health problems experienced by children of parents with SUDs can include anxiety disorders, attention-deficit/hyperactivity disorder, depression, oppositional defiant disorder, conduct disorder, truancy, and trauma and stress-related disorders.[49,50] It has been noted recently that among children whose parents have SUDs, children in rural populations have a greater risk of mental health problems.[33] Adverse childhood experiences include abuse (eg, emotional, physical, or sexual), neglect (eg, emotional or physical), and household dysfunction (eg, substance abuse, mental illness, intimate partner violence, incarceration, or separation or divorce), and these events may exceed the child's coping mechanisms, resulting in permanent changes in the developing brain.[51,52] These brain changes can manifest as behavior problems, violence, and substance use health risk behaviors by the child through the life span.[52]

Educational problems are especially common in children exposed to substance use.[53] These educational problems may be secondary to baseline cognitive limitations as a result of perinatal substance exposure or external distraction from a chaotic and unstructured home environment. Children affected by parental substance use may have a high absenteeism rate and impaired attention, compromising their academic productivity. Behavior problems place children at greater risk of suspension or expulsion from school.

Children are often distressed by their parents' substance use.[54] Children may blame themselves for the parents' behavior and may feel responsible for its cure. Children's prolonged exposure to inappropriate modeling of substance use increases their vulnerability to future substance use.[55] Children of alcoholics are nearly 4 times more likely to have an alcohol use disorder, with rates of hazardous use starting in the adolescent years and continuing into adulthood.[56–58]

METHODS TO ASSESS AND ENGAGE THE FAMILY AFFECTED BY PARENTAL SUBSTANCE USE

Pediatricians have a unique opportunity to identify and engage families affected by substance use. The opportunities for pediatricians to engage with a family begin with the transition of the mother from prenatal care to delivery of an infant. If the mother and family interact with a health care provider who demonstrates empathy and knowledge regarding the effects of prenatal substance use, the process of engagement has a better start. Many times, the likelihood of engagement depends on the confidence the family has that the health care providers meeting them at the intense period of birth will continue comprehensive care and that their issues will be incorporated into a care plan.

As an approach to engaging families, pediatricians may want to first ask about subjects remote from the substance use issue. Inquiring about other topics such as, "Do you have any medical problems? Are there any mental health problems such as depression or anxiety disorders in the family?" before moving to questions like, "Do you or anyone in your home smoke? Do you or anyone in your home drink alcohol? Do you or anyone in your home use drugs?" may be better received by parents, because it allows the provider to establish an initial rapport with parents around portions of their health that may be perceived as less threatening.

In the nursery setting, a new mother typically has a great interest in discussing all health issues that might affect her infant. Taking a history that includes questions such as, "Before you knew you were pregnant, how would you describe your use of alcohol?" and then asking, "After you knew of your pregnancy, how would you describe your use of alcohol?" allows the mother to discuss the changes she attempted and provides information to the pediatrician about either assisted or self-initiated harm reduction. Similarly, inquiring about tobacco, prescription medications with attention to opioids and sedative hypnotics, marijuana, cocaine, methamphetamine, and heroin could be included.

In the office setting, during the newborn period and first months of contact, pediatricians generally ask about feeding methods. Providing information to a mother with a history of substance use about possible transmission of substances, including ethanol, into human milk may open the door to a deeper discussion of the mother's substance use. Medically prescribed buprenorphine or methadone is not a contraindication to breastfeeding. Recommendations regarding the support of breastfeeding and potential effects on the newborn brain from passage of these substances warrant additional investigation and consensus.[59]

In a perfect health care system, the mother's health history would include sequential screening for alcohol, tobacco, and substance use throughout the pregnancy, and obstetric providers would communicate concerns to the pediatric team caring for the infant. With potentially concerning information, the discharging medical team might offer the mother resources to support her intentions of becoming a good parent for the infant with substance exposure. Those services might include home visiting, direction to home- and community-based services such as those that exist in Indian Health Service units, insurance company case managers, specialized clinics, developmental follow-up, and primary care settings that embrace the care of mothers with SUDs and infants with prenatal exposure.

Incorporating a short screening tool and directing parents who screen positive back to either their own primary care physician or a specialist is a practical approach. *Bright Futures: Guidelines for Health Supervision of Infants, Children, and Adolescents*[60] recommends developmental screening by a standardized instrument, such as the Ages & Stages Questionnaires, Third Edition (ASQ-3), matched with the clinical examination, to assess developmental delays possibly related to prenatal substance exposure or neglect of the child's nutrition and socioemotional needs.[61] For example, reports by parents of advanced communicative development may not be substantiated by verbal communication or capacity noted during the examination. In addition, attention to growth trends, particularly weight patterns, provides important information in early infancy about adequacy of feeding, particularly if the mother has initiated breastfeeding. Between 9 and 24 months of age, deceleration of weight gain can indicate family system stresses and inattention to the child's feeding in the home.

Some pediatricians can feel overwhelmed by what they perceive as their inability to screen parents and react to a positive screen successfully during a 15-minute appointment. To help, some brief screening questions could be incorporated into a routine health surveillance office visit. The National Institute on Alcohol Abuse and Alcoholism recommends the use of a single screening question to accurately identify unhealthy alcohol use. The question, "How many times in the past year have you had X or more drinks in a day?" (in which X is 5 for men and 4 for women, and a response of >1 is considered positive) has shown good sensitivity and specificity for detection of unhealthy alcohol use in a primary care population.[62] The National Institute on Drug Abuse (NIDA) has a single-question drug screen: "How many times in the past year have you used an illegal drug or used a prescription medication for nonmedical reasons?"[63] If the answer is "Never" for all drugs, NIDA recommends that the physician reinforce abstinence. However, if the answer is for any use of illegal or prescription drugs for nonmedical reasons, the parent needs to be

screened by a more comprehensive substance use instrument, probably by his or her primary care physician.

Once a parent has screened positive, a provider may use the time as a teaching moment to engage the parent, explain the results, express concern, provide a more structured brief intervention incorporating nonjudgmental, motivational interviewing-informed interactions, and suggest a more complete evaluation by the parent's primary care physician. If the results of a screen are positive and the parent would like more information about treatment locations, the Substance Abuse and Mental Health Services Administration has a searchable database of treatment locations throughout the United States (http://findtreatment.samhsa.gov).

As a reference, several short tools are available to screen for substance use by family members. The Alcohol Use Disorders Identification Test Consumption questions for alcohol and the Drug Abuse Screening Test for drugs are 2 tools that are short but garner vital information.[64–66] NIDA also provides a resource guide for substance use screening in the general medical setting that includes sample scripts.[63] As with the single-question screening tools, pediatricians using the short tools to screen need to be prepared to direct parents who screen positive to their primary care physician or another specialty provider for a more standardized brief intervention.

It is difficult to anticipate a parent's reaction to a discussion about their substance use. Therefore, providers are encouraged to secure a supportive and safe environment for the conversation to occur. When engaging in the conversation, a nonjudgmental, nonaccusatory tone will help to convey to parents the pediatrician's concern for them and their child. Objectively sharing the facts of the screen results and other observations will decrease

the opportunity for disagreement. Parents can be directed back to their primary care physician for management and services. Pediatricians may find it efficient to have a prepared list of community, regional, state, and national resources from which to choose and to offer to parents. Likewise, options for adult primary care physicians can be helpful for parents without an established medical home.

Parent screening for medical, psychiatric, psychosocial, and substance use disorders can help identify problems. If present, possible signs and symptoms associated with acute substance intoxication (eg, pinpoint pupils, frequent yawning, slurred speech, excessive attention to external stimuli, ataxic gait, or incoherent thought patterns) can be objectively documented in the child's medical record. Office staff could be encouraged to report any of these signs or symptoms to the pediatrician.[67] Additional guidance on dealing with the judgment-impaired parent in the pediatric office can be found in another clinical report from the American Academy of Pediatrics.[13] Indications of abuse or neglect would require a mandatory report to the child protective services agency.

Research has shown that parents who screened positive for substance use were open to the pediatrician discussing their use with them and presenting the parents with follow-up options.[67] With supportive care, parents often are willing to enter drug treatment or engage in harm reduction on behalf of their children. Even when parents do not go to treatment, they may reduce use of the substances that they view as more threatening, such as methamphetamine, but increase marijuana or tobacco use. Parents may also decrease their substance use even if they do not completely abstain. Therefore, pediatricians can feel empowered to address these topics when speaking with the parent.

In addition to screening of parents, a careful physical examination of the child should be performed in all situations in which abuse or neglect is suspected, because important cutaneous findings can be concealed easily by clothing (Tables 2 and 3). Although skin findings alone are not specific for maltreatment, their presence and the particular characteristics of findings, such as bruises, lacerations, abrasions, burns or thermal injuries, and bite marks, could raise suspicion for abuse. Any bruise without a plausible explanation or a skeletal injury in an infant who is not yet cruising can raise suspicion for abuse.[68] Bruises are common on young ambulatory children, with the most common sites being the anterior tibia or knee, forehead, scalp, and upper leg (ie, anterior surfaces and bony prominences). It is far less common for children to have bruising over posterior surfaces, the chest, the face (except for forehead), the buttocks, or hands.[68,69] Bruising in these areas as well as protected areas, such as the abdomen, genitalia, and ears, in infants and toddlers, although still nonspecific, is suspicious for inflicted trauma.[68-70] Patterned bruises might suggest a device or implement was used to cause the injury. Children struck with linear objects (eg, rods, rulers, belts) may present with linear configured scars. Likewise, flexible implements that are doubled over (eg, ropes, cords, chains) can leave a loop-configured bruise, abrasion, or scar at the site of contact. Slap marks may appear as a negative image such that an outline of the handprint is created on the skin as a result of blood extravasation from vessels into the surrounding interstitial space. Binding devices (eg, wires, ropes, cords) may manifest as circumferentially configured bruises, lacerations, or abrasions involving the neck, wrists, ankles, or oral

commissure. The combined presence of patterned cutaneous or skeletal injury appearing over unusual locations (eg, posterior surfaces, soft tissues, genitalia) may indicate additional inquiry or investigation to establish or allay suspicions of possible physical abuse and/or an underlying medical condition.[71,72] Similarly, any abnormality noted on physical examination of the genitals or anal area that is consistent with trauma may indicate additional inquiry to allay suspicion for possible sexual abuse.[73] However, in all states, suspected child abuse or neglect requires the filing of a mandated report with the state child protective services agency. All health care professionals need to become familiar with the specific reporting laws governing their state and know what exactly to report.

When a mandatory report to child protective services is necessary, health care professionals can engage the families in this process with a transparent and caring direct approach. To set the stage for a transparent interaction up front, a health care professional can discuss all of the following: the risks to and effects on children related to parental substance abuse, the requirements for mandated reporting to child protective services, the resources and services available to the family, and how child welfare can be a support to the family.

SUGGESTED PROFICIENCIES FOR PEDIATRICIANS INVOLVED IN THE CARE OF CHILDREN AND ADOLESCENTS OF FAMILIES AFFECTED BY SUBSTANCE USE

In 1999, Adger et al[74] defined potential levels of proficiencies for pediatricians that varied depending on their experience with substance use treatment. For the purpose of this report, those recommendations are updated and supplemented on the basis of more recent literature focusing on a reasonable level

of proficiency for a primary care provider who is not primarily managing substance use. Additional proficiencies are suggested (Table 4) for health care providers who accept responsibility for prevention, assessment, intervention, and coordination of care and those who accept responsibility for long-term treatment of children and adolescents in families affected by substance use.

Level 1 is a basic understanding of the biology of addiction, including recognition that drug and alcohol addiction are chronic and relapsing neurologic disorders that result from various drug effects on the brain's reward circuitries and neurotransmitter systems.[76] Chronic drug exposure may ultimately impair the function of brain regions involved with motivation and self-control.[76] Awareness of the medical, psychiatric, and behavioral signs and symptoms of substance use may assist health care providers in identifying affected families.[74]

Substance use screening that is age, sex, and culturally appropriate can be included in routine pediatric health maintenance care.[75] By using motivational interviewing techniques (asking screening questions, developing discrepancy, expressing empathy, avoiding argumentation, rolling with resistance, and supporting patient self-efficacy), a provider can assist families in identifying problems substance use can cause and reasons a person may want to quit or cut back.[75] Substance use screening could include review of the mother's prenatal medical information and screening by history and, when indicated, urine toxicologic testing in the newborn period before hospital discharge. It is helpful for the pediatrician to understand the interpretation of positive urine drug screens in the mother and infant. In addition, it is helpful for pediatricians to provide brief interventions to adolescent patients with positive screens for substance use.[75,77,78] Be able to direct families to community, regional, or state resources available for children and adolescents in families with substance use. Discussing identified concerns with the family and offering information, support, and follow-up are components of quality pediatric care.[74] It is important for pediatricians to develop respectful, compassionate approaches regardless of condition, ethnicity, age, or sexual orientation.[75]

Because health care providers are mandated reporters, they should understand obligatory child abuse reporting laws in their states and should know how to make a report to the responsible agency that investigates cases of alleged child abuse or neglect in their jurisdiction.[73]

COLLABORATING WITH OTHER PROVIDERS

Using a multidisciplinary approach, providers can do much to protect drug-endangered children when they work together across specialties and disciplines. It is important for the various professionals who have the opportunity to recognize a child at risk to understand their role in protecting and providing services to that child and the role of other professionals who may be involved with the same family. Reaching outside the silos of one's profession in a collaborative fashion greatly increases the chance for more informed decision-making regarding families affected by parental substance use.

SUMMARY

Substance use is a major public health concern in the United States, and substance use disorders are common. Pediatricians are likely to encounter families affected by parental substance use. Pediatricians are encouraged to screen parents for substance use,

TABLE 4 Suggested Proficiencies for Pediatricians

Level 1: For all health professionals with clinical responsibility for the care of children and adolescents:
  Be aware of the medical, psychiatric, and behavioral syndromes and symptoms with which children and adolescents in families with substance use present and of the potential benefit to both the child and the family of timely and early intervention.
  Be familiar with and able to direct families to community, regional, and state resources available for children and adolescents in families with substance use.
  As part of the general health assessment of children and adolescents, health professionals include appropriate screening for family history and current use of alcohol and other drugs by parents.
  Use motivational interviewing techniques (asking screening questions, developing discrepancy, expressing empathy, avoiding argumentation, rolling with resistance, and supporting patient self-efficacy), assist families in identifying problems substance use can cause and reasons a person may want to quit or cut back.[75]
  Assist parents who screen positive and identify treatment options.
  Offer information, support, and follow-up for parents who screen positive.
  Understand state mandatory child abuse reporting laws and know how to make a report to the responsible investigating agency.
Level II: In addition to Level I proficiencies, health care providers accepting responsibility for prevention, assessment, intervention, and coordination of care of children and adolescents in families with substance use may:
  Apprise the family of the nature of SUDs and their effects on all family members and strategies for achieving optimal health and recovery.
  Recognize and treat, or refer, all associated health problems in the child.
  Evaluate resources (physical health, economic, interpersonal, and social) to the degree necessary to formulate an initial management plan.
  Determine the need to involve extended family and other support people in the initial management plan.
  Develop a long-term management plan in consideration of the above standards and with the child's or adolescent's participation.
Level III: In addition to Level I and II proficiencies, the health care provider with additional training, who accepts responsibility for long-term treatment of children and adolescents in families with substance use, may:
  Acquire knowledge, by training or experience, in the medical and behavioral treatment of children in families affected by substance use.
  Throughout the course of health care treatment, continually monitor and treat, or refer for care, any health needs or psychiatric or behavioral disturbances of the child or adolescent.
  Acquire knowledge, by training or experience, of the recovery process and gain an understanding of how to establish and evaluate screening, brief intervention, and referral to treatment systems in practice.[75]
  Request consultation as needed.
  Be available to the child or adolescent and the family, as needed, for ongoing care and support.

Adapted with permission from Adger et al (1999).[74]

and for parents who screen positive, discuss options for access to treatment from their primary care physician or an appropriate specialist; be alert for signs of child abuse or neglect in children and families affected by substance use; monitor children for developmental delays and other academic difficulties; and be familiar with mandatory reporting requirements for suspected child abuse and neglect.

Government Web Sites

National Institute on Drug Abuse: www.drugabuse.gov

National Institute on Alcohol Abuse and Alcoholism: www.niaaa.nih.gov

Substance Abuse and Mental Health Services Administration: www.samhsa.gov

Massachusetts Department of Health and Human Services: www.mass.gov/eohhs/gov/departments/dcf/child-abuse-neglect

Child Welfare Information Gateway: www.childwelfare.gov

Drug Endangered Children: www.whitehouse.gov/ondcp/dec-info

National Web Sites

Monitoring the Future: www.monitoringthefuture.org

Youth Risk Behavior Surveillance: www.cdc.gov/HealthyYouth/yrbs

National Survey on Drug Use and Health: www.samhsa.gov/data/population-data-nsduh

National Resource Center for In-Home Services, *In-Home Programs for Drug Affected Families*: https://nrcihs-stage.icfwebservices.com/sites/default/files/drugaffectedmemo.pdf

Children and Family Futures: www.cffutures.org

National Alliance for Drug Endangered Children: www.nationaldec.org

National Association for Children of Alcoholics: www.nacoa.org

Bright Futures: brightfutures.aap.org

Street Drug Name Web Sites

www.drug-slang.com

www.streetlightpublications.net/misc/ondcp.htm

www.urban75.com/Drugs/drugterm.html

Office Safety Web Sites

Occupational Safety and Health Administration (OSHA): www.osha.gov

Treatment Locations

A searchable directory of 12 000 facilities with treatment programs for drug and alcohol abuse throughout the United States: http://findtreatment.samhsa.gov

LEAD AUTHORS

Vincent C. Smith, MD, MPH, FAAP
Celeste R. Wilson, MD, FAAP

COMMITTEE ON SUBSTANCE USE AND PREVENTION, 2015–2016

Sheryl A. Ryan, MD, FAAP, Chairperson
Pamela K. Gonzalez, MD, MS, FAAP
Stephen W. Patrick, MD, MPH, MS, FAAP
Joanna Quigley, MD, FAAP
Lorena Siqueira, MD, MSPH, FAAP
Leslie R. Walker, MD, FAAP

FORMER COMMITTEE MEMBER

Vincent C. Smith, MD, MPH, FAAP

LIAISONS

Vivian B. Faden, PhD – *National Institute of Alcohol Abuse and Alcoholism*
Gregory Tau, MD, PhD – *American Academy of Child and Adolescent Psychiatry*

STAFF

Renee Jarrett, MPH

ABBREVIATIONS

NIDA: National Institute on Drug Abuse
SUD: substance use disorder

REFERENCES

1. National Alliance for Drug Endangered Children. The problem. Available at: www.nationaldec.org/theproblem.html. Accessed November 3, 2015
2. Jessepe L. Abuse and neglect: the toxic lives of drug endangered children. *Indian Country Today Media Network*. July 21, 2014. Available at: http://indiancountrytodaymedianetwork.com. Accessed November 3, 2015
3. Callaghan T, Crimmins J, Schweitzer RD. Children of substance-using mothers: child health engagement and child protection outcomes. *J Paediatr Child Health*. 2011;47(4):223–227
4. Johnson JL, Leff M. Children of substance abusers: overview of research findings. *Pediatrics*. 1999;103(5 pt 2):1085–1099
5. Bailey JA, Hill KG, Oesterle S, Hawkins JD. Linking substance use and problem behavior across three generations. *J Abnorm Child Psychol*. 2006;34(3):263–292
6. Dore MM, Doris JM, Wright P. Identifying substance abuse in maltreating families: a child welfare challenge. *Child Abuse Negl*. 1995;19(5):531–543
7. Kulig JW; American Academy of Pediatrics Committee on Substance Abuse. Tobacco, alcohol, and other drugs: the role of the pediatrician in prevention, identification, and management of substance abuse. *Pediatrics*. 2005;115(3):816–821
8. Substance Abuse and Mental Health Services Administration. *Results From the 2013 National Survey on Drug Use and Health: Summary of National Findings. NSDUH Series H-48. HHS Publication No. (SMA) 14-4863.* Rockville, MD: Substance Abuse and Mental Health Services Administration; 2014
9. Miller TR, Hendrie D. *Substance Abuse Prevention Dollars and Cents: A Cost–Benefit Analysis*. Rockville, MD: US Department of Health and Human Services, Substance Abuse and Mental Health Services Administration, Center for Substance Abuse Prevention; 2009
10. Patrick SW, Davis MM, Lehmann CU, Cooper WO. Increasing incidence and geographic distribution of neonatal abstinence syndrome: United States 2009 to 2012 [published correction appears in *J Perinatol*. 2015;35(8):667]. *J Perinatol*. 2015;35(8):650–655
11. Behnke M, Smith VC; Committee on Substance Abuse; Committee on Fetus and Newborn. Prenatal substance abuse: short- and long-term effects on the exposed fetus. *Pediatrics*. 2013;131(3). Available at: www.pediatrics.org/cgi/content/full/131/3/e1009
12. Patrick SW, Dudley J, Martin PR, et al. Prescription opioid epidemic and infant outcomes. *Pediatrics*. 2015;135(5):842–850
13. Fraser JJ Jr, McAbee GN; American Academy of Pediatrics Committee on Medical Liability. Dealing with the parent whose judgment is impaired by alcohol or drugs: legal and ethical considerations. *Pediatrics*. 2004;114(3):869–873
14. Substance Abuse and Mental Health Services Administration, Office of Applied Studies. *The NSDUH Report: Children Living With Substance-Depending or Substance-Abusing Parents: 2002–2007*. Rockville, MD: Substance Abuse and Mental Health Services Administration; 2009
15. Hoyme HE, May PA, Kalberg WO, et al. A practical clinical approach to diagnosis of fetal alcohol spectrum disorders: clarification of the 1996 Institute of Medicine criteria. *Pediatrics*. 2005;115(1):39–47
16. Tortoriello G, Morris CV, Alpar A, et al. Miswiring the brain: Δ9-tetrahydrocannabinol disrupts

cortical development by inducing an SCG10/stathmin-2 degradation pathway. *EMBO J.* 2014;33(7):668–685

17. Williams JF, Smith VC; Committee on Substance Abuse. Fetal alcohol spectrum disorders. *Pediatrics.* 2015;136(5). Available at: www.pediatrics.org/cgi/content/full/136/5/e1395

18. Hsi A. Care of pregnant and parenting women and their children affected by substance use disorders: designing a care system around the family medical home. *Webinar presented at: Indian Health Services Clinical Rounds in collaboration with the American Academy of Pediatrics Committee on Native American Child Health, and the Indian Health Service Clinical Support Center;* December 11, 2014; Albuquerque, NM. Available at: http://ihs.adobeconnect.com/p4cq7qv69wy. Accessed August 12, 2015

19. Jaques SC, Kingsbury A, Henshcke P, et al. Cannabis, the pregnant woman and her child: weeding out the myths. *J Perinatol.* 2014;34(6):417–424

20. Konijnenberg C, Melinder A. Prenatal exposure to methadone and buprenorphine: a review of the potential effects on cognitive development. *Child Neuropsychol.* 2011;17(5):495–519

21. Altshuler SJ, Cleverly-Thomas A. What do we know about drug-endangered children when they are first placed into care? *Child Welfare.* 2011;90(3):45–68

22. Dube SR, Anda RF, Felitti VJ, Croft JB, Edwards VJ, Giles WH. Growing up with parental alcohol abuse: exposure to childhood abuse, neglect, and household dysfunction. *Child Abuse Negl.* 2001;25(12):1627–1640

23. Wolin SJ, Bennett LA, Noonan DL. Family rituals and the recurrence of alcoholism over generations. *Am J Psychiatry.* 1979;136(4B):589–593

24. Wolin SJ, Bennett LA, Noonan DL, Teitelbaum MA. Disrupted family rituals; a factor in the intergenerational transmission of alcoholism. *J Stud Alcohol.* 1980;41(3):199–214

25. Patterson GR, Stouthamer-Loeber M. The correlation of family management practices and delinquency. *Child Dev.* 1984;55(4):1299–1307

26. Testa M, Kubiak A, Quigley BM, et al. Husband and wife alcohol use as independent or interactive predictors of intimate partner violence. *J Stud Alcohol Drugs.* 2012;73(2):268–276

27. Woodin EM, Caldeira V, Sotskova A, Galaugher T, Lu M. Harmful alcohol use as a predictor of intimate partner violence during the transition to parenthood: interdependent and interactive effects. *Addict Behav.* 2014;39(12):1890–1897

28. Freisthler B, Gruenewald PJ. Where the individual meets the ecological: a study of parent drinking patterns, alcohol outlets, and child physical abuse. *Alcohol Clin Exp Res.* 2013;37(6):993–1000

29. Freisthler B. Alcohol use, drinking venue utilization, and child physical abuse: results from a pilot study. *J Fam Violence.* 2011;26(3):185–193

30. Freisthler B, Gruenewald PJ, Ring L, LaScala EA. An ecological assessment of the population and environmental correlates of childhood accident, assault, and child abuse injuries. *Alcohol Clin Exp Res.* 2008;32(11):1969–1975

31. Manly JT, Oshri A, Lynch M, Herzog M, Wortel S. Child neglect and the development of externalizing behavior problems: associations with maternal drug dependence and neighborhood crime. *Child Maltreat.* 2013;18(1):17–29

32. McGlade A, Ware R, Crawford M. Child protection outcomes for infants of substance-using mothers: a matched-cohort study. *Pediatrics.* 2009;124(1):285–293

33. Chasnoff IJ, Telford E, Wells AM, King L. Mental health disorders among children within child welfare who have prenatal substance exposure: rural vs. urban populations. *Child Welfare.* 2015;94(4):53–70

34. Slesnick N, Feng X, Brakenhoff B, Brigham GS. Parenting under the influence: the effects of opioids, alcohol and cocaine on mother-child interaction. *Addict Behav.* 2014;39(5):897–900

35. Cunningham S, Finlay K. Parental substance use and foster care: evidence from two methamphetamine supply shocks. *Econ Inq.* 2013;51(1):764–782

36. Semidei J, Radel LF, Nolan C. Substance abuse and child welfare: clear linkages and promising responses. *Child Welfare.* 2001;80(2):109–128

37. US Department of Health and Human Services. Blending perspectives and building common ground: a report to Congress on substance abuse and child protection. Washington, DC: US Government Printing Office; 1999. Available at: http://aspe.hhs.gov/execsum/blending-perspectives-and-building-common-ground. Accessed October 22, 2015

38. Seay K. How many families in child welfare services are affected by parental substance use disorders? A common question that remains unanswered. *Child Welfare.* 2015;94(4):19–51

39. Child Welfare Information Gateway. Parental substance use and the child welfare system. Washington, DC: US Department of Health and Human Services, Children's Bureau; 2014. Available at: https://www.childwelfare.gov/pubPDFs/parentalsubabuse.pdf. Accessed November 30, 2015

40. Street K, Whitlingum G, Gibson P, Cairns P, Ellis M. Is adequate parenting compatible with maternal drug use? A 5-year follow-up. *Child Care Health Dev.* 2008;34(2):204–206

41. US Department of Health and Human Services, Administration for Children and Families, Administration on Children, Youth and Families, Children's Bureau. Child maltreatment 2012. 2013. Available at: www.acf.hhs.gov/programs/cb/research-data-technology/statistics-research/child-maltreatment. Accessed August 12, 2015

42. Arria AM, Mericle AA, Meyers K, Winters KC. Parental substance use impairment, parenting and substance use disorder risk. *J Subst Abuse Treat.* 2012;43(1):114–122

43. Bijur PE, Kurzon M, Overpeck MD, Scheidt PC. Parental alcohol use,

problem drinking, and children's injuries. *JAMA*. 1992;267(23):3166–3171

44. Ammerman RT, Kolko DJ, Kirisci L, Blackson TC, Dawes MA. Child abuse potential in parents with histories of substance use disorder. *Child Abuse Negl*. 1999;23(12):1225–1238

45. Walsh C, MacMillan HL, Jamieson E. The relationship between parental substance abuse and child maltreatment: findings from the Ontario Health Supplement. *Child Abuse Negl*. 2003;27(12):1409–1425

46. Berger LM. Income, family characteristics, and physical violence toward children. *Child Abuse Negl*. 2005;29(2):107–133

47. Damashek A, Williams NA, Sher K, Peterson L. Relation of caregiver alcohol use to unintentional childhood injury. *J Pediatr Psychol*. 2009;34(4):344–353

48. Hildyard KL, Wolfe DA. Child neglect: developmental issues and outcomes. *Child Abuse Negl*. 2002;26(6-7):679–695

49. Kendler KS, Gardner CO, Edwards A, et al. Dimensions of parental alcohol use/ problems and offspring temperament, externalizing behaviors, and alcohol use/problems. *Alcohol Clin Exp Res*. 2013;37(12):2118–2127

50. Anda RF, Whitfield CL, Felitti VJ, et al. Adverse childhood experiences, alcoholic parents, and later risk of alcoholism and depression. *Psychiatr Serv*. 2002;53(8):1001–1009

51. Felitti VJ, Anda RF, Nordenberg D, et al. Relationship of childhood abuse and household dysfunction to many of the leading causes of death in adults. The Adverse Childhood Experiences (ACE) Study. *Am J Prev Med*. 1998;14(4):245–258

52. Shonkoff JP, Garner AS; Committee on Psychosocial Aspects of Child and Family Health; Committee on Early Childhood, Adoption, and Dependent Care; Section on Developmental and Behavioral Pediatrics. The lifelong effects of early childhood adversity and toxic stress. *Pediatrics*. 2012;129(1). Available at: www.pediatrics.org/cgi/content/full/129/1/e232

53. Torvik FA, Rognmo K, Ask H, Røysamb E, Tambs K. Parental alcohol use and adolescent school adjustment in the general population: results from the HUNT study. *BMC Public Health*. 2011;11:706

54. Duggan AK, Adger H Jr, McDonald EM, Stokes EJ, Moore R. Detection of alcoholism in hospitalized children and their families. *Am J Dis Child*. 1991;145(6):613–617

55. Yu J. The association between parental alcohol-related behaviors and children's drinking. *Drug Alcohol Depend*. 2003;69(3):253–262

56. Lieb R, Merikangas KR, Höfler M, Pfister H, Isensee B, Wittchen HU. Parental alcohol use disorders and alcohol use and disorders in offspring: a community study. *Psychol Med*. 2002;32(1):63–78

57. Dube SR, Felitti VJ, Dong M, Giles WH, Anda RF. The impact of adverse childhood experiences on health problems: evidence from four birth cohorts dating back to 1900. *Prev Med*. 2003;37(3):268–277

58. Sørensen HJ, Manzardo AM, Knop J, et al. The contribution of parental alcohol use disorders and other psychiatric illness to the risk of alcohol use disorders in the offspring. *Alcohol Clin Exp Res*. 2011;35(7):1315–1320

59. Sachs HC; Committee on Drugs. The transfer of drugs and therapeutics into human breast milk: an update on selected topics. *Pediatrics*. 2013;132(3). Available at: www.pediatrics.org/cgi/content/full/132/3/e796

60. Hagan JF, Shaw JS, Duncan P, eds. *Bright Futures: Guidelines for Health Supervision of Infants, Children, and Adolescents*. 3rd ed. Elk Grove Village, IL: American Academy of Pediatrics; 2008

61. Bricker D, Squires J. *Ages & Stages Questionnaires*. 3rd ed. Baltimore, MD: Paul H. Brookes; 2009

62. Smith PC, Schmidt SM, Allensworth-Davies D, Saitz R. Primary care validation of a single-question alcohol screening test. *J Gen Intern Med*. 2009;24(7):783–788

63. National Institute on Drug Abuse. Resource guide: screening for drug use in general medical settings. Available at: www.drugabuse. gov/publications/resource-guide-screening-drug-use-in-general-medical-settings/nida-quick-screen. Accessed November 3, 2015

64. Saunders JB, Aasland OG, Babor TF, de la Fuente JR, Grant M. Development of the Alcohol Use Disorders Identification Test (AUDIT): WHO Collaborative Project on Early Detection of Persons With Harmful Alcohol Consumption--II. *Addiction*. 1993;88(6):791–804

65. Bush K, Kivlahan DR, McDonell MB, Fihn SD, Bradley KA. The AUDIT alcohol consumption questions (AUDIT-C): an effective brief screening test for problem drinking. Ambulatory Care Quality Improvement Project (ACQUIP). Alcohol Use Disorders Identification Test. *Arch Intern Med*. 1998;158(16):1789–1795

66. Skinner HA. Assessment of substance abuse: Drug Abuse Screening Test (DAST). Encyclopedia of drugs, alcohol, and addictive behavior. 2001. Available at: www.encyclopedia.com/doc/1G2-3403100068.html. Accessed August 13, 2015

67. Wilson CR, Harris SK, Sherritt L, et al. Parental alcohol screening in pediatric practices. *Pediatrics*. 2008;122(5). Available at: www.pediatrics.org/cgi/content/full/122/5/e1022

68. Sugar NF, Taylor JA, Feldman KW; Puget Sound Pediatric Research Network. Bruises in infants and toddlers: those who don't cruise rarely bruise. *Arch Pediatr Adolesc Med*. 1999;153(4):399–403

69. Kemp AM, Dunstan F, Nuttall D, Hamilton M, Collins P, Maguire S. Patterns of bruising in preschool children: a longitudinal study. *Arch Dis Child*. 2015;100(5):426–431

70. Pierce MC, Kaczor K, Aldridge S, O'Flynn J, Lorenz DJ. Bruising characteristics discriminating physical child abuse from accidental trauma. *Pediatrics*. 2010;125(1):67–74

71. Christian CW; Committee on Child Abuse and Neglect, American Academy of Pediatrics. The evaluation of suspected child physical abuse. *Pediatrics*. 2015;135(5). Available at: www.pediatrics.org/cgi/content/full/135/2/e1337

72. Maguire S, Mann MK, Sibert J, Kemp A. Are there patterns of bruising in childhood which are diagnostic or suggestive of abuse? A systematic review. *Arch Dis Child*. 2005;90(2):182–186

73. Jenny C, Crawford-Jakubiak JE; Committee on Child Abuse and Neglect; American Academy of Pediatrics. The evaluation of children in the primary care setting when sexual abuse is suspected. *Pediatrics*. 2013;132(2). Available at: www.pediatrics.org/cgi/content/full/132/2/e558

74. Adger H Jr, Macdonald DI, Wenger S. Core competencies for involvement of health care providers in the care of children and adolescents in families affected by substance abuse. *Pediatrics*. 1999;103(5 pt 2):1083–1084

75. Seale JP, Shellenberger S, Clark DC. Providing competency-based family medicine residency training in substance abuse in the new millennium: a model curriculum. *BMC Med Educ*. 2010;10:33

76. Wood E, Samet JH, Volkow ND. Physician education in addiction medicine. *JAMA*. 2013;310(16):1673–1674

77. Jackson AH, Alford DP, Dubé CE, Saitz R. Internal medicine residency training for unhealthy alcohol and other drug use: recommendations for curriculum design. *BMC Med Educ*. 2010;10:22

78. American Academy of Pediatrics, Committee on Substance Use and Prevention. Substance use screening, brief intervention, and referral to treatment. *Pediatrics*. 2016;138(1):e20161210

Fathers' Roles in the Care and Development of Their Children: The Role of Pediatricians

- *Clinical Report*

CLINICAL REPORT Guidance for the Clinician in Rendering Pediatric Care

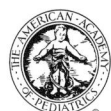

American Academy
of Pediatrics

DEDICATED TO THE HEALTH OF ALL CHILDREN™

Fathers' Roles in the Care and Development of Their Children: The Role of Pediatricians

Michael Yogman, MD, Craig F. Garfield, MD, COMMITTEE ON PSYCHOSOCIAL ASPECTS OF CHILD AND FAMILY HEALTH

abstract

Fathers' involvement in and influence on the health and development of their children have increased in a myriad of ways in the past 10 years and have been widely studied. The role of pediatricians in working with fathers has correspondingly increased in importance. This report reviews new studies of the epidemiology of father involvement, including nonresidential as well as residential fathers. The effects of father involvement on child outcomes are discussed within each phase of a child's development. Particular emphasis is placed on (1) fathers' involvement across childhood ages and (2) the influence of fathers' physical and mental health on their children. Implications and advice for all child health providers to encourage and support father involvement are outlined.

DOI: 10.1542/peds.2016-1128

PEDIATRICS (ISSN Numbers: Print, 0031-4005; Online, 1098-4275).

Copyright © 2016 by the American Academy of Pediatrics

FINANCIAL DISCLOSURE: The authors have indicated they do not have a financial relationship relevant to this article to disclose.

FUNDING: No external funding.

POTENTIAL CONFLICT OF INTEREST: The authors have indicated they have no potential conflicts of interest to disclose.

To cite: Yogman M, Garfield CF, AAP the COMMITTEE ON PSYCHOSOCIAL ASPECTS OF CHILD, HEALTH F. Fathers' Roles in the Care and Development of Their Children: The Role of Pediatricians. *Pediatrics.* 2016;138(1):e20161128

INTRODUCTION

In the decade that followed since the original clinical report on the father's role was published by the American Academy of Pediatrics in May 2004,[1] there has been a surge of attention and research on fathers and their role in the care and development of their children. Three areas (academic study, policy initiatives, and socioeconomic forces) have fueled this increase. First, high-quality studies, both qualitative and quantitative, have improved the conceptualization and understanding of the myriad of ways fathers are involved in and influence the health of their children, regardless of marital status. Of key import are several national, father-inclusive longitudinal studies in families, such as the Fragile Families and Child Wellbeing Study, the Early Childhood Longitudinal Study of Birth and Kindergarten, and Early Head Start, which for the first time allow for the reporting of nationally representative findings relating father involvement and child and family well-being over time.

In the public policy arena, shifts have occurred away from "deadbeat dads" and what men are not doing for their families to a focus on more supportive perspectives on positive involvement[2] and the unique ways fathers contribute to families and children. Another major policy development in the past decade is the adoption by several states (California, New Jersey, and Rhode Island) of paid family leave laws that were conceived as support for fathers' bonding and attachment with their newborn infants or young children.[3] In 2015, a Massachusetts law took effect that entitles male employees to take 8 weeks of unpaid leave for the birth or adoption of a child if they work for a company with at least 6 employees.[4] Despite this opportunity, men still face negative career effects if they take family leave time.[5]

Two major socioeconomic forces, the growth in women's educational achievement and the Great Recession of 2008, with its particularly severe impact on paternal employment, have led to more fathers having the opportunities to contribute at home or to become stay-at-home dads in families in which mothers are able to sustain family income. These influences, paired with the dramatic cross-cultural growth in academia, lay print, social media, television, and electronic publications focusing on fathers, have stimulated public discussion around fathers and their roles in families (eg, http://www.citydadsgroup.com/, https://www.facebook.com/groups/dadbloggers/, http://www.meetup.com/ChicagoDadsGroup/, https://www.thefatherhoodproject.org).[6-9]

The literature from the past decade and the increasing number of peer-reviewed studies published in major pediatric and medical journals focusing specifically on fathers[8,10-16] have painted a more nuanced picture of today's fathers' roles, married or not. Drawing on important contributions from such disciplines as infant mental health, sociology, and psychology, this literature offers a critical assessment of the central and unique role of fathers in the health of their children, their influence on maternal well-being,

and their interactions with the health care system. These studies reported that fathers are present at the birth of their children, frequently attend well-child or acute care visits across childhood, and have unique roles in child health that may differ from those of mothers. The involvement of fathers has important consequences for child well-being, especially with regard to issues of diet/nutrition, exercise, play, and parenting behaviors (eg, reading, discipline).[17] Barriers to health care involvement include systemic issues such as inconvenient office hours and lack of time off from work beyond the newborn period as well as individual issues, most notably employment, relationship quality with the mother and the potential of maternal "gatekeeping," and lack of parenting confidence.[14,17] Although many of these issues affect all parents, especially if they work swing shifts, they are more common barriers for fathers.

The field of pediatrics remains slow to incorporate these findings into practice and into the conceptualization of family-centered care. Although mothers continue to provide the majority of care for the well and sick child, fathers are more involved than ever before.[18] Yet, cultural and structural biases still play a role; pediatricians still see a majority of mothers at clinical encounters and therefore may not have changed their practices to be family-friendly in terms of available hours, comfort in interacting with men, and addressing fathers' unique concerns regarding their children. With few supportive parental leave programs in existence (at best for only 1 parent), fathers typically have to pit their workplace responsibilities against their home responsibilities at a very early stage in their transition to fatherhood. Pediatricians are often the first members of the health care team to engage fathers in their new role during this transition; failure to

make this connection may result in poorer downstream involvement and engagement. Given the changes in the stereotype of the father's exclusive role as breadwinner, child health care providers have an opportunity to have an even greater influence on child and family outcomes by supporting fathers and enhancing their involvement.[19]

The purpose of this report, therefore, is to update data on fathers' roles and to highlight the latest multidisciplinary findings related to fathers, children, and pediatrics. When possible, programs that are particularly innovative in supporting father involvement in children's health are highlighted as examples of approaches to family-friendly pediatric care.

FATHERS BY THE NUMBERS

Defining who is a father must account for the diversity of fathering that occurs. Most children have a father, whether he is currently residing with them or living separately. Some children have a single father or 2 parents who are both fathers. Children in a blended family may have both a biological nonresident father and a stepfather. Some gay men and lesbians have created families in which children have 3 or 4 adults in a parenting role, with 1 or 2 of them being fathers. Some children do not have a male figure involved in raising them (eg, those whose parent is a single mother, by choice or circumstance, and those whose parents are a lesbian couple). As in the previous report,[1] "father" is defined broadly as the male or males identified as most involved in caregiving and committed to the well-being of the child, regardless of living situation, marital status, or biological relation. A father may be a biological, foster, or adoptive father[20]; a stepfather; or a grandfather. He may or may not have legal custody and may be resident or nonresident. Data for many of these subgroups are quite limited and must not be extrapolated to all subgroups. Although parenthood status is usually straightforward, circumstances in which parenthood status and parental rights are unclear may involve complex legal issues, including implications in terms of parental access to the child's protected health information and ability to consent to care. Some states may legislate more restrictive definitions.

The number of fathers in the United States increased from 60.1 million in 2000, to 64.3 million in 2007, to 70.1 million in 2012.[18] The number of single fathers raising children was 1.96 million in 2012, approximately 10% of single parents, an increase of 60% in the past 10 years. Stay-at-home fathers were counted by the Census for the first time in 2003 and totaled 98 000. By 2007, the number of stay-at-home fathers increased by more than 60% to 159 000, and in the 2012 Census the number was 189 000. Fathers represent 3.4% of all stay-at-home parents, and 32% of these men are married to women working full-time. They care for more than 200 000 children full-time and almost 2 million preschoolers part-time. Fathers whose partners work full-time and stay-at-home fathers are 2 groups likely to take their child to the doctor and to be primarily responsible for their child's health care, recreation, and school-related activities. The census numbers may be underestimates, according to a recent Pew Center report that suggested that, in 2010, there were 2.2 million stay-at-home dads. One-quarter of these men were home because they were unemployed, 21% chose to stay home to care for their child (increased from 5% in 1989), and 35% were home because of illness or disability. Half of these fathers were poor, and they were more likely to be older. Low-income minority fathers had great difficulty

finding available jobs. Although most stay-at-home parents are mothers, fathers' share of stay-at-home parenting increased from 10% in 1989 to 16% in 2012.[21–23] Although 1 in 6 fathers are nonresidential, only 1% to 2% of them do not participate at all with their children,[24] sometimes because they meet a new partner and father new children.

FATHERS' TIME SPENT WITH CHILDREN

Researchers have long suggested that a "new fatherhood" is emerging, one that allows for balance between workplace and home responsibilities. Although no state offers a distinct paternity leave, several states have addressed 1 of the major barriers for fathers in taking leave to care for children and family by establishing paid family leave policies. In 1 study in fathers working for Fortune 500 companies, 85% took some time off after the birth of the child, generally for 1 to 2 weeks (unpaid), and reported feeling more stressed about coordinating family-work conflicts than mothers did.[25] Generally speaking, in families, work and time with children often compete with one another, with parents spending more time in the workplace than they are able to spend at home. With the use of time-use diaries such as the American Time Use Survey, the Pew Research on Social and Demographic Trends reported that although mothers continue to do the majority of work at home and with children, fathers have increased their time in both categories over the years. Comparing 1965 with 2011, fathers more than doubled their time spent on housework (4 vs 10 hours/week) and child care (2.5 vs 7 hours/week).[26] Researchers point to this increase as evidence of a subgroup of "new fathers" who appear to preserve time with children, likely by cutting back on, or incorporating their children into, their leisure time, especially on weekends.[27,28]

FATHER INVOLVEMENT AND CHILD OUTCOMES ACROSS THE CHILDHOOD LIFE SPAN

Perinatal and Newborn Period

The father's relationship with his child's health care provider is likely to begin in the early childhood years and can grow over time to a long-term relationship. Early encounters with pediatricians may occur as prenatal visits, visits in the newborn nursery, or any number of the well- or acute-care visits. Fathers have been shown to be involved prenatally by attending health care visits and assisting their pregnant partners; regardless of marital status, the vast majority of fathers are present at their child's birth.[29] Fathers have even been noted to have Couvade syndrome, wherein they experience insomnia, restlessness, and excess weight gain during their partner's pregnancy.[30] Prenatal involvement and residence at birth were the strongest predictors of paternal involvement by the time a child reached 5 years.[31] Father involvement during pregnancy correlated with mothers being 1.5 times more likely to receive first-trimester prenatal care[29] and with reductions in prematurity and infant mortality.[32,33] Among mothers who smoked, father involvement was associated with a smoking reduction of 36% compared with mothers whose partners were not involved.[34] Fathers' mental health/psychological distress during pregnancy has been correlated with adverse childhood emotional problems at 36 months of age. In a study comparing father skin-to-skin care with conventional cot care during the first 2 hours after birth, newborn infants in the father skin-to-skin group cried less, became drowsy sooner, and had less rooting, sucking, and wakefulness.[35] Simple interventions such as bathing demonstrations in the newborn period have been shown to have long-lasting effects on enhancing paternal involvement, as have paternal support groups in a variety of contexts.[16] Fathers can play a critical role in supporting maternal breastfeeding and, conversely, if feeling excluded and competitive, can undermine it. Many birthing hospitals have instituted programming designed for and marketed directly to expectant fathers to offer resources for them as key partners.

During infancy, fathers have been shown to be competent and capable of similar successful interactions with young infants and to have similar psychological experiences as mothers.[16] However, their relationship is not redundant; the father is more likely to be the infant's play partner than the mother, and father's play tends to be more stimulating, vigorous, and arousing for the infant.[16,36] Fathers were equally successful in matching emotions with their children (during social interactions, fathers were able to synchronize arousal rhythms with their infants just as successfully as mothers), but the quality of interactions (especially play) was more intense with fathers.[37,38] These high-intensity interactions with fathers may encourage childrens' exploration and independence, whereas the less-intensive interactions with mothers provide safety and balance.[9,16] Interestingly, it has now been shown in human males that testosterone levels are higher during conception and decrease during child rearing.[39,40] Correlations between fathers' responses to their own versus other 2- to 4-month-olds have been shown between salivary testosterone levels and functional MRI responses in prefrontal and subcortical areas.[41] Changes in paternal oxytocin levels have been correlated with exploratory play, and changes in prolactin levels have been correlated with affective synchrony during fathers' interaction with their 2- to 6-month-olds.[42,43] Paternal plasma and salivary oxytocin levels were uniquely

associated with stimulatory contact but not with affectionate touch as with mothers. Previous contact with infants had a greater impact on fathers compared with mothers.[44] Responses on functional MRI in mothers and fathers in response to seeing their own infants on video are also different: mothers show more activation in the amygdala but fathers show more activation in the superior temporal sulcus (temporoparietal and frontal regions), a key structure of the mentalizing network.[45]

Fathers' involvement during the newborn period is strongly associated with marital status. Forty percent of births are to unmarried couples, which has been accompanied by an increase in the number of nonresident fathers.[46] Although many unmarried couples are cohabitating at the time of the child's birth, recent studies showed that 63% of unmarried fathers are no longer living with the mother and their child after 5 years.[47] These nonresident fathers have less contact and involvement with their children than do resident fathers.[48] Several factors influence the level of involvement of nonresident fathers with their children, including age, level of education, employment status, geographical distance from their child, mental health status, and social support.[48–50] The relationship with the mother, including the maintenance of a coparenting relationship, is also a major indicator of nonresident father involvement.[47,51] Although nonresident father involvement has traditionally been thought to decrease over time, recent work shows that involvement can follow several different trajectories, including remaining stable and, in some cases, even increasing.[48] Increasing ongoing nonresident father involvement in a child's life can play an important role in child and adolescent well-being, even assuming traditional father responsibilities.[52] Recent commentaries have disputed

the inaccurate stereotype that black fathers desert their offspring; in fact, most black fathers in the United States live with their child (2.3 million live with their child and 1.7 million do not). The fact that 72% of black children are parented by single women reflects several influences, including the following: (1) 600 000 of the 1.5 million black men not living with their child are incarcerated, (2) many black couples live together but do not marry, and (3) some men have children with more than 1 woman.[53]

Given the increase in both nonmarital childbirths and nonresident father involvement, it is especially important to note that nontraditional forms of positive father involvement have been associated with children's academic achievement, emotional well-being, and behavioral adjustment.[54] Fostering father involvement in fragile single-parent families may reduce behavioral problems.[55] However, having a father move out of the house by 3 years of age was associated with infant temperament (ie, irregular schedule, difficult infant behavior), and it is not clear which is the precipitating factor.[56] Nonmarital father involvement drops sharply after the parents' relationship ends, especially when they enter subsequent relationships and have children with new partners.[57] Policy makers advocating for programs to strengthen low-income families have specifically called for better research on programs to enhance paternal involvement.[58]

Early Childhood

Father involvement in the early childhood years is associated with positive child developmental and psychological outcomes over time, although most studies do not differentiate the benefits of having 2 parents from a specifically male presence as the second parent. For example, at 3 years of age, father-child communication was a significant and unique predictor of advanced language development in the child but mother-child communication was not.[59] Despite this finding, infants from birth to 7 months of age were exposed to significantly more language from mothers compared with fathers.[60] Mothers tailor word choice to the child's known vocabulary, whereas fathers are more likely to introduce new words.[9] Child health care providers have an opportunity to encourage fathers to speak to their infants more.

In a prospective study, when fathers were more involved (caring, playing, communicating) in infancy, children had decreased mental health symptomatology at 9 years of age.[61] Fathers engaged in more roughhouse play, and their involvement in play with preschoolers predicted decreased externalizing and internalizing behavior problems and enhanced social competence.[62] In a nationally representative household sample, positive father involvement was inversely associated with child behavior trajectories, such that more involvement was accompanied by less child maladaptive behavior; furthermore, the influence of maternal depressive symptoms on child problem behaviors varied by the level of the father's positive involvement.[63] This information suggests that the influence of involved fathers may compensate for the negative influence of maternal depression (eg, reduced responsiveness to a child's socioemotional needs), thereby reducing the risk of child problem behaviors and development.

Definitions of masculinity are in flux, from an emphasis on toughness to an emphasis on tenderness; racial/ethnic differences still persist in this domain. In 1 study, white fathers were more demonstrative with children younger than 13 years than were black fathers, hugging their children more and telling them they

loved them.[64] Intervention programs with 8- to 12-year-old black boys that enhanced the parenting skills of nonresidential fathers were associated with reduced aggressive behavior of the boys.[65]

Adolescence

During adolescence, several recent national longitudinal studies have shown that father involvement is associated with a decrease in the likelihood of adolescent risk behaviors (even more strongly for boys)[66,67] and predicts less adolescent depressive symptoms for both genders.[68] A recent meta-analysis of longitudinal studies of father involvement showed that father engagement was correlated with enhanced cognitive development, reduced behavioral problems in male adolescents, decreased psychological problems in female adolescents, and decreased delinquency and economic disadvantage in families of low socioeconomic status.[8] Early father involvement with daughters has been associated with a decreased risk of early puberty, decreased early sexual experiences, and decreased teen pregnancy.[9,69] Extrapolating from animal studies, exposure to fathers' pheromones may slow female pubertal development.[9] Adolescents whose nonresident fathers are involved have been shown to be less likely to begin smoking regularly.[70] In general, increased father involvement has been associated with improved cognitive development, social responsiveness, independence, and gender role development, particularly in females.[16] Fathers can now be seen to have a role expanded far beyond that of stereotypic disciplinarian, breadwinner, and masculine role model to that of care provider, companion, teacher, role model for parenting, and supportive spouse. The unique and complementary role of fathers is beginning to be understood. More

research is needed on fathers' role in promoting resiliency.

FATHER INVOLVEMENT WITH CHILDREN WITH SPECIAL HEALTH CARE NEEDS

Mothers are typically the primary caregivers when children have physical illness or developmental delay, and medical information passed on to the father may be interpreted or selected by the mother. Over time, the mother becomes the conduit to the health care provider and indirectly in charge of the child's care. This indirect communication can be frustrating for the father and can affect the parental relationship. Fathers of children with special health care needs have been found to be highly involved in the care of their children. Fathers have been shown to increase involvement with children with chronic illnesses, often advocating for their children's medical needs even if it means positioning themselves in the health care system as "unpopular" family members.[71,72] Although mothers are generally more involved with their children's direct care, a father's participation in care has been linked to higher adherence to treatment, better child psychological adjustment, and improved health status compared with families with nonparticipating fathers.[73] Fathers of children with cancer and of infants recovering from cardiac surgery have been found, not surprisingly, to experience intense emotional reactions to their child's health and treatment.[74,75] Intervention programs with parents of developmentally delayed children have far better child outcomes when fathers participate in the parent training along with mothers.[76] Among preterm infants in the NICU (especially those with low-income black fathers), increased paternal involvement was associated with improved cognitive outcome at 3 years of age, even after adjusting for family income, neonatal health, and paternal age.[77,78] The population of children with special health care needs has not been well studied and needs better research.

IMPROVED UNDERSTANDING OF OTHER GROUPS OF FATHERS

With the growing understanding of the role of fathers, there has been an appreciation of the context within which fathering occurs. Although there are many universalities for fathers in terms of how men see their roles in caring for their children, the diversity of cultural and social norms and expectations is wide. As physicians who care for children from many backgrounds, pediatricians need to be aware of the issues relevant to these particular groups.

An emerging sociodemographic trend currently under study is the increasingly common family phenomenon in which parents have biological children with multiple partners (multipartner fertility). Almost 1 in 5 fathers between the ages of 15 and 44 years have children with more than 1 partner.[79] The prevalence of births with multiple partners varies significantly with demographics, with a higher rate of multipartner fertility among racial and ethnic minorities and those who are economically disadvantaged.[79,80] Age at first sexual experience, age at birth of the first child, and relationship status of partners are also indicators of multipartner fertility.[80,81] Men whose first children are born outside of marriage are 3 times as likely to experience multipartner fertility than are men who are married to the mother of their first child at the time of birth.[79] Children are affected by their fathers' multipartner fertility, because it leads to complex family structures and diminished resources for each child.[82,83] Children with nonresident fathers with multipartner fertility experience less overall parent-child interaction than children

with nonresident fathers without multipartner fertility.[84] Nonresident fathers also provide less monetary support for their children when they have a child with a new partner.[83] A link exists between multipartner fertility and depression in fathers, although the causal direction of this association is unclear.[85]

A variety of other groups of fathers are benefiting from the growth in fathering research. For example, in military families, not only have more fathers been deployed overseas in the past 10 years[86,87] but more mothers have also been deployed, leaving fathers to be the single parents of children while their mothers are away. Researchers who have described the sources of support for deployed fathers are currently testing a smartphone app designed to bolster support while a parent is serving overseas.[88]

Another population that is the subject of increased study is black fathers. Although black fathers have been noted to be less likely to marry and more likely to live apart from their children than white fathers (24% vs 8%),[24,89] black nonresidential fathers are more likely to provide daily child care support, such as bathing, dressing, and reading to their children, than white nonresidential fathers.[24] Interventions with nonresident black fathers designed to prevent risky youth behaviors by preschool-aged children showed some success in paternal monitoring and intentions to avoid violence but no effect on reducing aggressive behavior.[90] Black fathers involved in raising their preschool-aged children note unique concerns about keeping their children safe in violent neighborhoods and seek strategies for monitoring and educating children about safety and ways to improve community life.[91] Pediatric health care providers should be aware that, although black fathers are indeed eager to learn about child rearing, researchers report

they prefer to receive information from relatives or community-based organizations rather than from health care providers,[92] so making connections within the community may be the best way to reach fathers and families. More data are now available on the diversity of Hispanic fathers and the importance of understanding cultural differences, but there are still large research gaps in our understanding of at-risk children of non–English-speaking fathers or displaced undocumented immigrant fathers and of cultural differences more broadly.[93]

According to 2010 census data, there are 352 000 gay male couples in the United States, and approximately 10% of them are raising children.[94] This number does not include gay fathers who share custody with a child's mother after a divorce or single fathers parenting alone, who are not counted in the census. Many gay fathers became fathers in the context of a heterosexual relationship, although increasingly, gay male couples are adopting children, partnering with lesbian mothers, or using surrogate carriers to father children.[95,96] Children with gay parents are comparable to children with heterosexual parents on key psychosocial developmental outcomes.[97–99] Large sample surveys from the 2003–2013 American Time Use Survey ($N = 44 188$) showed that women with same-sex partners as well as opposite-sex partners and men with same-sex partners spent more time with their children than did men with opposite-sex partners.[100] Same-sex couples (both men and women) also reported more equal sharing of child care compared with heterosexual couples, who tend to specialize care (ie, mothers provide more child care than fathers).[98] A study from the United Kingdom examining adopted children 3 to 9 years old in gay father, lesbian mother, and heterosexual parent families found more positive parental well-being and parenting in gay father families and fewer externalizing behaviors compared with heterosexual families.[101] With continued focus on families with gay male parents and improved data collection allowing for more generalizability across the population, a greater understanding of the family dynamics and contributions to child development in families that include 2 fathers is certain to evolve.

Vulnerable and marginalized fathers, such as those who are socially or economically disadvantaged, adolescent, immigrant, or incarcerated but who wish to remain connected with their children, are especially important for pediatric outreach. More than 750 000 fathers are absent serving time in prison.[102] A new program at the Boston Children's Museum called Father's Uplift brings previously incarcerated fathers to the museum to reengage with their children in a welcoming, imaginative, child-centered learning environment that supports diverse families in nurturing their children's creativity and curiosity through joyful play. In a qualitative study, previously incarcerated black fathers expressed a need for employment, social support, and health care to rebuild healthy relationships with their children.[102,103] Increasingly, the relationship of children and incarcerated fathers is an area of study.[104] The fathers of children born to unmarried teenaged mothers (resident or nonresident) may be an important protective factor if they remain involved in their children's lives. The involvement of these fathers during their partners' pregnancy has been associated with improved outcomes such as low birth weight and infant mortality and has become an increasing area of research.[33]

INFLUENCE OF FATHERS' MENTAL AND PHYSICAL WELL-BEING ON CHILDREN'S AND FAMILIES' HEALTH

A father's own well-being can also influence the well-being of the child. Since the initial clinical report from the American Academy of Pediatrics was published, major research advances have been made in understanding paternal mental health problems.

Reviews of the literature in the postpartum period established a prevalence of depressed fathers that ranged from 2% to 25%, with an increase to 50% when mothers experienced postpartum depression.[105–110] New fathers were 1.38 times as likely to be depressed as comparably aged males.[111] A recent study found that nonresident fathers reported higher depression symptoms during the transition to fatherhood, but resident fathers had a 68% increase in their depressive symptoms in the first 5 years of fatherhood.[112] Because of higher rates of several stressors (eg, racism, unemployment, poverty, incarceration, and homelessness) not as commonly associated with white fathers, black fathers may be at higher risk of depression and other poor mental health outcomes.[49,113,114] Screening for postpartum depression by using the Edinburgh Postnatal Depression Scale has been validated for fathers as well as for mothers.[115]

The onset of depression in the postpartum period also occurs later for fathers (ie, up to a year postpartum) than mothers (ie, first 3 months postpartum).[106] The expression of depression is different in men than in women, with men more likely to avoid emotional expression, deny vulnerability, and not seek help, which explains the discrepancy in prevalences between men and women.[116,117] Psychology researchers who study men and masculinity also contend that men experience depression in uncharacteristic ways, such as alcohol- and drug-related comorbidity, compulsive and antisocial behavior, and interpersonal conflict marked with anger and defensive assertions.[118]

This behavior can lead to marital stress and domestic violence, can undermine breastfeeding, and can increase the risk of marital breakup. Conversely, a healthy father can mitigate the adverse effects of maternal depression on the infant. This example is only 1 of the ways in which fathers can buffer toxic stress, such as maternal substance abuse, a family death, or previous abuse. Recent research has shown that depressed fathers are 4 times as likely to spank their infants than nondepressed fathers and less likely to read to them.[105,119] Fathers' ratings of 16 domains/activities of their lives ranked the emotional experience of parenting along with work-life conflict as the most negative and the most tiring activities.[120] Longitudinal studies of paternal depression scores from the National Longitudinal Health Survey showed the highest score for nonresident fathers on entry to fatherhood.[112] Resident fathers have increased depression scores during early fatherhood (children 0–5 years of age), with a 68% increase by the time the children reach 5 years of age.[112] More than one-fifth of fathers have experienced depression by the time their child is 12 years of age.[121] Child health care providers may find it useful to ask fathers with a history of mental illness how being with their children affects their mental illness and how their symptoms affect the way they interact with their children.[122,123]

Like maternal depression, which has long been known to affect the mother-infant relationship and child development, recent data reveal that paternal depression also has negative effects on child behavior, mood, and development. Depression in fathers is a risk factor for excessive infant crying.[9] The Avon Longitudinal Study of Parents and Children, a sample of 12 884 fathers, showed that paternal depression in the postpartum period was associated with an increase in child conduct problems at ages 3 and 5 years, even when maternal depression and other sociodemographic correlates were controlled for.[124] Depressed fathers affect child outcomes by way of mothers (ie, both mothers' depression and couple's conflict), which, in turn, adversely affects the child's emotional and behavioral outcome.[125] In a study in a community sample of parents and adolescents ($N = 775$), maternal depression and paternal depression were both significantly associated with depression in adolescents.[126] A meta-analysis of fathers' mental health and child psychopathology found that paternal depression was significantly correlated with child and adolescent internalizing symptoms.[127] Other studies have shown that father involvement is associated with a decrease in externalizing behavior problems.[8] Recent research highlights the epigenetic risk for older fathers, who are at higher risk of conceiving children with autism or schizophrenia,[128] attention-deficit/hyperactivity disorder, academic problems, Marfan syndrome, dwarfism, and substance abuse.[9,129]

Mental health problems of parents have predictable and negative consequences on parental child care habits, father involvement, and coparenting. Depressed parents tend to spend less time with their children (aged 3 years and younger) and limit physical contact (ie, hugging and cuddling) and are more likely to express frustration in child rearing.[105,130] In a study in families of children enrolled in Head Start, nondepressed fathers were more involved with infants than were depressed fathers.[131] Similarly, depressed fathers in the Fragile Families and Child Wellbeing Study reported less father-child activities (engagement and reciprocal play), lower levels of relationship quality with the mother,

and lower levels of coparental relationship supportiveness than did nondepressed fathers.[132] Conflict in the coparental relationship may heighten the risk of the development of depression in fathers,[106,108,125] but more research is needed in this aspect of family life and paternal depression. Mental health problems in fathers are also highly correlated with later emotional disorders in their children.[133,134]

Becoming a father can be a transformative experience for men's physical health as well, during which men become motivated to take better care of themselves. President Barack Obama, in his Father's Day 2008 speech,[135] said, "When I was a young man, I thought life was all about me—how do I make my way in the world, and how do I become successful and how do I get the things that I want. But now, my life revolves around my 2 little girls." Research shows that many men credit becoming a father as a reason to improve their diet, decrease risky behaviors and alcohol use, and increase physical activity.[136] For children and families, this commitment to improved health behaviors bodes well, because a healthy father can protect against poverty by contributing to the family finances, sharing in child rearing, and often serving to introduce their offspring to the workplace in the form of first-time or summer jobs.

Just as children serve as motivation for fathers to improve their own health, 1 example of how a father's physical well-being may affect a child's well-being is obesity. Current research now suggests that when only 1 member of the parenting couple is in a higher weight status category, it is the father's and not the mother's weight status that is a significant predictor of later child overweight and obesity.[137,138] In fact, the odds of a healthy mother and overweight father having an obese child 4 years later were 4.18 (95% confidence interval: 1.01–17.33),

and the odds of a healthy mother and obese father having an obese child 4 years later were 14.88.[139] These results suggest that fathers are a key influence in shaping the family environment that leads to the development of child obesity.

Another example of how fathers can influence their children's health and well-being is pertussis immunization. Pertussis continues to infect, on average, more than 3000 infants and results in more than 19 deaths per year,[140] with the majority of cases, hospitalizations, and deaths occurring in infants younger than 2 months who are too young to be vaccinated. In 1 report, fathers were the source of 15% of infant infections.[141] The Centers for Disease Control and Prevention recommends that infants be protected before they receive the first pertussis vaccine at 6 to 8 weeks of age by vaccinating pregnant women and their close contacts in the peripartum period, but this recommendation has had limited success among fathers.[140] A paternal pertussis vaccine is reported to avert 16% of pertussis cases.[142] Because of the need to reach fathers, some hospitals and health care providers have successfully provided the vaccination in the maternity ward or during pediatric encounters,[143,144] further emphasizing the need to include the consideration of fathers when considering the health of children.

The increases in fathering research outlined in this clinical report yield new understanding and insight into the important role and influence of fathers in the health, care, and development of their children and, in turn, have resulted in innovative approaches to support fathers. For example, New York City introduced a Young Men's Initiative in 2011, committing $3 million, part of which established a City University of New York Fatherhood Academy to boost fathers' parenting skills, resulting in a 15% decrease in teenage pregnancies.[145] The White House launched My Brother's Keeper,[146] an initiative aimed at bettering outcomes for some of the nation's most at-risk young men. In addition, the White House recently expressed support for paid parental leave and held a White House summit on working fathers.[147] A Dad 2.0 Summit was held in Houston[148] in the winter of 2014 to link multiple bloggers on fatherhood to corporations interested in marketing to a previously ignored group of men. The message is clear: fathers do not parent like mothers, nor are they a replacement for mothers when they are not at home; they provide a unique, dynamic, and important contribution to their families and children. Parenting interventions to encourage father involvement seldom acknowledge fathers' coparenting role and need fundamental change.[149] Pediatricians are encouraged to stay abreast of this information and take advantage of specific opportunities to intervene[150] to support the overall family as a way to ultimately improve child outcomes.

ADVICE FOR PEDIATRICIANS/CHILD HEALTH CARE PROVIDERS

Pediatricians are likely to see a growing number of fathers involved in the health and health care of their children. With so many advances in the understanding of the roles fathers play with their children, a number of suggestions on how to encourage and support fathers in a pediatric setting are provided. Pediatricians can begin by adopting 1 or 2 suggestions the next time they see a father with his child.

Fourteen Pediatric Opportunities to Involve Fathers in Ongoing Care

1. Welcome fathers and express appreciation for their attendance. Speak directly to the father as well as the mother or partner and solicit his opinions. Encourage office staff and nurses to actively encourage father involvement at all pediatric office visits, especially during the early critical years. Starting with the prenatal visit, actively engage the father (eg, at the prenatal visit, ask the father about his decision whether to circumcise the infant if male).

2. Introduce yourself to the father and the mother or other parent, especially if this is the first visit. Politely explore the father's relationship to the other parent (eg, married, living together or not) and his cultural traditions and personal beliefs about his role in caring for the child. Assess differences in parenting beliefs and help parents negotiate, if necessary.

3. Recognize that mothers and fathers may not always agree on how best to raise a child. For example, parents may disagree on the approach to discipline or issues of firearm safety. Pediatricians can serve as a mediator in such discussions, meeting with both parents or caregivers together to discuss these and other behavior-management issues, and should avoid (whenever possible) siding with 1 parent or the other on important parenting issues.

4. Emphasize how children look to their fathers as role models of behavior and are likely to imitate behaviors they see. Use this in a positive way to encourage the increased use of seat belts and helmets for bike riding and decreased tobacco, alcohol, and other substance use.

5. Screen fathers for perinatal depression. Useful screens include the Edinburgh Postpartum Depression Scale (EPDS) or the version that uses the partners report (EPDS-P), the Gotland Male Depression Scale (GMDS), and the more general Center for Epidemiological Studies Depression Scale (CES-D) and Patient Health Questionnaire-9 (PHQ-9). As with maternal depression screening, have a plan in place (referral to own physician) if either parent screens positive or exhibits depressive symptoms.

6. Review the need for parents to keep up to date on adult vaccines and recommend any needed updates for vaccines, such as pertussis and influenza immunizations.

7. Stress the unique role many fathers play in encouraging age-appropriate physical play and modeling physical activity such as exercise.

8. Explore the family composition, cultural beliefs about fathering and men's roles in families, physical health of both parents, and the division of child care tasks within the family. If parents are not both living in the household, discuss living and visiting arrangements, time together, and custody arrangements. In the event of a parental separation or divorce, encourage both fathers as well as mothers to continue to communicate individually with the pediatrician.

9. Encourage fathers to assume some roles early on in the care of the child, and encourage the mother to let the father be involved and learn from his own mistakes. Early time alone with the child helps a father gain confidence and develop his own style of interaction and provides a mother or other parent with much-needed time alone. Ask fathers what skills they feel are lacking and develop a list of local or online resources to support fathers in gaining confidence and skills in parenting.

10. Inform the family about the normal elation, fatigue, and challenges of being a father. Discuss openly the usual interruptions in sleep for the whole family, the decreases in sleep for the whole family, the decrease in energy, the alterations in time together as a couple and individual free time, and the changes in intimacy and the sexual relationship. This may be the first time some fathers will have discussed these issues openly.

11. Educate fathers about the practicalities of breastfeeding and how to support mothers' nursing. If mothers plan to return to work after the first few months at home, they may need the infant to be flexible about taking a bottle while they are at work. If so, this represents an opportunity for fathers to participate in feeding by offering a daily bottle of the mother's milk (once breastfeeding is well established) to foster the necessary infant flexibility to take a bottle in addition to continuing to breastfeed whenever possible. In addition, fathers provide important skin-to-skin care and help the mother in routine tasks that facilitate rest, bonding, and continued breastfeeding.

12. Discuss how the couple is adapting to parenthood (with each child). Asking questions such as "How is your relationship (or the family) adjusting to the new infant?" or "How is it now that your child is older?" opens the door to reflection and discussion and can remind parents of the importance of their own partner relationship and the need to nurture and maintain it. Encourage parents to continue to dedicate time for adult activities without children.

13. As advocates for children and families, pediatricians can identify current and necessary future public policies that support fathers' involvement with their children. Promote the use of policies such as the Family Medical Leave Act (codified at 29 CFR S825 [1993]) and flexible work schedules as ways to balance employment and family responsibilities. "Use it or lose it" paternity leave policies abroad have resulted in more than 90% of new fathers taking brief paternity leave to bond with their newborn infants.

14. In most cases, permission for medical procedures can be granted by either legal parent, but in some cases it may be important to include both parents in such discussions and even legal documents. Even if not legally required, it is usually advisable for pediatricians to include fathers who share custody, whether residing with the child or not, in written communications about the child, such as results of testing or subspecialist evaluations.

LEAD AUTHORS

Michael W. Yogman, MD, FAAP (myogman@massmed.org)
Craig Garfield, MD, FAAP

COMMITTEE ON PSYCHOSOCIAL ASPECTS OF CHILD AND FAMILY HEALTH, 2015–2016

Michael W. Yogman, MD, FAAP, Chairperson
Nerissa S. Bauer, MD, FAAP
Thresia B. Gambon, MD, FAAP
Arthur Lavin, MD, FAAP
Keith M. Lemmon, MD, FAAP
Gerri Mattson, MD, FAAP
Jason Richard Rafferty, MD, MPH, EdM
Lawrence Sagin Wissow, MD, MPH, FAAP

LIAISONS

Sharon Berry, PhD, LP – *Society of Pediatric Psychology*
Terry Carmichael, MSW – *National Association of Social Workers*
Ed Christophersen, PhD, FAAP – *Society of Pediatric Psychology*

Norah L. Johnson, PhD, RN, CPNP-BC – *National Association of Pediatric Nurse Practitioners*
Leonard Read Sulik, MD, FAAP – *American Academy of Child and Adolescent Psychiatry*

CONSULTANT

George J. Cohen, MD, FAAP

STAFF

Stephanie Domain, MS, CHES

REFERENCES

1. Coleman WL, Garfield C; American Academy of Pediatrics Committee on Psychosocial Aspects of Child and Family Health. Fathers and pediatricians: enhancing men's roles in the care and development of their children. *Pediatrics.* 2004;113(5):1406–1411

2. Ad Council. Fatherhood involvement. Available at: www.adcouncil.org/Our-Campaigns/Family-Community/Fatherhood-Involvement. Accessed March 19, 2015

3. National Conference of State Legislatures. Labor and employment. Available at: www.ncsl.org/research/labor-and-employment/state-family-and -medical-leave-laws.aspx. Accessed March 24, 2015

4. An Act Relative to Parental Leave. Mass Gen Laws, 151B, Chapter 149, section 105D (2015)

5. Halverson C. From here to paternity: why men are not taking paternity leave under the Family Medical Leave Act. *Wis Womens Law J.* 2003;18(2):257–259

6. Roopnarine L, ed. Fathering: a journal of research, theory, and practice. Available at: http://fatheringjournal.com/default.aspx. Accessed March 19, 2015

7. Weinfield NS. Father recruitment and retention in longitudinal research: a quantitative and qualitative analysis. Presented at: *American Public Health Association Annual Meeting and Exposition*; October 29–November 2, 2011; Washington, DC

8. Sarkadi A, Kristiansson R, Oberklaid F, Bremberg S. Fathers' involvement and children's developmental outcomes: a systematic review of longitudinal studies. *Acta Paediatr.* 2008;97(2):153–158

9. Raeburn P. *Do Fathers Matter?* New York, NY: Farrar, Straus, Giroux; 2014

10. Garfield CF, Isacco A. Fathers and the well-child visit. *Pediatrics.* 2006;117(4). Available at: www.pediatrics.org/cgi/content/full/117/4/e637

11. Garfield CF, Clark-Kauffman E, Davis MM. Fatherhood as a component of men's health. *JAMA.* 2006;296(19):2365–2368

12. Garfield CF, Chung PJ. A qualitative study of early differences in fathers' expectations of their child care responsibilities. *Ambul Pediatr.* 2006;6(4):215–220

13. Dubowitz H, Lane W, Ross K, Vaughan D. The involvement of low-income African American fathers in their children's lives, and the barriers they face. *Ambul Pediatr.* 2004;4(6):505–508

14. Moore T, Kotelchuck M. Predictors of urban fathers' involvement in their child's health care. *Pediatrics.* 2004;113(3 pt 1):574–580

15. Yogman MW. The father's influence on infant health. In: Macfarlane A, ed. *Progress in Child Health.* London, United Kingdom: Churchill Livingstone; 1984:146–156

16. Yogman MW. Development of the father-infant relationship. In: Fitzgerald H, Lester BM, Yogman MW, eds. *Theory and Research in Behavioral Pediatrics.* Vol 1. New York, NY: Plenum Press; 1982:221–279

17. Garfield CF, Isacco AJ. Urban fathers involvement in their child's health and health care. *Psychol Men Masc.* 2012;13(1):32–48

18. US Census Bureau. Facts for features: Father's Day, June 16, 2013. Available at: www.census.gov/newsroom/facts-for-features/2013/cb13-ff13.html. Accessed March 24, 2015

19. Doherty WJ, Kouneski EF, Erickson MF. Responsible fathering: an overview and conceptual frame work. *J Marriage Fam.* 1998;60(2):277–292

20. Gogineni R, Fallon AE. The adoptive father. In: Brabender VM, Fallon AE, eds. *Working With Adoptive Parents.* Hoboken, NJ: John Wiley and Sons; 2013:89–104

21. Livingston G. Growing number of dads home with the kids. Washington, DC: Pew Research Center Social and Demographic Trends Project Blog; 2014. Available at: www.pewsocialtrends.org/2014/06/05. Accessed March 24, 2015

22. Livingston G. Why are dads staying home? Analysis of March Current Population Surveys Integrated Public Use Micro Data Series (IPUMS-CPS). Washington, DC: Pew Research Center; 1990–2013

23. Livingston G, Parker K. *A Tale of Two Fathers.* Washington, DC: Pew Research Center; 2011

24. Jones J, Mosher WD. Fathers' involvement with their children: United States, 2006-2010. *Natl Health Stat Rep.* 2013;(71):1–21

25. Harrington B, Van Deusen F, Sabatini Fraone J. *The New Dad: A Work (and Life).* Boston, MA: Boston College Center for Work and Family; 2013

26. Parker K, Wang W. *Modern Parenthood: Roles of Moms and Dads Converge as They Balance Work and Family.* Washington, DC: Pew Research Center; 2013. Available at: www.pewsocialtrends.org/2013/03/14/modern-parenthood-roles-of-moms-and-dads-converge-as-they-balance-work-and-family/. Accessed March 24, 2015

27. McGill BS. Navigating new norms of involved fatherhood: employment, fathering attitudes, and father involvement. *J Fam Issues.* 2014;35(8):1089–1106

28. Hook JL, Wolfe CM. New fathers? Residential fathers' time with children in four countries. *J Fam Issues.* 2012;33(4):415–450

29. Teitler JO. Father involvement, child health and maternal health behavior. *Child Youth Serv Rev.* 2001;23(4–5):403–425

30. Conner GK, Denson V. Expectant fathers' response to pregnancy: review of literature and implications for research in high-risk pregnancy. *J Perinat Neonatal Nurs.* 1990;4(2):33–42

31. Shannon JD, Cabrera NJ, Tamis-Lemonda C, Lamb ME. Who stays and who leaves: father accessibility across children's first 5 years. *Parent Sci Pract.* 2009;9(1–2):78–100

32. Alio AP, Mbah AK, Grunsten RA, Salihu HM. Teenage pregnancy and the influence of paternal involvement on fetal outcomes. *J Pediatr Adolesc Gynecol.* 2011;24(6):404–409

33. Alio AP, Mbah AK, Kornosky JL, Wathington D, Marty PJ, Salihu HM. Assessing the impact of paternal involvement on racial/ethnic disparities in infant mortality rates. *J Community Health.* 2011;36(1):63–68

34. Martin MA, Shalowitz MU, Mijanovich T, Clark-Kauffman E, Perez E, Berry CA. The effects of acculturation on asthma burden in a community sample of Mexican American schoolchildren. *Am J Public Health.* 2007;97(7):1290–1296

35. Erlandsson K, Dsilna A, Fagerberg I, Christensson K. Skin-to-skin care with the father after cesarean birth and its effect on newborn crying and prefeeding behavior. *Birth.* 2007;34(2):105–114

36. Yogman MW. Games fathers and mothers play with their infants. *Infant Ment Health J.* 1981;2:241–248

37. Feldman R. Infant mother and infant father synchrony: the coregulation of positive arousal. *Infant Ment Health J.* 2003;24(1):1–23

38. Yogman YW, Lester BM, Hoffman J. Behavioral and cardiac rhythmicity during mother-father-stranger infant social interaction. *Pediatr Res.* 1983;17(11):872–876

39. Gettler LT, McDade TW, Feranil AB, Kuzawa CW. Longitudinal evidence that fatherhood decreases testosterone in human males. *Proc Natl Acad Sci USA.* 2011;108(39):16194–16199

40. Perini T, Ditzen B, Hengartner M, Ehlert U. Sensation seeking in fathers: the impact on testosterone and paternal investment. *Horm Behav.* 2012;61(2):191–195

41. Kuo PX, Carp J, Light KC, Grewen KM. Neural responses to infants linked with behavioral interactions and testosterone in fathers. *Biol Psychol.* 2012;91(2):302–306

42. Gordon I, Zagoory-Sharon O, Leckman JF, Feldman R. Prolactin, oxytocin, and the development of paternal behavior across the first six months of fatherhood. *Horm Behav.* 2010;58(3):513–518

43. Weisman O, Zagoory-Sharon O, Feldman R. Oxytocin administration, salivary testosterone, and father-infant social behavior. *Prog Neuropsychopharmacol Biol Psychiatry.* 2014;49:47–52

44. Feldman R, Gordon I, Schneiderman I, Weisman O, Zagoory-Sharon O. Natural variations in maternal and paternal care are associated with systematic changes in oxytocin following parent-infant contact. *Psychoneuroendocrinology.* 2010;35(8):1133–1141

45. Feldman R. The adaptive human parental brain: implications for children's social development. *Trends Neurosci.* 2015;38(6):387–399

46. Martin JA, Hamilton BE, Osterman MJ, Curtin SC, Matthews TJ. Births: final data for 2012. *Natl Vital Stat Rep.* 2013;62(9):1–68

47. Carlson MJ, McLanahan SS, Brooks-Gunn J. Coparenting and nonresident fathers' involvement with young children after a nonmarital birth. *Demography.* 2008;45(2):461–488

48. Cheadle JE, Amato PR, King V. Patterns of nonresident father contact. *Demography.* 2010;47(1):205–225

49. Davis RN, Caldwell CH, Clark SJ, Davis MM. Depressive symptoms in nonresident African American fathers and involvement with their sons. *Pediatrics.* 2009;124(6):1611–1618

50. Castillo JT, Sarver CM. Non-resident fathers' social networks: the relationship between social support and father involvement. *Pers Relatsh.* 2012;19(4):759–774

51. Ryan RM, Kalil A, Ziol-Guest KM. Longitudinal patterns of nonresident fathers' involvement: the role of resources and relations. *J Marriage Fam.* 2008;70(4):962–977

52. King V, Sobolewski JM. Nonresident fathers' contributions to adolescent well-being. *J Marriage Fam.* 2006;68(3):537–557

53. Kotila LE, Kamp Dush CM. Another baby? Father involvement and childbearing in fragile families. *J Fam Psychol.* 2012;26(6):976–986

54. Adamsons K, Johnson SK. An updated and expanded meta-analysis of nonresident fathering and child well-being. *J Fam Psychol.* 2013;27(4):589–599

55. Waldfogel J, Craigie TA, Brooks-Gunn J. Fragile families and child wellbeing. *Future Child.* 2010;20(2):87–112

56. Flouri E, Malmberg LE. Child temperament and paternal transition to non-residence. *Infant Behav Dev.* 2010;33(4):689–694

57. Edin K, Tach L, Mincy R. Claiming fatherhood: race and the dynamics of paternal involvement among unmarried men. *Ann Am Acad Pol Soc Sci.* 2009;621(1):149–177

58. MDRC. Strengthening low-income families: a research agenda for parenting, relationship, and fatherhood programs. New York, NY: MDRC; 2013. Available at: www.mdrc.org/sites/default/files/Strengthening_Families_020113.pdf. Accessed March 24, 2015

59. Pancsofar N, Vernon-Feagans L. Mother and father language input to young children: contributions to later language. *J Appl Dev Psychol.* 2006;27(6):571–587

60. Johnson K, Caskey M, Rand K, Tucker R, Vohr B. Gender differences in adult-infant communication in the first months of life. *Pediatrics.* 2014;134(6). Available at: www.pediatrics.org/cgi/content/full/134/6/e1603

61. Boyce WT, Essex MJ, Alkon A, Goldsmith HH, Kraemer HC, Kupfer DJ. Early father involvement moderates biobehavioral susceptibility to mental health problems in middle childhood. *J Am Acad Child Adolesc Psychiatry.* 2006;45(12):1510–1520

62. Jia R, Kotila LE, Schoppe-Sullivan SJ. Transactional relations between father involvement and preschoolers' socioemotional adjustment. *J Fam Psychol.* 2012;26(6):848–857

63. Chang JJ, Halpern CT, Kaufman JS. Maternal depressive symptoms, father's involvement, and the trajectories of child problem behaviors in a US national sample. *Arch Pediatr Adolesc Med.* 2007;161(7):697–703

64. Child Trends Data Bank. Parental warmth and affection. 2002. Available at: www.childtrends.org/?indicators=parental-warmth-and-affection. Accessed March 24, 2015

65. Howard Caldwell C, Antonakos CL, Assari S, Kruger D, De Loney EH, Njai R. Pathways to prevention: improving nonresident African American fathers' parenting skills and behaviors to reduce sons' aggression. *Child Dev.* 2014;85(1):308–325

66. Bronte-Tinkew J, Moore KA, Carrano J. The father-child relationship, parenting styles, and adolescent risk behaviors in intact families. *J Fam Issues.* 2006;27(6):850–881

67. Carlson C, Trapani JN. Single parenting and step parenting. In: Bear GG, Minke KM, eds. *Children's Needs III: Development, Prevention and Intervention.* Bethesda, MD: National Association of School Psychologists; 2006:783–797

68. Cookston JT, Finlay AK. Father involvement and adolescent adjustment longitudinal findings from Add Health. *Fathering.* 2006;4(2):137–158

69. Ellis BJ, Schlomer GL, Tilley EH, Butler EA. Impact of fathers on risky sexual behavior in daughters: a genetically and environmentally controlled sibling study. *Dev Psychopathol.* 2012;24(1):317–332

70. Menning CL. Nonresident fathers' involvement and adolescents' smoking. *J Health Soc Behav.* 2006;47(1):32–46

71. Chesler MA, Parry C. Gender roles and/or styles in crisis: an integrative analysis of the experiences of fathers of children with cancer. *Qual Health Res.* 2001;11(3):363–384

72. McNeill T. Fathers' experience of parenting a child with juvenile rheumatoid arthritis. *Qual Health Res.* 2004;14(4):526–545

73. Wysocki T, Gavin L. Psychometric properties of a new measure of fathers' involvement in the management of pediatric chronic diseases. *J Pediatr Psychol.* 2004;29(3):231–240

74. Ogg M. The effects of pediatric cancer on fathers during the diagnostic and initial treatment phases. *Diss Abstr Int B Sci Eng.* 1997;58(9-B):5135

75. Bright MA, Franich-Ray C, Anderson V, et al. Infant cardiac surgery and the father-infant relationship: feelings of strength, strain, and caution. *Early Hum Dev.* 2013;89(8):593–599

76. Bagner DM. Father's role in parent training for children with developmental delay. *J Fam Psychol.* 2013;27(4):650–657

77. Yogman MW, Kindlon D, Earls F. Father involvement and cognitive/behavioral outcomes of preterm infants. *J Am Acad Child Adolesc Psychiatry.* 1995;34(1):58–66

78. Yogman MW. The father's role with preterm and full term infants. In: Call J, Galenson E, Tyson R, eds. *Frontiers in Infant Psychiatry.* Vol 2. New York, NY: Basic Books, Inc; 1985:363–374

79. Guzzo KB, Furstenberg FF Jr. Multipartnered fertility among American men. *Demography.* 2007;44(3):583–601

80. Carlson MJ, Furstenberg FF. The prevalence and correlates of multipartnered fertility among urban U.S. parents. *J Marriage Fam.* 2006;68(3):718–732

81. Manlove J, Logan C, Ikramullah E, Holcombe E. Factors associated with multiple-partner fertility among fathers. *J Marriage Fam.* 2008;70(2):536–548

82. Cancian M, Meyer DR, Cook ST. The evolution of family complexity from the perspective of nonmarital children. *Demography.* 2011;48(3):957–982

83. Manning WD, Smock PJ. "Swapping" families: serial parenting and economic support for children. *J Marriage Fam.* 2000;62(1):111–122

84. Carlson MJ, Berger LM. What kids get from parents: packages of parental involvement across complex family forms. *Soc Serv Rev.* 2013;87(2):213–249

85. Turney K, Carlson MJ. Multipartnered fertility and depression among fragile families. *J Marriage Fam.* 2011;73(3):570–587

86. Pfefferbaum B, Houston JB, Allen SF. Perception of change and burden in children of National Guard troops deployed as part of the global war on terror. *Int J Emerg Ment Health.* 2012;14(3):189–196

87. Willerton E, Schwarz RL, Wadsworth SM, Oglesby MS. Military fathers' perspectives on involvement. *J Fam Psychol.* 2011;25(4):521–530

88. Lee SJ, Neugut TB, Rosenblum KL, Tolman RM, Travis WJ, Walker MH. Sources of parenting support in early fatherhood: perspectives of United States Air Force members. *Child Youth Serv Rev.* 2013;35(5):908–915

89. Edin K, Nelson TJ. *Doing the Best I Can.* Berkeley, CA: University of California Press; 2013

90. Caldwell CH, Rafferty J, Reischl TM, De Loney EH, Brooks CL. Enhancing parenting skills among nonresident African American fathers as a strategy for preventing youth risky behaviors. *Am J Community Psychol.* 2010;45(1–2):17–35

91. Lettiecq B, Koblinsky SA. Parenting in violent neighborhoods. *J Fam Issues.* 2004;25(6):715–734

92. Smith TK, Tandon SD, Bair-Merritt MH, Hanson JL. Parenting needs of urban African American fathers. *Am J Men Health.* 2015;9(4):317–331

93. Cabrera NJ, Bradley RH. Latino fathers and their children. *Child Dev Perspect.* 2012;6(3):232–238

94. US Census Bureau, Fertility and Family Statistics Branch. Frequently asked questions about same-sex couple households. August 2013. Available at: www.census.gov/hhes/samesex/files/SScplfactsheet_final.pdf. Accessed January 11, 2016

95. Tornello SL, Farr RH, Patterson CJ. Predictors of parenting stress among gay adoptive fathers in the United States. *J Fam Psychol.* 2011;25(4):591–600

96. Gates GJ, Badgett MVL, Macomber JE, Chambers K. *Adoption and Foster Care by Gay and Lesbian Parents in the United States.* Los Angeles, CA: The Williams Institute, University of California at Los Angeles; 2007

97. Tasker F. Lesbian mothers, gay fathers, and their children: a review. *J Dev Behav Pediatr.* 2005;26(3):224–240

98. Farr RH, Patterson CJ. Coparenting among lesbian, gay, and heterosexual couples: associations with adopted children's outcomes. *Child Dev.* 2013;84(4):1226–1240

99. American Academy of Pediatrics Committee on Psychosocial Aspects of Child and Family Health. Promoting the well-being of children whose parents are gay or lesbian. *Pediatrics.* 2013;131(4):827–830

100. Prickett KC, Martin-Storey A, Crosnoe R. A research note on time with children in different-and same-sex two-parent families. *Demography.* 2015;52(3):905–918

101. Golombok S, Mellish L, Jennings S, Casey P, Tasker F, Lamb ME. Adoptive gay father families: parent-child relationships and children's psychological adjustment. *Child Dev.* 2014;85(2):456–468

102. Geller A, Cooper CE, Garfinkel I, Schwartz-Soicher O, Mincy RB. Beyond absenteeism: father incarceration and child development. *Demography.* 2012;49(1):49–76

103. Dill LJ, Mahaffey C, Mosley T, Treadwell H, Barkwell F, Barnhill S. "I want a second chance":Experiences of African American fathers in reentry. *Am J Mens Health.* 2015;9(1):1–8

104. Geller A. Paternal incarceration and father child contact in fragile families. *J Marriage Fam.* 2013;75(5):1288–1303

105. Davis RN, Davis MM, Freed GL, Clark SJ. Fathers' depression related to positive and negative parenting behaviors with 1-year-old children. *Pediatrics.* 2011;127(4):612–618

106. Goodman JH. Paternal postpartum depression, its relationship to maternal postpartum depression, and implications for family health. *J Adv Nurs.* 2004;45(1):26–35

107. Edmondson OJ, Psychogiou L, Vlachos H, Netsi E, Ramchandani PG. Depression in fathers in the postnatal period: assessment of the Edinburgh Postnatal Depression Scale as a screening measure. *J Affect Disord.* 2010;125(1–3):365–368

108. Ramchandani PG, Psychogiou L, Vlachos H, et al. Paternal depression: an examination of its links with father, child and family functioning in the postnatal period. *Depress Anxiety.* 2011;28(6):471–477

109. Paulson JF, Bazemore SD. Prenatal and postpartum depression in fathers and its association with maternal

depression: a meta-analysis. *JAMA*. 2010;303(19):1961–1969

110. Gawlik S, Muller M, Hoffmann L, et al. Prevalence of paternal perinatal depressiveness and its link to partnership satisfaction and birth concerns. *Arch Women Ment Health*. 2014;17(1):49–56

111. Giallo R, D'Esposito F, Christensen D, et al. Father mental health during the early parenting period: results of an Australian population based longitudinal study. *Soc Psychiatry Psychiatr Epidemiol*. 2012;47(12):1907–1966

112. Garfield CF, Duncan G, Rutsohn J, et al. A longitudinal study of paternal mental health during transition to fatherhood as young adults. *Pediatrics*. 2014;133(5):836–843

113. Anderson EA, Kohler JK, Letiecq BL. Predictors of depression among low-income, nonresidential fathers. *J Fam Issues*. 2005;26(5):547–567

114. Reinherz HZ, Giaconia RM, Hauf AM, Wasserman MS, Silverman AB. Major depression in the transition to adulthood: risks and impairments. *J Abnorm Psychol*. 1999;108(3):500–510

115. Matthey S, Barnett B, Kavanagh DJ, Howie P. Validation of the Edinburgh Postnatal Depression Scale for men, and comparison of item endorsement with their partners. *J Affect Disord*. 2001;64(2–3):175–184

116. Mansfield AK, Addis ME, Mahalik JR. "Why won't he go to the doctor?": the psychology of men's help seeking. *Int J Mens Health*. 2003;2(2):93–109

117. Rochlen AB. Men in (and out of) therapy: central concepts, emerging directions, and remaining challenges. *J Clin Psychol*. 2005;61(6):627–631

118. Cochran SV. Assessing and treating depression in men. In: Brooks GR, Good GE, eds. *The New Handbook of Psychotherapy and Counseling With Men*. Vol 1. San Francisco, CA: Jossey-Bass; 2001:3–21

119. Fletcher RJ, Feeman E, Garfield C, Vimpani G. The effects of early paternal depression on children's development. *Med J Aust*. 2011;195(11–12):685–689

120. Kahneman D, Krueger AB, Schkade DA, Schwarz N, Stone AA. A survey method for characterizing daily life experience: the day reconstruction method. *Science*. 2004;306(5702):1776–1780

121. Davé S, Petersen I, Sherr L, Nazareth I. Incidence of maternal and paternal depression in primary care: a cohort study using a primary care database. *Arch Pediatr Adolesc Med*. 2010;164(11):1038–1044

122. Garfield CF, Fletcher R. Sad dads: a challenge for pediatrics. *Pediatrics*. 2011;127(4):781–782

123. Fletcher RJ, Maharaj ON, Fletcher Watson CH, May C, Skeates N, Gruenert S. Fathers with mental illness: implications for clinicians and health services. *Med J Aust*. 2013;199(3 suppl):S34–S36

124. Ramchandani P, Stein A, Evans J, O'Connor TG; ALSPAC Study Team. Paternal depression in the postnatal period and child development: a prospective population study. *Lancet*. 2005;365(9478):2201–2205

125. Gutierrez-Galve L, Stein A, Hanington L, Heron J, Ramchandani P. Paternal depression in the postnatal period and child development: mediators and moderators. *Pediatrics*. 2015;135(2). Available at: www.pediatrics.org/cgi/content/full/135/2/e339

126. Shone LP, Dick AW, Klein JD, Zwanziger J, Szilagyi PG. Reduction in racial and ethnic disparities after enrollment in the State Children's Health Insurance Program. *Pediatrics*. 2005;115(6). Available at: www.pediatrics.org/cgi/content/full/115/2/e697

127. Kane P, Garber J. The relations among depression in fathers, children's psychopathology, and father-child conflict: a meta-analysis. *Clin Psychol Rev*. 2004;24(3):339–360

128. Kong A, Frigge ML, Masson G, et al. Rate of de novo mutations and the importance of father's age to disease risk. *Nature*. 2012;488(7412):471–475

129. D'Onofrio BM, Rickert ME, Frans E, et al. Paternal age at childbearing and offspring psychiatric and academic morbidity. *JAMA Psychiatry*. 2014;71(4):432–438

130. Lyons-Ruth K, Wolfe R, Lyubchik A, Steingard R. Depressive symptoms in parents of children under age 3: sociodemographic predictors, current correlates, and associated parenting behaviors. In: Halfon N, McLearn KT, eds. *Child Rearing in America: Challenges Facing Parents With Young Children*. New York, NY: Cambridge University Press; 2002:217–259

131. Roggman LA, Boyce LK, Cook GA, Cook J. Getting dads involved: predictors of father involvement in Early Head Start and with their children. *Infant Ment Health J*. 2002;23(1):62–78

132. Bronte-Tinkew JPD. Resident fathers' pregnancy intentions, prenatal behaviors, and links to involvement with infants. *J Marriage Fam*. 2007;69(4):977–990

133. Weitzman M, Rosenthal DG, Liu YH. Paternal depressive symptoms and child behavioral or emotional problems in the United States. *Pediatrics*. 2011;128(6):1126–1134

134. Kvalevaag AL, Ramchandani PG, Hove O, Assmus J, Eberhard-Gran M, Biringer E. Paternal mental health and socioemotional and behavioral development in their children. *Pediatrics*. 2013;131(2). Available at: www.pediatrics.org/cgi/content/full/131/2/e463

135. Obama's Father's Day remarks. *New York Times*. June 15, 2008. Available at: www.nytimes.com/2008/06/15/us/politics/15text-obama.html?pagewanted=all. Accessed March 24, 2015

136. Garfield CF, Isacco A, Bartlo WD. Men's health and fatherhood in the urban Midwestern United States. *Int J Mens Health*. 2010;9(3):161–174

137. Brophy S, Rees A, Knox G, Baker JS, Thomas NE. Child fitness and father's BMI are important factors in childhood obesity: a school based cross-sectional study. *PLoS One*. 2012;8(5):e36597

138. Freeman E, Fletcher R, Collins CE, Morgan PJ, Burrows T, Callister R. Preventing and treating childhood obesity: time to target fathers. *Int J Obes*. 2012;36(1):12–15

139. Flegal KM, Carroll MD, Kit BK, Ogden CL. Prevalence of obesity and trends in the distribution of body mass index among US adults, 1999-2010. *JAMA*. 2012;307(5):491–497

140. Centers for Disease Control and Prevention. Updated recommendations for use of tetanus toxoid, reduced

diphtheria toxoid and acellular pertussis vaccine (Tdap) in pregnant women and persons who have or anticipate having close contact with an infant aged <12 months—Advisory Committee on Immunization Practices (ACIP), 2011. *MMWR Morb Mortal Wkly Rep.* 2011;60(41):1424–1426

141. Bisgard KM, Pascual FB, Ehresmann KR, et al. Infant pertussis: who was the source? *Pediatr Infect Dis J.* 2004;23(11):985–989

142. Terranella A, Asay GR, Messonnier ML, Clark TA, Liang JL. Pregnancy dose Tdap and postpartum cocooning to prevent infant pertussis: a decision analysis. *Pediatrics.* 2013;131(6). Available at: www.pediatrics.org/cgi/content/full/131/6/e1748

143. Frère J, De Wals P, Ovetchkine P, Coïc L, Audibert F, Tapiero B. Evaluation of several approaches to immunize parents of neonates against B. pertussis. *Vaccine.* 2013;31(51):6087–6091

144. Walter EB, Allred N, Rowe-West B, Chmielewski K, Kretsinger K, Dolor RJ. Cocooning infants: Tdap immunization for new parents in the pediatric office. *Acad Pediatr.* 2009;9(5):344–347

145. Young Men's Initiative. Available at: www.nyc.gov/html/ymi/html/home/home.shtml. Accessed March 24, 2015

146. The White House. My Brother's Keeper. Available at: https://www.whitehouse.gov/my-brothers-keeper. Accessed March 24, 2015

147. White House Summit on Working Families. Available at: http://workingfamiliessummit.org/. Accessed March 24, 2015

148. Dad 2.0 Summit. Available at: www.dad2summit.com/. Accessed March 24, 2015

149. Panter-Brick C, Burgess A, Eggerman M, McAllister F, Pruett K, Leckman JF. Practitioner review: engaging fathers—recommendations for a game change in parenting interventions based on a systematic review of the global evidence. *J Child Psychol Psychiatry.* 2014;55(11):1187–1212

150. Yogman MW, Kindlon D. Pediatric opportunities with fathers and children. *Pediatr Ann.* 1998;27(1):16–22

The Female Athlete Triad

- *Clinical Report*

CLINICAL REPORT   Guidance for the Clinician in Rendering Pediatric Care

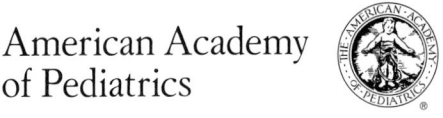

American Academy
of Pediatrics

DEDICATED TO THE HEALTH OF ALL CHILDREN™

The Female Athlete Triad

Amanda K. Weiss Kelly, MD, FAAP, Suzanne Hecht, MD, FACSM, COUNCIL ON SPORTS MEDICINE AND FITNESS

abstract

The number of girls participating in sports has increased significantly since the introduction of Title XI in 1972. As a result, more girls have been able to experience the social, educational, and health-related benefits of sports participation. However, there are risks associated with sports participation, including the female athlete triad. The triad was originally recognized as the interrelationship of amenorrhea, osteoporosis, and disordered eating, but our understanding has evolved to recognize that each of the components of the triad exists on a spectrum from optimal health to disease. The triad occurs when energy intake does not adequately compensate for exercise-related energy expenditure, leading to adverse effects on reproductive, bone, and cardiovascular health. Athletes can present with a single component or any combination of the components. The triad can have a more significant effect on the health of adolescent athletes than on adults because adolescence is a critical time for bone mass accumulation. This report outlines the current state of knowledge on the epidemiology, diagnosis, and treatment of the triad conditions.

Clinical reports from the American Academy of Pediatrics benefit from expertise and resources of liaisons and internal (AAP) and external reviewers. However, clinical reports from the American Academy of Pediatrics may not reflect the views of the liaisons or the organizations or government agencies that they represent.

The guidance in this report does not indicate an exclusive course of treatment or serve as a standard of medical care. Variations, taking into account individual circumstances, may be appropriate.

All clinical reports from the American Academy of Pediatrics automatically expire 5 years after publication unless reaffirmed, revised, or retired at or before that time.

DOI: 10.1542/peds.2016-0922

PEDIATRICS (ISSN Numbers: Print, 0031-4005; Online, 1098-4275).

FINANCIAL DISCLOSURE: The authors have indicated they have no financial relationships relevant to this article to disclose.

FUNDING: No external funding.

POTENTIAL CONFLICT OF INTEREST: The authors have indicated they have no potential conflicts of interest to disclose.

To cite: Weiss Kelly AK, Hecht S, AAP COUNCIL ON SPORTS MEDICINE AND FITNESS. The Female Athlete Triad. *Pediatrics.* 2016;137(6):e20160922

INTRODUCTION

The benefits of exercise in adolescents are well established, including improved self-esteem, fewer risk-taking behaviors, increased bone mineral density (BMD), and decreased obesity.[1-3] However, when exercise occurs without adequate energy intake to compensate for exercise-related energy expenditure, there may be adverse effects on reproductive, bone, and cardiovascular health. The female athlete triad (referred to hereafter as the "triad") was first widely acknowledged as the 3 interrelated conditions of amenorrhea, osteoporosis, and disordered eating in an American College of Sports Medicine position statement published in 1997.[4] Since that time, a more inclusive definition has evolved because it has become clear that each component of the triad exists on a spectrum; the 3 components were renamed menstrual function, BMD, and energy availability (EA) to more accurately represent the spectrum, which can range from optimal health to disease in each component.[5] In addition, athletes may present with 1, 2, or all 3 of the components.

Adolescent athletes are in a critical period of bone mass accumulation, so the triad disorders can be particularly harmful in this group.[6] Appropriate intervention during the adolescent years may improve peak bone mass accrual, an important predictor of postmenopausal osteoporosis, potentially preventing low BMD, postmenopausal osteoporosis, and fractures in adulthood. Two investigators have also identified lower BMD as a risk factor for stress fracture in athletes.[7,8] It is difficult to estimate the true prevalence of the triad because of the complexity of evaluation of each of the components. Reports have indicated that the prevalence of individuals with all 3 components simultaneously is only 1% to 1.2% in high school girls[9,10] and 0% to 16% in all female athletes. In high school–aged female athletes, the prevalence of 2 concurrent components of the triad is 4% to 18% and of any 1 component is as high as 16% to 54%.[9–15]

Education of pediatricians, who are most likely to encounter adolescents with triad-related disorders, is especially important. Unfortunately, a 2009 study found that only 20% of pediatricians were able to correctly identify all 3 components of the triad, compared with 50% of family medicine physicians and 41% of orthopedic surgeons.[16] Most physicians reported receiving no education in medical school or through continuing medical education on triad-related issues.[16]

RISK FACTORS

Although the triad disorders may occur in any sport, athletes participating in sports with endurance, aesthetic, or weight-class components or sports that emphasize and reward leanness are at increased risk (see Table 1).[5,17] Other identified risk factors for the triad include early

age at sport specialization, family dysfunction, abuse, and dieting.[5,17]

Energy Availability

EA is defined as daily dietary energy intake minus daily exercise energy expenditure corrected for fat-free mass (FFM).[5] Optimal EA has been identified to be 45 kcal/kg FFM per day in female adults but may be even higher in adolescents who are still growing and developing. The spectrum of EA ranges from optimal EA to inadequate EA, with or without the presence of disordered eating/eating disorder. Recently, it has become clear that many athletes affected by the triad do not exhibit pathologic eating behaviors, and their low EA is unintentional. Low EA adversely affects bone remodeling, and EA <30 kcal/kg FFM per day disrupts menstrual function and bone mineralization.[18–20] Disruptions in luteinizing hormone can be seen after only 5 days of reduction in EA to 30 kcal/kg FFM per day.[18] The only study of EA in adolescent females found that, although athletes were more likely to have suboptimal EA, both athletes and controls restricted intake, with 6% of female athletes and 4% of sedentary controls having an EA <30 kcal/kg FFM per day. Furthermore, 39% of athletes and 36% of controls had an EA <45 kcal/kg FFM per day.[9]

Disordered eating in adolescent athletes has been evaluated by using a variety of survey tools, such as the Eating Disorder Exam Questionnaire, the Eating Disorder Inventory, and the Three-Factor Eating Questionnaire. Studies that used these tools provide estimates of disordered eating ranging from 0% to 54%.[9,10,21–23] The use of pathologic weight-control techniques, such as vomiting, diuretics, or laxatives, ranges from 0% to 54% in recent studies.[9,10,24]

Even in the absence of amenorrhea, disordered eating is associated with lower BMD in athletes.[5,25] Low BMI

TABLE 1 Examples of Sports Emphasizing Leanness and Endurance

Wrestling
Light-weight rowing
Gymnastics
Dance
Figure skating
Cheerleading
Long and middle distance running
Pole vaulting

is also a strong predictor for low BMD.[13] Athletes with a high drive for thinness or increased dietary restraint (an intention to restrict food intake to control weight) are significantly more likely to have low BMD or to sustain a musculoskeletal injury than are athletes with normal eating behaviors.[26,27]

Many triggers for the onset of disordered eating in athletes have been identified.[17,28] Sundgot-Borgen[17] found that prolonged periods of dieting, weight fluctuations, coaching changes, injury, and casual comments made about weight by coaches, parents, and friends were the most common reasons given by athletes for the development of disordered eating. Rosen and Hough[28] found that 75% of gymnasts who were told by coaches that they were overweight resorted to pathogenic weight-control techniques. Beals[21] found that 13% to 17% of adolescent volleyball players felt pressured by their coaches or parents to achieve or maintain a particular body weight. Pediatricians can help coaches and families understand that comments and recommendations they make to young athletes regarding weight may increase the risk of disordered eating. If an athlete, her parents, or her coach believes that changes in weight are indicated, they should seek medical assessment and nutritional supervision before initiating a weight-loss plan.

Menstrual Function

The spectrum of menstrual disturbances associated with the

triad can range from anovulation and luteal dysfunction to oligomenorrhea and amenorrhea (primary or secondary). Primary amenorrhea is defined as the absence of menarche by the age of 15 years.[29] The absence of other signs of pubertal development by 14 years of age or a failure to achieve menarche within 3 years of thelarche is also abnormal.[29,30] Secondary amenorrhea is defined as the absence of menses for 3 consecutive months or longer in a female after menarche. Oligomenorrhea is defined as menstrual cycles longer than 35 days. Luteal phase deficiency is defined as a menstrual cycle with a luteal phase shorter than 11 days in length or with a low concentration of progesterone. Menstrual disturbances, such as anovulation and luteal phase deficiency, are asymptomatic, making them difficult to diagnose by history alone. After excluding other causes of amenorrhea (Table 2), amenorrhea in the setting of inadequate EA is diagnosed as functional hypothalamic amenorrhea.[5] The word "functional" indicates suppression, attributable to lack of energy, of an otherwise intact reproductive endocrine axis.

Menstrual irregularities are common during adolescence and are significantly more common in adolescent athletes. Of the published studies of menstrual disturbances in adolescent athletes, only 1 study included a sedentary control group. That study reported an incidence of menstrual irregularity of 21% in sedentary adolescents compared with 54% in adolescent athletes.[9] Other studies reported menstrual disturbances in adolescent athletes ranging from 12% to 54% for any menstrual irregularity (primary or secondary amenorrhea or oligomenorrhea).[9–11,21,22,24,31,32] When evaluating specific types of menstrual irregularity, primary amenorrhea in athletes ranges from 1.2% to 6%, secondary amenorrhea ranges from 5.3% to 30%, and

TABLE 2 Causes of Secondary Amenorrhea in Adolescents

Pregnancy
Polycystic ovarian syndrome
Pituitary tumor
Prolactinoma
Hyperthyroidism
Liver/kidney disease
Medications: oral contraceptive pills, chemotherapy, antipsychotics, antidepressants, corticosteroids
Eating disorders

oligomenorrhea ranges from 5.4% to 18%.[10,15,21,22,24,31] The prevalence of anovulation and luteal phase deficiency has not been evaluated in adolescent athletes but ranges from 5.9% to 30% in adult athletes.[11]

Amenorrheic adolescent athletes have a significantly lower BMD than eumenorrheic adolescent athletes or sedentary controls.[13,31,33] Some studies have found that athletes with menstrual irregularities are as much as 3 times more likely to sustain bone stress injury and other musculoskeletal injury than are eumenorrheic athletes,[26,34–36] but this finding has not been consistent.[37] Oligomenorrhea and amenorrhea have also been associated with cardiovascular risk factors, including increased cholesterol and abnormal endothelial function.[38,39] In addition, menstrual disturbance has recently been related to decreased performance in swimmers with evidence of ovarian suppression compared with those without ovarian suppression.[40]

Bone Health

The decreased rate of bone acquisition that can be associated with the triad in adolescent athletes is particularly concerning, because bone mass gains during childhood and adolescence are critical for the attainment of maximal peak bone mass and the prevention of osteoporosis in adulthood.[6,41] The maximum rate of bone formation usually occurs between the ages of 10 and 14 years, and peak bone mass

is likely attained between the ages of 20 and 30 years.[42,43] By the end of adolescence, almost 90% of adult bone mass has been obtained.[43]

Genetics, participation in weight-bearing activities, and diet all influence bone mass in children.[44] Appropriate dietary intake and weight-bearing exercise can positively influence maximum bone mass gains during childhood and adolescence. With improved EA and resumption of menses, some "catch up" bone mass accrual may be possible in athletes with the triad; however, some will have persistently lower BMD than their genetic potential, highlighting the need for early, aggressive intervention in adolescent athletes identified with triad components.[45]

BMD in children and adolescents is typically evaluated by using dual-energy radiograph absorptiometry (DXA), which is best performed and interpreted by centers with certified clinical densitometrists with knowledge of the official pediatric positions of the International Society for Clinical Densitometry.[6,46,47] Because athletes participating in weight-bearing sports are expected to have higher BMDs than nonathletes, the American College of Sports Medicine recommends different criteria than the International Society for Clinical Densitometry, as shown in Table 3. In athletes, a Z-score below –1.0 is considered lower than expected and indicates that, even in the absence of previous fracture, secondary causes of low BMD may be present.[5] A full discussion of the secondary causes of low BMD is beyond the scope of this report, but evaluations for secondary causes typically include the items in Table 4.[48]

Measures of bone microarchitecture, although primarily used for research purposes at this juncture, can add additional information regarding bone quality beyond that of BMD. Favorable changes in bone microarchitecture are associated

TABLE 3 Definition of BMD Criteria in Adolescents

	ISCD Official Position for Children and Adolescents[46]	ACSM Guidelines for Athletes[5]
Osteoporosis	Vertebral compression fracture or Z-score ≤ −2 and clinically significant fracture history[a]	Z-Score ≤2 and clinical risk factors[b]
Low BMD	—	Z-Score −1.0 to −1.9 and clinical risk factors
Lower BMD than expected	—	Z-Score ≤ −1.0

ACSM, American College of Sports Medicine; ISCD, International Society for Clinical Densitometry.
[a] Two or more long bone fractures by age 10 or ≥3 long bone fractures at any age up to 19 years.
[b] Nutritional deficiencies, hypoestrogenism, or stress fracture.

with sports participation in female adolescents. Weight-bearing athletic activity is associated with greater total trabecular area and greater cortical perimeter in the tibia.[49] Conversely, oligomenorrhea and amenorrhea are associated with unfavorable bone microarchitecture, including lower total density, lower trabecular number, and greater trabecular separation at the tibia.[49] Estimations of bone strength indicate that eumenorrheic, but not amenorrheic, athletes have greater stiffness and load-to-failure thresholds, which are associated with decreased fracture risk, compared with nonathlete controls.[11,50]

Although it is well known that exercise is a stimulus for bone formation, data support that different types of exercise can have differing effects on bone formation. For example, adolescent and collegiate swimmers have been shown to have a similar BMD compared with nonathlete controls and to have a lower BMD compared with athletes in other sports.[48] In fact, a longitudinal BMD study in swimmers, gymnasts, and nonathlete controls over an 8-month competitive season showed that swimmers and controls had no improvement in BMD, whereas gymnasts showed significant BMD gains despite more body dissatisfaction and menstrual disturbance.[51]

Numerous studies have shown running to have a positive effect on BMD compared with inactive controls,[48] but there is emerging concern, predominantly from cross-sectional studies, that endurance

TABLE 4 Evaluation for Low BMD (BMD < −1.0)

- Serum 25-hydroxyvitamin D
- Serum calcium
- Complete blood count with differential
- Thyroid-stimulating hormone
- Parathyroid hormone
- Bone-specific alkaline phosphatase
- 24-h urine for calcium
- Screening for cortisol excess: morning cortisol or 24-h urine for cortisol
- Celiac disease: serum tissue transglutaminase antibodies, total IgA, tissue transglutaminase IgG (in the IgA-deficient adolescent)
- Markers of bone formation and resorption: serum osteocalcin and urine N-telopeptide
- Reproductive hormone evaluation: estradiol, FSH, LH in girls, testosterone in boys

FSH, follicle-stimulating hormone; IgA, immunoglobulin A; IgG, immunoglobulin G; LH, luteinizing hormone.

runners have lower BMDs than sprinters, gymnasts, and ball sport athletes.[31,51–56] Barrack et al[53] reported a higher prevalence of low BMD in adolescent endurance runners (40%) than in ball or power sport athletes (10%). This study also showed that runners 17 to 18 years of age had similar bone mineral content (BMC) compared with 13- to 14-year-old runners, whereas BMC in nonrunner athletes showed a significantly higher BMC in the older group compared with the younger group. These findings suggest a possible suppression of bone accumulation in adolescent runners, although other factors may be contributing to this finding, including possible variable bone accrual patterns attributable to genetics, rate of maturation, specific type of current and previous physical activity, and EA and menstrual differences often found between endurance runners and nonendurance athletes.[53]

Many factors are associated with an increased risk of low BMD in female adolescent athletes, including late menarche, oligomenorrhea, amenorrhea, elevated dietary

restraint, greater length of time participating in endurance sports, lower body weight, and lower BMI.[1,13,31,32,52] The deficits in BMD seen with the triad are associated with low estrogen levels and energy deficiency. Levels of bone formation and resorption markers are significantly lower in amenorrheic adolescent athletes than in nonendurance athlete controls, indicating a state of overall decreased bone turnover.[33] The restriction of EA has been shown to cause estradiol suppression and increased bone resorption as well as suppression of bone formation.[19]

A recent multisite prospective study[34] identified the contribution of single and multiple triad-related risk factors for bone stress injury in 259 female adolescents and young adults participating in competitive or recreational exercise. The authors found an increased risk of bone stress injuries as the number of triad-related risk factors increased.[34]

Cardiovascular Health

Endothelial dysfunction, measured by brachial artery flow-mediated dilation (FMD), is an important predictor of coronary endothelial dysfunction, atherosclerotic disease progression, and cardiovascular event rates.[38,57,58] Endothelial dysfunction has been correlated with low whole-body and lumbar BMD, menstrual dysfunction, and low estrogen levels in dancers and endurance athletes.[38,39] In endurance athletes, oligomenorrheic and amenorrheic athletes had impaired FMD compared with eumenorrheic athletes, with amenorrheic athletes showing the greatest impairment.[39] In this group, amenorrhea was also associated with increased total cholesterol and low-density lipoprotein levels.[39] Among professional dancers, endothelial dysfunction alone was present in 64%, whereas the prevalence of dancers with endothelial dysfunction and all 3 components of the triad was 14%.[38] All of the dancers who reported current menstrual dysfunction (36%) had reduced FMD.[38] Amenorrheic runners and dancers treated with 4 weeks of folic acid supplementation showed improvements in FMD.[15,59] Although these studies were not exclusive to adolescents, adolescents were included in the study populations. These results raise concern that an athlete diagnosed with the triad could be at risk of developing cardiovascular disease.

MALE ATHLETES

Although female athletes have been the exclusive focus of research on the triad, low EA resulting in the suppression of the neuroendocrine reproductive axis is likely not gender selective. Low testosterone and estradiol levels have been documented in adolescent males diagnosed with anorexia nervosa.[60] This finding begs the question: is there a male athlete triad? Male athletes do not have an easily noted symptom such as missed

TABLE 5 The Female Athlete Triad Coalition's Recommended Screening Questions for the Female Athlete Triad[68]

Question	Included on the Fourth-Edition PPE Form[69]
1. Do you worry about your weight or body composition?	√
2. Do you limit or carefully control the foods that you eat?	√
3. Do you try to lose weight to meet weight or image/appearance requirements in your sport?	√
4. Does your weight affect the way you feel about yourself?	—
5. Do you worry that you have lost control over how much you eat?	—
6. Do you make yourself vomit or use diuretics or laxatives after you eat?	—
7. Do you currently or have you ever suffered from an eating disorder?	√
8. Do you ever eat in secret?	
9. What age was your first menstrual period?	√
10. Do you have monthly menstrual cycles?	√
11. How many menstrual cycles have you had in the last year?	√
12. Have you ever had a stress fracture?	√

menstrual cycles, but they may show suppression of reproductive function nonetheless. There is a small body of data suggesting that male athletes with inadequate EA may also suffer from hormonal changes and low BMD. Lower testosterone levels have been found in male runners compared with inactive controls.[61] Similar to female athletes, male endurance runners have been found to have lower BMD than male athletes in power or ball sports.[62] Adolescent males with anorexia nervosa display low BMD at multiple skeletal sites.[60,63] Although the body of scientific evidence is still developing, it is important to consider that adolescent males participating in sports that emphasize and reward leanness may be at risk of a constellation of findings similar to those seen in females with components of the triad.[64–66]

SCREENING

It is convenient to screen for the triad at the time of a well-child visit and/or the preparticipation physical evaluation (PPE). The Female Athlete Triad Coalition has developed 12 questions for screening (Table 5).[67–69] Another screening tool is found in the fourth-edition PPE consensus monograph.[69] This form contains 8 of the 12 questions suggested by the

Female Athlete Triad Coalition and has been endorsed by the American Academy of Pediatrics (AAP) for use when performing the PPE (Table 5). If an athlete answers "yes" to any of the triad questions on the PPE form, the remaining questions from the Female Athlete Triad Coalition[68] can be used for further evaluation.

A sports level of participation and return-to-play medical risk stratification scoring rubric has been developed by the Female Athlete Triad Coalition Consensus Panel to help the clinician assess an athlete with triad-related risk factors into low-, moderate-, or high-risk categories. Decisions regarding sports participation, level of participation permitted, and return-to-play are made on the basis of the risk category that the athlete falls into and can be reassessed as the athlete progresses through treatment.[68]

DIAGNOSIS

Obtaining a complete nutritional, menstrual, fracture, and exercise history is the first step in diagnosis. Vital signs may reveal bradycardia, which can also be a normal finding in well-trained athletes; orthostatic hypotension; low body weight (<85% expected body weight, which is 50% for height); or low BMI (less than the fifth percentile).[68] In athletes with eating disorders, cold/discolored hands and feet, hypercarotenemia, lanugo hair, and parotid gland enlargement may be found.[5] However, the physical examination is often normal and unrevealing in athletes with the triad, especially in those who do not intentionally restrict EA.[5]

Laboratory assessment aims to evaluate for other causes of oligomenorrhea/amenorrhea, including pregnancy, polycystic ovarian syndrome, prolactinoma, and thyroid disorders, as reviewed in Table 2. In athletes with an eating disorder, a chemistry profile and electrocardiography can be used to evaluate for possible arrhythmia or metabolic disturbance. BMD testing by DXA is indicated in athletes with any of the following: eating disorder (diagnosed by using criteria of the *Diagnostic and Statistical Manual of Mental Disorders, Fifth Edition*[70]), weight <85% of expected, recent weight loss of ≥10%, menstrual dysfunction or low EA ≥6 months, and/or a history of stress or insufficiency fracture.[5,68] Table 6 lists other factors that, when coupled with a single stress fracture, increase the risk of low BMD.[48]

TREATMENT

Improving EA is the cornerstone of treatment of the triad disorders and has been associated with the return of normal menses and improvements in BMD.[5,48,60] A multidisciplinary team approach is suggested and may include a physician, a dietitian, a certified athletic trainer, a behavioral health clinician, and, at times, an exercise physiologist. It is preferable that the medical team be familiar with treating athletes. For athletes with an unintentionally low EA without features of disordered eating or an eating disorder, a behavioral health clinician may not be needed.

Improvements in EA can be accomplished by both decreasing

TABLE 6 Factors Prompting BMD Evaluation in Athletes With Stress Fracture

Low BMI (<18.5 kg/m^2)
Recurrent stress fractures
Oligo- or amenorrhea ≤6 months
A history of an ED, DE, or low EA
Chronic medical conditions associated with bone loss
Medications associated with adverse effects on bone health
Cancellous versus cortical bone fractures, particularly proximal femur, tibial plateau, and calcaneus
Cyclists, swimmers
No recent change in activity level or training intensity

ED indicates eating disorder; DE, disordered eating.
Reproduced with permission from Scofield KL, Hecht S. Bone health in endurance athletes: runners, cyclists, and swimmers. *Curr Sports Med Rep.* 2012;11(6):328–334. Copyright © 2012 by the American College of Sports Medicine.

exercise expenditure and increasing dietary intake, with the goal of restoration of normal menses and weight. Improving EA to >30 kcal/kg FFM per day can restore menses, although an EA >45 kcal/kg FFM per day is optimal.[5,71] FFM can be measured by using DXA, air-displacement plethysmography (ie, BodPod analysis [National Institute for Fitness and Sport, Indianapolis, IN]), bioelectrical impedance analysis, or skinfold caliper measurements. Evaluation by an experienced sports dietitian or exercise physiologist can be helpful in determining EA and FFM. Because the assessment of EA can be challenging, other goals of treatment can include the reversal of recent weight loss (if present), return to a body weight associated with normal menses, attainment of BMI ≥18.5 or >85% expected weight, and a minimum daily energy intake of 2000 kcal.[48,60] A gradual increase of 200 to 600 kcal/day and a reduction in training volume of 1 day per week are usually sufficient to attain the needed improvements in weight and EA.[48,71] It is important to recognize that the resumption of menses may take up to 1 year or longer after restoration of appropriate EA.[48] A written treatment plan (contract) signed by the providers and athlete/parent(s) can be a useful tool to outline and define the treatment plan and expectations on the part of the athlete, parent(s), and medical providers (for a sample contract, see the Supplementary Data in ref 48).

Studies of the effects of oral contraceptive pills on BMD have produced mixed results,[5,6,72–74] and they may give the athlete a false sense of security that EA has been restored, so their use is typically avoided unless they are being prescribed for other indications. It is important to recognize that the hormonal environment provided by oral contraceptive pills is not the same as a naturally occurring menstrual cycle. Misra et al[75] reported a significant improvement in spine and hip BMD with the use of a transdermal estrogen patch in anorexic female adolescents, indicating that the transdermal route may be a more favorable method. However, this method has not yet been studied in athletes with the triad.

Optimizing calcium and vitamin D intake is an important part of treatment.[5,6] Significantly more athletes with stress fractures have low calcium intakes than do athletes without stress fractures.[35] Assessing 25-hydroxyvitamin D concentration is useful in athletes presenting with components of the triad.[1,46] The AAP currently recommends a daily intake of 1300 mg calcium for children and adolescents ages 9 to 18 years and 600 IU vitamin D for children and adolescents ages 1 to 18 years, although many experts recommend higher intakes of vitamin D, particularly in climates where sun exposure is limited.[1] The International Osteoporosis Foundation calcium calculator can be used as a tool to estimate calcium intake from dietary sources (www. iof.org). In addition to calcium and vitamin D, other vitamins and minerals are known to play a role in bone health (B vitamins, vitamin K, and iron), thus underscoring the importance of a well-balanced diet.

Bisphosphonates are antiresorptive agents frequently used in the treatment of postmenopausal osteoporosis. Unlike postmenopausal osteoporosis, the mechanism of low BMD in athletes affected by the triad is predominantly attributable to decreased bone formation rather than increased bone resorption. Therefore, bisphosphonates would likely be less effective in athletes with the triad.[20] Other concerns regarding treatment with bisphosphonates include their long half-life and potential teratogenic effects, thus making it prudent to avoid them in females of childbearing age.[6] It is important to note that the US Food and Drug Administration has not approved any pharmacologic interventions for the treatment of osteoporosis in premenopausal females.

PREVENTION

Athletes and parents often need education regarding the importance of EA and regular menstrual cycles. Many are unaware that amenorrhea is associated with low BMD and stress fractures and how appropriate EA plays an important role in the prevention of bone health consequences.[76] The ATHENA (Athletes Targeting Healthy Exercise and Nutrition Alternatives) study evaluated the usefulness of a peer intervention on the prevention of disordered eating, pathogenic weight-control behaviors, drug use, and risk-taking behaviors.[77] This randomized controlled intervention included eight 45-minute, small-group classroom sessions guided by peer leaders. The curriculum included education regarding substance use, nutrition, and

unhealthy behaviors. Refusal skills were practiced, and healthy norms were reinforced. The control schools received pamphlets regarding disordered eating, drug use, and sports nutrition. Questionnaires administered before and after the program revealed decreased use of diet pills, decreased intent to vomit to lose weight, and improved healthy eating behaviors in the teenagers in intervention schools. This trial shows that primary intervention techniques that use education with peer leaders can reduce the risk of disordered eating and other risk-taking behaviors.

CONCLUSIONS AND GUIDANCE FOR THE CLINICIAN

1. The well-child visit or PPE provides an opportune time for the pediatrician to screen for and provide education and guidance regarding the components of the female athlete triad and the risks of inadequate EA for athletes. The AAP has published a PPE form that includes a comprehensive preparticipation history and physical evaluation (sports physical).[69] If the athlete responds "yes" to any of the triad screening questions included on the PPE history form, further screening can be performed with the use of the remaining questions suggested by the Female Athlete Triad Coalition (see Table 5).

2. Athletes presenting with 1 component of the triad are at risk of having or developing the other triad conditions.

3. Menstrual dysfunction in adolescents may be a sign of inadequate energy intake. Patients presenting with menstrual dysfunction provide an opportunity for the pediatrician to counsel parents and adolescent athletes that menstrual dysfunction and restricted energy intake are not

normal in athletes and may be detrimental to their health and performance.

4. Functional hypothalamic amenorrhea is a diagnosis of exclusion made after other causes for primary and secondary amenorrhea have been evaluated. The restoration of optimal EA is the cornerstone of treatment of functional hypothalamic amenorrhea.

5. The resumption of menses may take up to 1 year or longer after restoration of appropriate EA.

6. Oral contraceptive pills are not the first-line intervention for an athlete with functional hypothalamic amenorrhea.

7. Weight-bearing exercise in the context of appropriate nutritional intake is important for the enhancement of bone mass accrual.

8. The criteria for performing DXA to measure BMD in athletes include menstrual dysfunction or low EA (<45 kcal/kg FFM per day) for ≥6 months and/or a history of stress or insufficiency fractures. Z-Scores are used to assess BMD in adolescents, and a Z-score of < –1.0 is the threshold to prompt further evaluation (see Table 4).

9. Regular physical activity plays an important role in optimizing bone health. Patients and parents can be reassured that as long as exercise-related energy expenditures are appropriately replaced with caloric intake, menstrual, bone, and cardiovascular health should not be adversely affected. The target EA is >45 kcal/kg FFM per day. FFM can be determined by using DXA, biometrical impedance measurements, or skinfold measurements.

10. When treating athletes with the triad, a multidisciplinary team capable of addressing the medical, nutritional,

psychological, and sports participation–related issues of the triad is helpful. Weight-gain or -loss concerns in an athlete are better addressed by medical and nutritional professionals rather than athletic coaching staff.

11. Adequate intakes of calcium (1300 mg/day) and vitamin D (600 IU/day) play an important role in bone mass accrual for all adolescents. Athletes with greater dietary intake of calcium will require less supplemental calcium. When determining the amount of calcium supplementation needed, some adolescents may require higher vitamin D intakes than others to achieve normal vitamin D levels.

12. Bisphosphonate use in adolescent females with a low BMD related to the triad is not supported by current literature.

13. Educational opportunities regarding the recognition, prevention, and treatment of issues related to the triad should be available for practicing pediatricians, pediatric residents, and medical students.

LEAD AUTHORS

Amanda K. Weiss Kelly, MD, FAAP
Suzanne Hecht, MD, FACSM

COUNCIL ON SPORTS MEDICINE AND FITNESS EXECUTIVE COMMITTEE, 2014–2015

Joel S. Brenner, MD, MPH, FAAP, Chairperson
Cynthia R. LaBella, MD, FAAP, Chairperson-Elect
Margaret A. Brooks, MD, FAAP
Alex Diamond, DO, FAAP
William Hennrikus, MD, FAAP
Michele LaBotz, MD, FAAP
Kelsey Logan, MD, FAAP
Keith J. Loud, MDCM, MSc, FAAP
Kody A. Moffatt, MD, FAAP
Blaise Nemeth, MD, FAAP
Brooke Pengel, MD, FAAP
Amanda K. Weiss Kelly, MD, FAAP

LIAISONS

Andrew J.M. Gregory, MD, FAAP – *American College of Sports Medicine*
Mark Halstead, MD, FAAP – *American Medical Society for Sports Medicine*

Lisa K. Kluchurosky, MEd, ATC – *National Athletic Trainers Association*

CONSULTANTS

Neeru A. Jayanthi, MD
Rebecca Carl, MD, FAAP
Sally Harris, MD, FAAP

STAFF

Anjie Emanuel, MPH

ABBREVIATIONS

AAP: American Academy of Pediatrics
BMC: bone mineral content
BMD: bone mineral density
DXA: dual-energy radiograph absorptiometry
EA: energy availability
FFM: fat-free mass
FMD: flow-mediated dilation
PPE: preparticipation physical evaluation

REFERENCES

1. Ackerman KE, Misra M. Bone health and the female athlete triad in adolescent athletes. *Phys Sportsmed*. 2011;39(1):131–141

2. Bailey DA, McKay HA, Mirwald RL, Crocker PR, Faulkner RA. A six-year longitudinal study of the relationship of physical activity to bone mineral accrual in growing children: the University of Saskatchewan Bone Mineral Accrual Study. *J Bone Miner Res*. 1999;14(10):1672–1679

3. Sabo DF, Miller KE, Farrell MP, Melnick MJ, Barnes GM. High school athletic participation, sexual behavior and adolescent pregnancy: a regional study. *J Adolesc Health*. 1999;25(3):207–216

4. Otis CL, Drinkwater B, Johnson M, Loucks A, Wilmore J. American College of Sports Medicine position stand: the Female Athlete Triad. *Med Sci Sports Exerc*. 1997;29(5):i–ix

5. Nattiv A, Loucks AB, Manore MM, Sanborn CF, Sundgot-Borgen J, Warren MP; American College of Sports Medicine. American College of Sports Medicine position stand: the female athlete triad. *Med Sci Sports Exerc*. 2007;39(10):1867–1882

6. Golden NH, Abrams SA; Committee on Nutrition. Optimizing bone health in children and adolescents. *Pediatrics*. 2014;134(4). Available at: www.pediatrics. org/cgi/content/full/134/4/e1229

7. Bennell, Malcolm SA, Thomas SA, et al. Risk factors for stress fractures in track and field athletes: a twelve-month prospective study. *Am J Sports Med*. 1996;24(2):810–818

8. Nattiv A, Puffer JC, Casper J, Dorey F. Stress fracture risk factors, incidence and distribution: a 3-year prospective study in collegiate runners [abstract]. *Med Sci Sports Exerc*. 2000;5(Suppl):S347

9. Hoch AZ, Pajewski NM, Moraski L, et al. Prevalence of the female athlete triad in high school athletes and sedentary students. *Clin J Sport Med*. 2009;19(5):421–428

10. Nichols JF, Rauh MJ, Lawson MJ, Ji M, Barkai HS. Prevalence of the female athlete triad syndrome among high school athletes. *Arch Pediatr Adolesc Med*. 2006;160(2):137–142

11. Barrack MT, Ackerman KE, Gibbs JC. Update on the female athlete triad. *Curr Rev Musculoskelet Med*. 2013;6(2):195–204

12. Fredericson M, Kent K. Normalization of bone density in a previously amenorrheic runner with osteoporosis. *Med Sci Sports Exerc*. 2005;37(9):1481–1486

13. Gibbs JC, Williams NI, De Souza MJ. Prevalence of individual and combined components of the female athlete triad. *Med Sci Sports Exerc*. 2013;45(5):985–996

14. Hind K. Recovery of bone mineral density and fertility in a former amenorrheic athlete. *J Sports Sci Med*. 2008;7(3):415–418

15. Hoch AZ, Papanek PE, Havlik HS, Raasch WG, Widlansky ME, Schimke JE. Prevalence of the female athlete triad/tetrad in professional ballet dancers [abstract]. *Med Sci Sports Exerc*. 2009;41(5):524

16. Porucanik CA, Sullivan MM, Nunu J, Joy E. Physician recognition, evaluation and treatment of the female athlete triad [abstract]. *Med Sci Sports Exerc*. 2009;41(5):83

17. Sundgot-Borgen J. Risk and trigger factors for the development of eating disorders in female elite athletes. *Med Sci Sports Exerc.* 1994;26(4):414–419

18. Loucks AB, Thuma JR. Luteinizing hormone pulsatility is disrupted at a threshold of energy availability in regularly menstruating women. *J Clin Endocrinol Metab.* 2003;88(1):297–311

19. Ihle R, Loucks AB. Dose-response relationships between energy availability and bone turnover in young exercising women. *J Bone Miner Res.* 2004;19(8):1231–1240

20. Misra M, Klibanski A. Bone metabolism in adolescents with anorexia nervosa. *J Endocrinol Invest.* 2011;34(4):324–332

21. Beals KA. Eating behaviors, nutritional status, and menstrual function in elite female adolescent volleyball players. *J Am Diet Assoc.* 2002;102(9):1293–1296

22. Nichols JF, Rauh MJ, Barrack MT, Barkai HS, Pernick Y. Disordered eating and menstrual irregularity in high school athletes in lean-build and nonlean-build sports. *Int J Sport Nutr Exerc Metab.* 2007;17(4):364–377

23. Rosendahl J, Bormann B, Aschenbrenner K, Aschenbrenner F, Strauss B. Dieting and disordered eating in German high school athletes and non-athletes. *Scand J Med Sci Sports.* 2009;19(5):731–739

24. Havemann L, DeLange Z, Pieterse K, Wright HH. Disordered eating and menstrual patterns in female university netball players. *South African J Sports Med.* 2011;23(3):68–72

25. Cobb KL, Bachrach LK, Greendale G, et al. Disordered eating, menstrual irregularity, and bone mineral density in female runners. *Med Sci Sports Exerc.* 2003;35(5):711–719

26. Rauh MJ, Nichols JF, Barrack MT. Relationships among injury and disordered eating, menstrual dysfunction, and low bone mineral density in high school athletes: a prospective study. *J Athl Train.* 2010;45(3):243–252

27. Thein-Nissenbaum JM, Rauh MJ, Carr KE, Loud KJ, McGuine TA. Associations between disordered eating, menstrual dysfunction, and musculoskeletal injury among high school athletes. *J Orthop Sports Phys Ther.* 2011;41(2):60–69

28. Rosen LW, Hough DO. Pathogenic weight-control behavior of female college gymnasts. *Phys Sportsmed.* 1988;16(9):141–144

29. American College of Obstetricians and Gynecologists Committee on Adolescent Health Care. ACOG Committee Opinion No. 349, November 2006: menstruation in girls and adolescents: using the menstrual cycle as a vital sign. *Obstet Gynecol.* 2006;108(5):1323–1328

30. Diaz A, Laufer MR, Breech LL; American Academy of Pediatrics Committee on Adolescence; American College of Obstetricians and Gynecologists Committee on Adolescent Health Care. Menstruation in girls and adolescents: using the menstrual cycle as a vital sign. *Pediatrics.* 2006;118(5):2245–2250

31. Barrack MT, Rauh MJ, Nichols JF. Prevalence of and traits associated with low BMD among female adolescent runners. *Med Sci Sports Exerc.* 2008;40(12):2015–2021

32. Gibbs JC, Nattiv A, Barrack MT, et al. Low bone density risk is higher in exercising women with multiple triad risk factors. *Med Sci Sports Exerc.* 2014;46(1):167–176

33. Christo K, Prabhakaran R, Lamparello B, et al. Bone metabolism in adolescent athletes with amenorrhea, athletes with eumenorrhea, and control subjects. *Pediatrics.* 2008;121(6):1127–1136

34. Barrack MT, Gibbs JC, De Souza MJ, et al. Higher incidence of bone stress injuries with increasing female athlete triad-related risk factors: a prospective multisite study of exercising girls and women. *Am J Sports Med.* 2014;42(4):949–958

35. Myburgh KH, Hutchins J, Fataar AB, Hough SF, Noakes TD. Low bone density is an etiologic factor for stress fractures in athletes. *Ann Intern Med.* 1990;113(10):754–759

36. Thein-Nissenbaum JM, Rauh MJ, Carr KE, Loud KJ, McGuine TA. Menstrual irregularity and musculoskeletal injury in female high school athletes. *J Athl Train.* 2012;47(1):74–82

37. Duckham RL, Peirce N, Meyer C, Summers GD, Cameron N, Brooke-Wavell K. Risk factors for stress fracture in female endurance athletes: a cross-sectional study. *BMJ Open.* 2012;2(6):e001920

38. Hoch AZ, Papanek P, Szabo A, Widlansky ME, Schimke JE, Gutterman DD. Association between the female athlete triad and endothelial dysfunction in dancers. *Clin J Sport Med.* 2011;21(2):119–125

39. Rickenlund A, Eriksson MJ, Schenck-Gustafsson K, Hirschberg AL. Amenorrhea in female athletes is associated with endothelial dysfunction and unfavorable lipid profile. *J Clin Endocrinol Metab.* 2005;90(3):1354–1359

40. Vanheest JL, Rodgers CD, Mahoney CE, De Souza MJ. Ovarian suppression impairs sport performance in junior elite female swimmers. *Med Sci Sports Exerc.* 2014;46(1):156–166

41. NIH Consensus Development Panel on Osteoporosis Prevention, Diagnosis, and Therapy. Osteoporosis prevention, diagnosis, and therapy. *JAMA.* 2001;285(6):785–795

42. Bonjour JP, Theintz G, Buchs B, Slosman D, Rizzoli R. Critical years and stages of puberty for spinal and femoral bone mass accumulation during adolescence. *J Clin Endocrinol Metab.* 1991;73(3):555–563

43. Sabatier JP, Guaydier-Souquières G, Laroche D, et al. Bone mineral acquisition during adolescence and early adulthood: a study in 574 healthy females 10-24 years of age. *Osteoporos Int.* 1996;6(2):141–148

44. Slemenda CW, Miller JZ, Hui SL, Reister TK, Johnston CC Jr. Role of physical activity in the development of skeletal mass in children. *J Bone Miner Res.* 1991;6(11):1227–1233

45. Barrack MT, Van Loan MD, Rauh MJ, Nichols JF. Body mass, training, menses, and bone in adolescent runners: a 3-yr follow-up. *Med Sci Sports Exerc.* 2011;43(6):959–966

46. Gordon CM, Leonard MB, Zemel BS; International Society for Clinical Densitometry. 2013 Pediatric Position Development Conference: executive summary and reflections. *J Clin Densitom.* 2014;17(2):219–224

47. Schousboe JT, Shepherd JA, Bilezikian JP, Baim S. Executive summary of the 2013 International Society for Clinical Densitometry Position Development

Conference on bone densitometry. *J Clin Densitom*. 2013;16(4):455–466

48. Scofield KL, Hecht S. Bone health in endurance athletes: runners, cyclists, and swimmers. *Curr Sports Med Rep*. 2012;11(6):328–334

49. Ackerman KE, Nazem T, Chapko D, et al. Bone microarchitecture is impaired in adolescent amenorrheic athletes compared with eumenorrheic athletes and nonathletic controls. *J Clin Endocrinol Metab*. 2011;96(10):3123–3133

50. Boutroy S, Bouxsein ML, Munoz F, Delmas PD. In vivo assessment of trabecular bone microarchitecture by high-resolution peripheral quantitative computed tomography. *J Clin Endocrinol Metab*. 2005;90(12):6508–6515

51. Taaffe DR, Robinson TL, Snow CM, Marcus R. High-impact exercise promotes bone gain in well-trained female athletes. *J Bone Miner Res*. 1997;12(2):255–260

52. Barrack MT, Rauh MJ, Barkai HS, Nichols JF. Dietary restraint and low bone mass in female adolescent endurance runners. *Am J Clin Nutr*. 2008;87(1):36–43

53. Barrack MT, Rauh MJ, Nichols JF. Cross-sectional evidence of suppressed bone mineral accrual among female adolescent runners. *J Bone Miner Res*. 2010;25(8):1850–1857

54. Mudd LM, Fornetti W, Pivarnik JM. Bone mineral density in collegiate female athletes: comparisons among sports. *J Athl Train*. 2007;42(3):403–408

55. Nichols JF, Rauh MJ, Barrack MT, Barkai HS. Bone mineral density in female high school athletes: interactions of menstrual function and type of mechanical loading. *Bone*. 2007;41(3):371–377

56. Tenforde AS, Fredericson M. Influence of sports participation on bone health in the young athlete: a review of the literature. *PM R*. 2011;3(9):861–867

57. Anderson TJ, Uehata A, Gerhard MD, et al. Close relation of endothelial function in the human coronary and peripheral circulations. *J Am Coll Cardiol*. 1995;26(5):1235–1241

58. Schächinger V, Britten MB, Zeiher AM. Prognostic impact of coronary vasodilator dysfunction on adverse long-term outcome of coronary heart disease. *Circulation*. 2000;101(16):1899–1906

59. Hoch AZ, Lynch SL, Jurva JW, Schimke JE, Gutterman DD. Folic acid supplementation improves vascular function in amenorrheic runners. *Clin J Sport Med*. 2010;20(3):205–210

60. Misra M, Prabhakaran R, Miller KK, et al. Weight gain and restoration of menses as predictors of bone mineral density change in adolescent girls with anorexia nervosa-1. *J Clin Endocrinol Metab*. 2008;93(4):1231–1237

61. De Souza MJ, Arce JC, Pescatello LS, Scherzer HS, Luciano AA. Gonadal hormones and semen quality in male runners: a volume threshold effect of endurance training. *Int J Sports Med*. 1994;15(7):383–391

62. Fredericson M, Chew K, Ngo J, Cleek T, Kiratli J, Cobb K. Regional bone mineral density in male athletes: a comparison of soccer players, runners and controls. *Br J Sports Med*. 2007;41(10):664–668

63. Castro J, Toro J, Lazaro L, Pons F, Halperin I. Bone mineral density in male adolescents with anorexia nervosa. *J Am Acad Child Adolesc Psychiatry*. 2002;41(5):613–618

64. Miller BE, Hackney AC, De Souza MJ. The endurance training on hormone and semen profiles in marathon runners. *Fertil Steril*. 1997;67(3):585–586; author reply: 586–587

65. Hackney AC. Endurance exercise training and reproductive endocrine dysfunction in men: alterations in the hypothalamic-pituitary-testicular axis. *Curr Pharm Des*. 2001;7(4):261–273

66. Hackney AC. Effects of endurance exercise on the reproductive system of men: the "exercise-hypogonadal male condition". *J Endocrinol Invest*. 2008;31(10):932–938

67. Mountjoy M, Hutchinson M, Cruz L, Lebrun C. Female athlete triad screening questionnaire. Female Athlete Triad Coalition. Available at: www.femaleathletetriad.org/~triad/wp-content/uploads/2008/11/ppe_for_website.pdf. Accessed July 15, 2015

68. De Souza MJ, Nattiv A, Joy E, et al; Expert Panel. 2014 Female Athlete Triad Coalition consensus statement on treatment and return to play of the female athlete triad. *Br J Sports Med*. 2014;48(4):289–309

69. American Academy of Family Physicians; American Academy of Pediatrics; American College of Sports Medicine. In: Roberts W, Bernhardt D, eds. *Preparticipation Physical Evaluation*. 4th ed. Elk Grove Village, IL: American Academy of Pediatrics; 2010

70. American Psychiatric Association. *Diagnostic and Statistical Manual of Mental Disorders, Fifth Edition*. Washington, DC: American Psychiatric Publishing; 2013

71. Kopp-Woodroffe SA, Manore MM, Dueck CA, Skinner JS, Matt KS. Energy and nutrient status of amenorrheic athletes participating in a diet and exercise training intervention program. *Int J Sport Nutr*. 1999;9(1):70–88

72. Cobb KL, Bachrach LK, Sowers M, et al. The effect of oral contraceptives on bone mass and stress fractures in female runners. *Med Sci Sports Exerc*. 2007;39(9):1464–1473

73. Golden NH, Lanzkowsky L, Schebendach J, Palestro CJ, Jacobson MS, Shenker IR. The effect of estrogen-progestin treatment on bone mineral density in anorexia nervosa. *J Pediatr Adolesc Gynecol*. 2002;15(3):135–143

74. Warren MP, Brooks-Gunn J, Fox RP, et al. Persistent osteopenia in ballet dancers with amenorrhea and delayed menarche despite hormone therapy: a longitudinal study. *Fertil Steril*. 2003;80(2):398–404

75. Misra M, Katzman D, Miller KK, et al. Physiologic estrogen replacement increases bone density in adolescent girls with anorexia nervosa. *J Bone Miner Res*. 2011;26(10):2430–2438

76. Feldmann JM, Belsha JP, Eissa MA, Middleman AB. Female adolescent athletes' awareness of the connection between menstrual status and bone health. *J Pediatr Adolesc Gynecol*. 2011;24(5):311–314

77. Elliot DL, Goldberg L, Moe EL, et al. Long-term outcomes of the ATHENA (Athletes Targeting Healthy Exercise & Nutrition Alternatives) program for female high school athletes. *J Alcohol Drug Educ*. 2008;52(2):73–92

Financing Graduate Medical Education to Meet the Needs of Children and the Future Pediatrician Workforce

- *Policy Statement*

POLICY STATEMENT Organizational Principles to Guide and Define the Child Health
Care System and/or Improve the Health of all Children

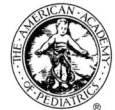

American Academy
of Pediatrics

DEDICATED TO THE HEALTH OF ALL CHILDREN™

Financing Graduate Medical Education to Meet the Needs of Children and the Future Pediatrician Workforce

COMMITTEE ON PEDIATRIC WORKFORCE

abstract

The American Academy of Pediatrics (AAP) believes that an appropriately financed graduate medical education (GME) system is critical to ensuring that sufficient numbers of trained pediatricians are available to provide optimal health care to all children. A shortage of pediatric medical subspecialists and pediatric surgical specialists currently exists in the United States, and this shortage is likely to intensify because of the growing numbers of children with chronic health problems and special health care needs. It is equally important to maintain the supply of primary care pediatricians. The AAP, therefore, recommends that children's hospital GME positions funded by the Health Resources and Services Administration be increased to address this escalating demand for pediatric health services. The AAP also recommends that GME funding for pediatric physician training provide full financial support for all years of training necessary to meet program requirements. In addition, all other entities that gain from GME training should participate in its funding in a manner that does not influence curriculum, requirements, or outcomes. Furthermore, the AAP supports funding for training innovations that improve the health of children. Finally, the AAP recommends that all institutional recipients of GME funding allocate these funds directly to the settings where training occurs in a transparent manner.

DOI: 10.1542/peds.2016-0211

PEDIATRICS (ISSN Numbers: Print, 0031-4005; Online, 1098-4275).

Copyright © 2016 by the American Academy of Pediatrics

To cite: AAP COMMITTEE ON PEDIATRIC WORKFORCE. Financing Graduate Medical Education to Meet the Needs of Children and the Future Pediatrician Workforce. *Pediatrics.* 2016;137(4):e20160211

Graduate medical education (GME) is a public good that ensures the sustained availability of a highly skilled pediatric workforce, including primary care pediatricians, pediatric medical subspecialists, and pediatric surgical specialists (as a group henceforth referred to as "pediatric physicians"), and increases the availability of health care for all children. It is the "hands-on" training phase of physician education that occurs after graduation from medical school before entering clinical practice. At least 3 years of GME training are required to be eligible for board certification in general pediatrics, and additional years of fellowship training are required to be eligible for certification in pediatric medical subspecialties. Pediatric surgical specialists begin their GME training in surgery but must also complete fellowship training in their desired pediatric surgical specialty. Fellowship training requirements vary by specialty, but at least 3 years of training are usually required. Although the Accreditation Council for Graduate Medical Education broadly determines the curriculum for GME training, GME funding policies affect the availability of training positions. Funding for GME also plays an essential role in improving access to pediatric care, because trainees provide valuable medical services under faculty supervision, frequently to underserved populations, during their training. Teaching hospitals are a safety net for the poor and uninsured and provide approximately 37% of all charity care nationwide.[1] Without adequate GME funding, there will be insufficient GME positions to remediate current, and prevent future, pediatric physician workforce shortages and provide the opportunity for all US medical graduates to complete their GME training.[2] Although US medical schools have increased their enrollment to address workforce shortages, there has not been a commensurate increase in GME positions. Without an increase in GME positions, it is likely that the increased competition for the limited number of GME positions will decrease the opportunities for international medical graduates (IMGs) to enter GME training as well, which has several implications for the physician workforce. For example, IMGs are more likely to practice in medically underserved areas than are graduates of US medical schools. IMGs also increase the diversity of the physician workforce, because they are more

likely to be of Asian or Hispanic descent than are US medical school graduates. It has also been suggested that decreased opportunities for IMGs will have a detrimental effect on countries that have benefited from returning physicians who have been trained in the United States.[3]

CURRENT SOURCES OF GME FUNDING

Although GME is an essential public investment in the future physician workforce, less than 1% of the $1.4 trillion in federal and state expenditures on health care is allocated to GME.[4] It is estimated that the cost to hospitals for training a resident averages $100 000 or more per year.[5] For most teaching hospitals in the United States, the largest source of GME funding is from the Centers for Medicare and Medicaid Services (CMS), but for pediatric training programs that are based at a children's hospital the major sources of GME funding are the Children's Hospital Graduate Medical Education (CHGME) Payment Program and Medicaid. All of these sources of funding are considered in this policy statement.

Total federal GME funding amounts to nearly $16 billion annually. Medicare is the largest federal government contributor to GME, providing $9.5 billion (almost $3 billion for direct graduate medical education [DGME]) to pay the salaries of residents and supervising physicians, and approximately $6.5 billion for indirect medical education (IME) to subsidize the higher costs that hospitals incur when they run training programs. Federal Medicaid spending adds another $2 billion for GME, and an additional $4 billion comes from the Veterans Health Administration and the Health Resources and Services Administration.[6]

In fiscal year 2012, the CMS provided $2.7 billion in DGME funding and $6.7 billion in IME to teaching

hospitals.[7] The DGME funding is hospital-specific and based on the institution's Medicare patient population and its resident-to-bed ratio. The CMS only provides "full" DGME payments for the initial residency period (IRP) required for a trainee to become eligible for board certification in the specialty in which the resident first begins training. IRP for a specialty is based on the minimum accredited length of a residency program, as determined by the Accreditation Council for Graduate Medical Education, which is 3 years for general pediatrics. After this IRP, any additional training, such as fellowship training (eg, in a pediatric medical subspecialty or surgical subspecialty), is funded at the 50% level. The IME payments are based, in part, on the number of trainees and the number of Medicare patients receiving care at the teaching hospital. Training outside of the teaching hospital and its clinics (eg, private physician offices) or time spent in scholarly and didactic activities usually does not qualify for payment even when such training is mandated by training requirements.

Despite increasing evidence of physician shortages in the United States, the Balanced Budget Act of 1997 (Pub L No. 105-33) capped the number of residents funded by Medicare at the number of full-time equivalent residents enrolled in a hospital's training program in 1996.[8,9] The Institute of Medicine (IOM), in its 2014 report, "Graduate Medical Education That Meets the Nation's Health Needs," called for maintaining GME support at the current level.[10] In contrast, the American Medical Association, Council on Graduate Medical Education, and Council of Medical Specialty Societies have all recommended increased funding for GME and expanding the number of GME trainee positions funded by Medicare. In its 21st report, the Council on Graduate Medical Education recommended that the number of trainee positions be increased to provide GME training for the additional 3000 medical school graduates who will need trainee positions because of the expansion of medical school enrollment in the United States.[11,12] The Association of American Medical Colleges has recommended that the number of federally supported GME training positions be increased by at least 4000 and that half of these positions be allocated to primary care.[13] The American Academy of Family Physicians (AAFP) has also recommended preferentially funding increased trainee positions for generalist physicians, particularly family physicians, with concomitantly less funding for the training of other physicians.[14] The American College of Physicians (ACP) also has recommended that GME funding by CMS place a priority on primary care.[15]

States support GME through nearly $4 billion in Medicaid spending. The federal government does not require state Medicaid programs to provide GME funding, but in 42 states and the District of Columbia Medicaid programs made GME payments in 2012. The federal government also does not have explicit guidelines on how these payments should be made. However, a number of states link Medicaid DGME and IME payments to state policy goals, such as encouraging training in primary care, increasing the supply of physicians who care for those insured by Medicaid, and improving the geographic distribution of the physician workforce. Attention to these state goals has been emphasized as states work to implement the Affordable Care Act (Pub L No. 111-148 [2010]).[10] In 2012, 40 states and the District of Columbia made GME payments under the Medicaid fee-for-service program, and 12 of these states used methods similar to those of the Medicare program to allocate

funding. Sixty-five percent of the 36 states and the District of Columbia with risk-based Medicaid managed care programs also provide some GME funding through a variety of methodologies (for current information on your state, please contact the American Academy of Pediatrics' [AAP's] Division of State Government Affairs at stgov@aap. org). These payments are primarily made directly to teaching hospitals, but a few states also make payments to nonhospital teaching sites or medical schools.[16]

Freestanding children's hospitals receive little or no GME support from Medicare, because they do not provide care for the elderly. In 1999, the CHGME program was enacted to address this disparity in federal GME support between freestanding children's hospitals and other teaching hospitals. Since its enactment, funding from the CHGME program has helped support the training of primary care pediatricians, pediatric medical subspecialists, and pediatric surgical subspecialists through an annual appropriation. More than 50 US children's hospitals currently participate in the program,[17] which is critical for maintaining an adequate pediatrician workforce, because 49% of primary care pediatricians and 51% of pediatric medical subspecialists receive their GME training at children's hospitals.[18]

Unfortunately, unlike Medicare GME funding, Congress must appropriate funds annually for the CHGME program, and each year established programs are unsure whether sufficient funds will be available to continue their programs. Because the duration of pediatric GME training is 3 to 6 years, trainees in children's hospitals could potentially lose their positions if there is a decrease in appropriations for CHGME. This lack of stable funding (eg, time-limited grant funding) is also a disincentive for children's hospitals to maintain

or expand their training programs. These issues are also noted in the IOM report on financing GME, which supported a stable and equitable source of Medicare funding for pediatric residents in freestanding children's hospitals.[10]

Title VII of the Public Health Service Act (42 USC 6A §201 [1944]) helps fund residency education in general pediatrics, internal medicine, and family practice by providing training grants in primary care medicine and dentistry. These grants provide the authority and funding for faculty development, academic administrative units, predoctoral training, and intensive primary care training for residents in diverse ambulatory settings. In 2012, $38.9 million was provided for these programs.[7]

Other federal sources for GME funding include the Teaching Health Centers GME Payment Program, which provides DME and IME funding for primary care residency programs that are sponsored by qualified teaching health centers. The Teaching Health Centers GME Payment Program is a $230-million, 5-year initiative that began in 2011 to support more primary care residents and dentists trained in community-based ambulatory patient care settings. Payments are made for direct expenses associated with sponsoring an approved graduate medical or dental residency training program and for indirect expenses associated with the additional costs relating to training residents in such programs. As of August 2014, however, only 3 of the >60 programs funded have been in pediatrics.[18,19] The Maternal and Child Health Bureau also provides funding to institutions of higher learning for leadership training of physicians and other health care professionals in the areas of teaching, research, clinical practice, public health administration and policy making, and community-based programs in maternal and child health.[20] In fiscal year 2013, the Division of Maternal and Child Health Workforce Development awarded 151 grants, an investment of $47 million. The National Institutes of Health sponsors a limited number of subspecialty training positions and, through research grants, provides funding for some resident research activities. The federal government also indirectly supports GME training through a variety of scholarships and loan repayment programs. Other nonfederal sources of pediatric GME funding include teaching institutions as well as payments for medical services to medical school practice plans and physician groups associated with teaching hospitals that fund GME positions that exceed the Medicare cap or trainees in fellowship programs that are not fully funded. States may also provide additional funding not tied to Medicaid, such as resident scholarships and funding to begin or expand training programs.

The current system of funding GME relies heavily on federal support from the CMS and provides insufficient financial support to ensure that all children have access to optimal health care provided by a pediatric physician. Therefore, additional sources of revenue are needed. Because the health care industry gains from a well-trained pediatrician workforce, funding sources logically should include hospitals, health care systems, health maintenance organizations, the pharmaceutical industry, private and public insurers, durable medical equipment companies, health care information technology companies, and others.

THE EFFECT OF GME FINANCING POLICY ON THE PHYSICIAN WORKFORCE

In its recent report, the Macy Foundation recommended that the goal of GME funding should be to produce an adequate and competent physician workforce

with the appropriate specialty mix.[21] Both the ACP and the AAFP also have recommended that GME funding be allocated in a manner that addresses the nation's physician workforce needs.[14,15] Under the current Medicare guidelines, training programs can use their GME funding for any accredited program, regardless of the physician workforce needs in their community. In addition, there is no requirement that training programs provide data on their program graduates, which could be used to assess the effectiveness of each program's efforts to address physician shortages. A recent analysis of the trainee positions that were expanded as a result of the redistribution of Medicare GME funding under the Medicare Modernization Act (Pub L No. 108-173 [2003]) revealed that these positions were allocated by teaching hospitals to non–primary care positions rather than the primary care specialties, which have the greatest shortages of physicians. This trend in allocation of GME positions shows that, without guidelines, teaching hospitals may not use additional GME funding in a manner that addresses the physician workforce needs of their community or the nation but rather expand positions in specialties that serve the needs of the teaching hospital.[22] Under the Affordable Care Act, redistribution of unused positions now must be prioritized to training positions in primary care and general surgery programs, which are specialties with physician shortages.

The IOM report listed 6 important goals, some of which are, at least in part, in concert with the positions of the Macy Foundation, the AAFP, and the ACP. In brief, these goals aim to achieve the following:

1. to encourage the production of a physician workforce that is better prepared to work within, lead, and improve the health care delivery

system that provides better care at a lower cost;

2. to encourage innovation in GME programs;

3. to create transparency and accountability of GME programs with respect to the stewardship of public funding;

4. to clarify and strengthen public policy planning and oversight of GME with reference to public funding;

5. to use public funds for GME in a rational, efficient, and effective manner; and

6. to avoid unintended negative effects of planned transitions in GME funding methods.[10]

These IOM goals, especially the ones pertaining to innovations in GME training, as well as improved transparency and accountability, should be encouraged.

From these laudable goals stemmed 5 complex recommendations that focus on GME training from the prevailing adult medicine perspective. The IOM recommendations, and not the goals, are intended to influence congressional proposals for GME reform and would require enabling legislation before they could be implemented. Because the AAP believes that any changes in public policy pertaining to financing GME must address current and future pediatric training needs and the IOM recommendations do not directly address pediatric GME funding issues or pediatric physician workforce shortages, the AAP is, therefore, unable to support all of the IOM recommendations at this time.

There is currently a shortage of pediatric medical subspecialists and pediatric surgical specialists in the United States, and this shortage is likely to increase because of the increasing number of children who have significant chronic health problems and special health care needs.[23] Despite this shortage, the current limitation on the duration of full Medicare GME funding to the IRP has created a financial barrier to expanding pediatric medical subspecialty and surgical specialty trainee positions, because the DME funding from Medicare that is available for these fellowship training years is 50% of the level provided for their IRP in general pediatrics or surgery. For similar reasons, direct GME payments from Medicare for some combined specialty programs that are recognized by the American Board of Pediatrics and other specialty boards to provide GME (eg, Pediatrics-Genetics) are limited, because the duration of these programs is longer than the IRP of 3 years that is required for certification in general pediatrics. This lack of support requires teaching institutions to find funding for these positions from patient care revenues, grants, and private sources. Unfortunately, these alternative sources are most likely to result in additional trainee positions in adult medicine specialties and subspecialties, which generate the largest amount of revenue for the teaching institution, rather than fields in which there are the greatest physician shortages. The AAP maintains that increasing the number of fully funded residency training positions directed toward pediatric surgical specialties, child psychiatry, pediatric medical subspecialties, and general pediatrics (a pipeline to further pediatric medical subspecialty training) could improve access to care and enhance pediatric health.

THE EFFECT OF GME FINANCING POLICY ON EDUCATIONAL EXPERIENCES

The current GME funding structure creates a financial barrier to providing trainees with all of the educational activities that contribute to a high-quality graduate training experience. Because most GME funding is based, in part, on the number of trainees and the number of Medicare patients receiving care at the teaching hospitals of the sponsoring institution, there is a financial disincentive for training institutions to allow residents to train outside of their teaching hospital and to appropriately fund the faculty and institutions that provide these nonhospital educational experiences, including private physician practices, public health clinics, and international health care sites. GME funding should flow to the site where training occurs on the basis of the amount of time a resident spends in each setting so that these nonhospital training opportunities can offset the costs they incur for GME training and have sufficient resources to provide a high-quality educational experience. There is also a financial disincentive for sponsoring institutions to provide residents with nonclinical scholarly and didactic experiences, even though these experiences are required for accreditation and are essential aspects of training.

Finally, there is no requirement that training programs provide outcome data that could determine their effectiveness in addressing physician shortages by graduating residents who ultimately practice in underserved communities, including rural areas. Without this information, it is difficult to redirect GME funding to programs that are most successful in addressing physician shortages. In addition, training institutions are not required to provide data on how the funding they receive is used. For example, a portion of GME funding should be used to support the training of faculty in both academic and nonacademic settings and the infrastructure needed to provide high-quality educational experiences, such as simulation laboratories, telemedicine experiences, and public health opportunities. Unless training institutions are required to provide utilization data, it is not possible to know whether GME funding is adequately used to support teaching faculty and provide high-quality educational opportunities as well as other activities that are directly related to the education of residents, payment of faculty, and clinical training sites rather than for other unrelated hospital purposes.

SUMMARY

GME is a public good that ensures the sustained availability of a highly skilled pediatric workforce and increases the availability of health care for all children. The current system of funding GME (including backing from both the CMS and the Health Resources and Services Administration for CHGME) provides insufficient financial support to address the current and future pediatrician workforce needs of the nation's infants, children, adolescents, and young adults. Current GME funding also fails to meet the increasing demand for pediatric services and does not adequately support training in all settings. Current shortages of pediatric physicians are likely to continue if funding remains at current levels. To address this potential shortage and ensure a well-trained pediatric physician workforce, the AAP recommends increased public funding of GME so that all pediatric physician trainees, including pediatric medical and surgical subspecialty fellows, are fully funded for the duration of their training. Entities that gain from an appropriately trained pediatrician workforce should contribute funding for GME training without an expectation of being able to influence curriculum or training requirements or outcomes of GME. The allocation of both the public and private GME funding must be transparent and documented to ensure that the funds are being used appropriately for GME training and distributed in a manner that addresses the current and future pediatrician workforce needs of the United States.

RECOMMENDATIONS

Because GME training is a public good that is essential to the production of pediatricians who practice the highest-quality patient-centered care and to increase the availability of health care for all children and their families, including the underserved and those with special health care needs, the AAP recommends that

1. GME training for all pediatric physician trainees, including pediatric medical subspecialists and pediatric surgical specialists, be fully funded for the full length of training required to meet the standards of each of these pediatric and pediatric medical subspecialty and pediatric surgical specialty programs;

2. all entities in the health care industry that gain from a well-trained pediatrician workforce, including government, hospitals, health care systems, health maintenance organizations, the pharmaceutical industry, private and public insurers, medical device and equipment companies, health information technology companies, and others, contribute funding for GME training without being able to influence the curriculum, training requirements, or outcomes of GME;

3. funding for GME programs that are sponsored by freestanding children's hospitals be provided in a stable manner and at a similar level as GME programs that are sponsored by other teaching hospitals and related institutions;

4. GME funding be allocated in a manner that addresses the current and future pediatrician workforce needs to meet the current and future health care needs of children in the United States;

5. GME funding from Medicare, Medicaid, CHGME, and all others who gain from GME be allocated for the time trainees spend in their scholarly and didactic activities and all clinical experiences (inpatient and ambulatory), including all educational activities required by accrediting agencies;

6. full GME funding be available for combined specialty programs that are recognized by the American Board of Pediatrics and other specialty boards to provide GME in a particular combined specialty (eg, Internal Medicine-Pediatrics, Pediatrics-Genetics);

7. funding for GME support the education of trainees in all settings and flow to the site where the training occurs;

8. GME funding be allocated in a transparent manner so that funders can assess whether the funds have been used appropriately for GME training;

9. the number of funded pediatric GME positions be increased to address the current and ongoing pediatrician workforce needs of the nation and the increasing demand for pediatric services; and

10. changes in public policy pertaining to financing GME address current and future pediatric training needs.

LEAD AUTHOR

Mary Ellen Rimsza, MD, FAAP

CONTRIBUTING AUTHORS

Andrew J. Hotaling, MD, FAAP
Harold K. Simon, MD, FAAP

COMMITTEE ON PEDIATRIC WORKFORCE, 2015-2016

William B. Moskowitz, MD, FAAP, Chairperson
Christopher E. Harris, MD, FAAP
Andrew J. Hotaling, MD, FAAP
James P. Marcin, MD, MPH, FAAP
Thomas W. Pendergrass, MD, MSPH, FAAP
Harold K. Simon, MD, FAAP

LIAISONS

Michelle M. Macias, MD, FAAP – *AAP Section Forum Management Committee*
Laurel K. Leslie MD, MPH, FAAP – *American Board of Pediatrics*

PAST COMMITTEE MEMBERS

William T. Basco, MD, MS, FAAP
Mary E. Keown, MD, FAAP
Mary Ellen Rimsza, MD, FAAP
Ted D. Sigrest, MD, FAAP
Gail A. McGuinness, MD, FAAP - Liaison, American Board of Pediatrics

STAFF

Holly J. Mulvey, MA

ABBREVIATIONS

AAFP: American Academy of Family Physicians
AAP: American Academy of Pediatrics
ACP: American College of Physicians
CHGME: children's hospital graduate medical education
CMS: Centers for Medicare and Medicaid Services
DGME: direct graduate medical education
GME: graduate medical education
IME: indirect medical education
IMG: international medical graduate
IOM: Institute of Medicine
IRP: initial residency period

REFERENCES

1. Association of American Medical Colleges. Proportion of charity care provided at COTH, other teaching, and non-teaching hospitals, 2012. Updated 2014. Available at: https://www.aamc.org/download/376938/data/proportionofcharitycareprovidedatcothotherteachingandnonteachin.pptx. Accessed April 8, 2015

2. Center for Workforce Studies. *Results of the 2013 Medical School Enrollment Survey*. Washington, DC: Association of American Medical Colleges; 2014

3. Traverso G, McMahon GT. Residency training and international medical graduates: coming to America no more. *JAMA*. 2012;308(21):2193–2194

4. Hartman M, Martin AB, Benson J, Catlin A; National Health Expenditure Accounts Team. National health spending in 2011: overall growth remains low, but some payers and services show signs of acceleration. *Health Aff (Millwood)*. 2013;32(1):87–99

5. Association of American Medical Colleges. What does Medicare have to do with graduate medical education? Available at: https://www.aamc.org/download/253380/data/medicare-gme.pdf. Accessed April 8, 2015

6. Chandra A, Khullar D, Wilensky GR. The economics of graduate medical education. *N Engl J Med*. 2014;370(25):2357–2360

7. US Government Accountability Office. Letter to Congress. Health care workforce: federally funded training programs in fiscal year 2012. Washington, DC: US Government Accountability Office; August 15, 2013. Publication GAO-13-709R. Available at: http://gao.gov/assets/660/656960.pdf. Accessed April 8, 2015

8. Council on Graduate Medical Education. Resource paper: the effects of the Balanced Budget Act of 1997 on graduate medical education. March 2000. Available at: www.hrsa.gov/advisorycommittees/bhwadvisory/cogme/Publications/budgetact.pdf. Accessed April 8, 2015

9. Sklar DP. How many physicians do we need? A special issue on the physician workforce. *Acad Med*. 2013;88(12):1785–1787

10. Institute of Medicine. *Graduate Medical Education That Meets the Nation's Health Needs*. Washington, DC: The National Academies Press; 2014

11. Council on Graduate Medical Education. Twenty-first report: improving value in graduate medical education. August 2013. Available at: www.hrsa.gov/advisorycommittees/bhpradvisory/cogme/Reports/twentyfirstreport.pdf. Accessed April 8, 2015

12. Council on Medical Specialty Societies. Position recommending increased financial support for GME funding. December 2011. Available at: www.cmss.org/DefaultTwoColumn.aspx?id=496. Accessed April 8, 2015

13. Association of American Medical Colleges. AAMC physician workforce policy recommendations. September 2012. Available at: www.aafp.org/about/policies/all/workforce-reform.html. Accessed April 8, 2015

14. American Academy of Family Physicians. Family physician workforce reform: recommendations of the American Academy of Family Physicians. Available at: www.aafp.org/about/policies/all/workforce-reform.html. Accessed April 8, 2015

15. American College of Physicians. Aligning GME policy with the nation's health care workforce needs: a position paper. 2011. Available at: www.acponline.org/acp_policy/policies/aligning_gme_policy_with_nations_healthcare_workforce_needs_2011.pdf. Accessed April 8, 2015

16. Association of American Medical Colleges. Medicaid graduate medical education payments: a 50-state survey. Available at: https://members.aamc.org/eweb/DynamicPage.aspx?Action=Add&ObjectKeyFrom=1A83491A-9853-4C87-86A4-F7D95601C2E2&WebCode=PubDetailAdd&DoNotSave=yes&ParentObject=CentralizedOrderEntry&ParentDataObject=Invoice%20Detail&ivd_formkey=69202792-63d7-4ba2-bf4e-a0da41270555&ivd_prc_prd_key=6545613C-9BDA-46C2-8126-7D41209D52C1. Accessed April 8, 2015

17. Department of Health and Human Services, Bureau of Health Professions. Children's Hospitals Graduate Medical Education Payment Program. Available at: http://bhpr.hrsa.gov/childrenshospitalgme/. Accessed April 8, 2015

18. Children's Hospital Association. Children's hospitals graduate medical education (CHGME)/workforce. Available at: www.childrenshospitals.net/AM/Template.cfm?Section=CHGME Accessed April 8, 2015

19. Department of Health and Human Services, Bureau of Health Professions. Teaching Health Center Graduate Medical Education (THCGME). Available at: http://bhpr.hrsa.gov/grants/teachinghealthcenters/index.html. Accessed April 8, 2015

20. Health Resources and Services Administration, Division of Maternal and Child Health Workforce Development. About the Division of Maternal and Child Health Workforce Development (DMCHWD). Available at: http://mchb.hrsa.gov/training/about.asp. Accessed April 8, 2015

21. Josiah Macy Jr Foundation. Conference summary: ensuring an effective physician workforce for the United States: recommendations for reforming graduate medical education to meet the needs of the public. May 2011. Available at: http://macyfoundation.org/docs/macy_pubs/Macy_GME_Report,_Aug_2011.pdf. Accessed April 8, 2015

22. Chen C, Xierali I, Piwnica-Worms K, Phillips R. The redistribution of graduate medical education positions in 2005 failed to boost primary care or rural training. *Health Aff (Millwood)*. 2013;32(1):102–110

23. Basco WT, Rimsza ME; American Academy of Pediatrics Committee on Pediatric Workforce. Pediatrician workforce policy statement. *Pediatrics*. 2013;132(2):390–397

Guidelines for Monitoring and Management of Pediatric Patients Before, During, and After Sedation for Diagnostic and Therapeutic Procedures: Update 2016

• •

- *Clinical Report*

CLINICAL REPORT Guidance for the Clinician in Rendering Pediatric Care

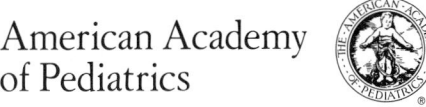

American Academy
of Pediatrics

DEDICATED TO THE HEALTH OF ALL CHILDREN™

Guidelines for Monitoring and Management of Pediatric Patients Before, During, and After Sedation for Diagnostic and Therapeutic Procedures: Update 2016

Charles J. Coté, MD, FAAP, Stephen Wilson, DMD, MA, PhD, AMERICAN ACADEMY OF PEDIATRICS, AMERICAN ACADEMY OF PEDIATRIC DENTISTRY

abstract

The safe sedation of children for procedures requires a systematic approach that includes the following: no administration of sedating medication without the safety net of medical/dental supervision, careful presedation evaluation for underlying medical or surgical conditions that would place the child at increased risk from sedating medications, appropriate fasting for elective procedures and a balance between the depth of sedation and risk for those who are unable to fast because of the urgent nature of the procedure, a focused airway examination for large (kissing) tonsils or anatomic airway abnormalities that might increase the potential for airway obstruction, a clear understanding of the medication's pharmacokinetic and pharmacodynamic effects and drug interactions, appropriate training and skills in airway management to allow rescue of the patient, age- and size-appropriate equipment for airway management and venous access, appropriate medications and reversal agents, sufficient numbers of staff to both carry out the procedure and monitor the patient, appropriate physiologic monitoring during and after the procedure, a properly equipped and staffed recovery area, recovery to the presedation level of consciousness before discharge from medical/dental supervision, and appropriate discharge instructions. This report was developed through a collaborative effort of the American Academy of Pediatrics and the American Academy of Pediatric Dentistry to offer pediatric providers updated information and guidance in delivering safe sedation to children.

This document is copyrighted and is property of the American Academy of Pediatrics and its Board of Directors. All authors have filed conflict of interest statements with the American Academy of Pediatrics. Any conflicts have been resolved through a process approved by the Board of Directors. The American Academy of Pediatrics has neither solicited nor accepted any commercial involvement in the development of the content of this publication.

Clinical reports from the American Academy of Pediatrics benefit from expertise and resources of liaisons and internal (AAP) and external reviewers. However, clinical reports from the American Academy of Pediatrics may not reflect the views of the liaisons or the organizations or government agencies that they represent.

The guidance in this report does not indicate an exclusive course of treatment or serve as a standard of medical/dental care. Variations, taking into account individual circumstances, may be appropriate.

All clinical reports from the American Academy of Pediatrics automatically expire 5 years after publication unless reaffirmed, revised, or retired at or before that time.

DOI: 10.1542/peds.2016-1212

PEDIATRICS (ISSN Numbers: Print, 0031-4005; Online, 1098-4275).

To cite: Coté CJ, Wilson S, AMERICAN ACADEMY OF PEDIATRICS, AMERICAN ACADEMY OF PEDIATRIC DENTISTRY. Guidelines for Monitoring and Management of Pediatric Patients Before, During, and After Sedation for Diagnostic and Therapeutic Procedures: Update 2016. Pediatrics. 2016; 138(1):e20161212

INTRODUCTION

The number of diagnostic and minor surgical procedures performed on pediatric patients outside of the traditional operating room setting has increased in the past several decades. As a consequence of this change and the increased awareness of the importance of providing analgesia and anxiolysis, the need for sedation for procedures in physicians' offices, dental offices, subspecialty procedure suites, imaging facilities, emergency departments, other inpatient hospital settings, and ambulatory surgery centers also has increased markedly.[1-52] In recognition of this need for both elective and emergency use of sedation in nontraditional settings, the American Academy of Pediatrics (AAP) and the American Academy of Pediatric Dentistry (AAPD) have published a series of guidelines for the monitoring and management of pediatric patients during and after sedation for a procedure.[53-58] The purpose of this updated report is to unify the guidelines for sedation used by medical and dental practitioners; to add clarifications regarding monitoring modalities, particularly regarding continuous expired carbon dioxide measurement; to provide updated information from the medical and dental literature; and to suggest methods for further improvement in safety and outcomes. This document uses the same language to define sedation categories and expected physiologic responses as The Joint Commission, the American Society of Anesthesiologists (ASA), and the AAPD.[56,57,59-61]

This revised statement reflects the current understanding of appropriate monitoring needs of pediatric patients both during and after sedation for a procedure.[3,4,11,18,20,21,23,24,33,39,41,44,47,51,62-73] The monitoring and care outlined may be exceeded at any time on the basis of the judgment of the responsible practitioner. Although intended to encourage high-quality patient care, adherence to the recommendations in this document cannot guarantee a specific patient outcome. However, structured sedation protocols designed to incorporate these safety principles have been widely implemented and shown to reduce morbidity.[11,23,24,27,30-33,35,39,41,44,47,51,74-84] These practice recommendations are proffered with the awareness that, regardless of the intended level of sedation or route of drug administration, the sedation of a pediatric patient represents a continuum and may result in respiratory depression, laryngospasm, impaired airway patency, apnea, loss of the patient's protective airway reflexes, and cardiovascular instability.[38,43,45,47,48,59,62,63,85-112]

Procedural sedation of pediatric patients has serious associated risks.[2,5,38,43,45,47,48,62,63,71,83,85,88-105,107-138] These adverse responses during and after sedation for a diagnostic or therapeutic procedure may be minimized, but not completely eliminated, by a careful preprocedure review of the patient's underlying medical conditions and consideration of how the sedation process might affect or be affected by these conditions: for example, children with developmental disabilities have been shown to have a threefold increased incidence of desaturation compared with children without developmental disabilities.[74,78,103] Appropriate drug selection for the intended procedure, a clear understanding of the sedating medication's pharmacokinetics and pharmacodynamics and drug interactions, as well as the presence of an individual with the skills needed to rescue a patient from an adverse response are critical.[42,48,62,63,92,97,99,125-127,132,133,139-158]

Appropriate physiologic monitoring and continuous observation by personnel not directly involved with the procedure allow for the accurate and rapid diagnosis of complications and initiation of appropriate rescue interventions.[44,63,64,67,68,74,90,96,110,159-174] The work of the Pediatric Sedation Research Consortium has improved the sedation knowledge base, demonstrating the marked safety of sedation by highly motivated and skilled practitioners from a variety of specialties practicing the above modalities and skills that focus on a culture of sedation safety.[45,83,95,128-138] However, these groundbreaking studies also show a low but persistent rate of potential sedation-induced life-threatening events, such as apnea, airway obstruction, laryngospasm, pulmonary aspiration, desaturation, and others, even when the sedation is provided under the direction of a motivated team of specialists.[129] These studies have helped define the skills needed to rescue children experiencing adverse sedation events.

The sedation of children is different from the sedation of adults. Sedation in children is often administered to relieve pain and anxiety as well as to modify behavior (eg, immobility) so as to allow the safe completion of a procedure. A child's ability to control his or her own behavior to cooperate for a procedure depends both on his or her chronologic age and cognitive/emotional development. Many brief procedures, such as suture of a minor laceration, may be accomplished with distraction and guided imagery techniques, along with the use of topical/local anesthetics and minimal sedation, if needed.[175-181] However, longer procedures that require immobility involving children younger than 6 years or those with developmental delay often require an increased depth of sedation to gain control of their behavior.[86,87,103] Children younger than 6 years (particularly those younger than 6 months) may be at greatest risk of an adverse event.[129] Children in this age group are particularly vulnerable

Suggested Management of Airway Obstructions

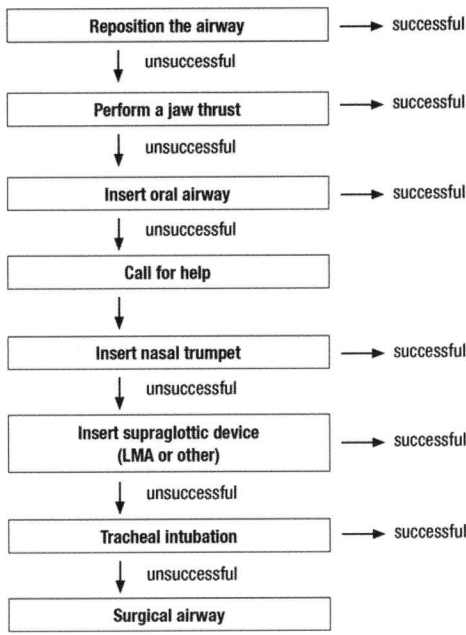

FIGURE 1
Suggested management of airway obstruction.

to the sedating medication's effects on respiratory drive, airway patency, and protective airway reflexes.[62,63] Other modalities, such as careful preparation, parental presence, hypnosis, distraction, topical local anesthetics, electronic devices with age-appropriate games or videos, guided imagery, and the techniques advised by child life specialists, may reduce the need for or the needed depth of pharmacologic sedation.[29,46,49,182–211]

Studies have shown that it is common for children to pass from the intended level of sedation to a deeper, unintended level of sedation,[85,88,212,213] making the concept of rescue essential to safe sedation. Practitioners of sedation must have the skills to rescue the patient from a deeper level than that intended for the procedure. For example, if the intended level of sedation is "minimal," practitioners must be able to rescue from "moderate sedation"; if the intended level of sedation is "moderate," practitioners must have the skills to rescue from "deep sedation"; if the

intended level of sedation is "deep," practitioners must have the skills to rescue from a state of "general anesthesia." The ability to rescue means that practitioners must be able to recognize the various levels of sedation and have the skills and age- and size-appropriate equipment necessary to provide appropriate cardiopulmonary support if needed.

These guidelines are intended for all venues in which sedation for a procedure might be performed (hospital, surgical center, freestanding imaging facility, dental facility, or private office). Sedation and anesthesia in a nonhospital environment (eg, private physician's or dental office, freestanding imaging facility) historically have been associated with an increased incidence of "failure to rescue" from adverse events, because these settings may lack immediately available backup. Immediate activation of emergency medical services (EMS) may be required in such settings, but the practitioner is responsible for life-support measures while awaiting

EMS arrival.[63,214] Rescue techniques require specific training and skills.[63,74,215,216] The maintenance of the skills needed to rescue a child with apnea, laryngospasm, and/or airway obstruction include the ability to open the airway, suction secretions, provide continuous positive airway pressure (CPAP), perform successful bag-valve-mask ventilation, insert an oral airway, a nasopharyngeal airway, or a laryngeal mask airway (LMA), and, rarely, perform tracheal intubation. These skills are likely best maintained with frequent simulation and team training for the management of rare events.[128,130,217–220] Competency with emergency airway management procedure algorithms is fundamental for safe sedation practice and successful patient rescue (see Figs 1, 2, and 3).[215,216,221–223]

Practitioners should have an in-depth knowledge of the agents they intend to use and their potential complications. A number of reviews and handbooks for sedating pediatric patients are available.[30,39,65,75,171,172,201,224–233] There are specific situations that are beyond the scope of this document. Specifically, guidelines for the delivery of general anesthesia and monitored anesthesia care (sedation or analgesia), outside or within the operating room by anesthesiologists or other practitioners functioning within a department of anesthesiology, are addressed by policies developed by the ASA and by individual departments of anesthesiology.[234] In addition, guidelines for the sedation of patients undergoing mechanical ventilation in a critical care environment or for providing analgesia for patients postoperatively, patients with chronic painful conditions, and patients in hospice care are beyond the scope of this document.

Suggested Management of Laryngospasm

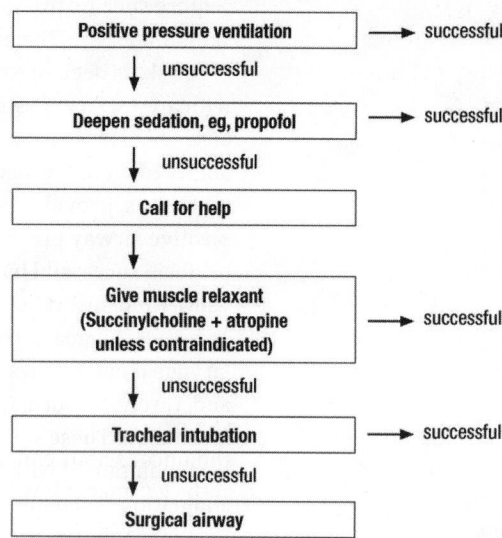

FIGURE 2
Suggested management of laryngospasm.

Suggested Management of Apnea

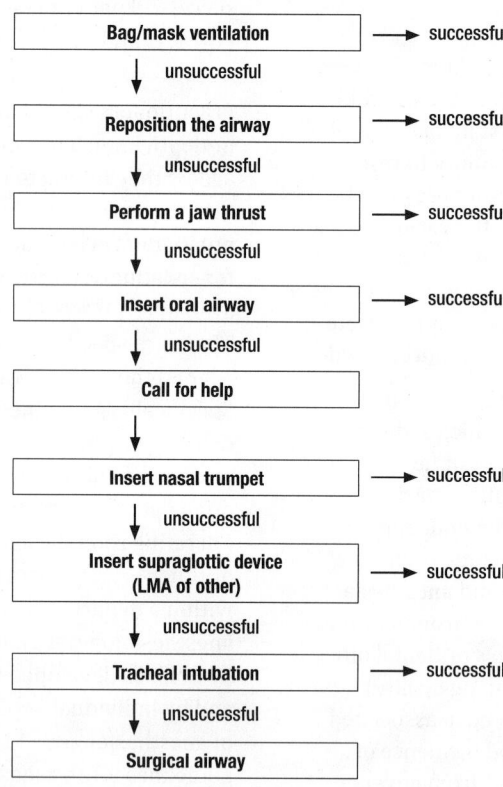

FIGURE 3
Suggested management of apnea.

GOALS OF SEDATION

The goals of sedation in the pediatric patient for diagnostic and therapeutic procedures are as follows: (1) to guard the patient's safety and welfare; (2) to minimize physical discomfort and pain; (3) to control anxiety, minimize psychological trauma, and maximize the potential for amnesia; (4) to modify behavior and/or movement so as to allow the safe completion of the procedure; and (5) to return the patient to a state in which discharge from medical/dental supervision is safe, as determined by recognized criteria (Supplemental Appendix 1).

These goals can best be achieved by selecting the lowest dose of drug with the highest therapeutic index for the procedure. It is beyond the scope of this document to specify which drugs are appropriate for which procedures; however, the selection of the fewest number of drugs and matching drug selection to the type and goals of the procedure are essential for safe practice. For example, analgesic medications, such as opioids or ketamine, are indicated for painful procedures. For nonpainful procedures, such as computed tomography or magnetic resonance imaging (MRI), sedatives/hypnotics are preferred. When both sedation and analgesia are desirable (eg, fracture reduction), either single agents with analgesic/sedative properties or combination regimens are commonly used. Anxiolysis and amnesia are additional goals that should be considered in the selection of agents for particular patients. However, the potential for an adverse outcome may be increased when 2 or more sedating medications are administered.[62,127,136,173,235] Recently, there has been renewed interest in noninvasive routes of medication administration, including intranasal and inhaled routes (eg, nitrous oxide; see below).[236]

Knowledge of each drug's time of onset, peak response, and duration of action is important (eg, the peak electroencephalogram [EEG] effect of intravenous midazolam occurs at ~4.8 minutes, compared with that of diazepam at ~1.6 minutes[237–239]). Titration of drug to effect is an important concept;

one must know whether the previous dose has taken full effect before administering additional drugs.[237] Drugs that have a long duration of action (eg, intramuscular pentobarbital, phenothiazines) have fallen out of favor because of unpredictable responses and prolonged recovery. The use of these drugs requires a longer period of observation even after the child achieves currently used recovery and discharge criteria.[62,238–241] This concept is particularly important for infants and toddlers transported in car safety seats; re-sedation after discharge attributable to residual prolonged drug effects may lead to airway obstruction.[62,63,242] In particular, promethazine (Phenergan; Wyeth Pharmaceuticals, Philadelphia, PA) has a "black box warning" regarding fatal respiratory depression in children younger than 2 years.[243] Although the liquid formulation of chloral hydrate is no longer commercially available, some hospital pharmacies now are compounding their own formulations. Low-dose chloral hydrate (10–25 mg/kg), in combination with other sedating medications, is used commonly in pediatric dental practice.

GENERAL GUIDELINES

Candidates

Patients who are in ASA classes I and II are frequently considered appropriate candidates for minimal, moderate, or deep sedation (Supplemental Appendix 2). Children in ASA classes III and IV, children with special needs, and those with anatomic airway abnormalities or moderate to severe tonsillar hypertrophy present issues that require additional and individual consideration, particularly for moderate and deep sedation.[68,244–249] Practitioners are encouraged to consult with appropriate subspecialists and/ or an anesthesiologist for patients at increased risk of experiencing adverse sedation events because of their underlying medical/surgical conditions.

Responsible Person

The pediatric patient shall be accompanied to and from the treatment facility by a parent, legal guardian, or other responsible person. It is preferable to have 2 adults accompany children who are still in car safety seats if transportation to and from a treatment facility is provided by 1 of the adults.[250]

Facilities

The practitioner who uses sedation must have immediately available facilities, personnel, and equipment to manage emergency and rescue situations. The most common serious complications of sedation involve compromise of the airway or depressed respirations resulting in airway obstruction, hypoventilation, laryngospasm, hypoxemia, and apnea. Hypotension and cardiopulmonary arrest may occur, usually from the inadequate recognition and treatment of respiratory compromise.[42,48,92,97,99,125,132,139–155,] Other rare complications also may include seizures, vomiting, and allergic reactions. Facilities providing pediatric sedation should monitor for, and be prepared to treat, such complications.

Back-up Emergency Services

A protocol for immediate access to back-up emergency services shall be clearly outlined. For nonhospital facilities, a protocol for the immediate activation of the EMS system for life-threatening complications must be established and maintained.[44] It should be understood that the availability of EMS does not replace the practitioner's responsibility to provide initial rescue for life-threatening complications.

On-site Monitoring, Rescue Drugs, and Equipment

An emergency cart or kit must be immediately accessible. This cart or kit must contain the necessary age- and size-appropriate equipment (oral and nasal airways, bag-valve-mask device, LMAs or other supraglottic devices, laryngoscope blades, tracheal tubes, face masks, blood pressure cuffs, intravenous catheters, etc) to resuscitate a nonbreathing and unconscious child. The contents of the kit must allow for the provision of continuous life support while the patient is being transported to a medical/dental facility or to another area within the facility. All equipment and drugs must be checked and maintained on a scheduled basis (see Supplemental Appendices 3 and 4 for suggested drugs and emergency life support equipment to consider before the need for rescue occurs). Monitoring devices, such as electrocardiography (ECG) machines, pulse oximeters with size-appropriate probes, end-tidal carbon dioxide monitors, and defibrillators with size-appropriate patches/ paddles, must have a safety and function check on a regular basis as required by local or state regulation. The use of emergency checklists is recommended, and these should be immediately available at all sedation locations; they can be obtained from http://www.pedsanesthesia.org/.

Documentation

Documentation prior to sedation shall include, but not be limited to, the following recommendations:

1. Informed consent: The patient record shall document that appropriate informed consent was obtained according to local, state, and institutional requirements.[251,252]

2. Instructions and information provided to the responsible

person: The practitioner shall provide verbal and/or written instructions to the responsible person. Information shall include objectives of the sedation and anticipated changes in behavior during and after sedation.[163,253–255] Special instructions shall be given to the adult responsible for infants and toddlers who will be transported home in a car safety seat regarding the need to carefully observe the child's head position to avoid airway obstruction. Transportation in a car safety seat poses a particular risk for infants who have received medications known to have a long half-life, such as chloral hydrate, intramuscular pentobarbital, or phenothiazine because deaths after procedural sedation have been reported.[62,63,238,242,256,257] Consideration for a longer period of observation shall be given if the responsible person's ability to observe the child is limited (eg, only 1 adult who also has to drive). Another indication for prolonged observation would be a child with an anatomic airway problem, an underlying medical condition such as significant obstructive sleep apnea (OSA), or a former preterm infant younger than 60 weeks' postconceptional age. A 24-hour telephone number for the practitioner or his or her associates shall be provided to all patients and their families. Instructions shall include limitations of activities and appropriate dietary precautions.

Dietary Precautions

Agents used for sedation have the potential to impair protective airway reflexes, particularly during deep sedation. Although a rare occurrence, pulmonary aspiration may occur if the child regurgitates and cannot protect his or her airway.[95,127,258] Therefore, the practitioner should evaluate preceding food and fluid intake before administering sedation. It is likely that the risk of aspiration during procedural sedation differs from that during general anesthesia involving tracheal intubation or other airway manipulations.[259,260] However, the absolute risk of aspiration during elective procedural sedation is not yet known; the reported incidence varies from ~1 in 825 to ~1 in 30 037.[95,127,129,173,244,261] Therefore, standard practice for fasting before elective sedation generally follows the same guidelines as for elective general anesthesia; this requirement is particularly important for solids, because aspiration of clear gastric contents causes less pulmonary injury than aspiration of particulate gastric contents.[262,263]

For emergency procedures in children undergoing general anesthesia, the reported incidence of pulmonary aspiration of gastric contents from 1 institution is ~1 in 373 compared with ~1 in 4544 for elective anesthetics.[262] Because there are few published studies with adequate statistical power to provide guidance to the practitioner regarding the safety or risk of pulmonary aspiration of gastric contents during procedural sedation,[95,127,129,173,244,259–261,264–268,] it is unknown whether the risk of aspiration is reduced when airway manipulation is not performed/anticipated (eg, moderate sedation). However, if a deeply sedated child requires intervention for airway obstruction, apnea, or laryngospasm, there is concern that these rescue maneuvers could increase the risk of pulmonary aspiration of gastric contents. For children requiring urgent/emergent sedation who do not meet elective fasting guidelines, the risks of sedation and possible aspiration are as-yet unknown and must be balanced against the benefits of performing the procedure promptly. For example, a prudent practitioner would be unlikely to administer deep sedation to a child with a minor condition who just ate a large meal; conversely, it is not justifiable to withhold sedation/analgesia from the child in significant pain from a displaced fracture who had a small snack a few hours earlier. Several emergency department studies have reported a low to zero incidence of pulmonary aspiration despite variable fasting periods[260,264,268]; however, each of these reports has, for the most part, clearly balanced the urgency of the procedure with the need for and depth of sedation.[268,269] Although emergency medicine studies and practice guidelines generally support a less restrictive approach to fasting for brief urgent/emergent procedures, such as care of wounds, joint dislocation, chest tube placement, etc, in healthy children, further research in many thousands of patients would be desirable to better define the relationships between various fasting intervals and sedation complications.[262–270]

Before Elective Sedation

Children undergoing sedation for elective procedures generally should follow the same fasting guidelines as those for general anesthesia (Table 1).[271] It is permissible for routine necessary medications (eg, antiseizure medications) to be taken with a sip of clear liquid or water on the day of the procedure.

For the Emergency Patient

The practitioner must always balance the possible risks of sedating nonfasted patients with the benefits of and necessity for completing the procedure. In particular, patients with a history of recent oral intake or with other known risk factors, such as trauma, decreased level of consciousness, extreme obesity (BMI ≥95% for age and sex), pregnancy, or bowel motility dysfunction, require careful evaluation before the administration of sedatives. When proper fasting has not been ensured, the increased risks of sedation must be carefully weighed against its benefits, and the lightest effective sedation should be used. In this circumstance, additional techniques for achieving analgesia and patient cooperation, such as distraction, guided imagery, video games, topical and local anesthetics, hematoma block or nerve blocks, and other techniques advised by child life specialists, are particularly helpful and should be considered.[29,49,182–201, 274,275]

The use of agents with less risk of depressing protective airway reflexes, such as ketamine, or moderate sedation, which would also maintain protective reflexes, may be preferred.[276] Some emergency patients requiring deep sedation (eg, a trauma patient who just ate a full meal or a child with a bowel obstruction) may need to be intubated to protect their airway before they can be sedated.

Use of Immobilization Devices (Protective Stabilization)

Immobilization devices, such as papoose boards, must be applied in such a way as to avoid airway obstruction or chest restriction.[277–281] The child's head position and respiratory excursions should be checked frequently to ensure airway patency. If an immobilization device is used, a hand or foot should be kept exposed, and the child should never be left unattended. If sedating medications are administered in conjunction with an immobilization device, monitoring must be used at a level consistent with the level of sedation achieved.

Documentation at the Time of Sedation

1. Health evaluation: Before sedation, a health evaluation shall be performed by an appropriately licensed practitioner and reviewed by the sedation team at the time of treatment for possible interval changes.[282] The purpose of this evaluation is not only to document baseline status

TABLE 1 Appropriate Intake of Food and Liquids Before Elective Sedation

Ingested Material	Minimum Fasting Period, h
Clear liquids: water, fruit juices without pulp, carbonated beverages, clear tea, black coffee	2
Human milk	4
Infant formula	6
Nonhuman milk: because nonhuman milk is similar to solids in gastric emptying time, the amount ingested must be considered when determining an appropriate fasting period.	6
Light meal: a light meal typically consists of toast and clear liquids. Meals that include fried or fatty foods or meat may prolong gastric emptying time. Both the amount and type of foods ingested must be considered when determining an appropriate fasting period.	6

Source: American Society of Anesthesiologists. Practice guidelines for preoperative fasting and the use of pharmacologic agents to reduce the risk of pulmonary aspiration: application to healthy patients undergoing elective procedures. An updated report by the American Society of Anesthesiologists Committee on Standards and Practice Parameters. Available at: https://www.asahq.org/For-Members/Practice-Management/Practice-Parameters.aspx. For emergent sedation, the practitioner must balance the depth of sedation versus the risk of possible aspiration; see also Mace et al[272] and Green et al.[273]

but also to determine whether the patient has specific risk factors that may warrant additional consultation before sedation. This evaluation also facilitates the identification of patients who will require more advanced airway or cardiovascular management skills or alterations in the doses or types of medications used for procedural sedation.

An important concern for the practitioner is the widespread use of medications that may interfere with drug absorption or metabolism and therefore enhance or shorten the effect time of sedating medications. Herbal medicines (eg, St John's wort, ginkgo, ginger, ginseng, garlic) may alter drug pharmacokinetics through inhibition of the cytochrome P450 system, resulting in prolonged drug effect and altered (increased or decreased) blood drug concentrations (midazolam, cyclosporine, tacrolimus).[283–292] Kava may increase the effects of sedatives by potentiating γ-aminobutyric acid inhibitory neurotransmission and may increase acetaminophen-induced liver toxicity.[293–295] Valerian may itself produce sedation that apparently is mediated through the modulation of γ-aminobutyric acid neurotransmission and receptor function.[291,296–299] Drugs such as erythromycin, cimetidine, and others may also inhibit the cytochrome

P450 system, resulting in prolonged sedation with midazolam as well as other medications competing for the same enzyme systems.[300–304] Medications used to treat HIV infection, some anticonvulsants, immunosuppressive drugs, and some psychotropic medications (often used to treat children with autism spectrum disorder) may also produce clinically important drug-drug interactions.[305–314] Therefore, a careful drug history is a vital part of the safe sedation of children. The practitioner should consult various sources (a pharmacist, textbooks, online services, or handheld databases) for specific information on drug interactions.[315–319] The US Food and Drug Administration issued a warning in February 2013 regarding the use of codeine for postoperative pain management in children undergoing tonsillectomy, particularly those with OSA. The safety issue is that some children have duplicated cytochromes that allow greater than expected conversion of the prodrug codeine to morphine, thus resulting in potential overdose; codeine should be avoided for postprocedure analgesia.[320–324]

The health evaluation should include the following:

• age and weight (in kg) and gestational age at birth (preterm infants may have associated sequelae such as apnea of prematurity); and

- health history, including (1) food and medication allergies and previous allergic or adverse drug reactions; (2) medication/drug history, including dosage, time, route, and site of administration for prescription, over-the-counter, herbal, or illicit drugs; (3) relevant diseases, physical abnormalities (including genetic syndromes), neurologic impairments that might increase the potential for airway obstruction, obesity, a history of snoring or OSA,[325–328] or cervical spine instability in Down syndrome, Marfan syndrome, skeletal dysplasia, and other conditions; (4) pregnancy status (as many as 1% of menarchal females presenting for general anesthesia at children's hospitals are pregnant)[329–331] because of concerns for the potential adverse effects of most sedating and anesthetic drugs on the fetus[329,332–338]; (5) history of prematurity (may be associated with subglottic stenosis or propensity to apnea after sedation); (6) history of any seizure disorder; (7) summary of previous relevant hospitalizations; (8) history of sedation or general anesthesia and any complications or unexpected responses; and (9) relevant family history, particularly related to anesthesia (eg, muscular dystrophy, malignant hyperthermia, pseudocholinesterase deficiency).

The review of systems should focus on abnormalities of cardiac, pulmonary, renal, or hepatic function that might alter the child's expected responses to sedating/analgesic medications. A specific query regarding signs and symptoms of sleep-disordered breathing and OSA may be helpful. Children with severe OSA who have experienced repeated episodes of desaturation will likely have altered mu receptors and be

analgesic at opioid levels one-third to one-half those of a child without OSA[325–328,339,340]; lower titrated doses of opioids should be used in this population. Such a detailed history will help to determine which patients may benefit from a higher level of care by an appropriately skilled health care provider, such as an anesthesiologist. The health evaluation should also include:

- vital signs, including heart rate, blood pressure, respiratory rate, room air oxygen saturation, and temperature (for some children who are very upset or noncooperative, this may not be possible and a note should be written to document this circumstance);

- physical examination, including a focused evaluation of the airway (tonsillar hypertrophy, abnormal anatomy [eg, mandibular hypoplasia], high Mallampati score [ie, ability to visualize only the hard palate or tip of the uvula]) to determine whether there is an increased risk of airway obstruction[74,341–344];

- physical status evaluation (ASA classification [see Appendix 2]); and

- name, address, and telephone number of the child's home or parent's, or caregiver's cell phone; additional information such as the patient's personal care provider or medical home is also encouraged.

For hospitalized patients, the current hospital record may suffice for adequate documentation of presedation health; however, a note shall be written documenting that the chart was reviewed, positive findings were noted, and a management plan was formulated. If the clinical or emergency condition of the patient precludes acquiring complete information before sedation, this health evaluation should be obtained as soon as feasible.

2. Prescriptions. When prescriptions are used for sedation, a copy of the prescription or a note describing the content of the prescription should be in the patient's chart along with a description of the instructions that were given to the responsible person. **Prescription medications intended to accomplish procedural sedation must not be administered without the safety net of direct supervision by trained medical/dental personnel.** The administration of sedating medications at home poses an unacceptable risk, particularly for infants and preschool-aged children traveling in car safety seats because deaths as a result of this practice have been reported.[63,257]

Documentation During Treatment

The patient's chart shall contain a time-based record that includes the name, route, site, time, dosage/kilogram, and patient effect of administered drugs. Before sedation, a "time out" should be performed to confirm the patient's name, procedure to be performed, and laterality and site of the procedure.[59] During administration, the inspired concentrations of oxygen and inhalation sedation agents and the duration of their administration shall be documented. Before drug administration, special attention must be paid to the calculation of dosage (ie, mg/kg); for obese patients, most drug doses should likely be adjusted lower to ideal body weight rather than actual weight.[345] When a programmable pump is used for the infusion of sedating medications, the dose/kilogram per minute or hour and the child's weight in kilograms should be double-checked and confirmed by a separate individual. The patient's chart shall contain documentation at the time of treatment that the patient's level of consciousness and responsiveness, heart rate, blood pressure, respiratory rate, expired carbon dioxide values, and oxygen saturation were monitored. Standard vital signs should be further documented at appropriate intervals during recovery until the patient attains predetermined discharge criteria (Appendix 1). A variety of sedation scoring systems are available that may aid this process.[212,238,346–348] Adverse events and their treatment shall be documented.

Documentation After Treatment

A dedicated and properly equipped recovery area is recommended (see Appendices 3 and 4). The time and condition of the child at discharge from the treatment area or facility shall be documented, which should include documentation that the child's level of consciousness and oxygen saturation in room air have returned to a state that is safe for discharge by recognized criteria (see Appendix 1). Patients receiving supplemental oxygen before the procedure should have a similar oxygen need after the procedure. Because some sedation medications are known to have a long half-life and may delay a patient's complete return to baseline or pose the risk of re-sedation[62,104,256,349,350] and because some patients will have complex multiorgan medical conditions, a longer period of observation in a less intense observation area (eg, a step-down observation area) before discharge from medical/dental supervision may be indicated.[239] Several scales to evaluate recovery have been devised and validated.[212,346–348,351,352] A simple evaluation tool may be the ability of the infant or child to remain awake for at least 20 minutes when placed in a quiet environment.[238]

CONTINUOUS QUALITY IMPROVEMENT

The essence of medical error reduction is a careful examination of index events and root-cause analysis of how the event could be avoided in the future.[353–359]

Therefore, each facility should maintain records that track all adverse events and significant interventions, such as desaturation; apnea; laryngospasm; need for airway interventions, including the need for placement of supraglottic devices such as an oral airway, nasal trumpet, or LMA; positive-pressure ventilation; prolonged sedation; unanticipated use of reversal agents; unplanned or prolonged hospital admission; sedation failures; inability to complete the procedure; and unsatisfactory sedation, analgesia, or anxiolysis.[360] Such events can then be examined for the assessment of risk reduction and improvement in patient/family satisfaction.

PREPARATION FOR SEDATION PROCEDURES

Part of the safety net of sedation is using a systematic approach so as to not overlook having an important drug, piece of equipment, or monitor immediately available at the time of a developing emergency. To avoid this problem, it is helpful to use an acronym that allows the same setup and checklist for every procedure. A commonly used acronym useful in planning and preparation for a procedure is **SOAPME**, which represents the following:

S = Size-appropriate suction catheters and a functioning suction apparatus (eg, Yankauer-type suction)

O = an adequate Oxygen supply and functioning flow meters or other devices to allow its delivery

A = size-appropriate Airway equipment (eg, bag-valve-mask or equivalent device [functioning]), nasopharyngeal and oropharyngeal airways, LMA, laryngoscope blades (checked and functioning), endotracheal tubes, stylets, face mask

P = Pharmacy: all the basic drugs needed to support life during an emergency, including antagonists as indicated

M = Monitors: functioning pulse oximeter with size-appropriate oximeter probes,[361,362] end-tidal carbon dioxide monitor, and other monitors as appropriate for the procedure (eg, noninvasive blood pressure, ECG, stethoscope)

E = special Equipment or drugs for a particular case (eg, defibrillator)

SPECIFIC GUIDELINES FOR INTENDED LEVEL OF SEDATION

Minimal Sedation

Minimal sedation (old terminology, "anxiolysis") is a drug-induced state during which patients respond normally to verbal commands. Although cognitive function and coordination may be impaired, ventilatory and cardiovascular functions are unaffected. Children who have received minimal sedation generally will not require more than observation and intermittent assessment of their level of sedation. Some children will become moderately sedated despite the intended level of minimal sedation; should this occur, then the guidelines for moderate sedation apply.[85,363]

Moderate Sedation

Moderate sedation (old terminology, "conscious sedation" or "sedation/ analgesia") is a drug-induced depression of consciousness during which patients respond purposefully to verbal commands or after light tactile stimulation. No interventions are required to maintain a patent airway, and spontaneous ventilation is adequate. Cardiovascular function is usually maintained. The caveat that loss of consciousness should be unlikely is a particularly important aspect of the definition of moderate sedation; drugs and techniques used should carry a margin of safety wide enough to render unintended loss of consciousness unlikely. Because the patient who receives moderate sedation may progress into a state of deep sedation and obtundation, the practitioner should be prepared to increase the level of vigilance corresponding to what is necessary for deep sedation.[85]

Personnel

THE PRACTITIONER. The practitioner responsible for the treatment of the patient and/or the administration of drugs for sedation must be competent to use such techniques, to provide the level of monitoring described in these guidelines, and to manage complications of these techniques (ie, to be able to rescue the patient). Because the level of intended sedation may be exceeded, the practitioner must be sufficiently skilled to rescue a child with apnea, laryngospasm, and/or airway obstruction, including the ability to open the airway, suction secretions, provide CPAP, and perform successful bag-valve-mask ventilation should the child progress to a level of deep sedation. Training in, and maintenance of, advanced pediatric airway skills is required (eg, pediatric advanced life support [PALS]); regular skills reinforcement with simulation is strongly encouraged.[79,80,128,130,217–220, 364]

SUPPORT PERSONNEL. The use of moderate sedation shall include the provision of a person, in addition to the practitioner, whose responsibility is to monitor appropriate physiologic parameters and to assist in any supportive or resuscitation measures, if required. This individual may also be responsible for assisting with interruptible patient-related tasks of short duration, such as holding an instrument or troubleshooting equipment.[60] This individual should be trained in and capable of providing advanced airway skills (eg, PALS). The support person shall have specific assignments in the event of an emergency and current knowledge of the emergency cart inventory. The practitioner and all ancillary personnel should participate in periodic reviews, simulation of rare emergencies, and practice drills of the facility's emergency protocol to ensure proper function of the equipment and coordination of staff roles in such emergencies.[133,365–367] It is recommended that at least 1 practitioner be skilled in obtaining vascular access in children.

Monitoring and Documentation

BASELINE. Before the administration of sedative medications, a baseline determination of vital signs shall be documented. For some children who are very upset or uncooperative, this may not be possible, and a note should be written to document this circumstance.

DURING THE PROCEDURE The physician/dentist or his or her designee shall document the name, route, site, time of administration, and dosage of all drugs administered. If sedation is being directed by a physician who is not personally administering the medications, then recommended practice is for the qualified health care provider administering the medication to confirm the dose verbally before administration. There shall be continuous monitoring of oxygen saturation and heart rate; when bidirectional verbal communication between the provider and patient is appropriate and possible (ie, patient is developmentally able and purposefully communicates), monitoring of ventilation by (1) capnography (preferred) or (2) amplified, audible pretracheal stethoscope (eg, Bluetooth technology)[368–371] or precordial stethoscope is strongly recommended. If bidirectional verbal communication is not appropriate or not possible, monitoring of ventilation by capnography (preferred), amplified, audible pretracheal stethoscope, or precordial stethoscope is required. Heart rate, respiratory rate, blood pressure, oxygen saturation, and expired carbon dioxide values should be recorded, at minimum, every 10 minutes in a time-based record. Note that the exact value of expired carbon dioxide is less important than simple assessment of continuous respiratory gas exchange. In some situations in which there is excessive patient agitation or lack of cooperation or during certain procedures such as bronchoscopy, dentistry, or repair of facial lacerations capnography may not be feasible, and this situation should be documented. For uncooperative children, it is often helpful to defer the initiation of capnography until the child becomes sedated. Similarly, the stimulation of blood pressure cuff inflation may cause arousal or agitation; in such cases, blood pressure monitoring may be counterproductive and may be documented at less frequent intervals (eg, 10–15 minutes, assuming the patient remains stable, well oxygenated, and well perfused). Immobilization devices (protective stabilization) should be checked to prevent airway obstruction or chest restriction. If a restraint device is used, a hand or foot should be kept exposed. The child's head position should be continuously assessed to ensure airway patency.

AFTER THE PROCEDURE. The child who has received moderate sedation must be observed in a suitably equipped recovery area, which must have a functioning suction apparatus as well as the capacity to deliver >90% oxygen and positive-pressure ventilation (bag-valve mask) with an adequate oxygen capacity as well as age- and size-appropriate rescue equipment and devices. The patient's vital signs should be recorded at specific intervals (eg, every 10–15 minutes). If the patient is not fully alert, oxygen saturation and heart rate monitoring shall be used continuously until appropriate discharge criteria are met (see Appendix 1). Because sedation medications with a long half-life may delay the patient's complete return to baseline or pose the risk of re-sedation, some patients might benefit from a longer period of less intense observation (eg, a step-down observation area where multiple patients can be observed simultaneously) before discharge from medical/dental supervision (see section entitled "Documentation Before Sedation" above).[62,256,349,350] A simple evaluation tool may be the ability of the infant or child to remain awake for at least 20 minutes when placed in a quiet environment.[238] Patients who have received reversal agents, such as flumazenil or naloxone, will require a longer period of observation, because the duration of the drugs administered may exceed the duration of the antagonist, resulting in re-sedation.

Deep Sedation/General Anesthesia

"Deep sedation" ("deep sedation/ analgesia") is a drug-induced depression of consciousness during which patients cannot be easily aroused but respond purposefully after repeated verbal or painful stimulation (eg, purposefully pushing away the noxious stimuli). Reflex withdrawal from a painful stimulus is not considered a purposeful response and is more consistent with a state of general anesthesia. The ability to independently maintain ventilatory function may be impaired. Patients may require assistance in maintaining a patent airway, and spontaneous ventilation may be inadequate. Cardiovascular function is usually maintained. A state of deep sedation may be accompanied by partial or complete loss of protective airway reflexes. Patients may pass from a state of deep sedation to the state of general anesthesia. In some situations, such as during MRI, one is not usually able to assess responses to stimulation, because this would defeat the purpose of sedation, and one should assume that such patients are deeply sedated.

"General anesthesia" is a drug-induced loss of consciousness during which patients are not arousable, even by painful stimulation. The ability to independently maintain ventilatory function is often impaired. Patients often require assistance in maintaining a patent airway, and positive-pressure ventilation may be required because of depressed spontaneous ventilation or drug-induced depression of neuromuscular function. Cardiovascular function may be impaired.

Personnel

During deep sedation, there must be 1 person whose only responsibility is to constantly observe the patient's vital signs, airway patency, and adequacy of ventilation and to either administer drugs or direct their administration. This individual must, at a minimum, be trained in PALS and capable of assisting with any emergency event. At least 1 individual must be present who is trained in and capable of providing advanced pediatric life support and who is skilled to rescue a child with apnea, laryngospasm, and/or airway obstruction. Required skills include the ability to open the airway, suction secretions, provide CPAP, insert supraglottic devices (oral airway, nasal trumpet, LMA), and perform successful bag-valve-mask ventilation, tracheal intubation, and cardiopulmonary resuscitation.

Equipment

In addition to the equipment needed for moderate sedation, an ECG monitor and a defibrillator for use in pediatric patients should be readily available.

Vascular Access

Patients receiving deep sedation should have an intravenous line placed at the start of the procedure or

have a person skilled in establishing vascular access in pediatric patients immediately available.

Monitoring

A competent individual shall observe the patient continuously. Monitoring shall include all parameters described for moderate sedation. Vital signs, including heart rate, respiratory rate, blood pressure, oxygen saturation, and expired carbon dioxide, must be documented at least every 5 minutes in a time-based record. Capnography should be used for almost all deeply sedated children because of the increased risk of airway/ventilation compromise. Capnography may not be feasible if the patient is agitated or uncooperative during the initial phases of sedation or during certain procedures, such as bronchoscopy or repair of facial lacerations, and this circumstance should be documented. For uncooperative children, the capnography monitor may be placed once the child becomes sedated. Note that if supplemental oxygen is administered, the capnograph may underestimate the true expired carbon dioxide value; of more importance than the numeric reading of exhaled carbon dioxide is the assurance of continuous respiratory gas exchange (ie, continuous waveform). Capnography is particularly useful for patients who are difficult to observe (eg, during MRI or in a darkened room).[64,67,72,90,96,110, 159–162,164–166,167–170,372–375]

The physician/dentist or his or her designee shall document the name, route, site, time of administration, and dosage of all drugs administered. If sedation is being directed by a physician who is not personally administering the medications, then recommended practice is for the nurse administering the medication to confirm the dose verbally before administration. The inspired concentrations of inhalation sedation agents and oxygen and the duration of administration shall be documented.

Postsedation Care

The facility and procedures followed for postsedation care shall conform to those described under "moderate sedation." The initial recording of vital signs should be documented at least every 5 minutes. Once the child begins to awaken, the recording intervals may be increased to 10 to 15 minutes. Table 2 summarizes the equipment, personnel, and monitoring requirements for moderate and deep sedation.

Special Considerations

Neonates and Former Preterm Infants

Neonates and former preterm infants require specific management, because immaturity of hepatic and renal function may alter the ability to metabolize and excrete sedating medications,[376] resulting in prolonged sedation and the need for extended postsedation monitoring. Former preterm infants have an increased risk of postanesthesia apnea,[377] but it is unclear whether a similar risk is associated with sedation, because this possibility has not been systematically investigated.[378]

Other concerns regarding the effects of anesthetic drugs and sedating medications on the developing brain are beyond the scope of this document. At this point, the research in this area is preliminary and inconclusive at best, but it would seem prudent to avoid unnecessary exposure to sedation if the procedure is unlikely to change medical/dental management (eg, a sedated MRI purely for screening purposes in preterm infants).[379-382]

Local Anesthetic Agents

All local anesthetic agents are cardiac depressants and may

cause central nervous system excitation or depression. Particular weight-based attention should be paid to cumulative dosage in all children.[118,120,125,383-386] To ensure that the patient will not receive an excessive dose, the maximum allowable safe dosage (eg, mg/kg) should be calculated before

administration. There may be enhanced sedative effects when the highest recommended doses of local anesthetic drugs are used in combination with other sedatives or opioids (see Tables 3 and 4 for limits and conversion tables of commonly used local anesthetics).[118,125,387-400] In general, when administering local

TABLE 2 Comparison of Moderate and Deep Sedation Equipment and Personnel Requirements

	Moderate Sedation	Deep Sedation
Personnel	An observer who will monitor the patient but who may also assist with interruptible tasks; should be trained in PALS	An independent observer whose only responsibility is to continuously monitor the patient; trained in PALS
Responsible practitioner	Skilled to rescue a child with apnea, laryngospasm, and/or airway obstruction including the ability to open the airway, suction secretions, provide CPAP, and perform successful bag-valve-mask ventilation; recommended that at least 1 practitioner should be skilled in obtaining vascular access in children; trained in PALS	Skilled to rescue a child with apnea, laryngospasm, and/or airway obstruction, including the ability to open the airway, suction secretions, provide CPAP, perform successful bag-valve-mask ventilation, tracheal intubation, and cardiopulmonary resuscitation; training in PALS is required; at least 1 practitioner skilled in obtaining vascular access in children immediately available
Monitoring	Pulse oximetry; ECG recommended; Heart rate; Blood pressure; Respiration; Capnography recommended	Pulse oximetry; ECG required; Heart rate; Blood pressure; Respiration; Capnography required
Other equipment	Suction equipment, adequate oxygen source/supply	Suction equipment, adequate oxygen source/supply, defibrillator required
Documentation	Name, route, site, time of administration, and dosage of all drugs administered; Continuous oxygen saturation, heart rate, and ventilation (capnography recommended); parameters recorded every 10 minutes	Name, route, site, time of administration, and dosage of all drugs administered; continuous oxygen saturation, heart rate, and ventilation (capnography required); parameters recorded at least every 5 minutes
Emergency checklists	Recommended	Recommended
Rescue cart properly stocked with rescue drugs and age- and size-appropriate equipment (see Appendices 3 and 4)	Required	Required
Dedicated recovery area with rescue cart properly stocked with rescue drugs and age- and size-appropriate equipment (see Appendices 3 and 4) and dedicated recovery personnel; adequate oxygen supply	Recommended; initial recording of vital signs may be needed at least every 10 minutes until the child begins to awaken, then recording intervals may be increased	Recommended; initial recording of vital signs may be needed for at least 5-minute intervals until the child begins to awaken, then recording intervals may be increased to 10–15 minutes
Discharge criteria	See Appendix 1	See Appendix 1

TABLE 3 Commonly Used Local Anesthetic Agents for Nerve Block or Infiltration: Doses, Duration, and Calculations

Local Anesthetic	Maximum Dose With Epinephrine,[a] mg/kg		Maximum Dose Without Epinephrine, mg/kg		Duration of Action,[b] min
	Medical	Dental	Medical	Dental	
Esters					
Procaine	10.0	6	7	6	60–90
Chloroprocaine	20.0	12	15	12	30–60
Tetracaine	1.5	1	1	1	180–600
Amides					
Lidocaine	7.0	4.4	4	4.4	90–200
Mepivacaine	7.0	4.4	5	4.4	120–240
Bupivacaine	3.0	1.3	2.5	1.3	180–600
Levobupivacaine[c]	3.0	2	2	2	180–600
Ropivacaine	3.0	2	2	2	180–600
Articaine[d]	—	7	—	7	60–230

Maximum recommended doses and durations of action are shown. Note that lower doses should be used in very vascular areas.

[a] These are maximum doses of local anesthetics combined with epinephrine; lower doses are recommended when used without epinephrine. Doses of amides should be decreased by 30% in infants younger than 6 mo. When lidocaine is being administered intravascularly (eg, during intravenous regional anesthesia), the dose should be decreased to 3 to 5 mg/kg; long-acting local anesthetic agents should not be used for intravenous regional anesthesia.

[b] Duration of action is dependent on concentration, total dose, and site of administration; use of epinephrine; and the patient's age.

[c] Levobupivacaine is not available in the United States.

[d] Use in pediatric patients under 4 years of age is not recommended.

TABLE 4 Local Anesthetic Conversion Chart

Concentration, %	mg/mL
4.0	40
3.0	30
2.5	25
2.0	20
1.0	10
0.5	5
0.25	2.5
0.125	1.25

TABLE 5 Treatment of Local Anesthetic Toxicity

1. Get help. Ventilate with 100% oxygen. Alert nearest facility with cardiopulmonary bypass capability.
2. Resuscitation: airway/ventilatory support, chest compressions, etc. Avoid vasopressin, calcium channel blockers, β-blockers, or additional local anesthetic. Reduce epinephrine dosages. Prolonged effort may be required.
3. Seizure management: benzodiazepines preferred (eg, intravenous midazolam 0.1–0.2 mg/kg); avoid propofol if cardiovascular instability.
4. Administer 1.5 mL/kg 20% lipid emulsion over ~1 minute to trap unbound amide local anesthetics. Repeat bolus once or twice for persistent cardiovascular collapse.
5. Initiate 20% lipid infusion (0.25 mL/kg per minute) until circulation is restored; double the infusion rate if blood pressure remains low. Continue infusion for at least 10 minutes after attaining circulatory stability. Recommended upper limit of ~10 mL/kg.
6. A fluid bolus of 10–20 mL/kg balanced salt solution and an infusion of phenylephrine (0.1 μg/kg per minute to start) may be needed to correct peripheral vasodilation.

Source: https://www.asra.com/advisory-guidelines/article/3/checklist-for-treatment-of-local-anesthetic-systemic-toxicity.

anesthetic drugs, the practitioner should aspirate frequently to minimize the likelihood that the needle is in a blood vessel; lower doses should be used when injecting into vascular tissues.[401] If high doses or injection of amide local anesthetics (bupivacaine and ropivacaine) into vascular tissues is anticipated, then the immediate availability of a 20% lipid emulsion for the treatment of local anesthetic toxicity is recommended (Tables 3 and 5).[402-409] Topical local anesthetics are commonly used and encouraged, but the practitioner should avoid applying excessive doses to mucosal surfaces where systemic uptake and possible toxicity (seizures, methemoglobinemia) could result and to remain within the manufacturer's recommendations regarding allowable surface area application.[410-415]

Pulse Oximetry

Newer pulse oximeters are less susceptible to motion artifacts and may be more useful than older oximeters that do not contain updated software.[416-420] Oximeters that change tone with changes in hemoglobin saturation provide immediate aural warning to everyone within hearing distance. The oximeter probe must be properly positioned; clip-on devices are easy to displace, which may produce artifactual data (under- or overestimation of oxygen saturation).[361,362]

Capnography

Expired carbon dioxide monitoring is valuable to diagnose the simple presence or absence of respirations, airway obstruction, or respiratory depression, particularly in patients sedated in less-accessible locations, such as in MRI machines or darkened rooms.[64,66,67,72,90,96,110,159-162,164-170, 372-375,421-427] In patients receiving supplemental oxygen, capnography facilitates the recognition of apnea or airway obstruction several minutes before the situation would be detected just by pulse oximetry. In this situation, desaturation would be delayed due to increased oxygen reserves; capnography would enable earlier intervention.[161] One study in children sedated in the emergency department found that the use of capnography reduced the incidence of hypoventilation and desaturation

(7% to 1%).[174] The use of expired carbon dioxide monitoring devices is now required for almost all deeply sedated children (with rare exceptions), particularly in situations in which other means of assessing the adequacy of ventilation are limited. Several manufacturers have produced nasal cannulae that allow simultaneous delivery of oxygen and measurement of expired carbon dioxide values.[421,422,427] Although these devices can have a high degree of false-positive alarms, they are also very accurate for the detection of complete airway obstruction or apnea.[164,168,169] Taping the sampling line under the nares under an oxygen face mask or nasal hood will provide similar information. The exact measured value is less important than the simple answer to the question: Is the child exchanging air with each breath?

Processed EEG (Bispectral Index)

Although not new to the anesthesia community, the processed EEG (bispectral index [BIS]) monitor is slowly finding its way into the sedation literature.[428] Several studies have attempted to use BIS monitoring as a means of noninvasively assessing the depth of sedation. This technology was designed to examine EEG signals and, through a variety of algorithms, correlate a number with depth of unconsciousness: that is, the lower the number, the deeper the sedation. Unfortunately, these algorithms are based on adult patients and have not been validated in children of varying ages and varying brain development. Although the readings correspond quite well with the depth of propofol sedation, the numbers may paradoxically go up rather than down with sevoflurane and ketamine because of central excitation despite a state of general anesthesia or deep sedation.[429,430] Opioids and benzodiazepines have minimal and variable effects on the BIS. Dexmedetomidine has minimal effect with EEG patterns, consistent

with stage 2 sleep.[431] Several sedation studies have examined the utility of this device and degree of correlation with standard sedation scales.[347,363,432–435] It appears that there is some correlation with BIS values in moderate sedation, but there is not a reliable ability to distinguish between deep sedation and moderate sedation or deep sedation from general anesthesia.[432] Presently, it would appear that BIS monitoring might provide useful information only when used for sedation with propofol[363]; in general, it is still considered a research tool and not recommended for routine use.

Adjuncts to Airway Management and Resuscitation

The vast majority of sedation complications can be managed with simple maneuvers, such as supplemental oxygen, opening the airway, suctioning, placement of an oral or nasopharyngeal airway, and bag-mask-valve ventilation. Rarely, tracheal intubation is required for more prolonged ventilatory support. In addition to standard tracheal intubation techniques, a number of supraglottic devices are available for the management of patients with abnormal airway anatomy or airway obstruction. Examples include the LMA, the cuffed oropharyngeal airway, and a variety of kits to perform an emergency cricothyrotomy.[436,437]

The largest clinical experience in pediatrics is with the LMA, which is available in multiple sizes, including those for late preterm and term neonates. The use of the LMA is now an essential addition to advanced airway training courses, and familiarity with insertion techniques can be life-saving.[438–442] The LMA can also serve as a bridge to secure airway management in children with anatomic airway abnormalities.[443,444] Practitioners are encouraged to gain

experience with these techniques as they become incorporated into PALS courses.

Another valuable emergency technique is intraosseous needle placement for vascular access. Intraosseous needles are available in several sizes; insertion can be life-saving when rapid intravenous access is difficult. A relatively new intraosseous device (EZ-IO Vidacare, now part of Teleflex, Research Triangle Park, NC) is similar to a hand-held battery-powered drill. It allows rapid placement with minimal chance of misplacement; it also has a low-profile intravenous adapter.[445–450] Familiarity with the use of these emergency techniques can be gained by keeping current with resuscitation courses, such as PALS and advanced pediatric life support.

Patient Simulators

High-fidelity patient simulators are now available that allow physicians, dentists, and other health care providers to practice managing a variety of programmed adverse events, such as apnea, bronchospasm, and laryngospasm.[133,220,450–452] The use of such devices is encouraged to better train medical professionals and teams to respond more effectively to rare events.[128,131,451,453–455] One study that simulated the quality of cardiopulmonary resuscitation compared standard management of ventricular fibrillation versus rescue with the EZ-IO for the rapid establishment of intravenous access and placement of an LMA for establishing a patent airway in adults; the use of these devices resulted in more rapid establishment of vascular access and securing of the airway.[456]

Monitoring During MRI

The powerful magnetic field and the generation of radiofrequency emissions necessitate the use of special equipment to provide continuous patient monitoring throughout the MRI scanning procedure.[457–459] MRI-compatible pulse oximeters and capnographs capable of continuous function during scanning should be used in any sedated or restrained pediatric patient. Thermal injuries can result if appropriate precautions are not taken; the practitioner is cautioned to avoid coiling of all wires (oximeter, ECG) and to place the oximeter probe as far from the magnetic coil as possible to diminish the possibility of injury. ECG monitoring during MRI has been associated with thermal injury; special MRI-compatible ECG pads are essential to allow safe monitoring.[460–463] If sedation is achieved by using an infusion pump, then either an MRI-compatible pump is required or the pump must be situated outside of the room with long infusion tubing so as to maintain infusion accuracy. All equipment must be MRI compatible, including laryngoscope blades and handles, oxygen tanks, and any ancillary equipment. All individuals, including parents, must be screened for ferromagnetic materials, phones, pagers, pens, credit cards, watches, surgical implants, pacemakers, etc, before entry into the MRI suite.

Nitrous Oxide

Inhalation sedation/analgesia equipment that delivers nitrous oxide must have the capacity of delivering 100% and never less than 25% oxygen concentration at a flow rate appropriate to the size of the patient. Equipment that delivers variable ratios of nitrous oxide >50% to oxygen that covers the mouth and nose must be used in conjunction with a calibrated and functional oxygen analyzer. All nitrous oxide-to-oxygen inhalation devices should be calibrated in accordance with appropriate state and local requirements. Consideration should be given to the National Institute of Occupational Safety and Health Standards for the scavenging of waste gases.[464] Newly constructed or reconstructed treatment facilities, especially those with piped-in nitrous oxide and oxygen, must have appropriate state or local inspections to certify proper function of inhalation sedation/analgesia systems before any delivery of patient care.

Nitrous oxide in oxygen, with varying concentrations, has been successfully used for many years to provide analgesia for a variety of painful procedures in children.[14,36,49,98,465–493] The use of nitrous oxide for minimal sedation is defined as the administration of nitrous oxide of ≤50% with the balance as oxygen, without any other sedative, opioid, or other depressant drug before or concurrent with the nitrous oxide to an otherwise healthy patient in ASA class I or II. The patient is able to maintain verbal communication throughout the procedure. It should be noted that although local anesthetics have sedative properties, for purposes of this guideline they are not considered sedatives in this circumstance. If nitrous oxide in oxygen is combined with other sedating medications, such as chloral hydrate, midazolam, or an opioid, or if nitrous oxide is used in concentrations >50%, the likelihood for moderate or deep sedation increases.[107,197,492,494,495]

In this situation, the practitioner is advised to institute the guidelines for moderate or deep sedation, as indicated by the patient's response.[496]

ACKNOWLEDMENTS

The lead authors thank Dr Corrie Chumpitazi and Dr Mary Hegenbarth for their contributions to this document.

LEAD AUTHORS

Charles J. Coté, MD, FAAP
Stephen Wilson, DMD, MA, PhD

AMERICAN ACADEMY OF PEDIATRICS

AMERICAN ACADEMY OF PEDIATRIC DENTISTRY

STAFF

Jennifer Riefe, MEd
Raymond J. Koteras, MHA

ABBREVIATIONS

AAP: American Academy of Pediatrics
AAPD: American Academy of Pediatric Dentistry
ASA: American Society of Anesthesiologists
BIS: bispectral index
CPAP: continuous positive airway pressure
ECG: electrocardiography
EEG: electroencephalogram/electroencephalography
EMS: emergency medical services
LMA: laryngeal mask airway
MRI: magnetic resonance imaging
OSA: obstructive sleep apnea
PALS: pediatric advanced life support

FINANCIAL DISCLOSURE: The authors have indicated they do not have a financial relationship relevant to this article to disclose.

FUNDING: No external funding.

POTENTIAL CONFLICT OF INTEREST: The authors have indicated they have no potential conflicts of interest to disclose.

REFERENCES

1. Milnes AR. Intravenous procedural sedation: an alternative to general anesthesia in the treatment of early childhood caries. *J Can Dent Assoc.* 2003;69:298–302

2. Law AK, Ng DK, Chan KK. Use of intramuscular ketamine for endoscopy sedation in children. *Pediatr Int.* 2003;45(2):180–185

3. Flood RG, Krauss B. Procedural sedation and analgesia for children in the emergency department. *Emerg Med Clin North Am.* 2003;21(1):121–139

4. Jaggar SI, Haxby E. Sedation, anaesthesia and monitoring for bronchoscopy. *Paediatr Respir Rev.* 2002;3(4):321–327

5. de Blic J, Marchac V, Scheinmann P. Complications of flexible bronchoscopy in children: prospective study of 1,328 procedures. *Eur Respir J.* 2002;20(5):1271–1276

6. Mason KP, Michna E, DiNardo JA, et al. Evolution of a protocol for ketamine-induced sedation as an alternative to general anesthesia for interventional radiologic procedures in pediatric patients. *Radiology.* 2002;225(2):457–465

7. Houpt M. Project USAP 2000—use of sedative agents by pediatric dentists: a 15-year follow-up survey. *Pediatr Dent.* 2002;24(4):289–294

8. Vinson DR, Bradbury DR. Etomidate for procedural sedation in emergency medicine. *Ann Emerg Med.* 2002;39(6):592–598

9. Everitt IJ, Barnett P. Comparison of two benzodiazepines used for sedation of children undergoing suturing of a laceration in an emergency department. *Pediatr Emerg Care.* 2002;18(2):72–74

10. Karian VE, Burrows PE, Zurakowski D, Connor L, Poznauskis L, Mason KP. The development of a pediatric radiology sedation program. *Pediatr Radiol.* 2002;32(5):348–353

11. Kaplan RF, Yang CI. Sedation and analgesia in pediatric patients for procedures outside the operating room. *Anesthesiol Clin North America.* 2002;20(1):181–194, vii

12. Wheeler DS, Jensen RA, Poss WB. A randomized, blinded comparison of chloral hydrate and midazolam sedation in children undergoing echocardiography. *Clin Pediatr (Phila).* 2001;40(7):381–387

13. Hain RD, Campbell C. Invasive procedures carried out in conscious children: contrast between North American and European paediatric oncology centres. *Arch Dis Child.* 2001;85(1):12–15

14. Kennedy RM, Luhmann JD. Pharmacological management of pain and anxiety during emergency procedures in children. *Paediatr Drugs.* 2001;3(5):337–354

15. Kanagasundaram SA, Lane LJ, Cavalletto BP, Keneally JP, Cooper MG. Efficacy and safety of nitrous oxide in alleviating pain and anxiety during painful procedures. *Arch Dis Child.* 2001;84(6):492–495

16. Younge PA, Kendall JM. Sedation for children requiring wound repair: a randomised controlled double blind comparison of oral midazolam and oral ketamine. *Emerg Med J.* 2001;18(1):30–33

17. Ljungman G, Gordh T, Sörensen S, Kreuger A. Lumbar puncture in pediatric oncology: conscious sedation vs. general anesthesia. *Med Pediatr Oncol.* 2001;36(3):372–379

18. Poe SS, Nolan MT, Dang D, et al. Ensuring safety of patients receiving sedation for procedures: evaluation of clinical practice guidelines. *Jt Comm J Qual Improv.* 2001;27(1):28–41

19. D'Agostino J, Terndrup TE. Chloral hydrate versus midazolam for sedation of children for neuroimaging: a randomized clinical trial. *Pediatr Emerg Care.* 2000;16(1):1–4

20. Green SM, Kuppermann N, Rothrock SG, Hummel CB, Ho M. Predictors of adverse events with intramuscular ketamine sedation in children. *Ann Emerg Med.* 2000;35(1):35–42

21. Hopkins KL, Davis PC, Sanders CL, Churchill LH. Sedation for pediatric imaging studies. *Neuroimaging Clin N Am.* 1999;9(1):1–10

22. Bauman LA, Kish I, Baumann RC, Politis GD. Pediatric sedation with analgesia. *Am J Emerg Med.* 1999;17(1):1–3

23. Bhatt-Mehta V, Rosen DA. Sedation in children: current concepts. *Pharmacotherapy.* 1998;18(4):790–807

24. Morton NS, Oomen GJ. Development of a selection and monitoring protocol for safe sedation of children. *Paediatr Anaesth.* 1998;8(1):65–68

25. Murphy MS. Sedation for invasive procedures in paediatrics. *Arch Dis Child.* 1997;77(4):281–284

26. Webb MD, Moore PA. Sedation for pediatric dental patients. *Dent Clin North Am.* 2002;46(4):803–814, xi

27. Malviya S, Voepel-Lewis T, Tait AR, Merkel S. Sedation/analgesia for diagnostic and therapeutic procedures in children. *J Perianesth Nurs.* 2000;15(6):415–422

28. Zempsky WT, Schechter NL. Office-based pain managemen: the 15-minute consultation. *Pediatr Clin North Am.* 2000;47(3):601–615

29. Kennedy RM, Luhmann JD. The "ouchless emergency department": getting closer: advances in decreasing distress during painful procedures in the emergency department. *Pediatr Clin North Am.* 1999;46(6):1215–1247, vii–viii

30. Rodriguez E, Jordan R. Contemporary trends in pediatric sedation and analgesia. *Emerg Med Clin North Am.* 2002;20(1):199–222

31. Ruess L, O'Connor SC, Mikita CP, Creamer KM. Sedation for pediatric diagnostic imaging: use of pediatric and nursing resources as an alternative to a radiology department sedation team. *Pediatr Radiol.* 2002;32(7):505–510

32. Weiss S. Sedation of pediatric patients for nuclear medicine procedures. *Semin Nucl Med.* 1993;23(3):190–198

33. Wilson S. Pharmacologic behavior management for pediatric dental treatment. *Pediatr Clin North Am.* 2000;47(5):1159–1175

34. McCarty EC, Mencio GA, Green NE. Anesthesia and analgesia for the ambulatory management of fractures in children. *J Am Acad Orthop Surg.* 1999;7(2):81–91

35. Egelhoff JC, Ball WS Jr, Koch BL, Parks TD. Safety and efficacy of sedation in children using a structured sedation

program. *AJR Am J Roentgenol.* 1997;168(5):1259–1262

36. Heinrich M, Menzel C, Hoffmann F, Berger M, Schweinitz DV. Self-administered procedural analgesia using nitrous oxide/oxygen (50:50) in the pediatric surgery emergency room: effectiveness and limitations. *Eur J Pediatr Surg.* 2015;25(3):250–256

37. Hoyle JD Jr, Callahan JM, Badawy M, et al; Traumatic Brain Injury Study Group for the Pediatric Emergency Care Applied Research Network (PECARN). Pharmacological sedation for cranial computed tomography in children after minor blunt head trauma. *Pediatr Emerg Care.* 2014;30(1):1–7

38. Chiaretti A, Benini F, Pierri F, et al. Safety and efficacy of propofol administered by paediatricians during procedural sedation in children. *Acta Paediatr.* 2014;103(2):182–187

39. Pacheco GS, Ferayorni A. Pediatric procedural sedation and analgesia. *Emerg Med Clin North Am.* 2013;31(3):831–852

40. Griffiths MA, Kamat PP, McCracken CE, Simon HK. Is procedural sedation with propofol acceptable for complex imaging? A comparison of short vs. prolonged sedations in children. *Pediatr Radiol.* 2013;43(10):1273–1278

41. Doctor K, Roback MG, Teach SJ. An update on pediatric hospital-based sedation. *Curr Opin Pediatr.* 2013;25(3):310–316

42. Alletag MJ, Auerbach MA, Baum CR. Ketamine, propofol, and ketofol use for pediatric sedation. *Pediatr Emerg Care.* 2012;28(12):1391–1395; quiz: 1396–1398

43. Jain R, Petrillo-Albarano T, Parks WJ, Linzer JF Sr, Stockwell JA. Efficacy and safety of deep sedation by non-anesthesiologists for cardiac MRI in children. *Pediatr Radiol.* 2013;43(5):605–611

44. Nelson T, Nelson G. The role of sedation in contemporary pediatric dentistry. *Dent Clin North Am.* 2013;57(1):145–161

45. Monroe KK, Beach M, Reindel R, et al. Analysis of procedural sedation provided by pediatricians. *Pediatr Int.* 2013;55(1):17–23

46. Alexander M. Managing patient stress in pediatric radiology. *Radiol Technol.* 2012;83(6):549–560

47. Macias CG, Chumpitazi CE. Sedation and anesthesia for CT: emerging issues for providing high-quality care. *Pediatr Radiol.* 2011;41(suppl 2):S17–S22

48. Andolfatto G, Willman E. A prospective case series of pediatric procedural sedation and analgesia in the emergency department using single-syringe ketamine-propofol combination (ketofol). *Acad Emerg Med.* 2010;17(2):194–201

49. Brown SC, Hart G, Chastain DP, Schneeweiss S, McGrath PA. Reducing distress for children during invasive procedures: randomized clinical trial of effectiveness of the PediSedate. *Paediatr Anaesth.* 2009;19(8):725–731

50. Yamamoto LG. Initiating a hospital-wide pediatric sedation service provided by emergency physicians. *Clin Pediatr (Phila).* 2008;47(1):37–48

51. Doyle L, Colletti JE. Pediatric procedural sedation and analgesia. *Pediatr Clin North Am.* 2006;53(2):279–292

52. Todd DW. Pediatric sedation and anesthesia for the oral surgeon. *Oral Maxillofac Surg Clin North Am.* 2013;25(3):467–478, vi–vii

53. Committee on Drugs, Section on Anesthesiology, American Academy of Pediatrics. Guidelines for the elective use of conscious sedation, deep sedation, and general anesthesia in pediatric patients. *Pediatrics.* 1985;76(2):317–321

54. American Academy of Pediatric Dentistry. Guidelines for the elective use of conscious sedation, deep sedation, and general anesthesia in pediatric patients. *ASDC J Dent Child.* 1986;53(1):21–22

55. Committee on Drugs, American Academy of Pediatrics. Guidelines for monitoring and management of pediatric patients during and after sedation for diagnostic and therapeutic procedures. *Pediatrics.* 1992;89(6 pt 1):1110–1115

56. Committee on Drugs, American Academy of Pediatrics. Guidelines for monitoring and management of pediatric patients during and after sedation for diagnostic and therapeutic procedures: addendum. *Pediatrics.* 2002;110(4):836–838

57. American Academy of Pediatrics, American Academy of Pediatric Dentistry. Guidelines on the elective use of minimal, moderate, and deep sedation and general anesthesia for pediatric dental patients. 2011. Available at: http://www.aapd.org/media/policies_guidelines/g_sedation.pdf. Accessed May 27, 2016

58. Coté CJ, Wilson S; American Academy of Pediatrics; American Academy of Pediatric Dentistry; Work Group on Sedation. Guidelines for monitoring and management of pediatric patients during and after sedation for diagnostic and therapeutic procedures: an update. *Pediatrics.* 2006;118(6):2587–2602

59. The Joint Commission. Comprehensive Accreditation Manual for Hospitals (CAMH): the official handbook. Oakbrook Terrace, IL: The Joint Commission; 2014

60. American Society of Anesthesiologists Task Force on Sedation and Analgesia by Non-Anesthesiologists. Practice guidelines for sedation and analgesia by non-anesthesiologists. *Anesthesiology.* 2002;96(4):1004–1017

61. Committee of Origin: Ad Hoc on Non-Anesthesiologist Privileging. Statement on granting privileges for deep sedation to non-anesthesiologist sedation practitioners. 2010. Available at: http://www.asahq.org/~/media/sites/asahq/files/public/resources/standards-guidelines/advisory-on-granting-privileges-for-deep-sedation-to-non-anesthesiologist.pdf. Accessed May 27, 2016

62. Coté CJ, Karl HW, Notterman DA, Weinberg JA, McCloskey C. Adverse sedation events in pediatrics: analysis of medications used for sedation. *Pediatrics.* 2000;106(4):633–644

63. Coté CJ, Notterman DA, Karl HW, Weinberg JA, McCloskey C. Adverse sedation events in pediatrics: a critical incident analysis of contributing factors. *Pediatrics.* 2000;105(4 pt 1):805–814

64. Kim G, Green SM, Denmark TK, Krauss B. Ventilatory response during

dissociative sedation in children-a pilot study. *Acad Emerg Med.* 2003;10(2):140–145

65. Coté CJ. Sedation for the pediatric patient: a review. *Pediatr Clin North Am.* 1994;41(1):31–58

66. Mason KP, Burrows PE, Dorsey MM, Zurakowski D, Krauss B. Accuracy of capnography with a 30 foot nasal cannula for monitoring respiratory rate and end-tidal CO2 in children. *J Clin Monit Comput.* 2000;16(4):259–262

67. McQuillen KK, Steele DW. Capnography during sedation/analgesia in the pediatric emergency department. *Pediatr Emerg Care.* 2000;16(6):401–404

68. Malviya S, Voepel-Lewis T, Tait AR. Adverse events and risk factors associated with the sedation of children by nonanesthesiologists. *Anesth Analg.* 1997;85(6):1207–1213

69. Coté CJ, Rolf N, Liu LM, et al. A single-blind study of combined pulse oximetry and capnography in children. *Anesthesiology.* 1991;74(6):980–987

70. Guideline SIGN; Scottish Intercollegiate Guidelines Network. SIGN Guideline 58: safe sedation of children undergoing diagnostic and therapeutic procedures. *Paediatr Anaesth.* 2008;18(1):11–12

71. Peña BM, Krauss B. Adverse events of procedural sedation and analgesia in a pediatric emergency department. *Ann Emerg Med.* 1999;34(4 pt 1):483–491

72. Smally AJ, Nowicki TA. Sedation in the emergency department. *Curr Opin Anaesthesiol.* 2007;20(4):379–383

73. Ratnapalan S, Schneeweiss S. Guidelines to practice: the process of planning and implementing a pediatric sedation program. *Pediatr Emerg Care.* 2007;23(4):262–266

74. Hoffman GM, Nowakowski R, Troshynski TJ, Berens RJ, Weisman SJ. Risk reduction in pediatric procedural sedation by application of an American Academy of Pediatrics/American Society of Anesthesiologists process model. *Pediatrics.* 2002;109(2):236–243

75. Krauss B. Management of acute pain and anxiety in children undergoing procedures in the emergency department. *Pediatr Emerg Care.* 2001;17(2):115–122; quiz: 123–125

76. Slovis TL. Sedation and anesthesia issues in pediatric imaging. *Pediatr Radiol.* 2011;41(suppl 2):514–516

77. Babl FE, Krieser D, Belousoff J, Theophilos T. Evaluation of a paediatric procedural sedation training and credentialing programme: sustainability of change. *Emerg Med J.* 2010;27(8):577–581

78. Meredith JR, O'Keefe KP, Galwankar S. Pediatric procedural sedation and analgesia. *J Emerg Trauma Shock.* 2008;1(2):88–96

79. Priestley S, Babl FE, Krieser D, et al. Evaluation of the impact of a paediatric procedural sedation credentialing programme on quality of care. *Emerg Med Australas.* 2006;18(5–6):498–504

80. Babl F, Priestley S, Krieser D, et al. Development and implementation of an education and credentialing programme to provide safe paediatric procedural sedation in emergency departments. *Emerg Med Australas.* 2006;18(5–6):489–497

81. Cravero JP, Blike GT. Pediatric sedation. *Curr Opin Anaesthesiol.* 2004;17(3):247–251

82. Shavit I, Keidan I, Augarten A. The practice of pediatric procedural sedation and analgesia in the emergency department. *Eur J Emerg Med.* 2006;13(5):270–275

83. Langhan ML, Mallory M, Hertzog J, Lowrie L, Cravero J; Pediatric Sedation Research Consortium. Physiologic monitoring practices during pediatric procedural sedation: a report from the Pediatric Sedation Research Consortium. *Arch Pediatr Adolesc Med.* 2012;166(11):990–998

84. Primosch RE. Lidocaine toxicity in children—prevention and intervention. *Todays FDA.* 1992;4:4C–5C

85. Dial S, Silver P, Bock K, Sagy M. Pediatric sedation for procedures titrated to a desired degree of immobility results in unpredictable depth of sedation. *Pediatr Emerg Care.* 2001;17(6):414–420

86. Maxwell LG, Yaster M. The myth of conscious sedation. *Arch Pediatr Adolesc Med.* 1996;150(7):665–667

87. Coté CJ. "Conscious sedation": time for this oxymoron to go away! *J Pediatr.* 2001;139(1):15–17; discussion: 18–19

88. Motas D, McDermott NB, VanSickle T, Friesen RH. Depth of consciousness and deep sedation attained in children as administered by nonanaesthesiologists in a children's hospital. *Paediatr Anaesth.* 2004;14(3):256–260

89. Cudny ME, Wang NE, Bardas SL, Nguyen CN. Adverse events associated with procedural sedation in pediatric patients in the emergency department. *Hosp Pharm.* 2013;48(2):134–142

90. Mora Capín A, Míguez Navarro C, López López R, Marañón Pardillo R. Usefulness of capnography for monitoring sedoanalgesia: influence of oxygen on the parameters monitored [in Spanish]. *An Pediatr (Barc).* 2014;80(1):41–46

91. Frieling T, Heise J, Kreysel C, Kuhlen R, Schepke M. Sedation-associated complications in endoscopy—prospective multicentre survey of 191142 patients. *Z Gastroenterol.* 2013;51(6):568–572

92. Khutia SK, Mandal MC, Das S, Basu SR. Intravenous infusion of ketamine-propofol can be an alternative to intravenous infusion of fentanyl-propofol for deep sedation and analgesia in paediatric patients undergoing emergency short surgical procedures. *Indian J Anaesth.* 2012;56(2):145–150

93. Kannikeswaran N, Chen X, Sethuraman U. Utility of endtidal carbon dioxide monitoring in detection of hypoxia during sedation for brain magnetic resonance imaging in children with developmental disabilities. *Paediatr Anaesth.* 2011;21(12):1241–1246

94. McGrane O, Hopkins G, Nielson A, Kang C. Procedural sedation with propofol: a retrospective review of the experiences of an emergency medicine residency program 2005 to 2010. *Am J Emerg Med.* 2012;30(5):706–711

95. Mallory MD, Baxter AL, Yanosky DJ, Cravero JP; Pediatric Sedation Research Consortium. Emergency physician-administered propofol sedation: a report on 25,433 sedations from the Pediatric Sedation Research

Consortium. *Ann Emerg Med.* 2011;57(5):462–468.e1

96. Langhan ML, Chen L, Marshall C, Santucci KA. Detection of hypoventilation by capnography and its association with hypoxia in children undergoing sedation with ketamine. *Pediatr Emerg Care.* 2011;27(5):394–397

97. David H, Shipp J. A randomized controlled trial of ketamine/propofol versus propofol alone for emergency department procedural sedation. *Ann Emerg Med.* 2011;57(5):435–441

98. Babl FE, Belousoff J, Deasy C, Hopper S, Theophilos T. Paediatric procedural sedation based on nitrous oxide and ketamine: sedation registry data from Australia. *Emerg Med J.* 2010;27(8):607–612

99. Lee-Jayaram JJ, Green A, Siembieda J, et al. Ketamine/midazolam versus etomidate/fentanyl: procedural sedation for pediatric orthopedic reductions. *Pediatr Emerg Care.* 2010;26(6):408–412

100. Melendez E, Bachur R. Serious adverse events during procedural sedation with ketamine. *Pediatr Emerg Care.* 2009;25(5):325–328

101. Misra S, Mahajan PV, Chen X, Kannikeswaran N. Safety of procedural sedation and analgesia in children less than 2 years of age in a pediatric emergency department. *Int J Emerg Med.* 2008;1(3):173–177

102. Green SM, Roback MG, Krauss B, et al; Emergency Department Ketamine Meta-Analysis Study Group. Predictors of airway and respiratory adverse events with ketamine sedation in the emergency department: an individual-patient data meta-analysis of 8,282 children. *Ann Emerg Med.* 2009;54(2):158–168.e1–e4

103. Kannikeswaran N, Mahajan PV, Sethuraman U, Groebe A, Chen X. Sedation medication received and adverse events related to sedation for brain MRI in children with and without developmental disabilities. *Paediatr Anaesth.* 2009;19(3):250–256

104. Ramaswamy P, Babl FE, Deasy C, Sharwood LN. Pediatric procedural sedation with ketamine: time to discharge after intramuscular versus intravenous administration. *Acad Emerg Med.* 2009;16(2):101–107

105. Vardy JM, Dignon N, Mukherjee N, Sami DM, Balachandran G, Taylor S. Audit of the safety and effectiveness of ketamine for procedural sedation in the emergency department. *Emerg Med J.* 2008;25(9):579–582

106. Capapé S, Mora E, Mintegui S, García S, Santiago M, Benito J. Prolonged sedation and airway complications after administration of an inadvertent ketamine overdose in emergency department. *Eur J Emerg Med.* 2008;15(2):92–94

107. Babl FE, Oakley E, Seaman C, Barnett P, Sharwood LN. High-concentration nitrous oxide for procedural sedation in children: adverse events and depth of sedation. *Pediatrics.* 2008;121(3). Available at: www.pediatrics.org/cgi/content/full/121/3/e528

108. Mahar PJ, Rana JA, Kennedy CS, Christopher NC. A randomized clinical trial of oral transmucosal fentanyl citrate versus intravenous morphine sulfate for initial control of pain in children with extremity injuries. *Pediatr Emerg Care.* 2007;23(8):544–548

109. Sacchetti A, Stander E, Ferguson N, Maniar G, Valko P. Pediatric Procedural Sedation in the Community Emergency Department: results from the ProSCED registry. *Pediatr Emerg Care.* 2007;23(4):218–222

110. Anderson JL, Junkins E, Pribble C, Guenther E. Capnography and depth of sedation during propofol sedation in children. *Ann Emerg Med.* 2007;49(1):9–13

111. Luhmann JD, Schootman M, Luhmann SJ, Kennedy RM. A randomized comparison of nitrous oxide plus hematoma block versus ketamine plus midazolam for emergency department forearm fracture reduction in children. *Pediatrics.* 2006;118(4). Available at: www.pediatrics.org/cgi/content/full/118/4/e1078

112. Waterman GD Jr, Leder MS, Cohen DM. Adverse events in pediatric ketamine sedations with or without morphine pretreatment. *Pediatr Emerg Care.* 2006;22(6):408–411

113. Moore PA, Goodson JM. Risk appraisal of narcotic sedation for children. *Anesth Prog.* 1985;32(4):129–139

114. Nahata MC, Clotz MA, Krogg EA. Adverse effects of meperidine, promethazine, and chlorpromazine for sedation in pediatric patients. *Clin Pediatr (Phila).* 1985;24(10):558–560

115. Brown ET, Corbett SW, Green SM. Iatrogenic cardiopulmonary arrest during pediatric sedation with meperidine, promethazine, and chlorpromazine. *Pediatr Emerg Care.* 2001;17(5):351–353

116. Benusis KP, Kapaun D, Furnam LJ. Respiratory depression in a child following meperidine, promethazine, and chlorpromazine premedication: report of case. *ASDC J Dent Child.* 1979;46(1):50–53

117. Garriott JC, Di Maio VJ. Death in the dental chair: three drug fatalities in dental patients. *J Toxicol Clin Toxicol.* 1982;19(9):987–995

118. Goodson JM, Moore PA. Life-threatening reactions after pedodontic sedation: an assessment of narcotic, local anesthetic, and antiemetic drug interaction. *J Am Dent Assoc.* 1983;107(2):239–245

119. Jastak JT, Pallasch T. Death after chloral hydrate sedation: report of case. *J Am Dent Assoc.* 1988;116(3):345–348

120. Jastak JT, Peskin RM. Major morbidity or mortality from office anesthetic procedures: a closed-claim analysis of 13 cases. *Anesth Prog.* 1991;38(2):39–44

121. Kaufman E, Jastak JT. Sedation for outpatient dental procedures. *Compend Contin Educ Dent.* 1995;16(5):462–466; quiz: 480

122. Wilson S. Pharmacological management of the pediatric dental patient. *Pediatr Dent.* 2004;26(2):131–136

123. Sams DR, Thornton JB, Wright JT. The assessment of two oral sedation drug regimens in pediatric dental patients. *ASDC J Dent Child.* 1992;59(4):306–312

124. Geelhoed GC, Landau LI, Le Souëf PN. Evaluation of SaO2 as a predictor of outcome in 280 children presenting

with acute asthma. *Ann Emerg Med.* 1994;23(6):1236–1241

125. Chicka MC, Dembo JB, Mathu-Muju KR, Nash DA, Bush HM. Adverse events during pediatric dental anesthesia and sedation: a review of closed malpractice insurance claims. *Pediatr Dent.* 2012;34(3):231–238

126. Lee HH, Milgrom P, Starks H, Burke W. Trends in death associated with pediatric dental sedation and general anesthesia. *Paediatr Anaesth.* 2013;23(8):741–746

127. Sanborn PA, Michna E, Zurakowski D, et al. Adverse cardiovascular and respiratory events during sedation of pediatric patients for imaging examinations. *Radiology.* 2005;237(1):288–294

128. Shavit I, Keidan I, Hoffmann Y, et al. Enhancing patient safety during pediatric sedation: the impact of simulation-based training of nonanesthesiologists. *Arch Pediatr Adolesc Med.* 2007;161(8):740–743

129. Cravero JP, Beach ML, Blike GT, Gallagher SM, Hertzog JH; Pediatric Sedation Research Consortium. The incidence and nature of adverse events during pediatric sedation/anesthesia with propofol for procedures outside the operating room: a report from the Pediatric Sedation Research Consortium. *Anesth Analg.* 2009;108(3):795–804

130. Blike GT, Christoffersen K, Cravero JP, Andeweg SK, Jensen J. A method for measuring system safety and latent errors associated with pediatric procedural sedation. *Anesth Analg.* 2005;101(1):48–58

131. Cravero JP, Havidich JE. Pediatric sedation—evolution and revolution. *Paediatr Anaesth.* 2011;21(7):800–809

132. Havidich JE, Cravero JP. The current status of procedural sedation for pediatric patients in out-of-operating room locations. *Curr Opin Anaesthesiol.* 2012;25(4):453–460

133. Hollman GA, Banks DM, Berkenbosch JW, et al. Development, implementation, and initial participant feedback of a pediatric sedation provider course. *Teach Learn Med.* 2013;25(3):249–257

134. Scherrer PD, Mallory MD, Cravero JP, Lowrie L, Hertzog JH, Berkenbosch JW; Pediatric Sedation Research Consortium. The impact of obesity on pediatric procedural sedation-related outcomes: results from the Pediatric Sedation Research Consortium. *Paediatr Anaesth.* 2015;25(7):689–697

135. Emrath ET, Stockwell JA, McCracken CE, Simon HK, Kamat PP. Provision of deep procedural sedation by a pediatric sedation team at a freestanding imaging center. *Pediatr Radiol.* 2014;44(8):1020–1025

136. Kamat PP, McCracken CE, Gillespie SE, et al. Pediatric critical care physician-administered procedural sedation using propofol: a report from the Pediatric Sedation Research Consortium Database. *Pediatr Crit Care Med.* 2015;16(1):11–20

137. Couloures KG, Beach M, Cravero JP, Monroe KK, Hertzog JH. Impact of provider specialty on pediatric procedural sedation complication rates. *Pediatrics.* 2011;127(5). Available at: www.pediatrics.org/cgi/content/full/127/5/e1154

138. Metzner J, Domino KB. Risks of anesthesia or sedation outside the operating room: the role of the anesthesia care provider. *Curr Opin Anaesthesiol.* 2010;23(4):523–531

139. Patel KN, Simon HK, Stockwell CA, et al. Pediatric procedural sedation by a dedicated nonanesthesiology pediatric sedation service using propofol. *Pediatr Emerg Care.* 2009;25(3):133–138

140. Koo SH, Lee DG, Shin H. Optimal initial dose of chloral hydrate in management of pediatric facial laceration. *Arch Plast Surg.* 2014;41(1):40–44

141. Ivaturi V, Kriel R, Brundage R, Loewen G, Mansbach H, Cloyd J. Bioavailability of intranasal vs. rectal diazepam. *Epilepsy Res.* 2013;103(2–3):254–261

142. Mandt MJ, Roback MG, Bajaj L, Galinkin JL, Gao D, Wathen JE. Etomidate for short pediatric procedures in the emergency department. *Pediatr Emerg Care.* 2012;28(9):898–904

143. Tsze DS, Steele DW, Machan JT, Akhlaghi F, Linakis JG. Intranasal ketamine for procedural sedation in pediatric laceration repair: a preliminary report. *Pediatr Emerg Care.* 2012;28(8):767–770

144. Jasiak KD, Phan H, Christich AC, Edwards CJ, Skrepnek GH, Patanwala AE. Induction dose of propofol for pediatric patients undergoing procedural sedation in the emergency department. *Pediatr Emerg Care.* 2012;28(5):440–442

145. McMorrow SP, Abramo TJ. Dexmedetomidine sedation: uses in pediatric procedural sedation outside the operating room. *Pediatr Emerg Care.* 2012;28(3):292–296

146. Sahyoun C, Krauss B. Clinical implications of pharmacokinetics and pharmacodynamics of procedural sedation agents in children. *Curr Opin Pediatr.* 2012;24(2):225–232

147. Sacchetti A, Jachowski J, Heisler J, Cortese T. Remifentanil use in emergency department patients: initial experience. *Emerg Med J.* 2012;29(11):928–929

148. Shah A, Mosdossy G, McLeod S, Lehnhardt K, Peddle M, Rieder M. A blinded, randomized controlled trial to evaluate ketamine/propofol versus ketamine alone for procedural sedation in children. *Ann Emerg Med.* 2011;57(5):425–433.e2

149. Herd DW, Anderson BJ, Keene NA, Holford NH. Investigating the pharmacodynamics of ketamine in children. *Paediatr Anaesth.* 2008;18(1):36–42

150. Shcarieff GQ, Trocinski DR, Kanegaye JT, Fisher B, Harley JR. Ketamine-propofol combination sedation for fracture reduction in the pediatric emergency department. *Pediatr Emerg Care.* 2007;23(12):881–884

151. Herd DW, Anderson BJ, Holford NH. Modeling the norketamine metabolite in children and the implications for analgesia. *Paediatr Anaesth.* 2007;17(9):831–840

152. Herd D, Anderson BJ. Ketamine disposition in children presenting for procedural sedation and analgesia in a children's emergency department. *Paediatr Anaesth.* 2007;17(7):622–629

153. Heard CM, Joshi P, Johnson K. Dexmedetomidine for pediatric MRI

sedation: a review of a series of cases. *Paediatr Anaesth.* 2007;17(9):888–892

154. Heard C, Burrows F, Johnson K, Joshi P, Houck J, Lerman J. A comparison of dexmedetomidine-midazolam with propofol for maintenance of anesthesia in children undergoing magnetic resonance imaging. *Anesth Analg.* 2008;107(6):1832–1839

155. Hertzog JH, Havidich JE. Non-anesthesiologist-provided pediatric procedural sedation: an update. *Curr Opin Anaesthesiol.* 2007;20(4):365–372

156. Petroz GC, Sikich N, James M, et al. A phase I, two-center study of the pharmacokinetics and pharmacodynamics of dexmedetomidine in children. *Anesthesiology.* 2006;105(6):1098–1110

157. Potts AL, Anderson BJ, Warman GR, Lerman J, Diaz SM, Vilo S. Dexmedetomidine pharmacokinetics in pediatric intensive care—a pooled analysis. *Paediatr Anaesth.* 2009;19(11):1119–1129

158. Mason KP, Lerman J. Dexmedetomidine in children: current knowledge and future applications [review]. *Anesth Analg.* 2011;113(5):1129–1142

159. Sammartino M, Volpe B, Sbaraglia F, Garra R, D'Addessi A. Capnography and the bispectral index—their role in pediatric sedation: a brief review. *Int J Pediatr.* 2010;2010:828347

160. Yarchi D, Cohen A, Umansky T, Sukhotnik I, Shaoul R. Assessment of end-tidal carbon dioxide during pediatric and adult sedation for endoscopic procedures. *Gastrointest Endosc.* 2009;69(4):877–882

161. Lightdale JR, Goldmann DA, Feldman HA, Newburg AR, DiNardo JA, Fox VL. Microstream capnography improves patient monitoring during moderate sedation: a randomized, controlled trial. *Pediatrics.* 2006;117(6). Available at: www.pediatrics.org/cgi/content/full/117/6/e1170

162. Yldzdaş D, Yapcoglu H, Ylmaz HL. The value of capnography during sedation or sedation/analgesia in pediatric minor procedures. *Pediatr Emerg Care.* 2004;20(3):162–165

163. Connor L, Burrows PE, Zurakowski D, Bucci K, Gagnon DA, Mason KP.

Effects of IV pentobarbital with and without fentanyl on end-tidal carbon dioxide levels during deep sedation of pediatric patients undergoing MRI. *AJR Am J Roentgenol.* 2003;181(6):1691–1694

164. Primosch RE, Buzzi IM, Jerrell G. Monitoring pediatric dental patients with nasal mask capnography. *Pediatr Dent.* 2000;22(2):120–124

165. Tobias JD. End-tidal carbon dioxide monitoring during sedation with a combination of midazolam and ketamine for children undergoing painful, invasive procedures. *Pediatr Emerg Care.* 1999;15(3):173–175

166. Hart LS, Berns SD, Houck CS, Boenning DA. The value of end-tidal CO2 monitoring when comparing three methods of conscious sedation for children undergoing painful procedures in the emergency department. *Pediatr Emerg Care.* 1997;13(3):189–193

167. Marx CM, Stein J, Tyler MK, Nieder ML, Shurin SB, Blumer JL. Ketamine-midazolam versus meperidine-midazolam for painful procedures in pediatric oncology patients. *J Clin Oncol.* 1997;15(1):94–102

168. Croswell RJ, Dilley DC, Lucas WJ, Vann WF Jr. A comparison of conventional versus electronic monitoring of sedated pediatric dental patients. *Pediatr Dent.* 1995;17(5):332–339

169. Iwasaki J, Vann WF Jr, Dilley DC, Anderson JA. An investigation of capnography and pulse oximetry as monitors of pediatric patients sedated for dental treatment. *Pediatr Dent.* 1989;11(2):111–117

170. Anderson JA, Vann WF Jr. Respiratory monitoring during pediatric sedation: pulse oximetry and capnography. *Pediatr Dent.* 1988;10(2):94–101

171. Rothman DL. Sedation of the pediatric patient. *J Calif Dent Assoc.* 2013;41(8):603–611

172. Scherrer PD. Safe and sound: pediatric procedural sedation and analgesia. *Minn Med.* 2011;94(3):43–47

173. Srinivasan M, Turmelle M, Depalma LM, Mao J, Carlson DW. Procedural sedation for diagnostic imaging in children by pediatric hospitalists

using propofol: analysis of the nature, frequency, and predictors of adverse events and interventions. *J Pediatr.* 2012;160(5):801–806.e1

174. Langhan ML, Shabanova V, Li FY, Bernstein SL, Shapiro ED. A randomized controlled trial of capnography during sedation in a pediatric emergency setting. *Am J Emerg Med.* 2015;33(1):25–30

175. Vetri Buratti C, Angelino F, Sansoni J, Fabriani L, Mauro L, Latina R. Distraction as a technique to control pain in pediatric patients during venipuncture: a narrative review of literature. *Prof Inferm.* 2015;68(1):52–62

176. Robinson PS, Green J. Ambient versus traditional environment in pediatric emergency department. *HERD.* 2015;8(2):71–80

177. Singh D, Samadi F, Jaiswal J, Tripathi AM. Stress reduction through audio distraction in anxious pediatric dental patients: an adjunctive clinical study. *Int J Clin Pediatr Dent.* 2014;7(3):149–152

178. Attar RH, Baghdadi ZD. Comparative efficacy of active and passive distraction during restorative treatment in children using an iPad versus audiovisual eyeglasses: a randomised controlled trial. *Eur Arch Paediatr Dent.* 2015;16(1):1–8

179. McCarthy AM, Kleiber C, Hanrahan K, et al. Matching doses of distraction with child risk for distress during a medical procedure: a randomized clinical trial. *Nurs Res.* 2014;63(6):397–407

180. Guinot Jimeno F, Mercadé Bellido M, Cuadros Fernández C, Lorente Rodríguez AI, Llopis Pérez J, Boj Quesada JR. Effect of audiovisual distraction on children's behaviour, anxiety and pain in the dental setting. *Eur J Paediatr Dent.* 2014;15(3):297–302

181. Gupta HV, Gupta VV, Kaur A, et al. Comparison between the analgesic effect of two techniques on the level of pain perception during venipuncture in children up to 7 years of age: a quasi-experimental study. *J Clin Diagn Res.* 2014;8(8):PC01–PC04

182. Newton JT, Shah S, Patel H, Sturmey P. Non-pharmacological approaches to

behaviour management in children. *Dent Update.* 2003;30(4):194–199

183. Peretz B, Bimstein E. The use of imagery suggestions during administration of local anesthetic in pediatric dental patients. *ASDC J Dent Child.* 2000;67(4):263–267, 231

184. Iserson KV. Hypnosis for pediatric fracture reduction. *J Emerg Med.* 1999;17(1):53–56

185. Rusy LM, Weisman SJ. Complementary therapies for acute pediatric pain management. *Pediatr Clin North Am.* 2000;47(3):589–599

186. Langley P. Guided imagery: a review of effectiveness in the care of children. *Paediatr Nurs.* 1999;11(3):18–21

187. Ott MJ. Imagine the possibilities! Guided imagery with toddlers and pre-schoolers. *Pediatr Nurs.* 1996;22(1):34–38

188. Singer AJ, Stark MJ. LET versus EMLA for pretreating lacerations: a randomized trial. *Acad Emerg Med.* 2001;8(3):223–230

189. Taddio A, Gurguis MG, Koren G. Lidocaine-prilocaine cream versus tetracaine gel for procedural pain in children. *Ann Pharmacother.* 2002;36(4):687–692

190. Eichenfield LF, Funk A, Fallon-Friedlander S, Cunningham BB. A clinical study to evaluate the efficacy of ELA-Max (4% liposomal lidocaine) as compared with eutectic mixture of local anesthetics cream for pain reduction of venipuncture in children. *Pediatrics.* 2002;109(6):1093–1099

191. Shaw AJ, Welbury RR. The use of hypnosis in a sedation clinic for dental extractions in children: report of 20 cases. *ASDC J Dent Child.* 1996;63(6):418–420

192. Stock A, Hill A, Babl FE. Practical communication guide for paediatric procedures. *Emerg Med Australas.* 2012;24(6):641–646

193. Barnea-Goraly N, Weinzimer SA, Ruedy KJ, et al; Diabetes Research in Children Network (DirecNet). High success rates of sedation-free brain MRI scanning in young children using simple subject preparation protocols with and without a commercial mock scanner—the Diabetes Research in Children Network (DirecNet) experience. *Pediatr Radiol.* 2014;44(2):181–186

194. Ram D, Shapira J, Holan G, Magora F, Cohen S, Davidovich E. Audiovisual video eyeglass distraction during dental treatment in children. *Quintessence Int.* 2010;41(8):673–679

195. Lemaire C, Moran GR, Swan H. Impact of audio/visual systems on pediatric sedation in magnetic resonance imaging. *J Magn Reson Imaging.* 2009;30(3):649–655

196. Nordahl CW, Simon TJ, Zierhut C, Solomon M, Rogers SJ, Amaral DG. Brief report: methods for acquiring structural MRI data in very young children with autism without the use of sedation. *J Autism Dev Disord.* 2008;38(8):1581–1590

197. Denman WT, Tuason PM, Ahmed MI, Brennen LM, Cepeda MS, Carr DB. The PediSedate device, a novel approach to pediatric sedation that provides distraction and inhaled nitrous oxide: clinical evaluation in a large case series. *Paediatr Anaesth.* 2007;17(2):162–166

198. Harned RK II, Strain JD. MRI-compatible audio/visual system: impact on pediatric sedation. *Pediatr Radiol.* 2001;31(4):247–250

199. Slifer KJ. A video system to help children cooperate with motion control for radiation treatment without sedation. *J Pediatr Oncol Nurs.* 1996;13(2):91–97

200. Krauss BS, Krauss BA, Green SM. Videos in clinical medicine: procedural sedation and analgesia in children. *N Engl J Med.* 2014;370(15):e23

201. Wilson S. Management of child patient behavior: quality of care, fear and anxiety, and the child patient. *Pediatr Dent.* 2013;35(2):170–174

202. Kamath PS. A novel distraction technique for pain management during local anesthesia administration in pediatric patients. *J Clin Pediatr Dent.* 2013;38(1):45–47

203. Asl Aminabadi N, Erfanparast L, Sohrabi A, Ghertasi Oskouei S, Naghili A. The impact of virtual reality distraction on pain and anxiety during dental treatment in 4-6 year-old children: a randomized controlled clinical trial. *J Dent Res Dent Clin Dent Prospect.* 2012;6(4):117–124

204. El-Sharkawi HF, El-Housseiny AA, Aly AM. Effectiveness of new distraction technique on pain associated with injection of local anesthesia for children. *Pediatr Dent.* 2012;34(2):e35–e38

205. Adinolfi B, Gava N. Controlled outcome studies of child clinical hypnosis. *Acta Biomed.* 2013;84(2):94–97

206. Peretz B, Bercovich R, Blumer S. Using elements of hypnosis prior to or during pediatric dental treatment. *Pediatr Dent.* 2013;35(1):33–36

207. Huet A, Lucas-Polomeni MM, Robert JC, Sixou JL, Wodey E. Hypnosis and dental anesthesia in children: a prospective controlled study. *Int J Clin Exp Hypn.* 2011;59(4):424–440

208. Al-Harasi S, Ashley PF, Moles DR, Parekh S, Walters V. Hypnosis for children undergoing dental treatment. *Cochrane Database Syst Rev.* 2010;8:CD007154

209. McQueen A, Cress C, Tothy A. Using a tablet computer during pediatric procedures: a case series and review of the "apps". *Pediatr Emerg Care.* 2012;28(7):712–714

210. Heilbrunn BR, Wittern RE, Lee JB, Pham PK, Hamilton AH, Nager AL. Reducing anxiety in the pediatric emergency department: a comparative trial. *J Emerg Med.* 2014;47(6):623–631

211. Tyson ME, Bohl DD, Blickman JG. A randomized controlled trial: child life services in pediatric imaging. *Pediatr Radiol.* 2014;44(11):1426–1432

212. Malviya S, Voepel-Lewis T, Tait AR, Merkel S, Tremper K, Naughton N. Depth of sedation in children undergoing computed tomography: validity and reliability of the University of Michigan Sedation Scale (UMSS). *Br J Anaesth.* 2002;88(2):241–245

213. Gamble C, Gamble J, Seal R, Wright RB, Ali S. Bispectral analysis during procedural sedation in the pediatric emergency department. *Pediatr Emerg Care.* 2012;28(10):1003–1008

214. Domino KB. Office-based anesthesia: lessons learned from the closed claims project. *ASA Newsl.* 2001;65:9–15

215. American Heart Association. *Pediatric Advance Life Support Provider Manual*. Dallas, TX: American Heart Association; 2011

216. American Academy of Pediatrics, American College of Emergency Physicians. *Advanced Pediatric Life Support*, 5th ed.. Boston, MA: Jones and Bartlett Publishers; 2012

217. Cheng A, Brown LL, Duff JP, et al; International Network for Simulation-Based Pediatric Innovation, Research, and Education (INSPIRE) CPR Investigators. Improving cardiopulmonary resuscitation with a CPR feedback device and refresher simulations (CPR CARES Study): a randomized clinical trial. *JAMA Pediatr*. 2015;169(2):137–144

218. Nishisaki A, Nguyen J, Colborn S, et al. Evaluation of multidisciplinary simulation training on clinical performance and team behavior during tracheal intubation procedures in a pediatric intensive care unit. *Pediatr Crit Care Med*. 2011;12(4):406–414

219. Howard-Quijano KJ, Stiegler MA, Huang YM, Canales C, Steadman RH. Anesthesiology residents' performance of pediatric resuscitation during a simulated hyperkalemic cardiac arrest. *Anesthesiology*. 2010;112(4):993–997

220. Chen MI, Edler A, Wald S, DuBois J, Huang YM. Scenario and checklist for airway rescue during pediatric sedation. *Simul Healthc*. 2007;2(3):194–198

221. Wheeler M. Management strategies for the difficult pediatric airway. In: Riazi J, ed. *The Difficult Pediatric Airway*. 16th ed. Philadelphia, PA: W.B. Saunders Company; 1998:743–761

222. Sullivan KJ, Kissoon N. Securing the child's airway in the emergency department. *Pediatr Emerg Care*. 2002;18(2):108–121; quiz: 122–124

223. Levy RJ, Helfaer MA. Pediatric airway issues. *Crit Care Clin*. 2000;16(3):489–504

224. Krauss B, Green SM. Procedural sedation and analgesia in children. *Lancet*. 2006; 367(9512):766–780

225. Krauss B, Green SM. Sedation and analgesia for procedures in children. *N Engl J Med*. 2000;342(13):938–945

226. Ferrari L, ed . *Anesthesia and Pain Management for the Pediatrician*, 1st ed. Baltimore, MD: John Hopkins University Press; 1999

227. Malvyia S. *Sedation Analgesia for Diagnostic and Therapeutic Procedures*, 1st ed. Totowa, NJ: Humana Press; 2001

228. Yaster M, Krane EJ, Kaplan RF, Coté CJ, Lappe DG. *Pediatric Pain Management and Sedation Handbook*. 1st ed. St. Louis, MO: Mosby-Year Book, Inc.; 1997

229. Cravero JP, Blike GT. Review of pediatric sedation. *Anesth Analg*. 2004;99(5):1355–1364

230. Deshpande JK, Tobias JD. *The Pediatric Pain Handbook*. 1st ed. St. Louis, MO: Mosby; 1996

231. Mace SE, Barata IA, Cravero JP, et al; American College of Emergency Physicians. Clinical policy: evidence-based approach to pharmacologic agents used in pediatric sedation and analgesia in the emergency department. *Ann Emerg Med*. 2004;44(4):342–377

232. Alcaino EA. Conscious sedation in paediatric dentistry: current philosophies and techniques. *Ann R Australas Coll Dent Surg*. 2000;15:206–210

233. Tobias JD, Cravero JP. *Procedural Sedation for Infants, Children, and Adolescents*. Elk Grove Village, IL: American Academy of Pediatrics; 2015

234. Committee on Standards and Practice Parameters. *Standards for Basic Anesthetic Monitoring*. Chicago, IL: American Society of Anesthesiologists; 2011

235. Mitchell AA, Louik C, Lacouture P, Slone D, Goldman P, Shapiro S. Risks to children from computed tomographic scan premedication. *JAMA*. 1982;247(17):2385–2388

236. Wolfe TR, Braude DA. Intranasal medication delivery for children: a brief review and update. *Pediatrics*. 2010;126(3):532–537

237. Bührer M, Maitre PO, Crevoisier C, Stanski DR. Electroencephalographic effects of benzodiazepines. II.

Pharmacodynamic modeling of the electroencephalographic effects of midazolam and diazepam. *Clin Pharmacol Ther*. 1990;48(5):555–567

238. Malviya S, Voepel-Lewis T, Ludomirsky A, Marshall J, Tait AR. Can we improve the assessment of discharge readiness? A comparative study of observational and objective measures of depth of sedation in children. *Anesthesiology*. 2004;100(2):218–224

239. Coté CJ. Discharge criteria for children sedated by nonanesthesiologists: is "safe" really safe enough? *Anesthesiology*. 2004;100(2):207–209

240. Pershad J, Palmisano P, Nichols M. Chloral hydrate: the good and the bad. *Pediatr Emerg Care*. 1999;15(6):432–435

241. McCormack L, Chen JW, Trapp L, Job A. A comparison of sedation-related events for two multiagent oral sedation regimens in pediatric dental patients. *Pediatr Dent*. 2014;36(4):302–308

242. Kinane TB, Murphy J, Bass JL, Corwin MJ. Comparison of respiratory physiologic features when infants are placed in car safety seats or car beds. *Pediatrics*. 2006;118(2):522–527

243. Wyeth Pharmaceuticals. *Wyeth Phenergan (Promethazine HCL) Tablets and Suppositories* [package insert]. Philadelphia, PA: Wyeth Pharmaceuticals; 2012

244. Caperell K, Pitetti R. Is higher ASA class associated with an increased incidence of adverse events during procedural sedation in a pediatric emergency department? *Pediatr Emerg Care*. 2009;25(10):661–664

245. Dar AQ, Shah ZA. Anesthesia and sedation in pediatric gastrointestinal endoscopic procedures: a review. *World J Gastrointest Endosc*. 2010;2(7):257–262

246. Kiringoda R, Thurm AE, Hirschtritt ME, et al. Risks of propofol sedation/ anesthesia for imaging studies in pediatric research: eight years of experience in a clinical research center. *Arch Pediatr Adolesc Med*. 2010;164(6):554–560

247. Thakkar K, El-Serag HB, Mattek N, Gilger MA. Complications of pediatric EGD: a 4-year experience

in PEDS-CORI. *Gastrointest Endosc.* 2007;65(2):213–221

248. Jackson DL, Johnson BS. Conscious sedation for dentistry: risk management and patient selection. *Dent Clin North Am.* 2002;46(4):767–780

249. Malviya S, Voepel-Lewis T, Eldevik OP, Rockwell DT, Wong JH, Tait AR. Sedation and general anaesthesia in children undergoing MRI and CT: adverse events and outcomes. *Br J Anaesth.* 2000;84(6):743–748

250. O'Neil J, Yonkman J, Talty J, Bull MJ. Transporting children with special health care needs: comparing recommendations and practice. *Pediatrics.* 2009;124(2):596–603

251. Committee on Bioethics, American Academy of Pediatrics. Informed consent, parental permission, and assent in pediatric practice *Pediatrics.* 1995;95(2):314–317

252. Committee on Pediatric Emergency Medicine; Committee on Bioethics. Consent for emergency medical services for children and adolescents. *Pediatrics.* 2011;128(2):427–433

253. Martinez D, Wilson S. Children sedated for dental care: a pilot study of the 24-hour postsedation period. *Pediatr Dent.* 2006;28(3):260–264

254. Kaila R, Chen X, Kannikeswaran N. Postdischarge adverse events related to sedation for diagnostic imaging in children. *Pediatr Emerg Care.* 2012;28(8):796–801

255. Treston G, Bell A, Cardwell R, Fincher G, Chand D, Cashion G. What is the nature of the emergence phenomenon when using intravenous or intramuscular ketamine for paediatric procedural sedation? *Emerg Med Australas.* 2009;21(4):315–322

256. Malviya S, Voepel-Lewis T, Prochaska G, Tait AR. Prolonged recovery and delayed side effects of sedation for diagnostic imaging studies in children. *Pediatrics.* 2000;105(3):E42

257. Nordt SP, Rangan C, Hardmaslani M, Clark RF, Wendler C, Valente M. Pediatric chloral hydrate poisonings and death following outpatient procedural sedation. *J Med Toxicol.* 2014;10(2):219–222

258. Walker RW. Pulmonary aspiration in pediatric anesthetic practice

in the UK: a prospective survey of specialist pediatric centers over a one-year period. *Paediatr Anaesth.* 2013;23(8):702–711

259. Babl FE, Puspitadewi A, Barnett P, Oakley E, Spicer M. Preprocedural fasting state and adverse events in children receiving nitrous oxide for procedural sedation and analgesia. *Pediatr Emerg Care.* 2005;21(11):736–743

260. Roback MG, Bajaj L, Wathen JE, Bothner J. Preprocedural fasting and adverse events in procedural sedation and analgesia in a pediatric emergency department: are they related? *Ann Emerg Med.* 2004;44(5):454–459

261. Vespasiano M, Finkelstein M, Kurachek S. Propofol sedation: intensivists' experience with 7304 cases in a children's hospital. *Pediatrics.* 2007;120(6). Available at: www.pediatrics.org/cgi/content/full/120/6/e1411

262. Warner MA, Warner ME, Warner DO, Warner LO, Warner EJ. Perioperative pulmonary aspiration in infants and children. *Anesthesiology.* 1999;90(1):66–71

263. Borland LM, Sereika SM, Woelfel SK, et al. Pulmonary aspiration in pediatric patients during general anesthesia: incidence and outcome. *J Clin Anesth.* 1998;10(2):95–102

264. Agrawal D, Manzi SF, Gupta R, Krauss B. Preprocedural fasting state and adverse events in children undergoing procedural sedation and analgesia in a pediatric emergency department. *Ann Emerg Med.* 2003;42(5):636–646

265. Green SM. Fasting is a consideration—not a necessity—for emergency department procedural sedation and analgesia. *Ann Emerg Med.* 2003;42(5):647–650

266. Green SM, Krauss B. Pulmonary aspiration risk during emergency department procedural sedation—an examination of the role of fasting and sedation depth. *Acad Emerg Med.* 2002;9(1):35–42

267. Treston G. Prolonged pre-procedure fasting time is unnecessary when using titrated intravenous ketamine for paediatric procedural

sedation. *Emerg Med Australas.* 2004;16(2):145–150

268. Pitetti RD, Singh S, Pierce MC. Safe and efficacious use of procedural sedation and analgesia by nonanesthesiologists in a pediatric emergency department. *Arch Pediatr Adolesc Med.* 2003;157(11):1090–1096

269. Thorpe RJ, Benger J. Pre-procedural fasting in emergency sedation. *Emerg Med J.* 2010;27(4):254–261

270. Paris PM, Yealy DM. A procedural sedation and analgesia fasting consensus advisory: one small step for emergency medicine, one giant challenge remaining. *Ann Emerg Med.* 2007;49(4):465–467

271. American Society of Anesthesiologists Committee. Practice guidelines for preoperative fasting and the use of pharmacologic agents to reduce the risk of pulmonary aspiration: application to healthy patients undergoing elective procedures: an updated report by the American Society of Anesthesiologists Committee on Standards and Practice Parameters. *Anesthesiology.* 2011;114(3):495–511

272. Mace SE, Brown LA, Francis L, et al Clinical policy: Critical issues in the sedation of pediatric patients in the emergency department. *Ann Emerg Med.* 2008;51:378–399

273. Green SM, Roback MG, Miner JR, Burton JH, Krauss B. Fasting and emergency department procedural sedation and analgesia: a consensus-based clinical practice advisory. *Ann Emerg Med.* 2007;49(4):454–461

274. Duchicela S, Lim A. Pediatric nerve blocks: an evidence-based approach. *Pediatr Emerg Med Pract.* 2013;10(10):1–19; quiz: 19–20

275. Beach ML, Cohen DM, Gallagher SM, Cravero JP. Major adverse events and relationship to nil per os status in pediatric sedation/anesthesia outside the operating room: a report of the Pediatric Sedation Research Consortium. *Anesthesiology.* 2016;124(1):80–88

276. Green SM, Krauss B. Ketamine is a safe, effective, and appropriate technique for emergency department

paediatric procedural sedation. *Emerg Med J.* 2004;21(3):271–272

277. American Academy of Pediatrics Committee on Pediatric Emergency Medicine. The use of physical restraint interventions for children and adolescents in the acute care setting. *Pediatrics.* 1997;99(3):497–498

278. American Academy of Pediatrics Committee on Child Abuse and Neglect. Behavior management of pediatric dental patients. *Pediatrics.* 1992;90(4):651–652

279. American Academy of Pediatric Dentistry. Guideline on protective stabilization for pediatric dental patients. *Pediatr Dent.* 2013;35(5):E169–E173

280. Loo CY, Graham RM, Hughes CV. Behaviour guidance in dental treatment of patients with autism spectrum disorder. *Int J Paediatr Dent.* 2009;19(6):390–398

281. McWhorter AG, Townsend JA; American Academy of Pediatric Dentistry. Behavior symposium workshop A report—current guidelines/revision. *Pediatr Dent.* 2014;36(2):152–153

282. American Society of Anesthesiologists CoSaPP. Practice advisory for preanesthesia evaluation an updated report by the American Society of Anesthesiologists Task Force on Preanesthesia Evaluation. *Anesthesiology.* 2012;116:1–17

283. Gorski JC, Huang SM, Pinto A, et al. The effect of echinacea (Echinacea purpurea root) on cytochrome P450 activity in vivo. *Clin Pharmacol Ther.* 2004;75(1):89–100

284. Hall SD, Wang Z, Huang SM, et al. The interaction between St John's wort and an oral contraceptive. *Clin Pharmacol Ther.* 2003;74(6):525–535

285. Markowitz JS, Donovan JL, DeVane CL, et al. Effect of St John's wort on drug metabolism by induction of cytochrome P450 3A4 enzyme. *JAMA.* 2003;290(11):1500–1504

286. Spinella M. Herbal medicines and epilepsy: the potential for benefit and adverse effects. *Epilepsy Behav.* 2001;2(6):524–532

287. Wang Z, Gorski JC, Hamman MA, Huang SM, Lesko LJ, Hall SD. The effects of St John's wort (Hypericum perforatum) on human cytochrome P450 activity. *Clin Pharmacol Ther.* 2001;70(4):317–326

288. Xie HG, Kim RB. St John's wort-associated drug interactions: short-term inhibition and long-term induction? *Clin Pharmacol Ther.* 2005;78(1):19–24

289. Chen XW, Sneed KB, Pan SY, et al. Herb-drug interactions and mechanistic and clinical considerations. *Curr Drug Metab.* 2012;13(5):640–651

290. Chen XW, Serag ES, Sneed KB, et al. Clinical herbal interactions with conventional drugs: from molecules to maladies. *Curr Med Chem.* 2011;18(31):4836–4850

291. Shi S, Klotz U. Drug interactions with herbal medicines. *Clin Pharmacokinet.* 2012;51(2):77–104

292. Saxena A, Tripathi KP, Roy S, Khan F, Sharma A. Pharmacovigilance: effects of herbal components on human drugs interactions involving cytochrome P450. *Bioinformation.* 2008;3(5):198–204

293. Yang X, Salminen WF. Kava extract, an herbal alternative for anxiety relief, potentiates acetaminophen-induced cytotoxicity in rat hepatic cells. *Phytomedicine.* 2011;18(7):592–600

294. Teschke R. Kava hepatotoxicity: pathogenetic aspects and prospective considerations. *Liver Int.* 2010;30(9):1270–1279

295. Izzo AA, Ernst E. Interactions between herbal medicines and prescribed drugs: an updated systematic review. *Drugs.* 2009;69(13):1777–1798

296. Ang-Lee MK, Moss J, Yuan CS. Herbal medicines and perioperative care. *JAMA.* 2001;286(2):208–216

297. Abebe W. Herbal medication: potential for adverse interactions with analgesic drugs. *J Clin Pharm Ther.* 2002;27(6):391–401

298. Mooiman KD, Maas-Bakker RF, Hendrikx JJ, et al. The effect of complementary and alternative medicines on CYP3A4-mediated metabolism of three different substrates: 7-benzyloxy-4-trifluoromethyl-coumarin, midazolam and docetaxel. *J Pharm Pharmacol.* 2014;66(6):865–874

299. Carrasco MC, Vallejo JR, Pardo-de-Santayana M, Peral D, Martín MA, Altimiras J. Interactions of Valeriana officinalis L. and Passiflora incarnata L. in a patient treated with lorazepam. *Phytother Res.* 2009;23(12):1795–1796

300. von Rosensteil NA, Adam D. Macrolide antibacterials: drug interactions of clinical significance. *Drug Saf.* 1995;13(2):105–122

301. Hiller A, Olkkola KT, Isohanni P, Saarnivaara L. Unconsciousness associated with midazolam and erythromycin. *Br J Anaesth.* 1990;65(6):826–828

302. Mattila MJ, Idänpään-Heikkilä JJ, Törnwall M, Vanakoski J. Oral single doses of erythromycin and roxithromycin may increase the effects of midazolam on human performance. *Pharmacol Toxicol.* 1993;73(3):180–185

303. Olkkola KT, Aranko K, Luurila H, et al. A potentially hazardous interaction between erythromycin and midazolam. *Clin Pharmacol Ther.* 1993;53(3):298–305

304. Senthilkumaran S, Subramanian PT. Prolonged sedation related to erythromycin and midazolam interaction: a word of caution. *Indian Pediatr.* 2011;48(11):909

305. Flockhart DA, Oesterheld JR. Cytochrome P450-mediated drug interactions. *Child Adolesc Psychiatr Clin N Am.* 2000;9(1):43–76

306. Yuan R, Flockhart DA, Balian JD. Pharmacokinetic and pharmacodynamic consequences of metabolism-based drug interactions with alprazolam, midazolam, and triazolam. *J Clin Pharmacol.* 1999;39(11):1109–1125

307. Young B. Review: mixing new cocktails: drug interactions in antiretroviral regimens. *AIDS Patient Care STDS.* 2005;19(5):286–297

308. Gonçalves LS, Gonçalves BM, de Andrade MA, Alves FR, Junior AS. Drug interactions during periodontal therapy in HIV-infected subjects. *Mini Rev Med Chem.* 2010;10(8):766–772

309. Brown KC, Paul S, Kashuba AD. Drug interactions with new and investigational antiretrovirals. *Clin Pharmacokinet.* 2009;48(4):211–241

310. Pau AK. Clinical management of drug interaction with antiretroviral agents. *Curr Opin HIV AIDS.* 2008;3(3):319–324

311. Moyal WN, Lord C, Walkup JT. Quality of life in children and adolescents with autism spectrum disorders: what is known about the effects of pharmacotherapy? *Paediatr Drugs.* 2014;16(2):123–128

312. van den Anker JN. Developmental pharmacology. *Dev Disabil Res Rev.* 2010;16(3):233–238

313. Pichini S, Papaseit E, Joya X, et al. Pharmacokinetics and therapeutic drug monitoring of psychotropic drugs in pediatrics. *Ther Drug Monit.* 2009;31(3):283–318

314. Tibussek D, Distelmaier F, Schönberger S, Göbel U, Mayatepek E. Antiepileptic treatment in paediatric oncology—an interdisciplinary challenge. *Klin Padiatr.* 2006;218(6):340–349

315. Wilkinson GR. Drug metabolism and variability among patients in drug response. *N Engl J Med.* 2005;352(21):2211–2221

316. Salem F, Rostami-Hodjegan A, Johnson TN. Do children have the same vulnerability to metabolic drug–drug interactions as adults? A critical analysis of the literature. *J Clin Pharmacol.* 2013;53(5):559–566

317. Funk RS, Brown JT, Abdel-Rahman SM. Pediatric pharmacokinetics: human development and drug disposition. *Pediatr Clin North Am.* 2012;59(5):1001–1016

318. Anderson BJ. My child is unique: the pharmacokinetics are universal. *Paediatr Anaesth.* 2012;22(6):530–538

319. Elie V, de Beaumais T, Fakhoury M, Jacqz-Aigrain E. Pharmacogenetics and individualized therapy in children: immunosuppressants, antidepressants, anticancer and anti-inflammatory drugs. *Pharmacogenomics.* 2011;12(6):827–843

320. Chen ZR, Somogyi AA, Reynolds G, Bochner F. Disposition and metabolism of codeine after single and chronic doses in one poor and seven extensive metabolisers. *Br J Clin Pharmacol.* 1991;31(4):381–390

321. Gasche Y, Daali Y, Fathi M, et al. Codeine intoxication associated with ultrarapid CYP2D6 metabolism. *N Engl J Med.* 2004;351(27):2827–2831

322. Kirchheiner J, Schmidt H, Tzvetkov M, et al. Pharmacokinetics of codeine and its metabolite morphine in ultra-rapid metabolizers due to CYP2D6 duplication. *Pharmacogenomics J.* 2007;7(4):257–265

323. Voronov P, Przybylo HJ, Jagannathan N. Apnea in a child after oral codeine: a genetic variant—an ultra-rapid metabolizer. *Paediatr Anaesth.* 2007;17(7):684–687

324. Kelly LE, Rieder M, van den Anker J, et al. More codeine fatalities after tonsillectomy in North American children. *Pediatrics.* 2012;129(5). Available at: www.pediatrics.org/cgi/content/full/129/5/e1343

325. Farber JM. Clinical practice guideline: diagnosis and management of childhood obstructive sleep apnea syndrome. *Pediatrics.* 2002;110(6):1255–1257; author reply: 1255–1257

326. Schechter MS; Section on Pediatric Pulmonology, Subcommittee on Obstructive Sleep Apnea Syndrome. Technical report: diagnosis and management of childhood obstructive sleep apnea syndrome. *Pediatrics.* 2002;109(4). Available at: www.pediatrics.org/cgi/content/full/109/4/e69

327. Marcus CL, Brooks LJ, Draper KA, et al; American Academy of Pediatrics. Diagnosis and management of childhood obstructive sleep apnea syndrome. *Pediatrics.* 2012;130(3):576–584

328. Coté CJ, Posner KL, Domino KB. Death or neurologic injury after tonsillectomy in children with a focus on obstructive sleep apnea: Houston, we have a problem! *Anesth Analg.* 2014;118(6):1276–1283

329. Wheeler M, Coté CJ. Preoperative pregnancy testing in a tertiary care children's hospital: a medico-legal conundrum. *J Clin Anesth.* 1999;11(1):56–63

330. Neuman G, Koren G. Safety of procedural sedation in pregnancy. *J Obstet Gynaecol Can.* 2013;35(2):168–173

331. Larcher V. Developing guidance for checking pregnancy status in adolescent girls before surgical, radiological or other procedures. *Arch Dis Child.* 2012;97(10):857–860

332. August DA, Everett LL. Pediatric ambulatory anesthesia. *Anesthesiol Clin.* 2014;32(2):411–429

333. Maxwell LG. Age-associated issues in preoperative evaluation, testing, and planning: pediatrics. *Anesthesiol Clin North America.* 2004;22(1):27–43

334. Davidson AJ. Anesthesia and neurotoxicity to the developing brain: the clinical relevance. *Paediatr Anaesth.* 2011;21(7):716–721

335. Reddy SV. Effect of general anesthetics on the developing brain. *J Anaesthesiol Clin Pharmacol.* 2012;28(1):6–10

336. Nemergut ME, Aganga D, Flick RP. Anesthetic neurotoxicity: what to tell the parents? *Paediatr Anaesth.* 2014;24(1):120–126

337. Olsen EA, Brambrink AM. Anesthesia for the young child undergoing ambulatory procedures: current concerns regarding harm to the developing brain. *Curr Opin Anaesthesiol.* 2013;26(6):677–684

338. Green SM, Coté CJ. Ketamine and neurotoxicity: clinical perspectives and implications for emergency medicine. *Ann Emerg Med.* 2009;54(2):181–190

339. Brown KA, Laferrière A, Moss IR. Recurrent hypoxemia in young children with obstructive sleep apnea is associated with reduced opioid requirement for analgesia. *Anesthesiology.* 2004;100(4):806–810; discussion: 5A

340. Moss IR, Brown KA, Laferrière A. Recurrent hypoxia in rats during development increases subsequent respiratory sensitivity to fentanyl. *Anesthesiology.* 2006;105(4):715–718

341. Litman RS, Kottra JA, Berkowitz RJ, Ward DS. Upper airway obstruction during midazolam/nitrous oxide sedation in children with enlarged tonsils. *Pediatr Dent.* 1998;20(5):318–320

342. Fishbaugh DF, Wilson S, Preisch JW, Weaver JM II. Relationship of tonsil size on an airway blockage maneuver in children during sedation. *Pediatr Dent.* 1997;19(4):277–281

343. Heinrich S, Birkholz T, Ihmsen H, Irouschek A, Ackermann A, Schmidt J. Incidence and predictors of difficult laryngoscopy in 11,219 pediatric

anesthesia procedures. *Paediatr Anaesth.* 2012;22(8):729–736

344. Kumar HV, Schroeder JW, Gang Z, Sheldon SH. Mallampati score and pediatric obstructive sleep apnea. *J Clin Sleep Med.* 2014;10(9):985–990

345. Anderson BJ, Meakin GH. Scaling for size: some implications for paediatric anaesthesia dosing. *Paediatr Anaesth.* 2002;12(3):205–219

346. Ramsay MA, Savege TM, Simpson BR, Goodwin R. Controlled sedation with alphaxalone-alphadolone. *BMJ.* 1974;2(5920):656–659

347. Agrawal D, Feldman HA, Krauss B, Waltzman ML. Bispectral index monitoring quantifies depth of sedation during emergency department procedural sedation and analgesia in children. *Ann Emerg Med.* 2004;43(2):247–255

348. Cravero JP, Blike GT, Surgenor SD, Jensen J. Development and validation of the Dartmouth Operative Conditions Scale. *Anesth Analg.* 2005;100(6):1614–1621

349. Mayers DJ, Hindmarsh KW, Sankaran K, Gorecki DK, Kasian GF. Chloral hydrate disposition following single-dose administration to critically ill neonates and children. *Dev Pharmacol Ther.* 1991;16(2):71–77

350. Terndrup TE, Dire DJ, Madden CM, Davis H, Cantor RM, Gavula DP. A prospective analysis of intramuscular meperidine, promethazine, and chlorpromazine in pediatric emergency department patients. *Ann Emerg Med.* 1991;20(1):31–35

351. Macnab AJ, Levine M, Glick N, Susak L, Baker-Brown G. A research tool for measurement of recovery from sedation: the Vancouver Sedative Recovery Scale. *J Pediatr Surg.* 1991;26(11):1263–1267

352. Chernik DA, Gillings D, Laine H, et al. Validity and reliability of the Observer's Assessment of Alertness/Sedation Scale: study with intravenous midazolam. *J Clin Psychopharmacol.* 1990;10(4):244–251

353. Bagian JP, Lee C, Gosbee J, et al. Developing and deploying a patient safety program in a large health care delivery system: you can't fix what you don't know about. *Jt Comm J Qual Improv.* 2001;27(10):522–532

354. May T, Aulisio MP. Medical malpractice, mistake prevention, and compensation. *Kennedy Inst Ethics J.* 2001;11(2):135–146

355. Kazandjian VA. When you hear hoofs, think horses, not zebras: an evidence-based model of health care accountability. *J Eval Clin Pract.* 2002;8(2):205–213

356. Connor M, Ponte PR, Conway J. Multidisciplinary approaches to reducing error and risk in a patient care setting. *Crit Care Nurs Clin North Am.* 2002;14(4):359–367, viii

357. Gosbee J. Human factors engineering and patient safety. *Qual Saf Health Care.* 2002;11(4):352–354

358. Tuong B, Shnitzer Z, Pehora C, et al. The experience of conducting Mortality and Morbidity reviews in a pediatric interventional radiology service: a retrospective study. *J Vasc Interv Radiol.* 2009;20(1):77–86

359. Tjia I, Rampersad S, Varughese A, et al. Wake Up Safe and root cause analysis: quality improvement in pediatric anesthesia. *Anesth Analg.* 2014;119(1):122–136

360. Bhatt M, Kennedy RM, Osmond MH, et al; Consensus Panel on Sedation Research of Pediatric Emergency Research Canada (PERC); Pediatric Emergency Care Applied Research Network (PECARN). Consensus-based recommendations for standardizing terminology and reporting adverse events for emergency department procedural sedation and analgesia in children. *Ann Emerg Med.* 2009;53(4):426–435.e4

361. Barker SJ, Hyatt J, Shah NK, Kao YJ. The effect of sensor malpositioning on pulse oximeter accuracy during hypoxemia. *Anesthesiology.* 1993;79(2):248–254

362. Kelleher JF, Ruff RH. The penumbra effect: vasomotion-dependent pulse oximeter artifact due to probe malposition. *Anesthesiology.* 1989;71(5):787–791

363. Reeves ST, Havidich JE, Tobin DP. Conscious sedation of children with propofol is anything but conscious. *Pediatrics.* 2004;114(1). Available at: www.pediatrics.org/cgi/content/full/114/1/e74

364. Maher EN, Hansen SF, Heine M, Meers H, Yaster M, Hunt EA. Knowledge of procedural sedation and analgesia of emergency medicine physicians. *Pediatr Emerg Care.* 2007;23(12):869–876

365. Fehr JJ, Boulet JR, Waldrop WB, Snider R, Brockel M, Murray DJ. Simulation-based assessment of pediatric anesthesia skills. *Anesthesiology.* 2011;115(6):1308–1315

366. McBride ME, Waldrop WB, Fehr JJ, Boulet JR, Murray DJ. Simulation in pediatrics: the reliability and validity of a multiscenario assessment. *Pediatrics.* 2011;128(2):335–343

367. Fehr JJ, Honkanen A, Murray DJ. Simulation in pediatric anesthesiology. *Paediatr Anaesth.* 2012;22(10):988–994

368. Martinez MJ, Siegelman L. The new era of pretracheal/precordial stethoscopes. *Pediatr Dent.* 1999;21(7):455–457

369. Biro P. Electrically amplified precordial stethoscope. *J Clin Monit.* 1994;10(6):410–412

370. Philip JH, Raemer DB. An electronic stethoscope is judged better than conventional stethoscopes for anesthesia monitoring. *J Clin Monit.* 1986;2(3):151–154

371. Hochberg MG, Mahoney WK. Monitoring of respiration using an amplified pretracheal stethoscope. *J Oral Maxillofac Surg.* 1999;57(7):875–876

372. Fredette ME, Lightdale JR. Endoscopic sedation in pediatric practice. *Gastrointest Endosc Clin N Am.* 2008;18(4):739–751, ix

373. Deitch K, Chudnofsky CR, Dominici P. The utility of supplemental oxygen during emergency department procedural sedation and analgesia with midazolam and fentanyl: a randomized, controlled trial. *Ann Emerg Med.* 2007;49(1):1–8

374. Burton JH, Harrah JD, Germann CA, Dillon DC. Does end-tidal carbon dioxide monitoring detect respiratory events prior to current sedation monitoring practices? *Acad Emerg Med.* 2006;13(5):500–504

375. Wilson S, Farrell K, Griffen A, Coury D. Conscious sedation experiences in graduate pediatric dentistry programs. *Pediatr Dent.* 2001;23(4):307–314

376. Allegaert K, van den Anker JN. Clinical pharmacology in neonates: small size, huge variability. *Neonatology.* 2014;105(4):344–349

377. Coté CJ, Zaslavsky A, Downes JJ, et al. Postoperative apnea in former preterm infants after inguinal herniorrhaphy: a combined analysis. *Anesthesiology.* 1995;82(4):809–822

378. Havidich JE, Beach M, Dierdorf SF, Onega T, Suresh G, Cravero JP. Preterm versus term children: analysis of sedation/anesthesia adverse events and longitudinal risk. *Pediatrics.* 2016;137(3):1–9

379. Nasr VG, Davis JM. Anesthetic use in newborn infants: the urgent need for rigorous evaluation. *Pediatr Res.* 2015;78(1):2–6

380. Sinner B, Becke K, Engelhard K. General anaesthetics and the developing brain: an overview. *Anaesthesia.* 2014;69(9):1009–1022

381. Yu CK, Yuen VM, Wong GT, Irwin MG. The effects of anaesthesia on the developing brain: a summary of the clinical evidence. *F1000 Res.* 2013;2:166

382. Davidson A, Flick RP. Neurodevelopmental implications of the use of sedation and analgesia in neonates. *Clin Perinatol.* 2013;40(3):559–573

383. Lönnqvist PA. Toxicity of local anesthetic drugs: a pediatric perspective. *Paediatr Anaesth.* 2012;22(1):39–43

384. Wahl MJ, Brown RS. Dentistry's wonder drugs: local anesthetics and vasoconstrictors. *Gen Dent.* 2010;58(2):114–123; quiz: 124–125

385. Bernards CM, Hadzic A, Suresh S, Neal JM. Regional anesthesia in anesthetized or heavily sedated patients. *Reg Anesth Pain Med.* 2008;33(5):449–460

386. Ecoffey C. Pediatric regional anesthesia—update. *Curr Opin Anaesthesiol.* 2007;20(3):232–235

387. Aubuchon RW. Sedation liabilities in pedodontics. *Pediatr Dent.* 1982;4:171–180

388. Fitzmaurice LS, Wasserman GS, Knapp JF, Roberts DK, Waeckerle JF, Fox M. TAC use and absorption of cocaine in a pediatric emergency department. *Ann Emerg Med.* 1990;19(5):515–518

389. Tipton GA, DeWitt GW, Eisenstein SJ. Topical TAC (tetracaine, adrenaline, cocaine) solution for local anesthesia in children: prescribing inconsistency and acute toxicity. *South Med J.* 1989;82(11):1344–1346

390. Gunter JB. Benefit and risks of local anesthetics in infants and children. *Paediatr Drugs.* 2002;4(10):649–672

391. Resar LM, Helfaer MA. Recurrent seizures in a neonate after lidocaine administration. *J Perinatol.* 1998;18(3):193–195

392. Yagiela JA. Local anesthetics. In: Yagiela JA, Dowd FJ, Johnson BS, Mariotti AJ, Neidle EA, eds. *Pharmacology and Therapeutics for Dentistry.* 6th ed. St. Louis, MO: Mosby, Elsevier; 2011:246–265

393. Haas DA. An update on local anesthetics in dentistry. *J Can Dent Assoc.* 2002;68(9):546–551

394. Malamed SF. Anesthetic considerations in dental specialties. In: Malamed SF, ed. *Handbook of Local Anesthesia.* 6th ed. St. Louis, MO: Elsevier; 2013:277–291

395. Malamed SF. The needle. In: Malamed SF, ed. *Handbook of Local Anesthetics.* 6th ed. St Louis, MO: Elsevier; 2013:92–100

396. Malamed SF. Pharmacology of local anesthetics. In: Malamed SF, ed. *Handbook of Local Anesthesia.* 6th ed. St. Louis, MO: Elsevier; 2013:25–38

397. Ram D, Amir E. Comparison of articaine 4% and lidocaine 2% in paediatric dental patients. *Int J Paediatr Dent.* 2006;16(4):252–256

398. Jakobs W, Ladwig B, Cichon P, Ortel R, Kirch W. Serum levels of articaine 2% and 4% in children. *Anesth Prog.* 1995;42(3–4):113–115

399. Wright GZ, Weinberger SJ, Friedman CS, Plotzke OB. Use of articaine local anesthesia in children under 4 years of age—a retrospective report. *Anesth Prog.* 1989;36(6):268–271

400. Malamed SF, Gagnon S, Leblanc D. A comparison between articaine HCl and lidocaine HCl in pediatric dental patients. *Pediatr Dent.* 2000;22(4):307–311

401. American Academy of Pediatric Dentistry, Council on Clinical Affairs. Guidelines on use of local anesthesia for pediatric dental patients. Chicago, IL: American Academy of Pediatric Dentistry; 2015. Available at: http://www.aapd.org/media/policies_guidelines/g_localanesthesia.pdf. Accessed May 27, 2016

402. Ludot H, Tharin JY, Belouadah M, Mazoit JX, Malinovsky JM. Successful resuscitation after ropivacaine and lidocaine-induced ventricular arrhythmia following posterior lumbar plexus block in a child. *Anesth Analg.* 2008;106(5):1572–1574

403. Eren CS, Tasyurek T, Guneysel O. Intralipid emulsion treatment as an antidote in lipophilic drug intoxications: a case series. *Am J Emerg Med.* 2014;32(9):1103–1108

404. Evans JA, Wallis SC, Dulhunty JM, Pang G. Binding of local anaesthetics to the lipid emulsion Clinoleic™ 20%. *Anaesth Intensive Care.* 2013;41(5):618–622

405. Presley JD, Chyka PA. Intravenous lipid emulsion to reverse acute drug toxicity in pediatric patients. *Ann Pharmacother.* 2013;47(5):735–743

406. Li Z, Xia Y, Dong X, et al. Lipid resuscitation of bupivacaine toxicity: long-chain triglyceride emulsion provides benefits over long- and medium-chain triglyceride emulsion. *Anesthesiology.* 2011;115(6):1219–1228

407. Maher AJ, Metcalfe SA, Parr S. Local anaesthetic toxicity. *Foot.* 2008;18(4):192–197

408. Corman SL, Skledar SJ. Use of lipid emulsion to reverse local anesthetic-induced toxicity. *Ann Pharmacother.* 2007;41(11):1873–1877

409. Litz RJ, Popp M, Stehr SN, Koch T. Successful resuscitation of a patient with ropivacaine-induced asystole after axillary plexus block using lipid infusion. *Anaesthesia.* 2006;61(8):800–801

410. Raso SM, Fernandez JB, Beobide EA, Landaluce AF. Methemoglobinemia and CNS toxicity after topical application of EMLA to a 4-year-old girl with

molluscum contagiosum. *Pediatr Dermatol.* 2006;23(6):592–593

411. Larson A, Stidham T, Banerji S, Kaufman J. Seizures and methemoglobinemia in an infant after excessive EMLA application. *Pediatr Emerg Care.* 2013;29(3):377–379

412. Tran AN, Koo JY. Risk of systemic toxicity with topical lidocaine/prilocaine: a review. *J Drugs Dermatol.* 2014;13(9):1118–1122

413. Young KD. Topical anaesthetics: what's new? *Arch Dis Child Educ Pract Ed.* 2015;100(2):105–110

414. Gaufberg SV, Walta MJ, Workman TP. Expanding the use of topical anesthesia in wound management: sequential layered application of topical lidocaine with epinephrine. *Am J Emerg Med.* 2007;25(4):379–384

415. Eidelman A, Weiss JM, Baldwin CL, Enu IK, McNicol ED, Carr DB. Topical anaesthetics for repair of dermal laceration. *Cochrane Database Syst Rev.* 2011;6:CD005364

416. Next-generation pulse oximetry. *Health Devices.* 2003;32(2):49–103

417. Barker SJ. "Motion-resistant" pulse oximetry: a comparison of new and old models. *Anesth Analg.* 2002;95(4):967–972

418. Malviya S, Reynolds PI, Voepel-Lewis T, et al. False alarms and sensitivity of conventional pulse oximetry versus the Masimo SET technology in the pediatric postanesthesia care unit. *Anesth Analg.* 2000;90(6):1336–1340

419. Barker SJ, Shah NK. Effects of motion on the performance of pulse oximeters in volunteers. *Anesthesiology.* 1996;85(4):774–781

420. Barker SJ, Shah NK. The effects of motion on the performance of pulse oximeters in volunteers (revised publication). *Anesthesiology.* 1997;86(1):101–108

421. Colman Y, Krauss B. Microstream capnograpy technology: a new approach to an old problem. *J Clin Monit Comput.* 1999;15(6):403–409

422. Wright SW. Conscious sedation in the emergency department: the value of capnography and pulse oximetry. *Ann Emerg Med.* 1992;21(5):551–555

423. Roelofse J. Conscious sedation: making our treatment options safe and sound. *SADJ.* 2000;55(5):273–276

424. Wilson S, Creedon RL, George M, Troutman K. A history of sedation guidelines: where we are headed in the future. *Pediatr Dent.* 1996;18(3):194–199

425. Miner JR, Heegaard W, Plummer D. End-tidal carbon dioxide monitoring during procedural sedation. *Acad Emerg Med.* 2002;9(4):275–280

426. Vascello LA, Bowe EA. A case for capnographic monitoring as a standard of care. *J Oral Maxillofac Surg.* 1999;57(11):1342–1347

427. Coté CJ, Wax DF, Jennings MA, Gorski CL, Kurczak-Klippstein K. Endtidal carbon dioxide monitoring in children with congenital heart disease during sedation for cardiac catheterization by nonanesthesiologists. *Paediatr Anaesth.* 2007;17(7):661–666

428. Bowdle TA. Depth of anesthesia monitoring. *Anesthesiol Clin.* 2006;24(4):793–822

429. Rodriguez RA, Hall LE, Duggan S, Splinter WM. The bispectral index does not correlate with clinical signs of inhalational anesthesia during sevoflurane induction and arousal in children. *Can J Anaesth.* 2004;51(5):472–480

430. Overly FL, Wright RO, Connor FA Jr, Fontaine B, Jay G, Linakis JG. Bispectral analysis during pediatric procedural sedation. *Pediatr Emerg Care.* 2005;21(1):6–11

431. Mason KP, O'Mahony E, Zurakowski D, Libenson MH. Effects of dexmedetomidine sedation on the EEG in children. *Paediatr Anaesth.* 2009;19(12):1175–1183

432. Malviya S, Voepel-Lewis T, Tait AR, Watcha MF, Sadhasivam S, Friesen RH. Effect of age and sedative agent on the accuracy of bispectral index in detecting depth of sedation in children. *Pediatrics.* 2007;120(3). Available at: www.pediatrics.org/cgi/content/full/120/3/e461

433. Sadhasivam S, Ganesh A, Robison A, Kaye R, Watcha MF. Validation of the bispectral index monitor for measuring the depth of

sedation in children. *Anesth Analg.* 2006;102(2):383–388

434. Messieha ZS, Ananda RC, Hoffman WE, Punwani IC, Koenig HM. Bispectral Index System (BIS) monitoring reduces time to discharge in children requiring intramuscular sedation and general anesthesia for outpatient dental rehabilitation. *Pediatr Dent.* 2004;26(3):256–260

435. McDermott NB, VanSickle T, Motas D, Friesen RH. Validation of the bispectral index monitor during conscious and deep sedation in children. *Anesth Analg.* 2003;97(1):39–43

436. Schmidt AR, Weiss M, Engelhardt T. The paediatric airway: basic principles and current developments. *Eur J Anaesthesiol.* 2014;31(6):293–299

437. Nagler J, Bachur RG. Advanced airway management. *Curr Opin Pediatr.* 2009;21(3):299–305

438. Berry AM, Brimacombe JR, Verghese C. The laryngeal mask airway in emergency medicine, neonatal resuscitation, and intensive care medicine. *Int Anesthesiol Clin.* 1998;36(2):91–109

439. Patterson MD. Resuscitation update for the pediatrician. *Pediatr Clin North Am.* 1999;46(6):1285–1303

440. Diggs LA, Yusuf JE, De Leo G. An update on out-of-hospital airway management practices in the United States. *Resuscitation.* 2014;85(7):885–892

441. Wang HE, Mann NC, Mears G, Jacobson K, Yealy DM. Out-of-hospital airway management in the United States. *Resuscitation.* 2011;82(4):378–385

442. Ritter SC, Guyette FX. Prehospital pediatric King LT-D use: a pilot study. *Prehosp Emerg Care.* 2011;15(3):401–404

443. Selim M, Mowafi H, Al-Ghamdi A, Adu-Gyamfi Y. Intubation via LMA in pediatric patients with difficult airways. *Can J Anaesth.* 1999;46(9):891–893

444. Munro HM, Butler PJ, Washington EJ. Freeman-Sheldon (whistling face) syndrome: anaesthetic and airway management. *Paediatr Anaesth.* 1997;7(4):345–348

445. Horton MA, Beamer C. Powered intraosseous insertion provides safe

and effective vascular access for pediatric emergency patients. *Pediatr Emerg Care*. 2008;24(6):347–350

446. Gazin N, Auger H, Jabre P, et al. Efficacy and safety of the EZ-IO™ intraosseous device: out-of-hospital implementation of a management algorithm for difficult vascular access. *Resuscitation*. 2011;82(1):126–129

447. Frascone RJ, Jensen J, Wewerka SS, Salzman JG. Use of the pediatric EZ-IO needle by emergency medical services providers. *Pediatr Emerg Care*. 2009;25(5):329–332

448. Neuhaus D. Intraosseous infusion in elective and emergency pediatric anesthesia: when should we use it? *Curr Opin Anaesthesiol*. 2014;27(3):282–287

449. Oksan D, Ayfer K. Powered intraosseous device (EZ-IO) for critically ill patients. *Indian Pediatr*. 2013;50(7):689–691

450. Santos D, Carron PN, Yersin B, Pasquier M. EZ-IO(®) intraosseous device implementation in a pre-hospital emergency service: a prospective study and review of the literature. *Resuscitation*. 2013;84(4):440–445

451. Tan GM. A medical crisis management simulation activity for pediatric dental residents and assistants. *J Dent Educ*. 2011;75(6):782–790

452. Schinasi DA, Nadel FM, Hales R, Boswinkel JP, Donoghue AJ. Assessing pediatric residents' clinical performance in procedural sedation: a simulation-based needs assessment. *Pediatr Emerg Care*. 2013;29(4):447–452

453. Rowe R, Cohen RA. An evaluation of a virtual reality airway simulator. *Anesth Analg*. 2002;95(1):62–66

454. Medina LS, Racadio JM, Schwid HA. Computers in radiology—the sedation, analgesia, and contrast media computerized simulator: a new approach to train and evaluate radiologists' responses to critical incidents. *Pediatr Radiol*. 2000;30(5):299–305

455. Blike G, Cravero J, Nelson E. Same patients, same critical events—different systems of care, different outcomes: description of a human

factors approach aimed at improving the efficacy and safety of sedation/analgesia care. *Qual Manag Health Care*. 2001;10(1):17–36

456. Reiter DA, Strother CG, Weingart SD. The quality of cardiopulmonary resuscitation using supraglottic airways and intraosseous devices: a simulation trial. *Resuscitation*. 2013;84(1):93–97

457. Schulte-Uentrop L, Goepfert MS. Anaesthesia or sedation for MRI in children. *Curr Opin Anaesthesiol*. 2010;23(4):513–517

458. Schmidt MH, Downie J. Safety first: recognizing and managing the risks to child participants in magnetic resonance imaging research. *Account Res*. 2009;16(3):153–173

459. Chavhan GB, Babyn PS, Singh M, Vidarsson L, Shroff M. MR imaging at 3.0 T in children: technical differences, safety issues, and initial experience. *Radiographics*. 2009;29(5):1451–1466

460. Kanal E, Shellock FG, Talagala L. Safety considerations in MR imaging. *Radiology*. 1990;176(3):593–606

461. Shellock FG, Kanal E. Burns associated with the use of monitoring equipment during MR procedures. *J Magn Reson Imaging*. 1996;6(1):271–272

462. Shellock FG. Magnetic resonance safety update 2002: implants and devices. *J Magn Reson Imaging*. 2002;16(5):485–496

463. Dempsey MF, Condon B, Hadley DM. MRI safety review. *Semin Ultrasound CT MR*. 2002;23(5):392–401

464. Department of Health and Human Services, Centers for Disease Control and PreventionCriteria for a Recommended Standard: Waste Anesthetic Gases: Occupational Hazards in Hospitals. 2007. Publication 2007-151. Available at: http://www.cdc.gov/niosh/docs/2007-151/pdfs/2007-151.pdf. Accessed May 27, 2016

465. O'Sullivan I, Benger J. Nitrous oxide in emergency medicine. *Emerg Med J*. 2003;20(3):214–217

466. Kennedy RM, Luhmann JD, Luhmann SJ. Emergency department management of pain and anxiety related to orthopedic fracture care: a guide to analgesic techniques and procedural sedation in children. *Paediatr Drugs*. 2004;6(1):11–31

467. Frampton A, Browne GJ, Lam LT, Cooper MG, Lane LG. Nurse administered relative analgesia using high concentration nitrous oxide to facilitate minor procedures in children in an emergency department. *Emerg Med J*. 2003;20(5):410–413

468. Everitt I, Younge P, Barnett P. Paediatric sedation in emergency department: what is our practice? *Emerg Med (Fremantle)*. 2002;14(1):62–66

469. Krauss B. Continuous-flow nitrous oxide: searching for the ideal procedural anxiolytic for toddlers. *Ann Emerg Med*. 2001;37(1):61–62

470. Otley CC, Nguyen TH. Conscious sedation of pediatric patients with combination oral benzodiazepines and inhaled nitrous oxide. *Dermatol Surg*. 2000;26(11):1041–1044

471. Luhmann JD, Kennedy RM, Jaffe DM, McAllister JD. Continuous-flow delivery of nitrous oxide and oxygen: a safe and cost-effective technique for inhalation analgesia and sedation of pediatric patients. *Pediatr Emerg Care*. 1999;15(6):388–392

472. Burton JH, Auble TE, Fuchs SM. Effectiveness of 50% nitrous oxide/50% oxygen during laceration repair in children. *Acad Emerg Med*. 1998;5(2):112–117

473. Gregory PR, Sullivan JA. Nitrous oxide compared with intravenous regional anesthesia in pediatric forearm fracture manipulation. *J Pediatr Orthop*. 1996;16(2):187–191

474. Hennrikus WL, Shin AY, Klingelberger CE. Self-administered nitrous oxide and a hematoma block for analgesia in the outpatient reduction of fractures in children. *J Bone Joint Surg Am*. 1995;77(3):335–339

475. Hennrikus WL, Simpson RB, Klingelberger CE, Reis MT. Self-administered nitrous oxide analgesia for pediatric fracture reductions. *J Pediatr Orthop*. 1994;14(4):538–542

476. Wattenmaker I, Kasser JR, McGravey A. Self-administered nitrous oxide for fracture reduction in children in an emergency room setting. *J Orthop Trauma*. 1990;4(1):35–38

477. Gamis AS, Knapp JF, Glenski JA. Nitrous oxide analgesia in a pediatric emergency department. *Ann Emerg Med*. 1989;18(2):177–181

478. Kalach N, Barbier C, el Kohen R, et al. Tolerance of nitrous oxide-oxygen sedation for painful procedures in emergency pediatrics: report of 600 cases [in French]. *Arch Pediatr.* 2002;9(11):1213–1215

479. Michaud L, Gottrand F, Ganga-Zandzou PS, et al. Nitrous oxide sedation in pediatric patients undergoing gastrointestinal endoscopy. *J Pediatr Gastroenterol Nutr.* 1999;28(3):310–314

480. Baskett PJ. Analgesia for the dressing of burns in children: a method using neuroleptanalgesia and Entonox. *Postgrad Med J.* 1972;48(557):138–142

481. Veerkamp JS, van Amerongen WE, Hoogstraten J, Groen HJ. Dental treatment of fearful children, using nitrous oxide. Part I: treatment times. *ASDC J Dent Child.* 1991;58(6):453–457

482. Veerkamp JS, Gruythuysen RJ, van Amerongen WE, Hoogstraten J. Dental treatment of fearful children using nitrous oxide. Part 2: the parent's point of view. *ASDC J Dent Child.* 1992;59(2):115–119

483. Veerkamp JS, Gruythuysen RJ, van Amerongen WE, Hoogstraten J. Dental treatment of fearful children using nitrous oxide. Part 3: anxiety during sequential visits. *ASDC J Dent Child.* 1993;60(3):175–182

484. Veerkamp JS, Gruythuysen RJ, Hoogstraten J, van Amerongen WE. Dental treatment of fearful children using nitrous oxide. Part 4: anxiety after two years. *ASDC J Dent Child.* 1993;60(4):372–376

485. Houpt MI, Limb R, Livingston RL. Clinical effects of nitrous oxide conscious sedation in children. *Pediatr Dent.* 2004;26(1):29–36

486. Shapira J, Holan G, Guelmann M, Cahan S. Evaluation of the effect of nitrous oxide and hydroxyzine in controlling the behavior of the pediatric dental patient. *Pediatr Dent.* 1992;14(3):167–170

487. Primosch RE, Buzzi IM, Jerrell G. Effect of nitrous oxide-oxygen inhalation with scavenging on behavioral and physiological parameters during routine pediatric dental treatment. *Pediatr Dent.* 1999;21(7):417–420

488. McCann W, Wilson S, Larsen P, Stehle B. The effects of nitrous oxide on behavior and physiological parameters during conscious sedation with a moderate dose of chloral hydrate and hydroxyzine. *Pediatr Dent.* 1996;18(1):35–41

489. Wilson S, Matusak A, Casamassimo PS, Larsen P. The effects of nitrous oxide on pediatric dental patients sedated with chloral hydrate and hydroxyzine. *Pediatr Dent.* 1998;20(4):253–258

490. Pedersen RS, Bayat A, Steen NP, Jacobsson ML. Nitrous oxide provides safe and effective analgesia for minor paediatric procedures—a systematic review [abstract]. *Dan Med J.* 2013;60(6):A4627

491. Lee JH, Kim K, Kim TY, et al. A randomized comparison of nitrous oxide versus intravenous ketamine for laceration repair in children. *Pediatr Emerg Care.* 2012;28(12):1297–1301

492. Seith RW, Theophilos T, Babl FE. Intranasal fentanyl and high-concentration inhaled nitrous oxide for procedural sedation: a prospective observational pilot study of adverse events and depth of sedation. *Acad Emerg Med.* 2012;19(1):31–36

493. Klein U, Robinson TJ, Allshouse A. End-expired nitrous oxide concentrations compared to flowmeter settings during operative dental treatment in children. *Pediatr Dent.* 2011;33(1):56–62

494. Litman RS, Kottra JA, Berkowitz RJ, Ward DS. Breathing patterns and levels of consciousness in children during administration of nitrous oxide after oral midazolam premedication. *J Oral Maxillofac Surg.* 1997;55(12):1372–1377; discussion: 1378–1379

495. Litman RS, Kottra JA, Verga KA, Berkowitz RJ, Ward DS. Chloral hydrate sedation: the additive sedative and respiratory depressant effects of nitrous oxide. *Anesth Analg.* 1998;86(4):724–728

496. American Academy of Pediatric Dentistry, Council on Clinical Affairs. Guideline on use of nitrous oxide for pediatric dental patients. Chicago, IL: American Academy of Pediatric Dentistry; 2013. Available at: http://www.aapd.org/media/policies_guidelines/g_nitrous.pdf. Accessed May 27, 2016

Handoffs: Transitions of Care for Children in the Emergency Department

• •

- *Policy Statement*

POLICY STATEMENT   Organizational Principles to Guide and Define the Child Health
Care System and/or Improve the Health of all Children

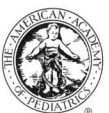

American Academy
of Pediatrics

DEDICATED TO THE HEALTH OF ALL CHILDREN™

Handoffs: Transitions of Care for Children in the Emergency Department

AMERICAN ACADEMY OF PEDIATRICS Committee on Pediatric Emergency Medicine, AMERICAN COLLEGE OF EMERGENCY PHYSICIANS Pediatric Emergency Medicine Committee, EMERGENCY NURSES ASSOCIATION Pediatric Committee

abstract

Transitions of care (ToCs), also referred to as handoffs or sign-outs, occur when the responsibility for a patient's care transfers from 1 health care provider to another. Transitions are common in the acute care setting and have been noted to be vulnerable events with opportunities for error. Health care is taking ideas from other high-risk industries, such as aerospace and nuclear power, to create models of structured transition processes. Although little literature currently exists to establish 1 model as superior, multiorganizational consensus groups agree that standardization is warranted and that additional work is needed to establish characteristics of ToCs that are associated with clinical or practice outcomes. The rationale for structuring ToCs, specifically those related to the care of children in the emergency setting, and a description of identified strategies are presented, along with resources for educating health care providers on ToCs. Recommendations for development, education, and implementation of transition models are included.

DOI: 10.1542/peds.2016-2680

PEDIATRICS (ISSN Numbers: Print, 0031-4005; Online, 1098-4275).

Copyright © 2016 by the American Academy of Pediatrics

FINANCIAL DISCLOSURE: The authors have indicated they have no financial relationships relevant to this article to disclose.

FUNDING: No external funding.

POTENTIAL CONFLICT OF INTEREST: The authors have indicated they have no potential conflicts of interest to disclose.

To cite: AMERICAN ACADEMY OF PEDIATRICS Committee on Pediatric Emergency Medicine, AMERICAN COLLEGE OF EMERGENCY PHYSICIANS Pediatric Emergency Medicine Committee, EMERGENCY NURSES ASSOCIATION Pediatric Committee. Handoffs: Transitions of Care for Children in the Emergency Department. *Pediatrics.* 2016;138(5):e20162680

INTRODUCTION

Patients who require emergency care for illness or injury may move among several areas of care, including the prehospital setting, the emergency department (ED), inpatient units, and operating rooms or procedure suites, before being transitioned back to the medical home. During transitions between care areas or even during care in a single area, a patient may be cared for by multiple health care personnel. It is likely that transitions of care (ToCs) occur more often in the ED than in any other hospital setting.[1] To provide the highest quality and safety, a patient's care is supposed to be seamless, despite multiple care providers and potentially multiple care areas.

At each patient care transition point, responsibility for the patient's care passes from 1 care provider to another, requiring accurate and timely transmission of important information. Referred to as a "handoff," "handover," "report," or "sign-out," a ToC occurs when ≥2 health care providers exchange information that is a summary of the patient's situation, specific to the mission of shaping subsequent treatment and decision-making; and the control over, or responsibility for, the patient is transferred from 1 care provider to another.[2,3] ToC entails the exchange of the following:

1. mission-specific information;

2. responsibility for patient care; and

3. authority for treatment and procedures.

ToC can occur between prehospital and ED providers, between ED providers at shift change, between ED and hospital providers when patients are transferred out of the ED or to another facility, and between ED providers and the patient's medical home when patients are discharged from the ED. All types of health care providers, including but not limited to physicians, nurses, advanced-practice nurses, physician assistants, respiratory therapists, paramedics, emergency medical technicians, social workers, and transporters, can be expected to participate in the transition of a patient's care. In an environment characterized by high patient volume, variable acuity, shift changes, and inopportune interruptions, maintaining focus on communication is especially challenging; however, intradepartmental, interdepartmental, prehospital, and interfacility processes can be designed to address these challenges systematically. These processes can include creating a structured and consistent ToC procedure that acknowledges human factors, operational procedures, team coordination, and care delivery systems.[4]

Published evidence is insufficient to define which system is the best approach to transitioning the care of patients in emergency and acute care settings. Current ToC practices have been criticized as being highly variable and unreliable. Results of a questionnaire and follow-up observation study revealed that ToC processes were unstructured, informal, and error prone, consistent with findings from other studies.[5] In another analysis of ToC processes, nonstandardized approaches led to adverse clinical consequences, near misses, and inefficient or duplicative care.[6]

In other high-risk industries, sign-outs have received considerable research attention, but only recently has the transfer of patient care been studied systematically and findings published in the health care literature. A systematic review of 18 studies that (1) had patient handoffs in hospitals as their explicit research focus and (2) reported at least 1 statistical test of an association between a handoff characteristic and outcome noted that research is highly diverse and quality is preliminary, so drawing general conclusions about ToC strategies is difficult.[7] Similarly, a clinical evidence review of nursing literature noted that ToC practices are in need of rigorous evaluation to determine which features lead to the best outcomes for patients in varied settings.[8] In addition to the need for more evidence gathering, surveys of graduate medical education program directors have concluded that there is a perceived need for emergency medicine and pediatric emergency medicine training programs to provide specific guidance to trainees regarding ToC processes.[9] A new clinical report from the Committee on Hospital Care of the American Academy of Pediatrics, "Standardization of Inpatient Handoff Communication," is published simultaneously in this issue of the Journal (http://www.pediatrics.org/cgi/doi/10.1542/peds.2016-2681).

IMPACT OF ToCs

Communication failures have been implicated as the root cause of more than 60% of sentinel events reported to The Joint Commission (formerly Joint Commission on Accreditation of Health Care Organizations).[10] The Institute of Medicine report "To Err Is Human" noted that 84% of treatment delays were later judged to be attributable to miscommunication, and 62% of these were continuum-of-care issues associated with shift changes.[11]

When care is transitioned, the patient is vulnerable to the cognitive biases of multiple providers.[12] Examples of cognitive biases include the following.[13-16]

- Framing effect: A decision is influenced by the way the scenario is presented.

- Diagnosis momentum: A particular diagnosis is established despite other evidence.

- Confirmation bias/ascertainment effect: Thinking is preshaped by expectations, and providers seek confirmatory data while ignoring data that may lead to the correct diagnosis.

- Triage cueing: Judgments made early in the patient care process predispose subsequent providers toward a particular decision.

BARRIERS TO EFFECTIVE ToCs

Numerous factors predictably lead to errors when humans work in complex systems, including memory, vigilance, and attention to detail. These factors can be exacerbated when people are fatigued or stressed,[17] as happens often when providing emergency care to children. The emergency setting is especially prone to errors because of human as well as environmental factors,[4,18-21] such as the following:

- simultaneous management of multiple ill patients;

- frequent workflow interruptions;
- wide fluctuations in patient volume;
- shift work, staff changes;
- authority gradients;
- experience gradients within the health care environment;
- limited knowledge of patients' history and preexisting conditions;
- high levels of diagnostic uncertainty; and
- high decision density.

When performed suitably, ToC practice promotes quality of care and protects patient safety by providing "audit points" for the detection and mitigation of failure,[22] for example, when the receiving health care provider may notice something overlooked by current providers.[23] Adequate ToC procedures offer the opportunity for rescue and recovery when situations are unclear or a practitioner's thinking is incomplete.[1] Allowing patients to be a part of the ToC process by using "bedside" handoffs has been shown to have positive outcomes for patients and the health care team, including increased patient satisfaction and patient involvement in their own care, with the potential for improved patient safety.[24–26] A physician exchange of information at bedside was shown to be a patient-preferred methodology that encourages patients to participate in their care.[27]

WHY STRUCTURE ToCs?

Consistently structuring 2-way, open, and concise communication provides a means for ensuring consistent, high-quality ToCs.[4] By using information from other high-risk industries, such as aerospace, nuclear power, and aviation, health care providers may learn the value of scripted, precise, unambiguous, impersonal, and efficient language embedded within a framework that allows opportunity for reassessing

clinical reasoning and providing read-back of information. Benefits include the following:

- Memory trigger: Omitted information and faulty communication processes were identified as the root cause of most errors linked to ToCs.[10] Structured and consistent processes and the use of checklists serve as a memory trigger during ToCs.

- Opportunity to ask and respond to questions: As part of the 2008 National Patient Safety Goals, The Joint Commission published specific recommendations on physician ToCs, including the need for a standardized ToC process involving certain elements and the opportunity to ask and respond to questions.[28]

- Mitigation of authority gradients: Authority gradients in the workplace can stand in the way of communication.[29] Adopting structured and consistent communication strategies helps put all team members on a level playing field while they work together to keep patients safe.[1] One study found that role variability (information provider versus receiver) created conflicts that made quality-improvement efforts challenging, and the research team hypothesized that these challenges would transfer to different contexts and health care professions.[14]

- Mitigation of experience gradients: Experience gradients can also pose challenges because of varying opinions regarding the best method for ToCs. The results of a multimethod study of ToCs during nursing shift changes by Carroll et al[20] showed "considerable variability" in ToC practices originating from novice versus more experienced nurses.

- Limiting diagnosis momentum: ToCs very frequently transmit judgments about severity of illness, diagnostic considerations, or

patient prospects.[2] A structured and consistent ToC that explicitly states the severity of illness and cardinal features with diagnostic considerations will prevent transmitting certainty in diagnosis when uncertainty remains.[21] The opportunity to question or discuss these judgments in a structured, nonthreatening ToC setting can prevent bias in the continuation of care.[30]

- Promotion of family-centered care: Because pediatric patients may lack the communication skills, knowledge, and/or intelligence to participate meaningfully in their own care, it is especially important to consider family presence as a standard means to involving patients in their own care. Honoring the context of the patient's family, culture, values, and goals will result in better health care, safety, and patient satisfaction.[31] Structuring ToC processes to be clear, concise, and nonjudgmental will facilitate patient- and family-centered care in the ED.

IDENTIFIED STRATEGIES FOR ToCs

ToCs in the ED ought to adhere to Grice's maxims of quality, quantity, relevance, and clarity.[32] Little evidence supports the superiority of any 1 model of ToC. In general, strategies will define the following components in each setting:

- who (participants [single, multidisciplinary]),
- where (location [central, bedside]),
- what (method of information exchange [written, oral]), and
- how (use of adjuncts [templates, mnemonics, computers]).

Recognizing barriers to effective communication at the time of a ToC, such as environmental distractions or interruptions, is crucial to enhancing the process. Mitigating these barriers may include transitioning care in a separate or protected area, performing the ToC in the presence of patients and families, or assigning shift overlap periods to be devoted to ToCs.[18] Allowing multiple concurrent conversations between individuals also is a barrier to effective ToC communication.[33] Other recommendations to improve the ToC process include training sessions, senior supervision, and the use of electronic aids.[34] The following 5 principles reflect effective ToCs[23]:

- assigned accountability for tasks and outcomes;

- clear and direct communication of treatment plans, follow-up expectations, and contingency plans;

- timely feedback and feed-forward with read-back of information;

- involvement of the patient and family members, unless inappropriate; and

- respect of the hub of coordination of care, which is patient centered and could be the medical home or admitting service, specifically when transitioning care out of the emergency setting.

Assigning accountability is important to avoid duplication or omission of care. A structured ToC process will define the point at which 1 provider stops providing care and the next provider begins providing care. One example of a shift-to-shift ToC strategy that has been tested in the pediatric setting is the I-PASS (Illness severity, Patient summary, Action list, Situation awareness and contingency plans, Synthesis by receiver) handoff model. A prospective intervention study on inpatient units at 9 pediatric residency training programs in the United States showed reductions in medical errors, reductions in preventable adverse events, and improvements in communication.[35]

Increasing the adoption of electronic health records (EHRs) has led to

further innovation in ToC procedures, and increased ToC accuracy has been shown.[36] Pediatric trainees who were introduced to a ToC bundle, including training, a mnemonic, and a new team structure, were noted to decrease medication errors and preventable adverse events in pediatric patients admitted to the hospital, whereas a computerized ToC tool linked to the EHR was noted to further reduce omissions of key ToC information.[37] Consensus groups suggest that the short-term target of efforts to establish electronic transfers of information will focus on defining some universally, nationally defined set of core transfer information.[23]

One area in which the EHR may be expected to be used effectively is during the transition from the ED to an inpatient unit. An examination of ToC practices at 1 institution revealed the emerging practice of "chart biopsy."[38] This phenomenon, which occurs after receiving notification of an admission, entails reviewing information by the receiving provider about the patient from the EHR before the live ToC process begins. Chart biopsy was noted to serve 3 functions:

1. provide an overview of the patient;

2. prepare for ToC process and subsequent care; and

3. defend against potential cognitive biases by allowing independent perspectives to emerge; for instance, reviewing the chart allows the admitting provider to develop his or her own understanding of the patient and may reveal laboratory test data that just became available, which may change the appropriateness of admitting the patient or placing the patient on a particular service.

It is postulated that "chart biopsy" may enrich the quality of the ToC by allowing receiving providers to enter the ToC as active participants

rather than as passive recipients of information.

An alternate view is to decrease the number of ToCs altogether, which could be accomplished by allowing a buffer of time between shift changes, either by scheduling overlapping shifts or by protecting the departing provider from acquiring new patients at the end of the shift.[3] Methods to encourage quality ToCs, such as compensation for the time spent signing out or development of incentivized performance-based quality metrics, can be considered.

Although standardizing ToC practices is important for quality transitioning of care, individual institutions may need to tailor the recommended techniques to fit their unique settings. Institutions are encouraged to choose a structured and consistent ToC model that can be adopted across the entire enterprise, with location-specific modifications, to further emphasize the benefits of standardization. ED provider groups are encouraged to establish a consensus on near-end-of-shift practices, and outgoing providers would pattern their patient involvement during the pretransition period in a like manner.[39]

The Supplemental Information contains lists of standardized ToC models. Models that have been developed or studied in the emergency or acute care setting include Safer Sign Out (from the Emergency Medicine Patient Safety Foundation),[40] ASHICE, CUBAN, DeMIST, MIST, ISBARQ, SHARED, and SOAP.

MANAGING SPECIFIC ToC SITUATIONS

Prehospital to ED

Emergency medical services (EMS) providers usually have only 1 opportunity to convey information about a patient to ED personnel. If this ToC detailing initial vital signs and the events leading up to the ED visit is not received in real time, ED clinicians track down run sheets or wait for patient care records to be printed or downloaded.[41] ED staff receiving patients from ambulance crews will naturally be focused on their own initial assessment of the patient, which often distracts them from listening carefully to the ambulance crew's ToC. Any information that was not handed over verbally, not recorded on the patient report form, or not retained by ED staff may be lost forever after the ambulance crew leaves.[33] A review of a quality-improvement database in which ToC from EMS to ED was observed revealed that a significant amount of basic and key clinical information was not passed from EMS to ED staff.[42]

Information that is strongly encouraged to be included in a ToC from EMS to ED includes the following:

- vital signs;
- attempts at procedures;
- medications administered;
- clinical status and examination findings, including changes in patient condition during transport;
- health history and preexisting conditions;
- allergies; and
- estimated weight (by length-based tape or parental report).

Focus groups of EMS providers have identified 4 potential ways to improve the structure and process of ToCs[43]:

- communicate directly with the ED provider responsible for the patient's care;
- increase interdisciplinary feedback, transparency, and shared understanding of scope of practice;
- standardize some (but not all) aspects of the handoff; and
- harness technology to close gaps in information exchange.

When transporting a patient from a nonhome setting, such as a school, child care, or medical office, EMS providers may bring consent or health history documents maintained at that location. In the setting of trauma, the mechanism of injury reported to EMS personnel is an important data point. Especially important are pieces of information or visual clues to potential nonaccidental trauma or neglect that may be noted at the scene by prehospital providers. To aid in family reunification, it is important for the ToC from EMS providers to include information about the condition and destination of family members. EMS providers also can serve a valuable role in triage and disaster resource utilization during mass casualty incidents by relaying information regarding scene information and number of potential victims.

Provider to Provider Within the ED

Health care providers working in EDs can be expected to transition the care of all patients under their care frequently, during or at the end of shifts. Maintaining low rates of error and harm in this high-risk environment necessitates that any ToC be accomplished in an effective, orderly, and predictable manner. It is important for a ToC to reflect the multidisciplinary needs of ED patients, and the most favorable environment may include the presence of physician and nursing providers as well as other relevant ancillary staff to discuss ToC information as a team.[44] Recognized models for effective team communication include SHARED (Situation, History, Assessment, Requirements, Evaluation, Documentation), TeamSTEPPS (Team Strategies and Tools to Enhance Performance and Patient Safety), iSoBAR (Identify, Situation, Observations, Background, Agreed Plan & Accountability, Read Back),

and SBAR (Situation, Background, Assessment, Recommendation) models.[45,46] An important consideration is that systematic studies have noted that, until further evidence is gathered, no model can be recommended over another, and ToC processes at shift change or change-of-duty will follow the overarching principles discussed throughout this statement.

Bedside handoffs respond directly to several of The Joint Commission's National Patient Safety Goals, which address patient identification, communication among health care providers, and patients' involvement in their own care.[47,48] Embedding bedside handoffs into institutional culture and into individual practice has been challenging.[49] A 2007 survey reported that bedside rounds during shift changes took place in only 24% of EDs participating in the Pediatric Emergency Care Applied Research Network.[50]

An algorithm presented by the Council of Emergency Medicine Residency Directors' Transitions of Care Task Force describes the execution of the ToC process, based on survey responses from emergency medicine faculty and residents and ED nurses.[51] Steps include the following:

- setting an uninterrupted time and space with access to medical records;
- presence of as many health care team members as possible;
- prioritizing discussion of high-risk patients first;
- structured sign-out to identified receiving provider for each patient; and
- closing the loop (invitation for questions, documentation of ToC).

The Australasian College of Emergency Medicine Guideline also notes that scheduling should allow protected time for ToC rounds to occur during working hours.[45]

ED to Consultant

The lack of proper and timely communication between the ED and consultants also can place patients at risk. Although there is transfer of information between 2 services regarding patient information as well as shared responsibility for a patient, consultations are distinctly different from patient ToC, in which the responsibility of care is completely transferred. Furthermore, there is no accepted standard of ED provider to consultant communication. This situation has prompted researchers to consider a "taxonomy" of ED consultations and conceptual flow for engaging outside expertise.[52] Because of the implied sharing of responsibility for the patient, structured and consistent ToC processes will delineate the responsibility of each provider for patient care, whether that includes collaborative care, comanagement, or solely recommendations to the ED provider. If patients are transported out of the ED for specialist consultation, evaluation, or testing, another ToC will occur at the time that the patient returns to the ED setting. Communication between ED providers and consultants is an area for future investigation.

Transfer From ED to Receiving Facility

Transferring patients from the ED to outside facilities will nearly always preclude face-to-face communication; however, it need not preclude 2-way communication and the opportunity to answer questions. There are aspects of interfacility transfer of patients that are governed by the Emergency Medical Treatment and Labor Act,[53] and hospitals are encouraged to be familiar with these obligations.[54] Safe interfacility transfer of patients out of the ED will be aided by having interfacility transfer guidelines in place. Sample transfer checklists, which could be used to script a transfer ToC that is

inclusive of information necessary for the EMS transport service, as well as the accepting facility's service, are available from the EMS for Children National Resource Center.[55]

ED to Inpatient Setting

There is a paucity of pediatric specific literature regarding ED to inpatient transitions; however, many of the same challenges existing in general emergency care apply to pediatric patients. In addition, the inability of young pediatric patients to verbalize their condition invites further opportunity for adverse events. The general concepts of transfer of information, responsibility, and authority[56] apply to ToCs from ED to inpatient units as well as intradepartmental ToCs or transfers to outside facilities.

An ineffective ToC from the ED is a well-identified source of adverse events and near misses for inpatients[57] and is implicated in nearly one-quarter of ED malpractice claims.[58] Communication defects between the ED and inpatient team are the primary source of faulty ToCs, with up to 50% to 60% of handoffs omitting vital information,[59,60] regardless of provider experience. Poor communication may occur because of lack of communication and ToC training,[59-61] uncertain diagnoses, lack of complete results of testing, discrepancies of expectations, and potentially contradictory goals of the ED and inpatient providers[44,62,63] as well as cognitive errors caused by inheriting the thoughts of others about the patient's condition.[64] Workplace and human factors engineering within the ED and pediatric ED, such as frequency of interruptions,[65] background noise,[66,67] and the wide variety of patient conditions and unique patient needs, further complicate the ToC from ED to inpatient units.

When admitting a patient from the ED to the inpatient setting, information may be shared between

clinicians, but the patient's physical location may make it difficult for the clinician who has assumed responsibility for patient care to assume control at the same time. For instance, when admitted patients are boarded in the ED or when the inpatient provider is not free to attend to the patient promptly, confusion may exist as to the actual transfer of responsibility for care. Furthermore, a ToC may occur separately for each provider type (physician, nurse, etc). The lack of a coordinated transition between health care providers may result in communication of different depth and content of information, which could cause delays in care. Laboratory and imaging results may not be available until after the ToC, and patients may have a continued need for "as needed" medications.[2] Structured and consistent ToC processes that include an unambiguous transfer of authority and responsibility for pending and future care would delineate how to proceed in such cases, thereby avoiding confusion.

The American College of Emergency Physicians offers several suggestions to improve ToCs from EDs to inpatient units. These include reducing interruptions and distractions during ToCs, incorporating 2-way communication with read-back to confirm understanding, promoting formal education for trainees and attending physicians, practicing and evaluating department-specific ToCs, and considering standardized ToC procedures specific to the needs of each facility,[12] recognizing that no single ToC method will meet the needs of all departments.[7,68] A subsequent 2014 survey of 8 teaching hospitals revealed the use of standardized tools in 18% of ToCs from EDs to inpatient units and formal education of less than one-third of physicians.[69]

Specific to pediatric patients, Bigham et al[70] used several of these processes when studying pediatric transfers from EDs to inpatient units within a broader handoff project involving 23 children's hospitals. The study focused on interventions addressing defined ToC intent, content, and process, the latter including the use of standard format, tools, and clear and timely transition of responsibility. Results revealed a significant decrease in ToC-related care failures, from 37.2% to 13.4%, with an accompanying increase in staff satisfaction.

ED to Medical Home

Although literature exists on ToCs from the inpatient to the outpatient setting, effective means of transferring care back to the medical home after an acute care visit has not been well studied. Examples of communication from the ED to the medical home include phone calls and automated faxes or e-mails with details of the patient visit.

Two-way ToC processes may not be feasible for every patient seen in the ED; however, patients discharged with pending studies or consults may warrant such communication, and this ToC is especially important for medically complex patients. Direct provider-to-provider communications may be the expectation based on the complexity or severity of the patient's condition. If the patient's status is critical (ie, requiring admission to an ICU or a grave new diagnosis made) or if the patient dies, a phone call between the ED and primary care provider may enable the primary care provider to support the patient or family.

It is important for the acute care setting to perform medication reconciliation at the time of discharge and to communicate newly prescribed medications to the medical home. EDs may consider adding the resources necessary to accomplish this. EHRs may be able to generate ED visit summaries that provide adequate 1-way ToC information, including date of service, treatments received, study results, diagnosis, and follow-up plan. Institutions are encouraged to inquire about how the use of the EHR for communication with the medical home may qualify as "meaningful use" in the Medicare and Medicaid EHR Incentive Programs.

Transferring care back to the medical home is a shared responsibility between the acute care setting and outpatient setting. The American Medical Association published a consensus report on the responsibilities of ambulatory practices in ToCs.[71] This report focused mainly on inpatient teams to ambulatory teams but emphasized the importance of both teams being responsible and accountable for communication that would ensure a safe care transition. The report states that, in most instances, the ambulatory practice is best situated to take lead responsibility for these tasks, because the ambulatory practice will be responsible for providing ongoing care to the patient.

TEACHING ToCs

A standardized procedure needs to be developed for trainees within emergency medicine residency and fellowship programs[72] as well as nursing and allied health training programs. With the initiation of resident duty hour limits, more frequent ToCs in academic medicine raise the potential for more safety concerns.[73] A survey of emergency residency programs revealed that 75% had no formal didactic training and 90% had no written policy about ToCs.[9]

Numerous organizations, including The Joint Commission[74] and the Institute of Medicine,[75] call for formal attention to ToCs involving trainees. The Emergency Medicine Milestones Project, supported by the Society for Academic Emergency Medicine and the American Board of Emergency Medicine, along with the Accreditation Council for Graduate Medical Education (ACGME), identifies effective ToCs as a competency of all graduating emergency medicine residents.[76] The ACGME, a professional organization responsible for the accreditation of numerous residency education programs, requires specific attention to ToC procedures in both residency and fellowship training programs, creating common standards for all training programs.[77] The American Association of Colleges of Nursing also includes knowledge of and ability to perform appropriate ToC practices as a competency for graduate nursing.[78] Despite the recognized need for standardized tools and procedures at each site, the ACGME recognizes that each site may have different needs and will not use the same templates or tools.[68]

ToC concepts apply to practitioners beyond the training period. With the use of learner-identified ToC milestones, a longitudinal education and evaluation curriculum that uses tool- and simulation-based education modules has been developed for all levels of learners, from medical student through faculty.[79] The American Board of Pediatrics offers a handoff improvement project for pediatric emergency physicians within its Maintenance of Certification category 4 program.[80] Future professional development programs may offer further opportunity to train providers.

ADDRESSING AUTHORITY GRADIENTS WITHIN SIMULATIONS

The concept of authority gradients was introduced to the health care community in "To Err Is Human: Building a Safer Health System,"[11] yet the role of authority gradients in communication breakdowns and in resulting medical error has only recently received attention in the health care literature.[21] In acknowledgment of this concept, research has been conducted that incorporates the authority gradient into simulation exercises. Two such studies showed that when a health care team was presented with an acute situation in which patient safety was at risk, neither nurses nor resident physicians usually were successful in challenging erroneous orders given by the attending physician, even when they recognized the orders as potentially harmful.[81,82] The results of these studies were consistent with the current literature on the effects of authority gradients and suggest that incorporating the concept into multidisciplinary simulations may be beneficial to building team communication skills and strengthening handoff processes.

RECOMMENDATIONS

1. All EDs that care for children are strongly encouraged to implement a structured and consistent approach to ToC communications, spanning the entire continuum of patient acute care, including prehospital care, ED shift changes, consultations with specialists, admitting patients to the hospital, and transferring care back to the medical home.

2. ToC communication should attempt to be patient- and family-centered, involving patients and/or caregivers at every transition along the continuum of acute care.

3. ED staff members who provide care for children should receive training and education on structured ToC processes as part of the institution's implementation process.

4. Trainees in programs including pediatrics, pediatric emergency medicine, emergency medicine, family medicine, physician assistant, advanced practice nursing, paramedicine, respiratory therapy, and nursing should receive formal training and education on structured and consistent ToC practices. ToC training in pediatric emergency medicine education programs should be structured; the use of simulation training should be considered. Nontrainees should be offered training in ToC advancements via maintenance of certification or other continuing education activities.

5. EDs that provide care for children are encouraged to work with local EMS agencies to develop a structured and consistent ToC process or script that encompasses vital signs, clinical status, patient care, pertinent history and examination findings, mechanism of injury, and scene safety information.

6. EDs that provide care for children should have interfacility transfer guidelines in place.

7. Studies comparing ToC models in the ED setting are encouraged. Standardized, validated process and outcome metrics are recommended to evaluate the effectiveness of ToC processes of care.

8. Institutions should keep their information technology department included in the planning and implementation of structured and consistent ToC processes and abreast of developments in EHR technologies.

LEAD AUTHORS

Toni K. Gross, MD, MPH, FAAP
Lee S. Benjamin, MD, FAAP, FACEP
Elizabeth Stone, MSN

AMERICAN ACADEMY OF PEDIATRICS, COMMITTEE ON PEDIATRIC EMERGENCY MEDICINE, 2014–2015

Joan E. Shook, MD, MBA, FAAP, Chairperson
Thomas H. Chun, MD, MPH, FAAP
Gregory P. Conners, MD, MPH, MBA, FAAP
Edward E. Conway Jr, MD, MS, FAAP
Nanette C. Dudley, MD, FAAP
Susan M. Fuchs, MD, FAAP
Natalie E. Lane, MD, FAAP
Charles G. Macias, MD, MPH, FAAP
Brian R. Moore, MD, FAAP
Joseph L. Wright, MD, MPH, FAAP

LIAISONS

Kim Bullock, MD – *American Academy of Family Physicians*
Elizabeth Edgerton, MD, MPH, FAAP – *Maternal and Child Health Bureau*
Toni K. Gross, MD, MPH, FAAP – *National Association of EMS Physicians*
Tamar Magarik Haro – *American Academy of Pediatrics Department of Federal Affairs*
Lee Benjamin, MD, FAAP – *American College of Emergency Physicians*
Angela Mickalide, PhD, MCHES – *EMS for Children National Resource Center*
Paul Sirbaugh, DO, MBA, FAAP – *National Association of Emergency Medical Technicians*
Sally K. Snow, RN, BSN, CPEN, FAEN – *Emergency Nurses Association*
David W. Tuggle, MD, FAAP – *American College of Surgeons*
Cynthia Wright, MSN, RNC – *National Association of State EMS Officials*

STAFF

Sue Tellez

AMERICAN COLLEGE OF EMERGENCY PHYSICIANS, PEDIATRIC EMERGENCY MEDICINE COMMITTEE, 2013–2014

Lee S. Benjamin, MD, FACEP, Chairperson
Isabel A. Barata, MD, FACEP, FAAP
Kiyetta Alade, MD
Joseph Arms, MD
Jahn T. Avarello, MD, FACEP
Steven Baldwin, MD
Kathleen Brown, MD, FACEP
Richard M. Cantor, MD, FACEP
Ariel Cohen, MD
Ann Marie Dietrich, MD, FACEP
Paul J. Eakin, MD
Marianne Gausche-Hill, MD, FACEP, FAAP
Michael Gerardi, MD, FACEP, FAAP
Charles J. Graham, MD, FACEP
Doug K. Holtzman, MD, FACEP
Jeffrey Hom, MD, FACEP
Paul Ishimine, MD, FACEP
Hasmig Jinivizian, MD
Madeline Joseph, MD, FACEP
Sanjay Mehta, MD, Med, FACEP
Aderonke Ojo, MD, MBBS
Audrey Z. Paul, MD, PhD
Denis R. Pauze, MD, FACEP
Nadia M. Pearson, DO
Brett Rosen, MD
W. Scott Russell, MD, FACEP
Mohsen Saidinejad, MD
Harold A. Sloas, DO

ABBREVIATIONS

ACGME: Accreditation Council for Graduate Medical Education
ED: emergency department
EHR: electronic health record
EMS: emergency medical services
ToC: transition of care

REFERENCES

1. Pruitt CM, Liebelt EL. Enhancing patient safety in the pediatric emergency department: teams, communication, and lessons from crew resource management. *Pediatr Emerg Care.* 2010;26(12):942–948; quiz 949–951

2. Cohen MD, Hilligoss PB. The published literature on handoffs in hospitals: deficiencies identified in an extensive review. *Qual Saf Health Care.* 2010;19(6):493–497

3. Cheung DS, Kelly JJ, Beach C, et al; Section of Quality Improvement and Patient Safety, American College of Emergency Physicians. Improving handoffs in the emergency department. *Ann Emerg Med.* 2010;55(2):171–180

4. Dhingra KR, Elms A, Hobgood C. Reducing error in the emergency department: a call for standardization of the sign-out process. *Ann Emerg Med.* 2010;56(6):637–642

5. Bomba DT, Prakash R. A description of handover processes in an Australian public hospital. *Aust Health Rev.* 2005;29(1):68–79

6. Horwitz LI, Moin T, Krumholz HM, Wang L, Bradley EH. Consequences of inadequate sign-out for patient care. *Arch Intern Med.* 2008;168(16):1755–1760

7. Foster S, Manser T. The effects of patient handoff characteristics on subsequent care: a systematic review and areas for future research. *Acad Med.* 2012;87(8):1105–1124

8. Halm MA. Nursing handoffs: ensuring safe passage for patients. *Am J Crit Care.* 2013;22(2):158–162

9. Sinha M, Shriki J, Salness R, Blackburn PA. Need for standardized sign-out in the emergency department: a survey of emergency medicine residency and pediatric emergency medicine fellowship program directors. *Acad Emerg Med.* 2007;14(2):192–196

10. Arora V, Johnson J, Lovinger D, Humphrey HJ, Meltzer DO. Communication failures in patient sign-out and suggestions for improvement: a critical incident analysis. *Qual Saf Health Care.* 2005;14(6):401–407

11. Institute of Medicine, Committee on Quality of Health Care in America. In: Kohn LT, Corrigan J, Donaldson MS, eds. *To Err Is Human: Building a Safer Health System.* Washington, DC: National Academies Press; 2000

12. American College of Emergency Physicians. Available at: www.acep.org/ workarea/DownloadAsset.aspx?id= 91206. Accessed September 28, 2015

13. Croskerry P. From mindless to mindful practice--cognitive bias and clinical decision making. *N Engl J Med.* 2013;368(26):2445–2448

14. Croskerry P, Singhal G, Mamede S. Cognitive debiasing 1: origins of bias and theory of debiasing. *BMJ Qual Saf.* 2013;22(suppl 2):ii58–ii64

15. Croskerry P, Singhal G, Mamede S. Cognitive debiasing 2: impediments to and strategies for change. *BMJ Qual Saf.* 2013;22(suppl 2):ii65–ii72

16. Beach C, Croskerry P, Shapiro M; Center for Safety in Emergency Care. Profiles in patient safety: emergency care transitions. *Acad Emerg Med.* 2003;10(4):364–367

17. Reason JT. *Human Error.* New York, NY: Cambridge University Press; 1990

18. Krug SE, Frush K; Committee on Pediatric Emergency Medicine. Patient safety in the pediatric emergency care setting. *Pediatrics.* 2007;120(6):1367–1375

19. Croskerry P, Sinclair D. Emergency medicine: a practice prone to error? *CJEM.* 2001;3(4):271–276

20. Carroll JS, Williams M, Gallivan TM. The ins and outs of change of shift handoffs between nurses: a communication challenge. *BMJ Qual Saf.* 2012;21(7):586–593

21. Cosby KS, Croskerry P. Profiles in patient safety: authority gradients in medical error. *Acad Emerg Med.* 2004;11(12):1341–1345

22. Manser T, Foster S, Gisin S, Jaeckel D, Ummenhofer W. Assessing the quality of patient handoffs at care transitions. *Qual Saf Health Care.* 2010;19(6):e44

23. Snow V, Beck D, Budnitz T, et al; American College of Physicians; Society of General Internal Medicine; Society of Hospital Medicine; American Geriatrics Society; American College of Emergency Physicians; Society of Academic Emergency Medicine. Transitions of care consensus policy statement: American College of Physicians-Society of General Internal Medicine-Society of Hospital Medicine-American Geriatrics Society-American College of Emergency Physicians-Society of Academic

Emergency Medicine. *J Gen Intern Med.* 2009;24(8):971–976

24. Tidwell T, Edwards J, Snider E, et al. A nursing pilot study on bedside reporting to promote best practice and patient/family-centered care. *J Neurosci Nurs.* 2011;43(4):E1–E5

25. Maxson PM, Derby KM, Wrobleski DM, Foss DM. Bedside nurse-to-nurse handoff promotes patient safety. *Medsurg Nurs.* 2012;21(3):140–144; quiz 145

26. Chaboyer W, McMurray A, Johnson J, Hardy L, Wallis M, Sylvia Chu FY. Bedside handover: quality improvement strategy to "transform care at the bedside". *J Nurs Care Qual.* 2009;24(2):136–142

27. Lehmann LS, Brancati FL, Chen MC, Roter D, Dobs AS. The effect of bedside case presentations on patients' perceptions of their medical care. *N Engl J Med.* 1997;336(16):1150–1155

28. Revere A, Eldridge N; VA National Center for Patient Safety. Joint Commission National Patient Safety Goals for 2008. *Topics in Patient Safety.* 2008: 12(1):1-4. Available at: www.patientsafety.va.gov/docs/TIPS/TIPS_JanFeb08.pdf. Accessed September 16, 2015

29. Cosby KS, Roberts R, Palivos L, et al. Characteristics of patient care management problems identified in emergency department morbidity and mortality investigations during 15 years. *Ann Emerg Med.* 2008;51(3):251–261, 261.e1

30. Angela Munasque. Thinking about thinking: heuristics and the emergency physician. *Emergency Medicine News.* October 2009. Available at: http://journals.lww.com/em-news/Documents/Cognitiveautopsy.pdf. Accessed September 16, 2015

31. O'Malley PJ, Brown K, Krug SE; Committee on Pediatric Emergency Medicine. Patient- and family-centered care of children in the emergency department. *Pediatrics.* 2008;122(2). Available at: www.pediatrics.org/cgi/content/full/122/2/e511

32. Cole P, Morgan J, eds. Logic and conversation: syntax and semantics. Vol. 3. In: *Speech Acts.* New York, NY: Academic Press; 1975:41–58

33. Talbot R, Bleetman A. Retention of information by emergency department staff at ambulance handover: do standardised approaches work? *Emerg Med J.* 2007;24(8):539–542

34. Thompson JE, Collett LW, Langbart MJ, et al. Using the ISBAR handover tool in junior medical officer handover: a study in an Australian tertiary hospital. *Postgrad Med J.* 2011;87(1027):340–344

35. Starmer AJ, Spector ND, Srivastava R, et al; I-PASS Study Group. Changes in medical errors after implementation of a handoff program. *N Engl J Med.* 2014;371(19):1803–1812

36. Palma JP, Sharek PJ, Longhurst CA. Impact of electronic medical record integration of a handoff tool on sign-out in a newborn intensive care unit. *J Perinatol.* 2011;31(5):311–317

37. Starmer AJ, Sectish TC, Simon DW, et al. Rates of medical errors and preventable adverse events among hospitalized children following implementation of a resident handoff bundle. *JAMA.* 2013;310(21):2262–2270

38. Hilligoss B, Zheng K. Chart biopsy: an emerging medical practice enabled by electronic health records and its impacts on emergency department-inpatient admission handoffs. *J Am Med Inform Assoc.* 2013;20(2):260–267

39. Singer JI, Dean J. Emergency physician intershift handovers: an analysis of our transitional care. *Pediatr Emerg Care.* 2006;22(10):751–754

40. Emergency Medicine Patient Safety Foundation. Safer sign out. Available at: http://safersignout.com/. Accessed September 16, 2015

41. Landman ABLC, Lee CH, Sasson C, Van Gelder CM, Curry LA. Prehospital electronic patient care report systems: early experiences from emergency medical services agency leaders. *PLoS One.* 2012;7(3):e32692

42. Panchal AR, Gaither JB, Svirsky I, Prosser B, Stolz U, Spaite DW. The impact of professionalism on transfer of care to the emergency department. *J Emerg Med.* 2015;49(1):18–25

43. Meisel ZF, Shea JA, Peacock NJ, et al. Optimizing the patient handoff between emergency medical services and the

emergency department. *Ann Emerg Med.* 2015;65(3):310–317.e1

44. Patterson ES, Roth EM, Woods DD, Chow R, Gomes JO. Handoff strategies in settings with high consequences for failure: lessons for health care operations. *Int J Qual Health Care.* 2004;16(2):125–132

45. Australasian College for Emergency Medicine. *Guideline on Clinical Handover in the Emergency Department.* Melbourne, Australia: Australasian College for Emergency Medicine; 2010

46. Emergency Nurses Association. *Position Statement: Patient Handoff/Transfer.* Des Plaines, IL: Emergency Nurses Association; 2013

47. The Joint Commission. 2015 National Patient Safety Goals. Available at: www.jointcommission.org/standards_information/npsgs.aspx. Accessed September 16, 2015

48. Baker SJ. Bedside shift report improves patient safety and nurse accountability. *J Emerg Nurs.* 2010;36(4):355–358

49. Gregory S, Tan D, Tilrico M, Edwardson N, Gamm L. Bedside shift reports: what does the evidence say? *J Nurs Adm.* 2014;44(10):541–545

50. Shaw KN, Ruddy RM, Olsen CS, et al; Pediatric Emergency Care Applied Research Network. Pediatric patient safety in emergency departments: unit characteristics and staff perceptions. *Pediatrics.* 2009;124(2):485–493

51. Kessler C, Shakeel F, Hern HG, et al. An algorithm for transition of care in the emergency department. *Acad Emerg Med.* 2013;20(6):605–610

52. Kessler CS, Asrow A, Beach C, et al. The taxonomy of emergency department consultations—results of an expert consensus panel. *Ann Emerg Med.* 2013;61(2):161–166

53. Centers for Medicare and Medicaid Services. Emergency Medical Treatment and Labor Act (EMTALA). Available at: https://www.cms.gov/Regulations-and-Guidance/Legislation/EMTALA/index.html. Accessed August 21, 2015

54. Centers for Medicare and Medicaid Services. Emergency Medical Treatment and Labor Act (EMTALA).

Available at: www.acep.org/Clinical—Practice-Management/Focus-On—The-Emergency-Medical-Treatment-and-Labor-Act/. Accessed September 16, 2015

55. Emergency Medical Services for Children National Resource Center. Healthcare provider resources. Available at: www.emscnrc.org/EMSC_Resources/Interfacility_Transfer_Toolbox.aspx#resources. Accessed September 16, 2015

56. Behara R, Wears RL, Perry SJ, et al. A conceptual framework for studying the safety of transitions in emergency care. In: Henriksen K, Battles JB, Marks ES, Lewin DI, eds. *Advances in Patient Safety: From Research to Implementation. Volume 2: Concepts and Methodology.* Rockville, MD: Agency for Healthcare Research and Quality; 2005

57. Horwitz LI, Meredith T, Schuur JD, Shah NR, Kulkarni RG, Jenq GY. Dropping the baton: a qualitative analysis of failures during the transition from emergency department to inpatient care. *Ann Emerg Med.* 2009;53(6):701.e4–710.e4

58. Kachalia A, Gandhi TK, Puopolo AL, et al. Missed and delayed diagnoses in the emergency department: a study of closed malpractice claims from 4 liability insurers. *Ann Emerg Med.* 2007;49(2):196–205

59. Maughan BC, Lei L, Cydulka RK. ED handoffs: observed practices and communication errors. *Am J Emerg Med.* 2011;29(5):502–511

60. Chang VY, Arora VM, Lev-Ari S, D'Arcy M, Keysar B. Interns overestimate the effectiveness of their hand-off communication. *Pediatrics.* 2010;125(3):491–496

61. Farhan M, Brown R, Woloshynowych M, Vincent C. The ABC of handover: a qualitative study to develop a new tool for handover in the emergency department. *Emerg Med J.* 2012;29(12):941–946

62. Beach C, Cheung DS, Apker J, et al. Improving interunit transitions of care between emergency physicians and hospital medicine physicians: a conceptual approach. *Acad Emerg Med.* 2012;19(10):1188–1195

63. Apker J, Mallak LA, Applegate EB III, et al. Exploring emergency physician-hospitalist handoff interactions: development of the Handoff Communication Assessment. *Ann Emerg Med.* 2010;55(2):161–170

64. Campbell SG, Croskerry P, Bond WF. Profiles in patient safety: a "perfect storm" in the emergency department. *Acad Emerg Med.* 2007;14(8):743–749

65. Chisholm CD, Dornfeld AM, Nelson DR, Cordell WH. Work interrupted: a comparison of workplace interruptions in emergency departments and primary care offices. *Ann Emerg Med.* 2001;38(2):146–151

66. Buelow M. Noise level measurements in four Phoenix emergency departments. *J Emerg Nurs.* 2001;27(1):23–26

67. Ratnapalan S, Cieslak P, Mizzi T, McEvoy J, Mounstephen W. Physicians' perceptions of background noise in a pediatric emergency department. *Pediatr Emerg Care.* 2011;27(9):826–833

68. Riesenberg LA, Leitzsch J, Little BW. Systematic review of handoff mnemonics literature. *Am J Med Qual.* 2009;24(3):196–204

69. Kessler C, Scott NL, Siedsma M, Jordan J, Beach C, Coletti CM. Interunit handoffs of patients and transfers of information: a survey of current practices. *Ann Emerg Med.* 2014;64(4):343.e5–349.e5

70. Bigham MT, Logsdon TR, Manicone PE, et al. Decreasing handoff-related care failures in children's hospitals. *Pediatrics.* 2014;134(2). Available at: www.pediatrics.org/cgi/content/full/134/2/e572

71. Sokol PE, Wynia MK; American Medical Association, Expert Panel on Care Transitions. *There and Home Again, Safely: Five Responsibilities of Ambulatory Practices in High Quality Care Transitions.* Chicago, IL: American Medical Association; 2013. Available at: http://selfmanagementalliance.org/wp-content/uploads/2013/11/There-and-Home-Safely_ambulatory-practices.pdf. Accessed September 16, 2015

72. Volpp KG, Grande D. Residents' suggestions for reducing errors in

teaching hospitals. *N Engl J Med.* 2003;348(9):851–855

73. Philibert I, Chang B, Flynn T, et al. The 2003 common duty hour limits: process, outcome, and lessons learned. *J Grad Med Educ.* 2009;1(2):334–337

74. Arora V, Johnson J. A model for building a standardized hand-off protocol. *Jt Comm J Qual Patient Saf.* 2006;32(11):646–655

75. Institute of Medicine, Committee on Optimizing Graduate Medical Trainee. (Resident) Hours and work schedules to improve patient safety. In: Ulmer C, Wolman D, Johns M, eds. *Resident Duty Hours: Enhancing Sleep, Supervision, and Safety.* Washington, DC: National Academies Press; 2008

76. Accreditation Council on Graduate Medical Education, American Board of Emergency Medicine. Emergency medicine milestones. 2011. Available at: https://www.abem.org/public/publications/emergency-medicine-milestones. Accessed September 28, 2015

77. Riebschleger M, Philibert I. New standards for transitions of care: discussion and justification. In: Philibert I, Amis S, eds. *The ACGME 2011 Duty Hour Standards: Enhancing Quality of Care, Supervision, and Resident Professional Development.* Chicago, IL: Accreditation Council for Graduate Medical Education; 2011

78. American Association of Colleges of Nursing Education Consortium. Graduate-level QSEN competencies: knowledge, skills and attitudes. 2012. Available at: www.aacn.nche.edu/faculty/qsen/competencies.pdf. Accessed September 16, 2015

79. Farnan JM, Arora VM. A longitudinal approach to handoff training. *Virtual Mentor.* 2012;14(5):383–388

80. American Academy of Pediatrics. Improving shift transitions with briefing checklists in the Emergency Department. Available at: https://qidata.aap.org/briefingchecklists/welcome?sso=true&nfstatus=401&nftoken=00000000-0000-0000-0000-000000000000&nfstatusdescription=ERROR%3a+No+local+token. Accessed September 19, 2016

81. Calhoun AW, Boone MC, Porter MB, Miller KH. Using simulation to address hierarchy-related errors in medical practice. *Perm J.* 2014;18(2):14–20

82. St Pierre M, Scholler A, Strembski D, Breuer G. Do residents and nurses communicate safety relevant concerns? Simulation study on the influence of the authority gradient [in German]. *Anaesthesist.* 2012;61(10):857–866

83. Dekosky AS, Gangopadhyaya A, Chan B, Arora VM. Improving written sign-outs through education and structured audit: the UPDATED approach. *J Grad Med Educ.* 2013;5(2):335–336

84. Connor MP, Bush AC, Brennan J. IMOUTA: a proposal for patient care handoffs. *Laryngoscope.* 2013;123(11):2649–2653

85. Turner P. Implementation of TeamSTEPPS in the emergency department. *Crit Care Nurs Q.* 2012;35(3):208–212

Helping Children and Families Deal With Divorce and Separation

- *Clinical Report*

CLINICAL REPORT   Guidance for the Clinician in Rendering Pediatric Care

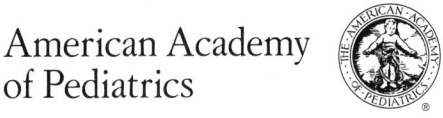

American Academy
of Pediatrics

DEDICATED TO THE HEALTH OF ALL CHILDREN™

Helping Children and Families Deal With Divorce and Separation

George J. Cohen, MD, FAAP, Carol C. Weitzman, MD, FAAP, COMMITTEE ON PSYCHOSOCIAL ASPECTS OF CHILD AND FAMILY HEALTH, SECTION ON DEVELOPMENTAL AND BEHAVIORAL PEDIATRICS

abstract

For the past several years in the United States, there have been more than 800 000 divorces and parent separations annually, with over 1 million children affected. Children and their parents can experience emotional trauma before, during, and after a separation or divorce. Pediatricians can be aware of their patients' behavior and parental attitudes and behaviors that may indicate family dysfunction and that can indicate need for intervention. Age-appropriate explanation and counseling for the child and advice and guidance for the parents, as well as recommendation of reading material, may help reduce the potential negative effects of divorce. Often, referral to professionals with expertise in the social, emotional, and legal aspects of the separation and its aftermath may be helpful for these families.

DOI: 10.1542/peds.2016-3020

PEDIATRICS (ISSN Numbers: Print, 0031-4005; Online, 1098-4275).

FINANCIAL DISCLOSURE: The authors have indicated they do not have a financial relationship relevant to this article to disclose.

FUNDING: No external funding.

POTENTIAL CONFLICT OF INTEREST: The authors have indicated they have no potential conflicts of interest to disclose.

To cite: Cohen GJ, Weitzman CC, AAP COMMITTEE ON PSYCHOSOCIAL ASPECTS OF CHILD AND FAMILY HEALTH, AAP SECTION ON DEVELOPMENTAL AND BEHAVIORAL PEDIATRICS. Helping Children and Families Deal With Divorce and Separation. *Pediatrics.* 2016;138(6):e20163020

INTRODUCTION

Every year, more than 1 million American children experience the divorce or separation of their parents. Poverty, lower levels of parent education, and parents being children of divorce can be factors in divorce.[1] Parents of children with chronic or serious illnesses and neurodevelopmental disorders such as cancer and autism spectrum disorders are often at higher risk of divorce, although some studies have shown this is not always the case.[2] The separation itself is usually the culmination of other stressors in the family to which the child has been exposed; parental conflict and tension often precede and may lead to behavior problems in the child.[1]

Many children show behavior changes in the first year of parent separation. Although most adjustment problems resolve in 2 to 3 years after the separation,[1] the child's sense of loss may last for years, with exacerbation on holidays, birthdays, and other special events. Adjustment to a new living situation, continuing parental tensions, and alienation can cause distress in the child.[3,4]

CHILDREN'S REACTIONS

Children's manifestations of reaction to parental divorce are related to many factors, including the stage of development of the child,[5] the parents' ability to focus on the child's needs and feelings, the child's temperament, and the child's and parents' pre- and postseparation psychosocial functioning.[1,3]

Infants

Although infants cannot understand the separation, they react to changes in routine and caregivers and the break in attachment. They may be fussier, irritable, or listless and have sleep and feeding disturbances. At approximately 6 months of age, normal separation and stranger anxiety may be increased.[6–9]

Toddlers

Separation anxiety is a frequent manifestation of distress at this age, and children may be reluctant to separate from parents even in familiar settings, such as child care or a grandparent's home. Developmental regression, including loss of toileting and language skills, is not uncommon. Eating and sleep disorders are also common.[10,11]

Preschool-Aged Children

At this age, children do not understand the permanence of the separation and will repeatedly ask for the absent parent. They may be demanding and defiant and may have sleeping and eating problems as well as regression in developmental milestones. They often test and manipulate differences in limit setting by the 2 parents. By age 4 to 5 years, they may blame themselves for the separation, begin acting out, have nightmares, have more reluctance to separate, and fear that they may be abandoned.[1,3]

School-Aged Children

Self-blame and asking and fantasizing about the reunion of the parents are not uncommon. At this age, mood and behavior changes, such as withdrawal and anger, are frequent, school performance may decline, and the child may feel abandoned by the parent no longer living in the home.[1,3]

Adolescents

Although by this age, children may understand some of the reasons for the family breakup, they may still have difficulty accepting the situation and may try to take on adult roles.[1,3,8,9] They may de-idealize 1 or both parents and still believe that they can reunite the parents. Aggressive delinquent behavior, withdrawal, substance abuse, inappropriate sexual behavior, and poor school performance are frequent responses to the change in family structure.[12] Suicidal ideation is increased in junior high school–aged boys of separated mothers[13] and is more frequent in men than in women of divorced parents.[14] Girls living with divorced fathers are more likely to make suicide attempts than girls living with their divorced mothers.[15]

Parents' Reactions

Parents also suffer negative effects of separation and divorce. Mothers are likely to feel stressed and humiliated, to use alcohol, and to seek mental health services compared with divorced fathers. Mothers' problems can persist for prolonged periods after divorce. However, fathers often feel alienated, seem less accepting of their children, and may become depressed and anxious and abuse substances. Grandparents, too, may feel a decreased quality of relationship with their grandchildren, especially in relation to custody arrangements that favor their ex–son-in-law or ex–daughter-in-law.[3]

MODIFYING FACTORS

Different situations and activities can have different effects on the children of divorce and separation. However, if the parent does not understand the child's individual need, the child is likely to be frustrated and demonstrate externalizing behaviors, such as tantrums, oppositional behavior, and general acting out.[10] Moving away from a familiar milieu may be a negative factor in the child's adjustment; children who move away from their former home are likely to feel more distress. As adolescents, girls show more hostility and boys are less hostile when they moved as children with the custodial father.[16]

Paternal Involvement

Nonresidential fathers believed they were more involved with their children than was perceived by the custodial mother but also felt a more negative change over time in their relationship with the children. The custodial mother's feelings about the relationship with her children were less likely to change.[17] Prolonged legal action in the divorce leads to worse coparenting relationships and more negative feelings in the father. However, if the father is the initiator of the divorce, he is likely to feel more fulfilled in his parenting role.[18] If the child spends more time living with the father after the separation, the child-father relationship is likely to be more positive regardless of continuing parental conflict.[19] Fathers' greater involvement with their sons has been shown to be important for the sons' development. The father's behavior and reactions to the separation, however, are specific areas that often require professional involvement.[20,21]

Children who end up living in nonnuclear (ie, other than 2 married parents) families are more likely to have a higher incidence of poor health, learning difficulties, attention-deficit/hyperactivity disorder, emotional and behavioral difficulties, and emergency department visits than those in nuclear families.[22] Interventions, such as counseling of the mother, that foster positive changes in the mother-child relationship and consistent discipline practices have resulted in increased coping efficacy in children at 6 months and at 6 years after the intervention, including in divorced, separated, and single-parent families.[23]

Financial Considerations

Low-income families are more likely to separate, and if the mother is in a new relationship, there is often a decrease in supportive coparenting.[24] When there is parental separation, fathers usually have more financial resources than the mothers. This disparity tends to increase the inequality of money available for children and thus results in a significant increase in child poverty.[25] After divorce, women are more likely than men to face significant financial challenges, receive public assistance, lose health insurance, and have decreased earning potential. In the recent US Census Bureau report on marriage, 28% of children in divorced families lived below the poverty threshold, compared with 15.9% of the total population. This situation puts children of divorced parents at a higher risk of a number of adverse outcomes.[26]

History of Child Abuse

Divorce in a family with a history of child abuse is related to a greater incidence of conduct disorder, posttraumatic stress disorder, and suicide attempts in children than does either divorce or child abuse alone.[27]

Family Conflict

Legal sources suggest that mandated parenting classes, recommended by divorce courts, could improve outcomes for all members of the family.[1] Adolescents' rating of family harmony predicted their own self-image and emotional development. Ten years after the divorce, daughters of high-conflict families

reported more depression. Wariness regarding relationships was higher in children from divorced homes or homes with parental conflict.[28] Alienation of the child and the targeted parent is a frequent problem that needs practical professional input to correct the negative effects on all parties.[29] The father's reactions and behavior to the separation is a specific area that needs professional involvement.[19]

The divorce patterns of service members and veterans further highlight the potential positive effects of the support for families that the military provides. While they are in the military, couples are less likely to divorce than their civilian counterparts. Once they leave the military, however, this trend reverses. Veterans are 3 times as likely to be divorced as those who have never served in the military. Research indicates that the military environment protects families from the stresses that often lead to divorce and that veterans' marriages become less stable once they leave the supportive military setting.[30,31]

Legal Considerations

The legal profession reports that there is momentum building for more focus on the child in divorce disputes.[32] Courts and legislators also are looking at divorce as a sign of problems in parenting and the need to improve education of parents about the effects on the child of parental discord.[33] Attention can be given to the child's reactions as he or she becomes an adolescent and also to the changes in parents' lives.[34] Legal research internationally is looking at past, present, and future relocation as related to children in divorced and separated families.[35] Research suggests that previous moves and changes in family structure may cause more psychological risk to children.

Although not a common aspect of pediatric practice, pediatricians may

be subpoenaed by a court or asked by a parent to provide testimony in a child custody hearing. In such circumstances, pediatricians should be cognizant of the following information. A "subpoena" is a legal document that notifies a witness that he or she is needed to present evidence in court. A subpoena might require testimony (subpoena ad testificandum), the production of documents (subpoena duces tecum), or both. Because a subpoena suspends typical rules regarding medical confidentiality, it is important for the pediatrician to read carefully what disclosures are commanded (and therefore allowed) by the subpoena. A provider receiving a subpoena for a medical record that he or she did not create should notify the attorney issuing the subpoena of the appropriate custodian instead of disclosing the record. On receiving any subpoena, the wisest course is to call the attorney who issued the subpoena and discuss with that attorney what testimony or documents are required and what facts or opinions the attorney hopes to elicit.

If a pediatrician is requested by a parent (or a particular party to a custody hearing) to provide testimony, in furtherance of the best interests of children of divorced families and maintenance of good physician-family relationships it may be prudent for the pediatrician to defer those requests to child-abuse pediatric experts (where available) or consult with them before providing any testimony. It is important for the pediatrician to remember that he or she should consider himself or herself an impartial educator of the court about the topic of his or her expertise. A physician has an ethical obligation to provide accurate, unbiased testimony based on sound scientific principles.[36] Pediatricians should make every effort to avoid taking sides and testifying on behalf of either parent about the appropriateness of parenting skills. One should seek legal advice from hospital-based forensic teams to explore alternative responses to a subpoena to testify. In the long term, the child's relationship with the pediatrician is best served by maintaining good relationships with both parents if possible.

When providing testimony in court, the court may deem the pediatrician as a "fact" or "expert" witness. If the pediatrician is providing only "fact" testimony, then exploration/ questions into the physician's qualifications are unnecessary, and a "fact" witness will provide testimony only to the specific facts that the witness has seen, heard, felt, etc. If the pediatrician is to be deemed an "expert" witness, then a formal courtroom procedure of qualifying the witness as an "expert" will be conducted. This legal procedure is a series of questions that demonstrates to the court that the witness has sufficient training, research, writing, professional activities, or other qualifications to serve as an "expert." Being qualified as an expert on a particular subject matter entitles the expert to offer opinions in court.[37] One need not be the foremost authority on the subject matter nor understand every nuance of the subject to qualify.[38]

The best preparation for any kind of court testimony is to be thoroughly familiar with the medical facts of the case. Although many courts will permit a witness to refer to notes during testimony, the witness should be able to recite the basic facts of the case (patient's name, age, dates seen, high points of the history, and injuries found) from memory. The expert should be familiar with the patient's entire chart, because questions may be asked about the patient's medical conditions unrelated to the issue of custody. If the pediatrician is asked to opine about a matter with which he or she is uncomfortable (ie, rendering

TABLE 1 American Academy of Pediatrics–Recommended Qualifications for Physician Expert Witnesses

1. Licensed in the state where the expert practices medicine.
2. Board certification in the area relevant to the testimony.
3. Actively engaged in clinical practice of medicine relevant to the testimony.
4. Unless retired from clinical practice, most of a physician's professional time should not be devoted to expert witness work. If retired, a physician should only testify on cases that occurred when he or she was in active practice.

an abuse or neglect diagnosis), the pediatrician may either confer with a specialist in that field (ie, a child-abuse pediatrician) before providing that testimony or inform the court of his or her discomfort in rendering a formal opinion on that subject matter. It is important that the pediatrician be cognizant of not providing irresponsible testimony.[39] Irresponsible testimony includes testimony for which the expert is insufficiently qualified or testimony based on idiosyncratic theories that have either not been substantiated by well-conducted medical studies or have not gained wide acceptance in the medical community.[36] Recommendations from the American Academy of Pediatrics for expert witnesses are listed in Table 1.[36]

THE LEGAL FRAMEWORK

Divorce is a legal term that means the dissolution or legal conclusion of a marriage. For children of married parents, the divorce process includes legal protections for children. For unmarried parents, state laws may provide similar protections for children through a custody/ visitation action. Specifically, family courts during a divorce or custody/ visitation action are charged with determining and securing the best interests of children. This assessment includes the financial and psychosocial needs of the children and typically leads to an agreement or order specifying the amount of time children will spend with each parent and which parent (or parents) is responsible for decision-making

with regard to education, health care, family values, and related matters. Some states have marital equivalents such as civil unions or domestic partnerships. Children of parents in civil union or domestic partnership relationships ideally should have the same legal protections as children born to married parents. The nonmedical literature has reported on the variability of legal decisions in cases involving same-sex parents and their children.[40]

The touchstone for determining whether a person who raises a child has a legal status as parent to that child is biology, marriage, or adoption. Although parenthood status is usually straightforward, circumstances in which parenthood status and parental rights are unclear may involve complex issues of law. A person with a biological or legal adoptive relationship to a child is that child's legal parent. Similarly, a person whose spouse bears a child is presumed to be a parent of that child. In any case involving a relationship dissolution involving a biological, marital, or adoptive parent, a court is expected to assess the best interests of the child.

A person who raises a child but who does not have a legal relationship to that child through biology, marriage, or adoption may not have the same protections for a continued relationship with the child despite the fact that the effect on the child can be as significant.[1] The courts have increasingly found ways to protect such relationships by recognizing them as psychological, de facto, or equitable parenting relationships.

These developments vary state by state. As families that formed through the expanding capacity of human reproductive technology separate and divorce, there will continue to be legal challenges and areas without legal precedent regarding custody determinations of the child.

Another area that is important to consider that is far more common than divorce is the issue of the separation of nonmarried heterosexual partners. In 2006, approximately 38% of all births were to nonmarried women. Although nearly 50% of partners were living together at the time of the child's birth, approximately 45% were separated 5 years later. Less attention is often given to these separations as when there is a legal divorce, but the psychological effect on children is likely as significant.[41]

THE PEDIATRICIAN'S ROLE

Prevention

Pediatricians may only learn about divorce or separation from the children's behavioral changes, family moves, and changes in family financial responsibility. Inquiring about family stressors, including parental difficulties, can be a routine part of the pediatric health supervision visit, as noted in the third edition of Bright Futures.[42] When pediatricians counsel the family regarding issues of child development and behavior, areas of marital discord or stress are often uncovered. Being aware of these stressors and referring for marital counseling are appropriate and may preserve the marital relationship. Pediatricians are encouraged to consider their own attitudes, religious beliefs, and ethical positions concerning divorce, especially if they have experienced divorce in their own families. Being as objective as possible in counseling children and parents is important. If the separation appears to be definite,

early interventions, such as referral to a family counselor, may decrease parental hostility and assist the child and parents in coping with family disruptions to come.

In cases of marital discord, the potential role of pediatricians includes carefully considering the child's physical and emotional needs and communicating this to parents, listening to each parent's perspective, and suggesting that they consider consulting a marriage/divorce counselor to develop strategies to address the discord or to help the child through the dissolution of the marriage. A positive, neutral relationship with both parents after a divorce and being the child's advocate are appropriate goals.

Anticipatory Guidance

The pediatrician can assess the child's reactions, the parents' reactions and levels of hostility, their abilities to understand and meet the child's physical and emotional needs, their support systems, and any indication of parental mental illness or possible substance use.[43,44] Understanding the child's experience of divorce is essential if the pediatrician is to advise the family. The works of several authors can be particularly helpful.[8,35,45–48] Wallerstein[49] correctly notes that the family divorce is a process, not simply a single event. Consequently, a child's understanding of and adjustment to divorce or separation occurs in stages.

Acute parental separation, which may precede the legal divorce by months or years, is typically the time of highest vulnerability for the child. Parental distress is high. One parent may be physically absent and often temporarily lost to the child. The custodial parent may find parenting responsibilities more difficult because of his or her own distress. At a time when children's needs are increased, parents are at an emotional disadvantage and are

often less emotionally available and less able to address the needs of their children.

Decreasing school performance, behavioral difficulties, social withdrawal, and somatic complaints are common reactions of children and accompaniments of divorce that require intervention. A heightened level of sadness is typical, and depression is not uncommon in both children and parents.[8,9]

A parent conference at this stage might be scheduled. The pediatrician can meet with the parents together, ideally, or separately, if necessary, to assess the current situation and to assist in future planning for the children's needs. It is important that pediatricians establish appropriate boundaries with parents at this point, clearly informing them that their role is to understand and meet the child's needs as much as possible, and that the pediatrician is unwilling to take sides in a contentious divorce or be a conduit of information between parents. However, if a pediatrician becomes concerned that living with a particular parent presents a significant risk of current or future abuse or neglect for the child, the pediatrician should make a report to child protective services. If a pediatrician is uncertain whether the family psychosocial dynamics pose sufficient risk to warrant a report to child protective services, it may be prudent to consult a local child-abuse pediatrician. The pediatrician can offer each parent an opportunity to discuss the separation as it affects the child.

The discussion can begin by inquiring how each member of the family is doing at this time of family stress and transition. Do both parents have adequate support systems, such as extended family, clergy, or a personal physician to help meet their own physical and emotional needs? Are there supports that can help parents in their parenting roles? What is the apparent emotional reaction of the children? It may be helpful to interpret these reactions to the parents on the basis of the child's developmental level and perspective.

Pediatricians can help parents understand their children's reactions and encourage them to discuss the divorce process with their children. Parents can be helped to answer the children's questions honestly at their level of understanding. The children's routines of school, extracurricular activities, contact with family and friends, discipline, and responsibilities ideally should remain as normal and unchanged as possible. Children can be given permission for their feelings and opportunities to express them. Children must understand that they did not cause the divorce and cannot bring the parents back together. It is hoped that they can be told that each parent will continue to love and care for them, but if they cannot be provided with this reassurance, pediatricians can help the involved parent develop strategies to help the child articulate feelings of loss and identify resources to assist the child. The pediatrician can offer families pertinent written material on divorce directed at parents and children (see the reading lists at the end of this report). These resources can be informative for the pediatrician as well. Ideally, children would not be "put in the middle" between divorcing or divorced parents, such as being asked to provide information about 1 parent to the other or when 1 or both parents are seen to be demonizing the other parent. These situations can result in children feeling disloyal to a parent and feeling that they need to choose 1 parent over the other and can result in feelings of guilt, sorrow, and anger. If this is happening, pediatricians need to be comfortable having frank, nonjudgmental, and open discussions with parents and exploring ways to help the family manage these challenges.

Custody options can be discussed, and the parents' plan may be explored. It may be helpful to remind parents that professional help can aid them in a nonbiased evaluation of the situation and approaches to resolution. If there are legal issues, including custody, finding an attorney who considers the child's best interest of highest importance is essential. Legal custody and parental rights and responsibilities can vary in their physical and legal arrangements, from sole 1-parent custody, to various forms of shared arrangements, to equal or joint custody.[3] Varying statutory requirements exist to protect the interests of children.

More important for the child's mental health than the type of custody is the quality of parenting that the child receives from each parent through the divorce and postdivorce periods as well as the child's own resilience. Regardless of the type of custody arrangement, it is important that the pediatrician be informed in writing by both parents of who has legal permission for access to the child's medical record, who is responsible for informed consent, who is to pay for the child's health care, and with whom the pediatrician may discuss health information about the child in accordance with regulations of the Health Insurance Portability and Accountability Act. If the noncustodial parent has legal visiting rights and access to health information, it is important that immunization and other pertinent health records be given to both parents in case of an emergency or urgent situation. Any conflict between parents about these issues should be resolved in accordance with legal custody agreements and may require written authorization by both parents. In an emergency situation, the pediatrician can always act to protect the child. It is a good idea for parents to inform the child's school of the change in

the family structure, request that report cards be sent to both parents, and identify which parent has the authority to grant permission for the child's school-related activities. For additional guidance, pediatricians can refer to the existing American Academy of Pediatrics' clinical report "Consent by Proxy for Nonurgent Pediatric Care."[50]

Long-term Follow-up

Although many children have long-lasting emotional and adjustment problems associated with their parents' divorce, most adjust and function well over time, particularly those who have supportive relationships and are well adjusted before the separation/divorce. Professional counseling may be necessary and has shown to be effective in helping children adjust to divorce and separation.[34,37,38,51,52] It is important that pediatricians recognize that a divorce is a process and not an event; substantive periods of change during the process can demand new adjustments on the part of children and parents. Although the legal divorce is an important issue for parents, it may be insignificant to a younger child who knows little of the legal process or very significant for the older child who experiences further proof that his parents will not reconcile. Among troublesome issues for children may be the parents' dating and sexual activities. Parental discretion and truthfulness are important for the maintenance of respect for the parents. Stepfamilies introduce another adjustment challenge for children and their parents.

As children develop and mature, their emotions, behaviors, and needs with regard to the divorce are likely to change. A custody arrangement that made sense for a younger child may need adjustment for a preadolescent or adolescent. For adolescents, with their advancing maturity, awakening sexuality, and important steps toward their own adulthood, their parents' divorce is reinterpreted and may require rediscussion and readjustment. Many behavioral and emotional reactions from the separation can be reawakened at times of subsequent loss, at anniversaries, with the child's advancing maturity, and with the need to adjust to new and different family structures.[49] Ideally, the pediatrician will be able to maintain a professional relationship with both parents so as to continue to help them care for their children in a comfortable and positive manner.

SUGGESTIONS FOR ASSISTING CHILDREN AND FAMILIES

1. Be alert to warning signs of dysfunctional marriage or coparenting relationships and impending separation. Consider inquiring orally or by written questionnaire about family changes or problems at each visit.

2. Discuss family functioning in anticipatory guidance and offer advice pertinent to divorce, as appropriate. Remind parents that what they do during and after a divorce is very important in terms of their child's adjustment.

3. Always be the child's advocate, offering support and age-appropriate advice to the child and parents regarding reactions to divorce, especially guilt, anger, sadness, and perceived loss of love. The child needs to be reassured that he or she did not cause the separation and cannot solve the problem.

4. Establish clear boundaries around divorce and define what role a pediatrician can play in divorce. Try to maintain positive relationships with both parents by not taking sides with 1 parent or the other. If there is concern for an ongoing or future abusive or neglectful situation, referral to child protective services is

indicated. If a pediatrician is uncertain whether his or her statutory obligation to report has been met, discussion of the case-specific situation with a child-abuse pediatrician may be prudent. Encourage open discussion about separation and divorce with and between parents, emphasizing ways to help the child adjust to the situation and identifying appropriate reading materials.

5. Refer families to mental health and child-oriented resources with expertise in divorce if necessary.

READINGS FOR PARENTS

1. Barnes RG. *You're Not My Daddy: Winning the Heart of Your Stepchild*. Grand Rapids, MI: Zondervan Publishing House; 1997

2. Benedek EP, Brown CF. *How to Help Your Child Overcome Your Divorce*. Washington, DC: American Psychiatric Press; 1995

3. Davis RF, Borns NF. *Solo Dad Survival Guide: Raising Your Kids on Your Own*. Chicago, IL: Contemporary Books; 1999

4. Engber A, Klungness L. *The Complete Single Mother: Reassuring Answers to Your Most Challenging Concerns*. Holbrook, MA: Adams Media; 2000

5. Ricci I. *Mom's House, Dad's House: A Complete Guide for Parents Who Are Separated, Divorced or Remarried*. New York, NY: Simon & Schuster; 1997

6. Stahl PM. *Parenting After Divorce: Resolving Conflicts*. Atascadera, CA: Impact Publishers; 2007

7. Stoner KE. *Divorce Without Court*. Berkeley, CA: Nolo, Inc; 2006

8. Teyber E. *Helping Children Cope With Divorce*. New York, NY: John Wiley & Sons; 2001

9. Zero to Three. *Talking to Very Young Children About Divorce*. Washington, DC: Zero to Three; 2012. Available at: http://main.zerotothree.org/site/DocServer/ONE_PAGE_FINAL_5-14-12.pdf?docID=13461

10. Emery RE. *The Truth About Children and Divorce*. New York, NY: Viking-Penguin; 2004

11. Long N, Forehand R. *Making Divorce Easier on Your Children*. New York, NY: McGraw Hill; 2002

READINGS FOR CHILDREN

1. Blume J. *It's Not the End of the World*. Scarsdale, NY: Bradbury Press; 1972

2. Cole J. *How Do I Feel About My Parents' Divorce?* Brookfield, CT: The Millbrook Press; 1998

3. Holyoke N. *A Smart Girl's Guide to Her Parents' Divorce*. Middleton, WI: American Girl Publishing Co; 2009

4. Lindsay JW. *Do I Have A Daddy?* Buena Park, CA: Morning Glory Express; 2000

5. Rogers F. *Let's Talk About It: Divorce*. New York, NY: G.P. Putnam Sons; 1996

6. Rogers F. *Let's Talk About It: Step Families*. New York, NY: G.P. Putnam Sons; 1997

LEAD AUTHORS

George J. Cohen, MD, FAAP
Carol C. Weitzman, MD, FAAP

COMMITTEE ON PSYCHOSOCIAL ASPECTS OF CHILD AND FAMILY HEALTH, 2015–2016

Michael Yogman, MD, FAAP, Chairperson
Nerissa Bauer, MD, MPH, FAAP
Thresia B. Gambon, MD, FAAP
Arthur Lavin, MD, FAAP
Keith M. Lemmon, MD, FAAP
Gerri Mattson, MD, FAAP

Jason Richard Rafferty, MD
Lawrence Sagin Wissow, MD, MPH, FAAP

LIAISONS

Sharon Berry, PhD, LP – *Society of Pediatric Psychology*
Terry Carmichael, MSW – *National Association of Social Workers*
Ed Christophersen, PhD, FAAP – *Society of Pediatric Psychology*
Norah Johnson, PhD, RN, CPNP-BC – *National Association of Pediatric Nurse Practitioners*
Leonard Read Sulik, MD, FAAP – *American Academy of Child and Adolescent Psychiatry*

CONSULTANT

George J. Cohen, MD, FAAP

STAFF

Stephanie Domain, MS

SECTION ON DEVELOPMENTAL AND BEHAVIORAL PEDIATRICS EXECUTIVE COMMITTEE, 2015–2016

Nathan J. Blum, MD, FAAP, Chairperson
Michelle M. Macias, MD, FAAP, Immediate Past Chairperson
Nerissa S. Bauer, MD, MPH, FAAP
Carolyn Bridgemohan, MD, FAAP
Edward Goldson, MD, FAAP
Laura J. McGuinn, MD, FAAP
Peter J. Smith, MD, MA, FAAP
Carol C. Weitzman, MD, FAAP
Stephen H. Contompasis, MD, FAAP, Web site Editor
Damon R. Korb, MD, FAAP, Discussion Board Moderator
Michael I. Reiff, MD, FAAP, Newsletter Editor
Robert G. Voigt, MD, FAAP, Program Chairperson

LIAISONS

Pamela C. High, MD, MS, FAAP – *Society for Developmental and Behavioral Pediatrics*
Beth Ellen Davis, MD, MPH, FAAP – *Council on Children With Disabilities*

STAFF

Linda Paul, MPH

REFERENCES

1. Kleinsorge C, Covitz LM. Impact of divorce on children: developmental considerations. *Pediatr Rev.* 2012;33(4):147–154; quiz: 154–155
2. Urbano RC, Hodapp RM. Divorce in families of children with Down syndrome: a population-based study. *Am J Ment Retard.* 2007;112(4):261–274
3. Cohen GJ; American Academy of Pediatrics Committee on Psychosocial Aspects of Child and Family Health. Helping children and families deal with divorce and separation. *Pediatrics.* 2002;110(5):1019–1023
4. Darnall D. The psychosocial treatment of parental alienation. *Child Adolesc Psychiatr Clin N Am.* 2011;20(3):479–494
5. Lansford JE. Parental divorce and children's adjustment. *Perspect Psychol Sci.* 2009;4(2):140–152
6. Wallerstein JS, Kelly JB. The effects of parental divorce: experiences of the preschool child. *J Am Acad Child Psychiatry.* 1975;14(4):600–616
7. Wallerstein JS, Kelly JB. The effects of parental divorce: experiences of the child in later latency. *Am J Orthopsychiatry.* 1976;46(2):256–269
8. Clarke-Stewart KA, Vandell DL, McCartney K, Owen MT, Booth C. Effects of parental separation and divorce on very young children. *J Fam Psychol.* 2000;14(2):304–326
9. Clarke-Stewart KA, Brentano C. *Divorce: Causes and Consequences.* New Haven, CT: Yale University Press; 2006
10. Mrazek D, Garrison W. *A to Z Guide to Your Child's Behavior.* New York, NY: Putnam Publishing Group; 1993
11. Canada Department of Justice, Research and Statistics Division. The effects of divorce on children: a selected literature review. Ottawa, Canada: Canada Department of Justice; 1997. Available at: www.justice.gc.ca/eng/rp-pr/fl-lf/divorce/wd98_2-dt98_2/wd98_2.pdf. Accessed June 17, 2015
12. Sentse M, Ormel J, Veenstra R, Verhulst FC, Oldehinkel AJ. Child temperament moderates the impact of parental separation on adolescent mental health: The Trails Study. *J Fam Psychol.* 2011;25(1):97–106
13. Hayatbakhsh MR, Najman JM, Jamrozik K, Mamun AA, Williams GM, Alati R. Changes in maternal marital status are associated with young adults' cannabis use: evidence from a 21-year follow-up of a birth cohort. *Int J Epidemiol.* 2006;35(3):673–679
14. Ang RP, Ooi YP. Impact of gender and parents' marital status on adolescents' suicidal ideation. *Int J Soc Psychiatry.* 2004;50(4):351–360
15. Lizardi D, Thompson RG, Keyes K, Hasin D. Parental divorce, parental depression, and gender differences in adult offspring suicide attempt. *J Nerv Ment Dis.* 2009;197(12):899–904
16. Braver SL, Ellman IM, Fabricius WV. Relocation of children after divorce and children's best interests: new evidence and legal considerations. *J Fam Psychol.* 2003;17(2):206–219
17. Pruett MK, Williams TY, Insabella G, Little TD. Family and legal indicators of child adjustment to divorce among families with young children. *J Fam Psychol.* 2003;17(2):169–180
18. Baum N. Divorce process variables and the co-parental relationship and parental role fulfillment of divorced parents. *Fam Process.* 2003;42(1):117–131
19. Fabricius WV, Luecken LJ. Postdivorce living arrangements, parent conflict, and long-term physical health correlates for children of divorce. *J Fam Psychol.* 2007;21(2):195–205
20. Hetherington EM, Stanley-Hagan M. The adjustment of children with divorced parents: a risk and resiliency perspective. *J Child Psychol Psychiatry.* 1999;40(1):129–140
21. Kruk E. Parental and social institutional responsibilities to children's needs in the divorce transition: fathers' perspectives. *J Mens Stud.* 2010;18(2):159–178
22. Blackwell DL. Family structure and children's health in the United States: findings from the National Health Interview Survey, 2001-2007. *Vital Health Stat 10.* 2010; (246):1–166
23. Vélez CE, Wolchik SA, Tein JY, Sandler I. Protecting children from the consequences of divorce: a longitudinal study of the effects of parenting on children's coping processes. *Child Dev.* 2011;82(1):244–257
24. Kamp Dush CM, Kotila LE, Schoppe-Sullivan SJ. Predictors of supportive coparenting after relationship dissolution among at-risk parents. *J Fam Psychol.* 2011;25(3):356–365
25. Lerman R. The impact of the changing US family structure on child poverty and income inequality. *Economica.* 1996;63(250 suppl):119–139

26. Elliot DB, Simmons T. *Marital Events of Americans 2009. The American Community Survey Reports*. Washington, DC: US Census Bureau; 2011

27. Afifi TO, Boman J, Fleisher W, Sareen J. The relationship between child abuse, parental divorce, and lifetime mental disorders and suicidality in a nationally representative adult sample. *Child Abuse Negl.* 2009;33(3):139–147

28. Burns A, Dunlop R. Parental marital quality and family conflict: longitudinal effects on adolescents from divorcing and non-divorcing families. *J Divorce Remarriage.* 2002;37(1–2):57–74

29. Andre K, Baker AJL. Working with alienated children and their targeted parents; suggestions for sound practices for mental health professionals. *Ann Am Psychother Assoc.* 2008;11:10–17

30. Hogan PF, Seifert RF. Marriage and the military: evidence that those who serve marry earlier and divorce earlier. *Armed Forces Soc.* 2010;36(3):420–438

31. Karney BR, Crown JA. *Families Under Stress: An Assessment of Data, Theory, and Research on Marriage and Divorce in the Military. MG-599-OSD.* Arlington, VA: Rand Corporation; 2007. http://www.rand.org/pubs/monographs/MG599.html.http://www.rand.org/pubs/monographs/MG599.html. Accessed June 17, 2015

32. Elrod LD. National and international momentum builds for more child focus in relocation disputes. *Fam Law Q.* 2010;44(3):341–374

33. Schaefer T. Saving children or blaming parents? Lessons from mandated parenting classes. *Columbia J Gend Law.* 2010;19(2):491–537

34. Lux JG. Growing pains that cannot be ignored: automatic reevaluation

of custody arrangements at child's adolescence. *Fam Law Q.* 2010;44(3):445–468

35. Taylor N, Freeman M. International research on relocation: past, present and future. *Fam Law Q.* 2010;44(3):317–339

36. Committee on Medical Liability and Risk Management. Policy statement: expert witness participation in civil and criminal proceedings. *Pediatrics.* 2009;124(1):428–438

37. Legal Information Institute. Article VII. Opinions and Expert Testimony. Rule 703: Bases of an Expert. Available at: www.law.cornell.edu/rules/fre/rule_703. Accessed June 17, 2015

38. *State v Wakisaka*, 78 P3d 317, 333 (2003)

39. Chadwick DL, Krous HF. Irresponsible testimony by medical experts in cases involving the physical abuse and neglect of children. *Child Maltreat.* 1997;2(4):313–321

40. Silverstein & Ostovitz LLC. Same-sex parents' standing in Maryland custody determination. Available at: http://mddivorce.com/2013/08/28/same-sex-parents-standing-in-maryland-custody-determinations.html. Accessed July 26, 2015

41. Melnyk BM, Alpert-Gillis LJ. Coping with marital separation: smoothing the transition for parents and children. *J Pediatr Health Care.* 1997;11(4):165–174

42. Hagan J, Shaw J, Duncan P, eds. *Bright Futures: Guidelines for Health Supervision of Infants, Children, and Adolescents.* 3rd ed. Elk Grove Village, IL: American Academy of Pediatrics; 2008

43. Amato P, Doruis C. Fathers, children, and divorce. In: Lamb M, ed. *The Role*

of the Father in Child Development. Hoboken, NJ: John Wiley & Sons; 2010:177–200

44. Delaney SE. Divorce mediation and children's adjustment to parental divorce. *Pediatr Nurs.* 1995;21(5):434–437

45. Pruett KD, Pruett MK. "Only God decides": young children's perceptions of divorce and the legal system. *J Am Acad Child Adolesc Psychiatry.* 1999;38(12):1544–1550

46. Emery RE, Laumann-Billings L. Practical and emotional consequences of parental divorce. *Adolesc Med.* 1998;9(2):271–282, vi

47. Wallerstein JS, Johnston JR. Children of divorce: recent findings regarding long-term effects and recent studies of joint and sole custody. *Pediatr Rev.* 1990;11(7):197–204

48. Whiteside MF, Becker BJ. Parental factors and the young child's postdivorce adjustment: a meta-analysis with implications for parenting arrangements. *J Fam Psychol.* 2000;14(1):5–26

49. Wallerstein JS. Children of divorce: the psychological tasks of the child. *Am J Orthopsychiatry.* 1983;53(2):230–243

50. McAbee GN; American Academy of Pediatrics Committee on Medical Liability and Risk Management. Consent by proxy for nonurgent pediatric care. *Pediatrics.* 2010;126(5):1022–1031

51. Allen KR. Ambiguous loss after lesbian couples with children break up: a case for same gender divorce. *Fam Relat.* 2007;56(2):175–183

52. Sammons WA, Lewis J. Helping children survive divorce. *Contemp Pediatr.* 2001;18(3):103–114

Indoor Environmental Control Practices and Asthma Management

• •

- *Clinical Report*

CLINICAL REPORT Guidance for the Clinician in Rendering Pediatric Care

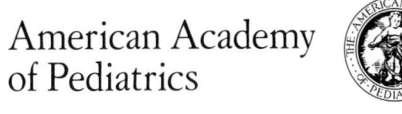

American Academy
of Pediatrics

DEDICATED TO THE HEALTH OF ALL CHILDREN™

Indoor Environmental Control Practices and Asthma Management

Elizabeth C. Matsui, MD, MHS, FAAP, Stuart L. Abramson, MD, PhD, AE-C, FAAP, Megan T. Sandel, MD, MPH, FAAP, SECTION ON ALLERGY AND IMMUNOLOGY, COUNCIL ON ENVIRONMENTAL HEALTH

abstract

Indoor environmental exposures, particularly allergens and pollutants, are major contributors to asthma morbidity in children; environmental control practices aimed at reducing these exposures are an integral component of asthma management. Some individually tailored environmental control practices that have been shown to reduce asthma symptoms and exacerbations are similar in efficacy and cost to controller medications. As a part of developing tailored strategies regarding environmental control measures, an environmental history can be obtained to evaluate the key indoor environmental exposures that are known to trigger asthma symptoms and exacerbations, including both indoor pollutants and allergens. An environmental history includes questions regarding the presence of pets or pests or evidence of pests in the home, as well as knowledge regarding whether the climatic characteristics in the community favor dust mites. In addition, the history focuses on sources of indoor air pollution, including the presence of smokers who live in the home or care for children and the use of gas stoves and appliances in the home. Serum allergen-specific immunoglobulin E antibody tests can be performed or the patient can be referred for allergy skin testing to identify indoor allergens that are most likely to be clinically relevant. Environmental control strategies are tailored to each potentially relevant indoor exposure and are based on knowledge of the sources and underlying characteristics of the exposure. Strategies include source removal, source control, and mitigation strategies, such as high-efficiency particulate air purifiers and allergen-proof mattress and pillow encasements, as well as education, which can be delivered by primary care pediatricians, allergists, pediatric pulmonologists, other health care workers, or community health workers trained in asthma environmental control and asthma education.

DOI: 10.1542/peds.2016-2589

PEDIATRICS (ISSN Numbers: Print, 0031-4005; Online, 1098-4275).

FINANCIAL DISCLOSURE: The authors have indicated they do not have a financial relationship relevant to this article to disclose.

FUNDING: No external funding.

POTENTIAL CONFLICT OF INTEREST: The authors have indicated they have no potential conflicts of interest to disclose.

To cite: Matsui EC, Abramson SL, Sandel MT, AAP SECTION ON ALLERGY AND IMMUNOLOGY AAP COUNCIL ON ENVIRONMENTAL HEALTH. Indoor Environmental Control Practices and Asthma Management. *Pediatrics.* 2016;138(5):e20162589

INTRODUCTION

Asthma is one of the most common chronic childhood illnesses, affecting as many as 10% of children across the United States, with prevalence rates as high as 25% in some communities.[1] Self-reported black race, Puerto Rican ethnicity, and poverty are the major risk factors for asthma in US populations.[1] Children with asthma who are sensitized and exposed to indoor allergens, including dust mite,[2] rodent,[3,4] cockroach, and pet allergens,[5,6] have worse asthma control and lung function and greater airway inflammation and morbidity than those who are either not sensitized or not exposed to these allergens. In addition, exposure to common indoor pollutants, including secondhand smoke (SHS)[7] and nitrogen dioxide (NO_2),[8] exacerbates asthma, regardless of the presence of allergic sensitization.

Children may be vulnerable to these environmental exposures for several potential reasons. First, perhaps because of their airway physiology, they may be exposed to larger doses of airborne pollutants.[9-11] Second, it is possible that their exposure to pollutants, chemicals, and/or allergens is greater because of their proximity to the floor, which can be a reservoir for these exposures.[12] It is also noteworthy that most children with asthma who are at least school-aged have evidence of allergic sensitization, so that allergen exposure likely plays a significant role in childhood asthma. However, an estimated 20% of school-aged children with persistent asthma are not atopic,[13-15] and although they are not susceptible to allergen exposure, they are susceptible to pollutants and irritants, as are children with atopic diseases. For all children with asthma, viruses are a major trigger of exacerbations.

The purpose of this report is to raise awareness among pediatricians regarding the need to assess for and implement indoor environmental control practice measures in the management of asthma and, thereof, to provide guidance. The recently published manual *Pediatric Environmental Health*, known as the "Green Book" (third edition, 2012) from the American Academy of Pediatrics (AAP), has 2 chapters devoted to the discussion of topics included in this report: chapter 20, "Air Pollutants, Indoor," and chapter 43, "Asthma."[16] These chapters provide additional reference material that supports a number of findings discussed in this report. There are no contradictions evident between the 2 resources, but the current report includes some updated references and commentary (eg, electronic nicotine delivery systems [e-cigarettes], practice parameters regarding environmental assessment of and exposure reduction to rodent and cockroach allergens, etc).

Environmental control strategies are tailored to each potentially relevant indoor exposure on the basis of knowledge of the patient's allergic sensitivities and relevant indoor exposures. Serum allergen-specific immunoglobulin E (IgE) antibody tests may be performed, or the patient may be referred to a board-certified allergist for allergy skin testing to identify indoor allergens that are most likely to be clinically relevant for a patient who meets National Asthma Education and Prevention Program criteria for persistent asthma, which include patients taking a long-term controller medication as well as patients having symptoms >2 days per week or nocturnal symptoms more than twice per month.[17] Serum IgE testing and allergy skin testing are both appropriate methods of assessing allergic sensitivities; neither is clearly better than the other in identifying clinically important sensitizations,[18] and there is no lower age limit for either of these tests.

For allergic children, an environmental history includes questions regarding the presence of furry pets or pests or evidence of pests in the home. Understanding whether the climatic characteristics of a community favor dust mite growth is important for assessing the likelihood that the patient has significant exposure to dust mites. Except for arid climates, exposure to dust mites is an important consideration. For all children, both allergic and nonallergic, the environmental history focuses on nonallergen exposures as well. Allergens only affect a subset of those who are sensitized to the specific allergen(s), whereas irritants affect all children to variable degrees. For pollutants, the history focuses on sources of indoor air pollution, including smokers who live in the home or care for the child and the use of gas stoves and appliances. Household chemicals, such as those found in air fresheners and cleaning agents, also can be respiratory irritants and trigger asthma symptoms.[16] The specific strategies used to target an exposure depend on knowledge about the sources and underlying characteristics of the exposure. Environmental control strategies include source removal (eradication of the allergen source), source control (controlling the population/amount of the allergen source), and mitigation strategies (reducing the amount of allergen in the air, dust, bedding, etc, that is produced by the source), such as using high-efficiency particulate air (HEPA) purifiers and allergen-proof mattress/box spring and pillow encasements. Individually tailored, multifaceted environmental interventions are endorsed by the National Asthma Education and Prevention Program guidelines and may be similar in terms of efficacy to controller medications.[9] Although a multifaceted approach makes intuitive sense and reflects clinical practice, much of the foundational research has focused on single allergens; therefore, each allergen will be discussed individually in this report.

INDOOR ALLERGENS

Dust Mites

The major dust mite allergens are Der f 1 and Der p 1, from the 2 most common house dust mite species, *Dermatophagoides farinae* and *Dermatophagoides pteronyssinus*, respectively. Dust mites, microscopic members of the Arachnid class, are rare in arid environments, because they require moisture to survive; humid environments such as those found in the southeastern United States and along the coasts are most conducive to dust mite growth. In more humid climates, dust mites are found not only in homes but also in public places such as schools.

Dust mite allergen exposure has been repeatedly linked to worse asthma among those who are dust mite sensitized[2]; and many, but not all, studies indicate that effective reduction in dust mite allergen exposure improves asthma in this patient group.[2,19-21] Approximately 30% to 62% of children with persistent asthma are sensitized to dust mite allergens,[2,22,23] and it is this population who are susceptible to the effects of dust mite allergen exposure. Unlike patients who may describe allergic reactions to furry pet exposure, patients who are allergic to dust mites are unable to identify dust mites, which are microscopic, as an allergic trigger. Therefore, the pediatrician can only rely on an understanding of whether the climatic conditions of the community are conducive to dust mite growth. As an alternative, a family can have a home dust sample tested for dust mite content with the use of a commercially available kit, although this test is not currently reimbursed by third-party payers.

Dust mite allergen exposure reduction strategies focus on source removal (ie, killing the dust mites) and/or removal of the allergen. Strategies that have been attempted include measures that target the bed, including frequent washing of all bed linens in hot water and the use of allergen-impermeable mattress and pillow encasements, and measures that target other allergen reservoirs, such as vacuuming, removal of carpet and stuffed toys from the bed, and application of acaricides or allergen-denaturing agents.[24] Applications of acaricides and allergen-denaturing agents are cumbersome and ineffective, sustained reduction in indoor relative humidity is difficult to achieve, and carpet removal is expensive and of unclear benefit.[24] There are also potential risks when applying chemicals to the indoor environment, and although these risks are small when the agents are handled according to instructions, they are an important consideration. More information about the risks of chemical agents, including pesticides, can be found in the AAP publication *Pediatric Environmental Health*.[16] Because the major dust mite allergens are carried on larger particles (>10 µm), they quickly settle to dependent surfaces after disturbance of the reservoir. For this reason, air filtration is not likely to have any meaningful effect on dust mite allergen exposure. Because dust mites feed on shed human skin, which is abundant in the bed, first-line approaches to reduce dust mite allergen exposure include washing of bed linens and the use of allergen-impermeable mattress and pillow encasements, which can be highly effective in reducing dust mite allergen in the bed.

Although the most recent meta-analysis of dust mite interventions concluded that dust mite interventions had no effect on asthma, this meta-analysis included studies whose interventions had little to no effect on dust mite exposure and whose populations may not have been dust mite allergic.[25] In contrast, most of the studies in children who are very likely to have dust mite–driven asthma found that dust mite interventions that resulted in a substantial reduction in dust mite allergen levels had a beneficial clinical effect. For example, of the 15 studies of bedding encasements in dust mite–sensitized children included in the meta-analysis, 14 included assessments of dust mite allergen exposure, and 7 found at least an 80% reduction in dust mite allergen in the active intervention groups. Of these 7 studies, 5 found that the active intervention group had improvements in asthma.[21,24,26–29]

Cat and Dog Allergens

The most common furry pets found in homes are cats and dogs; the major dog allergen is Can f 1 and the major cat allergen is Fel d 1. Exposure to these allergens has been linked to worse asthma among pet-sensitized asthmatics, and approximately 25% to 65% of children with persistent asthma are sensitized to cat or dog allergens.[2,3,22,23] When patients are asked about the presence of a pet in the home (or in other places where the child spends significant time), an affirmative response confirms significant exposure, but the absence of a pet does not ensure that the patient does not have clinically meaningful pet allergen exposure. It is also important to note that a child with clinically relevant pet sensitization may not have acute allergic symptoms with exposure, so that the absence of these symptoms does not rule out a role for the pet in the child's asthma. Although pet allergens are found in higher concentrations in homes with pets, they are ubiquitous and detected in places such as schools, child care centers, and public transportation. Furry animal allergens adhere to clothing, walls, furniture, etc, and, in contrast to dust mite and cockroach allergens, are predominantly carried on smaller particles (<10–20 µm), so they remain airborne for long periods of time. As a result, they are carried on clothing of people who have a cat or dog and are transferred to environments that do not contain a cat or dog. Indirect exposure to pet allergens through this mechanism can also cause asthma symptoms in sensitized children. For example, cat allergen brought into classrooms by students with cats has been linked to worsening of asthma in cat-sensitized classmates with asthma.[5]

Clinically significant reductions in animal allergen levels require source removal, or relocating the pet.[30] Even after removing the pet from the home, it can take several months before significant reductions in allergen levels are observed,[31] so it is important that parents are counseled accordingly. In the only prospective (but nonrandomized) study of pet removal, asthma improved significantly and controller medication needs were reduced substantially in the group who removed the pet but not in the group who kept the pet.[32] Because of the reluctance of patients to give up their pets, there have been several studies examining the efficacy of air filtration in reducing airborne pet allergen levels and improving asthma in sensitized patients.[33–35] Overall, these studies have found that this approach is ineffective at improving asthma outcomes and, at best, only modestly reduces airborne allergen levels. A common patient question is whether certain dog breeds are "hypoallergenic." A recent study found that homes with dogs believed to be hypoallergenic had levels of dog allergen similar to homes with dogs that were not considered to be hypoallergenic.[36] The "Thanksgiving effect" refers to the phenomenon when cat-allergic asthma patients living with, and apparently tolerating, a cat go away to college in the fall and then return home for Thanksgiving and, on reexposure to the cat, develop significant asthma symptoms.[37] Sustained animal

allergen exposure as an attempt at inducing tolerance is unlikely to be effective, but pet removal is quite effective.[32]

Rodents

Rodent allergens have been recognized as a cause of occupational allergy and asthma for many decades but have only recently been recognized as an exacerbator of asthma in rodent-sensitized community populations.[38] Mus m 1, the major mouse allergen, is found primarily on small particles, like other furred animal allergens, so it is readily airborne.[39,40] It is found in virtually all inner-city homes, particularly in the northeastern and Midwestern United States.[41–43] Although 75% to 80% of US homes have detectable mouse allergen, concentrations in inner-city homes are as much as 1000-fold higher than those found in suburban homes.[44,45] A report of any evidence of infestation, particularly from a patient living in an urban neighborhood, suggests that there are clinically significant levels of mouse allergen in the home. However, a report of absence of infestation is not a reassurance that there is not clinically significant exposure when the patient resides in an urban neighborhood. Mouse allergen exposure has repeatedly been linked to an increased risk of a range of markers of uncontrolled and more severe asthma among sensitized children.[3,4,42,43]

A substantial reduction in mouse allergen levels can be achieved with a professionally delivered integrated pest-management intervention that includes trap placement, sealing of holes and cracks that can serve as entry points into the home, and application of rodenticide.[46] It is important to weigh the potential benefits of rodenticide against the potential risks, and a discussion of these risks can be found in *Pediatric Environmental Health*.[16] Although

a minor mouse infestation can be handled without rodenticide, some homes with serious infestation may require a rodenticide; in this circumstance, bait blocks may be associated with the risk of accidental ingestion by children and pets, and families may have greater benefit from professionally applied rodenticide.

Although there has yet to be a study testing the clinical efficacy of intervention on mouse allergen, mouse-sensitized patients who have any evidence of infestation may benefit from integrated pest management, because reducing mouse allergen would be expected to be clinically efficacious. Integrated pest management targets mice and other pests, such as cockroaches, and includes sealing up entry points for pests and removing sources of food, shelter, and water for pests by storing food in chew-proof containers, cleaning up immediately after eating, fixing leaky faucets and pipes, and taking the trash out on a regular basis. For patients living in rental units, families can work with landlords and/or property managers to address the infestation. Patients with mouse sensitization are very likely to be cat sensitized as well, so the acquisition of a cat may not be a prudent approach to mouse infestation. Rat allergen exposure is less common, because it is detected in approximately one-third of inner-city homes; so, although it is associated with worse asthma, a smaller proportion of children are affected by rat allergen exposure than mouse allergen exposure.

Rodents are also kept as pets, and the more common rodent pets are gerbils, guinea pigs, and hamsters. Rabbits and ferrets, which are not rodents, are also common furry pets. Exposure to these animals can contribute to worse asthma among patients who are sensitized.

Cockroach

The most common cockroaches in US inner cities are the German and American cockroaches; the major German cockroach allergens, Bla g 1 and Bla g 2, are the best studied in terms of health effects. Cockroach allergen exposure among sensitized inner-city children with asthma was first linked to asthma morbidity in the National Cooperative Inner-City Asthma Study report published in 1997.[47] Since then, the link with asthma morbidity has been replicated, and highly effective methods based on integrated pest-management principles to reduce cockroach allergen levels have been identified. Pesticides that come in gel form are preferred to aerosolized pesticides, which likely result in greater pesticide exposure.[48,49] Moreover, in a successful multifaceted environmental intervention in inner-city children with asthma, the degree of reduction in cockroach allergen was correlated with the degree of improvement in asthma symptoms, providing support for cockroach allergen environmental control measures, which include integrated pest management, as an integral part of asthma management in cockroach-sensitized children with asthma.[19,50]

Dampness and Mold

Excessive moisture in homes can contribute to asthma through an increase in mold exposure as well as increased cockroach and dust mite allergen. Excessive moisture may be present because of inadequate ventilation or other building problems or because of a flooding event. Mold exposure occurs mainly as spores become aerosolized, and a substantial number of asthma cases may be attributed to dampness and mold exposure.[51] The prevalence of mold sensitization in children with persistent asthma is approximately 50%, and the most common species to which children are sensitized and

exposed are *Alternaria*, *Aspergillus*, *Cladosporium*, and *Penicillium*.[52] Although *Alternaria* and *Aspergillus* are derived from outdoor sources, they are present indoors and may be clinically relevant.[53] The National Survey of Lead and Allergens in Housing found that 56% of homes had levels of some molds above thresholds observed to be associated with asthma symptoms.[54] Children sensitized and exposed to the major indoor molds appear to be at greater risk of asthma exacerbations.[52] Remediation of mold has been shown to reduce symptoms and medication use in several populations, and its effects may not depend on whether the population is sensitized to mold.[55,56]

The evaluation of a patient with persistent asthma includes an assessment of sensitization to the major indoor molds, which can be accomplished with specific IgE testing performed on a blood sample or through referral to a board-certified allergist for skin testing. Air sampling, thermography, moisture meters, environmental history, and direct observation are all useful techniques to identify moisture problems. Although more sophisticated techniques for assessing home dampness and mold exposure are ideal, parental report of dampness, leaks, or mold is helpful and, in a child with sensitization to the major indoor molds, suggests that the parents be counseled to intervene on the home environment (some simple measures are listed in the Supplemental Appendix). A common tool used to assess home mold exposure is air sampling, but it is important to note that molds are ubiquitous, so reports from air sampling are uninterpretable without concomitant indoor and outdoor sampling. More detailed information about dampness and mold can be found in the Institute of Medicine's report *Damp Indoor Spaces and Health*[57] and the World Health

Organization's *Guidelines for Indoor Air Quality: Dampness and Mould*.[58]

INDOOR POLLUTANTS

Particulate Matter and SHS Exposure

Particulate matter (PM) simply means airborne particles, and it is often expressed as either $PM_{2.5}$, which is the portion of PM that is 2.5 μm in diameter or less, or PM_{10}, which is the portion of PM that is 10 μm or less. Both allergic and nonallergic children with asthma are susceptible to the effects of indoor PM and SHS.[59] $PM_{2.5}$, also known as fine PM, penetrates further into the airways than larger-sized particles and is capable of entering the alveoli. Indoor PM is composed partly of outdoor PM but mostly of particles generated indoors by smoking and other activities, such as cooking and sweeping.[60-63] PM exposure is associated with lung inflammation, decreased lung function, and respiratory symptoms in children with asthma, regardless of whether they have allergic sensitization. Other sources of indoor PM include wood-burning stoves, fireplaces, biomass burning, electronic nicotine delivery systems (e-cigarettes),[64] cigar smoke, incense, bus idling outside of school, and other substances that are smoked, such as marijuana.[16]

SHS

Cigarette smoke is a major contributor to indoor PM in US homes, because each half-pack of cigarettes smoked in the home is estimated to contribute 4.0 μg/m³ of PM,[7,60] and approximately 30% of all US children and 40% to 60% of US children in low-income households are exposed to SHS in their homes.[7,65,66] Smoking cessation by close family members and caregivers is the most effective way to reduce or eliminate tobacco smoke exposure. Although tobacco dependence can be a very severe addiction, tobacco-dependence treatment medications approved by the US Food and Drug Administration are very effective in treating tobacco dependence and allowing the tobacco smoker to stop smoking.[67] State-of-the-art approaches to treating tobacco dependence initiate therapy on the basis of severity of the tobacco dependence and adjust therapy to control nicotine withdrawal symptoms. The AAP Section on Tobacco Control recently published documents that address clinical practice policy as well as public policy to protect children from tobacco, nicotine, and tobacco smoke and provided an accompanying technical report to support evidence-based approaches.[68–70]

If tobacco-dependent family members are not ready to stop smoking or initiate tobacco-dependence treatment, smoke-free home and car policies can reduce but not eliminate a child's tobacco smoke exposure. For families who are not willing to consider smoking cessation, starting tobacco-dependence treatment, or keeping the home smoke free, 2 randomized controlled trials suggest that the use of portable HEPA purifiers in the home may be of some benefit[7,71] but would not be as effective as if occupants of the home stopped smoking or instituted a home smoking ban. HEPA purifiers are also costly, so whether the expenditure is worth the benefit will vary depending on the child's clinical picture, progress in smoking cessation or institution of a home smoking ban, and the financial resources available. It is also important to note that homes are not the only indoor spaces where children are exposed to SHS. SHS exposure in public places has been targeted by legislation that bans smoking in public places, and this legislation has been associated with significant decreases in asthma morbidity in children, including asthma hospitalizations.[72]

Portable HEPA Purifiers

The use of portable HEPA purifiers has been shown to reduce indoor PM concentrations by approximately 25% to 50% and to reduce asthma symptoms and exacerbations.[7,71] Portable HEPA purifiers appear to be effective in reducing PM from tobacco and nontobacco smoke sources, but there is little evidence to support their efficacy in reducing airborne animal allergens or pollen. Although HEPA purifiers are expected to be much less effective than the first-line approach of source removal, if they are suggested, nonionizing HEPA purifiers with clean air delivery rates that are appropriate for the size of the room in which they will be used may be most effective. This information is indicated on the air purifier packaging. It is important to note that cigarette smoke also produces nonparticle, gaseous pollutants, such as nicotine and others, and that HEPA purifiers do not appear to have any effect on air nicotine and possibly other gaseous components of tobacco smoke.[7] As a result, HEPA purifiers will not offer any protection from the adverse health effects of these nonparticle components of SHS.

NO_2

NO_2 is a gas that is a byproduct of combustion, so it is found outdoors as a result of traffic and other combustion activities, and affects both allergic and nonallergic children with asthma.[73] It can be found in concentrations associated with adverse health effects in homes, where the most important source is gas heat and appliances.[8,73] In addition, older wood-burning stoves, unvented space heaters, and other sources of combustion can produce NO_2 and other pollutants. Higher indoor NO_2 concentrations have been linked to worse asthma in children with asthma,[8] although 1 study found that only nonatopic children with asthma were affected.[73]

Although data are scant regarding effective interventions for reducing indoor NO_2, ensuring that the stove is properly vented and using the vent while the stove is in use would be expected to reduce indoor NO_2 concentrations. One randomized controlled trial found reductions of 40% to 50% in indoor NO_2 concentrations when a gas stove was replaced with an electric one.[74] Whether this degree of indoor NO_2 reduction results in improvements in asthma remains unclear, however.

ENVIRONMENTAL EVALUATION AND MANAGEMENT FOR THE PEDIATRIC PATIENT WITH ASTHMA

An assessment of environmental triggers and education regarding evidence-based approaches to exposure reduction are an integral part of asthma management in the pediatric patient.[75] Children are vulnerable to the respiratory effects of indoor environmental exposures because of their respiratory physiology and because any pulmonary effects from these exposures may affect their respiratory health in adulthood. An assessment of allergic sensitization to a panel of indoor allergens is useful for determining whether indoor allergens may be clinically relevant for a patient and, if so, for identifying which allergens may be relevant. Allergen-specific IgE tests can be performed at commercial laboratories, so they can be ordered by a primary care provider. Testing to large panels of allergens is not helpful, because there may be many positive results to allergens that are not relevant to the individual patient's environment and history; instead, testing to selected relevant allergens is preferred. The clinical scenario guides which allergens to include in testing; for pediatric patients with persistent asthma, testing to common indoor allergens, including cat, dog, dust mites (if in a nonarid area of the country), and molds, is appropriate. For children living in a community in which pest infestation is common, testing for mouse and cockroach sensitization would also be appropriate. More information about allergy testing can be found in a recent AAP clinical report on the subject.[18] Alternatively, the patient can be referred to an allergist-immunologist for allergy skin testing, interpretation of results, and education of the family about environmental triggers.

In most cases, a careful exposure history, combined with knowledge about the community and allergy testing, is sufficient to identify the major exposures that may be clinically relevant. The history includes asking parents and patients about exposure to pets, dampness, or mold and whether they have seen evidence of pest infestation. Relevant exposures occur at schools, child care centers, cars/transportation, and relatives' homes, so these other locations of potential exposure are included in the environmental history. Understanding whether the patient lives in an area conducive to dust mite growth or to mouse or cockroach infestation is also an important component of determining the potentially relevant allergens for the patient. For pollutants, which are relevant for both allergic and nonallergic children with asthma, the history includes asking parents and patients first about SHS exposure. An additional history elicits the presence of gas heat and/or appliances, because this finding would suggest that the patient may have clinically relevant NO_2 exposure. Because relevant exposures occur in schools and child care centers, it is important to elicit potential relevant exposures that occur in other settings outside of the home. Often, families can work with schools and child care centers to address relevant exposures, and both the Environmental Protection Agency and the Centers for Disease Control and Prevention have online

resources for addressing the school environment (http://www.epa.gov/iaq/schools/managingasthma.html and http://www.cdc.gov/HealthyYouth/asthma/creatingafs/, respectively).

The environmental history and assessment of allergic sensitization will inform a tailored environmental control plan for the patient. It is important to note that environmental interventions that target all relevant exposures are more likely to be successful than those that target only 1 or 2 exposures. For patients sensitized to an allergen, the first-line strategies for targeting indoor exposures discussed previously are likely to result in a reduction in relevant indoor exposures and improvements in asthma. Although the role of allergen-proof mattress and pillow encasements has been debated,[76,77] their efficacy may be greater for children than for adults,[20,21,26-28] and they have been an integral part of successful, individually tailored, multifaceted home environmental interventions.[19] For patients with SHS exposure, helping the smoker obtain effective tobacco-dependence treatment so that he or she can stop smoking is the most effective approach, because it eliminates the source of the tobacco smoke. A home smoking ban can reduce, but does not eliminate, the tobacco smoke exposure. In some cases, the parent may not be able to influence the smoking behavior of household members and may not be able to move to another home. In that situation, the use of portable HEPA purifiers may be better than no intervention. Insurance coverage for air purifiers and other goods and services for environmental control is being reevaluated and may be more widespread in the future. For patients with gas heat and appliances, the first-line environmental control strategies would include ensuring that the gas stove is properly vented and the vent is used when the stove is on.

Because each child has his or her own profile of relevant exposures, it is important that the strategies regarding environmental control be tailored to each patient. In addition, each of the child's exposures affects his or her asthma, so targeting all of the exposures, to the extent possible, is important to achieve the maximal benefit. A sample environmental control plan is provided (Supplemental Appendix), which can be used to indicate the child's allergic status, to provide basic background information about indoor environmental exposures, and to list the environmental control practices that the family can implement to reduce the child's exposure to indoor allergens and irritants that are contributing to the child's asthma.

Although public and private insurers may cover environmental assessments and control measures, most do not, despite evidence of their cost-effectiveness. Public and private resources are available, including legal assistance (such as through medical-legal partnerships; www.medical-legalpartnerships.org), to help primary care pediatricians, asthma and allergy specialists, and patients with environmental remediation efforts pertinent to various residential settings. In some states, Medicaid may cover some components of an environmental intervention, such as a home visit for an environmental assessment and education, which can be delivered by health care workers or community health workers trained in asthma environmental control. It is important to note, however, that insurance coverage differs from state to state and among insurers and is expected to change over time, so it is best to seek information from your AAP Chapter, the AAP Department of Practice, or the Asthma and Allergy Foundation to understand what resources, including insurance coverage, are available to support environmental control goods and services.

KEY POINTS

1. Individually tailored environmental control measures have been shown to reduce asthma symptoms and exacerbations, are similar in efficacy to controller medications, and appear to be cost-effective when the aim is to reduce days of symptoms and their associated costs.[75,78] The efficacy of environmental control measures has been sustained for up to 1 year after the intervention.[19]

2. As a part of developing tailored strategies regarding environmental control measures, an environmental history may be obtained to evaluate the key indoor environmental exposures that are known to trigger asthma symptoms and exacerbations, including both indoor pollutants and allergens.

3. The leading indoor environmental contributors to asthma symptoms are indoor allergens (pets, dust mites, mice, rats, cockroaches, molds) and pollutants (airborne PM, SHS, NO_2).

4. An environmental history may include questions regarding the presence of pets or pests, or evidence of pests in the home, as well as knowledge regarding whether the climatic characteristics in the community favor dust mites. In addition, the history may focus on sources of indoor air pollution, including smokers in the home, use of gas stoves and appliances, and presence of mold in the home.

5. Serum allergen-specific IgE antibody tests may be performed or the patient may be referred to a board-certified allergist for evaluation and allergy skin testing to identify indoor allergens that are most likely to be clinically relevant.

6. Environmental control strategies are tailored to each potentially relevant indoor exposure and are based on knowledge of the sources and underlying characteristics of the exposure. Strategies include source removal, source control, and mitigation strategies.

LEAD AUTHORS

Elizabeth C. Matsui, MD, MHS, FAAP
Stuart L. Abramson, MD, PhD, AE-C, FAAP
Megan T. Sandel, MD, MPH, FAAP

SECTION ON ALLERGY AND IMMUNOLOGY EXECUTIVE COMMITTEE, 2015–2016

Elizabeth C. Matsui, MD, MHS, FAAP, Chair
Stuart L. Abramson, MD, PhD, AE-C, FAAP
Chitra Dinakar, MD, FAAP
Anne-Marie Irani, MD, FAAP
Jennifer S. Kim, MD, FAAP
Todd A. Mahr, MD, FAAP, Immediate Past Chair
Michael Pistiner, MD, FAAP
Julie Wang, MD, FAAP

FORMER EXECUTIVE COMMITTEE MEMBERS

Thomas A. Fleisher, MD, FAAP
Scott H. Sicherer, MD, FAAP
Paul V. Williams, MD, FAAP

STAFF

Debra L. Burrowes, MHA

COUNCIL ON ENVIRONMENTAL HEALTH EXECUTIVE COMMITTEE, 2015–2016

Jennifer A. Lowry, MD, FAAP, Chair
Samantha Ahdoot, MD, FAAP
Carl R. Baum, MD, FAAP
Aaron S. Bernstein, MD, MPH, FAAP
Aparna Bole, MD, FAAP
Heather L. Brumberg, MD, MPH, FAAP
Carla C. Campbell, MD, MS, FAAP
Bruce P. Lanphear, MD, MPH, FAAP
Susan E. Pacheco, MD, FAAP
Adam J. Spanier, MD, PhD, MPH, FAAP
Leonardo Trasande, MD, MPP, FAAP

FORMER EXECUTIVE COMMITTEE MEMBERS

Kevin C. Osterhoudt, MD, MSCE, FAAP
Jerome A. Paulson, MD, FAAP
Megan T. Sandel, MD, MPH, FAAP

LIAISONS

John M. Balbus, MD, MPH – *National Institute of Environmental Health Sciences*
Todd Brubaker, DO – *AAP Section on Medical Students, Residents, and Fellowship Trainees*
Ruth A. Etzel, MD, PhD, FAAP – *US Environmental Protection Agency*
Mary Ellen Mortensen, MD, MS – *Centers for Disease Control and Prevention/National Center for Environmental Health*
Nathaniel G. DeNicola, MD, MSC – *American Congress of Obstetricians and Gynecologists*
Mary H. Ward, PhD – *National Cancer Institute*

STAFF

Paul Spire

ABBREVIATIONS

AAP: American Academy of Pediatrics
HEPA: high-efficiency particulate air
IgE: immunoglobulin E
NO_2: nitrogen dioxide
PM: particulate matter
SHS: secondhand smoke

REFERENCES

1. Keet CA, McCormack MC, Pollack CE, Peng RD, McGowan E, Matsui EC. Neighborhood poverty, urban residence, race/ethnicity, and asthma: rethinking the inner-city asthma epidemic. *J Allergy Clin Immunol.* 2015;135(3):655–662

2. Gruchalla RS, Pongracic J, Plaut M, et al. Inner City Asthma Study: relationships among sensitivity, allergen exposure, and asthma morbidity. *J Allergy Clin Immunol.* 2005;115(3):478–485

3. Ahluwalia SK, Peng RD, Breysse PN, et al Mouse allergen is the major allergen of public health relevance in Baltimore City. *J Allergy Clin Immunol.* 2013;132(4):830–835, e831–e832

4. Torjusen EN, Diette GB, Breysse PN, Curtin-Brosnan J, Aloe C, Matsui EC. Dose-response relationships between mouse allergen exposure and asthma morbidity among urban children and adolescents. *Indoor Air.* 2013;23(4):268–274

5. Almqvist C, Wickman M, Perfetti L, et al. Worsening of asthma in children allergic to cats, after indirect exposure

to cat at school. *Am J Respir Crit Care Med.* 2001;163(3 pt 1):694–698

6. Matsui EC, Sampson HA, Bahnson HT, et al; Inner-city Asthma Consortium. Allergen-specific IgE as a biomarker of exposure plus sensitization in inner-city adolescents with asthma. *Allergy.* 2010;65(11):1414–1422

7. Butz AM, Matsui EC, Breysse P, et al. A randomized trial of air cleaners and a health coach to improve indoor air quality for inner-city children with asthma and secondhand smoke exposure. *Arch Pediatr Adolesc Med.* 2011;165(8):741–748

8. Hansel NN, Breysse PN, McCormack MC, et al. A longitudinal study of indoor nitrogen dioxide levels and respiratory symptoms in inner-city children with asthma. *Environ Health Perspect.* 2008;116(10):1428–1432

9. Bennett WD, Zeman KL. Deposition of fine particles in children spontaneously breathing at rest. *Inhal Toxicol.* 1998;10(9):831–842

10. Bennett WD, Zeman KL, Jarabek AM. Nasal contribution to breathing and fine particle deposition in children versus adults. *J Toxicol Environ Health A.* 2008;71(3):227–237

11. Foos B, Marty M, Schwartz J, et al. Focusing on children's inhalation dosimetry and health effects for risk assessment: an introduction. *J Toxicol Environ Health A.* 2008;71(3):149–165

12. Miller MD, Marty MA, Arcus A, Brown J, Morry D, Sandy M. Differences between children and adults: implications for risk assessment at California EPA. *Int J Toxicol.* 2002;21(5):403–418

13. Childhood Asthma Management Program Research Group. Long-term effects of budesonide or nedocromil in children with asthma. *N Engl J Med.* 2000;343(15):1054–1063

14. Covar RA, Spahn JD, Murphy JR, Szefler SJ; Childhood Asthma Management Program Research Group. Progression of asthma measured by lung function in the childhood asthma management program. *Am J Respir Crit Care Med.* 2004;170(3):234–241

15. Eggleston PA, Rosenstreich D, Lynn H, et al. Relationship of indoor allergen exposure to skin test sensitivity in inner-city children with asthma. *J Allergy Clin Immunol.* 1998;102(4 pt 1):563–570

16. Etzel RA, Balk SJ, eds. *Pediatric Environmental Health.* 3rd ed. Elk Grove Village, IL: American Academy of Pediatrics; 2012

17. National Asthma Education and Prevention Program. Expert Panel Report 3 (EPR-3): guidelines for the diagnosis and management of asthma—summary report 2007. *J Allergy Clin Immunol.* 2007;120(5 suppl):S94–S138

18. Sicherer SH, Wood RA; American Academy of Pediatrics Section on Allergy and Immunology. Allergy testing in childhood: using allergen-specific IgE tests. *Pediatrics.* 2012;129(1):193–197

19. Morgan WJ, Crain EF, Gruchalla RS, et al; Inner-City Asthma Study Group. Results of a home-based environmental intervention among urban children with asthma. *N Engl J Med.* 2004;351(11):1068–1080

20. Carswell F, Birmingham K, Oliver J, Crewes A, Weeks J. The respiratory effects of reduction of mite allergen in the bedrooms of asthmatic children—a double-blind controlled trial. *Clin Exp Allergy.* 1996;26(4):386–396

21. Halken S, Høst A, Niklassen U, et al. Effect of mattress and pillow encasings on children with asthma and house dust mite allergy. *J Allergy Clin Immunol.* 2003;111(1):169–176

22. Weiss ST, Horner A, Shapiro G, Sternberg AL; Childhood Asthma Management Program Research Group. The prevalence of environmental exposure to perceived asthma triggers in children with mild-to-moderate asthma: data from the Childhood Asthma Management Program (CAMP). *J Allergy Clin Immunol.* 2001;107(4):634–640

23. Kattan M, Mitchell H, Eggleston P, et al. Characteristics of inner-city children with asthma: the National Cooperative Inner-City Asthma Study. *Pediatr Pulmonol.* 1997;24(4):253–262

24. Portnoy J, Miller JD, Williams PB, et al; Joint Taskforce on Practice Parameters; Practice Parameter Workgroup. Environmental assessment and exposure control of dust mites: a practice parameter. *Ann Allergy Asthma Immunol.* 2013;111(6):465–507

25. Gøtzsche PC, Johansen HK. House dust mite control measures for asthma. *Cochrane Database Syst Rev.* 2008;2:CD001187

26. Ehnert B, Lau-Schadendorf S, Weber A, Buettner P, Schou C, Wahn U. Reducing domestic exposure to dust mite allergen reduces bronchial hyperreactivity in sensitive children with asthma. *J Allergy Clin Immunol.* 1992;90(1):135–138

27. Rijssenbeek-Nouwens LH, Oosting AJ, de Bruin-Weller MS, Bregman I, de Monchy JG, Postma DS. Clinical evaluation of the effect of anti-allergic mattress covers in patients with moderate to severe asthma and house dust mite allergy: a randomised double blind placebo controlled study. *Thorax.* 2002;57(9):784–790

28. Rijssenbeek-Nouwens LH, Oosting AJ, De Monchy JG, Bregman I, Postma DS, De Bruin-Weller MS. The effect of anti-allergic mattress encasings on house dust mite-induced early- and late-airway reactions in asthmatic patients: a double-blind, placebo-controlled study. *Clin Exp Allergy.* 2002;32(1):117–125

29. Colloff MJ, Ayres J, Carswell F, et al. The control of allergens of dust mites and domestic pets: a position paper. *Clin Exp Allergy.* 1992;22(suppl 2):1–28

30. Portnoy J, Kennedy K, Sublett J, et al. Environmental assessment and exposure control: a practice parameter - furry animals. *Ann Allergy Asthma Immunol.* 2012;108(4):223. e1–223.15

31. Wood RA, Chapman MD, Adkinson NF Jr, Eggleston PA. The effect of cat removal on allergen content in household-dust samples. *J Allergy Clin Immunol.* 1989;83(4):730–734

32. Shirai T, Matsui T, Suzuki K, Chida K. Effect of pet removal on pet allergic asthma. *Chest.* 2005;127(5):1565–1571

33. Wood RA, Johnson EF, Van Natta ML, Chen PH, Eggleston PA. A

placebo-controlled trial of a HEPA air cleaner in the treatment of cat allergy. *Am J Respir Crit Care Med.* 1998;158(1):115–120

34. van der Heide S, van Aalderen WM, Kauffman HF, Dubois AE, de Monchy JG. Clinical effects of air cleaners in homes of asthmatic children sensitized to pet allergens. *J Allergy Clin Immunol.* 1999;104(2 pt 1):447–451

35. Sulser C, Schulz G, Wagner P, et al. Can the use of HEPA cleaners in homes of asthmatic children and adolescents sensitized to cat and dog allergens decrease bronchial hyperresponsiveness and allergen contents in solid dust? *Int Arch Allergy Immunol.* 2009;148(1):23–30

36. Vredegoor DW, Willemse T, Chapman MD, Heederik DJ, Krop EJ. Can f 1 levels in hair and homes of different dog breeds: lack of evidence to describe any dog breed as hypoallergenic. *J Allergy Clin Immunol.* 2012;130(4):904–909, e907

37. Erwin EA, Woodfolk JA, Ronmark E, Perzanowski M, Platts-Mills TAE. The long-term protective effects of domestic animals in the home. *Clin Exp Allergy.* 2011;41(7):920–922

38. Phipatanakul W, Matsui E, Portnoy J, et al; Joint Task Force on Practice Parameters. Environmental assessment and exposure reduction of rodents: a practice parameter. *Ann Allergy Asthma Immunol.* 2012;109(6):375–387

39. Ohman JL Jr, Hagberg K, MacDonald MR, Jones RR Jr, Paigen BJ, Kacergis JB. Distribution of airborne mouse allergen in a major mouse breeding facility. *J Allergy Clin Immunol.* 1994;94(5):810–817

40. Matsui EC, Simons E, Rand C, et al. Airborne mouse allergen in the homes of inner-city children with asthma. *J Allergy Clin Immunol.* 2005;115(2):358–363

41. Phipatanakul W, Eggleston PA, Wright EC, Wood RA. Mouse allergen. I. The prevalence of mouse allergen in inner-city homes. The National Cooperative Inner-City Asthma Study. *J Allergy Clin Immunol.* 2000;106(6):1070–1074

42. Pongracic JA, Visness CM, Gruchalla RS, Evans R III, Mitchell HE. Effect of mouse allergen and rodent environmental intervention on asthma in inner-city children. *Ann Allergy Asthma Immunol.* 2008;101(1):35–41

43. Matsui EC, Eggleston PA, Buckley TJ, et al. Household mouse allergen exposure and asthma morbidity in inner-city preschool children. *Ann Allergy Asthma Immunol.* 2006;97(4):514–520

44. Matsui EC, Wood RA, Rand C, Kanchanaraksa S, Swartz L, Eggleston PA. Mouse allergen exposure and mouse skin test sensitivity in suburban, middle-class children with asthma. *J Allergy Clin Immunol.* 2004;113(5):910–915

45. Cohn RD, Arbes SJ Jr, Yin M, Jaramillo R, Zeldin DC. National prevalence and exposure risk for mouse allergen in US households. *J Allergy Clin Immunol.* 2004;113(6):1167–1171

46. Phipatanakul W, Cronin B, Wood RA, et al. Effect of environmental intervention on mouse allergen levels in homes of inner-city Boston children with asthma. *Ann Allergy Asthma Immunol.* 2004;92(4):420–425

47. Rosenstreich DL, Eggleston P, Kattan M, et al. The role of cockroach allergy and exposure to cockroach allergen in causing morbidity among inner-city children with asthma. *N Engl J Med.* 1997;336(19):1356–1363

48. Arbes SJ Jr, Sever M, Mehta J, et al. Abatement of cockroach allergens (Bla g 1 and Bla g 2) in low-income, urban housing: month 12 continuation results. *J Allergy Clin Immunol.* 2004;113(1):109–114

49. Wood RA, Eggleston PA, Rand C, Nixon WJ, Kanchanaraksa S. Cockroach allergen abatement with extermination and sodium hypochlorite cleaning in inner-city homes. *Ann Allergy Asthma Immunol.* 2001;87(1):60–64

50. Portnoy J, Chew GL, Phipatanakul W, et al Environmental assessment and exposure reduction of cockroaches: a practice parameter. *J Allergy Clin Immunol.* 2013;132(4):802–808, e801–e825

51. Dales R, Liu L, Wheeler AJ, Gilbert NL. Quality of indoor residential air and health. *CMAJ.* 2008;179(2):147–152

52. Pongracic JA, O'Connor GT, Muilenberg ML, et al. Differential effects of outdoor versus indoor fungal spores on asthma morbidity in inner-city children. *J Allergy Clin Immunol.* 2010;125(3):593–599

53. Salo PM, Arbes SJ Jr, Sever M, et al. Exposure to *Alternaria alternata* in US homes is associated with asthma symptoms. *J Allergy Clin Immunol.* 2006;118(4):892–898

54. Salo PM, Arbes SJ Jr, Crockett PW, Thorne PS, Cohn RD, Zeldin DC. Exposure to multiple indoor allergens in US homes and its relationship to asthma. *J Allergy Clin Immunol.* 2008;121(3):678–684, e672

55. Kercsmar CM, Dearborn DG, Schluchter M, et al. Reduction in asthma morbidity in children as a result of home remediation aimed at moisture sources. *Environ Health Perspect.* 2006;114(10):1574–1580

56. Burr ML, Matthews IP, Arthur RA, et al. Effects on patients with asthma of eradicating visible indoor mould: a randomised controlled trial. *Thorax.* 2007;62(9):767–772

57. Institute of Medicine, Board on Health Promotion and Disease Prevention, Committee on Damp Indoor Spaces and Health. *Damp Indoor Spaces and Health.* Washington, DC: National Academies Press; 2004. Available at: www.iom.edu/Reports/2004/Damp-Indoor-Spaces-and-Health.aspx. Accessed January 25, 2016

58. World Health Organization Regional Office for Europe. Guidelines for Indoor Air Quality: Dampness and Mould. Geneva, Switzerland: World Health Organization; 2009. Available at: www.who.int/indoorair/publications/7989289041683/en/. Accessed January 25, 2016

59. McCormack MC, Breysse PN, Matsui EC, et al; Center for Childhood Asthma in the Urban Environment. Indoor particulate matter increases asthma morbidity in children with non-atopic and atopic asthma. *Ann Allergy Asthma Immunol.* 2011;106(4):308–315

60. McCormack MC, Breysse PN, Hansel NN, et al. Common household activities are associated with elevated particulate matter concentrations in bedrooms of inner-city Baltimore pre-school children. *Environ Res.* 2008;106(2):148–155

61. Koenig JQ, Mar TF, Allen RW, et al. Pulmonary effects of indoor- and outdoor-generated particles in children with asthma. *Environ Health Perspect.* 2005;113(4):499–503

62. Delfino RJ, Quintana PJ, Floro J, et al. Association of FEV1 in asthmatic children with personal and microenvironmental exposure to airborne particulate matter. *Environ Health Perspect.* 2004;112(8):932–941

63. Weinmayr G, Romeo E, De Sario M, Weiland SK, Forastiere F. Short-term effects of PM10 and NO2 on respiratory health among children with asthma or asthma-like symptoms: a systematic review and meta-analysis. *Environ Health Perspect.* 2010;118(4):449–457

64. Schober W, Szendrei K, Matzen W, et al. Use of electronic cigarettes (e-cigarettes) impairs indoor air quality and increases FeNO levels of e-cigarette consumers. *Int J Hyg Environ Health.* 2014;217(6):628–637

65. Morkjaroenpong V, Rand CS, Butz AM, et al. Environmental tobacco smoke exposure and nocturnal symptoms among inner-city children with asthma. *J Allergy Clin Immunol.* 2002;110(1):147–153

66. Eggleston PA, Butz A, Rand C, et al. Home environmental intervention in inner-city asthma: a randomized controlled clinical trial. *Ann Allergy Asthma Immunol.* 2005;95(6):518–524

67. 2008 PHS Guideline Update Panel, Liaisons, and Staff. Treating tobacco use and dependence: 2008 update U.S. Public Health Service Clinical Practice Guideline executive summary. *Respir Care.* 2008;53(9):1217–1222

68. Farber HJ, Groner J, Walley S, Nelson K; Section on Tobacco Control. Protecting children from tobacco, nicotine, and tobacco smoke [technical report]. *Pediatrics.* 2015;136(5). Available at: www.pediatrics.org/cgi/content/full/136/5/e1439

69. Farber HJ, Walley SC, Groner JA, Nelson KE; Section on Tobacco Control. Clinical practice policy to protect children from tobacco, nicotine, and tobacco smoke [policy statement]. *Pediatrics.* 2015;136(5):1008–1017

70. Farber HJ, Nelson KE, Groner JA, Walley SC; Section on Tobacco Control. Public policy to protect children from tobacco, nicotine, and tobacco smoke [policy statement]. *Pediatrics.* 2015;136(5):998–1007

71. Lanphear BP, Hornung RW, Khoury J, Yolton K, Lierl M, Kalkbrenner A. Effects of HEPA air cleaners on unscheduled asthma visits and asthma symptoms for children exposed to secondhand tobacco smoke. *Pediatrics.* 2011;127(1):93–101

72. Been JV, Nurmatov U, van Schayck CP, Sheikh A. The impact of smoke-free legislation on fetal, infant and child health: a systematic review and meta-analysis protocol. *BMJ Open.* 2013;3(2):e002261

73. Kattan M, Gergen PJ, Eggleston P, Visness CM, Mitchell HE. Health effects of indoor nitrogen dioxide and passive smoking on urban asthmatic children. *J Allergy Clin Immunol.* 2007;120(3):618–624

74. Paulin LM, Diette GB, Scott M, et al. Home interventions are effective at decreasing indoor nitrogen dioxide concentrations. *Indoor Air.* 2014;24(4):416–424

75. Wu F, Takaro TK. Childhood asthma and environmental interventions. *Environ Health Perspect.* 2007;115(6):971–975

76. Woodcock A, Forster L, Matthews E, et al; Medical Research Council General Practice Research Framework. Control of exposure to mite allergen and allergen-impermeable bed covers for adults with asthma. *N Engl J Med.* 2003;349(3):225–236

77. Platts-Mills TA. Allergen avoidance in the treatment of asthma: problems with the meta-analyses. *J Allergy Clin Immunol.* 2008;122(4):694–696

78. Kattan M, Stearns SC, Crain EF, et al. Cost-effectiveness of a home-based environmental intervention for inner-city children with asthma. *J Allergy Clin Immunol.* 2005;116(5):1058–1063

Infectious Complications With the Use of Biologic Response Modifiers in Infants and Children

- *Clinical Report*

CLINICAL REPORT   Guidance for the Clinician in Rendering Pediatric Care

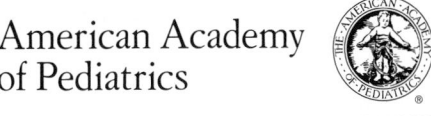

American Academy
of Pediatrics

DEDICATED TO THE HEALTH OF ALL CHILDREN™

Infectious Complications With the Use of Biologic Response Modifiers in Infants and Children

H. Dele Davies, MD, FAAP, COMMITTEE ON INFECTIOUS DISEASES

abstract

Biologic response modifiers (BRMs) are substances that interact with and modify the host immune system. BRMs that dampen the immune system are used to treat conditions such as juvenile idiopathic arthritis, psoriatic arthritis, or inflammatory bowel disease and often in combination with other immunosuppressive agents, such as methotrexate and corticosteroids. Cytokines that are targeted include tumor necrosis factor α; interleukins (ILs) 6, 12, and 23; and the receptors for IL-1α (IL-1A) and IL-1β (IL-1B) as well as other molecules. Although the risk varies with the class of BRM, patients receiving immune-dampening BRMs generally are at increased risk of infection or reactivation with mycobacterial infections (*Mycobacterium tuberculosis* and nontuberculous mycobacteria), some viral (herpes simplex virus, varicella-zoster virus, Epstein-Barr virus, hepatitis B) and fungal (histoplasmosis, coccidioidomycosis) infections, as well as other opportunistic infections. The use of BRMs warrants careful determination of infectious risk on the basis of history (including exposure, residence, and travel and immunization history) and selected baseline screening test results. Routine immunizations should be given at least 2 weeks (inactivated or subunit vaccines) or 4 weeks (live vaccines) before initiation of BRMs whenever feasible, and inactivated influenza vaccine should be given annually. Inactivated and subunit vaccines should be given when needed while taking BRMs, but live vaccines should be avoided unless under special circumstances in consultation with an infectious diseases specialist. If the patient develops a febrile or serious respiratory illness during BRM therapy, consideration should be given to stopping the BRM while actively searching for and treating possible infectious causes.

DOI: 10.1542/peds.2016-1209

PEDIATRICS (ISSN Numbers: Print, 0031-4005; Online, 1098-4275).

Copyright © 2016 by the American Academy of Pediatrics

FINANCIAL DISCLOSURE: The author has indicated he does not have a financial relationship relevant to this article to disclose.

FUNDING: No external funding.

POTENTIAL CONFLICT OF INTEREST: The author has indicated he has no potential conflicts of interest to disclose.

To cite: Davies HD and AAP COMMITTEE ON INFECTIOUS DISEASES. Infectious Complications With the Use of Biologic Response Modifiers in Infants and Children. *Pediatrics.* 2016;138(2):e20161209

INTRODUCTION

Biologic response modifiers (BRMs) refer to substances that interact with the host immune system and modify it. Several BRMs, such as cytokines, chemokines, and antibodies, occur naturally in the body and help to protect against infections. Depending on the condition, synthetic BRMs mimicking natural cytokines or inhibitors, including humanized monoclonal antibodies against a cytokine or its receptor, have been used in treatment to restore, boost, or dampen the host immune response. The focus of this clinical report is on cytokine-inhibiting BRMs that dampen the immune response and treat immune-mediated conditions, such as juvenile idiopathic arthritis (JIA), inflammatory bowel disease, graft-versus-host disease associated with hematopoietic stem cell transplant (HSCT), and scleritis. Cytokines that have been targeted include tumor necrosis factor (TNF) α; interleukins (ILs) 6, 12, and 23; and the receptors for IL-1α (IL-1A) and IL-1β (IL-1B) as well as other molecules described below. These medications are increasingly being used in pediatric populations in combination with other immunosuppressive agents, such as methotrexate and corticosteroids. Although they have been very effective in treating the symptoms of the underlying immune-mediated conditions and lessening disability, the immunosuppressive effect of the cytokine-inhibiting BRMs can persist for weeks to months after the last dose.[1] There is strong evidence of an association of the use of these drugs with an elevated risk of infection with viral and mycobacterial pathogens and weaker evidence for fungal and other intracellular pathogens.[2-4]

This clinical report aims to summarize the infectious disease complications associated with BRMs to guide subspecialists and to familiarize pediatricians, family physicians, and other primary care practitioners who may care for, diagnose, and manage infections in children treated with BRMs. A summary of key points for primary care providers is given in Table 1. It should be noted that experience with the use of BRMs varies by product, with infliximab having the most data available for its use. Data for children are mostly extrapolated from studies in adults,[5-9] with mostly small case series and cohort studies reported,[2,10-15] and thus suggested practices are consensus driven on the basis of knowledge of the impact of BRMs on the immune system. Finally, patients are usually prescribed BRMs in conjunction with other immunosuppressive agents, such as methotrexate and prednisone, which also have immunomodulatory effects that must be considered when the data are being reviewed. In general, the combinations should be considered at least as immunosuppressive as the most immunosuppressive agent in the combination. Table 2 summarizes the BRMs that are currently approved by the US Food and Drug Administration (FDA) along with their mechanisms of action, route of administration, half-lives, and indications. There are also several other products under consideration or in clinical trials. Some currently licensed BRMs are being tested for many new indications, and unlicensed BRMs are also being tested for various indications either as sole agents or in combinations.

FDA-APPROVED BRMS

TNF-α Blockers

Two classes of TNF-α blocking agents are currently used in managing rheumatologic conditions: (1) monoclonal anti-TNF antibodies (includes infliximab [Remicade; Janssen Biotech, Horsham, PA],[21,37-39] adalimumab [Humira; AbbVie, North Chicago, IL],[38,40-43] golimumab [Simponi; Janssen Biotech, Horsham, PA],[24,44,45] and certolizumab pegol

[Cimzia; UCB, Smyrna, GA][25]) and (2) soluble TNF receptors (etanercept [Enbrel; Immunex, Thousand Oaks, CA]).[22,46,47] Infliximab, the first to be licensed in its class, is a chimeric mouse/human protein, and the other monoclonal anti-TNF agents are fully composed of human amino acid sequences. Certolizumab pegol is unique in also being pegylated, which improves its pharmacokinetics and bioavailability.[48] Etanercept is composed of 2 extracellular domains of human TNF-R2 fused to the fragment-crystallizable (Fc) fragment of human immunoglobulin (Ig) G1 (Fig 1).[48]

Non–TNF-α Blockers

The other classes of BRMs consist of monoclonal antibodies and other proteins that antagonize IL-1, IL-6, IL-12, and IL-23 or other molecules, which are important in the inflammatory cascade.

Monoclonal Antibodies

Tocilizumab (Actemra [IL-6]; Genentech, South San Francisco, CA), ustekinumab (Stelara [IL-12 and IL-23]; Janssen Biotech, Horsham, PA), and canakinumab (Ilaris [IL-1B]; Novartis Pharma, Basil, Switzerland) are all humanized monoclonal antibodies against the interleukins noted. Natalizumab (Tysabri, Biogen, Cambridge, MA) is a recombinant human monoclonal antibody against the cell adhesion molecule α-4-integrin, which acts by preventing the adhesion of leukocytes to endothelial cells. Rituximab (Rituxan; Genentech, South San Francisco, CA) is a chimeric monoclonal antibody against the CD20 protein, primarily found on the surface of B cells, which acts by inducing B-cell destruction through mechanisms that could include complement-dependent cytotoxicity, apoptosis, or antibody-dependent cytotoxicity. Belimumab (Benlysta; GlaxoSmithKline, Rockville, MD) is a human IgG1-λ

TABLE 1 Summary of Suggested Screening/Immunizations Before and After BRM Therapy

Suggested screening/immunizations before BRM started
Thorough history
Document previous vaccines, antibody testing when indicated (routine antibody testing not recommended for varicella)
Query about possible exposure and epidemiologic risk factors for histoplasmosis and coccidioidomycosis
Query about history of recurrent HSV
Consider serologic testing for EBV
Screen for past hepatitis B and determine need for vaccine (Table 3)
Routine immunizations
Follow current AAP, Centers for Disease Control and Prevention, and American Academy of Family Physicians guidelines[16,17]
Give recommended vaccines, inactivated, or subunit vaccines 2 weeks before initiation of BRM
Consider safety of giving live vaccine; if appropriate, give 4 weeks before initiating BRM[18]
TB
Test for latent TB and manage based on result (see ref 19 for algorithm)
Suggested screening/immunizations after BRM started
Routine immunizations
May still receive routine inactivated, polysaccharide, recombinant, or subunit vaccine[a]
Give annual inactivated influenza vaccine[18]
Avoid live vaccines, unless under special circumstances with help of infectious diseases specialist[18]
Immunizing immunocompetent household contacts (before or during treatment)?
Follow AAP guidelines for immunizing household contacts of immunocompromised patients[18]
Risk of listeriosis
Avoid unpasteurized milk and milk products, uncooked meats[20]
Febrile or serious respiratory illness during BRM therapy
Consider stopping BRM and actively search for infections including bacterial, mycobacterial, and opportunistic infections
Suggested screening/immunizations after BRM stopped
Routine immunizations
May still receive routine inactivated, polysaccharide, recombinant, or subunit vaccine[a]
Timing of giving live vaccines after stoppage of BRM ± other immunosuppressive agents?
Consult infectious diseases specialist

These are suggestions only. Each situation should be guided by clinical scenario, and the help of an infectious diseases consultant may be sought.

[a] If receiving rituximab, may not respond.

monoclonal antibody against soluble human B lymphocyte stimulator protein (BLyS; also known as BAFF and TNFSF13B). It does not bind B cells directly but blocks the binding of soluble BLyS to its receptors on B cells, thereby inhibiting B-cell survival and differentiation into immunoglobulin-producing plasma cells.[34]

Recombinant IL1 Antagonist

Anakinra (Kineret; Swedish Orphan Biovitrum AB, Stockholm, Sweden) is a recombinant, nonglycosylated human IL-1 receptor (IL-1R) antagonist that blocks the biologic activity of both IL-1A and IL-1B by competitively inhibiting IL-1 binding to the IL-1 type 1 receptor found in a wide range of organs and tissues.

Fusion Proteins

Abatacept (Orencia; Bristol Myers Squibb, Princeton, NJ) and rilonacept (Arcalyst; Regeneron Pharmaceuticals, Tarrytown, NY) are both fusion proteins composed of Fc regions of IgG1 fused with another molecule. Abatacept is a fusion protein of the Fc region of IgG1 fused to the extracellular domain of cytotoxic T-lymphocyte antigen 4. Abatacept has strong affinity and binds to the B7 protein on the antigen-presenting cells, which would normally bind to the CD28 protein on T cells, preventing the antigen-presenting cells from delivering the costimulatory signals needed to fully activate the T cells. Rilonacept (Arcalyst; Regeneron Pharmaceuticals, Tarrytown, NY) is a dimeric fusion protein made of the Fc region of human IgG1 that binds IL-1 linked to the ligand binding domains of the extracellular portions of human IL-1R1 and the IL-1R accessory protein (IL-1RAcP).

Tofacitinib (Xeljanz; Pfizer, New York, NY) is an oral, small-molecule protein kinase inhibitor of the enzyme Janus kinase (JAK) 3 and 1 (JAK3 and JAK1, respectively) that interferes with the JAK-STAT signaling pathway, which transmits extracellular information into the cell nucleus, influencing DNA transcription. Functionally, tofacitinib affects both innate and adaptive immune responses by inhibiting pathogenic T helper (Th) 17 cells and Th-1 and Th-2 cell differentiation (Table 2).[49-52]

INFECTIONS ASSOCIATED WITH THE USE OF BRMS

Overall Rate of Serious Infections

BRM use has been associated with an increased risk of developing certain infections. In addition to the immunosuppressive effects of these agents, concomitant use of other immunosuppressive agents, such as steroids and methotrexate, and the

TABLE 2 FDA-Approved BRMs and Indications

Generic Name (Year[s] FDA Approved for Indications)	Trade Name	Mechanism of Action	Usual Route, Half-life	FDA-Approved Indication[a]
Infliximab (1999, 2009)	Remicade[21]	TNF-α inhibitor (anti–TNF-α chimeric monoclonal IgG1κ antibody)	IV, 7.5–9.5 d	Crohn disease [RA, plaque psoriasis, psoriatic arthritis, ankylosing spondylitis, ulcerative colitis]
Etanercept (1998)	Enbrel[22]	TNF-α inhibitor (soluble TNF-α receptor fusion protein)	SQ, 70–132 h	JIA [RA, plaque psoriasis, psoriatic arthritis, ankylosing spondylitis]
Adalimumab (2002)	Humira[23]	TNF-α inhibitor (anti–TNF-α humanized monoclonal IgG1 antibody)	SQ, 10–20 d	JIA [RA, plaque psoriasis, psoriatic arthritis, ankylosing spondylitis, Crohn disease]
Golimumab (2009)	Simponi[24]	TNF-α inhibitor (anti–TNF-α IgG1κ antibody)	SQ, 7–20 d	[RA, psoriatic arthritis, ankylosing spondylitis]
Certolizumab pegol (2009)	Cimzia[25]	TNF-α inhibitor (PEGylated human Fab antigen binding)	SQ, 14 d	[RA, Crohn disease]
Abatacept (2005, 2009)	Orencia[26]	Anti-CTLA4 selective T-cell costimulation modulator protein (blocks TNF-α, IL-2, and interferon-γ production)	IV or SQ, 8–25 d	JIA [RA]
Anakinra (2001)	Kineret[27]	Recombinant anti-IL-1 receptor antagonist	SQ, 4–6 h	[RA]
Rituximab (2006)	Rituxan[28]	Anti-CD20 therapy	IV, 14–62 d	[RA, non-Hodgkin's lymphoma]
Tocilizumab (2010)	Actemra[29]	Anti-IL-6 humanized monoclonal antibody	IV, 8–14 d	[RA]
Ustekinumab (2013)	Stelara[30]	Anti-IL-12 and IL-23 humanized monoclonal antibody	SQ, 20–24 d	[Psoriatic arthritis, plaque psoriasis]
Canakinumab (2009, 2013)	Ilaris[31,32]	Anti-IL-1B human monoclonal antibody	SQ, 26 d	CAPS, JIA
Natalizumab (2008, 2013)	Tysabri[33]	Humanized anti–integrin α 4 subunit monoclonal antibody (reduces leukocyte adhesion and transmigration)	IV, 11 d	[Crohn disease, multiple sclerosis]
Belimumab (2011)	Benlysta[34]	Human IgG1λ monoclonal antibody against soluble human B lymphocyte stimulator protein	IV, 19 d	[Systemic lupus erythematosus]
Rilonacept (2008, orphan drug)	Arcalyst[35]	IL-1 receptor fusion protein	SQ, 8.6 d	CAPS
Tofacitinib (2012)	Xeljanz[36]	Small molecule protein kinase inhibitor of JAK3 and JAK1	Oral, 3 h	[RA]

CAPS, cryopyrin-associated periodic syndromes (consisting of familial cold autoinflammatory syndrome and Muckle-Wells syndrome); IV, intravenous; SQ, subcutaneous.
[a] For underlined conditions, safety and efficacy have been established in children <18 y; for bracketed indications, safety and efficacy have only been shown in adults. Infliximab, etanercept, and adalimumab have been used off-label for scleritis, but none are FDA approved for this condition.

underlying inflammatory disease likely contribute to increased infectious risk.[47,53,54]

A 2011 Cochrane review examined adverse events identified in randomized controlled trials, controlled clinical trials, and open-label extension studies involving >60 000 participants (primarily adults) receiving 9 BRMs (adalimumab, certolizumab, etanercept, golimumab, infliximab, anakinra, tocilizumab, abatacept, and rituximab) for treatment of either rheumatoid arthritis (RA) or cancer.[55] Serious infections were defined as infections associated with death, hospitalization, and/or use of intravenous antibiotics. The review identified an overall increased risk of serious infections (odds ratio [OR]: 1.37; 95% confidence interval [CI]: 1.04–1.82) among participants receiving BRMs compared with placebo recipients.[55] The drugs most commonly associated with serious infection were certolizumab (OR: 4.75; 95% CI: 1.52–18.5) and anakinra (OR: 4.05; 95% CI: 1.22–16.8). Overall, patients receiving TNF-α inhibitors had a greater risk of developing a serious infection versus patients receiving other BRMs (OR: 1.4; 95% CI: 1.13–1.75). However, patients receiving any

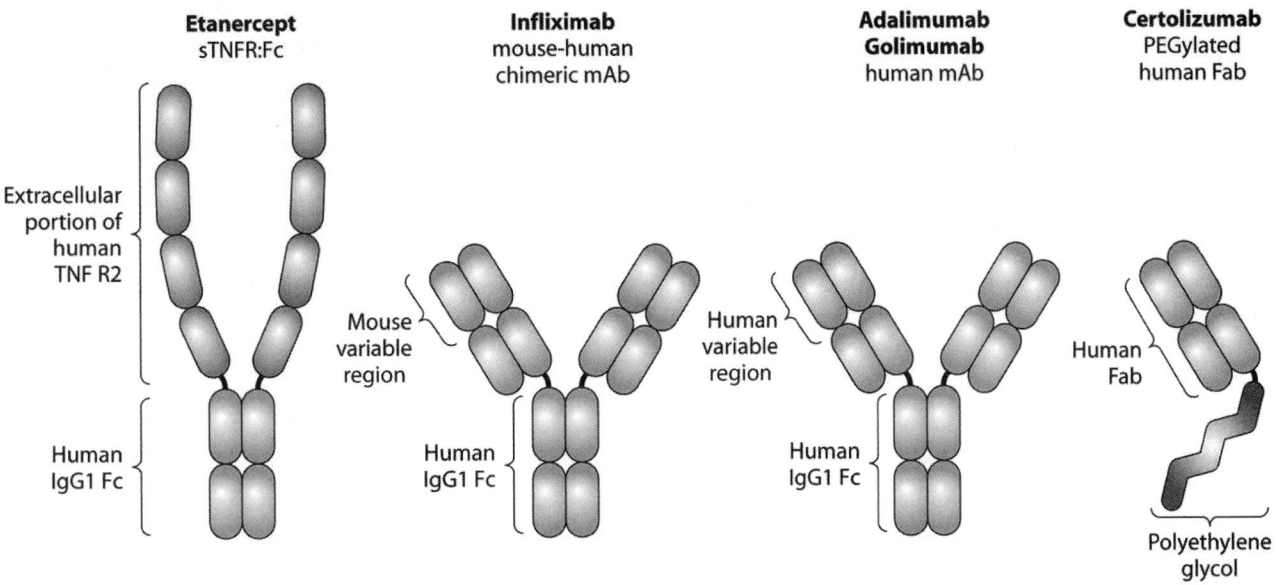

FIGURE 1
Structures of the TNF-α antagonists. (Adapted from Wallis RS. Biologics and infections: lessons from tumor necrosis factor blocking agents. *Infect Dis Clin North Am.* 2011;25(4):896, with permission from Elsevier Limited.) Fab, Fragment antibody binding; mAb, monoclonal antibody; sTNFR, soluble TNF receptor.

of the other BRMs also had an increased overall risk of serious infection when compared with those receiving placebo. There was evidence of an increased risk of reactivation of tuberculosis (TB) among patients receiving BRMs compared with those receiving placebo (see section titled "TB").

Although the risk of serious infections is increased, there is no clear evidence of overall increased risk of bacterial infections, other than mycobacteria, with the use of BRMs. Before the BRM era, the rate of serious bacterial infections requiring hospitalization or parenteral antibiotics in patients with RA (primarily adults) was reported to be between 0.02 and 0.12 per patient-year.[56,57] In contrast, the incidence of infection noted for patients with RA treated with etanercept has ranged from 0.017 to 0.050 per patient-year, a rate that is not significantly different from the general population.[58] One hypothesis would be that even though BRMs temporarily increase the risk of serious infections, their

profound positive effects on the underlying disease counterbalances this effect.

In head-to-head trials, the rates of upper respiratory infections (20%) were similar among recipients of etanercept and control patients with RA.[47] Among studies involving children alone, etanercept has not been shown to increase the risk of serious nonmycobacterial infection compared with etanercept plus conventional disease-modifying antirheumatic drugs (DMARDs) such as methotrexate,[22,46,59–66] with rates ranging from 0.007 to 0.035 per patient-year. Children receiving infliximab[12,31,61,67–70] and adalimumab[38,42,43,64,71] had higher rates of serious nonmycobacterial infections, ranging from 0.027 to 0.086 per patient-year, but there were no data presented to suggest that these rates were higher than those observed for patients receiving DMARDs alone or DMARDs in combination with the BRMs. Infections related to these BRMs were primarily lower respiratory tract and gastrointestinal infections,

sepsis, and abscesses. Although there is no clear increased risk compared with patients receiving DMARDs alone, case reports of sepsis and even death among patients receiving these drugs necessitate caution in instituting therapy in patients who have active infections.

Studies involving children treated with the other classes of BRMs (IL-1 [anakinra], IL-6 [tocilizumab], and T-cell costimulation [abatacept] inhibitors) are limited and generally showed few serious infections. Similarly, infection rates have been low in adult patients treated with ustekinumab, canakinumab, and rilonacept. When infections are identified, they have primarily been viral, gastrointestinal tract, or skin infections. However, there are no data to suggest that the overall incidence of infection is increased compared with the incidence in patients taking DMARDs alone. More studies are needed on the rates of infections for patients receiving these classes of BRMs.

Rituximab-Associated Neutropenia

Rituximab-associated neutropenia is prolonged neutropenia described during or after the completion of therapy, primarily in adult patients being treated for lymphomas.[72-80] The incidence ranges mostly from 0.02% to 6%, although it has been described to be as high as 25% in 1 series and has involved admission to the hospital with fever and neutropenia and sometimes sepsis with bacterial pathogens including *Pseudomonas* species. The duration of the neutropenia has ranged from 4 days to 1 year. The mechanism is unknown, but circulating antibodies against neutrophils were postulated in 1 study.[80] In 1 open-label cohort study in which rituximab was used to treat JIA in 55 children who had failed to respond to infliximab and other DMARDs, 8 serious infections, all lower respiratory tract infections including *Pneumocystis jirovecii* and *Mycoplasma* pneumonia, were identified during a 96-week follow-up period.[81] Of interest, neutropenia occurred in 17 (31%) of these patients between weeks 6 and 28 of treatment. The neutrophil count did not exceed 1500 per μL in 9 (16%) of the patients, was <1000 per μL in 5 (9%) of the patients, and was <500 per μL in 3 (6%) of the patients. All patients were treated with granulocyte-macrophage colony–stimulating factor (5 μg/kg), and no cases of sepsis or febrile neutropenia were described. Not surprisingly given the mechanism of action (anti-CD20 monoclonal antibody), 80% of the patients had a complete depletion of their B cells (CD20+ cells), which remained low throughout the 96 weeks of follow-up, but the level or duration of depletion did not correlate with any specific infection. Eleven (20%) patients also had a reduction in their serum immunoglobulin (IgM and IgG) levels below the age-related lower limits of normal. The most common (mild) infections noted were ear, nose, and throat (14%) as well as skin (11%) infections. Four cases of herpetic infections were also reported among the mild infections.

Specific Infections

TB

Reactivation infections caused by organisms in the *Mycobacterium tuberculosis* complex have been associated with use of TNF inhibitors. TNF-α has been shown in mouse models to contribute to granuloma formation and to induce and maintain latency of TB infection.[82] In contrast, blockage of this cytokine results in failure to control bacillary growth and form protective granulomata.[83-86] In the Cochrane review by Singh et al,[55] the overall OR of TB reactivation was 4.7 (95% CI: 1.2–18.6) among patients receiving BRMs compared with those receiving placebo, with the absolute risk measured at 20 cases per 10 000 compared with 4 per 10 000 patients receiving placebo. However, there were insufficient data in that study to compare risk of TB activation in patients receiving 1 BRM versus another.

In other studies conducted in adults, the risk of TB reactivation appeared to be related to the class of TNF inhibitor. TNF antibodies (eg, infliximab and adalimumab) are associated with the highest risk, whereas soluble TNF receptor antibodies (eg, etanercept) appear to have the lowest risks.[87] One study counted the rates of opportunistic infections associated with infliximab use by analysis of the Adverse Event Reporting System (AERS) of MedWatch, a spontaneous reporting system of the FDA.[4] Although the baseline rate of TB in adults was estimated at 6.2 per 100 000, the rate among the estimated 147 000 patients receiving infliximab was found to range from ~10 per 100 000[88] to 24.4 per 100 000.[4] In contrast, there were many fewer cases of TB reported in relation to etanercept, with 9 cases identified among ~102 000 patients treated in the same database. Similar results were reported by Dixon et al,[89] based on analysis of 10 712 patients treated with anti-TNF BRMs (3913 etanercept, 3295 infliximab, 3504 adalimumab). The rates of TB were much higher in patients receiving either of the monoclonal antibodies (adalimumab: 144 events per 100 000 person-years; infliximab: 136 per 100 000 person-years) versus those taking etanercept (39 per 100 000 person-years). Other data suggest that adalimumab is associated with TB in patients with RA in a dose-related manner, with higher doses associated with greater risk.[90]

Although the risk appears to be lower with etanercept, since its approval many cases of TB have been described among patients receiving the drug. The estimated incidence noted in studies of 10 to 14.3 cases per 100 000 etanercept-treated patients is more than the Centers for Disease Control and Prevention–estimated rate of TB in the general US population of 6.2 per 100 000.[88,90,91] Most cases have localized disease, although disseminated infections have been reported. Other cohort[92] and case-control[93,94] studies noted rates of 6 to 39 cases of TB for etanercept, compared with 71 to 100 cases for infliximab and adalimumab per 100 000 patient-years.

Risk of Extrapulmonary and Disseminated TB Of note is the significant increase in the incidence of extrapulmonary and disseminated disease among the TB cases detected in adult patients receiving BRMs, with many cases requiring an invasive procedure for diagnosis.[95] For example, in the Keane et al study,[4] 56% of patients receiving infliximab who developed TB had extrapulmonary TB, and 24% had disseminated disease, compared with an expected background rate of 18% and 2%, respectively, in patients with non–HIV-related TB. Similarly, in the study by Dixon et al,[89] 62% of all cases were extrapulmonary TB, with 28% with disseminated disease. A high proportion of patients do not develop granulomas, which is consistent with diminished host response against the mycobacteria. In general, the median time to presentation is fastest with infliximab (12 weeks) versus adalimumab (30 weeks) and etanercept (46 weeks), suggesting different pharmacokinetics or pharmacodynamics or different levels of modulation of the immune system for each medication.[94]

Although there are fewer data available in children, the increased risk of TB reactivation with infliximab and etanercept has been corroborated in several case reports[88,96,97] and at least 1 randomized controlled trial.[31,68] However, it is important to note that the risk of TB reactivation associated with the underlying autoimmune/inflammatory conditions alone without medications has been estimated to be twice the baseline rate for the normal population.[98]

Screening to Reduce TB Infections During BRM Therapy There is fair evidence that screening for TB and treating before starting BRMs substantially reduces the risk of TB reactivation. In a small case series, 36 children from Turkey with JIA were treated with etanercept for a median duration of 11.5 months after careful screening with the use of chest radiography, tuberculin skin test (TST), clinical histories, family screening, and physical examination.[99] It was noted that Turkey has a moderate baseline prevalence of TB of 27 per 100 000 population. Patients with TST results of >10 mm who had received bacille

Calmette-Guérin (BCG) vaccine or those suspected of having latent TB for other reasons underwent computed tomography of the chest and/or had cultures performed if specimens were available. Those identified as having only latent TB (no evidence of abnormalities on computed tomography and/or sputum specimens) received 4 to 8 weeks of "treatment doses" of isoniazid followed by 9 months of "lower prophylactic doses." The investigators did not indicate the actual doses used for either isoniazid treatment or prophylaxis, and North American authorities do not normally make a distinction between prophylaxis and treatment doses. Treatment with etanercept was started only during the "prophylaxis stage" of the treatment in 7 of the 36 children meeting the criteria, and none of the 36 developed active TB. Similarly, among 2210 adult patients with different rheumatologic conditions who were treated worldwide with golimumab, no cases of TB developed among the 317 who were assessed and treated for latent TB with isoniazid, whereas 5 cases developed in patients not assessed and treated by week 52.[44]

Nontuberculous Mycobacteria

Although *M tuberculosis* has received the most attention, some reports suggest that nontuberculous mycobacteria (NTM) may be twice as common as TB in adult patients receiving BRMs.[100-102] With the use of the FDA MedWatch database, 239 patients with NTM were identified among patients taking BRMs.[102] Although pulmonary disease was most common (56%), a substantial number of presentations were extrapulmonary (44%), which is similar to the cases seen for patients developing TB while receiving BRMs. Most of the cases occurred during treatment with infliximab (75%), but this

finding may be more indicative of the overall usage of this agent compared with the others. *Mycobacterium avium* was the organism most commonly isolated. Actual rates of disease could not be calculated from the data presented because the total numbers of patients in the database were not reported. Even though NTM may be common, there is no consensus on baseline screening, because there is no accurate (sensitive and specific) screening test.[102] Furthermore, the treatment of NTM is not as clearly delineated as for TB.

Varicella and Herpes Zoster Infections

Varicella-zoster virus (VZV) infections (primary or reactivated) are a frequently reported complication among patients receiving BRMs. For patients receiving anti–TNF-α BRMs, reactivation of VZV is the most common infection.[2,60,63,103] However, primary VZV infections have also been reported.Varicella.

In a retrospective cohort study of etanercept use among 25 Italian children younger than 4 years treated for a mean period of 23 months, 2 unimmunized patients developed primary VZV infections at 40 and 24 months, respectively,[60] with 1 case being complicated with necrotizing fasciitis. Similarly, Lovell et al[63] described 3 patients (ages 13, 10, and 8 years) with primary VZV among 58 children (ages 4–17 years) enrolled in a North American open-label trial of treatment of JIA with etanercept. Although there was no report of their immunization status, all 3 were antibody negative at the time of diagnosis and seroconverted after infection, suggesting that these were primary wild-type infections. One of these 3 patients' courses was complicated by aseptic meningitis, but all 3 recovered with acyclovir therapy and discontinuation of etanercept. These data support the importance of appropriate varicella immunization and the recognition of exposures in patients taking all BRMs.

Herpes Zoster There is mixed evidence of an increase in zoster infections with the use of BRMs. The data for this evidence are almost exclusively from adult patients. In a large German registry in which 5040 patients receiving anti–TNF-α BRMs or DMARDs were enrolled prospectively to monitor their outcomes, there was a significant increase in the risk of herpes zoster infections in patients treated with monoclonal antibodies (infliximab or adalimumab) but no increase noted for those receiving etanercept or DMARDs.[104] Similarly, Smitten et al,[105] Galloway et al,[106] and Winthrop et al,[107] analyzing large databases in the United States and United Kingdom, found an increased risk of VZV reactivation in patients receiving BRMs compared with those receiving DMARDs alone. In contrast, another study[108] involving the National Data Bank for Rheumatic Diseases did not find an increased risk of zoster for infliximab, etanercept, or adalimumab. Encephalitis and meningitis attributable to herpes simplex virus (HSV) and VZV have also been described in postmarketing surveillance of patients receiving natalizumab.[33]

Herpes Simplex Although uncommon, HSV encephalitis, disseminated cutaneous HSV, and localized disease have been described primarily in case series as a complication of treatment with TNF-α inhibitors.[5,109-113] There is at least 1 case report in which infliximab was successfully used along with valacyclovir prophylaxis in a girl with Crohn disease who had relapsing peribuccal herpes labialis attributable to HSV type 1.[114]

Hepatitis B

There have been reports of an increased risk of hepatitis B reactivation for patients receiving BRMs.[115,116] As expected, the risk is greatest in patients who are hepatitis B surface antigen (HBsAg) positive. However, the presence of hepatitis B core antibody (HBcAb) in HBsAg-negative patients (indicating immunity on the basis of infection rather than vaccine) has been associated with HBV reactivation in some patients up to 2 years after immunosuppression with BRMs.[117] In 1 study involving 257 patients infected with hepatitis B and treated with TNF inhibitors, 39% of patients who were HBsAg positive and 5% of those who were HBcAb positive had reactivation of hepatitis B.[45] Increased risk of reactivation correlates with low levels of hepatitis B surface antibody (HbsAb) for patients taking rituximab or TNF-α antagonists,[115,116] suggesting that reactivation is a direct result of the BRM decreasing antibody levels.

Endemic Mycoses and Other Fungi

Fungal infections (*Aspergillus*,[111,113,118] *Coccidioides*,[119-121] *Histoplasma*, *Cryptococcus*, *Sporothrix*, and *Candida*)[3,5,70,101,111,118,122-124] have been noted, primarily in case reports or series during treatment with BRMs. *Histoplasma* is the most common invasive fungal organism identified[3,122,123] and is especially important to diagnose, because the symptoms, signs, and chest radiography findings are virtually indistinguishable from those of acute TB (cough, fever, chills, night sweats, weight loss, and possible skin or mouth lesions). In at least 1 series, histoplasmosis was diagnosed 3 times more commonly than TB among recipients of BRMs.[101] The presentation of histoplasmosis generally includes fever of unknown origin with disseminated disease in

approximately three-fourths of patients, and pulmonary disease is less common. Because the signs and symptoms are nonspecific, diagnosis is usually more challenging. Furthermore, the case fatality rate of patients with disseminated disease receiving BRMs is very high (50%).[122] Pancytopenia and liver dysfunction are often noted. Antigen detection in urine and serum is most useful for diagnosis, although culture of bone marrow could be considered.

Other fungi are less common. In an observational study of AERS data by Keane et al,[4] although actual incidence rates were not given, there were 12 patients with *P jirovecii* pneumonia (PCP), 7 with histoplasmosis, 6 with aspergillosis, and 7 with severe *Candida* infections in association with infliximab treatment among the cohort of ~147 000 patients treated.

HIV

There have been no studies showing an increased rate of HIV infections among patients receiving BRMs.

Progressive Multifocal Leukoencephalopathy

Progressive multifocal leukoencephalopathy (PML), an opportunistic viral infection of the brain associated with JC virus (a human polyomavirus named after the initials of the first patient in whom it was identified) infection in immunocompromised hosts, has been reported in adult patients receiving natalizumab, either as monotherapy or in conjunction with other immunomodulators or immunosuppressors.[33] Risk factors associated with the development of PML include the duration of therapy, previous use of immunosuppressants, and presence of anti–JC virus antibodies. For this reason, natalizumab is only available through a restricted distribution program that also involves close monitoring known as the TOUCH prescribing program (https://www.touchprogram.com/TTP/).[33]

Other Infections

Other opportunistic-type infections that have been noted (mostly case reports or case series) during treatment with BRMs used alone or with other immunosuppressive agents include viral (cytomegalovirus, Epstein-Barr virus [EBV]),[111] protozoal (*Pneumocystis*),[4,111] and bacterial (*Listeria*[125-127] and *Legionella*[128,129]) during postmarketing surveillance[47] or in national or regional databases. In studies in which EBV or cytomegalovirus viral load was measured or polymerase chain reaction assay was performed before and during infliximab treatment over a period of 6 weeks to 5 years, there was no evidence of viral reactivation.[130,131] In the adult US population older than 60 years, the annual risk of *Listeria* was identified as 43 per 1 000 000 among people receiving anti-TNF regimens versus 13 million in the general population.[127] Similarly, a Spanish registry identified rates of 26.5 per 100 000 patient-years versus 0.34 per 100 000 patient-years in the general population.[126]

P jirovecii colonization has been identified in 16% to 29% of adult patients with systemic autoimmune inflammatory diseases.[132-134] In mouse models, B cells play an antibody-independent role in clearing a murine form of *Pneumocystis* (*Pneumocystis carinii* f sp *muris*) by presenting antigen to CD4 T cells.[135] Rituximab depletes B cells, and there have been reports of an increased risk of PCP in the population of patients receiving this BRM, primarily those patients receiving it for hematologic malignancies.[136] Despite this report, the benefit of using induced

sputum to screen for *P jirovecii* or chemoprophylaxis for PCP in patients receiving rituximab is unclear.[133,137] Although some experts have recommended PCP prophylaxis in the setting of rituximab therapy,[138] there are concerns that the PCP risk is lower than the target of 3.5% for the benefits to outweigh the adverse effects of chemoprophylaxis in non–HIV-infected patients.[139,140] PCP infections have also been identified in 84 patients receiving infliximab identified through the AERS database[141] and in those receiving other BRMs.[142,143] However, virtually all of the patients were also receiving concomitant immunosuppressive agents that included methotrexate, prednisone, azathioprine, 6-mercaptopurine, and cyclosporine. As a result, it is unclear whether there is an increased risk for PCP beyond that attributable to the underlying DMARDs.

INFECTIOUS CONSIDERATIONS FOR PATIENTS BEFORE INITIATION AND WHILE RECEIVING BRMS

General Precautions

The indications for intervening with biologics are often to reverse a serious clinical condition. Thus, deferring BRMs to provide protection against vaccine-preventable diseases often involves trading risks. Although, at times, it is clearly appropriate to defer BRMs so the patient can receive an immunization, it may not always be the case, and deferral of BRMs should generally be undertaken in consultation with the relevant specialist managing the patient (eg, rheumatologist, gastroenterologist, dermatologist). However, some basic principles can be applied to reduce the risk of serious infections for patients taking BRMs. All patients with a newly diagnosed rheumatologic or immune-mediated condition, including Crohn disease and graft-versus-host disease after HSCT should be considered

as a current or future candidate for a BRM and should be screened for potential opportunistic infections at the time of diagnosis before initiation of any immunosuppressive agents. Although the guidelines in this statement are applicable, patients with HSCT with or without graft-versus-host disease generally need to have several other considerations before and after their transplantation that are beyond the scope of this statement, and consultation with an infectious diseases specialist is warranted. These agents should not be given to any patients while they have clinically significant acute infections. Furthermore, restraint should be shown in prescribing BRMs to children who are being treated for chronic infections, those with a history of recurrent infections, or those with conditions (including HIV infection) that predispose them to such infections.[89] For such children, it is prudent to involve an infectious diseases specialist to help guide and advocate that all risks are assessed and that appropriate screening tests before treatment and monitoring during and after treatment occur. Risks associated with potential opportunistic infections that are endemic in the area of residence (eg, histoplasmosis, coccidioidomycosis, etc) should be thoroughly considered before starting a BRM. Part of the consideration for such children will include the determination of underlying previous exposure to the infectious agent and associated risk of reactivation or infection during treatment with the BRM. If a decision is made to treat such children with a BRM, close monitoring will be required, ideally in conjunction with an infectious diseases specialist. Special consideration should always be given to the risk of TB. The development of symptoms suggestive of an opportunistic infection should lead to immediate cessation of the BRM pending confirmation of the infection, appropriate management of the infection, and resolution of symptoms. Serum neutrophil counts should be monitored regularly (weekly) in patients receiving rituximab, and episodes of recurrent ear, nose, or throat infections in these patients should lead to measurement of serum immunoglobulin concentrations.

Screening for and Facilitating Adequacy of Immunizations

Immunization Before a BRM Is Started

Immunizations of children about to receive a BRM should follow the current recommendations of the American Academy of Pediatrics (AAP), Centers for Disease Control and Prevention, and American Academy of Family Physicians for persons 0 through 18 years of age[16] (available at: http://aapredbook.aappublications. org/site/resources/IZSchedule. pdf[144]). Before the initiation of BRM therapy, a thorough history should be taken for documentation of previous receipt of appropriate inactivated and live vaccines or history of having had the disease, with testing for specific antibody concentrations where documentation is inadequate. For varicella, if there is a reported history of vaccination but not confirmed by documentation, serologic testing is not indicated and vaccination is recommended if there is sufficient time to safely administer it (4 weeks minimum) before initiating the BRM (Table 2).

All recommended inactivated vaccines should be given at least 2 weeks before the initiation of BRMs to enhance immunogenicity. Live vaccines (rotavirus, live-attenuated influenza, varicella, measles, mumps, and rubella) should be given a minimum of 4 weeks in advance of beginning BRMs. The measles-mumps-rubella (MMR) vaccine can be given on the same day as a TST is administered. If the MMR vaccine is given before administering the TST, the latter should be delayed for 4 to 6 weeks because of temporary suppression of the TST test by the MMR vaccine.[145] Inactivated vaccines, polysaccharide vaccines, and recombinant or subunit vaccines and toxoids do not interfere with TST interpretation. The determination of which vaccines are safe to give for patients receiving steroids should be made in concert with an infectious diseases specialist. The Committee on Infectious Diseases of the AAP recommends that children who have diseases such as systemic lupus erythematosus, which are, in themselves, considered to be suppressive of the immune system, and/or who are receiving immunosuppressive medications other than corticosteroids and who are receiving systemic or locally administered corticosteroids should not be given live-virus vaccines except in special circumstances.[18] Patients receiving higher doses of steroids ($\geq$2 mg/kg per day of prednisone or its equivalent or $\geq$20 mg/day for $\geq$14 days for those weighing >10 kg) should not receive any live-virus vaccines until corticosteroid therapy has been discontinued for at least 1 month.[18]

Immunization After a BRM Is Started

If the patient is already receiving a BRM, he or she may still receive any inactivated, polysaccharide, recombinant, or subunit vaccine that is due. There is evidence that adult patients receiving BRM therapy develop a diminished but adequate response to such vaccines, including the annual inactivated influenza immunizations.[146-149] A possible exception to this may be if the child is receiving rituximab, which has been shown to significantly impair antibody response, especially to pneumococcal vaccines.[150-154] These impairments may persist for up to 6 months after the discontinuation of rituximab and highlight the importance of immunizing such patients who are to receive this or other BRMs before they begin BRM therapy. Where there is a test available for a known antibody correlate of protection in patients who are immunized while receiving a BRM, specific postimmunization serum antibody titers can be measured 4 to 6 weeks after immunization to assess immune response and to guide further immunization and management of future exposures.[18] All children receiving BRMs should receive annual immunization with inactivated influenza vaccine. Live vaccines, including the live-attenuated influenza vaccines, should not be given to any patients receiving BRMs or other immunosuppressive drugs during treatment because of the risk of dissemination and adverse outcomes, except in special circumstances as recommended by an infectious diseases specialist.[18]

Immunization After a BRM is Stopped

Because patients receiving BRMs may have prolonged periods of immunosuppression after the discontinuation of the agent, there are currently no clear data to guide how soon a live vaccine may be administered, and studies of duration of suppression are needed.[18] Any consideration for giving a live vaccine after the cessation of a BRM should be made in consultation with an infectious diseases specialist.

Immunizing Immunocompetent Household Contacts of Patients Receiving BRMs

The immunization history of household members of patients receiving BRMs should also be assessed, because they may pose a risk of transmitting vaccine-preventable conditions. Household members should all be up to date with the recommended inactivated vaccines. The principles of vaccination of household contacts of patients receiving BRMs should follow the same principles recommended by the AAP for household contacts of immunocompromised patients.[18] All household contacts aged ≥6 months should also receive influenza immunization annually.[18] With regard to live vaccines, oral polio vaccine (no longer given in the United States) should not be administered to household contacts of persons receiving BRMs. However, susceptible household contacts can and should receive both MMR and rotavirus vaccines, because the vaccine-strain viruses are rarely transmitted. Similarly, varicella vaccine should be given to susceptible household contacts, because vaccine-strain virus is also rarely transmitted. In the event a household contact of a patient receiving a BRM who is thought to be susceptible to VZV develops a vesicular rash after receiving the varicella vaccine, efforts should be made to separate him or her from the person receiving a BRM for the duration of the rash. However, because the risk of transmission of the vaccine strain is very low and disease associated with the virus is expected to be mild, VariZIG (varicella-zoster immune globulin) is not indicated if contact does occur. For further guidance on immunizing parents and other household contacts in the pediatric office setting, including medico-legal, financial, and logistic considerations, please see the AAP's technical report "Immunizing Parents and Other Households Contacts in the Pediatric Office Setting" (http://pediatrics. aappublications.org/content/129/ 1/e247.full; accessed September 10, 2015).

Screening and Treatment Recommendations for TB

As soon as a patient is diagnosed with a rheumatologic or inflammatory/ autoimmune condition for which BRMs may be later needed for treatment, TB screening and appropriate treatment should be initiated[155–157] using the principles outlined as follows:

- All patients, regardless of specific TB risk factors, who will be taking an immunomodulating biologic agent should be tested for latent TB infection (LTBI) before starting the therapy.

- There are 2 options that should be considered for screening, depending on the clinical scenario: either TST or use of an interferon-γ release assay (IGRA) or both. There are 2 choices for IGRA, the QuantiFERON-TB Gold In-Tube assay (Cellestis/Qiagen, Carnegie, Australia) and the T-SPOT.TB assay (Oxford Immunotec, Abingdon, United Kingdom). Both are considered acceptable.[19,157]

- For children without risk factors for LTBI (previous history of TB, previous history of positive TST result, history of exposure to someone with active TB, travel to an area with endemic TB in the past 12 months, or foreign-born patient or parents from area with endemic TB) and without any symptoms suggestive of TB, the decision as to which screening method to use at baseline should be based on age. Children younger than 5 years, in general, should be screened with TST, whereas an IGRA is preferred for children older than 5 years.[19]

- For patients with any risk factor for LTBI (previous history of TB, previous history of positive TST result, history of exposure to someone with active TB, or travel to an area with endemic TB in the past 12 months) or any symptoms suggestive of TB, both the TST and an IGRA should be performed and appropriate treatment of LTBI should be started if either test result is positive once TB disease has been ruled out.[19] Most experts do not currently use an IGRA when testing for LTBI for children younger than 2 years because of a lack of data for this age group and a high risk of progression to disease but will still use an IGRA in children 2 years or older, especially if they have received a bacille Calmette-Guerin vaccine.[19] Although most of the data available are for children 5 years and older, there are increasing data also available for children 2 to 5 years of age.[19]

- Patients with a positive TST or an IGRA result or any risk factor as stated previously for LTBI should also have chest radiography (postanterior and lateral) performed.

- Routine annual TST or IGRA is not recommended, but patients should be asked at least annually about TB symptoms and risk factors.

- If there is a change in risk or new symptoms suggestive of TB infection while receiving treatment, there should be further evaluation and risk assessment, including a repeat of both TST and IGRA (if the baseline was negative) as well as chest radiography.

- If LTBI is diagnosed, the patient needs treatment to prevent TB disease.[155,156]

- Patients suspected of having active TB should have their BRM and other immunosuppressive agents discontinued until TB is ruled out or under control. Guidance from an infectious diseases specialist is recommended in this setting for possible isolation precautions and management. Risk factors for drug-resistant TB (previous history of treatment of TB disease, contact with a patient with known drug-resistant TB, country of origin or current residence in geographic area with a high prevalence of drug-resistant TB, or contact with a source case who has positive smears for acid-fast bacilli or cultures after

2 months of appropriate anti-TB therapy) should be considered in formulating empirical therapy.[158] There will need to be an intensive investigation to examine for disseminated or extrapulmonary disease guided by an expert in TB management.

NTM

There are no recommendations or tests at the present time for screening for NTM. However, NTM should be considered in the differential diagnosis of patients receiving BRMs with febrile illnesses, cervical or unexplained lymphadenitis, or other focal infections or anytime TB is being considered.

Screening for Histoplasmosis and Other Fungi

All patients should be queried about possible exposure and epidemiologic risk factors for potentially invasive fungal infections, especially histoplasmosis and coccidioidomycosis, which have symptoms and signs that significantly overlap with TB. The main epidemiologic determinants of risk for histoplasmosis include the following[122,124,159-161]: geographic location of residence near river beds (Mississippi River Valley, Ohio River Valley, Chesapeake Bay area, eastern Oklahoma, and eastern Texas). Anyone who lives in a histoplasmosis belt is potentially infected; estimates are that 90% of residents acquire histoplasmosis and self-resolve before adulthood; thus, routine laboratory screening is not indicated. Furthermore, negative serologic test results before the initiation of BRMs does not predict patients at risk of development of histoplasmosis, especially among patients already receiving DMARDs.[122] Immunosuppression and extremes of age are also major risk factors. Residence in geographic areas where coccidioidomycosis is endemic (eg, southwestern

United States and southern California) is an epidemiologic risk factor for developing coccidioidomycosis,[119,120,161-164] and Filipino, Hispanic, black, American Indian, and Asian persons and pregnant women during the third trimester and women in the immediate postpartum period are at risk for more severe disease. Any form of immunosuppression also leads to an increased risk of invasive and disseminated disease. Up to 2% of patients receiving BRMs will develop coccidioidomycosis if they reside in an at-risk region.

Patients suspected of having signs or symptoms compatible with acute histoplasmosis[122,124,159,160] or coccidioidomycosis[119-121,162-164] during therapy with BRMs should have the BRM discontinued immediately and require evaluation with a combination of chest radiography and serologic, antigen detection, and culture tests. These tests and treatment options are best conducted in consultation with an infectious diseases expert.

Screening for HSV, VZV, EBV, Hepatitis B, and PML

VZV and HSV

As noted previously in the immunization section, all patients should be screened by history, immunization, and possibly laboratory serologic records to facilitate documentation that they are either immune or have received the age-appropriate dose(s) of varicella vaccine at presentation. Routine testing for VZV is not recommended because of the variability in sensitivity of the assays, particularly in assessing immunity after VZV immunization; and where there is doubt about immunity on the basis of history or inadequacy of records, vaccination is recommended. If VZV vaccine is needed, because it is a live-virus vaccine it should be given at least 4 weeks before the initiation of BRM therapy.[165]

Patients suspected of having VZV or HSV infection during BRM therapy should stop taking the BRM. Diagnosis should be sought by a combination of clinical, serologic, and polymerase chain reaction tests from skin lesions (ie, vesicles or papules), and acyclovir or valacyclovir therapy should be started pending confirmation of diagnosis. Patients with recurrent HSV who are being considered for BRM therapy should be given consideration for prophylaxis with valacyclovir or acyclovir.

EBV

Consideration should be given to baseline serologic testing for EBV at the time of diagnosis of the underlying rheumatologic condition. Further serologic testing should be considered if the patient develops signs or symptoms that have been associated with EBV, including mononucleosis-like illness or excessive fatigue.

Hepatitis B

Patients being considered for BRM therapy should be screened for past hepatitis B infection with both immunization records and serologic testing for HBsAg, HbcAb (total and IgM), and quantitative HBsAb[166] (Table 3). It is advisable to obtain baseline liver function tests (LFTs) at the same time.[167-172] Patients who are negative for HBsAg, HBcAb, and HBsAb are considered uninfected and nonimmune. They should be immunized with the first dose of hepatitis B vaccine at least 2 weeks before initiation of the BRM.[173] Consideration of whether the full series of HBV vaccinations is given before initiation of the BRM should be made in conjunction with the specialist initiating the BRM, weighing the risks and benefit of delaying BRM therapy. Patients who are only HBsAb positive are likely immune and can be safely treated with BRMs. If their antibody

TABLE 3 Screening Tests for HBV Infection, Interpretation, and Recommendations Before BRM Therapy

HBV Infection	HBsAg	HBsAb	HBcAb	HBcIgM	Abnormal LFTs and/or Symptoms	Additional Testing	Management	Comments
Uninfected, nonimmune	−	−	−	−	−	Not needed	Safely treat with BRM	Administer hepatitis B vaccine before BRM therapy
Vaccinated	−	+	−	−	−	Not needed	Safely treat with BRM	For HBsAb <10 mIU/mL, suggest HBV booster
Acute	+	−	+	+	+	Not needed	Defer BRM therapy	
Chronic	+	−	+	−	+/−	HBeAg, HBeAb, HBV DNA	Treat with BRM in consultation with ID consultant or hepatologist	
Resolved	−	+	+	−	−	HBV DNA	Treat with BRM in consultation with ID consultant or hepatologist	
Occult	−	−	+	−	−	HBV DNA	Treat with BRM in consultation with ID consultant or hepatologist	

Adapted with permission from ref 117. HBcIgM, hepatitis B core IgM antibody; HBeAb, hepatitis B core e antibody; HBeAg, hepatitis B core e antigen; ID, infectious diseases; −, negative; +, positive.

titer is low (<10 mIU/mL), strong consideration should be given to giving a booster dose of hepatitis B vaccine before initiation of treatment.[148,166] Recent receipt of Immune Globulin Intravenous (IGIV) may be associated with a transiently positive serologic test result. Patients who have acute HBV infection (HBsAg positive, total HBcAb positive, hepatitis B core IgM positive, and elevated LFTs) should not receive a BRM. Patients who show evidence of chronic HBV infection (HBsAg positive, HBcAb positive, hepatitis B core IgM negative, and persistently or intermittently high LFT results) should be evaluated by either an infectious diseases specialist or a hepatologist for further testing to determine their status.[169] This testing will likely involve measuring HBV DNA levels to determine the likelihood of clearance with antiviral treatment. In general, chronic carriers with a high viral load (HBV DNA >10^5 copies per mL) and abnormal LFTs will need to be treated with antiviral agents effective against HBV, but guidance by an infectious diseases specialist or hepatologist is strongly recommended. Patients who are HBsAg negative, HBsAb positive, and HBcAb positive are considered to have "resolved HBV infection" and can likely be treated with close monitoring by an infectious diseases expert or hepatologist. In this scenario, it is advisable to first obtain a baseline HBV DNA quantitative level as well as LFTs that can be monitored in follow-up. Finally, some patients will only be positive for HBcAb and are generally considered to have "occult HBV." Some of these patients may also have a false-positive test result or may have resolving infection. They may or may not be at risk of HBV reactivation. Most can be treated with the BRM under the guidance of an infectious diseases expert or a hepatologist.

Long-term Monitoring for HBV

All patients at risk of HBV reactivation (chronic, resolved, or occult) should have regular (every 1–3 months, depending on underlying HBV infection) monitoring of their LFTs, HBsAg, hepatitis B e antigen, and HBV DNA counts. This monitoring should continue for at least 6 months after termination of the BRM.

PML

All patients receiving natalizumab should be monitored regularly (3 and 6 months after the first infusion and every 6 months after and for at least 6 months after discontinuation) for PML, and the medication should be withheld immediately with any signs or symptoms of the condition.[174] Diagnosis of PML involves a gadolinium-enhanced MRI brain scan and cerebrospinal fluid analysis for JC viral DNA when indicated. An algorithm has been proposed for risk profiling and management of PML for patients receiving natalizumab.[174]

CONCLUSIONS

BRMs have become an important component of effective management of patients with a variety of autoimmune/inflammatory conditions. However, there is an increased risk of certain serious and opportunistic infections for patients receiving these biologic agents, especially the risks of TB and viral infections. It is important for pediatricians, family physicians, and other primary care practitioners managing patients who receive these important treatments to be aware of the potential infections complications and to practice anticipatory guidance between visits to reduce the risk of occurrence or of negative outcomes if the complications do occur. In most scenarios, a close working relationship among the pediatrician, the pediatric medical subspecialist prescribing the BRM, and an infectious diseases specialist is warranted.

COMMITTEE ON INFECTIOUS DISEASES, 2015–2016

Carrie L. Byington, MD, FAAP, Chairperson
Yvonne A. Maldonado, MD, FAAP, Vice Chairperson
Elizabeth D. Barnett, MD, FAAP
H. Dele Davies, MD, FAAP
Kathryn M. Edwards, MD, FAAP
Ruth Lynfield, MD, FAAP
Flor M. Munoz-Rivas, MD, FAAP
Dawn L. Nolt, MD, FAAP
Ann-Christine Nyquist, MD, MSPH, FAAP
Mobeen H. Rathore, MD, FAAP
Mark H. Sawyer, MD, FAAP
William J. Steinbach, MD, FAAP
Tina Q. Tan, MD, FAAP
Theoklis E. Zaoutis, MD, MSCE, FAAP

FORMER COMMITTEE MEMBERS

Dennis L. Murray, MD, FAAP
Gordon E. Schutze, MD, FAAP
Rodney E. Willoughby, MD, FAAP

EX OFFICIO

Henry H. Bernstein, DO, MHCM, FAAP – *Red Book Online* Associate Editor
Michael T. Brady, MD, FAAP – *Red Book* Associate Editor
Mary Anne Jackson, MD, FAAP, *Red Book* Associate Editor
David W. Kimberlin, MD, FAAP – *Red Book* Editor
Sarah S. Long, MD, FAAP – *Red Book* Associate Editor
H. Cody Meissner, MD, FAAP – Visual *Red Book* Associate Editor

LIAISONS

Douglas Campos-Outcalt, MD, MPH – *American Academy of Family Physicians*
Karen M. Farizo, MD – *Food and Drug Administration*
Marc Fischer, MD, FAAP – *Centers for Disease Control and Prevention*
Bruce Gellin, MD, MPH – *National Vaccine Program Office*
Richard L. Gorman, MD, FAAP – *National Institutes of Health*
Natasha B. Halasa, MD, MPH, FAAP – *Pediatric Infectious Diseases Society*
Joan L. Robinson, MD – *Canadian Paediatric Society*
Marco Aurelio Palazzi Safadi, MD – *Sociedad Latinoamericana de Infectologia Pediatrica*
Jane F. Seward, MBBS, MPH, FAAP – *Centers for Disease Control and Prevention*
Geoffrey Simon, MD, FAAP – *Committee on Practice Ambulatory Medicine*

Jeffrey R. Starke, MD, FAAP – *American Thoracic Society*

STAFF

Jennifer M. Frantz, MPH

ABBREVIATIONS

AAP: American Academy of Pediatrics
AERS: Adverse Event Reporting System
BRM: biologic response modifier
CI: confidence interval
DMARD: disease-modifying antirheumatic drug
EBV: Epstein-Barr virus
Fc: fragment-crystallizable
FDA: Food and Drug Administration
HBcAb: hepatitis B core antibody
HBsAb: hepatitis B surface antibody
HBsAg: hepatitis B surface antigen
HBV: hepatitis B virus
HSCT: hematopoietic stem cell transplant
HSV: herpes simplex virus
Ig: immunoglobulin
IGRA: interferon-γ release assay
IL: interleukin
JAK: Janus kinase
JIA: juvenile idiopathic arthritis
LFT: liver function test
LTBI: latent tuberculosis infection
MMR: measles-mumps-rubella
NTM: nontuberculous mycobacteria
OR: odds ratio
PCP: *Pneumocystis jirovecii* (previously *carinii*) pneumonia
PML: progressive multifocal leukoencephalopathy
RA: rheumatoid arthritis
TB: tuberculosis
Th: T helper
TNF: tumor necrosis factor
TST: tuberculin skin test
VZV: varicella-zoster virus

REFERENCES

1. Saag KG, Teng GG, Patkar NM, et al; American College of Rheumatology. American College of Rheumatology 2008 recommendations for the use of nonbiologic and biologic disease-modifying antirheumatic drugs in rheumatoid arthritis. *Arthritis Rheum*. 2008;59(6):762–784

2. Toussi SS, Pan N, Walters HM, Walsh TJ. Infections in children and adolescents with juvenile idiopathic arthritis and inflammatory bowel disease treated with tumor necrosis factor-α inhibitors: systematic review of the literature. *Clin Infect Dis*. 2013;57(9):1318–1330

3. Giles JT, Bathon JM. Serious infections associated with anticytokine therapies in the rheumatic diseases. *J Intensive Care Med*. 2004;19(6):320–334

4. Keane J, Gershon S, Wise RP, et al. Tuberculosis associated with infliximab, a tumor necrosis factor alpha-neutralizing agent. *N Engl J Med*. 2001;345(15):1098–1104

5. Ford AC, Peyrin-Biroulet L. Opportunistic infections with anti-tumor necrosis factor-α therapy in inflammatory bowel disease: meta-analysis of randomized controlled trials. *Am J Gastroenterol*. 2013;108(8):1268–1276

6. Lichtenstein GR, Feagan BG, Cohen RD, et al. Serious infections and mortality in association with therapies for Crohn's disease: TREAT registry. *Clin Gastroenterol Hepatol*. 2006;4(5):621–630

7. Rahier JF, Ben-Horin S, Chowers Y, et al; European Crohn's and Colitis Organisation. European evidence-based consensus on the prevention, diagnosis and management of opportunistic infections in inflammatory bowel disease. *J Crohn's Colitis*. 2009;3(2):47–91

8. Rahier JF, Yazdanpanah Y, Colombel JF, Travis S. The European (ECCO) consensus on infection in IBD: what does it change for the clinician? *Gut*. 2009;58(10):1313–1315

9. Viget N, Vernier-Massouille G, Salmon-Ceron D, Yazdanpanah Y, Colombel JF. Opportunistic infections in patients with inflammatory bowel disease: prevention and diagnosis. *Gut*. 2008;57(4):549–558

10. Beukelman T, Patkar NM, Saag KG, et al. 2011 American College of Rheumatology recommendations for the treatment of juvenile idiopathic arthritis: initiation and safety monitoring of therapeutic agents for the treatment of arthritis and systemic features. *Arthritis Care Res (Hoboken)*. 2011;63(4):465–482

11. Beukelman T, Xie F, Baddley JW, et al; SABER Collaboration. Brief report: incidence of selected opportunistic infections among children with juvenile idiopathic arthritis. *Arthritis Rheum*. 2013;65(5):1384–1389

12. Hyams J, Walters TD, Crandall W, et al. Safety and efficacy of maintenance infliximab therapy for moderate-to-severe Crohn's disease in children: REACH open-label extension. *Curr Med Res Opin*. 2011;27(3):651–662

13. Le Saux N; Canadian Paediatric Society, Infectious Diseases and Immunization Committee. Biologic response modifiers to decrease inflammation: focus on infection risks. *Paediatr Child Health*. 2012;17(3):147–154

14. Veereman-Wauters G, de Ridder L, Veres G, et al; ESPGHAN IBD Porto Group. Risk of infection and prevention in pediatric patients with IBD: ESPGHAN IBD Porto Group commentary. *J Pediatr Gastroenterol Nutr*. 2012;54(6):830–837

15. Woerner A, Ritz N. Infections in children treated with biological agents. *Pediatr Infect Dis J*. 2013;32(3):284–288

16. Centers for Disease Control and Prevention, Advisory Committee on Immunization Practices;. Recommended immunization schedules for persons aged 0 through 18 years—United States, 2013. *MMWR Morb Mortal Wkly Rep*. 2013;62(1):2–8

17. Centers for Disease Control and Prevention, Advisory Committee on Immunization Practices; American Academy of Pediatrics; American Academy of Family Physicians. Recommended immunization schedules for persons aged 0 through 18 years--United States, 2013. *MMWR Morb Mortal Wkly Rep*. 2013;62(1):1–19

18. American Academy of Pediatrics. Immunization in special clinical circumstances. In: Pickering LK, Baker CJ, Kimberlin DW, Long SS, eds. *Red Book: 2012 Report of the Committee on Infectious Diseases*. Elk Grove Village, IL: American Academy of Pediatrics; 2012:69–109

19. Starke JR; Committee on Infectious Diseases. Interferon-γ release assays for diagnosis of tuberculosis infection and disease in children. *Pediatrics*. 2014;134(6). Available at: www.pediatrics.org/cgi/content/full/134/6/e1763

20. American Academy of Pediatrics. *Listeria monocytogenes* infections (listeriosis). In: Pickering LK, Baker CJ, Kimberlin DW, Long SS, eds. *Red Book: 2012 Report of the Committee on Infectious Diseases*. Elk Grove Village, IL: American Academy of Pediatrics; 2012:471–474

21. Remicade (infliximab) [package insert]. Horsham, PA: Janssen Biotech; 2013. Available at: www.remicade.com/shared/product/remicade/prescribing-information.pdf. Accessed October 22, 2014

22. Horneff G, De Bock F, Foeldvari I, et al; German and Austrian Paediatric Rheumatology Collaborative Study Group. Safety and efficacy of combination of etanercept and methotrexate compared to treatment with etanercept only in patients with juvenile idiopathic arthritis (JIA): preliminary data from the German JIA Registry. *Ann Rheum Dis*. 2009;68(4):519–525

23. Humira (adalimunab) [package insert]. North Chicago, IL: AbbVie; 2013. Available at: www.rxabbvie.com/pdf/humira.pdf. Accessed October 22, 2014

24. Simponi (golimumab) [package insert]. Horsham, PA: Jannsen Biotech; 2013. Available at: www.simponiaria.com/shared/product/simponiaria/prescribing-information.pdf. Accessed October 22, 2014

25. Cimzia (certolizumab pegol) [package insert]. Smyrna, GA: UCB; 2012. Available at: www.cimzia.com/assets/pdf/Prescribing_Information.pdf. Accessed October 22, 2014

26. Orencia (abatacept) [package insert]. Princeton, NJ: Bristol Myers Squibb; 2013. Available at: http://packageinserts.bms.com/pi/pi_orencia.pdf. Accessed October 22, 2014

27. Kineret (anakinra) [package insert]. Stockholm, Sweden: Swedish Orphan Biovitrum AB; 2013. Available at: www.kineretrx.com/fileadmin/user_upload/kineretus/documents/Kineret_Full_Prescribing_Information.pdf. Accessed October 22, 2014

28. Rituxan (rituximab) [package insert]. South San Francisco, CA: Genentech; 2013. Available at: www.gene.com/download/pdf/rituxan_prescribing.pdf. Accessed October 22, 2014

29. Actemra (tocilizumab) [package insert]. South San Francisco, CA: Genentech; 2013. Available at: www.gene.com/download/pdf/actemra_prescribing.pdf. Accessed October 22, 2014

30. Stelara (ustekinumab) [package insert]. Horsham, PA: Janssen Biotech; 2013. Available at: www.stelarainfo.com/pdf/PrescribingInformation.pdf. Accessed October 22, 2014

31. Ruperto N, Lovell DJ, Cuttica R, et al; Paediatric Rheumatology International Trials Organisation; Pediatric Rheumatology Collaborative Study Group. A randomized, placebo-controlled trial of infliximab plus methotrexate for the treatment of polyarticular-course juvenile rheumatoid arthritis. *Arthritis Rheum.* 2007;56(9):3096–3106

32. Ilaris (canakinumab) [package insert]. East Hanover, NJ: Novartis; 2013. Available at: www.pharma.us.novartis.com/product/pi/pdf/ilaris.pdf. Accessed October 22, 2014

33. Tysabri (natalizumab) [package insert]. Cambridge, MA: Biogen Idec; 2013. Available at: www.tysabri.com/pdfs/I61061-13_PI.pdf. Accessed October 22, 2014

34. Benlysta (belimumab) [package insert]. GlaxoSmithKline, Mississauga, Ontario, Canada; 2014. Available at: www.gsksource.com/gskprm/en/US/adirect/gskprm?cmd=ProductDetailPage&product_id=1300455676143&featureKey=602522&tab=tab1&footer=yes&pTab=

one#nlmhighlights. Accessed October 22, 2014

35. Arcalyst (rilonacept) [package insert]. Tarrytown, NY: Regeneron Pharmaceuticals; 2013. Available at: www.arcalyst.com/images/pdf/ARCALYST-fpi.pdf?phpMyAdmin=e99e09ae33c1fdbbafd69c8883f97963. Accessed October 22, 2014

36. Xeljanz (tofacitinib) [package insert]. New York, NY: Pfizer; 2014. Available at: http://labeling.pfizer.com/ShowLabeling.aspx?id=959. Accessed October 22, 2014

37. Bray V. The safety of infliximab (Remicade(R)) infusion in clinical practice [abstract 153]. *Arthritis Rheum.* 2001;(suppl 9):S83

38. Hyams JS, Griffiths A, Markowitz J, et al Safety and efficacy of adalimumab for moderate to severe Crohn's disease in children. *Gastroenterology.* 2012;143(2):365.e2–374.e2

39. Lipsky PE, van der Heijde DM, St Clair EW, et al; Anti-Tumor Necrosis Factor Trial in Rheumatoid Arthritis with Concomitant Therapy Study Group. Infliximab and methotrexate in the treatment of rheumatoid arthritis. *N Engl J Med.* 2000;343(22):1594–1602

40. Furst D, Schiff M, Fleischmann R, et al. Safety and efficacy of adalimumab (D2E7), a fully human anti-TNF-alpha monoclonal antibody, given in combination with standard antirheumatic therapy: safety trial of adalimumab in rheumatoid arthritis (RA) [abstract]. *Arthritis Rheum.* 2002;46(suppl):S572

41. Keystone E, Kavanaugh A, Sharp J, et al. Adalimumab (D2E7), a fully human anti-TNF-alpha monoclonal antibody, inhibits the progression of structural joint damage in patients with active RA despite concomitant methotrexate therapy [abstract]. *Arthritis Rheum.* 2002;46(suppl 9):S205

42. Lovell DJ, Ruperto N, Goodman S, et al; Pediatric Rheumatology Collaborative Study Group; Pediatric Rheumatology International Trials Organisation. Adalimumab with or without methotrexate in juvenile rheumatoid arthritis. *N Engl J Med.* 2008;359(8):810–820

43. Trachana M, Pratsidou-Gertsi P, Pardalos G, Kozeis N, Badouraki M, Kanakoudi-Tsakalidou F. Safety and efficacy of adalimumab treatment in Greek children with juvenile idiopathic arthritis. *Scand J Rheumatol.* 2011;40(2):101–107

44. Hsia EC, Cush JJ, Matteson EL, et al. Comprehensive tuberculosis screening program in patients with inflammatory arthritides treated with golimumab, a human anti-tumor necrosis factor antibody, in phase III clinical trials. *Arthritis Care Res (Hoboken).* 2013;65(2):309–313

45. Pérez-Alvarez R, Díaz-Lagares C, García-Hernández F, et al; BIOGEAS Study Group. Hepatitis B virus (HBV) reactivation in patients receiving tumor necrosis factor (TNF)-targeted therapy: analysis of 257 cases. *Medicine (Baltimore).* 2011;90(6):359–371

46. Giannini EH, Ilowite NT, Lovell DJ, et al; Pediatric Rheumatology Collaborative Study Group. Long-term safety and effectiveness of etanercept in children with selected categories of juvenile idiopathic arthritis. *Arthritis Rheum.* 2009;60(9):2794–2804

47. Enbrel (etanercept) [package insert]. Thousand Oaks, CA: Immunex; 2013. Available at: http://pi.amgen.com/united_states/enbrel/derm/enbrel_pi.pdf. Accessed October 22, 2014

48. Wallis RS. Biologics and infections: lessons from tumor necrosis factor blocking agents. *Infect Dis Clin North Am.* 2011;25(4):895–910

49. Cutolo M. The kinase inhibitor tofacitinib in patients with rheumatoid arthritis: latest findings and clinical potential. *Ther Adv Musculoskelet Dis.* 2013;5(1):3–11

50. Ghoreschi K, Laurence A, O'Shea JJ. Selectivity and therapeutic inhibition of kinases: to be or not to be? *Nat Immunol.* 2009;10(4):356–360

51. Ghoreschi K, Laurence A, O'Shea JJ. Janus kinases in immune cell signaling. *Immunol Rev.* 2009;228(1):273–287

52. Riese RJ, Krishnaswami S, Kremer J. Inhibition of JAK kinases in patients with rheumatoid arthritis: scientific rationale and clinical outcomes.

Best Pract Res Clin Rheumatol. 2010;24(4):513–526

53. Bongartz T, Sutton AJ, Sweeting MJ, Buchan I, Matteson EL, Montori V. Anti-TNF antibody therapy in rheumatoid arthritis and the risk of serious infections and malignancies: systematic review and meta-analysis of rare harmful effects in randomized controlled trials. *JAMA.* 2006;295(19):2275–2285

54. Thompson AE, Rieder SW, Pope JE. Tumor necrosis factor therapy and the risk of serious infection and malignancy in patients with early rheumatoid arthritis: a meta-analysis of randomized controlled trials. *Arthritis Rheum.* 2011;63(6):1479–1485

55. Singh JA, Wells GA, Christensen R, et al. Adverse effects of biologics: a network meta-analysis and Cochrane overview. *Cochrane Database Syst Rev.* 2011;2:CD008794

56. Doran MF, Crowson CS, Pond GR, O'Fallon WM, Gabriel SE. Predictors of infection in rheumatoid arthritis. *Arthritis Rheum.* 2002;46(9):2294–2300

57. Jeurissen ME, Boerbooms AM, van de Putte LB, et al. Methotrexate versus azathioprine in the treatment of rheumatoid arthritis: a forty-eight-week randomized, double-blind trial. *Arthritis Rheum.* 1991;34(8):961–972

58. Immunex Corporation. *Enbrel: serious and opportunistic infection rates.* Thousand Oaks, CA: Immunex; 2013. Available at: www.enbrel.com/RheumPro/infection-rates.jspx. Accessed October 22, 2014

59. Beukelman T, Xie F, Chen L, et al; SABER Collaboration. Rates of hospitalized bacterial infection associated with juvenile idiopathic arthritis and its treatment. *Arthritis Rheum.* 2012;64(8):2773–2780

60. Bracaglia C, Buonuomo PS, Tozzi AE, et al. Safety and efficacy of etanercept in a cohort of patients with juvenile idiopathic arthritis under 4 years of age. *J Rheumatol.* 2012;39(6):1287–1290

61. Gerloni V, Pontikaki I, Gattinara M, Fantini F. Focus on adverse events of tumour necrosis factor alpha blockade in juvenile idiopathic arthritis

in an open monocentric long-term prospective study of 163 patients. *Ann Rheum Dis.* 2008;67(8):1145–1152

62. Lovell DJ, Giannini EH, Reiff A, et al; Pediatric Rheumatology Collaborative Study Group. Etanercept in children with polyarticular juvenile rheumatoid arthritis. *N Engl J Med.* 2000;342(11):763–769

63. Lovell DJ, Giannini EH, Reiff A, et al; Pediatric Rheumatology Collaborative Study Group. Long-term efficacy and safety of etanercept in children with polyarticular-course juvenile rheumatoid arthritis: interim results from an ongoing multicenter, open-label, extended-treatment trial. *Arthritis Rheum.* 2003;48(1):218–226

64. Lovell DJ, Reiff A, Ilowite NT, et al; Pediatric Rheumatology Collaborative Study Group. Safety and efficacy of up to eight years of continuous etanercept therapy in patients with juvenile rheumatoid arthritis. *Arthritis Rheum.* 2008;58(5):1496–1504

65. Lovell DJ, Reiff A, Jones OY, et al; Pediatric Rheumatology Collaborative Study Group. Long-term safety and efficacy of etanercept in children with polyarticular-course juvenile rheumatoid arthritis. *Arthritis Rheum.* 2006;54(6):1987–1994

66. Prince FH, Twilt M, ten Cate R, et al. Long-term follow-up on effectiveness and safety of etanercept in juvenile idiopathic arthritis: the Dutch national register. *Ann Rheum Dis.* 2009;68(5):635–641

67. Hyams J, Damaraju L, Blank M, et al; T72 Study Group. Induction and maintenance therapy with infliximab for children with moderate to severe ulcerative colitis. *Clin Gastroenterol Hepatol.* 2012;10(4):391–399.e1

68. Ruperto N, Lovell DJ, Cuttica R, et al; Paediatric Rheumatology INternational Trials Organization (PRINTO); Pediatric Rheumatology Collaborative Study Group (PRCSG). Long-term efficacy and safety of infliximab plus methotrexate for the treatment of polyarticular-course juvenile rheumatoid arthritis: findings from an open-label treatment extension. *Ann Rheum Dis.* 2010;69(4):718–722

69. Stephens MC, Shepanski MA, Mamula P, Markowitz JE, Brown KA, Baldassano RN. Safety and steroid-sparing

experience using infliximab for Crohn's disease at a pediatric inflammatory bowel disease center. *Am J Gastroenterol.* 2003;98(1):104–111

70. Tschudy J, Michail S. Disseminated histoplasmosis and pneumocystis pneumonia in a child with Crohn disease receiving infliximab. *J Pediatr Gastroenterol Nutr.* 2010;51(2):221–222

71. Imagawa T, Takei S, Umebayashi H, et al. Efficacy, pharmacokinetics, and safety of adalimumab in pediatric patients with juvenile idiopathic arthritis in Japan. *Clin Rheumatol.* 2012;31(12):1713–1721

72. Chaiwatanatorn K, Lee N, Grigg A, Filshie R, Firkin F. Delayed-onset neutropenia associated with rituximab therapy. *Br J Haematol.* 2003;121(6):913–918

73. Dunleavy K, Hakim F, Kim HK, et al. B-cell recovery following rituximab-based therapy is associated with perturbations in stromal derived factor-1 and granulocyte homeostasis. *Blood.* 2005;106(3):795–802

74. Fukuno K, Tsurumi H, Ando N, et al. Late-onset neutropenia in patients treated with rituximab for non-Hodgkin's lymphoma. *Int J Hematol.* 2006;84(3):242–247

75. Hofer S, Viollier R, Ludwig C. Delayed-onset and long-lasting severe neutropenia due to rituximab. *Swiss Med Wkly.* 2004;134(5-6):79–80

76. Mitsuhata N, Fujita R, Ito S, Mannami M, Keimei K. Delayed-onset neutropenia in a patient receiving rituximab as treatment for refractory kidney transplantation. *Transplantation.* 2005;80(9):1355

77. Nitta E, Izutsu K, Sato T, et al. A high incidence of late-onset neutropenia following rituximab-containing chemotherapy as a primary treatment of CD20-positive B-cell lymphoma: a single-institution study. *Ann Oncol.* 2007;18(2):364–369

78. Terrier B, Ittah M, Tourneur L, et al. Late-onset neutropenia following rituximab results from a hematopoietic lineage competition due to an excessive BAFF-induced B-cell recovery. *Haematologica.* 2007;92(2):e20–e23

79. Voog E, Morschhauser F, Solal-Céligny P. Neutropenia in patients

treated with rituximab. *N Engl J Med.* 2003;348(26):2691–2694; discussion: 2691–2694

80. Weissmann-Brenner A, Brenner B, Belyaeva I, Lahav M, Rabizadeh E. Rituximab associated neutropenia: description of three cases and an insight into the underlying pathogenesis. *Med Sci Monit.* 2011;17(11):CS133–CS137

81. Alexeeva EI, Valieva SI, Bzarova TM, et al. Efficacy and safety of repeat courses of rituximab treatment in patients with severe refractory juvenile idiopathic arthritis. *Clin Rheumatol.* 2011;30(9):1163–1172

82. Flynn JL, Goldstein MM, Chan J, et al. Tumor necrosis factor-alpha is required in the protective immune response against Mycobacterium tuberculosis in mice. *Immunity.* 1995;2(6):561–572

83. Wagner TE, Huseby ES, Huseby JS. Exacerbation of *Mycobacterium tuberculosis* enteritis masquerading as Crohn's disease after treatment with a tumor necrosis factor-alpha inhibitor. *Am J Med.* 2002;112(1):67–69

84. Fallahi-Sichani M, Schaller MA, Kirschner DE, Kunkel SL, Linderman JJ. Identification of key processes that control tumor necrosis factor availability in a tuberculosis granuloma. *PLOS Comput Biol.* 2010;6(5):e1000778

85. Marino S, Myers A, Flynn JL, Kirschner DE. TNF and IL-10 are major factors in modulation of the phagocytic cell environment in lung and lymph node in tuberculosis: a next-generation two-compartment model. *J Theor Biol.* 2010;265(4):586–598

86. Mata-Espinosa DA, Mendoza-Rodríguez V, Aguilar-León D, Rosales R, López-Casillas F, Hernández-Pando R. Therapeutic effect of recombinant adenovirus encoding interferon-gamma in a murine model of progressive pulmonary tuberculosis. *Mol Ther.* 2008;16(6):1065–1072

87. Salgado E, Gómez-Reino JJ. The risk of tuberculosis in patients treated with TNF antagonists. *Expert Rev Clin Immunol.* 2011;7(3):329–340

88. Mohan AK, Coté TR, Block JA, Manadan AM, Siegel JN, Braun MM. Tuberculosis following the use of etanercept, a tumor necrosis factor inhibitor. *Clin Infect Dis.* 2004;39(3):295–299

89. Dixon WG, Hyrich KL, Watson KD, et al; BSRBR Control Centre Consortium; BSR Biologics Register. Drug-specific risk of tuberculosis in patients with rheumatoid arthritis treated with anti-TNF therapy: results from the British Society for Rheumatology Biologics Register (BSRBR). *Ann Rheum Dis.* 2010;69(3):522–528

90. Fleischmann R, Yocum D. Does safety make a difference in selecting the right TNF antagonist? *Arthritis Res Ther.* 2004;6(suppl 2):S12–S18

91. Dye C, Scheele S, Dolin P, Pathania V, Raviglione MC. Global burden of tuberculosis: estimated incidence, prevalence, and mortality by country [consensus statement]. WHO Global Surveillance and Monitoring Project. *JAMA.* 1999;282(7):677–686

92. Dixon WG, Watson K, Lunt M, Hyrich KL, Silman AJ, Symmons DP; British Society for Rheumatology Biologics Register. Rates of serious infection, including site-specific and bacterial intracellular infection, in rheumatoid arthritis patients receiving anti-tumor necrosis factor therapy: results from the British Society for Rheumatology Biologics Register. *Arthritis Rheum.* 2006;54(8):2368–2376

93. Tubach F, Salmon D, Ravaud P, et al; Research Axed on Tolerance of Biotherapies Group. Risk of tuberculosis is higher with anti-tumor necrosis factor monoclonal antibody therapy than with soluble tumor necrosis factor receptor therapy: the three-year prospective French Research Axed on Tolerance of Biotherapies Registry [published correction appears in *Arthritis Rheum.* 2009;60(8):2540. *Arthritis Rheum.* 2009;60(7):1884–1894

94. Imperato AK, Smiles S, Abramson SB. Long-term risks associated with biologic response modifiers used in rheumatic diseases. *Curr Opin Rheumatol.* 2004;16(3):199–205

95. Gómez-Reino JJ, Carmona L, Angel Descalzo M; Biobadaser Group. Risk of tuberculosis in patients treated with tumor necrosis factor antagonists due to incomplete prevention of reactivation of latent infection. *Arthritis Rheum.* 2007;57(5):756–761

96. Myers A, Clark J, Foster H. Tuberculosis and treatment with infliximab. *N Engl J Med.* 2002;346(8):623–626

97. Armbrust W, Kamphuis SSM, Wolfs TWF, et al. Tuberculosis in a nine-year-old girl treated with infliximab for systemic juvenile idiopathic arthritis. *Rheumatology (Oxford).* 2004;43(4):527–529

98. Askling J, Fored CM, Brandt L, et al. Risk and case characteristics of tuberculosis in rheumatoid arthritis associated with tumor necrosis factor antagonists in Sweden. *Arthritis Rheum.* 2005;52(7):1986–1992

99. Ayaz NA, Demirkaya E, Bilginer Y, et al. Preventing tuberculosis in children receiving anti-TNF treatment. *Clin Rheumatol.* 2010;29(4):389–392

100. Winthrop KL, Daley CL, Griffith D. Nontuberuclous mycobacterial disease: updated diagnostic criteria for an under-recognized infectious complication of anti-tumor necrosis factor therapy. *Nat Clin Pract Rheumatol.* 2007;3(10):E1

101. Winthrop KL, Yamashita S, Beekmann SE, Polgreen PM; Infectious Diseases Society of America Emerging Infections Network. Mycobacterial and other serious infections in patients receiving anti-tumor necrosis factor and other newly approved biologic therapies: case finding through the Emerging Infections Network. *Clin Infect Dis.* 2008;46(11):1738–1740

102. Winthrop KL, Chang E, Yamashita S, Iademarco MF, LoBue PA. Nontuberculous mycobacteria infections and anti-tumor necrosis factor-alpha therapy. *Emerg Infect Dis.* 2009;15(10):1556–1561

103. Cullen G, Baden RP, Cheifetz AS. Varicella zoster virus infection in inflammatory bowel disease. *Inflamm Bowel Dis.* 2012;18(12):2392–2403

104. Strangfeld A, Listing J, Herzer P, et al. Risk of herpes zoster in patients with rheumatoid arthritis treated with anti-TNF-alpha agents. *JAMA.* 2009;301(7):737–744

105. Smitten AL, Choi HK, Hochberg MC, et al. The risk of herpes zoster in patients

with rheumatoid arthritis in the United States and the United Kingdom. *Arthritis Rheum.* 2007;57(8):1431–1438

106. Galloway JB, Mercer LK, Moseley A, et al. Risk of skin and soft tissue infections (including shingles) in patients exposed to anti-tumour necrosis factor therapy: results from the British Society for Rheumatology Biologics Register. *Ann Rheum Dis.* 2013;72(2):229–234

107. Winthrop KL, Baddley JW, Chen L, et al. Association between the initiation of anti-tumor necrosis factor therapy and the risk of herpes zoster. *JAMA.* 2013;309(9):887–895

108. Wolfe F, Michaud K, Chakravarty EF. Rates and predictors of herpes zoster in patients with rheumatoid arthritis and non-inflammatory musculoskeletal disorders. *Rheumatology (Oxford).* 2006;45(11):1370–1375

109. Bradford RD, Pettit AC, Wright PW, et al. Herpes simplex encephalitis during treatment with tumor necrosis factor-alpha inhibitors. *Clin Infect Dis.* 2009;49(6):924–927

110. Justice EA, Khan SY, Logan S, Jobanputra P. Disseminated cutaneous herpes simplex virus-1 in a woman with rheumatoid arthritis receiving infliximab: a case report. *J Med Case Reports.* 2008;2:282

111. Salmon-Ceron D, Tubach F, Lortholary O, et al; RATIO Group. Drug-specific risk of non-tuberculosis opportunistic infections in patients receiving anti-TNF therapy reported to the 3-year prospective French RATIO registry. *Ann Rheum Dis.* 2011;70(4):616–623

112. Sciaudone G, Pellino G, Guadagni I, Selvaggi F. Education and imaging: gastrointestinal: herpes simplex virus-associated erythema multiforme (HAEM) during infliximab treatment for ulcerative colitis. *J Gastroenterol Hepatol.* 2011;26(3):610

113. van der Klooster JM, Bosman RJ, Oudemans-van Straaten HM, van der Spoel JI, Wester JP, Zandstra DF. Disseminated tuberculosis, pulmonary aspergillosis and cutaneous herpes simplex infection in a patient with infliximab and methotrexate. *Intensive Care Med.* 2003;29(12):2327–2329

114. Checchin D, Buda A, Sgarabotto D, Sturniolo GC, D'Incà R. Successful prophylaxis with valaciclovir for relapsing HSV-1 in a girl treated with infliximab for moderate Crohn's disease. *Eur J Gastroenterol Hepatol.* 2009;21(9):1095–1096

115. Carroll MB. The impact of biologic response modifiers on hepatitis B virus infection. *Expert Opin Biol Ther.* 2011;11(4):533–544

116. Zachou K, Sarantopoulos A, Gatselis NK, et al. Hepatitis B virus reactivation in hepatitis B virus surface antigen negative patients receiving immunosuppression: a hidden threat. *World J Hepatol.* 2013;5(7):387–392

117. Motaparthi K, Stanisic V, Van Voorhees AS, Lebwohl MG, Hsu S; Medical Board of the National Psoriasis Foundation. From the Medical Board of the National Psoriasis Foundation: recommendations for screening for hepatitis B infection prior to initiating anti-tumor necrosis factor-alfa inhibitors or other immunosuppressive agents in patients with psoriasis. *J Am Acad Dermatol.* 2014;70(1):178–186

118. Tsiodras S, Samonis G, Boumpas DT, Kontoyiannis DP. Fungal infections complicating tumor necrosis factor alpha blockade therapy. *Mayo Clin Proc.* 2008;83(2):181–194

119. Ampel NM. Coccidioidomycosis: a review of recent advances. *Clin Chest Med.* 2009;30(2):241–251

120. Bergstrom L, Yocum DE, Ampel NM, et al. Increased risk of coccidioidomycosis in patients treated with tumor necrosis factor alpha antagonists. *Arthritis Rheum.* 2004;50(6):1959–1966

121. Taroumian S, Knowles SL, Lisse JR, et al. Management of coccidioidomycosis in patients receiving biologic response modifiers or disease-modifying antirheumatic drugs. *Arthritis Care Res (Hoboken).* 2012;64(12):1903–1909

122. Hage CA, Bowyer S, Tarvin SE, Helper D, Kleiman MB, Wheat LJ. Recognition, diagnosis, and treatment of histoplasmosis complicating tumor necrosis factor blocker therapy. *Clin Infect Dis.* 2010;50(1):85–92

123. Winthrop KL, Chiller T. Preventing and treating biologic-associated opportunistic infections. *Nat Rev Rheumatol.* 2009;5(7):405–410

124. Lee JH, Slifman NR, Gershon SK, et al. Life-threatening histoplasmosis complicating immunotherapy with tumor necrosis factor alpha antagonists infliximab and etanercept. *Arthritis Rheum.* 2002;46(10):2565–2570

125. Bodro M, Paterson DL. Listeriosis in patients receiving biologic therapies. *Eur J Clin Microbiol Infect Dis.* 2013;32(9):1225–1230

126. Peña-Sagredo JL, Hernández MV, Fernandez-Llanio N, et al; Biobadaser Group. *Listeria monocytogenes* infection in patients with rheumatic diseases on TNF-alpha antagonist therapy: the Spanish Study Group experience. *Clin Exp Rheumatol.* 2008;26(5):854–859

127. Slifman NR, Gershon SK, Lee JH, Edwards ET, Braun MM. Listeria monocytogenes infection as a complication of treatment with tumor necrosis factor alpha-neutralizing agents. *Arthritis Rheum.* 2003;48(2):319–324

128. Lanternier F, Tubach F, Ravaud P, et al; Research Axed on Tolerance of Biotherapies Group. Incidence and risk factors of Legionella pneumophila pneumonia during anti-tumor necrosis factor therapy: a prospective French study. *Chest.* 2013;144(3):990–998

129. Tubach F, Ravaud P, Salmon-Céron D, et al; Recherce Axée sur la Tolérance des Biothérapies Group. Emergence of Legionella pneumophila pneumonia in patients receiving tumor necrosis factor-alpha antagonists. *Clin Infect Dis.* 2006;43(10):e95–e100

130. Torre-Cisneros J, Del Castillo M, Castón JJ, Castro MC, Pérez V, Collantes E. Infliximab does not activate replication of lymphotropic herpesviruses in patients with refractory rheumatoid arthritis. *Rheumatology (Oxford).* 2005;44(9):1132–1135

131. Balandraud N, Guis S, Meynard JB, Auger I, Roudier J, Roudier C. Long-term treatment with methotrexate or tumor necrosis factor alpha inhibitors does not increase

Epstein-Barr virus load in patients with rheumatoid arthritis. *Arthritis Rheum*. 2007;57(5):762–767

132. Fritzsche C, Riebold D, Munk-Hartig A, Klammt S, Neeck G, Reisinger E. High prevalence of Pneumocystis jirovecii colonization among patients with autoimmune inflammatory diseases and corticosteroid therapy. *Scand J Rheumatol*. 2012;41(3):208–213

133. Mekinian A, Durand-Joly I, Hatron PY, et al. *Pneumocystis jirovecii* colonization in patients with systemic autoimmune diseases: prevalence, risk factors of colonization and outcome. *Rheumatology (Oxford)*. 2011;50(3):569–577

134. Mori S, Cho I, Sugimoto M. A cluster of Pneumocystis jirovecii infection among outpatients with rheumatoid arthritis. *J Rheumatol*. 2010;37(7):1547–1548

135. Lund FE, Hollifield M, Schuer K, Lines JL, Randall TD, Garvy BA. B cells are required for generation of protective effector and memory CD4 cells in response to Pneumocystis lung infection. *J Immunol*. 2006;176(10):6147–6154

136. Martin-Garrido I, Carmona EM, Specks U, Limper AH. Pneumocystis pneumonia in patients treated with rituximab. *Chest*. 2013;144(1):258–265

137. Mori S, Cho I, Sugimoto M. A followup study of asymptomatic carriers of Pneumocystis jiroveci during immunosuppressive therapy for rheumatoid arthritis. *J Rheumatol*. 2009;36(8):1600–1605

138. Specks U. Biologic agents in the treatment of granulomatosis with polyangiitis. *Cleve Clin J Med*. 2012;79(suppl 3):S50–S53

139. Besada E, Nossent JC. Should Pneumocystis jiroveci prophylaxis be recommended with rituximab treatment in ANCA-associated vasculitis? *Clin Rheumatol*. 2013;32(11):1677–1681

140. Green H, Paul M, Vidal L, Leibovici L. Prophylaxis of Pneumocystis pneumonia in immunocompromised non-HIV-infected patients: systematic review and meta-analysis of randomized controlled trials. *Mayo Clin Proc*. 2007;82(9):1052–1059

141. Kaur N, Mahl TC. Pneumocystis jiroveci (carinii) pneumonia after infliximab

therapy: a review of 84 cases. *Dig Dis Sci*. 2007;52(6):1481–1484

142. Tanaka M, Sakai R, Koike R, et al. Pneumocystis jirovecii pneumonia associated with etanercept treatment in patients with rheumatoid arthritis: a retrospective review of 15 cases and analysis of risk factors. *Mod Rheumatol*. 2012;22(6):849–858

143. Watanabe K, Sakai R, Koike R, et al. Clinical characteristics and risk factors for Pneumocystis jirovecii pneumonia in patients with rheumatoid arthritis receiving adalimumab: a retrospective review and case-control study of 17 patients. *Mod Rheumatol*. 2013;23(6):1085–1093

144. Rubin LG, Levin MJ, Ljungman P, et al; Infectious Diseases Society of America. 2013 IDSA clinical practice guideline for vaccination of the immunocompromised host. *Clin Infect Dis*. 2014;58(3):309–318

145. American Academy of Pediatrics. Testing for *Mycobacterium tuberculosis* infection. In: Pickering LK, Baker CJ, Kimberlin DW, Long SS, eds. *Red Book: 2012 Report of the Committee on Infectious Diseases*. Elk Grove Village, IL: American Academy of Pediatrics; 2012:39

146. Elkayam O, Bashkin A, Mandelboim M, et al. The effect of infliximab and timing of vaccination on the humoral response to influenza vaccination in patients with rheumatoid arthritis and ankylosing spondylitis. *Semin Arthritis Rheum*. 2010;39(6):442–447

147. Glück T, Müller-Ladner U. Vaccination in patients with chronic rheumatic or autoimmune diseases. *Clin Infect Dis*. 2008;46(9):1459–1465

148. Moses J, Alkhouri N, Shannon A, et al. Hepatitis B immunity and response to booster vaccination in children with inflammatory bowel disease treated with infliximab. *Am J Gastroenterol*. 2012;107(1):133–138

149. Visvanathan S, Keenan GF, Baker DG, Levinson AI, Wagner CL. Response to pneumococcal vaccine in patients with early rheumatoid arthritis receiving infliximab plus methotrexate or methotrexate alone. *J Rheumatol*. 2007;34(5):952–957

150. Bingham CO III, Looney RJ, Deodhar A, et al. Immunization responses

in rheumatoid arthritis patients treated with rituximab: results from a controlled clinical trial. *Arthritis Rheum*. 2010;62(1):64–74

151. Crnkic Kapetanovic M, Saxne T, Jönsson G, Truedsson L, Geborek P. Rituximab and abatacept but not tocilizumab impair antibody response to pneumococcal conjugate vaccine in patients with rheumatoid arthritis. *Arthritis Res Ther*. 2013;15(5):R171

152. Nazi I, Kelton JG, Larché M, et al. The effect of rituximab on vaccine responses in patients with immune thrombocytopenia. *Blood*. 2013;122(11):1946–1953

153. van Assen S, Holvast A, Benne CA, et al. Humoral responses after influenza vaccination are severely reduced in patients with rheumatoid arthritis treated with rituximab. *Arthritis Rheum*. 2010;62(1):75–81

154. van der Kolk LE, Baars JW, Prins MH, van Oers MH. Rituximab treatment results in impaired secondary humoral immune responsiveness. *Blood*. 2002;100(6):2257–2259

155. Centers for Disease Control and Prevention. Latent tuberculosis infection: a guide for primary health care providers. Atlanta, GA: Centers for Disease Control and Prevention; 2013. Available at: www.cdc.gov/tb/publications/ltbi/diagnosis.htm. Accessed October 22, 2014

156. Centers for Disease Control and Prevention. TB guidelines, treatment. Atlanta, GA: Centers for Disease Control and Prevention; 2013. Available at: www.cdc.gov/tb/publications/guidelines/treatment.htm. Accessed October 22, 2014

157. Mazurek GH, Jereb J, Vernon A, LoBue P, Goldberg S, Castro K; IGRA Expert Committee; Centers for Disease Control and Prevention. Updated guidelines for using interferon gamma release assays to detect Mycobacterium tuberculosis infection—United States, 2010. *MMWR Recomm Rep*. 2010;59(RR-5):1–25

158. American Academy of Pediatrics. Tuberculosis. In: Pickering LK, Baker CJ, Kimberlin DW, Long SS, eds. *Red Book: 2012 Report of the Committee on Infectious Diseases*. Elk Grove Village, IL: American Academy of Pediatrics; 2012:736–759

159. Chamany S, Mirza SA, Fleming JW, et al. A large histoplasmosis outbreak among high school students in Indiana, 2001. *Pediatr Infect Dis J.* 2004;23(10):909–914

160. National Institute for Occupational Safety and Health. Histoplasmosis, protecting workers at risk. Atlanta, GA: National Institute for Occupational Safety and Health, Department of Health and Human Services; 2004. Available at: www.cdc.gov/niosh/docs/2005-109/. Accessed October 22, 2014

161. Jassal MS, Bishai WR. The risk of infections with tumor necrosis factor-alpha inhibitors. *J Clin Rheumatol.* 2009;15(8):419–426

162. Chiller TM, Galgiani JN, Stevens DA. Coccidioidomycosis. *Infect Dis Clin North Am.* 2003;17(1):41–57, viii

163. Crum NF, Lederman ER, Stafford CM, Parrish JS, Wallace MR. Coccidioidomycosis: a descriptive survey of a reemerging disease—clinical characteristics and current controversies. *Medicine (Baltimore).* 2004;83(3):149–175

164. Rosenstein NE, Emery KW, Werner SB, et al. Risk factors for severe pulmonary and disseminated coccidioidomycosis: Kern County, California, 1995-1996. *Clin Infect Dis.* 2001;32(5):708–715

165. American Academy of Pediatrics. Varicella-zoster infections. In: Pickering LK, Baker CJ, Kimberlin DW, Long SS, eds. *Red Book: 2012 Report of the Committee on Infectious Diseases.* Elk Grove Village, IL: American Academy of Pediatrics; 2012:774–789

166. Centers for Disease Control and Prevention. Hepatitis B information for health professionals. Atlanta, GA: Centers for Disease Control and Prevention; 2013. Available at: www.cdc.gov/hepatitis/hbv/hbvfaq.htm. Accessed October 22, 2014

167. Carroll MB, Bond MI. Use of tumor necrosis factor-alpha inhibitors in patients with chronic hepatitis B infection. *Semin Arthritis Rheum.* 2008;38(3):208–217

168. Kato M, Atsumi T, Kurita T, et al. Hepatitis B virus reactivation by immunosuppressive therapy in patients with autoimmune diseases: risk analysis in hepatitis B surface antigen-negative cases. *J Rheumatol.* 2011;38(10):2209–2214

169. Lok AS, McMahon BJ. Chronic hepatitis B. *Hepatology.* 2007;45(2):507–539

170. Post A, Nagendra S. Reactivation of hepatitis B: pathogenesis and clinical implications. *Curr Infect Dis Rep.* 2009;11(2):113–119

171. Yeo W, Chan PK, Zhong S, et al. Frequency of hepatitis B virus reactivation in cancer patients undergoing cytotoxic chemotherapy: a prospective study of 626 patients with identification of risk factors. *J Med Virol.* 2000;62(3):299–307

172. Yeo W, Johnson PJ. Diagnosis, prevention and management of hepatitis B virus reactivation during anticancer therapy. *Hepatology.* 2006;43(2):209–220

173. Rahier JF, Moutschen M, Van Gompel A, et al. Vaccinations in patients with immune-mediated inflammatory diseases. *Rheumatology (Oxford).* 2010;49(10):1815–1827

174. Hunt D, Giovannoni G. Natalizumab-associated progressive multifocal leucoencephalopathy: a practical approach to risk profiling and monitoring. *Pract Neurol.* 2012;12(1):25–35

Informed Consent in Decision-Making in Pediatric Practice

• *Policy Statement*

POLICY STATEMENT Organizational Principles to Guide and Define the Child Health Care System and/or Improve the Health of all Children

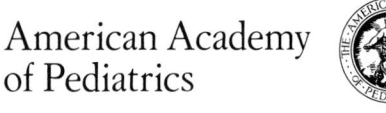

American Academy of Pediatrics

DEDICATED TO THE HEALTH OF ALL CHILDREN™

Informed Consent in Decision-Making in Pediatric Practice

COMMITTEE ON BIOETHICS

abstract

Informed consent should be seen as an essential part of health care practice; parental permission and childhood assent is an active process that engages patients, both adults and children, in health care. Pediatric practice is unique in that developmental maturation allows, over time, for increasing inclusion of the child's and adolescent's opinion in medical decision-making in clinical practice and research.

INTRODUCTION

Since the publication of previous American Academy of Pediatrics (AAP) statements on informed consent in 1976[1] and 1995,[2] obtaining informed permission from parents or legal guardians before medical interventions on pediatric patients has become standard within our medical and legal culture. The 1995 statement also championed, as pediatrician William Bartholome stated, "the experience, perspective and power of children" in the collaboration between pediatricians, their patients, and parents and remains an essential guide for modern ethical pediatric practice.[2] As recommended in the 1995 publication, this revised statement affirms that patients should participate in decision-making commensurate with their development; they should provide assent to care whenever reasonable. Pediatric decision-making continues to evolve in response to changes in information technology, scientific discoveries, and legal rulings. Continuing limits on the widespread use of pediatric assent/refusal makes this review and restatement of AAP policy important.[3]

This policy statement provides a brief review of informed consent, including the ethical and legal roots, frameworks for surrogate decision-making, and information on special issues in informed consent in pediatric care. Recommendations on informed consent or refusal, parental permission, and assent in clinical practice and research are summarized at the end of this statement. A more detailed review of pediatric consent and decision-making can be found in the accompanying technical report to this policy statement.[4]

Policy statements from the American Academy of Pediatrics benefit from expertise and resources of liaisons and internal (American Academy of Pediatrics) and external reviewers. However, policy statements from the American Academy of Pediatrics may reflect the views of the liaisons or the organizations or government agencies that they represent.

The guidance in this statement does not indicate an exclusive course of treatment or serve as a standard of medical care. Variations, taking into account individual circumstances, may be appropriate.

All policy statements from the American Academy of Pediatrics automatically expire 5 years after publication unless reaffirmed, revised, or retired at or before that time.

DOI: 10.1542/peds.2016-1484

PEDIATRICS (ISSN Numbers: Print, 0031-4005; Online, 1098-4275).

To cite: AAP COMMITTEE ON BIOETHICS. Informed Consent in Decision-Making in Pediatric Practice. *Pediatrics.* 2016; 138(2):e20161484

PURPOSE OF INFORMED CONSENT

The current concept of informed consent in medical practice has roots within both ethical theory and law. The support for informed consent in ethical theory is most commonly found in the concept of autonomy. The legal concept of informed consent has its roots in case law addressing issues of battery and medical malpractice. The law has evolved to require a full disclosure to the patient of the facts necessary to form the basis of a reasonable, informed consent. Informed consent incorporates 3 duties: disclosure of information to patients and their surrogates, assessment of patient and surrogate understanding of the information and their capacity for medical decision-making, and obtaining informed consent before treatments and interventions.

This background helps us understand the conceptual difficulties encountered in trying to apply the framework of informed consent in the pediatric setting, in which most patients either lack the ability to act independently or have limited or no capacity for medical decision-making. Nevertheless, the goals of the informed consent process (protecting and promoting health-related interests and incorporating the patient and/or the family in health care decision-making) are the same in the pediatric and adult population and are grounded by the same ethical principles of beneficence, justice, and respect for autonomy.

FRAMEWORK FOR INFORMED CONSENT/PERMISSION/ASSENT

Knowledge about a medical condition is critical to making informed health care decisions. Informed consent regarding medical care must consistently incorporate several key components (see Table 1).

Pediatricians should be adept at using developmentally appropriate

TABLE 1 Elements of Informed Consent for Medical Decision-Making

- Provision of information about the following:
  - o nature of the illness or condition
  - o proposed diagnostic steps and/or treatments and the probability of their success
  - o the potential risks, benefits, and uncertainties of the proposed treatment and alternative treatments, including the option of no treatment other than comfort measures
- Assessment of patient and surrogate understanding and medical decision-making capacity, including assurance of time for questions by patient and surrogate
- Ensure that there is voluntary agreement with the plan

TABLE 2 Practical Aspects of Assent by Pediatric Patients for Medical Decision-Making

- Help the patient achieve a developmentally appropriate awareness of the nature of his or her condition
- Tell the patient what he or she can expect with tests and treatments
- Make a clinical assessment of the patient's understanding of the situation and the factors influencing how he or she is responding (including whether there is inappropriate pressure to accept testing or therapy)
- Solicit an expression of the patient's willingness to accept the proposed care

language during discussions with minors, and information must be provided in a manner that respects the cognitive abilities of the child or adolescent. Clinicians should use these opportunities to elicit information regarding their pediatric patient's value-based treatment goals and to assess whether there is adequate capacity for understanding and decision-making. Only patients who have appropriate decisional capacity and who meet legal requirements can give their informed consent to medical care. Parents or other surrogates technically provide "informed permission" for diagnosis and treatment, with the assent of the child whenever appropriate.[2] When defined as agreement with proposed interventions, assent from children even as young as 7 years can foster the moral growth and development of autonomy in young patients.[2,5–7] This consideration is based on an understanding that, starting around 7 years of age, children enter the concrete operations stage of development, allowing for limited logical thought processes and the ability to develop a reasoned decision.[8–11]

A stricter interpretation of assent requires that the minor meet all of the elements of an adult informed consent, a requirement

that challenges obtaining assent at younger ages. Alternatively, a developmental approach to assent anticipates different levels of understanding from children as they age.[6] At a minimum, assent should include the elements listed in Table 2. Note that one should not solicit a child's assent if the treatment or intervention is required to satisfy goals of care agreed on by the physician and parent or surrogate, but the patient should be told that fact and should not be deceived. Providing disclosure of appropriate diagnostic and treatment information and allowing choices about aspects of care, when possible, should be a consistent part of the care plan for children.

Completely voluntary choice in treatments may be illusory in general, but is particularly so in pediatric care. Clinicians should be aware that parental decision-making can be influenced by the quality of the clinician-patient relationship, previous medical knowledge, emotional distress, faith, and critical changes in a child's health status.[12] Decision-making by children and adolescents is usually influenced by their parents' point of view and may not be entirely voluntary or autonomous. Unless there is significant coercion perceived

TABLE 3 Standards for Surrogate Decision-Making in Pediatrics

Best-interest standard	Surrogate should aim to maximize benefits and minimize harms to the patient, while using a holistic view of the patient's interests
Harm principle	Identify a harm threshold below which parental decisions will not be tolerated
Constrained parental autonomy	Parents may balance the best interest of the patient with the family's best interest if the patient's basic needs are met
Shared, family-centered decision-making	Process that builds on collaborative mechanism between families and clinicians

by clinicians, this situation is not unacceptable, because medical decision-making cannot, and should not, occur in a vacuum, isolated from all other concerns. Medical decision-making is not a discrete event but evolves over time among the health care team, family, and pediatric patient as new information becomes available.

FRAMEWORK FOR DECISION-MAKING

Although commonly used in adult practice, substituted judgment is an uncommon standard for decision-making in the pediatric setting. An exception occurs when mature adolescents, usually those with chronic diseases, have expressed wishes about goals of care before deterioration of cognitive function. These wishes may be respected by parents and physicians in a manner similar to surrogate decision-making for adults. The opportunity to provide guidance about their future medical care should be discussed during their ongoing health care in a manner consistent with their cognitive development and maturity.

Parents generally are better situated than others to understand the unique needs of their children and to make appropriate, caring decisions regarding their children's health care. This is not an absolute legal right, however, because the state also has a societal interest in protecting the child from harm (the doctrine of *parens patriae*) and can challenge parental authority in situations in which a minor is put at significant risk of serious harm or neglect. Parental decision-making should primarily be understood as

parents' responsibility to support the interests of their child and to preserve family relationships, rather than being focused on their rights to express their own autonomous choices. By moving the conversation from parental rights toward parental responsibility, clinicians may help families minimize conflicts encountered in the course of more serious and difficult medical decision-making.

Medical decision-making in pediatrics is informed by the cultural, social, and religious diversity of physicians, patients, and families. The AAP recommends that infants, children, and adolescents, regardless of parental religious beliefs, receive effective medical treatment when such treatment is likely to prevent substantial harm, serious disability, or death.[13] Clinicians must balance the need to work collaboratively with all parents/families, respecting their cultures, religions, and the importance of the families' autonomy and intimacy with the need to protect children from serious and imminent harm. For some mature adolescents, it must be recognized that they may either endorse or reject the tenets of their parent's faith over time.

Several standards for pediatric decision-making have emerged in the literature (see Table 3). Historically, medical decision-making in minors has centered on the best-interest standard, which directs the surrogate to maximize benefits and minimize harms to the minor.[14] A broader approach for using the best-interest standard is to acknowledge the pediatric patient's emotional, social, and medical concerns along with the

interests of the child's family in the process of medical decision-making.

The harm principle may be seen as a more realistic standard to apply in pediatric surrogate medical decision-making. The intent of the harm principle is not to identify a single course of action that is in the minor's best interest or is the physician's preferred approach, but to identify a harm threshold below which parental decisions will not be tolerated and outside intervention is indicated to protect the child.[15]

The model of constrained parental autonomy[16] allows parents, as surrogate decision-makers, to balance the "best interest" of the minor patient with his or her understanding of the family's best interests as long as the child's basic needs, medical and otherwise, are met. A parent's authority is not absolute but constrained by respect for the child.

Shared, family-centered decision-making, although not a standard, is an increasingly used process for pediatric medical decision-making and builds on collaborative communication between families and clinicians.[17]

THE CHILD/ADOLESCENT AS MEDICAL DECISION-MAKER

Pediatric practice is unique in that developmental maturation of the child allows for increasing longitudinal inclusion of the child's opinion in the decision-making process. Encouraging pediatric patients to actively explore options and to take on a greater role in their health care may promote empowerment and compliance with a treatment plan. With this in mind, informed consent/assent should be recognized as an essential part of health care practice.

Adolescent decision-making is dependent on several factors, including cognitive ability, maturity of judgment, and moral authority, which may not all proceed to maturation along the same timeline. Many minors reach the formal operational stage of cognitive development that allows abstract thinking and the ability to handle complex tasks by midadolescence.[18,19] Brain remodeling with enhanced connectivity generally proceeds through the third decade of life, with the prefrontal cortex, the site of executive functions and impulse control, among the last to mature. In contrast, the risk-taking and sensation-seeking areas (limbic and paralimbic regions) develop around puberty. This temporal imbalance or "gap" between the 2 systems can lead to the risky behavior seen in adolescence.[20] A detailed discussion of the neurologic maturation of the adolescent brain is beyond the scope of this policy statement, and the reader is referred to the accompanying technical report.[4]

The implications for decision-making by adolescents in stressful health care environments are that they may rely more on their mature limbic system (socioemotional) rather than on the impulse-controlling, less-developed prefrontal cognitive system.[21]

Dissent by the pediatric patient should carry considerable weight when the proposed intervention is not essential and/or can be deferred without substantial risk.

If the likely benefits of treatment in conditions with a good prognosis outweigh the burdens, parents should choose a treatment plan over the objections or dissent of the minor, as in choosing an appendectomy for acute appendicitis. In general, adolescents should not be allowed to refuse life-saving treatment even when parents agree with the child.[22-24] In medical scenarios with a poor prognosis and burdensome or unproven interventions, more consideration should be given by the physician to advocating for the cognitively mature teenager who wants to refuse treatment and uphold an adolescent's assent or refusal for further attempts at curative treatments.[25]

Although there is still no bright line demarcating when a minor becomes "mature" enough to independently satisfy the decision-making criteria for informed consent or refusal, the courts have weighed in on this issue with a variety of outcomes, which are detailed in the accompanying technical report.[4]

When conflicts about goals of treatment persist despite guidance by the physician and a collaborative approach with the patient and family, the primary health care team should enlist the involvement of consultants, including ethics consultation, psychologists, psychiatrists, chaplains, and, when appropriate, an integrated palliative care team. Seeking legal intervention should be a last resort.

EXCEPTIONS TO LIMITATIONS ON ADOLESCENT MEDICAL DECISION-MAKING

There are 3 broad categories of when a minor can legally make decisions regarding his or her own health care: exceptions based on specific diagnostic/care categories, the "mature minor" exception, and legal emancipation. The legal ability of adolescents to consent for health care needs related to sexual activity, including treatment of sexually transmitted infections, contraceptive services, and prenatal care, is recognized in all states. There has been a similar expansion regarding adolescents' access to mental health and substance abuse prevention and treatment services. These changes reflect a public health concern that adolescents will not access these services if parental consent is required. However, state statutes that permit adolescents to consent to these services do not always protect their confidentiality. Practitioners should become familiar with their state statutes on these issues and consider promoting changes in legislation to improve adolescent confidentiality protection where appropriate.[26]

The mature-minor doctrine recognizes that there is a subset of adolescents who have adequate maturity and intelligence to understand and appreciate an intervention's benefits, risks, likelihood of success, and alternatives and can reason and choose voluntarily. Most states have mature-minor statutes in which the minor's age, overall maturity, cognitive abilities, and social situation as well as the gravity of the medical situation are considered in a judicial determination, finding that an otherwise legally incompetent minor is sufficiently mature to make a legally binding decision and provide his or her own consent for medical care.

In distinction, emancipated minor statutes do not address decision-making ability, but rather, the legal and social status of the minor. Adolescents living separately from their parents and self-supporting, married, or on active duty with the armed forces are generally considered legally emancipated and able to provide informed consent or refusal for their own medical care.

In all states, adolescent parents, similar to other parents, are presumed to be the appropriate decision-makers for their children and may give informed consent for their child's medical care. This right reflects the adolescent's status as a parent. There is clearly a concerning paradox encountered when adolescents are allowed to make complex medical decisions for their child but cannot legally direct their own medical care.[27]

EMERGENCY EXCEPTIONS TO INFORMED CONSENT

Children may present with emergency medical conditions without a parent or legal guardian available to provide consent.[28] In addition to common and statutory law generally supporting the provision of emergently needed care, the Emergency Medical Treatment and Active Labor Act mandates that a medical screening examination and delivery of appropriate medical care for the pediatric patient with an urgent or emergent condition should never be withheld or delayed because of problems with obtaining consent in these situations in which a parent or guardian is not available.

INFORMED CONSENT/ASSENT/REFUSAL IN RESEARCH INVOLVING CHILDREN AND ADOLESCENTS

In distinction from clinical practice, there are clear federal mandates in research to obtain assent from the child research subject and informed permission from a subject's parent(s). A minor's dissent from study participation is also respected. Although assent is mandated, guidelines for how to obtain assent for research and at what age are not explicit. Similar to concerns raised regarding adolescent refusal of life-saving therapy in the clinical arena, the institutional review board can provide a waiver from requiring assent if the research has the potential for an important direct benefit that is only available in the context of research.[29]

RECOMMENDATIONS

1. Physicians should involve pediatric patients in their health care decision-making by providing information on their illness and options for diagnosis and treatment in a developmentally appropriate manner and seeking assent to medical care whenever appropriate.

2. Parents should generally be recognized as the appropriate ethical and legal surrogate medical decision-makers for their children and adolescents. This recognition affirms parents' intimate understanding of their children's interests and respects the importance of family autonomy.

3. Surrogate decision-making by parents or guardians for pediatric patients should seek to maximize benefits for the child by balancing health care needs with social and emotional needs within the context of overall family goals, religious and cultural beliefs, and values.

4. Physicians should recognize that some pediatric patients, especially older adolescents and those with medical experience because of chronic illness, may possess adequate capacity, cognitive ability, and judgment to engage effectively in the informed consent or refusal process for proposed goals of care.

5. The dilemma of an adolescent treatment refusal is ethically and emotionally challenging. Instances in which treatment burdens may outweigh benefits and fail to achieve a curative end should mandate thoughtful guidance from the physician, with continued communication among the patient, surrogates, and health care team to clarify values and treatment goals. Knowledge of individual state laws on adolescent treatment refusals is critical in these situations.

6. Physicians have both a moral obligation and a legal responsibility to question and, if necessary, to contest both the surrogate's and the patient's medical decisions if they put the patient at significant risk of serious harm.

7. Physicians must realize that informed consent/permission/assent/refusal constitutes a process, not a discrete event, and requires the sharing of information in ongoing physician-patient-family communication and education.

8. Physicians must have access to and understanding of their specific state statutes governing the care of sexually transmitted infections, provision of contraceptive and abortion services, mental health and substance abuse treatment, and the definition and care of the emancipated minor and adolescents who possess decision-making capacity (mature minors). These statutes may not include protection of adolescent confidentiality.

9. Physicians who are involved in clinical research must understand both the special place of assent in the process of enrolling children in clinical research trials and the specific additional protections that regulate the participation of children and adolescents as research subjects.

LEAD AUTHORS

Aviva L. Katz, MD, FAAP
Sally A. Webb, MD, FAAP

COMMITTEE ON BIOETHICS, 2015–2016

Aviva L. Katz, MD, FAAP, Chairperson
Robert C. Macauley, MD, FAAP
Mark R. Mercurio, MD, MA, FAAP
Margaret R. Moon, MD, FAAP

Alexander L. Okun, MD, FAAP
Douglas J. Opel, MD, MPH, FAAP
Mindy B. Statter, MD, FAAP

CONTRIBUTING FORMER COMMITTEE MEMBERS

Mary E. Fallat, MD, FAAP, Past Chairperson
Sally A. Webb, MD
Kathryn L. Weise, MD

LIAISONS

Mary Lynn Dell, MD, DMin — *American Academy of Child and Adolescent Psychiatry*

Douglas S. Diekema, MD, MPH — *American Board of Pediatrics*
Dawn Davies, MD, FRCPC, MA — *Canadian Pediatric Society*
Sigal Klipstein, MD — *American College of Obstetricians and Gynecologists*

FORMER LIAISONS

Kevin W. Coughlin, MD, FAAP — *Canadian Pediatric Society*
Steven J. Ralston, MD — *American College of Obstetricians and Gynecologists*
Monique A. Spillman, MD, PhD — *American College of Obstetricians and Gynecologists*

LEGAL CONSULTANTS

Nanette Elster, JD, MPH
Jessica Wilen Berg, JD, MPH

STAFF

Florence Rivera, MPH
Alison Baker, MS

ABBREVIATION

AAP: American Academy of Pediatrics

FINANCIAL DISCLOSURE: The authors have indicated they do not have a financial relationship relevant to this article to disclose.

FUNDING: No external funding.

POTENTIAL CONFLICT OF INTEREST: The authors have indicated they have no potential conflicts of interest to disclose.

REFERENCES

1. American Academy of Pediatrics. Consent. *Pediatrics*. 1976;57(3):414–416

2. American Academy of Pediatrics, Committee on Bioethics. Informed consent, parental permission, and assent in pediatric practice. *Pediatrics*. 1995;95(2):314–317

3. Lee KJ, Havens PL, Sato TT, Hoffman GM, Leuthner SR. Assent for treatment: clinician knowledge, attitudes, and practice. *Pediatrics*. 2006;118(2):723–730

4. American Academy of Pediatrics, Committee on Bioethics. Informed consent in decision making in pediatrics. *Pediatrics*. 2016;138(2):e20161485

5. Denham EJ, Nelson RM. Self-determination is not an appropriate model for understanding parental permission and child assent. *Anesth Analg*. 2002;94(5):1049–1051

6. Miller VA, Nelson RM. A developmental approach to child assent for nontherapeutic research. *J Pediatr*. 2006;149(1 suppl):S25–S30

7. Unguru Y, Coppes MJ, Kamani N. Rethinking pediatric assent: from requirement to ideal. *Pediatr Clin North Am*. 2008;55(1):211–222, xii

8. Pretzlaff RK. Should age be a deciding factor in ethical decision-making? *Health Care Anal*. 2005;13(2):119–128

9. Ruhe KM, Wangmo T, Badarau DO, Elger BS, Niggli F. Decision-making capacity of children and adolescents—suggestions for advancing the concept's implementation in pediatric healthcare. *Eur J Pediatr*. 2015;174(6):775–782

10. Moore L, Kirk S. A literature review of children's and young people's participation in decisions relating to health care. *J Clin Nurs*. 2010;19(15–16):2215–2225

11. Miller VA, Drotar D, Kodish E. Children's competence for assent and consent: a review of empirical findings. *Ethics Behav*. 2004;14(3):255–295

12. Lipstein EA, Brinkman WB, Britto MT. What is known about parents' treatment decisions? A narrative review of pediatric decision making. *Med Decis Making*. 2012;32(2):246–258

13. American Academy of Pediatrics Committee on Bioethics. Religious objections to medical care. *Pediatrics*. 1997;99(2):279–281

14. Kopelman LM. The best-interests standard as threshold, ideal, and standard of reasonableness. *J Med Philos*. 1997;22(3):271–289

15. Diekema DS. Parental refusals of medical treatment: the harm principle as threshold for state intervention. *Theor Med Bioeth*. 2004;25(4):243–264

16. Ross L. *Children, Families, and Health Care Decision-Making*. New York, NY: Oxford University Press; 1998

17. Committee on Hospital Care, American Academy of Pediatrics. Family-centered care and the pediatrician's role. *Pediatrics*. 2003;112(3 pt 1):691–697

18. Weithorn LA, Campbell SB. The competency of children and adolescents to make informed treatment decisions. *Child Dev*. 1982;53(6):1589–1598

19. McCabe MA. Involving children and adolescents in medical decision making: developmental and clinical considerations. *J Pediatr Psychol*. 1996;21(4):505–516

20. Steinberg L. A dual systems model of adolescent risk-taking. *Dev Psychobiol*. 2010;52(3):216–224

21. Johnson SB, Blum RW, Giedd JN. Adolescent maturity and the brain: the promise and pitfalls of neuroscience research in adolescent health policy. *J Adolesc Health*. 2009;45(3):216–221

22. Diekema DS. Adolescent refusal of lifesaving treatment: are we asking the right questions? *Adolesc Med State Art Rev*. 2011;22(2):213–228, viii

23. De Lourdes Levy M, Larcher V, Kurz R; Ethics Working Group of the Confederation of European Specialists in Paediatrics. Statement of the Ethics Working Group of the Confederation

of European Specialists in Paediatrics (CESP). Informed consent/assent in children. *Eur J Pediatr.* 2003;162(9):629–633

24. Ross LF. Against the tide: arguments against respecting a minor's refusal of efficacious life-saving treatment. *Camb Q Healthc Ethics.* 2009;18(3):302–315; discussion: 315–322

25. Pousset G, Bilsen J, De Wilde J, et al. Attitudes of adolescent cancer survivors toward end-of-life decisions for minors. *Pediatrics.* 2009;124(6).

Available at: www.pediatrics.org/cgi/content/full/124/6/e1142

26. Guttmacher Institute. Preventing cervical cancer: new resources to advance the domestic and global fight. *Guttmacher Policy Review.* Winter 2012;15:1. Available at: www.guttmacher.org/pubs/gpr/15/1/gpr150108.html. Accessed October 28, 2013

27. Mercurio MR. Adolescent mothers of critically ill newborns: addressing the rights of parent and child. *Adolesc*

Med State Art Rev. 2011;22(2): 240–250, ix

28. Committee on Pediatric Emergency Medicine; Committee on Bioethics. Consent for emergency medical services for children and adolescents. *Pediatrics.* 2011;128(2):427–433

29. Wendler D, Belsky L, Thompson KM, Emanuel EJ. Quantifying the federal minimal risk standard: implications for pediatric research without a prospect of direct benefit. *JAMA.* 2005;294(7):826–832

Informed Consent in Decision-Making in Pediatric Practice

● ●

- *Technical Report*

TECHNICAL REPORT

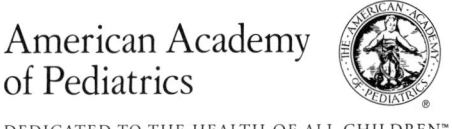

American Academy
of Pediatrics

DEDICATED TO THE HEALTH OF ALL CHILDREN™

Informed Consent in Decision-Making in Pediatric Practice

Aviva L. Katz, MD, FAAP, Sally A. Webb, MD, FAAP, COMMITTEE ON BIOETHICS

abstract

Informed consent should be seen as an essential part of health care practice; parental permission and childhood assent is an active process that engages patients, both adults and children, in their health care. Pediatric practice is unique in that developmental maturation allows, over time, for increasing inclusion of the child's and adolescent's opinion in medical decision-making in clinical practice and research. This technical report, which accompanies the policy statement "Informed Consent in Decision-Making in Pediatric Practice" was written to provide a broader background on the nature of informed consent, surrogate decision-making in pediatric practice, information on child and adolescent decision-making, and special issues in adolescent informed consent, assent, and refusal. It is anticipated that this information will help provide support for the recommendations included in the policy statement.

DOI: 10.1542/peds.2016-1485

PEDIATRICS (ISSN Numbers: Print, 0031-4005; Online, 1098-4275).

FINANCIAL DISCLOSURE: The authors have indicated they do not have a financial relationship relevant to this article to disclose.

FUNDING: No external funding.

POTENTIAL CONFLICT OF INTEREST: The authors have indicated they have no potential conflicts of interest to disclose.

To cite: Katz AL, Webb SA, AAP COMMITTEE ON BIOETHICS. Informed Consent in Decision-Making in Pediatric Practice. *Pediatrics.* 2016;138(2):e20161485

Since the publication of previous American Academy of Pediatrics (AAP) statements on informed consent in 1976[1] and 1995,[2] obtaining informed permission from parents or legal guardians before medical interventions on pediatric patients is now standard within our medical and legal culture. The 1995 statement also championed, as pediatrician William Bartholome stated, "the experience, perspective and power of children" in the collaboration between pediatricians, their patients, and parents and remains an essential guide for modern ethical pediatric practice.[2] As recommended in the 1995 publication, the revised policy statement[3] affirms that patients should participate in decision-making commensurate with their development; they should provide assent to care whenever reasonable.

Although some aspects of decision-making in pediatrics are evolving in response to changes in information technology, scientific discoveries, and legal rulings, recent reports have noted that change can be slow. Despite the long-standing stance of the AAP that older children and adolescents should be involved in the medical decision-making and consent process, there still has not been widespread understanding and endorsement among practitioners of the concept of pediatric assent or refusal.[4-6]

The discordance between current clinical practice and previously published guidance may reflect the gradual evolution of change within the culture of medicine or perhaps suggests a need to build on the discussion of informed consent, assent, and refusal for children and adolescents. The purpose of this technical report is to provide a firm grounding of the concept of informed consent, addressing both the legal and philosophical roots, to provide information on a variety of standards applicable for decision-making by surrogates for pediatric patients and to discuss how issues of assent, refusal, and consent affect the care of children and adolescents in a variety of clinical and research settings.

For purposes of this report, we will define and use the following terms: a pediatric patient or a minor who has not reached the legal age of majority (in most states, 18 years of age) is a patient younger than 18 years; an adolescent refers to a person in the transition between childhood and adulthood, classically defined as 13 to 18 years of age; a child refers to a person from the ages of 1 through 12 years; and an infant refers to a person in the first year of life.

HISTORY AND NATURE OF INFORMED CONSENT

The current concept of informed consent in medical practice has roots within both ethical theory and law. The support for informed consent in ethical theory is most commonly found in the concept of autonomy, the right of an autonomous agent to make decisions as guided by his or her own reason.[7] As a brief description, informed consent incorporates 2 duties: disclosing information to patients and their surrogates and obtaining legal authorization before undertaking any interventions. The historical shift in US medical practice from paternalism to respect for individual

autonomy was shaped by events in the 20th century, such as the distrust of the medical profession after the Nuremburg trial of Nazi doctors, widespread publicity regarding research ethics violations, the turbulence of the civil rights and women's rights movements, and the long-standing American characteristic of individualism. This long-standing American emphasis on individualism correlated with an increased interest in and attention to the issue of informed consent.[8,9]

Autonomy (from the ancient Greek *autos* [self] and *nomos* [rule or law]) can be seen as derived from Kantian moral philosophy, with key elements of liberty, the capacity to live life according to your own reasons and motives, and agency, the rational capacity for intentional action. A formulation of Kant's categorical imperative notes that we are obliged to act out of fundamental respect for other persons by virtue of their personal autonomy. This imperative forms the moral basis to respect others and ourselves as moral equals and provides moral support for the concept of informed consent. Although many, if not most, patients in pediatric practice lack the agency required to be truly autonomous agents, this framework remains important in providing the background for continued respect of their moral potential.

In pediatrics, the duties to protect and promote health-related interests of the child and adolescent by the physician are also grounded in the fiduciary relationship (to act in the best interest of the patient and subordinating one's own interests) between the physician and patient, but these duties may conflict with the parent's or patient's wishes and set up tensions either within the family or between the family and the physician. Most believe that parents have an ethically parallel fiduciary obligation to protect and promote both the health-related and

the non–health-related interests of their child or adolescent, with the pediatrician and the parents acting as "co-fiduciaries" for health matters.[10] This provides a conceptual framework for moving the discussion from parental rights to parental responsibility when considering pediatric medical decision-making and informed consent.

Appropriate decisional capacity and legal empowerment are the determinants of decision-making authority in medicine. A reliance on individual liberties and autonomy in the pediatric patient is not realistic or legally accepted, so parents or other surrogates provide "informed permission" for diagnosis and treatment, with the assent of the child as developmentally appropriate.[2] However, the goals of the informed consent process (protecting and promoting health-related interests and incorporating the patient and/or the family in health care decision-making) are similar in the pediatric and adult population and are grounded by the same ethical principles of beneficence, justice, and respect for autonomy. As we will discuss further, in pediatric care we often need to expand our understanding of autonomy to recognize the autonomy of the family unit, allowing respect for both the privacy of the family unit, within limits, and parental authority and responsibility for medical decision-making.

Although the requirement of "simple" consent by patients for surgical procedures dates back to 18th-century English law, it was only in the 1950s that the American courts began to develop the doctrine of true "informed" consent from patients through disclosure of facts by physicians. The term "informed consent" is derived from the ruling in *Salgo v Leland Stanford Jr University Board of Trustees* in 1957.[11] This term was adopted verbatim from an *amicus curiae* brief filed by the

American College of Surgeons: "A physician violates his duty to his patient and subjects himself to liability if he withholds any facts which are necessary to form the basis of an intelligent consent... in discussing the element of risk a certain amount of discretion must be employed consistent with the full disclosure of facts necessary to an informed consent."

The judgment in this case identified the need for a full disclosure of the facts necessary to form an informed consent. Later cases (*Mitchell v Robinson, Natanson v Kline*)[8,9] shaped our modern understanding of the required elements of disclosure during the consent process by mandating disclosure of risks, the nature of the medical condition, details of the proposed treatment, the probability of success, and possible alternative treatments. The standard of what information must be included in discussions leading to informed consent or informed refusal of treatment has evolved over time and varies somewhat from state to state.[9]

THE PROCESS OF INFORMED CONSENT

Several different but common standards for the physician's disclosure obligation have emerged. The professional community standard defines adequate disclosure by what the trained and experienced physician tells his or her patient. The objective, reasonable person standard requires the physician to disclose information that a reasonable person in the patient's condition would need and want to know.[9] A small minority of states use the subjective standard of what a particular patient would need to know to make a decision to evaluate the extent of disclosure. Physicians should make substantial efforts to craft disclosures that maximize understanding by all surrogates or patients regardless of developmental maturity, severity of illness,

educational limitations, or language barriers.

Pediatricians should be adept at explaining information to their young patients in an age-appropriate and descriptive manner. This vital skill, if not a standard, enhances the assent and permission process in pediatrics. Although the ability of the child or adolescent to provide assent or consent changes along with cognitive development and maturation, disclosure of the medical condition and the anticipated interventions in a developmentally appropriate manner demonstrates respect for the patient's emerging autonomy and may help enhance cooperation with medical care. The pediatrician and pediatric medical subspecialist should have an understanding of the spectrum of intellectual disability encountered in childhood and adolescence and should be prepared to provide the individualized support needed to maximize understanding of the disease process and therapeutic options.

The content of the informed consent discussion is closely linked with professional experience. Disclosure of risks may differ between physicians in community and academic settings, between younger and older physicians, or among those who perform minimally invasive compared with open procedures.[12] During disclosure to the patient and/ or the surrogate regarding treatment options, many believe it is important for the physician to disclose his or her or the facility's own experience with the proposed intervention and periprocedural complications. The issue of disclosure of surgeon-specific outcome data has been addressed recently in the surgical literature.[13,14] Although the potential advantages of this disclosure may include enhanced patient autonomy and understanding during decision-making, some critics contend the accuracy of surgeon-specific performance rates is often illusory because of a variety of

limitations and generally not truly available for thoughtful discussion in the informed consent process.[13] Transparency and honesty in discussing provider experience with patients and families are critical, and there is case law on this issue, with the court finding that, in certain instances, physician-specific data may be material in allowing a fully informed consent.[15]

Although informed consent is usually thought of as linked to surgical or invasive interventions in health care, the same process of disclosure of potential diagnosis, options for evaluation and treatment, likely outcomes, and potential associated risks is also necessary to ensure that medical decision-making for routine or noninvasive clinical treatments is transparent to patients and families.

SEEKING INFORMED CONSENT

Knowledge about a medical condition is critical to making informed health care decisions by and for adults, adolescents, children, and infants. Informed consent is not satisfied by merely obtaining a signature on a form but is a process of dialog with a patient about a planned course of action. The first part of that dialog is determining whether the patient and/or his or her family/surrogate are capable of understanding the information one discloses. The terms "capacity" and "competence" are frequently blurred in medical discourse. Capacity is a clinical determination that addresses the integrity of mental abilities, and competence is a legal determination that addresses society's interest in restricting decision-making when capacity is in question.[16] Pediatricians can determine whether an adolescent is capable of making health care decisions, and the courts generally determine competence. It is also important to understand that an individual can still have decision-making capacity while being declared legally incompetent. This situation is typically illustrated when an adult with newly diagnosed dementia is still able to participate and make health care decisions but is incompetent to manage financial affairs, as determined by the courts. It is critical to recognize that capacity is not an all-or-none phenomenon and is relatively task specific. A patient may have the capacity to participate in certain areas of medical decision-making but may not have the capacity to contribute in more complex discussions, such as end-of-life decision-making. In addition, it is important to recognize that neither capacity nor competence is permanent and may fluctuate over time and should be reassessed over the course of illness, as indicated.

As informed consent and, more recently, assent in pediatrics have evolved over the 50 years since the Salgo case, certain elements of the process listed as follows serve as the framework for conversations with our patients and their families.[2] It is vital that throughout the process, the health care professional understands that providing information and obtaining permission, consent, or assent are 2 different, although linked, functions.

1. Provision of information: patients and their surrogates should be provided explanations, in understandable, developmentally appropriate language, of the nature of their illness or condition; the nature of the proposed diagnostic steps and/ or treatments and the probability of their success; the existence and nature of the risks and anticipated benefits involved; and the existence, potential benefits, and risks of potential alternative treatments, including the option of no treatment.

2. The patient's and/or surrogate's understanding of the above information should be assessed.

3. Because decisional capacity is a critical requirement in providing consent, the capacity of the patient and/or surrogate to make the necessary decisions should be assessed (often, assessment of the capacity to make decisions and the understanding of the pertinent medical information occurs simultaneously).

4. There should be assurance, insofar as is possible through ongoing dialog, that the consent is voluntary and that the patient and/or surrogate has the freedom to choose among the medical alternatives without undue influence, coercion, or manipulation. This condition recognizes that we are all subject to subtle pressures in decision-making and that medical decision0making cannot occur in isolation from other concerns and relationships.

The process of informed consent requires participation by the physician or health care provider of record. In teaching hospitals or clinics, it is ethically and legally inappropriate to permit medical students to obtain informed consent from parents or patients without the support and involvement of more senior, knowledgeable staff. Medical students lack the comprehensive medical knowledge required to provide adequate information for a truly informed consent. Junior house staff may also not have sufficient knowledge to satisfy condition number 1 listed above and will need education from more experienced physicians to assist in the dialog with patients and surrogates. Both medical students and junior house staff benefit from opportunities to observe attending physicians engage patients and families in informed consent discussions and may assist in providing initial information to patients and families and by answering questions that fall within their level of understanding.[17,18]

Patient or surrogate comprehension of procedural consent has been reported to be <50% in the adult surgical literature.[19] Similarly, studies of recall and comprehension by parents and pediatric research subjects after informed consent discussions reveal that parents and subjects have far greater understanding of their research rights than the clinical implications of the interventions.[20] New strategies to improve patient literacy and recall during consent are being developed and include multimedia presentations, requirements for "repeat back" elements of the proposed interventions, and trying to increase the time spent in the informed consent discussion.[19,20]

How one shares this information is also crucial to building a successful, trusting relationship with children, adolescents, and their parents/ guardians and is critical to achieving the goals of treatment. The event model, in which discrete interventions are seen as a one-shot encounter and patients and their surrogates are left to accept or reject a physician-formulated plan, is inferior to the process model, in which medical decision-making is a longitudinal process over time, with information shared between the physician and the patient/surrogate.[9] This process model, which recognizes that a multitude of decisions are made throughout the medical course as new information emerges, fosters better communication and understanding between clinicians and patients/surrogates. An example of the importance in framing medical decision-making as a longitudinal process that takes shape over time is the care of a critically ill child undergoing resuscitation and stabilization in the ICU. A broad discussion of the many elements that may be required for resuscitation is clearly required, but individualized consent for each element, especially in the likely condensed time frame is not, as long as there has been an overarching discussion and agreement on the goals of care and an understanding of the likely intensity of interventions required. A more interactive role for the decision-maker and/or patient in informed consent and pediatric assent may improve understanding and ownership of the medical condition and its management and often improves compliance with recommended care.

STANDARDS FOR SURROGATE DECISION-MAKING FOR CHILDREN AND ADOLESCENTS

A deeper understanding of the issue of assent and consent in childhood is facilitated by distancing oneself from the potentially confrontational and legalistic approach of respect for individual autonomy as an overarching principle in pediatrics. A more nuanced approach, incorporating respect for the pediatric patient's medical experience, for family dynamics, and for emerging data on adolescent cognitive development and decision-making, allows for alternative models for both child and surrogate decision-making.

Before discussing models and standards for decision-making in pediatrics, it is helpful to appreciate the complexity of how decisions are made by parents and surrogates. A recent literature review of 55 research articles on the process of treatment decision-making noted that decisions are influenced by such things as provider relationships, previous knowledge, changes in a child's health status, emotions, and faith.[21] Parental distress presents a challenge for good informed decision-making. Parents who receive new diagnoses of cancer or other life-threatening illnesses in their children report burdensome emotional and psychological stress that can interfere with

decision-making.[22-24] Parental coping mechanisms and their perceptions of undue external influence by clinicians or family members on decision-making may result in hostile and uncertain feelings about treatment goals for their seriously ill children.[24] Clinicians should be aware of the effects of stress and uncertainty on autonomous parental decision-making and choose effective communication strategies to limit these negative effects.

When compared with surrogate decision-making that uses substituted judgment for adults who have lost the capacity to make their own medical decisions, surrogate decision-making for infants, children, and adolescents draws from different constructs, such as the best-interest standard, harm principle, constrained parental autonomy, and shared, family-centered decision-making. With substituted judgment, a standard often used in surrogate decision-making for incapacitated adults who previously had the capacity for medical decision-making, surrogates "substitute" their understanding of the patient's known preferences and values in determining goals of treatment. It is important to note that this is an uncommon decision-making model in pediatrics, because most children and many adolescents cannot or have not stated known preferences that are based on their level of understanding and are reflective of core values that an adult with capacity may have had an opportunity to share. In cases in which adolescents, usually those with chronic debilitating diseases, have had the capacity to express wishes about goals of care before deterioration of cognitive function or the onset of overwhelming illness, the substituted judgment standard should be respected by families and the health care team. The opportunity to provide this guidance about their future medical care should be discussed with adolescents during

their ongoing health care in a manner consistent with their cognitive development and maturity.

Parents generally are better situated than others to understand the unique needs of their children and family and make appropriate, caring decisions regarding their children's health care. This parental responsibility for medical decision-making in caring for their child or young adult is not an absolute right, however, because the state also has a societal interest in protecting the child or young adult from harm and can challenge parental authority in situations in which the child or young adult is put at risk (the doctrine of *parens patriae*).

Pediatric health care providers have legal and ethical duties to provide a standard of care that meets the pediatric patient's needs and not necessarily what the parents desire or request. Parental decision-making should primarily be understood as parents' responsibility to support the interests of their child and to preserve family relationships, rather than being focused on their rights to express their own autonomous choices. It is important to note that parental authority regarding medical decision-making for their minor child or young adult who lacks the capacity for medical decision-making is constrained compared with the more robust autonomy in medical decision-making enjoyed by competent adults making decisions regarding their own care. By moving the conversation from parental rights toward parental responsibility, clinicians may help families minimize conflicts encountered in the course of difficult medical decision-making. It is important to recognize that just as there may be conflict between the family and the health care team, there may also be conflict between the patient's parents. Conflict between parents may predate the current health care concern or crisis or may reflect a different understanding of what medical intervention is in the best interest of their child. These issues must be acknowledged and addressed in the process of medical decision-making for the patient.

Since publication of the 1995 AAP statement, several frameworks providing guidance for pediatric decision-making have emerged in the literature. Historically and legally, medical decision-making in children has centered on the best-interest standard, which directs the surrogate to maximize benefits and minimize harms to the minor and sets a threshold for intervention in cases of abuse and neglect.[25] The focus is on the pediatric patient rather than on the interests of the caregiver and, as philosophers Buchanan and Brock[26] defined it, "acting so as to promote maximally the good of the individual." Confusion and concern regarding the use of this standard occur if it is interpreted this rigidly, asking the parent to consider the child's absolute best medical interest in isolation, without considering other interests such as finances or family.[25,27] A broader approach for using the best-interest standard acknowledges the pediatric patient's emotional, social, and medical concerns along with the interests of the child's family and strives to maximize benefits and minimize harms within this framework. Best-interest determination in this "ideal" framework may help establish prima facie, rather than absolute, duties to children. Another option is to view best interest as a standard of reasonableness wherein the benefit to burden ratio is balanced such that most rational people would agree with the choice of action.[25]

The harm principle may be seen as a more realistic framework to apply in pediatric surrogate medical decision-making, especially when there is a concern about the child's safety. The goal here is not to identify a single course of action that is in the child's best interest or represents the physician's preferred approach but to identify a harm threshold below which parental decisions will not be tolerated and outside intervention is indicated to protect the child.[27] In addition, when considering intervention, the potential harm to the child by the parental decision must be serious and imminent and a greater threat than the potential harm from state intervention. Diekema[27] stated that if a parental refusal places the child at significant risk of serious harm (eg, refusing a potentially life-saving therapy or a critical therapy of proven efficacy), other questions should be asked to justify state interference: Do the projected benefits of the proposed intervention outweigh the burdens more favorably than the parents' option? Would another option that is less intrusive to parental autonomy prevent the harm? Can state interference be generalized to all other similar cases? Would the public agree that state interference is reasonable? Proponents of the harm principle note that it is a more appropriate standard for determining when to interfere with parental decisions than the best-interest standard, because parents often make decisions that conflict with a child's best medical interest, and this situation is generally tolerated within the context of the overall care of the child and family. These concerns would also apply in considering parental decision-making for young adults who lack the capacity to participate in their own medical decision-making.

The model of constrained parental autonomy[28] allows parents, as surrogate decision-makers, to balance the "best interest" of the minor patient with their understanding of the family's best interests as long as the child's basic needs, medical and otherwise, are met. Rather than best interests, there is the promotion of basic interests, with medical care as a basic interest. This model reinforces that a parent's authority is not absolute but is constrained by their caring and responsibility for the child. An important focus in this model is family autonomy, with the goal of promoting long-term autonomy for the child throughout his or her development within the family setting.

Shared decision-making is a central tenet of the family-centered medical home, especially with respect to children with chronic health conditions. Shared, family-centered decision-making is an increasingly used process for pediatric medical decision-making.[29] This process is dependent on collaborative communication and the exchange of information between the medical team and the family. In addition to the medical team providing information about the patient's disease process and the risks and benefits of treatment options, it is important for family members to share information regarding their goals and values so that care decisions can meet these needs and address each stakeholder's perception of the disease process.

CULTURAL AND RELIGIOUS INFLUENCE ON DECISION-MAKING

Medical decision-making in pediatrics is informed by the cultural, social, and religious diversity of physicians, patients, and families. Understanding this tenet and embracing culturally effective pediatric health care may allow for better incorporation of family values in the informed consent process.[30] Occasionally, parental decisions based on culture or religion may conflict with the medical recommendations. Low health literacy in non–English-speaking families can lead to unfavorable health outcomes. The use of appropriately trained interpreters during the informed consent process is vital to obtain and share relevant information in an easily understandable fashion and to optimize medical treatment of pediatric patients.[30,31]

Other examples of the potential impact of religious and cultural beliefs on medical care include the risk associated with religious-based refusals, such as the refusal of blood transfusions as a life-saving therapy by patients who practice the Jehovah's Witnesses faith, and the refusal to seek medical care when medically necessary, or declining interventions, even in the face of serious illness, by patients who are Christian Scientists. Although adults with the capacity for medical decision-making have the freedom to make decisions that reflect their faith and religious values, even at the risk of serious harm or death, there is clearly a competing state interest in protecting a child from significant risk of serious harm, as noted in the 1944 US Supreme Court ruling *Prince v Massachusetts*.[32] The AAP statement on religious objections to medical care[33] endorses that children, regardless of parental religious beliefs, deserve effective medical treatment when such treatment is not overly burdensome and is likely to prevent substantial harm, serious disability, or death. Clinicians must balance the need to work collaboratively with all parents/families, respecting their culture, religion, and the importance of the family's autonomy and intimacy, with the need to protect children from serious and imminent harm. Clinicians must recognize that failure to provide appropriate care may constitute abuse or neglect, and this situation should not be unreported because of perceived state or federal exemptions for religious groups. This protection is extended until children are able to make such religious decisions for themselves, recognizing that some mature adolescents may either endorse or reject the tenets of their parent's faith over time.

THE CHILD/ADOLESCENT AS MEDICAL DECISION-MAKER

The value of involving children and adolescents in their own medical decision-making is increasingly recognized around the world.[34–37] The respect owed to pediatric patients as participants in the medical decision-making process is dependent on several factors, including cognitive abilities, maturity of judgment, and the respect owed to a moral agent, which may not all proceed to maturation along the same timeline. Children and adolescents are dependent on their parents for most aspects of their daily life and usually have limited experience with making any medical decisions. Although the child or adolescent should be recognized as a moral being with all of the appropriate dignity and rights, they are more vulnerable decision-makers than adults, in significant part because of both inexperience with decision-making and the slow process of maturation of judgment, as reviewed below.

Developmental research in the 1980s concluded that many minors reach the formal operational stage of cognitive development that allows abstract thinking and the ability to handle complex tasks by midadolescence.[38,39] During that time, the Tennessee Supreme Court, in deciding *Cardwell v Bechtol* in 1987,[40] used the "rule of sevens" to uphold the presumption of decision-making capacity for a 17-year-old girl receiving spinal manipulation. This "rule" stated that no capacity exists for children younger than the age of 7 years, a lack of capacity is presumed but may be rebutted with appropriate evidence between the ages 7 and 14 years, and capacity is presumed but may be rebutted at age 14 years and older. Newer insight into brain structure and function now makes the determination of which minors possess the maturity for decision-making much less clear-cut.

For more than a decade, considerable neurobiological research in animals and humans has focused on the complex interaction of brain development and remodeling with social, emotional, and cognitive processes during adolescence. Although the size of the brain nearly reaches its adult size in early childhood, we know from structural MRI studies that much of the brain has continued dynamic changes in gray matter volume and myelination into the third decade of life.[41–44] The prefrontal cortex, where many executive functions are coordinated, including the balancing of risks and rewards, is among the last areas of the brain to mature, with these functions continuing to develop and mature into young adulthood.

Neuropsychological research to link adolescent behaviors such as sensation seeking and risk taking to brain structure and function is ongoing but still speculative in many areas.[45–47] One theory is that adolescents have a dual-systems model of decision-making.[48,49] A "socioemotional" system located in the limbic and paralimbic brain regions is believed to develop around puberty, with increased dopaminergic activity, and manifests as reward-seeking behavior. The "cognitive control" system, which promotes self-regulation and impulse control, is in the prefrontal cortices and gradually develops into the third decade of life. This temporal imbalance or gap between the 2 systems can lead to the risky behavior seen in adolescence and has been analogized to starting a car engine without the benefit of a skilled driver.[50] Or, in other words, the circuitry of reward-related behavior develops earlier than the control-related brain regions.

Other contributors to the risky choices that some adolescents may make include peer pressure and highly complex or stressful situations. Although pubertal changes do affect behavior, as has been mentioned, all changes cannot be attributed to "raging hormones."

On the positive side, late adolescence is also a period during which youth develop a coherent sense of identity, with an increased understanding of their individual beliefs, values, and priorities.[51] The path toward autonomy in the journey from adolescence to adulthood is linked to both intellectual maturity and moral functioning.[52] Early life experiences are paramount in the shaping of moral functioning. With normal development, the integration of emotions, reasoning, and self-reflection with physical and social experiences helps determine the degree of moral intelligence in the transition to adulthood. A coherent sense of identity and stable, deep-seated values are key to making reflective, autonomous decisions required for true informed consent.

Some youth navigate this complex developmental process quite well despite the complex interactions of biology and social context. However, the research to date articulates that, in general, adolescents make decisions differently than adults do, and although they may have cognitive skills, they are more likely to underutilize these skills.[45,53,54] The implications for decision-making by adolescents in stressful health care environments are that they may rely more on their mature limbic system (socioemotional) rather than on the impulse-controlling, less developed prefrontal cognitive system. As clinicians, we should look for evidence of stable, internalized values in adolescent medical decision-making that is reflective of the patient's cognitive maturation. These values are key to the decision-making process and, in difficult situations, may help provide a foundation in developing goals of care.

Some adolescents and young adults with cognitive impairments and special health needs may never develop the capacity to allow meaningful participation in medical decision-making. Parents will need to continue to serve as surrogate decision-makers for these patients, even as these adolescents turn 18 years of age and become adults. The legal issues involved in securing guardianship are beyond the scope of this report.

ASSENT IN PEDIATRIC DECISION-MAKING

Pediatric practice is unique in that the developmental maturation of the child allows for increasing longitudinal inclusion of the child's voice in the decision-making process. Assent from children even as young as 7 years for medical interventions may help them become more involved in their medical care and can foster moral growth and development of autonomy in young patients.[2,55-59] The 1995 AAP statement on informed consent endorses pediatric assent in decision-making. However, the definition and application of assent have lacked consistency in both clinical and research arenas.[55,56] A strict interpretation of assent requires that the child meet all of the elements of an adult informed consent, a requirement that challenges obtaining assent at younger ages. Others seek a developmental approach that would require different levels of understanding from children as they age.[57] At the very least, assent should include the following elements[2]:

1. helping the patient achieve a developmentally appropriate awareness of the nature of his or her condition;

2. telling the patient what he or she can expect with tests and treatments;

3. making a clinical assessment of the patient's understanding of the situation and the factors influencing how he or she is responding (including whether there is inappropriate pressure to accept testing or therapy); and

4. soliciting an expression of the patient's willingness to accept the proposed care.

Note that one should not solicit a child's assent if the treatment or intervention is required; the patient should be told that fact and should not be deceived. A child is not the final decision-maker, the parent or surrogate is. Many recommended medical interventions come with the likelihood of associated pain, invasive procedures, or at a minimum, inconvenience. Parents should balance the anticipated benefits with the level of burdens and risks of such treatments when making decisions for their children about pursuing therapy. If the likely benefits of treatment in conditions with a good prognosis outweigh the burdens, parents may choose a treatment plan over the objections or dissent of the child. A common example of this situation is an appendectomy for acute appendicitis. Regardless of the child's degree of participation in and/or disagreement with the care plan, he or she should still be given as much control over the actual treatment as possible: for example, in determining the location for intravenous catheter placement.

Dissent by the pediatric patient should carry increased weight when the proposed intervention is not essential and/or can be deferred without substantial risk or discomfort to the patient or family. A perceived dilemma with assent is that parents and clinicians may resist incorporating assent into their practice when the stakes are too high if the child dissents, as in the case of an appendectomy for acute appendicitis. In 1 recent survey example, the majority of pediatricians would ignore an adolescent's refusal of treatment when parents are in favor and the prognosis is good.[4] As stated previously in this report, maintaining honesty in communications with patients and families helps to minimize this concern; information should always be provided in a developmentally appropriate manner, but assent should only be solicited if some element of refusal will be respected. In situations with a poor prognosis and interventions associated with a heavy patient burden, more consideration should be given to the adolescent's opportunity to provide assent or refusal.

Encouraging the patient to actively explore options and take on a greater role in his or her health care may promote empowerment and compliance with a treatment plan.[60] There is core philosophical and developmental support for the notion that we all need the opportunity to make choices to create ourselves as moral agents and create a coherent sense of identity.[61]

SPECIAL ISSUES IN ADOLESCENT INFORMED CONSENT/ASSENT/REFUSAL

There are 3 broad categories of circumstances in which a minor can legally make decisions regarding his or her own health care: exceptions based on specific diagnostic/care categories, the mature minor exception, and legal emancipation.

The legal ability of adolescents to consent for health care needs related to sexual activity, including treatment of sexually transmitted infections (STIs) and provision of contraceptive services, prenatal care, and abortion services, has expanded over the past several decades. This change is not specifically related to an acceptance of the adolescents' abilities in medical decision-making. Rather, this is a public health decision and reflects both the concern that adolescents will not seek care for issues that reflect sexual activity if required to involve their parents for consent and an extension of the broad US

Supreme Court rulings regarding the constitutional right to privacy for all on these matters. It is important for the clinician to note the significant variability between states in how the statutes are worded regarding access for these services. The Guttmacher Institute (www.guttmacher.org) is an excellent resource for reviewing state policies on sexual and reproductive health and can be accessed electronically.[62]

Although all states allow access to treatment of STIs, the protection of the adolescent's confidentiality is less widespread. Some states permit the practitioner to disclose information to parents/guardians if they believe it is in the minor's best interest. Many states, insurers, and electronic medical record systems do not make provisions for deferred billing and/or payment for STI services, thus endangering an adolescent's desire for confidentiality. Practitioners are best advised to become familiar with their state statutes and to consider promoting changes in legislation to improve adolescent confidentiality protection where appropriate.[63]

Human papillomavirus (HPV) infection is the most common STI, and several strains of HPV are known to cause cervical cancer, with new data also linking this virus to oral cancers. Primary prevention is available in the form of vaccination, which is recommended for both boys and girls ages 11 through 12 years by the Advisory Committee on Immunization Practices of the Centers for Disease Control and Prevention. It is unknown whether most states will include the HPV primary prevention vaccination in the category of protected STI treatment or general vaccination for which minors may not provide consent.

The majority of states allow some or all adolescents 12 years or older access to contraceptive services and usually do not require parental notification. In contrast,

minor consent to abortion without parental involvement is uncommon: currently, 37 states require parental involvement, although, in general, there is a mechanism by which the minor can petition the court for access to abortion services without parental knowledge or consent.

There is similar variability among the states regarding adolescents' access to mental health and substance abuse prevention and treatment services. The majority of states do allow adolescents to consent to treatment of substance abuse, and importantly, programs receiving federal funding are governed by federal confidentiality regulations that prohibit sharing information regarding treatment without the patient's consent.[64]

The mature minor doctrine recognizes that there is a subset of adolescents who have adequate maturity and capacity to understand and appreciate an intervention's benefits, risks, likelihood of success, and alternatives and can reason and can choose voluntarily. Under the mature minor doctrine, the age, overall maturity, cognitive abilities, and social situation of the minor are considered in a judicial determination, finding that an otherwise legally incompetent minor is sufficiently mature to make a legally binding decision and provide his or her own consent for medical care. In contrast, legally emancipated minor statutes do not address decision-making ability but rather the legal status of the minor. Adolescents who are living separately from their parents and are self-supporting, married, or on active duty with the armed forces are generally considered legally emancipated and competent to make their own decisions and provide consent for medical care.

Although there are significant limitations on adolescents' legal right to consent to their own medical care, all states presume adolescent parents to be the appropriate surrogate decision-makers for their children and allow them to give informed consent for their child's medical care. This right reflects the adolescent's status as a parent, rather than his or her decision-making capacity as a mature or emancipated minor. There is clearly a significant and concerning paradox encountered in allowing adolescents to take responsibility for complex medical decision-making for their infants and children while, in general, "protecting" adolescents from providing assent and directing their own medical care, even in more controlled, low-risk situations. The case of early adolescent parents of critically ill infants is particularly difficult with regard to consent. These parents, often the mother alone without the involvement or support of the infant's father, are generally charged with the responsibility of making important medical decisions for their infants that they would never be permitted to make for themselves or for other relatives.[65,66]

Although this arrangement meets the legal responsibility of recognizing and respecting the adolescent's status as a parent who has a right and responsibility for decision-making for his or her child, it does not appropriately address the ethical issues raised by young adolescent decision-making nor the physician's ethical responsibility to both the adolescent and his or her child. Adolescent parents are in a very vulnerable situation, facing the need to care for a child while still completing important developmental tasks for themselves. Many pediatricians and neonatologists seek permission from the adolescent parent to involve an adult relative, often the maternal grandparents, in crucial decisions regarding the care of the infant. This adult, selected by the mother as her co–decision-maker, can provide mentoring in shared decision-making to the adolescent

parent and may help safeguard the rights and well-being of the infant. Although not required by law, physicians should provide support for the adolescent mother, as needed, in selecting someone to help her provide informed permission for her infant's care.[65,66]

The informed consent process surrounding relatively higher risk, yet elective procedures, such as pectus excavatum repair and bariatric surgery, highlights the complex issue of adolescent medical decision-making. Surgery to repair pectus excavatum is most commonly undertaken in adolescent patients. The evidence to support significant physiologic improvement in cardiorespiratory function as a result of the surgery is limited, and the most common indication for surgery is distress regarding the appearance of the chest wall. Although the surgery is most often completed in a minimally invasive manner, it is not without the risk of complications, including significant postoperative pain, an extended period postoperatively of limitation of activities, the potential for recurrence of the pectus excavatum appearance, and rarely, the risk of cardiac injury and hemorrhage.[67-69] These can be extremely difficult concerns for the adolescent, especially the younger adolescent to consider and balance, because this deliberation includes the need to consider both acute and long-term risks and benefits. In this situation, the surgeon and the health care team must undertake thoughtful, developmentally appropriate conversations with both the adolescent patient and his or her family to provide the medical information needed to make an informed medical decision. In addition, the surgeon and the health care team must work to elicit from the family, but especially from the adolescent patient, their beliefs and concerns about the surgery and their cognitive understanding

of the associated risks and benefits and how these issues affect their medical decision-making. With this process, which includes input from both the family and the health care team, the adolescent should be able to be supported in making either an informed assent or refusal of the surgical procedure. This procedure provides an excellent example of a situation in which a major medical decision must be made but is best made by carefully supporting the adolescent's opportunity to provide assent or refusal, because only he or she can truly weight the risks and benefits as they apply to him or her. Throughout this process, the surgeon and the health care team must also be aware of balance between coercion by the family or health care team as well as the opportunity to support developmentally appropriate decision-making. A considered refusal of surgery by the adolescent should be respected, given the elective nature of the procedure and the associated postoperative pain and risks. Parental requests for surgical intervention must include the adolescent in the discussion, and the need to include the adolescent and respect his or her concerns must be discussed with the family. The surgeon and the health care team may also find themselves in the situation in which the adolescent is anxious to proceed with surgery, while the family/parents are reticent to provide consent. Continued discussion directed at having all participants clarify their goals for the surgery and their understanding of the risks may allow for a decision that all can respect.

INFORMED REFUSAL OF TREATMENT BY ADOLESCENTS

Adolescents or older children who have experienced serious and/ or chronic illnesses often have an enhanced capacity for decision-making when weighing the benefits and burdens of continued treatment, especially when the likelihood of a good outcome is low.[70] Refusal of life-sustaining therapy by such an adolescent should be given careful consideration by parents and the health care team. The pediatrician should work with the health care team, patient, and family in a collaborative approach to resolve any conflicts between the parents and adolescent, and the clinicians should generally advocate for the adolescent's wishes if they reflect an ethically acceptable treatment option. When conflicts about the goals of treatment persist, the health care team should enlist the involvement of secondary consultants, an integrated palliative care team, ethics consultation, psychologists, psychiatrists, or chaplains. Seeking legal intervention should be a last resort.

In general, it is also reasonable to respect an adolescent's refusal of nonurgent, non–life-threatening care as long as efforts are directed toward helping the physician and the family understand the basis of the refusal and providing appropriate education for any misconceptions.

Although age provides a clear legal definition of majority, there is still no bright line demarcating when a minor becomes "mature" enough to independently demonstrate the capacity for informed consent or refusal. Courts have weighed in on this issue with a variety of outcomes, detailed below. Recent pressure to generalize functional MRI neurobiological research to individual adolescents to prove criminal culpability is disturbing, because the science still struggles to separate social and environmental influences from biological determinants of behavior.[45]

One of the first mature-minor doctrine cases to rule on whether an adolescent has the right to make decisions about life-sustaining treatments is *In re E.G.* (1989).[71] In this case, the Illinois Supreme

Court ruled that a 17-year-old with leukemia and who was a member of the Jehovah's Witnesses faith was mature and had the right to refuse blood transfusions. Importantly, her mother agreed with her decision. The judges observed that the age of majority "is not an impenetrable barrier that magically precludes a minor from possessing and exercising certain rights normally associated with adulthood." A second case, *Belcher v Charleston Area Medical Center* (1992),[72] heard by the West Virginia Supreme Court of Appeals, also recognized the mature-minor doctrine and directed physicians to seek input from a mature minor before treatment. In this case, a physician wrote a do-not-resuscitate order for a 17-year-old with muscular dystrophy without discussion with the patient, despite the family's request that he do so. The patient, Larry Belcher, later had a cardiac arrest and died without resuscitation.

Case law continues to evolve on the issue of a minor's right to refuse medical treatment. A recent case[73] involved 13-year-old Daniel Hauser and his mother, Colleen Hauser. Daniel was found to have a very treatable form of Hodgkin lymphoma, with an estimated survival of 80% to 95% after standard chemotherapy and radiation therapy. Despite receiving an initial course of chemotherapy, Daniel and his mother refused further recommended chemotherapy, insisting instead on using "holistic" medicine based on Native American healing practices. One important aspect of this case was Daniel's inability to meet elements of informed assent/consent, because his limited cognitive abilities and illiteracy hampered his ability to comprehend his medical condition and its recommended treatments. A 2009 Minnesota court order in this case considered both a parent's right to raise a child free of interference and the constitutionally protected

right to religious belief but found both less compelling than the state's need to protect the child and to proceed with necessary medical therapy for a treatable, life-threatening illness.

This legal decision is in contrast to previous decisions, such as the case of Dennis Lindberg.[74] Dennis was a 14-year-old with leukemia who practiced the Jehovah's Witnesses faith and was allowed to refuse a blood transfusion after a 2007 court ruling by a Mt Vernon, Washington, judge who found him to be a mature minor. Although Dennis' biological parents objected to this ruling, his long-time guardian, who had raised him in the Jehovah's Witnesses faith, supported his refusal of transfusions. He died within hours of the ruling. In another prominent case in 2006, Abraham Starchild Cherrix, a 16-year-old with lymphoma, successfully deferred standard therapy for his lymphoma, supported by a Virginia court ruling. This ruling centered on the patient's maturity, understanding of his illness, and parental support of his refusal and quickly resulted in Virginia's 2007 "Abraham's Law" that allows adolescents 14 years of age and older a decision-making role in life-threatening conditions.[75]

Despite the legal rulings and ethical guidance, there is still much controversy about informed refusal by adolescents of life-sustaining treatments.[5,76–80] A recent statement from the Confederation of European Specialists in Pediatrics clearly states that pediatric patients may not refuse life-saving treatment.[35] Although the Confederation of European Specialists in Pediatrics references the United Nations Convention of the Rights of the Child, citing article 12, which provides for "the view of the child being given due weight in accordance with the age and maturity of the child," and finds that this clearly applies to medical treatment, they state that the physician has a duty to act in the best interest of the child.

Many bioethicists support limiting a child's or adolescent's short-term autonomy by overriding a treatment refusal to preserve long-term autonomous choice and an open future.[28,54] Although adolescents may possess the capacity for decision-making, as discussed earlier, it may be limited by lack of perspective or real-life experiences. Some also argue that parental responsibility in promoting and protecting their child's life does not abruptly end when an adolescent has decision-making capacity. They should not cede sole decision-making authority to their minor child.[77] Instead, parental authority and decision-making are constrained to identify and protect the best interests of their child when he or she refuses medical care.

In general, adolescents should not be allowed to refuse life-saving treatment, even when parents agree.[34,54,78] However, in circumstances of a life-limiting terminal illness when only unproven, overly burdensome or likely ineffective treatment options exist, some adolescents may make an informed choice to forgo interventions to address their underlying disease and instead focus on measures that provide comfort and support.

The dilemma of an adolescent treatment refusal is ethically and emotionally challenging. Pediatricians must ascertain the capacity of the minor for decision-making while recognizing that the "science" of that determination is still evolving. The presence of chronic illness can either enhance a child's decisional skills or contribute to regression, emotional immaturity, and anger when facing a choice. The involvement of psychiatric counselors, ethicists, child life specialists, social workers, or other consultants, such as an integrated palliative care service, may help the patient, family, and clinical team resolve conflict.

EMERGENCY EXCEPTIONS TO INFORMED CONSENT

Parental consent is usually required for the evaluation and medical treatment of pediatric patients. However, there are situations in which children may present with emergency medical conditions and a parent or legal guardian is not available to provide consent. The AAP policy statement "Consent for Emergency Medical Services for Children and Adolescents"[31] recommends that a medical screening examination and appropriate medical stabilization of the pediatric patient with an urgent or emergent condition should never be withheld or delayed because of problems with obtaining consent. Although clinicians, courts, and parents may differ on what constitutes an emergency, this standard should apply when urgent interventions to prevent imminent and significant harm are necessary and when reasonable efforts to find a surrogate are unsuccessful.

Clinicians should also be aware that current federal law, under the Emergency Medical Treatment and Active Labor Act, mandates a medical screening examination and, if indicated, treatment and stabilization of an emergency medical condition, regardless of consent issues, in any hospital that receives federal funding. If an emergency medical condition is not identified with a screening examination, then Emergency Medical Treatment and Active Labor Act regulations no longer apply and the physician should seek proper consent or assent before further nonurgent care is provided.[31]

There also may be situations in which practitioners seek consent by proxy for nonurgent care (eg, a babysitter brings a 6-year-old to the doctor's office). Guidance for clinicians in this area is found in the AAP policy statement "Consent by Proxy for Nonurgent Pediatric Care."[81]

INFORMED CONSENT/ASSENT/REFUSAL IN RESEARCH INVOLVING CHILDREN AND ADOLESCENTS

The informed consent process for both research and clinical care shares similar ethical foundations and also encounters similar problems in ensuring consistency across institutions and practices. Informed consent and assent obtained from children involved in research are clearly mandated, in contrast to the "recommended" guidance in place in clinical care. This process has been closely scrutinized for >3 decades since the publication of the *Belmont Report* in 1978.[82] Produced by the National Commission for the Protection of Human Subjects of Biomedical and Behavioral Research, the *Belmont Report* formed the basis of much of the work on informed consent in the research setting. Institutional review boards (IRBs) have incorporated the *Belmont Report*, the *Report and Recommendation: Research Involving Children*,[83] the NIH Policy and Guidelines on the Inclusion of Children as Participants in Research Involving Human Subjects,[84] and the appropriate federal guidelines (the "Common Rule" [45 CFR §46, 1991]) into the rules balancing the risk/benefit ratio that guide the review of research protocols including children as research subjects. The informed permission of the child subject's parent(s) must be obtained before enrolling the subject in the research protocol. In a distinction from the usual clinical practice, there are also clear guidelines on the need to obtain assent from the child subject in research and to respect a minor's dissent from study participation, with limited exceptions.

Although assent is mandated, federal guidelines on how to obtain assent and at what age are not explicit. This situation results in variability in requirements of local IRBs of the age at which assent should be obtained and what elements of the traditional informed consent process are required from children and adolescents.[2,55-59] Although the AAP and the National Commission for the Protection of Human Subjects of Biomedical and Behavioral Research recommend assent for children >7 years, there is still wide variation in the inclusion of children in the assent process.[85] The ability of the capable mature minor to consent to medical research depends on individual state laws, but generally, risks must be minimal and the research aim should center on a medical condition for which the minor can legally give consent. More detailed information is found in the AAP clinical report "Guidelines for the Ethical Conduct of Studies To Evaluate Drugs in Pediatric Populations."[86]

Most research into the assent or consent process has occurred in the pediatric oncology population, because up to 80% of pediatric patients with cancer are also enrolled as subjects in clinical research trials. Oncologists may neglect to include adolescents in the decision-making process because of perceived inability of the adolescent to comprehend information when facing a life-threatening situation and the presumed sufficiency of parental permission.[87] Children enrolled in clinical trials very often have limited awareness and appreciation of the research trial, do not recall having a role in deciding whether to enroll, and do not feel free to dissent.[59] Observational studies have noted variations in how often the physician addressed the child versus the parent during the assent/permission discussion.[70,88] Observed decision-making approaches during discussion of enrollment include patient-centered, parent-centered, or joint child-parent decisions. The latter or partnering approach may be the most successful in meeting the criteria for parental permission and child assent but may not be possible when families or physicians exercise authority over the child. A strong push toward endorsing a developmentally appropriate assent process in research may encourage more joint decision-making.

The IRB can provide a waiver from requiring assent if greater-than-minimal-risk research has the potential for an important direct benefit that is only available in the context of the research or the research carries only minimal risk and could not be carried out without the waiver.[89] This is a critical difference from the child's input into decision-making in the clinical world.

CONCLUSIONS

Informed consent should be seen as a constitutive part of health care practice; parental permission and childhood assent is an active process that engages patients, adults, and children in the health care process. Pediatric practice is unique in that developmental maturation of the child allows for increasing longitudinal inclusion of the child's opinion in medical decision-making in clinical and research practice. Although new research has shown that neurologic maturation continues into the third decade of life, seeking assent from children and adolescents for medical interventions can foster the moral growth and development of autonomy in young patients and is strongly recommended. Surrogate decision-making by parents or guardians for pediatric patients should seek to maximize the benefits for their child by balancing health care needs with social and emotional needs within the context of overall family goals, cultural beliefs, and values. Physicians should recognize that some pediatric patients, especially older adolescents and those with medical experience because of chronic illness, are minors with enough decision-making capacity, moral intelligence, and judgment to provide true informed consent, or, in non–life-threatening settings, informed refusal, for their proposed care plan. Clinicians have both a moral obligation and a legal responsibility to question and, if necessary, to contest surrogate and/or patient medical decisions that put the patient at significant risk of serious harm. Adolescent treatment refusals remain controversial and are ethically and emotionally challenging for families and clinicians.

LEAD AUTHORS

Aviva L. Katz, MD, FAAP
Sally A. Webb, MD, FAAP

COMMITTEE ON BIOETHICS, 2015–2016

Aviva L. Katz, MD, FAAP, Chairperson
Robert C. Macauley, MD, FAAP
Mark R. Mercurio, MD, MA, FAAP
Margaret R. Moon, MD, FAAP
Alexander L. Okun, MD, FAAP
Douglas J. Opel, MD, MPH, FAAP
Mindy B. Statter, MD, FAAP

CONTRIBUTING FORMER COMMITTEE MEMBERS

Mary E. Fallat, MD, FAAP, Past Chairperson
Sally A. Webb, MD
Kathryn L. Weise, MD

LIAISONS

Mary Lynn Dell, MD, DMin – *American Academy of Child and Adolescent Psychiatry*
Douglas S. Diekema, MD, MPH – *American Board of Pediatrics*
Dawn Davies, MD, FRCPC, MA – *Canadian Pediatric Society*
Sigal Klipstein, MD – *American College of Obstetricians and Gynecologists*

FORMER LIAISONS

Kevin W. Coughlin, MD, FAAP – *Canadian Pediatric Society*
Steven J. Ralston, MD – *American College of Obstetricians and Gynecologists*
Monique A. Spillman, MD, PhD – *American College of Obstetricians and Gynecologists*

LEGAL CONSULTANTS

Nanette Elster, JD, MPH
Jessica Wilen Berg, JD, MPH

STAFF

Florence Rivera, MPH
Alison Baker, MS

ABBREVIATIONS

AAP: American Academy of
        Pediatrics
HPV: human papillomavirus
IRB: institutional review board
STI: sexually transmitted
        infection

REFERENCES

1. American Academy of
   Pediatrics. Consent. *Pediatrics*.
   1976;57(3):414–416

2. American Academy of Pediatrics,
   Committee on Bioethics. Informed
   consent, parental permission, and
   assent in pediatric practice. *Pediatrics*.
   1995;95(2):314–317

3. American Academy of Pediatrics,
   Committee on Bioethics. Informed
   consent in decision-making in
   pediatric practice [policy statement].
   Pediatrics. 2016

4. Lee KJ, Havens PL, Sato TT, Hoffman
   GM, Leuthner SR. Assent for
   treatment: clinician knowledge,
   attitudes, and practice. *Pediatrics*.
   2006;118(2):723–730

5. Talati ED, Lang CW, Ross LF. Reactions
   of pediatricians to refusals of medical
   treatment for minors. *J Adolesc
   Health*. 2010;47(2):126–132

6. Duncan RE, Sawyer SM. Respecting
   adolescents' autonomy (as long as
   they make the right choice). *J Adolesc
   Health*. 2010;47(2):113–114

7. Beauchamp TL, Childress JF. *Principle
   of Biomedical Ethics*. 5th ed. New York,
   NY: Oxford University Press; 2001

8. Faden RR, Beauchamp TL. *A History and
   Theory of Informed Consent*. New York,
   NY: Oxford University Press; 1986

9. Berg JW, Appelbaum PS, Lidz PS, Parker
   LS. *Informed Consent: Legal Theory and
   Clinical Practice*, 2nd ed. New York, NY:
   Oxford University Press; 2001

10. McCullough LB. Contributions of
    ethical theory to pediatric ethics;
    pediatricians and parents as

co-fiduciaries of pediatric patients. In:
Miller G, ed. *Pediatric Bioethics*. New
York, NY: Cambridge University Press;
2010:11–21

11. *Salgo v Leland Stanford Jr University
    Board of Trustees*, 154 Cal App 2d 560
    (1957)

12. Berman L, Dardik A, Bradley EH,
    Gusberg RJ, Fraenkel L. Informed
    consent for abdominal aortic
    aneurysm repair: assessing
    variations in surgeon opinion through
    a national survey. *J Vasc Surg*.
    2008;47(2):287–295

13. Burger I, Schill K, Goodman S.
    Disclosure of individual surgeon's
    performance rates during informed
    consent: ethical and epistemological
    considerations. *Ann Surg*.
    2007;245(4):507–513

14. Jones JW, McCullough LB, Richman BW.
    The Ethics of Surgical Practice. New
    York, NY: Oxford University Press; 2008

15. *Johnson v Kokemoor*, 545 NW2d 495,
    199 Wis 2d 615 (Wis 1996)

16. Appelbaum PS, Grisso T. Assessing
    patients' capacities to consent
    to treatment. *N Engl J Med*.
    1988;319(25):1635–1638

17. Sherman HB, McGaghie WC, Unti
    SM, Thomas JX. Teaching pediatrics
    residents how to obtain informed
    consent. *Acad Med*. 2005;80(10
    suppl):S10–S13

18. Yap TY, Yamokoski A, Noll R, Drotar
    D, Zyzanski S, Kodish ED; Multi-Site
    Intervention Study to Improve Consent
    Research Team. A physician-directed
    intervention: teaching and measuring
    better informed consent. *Acad Med*.
    2009;84(8):1036–1042

19. Fink AS, Prochazka AV, Henderson WG,
    et al. Predictors of comprehension
    during surgical informed consent.
    J Am Coll Surg. 2010;210(6):919–926

20. O'Lonergan TA, Forster-Harwood JE.
    Novel approach to parental permission
    and child assent for research:
    improving comprehension. *Pediatrics*.
    2011;127(5):917–924

21. Lipstein EA, Brinkman WB, Britto
    MT. What is known about parents'
    treatment decisions? A narrative
    review of pediatric decision making.
    Med Decis Making. 2012;32(2):246–258

22. Pyke-Grimm KA, Stewart JL, Kelly KP,
    Degner LF. Parents of children with
    cancer: factors influencing their
    treatment decision making roles.
    J Pediatr Nurs. 2006;21(5):350–361

23. Benedict JM, Simpson C, Fernandez
    CV. Validity and consequence of
    informed consent in pediatric bone
    marrow transplantation: the parental
    experience. *Pediatr Blood Cancer*.
    2007;49(6):846–851

24. Miller VA, Luce MF, Nelson RM.
    Relationship of external influence
    to parental distress in decision
    making regarding children with a life-
    threatening illness. *J Pediatr Psychol*.
    2011;36(10):1102–1112

25. Kopelman LM. The best-interests
    standard as threshold, ideal, and
    standard of reasonableness. *J Med
    Philos*. 1997;22(3):271–289

26. Buchanan AE, Brock DW. *Deciding
    for Others: The Ethics of Surrogate
    Decision Making*. Cambridge, United
    Kingdom: Cambridge University Press;
    1990

27. Diekema DS. Parental refusals of
    medical treatment: the harm principle
    as threshold for state intervention.
    Theor Med Bioeth. 2004;25(4):243–264

28. Ross L. *Children, Families, and Health
    Care Decision-Making*. New York, NY:
    Oxford University Press; 1998

29. Committee on Hospital Care, American
    Academy of Pediatrics. Family-centered
    care and the pediatrician's role.
    Pediatrics. 2003;112(3 pt 1):691–697

30. Britton CV; American Academy of
    Pediatrics Committee on Pediatric
    Workforce. Ensuring culturally
    effective pediatric care: implications
    for education and health policy.
    Pediatrics. 2004;114(6):1677–1685

31. Committee on Pediatric Emergency
    Medicine and Committee on Bioethics.
    Consent for emergency medical
    services for children and adolescents.
    Pediatrics. 2011;128(2):427–433

32. *Prince v Massachusetts*, 321 US 158
    (1944)

33. American Academy of Pediatrics
    Committee on Bioethics. Religious
    objections to medical care. *Pediatrics*.
    1997;99(2):279–281

34. Canadian Pediatric Society. Treatment decisions regarding infants, children and adolescents. *Paediatr Child Health.* 2004;9(2):99–114

35. De Lourdes Levy M, Larcher V, Kurz R; Ethics Working Group of the Confederation of European Specialists in Paediatrics. Statement of the Ethics Working Group of the Confederation of European Specialists in Paediatrics (CESP). Informed consent/assent in children. *Eur J Pediatr.* 2003;162(9):629–633

36. Larcher V, Hutchinson A. How should paediatricians assess Gillick competence? *Arch Dis Child.* 2010;95(4):307–311

37. Michaud PA, Berg-Kelly K, Macfarlane A, Benaroyo L. Ethics and adolescent care: an international perspective. *Curr Opin Pediatr.* 2010;22(4):418–422

38. Weithorn LA, Campbell SB. The competency of children and adolescents to make informed treatment decisions. *Child Dev.* 1982;53(6):1589–1598

39. McCabe MA. Involving children and adolescents in medical decision making: developmental and clinical considerations. *J Pediatr Psychol.* 1996;21(4):505–516

40. *Cardwell v Bechtol*, 724 SW 2d 739, 745 (Tenn 1987)

41. Giedd JN, Blumenthal J, Jeffries NO, et al. Brain development during childhood and adolescence: a longitudinal MRI study. *Nat Neurosci.* 1999;2(10):861–863

42. Sowell ER, Thompson PM, Holmes CJ, Jernigan TL, Toga AW. In vivo evidence for post-adolescent brain maturation in frontal and striatal regions. *Nat Neurosci.* 1999;2(10):859–861

43. Sowell ER, Thompson PM, Tessner KD, Toga AW. Mapping continued brain growth and gray matter density reduction in dorsal frontal cortex: Inverse relationships during postadolescent brain maturation. *J Neurosci.* 2001;21(22):8819–8829

44. Giedd JN. The teen brain: insights from neuroimaging. *J Adolesc Health.* 2008;42(4):335–343

45. Johnson SB, Blum RW, Giedd JN. Adolescent maturity and the brain: the promise and pitfalls of neuroscience research in adolescent health policy. *J Adolesc Health.* 2009;45(3):216–221

46. Romer D. Adolescent risk taking, impulsivity, and brain development: implications for prevention. *Dev Psychobiol.* 2010;52(3):263–276

47. Van Leijenhorst L, Gunther Moor B, Op de Macks ZA, Rombouts SA, Westenberg PM, Crone EA. Adolescent risky decision-making: neurocognitive development of reward and control regions. *Neuroimage.* 2010;51(1):345–355

48. Dahl RE, Gunnar MR. Heightened stress responsiveness and emotional reactivity during pubertal maturation: implications for psychopathology. *Dev Psychopathol.* 2009;21(1):1–6

49. Steinberg L. A dual systems model of adolescent risk-taking. *Dev Psychobiol.* 2010;52(3):216–224

50. Steinberg L. Cognitive and affective development in adolescence. *Trends Cogn Sci.* 2005;9(2):69–74

51. Steinberg L, Cauffman E. Maturity of judgment in adolescence: psychosocial factors in adolescent decision-making. *Law Hum Behav.* 1996;20(3):249–272

52. Narvaez D. The emotional foundations of high moral intelligence. *New Dir Child Adolesc Dev.* 2010;2010(129):77–94

53. Silber TJ. Adolescent brain development and the mature minor doctrine. *Adolesc Med State Art Rev.* 2011;22(2):207–212, viii

54. Diekema DS. Adolescent refusal of lifesaving treatment: are we asking the right questions? *Adolesc Med State Art Rev.* 2011;22(2):213–228, viii

55. Denham EJ, Nelson RM. Self-determination is not an appropriate model for understanding parental permission and child assent. *Anesth Analg.* 2002;94(5):1049–1051

56. Kon AA. Assent in pediatric research. *Pediatrics.* 2006;117(5):1806–1810

57. Miller VA, Nelson RM. A developmental approach to child assent for nontherapeutic research. *J Pediatr.* 2006;149(1 suppl):S25–S30

58. Wendler DS. Assent in paediatric research: theoretical and practical considerations. *J Med Ethics.* 2006;32(4):229–234

59. Unguru Y, Coppes MJ, Kamani N. Rethinking pediatric assent: from requirement to ideal. *Pediatr Clin North Am.* 2008;55(1):211–222, xii

60. Waller BN. Patient autonomy naturalized. *Perspect Biol Med.* 2001;44(4):584–593

61. Korsgaard C. *Self Constitution, Agency, Identity and Integrity.* New York, NY: Oxford University Press; 2009

62. Guttmacher Institute. Preventing cervical cancer: new resources to advance the domestic and global fight. *Guttmacher Policy Review.* Winter 2012;15:1. Available at: www.guttmacher.org/pubs/gpr/15/1/gpr150108.html. Accessed October 28, 2013

63. Ford CA, English A. Limiting confidentiality of adolescent health services: what are the risks? *JAMA.* 2002;288(6):752–753

64. 42 CFR part 2, Implementing the Substance Abuse and Mental Health Administration (42 USC 290dd.2)

65. De Ville K. Adolescent parents and medical decision-making. *J Med Philos.* 1997;22(3):253–270

66. Mercurio MR. Adolescent mothers of critically ill newborns: addressing the rights of parent and child. *Adolesc Med State Art Rev.* 2011;22(2):240–250, ix

67. Nasr A, Fecteau A, Wales PW. Comparison of the Nuss and the Ravitch procedure for pectus excavatum repair: a meta-analysis. *J Pediatr Surg.* 2010;45(5):880–886

68. Papandria D, Arlikar J, Sacco Casamassima MG, et al. Increasing age at time of pectus excavatum repair in children: emerging consensus? *J Pediatr Surg.* 2013;48(1):191–196

69. Johnson JN, Hartman TK, Pianosi PT, Driscoll DJ. Cardiorespiratory function after operation for pectus excavatum. *J Pediatr.* 2008;153(3):359–364

70. Pousset G, Bilsen J, De Wilde J, et al. Attitudes of adolescent cancer survivors toward end-of-life decisions for minors. *Pediatrics.* 2009;124(6):e1142–e1148

71. *In re E.G.*, 133 Ill 2d 98105549 NE 2d 322325 (1989)

72. *Belcher v Charleston Area Med Ctr*, 422 SE 2d 827, 838 (W Va 1992)

73. In the Matter of the Welfare of the Child of Colleen Hauser and Anthony Hauser, JV-09-68, Minn, Brown County, 5th Judicial District (2009)

74. Ostrom CM. Mount Vernon leukemia patient, 14, dies after rejecting transfusions. The Seattle Times. November 29, 2007. Available at: http://www.seattletimes.com/seattle-news/health/mount-vernon-leukemia-patient-14-dies-after-rejecting-transfusions/. Accessed June 27, 2016

75. Abraham's Law, VA Code §63.2-100 (2007)

76. Doig C, Burgess E. Withholding life-sustaining treatment: are adolescents competent to make these decisions? *CMAJ*. 2000;162(11):1585–1588

77. Mercurio MR. An adolescent's refusal of medical treatment: implications of the Abraham Cherrix case. *Pediatrics*. 2007;120(6):1357–1358

78. Ross LF. Against the tide: arguments against respecting a minor's refusal of efficacious life-saving treatment. *Camb Q Healthc Ethics*. 2009;18(3):302–315; discussion: 315–322

79. Johnston C. Overriding competent medical treatment refusal by adolescents: when "no" means "no". *Arch Dis Child*. 2009;94(7):487–491

80. Alderson P. Competent children? Minors' consent to health care treatment and research. *Soc Sci Med*. 2007;65(11):2272–2283

81. McAbee GN; Committee on Medical Liability and Risk Management American, Academy of Pediatrics. Consent by proxy for nonurgent pediatric care. *Pediatrics*. 2010;126(5):1022–1031

82. US National Commission for the Protection of Human Subjects of Biomedical and Behavioral Research. *The Belmont Report: Ethical Principles and Guidelines for the Protection of Human Subjects of Research*. Washington, DC: US Government Printing Office; 1979. DHEW publication (OS) 78-0012-78-0014

83. US National Commission for the Protection of Human Subjects of Biomedical and Behavioral Research. *Report and Recommendation: Research Involving Children*. Washington, DC: US Government Printing Office; 1977. DHEW publication (OS) 77-0004

84. National Institutes of Health. NIH Policy and Guidelines on the Inclusion of Children as Participants in Research Involving Human Subjects. Available at: http://grants.nih.gov/grants/guide/notice-files/not98-024.html. Accessed October 28, 2013

85. Whittle A, Shah S, Wilfond B, Gensler G, Wendler D. Institutional review board practices regarding assent in pediatric research. *Pediatrics*. 2004;113(6):1747–1752

86. Shaddy RE, Denne SC; Committee on Drugs and Committee on Pediatric Research. Clinical report—guidelines for the ethical conduct of studies to evaluate drugs in pediatric populations. *Pediatrics*. 2010;125(4):850–860

87. de Vries MC, Wit JM, Engberts DP, Kaspers GJ, van Leeuwen E. Pediatric oncologists' attitudes towards involving adolescents in decision-making concerning research participation. *Pediatr Blood Cancer*. 2010;55(1):123–128

88. Olechnowicz JQ, Eder M, Simon C, Zyzanski S, Kodish E. Assent observed: children's involvement in leukemia treatment and research discussions. *Pediatrics*. 2002;109(5):806–814

89. Wendler D, Belsky L, Thompson KM, Emanuel EJ. Quantifying the federal minimal risk standard: implications for pediatric research without a prospect of direct benefit. *JAMA*. 2005;294(7):826–832

Management of Pediatric Trauma

- *Policy Statement*

POLICY STATEMENT Organizational Principles to Guide and Define the Child Health
Care System and/or Improve the Health of all Children

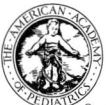

American Academy
of Pediatrics

DEDICATED TO THE HEALTH OF ALL CHILDREN™

Management of Pediatric Trauma

COMMITTEE ON PEDIATRIC EMERGENCY MEDICINE, COUNCIL ON INJURY, VIOLENCE, AND POISON PREVENTION,
SECTION ON CRITICAL CARE, SECTION ON ORTHOPAEDICS, SECTION ON SURGERY, SECTION ON TRANSPORT
MEDICINE, PEDIATRIC TRAUMA SOCIETY, AND SOCIETY OF TRAUMA NURSES, PEDIATRIC COMMITTEE

abstract

Injury is still the number 1 killer of children ages 1 to 18 years in the United
States (http://www.cdc.gov/nchs/fastats/children.htm). Children who sustain
injuries with resulting disabilities incur significant costs not only for their
health care but also for productivity lost to the economy. The families of
children who survive childhood injury with disability face years of emotional
and financial hardship, along with a significant societal burden. The entire
process of managing childhood injury is enormously complex and varies by
region. Only the comprehensive cooperation of a broadly diverse trauma
team will have a significant effect on improving the care of injured children.

INTRODUCTION

Unintentional and intentional injury and homicide cause more deaths
in children and adolescents ages 1 to 18 years than all other causes
combined.[1] Deaths caused by injuries, intentional or unintentional,
account for more years of potential life lost under 18 years than sudden
unexplained infant death, cancer, and infectious diseases combined. It is
estimated that 1 in 4 children sustain an unintentional injury requiring
medical care each year.[2] The direct cost of childhood injury is >$50
billion annually.[3] Survivors of childhood trauma may suffer lifelong
disability and require long-term skilled care. Improving outcomes for the
injured child requires an approach that recognizes childhood injury as a
significant public health problem. Additional topics related to the injured
child can be found in other publications from the American Academy of
Pediatrics (AAP).[4–9] These publications complement and enhance our
understanding of managing pediatric trauma.

TRAUMA SYSTEMS

Children are injured in a wide variety of geographic locations, and the
involvement of local and regional centers is paramount to optimizing
care for injured children. A pediatric trauma system functions best
as a part of the inclusive emergency medical services (EMS), trauma
system, and disaster response system at the local, regional, state, and

This document is copyrighted and is property of the American
Academy of Pediatrics and its Board of Directors. All authors have
filed conflict of interest statements with the American Academy
of Pediatrics. Any conflicts have been resolved through a process
approved by the Board of Directors. The American Academy of
Pediatrics has neither solicited nor accepted any commercial
involvement in the development of the content of this publication.

Policy statements from the American Academy of Pediatrics benefit
from expertise and resources of liaisons and internal (AAP) and
external reviewers. However, policy statements from the American
Academy of Pediatrics may not reflect the views of the liaisons or the
organizations or government agencies that they represent.

The guidance in this statement does not indicate an exclusive course
of treatment or serve as a standard of medical care. Variations, taking
into account individual circumstances, may be appropriate.

All policy statements from the American Academy of Pediatrics
automatically expire 5 years after publication unless reaffirmed,
revised, or retired at or before that time.

DOI: 10.1542/peds.2016-1569

PEDIATRICS (ISSN Numbers: Print, 0031-4005; Online, 1098-4275).

FINANCIAL DISCLOSURE: The authors have indicated they do
not have a financial relationship relevant to this article to
disclose.

FUNDING: No external funding.

POTENTIAL CONFLICT OF INTEREST: The authors have
indicated they have no potential conflicts of interest to
disclose.

To cite: AAP COMMITTEE ON PEDIATRIC EMERGENCY MEDICINE,
COUNCIL ON INJURY, VIOLENCE, AND POISON PREVENTION,
SECTION ON CRITICAL CARE, SECTION ON ORTHOPAEDICS,
SECTION ON SURGERY, SECTION ON TRANSPORT MEDICINE,
PEDIATRIC TRAUMA SOCIETY, SOCIETY OF TRAUMA NURSES,
PEDIATRIC COMMITTEE. Management of Pediatric Trauma.
Pediatrics. 2016;138(2):e20161569

national levels. The inclusive trauma system is defined as one in which all EMS providers, physicians, other caregivers, and hospitals participate in the care of injured patients. Regional adult trauma centers and regional pediatric trauma centers are the central components of such a system. These systems allow for prompt communication, earlier recognition of critical injuries, and continuing education for trauma and emergency care providers. An inclusive trauma system ranges from hospitals capable of initial stabilization to those that provide comprehensive trauma care. As was noted in the Institute of Medicine's report "Emergency Care for Children: Growing Pains,"[10] within any given EMS or trauma system, it is likely that not all hospitals will be completely equipped with appropriate pediatric resuscitation equipment or medications.[10,11] There may also be significant variability in pediatric training and experience among physicians and nurses working in hospital emergency departments (EDs).[12,13] However, pediatric readiness, including administrative support, quality improvement, education, equipment, supplies, medication, and continuing education, is important for all hospitals.

Approximately 80% of US children live within 50 miles of a level I or II trauma center. However, in many less populated states, the percentage of children living within 50 miles of a trauma center is much lower.[14] An estimated 17.4 million children do not have access to a pediatric trauma center within 60 minutes.[15,16] When the trauma system extends over a large geographic area, the outlying hospitals of the system must be able to undertake the stabilization and initial management of the injured child or children who present to the hospital. Optimally, each trauma system will also define the age range of the pediatric patient on the basis of specific hospital and trauma team resources that are available.

When a regional pediatric referral center is available within the trauma system, the most severely injured children may be transported to a facility with a level I or II pediatric trauma designation.[17] Trauma system administrators are key stakeholders to facilitate ways in which all hospitals with EDs may be required to evaluate and resuscitate injured children.[4,5,7,10] A mass casualty event, such as a tornado strike on 1 hospital in a system, highlights the need for such readiness. It has been recommended that a physician and nurse coordinator for pediatric emergency care be identified in each facility, with pediatric-specific policies, procedures, equipment, a quality-improvement process, and guidelines for care established.[7,10] These guidelines are outlined in the AAP/American College of Emergency Physicians/Emergency Nurses Association joint policy statement "Guidelines for Care of Children in the Emergency Department."[7] In addition, the Emergency Medical Services for Children performance measures that assess a state's operational capacity to provide pediatric emergency care are important adjuncts to managing a trauma system.[17]

Protocols for field and hospital triage, treatment, and transfer of victims of pediatric trauma are an important part of any trauma system.[18] Transfer recommendations and toolkits are available from many states and regional systems as well as from national organizations.[19,20] Ideally, the quality of care that is provided within the system is continuously evaluated by the trauma system administration through performance improvement processes. Benchmarking care by using risk-adjusted data is important for the ongoing improvement in pediatric care and system delivery models. The outcomes for pediatric trauma patients can be compared with available benchmarks such as the National Trauma Data Bank,[21] and information shared with specific providers so that an optimal environment for quality improvement in pediatric trauma care is promoted. The American College of Surgeons (ACS) has initiated a Pediatric Trauma Quality Improvement Project that will provide participating hospitals with additional pediatric specific benchmarking data.[22]

PREHOSPITAL PEDIATRIC TRAUMA CARE

Prehospital providers may not be as familiar with effective pediatric emergency care as they are with the care provided to adults,[23] because most prehospital providers are infrequently exposed to critically ill or injured children. Lack of experience with pediatric trauma patients is typically addressed by continuing education efforts for EMS providers through established courses supported by the AAP and the National Association of Emergency Medical Technicians or by practical experience in a children's hospital. Online and remote training may be an effective and reasonable alternative in largely rural states.[24] State and national certifying and licensing bodies can ensure that adequate continuing education units are obtained in pediatric trauma management by prehospital providers to maintain proficiency. No matter how continuing education is accomplished, mechanisms for assessing knowledge and skill retention and continuous evaluation of performance are crucial for prehospital personnel. The method for maintaining skills may include continuous evaluation of performance or collaboration with a pediatric health care system that provides opportunities to maintain and expand on pediatric acute care knowledge and skills. New projects that use simulation show promising results.[25] Direct feedback to field providers is an essential component for continual improvement in any trauma system to improve outcomes for injured children. This feedback can be provided by the receiving facility by using real-time reviews, case review presentations, or feedback to the referring prehospital agency.

There is a relative lack of data regarding the best practices for pediatric resuscitation in out-of-hospital traumatic cardiac arrest, including fluid administration, cervical spine stabilization, and airway management of children. The Broselow system does provide useful information for early resuscitation, and there are new recommendations for termination of resuscitation in the field.[26] Comprehensive support for research in this area needs to come from regional, state, and national organizations. Current examples of research support include the federally funded Emergency Medical Services for Children program,[27] the Pediatric Emergency Care Applied Research Network,[28] the Pediatric Emergency Research Network,[29] and the American Pediatric Surgical Association Outcomes and Clinical Trials Center.[30]

TRAUMA CENTERS

It has been shown that younger and more seriously injured children have improved outcomes at a trauma center within a children's hospital or at a trauma center that integrates pediatric and adult trauma services.[14,31-34] Data suggest that the presence of a pediatric trauma center within a state was associated with lower pediatric injury mortality rates.[35] The requirements for a hospital trauma program that cares for children vary by state. The most comprehensive description of the various levels of pediatric trauma care is provided

by the ACS "Optimal Care of the Injured Patient" document.[36] The ability to provide a broad range of pediatric services, including the presence of providers trained in pediatric emergency medicine, pediatric medical subspecialties and surgical specialties, pediatric anesthesiology, pediatric critical care, traumatic stress and substance abuse counseling, pediatric rehabilitation, and other specialized trauma care, is important. Nurses with demonstrated competency in the care of pediatric trauma patients are an important aspect of care as well.

Management of the injured child requires special considerations. Issues that are unique to children include reducing diagnostic radiation exposure, family presence during resuscitation,[37] the availability of child life specialists, fluid and electrolyte management, and blood transfusions, to name a few. Careful consideration of diagnostic radiation for trauma evaluation is always of primary importance because of the radiation dose that is often delivered.[38] Pediatric protocols for imaging and diagnostic testing[39] and a child- and family-centered environment of care for injured individuals and in mass casualty events[8,40] are important resources to proactively have in place at all hospitals, including pediatric and non–children's hospital trauma centers. Specific guidelines for implementing and facilitating family presence during pediatric trauma care are useful to facilitate safety and efficacy of family presence within a hospital.[8] Specific pain management protocols could allow the injured child timely control of pain. Competency and ability to provide a full range of pediatric pain strategies for children, including systemic analgesics, regional and local pain control options, and distraction techniques, are essential components for pediatric trauma care.[8] Pain management is important from

the time of injury and throughout the care continuum, including rehabilitation.

Continuing trauma education for hospital providers and trauma nurses is important and can be accomplished by current certification in the Advanced Trauma Life Support course from the ACS and courses in trauma nursing supported by the Society of Trauma Nurses and the Emergency Nurses Association.[8] Some trauma centers may not have the resources to care for all of the injured children within their referral region at any given time, especially in less populated states. Thus, the most seriously injured children may need to be stabilized in regional referral centers and transported to tertiary facilities with these resources. Pediatric critical care transport teams are often the best resource for such transfers.[41] Hospitals that seek regional or state designation or verification as a pediatric trauma center through the verification process of the ACS or similar state trauma designation processes are examples of facilities that have made an extraordinary effort to provide resources to care for injured children.

A well-equipped and staffed pediatric intensive care unit (PICU) is another essential component of a pediatric trauma center. PICUs offer a setting with the necessary monitoring devices, equipment, medications, and technology to support physiologic function and are staffed with professionals with the expertise to apply them to the pediatric patient. Data show that the availability of PICU beds within a region may improve survival in pediatric trauma.[34] Pediatric critical care physicians, surgeons, and anesthesiologists trained in the care of injured children working together are needed for optimal care of severely injured and unstable patients in the ICU setting. In addition to critically injured children, stable patients with the potential for deterioration may also require the specialized services of a PICU. Pediatric trauma care specialists, especially those with critical care training, are in short supply and are distributed irregularly in the population, thus endangering the nationwide delivery of pediatric trauma care.[42] Furthermore, the presence of experienced PICU nursing and allied health care personnel supports the environment necessary for frequent monitoring and assessment of injured children. Moreover, pediatric trauma care continues on inpatient floors. Once the child is stable and the possibility of rapid deterioration is decreased, a comprehensive evaluation of the child's physical function and psychological needs, pain management, and the rehabilitation process generally begins while still in the inpatient setting.

REHABILITATION AND THE MEDICAL HOME

It is the goal of a comprehensive trauma system to reintegrate the child into his or her community and to his or her primary care medical home. The availability of rehabilitation resources for pediatric patients is a vital component of pediatric trauma care. Returning the child to full, age-appropriate function, with the ability to reach his or her maximum adult potential, is the ultimate goal after injury. Early rehabilitation is especially crucial for those children suffering neurologic injuries. Physical, occupational, cognitive, speech, and play therapy, as well as psychological and social support, are all essential elements of a comprehensive rehabilitation effort for the injured child and his or her family. It is important to address acute stress and posttraumatic stress reactions in trauma patients.[43] In particular, crisis intervention and ongoing support can be offered to youth who are injured through interpersonal violence, because

they are especially at risk of repeat, violent injuries and psychosocial trauma. Some examples of support organizations are the National Network of Hospital-Based Violence Intervention Programs (www.nnhvip.org) and the National Child Traumatic Stress Network (www.nctsn.org).

PERFORMANCE IMPROVEMENT

The presence of active and effective performance improvement committees, with issues focused toward pediatrics, is an integral component for trauma centers. In any trauma center, these activities also include attention to patient safety. Periodic review of trauma care by the providers of that care is the process that is most likely to improve patient outcomes in any hospital. Trauma care review is facilitated by a comprehensive trauma registry that has ties with national databases so that outcomes can be benchmarked for improved quality of care. Mandatory systematic child death review processes are recommended to identify emerging trends and higher level risk factors for which interventions can be developed and evaluated. The ACS suggests that every facility that provides care for injured children have a quality-improvement process that leads to focused continuing education.[36]

Another unique aspect related to pediatric trauma care is the need for increased awareness for signs of potential child abuse.[44] Pediatric trauma center personnel need to be aware of state reporting requirements within their jurisdiction and remain vigilant to facilitate early detection of abuse and neglect. This is best accomplished by using a protocol or screening to detect child abuse in the ED that cares for children. It is the responsibility of all pediatric providers to be educated regarding the early detection, diagnosis, and

management of inflicted injuries. Community hospitals with limited pediatric services can identify resources for specialized child protection teams in their regional referral areas. Cooperation and collaboration between referring providers and hospital-based child protection teams are important for the management of cases of suspected abuse and neglect.

INJURY PREVENTION

Injury prevention is the cornerstone to any discussion concerning pediatric trauma. Injury-prevention initiatives do work.[45] For example, the Safe Kids program has been instrumental in decreasing deaths attributable to trauma. However, these initiatives are not promoted equally across the United States, often because of limited resources. There are methods to identify and refine the approach to injury-prevention initiatives that are specific to individual regions.[46] Trauma programs can use data from the trauma registry to identify high-risk injury-prevention needs. Injury-prevention activities can be identified by using local data and may focus on such things as fall prevention, alcohol and drug abuse recognition and intervention, child passenger safety, bike safety, water safety, and other regionally appropriate activities as endorsed by the Injury Free Coalition for Kids (www.injuryfree.org). Ideally EMS providers, hospitals, EDs, and trauma centers have injury-prevention content and information as well as activities incorporated into patient and staff education and as part of community-based injury-prevention programs. Primary care providers are encouraged to emphasize individual and community safety and injury-prevention programs such as The Injury Prevention Program from the AAP.[47]

PEDIATRIC DISASTER PREPAREDNESS AND SURGE

Disaster preparedness in the United States has improved significantly in the years since Hurricane Katrina. Hospital accreditation programs such as The Joint Commission have strengthened their disaster preparedness requirements. Children have unique needs for care in mass casualty incidents, especially if chemical, biological, or nuclear events occur. Along with physiologic considerations, triage, identification, decontamination, tracking, and reunification are all issues that must be considered during mass casualty events. A process for recruiting pediatric health care professionals when a surge response is needed is often included in any disaster plan. One model includes a calling tree within the various departments and sections to recruit providers for a surge response.

States and regions (facilitated by federal partners) can review current emergency operations and devise appropriate plans to address the population-based needs of infants and children in large-scale disasters. Action at the state, regional, and federal levels addresses legal, operational, and information systems to provide effective pediatric mass critical care through the following: (1) pre–disaster/mass casualty planning, management, and assessment with input from child health professionals; (2) close cooperation, agreements, public-private partnerships, and unique delivery systems; and (3) use of existing public health data to assess pediatric populations at risk and to model graded response plans on the basis of increasing patient volume and acuity.[48]

Ideally, attending to the psychological needs of injured children is considered in any such event. Although the needs of children in disasters can be anticipated, the capability of a trauma system to meet these needs will remain in question until the nation achieves an optimal level of emergency readiness for children on a daily basis.[49]

RECOMMENDATIONS

1. The unique needs of injured children need to be integrated specifically into trauma systems and disaster planning at the local, state, regional, and national levels.

2. Every state should identify appropriate facilities with the resources to care for injured children and establish continuous monitoring processes for care delivered to injured children. These facilities are especially important for the youngest and most severely injured children.

3. Evaluation and management of the injured child should begin with the providers at the bedside who have basic competency in pediatric trauma care.

4. Prehospital and hospital providers should make every effort to stay current in the emergency management of injured children. In addition, providers should actively participate in and cultivate an injury-prevention program within their service area to ultimately reduce the rate of children injured.

5. Pediatric providers should be familiar with the pediatric trauma services in their region and how to integrate the available services into their practice. Hospital-based providers who are not at regional pediatric centers should be able to evaluate, stabilize, and transfer acutely injured children.

6. Pediatric injury management should include an integrated public health approach from prevention through prehospital care, to emergency and acute hospital care, to rehabilitation and long-term follow–up, as indicated, for stress reactions associated with the injury.

7. Qualified pediatric critical care transport teams should be used when available in the interfacility transport of critically injured children.

8. Interfacility transfer agreements should be in place to facilitate rapid acceptance and transport of critically injured children to a facility with the appropriate level of care.

9. National organizations with a special interest in pediatric trauma, such as the AAP, the ACS, the American College of Emergency Physicians, the American Academy of Emergency Medicine, the Emergency Nurses Association, the Pediatric Trauma Society, the American Pediatric Surgery Association, the Pediatric Orthopaedic Society of North America, the American Pediatric Surgical Nurses Association, and the Society of Trauma Nurses, should collaborate to advocate for a higher quality of care across the nation.

10. Evidence-based protocols for the management of the injured child can be developed for essential aspects of care, including prehospital, acute resuscitation, and postdischarge through rehabilitation.

11. Research including data collection for best practices in isolated trauma and mass casualty events specifically addressing the needs of children should be supported.

12. State and federal financial support for research, advocacy, education, and trauma system development and maintenance must be provided.

13. Steps should be taken to increase the number of trainees in specialties that care for injured children to address key subspecialty service shortages in pediatric trauma care. Strategies should include increased funding for graduate medical education and appropriate reimbursement for pediatric trauma specialists.

14. Direct, constructive feedback to field providers and referring hospitals should occur from the pediatric trauma center to allow for continued education and improved pediatric care.

15. All health care providers should be aware that injured children and their families should be evaluated and referred for stress reactions related to injury.

16. All health care providers should be alert to signs of potential abuse when evaluating injured children and should report concerns to the appropriate authorities.

LEAD AUTHORS

David W. Tuggle, MD, FAAP, FACS
Sally K. Snow, RN, BSN, CPEN, FAEN

AAP COMMITTEE ON PEDIATRIC EMERGENCY MEDICINE, 2015–2016

Joan E. Shook, MD, MBA, FAAP, Chairperson
James M. Callahan, MD, FAAP
Thomas H. Chun, MD, MPH, FAAP
Gregory P. Conners, MD, MPH, MBA, FAAP
Edward E. Conway Jr, MD, MS, FAAP
Nanette C. Dudley, MD, FAAP
Toni K. Gross, MD, MPH, FAAP
Natalie E. Lane, MD, FAAP
Charles G. Macias, MD, MPH, FAAP
Nathan L. Timm, MD, FAAP

LIAISONS

Kim Bullock, MD – *American Academy of Family Physicians*
Elizabeth Edgerton, MD, MPH, FAAP – *Maternal and Child Health Bureau*
Tamar Magarik Haro – *AAP Department of Federal Affairs*
Madeline Joseph, MD, FACEP, FAAP – *American College of Emergency Physicians*
Angela Mickalide, PhD, MCHES – *Emergency Medical Services for Children National Resource Center*

Brian R. Moore, MD, FAAP – *National Association of EMS Physicians*
Katherine E. Remick, MD, FAAP – *National Association of Emergency Medical Technicians*
Sally K. Snow, RN, BSN, CPEN, FAEN – *Emergency Nurses Association*
David W. Tuggle, MD, FAAP – *American College of Surgeons*
Cynthia Wright-Johnson, MSN, RNC – *National Association of State EMS Officials*

FORMER MEMBERS AND LIAISONS, 2013–2015

Alice D. Ackerman, MD, MBA, FAAP
Lee Benjamin, MD, FACEP, FAAP - *American College of Physicians*
Susan M. Fuchs, MD, FAAP
Marc H. Gorelick, MD, MSCE, FAAP
Paul Sirbaugh, DO, MBA, FAAP - *National Association of Emergency Medical Technicians*
Joseph L. Wright, MD, MPH, FAAP

STAFF

Sue Tellez

AAP COUNCIL ON INJURY, VIOLENCE, AND POISON PREVENTION, 2015-2016

Kyran Quinlan, MD, MPH, FAAP, Chairperson
Phyllis F. Agran, MD, MPH, FAAP
Michele Burns, MD, FAAP
Sarah Denny, MD, FAAP
Michael Hirsh, MD, FAAP
Brian Johnston, MD, MPH, FAAP
Kathy Monroe, MD, FAAP
Elizabeth C. Powell, MD, FAAP
Judith Schaechter, MD, FAAP
Mark R. Zonfrillo, MD, FAAP

LIAISONS

Elizabeth Edgerton, MD, MPH, FAAP – *Health Resources and Services Administration*
Julie Gilchrist, MD, FAAP – *Centers for Disease Control and Prevention*
Lynne Haverkos, MD, MPH, FAAP – *National Institute of Child Health and Human Development*
Jonathan Midgett, PhD – *Consumer Product Safety Commission*
Alexander Sandy Sinclair – *National Highway Traffic Safety Administration*

STAFF

Bonnie Kozial

AAP SECTION ON CRITICAL CARE EXECUTIVE COMMITTEE, 2015–2016

Edward E. Conway Jr, MD, MS, FAAP, Chairperson
Michael S.D. Agus, MD, FAAP, Chair-Elect
Benson S. Hsu, MD, MBA, FAAP
Susan R. Hupp, MD
W. Bradley Poss, MD, MMM
Jana A. Stockwell, MD, FAAP
John P. Straumanis, MD, FAAP
Donald D. Vernon, MD, FAAP, Immediate Past Chair

FORMER EXECUTIVE COMMITTEE MEMBERS, 2013–2015

Mary W. Lieh-Lai, MD, FAAP
Richard B. Mink, MD, MACM, FAAP
Carley L. Riley, MD, MPP, MHS, FAAP
Richard A. Salerno, MD, MS, FAAP

STAFF

Sue Tellez

AAP SECTION ON ORTHOPAEDICS EXECUTIVE COMMITTEE, 2015–2016

Norman Y. Otsuka, MD, FAAP, Chairperson
Joshua M. Abzug, MD, FAAP
Theodore Ganley, MD, FAAP
Martin Herman, MD, FAAP
Joshua E. Hyman, MD, FAAP
Lee Segal, MD, FAAP
Brian A. Shaw, MD, FAAOS, FAAP
Richard M. Schwend, MD, FAAP, Immediate Past Chair

STAFF

S. Niccole Alexander, MPP

AAP SECTION ON SURGERY EXECUTIVE COMMITTEE, 2015–2016

Michael G. Caty, MD, FAAP, Chairperson
Gail Besner, MD, FAAP
Andrew Davidoff, MD, FAAP
Mary E. Fallat, MD, FAAP
Kurt F. Heiss, MD, FAAP
Rebecka L. Meyers, MD, FAAP
R. Lawrence Moss, MD, FAAP, Immediate Past Chair

STAFF

Vivian Thorne

AAP SECTION ON TRANSPORT MEDICINE EXECUTIVE COMMITTEE, 2015–2016

Keith Meyer, MD, FAAP, Chairperson
Howard S. Heiman, MD, FAAP
Robert G. Holcomb Jr, MD, FAAP
Michael T. Meyer, MD, FAAP
Jay K. Pershad, MD, MMM, FAAP
Michael H. Stroud, MD, FAAP
Michele M. Walsh, MD, FAAP
M. Michele Moss, MD, FAAP, Immediate Past Chairperson
Webra Price Douglas, PhD, CRNP, Affiliates Liaison

LIAISONS

Michael T. Bigham, MD, FAAP – *Air Medical Physician Association*
Tammy Rush, MSN, RN, C-NPT, EMT – *National Association of Neonatal Nurses*

STAFF

S. Niccole Alexander, MPP

PEDIATRIC TRAUMA SOCIETY, 2014–2015

Richard Falcone Jr, MD, MPH, 2015 President
Barbara Gaines, MD, 2014 President
Lynn Haas, RN, MSN, CNP, 2013 President
Laura Cassidy, MS, PhD
Terri Elsbernd, RN, MSN
Garet Free, EMT-P
Lisa Gray, RN, CNP
Jonathan Groner, MD
Kathy Haley, MS, BSN, RN
Robert Letton Jr, MD
William Millikan Jr, MD
Michael Nance, MD, FACS
Pina Violano, RN, MSPH

SOCIETY OF TRAUMA NURSES PEDIATRIC COMMITTEE, 2014–2015

Lisa Gray, MHA, BSN, CPN, Co-Chair
Linda Roney, MSN, RN-BC, CPEN, Co-Chair
Chris McKenna, MSN, RN, CRNP
Mary Jo Pedicino, MSN
Susan Rzucidlo, MSN, RN
Sally K. Snow, BSN, RN, CPEN, FAEN
Lisa Reichter, BSN, RN

EMERGENCY MEDICAL SERVICES FOR CHILDREN LIAISON

Diana Fendya, MSN(R), RN

BOARD LIAISONS

Tracy Rogers, MSN, RN, 2014
Diana J. Kraus, RN, BSN, TNS, 2015

STAFF

Kim Goff, Education and Committee Manager

ABBREVIATIONS

AAP: American Academy of Pediatrics
ACS: American College of Surgeons
ED: emergency department
EMS: emergency medical services
PICU: pediatric intensive care unit

REFERENCES

1. Hamilton BE, Hoyert DL, Martin JA, Strobino DM, Guyer B. Annual summary of vital statistics: 2010–2011. *Pediatrics.* 2013;131(3):548–558

2. Danseco ER, Miller TR, Spicer RS. Incidence and costs of 1987–1994 childhood injuries: demographic breakdowns. *Pediatrics.* 2000;105(2).

Available at: www.pediatrics.org/cgi/content/full/105/2/E27

3. Finklestein EA, Corso PS, Miller TR. *Incidence and Economic Burden of Injuries in the United States.* Oxford, United Kingdom: Oxford University Press; 2006

4. American Academy of Pediatrics, Committee on Pediatric Emergency Medicine, Committee on Medical Liability, Task Force on Terrorism. The pediatrician and disaster preparedness. *Pediatrics.* 2006;117(2):560–565. Reaffirmed September 2013

5. Knapp JF, Pyles LA; American Academy of Pediatrics, Committee on Pediatric Emergency Medicine. Role of pediatricians in advocating life support training courses for parents and the public. *Pediatrics.* 2004;114(6):1676. Reaffirmed August 2013

6. Jaimovich DG, ed. *Handbook of Pediatric and Neonatal Transport Medicine.* 2nd ed. Philadelphia, PA: Lippincott, Williams, and Wilkins; 2004

7. American Academy of Pediatrics Committee on Pediatric Emergency Medicine; American College of Emergency Physicians Pediatric Committee; Emergency Nurses Association Pediatric Committee. Joint policy statement—guidelines for care of children in the emergency department. *Pediatrics.* 2009;124(4):1233–1243

8. Fein JA, Zempsky WT, Cravero JP; American Academy of Pediatrics Committee on Pediatric Emergency Medicine and Section on Anesthesiology and Pain Medicine. Relief of pain and anxiety in pediatric patients in emergency medical systems. *Pediatrics.* 2012;130(5):e1391–e1405

9. Christian CW, Block R; American Academy of Pediatrics Committee on Child Abuse and Neglect. Abusive head trauma in infants and children. *Pediatrics.* 2009;123(5):1409–1411

10. Institute of Medicine, Committee on the Future of Emergency Care in the United States Health System. *Future of Emergency Care Series: Emergency Care for Children, Growing*

Pains. Washington, DC: The National Academies Press; 2007

11. Schappert SM, Bhuiya F. Availability of pediatric services and equipment in emergency departments: United States, 2006. *Natl Health Stat Rep.* 2012;(47):1–21

12. Yamamoto LG; American Academy of Pediatrics Committee on Pediatric Emergency Medicine. Access to optimal emergency care for children. *Pediatrics.* 2007;119(1):161–164. Reaffirmed July 2014

13. Carr BG, Nance ML. Access to pediatric trauma care: alignment of providers and health systems. *Curr Opin Pediatr.* 2010;22(3):326–331

14. Brantley MD, Lu H, Barfield WD, Holt JB. Visualizing pediatric mass critical care hospital resources by state, 2008. Available at: http://proceedings.esri.com/library/userconf/health10/docs/esri_hc_2010_op2.pdf. Accessed June 18, 2015

15. Brantley MD, Lu H, Barfield WD, Holt JB, Williams A. Mapping US pediatric hospitals and subspecialty critical care for public health preparedness and disaster response, 2008. *Disaster Med Public Health Prep.* 2012;6(2):117–125

16. Densmore JC, Lim HJ, Oldham KT, Guice KS. Outcomes and delivery of care in pediatric injury. *J Pediatr Surg.* 2006;41(1):92–98; discussion: 92–98

17. National Emergency Medical Services for Children Data Analysis Research Center. What are the EMSC performance measures? Available at: www.nedarc.org/performanceMeasures/index.html. Accessed June 18, 2015

18. Sasser SM, Hunt RC, Sullivent EE, et al; National Expert Panel on Field Triage, Centers for Disease Control and Prevention. Guidelines for field triage of injured patients: recommendations of the National Expert Panel on Field Triage. *MMWR Recomm Rep.* 2009;58(RR-1):1–35. Available at: www.cdc.gov/mmwr/preview/mmwrhtml/rr5801a1.htm. Accessed June 18, 2015

19. National Pediatric Readiness Project. Guidelines for policies, procedures, and protocols for the ED. Available at: www.pediatricreadiness.org/PRP_Resources/Policies_Procedures_Protocols.aspx. Accessed June 18, 2015

20. Sasser SM, Hunt RC, Faul M, et al; Centers for Disease Control and Prevention. Guidelines for field triage of injured patients: recommendations of the National Expert Panel on Field Triage, 2011. *MMWR Recomm Rep.* 2012;61(RR-1):1–20

21. American College of Surgeons. National Trauma Data Bank. Available at: www.facs.org/trauma/ntdb/index.html. Accessed June 18, 2015

22. American College of Surgeons. Trauma Quality Improvement Program. Available at: www.facs.org/trauma/ntdb/tqip.html. Accessed June 18, 2015

23. Lammers R, Byrwa M, Fales W. Root causes of errors in a simulated prehospital pediatric emergency. *Acad Emerg Med.* 2012;19(1):37–47

24. Warren L, Sapien R, Fullerton-Gleason L. Is online pediatric continuing education effective in a rural state? *Prehosp Emerg Care.* 2008;12(4):498–502

25. Eppich WJ, Nypaver MM, Mahajan P, et al. The role of high-fidelity simulation in training pediatric emergency medicine fellows in the United States and Canada. *Pediatr Emerg Care.* 2013;29(1):1–7

26. Fallat ME; American College of Surgeons Committee on Trauma; American College of Emergency Physicians Pediatric Emergency Medicine Committee; National Association of Ems Physicians; American Academy of Pediatrics Committee on Pediatric Emergency Medicine. Withholding or termination of resuscitation in pediatric out-of-hospital traumatic cardiopulmonary arrest. *Pediatrics.* 2014;133(4). Available at: www.pediatrics.org/cgi/content/full/133/4/e1104

27. Ball JW, Liao E, Kavanaugh D, Turgel C. The emergency medical services for children program: accomplishments and contributions. *Clin Pediatr Emerg Med.* 2006;7(1):6–14

28. Foltin GL, Dayan P, Tunik M, et al; Prehospital Working Group of the Pediatric Emergency Care Applied Research Network. Priorities for pediatric prehospital research. *Pediatr Emerg Care.* 2010;26(10):773–777

29. Klassen TP, Acworth J, Bialy L, et al. Pediatric emergency research networks: a global initiative in pediatric emergency medicine. *Pediatr Emerg Care.* 2010;26(8):541–543

30. American Pediatric Surgical Association Outcomes Committee. American Pediatric Surgical Association Outcomes and Clinical Trials Center. *Semin Pediatr Surg.* 2002;11(3):181–183

31. Stylianos S, Egorova N, Guice KS, Arons RR, Oldham KT. Variation in treatment of pediatric spleen injury at trauma centers versus nontrauma centers: a call for dissemination of American Pediatric Surgical Association benchmarks and guidelines. *J Am Coll Surg.* 2006;202(2):247–251

32. MacKenzie EJ, Rivara FP, Jurkovich GJ, et al. A national evaluation of the effect of trauma-center care on mortality. *N Engl J Med.* 2006;354(4):366–378

33. Amini R, Lavoie A, Moore L, Sirois MJ, Emond M. Pediatric trauma mortality by type of designated hospital in a mature inclusive trauma system. *J Emerg Trauma Shock.* 2011;4(1):12–19

34. Odetola FO, Miller WC, Davis MM, Bratton SL. The relationship between the location of pediatric intensive care unit facilities and child death from trauma: a county-level ecologic study. *J Pediatr.* 2005;147(1):74–77

35. Notrica DM, Weiss J, Garcia-Filion P, et al. Pediatric trauma centers: correlation of ACS-verified trauma centers with CDC statewide pediatric mortality rates. *J Trauma Acute Care Surg.* 2012;73(3):566–570; discussion: 570–572

36. American College of Surgeons. Resources for optimal care of the injured patient. . Available at: https://www.facs.org/~/media/files/quality programs/trauma/vrc resources/resources for optimal care 2014 v11.ashx. Accessed March 31, 2016

37. Kingsnorth J, O'Connell K, Guzzetta CE, et al. Family presence during trauma activations and medical resuscitations in a pediatric emergency department: an evidence-based practice project. *J Emerg Nurs.* 2010;36(2):115–121

38. Mueller DL, Hatab M, Al-Senan R, et al. Pediatric radiation exposure during the initial evaluation for blunt trauma. *J Trauma.* 2011;70(3):724–731

39. Sun R, Skeete D, Wetjen K, et al. A pediatric cervical spine clearance protocol to reduce radiation exposure in children. *J Surg Res.* 2013;183(1):341–346

40. Mason KE, Urbansky H, Crocker L, Connor M, Anderson MR, Kissoon N; Task Force for Pediatric Emergency Mass Critical Care. Pediatric emergency mass critical care: focus on family-centered care. *Pediatr Crit Care Med.* 2011;12(suppl 6):S157–S162

41. Orr RA, Felmet KA, Han Y, et al. Pediatric specialized transport teams are associated with improved outcomes. *Pediatrics.* 2009;124(1):40–48

42. Mayer ML, Skinner AC. Influence of changes in supply on the distribution of pediatric subspecialty care. *Arch Pediatr Adolesc Med.* 2009;163(12):1087–1091

43. Kassam-Adams N, Marsac ML, Hildenbrand A, Winston F. Posttraumatic stress following pediatric injury: update on diagnosis, risk factors, and intervention. *JAMA Pediatr.* 2013;167(12):1158–1165

44. Fang X, Brown DS, Florence CS, Mercy JA. The economic burden of child maltreatment in the United States and implications for prevention. *Child Abuse Negl.* 2012;36(2):156–165

45. Houston M, Cassabaum V, Matzick S, et al; Mile-High Regional Emergency Medical and Trauma Advisory Council. Teen traffic safety campaign: competition is the key. *J Trauma.* 2010;68(3):511–514

46. Rogers SC, Campbell BT, Saleheen H, Borrup K, Lapidus G. Using trauma registry data to guide injury prevention program activities. *J Trauma.* 2010;69(suppl 4):S209–S213

47. American Academy of Pediatrics. The Injury Prevention Program. Available at: http://patiented.solutions.aap.org/Handout-Collection.aspx?categoryid=32033. Accessed June 18, 2015

48. Barfield WD, Krug SE, Kanter RK, et al; Task Force for Pediatric

Emergency Mass Critical Care. Neonatal and pediatric regionalized systems in pediatric emergency mass critical care. *Pediatr Crit Care Med.* 2011;12(suppl 6): S128–S134

49. National Commission on Children and Disasters. *2010 Report to the President and Congress.* Rockville, MD: Agency for Healthcare Research and Quality; 2010. AHRQ Publication 10-M037

Media and Young Minds

- *Policy Statement*

POLICY STATEMENT   Organizational Principles to Guide and Define the Child Health Care System and/or Improve the Health of all Children

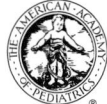

American Academy
of Pediatrics

DEDICATED TO THE HEALTH OF ALL CHILDREN™

Media and Young Minds

COUNCIL ON COMMUNICATIONS AND MEDIA

abstract

Infants, toddlers, and preschoolers are now growing up in environments saturated with a variety of traditional and new technologies, which they are adopting at increasing rates. Although there has been much hope for the educational potential of interactive media for young children, accompanied by fears about their overuse during this crucial period of rapid brain development, research in this area still remains limited. This policy statement reviews the existing literature on television, videos, and mobile/interactive technologies; their potential for educational benefit; and related health concerns for young children (0 to 5 years of age). The statement also highlights areas in which pediatric providers can offer specific guidance to families in managing their young children's media use, not only in terms of content or time limits, but also emphasizing the importance of parent–child shared media use and allowing the child time to take part in other developmentally healthy activities.

DOI: 10.1542/peds.2016-2591

PEDIATRICS (ISSN Numbers: Print, 0031-4005; Online, 1098-4275).

Copyright © 2016 by the American Academy of Pediatrics

FINANCIAL DISCLOSURE: The authors have indicated they do not have a financial relationship relevant to this article to disclose.

FUNDING: No external funding.

POTENTIAL CONFLICT OF INTEREST: The authors have indicated they have no potential conflicts of interest to disclose.

To cite: AAP COUNCIL ON COMMUNICATIONS AND MEDIA. Media and Young Minds. *Pediatrics.* 2016;138(5):e20162591

INTRODUCTION

Technologic innovation has transformed media and its role in the lives of infants and young children. More children, even in economically challenged households, are using newer digital technologies, such as interactive and mobile media, on a daily basis[1] and continue to be the target of intense marketing.[2] This policy statement addresses the influence of media on the health and development of children from 0 to 5 years of age, a time of critical brain development, building secure relationships, and establishing health behaviors.

INFANTS AND TODDLERS

Children younger than 2 years need hands-on exploration and social interaction with trusted caregivers to develop their cognitive, language, motor, and social-emotional skills. Because of their immature symbolic, memory, and attentional skills, infants and toddlers cannot learn from traditional digital media as they do from interactions with caregivers,[3] and they have difficulty transferring that knowledge to their 3-dimensional experience.[4] The chief factor that facilitates toddlers' learning from commercial media (starting around 15 months of age) is parents watching with them and reteaching the content.[5,6]

The interactivity of touchscreens enables applications (apps) to identify when a child responds accurately and then tailor its responses, thereby supporting children at their levels of competence. Emerging evidence shows that at 24 months of age, children can learn words from live video-chatting with a responsive adult[7] or from an interactive touchscreen interface that scaffolds the child to choose the relevant answers.[8] Starting at 15 months of age, toddlers can learn novel words from touchscreens in laboratory-based studies but have trouble transferring this knowledge to the 3-dimensional world.[9] However, it should be noted that these experiments used specially designed apps that are not commercially available.

Many parents now use video-chat (eg, Skype, FaceTime) as an interactive media form that facilitates social connection with distant relatives. New evidence shows that infants and toddlers regularly engage in video-chatting,[10] but the same principles regarding need for parental support would apply in order for infants and toddlers to understand what they are seeing.

In summary, for children younger than 2 years, evidence for benefits of media is still limited, adult interaction with the child during media use is crucial, and there continues to be evidence of harm from excessive digital media use, as described later in this statement.

PRESCHOOL MEDIA AND LEARNING

Well-designed television programs, such as Sesame Street, can improve cognitive, literacy, and social outcomes for children 3 to 5 years of age[11,12] and continue to create programming that addresses evolving child health and developmental needs (eg, obesity prevention, resilience). Evaluations of apps from Sesame Workshop and the Public Broadcasting Service (PBS) also have shown efficacy in teaching literacy skills to preschoolers.[2] Unfortunately, most apps parents find under the "educational" category in app stores have no such evidence of efficacy, target only rote academic skills, are not based on established curricula, and use little or no input from developmental specialists or educators.[2,13] Most apps also generally are not designed for a dual audience (ie, both parent and child).[2,14] It is important to emphasize to parents that the higher-order thinking skills and executive functions essential for school success, such as task persistence, impulse control, emotion regulation, and creative, flexible thinking, are best taught through unstructured and social (not digital) play,[15] as well as responsive parent–child interactions.[16]

Digital books (also called "eBooks," books that can be read on a screen) often come with interactive enhancements that, research suggests, may decrease child comprehension of content or parent dialogic reading interactions when visual effects are distracting.[17] Parents should, therefore, be instructed to interact with children during eBook reading, as they would a print book.

HEALTH AND DEVELOPMENTAL CONCERNS

Obesity

Heavy media use during preschool years is associated with small but significant increases in BMI,[18] may explain disparities in obesity risk in minority children,[19] and sets the stage for weight gain later in childhood.[20] Although many studies have used a 2-hour cutoff to examine obesity risk, a recent study of 2-year-olds found that BMI increased for every hour per week of media consumed.[21] It is believed that exposure to food advertising[22] and watching television while eating (which diminishes attention to satiety cues)[23] drives these associations.

Sleep

Increased duration of media exposure and the presence of a television, computer, or mobile device in the bedroom in early childhood have been associated with fewer minutes of sleep per night.[24]

Even infants exposed to screen media in the evening hours show significantly shorter night-time sleep duration than those with no evening screen exposure.[25] Mechanisms underlying this association include arousing content[26] and suppression of endogenous melatonin by blue light emitted from screens.[27]

Child Development

Population-based studies continue to show associations between excessive television viewing in early childhood and cognitive,[28–30] language,[31,32] and social/emotional delays,[33–36] likely secondary to decreases in parent–child interaction when the television is on[37] and poorer family functioning in households with high media use.[37] An earlier age of media use onset, greater cumulative hours of media use, and non-PBS content all are significant independent predictors of poor executive functioning in preschoolers.[38] Content is crucial: experimental evidence shows that switching from violent content to educational/prosocial content results in significant improvement in behavioral symptoms, particularly for low-income boys.[12] Notably, the quality of parenting can modify associations between media use and child development: one study found that inappropriate content and inconsistent parenting had cumulative negative effects on low-income preschoolers' executive function, whereas warm parenting and educational content interacted to produce additive benefits.[39]

Child characteristics also may influence how much media children consume: excessive television viewing is more likely in infants and toddlers with a difficult temperament[40,41] or self-regulation problems,[42] and toddlers with social-emotional delays are more likely to be given a mobile device to calm them down.[43]

Parental Media Use

Parents' background television use distracts from parent–child interactions[44] and child play.[45] Heavy parent use of mobile devices is associated with fewer verbal and nonverbal interactions between parents and children[46] and may be associated with more parent-child conflict.[47] Because parent media use is a strong predictor of child media habits,[48] reducing parental media use and enhancing parent–child interactions may be an important area of behavior change.

CONCLUSIONS: CLINICAL IMPLICATIONS

In summary, multiple developmental and health concerns continue to exist for young children using all forms of digital media to excess. Evidence is sufficient to recommend time limitations on digital media use for children 2 to 5 years to no more than 1 hour per day to allow children ample time to engage in other activities important to their health and development and to establish media viewing habits associated with lower risk of obesity later in life.[49] In addition, encouraging parents to change to educational and prosocial content and engage with their children around technology

will allow children to reap the most benefit from what they view.

As digital technologies become more ubiquitous, pediatric providers must guide parents not only on the duration and content of media their child uses, but also on (1) creating unplugged spaces and times in their homes, because devices can now be taken anywhere; (2) the ability of new technologies to be used in social and creative ways; and (3) the importance of not displacing sleep, exercise, play, reading aloud, and social interactions. Realistically, pediatric providers will need to know how to help parents find resources finding appropriate content, tools for monitoring or limiting child use, ideas for play or activities in which to engage rather than digital play, and how parents can limit their own media use (see HealthyChildren. org for examples); each of these can be built into the Family Media Use Plan (see the American Academy of Pediatrics guide to developing a plan at www.healthychildren.org/ MediaUsePlan).

RECOMMENDATIONS

Pediatricians

- Start the conversation early. Ask parents of infants and young children about family media use, their children's use habits, and media use locations.

- Help families develop a Family Media Use Plan (www.healthychildren.org/ MediaUsePlan) with specific guidelines for each child and parent.

- Educate parents about brain development in the early years and the importance of hands-on, unstructured, and social play to build language, cognitive, and social-emotional skills.

- For children younger than 18 months, discourage use of screen media other than video-chatting.

- For parents of children 18 to 24 months of age who want to introduce digital media, advise that they choose high-quality programming/apps and use them together with children, because this is how toddlers learn best. Letting children use media by themselves should be avoided.

- Guide parents to resources for finding quality products (eg, Common Sense Media, PBS Kids, Sesame Workshop).

- In children older than 2 years, limit media to 1 hour or less per day of high-quality programming. Recommend shared use between parent and child to promote enhanced learning, greater interaction, and limit setting.

- Recommend no screens during meals and for 1 hour before bedtime.

- Problem-solve with parents facing challenges, such as setting limits, finding alternate activities, and calming children.

Families

- Avoid digital media use (except video-chatting) in children younger than 18 to 24 months.

- For children ages 18 to 24 months of age, if you want to introduce digital media, choose high-quality programming and use media together with your child. Avoid solo media use in this age group.

- Do not feel pressured to introduce technology early; interfaces are so intuitive that children will figure them out quickly once they start using them at home or in school.

- For children 2 to 5 years of age, limit screen use to 1 hour per day of high-quality programming, coview with your children, help children understand what they are seeing, and help them apply what they learn to the world around them.

- Avoid fast-paced programs (young children do not understand them as well), apps with lots of distracting content, and any violent content.

- Turn off televisions and other devices when not in use.

- Avoid using media as the only way to calm your child. Although there are intermittent times (eg, medical procedures, airplane flights) when media is useful as a soothing strategy, there is concern that using media as strategy to calm could lead to problems with limit setting or the inability of children to develop their own emotion regulation. Ask your pediatrician for help if needed.

- Monitor children's media content and what apps are used or downloaded. Test apps before the child uses them, play together, and ask the child what he or she thinks about the app.

- Keep bedrooms, mealtimes, and parent–child playtimes screen free for children and parents. Parents can set a "do not disturb" option on their phones during these times.

- No screens 1 hour before bedtime, and remove devices from bedrooms before bed.

- Consult the American Academy of Pediatrics Family Media Use Plan, available at: www.healthychildren.org/MediaUsePlan.

Industry

- Work with developmental psychologists and educators to create design interfaces that are appropriate to child developmental abilities, that are not distracting, and that promote shared parent–child media use and application of skills to the real world. Cease making apps for children younger than 18 months until evidence of benefit is demonstrated.

- Formally and scientifically evaluate products before making educational claims.

- Make high-quality products accessible and affordable to low-income families and in multiple languages.

- Eliminate advertising and unhealthy messages on apps. Children at this age cannot differentiate between advertisements and factual information, and therefore, advertising to them is unethical.

- Help parents to set limits by stopping auto-advance of videos as the default setting. Develop systems embedded in devices that can help parents monitor and limit media use.

LEAD AUTHORS

Jenny Radesky, MD, FAAP
Dimitri Christakis, MD, MPH, FAAP

COUNCIL ON COMMUNICATIONS AND MEDIA EXECUTIVE COMMITTEE, 2016-2017

David Hill, MD, FAAP, Chairperson
Nusheen Ameenuddin, MD, MPH, FAAP
Yolanda (Linda) Reid Chassiakos, MD, FAAP
Corinn Cross, MD, FAAP
Jenny Radesky, MD, FAAP
Jeffrey Hutchinson, MD, FAAP
Rhea Boyd, MD, FAAP
Robert Mendelson, MD, FAAP
Megan A. Moreno, MD, MSEd, MPH, FAAP
Justin Smith, MD, FAAP
Wendy Sue Swanson, MD, MBE, FAAP

LIAISONS

Kris Kaliebe, MD — American Academy of Child and Adolescent Psychiatry
Jennifer Pomeranz, JD, MPH — American Public Health Association
Brian Wilcox, PhD — American Psychological Association

STAFF

Thomas McPheron

ABBREVIATIONS

app: application
PBS: Public Broadcasting Service

REFERENCES

1. Kabali HK, Irigoyen MM, Nunez-Davis R, et al. Exposure and use of mobile devices by young children. *Pediatrics.* 2015;136(6):1044–1050

2. Chiong C, Shuler C; The Joan Ganz Cooney Center at Sesame Workshop. Learning: Is there an app for that? Investigations of young children's usage of learning with mobile devices and apps. Available at: http://dmlcentral.net/wp-content/uploads/files/learningapps_final_110410.pdf. Accessed September 2, 2016

3. Anderson DR, Pempek TA. Television and very young children. *Am Behav Sci.* 2005;48(5):505–522

4. Barr R. Memory constraints on infant learning from picture books, television, and touchscreens. *Child Dev Perspect.* 2013;7(4):205–210

5. DeLoache JS, Chiong C, Sherman K, et al. Do babies learn from baby media? *Psychol Sci.* 2010;21(11):1570–1574

6. Richert RA, Robb MB, Fender JG, Wartella E. Word learning from baby videos. *Arch Pediatr Adolesc Med.* 2010;164(5):432–437

7. Roseberry S, Hirsh-Pasek K, Golinkoff RM. Skype me! Socially contingent interactions help toddlers learn language. *Child Dev.* 2014;85(3):956–970

8. Kirkorian HL, Choi K, Pempek TA. Toddlers' Word Learning From Contingent and Noncontingent Video on Touch Screens. *Child Dev.* 2016;87(2):405–413

9. Zack E, Gerhardstein P, Meltzoff AN, Barr R. 15-month-olds' transfer of learning between touch screen and real-world displays: language cues and cognitive loads. *Scand J Psychol.* 2013;54(1):20–25

10. McClure ER, Chentsova-Dutton YE, Barr RF, Holochwost SJ, Parrott WG. "Facetime doesn't count": video-chat as an exception to media restrictions for infants and toddlers. *Int J Child Comput Interact.* 2016;6:1–6

11. Anderson DR, Huston AC, Schmitt KL, Linebarger DL, Wright JC. Early childhood television viewing and adolescent behavior: the recontact

study. *Monogr Soc Res Child Dev.* 2001;66(1):I–VIII, 1–147

12. Christakis DA, Garrison MM, Herrenkohl T, et al. Modifying media content for preschool children: a randomized controlled trial. *Pediatrics.* 2013;131(3):431–438

13. Guernsey L, Levine MH. *Tap Click Read: Growing readers in a world of screens.* San Fransisco, CA: Jossey-Bass; 2015

14. Hirsh-Pasek K, Zosh JM, Golinkoff RM, Gray JH, Robb MB, Kaufman J. Putting education in "educational" apps: lessons from the science of learning. *Psychol Sci Public Interest.* 2015;16(1):3–34

15. Shaheen S. How child's play impacts executive function--related behaviors. *Appl Neuropsychol Child.* 2014;3(3):182–187

16. Blair C, Granger DA, Willoughby M, et al; FLP Investigators. Salivary cortisol mediates effects of poverty and parenting on executive functions in early childhood. *Child Dev.* 2011;82(6):1970–1984

17. Bus AG, Takacs ZK, Kegel CA. Affordances and limitations of electronic storybooks for young children's emergent literacy. *Dev Rev.* 2015;35:79–97

18. Cox R, Skouteris H, Rutherford L, Fuller-Tyszkiewicz M, Dell' Aquila D, Hardy LL. Television viewing, television content, food intake, physical activity and body mass index: a cross-sectional study of preschool children aged 2-6 years. *Health Promot J Austr.* 2012;23(1):58–62

19. Taveras EM, Gillman MW, Kleinman KP, Rich-Edwards JW, Rifas-Shiman SL. Reducing racial/ethnic disparities in childhood obesity: the role of early life risk factors. *JAMA Pediatr.* 2013;167(8):731–738

20. Suglia SF, Duarte CS, Chambers EC, Boynton-Jarrett R. Social and behavioral risk factors for obesity in early childhood. *J Dev Behav Pediatr.* 2013;34(8):549–556

21. Wen LM, Baur LA, Rissel C, Xu H, Simpson JM. Correlates of body mass index and overweight and obesity of children aged 2 years: findings from the healthy beginnings trial. *Obesity (Silver Spring).* 2014;22(7):1723–1730

22. Mazarello Paes V, Ong KK, Lakshman R. Factors influencing obesogenic dietary intake in young children (0-6 years): systematic review of qualitative evidence. *BMJ Open.* 2015;5(9):e007396

23. Bellissimo N, Pencharz PB, Thomas SG, Anderson GH. Effect of television viewing at mealtime on food intake after a glucose preload in boys. *Pediatr Res.* 2007;61(6):745–749

24. Cespedes EM, Gillman MW, Kleinman K, Rifas-Shiman SL, Redline S, Taveras EM. Television viewing, bedroom television, and sleep duration from infancy to mid-childhood. *Pediatrics.* 2014;133(5). Available at: www.pediatrics.org/cgi/content/full/133/5/e1163

25. Vijakkhana N, Wilaisakditipakorn T, Ruedeekhajorn K, Pruksananonda C, Chonchaiya W. Evening media exposure reduces night-time sleep. *Acta Paediatr.* 2015;104(3):306–312

26. Garrison MM, Liekweg K, Christakis DA. Media use and child sleep: the impact of content, timing, and environment. *Pediatrics.* 2011;128(1):29–35

27. Salti R, Tarquini R, Stagi S, et al. Age-dependent association of exposure to television screen with children's urinary melatonin excretion? *Neuroendocrinol Lett.* 2006;27(1-2):73–80

28. Tomopoulos S, Dreyer BP, Berkule S, Fierman AH, Brockmeyer C, Mendelsohn AL. Infant media exposure and toddler development. *Arch Pediatr Adolesc Med.* 2010;164(12):1105–1111

29. Schmidt ME, Rich M, Rifas-Shiman SL, Oken E, Taveras EM. Television viewing in infancy and child cognition at 3 years of age in a US cohort. *Pediatrics.* 2009;123(3). Available at: www.pediatrics.org/cgi/content/full/123/3/e370

30. Lin LY, Cherng RJ, Chen YJ, Chen YJ, Yang HM. Effects of television exposure on developmental skills among young children. *Infant Behav Dev.* 2015;38:20–26

31. Zimmerman FJ, Christakis DA, Meltzoff AN. Associations between media viewing and language development in children under age 2 years. *J Pediatr.* 2007;151(4):364–368

32. Duch H, Fisher EM, Ensari I, et al. Association of screen time use and

language development in Hispanic toddlers: a cross-sectional and longitudinal study. *Clin Pediatr (Phila).* 2013;52(9):857–865

33. Tomopoulos S, Dreyer BP, Valdez P, et al. Media content and externalizing behaviors in Latino toddlers. *Ambul Pediatr.* 2007;7(3):232–238

34. Hinkley T, Verbestel V, Ahrens W, et al; IDEFICS Consortium. Early childhood electronic media use as a predictor of poorer well-being: a prospective cohort study. *JAMA Pediatr.* 2014;168(5):485–492

35. Pagani LS, Fitzpatrick C, Barnett TA, Dubow E. Prospective associations between early childhood television exposure and academic, psychosocial, and physical well-being by middle childhood. *Arch Pediatr Adolesc Med.* 2010;164(5):425–431

36. Conners-Burrow NA, McKelvey LM, Fussell JJ. Social outcomes associated with media viewing habits of low-income preschool children. *Early Educ Dev.* 2011;22(2):256–273

37. Christakis DA, Gilkerson J, Richards JA, et al. Audible television and decreased adult words, infant vocalizations, and conversational turns: a population-based study. *Arch Pediatr Adolesc Med.* 2009;163(6):554–558

38. Nathanson AI, Aladé F, Sharp ML, Rasmussen EE, Christy K. The relation between television exposure and executive function among preschoolers. *Dev Psychol.* 2014;50(5):1497–1506

39. Linebarger DL, Barr R, Lapierre MA, Piotrowski JT. Associations between parenting, media use, cumulative risk, and children's executive functioning. *J Dev Behav Pediatr.* 2014;35(6):367–377

40. Thompson AL, Adair LS, Bentley ME. Maternal characteristics and perception of temperament associated with infant TV exposure. *Pediatrics.* 2013;131(2). Available at: www.pediatrics.org/cgi/content/full/131/2/e390

41. Sugawara M, Matsumoto S, Murohashi H, Sakai A, Isshiki N. Trajectories of early television contact in Japan: Relationship with preschoolers' externalizing problems. *J Child Media.* 2015;9(4):453–471

42. Radesky JS, Silverstein M, Zuckerman B, Christakis DA. Infant self-regulation and early childhood media exposure. *Pediatrics*. 2014;133(5). Available at: www.pediatrics.org/cgi/content/full/133/5/e1172

43. Radesky JS, Peacock-Chambers E, Zuckerman B, Silverstein M. Use of mobile technology to calm upset children: associations with social-emotional development. *JAMA Pediatr*. 2016;170(4):397–399

44. Kirkorian HL, Pempek TA, Murphy LA, Schmidt ME, Anderson DR. The impact of background television on parent-child interaction. *Child Dev*. 2009;80(5):1350–1359

45. Schmidt ME, Pempek TA, Kirkorian HL, Lund AF, Anderson DR. The effects of background television on the toy play behavior of very young children. *Child Dev*. 2008;79(4):1137–1151

46. Radesky J, Miller AL, Rosenblum KL, Appugliese D, Kaciroti N, Lumeng JC. Maternal mobile device use during a structured parent-child interaction task. *Acad Pediatr*. 2015;15(2):238–244

47. Radesky JS, Kistin CJ, Zuckerman B, et al. Patterns of mobile device use by caregivers and children during meals in fast food restaurants. *Pediatrics*. 2014;133(4). Available at: www.pediatrics.org/cgi/content/full/133/4/e843

48. Jago R, Stamatakis E, Gama A, et al. Parent and child screen-viewing time and home media environment. *Am J Prev Med*. 2012;43(2):150–158

49. American Academy of Pediatrics, Council on Communications and Media. Media use in school-aged children and adolescents. *Pediatrics*. 2016;138(5):e20162592

Media Use in School-Aged Children and Adolescents

• *Policy Statement*

POLICY STATEMENT   Organizational Principles to Guide and Define the Child Health
Care System and/or Improve the Health of all Children

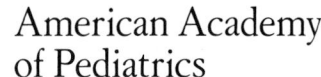
American Academy
of Pediatrics
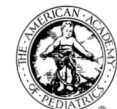

DEDICATED TO THE HEALTH OF ALL CHILDREN™

Media Use in School-Aged Children and Adolescents

COUNCIL ON COMMUNICATIONS AND MEDIA

abstract

This policy statement focuses on children and adolescents 5 through 18 years of age. Research suggests both benefits and risks of media use for the health of children and teenagers. Benefits include exposure to new ideas and knowledge acquisition, increased opportunities for social contact and support, and new opportunities to access health-promotion messages and information. Risks include negative health effects on weight and sleep; exposure to inaccurate, inappropriate, or unsafe content and contacts; and compromised privacy and confidentiality. Parents face challenges in monitoring their children's and their own media use and in serving as positive role models. In this new era, evidence regarding healthy media use does not support a one-size-fits-all approach. Parents and pediatricians can work together to develop a Family Media Use Plan (www.healthychildren.org/MediaUsePlan) that considers their children's developmental stages to individualize an appropriate balance for media time and consistent rules about media use, to mentor their children, to set boundaries for accessing content and displaying personal information, and to implement open family communication about media.

Policy statements from the American Academy of Pediatrics benefit from expertise and resources of liaisons and internal (AAP) and external reviewers. However, policy statements from the American Academy of Pediatrics may not reflect the views of the liaisons or the organizations or government agencies that they represent.

The guidance in this statement does not indicate an exclusive course of treatment or serve as a standard of medical care. Variations, taking into account individual circumstances, may be appropriate.

All policy statements from the American Academy of Pediatrics automatically expire 5 years after publication unless reaffirmed, revised, or retired at or before that time.

DOI: 10.1542/peds.2016-2592

PEDIATRICS (ISSN Numbers: Print, 0031-4005; Online, 1098-4275).

Copyright © 2016 by the American Academy of Pediatrics

FINANCIAL DISCLOSURE: The authors have indicated they do not have a financial relationship relevant to this article to disclose.

FUNDING: No external funding.

POTENTIAL CONFLICT OF INTEREST: The authors have indicated they have no potential conflicts of interest to disclose.

To cite: AAP COUNCIL ON COMMUNICATIONS AND MEDIA. Media Use in School-Aged Children and Adolescents. *Pediatrics.* 2016;138(5):e20162592

INTRODUCTION

Today's generation of children and adolescents are growing up immersed in media, including broadcast and social media. Broadcast media include television and movies. Interactive media include social media and video games in which users can both consume and create content. Interactive media allow information sharing and provide an engaging digital environment that becomes highly personalized.

Media Use Patterns

The most common broadcast medium continues to be TV. A recent study found that TV hours among school-aged children have decreased in the past decade for children younger than 8 years.[1] However, among children aged 8 years and older, average daily TV time remains over 2 hours per day.[2] TV viewing also has changed over the past decade, with content available via streaming or social media sites, such as YouTube and Netflix.

Overall media use among adolescents has continued to grow over the past decade, aided by the recent increase in mobile phone use among teenagers. Approximately three-quarters of teenagers today own a smartphone,[3] which allows access to the Internet, streaming TV/videos, and interactive "apps." Approximately one-quarter of teenagers describe themselves as "constantly connected" to the Internet.[3]

Social media sites and mobile apps provide platforms for users to create an online identity, communicate with others, and build social networks. At present, 76% of teenagers use at least 1 social media site.[3] Although Facebook remains the most popular social media site,[3] teenagers do not typically commit to just 1 social media platform; more than 70% maintain a "social media portfolio" of several selected sites, including Facebook, Twitter, and Instagram.[3] Mobile apps provide a breadth of functions, such as photo sharing, games, and video-chatting.

Video games remain very popular among families; 4 of 5 households own a device used to play video games.[4] Boys are the most avid video game players, with 91% of boys reporting having access to a game console and 84% reporting playing video games online or on a cell phone.[3]

Benefits of Media

Both traditional and social media can provide exposure to new ideas and information, raising awareness of current events and issues. Interactive media also can provide opportunities for the promotion of community participation and civic engagement. Students can collaborate with others on assignments and projects on many online media platforms. The use of social media helps families and friends who are separated geographically communicate across the miles.

Social media can enhance access to valuable support networks, which may be particularly helpful for patients with ongoing illnesses, conditions, or disabilities.[5] In 1 study, young adults described the benefits of seeking health information online and through social media, and recognized these channels as useful supplementary sources of information to health care visits.[6] Research also supports the use of social media to foster social inclusion among users who may feel excluded[7] or who are seeking a welcoming community: for example, those identifying as lesbian, gay, bisexual, transgender, questioning, or intersex. Finally, social media may be used to enhance wellness and promote healthy behaviors, such as smoking cessation and balanced nutrition.[8]

Risks of Media

A first area of health concern is media use and obesity, and most studies have focused on TV. One study found that the odds of being overweight were almost 5 times greater for adolescents who watch more than 5 hours of TV per day compared with those who watch 0 to 2 hours.[9] This study's findings contributed to recommendations by the American Academy of Pediatrics that children have 2 hours or less of sedentary screen time daily. More recent studies have provided new evidence that watching TV for more than 1.5 hours daily was a risk factor for obesity, but only for children 4 through 9 years of age.[10] Increased caloric intake via snacking while watching TV has been shown to be a risk factor for obesity, as is exposure to advertising for high-calorie foods and snacks.[11,12] Having a TV in the bedroom continues to be associated with the risk of obesity.[13]

Evidence suggests that media use can negatively affect sleep.[14] Studies show that those with higher social media use[15] or who sleep with mobile devices in their rooms[16] were at greater risk of sleep disturbances. Exposure to light (particularly blue light) and activity from screens before bed affects melatonin levels and can delay or disrupt sleep.[17] Media use around or after bedtime can disrupt sleep and negatively affect school performance.[13]

Children who overuse online media are at risk of problematic Internet use,[18] and heavy users of video games are at risk of Internet gaming disorder.[19] The *Diagnostic and Statistical Manual of Mental Disorders, Fifth Edition*,[20] lists both as conditions in need of further research. Symptoms can include a preoccupation with the activity, decreased interest in offline or "real life" relationships, unsuccessful attempts to decrease use, and withdrawal symptoms. The prevalence of problematic Internet use among children and adolescents is between 4% and 8%,[21,22] and up to 8.5% of US youth 8 to 18 years of age meet criteria for Internet gaming disorder.[23]

At home, many children and teenagers use entertainment media at the same time that they are engaged in other tasks, such as homework.[24] A growing body of evidence suggests that the use of media while engaged in academic tasks has negative consequences on learning.[25,26]

Media Influence

Evidence gathered over decades supports links between media exposure and health behaviors among teenagers.[27] The exposure of adolescents through media to alcohol,[28,29] tobacco use,[30,31] or sexual behaviors[32] is associated with earlier initiation of these behaviors.

Adolescents' displays on social media frequently include portrayal of health risk behaviors, such as substance use, sexual behaviors, self-injury, or disordered eating.[33-36] Peer viewers of such content may see these behaviors as normative and desirable.[37,38] Research from both the United States and the United Kingdom indicates that the major alcohol brands maintain a strong presence on Facebook, Twitter, and YouTube.[29,39]

Cyberbullying, Sexting, and Online Solicitation

Cyberbullying and traditional bullying overlap,[40] although online bullying presents unique challenges. These challenges include that perpetrators can be anonymous and bully at any time of day, that information can spread online rapidly,[41] and that perpetrator and target roles can be quite fluid in the online world. Cyberbullying can lead to short- and long-term negative social, academic, and health consequences for both the perpetrator and the target.[42] Fortunately, newer studies suggest that interventions that target bullying may reduce cyberbullying.[43]

"Sexting" is commonly defined as the electronic transmission of nude or seminude images as well as sexually explicit text messages. It is estimated that ~12% of youth aged 10 to 19 years have ever sent a sexual photo to someone else.[44] The Internet also has created opportunities for the exploitation of children by sex offenders through social networking, chat rooms, e-mail, and online games.[45]

Social Media and Mental Health

Research studies have identified both benefits and concerns regarding mental health and social media use. Benefits from the use of social media in moderation include the opportunity for enhanced social support and connection. Research has suggested a U-shaped relationship between Internet use

and depression, with increased risks of depression at both the high and low ends of Internet use.[46,47] One study found that older adolescents who used social media passively (eg, viewing others' photos) reported declines in life satisfaction, whereas those who interacted with others and posted content did not experience these declines.[48] Thus, in addition to the number of hours an individual spends on social media, a key factor is how social media is used.

Social Media and Privacy

Content that an adolescent chooses to post is shared with others, and the removal of such content once posted may be difficult or impossible. Adolescents vary in their understanding of privacy practices[49]; even those who know how to set privacy settings often don't believe they will work.[50] Despite efforts by some social media sites to protect privacy or to delete content after it is viewed, privacy violations and unwelcome distribution are always risks.[51,52]

Parent Media Use and Child Health

Social media can provide positive social experiences, such as opportunities for parents to connect with children via video-chat services. Unfortunately, some parents can be distracted by media and miss important opportunities for emotional connections that are known to improve child health.[53,54] One research study found that when a parent turned his or her attention to a mobile device while with a young child, the parent was less likely to talk with the child.[55] Parental engagement is critical in the development of children's emotional and social development, and these distractions may have short- and long-term negative effects.

CONCLUSIONS

The effects of media use are multifactorial and depend on the

type of media, the type of use, the amount and extent of use, and the characteristics of the individual child. Children today are growing up in an era of highly personalized media use experiences, so parents must develop personalized media use plans for their children that attend to each child's age, health, temperament, and developmental stage. Research evidence shows that children and teenagers need adequate sleep, physical activity, and time away from media. Pediatricians can help families develop a Family Media Use Plan (www.HealthyChildren.org/MediaUsePlan) that prioritizes these and other health goals.

RECOMMENDATIONS

Pediatricians

- Work with families and schools to promote understanding of the benefits and risks of media.

- Promote adherence to guidelines for adequate physical activity and sleep via a Family Media Use Plan (www.HealthyChildren.org/MediaUsePlan).

- Advocate for and promote information and training in media literacy.

- Be aware of tools to screen for sexting, cyberbullying, problematic Internet use, and Internet gaming disorder.

Families

- Develop, consistently follow, and routinely revisit a Family Media Use plan (see the plan from the American Academy of Pediatrics at www.HealthyChildren.org/MediaUsePlan).

  o Address what type of and how much media are used and what media behaviors are appropriate for each child or teenager, and for parents. Place consistent limits on hours per day of media use as well as types of media used.

- ○ Promote that children and adolescents get the recommended amount of daily physical activity (1 hour) and adequate sleep (8–12 hours, depending on age).

- ○ Recommend that children not sleep with devices in their bedrooms, including TVs, computers, and smartphones. Avoid exposure to devices or screens for 1 hour before bedtime.

- ○ Discourage entertainment media while doing homework.

- ○ Designate media-free times together (eg, family dinner) and media-free locations (eg, bedrooms) in homes. Promote activities that are likely to facilitate development and health, including positive parenting activities, such as reading, teaching, talking, and playing together.

- ○ Communicate guidelines to other caregivers, such as babysitters or grandparents, so that media rules are followed consistently.

- Engage in selecting and co-viewing media with your child, through which your child can use media to learn and be creative, and share these experiences with your family and your community.

- Have ongoing communication with children about online citizenship and safety, including treating others with respect online and offline, avoiding cyberbullying and sexting, being wary of online solicitation, and avoiding communications that can compromise personal privacy and safety.

- Actively develop a network of trusted adults (eg, aunts, uncles, coaches, etc) who can engage with children through social media and to whom children can turn when they encounter challenges.

Researchers, Governmental Organizations, and Industry

- Continue research into the risks and benefits of media.

- ○ Prioritize longitudinal and robust study designs, including new methodologies for understanding media exposure and use.

- ○ Prioritize interventions including reducing harmful media use and preventing and addressing harmful media experiences.

- Inform educators and legislators about research findings so they can develop updated guidelines for safe and productive media use.

LEAD AUTHORS

Megan A. Moreno, MD, MSEd, MPH, FAAP
Yolanda (Linda) Reid Chassiakos, MD, FAAP
Corinn Cross, MD, FAAP

COUNCIL ON COMMUNICATIONS AND MEDIA EXECUTIVE COMMITTEE, 2016–2017

David Hill, MD, FAAP, Chairperson
Nusheen Ameenuddin, MD, MPH, FAAP
Yolanda (Linda) Reid Chassiakos, MD, FAAP
Corinn Cross, MD, FAAP
Jenny Radesky, MD, FAAP
Jeffrey Hutchinson, MD, FAAP
Rhea Boyd, MD, FAAP
Robert Mendelson, MD, FAAP
Megan A. Moreno, MD, MSEd, MPH, FAAP
Justin Smith, MD, FAAP
Wendy Sue Swanson, MD, MBE, FAAP

LIAISONS

Kristopher Kaliebe, MD – *American Academy of Child and Adolescent Psychiatry*
Jennifer Pomeranz, JD, MPH – *American Public Health Association*
Brian Wilcox, PhD – *American Psychological Association*

STAFF

Thomas McPheron

REFERENCES

1. Loprinzi PD, Davis RE. Secular trends in parent-reported television viewing among children in the United States, 2001-2012. *Child Care Health Dev.* 2016;42(2):288–291

2. Rideout VJ. *Common Sense Census: Media Use by Tweets and Teens.* San Francisco, CA: Common Sense Media; 2015

3. Lenhart A. *Teens, Social Media & Technology Overview 2015.* Washington, DC: Pew Internet and American Life Project; 2015

4. Entertainment Software Association. *2015 Sales, Demographic and Usage Data: Essential Facts About the Computer and Video Game Industry.* Washington, DC: Entertainment Software Association; 2015

5. Naslund JA, Aschbrenner KA, Marsch LA, Bartels SJ. The future of mental health care: peer-to-peer support and social media. *Epidemiol Psychiatr Sci.* 2016;25(2):113–122

6. Briones R. Harnessing the Web: how e-health and e-health literacy impact young adults' perceptions of online health information. *Med 2 0.* 2015;4(2):e5

7. Krueger EA, Young SD. Twitter: a novel tool for studying the health and social needs of transgender communities. *JMIR Ment Health.* 2015;2(2)

8. Chou WY, Hunt YM, Beckjord EB, Moser RP, Hesse BW. Social media use in the United States: implications for health communication. *J Med Internet Res.* 2009;11(4):e48

9. Gortmaker SL, Must A, Sobol AM, Peterson K, Colditz GA, Dietz WH. Television viewing as a cause of increasing obesity among children in the United States, 1986-1990. *Arch Pediatr Adolesc Med.* 1996;150(4):356–362

10. de Jong E, Visscher TL,, HiraSing RA, Heymans MW, Seidell JC, Renders CM. Association between TV viewing, computer use and overweight, determinants and competing activities of screen time in 4- to 13-year-old children. *Int J Obes (Lond).* 2013;37(1):47–53

11. Goris JM, Petersen S, Stamatakis E, Veerman JL. Television food advertising and the prevalence of childhood overweight and obesity: a multicountry comparison. *Public Health Nutr.* 2010;13(7):1003–1012

12. Blass EM, Anderson DR, Kirkorian HL, Pempek TA, Price I, Koleini MF. On the

road to obesity: television viewing increases intake of high-density foods. *Physiol Behav.* 2006;88(4–5):597–604

13. Borghese MM, Tremblay MS, Katzmarzyk PT, et al. Mediating role of television time, diet patterns, physical activity and sleep duration in the association between television in the bedroom and adiposity in 10 year-old children. *Int J Behav Nutr Phys Act.* 2015;12:60–70

14. Bruni O, Sette S, Fontanesi L, Baiocco R, Laghi F, Baumgartner E. Technology use and sleep quality in preadolescence and adolescence. *J Clin Sleep Med.* 2015;11(12):1433–1441

15. Levenson JC, Shensa A, Sidani JE, Colditz JB, Primack BA. The association between social media use and sleep disturbance among young adults. *Prev Med.* 2016;85(Jan):36–41

16. Buxton OM, Chang AM, Spilsbury JC, Bos T, Emsellem H, Knutson KL. Sleep in the modern family: protective family routines for child and adolescent sleep. *Sleep Health.* 2015;1(1):15–27

17. Wahnschaffe A, Haedel S, Rodenbeck A, et al. Out of the lab and into the bathroom: evening short-term exposure to conventional light suppresses melatonin and increases alertness perception. *Int J Mol Sci.* 2013;14(2):2573–2589

18. Moreno MA, Jelenchick L, Cox E, Young H, Christakis DA. Problematic Internet use among US youth: a systematic review. *Arch Pediatr Adolesc Med.* 2011;165(9):797–805

19. Holtz P, Appel M. Internet use and video gaming predict problem behavior in early adolescence. *J Adolesc.* 2011;34(1):49–58

20. American Psychiatric Association. *Diagnostic and Statistical Manual of Mental Disorders, Fifth Edition.* Washington, DC: American Psychiatric Association; 2013

21. Liu TC, Desai RA, Krishnan-Sarin S, Cavallo DA, Potenza MN. Problematic Internet use and health in adolescents: data from a high school survey in Connecticut. *J Clin Psychiatry.* 2011;72(6):836–845

22. Jelenchick LA, Eickhoff J, Zhang C, Kraninger K, Christakis DA, Moreno MA. Screening for adolescent problematic Internet use: validation of the Problematic and Risky Internet Use Screening Scale (PRIUSS). *Acad Pediatr.* 2015;15(6):658–665

23. Gentile D. Pathological video-game use among youth ages 8 to 18: a national study. *Psychol Sci.* 2009;20(5):594–602

24. Brasel SA, Gips J. Media multitasking behavior: concurrent television and computer usage. *Cyberpsychol Behav Soc Netw.* 2011;14(9):527–534

25. Jacobsen WC, Forste R. The wired generation: academic and social outcomes of electronic media use among university students. *Cyberpsychol Behav Soc Netw.* 2011;14(5):275–280

26. Carrier LM, Rosen LD, Cheever NA, Lim AF. Causes, effects, and practicalities of everyday multitasking. Special issue: Living in the "Net" Generation: Multitasking, Learning, and Development. *Dev Rev.* 2015;35:64–78

27. Klein JD, Brown JD, Childers KW, Oliveri J, Porter C, Dykers C. Adolescents' risky behavior and mass media use. *Pediatrics.* 1993;92(1):24–31

28. Robinson TN, Chen HL, Killen JD. Television and music video exposure and risk of adolescent alcohol use. *Pediatrics.* 1998;102(5):E54

29. Winpenny EM, Marteau TM, Nolte E. Exposure of children and adolescents to alcohol marketing on social media websites. *Alcohol Alcohol.* 2014;49(2):154–159

30. Dalton MA, Beach ML, Adachi-Mejia AM, et al. Early exposure to movie smoking predicts established smoking by older teens and young adults. *Pediatrics.* 2009;123(4):e551–e558

31. Titus-Ernstoff L, Dalton MA, Adachi-Mejia AM, Longacre MR, Beach ML. Longitudinal study of viewing smoking in movies and initiation of smoking by children. *Pediatrics.* 2008;121(1):15–21

32. Ashby SL, Arcari CM, Edmonson MB. Television viewing and risk of sexual initiation by young adolescents. *Arch Pediatr Adolesc Med.* 2006;160(4):375–380

33. Hinduja S, Patchin JW. Personal information of adolescents on the Internet: a quantitative content analysis of MySpace. *J Adolesc.* 2008;31(1):125–146

34. Moreno MA, Parks MR, Zimmerman FJ, Brito TE, Christakis DA. Display of health risk behaviors on MySpace by adolescents: prevalence and associations. *Arch Pediatr Adolesc Med.* 2009;163(1):35–41

35. McGee JB, Begg M. What medical educators need to know about "Web 2.0". *Med Teach.* 2008;30(2):164–169

36. Moreno MA, Ton A, Selkie E, Evans Y. Secret Society 123: understanding the language of self-harm on Instagram. *J Adolesc Health.* 2016;58(1):78–84

37. Moreno MA, Briner LR, Williams A, Walker L, Christakis DA. Real use or "real cool": adolescents speak out about displayed alcohol references on social networking websites. *J Adolesc Health.* 2009;45(4):420–422

38. Litt DM, Stock ML. Adolescent alcohol-related risk cognitions: the roles of social norms and social networking sites. *Psychol Addict Behav.* 2011;25(4):708–713

39. Jernigan DH, Rushman AE. Measuring youth exposure to alcohol marketing on social networking sites: challenges and prospects. *J Public Health Policy.* 2014;35(1):91–104

40. Waasdorp TE, Bradshaw CP. The overlap between cyberbullying and traditional bullying. *J Adolesc Health.* 2015;56(5):483–488

41. Raskauskas J, Stoltz AD. Involvement in traditional and electronic bullying among adolescents. *Dev Psychol.* 2007;43(3):564–575

42. Vaillancourt T, Brittain HL, McDougall P, Duku E. Longitudinal links between childhood peer victimization, internalizing and externalizing problems, and academic functioning: developmental cascades. *J Abnorm Child Psychol.* 2013;41(8):1203–1215

43. Del Rey R, Casas JA, Ortega R. The impacts of the CONRED program on different cyberbullying roles [published online ahead of print 2015]. *Aggress Behav.* doi: 10.002/ab.21608

44. Temple JR, Choi H. Longitudinal association between teen sexting and sexual behavior. *Pediatrics.* 2014;134(5):e1287–e1292

45. Mitchell KJ, Finkelhor D, Wolak J. Youth Internet users at risk for the most

serious online sexual solicitations. *Am J Prev Med*. 2007;32(6):532–537

46. Bélanger RE, Akre C, Berchtold A, Michaud PA. A U-shaped association between intensity of Internet use and adolescent health. *Pediatrics*. 2011;127(2):e330–e335

47. Moreno MA, Jelenchick L, Koff R, Eickhoff J. Depression and internet use among older adolescents: an experience sampling approach. *Psychology (Irvine)*. 2012;3(9):743–748

48. Kross E, Verduyn P, Demiralp E, et al. Facebook use predicts declines in subjective well-being in young adults. *PLoS One*. 2013;8(8):e69841

49. Madden M, Lenhart A, Cortesi S, et alTeens, Social Media, and Privacy. Available at: http://www.pewinternet.org/2013/05/21/teens-social-media-and-privacy/. Accessed September 2, 2016

50. Marwick A, Boyd D. Networked privacy: How teenagers negotiate context in social media. *New Media Soc*. 2014;16(7):1051–1067

51. Hoadley CM, Xu H, Lee JJ, Rosson MB. Privacy as information access and illusory control: the case of the Facebook News Feed privacy outcry. *Electron Commer Res Appl*. 2010;9(1):50–60

52. Tsukayama H. Facebook draws fire from privacy advocates over ad changes. *The Washington Post*. June 12, 2014. Available at: https://www.washingtonpost.com/news/the-switch/wp/2014/06/12/privacy-experts-say-facebook-changes-open-up-unprecedented-data-collection/. Accessed September 2, 2016

53. Fiese BH. Family mealtime conversations in context. *J Nutr Educ Behav*. 2012;44(1):e1

54. Jago R, Thompson JL, Sebire SJ, et al. Cross-sectional associations between the screen-time of parents and young children: differences by parent and child gender and day of the week. *Int J Behav Nutr Phys Act*. 2014;11:54–62

55. Radesky J, Miller AL, Rosenblum KL, Appugliese D, Kaciroti N, Lumeng JC. Maternal mobile device use during a structured parent-child interaction task. *Acad Pediatr*. 2015;15(2):238–244

Mediators and Adverse Effects of Child Poverty in the United States

- *Technical Report*

TECHNICAL REPORT

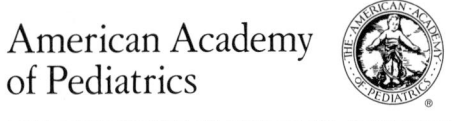

Mediators and Adverse Effects of Child Poverty in the United States

John M. Pascoe, MD, MPH, FAAP, David L. Wood, MD, MPH, FAAP, James H. Duffee, MD, MPH, FAAP, Alice Kuo, MD, PhD, MEd, FAAP, COMMITTEE ON PSYCHOSOCIAL ASPECTS OF CHILD AND FAMILY HEALTH, COUNCIL ON COMMUNITY PEDIATRICS

abstract

The link between poverty and children's health is well recognized. Even temporary poverty may have an adverse effect on children's health, and data consistently support the observation that poverty in childhood continues to have a negative effect on health into adulthood. In addition to childhood morbidity being related to child poverty, epidemiologic studies have documented a mortality gradient for children aged 1 to 15 years (and adults), with poor children experiencing a higher mortality rate than children from higher-income families. The global great recession is only now very slowly abating for millions of America's children and their families. At this difficult time in the history of our nation's families and immediately after the 50th anniversary year of President Lyndon Johnson's War on Poverty, it is particularly germane for the American Academy of Pediatrics, which is "dedicated to the health of all children," to publish a research-supported technical report that examines the mediators associated with the long-recognized adverse effects of child poverty on children and their families. This technical report draws on research from a number of disciplines, including physiology, sociology, psychology, economics, and epidemiology, to describe the present state of knowledge regarding poverty's negative impact on children's health and development. Children inherit not only their parents' genes but also the family ecology and its social milieu. Thus, parenting skills, housing, neighborhood, schools, and other factors (eg, medical care) all have complex relations to each other and influence how each child's genetic canvas is expressed. Accompanying this technical report is a policy statement that describes specific actions that pediatricians and other child advocates can take to attenuate the negative effects of the mediators identified in this technical report and improve the well-being of our nation's children and their families.

DOI: 10.1542/peds.2016-0340

PEDIATRICS (ISSN Numbers: Print, 0031-4005; Online, 1098-4275).

To cite: Pascoe JM, Wood DL, Duffee JH, et al. AAP Committee on Psychosocial Aspects of Child and Family Health, Council on Community Pediatrics. Mediators and Adverse Effects of Child Poverty in the United States. *Pediatrics.* 2016;137(4):e20160340

There is no keener revelation of a society's soul than the way in which it treats its children.

—Nelson Mandela

The advent of the Great Recession in December 2007 heralded an increase in child poverty from a prerecession 13.3 million children to 16.3 million children by 2010.[1,2] The Great Recession is only now very slowly abating for millions of this nation's families, and "full employment" is forecasted finally to return sometime in 2017.[3] In 2014, an estimated 21.1% of children, or 15.5 million, lived in poverty.[2]

Although medical care and access to medical care are important factors in the health of children as well as adults, a broader perspective of the social determinants of health throughout the life cycle is critically important if significant gains are to be realized in our efforts to improve the health of this nation's children. Research that examines mediators of health as well as the effects of poverty and other circumstances in which people grow, live, work, and age in childhood and throughout the life course is accumulating rapidly, and findings are providing critical insights that can inform these efforts.[4]

The environment in which a child develops is influenced by parents' health, the immediate and extended family, housing, and community. All these factors are related to a family's social, economic, and health status.[5] These multiple factors in both the social and the physical domains have dynamic influences that link them to the long-term physical and mental health of children, youth, and adults.[6,7] The interaction of these factors that ultimately influence children's health has been published as a figure within an earlier technical report from the American Academy of Pediatrics (AAP) on toxic stress.[8] The ongoing investigation of these factors creates the basic science of pediatrics (Fig 1).

A 1958 birth cohort longitudinal study from the United Kingdom recently reported that 45-year-old adults who experienced psychological distress during childhood were at

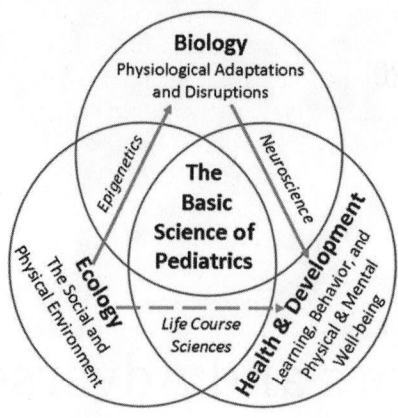

FIGURE 1

The basic science of pediatrics. An emerging, multidisciplinary science of development supports an ecobiodevelopmental framework for understanding the evolution of human health and disease across the life span. In recent decades, epidemiology, developmental psychology, and longitudinal studies of early childhood interventions have shown significant associations (dashed arrow) between the ecology of childhood and a wide range of developmental outcomes and life-course trajectories. Concurrently, advances in the biological sciences, particularly in developmental neuroscience and epigenetics, have made parallel progress in beginning to elucidate the biological mechanisms (solid arrows) underlying these important associations. The convergence of these diverse disciplines defines a promising new basic science of pediatrics.

increased risk of adult cardiovascular and metabolic disease even if the distress resolved during adulthood.[9] Another recent study from Europe reviewed 201 studies from 32 countries from all European regions. The investigators found that multiple social factors from different levels (eg, neighborhood, household) are sources of child health or development disadvantage. These findings support the necessity for effective interventions to target multiple social factors operating at different levels.[10]

The notion that development is affected by both biology and experience coactively is sometimes referred to as "canalization." This idea is a major tenet of the psychobiological model of growth and development and provides a framework to understand why

individuals do, or do not, develop specific sets of skills that reflect their genes as well as their life experiences.[11] This concept is very similar to the ecobiodevelopmental framework proposed in the AAP policy statement and technical report on toxic stress.[8,12] Although occasional stories appear of extraordinary disadvantaged youth who have overcome the myriad negative experiences of their childhood, for most children early adversity casts a long shadow into their adulthood and even into the next generation.[13] This technical report provides an analysis of the current research on child poverty and mechanisms by which poverty and other factors associated with disadvantage influence the health and well-being of children. This report is especially appropriate immediately after the 50th anniversary year of President Johnson's War on Poverty.[14,15]

OVERVIEW OF POVERTY, RELATIONAL HEALTH, AND TOXIC STRESS

Poor families experience a plethora of stressful challenges that influence health.[16] Housing and food insecurity are 2 examples of social determinants of health that contribute to health disparities in childhood.[17,18] Poverty is an independent determinant of health through its adverse effect on family relationships, also called relational health.[19] Relational health in early childhood is the ability to form secure attachments with engaged, responsive caregivers in a safe, stable, and nurturing emotional environment[20]; it is an essential protective factor for the development of emotional regulation and resilience and the ability to cope with adversity during an individual's lifetime.[21]

Family relational processes can be affected by both biological and psychosocial pathways. For example, parents' poverty-related stress can activate children's stress mechanisms or children's immune systems, and economic hardship has been associated with depressed parental mood and marital conflict.[22]

Poverty has direct negative effects on early brain development through the mechanism of toxic stress. The pathophysiology of toxic stress consists of frequent, unremitting activation of the hypothalamic-pituitary-adrenocortical (HPA) axis stress system and chronic elevation of cortisol as well as inflammatory mediators. The most common physiologic adaptive response to stress involves activation of the HPA axis and the sympathetic-adrenomedullary system. This activation results in increased levels of stress hormones, such as corticotropin-releasing hormone, cortisol, norepinephrine, and adrenaline. These changes occur at the same time that other mediators are released, such as inflammatory cytokines.[23,24] Although transient increases in these hormones are protective and may be necessary for survival, very high levels or prolonged exposures can be harmful and even toxic for the human body.[25] The dysregulation of this combination of physiologic mediators (eg, too much or too little cortisol or inflammatory response) can create a "wear and tear" effect on a number of organs, including the brain.[26] The overall stress-induced burden on body functioning and the aggregated physiologic and psychological costs required for coping and returning to homeostatic balance have been termed "allostatic load."

The chronic stress of poverty during early childhood development is associated with an impaired ability of the prefrontal cortex to suppress the amygdala, the "on switch" for the stress response.[27] Prefrontal lobe dysfunction impairs executive control[28] of affect regulation and impulsive behavior, and the epigenetic, anatomic, and

neuroendocrine disruption related to chronic toxic stress may impair learning, behavior, and interpersonal relationships.[29] This dysregulation adversely affects physical and mental illness throughout the life course. The combination of impaired self-regulation and chronic stress may lead to maladaptive behaviors, such as smoking, excessive alcohol intake, overeating, promiscuity, and substance abuse, that transiently turn off the stress response but over the life course may cause morbidity and early mortality.[30,31]

In summary, poverty and other social determinants of health adversely affect relational health. Poor relational health, particularly the absence of emotional support by a nurturing adult, increases the risk of childhood toxic stress and difficulties in emotional regulation, early child development, and eventually, lifelong health. Prolonged activation of the body's stress response becomes intolerable in the absence of the buffering effect of a supportive adult relationship.[32] On the other hand, with good relational health and family stability, a child who experiences stress is more likely to turn off the physiologic stress response in a timely manner and avoid the adverse consequences.[8,33] Programs focused on building self-regulation in impoverished children have been shown to improve executive function and decrease chronic stress.[34] Thus, poverty-related stress may be tolerable if good relational health is present as a protective factor. Recommendations made in the accompanying policy statement,[35] "Poverty and Child Health in the United States," are based on emerging research and evaluation findings that support the notion that the brain development of a child experiencing poverty and his or her health during the life course may be protected from harm by programs that foster improved parent engagement and relational

health within the family and help to buffer the chronic stress of poverty.[34,36]

DEFINING AND DESCRIBING POVERTY IN THE UNITED STATES

Poverty is defined as a state in which one lacks a usual or socially acceptable amount of money or material possessions to provide for his or her basic needs, which typically include food, water, sanitation, clothing, shelter, health care, and education.[37]

Federal Poverty Level

In the United States, the current method of operationalizing and measuring poverty is called the federal poverty level (FPL). Each year, the US Department of Health and Human Services develops a set of poverty guidelines and thresholds on the basis of family size and family composition. These guidelines and thresholds are based on census data and are loosely referred to as the FPL. The income and demographic data for FPL estimates are collected within the Current Population Survey, an annual and nationally representative household survey jointly conducted by the US Census Bureau and the US Bureau of Labor Statistics within the US Department of Labor.

The FPL was developed in the early 1960s on the basis of data from the US Department of Agriculture's 1955 Food Consumption Survey. That research in the 1950s found that the average US family spent one-third of its pretax income on food. By using the US Department of Agriculture's Economy Food Plan, a bare-bones plan designed to provide a healthy diet for a temporary period when funds are low, the federal poverty measure was determined by multiplying the budget for the basic food plan by 3.

The federal poverty measure has not changed fundamentally since 1969, except that it is adjusted annually for overall food price inflation, as measured by the Consumer Price Index. Thus, the FPL reflects 1950s living standards and has not been adjusted to reflect changes in needs associated with the dramatic increase in 2-parent working families and the improvement in the standards of living that have occurred over the past 45 years, which have significantly changed the composition of the family budget. Food now accounts for approximately 15% of the budget, and the proportion allocated to work-related costs, child care, housing, and transportation has increased substantially. If the same methodology of the basic food basket were applied today, the FPL would be more than 2 times higher than the current level.[38] However, it is also important to note that the FPL does not take into consideration government cash or near-cash subsidies, such as the Supplemental Nutrition Assistance Program (SNAP), the Special Supplemental Nutrition Program for Women, Infants, and Children (WIC), housing subsidies, low-income home energy assistance, or earned income and child tax credits. The FPL also does not account for variations in medical costs across population groups or geographic differences in the cost of living. To account for geographic variations in the cost of living and to include income-transfer programs listed above, in 2010 the National Academy of Sciences[39] conducted a study of current family budgets and developed the Supplemental Poverty Measure (SPM).[40]

Individuals and families living below the FPL are referred to as "poor" (in 2014, this was $15 379 for a 2-person family and $24 230 for a family of 4).[2] Research suggests that, on average, families need an income equal to at least 2 times the FPL to meet their basic needs.[41] Families with incomes up to 200% of the FPL are referred to as "low income" ($48 460 for a family of 4). Families at 50% of the

TABLE 1 Definitions of Poverty

Low-income: income at 150% to 200% of the FPL
Poverty: income less than 100% of the FPL
Extreme or deep poverty: income less than 50% of the FPL
Sources:
　　Low-income: http://datacenter.kidscount.org/data/tables/118-children-living-in-low-income-families-
　　　　below-200-percent-of-the-poverty-threshold-by-family-nativity?loc=1&loct=2#detailed/2/2-52/false/
　　　　36,868,867,133,38/78,79/451,452
　　Poverty: http://datacenter.kidscount.org/data/tables/52-population-in-poverty?loc=1&loct=2#detailed/
　　　　2/2-52/false/36,868,867,133,38/any/339,340
　　Deep poverty: http://datacenter.kidscount.org/data/tables/45-children-in-extreme-poverty-50-percent-
　　　　poverty#detailed/1/any/false/36,868,867,133,38/any/325,326; http://www.ers.usda.gov/amber-waves/
　　　　2014-march/poverty-and-deep-poverty-increasing-in-rural-america.aspx#.VSkziLrVQbA

FPL are considered to be living in "deep poverty"; in 2014, 9.3% of children younger than 18 years in the United States lived in deep poverty, representing 32.7% of people living in deep poverty (Table 1).[2]

Family income is not the only, or perhaps best, indicator of poverty. Family wealth, defined as the total value of family assets such as housing, monetary savings, investments, etc, may be a more important measure of both family financial stability and the capacity to sufficiently provide for children. The wealth gap has widened significantly since the recent economic downturn. In 1995, the disparity of median household wealth (net assets) between white families and for both black and Hispanic families was 7:1. By 2009, at the end of the Great Recession, the median household wealth for white families was 18 times that for Hispanic families and 20 times that for black families.[42] Other measures of financial status or stability include measures of educational achievement, quality of housing, and stability of employment, all of which contribute to quality of life more directly than does a moderate increase in income or net wealth.[43]

Challenges With the Poverty Measures

Current poverty measures all have inherent difficulties, and attempts have been made to compensate for them. For example, these measures are point-in-time or prevalence measures of poverty. However,

individual and family poverty and deprivation are not static; family income changes over time. Moreover, poverty and deprivation most strongly affect children and families over time. To measure the longitudinal dimension of poverty, researchers use recurring surveys, such as the Panel Study of Income Dynamics,[44] a nationally representative survey that interviewed respondents (including families with children) annually from 1968 to 1997 and biennially thereafter.[45]

Another problem with a federal measure of poverty is that the cost of living varies significantly by region. In 2012, the estimated cost of meeting a family's basic needs for a family of 4 was approximately $64 000 per year in Los Angeles, California; $57 000 in Newark, New Jersey; $46 000 in Indianapolis, Indiana; and $42 000 in Jackson, Mississippi.[46] This variation is not taken into account by the FPL but is taken into account by the SPM. As a result, in high-cost areas (eg, New Jersey, California), the SPM indicates higher poverty rates than does the FPL, and in lower-cost areas (eg, Mississippi) the SPM indicates lower poverty rates than does the FPL.[38]

PREVALENCE AND CHARACTERISTICS OF CHILD POVERTY IN THE UNITED STATES

By using the FPL, the percentage of children younger than 18 years living in poverty declined significantly during the 1950s and 1960s,[47] but from the mid-1970s until 2010 the proportion of children living in poverty increased, rising strongly during economic recessions and declining modestly during periods of economic growth.[38] From 2007 to 2010, the percentage of children in poverty increased from 18% to 22%, an increase of 3 million children living in poverty. From 2010 to 2014, the child poverty rate was stable and did not appreciably increase or decline.[2,48] In 2014, 9.3% of children lived in extreme poverty, with their families earning less than 50% of the FPL.[2,49,50]

Demographics

Age.

Younger children are more likely to be poor or low income than are older children. In 2013, 25% of children from birth to 5 years of age were poor and 48% were low income, compared with adolescents, 19% of whom were poor and 41% of whom were low income.[51,52] In other words, poverty and low income have the highest prevalence among the most vulnerable members of our society during the most critical time in their development.

Race, Ethnicity, and Immigrant Status.

Race and ethnicity are particularly strong determinants of both individual- and community-level poverty. In 2014, 12.3% of white children and 13.4% of Asian children lived below poverty level, compared with 37.1% of black children and 31.9% of Hispanic children.[2] In 2013, 25.8% of children in the United States had at least 1 immigrant parent. The poverty rate among children of immigrant parents in 2013 was 28.4%.[53]

Parental Education.

Higher levels of parental education decrease the likelihood that a child will live in a low-income or poor family. Among children with at least 1 parent with some college or additional education, 13% are poor and 31% are low income. By contrast, among children whose parents have less than a high school degree, 57% are poor and 86% are low income.[46]

Parental Employment Status.

Children with a parent who is employed full-time, year-round are less likely to live in poor families than are children with parents who work part-time or part of the year or who are not employed. Of children with 1 parent who works full-time, year-round, 9% are poor and 31% are low income. In contrast, of children in families with no parent who works full-time, 48% are poor and 74% are low income. It is important to note that almost half (49%) of low-income children and 28% of poor children have at least 1 parent employed full-time, year-round.[44,46]

Family Structure.

Single-parent families are more than 4 times more likely to be poor than are 2-parent families.[48] Among all single female-headed families, 42% are poor and 69% are low income compared with 12% and 32%, respectively, for 2-parent families.[46] A major contributor to poverty in the United States is the increase in the proportion of children who live in single-parent families. In 1960, 87.8% of children were living in 2-parent families, compared with 64.4% in 2014.[54] The absence of fathers in the home is associated with a fourfold risk of poverty. Children of single mothers are also at greater risk of infant mortality, child maltreatment, failure to graduate from high school, and incarceration.[55,56]

Children being raised by same-sex parents are twice as likely to live in poverty, compared with children living in households with heterosexual parents.[47,57] The average household income for families headed by same-sex parents is 20% lower than that of families headed by heterosexual parent couples.[57,58] Moreover, only 51% of same-sex parent couples with children own their homes, compared with 71% of married heterosexual parent couples with children. A higher proportion of same-sex parent couples raising children live in states with high poverty rates: Mississippi, Wyoming, Alaska, Arkansas, Texas, Louisiana, Oklahoma, Kansas, Alabama, Montana, South Dakota, and South Carolina. In the past, because of limited federal and state recognition of spousal relationships between same-sex couples, families headed by same-sex couples were denied access to many family-income support programs.[58] However, recent Supreme Court decisions invalidating section 3 of the Defense of Marriage Act (which provided federal definitions of marriage that precluded federal recognition of same-sex marriages)[59,60] and the June 26, 2015, Supreme Court decision (Obergefell et al v Hodges) upholding the legality of marriage between same-sex couples should improve access to federal income-support programs for same-sex married couples.[61]

Geography

The overall national child poverty estimates mask important geographic variation in poverty across states, cities, and neighborhoods. In 2014, the percentage of children living in poverty ranged from 13% in Maryland, New Hampshire, Utah, and Wyoming to 30% in New Mexico. As shown in Fig 2, the southern states have higher levels of child poverty than do the northern states.[62] More substantial variation in community poverty exists among large and small cities and neighborhoods. Among large metropolitan regions, the prevalence of poverty rates varies from a high of 36% (eg, McAllen-Edinburg-Mission, Texas, and Fresno, California) to a low of

8% (eg, Washington, DC-Arlington/ Alexandria, Virginia, and Bridgeport-Stamford-Norwalk, Connecticut). At the neighborhood level, poverty can be even more concentrated in particular areas. More than 4% of children live in neighborhoods of very concentrated poverty, defined as neighborhoods in which ≥40% of households are poor. Twenty percent of children live in "poverty areas," defined as neighborhoods in which 20% to 39% of households are poor.[63]

Black, Hispanic, and American Indian/Alaska Native children are more likely to live in neighborhoods of concentrated poverty than are either Asian or white non-Hispanic children. Almost two-thirds of black, Hispanic, and American Indian/Alaska Native children live in areas of concentrated poverty, compared with one-third of white children.[38] As the severity of poverty in areas increases, the disproportionate representation of black, Hispanic, and American Indian/Alaska Native families and children increases to between 33% and 43%, compared with only 14% for white families.[38] Consistent with these data, recent studies show that residential segregation by income has increased over the past 30 years. The analysis found that 28% of lower-income households in 2010 were located in a majority lower-income census tract, up from 23% in 1980, and that 18% of upper-income households were located in a majority upper-income census tract, up from 9% in 1980.[46,64] That is, poverty and wealth are becoming more concentrated in very different neighborhoods.

An additional aspect of the geography of child poverty is that rural poverty rates have been historically higher than urban poverty rates, and rural poverty has increased more substantially in

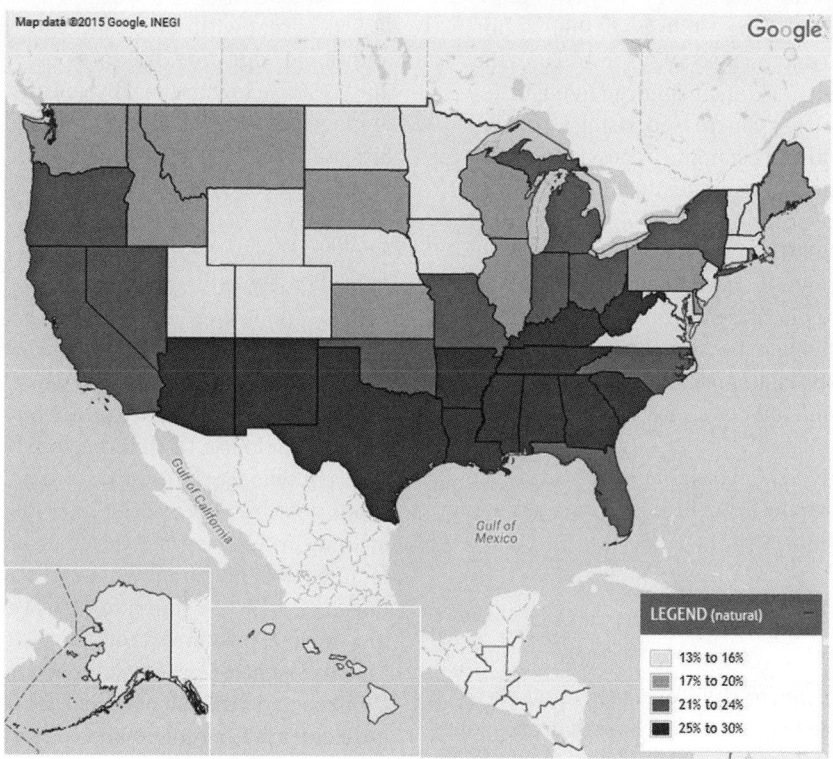

FIGURE 2

Children in Poverty 2014: analysis of Census Bureau American Community Survey data. (Reprinted with permission from the Kids Count Data Center, a project of the Annie E. Casey Foundation; http://datacenter.kidscount.org/data/Map/43-children-in-poverty-100-percent-poverty?loc=1&loct=1#2/any/false/869/any/322/Orange/.)

recent years, to 26.7% compared with 20.9% for metropolitan areas.[65] Since 2008, city suburbs have experienced the fastest growth in poverty of any population area. Children living in neighborhoods and communities characterized by concentrated poverty are more frequently exposed to environmental toxins, poorly performing schools and child care settings, community violence, and fewer community and social supports. The accumulation of multiple environmental risks found in areas of concentrated poverty undermines the healthy development of children.[66] Therefore, poor and minority children are in double jeopardy because of the lack of resources within their own families and the exposure to detrimental influences or lack of social supports in areas of concentrated poverty in urban, suburban, and rural areas.

Timing and Duration

Investigators from the Urban Institute studied the duration and severity of poverty among a sample of children over an interval of 18 years using data from the Panel Study of Income Dynamics. They found that 10% of children were persistently poor (more than 9 years) and another 10% were poor for 4 to 8 years. Persistent poverty differed significantly by race. Approximately 37% of black children were poor for more than 9 years of their childhood, whereas 5% of white children were persistently poor.[67] Children who experience poverty also tend to cycle into and out of poverty, and even the most persistently poor children spend intermittent years living above the FPL. The investigators also found that being poor at birth is a strong predictor of future poverty status: 31% of white children and 69% of black children who are poor at birth go on to spend at least half their childhood living in poverty.

Another important observation is that the effects of poverty are cumulative, and poverty in 1 period of a child's life hinders development in another stage or even into adulthood.[68] Shonkoff and colleagues[5] asserted that a "scientific consensus" has evolved on the origins of adult disease as a direct result of childhood adverse experiences and that childhood adverse experiences affect adult health either through "cumulative damage" or "biological embedding of adversities" that are related to adult disease.

THE PATHOPHYSIOLOGY OF POVERTY

Toxic Stress

An important concept in understanding the well-documented childhood gradient of morbidity and mortality is "toxic stress," a concept related to the change in stress hormones in response to experience over time.[69] For challenges of limited duration, the body's response is twofold: turning on a response that initiates a complex hormonal pathway and then shutting it off as the challenge resolves. The most common response involves the sympathetic nervous system and the HPA axis. Catecholamines are released from nerves and the adrenal medulla that stimulate a cascade within the HPA axis that results in the secretion of adrenocorticotropin from the pituitary gland. Adrenocorticotropin hormone stimulates cortisol secretion by the adrenal cortex. Although the immune-enhancing effects of acute stress have been observed to last 3 to 5 days, during the state of toxic stress the delayed hypersensitivity response is substantially blunted. When stress is chronic and continuous, such as the stress associated with chronic poverty, response systems, including the HPA axis and the sympathetic

adrenal system, are on "high alert." As a result, stress hormones, such as cortisol, are relatively high.

Appropriately labeled "a biology of misfortune" by Boyce,[70] the observation about toxic stress described above is supported by 2 recent studies. The Family Life Project was designed to follow young children and their families with high levels of poverty in eastern North Carolina and central Pennsylvania from the index child's birth through 4 years of age.[71] A representative sample of 1292 children were selected and home visited at approximately 7, 15, 24, 36, and 48 months of age. Salivary cortisol samples were collected at each home visit. During the first 4 years of the study, the statistically significant predictors of higher cortisol levels were black race, poor-quality housing, and 2 or more adults leaving the home before the index child's fourth birthday. Older children were studied by Evans and Kim,[72] who monitored overnight urinary cortisol concentrations to assess "chronic physiologic stress." Children were assessed in wave 1 at approximately 8 years of age and in wave 2 at 13 years of age with 12-hour overnight urinary free cortisol samples. After controlling for urinary cortisol concentrations in wave 1, urinary cortisol concentrations in wave 2 were significantly related to duration of family poverty. In addition, more time living in poverty for children aged 13 years old was related to a more attenuated cardiovascular response to an acute stressor. This pattern of chronic elevated HPA axis activity, muted cardiovascular response, and a gradient of cumulative risk for children living in poverty corroborates the findings of a large longitudinal British study that found the self-reported health of study participants aged 23 years old was related to a number of risk factors that began in childhood.[73]

Chronic Inflammation

Another biological process that may have a direct effect on the negative health outcomes observed in adults who experienced child poverty is chronic inflammation. Ziol-Guest et al[74] reported on a nationally representative sample of adults from the Panel Study of Income Dynamics. Adult study subjects (30–41 years of age) who experienced child poverty were more likely to report arthritis or hypertension and limitations in daily activities compared with adults who did not experience child poverty. Although the investigators noted the lack of direct measures of immune function in their study, earlier work has described a link between low social class early in life and chronic inflammation.[75] Facilitated by other exposures and genetic liabilities, chronic inflammation drives the pathogenic mechanisms that ultimately result in chronic disease.[76] In addition, animal research in mice has identified upregulation of inflammatory gene expression in the presence of social stress.[77]

THE ENVIRONMENT OF POVERTY

Children growing up in low-income families and low-income neighborhoods face a daunting array of psychosocial and environmental inequities that undermine their healthy development. The exposure to multiple stressors may be a unique, critically important feature of the environment of children growing up in poverty. Compared with their economically advantaged counterparts, children living in poor families and poor neighborhoods are exposed to more family turmoil, violence, and separation from their families.[65] Children from low-income families hear fewer words between age 1 and 3 years and the context of the language to which they are exposed is more negative and punitive compared with higher-income families.[78] More than one-quarter of poor children (28%) live in families with divorced or separated parents compared with less than 5% of children in the highest income group.[79] Almost half (45%) of children with single mothers live in poverty, compared with 13% of children from 2-parent families.[80] Low-income children also are much more likely to experience housing instability and multiple moves.[81,82] The physical environment of low-income children is more hazardous than that of higher-income children, because they are exposed more frequently to pollution, lower-quality homes, and dangerous neighborhoods.[83]

Unintentional Injuries and Child Maltreatment

Although mortality among US children has decreased over the past 15 years, injury and violence still account for nearly 50% of all childhood deaths after the first birthday.[84] Children from the lowest socioeconomic stratum have a death rate from unintentional injuries that is 5 times that of children from higher socioeconomic strata. Poor families are more likely to reside in homes without functional smoke detectors and with open fires, unprotected windows, and unsafe roofs or stairs. They may live close to dense, fast-moving traffic and lack safe areas in which to play.[85] Children in poor neighborhoods are at increased risk of cycling accidents, pedestrian injuries, falls, burns, poisonings, and chemical burns.[86] If children in the least healthy communities experienced mortality rates from unintentional injuries and homicide similar to those of the most resource-rich communities, overall US child mortality would decrease by one-third.[87]

Injuries from child maltreatment and developmental consequences of neglect also are risks for poor children. Recent survey data confirm that both poverty and income

inequality are positively associated with the rates of protective service referrals for child maltreatment.[88] Within families, poverty is associated with intimate partner violence, maternal depression, single-parent families, and parental substance abuse, all of which are risk factors for child maltreatment.[89] In 1998, Felitti et al[90] published the Adverse Childhood Experiences (ACE) Study, a landmark study that linked adverse childhood experiences, including childhood maltreatment, and mortality in adults. A recent study[88] corroborated the association between child poverty and child maltreatment at the county level for each of the 3142 counties in the United States. Child maltreatment is a global problem[91] that has a well-documented association with later negative physical and mental health outcomes in adults.[92] Although toxic stress has a role in the association between child maltreatment and later mental and physical health problems,[93] posttraumatic cognition (eg, an individual's appraisal or interpretation of the traumatic event or events) is another putative mediator.[94] Posttraumatic cognitions may act to either attenuate the adverse effects of child maltreatment or prevent healthy coping. Dysfunctional posttraumatic cognitions may lead to poorer health outcomes for the victims of child maltreatment.[95]

ADVERSE PSYCHOSOCIAL AND ENVIRONMENTAL EFFECTS OF POVERTY AND LOW INCOME ON CHILDREN

Inadequate Housing and Neighborhoods

Place matters. Where a child lives contributes to health disparities and predicts health inequities.[96] In addition to experiencing food insecurity, poor families may have difficulty maintaining adequate housing, heat, and utilities. In 2011, more than 45% of all households

with children reported housing problems, including multiple moves, overcrowding, and physically inadequate housing as well as inability to pay the rent.[97] An estimated 1.6 million American children experienced homelessness in 2010.[98] Household energy security (ie, the costs of home heating, cooling, and utilities) can present a constant struggle for low-income families. Researchers at the pediatric research center Children's Health Watch have identified energy insecurity as a risk to child health that is often found among families who are also food insecure.[99,100]

Poverty affects where and how families live. Housing options are often limited to urban areas with crowding, violence, and lack of safety; to rural areas that are isolated and lack social support[66, 101]; or to suburban neighborhoods that are either ethnic enclaves or affected by foreclosures and deteriorating housing stock. A large body of research has documented the relationship between neighborhood conditions and health.[102] For example, poverty is a risk factor for lead exposure in the home, and poor black children are twice as likely as poor Hispanic and white children to have concentrations of lead in their blood of at least 2.5 µg/dL (33% vs 17% and 13%, respectively).[103,104] There is an interaction between race and poverty, and not all poor children have the same experience. It appears that poor black children are more likely to be exposed to lead than poor children from other races.

Poor neighborhoods expose families to a variety of barriers and harms. Poor families often face elevated levels of crime, violence, and toxic exposure inherited from the days of racial segregation, now referred to as spatial racism, when communities of color were targeted for diminished resources and toxic industry. Areas of concentrated poverty also may lack quality schools, sustainable jobs, health care facilities, safe recreation spaces, and other resources that support healthy community activities.[105,106]

Limited Access to Developmentally Appropriate Experiences and High-Quality Educational Opportunities

Poor families may have difficulty obtaining resources that support child development and provide a nurturing and stimulating home environment. Data from the National Longitudinal Survey of Youth indicate that children in poor households have less access to learning materials and experiences, including books, stimulating toys, skill-building lessons, and other enriching experiences.[107]

In addition to individual family characteristics, funding and resources for schools make a difference in achievement. Forty-three percent of public school principals reported that the condition of their school facility interfered with classroom instruction.[108] Smaller class size, which requires more money, has been shown to produce lasting gains, particularly for economically disadvantaged students.[109] School funding formulas vary by state but are often dependent on property taxes, which can exacerbate economic disparities between communities. Unless the state has a formula that equalizes resources, poor communities tend to have less to spend per pupil than do wealthier communities. In 1 study, communities with 22% of students in poverty spent one-third as much per pupil as communities with 6% of students in poverty ($4000 vs $13 000 annually).[110]

Suboptimal Nutrition

Food insecurity is defined as limited or uncertain availability of nutritionally adequate and safe foods.[111] An estimated 20% of households with children in the United States experienced food insecurity during 2013.[112] The rate of food insecurity for children living in poverty is nearly 40%.[113] Although children are often shielded from very low food security, in approximately 10% of households with children (more than 3.9 million households), children did not have access to adequate, nutritious food at some time during the year. Food insecurity has a significant effect on both physical and cognitive development, because the lack of adequate, nutritious food increases the likelihood of iron-deficiency anemia, lower academic achievement, and behavioral problems.[114]

Paradoxically, US children from the poorest communities have the highest rates of obesity.[115,116] In fact, children from poor families are 7 times as likely to be obese as they are to be underweight.[117] The origins of this obesity paradox are likely multifactorial but may stem from the fact that foods high in calories, fats, and added sugars tend to cost less than do nutrient-dense foods, and many low-income families face challenges in obtaining high-quality, nutritious foods.

EFFECTS OF POVERTY

Infant Mortality, Adolescent Pregnancy, and Low Birth Weight

Higher infant mortality rates among the impoverished have been recognized as a societal problem in the United States for 140 years.[118] Children in the poorest 20% of urban populations in the United States are twice as likely to die before their first birthday compared with children in the richest 20% of the population.[119] The risk of teen pregnancy increases 10-fold for the lowest income level compared with the highest,[120] and teen pregnancy increases the risk of remaining in poverty in the future.[121]

Low birth weight is often used as a marker for infant and child outcomes and has been found to be a leading predictor of first-year mortality risk.[122] The increased risk of low birth weight in poor neighborhoods is associated with a high prevalence of teen pregnancy and inadequate prenatal care.[123] Low birth weight also may be related to the development of adult illness through epigenetic adaptation to intrauterine nutritional deficiencies (Barker hypothesis).[124]

Delayed Growth and Development

The effects of poverty on both growth and development manifest in early infancy. For example, low-income children have measurable gaps in language development beginning at the time of their first words, resulting in substantial differences in school readiness.[78] These differences may be mediated by aspects of the early home environments, including less reading aloud by parents and more exposure to electronic media.[125] The influence of poverty on physical growth also can be measured in early childhood. According to the 2009 Pediatric Nutrition Surveillance Survey, 6% of children qualifying for federal nutritional assistance from birth to age 4 years were of short stature, compared with 3.7% of all US children of the same age.[116]

Chronic Conditions

In addition to the high rate of obesity, poor children 6 to 18 years of age are more likely to be sedentary and exposed to tobacco when compared with their wealthiest counterparts, which may increase the risk of cardiovascular and pulmonary disease as adults.[126] Low family income during the first 2 years of life is associated with a twofold increase in the rate of hypertension in early adulthood.[74]

Chronic poverty also is associated with increased frequency of asthma attacks as well as worse overall health status reported by parents.[127,128] The neighborhood in which the family lives has a particularly strong effect on the prevalence of asthma, with asthma occurring much more frequently in neighborhoods with predominantly poor and nonwhite populations than in those with higher-income and white populations.[129] Characteristics of poor neighborhoods associated with the increase in asthma morbidity include crowding, air pollution, dampness, and the presence of pests.[130]

Untreated early childhood caries are 2.5 times more common in children in poor families than in families with incomes above the FPL. The application of dental sealants and the rate of visits to a dentist are also lower for poor children.[131]

Compromised Mental Health, Behavioral Health, and Relational Development

Children raised in poverty have been shown to have higher levels of depression and antisocial behavioral problems than those raised in families with adequate incomes. Depression in poor children younger than 18 years has been linked to substance abuse, poor academic performance, teen childbearing, and unemployment.[132] Poor children also are more likely to be diagnosed with conduct disorders[133] and attention-deficit/hyperactivity disorder.[134] Substance abuse, including alcohol and tobacco, is higher for poor adolescents, increasing the risk of emphysema and cirrhosis as well as cancer.[135] Parental depression and anxiety are common in low-income families and associated with well-documented adverse effects on children's relational and emotional development.[136–138]

Poor Academic Progress

Many observational studies confirm the link between low socioeconomic status and poor achievement in school, both in primary and secondary education.[139] This

association is mediated by factors such as school violence,[140] family structure,[141] parental involvement at school,[142] and parental involvement in education at home.[143] Early intervention is critically important in this domain, because the disparities between poor and nonpoor children are already apparent at school entry.[144]

Data from 2013 revealed that 89% of fourth-grade students from low-income families read below the proficiency level, compared with 49% of students from higher-income families.[145] The national high school drop-out rate is 7.4% for low-income students and 1.4% for high-income students.[146] For students taking the SAT in 2012, students from families at or below the FPL averaged in the 30th percentile on reading and students from families with incomes greater than $200 000/year scored in the 70th percentile.[147]

Studies that used functional MRI have shown that socioeconomic factors are associated with brain-behavior relationships in the acquisition of reading skills.[148] A longitudinal study that included multiple MRIs on 389 typically developing children found that childhood poverty was associated with structural differences in several areas of the brain important in the development of school readiness skills. The most significant changes were observed in children from the poorest families.[149] Adequate nutrition; a quiet, safe, toxin-free environment; and the effective, timely detection and treatment of chronic childhood health conditions are all factors that enable children to arrive at school each morning ready and able to learn.[129] Several putative mediators are well established in the relationship between poverty and school underachievement. Almost 17 million children are from families "at risk" of going hungry,[150] and even intermittent food insufficiency in

low-income children is associated with a number of adverse academic outcomes, including poor scores on achievement tests, grade repetition, and absenteeism, compared with children who are never hungry. In addition, chronic high-noise environments and exposure to indoor air pollution, especially passive smoking, have been associated with decreased academic performance. It is estimated that asthma accounts for approximately 10 million days of school missed each year, 3 times the amount of missed school for children without a chronic health condition.[151] In a recent analysis of data from the National Center for Health Statistics (2009–2011), asthma prevalence was associated with both urban and nonurban poverty.[152]

TRACKING IN HEALTH CARE SETTINGS

Compared with the *International Classification of Diseases, Ninth Revision, Clinical Modification*, the *International Classification of Diseases, 10th Revision, Clinical Modification* (ICD-10-CM)[153] provides a more robust classification system that enables clinicians to track socioeconomic factors in patient care that may be related to families' annual income level. By using the ICD-10-CM, child health clinicians can submit supplemental codes for their patient care that include not only diagnosis, such as acute asthma exacerbation, but additional socioeconomic factors related to the asthma exacerbation and treatment, such as childhood poverty or the family's inability to afford the recommended medical regimen. It will be important to capture this additional socioeconomic information with the use of ICD-10-CM codes to enable investigators to examine the putative impact of expanded codes on children's health care.

CONCLUSIONS

Knowledge about the effects of poverty on children and their development has increased dramatically since Brooks-Gunn and Duncan's often cited (over 65 000 citations) landmark study in 1997.[154] In the 21st century, Sir Michael Marmot has emerged as a global leader in studying the social determinants of health. Since 2005, Marmot has led the World Health Organization's Commission on Social Determinants of Health.[155] His 2009 article published in the *Journal of the American Medical Association*[156] noted that a global mortality gradient exists among poor and rich countries. Evidence supports the hypothesis that the slope of a health gradient is not fixed but responds to political, social, and economic changes.[157]

Research is rapidly accumulating that refines our understanding of the mediators of poverty's adverse effects on children and adults and informs the implementation of effective interventions to ameliorate poverty's adverse effects.[158] For example, recent research has strongly suggested that stress related to child poverty may be buffered by parent engagement and good relational health. The AAP policy statement that accompanies this technical report describes specific recommendations and population health strategies that could attenuate the adverse effects of child poverty and address many of the mediators of poverty that affect child health and development. Addressing the immediate needs of our youngest and poorest citizens is both the right thing to do for our children and an economically sound strategy for the future.[159]

ACKNOWLEDGMENTS

We appreciate the contributions from the following pediatric and internal medicine and pediatrics residents at University of California–Los Angeles who worked on parts of this statement during a 2-week child health policy elective in June 2013: Natalie Cerda, MD, Jeremy Lehman Fox, MD, Neil A. Gholkar, MD, Lydia Soo-Hyun Kim, MD, MPH, Rachel J. Klein, MD, Ashley E. Lewis Hunter, MD, Sarah J. Maufe, MD, Colin L. Robinson, MD, MPH, Joseph R. Rojas, MD, and Weiyi Tan, MD, MPH.

LEAD AUTHORS

John M. Pascoe, MD, MPH, FAAP
David Wood, MD, MPH, FAAP
James H. Duffee, MD, MPH, FAAP
Alice Kuo, MD, PhD, MEd, FAAP

COMMITTEE ON PSYCHOSOCIAL ASPECTS OF CHILD AND FAMILY HEALTH, 2015–2016

Michael Yogman, MD, FAAP, Chairperson
Nerissa Bauer, MD, MPH, FAAP
Thresia B Gambon, MD, FAAP
Arthur Lavin, MD, FAAP
Keith M. Lemmon, MD, FAAP
Gerri Mattson, MD, FAAP
Jason Richard Rafferty, MD, MPH, EdM
Lawrence Sagin Wissow, MD, MPH, FAAP

LIAISONS

Sharon Berry, PhD, LP – *Society of Pediatric Psychology*
Terry Carmichael, MSW – *National Association of Social Workers*
Edward Christophersen, PhD, FAAP – *Society of Pediatric Psychology*
Norah Johnson, PhD, RN, CPNP-BC – *National Association of Pediatric Nurse Practitioners*
Leonard Read Sulik, MD, FAAP – *American Academy of Child and Adolescent Psychiatry*

CONSULTANTS

George J. Cohen, MD, FAAP
Anne Brown Rodgers, Science Writer

STAFF

Stephanie Domain, MS, CHES

COUNCIL ON COMMUNITY PEDIATRICS EXECUTIVE COMMITTEE, 2015–2016

Benjamin A. Gitterman, MD, FAAP, Chairperson
Patricia J. Flanagan MD, FAAP, Vice-Chairperson
William H. Cotton, MD, FAAP
Kimberley J. Dilley, MD, MPH, FAAP
James H. Duffee, MD, MPH, FAAP
Andrea E. Green, MD, FAAP
Virginia A. Keane, MD, FAAP
Scott D. Krugman, MD, MS, FAAP
Julie M. Linton, MD, FAAP
Carla D. McKelvey, MD, MPH, FAAP
Jacqueline L. Nelson, MD, FAAP

LIAISONS

Jacqueline R. Dougé, MD, MPH, FAAP – *Chairperson, Public Health Special Interest Group*
Janna Gewirtz O'Brien, MD – *Section on Medical Students, Residents, and Fellowship Trainees*

FORMER EXECUTIVE COMMITTEE MEMBERS

Lance A. Chilton, MD, FAAP – Vice-Chairperson
Thresia B. Gambon, MD, FAAP
Alice A. Kuo, MD, PhD, FAAP
Gonzalo J. Paz-Soldan, MD, FAAP
Barbara Zind, MD, FAAP

FORMER LIAISONS

Toluwalase Ajayi, MD – *Section on Medical Students, Residents, and Fellowship Trainees*
Ricky Y. Choi, MD, MPH, FAAP – *Chairperson, Immigrant Health Special Interest Group*
Frances J. Dunston, MD, MPH, FAAP – *Commission to End Health Care Disparities*
M. Edward Ivancic, MD, FAAP – *Chairperson, Rural Health Special Interest Group*

ABBREVIATIONS

AAP: American Academy of Pediatrics
FPL: federal poverty level
HPA: hypothalamic-pituitary-adrenocortical
ICD-10-CM: *International Classification of Diseases, 10th Revision, Clinical Modification*
SPM: Supplemental Poverty Measure

REFERENCES

1. Sell K, Zlotnik S, Noonan K, Rubin D. *The Effect of Recession on Child Well-being: A Synthesis of the Evidence by PolicyLab, The Children's Hospital of Philadelphia.* Washington, DC: First Focus; 2010

2. DeNavas-Walt C, Proctor BD. *US Census Bureau. Current Population Reports, P60-252, Income and Poverty in the United States: 2014.* Washington, DC: US Government Printing Office; 2015

3. Seefeldt K, Abner G, Bolinger JA, Xu L, Graham JD. *At Risk: America's Poor During and After the Great Recession.* Bloomington, IN: Indiana University; 2012

4. Dreyer BP. To create a better world for children and families: the case for ending childhood poverty. *Acad Pediatr.* 2013;13(2):83–90

5. Shonkoff JP, Boyce WT, McEwen BS. Neuroscience, molecular biology, and the childhood roots of health disparities: building a new framework for health promotion and disease prevention. *JAMA.* 2009;301(21):2252–2259

6. Schreier HM, Chen E. Socioeconomic status and the health of youth: a multilevel, multidomain approach to conceptualizing pathways. *Psychol Bull.* 2013;139(3):606–654

7. Thompson RA, Haskins R. Early stress gets under the skin: promising initiatives to help children facing chronic adversity. Policy Brief. Princeton, NJ: *The Future of Children.* Spring 2014

8. Shonkoff JP, Garner AS; Committee on Psychosocial Aspects of Child and Family Health; Committee on Early Childhood, Adoption, and Dependent Care; Section on Developmental and Behavioral Pediatrics. The lifelong effects of early childhood adversity and toxic stress. *Pediatrics.* 2012;129(1). Available at: www.pediatrics.org/cgi/content/full/129/1/e232

9. Winning A, Glymour MM, McCormick MC, Gilsanz P, Kubzansky LD. Psychological distress across the life course and cardiometabolic risk: findings from the 1958 British birth cohort study. *J Am Coll Cardiol.* 2015;66(14):1577–1586

10. Pillas D, Marmot M, Naicker K, Goldblatt P, Morrison J, Pikhart H. Social inequalities in early childhood health and development: a European-wide systematic review. *Pediatr Res.* 2014;76(5):418–424

11. Blair C, Raver CC. Child development in the context of adversity: experiential canalization of brain and behavior. *Am Psychol.* 2012;67(4):309–318

12. Garner AS, Shonkoff JP; Committee on Psychosocial Aspects of Child and Family Health; Committee on Early Childhood, Adoption, and Dependent Care; Section on Developmental and Behavioral Pediatrics. Early childhood adversity, toxic stress, and the role of the pediatrician: translating

developmental science into lifelong health. *Pediatrics.* 2012;129(1). Available at: www.pediatrics.org/cgi/content/full/129/1/e224

13. Brent DA, Silverstein M. Shedding light on the long shadow of childhood adversity. *JAMA.* 2013;309(17):1777–1778

14. Bornstein D. In the long war on poverty, small victories that matter. *New York Times.* January 8, 2014. Available at: http://opinionator.blogs.nytimes.com/2014/01/08/in-the-long-war-on-poverty-small-victories-that-matter/. Accessed August 5, 2015

15. David RJ, Collins JW. Layers of inequality: power, policy, and health. *Am J Public Health.* 2014;104(suppl 1):S8–S10

16. Center on the Developing Child at Harvard University. *The Foundations of Lifelong Health Are Built in Early Childhood.* Cambridge, MA: Center on the Developing Child at Harvard University; 2010. Available at: http://developingchild.harvard.edu/resources/reports_and_working_papers/foundations-of-lifelong-health/. Accessed August 5, 2015

17. Braveman P, Barclay C. Health disparities beginning in childhood: a life-course perspective. *Pediatrics.* 2009;124(suppl 3):S163–S175

18. Insel TR. Mental disorders in childhood: shifting the focus from behavioral symptoms to neurodevelopmental trajectories. *JAMA.* 2014;311(17):1727–1728

19. Middlebrooks JS, Audage NC. *The Effects of Childhood Stress on Health Across the Lifespan.* Atlanta, GA: Centers for Disease Control and Prevention, National Center for Injury Prevention and Control; 2008

20. Crockenberg SB. Infant irritability, mother responsiveness, and social support influences on the security of infant-mother attachment. *Child Dev.* 1981;52(3):857–865

21. Luby J, Belden A, Botteron K, et al. The effects of poverty on childhood brain development: the mediating effect of caregiving and stressful life events. *JAMA Pediatr.* 2013;167(12):1135–1142

22. Yoshikawa H, Aber JL, Beardslee WR. The effects of poverty on the mental,

emotional, and behavioral health of children and youth: implications for prevention. *Am Psychol.* 2012;67(4):272–284

23. Danese A, Pariante CM, Caspi A, Taylor A, Poulton R. Childhood maltreatment predicts adult inflammation in a life-course study. *Proc Natl Acad Sci USA.* 2007;104(4):1319–1324

24. Haroon E, Raison CL, Miller AH. Psychoneuroimmunology meets neuropsychopharmacology: translational implications of the impact of inflammation on behavior. *Neuropsychopharmacology.* 2012;37(1):137–162

25. Reynolds RM. Glucocorticoid excess and the developmental origins of disease: two decades of testing the hypothesis—2012 Curt Richter Award Winner. *Psychoneuroendocrinology.* 2013;38(1):1–11

26. Barboza Solís C, Kelly-Irving M, Fantin R, et al. Adverse childhood experiences and physiological wear-and-tear in midlife: findings from the 1958 British birth cohort. *Proc Natl Acad Sci USA.* 2015;112(7):E738–E746

27. Kim P, Evans GW, Angstadt M, et al. Effects of childhood poverty and chronic stress on emotion regulatory brain function in adulthood. *Proc Natl Acad Sci USA.* 2013;110(46):18442–18447

28. Blair C, Granger DA, Willoughby M, et al; FLP Investigators. Salivary cortisol mediates effects of poverty and parenting on executive functions in early childhood. *Child Dev.* 2011;82(6):1970–1984

29. Hanson JL, Hair N, Shen DG, et al. Family poverty affects the rate of human infant brain growth. *PLoS One.* 2013;8(12):e80954

30. Najman JM, Hayatbakhsh MR, Heron MA, Bor W, O'Callaghan MJ, Williams GM. The impact of episodic and chronic poverty on child cognitive development. *J Pediatr.* 2009;154(2):284–289

31. Pulkki-Råback L, Elovainio M, Hakulinen C, et al. Cumulative effect of psychosocial factors in youth on ideal cardiovascular health in adulthood: the Cardiovascular Risk in Young Finns Study [published correction appears

in *Circulation*. 2015;131(14):e403]. *Circulation*. 2015;131(3):245–253

32. Maccari S, Krugers HJ, Morley-Fletcher S, Szyf M, Brunton PJ. The consequences of early-life adversity: neurobiological, behavioural and epigenetic adaptations. *J Neuroendocrinol*. 2014;26(10):707–723

33. Zeanah CH, Berlin LJ, Boris NW. Practitioner review: clinical applications of attachment theory and research for infants and young children. *J Child Psychol Psychiatry*. 2011;52(8):819–833

34. Blair C, Raver CC. Closing the achievement gap through modification of neurocognitive and neuroendocrine function: results from a cluster randomized controlled trial of an innovative approach to the education of children in kindergarten. *PLoS One*. 2014;9(11):e112393

35. American Academy of Pediatrics, Council on Community Pediatrics; Committee on Psychosocial Aspects of Child and Family Health. Poverty and Child Health in the United States. *Pediatrics*. 2016;137(4):e20160339

36. Larson K, Russ SA, Nelson BB, Olson LM, Halfon N. Cognitive ability at kindergarten entry and socioeconomic status. *Pediatrics*. 2015;135(2). Available at: www.pediatrics.org/cgi/content/full/135/2/e440

37. *Merriam-Webster Dictionary*. Accessed July 5, 2014

38. Gabe T. *Poverty in the United States: 2012. Congressional Research Service Report to Congress*. Washington, DC: Congressional Research Service; 2013

39. National Research Council, Panel on Poverty and Family Assistance. In: Citro CF, Michael RT, eds. *Measuring Poverty: A New Approach*. Washington, DC: National Academies Press; 1995

40. Economics and Statistics Administration. *Census Bureau to Develop Supplemental Poverty Level* [news release]. Washington, DC: Economics and Statistics Administration, US Department of Commerce; March 2, 2010

41. Cauthen NK, Fass S. *Measuring Income and Poverty in the United States*. New York, NY: National Center for Children

in Poverty, Columbia University, Mailman School of Public Health; 2008

42. Kochhar R, Fry R, Taylor P. Wealth gaps rise to record highs between whites, blacks, Hispanics twenty-to-one. Social and Demographic Trends. Washington, DC: Pew Research Center; 2011. Available at: www.pewsocialtrends.org/2011/07/26/wealth-gaps-rise-to-record-highs-between-whites-blacks-hispanics/. Accessed August 5, 2015

43. Kirwan Institute for the Study of Race and Ethnicity. *Using GIS to Support Advocacy and Social Justice*. Columbus, OH: Kirwan Institute for the Study of Race and Ethnicity; 2009. Available at: www.kirwaninstitute.osu.edu/reports/2009/06_2009_GIStoSupportSocialAdvocacyandJustice_Kirwan_JointCenter.pdf. Accessed August 5, 2015

44. Grieger LD, Schoeni RF, Danziger S. *Accurately Measuring the Trend in Poverty in the United States Using the Panel Study of Income Dynamics*. Ann Arbor, MI: Institute for Social Research, University of Michigan; 2008. Panel Study of Income Dynamics Technical Paper 08-04

45. Ratcliffe C, McKernan SM. *Childhood Poverty Persistence: Facts and Consequences*. Washington, DC: Urban Institute; June 2010. Brief 14

46. Jiang Y, Ekono M, Skinner C. *Basic Facts About Low-Income Children: Children Under 18 Years, 2013*. New York, NY: National Center for Children in Poverty, Mailman School of Public Health, Columbia University; 2015

47. Corcoran ME, Chaudry A. The dynamics of childhood poverty. *Future Child*. 1997;7(2):40–54

48. DeNavas-Walt C, Proctor BD. *Income and Poverty in the United States: 2013 Current Population Reports*. Washington, DC: US Department of Commerce, US Census Bureau; 2014

49. Addy S, Wright V. *Basic Facts About Low-Income Children, 2010: Children Under Age 18*. New York, NY: National Center for Children in Poverty; 2012. Available at: www.nccp.org/publications/pub_1049.html. Accessed August 5, 2015

50. DeNavas-Walt C, Proctor BD, Smith JC. *US Census Bureau, Current Population*

Reports: Income, Poverty and Health Insurance in the United States: 2009. Washington, DC: US Government Printing Office; 2010:60–238

51. Jiang Y, Ekono M, Skinner C. *Basic Facts About Low-Income Children: Children Under 6 Years, 2013*. New York, NY: National Center for Children in Poverty, Mailman School of Public Health, Columbia University; 2015

52. Jiang Y, Ekono M, Skinner C. *Basic Facts About Low-Income Children: Children 12 Through 17 Years, 2013*. New York, NY: National Center for Children in Poverty, Mailman School of Public Health, Columbia University; 2015

53. Child Health USA. 2014. Data source: US Census, Bureau of Labor Statistics, Current Population Survey, Annual Social and Economic Supplement. Available at: http://mchb.hrsa.gov/chusa14/population-characteristics/children-immigrant-parents.html, Accessed January 31, 2016

54. Child Trends. Databank: Family Structure, March, 2015. Available at: www.childtrends.org/?indicators=family-structure. Accessed August 5, 2015

55. Child Welfare Information Gateway. *The Importance of Fathers in the Healthy Development of Children*. Washington, DC: US Department of Health and Human Services, Children's Bureau; 2006

56. National Fatherhood Initiative. Father facts. Germantown, MD: National Fatherhood Initiative; 2014. Available at: www.fatherhood.org/father-absence-statistics. Accessed August 5, 2015

57. Albelda R, Badgett MVL, Schneebaum A, Gates G. *Poverty in the Lesbian, Gay, and Bisexual Community*. Los Angeles, CA: The Williams Institute, University of California-Los Angeles; 2009. Available at http://escholarship.org/uc/item/2509p8r5. Accessed August 5, 2015

58. Movement Advancement Project. All children matter: how legal and social inequalities hurt LGBT families. Denver, CO: Movement Advancement Project; 2011. Available at: www.lgbtmap.org/policy-and-issue-analysis/all-children-matter-full-report. Accessed August 5, 2015

59. Chamberlain A, Prante G. Who pays and who receives government spending? An analysis of federal, state and local tax and spending distributions, 1991-2004. Washington, DC: Tax Foundation; 2007, Available at http://taxfoundation.org/article/who-pays-taxes-and-who-receives-government-spending-analysis-federal-state-and-local-tax-and. Accessed August 5, 2015

60. United States v Windsor, 570 US 12, 133 S Ct (2013) (Docket No. 12-307)

61. Obergefell et al v Hodges, Director, Ohio Department of Health, et al, 576 US No. 14-556 (2015). Available at: www.supremecourt.gov/opinions/14pdf/14-556_3204.pdf. Accessed June 27, 2015

62. Wight VR, Chau M, Thampi K, Aratani Y. Examining the landscape of child poverty in the US today. *Curr Probl Pediatr Adolesc Health Care*. 2010;40(10):263–266

63. Bishaw A. Areas with concentrated poverty: 2006–2010. American Community Survey Briefs. December 2011. Available at: www.census.gov/prod/2011pubs/acsbr10-17.pdf. Accessed August 5, 2015

64. Fry R. *The Rise in Residential Segregation by Income*. Washington, DC: Pew Research Center; 2012

65. US Department of Agriculture, Economic Research Service. Poverty overview. Available at: www.ers.usda.gov/topics/rural-economy-population/rural-poverty-well-being/poverty-overview.aspx. Accessed August 5, 2015

66. Evans GW. The environment of childhood poverty. *Am Psychol*. 2004;59(2):77–92

67. Ratcliffe C, McKernan SM. *Childhood Poverty Persistence: Facts and Consequences*. Washington, DC: Urban Institute; June 2010. Brief 14

68. Conroy K, Sandel M, Zuckerman B. Poverty grown up: how childhood socioeconomic status impacts adult health. *J Dev Behav Pediatr*. 2010;31(2):154–160

69. McEwen BS. The neurobiology of stress: from serendipity to clinical relevance. *Brain Res*. 2000;886(1–2):172–189

70. Boyce WT. A biology of misfortune. *Focus*. 2012;29(1):1. Available at: www.

irp.wisc.edu/publications/focus/pdfs/foc291a.pdf. Accessed August 5, 2015

71. Blair C, Raver CC, Granger D, Mills-Koonce R, Hibel L; Family Life Project Key Investigators. Allostasis and allostatic load in the context of poverty in early childhood. *Dev Psychopathol*. 2011;23(3):845–857

72. Evans GW, Kim P. Childhood poverty and health: cumulative risk exposure and stress dysregulation. *Psychol Sci*. 2007;18(11):953–957

73. Power C, Matthews S. Origins of health inequalities in a national population sample. *Lancet*. 1997;350(9091):1584–1589

74. Ziol-Guest KM, Duncan GJ, Kalil A, Boyce WT. Early childhood poverty, immune-mediated disease processes, and adult productivity. *Proc Natl Acad Sci USA*. 2012;109(suppl 2):17289–17293

75. Miller GE, Chen E, Fok AK, et al. Low early-life social class leaves a biological residue manifested by decreased glucocorticoid and increased proinflammatory signaling. *Proc Natl Acad Sci USA*. 2009;106(34):14716–14721

76. Miller GE, Chen E, Parker KJ. Psychological stress in childhood and susceptibility to the chronic diseases of aging: moving toward a model of behavioral and biological mechanisms. *Psychol Bull*. 2011;137(6):959–997

77. Powell ND, Sloan EK, Bailey MT, et al. Social stress up-regulates inflammatory gene expression in the leukocyte transcriptome via β-adrenergic induction of myelopoiesis. *Proc Natl Acad Sci USA*. 2013;110(41):16574–16579

78. Hart B, Risley T. *Meaningful Differences in the Everyday Experience of Young American Children*. Baltimore, MD: Brookes Publishing; 1995

79. US Census Bureau. *Population Survey. March 2000, Supplement 162*. Washington, DC: US Government Printing Office; 2000

80. Mitchell J. About half of kids with single moms live in poverty. *Wall Street Journal*. November 25, 2013. Available at: http://blogs.wsj.com/economics/2013/11/25/about-half-of-kids-with-single-moms-live-in-poverty/. Accessed August 5, 2015

81. Weitzman M, Baten A, Rosenthal DG, Hoshino R, Tohn E, Jacobs DE. Housing and child health. *Curr Probl Pediatr Adolesc Health Care*. 2013;43(8):187–224

82. Cutts DB, Meyers AF, Black MM, et al. US housing insecurity and the health of very young children. *Am J Public Health*. 2011;101(8):1508–1514

83. Aratani Y. *Homeless Children and Youth*. New York, NY: National Center for Children in Poverty, Columbia University, Mailman School of Public Health; 2009

84. Centers for Disease Control and Prevention. Protect the ones you love: child injuries are preventable. Available at: www.cdc.gov/safechild/NAP/background.html. Accessed August 5, 2015

85. World Health Organization. 10 Facts on climate change and health. October 2012. Available at: www.who.int/features/factfiles/climate_change/en/. Accessed August 25, 2015

86. Hippisley-Cox J, Groom L, Kendrick D, Coupland C, Webber E, Savelyich B. Cross sectional survey of socioeconomic variations in severity and mechanism of childhood injuries in Trent 1992-7. *BMJ*. 2002;324(7346):1132–1134

87. Singh GK, Kogan MD. Widening socioeconomic disparities in US childhood mortality, 1969 2000. *Am J Public Health*. 2007;97(9):1658–1665

88. Eckenrode J, Smith EG, McCarthy ME, Dineen M. Income inequality and child maltreatment in the United States. *Pediatrics*. 2014;133(3):454–461

89. Wood D. Effect of child and family poverty on child health in the United States. *Pediatrics*. 2003;112(3 part 2):707–711

90. Felitti VJ, Anda RF, Nordenberg D, et al. Relationship of childhood abuse and household dysfunction to many of the leading causes of death in adults: the Adverse Childhood Experiences (ACE) Study. *Am J Prev Med*. 1998;14(4):245–258

91. Kadir A, Marais F, Desmond N. Community perceptions of the social determinants of child health in Western Cape, South Africa: neglect as a major indicator of child health and

wellness. *Paediatr Int Child Health.* 2013;33(4):310–321

92. Jonson-Reid M, Kohl PL, Drake B. Child and adult outcomes of chronic child maltreatment. *Pediatrics.* 2012;129(5):839–845

93. Lanier P, Jonson-Reid M, Stahlschmidt MJ, Drake B, Constantino J. Child maltreatment and pediatric health outcomes: a longitudinal study of low-income children. *J Pediatr Psychol.* 2010;35(5):511–522

94. Reichert E. Childhood maltreatment, posttraumatic cognitions, and health outcomes among young adults [dissertation]. University of Rhode Island. *Open Access Dissertations.* Paper 14. 2013. Available at: http://digitalcommons.uri.edu/oa_diss/14. Accessed August 5, 2015

95. Kendall-Tackett K, Klest B. Causal mechanisms and multidirectional pathways between trauma, dissociation, and health. *J Trauma Dissociation.* 2009;10(2):129–134

96. Unnatural Causes. Is inequality making us sick? Adelman L, creator and executive producer. Produced by California Newsreel with Vital Pictures, Inc; 2008. Available at: www.unnaturalcauses.org/episode_descriptions.php?page=5. Accessed August 5, 2015

97. America's children: key national indicators of well-being, 2013. Housing problems. Washington, DC: US Department of Housing and Urban Development; 2013. Available at: www.childstats.gov/pdf/ac2013/ac_13.pdf. Accessed February 7, 2014

98. Council on Community Pediatrics. Providing care for children and adolescents facing homelessness and housing insecurity. *Pediatrics.* 2013;131(6):1206–1210

99. Cook JT, Frank DA, Casey PH, et al. A brief indicator of household energy security: associations with food security, child health, and child development in US infants and toddlers. *Pediatrics.* 2008;122(4). Available at: www.pediatrics.org/cgi/content/full/122/4/e867

100. Children's Health Watch. Energy insecurity is a major threat to child health. Policy Action Brief.

February 2010. Available at: www.childrenshealthwatch.org/upload/resource/energy_brief_feb10.pdf. Accessed August 5, 2015

101. Kohen DE, Leventhal T, Dahinten VS, McIntosh CN. Neighborhood disadvantage: pathways of effects for young children. *Child Dev.* 2008;79(1):156–169

102. Macintyre S, Ellaway A. Neighborhoods and health: an overview. In: Kawachi I, Berkman LF, eds. *Neighborhoods and Health.* New York, NY: Oxford University Press; 2003:20–42

103. Mayer SE. Trends in the economic well-being and life chances of America's children. In: Duncan GJ, Brooks-Gunn J, eds. *Consequences of Growing Up Poor.* New York, NY: Russell Sage Foundation; 1997:49–69

104. Powell J. Dreaming of a self beyond whiteness and isolation. *Wash Univ J Law Policy.* 2005;18(13):13–45

105. Robert Wood Johnson Foundation. Beyond health care: new directions to a healthier America. Princeton, NJ: Robert Wood Johnson Foundation; 2009. Available at: www.rwjf.org/content/dam/farm/reports/reports/2009/rwjf40483. Accessed August 5, 2015

106. Kirwan Institute for the Study of Race and Ethnicity. The residual impact of history: connecting residential segregation, mortgage redlining, and the housing crisis. Columbus, OH: Kirwan Institute for the Study of Race and Ethnicity; 2010. Available at: http://kirwaninstitute.osu.edu/reports/2010/02_2010_RedliningHistorySubprime_Hernandez.pdf Accessed August 5, 2015

107. Bradley RH, Corwyn RF, McAdoo HP, Coll CG. The home environments of children in the United States part I: variations by age, ethnicity, and poverty status. *Child Dev.* 2001;72(6):1844–1867

108. US Department of Education, National Center for Education Statistics. Public school principals report on their school facilities: fall 2005. NCES 2007-007. US Department of Education, National Center for Education Statistics; 2007. Available at: http://nces.ed.gov/pubs2007/2007007.pdf. Accessed August 5, 2015

109. Word E, Johnston J, Bain HP, et al. *Student/Teacher Achievement Ratio (STAR): Tennessee's K–3 Class Size Study. Final Summary Report 1985–1990.* Nashville, TN: Tennessee Department of Education; 1990

110. National Center for Education Statistics. *Common Core of Data for School Years 1993/94 Through 1997/98.* Washington, DC: Office of Educational Research and Improvement, US Department of Education; 2000

111. Anderson SA. Core indicators of nutritional state for difficult-to-sample populations. *J Nutr.* 1990;120(suppl 11):1557S–1600S

112. US Department of Agriculture. Food security status of US households with children in 2011. Available at: www.ers.usda.gov/topics/food-nutrition-assistance/food-security-in-the-us/key-statistics-graphics.aspx#.UagrrGTF1yo. Accessed August 5, 2015

113. Gundersen C, Ziliak J. *Feeding America's Children: Food Insecurity and Poverty.* Washington, DC: The Brookings Institution; 2014. Available at: www.brookings.edu/blogs/social-mobility-memos/posts/2014/09/15-feeding-americas-children-poverty. Accessed August 5, 2015

114. Alaimo K, Olson CM, Frongillo EA Jr. Food insufficiency and American school-aged children's cognitive, academic, and psychosocial development. *Pediatrics.* 2001;108(1):44–53

115. Metallinos-Katsaras E, Must A, Gorman K. A longitudinal study of food insecurity on obesity in preschool children. *J Acad Nutr Diet.* 2012;112(12):1949–1958

116. Polhamus BDK, Borland E, Mackintosh H, Smith B, Grummer-Strawn L. *Pediatric Nutrition Surveillance 2009 Report.* Atlanta, GA: US Department of Health and Human Services, Centers for Disease Control and Prevention; 2011

117. Ludwig DS, Blumenthal SJ, Willett WC. Opportunities to reduce childhood hunger and obesity: restructuring the Supplemental Nutrition Assistance Program (the Food Stamp Program). *JAMA.* 2012;308(24):2567–2568

118. Hogue CJ, Hargraves MA. Class, race, and infant mortality in the United States. *Am J Public Health.* 1993;83(1):9–12

119. World Health Organization. Global Health Observatory data on infant mortality. Available at: www.who.int/gho/urban_health/outcomes/infant_mortality/en/. Accessed August 5, 2015

120. Smith T. Influence of socioeconomic factors on attaining targets for reducing teenage pregnancies. *BMJ.* 1993;306(6887):1232–1235

121. Nord CW, Moore KA, Morrison DR, Brown B, Myers DE. Consequences of teen-age parenting. *J Sch Health.* 1992;62(7):310–318

122. Collins JW Jr, Wambach J, David RJ, Rankin KM. Women's lifelong exposure to neighborhood poverty and low birth weight: a population-based study. *Matern Child Health J.* 2009;13(3):326–333

123. Gould JB, LeRoy S. Socioeconomic status and low birth weight: a racial comparison. *Pediatrics.* 1988;82(6):896–904

124. Langley-Evans SC, McMullen S. Developmental origins of adult disease. *Med Princ Pract.* 2010;19(2):87–98

125. Brooks-Gunn J, Markman LB. The contribution of parenting to ethnic and racial gaps in school readiness. *Future Child.* 2005;15(1):139–168

126. Ali MK, Bullard KM, Beckles GL, et al. Household income and cardiovascular disease risks in U.S. children and young adults: analyses from NHANES 1999-2008. *Diabetes Care.* 2011;34(9):1998–2004

127. Béatrice N, Lise G, Victoria ZM, Louise S. Longitudinal patterns of poverty and health in early childhood: exploring the influence of concurrent, previous, and cumulative poverty on child health outcomes. *BMC Pediatr.* 2012;12. Available at: http://bmcpediatr.biomedcentral.com/articles/10.1186/1471-2431-12-141.

128. Nikiéma B, Spencer N, Séguin L. Poverty and chronic illness in early childhood: a comparison between the United Kingdom and Quebec. *Pediatrics.* 2010;125(3). Available at: www.pediatrics.org/cgi/content/full/125/3/e499

129. Ben-Shlomo Y, Kuh D. A life course approach to chronic disease epidemiology: conceptual models, empirical challenges and interdisciplinary perspectives. *Int J Epidemiol.* 2002;31(2):285–293

130. Williams DR, Sternthal M, Wright RJ. Social determinants: taking the social context of asthma seriously. *Pediatrics.* 2009;123(suppl 3):S174–S184

131. Dye BA, Li X, Thorton-Evans G. Oral health disparities as determined by selected healthy people 2020 oral health objectives for the United States, 2009-2010. *NCHS Data Brief.* 2012; Aug(104):1–8

132. Tracy M, Zimmerman FJ, Galea S, McCauley E, Stoep AV. What explains the relation between family poverty and childhood depressive symptoms? *J Psychiatr Res.* 2008;42(14):1163–1175

133. Murali V, Oyebode F. Poverty, social inequality and mental health. *Adv Psychiatr Treat.* 2004;10(3):216–224

134. Davis E, Sawyer MG, Lo SK, Priest N, Wake M. Socioeconomic risk factors for mental health problems in 4-5-year-old children: Australian population study. *Acad Pediatr.* 2010;10(1):41–47

135. Lowry R, Kann L, Collins JL, Kolbe LJ. The effect of socioeconomic status on chronic disease risk behaviors among US adolescents. *JAMA.* 1996;276(10):792–797

136. Ackerman BP, Brown ED. Physical and psychosocial turmoil in the home and cognitive development. In: Evans G, Wachs TD, eds. *Chaos and Its Influence on Children's Development: An Ecological Perspective.* Washington, DC: American Psychological Association; 2010:35–47

137. Foster H, Brooks-Gunn J. Toward a stress process model of children's exposure to physical family and community violence. *Clin Child Fam Psychol Rev.* 2009;12(2):71–94

138. Molnar BE, Buka SL, Brennan RT, Holton JK, Earls F. A multilevel study of neighborhoods and parent-to-child physical aggression: results from the project on human development in Chicago neighborhoods. *Child Maltreat.* 2003;8(2):84–97

139. Stewart EB. School structural characteristics, student effort, peer associations, and parental involvement: the influence of school- and individual-level factors on academic achievement. *Educ Urban Soc.* 2008;40(2):179–204

140. Heaviside S, Rowand C, Williams C, Farris E. *Violence and Discipline Problems in U.S. Public Schools: 1996-1997.* Washington, DC: US Department of Education, National Center for Education Statistics; 1998. NCES Publication 98-030

141. Astone NM, McLanahan SS. Family structure, parental practices and high school completion. *Am Sociol Rev.* 1991;56(3):309–320

142. Desimone L. Linking parent involvement with student achievement: do race and income matter? *J Educ Res.* 1999;93(1):11–30

143. Christenson SL, Rounds T, Gorney D. Family factors and student achievement: an avenue to increase students' success. *Sch Psychol Q.* 1992;7(3):178–206

144. Ramey CT, Ramey SL. Early learning and school readiness. *Merrill-Palmer Q.* 2014;50(4):471–491

145. The Annie E. Casey Foundation. *Early Warning Confirmed: A Research Update on Third-Grade Reading.* Baltimore, MD: The Annie E. Casey Foundation; 2013

146. Aud S, Hussar W, Planty M, Snyder T. The condition of education 2010. NCES 2010-028. Washington, DC: National Center for Education Statistics, Institute of Education Sciences, US Department of Education; 2010. Available at: http://nces.ed.gov/pubs2010/2010028.pdf. Accessed August 5, 2015

147. The College Board. College-bound seniors 2012 total group profile report. Available at: http://research.collegeboard.org/programs/sat/data/cb-seniors-2012. Accessed August 5, 2015

148. Noble KG, Wolmetz ME, Ochs LG, Farah MJ, McCandliss BD. Brain-behavior relationships in reading acquisition are modulated by socioeconomic factors. *Dev Sci.* 2006;9(6):642–654

149. Hair NL, Hanson JL, Wolfe BL, Pollak SD. Association of child poverty, brain development, and academic

achievement. *JAMA Pediatr.* 2015;169(9):822–829

150. Seligman HK, Schillinger D. Hunger and socioeconomic disparities in chronic disease. *N Engl J Med.* 2010;363(1):6–9

151. Pascoe J, Shaikh U, Forbis S, Etzel RA. Health and nutrition as a foundation for success in school. In: Pianta RC, Cox RC, Snow KL, eds. *School Readiness and the Transition to Kindergarten in the Era of Accountability.* Baltimore, MD: Paul H. Brookes Publishing; 2007:99–101

152. Keet CA, McCormack MC, Pollack CE, Peng RD, McGowan E, Matsui EC. Neighborhood poverty, urban residence, race/ethnicity, and asthma: Rethinking the inner-city asthma epidemic. *J Allergy Clin Immunol.* 2015;135(3):655–662

153. World Health Organization. International Classification of Diseases, Tenth Revision, Clinical Modification (ICD-10-CM). Geneva, Switzerland: World Health Organization; 2016. Available at: www.cdc.gov/nchs/icd/icd10cm.htm. Accessed January 11, 2016

154. Brooks-Gunn J, Duncan GJ. The effects of poverty on children. *Future Child.* 1997;7(2):55–71

155. Commission on Social Determinants of Health. *CSDH Final Report: Closing the Gap in a Generation: Health Equity Through Action on the Social Determinants of Health.* Geneva, Switzerland: World Health Organization; 2008

156. Marmot MG, Bell R. Action on health disparities in the United States: commission on social determinants of health. *JAMA.* 2009;301(11):1169–1171

157. Singh GK, Siahpush M. Widening socioeconomic inequalities in US life expectancy, 1980-2000. *Int J Epidemiol.* 2006;35(4):969–979

158. Mistry KB, Minkovitz CS, Riley AW, et al. A new framework for childhood health promotion: the role of policies and programs in building capacity and foundations of early childhood health. *Am J Public Health.* 2012;102(9):1688–1696

159. Heckman JJ. Skill formation and the economics of investing in disadvantaged children. *Science.* 2006;312(5782):1900–1902

Medical Countermeasures for Children in Public Health Emergencies, Disasters, or Terrorism

• *Policy Statement*

POLICY STATEMENT Organizational Principles to Guide and Define the Child Health
Care System and/or Improve the Health of all Children

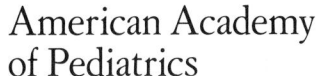

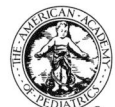

American Academy
of Pediatrics

DEDICATED TO THE HEALTH OF ALL CHILDREN™

Medical Countermeasures for Children in Public Health Emergencies, Disasters, or Terrorism

DISASTER PREPAREDNESS ADVISORY COUNCIL

abstract

Significant strides have been made over the past 10 to 15 years to develop medical countermeasures (MCMs) to address potential disaster hazards, including chemical, biological, radiologic, and nuclear threats. Significant and effective collaboration between the pediatric health community, including the American Academy of Pediatrics, and federal partners, such as the Office of the Assistant Secretary for Preparedness and Response, Centers for Disease Control and Prevention, Federal Emergency Management Agency, National Institutes of Health, Food and Drug Administration, and other federal agencies, over the past 5 years has resulted in substantial gains in addressing the needs of children related to disaster preparedness in general and MCMs in particular. Yet, major gaps still remain related to MCMs for children, a population highly vulnerable to the effects of exposure to such threats, because many vaccines and pharmaceuticals approved for use by adults as MCMs do not yet have pediatric formulations, dosing information, or safety information. As a result, the nation's stockpiles and other caches (designated supply of MCMs) where pharmacotherapeutic and other MCMs are stored are less prepared to address the needs of children compared with those of adults in the event of a disaster. This policy statement provides recommendations to close the remaining gaps for the development and use of MCMs in children during public health emergencies or disasters. The progress made by federal agencies to date to address the needs of children and the shared commitment of collaboration that characterizes the current relationship between the pediatric health community and the federal agencies responsible for MCMs should encourage all child advocates to invest the necessary energy and resources now to complete the process of remedying the remaining significant gaps in preparedness.

DOI: 10.1542/peds.2015-4273

Accepted for publication Nov 24, 2015

PEDIATRICS (ISSN Numbers: Print, 0031-4005; Online, 1098-4275).

To cite: AAP DISASTER PREPAREDNESS ADVISORY COUNCIL. Medical Countermeasures for Children in Public Health Emergencies, Disasters, or Terrorism. *Pediatrics*. 2016;137(2):e20154273

Events over the past 2 decades are a stark reminder that disasters, human-caused or natural, can affect children directly. Despite our best efforts to protect children, this population may be the chance target of natural disasters or the intended target for acts of violence or terrorism. Children represent a particularly vulnerable population during a pandemic, natural disaster, or act of terrorism. Medical countermeasures (MCMs), defined as medications, antitoxins, vaccines, immunoglobulins, medical devices, and pediatric age-appropriate life-saving medical equipment and supplies required to protect or treat children for possible chemical, biological, radiologic, or nuclear (CBRN) threats, are of paramount importance to the health security of children and the nation as a whole.[1-3]

Children have unique needs that must be taken into consideration for communities to be truly prepared to respond to disasters and public health emergencies and to remain resilient in their aftermath.[4] It has been well documented that children differ from adults by virtue of their unique anatomic, physiologic, and developmental/behavioral characteristics.[5] The National Commission on Children and Disasters examined the current state of pediatric disaster readiness in the United States and made recommendations in the *2010 Report to the President and Congress*.[5] In particular, this report included a recommendation that the US Department of Health and Human Services (DHHS) and the US Department of Homeland Security (DHS)/Federal Emergency Management Agency should ensure the availability of and access to pediatric MCMs at the federal, state, and local levels for CBRN threats.[2] Formed in 2014, the DHHS National Advisory Committee on Children and Disasters provides advice and consultation to the DHHS Secretary on issues related to the medical and public health needs of children as they relate to disasters.[6]

MCM RESEARCH, DEVELOPMENT, ACQUISITION, AND SUPPORT

The DHHS Office of the Assistant Secretary for Preparedness and Response (ASPR) leads the nation's preparedness efforts for response and recovery from the adverse health effects of emergencies and disasters. Within the ASPR, the Biomedical Advanced Research and Development Authority (BARDA) oversees the development and purchase of the necessary vaccines, drugs, therapies, and diagnostic tools for public health medical emergencies through advanced research, development, and acquisition contracts and grant awards.

The Public Health Emergency Medical Countermeasures Enterprise (PHEMCE) is a federal interagency body responsible for providing recommendations to the DHHS Secretary on MCM priorities and the development, acquisition, and distribution of MCMs within the Strategic National Stockpile (SNS). The SNS is a federally maintained cache of MCMs for rapid deployment and use in response to a public health emergency or disaster. The PHEMCE coordinates federal efforts to enhance preparedness for CBRN and emerging infectious disease threats with respect to MCMs and conducts an annual review of the SNS contents. The PHEMCE is led by the ASPR and includes 3 primary DHHS internal agency partners: the Centers for Disease Control and Prevention (CDC), the Food and Drug Administration (FDA), and the National Institutes of Health as well as several interagency partners, including the US Department of Defense (DoD), the Department of Veterans Affairs, the US Department of Agriculture, and the DHS (see www.phe.gov/Preparedness/mcm/phemce/Pages/mission.aspx).

The ongoing analysis of health security threats and the nation's MCM portfolio is informed by the efforts of 10 integrated program teams (IPTs). The IPTs provide an end-to-end vision of MCMs against a particular threat type (eg, chemical, radiologic, nuclear), capability (eg, diagnostics), or cross-cutting issues, such as at-risk populations. The Pediatric and Obstetric (PedsOB) IPT supports all threat-based PHEMCE IPTs with strategies for identifying, developing, acquiring, deploying, and utilizing high-priority MCMs for children and pregnant women. The PedsOB IPT serves as a subject matter expert (SME) community of practice for the interagency vetting and input on issues relevant to MCMs and pediatric readiness (see www.phe.gov/about/OPP/mcsr/Pages/threat-analysis.aspx).

The CDC provides clinical guidance to health care providers and facilities and coordinates the development of guidance to state, territorial, and local public health departments in support of efforts to detect and respond to public health emergencies. The CDC also oversees the distribution of MCMs from the SNS to individual states. The FDA ensures the safety and effectiveness of MCMs while regulating the approval, licensure, development, and certain postmarket surveillance of medical products. The FDA may authorize the emergency use of an unapproved or unlicensed medical product or an unapproved or unlicensed use (such as for a pediatric subpopulation) of an already approved product if certain public health emergency criteria are met or declarations are made.[7] The National Institutes of Health collaborates with other agencies to conduct research and provide funding necessary for the development of new or enhanced MCMs. The DHHS and PHEMCE MCM acquisition strategy is based on a multistep process that includes assessing the threat and potential public health consequences of CBRN agents, determining the type and quantity of needed MCMs, evaluating the public health response capability, and developing and acquiring countermeasures for the SNS. The Project BioShield Act (Pub L No. 108-276 [2004]) requires the DHHS to assess the public health consequences of exposure to CBRN agents that the DHS determines are material threats to the nation and to determine for which of these agents MCMs are necessary to protect the public's health.

EMERGENCY ACCESS TO UNAPPROVED MCMS

The FDA has several mechanisms to allow emergency access to unapproved medical products (see www.fda.gov/downloads/ Drugs/GuidanceComplianc eRegulatoryInformation/Guidances/ UCM351261.pdf). One mechanism is the Emergency Use Authorization (EUA).[8] Under section 564 of the Food, Drug, and Cosmetic Act (Pub L No. 110-85 [2007]), the FDA may authorize the emergency use of medical products (drugs, biologics, devices) including diagnostics that were not previously FDA approved, as well as the unapproved use of an approved product. These authorizations require a declaration that circumstances exist to justify the issuance of an EUA, on the basis of a determination made by the Secretary of DoD, DHS, or DHHS. This approach was used during the H1N1 influenza pandemic in 2009 to allow the emergency use of certain antiviral drugs in children and personal respiratory-protection devices. A modified EUA mechanism, emergency use instructions, was established under the Pandemic and All-Hazards Preparedness Reauthorization Act of 2013 (PAHPRA; Pub L No. 113-5), which allows the CDC, at the direction of the DHHS Secretary, to authorize

pediatric indications of MCMs for emergency use before an emergency is known or imminent. This process has become a useful tool in creating a more timely solution to emerging or perceived threats, especially for children, until sufficient research on pediatric use has been collected on an MCM already approved for adults and/or until research on new MCMs for children has been completed. Information on the EUA process and other resources may be found on the FDA Web site (see www.fda.gov/EmergencyPrepared ness/Counterterrorism/ MedicalCountermeasures/ MCMLegalRegulator yandPolicyFramework/ucm182568. htm). The general authorities within the PAHPRA are also useful in situations involving children. The link to the page with the listing of current EUAs is as follows: www. fda.gov/EmergencyPrepared ness/Counterterrorism/ MedicalCountermeasures/ MCMLegalRegulator yandPolicyFramework/ucm182568. htm#current.

SNS AND MCM DISTRIBUTION PLAN

To protect the health security of children and families during a public health emergency, the contents of the SNS ultimately need to reach the end user. The SNS, depending on the threat, is intended to supplement state and local supplies used for immediate care during the initial response, within 12 hours of notification/incident. Local and state funding challenges have resulted in decreases in state and local caches, underscoring further the need to ensure a well-stocked and rapidly deployed SNS. Because of the nature of certain threats, such as nerve agents, some MCMs are stored in local advance-deployed caches to allow for immediate access and administration to victims. Although the federal government maintains the

SNS and makes the ultimate decision to release SNS assets, the distribution of MCMs to the affected population is the responsibility of state and local government and public health and emergency management agencies. Each state and many local agencies have specific MCM distribution plans. It is critical that pediatricians (including primary care pediatricians and pediatric medical and surgical subspecialists) collaborate in advance with public health colleagues at the state and local levels to ensure that MCM distribution plans incorporate the needs of all children, including various subgroups such as infants, those with disabilities, and others with access and functional needs.

A broad array of potential MCM distribution strategies exist, ranging from utilizing the US Postal Service for home delivery in cities[9] to using large facilities as distribution centers or points of dispensing (PODs), thereby leveraging public and private sector partnerships. Each state has plans on file to receive and distribute MCMs to local communities as quickly as possible. The CDC Cities Readiness Initiative (see www.bt. cdc.gov/cri/) supports planning to respond to a large-scale bioterrorist event by dispensing antibiotics to a specific population within 48 hours. The POD system concept has been widely discussed and tested.[10–13] Many POD locations will likely be open-public sites, such as schools and community centers, visited by the population at risk who have been advised to report to that site for MCMs. Other PODs may be closed, dispensing MCMs to a select at-risk population (eg, employees of a large company, university students/ faculty/staff) and not to the general public.

Furthermore, all health care providers need to be knowledgeable of MCMs and their appropriate use so that they can effectively perform their role within their community and medical home and serve as reliable sources of information in the event of a public health emergency.[14,15] Pediatricians, pediatric health care providers, and others who will be providing medical care for children in the event of a disaster will need specialized education and training that includes knowledge on when and how MCMs should be used as well as possible adverse reactions (see www.aap. org/disasters/educationandtraining). At present, few, if any, pediatric office practices or medical homes[15] have made arrangements to be used as a POD for MCM distribution, although the medical home may be considered as a means of distribution for certain MCMs (eg, vaccines) or for some populations, such as children and youth with special health care needs. In any event, the medical home should be viewed as an entity that can be a vital component of any community's response to or recovery from a public health emergency.[16,17] Pediatricians can also advocate for the inclusion of considerations for children and families within the existing POD plan in their community.

THE SNS AND PEDIATRIC MCM CHALLENGES

When considering the stockpiling and rapid distribution of MCMs in response to a CBRN event, the unique requirements of the pediatric population pose several challenges. Liquid and other pediatric formulations of most MCMs are limited within stockpiles; liquid formulations are bulky, may be more expensive per dose, and cost more to store. Pediatric formulations also typically have a shorter shelf-life and are therefore more expensive to maintain. Certain critical MCMs are prepackaged in dose aliquots or in auto-injector devices to facilitate rapid delivery for victims in the field. For these same MCMs to be delivered safely and as efficiently

to children, pediatric-sized vials or auto-injectors must be available, although stockpiling both adult- and pediatric-sized delivery devices may also increase cost.

Moreover, until recently, there has been a relative lack of pediatric MCM development and procurement; many MCMs were initially developed for use by the military and have been evaluated and tested only in adults. Furthermore, the primary market for many MCMs has been the military. Outside of the DoD, the BARDA and the PHEMCE have federal responsibility to stimulate and drive the market for advanced research and for the development and procurement of MCMs, especially those for which there is not a commercial market. Reliance on traditional market mechanisms for public health preparedness and response to disasters is risky. In the specific circumstance of MCM development for children, traditional market mechanisms for preparedness and response would create a gap that can be life-threatening for children.

Developmental aspects of children also account for some of the challenges with pediatric MCMs. Children may have trouble swallowing pills and may refuse to consume formulations that are not palatable. Limited drug pharmacokinetic data and adverse reactions/sensitivities to medications (eg, antibiotics that stain teeth or disrupt growth plates) pose additional challenges.

PRACTICAL CONCERNS RELATED TO RESEARCH ON MCMS IN CHILDREN

There are reasonable concerns about conducting certain types of MCM research in the context of the special protections afforded to children as human subjects,[18–20] related in part to their relative vulnerability and general inability to provide their own informed consent.

These practical considerations and necessary additional protections often result in further financial costs and the perception of increased risk when conducting research with children instead of adults. Any additional cost that may result from including children in a meaningful way in clinical drug trials is not an appropriate rationale to limit or exclude them from such research. Likewise, the investigational or unlicensed use of an MCM in the pediatric population during a disaster imposes consent requirements that could impede timely distribution. An excellent example of this dilemma may be found in recommendations for the pre-event study of anthrax vaccine in children made by the DHHS National Biodefense Science Board (now known as the National Preparedness and Response Science Board) and the Presidential Commission for the Study of Bioethical Issues.[19,20]

PRIORITIZING PEDIATRIC PREPAREDNESS: WHAT DOES THE AMERICAN PUBLIC EXPECT?

As an organization devoted to advancing the needs of children and families, the mission of the American Academy of Pediatrics (AAP) includes public policy advocacy on a broad scope of concerns relevant to the health and well-being of children. In an effort to stimulate discussion on the use of resources related to disaster planning and response specific to children's issues, the AAP and Children's Health Fund collaborated on a 2010 telephone survey, conducted by the Marist College Institute for Public Opinion. The majority of people surveyed supported giving higher priority to children and their needs over adults. Opinions remained consistent across various demographics, including region, household income, education, age, race, gender, and political party.[21]

RECOMMENDATIONS FOR MCMS FOR CHILDREN EXPOSED TO PUBLIC HEALTH EMERGENCIES, DISASTERS, OR ACTS OF TERRORISM

Recommendations and key considerations regarding MCMs for children include the following:

In the interest of preparing to meet the needs of children exposed to public health emergencies, disasters, or acts of terrorism, federal, state, and local governments should acquire and maintain adequate amounts of MCMs appropriate for children of all ages in caches such as the SNS.

The SNS and other federal, state, and local caches should contain MCMs appropriate for children in quantities at least in proportion to the number of children in the intended population for protection by the cache. To meet the needs of children of all ages, stockpiles should include MCMs with appropriate formulations (eg, liquids), delivery devices (eg, pediatric auto-injectors), and age- or size-based dosing instructions. Concern for incremental cost, storage space, or inconvenience for MCMs intended for pediatric use must not be used as a rationale for lesser protection for children. As mentioned, ensuring protection for children is viewed as a priority by the US public.[22] To ensure the presence of appropriate MCMs, pediatric SMEs should be part of decision-making bodies, such as the PHEMCE and BARDA, on an ongoing basis. Such experts should be represented in sufficient numbers and in positions of authority so that their involvement can substantially determine the outcome of decision-making processes as appropriate.

Federal agencies, collaborating with industry, academia, and other BARDA partners, should research, develop, and procure pediatric MCMs for all public health emergency, disaster, and terrorism scenarios and report on progress made.

The federal government should make it a priority to develop MCMs appropriate for use in children (in terms of agent, dose, formulation, and necessary equipment and delivery devices) that ensures successful treatment while minimizing long-term medical and developmental consequences. The FDA should begin by taking full advantage of all pathways currently available to ensure that products can be tested in pediatric populations. Initial efforts might focus on MCMs presently available for use in adults that do not yet have approved pediatric formulations, dose ranges, or indications that cover the full spectrum of pediatric subpopulations, and target the highest priority gaps (ie, gaps for which a serious threat exists and alternative agents are unavailable). The federal government should create a strategic plan to eliminate all gaps in pediatric MCMs and provide an annual report to appropriate authorities on progress made.

All future MCMs developed or procured with the use of governmental funds should include provisions for use in pediatrics and/or sufficient study of pediatric indications that will facilitate emergency use before FDA approval unless there are compelling reasons, other than cost, for not doing so.

Biomedical research funded by the federal government that involves MCMs should include

reasonable steps to accommodate the special protections afforded to children as human subjects, but such protections should not justify the failure to identify pediatric indications for MCMs.

Standards of therapeutic evidence in children should be congruent with adult standards. Whenever feasible, guidance for the use and dosing of MCMs in the pediatric population should be based on evidence garnered from research. The MCM research should take reasonable steps to accommodate the special protections afforded to children as human subjects related to their relative vulnerability, but such protections and associated practical considerations should not be permitted as a rationale for the failure to identify pediatric indications for MCMs that may ultimately be life-saving, because this may only render children more vulnerable.[17] Likewise, the additional costs that may be inherent in clinical trials involving children as research subjects do not constitute an appropriate rationale to limit or exclude them from study, nor should those same factors preclude the stockpiling of pediatric formulations.

Research to develop pediatric dosing guidelines and formulations of MCMs already approved for adult use should be deemed a high priority. These endeavors may facilitate MCM administration in other at-risk populations, including the elderly and medically complex adults, especially those who have difficulty taking pills because of preexisting developmental or medical problems.

Federal, state, and local government, along with private sector and community stakeholders, should address the needs of children and families

in MCM implementation, distribution, and administration planning.

Mechanisms for the forward deployment and distribution of MCMs should consider the needs of children as a priority. Locations where children congregate (eg, schools and before- and after-school programs, Head Start and other early education and child care programs, camps, and other community programs) should be explored as opportunities for advance cache storage and rapid distribution to families with children. These sites may be well suited to handle the unique characteristics of pediatric dosing, such as weight-based dosing, and the possible need for suspension or other reformulating requirements or may better support the need to obtain informed consent from parents for the distribution of unlicensed or investigational MCMs to children. The distribution of MCMs to adults might also be accomplished at such sites. Such a plan could align with the CDC/state-local government public-private partnership closed PODs and potentially with increasing school-located vaccine efforts.[10–12] To facilitate their development, the costs of creating caches in such locations should be borne by public health and emergency preparedness budgets and not as an unfunded mandate imposed on schools, child care facilities, or community organizations.

Easy-to-follow instructions (eg, the use of pictograms, videos, and other visual aids) regarding proper preparation, dosing, and administration of MCMs for use by children should be developed before any incident in formats that can be readily understood by caregivers, who will undoubtedly be under great stress during an emergency and who may have limited health literacy themselves and/or an incomplete preexisting understanding of medication preparation, dosing, and administration.[8] These instructional materials should also be available translated in the languages of the population to be protected and modified to ensure access to children and adults with disabilities. The CDC has already engaged caregivers and pediatric SMEs in the development and pilot testing of such dosing aids; further efforts should be supported and expanded.

Consideration for the liberalization of FDA-approved dosing guidelines during a public health emergency for medications (such as dosing guidelines that would otherwise result in the administration of a portion of an adult pill, tablet, or capsule or liquid reformulation of pills/tablets/capsules that require complicated instructions to determine the appropriate volume for children on the basis of weight) will facilitate the ease and success of dosing in the context of a crisis. These adjustments should be considered when the risk of such dosing modifications is small when compared with the risk of contracting the illness if the medication is not administered because of the complexity of the instructions. The compounding of pills or capsules into liquids and dosing by families to a high level of specificity may be unrealistic in the midst of a public health emergency and certainly in the context of a crisis in which there are large-scale distribution challenges with limited medical supervision and support. If the instructions are overwhelming, they are likely to be ignored or misunderstood, resulting in improper dosing or poor compliance.

The federal government should proactively identify anticipated uses of MCMs in children during a public health emergency and, where pediatric FDA-approved indications do not exist, establish a plan to collect sufficient data to support the issuance of a pre-event EUA that includes

information such as safety and dosing information.

The AAP supports the continuing efforts of the DHHS, ASPR, CDC, FDA, and others to address this gap in pediatric dosing guidelines through the creation of a process that allows for the advance approval of off-label use of MCMs in children before the declaration of an imminent threat (ie, before an EUA can be issued). Specifically, the PAHPRA has stated that at the direction of the DHHS Secretary, authorization of pediatric indications of MCMs may occur for emergency use before an emergency is known or imminent. The government should continue actively engaging pediatric SMEs in the development of such recommendations. The AAP will continue its efforts to educate pediatric health care providers and others about its recommendations with regard to the off-label use of drugs in children.[22]

The federal government should use existing entities with pediatric SMEs, such as the PHEMCE, PedsOB IPT, and the DHHS National Advisory Committee on Children and Disasters, and continue to collaborate with private sector partners offering pediatric expertise to provide advice and consultation on pediatric MCMs and MCM distribution planning.

The DHHS National Advisory Committee on Children and Disasters was established by Congress under the PAHPRA as an expert body composed of nonfederal and federal SMEs to provide advice and consultation on all ASPR activities related to children, including MCMs, as well as state emergency preparedness and response activities pursuant to the recommendation of the National Commission on Children and Disasters.[2] Other entities, such as the PHEMCE PedsOB IPT,[23] exist to support and advance pediatric MCMs and MCM distribution planning within the federal government. To make meaningful and sustained progress to address gaps in pediatric MCMs, these expert entities should be maximized by the federal government, and others should be created as needed to ensure that sufficient sustained attention to the unique needs of children related to MCMs are addressed consistently. In addition to leveraging the pediatric expertise within government, the federal government should continue its collaboration with private sector partners as a means to access a broad array of subject matter expertise and as a mechanism to engage the support of those partners.

Pediatric health care professionals should be provided with access to current information on the appropriate use of MCMs and local distribution plans so that they can provide effective health care to children and advise families during a public health emergency.

Pediatricians and others who will be taking care of children in the event of a disaster will need requisite knowledge of when and how MCMs should be used. To best support the needs of children and families, health care providers must be familiar with appropriate dosing, drug/food interactions, and possible adverse reactions. Because MCM distribution plans may vary by location, it is important for pediatricians and other pediatric health care providers to collaborate with public health and emergency management officials so that these plans incorporate the needs of children of all ages, including preterm infants and children/youth with special health care needs. In

any event, the physician's office, the community health center, and the medical home should all be viewed as vital components of any community's response to a public health emergency and as a core asset toward resiliency.

CONCLUSIONS

Children represent nearly a quarter of the US population, but they are affected disproportionately by most disasters and public health emergencies. Children are highly vulnerable to the effects of CBRN agents and have unique anatomic, physiologic, and developmental characteristics that need to be addressed. The protection of children has also been identified by the US public as the highest priority. Although important progress has been made over the past decade in strengthening the nation's emergency and disaster preparedness for children, including considerations for the use of MCMs in children, meaningful gaps still exist. The recommendations outlined in this statement should be used to guide pediatricians; federal, state, and local government agencies; and others in addressing this need.

LEAD AUTHORS

Daniel B. Fagbuyi, MD, FAAP

David J. Schonfeld, MD, FAAP

DISASTER PREPAREDNESS ADVISORY COUNCIL

Steven E. Krug, MD, FAAP, Chairperson

Sarita Chung, MD, FAAP

Daniel B. Fagbuyi, MD, FAAP

Margaret C. Fisher MD, FAAP

Scott M. Needle, MD, FAAP

David J. Schonfeld, MD, FAAP

LIAISONS

John J. Alexander, MD, FAAP – *Food and Drug Administration*

Daniel Dodgen, PhD – *Office of the Assistant Secretary for Preparedness and Response*

Andrew L. Garrett, MD, MPH – *Office of the Assistant Secretary for Preparedness and Response*

Georgina Peacock, MD, MPH, FAAP – *Centers for Disease Control and Prevention*

Sally Phillips, RN, PhD – *Department of Homeland Security, Office of Health Affairs*

Erica Radden, MD – *Food and Drug Administration*

David A. Siegel, MD, FAAP – *National Institute of Child Health and Human Development*

STAFF

Laura Aird, MS

Sean Diederich

Tamar Magarik Haro

ABBREVIATIONS

AAP: American Academy of Pediatrics

ASPR: Assistant Secretary for Preparedness and Response

BARDA: Biomedical Advanced Research and Development Authority

CBRN: chemical, biological, radiologic, and nuclear

CDC: Centers for Disease Control and Prevention

DHHS: US Department of Health and Human Services

DHS: US Department of Homeland Security

DoD: US Department of Defense

EUA: Emergency Use Authorization

FDA: Food and Drug Administration

IPT: integrated program team

MCM: medical countermeasure

PAHPRA: Pandemic and All-Hazards Preparedness Reauthorization Act of 2013

PedsOB: Pediatric and Obstetric

PHEMCE: Public Health Emergency Medical Countermeasures Enterprise

POD: point of dispensing

SME: subject matter expert

SNS: Strategic National Stockpile

REFERENCES

1. Committee on Homeland Security and Governmental Affairs, US Senate. National preparedness: improvements needed for acquiring medical countermeasures to threats from terrorism and other sources. Washington, DC: US Government Accountability Office; October 26, 2011. Publication GAO-12-121. Available at: www.gao.gov/assets/520/511470.pdf. Accessed October 21, 2015

2. National Commission on Children and Disasters. National Commission on Children and Disasters, interim report. Washington, DC: National Commission on Children and Disasters; October 14, 2009. Available at: cybercemetery.unt.edu/archive/nccd/20110426214349/www.childrenanddisasters.acf.hhs.gov/20091014_508IR_partII.pdf. Accessed October 21, 2015

3. Office of Public Health Emergency Medical Countermeasures. HHS Public Health emergency medical countermeasure enterprise strategy for chemical, biological, radiological, and nuclear threats. Washington, DC: US Department of Health and Human Services; April, 2007. Available at: www.phe.gov/Preparedness/mcm/phemce/Documents/2007-phemce-implementation.pdf. Accessed October 21, 2015

4. US Department of Health and Human Services. National health security strategy of the United States of America. Washington, DC: US Department of Health and Human Services; December 2009. Available at: www.phe.gov/Preparedness/planning/authority/nhss/strategy/Documents/nhss-final.pdf. Accessed October 21, 2015

5. National Commission on Children and Disasters. 2010 Report to the President and Congress. Rockville, MD: Agency for Healthcare Research and Quality; 2010. AHRQ Publication 10-M037. Available at: archive.ahrq.gov/prep/nccdreport/. Accessed October 21, 2015

6. National Advisory Committee on Children and Disasters. US Department of Health and Human Services Web site. Available at: www.phe.gov/Preparedness/legal/boards/naccd/Pages/default.aspx. Accessed October 21, 2015

7. Nightingale SL, Prasher JM, Simonson S. Emergency Use Authorization (EUA) to enable use of needed products in civilian and military emergencies, United States. *Emerg Infect Dis*. 2007;13(7):1046–1051

8. Food and Drug Administration. Pandemic and All-Hazards Preparedness Reauthorization Act of 2013 (PAHPRA) Medical Countermeasure (MCM) Authorities: FDA questions and answers for public health preparedness and response stakeholders. January 2014. Available at: www.fda.gov/downloads/EmergencyPreparedness/Counterterrorism/MedicalCountermeasures/UCM380269.pdf. Accessed October 21, 2015

9. Cities Readiness Initiative. Centers for Disease Control and Prevention Web site. Available at: www.bt.cdc.gov/cri/. Updated May 20, 2010. Accessed October 21, 2015

10. Centers for Disease Control and Prevention. *Receiving, Distributing, and Dispensing Strategic National Stockpile Assets: A Guide to Preparedness, Version 11*. Atlanta, GA: Centers for Disease Control and Prevention; 2014

11. Institute of Medicine. Dispensing medical countermeasures for public health emergencies: workshop summary. Washington, DC: National Academies Press; 2008. Available at: www.nap.edu/catalog/12221.html. Accessed October 21, 2015

12. Strategic National Stockpile. Centers for Disease Control and Prevention Web site. Available at: www.cdc.gov/phpr/stockpile/stockpile.htm. Accessed October 21, 2015

13. Point of dispensing (POD) standards. Centers for Disease Control and Prevention Web site. April 2008. Available at: www.cdc.gov/phpr/documents/coopagreement-archive/FY2008/DispensingStandards.pdf. Accessed October 21, 2015

14. American Academy of Pediatrics, Council on Community Pediatrics. Community pediatrics: navigating the intersection of medicine, public health, and social determinants of children's health. *Pediatrics*. 2013;131(3):623–628

15. Medical Home Initiatives for Children With Special Needs Project Advisory Committee, American Academy of Pediatrics. The medical home. *Pediatrics*. 2002;110(1 pt 1):184–186

16. American Academy of Pediatrics. Preparedness checklist for pediatric practices. Elk Grove Village, IL: American Academy of Pediatrics; 2013. Available at: www.aap.org/en-us/advocacy-and-policy/aap-health-initiatives/Children-and-Disasters/Documents/PedPreparednessChecklist1b.pdf. Accessed October 21, 2015

17. Disaster Preparedness Advisory Council; Committee on Pediatric Emergency Medicine. Ensuring the health of children in disasters. *Pediatrics*. 2015;136(5):e1407–e1417

18. Challenges in the use of anthrax vaccine adsorbed (AVA) in the pediatric population as a component of post-exposure prophylaxis (PEP). National Biodefense Science Board. October 2011. Available at: www.phe.gov/Preparedness/legal/boards/nprsb/recommendations/Documents/avwgrpt1103.pdf. Accessed October 21, 2015

19. Presidential Commission for the Study of Bioethical Issues. Safeguarding children: pediatric medical countermeasure research. Washington, DC: Presidential Commission for the Study of Bioethical Issues; March 2013. Available at: bioethics.gov/node/833. Accessed October 21, 2015

20. Shaddy RE, Denne SC; Committee on Drugs and Committee on Pediatric Research. Clinical report—guidelines for the ethical conduct of studies to evaluate drugs in pediatric populations. *Pediatrics*. 2010;125(4):850–860

21. Opinion poll. American Academy of Pediatrics Children and Disasters Web site. Available at: www.aap.org/en-us/advocacy-and-policy/aap-health-initiatives/Children-and-Disasters/

Pages/Opinion-Poll.aspx. Accessed October 21, 2015

22. Frattarelli DA, Galinkin JL, Green TP, et al; American Academy of Pediatrics Committee on Drugs. Off-label use of drugs in children. *Pediatrics.* 2014;133(3):563–567

23. US Department of Health and Human Services Assistant Secretary for Preparedness and Response, BARDA Division of Medical Countermeasures. Threat analysis and portfolio management. Available at: www.phe. gov/about/OPP/mcsr/Pages/threat-analysis.aspx. Accessed October 21, 2015

Medical Versus Nonmedical Immunization Exemptions for Child Care and School Attendance

- *Policy Statement*

POLICY STATEMENT Organizational Principles to Guide and Define the Child Health
Care System and/or Improve the Health of all Children

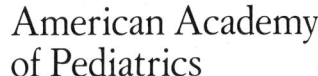
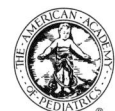

American Academy
of Pediatrics

DEDICATED TO THE HEALTH OF ALL CHILDREN™

Medical Versus Nonmedical Immunization Exemptions for Child Care and School Attendance

COMMITTEE ON PRACTICE AND AMBULATORY MEDICINE, COMMITTEE ON INFECTIOUS DISEASES, COMMITTEE ON STATE GOVERNMENT AFFAIRS, COUNCIL ON SCHOOL HEALTH, SECTION ON ADMINISTRATION AND PRACTICE MANAGEMENT

abstract

Routine childhood immunizations against infectious diseases are an integral part of our public health infrastructure. They provide direct protection to the immunized individual and indirect protection to children and adults unable to be immunized via the effect of community immunity. All 50 states, the District of Columbia, and Puerto Rico have regulations requiring proof of immunization for child care and school attendance as a public health strategy to protect children in these settings and to secondarily serve as a mechanism to promote timely immunization of children by their caregivers. Although all states and the District of Columbia have mechanisms to exempt school attendees from specific immunization requirements for medical reasons, the majority also have a heterogeneous collection of regulations and laws that allow nonmedical exemptions from childhood immunizations otherwise required for child care and school attendance. The American Academy of Pediatrics (AAP) supports regulations and laws requiring certification of immunization to attend child care and school as a sound means of providing a safe environment for attendees and employees of these settings. The AAP also supports medically indicated exemptions to specific immunizations as determined for each individual child. The AAP views nonmedical exemptions to school-required immunizations as inappropriate for individual, public health, and ethical reasons and advocates for their elimination.

DOI: 10.1542/peds.2016-2145

PEDIATRICS (ISSN Numbers: Print, 0031-4005; Online, 1098-4275).

Copyright © 2016 by the American Academy of Pediatrics

FINANCIAL DISCLOSURE: The authors have indicated they do not have a financial relationship relevant to this article to disclose.

FUNDING: No external funding.

POTENTIAL CONFLICT OF INTEREST: The authors have indicated they have no potential conflicts of interest to disclose.

To cite: AAP COMMITTEE ON PRACTICE AND AMBULATORY MEDICINE, AAP COMMITTEE ON INFECTIOUS DISEASES, AAP COMMITTEE ON STATE GOVERNMENT AFFAIRS, AAP COUNCIL ON SCHOOL HEALTH, AAP SECTION ON ADMINISTRATION AND PRACTICE MANAGEMENT. Medical Versus Nonmedical Immunization Exemptions for Child Care and School Attendance. *Pediatrics.* 2016;138(3):e20162145

BACKGROUND

Principles of Childhood Immunization and Community Immunity

Childhood immunization is one of the greatest accomplishments of modern medicine. In the United States 2009 birth cohort, routine childhood immunization will prevent approximately 42 000 early deaths and 20 million cases of disease, saving $13.5 billion in direct costs and $68.8 billion in societal costs.[1]

However, vaccines are not 100% effective in individuals receiving them. Certain infants, children, and adolescents cannot safely receive specific vaccines because of age or specific health conditions. These individuals benefit from the effectiveness of immunizations through a mechanism known as community immunity (also known as "herd" immunity). Community immunity occurs when nearly all individuals for whom vaccine is not contraindicated have been appropriately immunized, minimizing the risk of illness or spread of a vaccine-preventable infectious agent to those who do not have the direct benefit of immunization. Although there is variance for levels of immunization required to generate community immunity specific to each disease and vaccine, it is generally understood that population immunization rates of at least 90% are required, as reflected in the Healthy People 2020 goals.[2] Certain highly contagious diseases, such as pertussis and measles, require a population immunization rate of ≥95% to achieve community immunity.

School Immunization Requirements

Each of the 50 states and the District of Columbia and Puerto Rico have requirements for proof of immunization for attendees of child care centers and public schools, and nearly all have laws covering private schools as well.[3] Some states allow local school boards to set requirements for some vaccines, although the majority set requirements at the state level. These policies are designed to protect children attending child care and school from vaccine-preventable diseases by creating a learning environment with a very high rate of community immunity. In addition,

vocational schools, colleges, and universities also have immunization requirements. As an additional public health benefit, immunization requirements serve as a strong incentive for parents and families to immunize their children according to the schedule recommended by the Centers for Disease Control and Prevention and the American Academy of Pediatrics (AAP). Public health data show that vaccine requirements for child care and/or school entry result in increased community immunization rates[4] and decreased incidence of those vaccine-preventable diseases.[5,6]

Medical Immunization Exemptions

Although there are fairly consistent standards for required immunizations across the United States, every state, the District of Columbia, and Puerto Rico have allowances to exempt children from school-required immunization for medically indicated reasons. Examples of such include allergy to a vaccine component, previous significant adverse reaction to a vaccine or its components, or other underlying health condition such as an immunosuppressed organ transplant recipient.[7] Almost half of states have laws that distinguish between temporary and permanent medical contraindications,[3] with nearly another half of these states requiring annual or more frequent health care provider recertification for the medical exemptions. Because only a very small proportion of children have medical conditions prohibiting specific immunizations, medically indicated exemptions, when granted appropriately, typically do not compromise community immunity. It is this specific group of children that depends on community immunity for protection.

Nonmedical Immunization Exemptions

Although not required under current federal constitutional and

statutory law,[8] almost all states allow exemptions from school attendance immunization requirements on the basis of religious belief, and almost half of the states allow philosophical (also known as personal-belief) exemptions.

Although nearly ubiquitous, nonmedical exemption regulations are quite heterogeneous from state to state in terms of how they are granted, used, and maintained.[3] Some states explicitly exclude philosophical and personal-belief exemptions and define these as not falling under the scope of religious exemptions. More than half of the states legally allow for exclusion of exempted students or can withdraw nonmedical exemptions during outbreaks, epidemics, or emergencies. More than one-quarter of the states require parental notarization or affidavit confirming either a religious or personal-belief justification in applying for a nonmedical school immunization exemption. A number of states have laws requiring parent/guardian education by health departments or health care providers about the benefits of vaccines and the risks and consequences of not receiving recommended childhood immunizations.

PUBLIC HEALTH EFFECTS OF IMMUNIZATION EXEMPTIONS

Exemption Rates and Vaccine-Preventable Disease Incidence

Legislation requiring immunization before school entry increases immunization rates and dramatically decreases the incidence of vaccine-preventable diseases.[9] Examples of these include immunization against measles and chickenpox. Likewise, higher rates of immunization exemptions in communities correlate with higher rates of vaccine-preventable illnesses and disease outbreaks, such as pertussis and measles.[10-13]

Although overall rates of many required immunizations have increased or remained steady over the past 10 years, recent studies show that unvaccinated children are often geographically clustered within communities[14] and have corresponding higher rates of immunization exemption. This clustering reflects the fact that families with similar sociocultural beliefs often live near each other or attend the same schools which results in population clusters within larger communities with significantly lower immunization rates that are insufficient to sustain community immunity. This phenomenon results in disease outbreaks when a vaccine-preventable illness is introduced into these communities.

Exemption Rates and Legal Requirements

States with less rigorous requirements for nonmedical exemptions and those that grant permanent medical exemptions have significantly higher vaccine exemption rates than those states with more rigorous requirements or those that only grant temporary exemptions.[15]

States that offer personal-belief exemptions have had steady increases in the number of exemptions over time. Religious exemptions have increased for states that do not offer personal-belief/philosophical exemptions but have, through regulatory language, broadly defined religion for the purposes of obtaining vaccine exemption. The ease of requirements to obtain nonmedical exemptions, especially those of personal belief, can have a significant impact on the rate of exemptions and immunizations.[16] Oregon, which in 2014 began requiring parental completion of an educational module on the benefits of vaccines before allowing a certified exemption, saw a 17% decrease in the number of exemptions granted the following school year.

JUSTIFICATION FOR IMMUNIZATION REQUIREMENTS

Legal Justification

Resistance and legal challenges to compulsory vaccination laws have existed since the early 19th century. In *Jacobson versus Massachusetts*,[8] the court found legislative vaccine mandates to be constitutional as a means of protecting public health and public safety. In *Zucht versus King* in 1922, the Supreme Court upheld a local ordinance requiring vaccination as a condition for school attendance.[17] In the 1944 case *Prince versus Commonwealth of Massachusetts*, the court ruled that the constitutional rights of religion or parenthood were not beyond limitation and that states had the authority to protect the welfare of children and the community. Although the specific case was with regard to child labor laws, the court extended its language to encompass both religious and personal activities such that, "The right to practice religion freely does not include liberty to expose the community or the child to communicable disease or the latter to ill health or death."[18] Since these rulings, there have been numerous challenges to state and local immunization requirements (eg, *Workman versus Mingo County Schools, Phillips versus City of New York*). All of these challenges failed.

Ethical Considerations

Parents and the government both have a responsibility in maintaining the health of children. There is a societal interest in protecting the health of the individual child and society as a whole. Although society generally believes that parents or guardians are best situated to understand their child's unique needs, including health care needs, and should participate in caring and thoughtful medical decision-making, this parental responsibility is not an absolute right. With this in mind, it is critical to design childhood immunization exemption policies so that they clearly serve the best interests of both the individual child and the community.

Parents are expected to consider the best interest of their child in medical decision-making, focusing on their child's medical, emotional, and social needs, rather than their own social or emotional interests. In general, the state is empowered to overrule parental medical decision-making only when such decision-making or refusal of care places a child at significant risk of serious harm. Vaccination is unique within the realm of medical interventions because it not only provides a benefit to the patient who is vaccinated but also confers a significant public health benefit in terms of community immunity. Similarly, refusal of vaccination not only puts the individual child at risk but also increases societal risk by decreasing community immunity and adding to a population of unimmunized individuals within which vaccine-preventable disease may spread. Declining community immunity may be a significant risk for children and adults with medical contraindications to vaccination, who rely on community immunity for protection from vaccine-preventable diseases. Thus, nonmedical exemptions effectively disenfranchise people with medically indicated contraindications to vaccines from receiving equal protection under public health policy.

Several pediatric bioethicists have argued against the elimination of nonmedical exemptions by citing the ethical Principle of Least Restrictive Means for public health policy.[19] This principle recognizes that where multiple options exist to achieve public health goals, "that the full force of state authority and power should be reserved for exceptional circumstances and that more coercive methods should be employed only when less coercive methods have failed."[20] However, this principle was developed to protect individuals from serious deprivations of personal liberty. The current immunization requirements that some seek to avoid with nonmedical exemptions are limited in scope to attendance in child care or school settings and are not requirements for the mandatory vaccination or quarantine of individuals who are unimmunized. Neither is there an undue burden of health risk to the individual in that immunization safety is scientifically well established. The public health value and benefit from requiring childhood immunizations for child care and school attendance versus allowing nonmedical exemptions are not equal alternatives. Nonmedical exemptions negatively affect community immunity and have indeed failed, as documented in the medical literature.[12] In addition, the heterogeneous collections of regulations covering nonmedical exemptions, they actually present an ethical dilemma of unfair implementation and application to families.[21]

CONCLUSIONS

Immunization requirements for child care and school attendance are an effective means of protecting people from vaccine-preventable diseases, both by direct protection from the vaccine and indirect protection via community immunity. Immunization requirements also have a beneficial effect on timely immunization of children. Because rare medically recognized contraindications for specific individuals to receive specific vaccines exist, legitimate medical exemptions to immunization requirements are important to observe. However, nonmedical exemptions to immunization

requirements are problematic because of medical, public health, and ethical reasons and create unnecessary risk to both individual people and communities.

RECOMMENDATIONS

1. The AAP supports laws and regulatory measures that require certification of immunization to attend child care and school as a sound means of providing a safe environment for attendees and employees of these settings.

2. The AAP supports medically indicated exemptions to specific immunizations as determined for each individual student.

3. The AAP recommends that all states and the District of Columbia use their public health authority to eliminate nonmedical exemptions from immunization requirements.

4. The AAP recommends that all child care centers, schools, and other covered entities comply with state laws and regulations requiring current and accurate documentation of appropriate immunization status and appropriate medical exemptions of attendees and students.

5. The AAP recommends that the appropriate public health authorities provide the community with information about immunization rates in child care centers, schools, and other covered entities and determine whether there are risks to community immunity on the basis of this information.

LEAD AUTHORS

Geoffrey R. Simon, MD, FAAP
Carrie Byington, MD, FAAP
Christoph Diasio, MD, FAAP
Anne R. Edwards, MD, FAAP
Breena Holmes, MD, FAAP

COMMITTEE ON PRACTICE AND AMBULATORY MEDICINE, 2015–2016

Geoffrey R. Simon, MD, FAAP, Chairperson

Alexy D. Arauz Boudreau, MD, MPH, FAAP
Cynthia Baker, MD, FAAP
Graham A. Barden III, MD, FAAP
Jesse Hackell, MD, FAAP
Amy Hardin, MD, FAAP
Kelley Meade, MD, FAAP
Scot Moore, MD, FAAP
Julia E. Richerson, MD, FAAP

STAFF

Elizabeth Sobczyk, MPH, MSW

COMMITTEE ON INFECTIOUS DISEASES, 2015–2016

Carrie L. Byington, MD, FAAP, Chairperson
Yvonne A. Maldonado, MD, FAAP, Vice Chairperson
Elizabeth D. Barnett, MD, FAAP
H. Dele Davies, MD, MS, MHCM, FAAP
Kathryn M. Edwards, MD, FAAP
Ruth Lynfield, MD, FAAP
Flor M. Munoz, MD, FAAP
Dawn Nolt, MD, MPH
Ann-Christine Nyquist, MD, MSPH, FAAP
Mobeen H. Rathore, MD, FAAP
Mark H. Sawyer, MD, FAAP
William J. Steinbach, MD, FAAP
Tina Q. Tan, MD, FAAP
Theoklis E. Zaoutis, MD, MSCE, FAAP

EX OFFICIO

David W. Kimberlin, MD, FAAP – *Red Book* Editor
Michael T. Brady, MD, FAAP – *Red Book* Associate Editor
Mary Anne Jackson, MD, FAAP – *Red Book* Associate Editor
Sarah S. Long, MD, FAAP – *Red Book* Associate Editor
Henry H. Bernstein, DO, MHCM, FAAP – *Red Book* Online Associate Editor
H. Cody Meissner, MD, FAAP – Visual *Red Book* Associate Editor

LIAISONS

Douglas Campos-Outcalt, MD, MPA – *American Academy of Family Physicians*
Amanda C. Cohn, MD, FAAP – *Centers for Disease Control and Prevention*
Karen M. Farizo, MD – *US Food and Drug Administration*
Marc Fischer, MD, FAAP – *Centers for Disease Control and Prevention*
Bruce G. Gellin, MD, MPH – *National Vaccine Program Office*
Richard L. Gorman, MD, FAAP – *National Institutes of Health*
Natasha Halasa, MD, MPH, FAAP – *Pediatric Infectious Diseases Society*
Joan L. Robinson, MD – *Canadian Paediatric Society*
Jamie Deseda-Tous, MD – *Sociedad Latinoamericana de Infectologia Pediatrica*
Geoffrey R. Simon, MD, FAAP – *Committee on Practice Ambulatory Medicine*

REFERENCES

1. Zhou F, Shefer A, Wenger J, et al. Economic evaluation of the routine childhood immunization program in the United States, 2009. *Pediatrics.* 2014;133(4):577–585

2. HealthyPeople.gov. Immunization and infectious diseases. Available at: https://www.healthypeople.gov/2020/topics-objectives/topic/immunization-and-infectious-diseases/objectives

3. Centers for Disease Control and Prevention. State School and Childcare Vaccination Laws. Available at: http://www.cdc.gov/phlp/publications/topic/vaccinations.html. Accessed August 3, 2016

4. Davis MM, Gaglia MA. Associations of daycare and school entry vaccination requirements with varicella immunization rates. *Vaccine.* 2005;23(23):3053–3060

5. Ernst KC, Pogreba-Brown K, Rasmussen L, Erhart LM. The effect of policy changes on hepatitis A vaccine uptake in Arizona children, 1995-2008. *Public Health Rep.* 2011;126(suppl 2):87–96

6. Lopez AS, Kolasa MS, Seward JR. Status of school entry requirements for varicella vaccination and vaccination coverage 11 years after implementation of the Varicella Vaccination program. *J Infect Dis.* 2008;197(suppl 2):S76–S81

7. Centers for Disease Control and Prevention. Chart of Contraindications and Precautions to Commonly Used Vaccines. Available at: www.cdc.gov/vaccines/hcp/admin/contraindications-vacc.html. Accessed August 3, 2016

8. *Jacobson v Massachusetts*, 197 US 11 (1905)

9. Diekema DS. Personal belief exemptions from school vaccination requirements. *Annu Rev Public Health.* 2014;35:275–292

10. Omer SB, Pan WK, Halsey NA, et al. Nonmedical exemptions to school immunization requirements: secular trends and association of state policies with pertussis incidence. *JAMA.* 2006;296(14):1757–1763

11. Imdad A, Tserenpuntsag B, Blog DS, et al. Religious exemptions for immunization and risk of pertussis in New York State, 2000–2011. *Pediatrics.* 2013;132(1):37–43

12. Phadke VK, Bednarczyk RA, Salmon DA, Omer SB. Association between vaccine refusal and vaccine-preventable diseases in the United States: a review of measles and pertussis. *JAMA.* 2016;315(11):1149–1158

13. Atwell JE, Van Otterloo J, Zipprich J, et al. Nonmedical vaccine exemptions and pertussis in California, 2010. *Pediatrics.* 2013;132(4):624–630

14. Hill HA, Elam-Evans LD, Yankey D, Singleton JA, Kolasa M. National, state, and selected local area vaccination coverage among children aged 19-35 months—United States, 2014. *MMWR Morb Mortal Wkly Rep.* 2015;64(33):889–896

15. Blank NR, Caplan AL, Constable C. Exempting schoolchildren from immunizations: states with few barriers had highest rates of nonmedical exemptions. *Health Aff (Millwood).* 2013;32(7):1282–1290

16. Stadlin S, Bednarczyk RA, Omer SB. Medical exemptions to school immunization requirements in the United States—association of state policies with medical exemption rates (2004–2011). *J Infect Dis.* 2012;206(7):989–992

17. *Zucht v King*, 260 US 174 (1922)

18. *Prince v Commonwealth of Massachusetts*, 321 US 158 (1944)

19. Opel DJ, Kronman MP, Diekema DS, et al. Childhood vaccine exemption policy: the case for a less restrictive alternative. *Pediatrics.* 2016;137(4):e20154230

20. Upshur RE. Principles for the justification of public health intervention. *Can J Public Health.* 2002;93(2):101–103

21. Kass NE. An ethics framework for public health. *Am J Public Health.* 2001;91(11):1776–1782

Medication-Assisted Treatment of Adolescents With Opioid Use Disorders

• *Policy Statement*

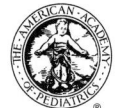

POLICY STATEMENT   Organizational Principles to Guide and Define the Child Health
Care System and/or Improve the Health of all Children

American Academy
of Pediatrics
DEDICATED TO THE HEALTH OF ALL CHILDREN™

Medication-Assisted Treatment of Adolescents With Opioid Use Disorders

COMMITTEE ON SUBSTANCE USE AND PREVENTION

abstract

Opioid use disorder is a leading cause of morbidity and mortality among US youth. Effective treatments, both medications and substance use disorder counseling, are available but underused, and access to developmentally appropriate treatment is severely restricted for adolescents and young adults. Resources to disseminate available therapies and to develop new treatments specifically for this age group are needed to save and improve lives of youth with opioid addiction.

BACKGROUND

With a renewed emphasis on treating pain directed by the US Department of Health and Human Services in 1992[1] and institutionalized by the Joint Commission on Accreditation of Hospitals in 2001,[2] combined with the development of potent oral opioid pain medications, exponential increases in the annual number of opioid prescriptions written by US physicians have occurred over the past 2 decades.[3] Between 1991 and 2012, the rate of "nonmedical use" (ie, use without a prescription or more than prescribed) of opioid medication by adolescents (12–17 years of age) and young adults (18–25 years of age) more than doubled,[4,5] and the rate of opioid use disorders, including heroin addiction, increased in parallel.[6] The rate of fatal opioid overdose more than doubled between 2000 and 2013.[7] In 2008, more than 16 000 people died of opioid pain reliever overdose.[7] Other serious adverse health outcomes result from intravenous drug use and include endocarditis,[8] abscesses,[9] and infection with hepatitis C.[10]

Severe opioid use disorder is a chronic condition in which neurologic changes in the reward center of the brain are responsible for cravings and compulsive substance use.[11] The associated behavioral disruptions and change in functioning range from modest to severe; remarkably, some adolescents may continue to do well in school and in other areas of life despite severe opioid use disorder. The rate of spontaneous remission is low; however, patients can recover. Three medications are currently indicated for treating severe opioid use disorder: methadone,

This document is copyrighted and is property of the American Academy of Pediatrics and its Board of Directors. All authors have filed conflict of interest statements with the American Academy of Pediatrics. Any conflicts have been resolved through a process approved by the Board of Directors. The American Academy of Pediatrics has neither solicited nor accepted any commercial involvement in the development of the content of this publication.

Policy statements from the American Academy of Pediatrics benefit from expertise and resources of liaisons and internal (AAP) and external reviewers. However, policy statements from the American Academy of Pediatrics may not reflect the views of the liaisons or the organizations or government agencies that they represent.

The guidance in this statement does not indicate an exclusive course of treatment or serve as a standard of medical care. Variations, taking into account individual circumstances, may be appropriate.

All policy statements from the American Academy of Pediatrics automatically expire 5 years after publication unless reaffirmed, revised, or retired at or before that time.

DOI: 10.1542/peds.2016-1893

PEDIATRICS (ISSN Numbers: Print, 0031-4005; Online, 1098-4275).

FINANCIAL DISCLOSURE: The authors have indicated they do not have a financial relationship relevant to this article to disclose.

FUNDING: No external funding.

POTENTIAL CONFLICT OF INTEREST: The authors have indicated they have no potential conflicts of interest to disclose.

To cite: AAP COMMITTEE ON SUBSTANCE USE AND PREVENTION. Medication-Assisted Treatment of Adolescents With Opioid Use Disorders. *Pediatrics.* 2016;138(3):e20161893

naltrexone, and buprenorphine. Methadone, a full opioid agonist with a long half-life that can ameliorate the cycle of intense euphoria followed by intense withdrawal associated with opioid use, has long been established as an effective treatment of opioid addiction, although federal regulations prohibit most methadone programs from admitting patients younger than 18 years. In 2000, the US Congress passed the Drug Addiction Treatment Act, which allows for physicians to complete 8 hours of training and apply for a waiver to prescribe buprenorphine, a partial opioid agonist, to treat opioid use disorders in general medical settings.[12] Naltrexone, an opioid antagonist with high affinity for the opioid receptor, has also proven to be an effective treatment of opioid addiction. Unlike opioid agonists, naltrexone has a very limited potential for misuse or diversion. The extended-release formulation may reduce patient adherence burden. Although there is not yet rigorous research support for efficacy in adolescents, growing experience and anecdotal reports support it as a promising practice. Naltrexone, which also reduces alcohol cravings, may be a good therapeutic option for adolescents and young adults with co-occurring alcohol use disorder, as well as those living in unstable or unsupervised housing.

In 2002, the US Food and Drug Administration approved the use of buprenorphine for patients 16 years and older.[13] Buprenorphine is a partial opioid agonist with high affinity for the opioid receptor. Buprenorphine binding results in gentle stimulation of the opioid system, which, like methadone, can ameliorate the highs and lows associated with full agonists with short and moderate half-lives. An expansive body of research has shown the effectiveness of buprenorphine for treating adults with opioid use disorders,[14] and

2 randomized controlled trials have examined the therapeutic efficacy of buprenorphine combined with substance use counseling in adolescents and young adults. Marsch et al[15] found that adolescents 13 to 18 years of age who received 2 weeks of buprenorphine treatment were more likely to continue medical care compared with those who received clonidine for the same period of time. A trial conducted by Woody et al[16] compared 2 detoxification regimens among adolescents and young adults 15 to 21 years of age. One group received 8 weeks of buprenorphine before tapering, and the second group received 2 weeks. Adolescents who received 8 weeks had lower rates of illicit opioid use while they were taking buprenorphine, and the differences quickly disappeared once the medication was discontinued. The findings led the authors to conclude that there is no obvious reason to stop medications in adolescent patients who are doing well on buprenorphine. Matson et al[17] found that continued buprenorphine compliance is associated with an increase in treatment and can help adolescents achieve long-term sobriety. In general, youth have lower rates of treatment retention compared with adults,[18–20] underscoring the need to deliver developmentally appropriate treatment to achieve best outcomes.

Buprenorphine has the potential for misuse and diversion because of its opioid agonist activity, although its "addiction potential" is thought to be much lower than that of full opioid agonists, such as oxycodone or heroin. Extensive experience with adults has established the evidence supporting the efficacy of buprenorphine, and although not as well studied among youth so far, research and clinical experience to date have not identified any age-specific safety concerns. Nonetheless, confusion, stigma, and limited resources severely restrict

access to buprenorphine for both adolescents and adults. Knudsen et al[21] found that less than 50% of a nationally representative sample of 345 addiction treatment programs serving adolescents and adults offer patients medication for the treatment of opioid use disorders, and even among programs that do offer it, medication is significantly underutilized. The same study found that only 34% of opioid-dependent patients in treatment receive medication. By comparison, 70% of patients with mental health disorders in these same programs received medication. Policies, attitudes, and messages that serve to prevent patients from accessing a medication that can effectively treat a life-threatening condition may be harmful to adolescent health.

RECOMMENDATIONS

1. Opioid addiction is a chronic relapsing neurologic disorder. Although rates of spontaneous recovery are low, outcomes can be improved with medication-assisted treatment. The American Academy of Pediatrics (AAP) advocates for increasing resources to improve access to medication-assisted treatment of opioid-addicted adolescents and young adults. This recommendation includes both increasing resources for medication-assisted treatment within primary care and access to developmentally appropriate substance use disorder counseling in community settings. Pediatricians have access to an AAP-endorsed buprenorphine waiver course at www.aap.org/mat.

2. The AAP recommends that pediatricians consider offering medication-assisted treatment to their adolescent and young adult patients with severe opioid use disorders or discuss referrals to other providers for this service.

3. The AAP supports further research focus on developmentally appropriate treatment of substance use disorders in adolescents and young adults, including primary and secondary prevention, behavioral interventions, and medication treatment.

LEAD AUTHORS

Sharon Levy, MD, MPH, FAAP

COMMITTEE ON SUBSTANCE USE AND PREVENTION, 2015–2016

Sheryl A. Ryan, MD, FAAP, Chairperson
Pamela K. Gonzalez, MD, FAAP
Stephen W. Patrick, MD, MPH, MS, FAAP
Joanna Quigley, MD, FAAP
Lorena Siqueira, MD, MSPH, FAAP
Leslie R. Walker, MD, FAAP

FORMER COMMITTEE MEMBER

Sharon Levy, MD, MPH, FAAP

LIAISONS

Vivian B. Faden, PhD – *National Institute of Alcohol Abuse and Alcoholism*
Gregory Tau, MD, PhD – *American Academy of Child and Adolescent Psychiatry*

STAFF

Renee Jarrett, MPH

ABBREVIATION

AAP: American Academy of Pediatrics

REFERENCES

1. Agency for Health Care Policy and Research Public Health Service. Acute pain management: operative or medical procedures and trauma (clinical practice guideline). Rockville, MD: Agency for Health Care Policy and Research; 1992. Available at: http://archive.ahrq.gov/clinic/medtep/acute.htm. Accessed November 11, 2014

2. The Joint Commission. Pain Management Fact Sheet. 2014. Available at: www.jointcommission.org/topics/pain_management.aspx. Accessed November 10, 2014

3. Volkow ND. America's addiction to opioids: heroin and prescription drug abuse. National Institute on Drug Abuse; May 14, 2014. Available at: www.drugabuse.gov/about-nida/legislative-activities/testimony-to-congress/2014/americas-addiction-to-opioids-heroin-prescription-drug-abuse. Accessed September 12, 2014

4. Substance Abuse and Mental Health Services Administration Office of Applied Studies. National Household Survey on Drug Abuse: Population Estimates 1992. Rockville, MD: Substance Abuse and Mental Health Services Administration; 1993. Available at: https://babel.hathitrust.org/cgi/pt?id=mdp.39015026207988;view=1up;seq=89. Accessed March 1, 2016

5. Substance Abuse and Mental Health Services Administration. *Results From the 2012 National Survey on Drug Use and Health: Summary of National Findings*. Rockville, MD: Substance Abuse and Mental Health Services Administration; 2013

6. Muhuri PK, Gfroerer JC, Davies MC. Associations of nonmedical pain reliever use and initiation of heroin use in the United States. Rockville, MD: Substance Abuse and Mental Health Services Administration; 2013. Available at: www.samhsa.gov/data/sites/default/files/DR006/DR006/nonmedical-pain-reliever-use-2013.htm. Accessed November 5, 2014

7. Hedegaard H, Chen L-H, Warner M. Drug-poisoning deaths involving heroin: United States, 2000–2013. Hyattsville, MD: Centers for Disease Control and Prevention; 2015. Available at: www.cdc.gov/nchs/data/databriefs/db190.htm. Accessed October 26, 2015

8. Moss R, Munt B. Injection drug use and right sided endocarditis. *Heart*. 2003;89(5):577–581. Available at: http://heart.bmj.com/content/89/5/577.short. Accessed October 26, 2015

9. Summanen PH, Talan DA, Strong C, et al. Bacteriology of skin and soft-tissue infections: comparison of infections in intravenous drug users and individuals with no history of intravenous drug use. *Clin Infect Dis*. 1995;20(suppl 2):S279–S282. Available at: http://cid.oxfordjournals.org/content/20/Supplement_2/S279.short. Accessed October 26, 2015

10. Tsui JI, Evans JL, Lum PJ, Hahn JA, Page K. Association of opioid agonist therapy with lower incidence of hepatitis C virus infection in young adult injection drug users. *JAMA Intern Med*. 2014;174(12):1974–1981. Available at: www.pubmedcentral.nih.gov/articlerender.fcgi?artid=4506774&tool=pmcentrez&rendertype=abstract. Accessed October 26, 2015

11. Kosten TR, George TP. The neurobiology of opioid dependence: implications for treatment. *Sci Pract Perspect*. 2002;1(1):13–20. Available at: www.pubmedcentral.nih.gov/articlerender.fcgi?artid=2851054&tool=pmcentrez&rendertype=abstract. Accessed November 10, 2014

12. Substance Abuse and Mental Health Services Administration. Drug Addiction Treatment Act of 2000: Title XXXV, Section 3502 of the Children's Health Act of 2000. 2014. Available at: http://buprenorphine.samhsa.gov/titlexxxv.html. Accessed November 12, 2014

13. McCormick C. *Suboxone and Subtex Approval Letter*, vol. 732. Rockville, MD: Center for Drug Evaluation and Research; Food and Drug Administration; 2002

14. Kraus ML, Alford DP, Kotz MM, et al; American Society of Addiction Medicine. Statement of the American Society of Addiction Medicine Consensus Panel on the use of buprenorphine in office-based treatment of opioid addiction. *J Addict Med*. 2011;5(4):254–263. Available at: www.ncbi.nlm.nih.gov/pubmed/22042215. Accessed November 11, 2014

15. Marsch LA, Bickel WK, Badger GJ, et al. Comparison of pharmacological treatments for opioid-dependent adolescents: a randomized controlled trial. *Arch Gen Psychiatry*. 2005;62(10):1157–1164

16. Woody GE, Poole SA, Subramaniam G, et al. Extended vs short-term buprenorphine-naloxone for treatment of opioid-addicted youth: a randomized trial. *JAMA*. 2008;300(17):2003–2011. Available at: www.pubmedcentral.nih.gov/articlerender.fcgi?artid=2610690&

tool=pmcentrez&rendertype=abstract. Accessed June 20, 2014

17. Matson SC, Hobson G, Abdel-Rasoul M, Bonny AE. A retrospective study of retention of opioid-dependent adolescents and young adults in an outpatient buprenorphine/naloxone clinic. *J Addict Med.* 2014;8(3):176–182

18. Schuman-Olivier Z, Weiss RD, Hoeppner BB, Borodovsky J, Albanese MJ. Emerging adult age status predicts poor buprenorphine treatment

retention. *J Subst Abuse Treat.* 2014;47(3):202–212

19. Dreifuss JA, Griffin ML, Frost K, et al. Patient characteristics associated with buprenorphine/naloxone treatment outcome for prescription opioid dependence: Results from a multisite study. *Drug Alcohol Depend.* 2013;131(1–2):112–118

20. Marsch LA, Stephens MAC, Mudric T, Strain EC, Bigelow GE, Johnson RE. Predictors of outcome in LAAM,

buprenorphine, and methadone treatment for opioid dependence. *Exp Clin Psychopharmacol.* 2005;13(4):293–302

21. Knudsen HK, Abraham AJ, Roman PM. Adoption and implementation of medications in addiction treatment programs. *J Addict Med.* 2011;5(1):21–27. Available at: www.pubmedcentral.nih.gov/articlerender.fcgi?artid=3045214&tool=pmcentrez&rendertype=abstract. Accessed October 30, 2014

Menstrual Management for Adolescents With Disabilities

• *Clinical Report*

CLINICAL REPORT   Guidance for the Clinician in Rendering Pediatric Care

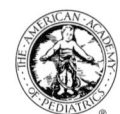

American Academy
of Pediatrics

DEDICATED TO THE HEALTH OF ALL CHILDREN™

Menstrual Management for Adolescents With Disabilities

Elisabeth H. Quint, MD, Rebecca F. O'Brien, MD, COMMITTEE ON ADOLESCENCE, The North American Society for Pediatric and Adolescent Gynecology

abstract

The onset of menses for adolescents with physical or intellectual disabilities can affect their independence and add additional concerns for families at home, in schools, and in other settings. The pediatrician is the primary health care provider to explore and assist with the pubertal transition and menstrual management. Menstrual management of both normal and abnormal cycles may be requested to minimize hygiene issues, premenstrual symptoms, dysmenorrhea, heavy or irregular bleeding, contraception, and conditions exacerbated by the menstrual cycle. Several options are available for menstrual management, depending on the outcome that is desired, ranging from cycle regulation to complete amenorrhea. The use of medications or the request for surgeries to help with the menstrual cycles in teenagers with disabilities has medical, social, legal, and ethical implications. This clinical report is designed to help guide pediatricians in assisting adolescent females with intellectual and/or physical disabilities and their families in making decisions related to successfully navigating menarche and subsequent menstrual cycles.

Clinical reports from the American Academy of Pediatrics benefit from expertise and resources of liaisons and internal (AAP) and external reviewers. However, clinical reports from the American Academy of Pediatrics may not reflect the views of the liaisons or the organizations or government agencies that they represent.

The guidance in this report does not indicate an exclusive course of treatment or serve as a standard of medical care. Variations, taking into account individual circumstances, may be appropriate.

All clinical reports from the American Academy of Pediatrics automatically expire 5 years after publication unless reaffirmed, revised, or retired at or before that time.

DOI: 10.1542/peds.2016-0295

PEDIATRICS (ISSN Numbers: Print, 0031-4005; Online, 1098-4275).

Copyright © 2016 by the American Academy of Pediatrics

FINANCIAL DISCLOSURE: The authors have indicated they do not have a financial relationship relevant to this article to disclose.

FUNDING: No external funding.

POTENTIAL CONFLICT OF INTEREST: The authors have indicated they have no potential conflict of interest to disclose.

To cite: Quint EH, O'Brien RF, AAP THE COMMITTEE ON ADOLESCENCE, AAP The North American Society for Pediatric and Adolescent Gynecology. Menstrual Management for Adolescents With Disabilities. *Pediatrics*. 2016;137(4): e20160295

The physical pubertal transition is a complicated time for most adolescents and their families and may be even more challenging for teenagers with disabilities. For the purpose of this report, "family" and "families" also refers to caregivers and guardians. Teenagers may have concerns about body image, sexuality, and how menses will affect their lives. Parents often worry about the impact of pubertal development on the lives and health of their daughters with disabilities.[1] A large Canadian study showed that parents' concerns for their adolescent daughters with intellectual disabilities include menstrual suppression, hygiene, parental burden, and menstrual symptoms.[2] The pediatrician and the medical home play a key role in anticipatory guidance with the family and teenager regarding emerging sexuality, physical changes of puberty and onset of menstruation, and the emotional and behavioral changes associated with puberty. Even before the onset of menses, the pediatrician could be asked to assist with anticipatory guidance and options for the menstrual cycle because of parental fear of menstrual periods or hormonal mood changes as well as the complex issues of sexuality, vulnerability, and fertility in the context of the disability. This clinical report briefly addresses pubertal issues in female adolescents with physical and/or intellectual disabilities and provides details on the options for menstruation management. The American Academy of Pediatrics (AAP) clinical report titled "Sexuality of Children and Adolescents With Developmental Disabilities" complements this report and includes Internet resources on this topic.[3]

PUBERTY IN ADOLESCENT GIRLS WITH DISABILITIES

Disabilities in children are common, with 2.8 million or 5.2% of US children and adolescents 5 through 17 years of age affected in 2010.[4] Approximately 3% of the general population has a significant intellectual disability, and 1.2 million of those affected are teenagers with varying levels of cognitive abilities (80% have mild disability, 12% have moderate disability, and 8% have severe intellectual disabilities).[5] This clinical report will not include specific discussions around teenagers with psychiatric illnesses.

For most adolescents with intellectual disabilities, although the pattern of pubertal maturation is similar to adolescents without disabilities, the tempo and timing of maturation may vary. Earlier sexual development may occur in girls with neurodevelopmental disabilities,[6] whereas some girls with autism spectrum disorders may experience a slight delay in the onset of menarche.[7] Adolescents with disabilities that compromise their nutrition or are associated with chronic inflammation may have a later onset of puberty. Premenarchal suppression is not recommended for most teenagers with intellectual

TABLE 1 General Principles for Approaching Menstruation in Adolescents With Disabilities

1. Initiate anticipatory guidance before the start of menses
2. Discuss concerns around sexual education and expression
3. Help families with guidance on safety and abuse prevention
4. Start menstrual management on the basis of issues related to interference with the teenager's activities, taking into consideration patient medical needs and mobility concerns
5. Help families understand menstrual management options and the benefits and limitations of the different methods

disabilities because expectant management allows for patients and families to determine whether they can cope, and suppressing menarche can result in premature closure of the epiphyses of the long bones, preventing the patient from reaching her full height potential.[2] Precocious puberty, however, should be addressed in the usual manner.

Menstrual management can begin if cycles are creating difficulties in the patient's life, as determined by health care providers, patients, and families. All teenagers may have irregular cycles initially, but by the third year after menarche, 60% to 80% of girls have cycles from 21 to 34 days long, consistent with those of adults.[8] However, there are some circumstances that can cause teenagers with disabilities to have more menstrual irregularities related to medical comorbidities and medication adverse effects. Medications that affect the dopaminergic system can cause high prolactin concentrations with subsequent anovulation and amenorrhea.[9] In adolescents with obesity and in teenagers with seizure disorders and polycystic ovary syndrome, anovulation is more common; independently, valproic acid can cause hormonal aberrations like those in polycystic ovary syndrome.[10] Medications that can cause elevated prolactin concentrations include risperidone, phenothiazines, amitriptyline, cimetidine, prostaglandins, methyldopa, benzodiazepines, haloperidol, cocaine, and metoclopramide.[11]

Irregular bleeding in all teenagers can lead patients and families to seek medical intervention, but more so in teenagers with intellectual and physical disabilities, who may be dependent on others for their hygiene needs. The impact of menses ranges from an inability to go to school because of heavy menses and inadequate assistance in managing menses to severe pre- and perimenstrual behavioral changes in teenagers with developmental delay, prohibiting normal activities and causing additional management challenges.[12,13]

INITIAL EVALUATION

As part of the initial evaluation, the pediatrician addresses the menstrual cycle, including regularity and heaviness of bleeding, associated dysmenorrhea, behavioral and mood changes, and the impact on the adolescent's life. Symptom calendars can be helpful in identifying noncyclical versus cyclical problems, such as catamenial seizures. Other reproductive topics may include assessment of sexual knowledge, interest in sexual activity, and the need for relationship safety education (Table 1).[3]

Although confidential discussions about sexuality and sexual activity are recommended for all teenagers by the AAP[14] and American College of Obstetricians and Gynecologists (ACOG),[8] teenagers with any disability are often incorrectly considered to be asexual or uninvolved in relationships, and confidential conversations with their pediatrician may not occur. Teenagers with physical disabilities

TABLE 2 Methods for Menstrual Management in Teens With Disabilities

Category	Method	Benefits	Cautions
Estrogen and progestin	COC	Extended use	Interaction with EI-AED
			Uncertain risk of VTE with limited mobility
	Ring	Monthly extended use	Interaction with EI-AED
			Uncertain risk of VTE with limited mobility
			Dexterity/privacy with insertion
	Patch	Weekly extended use	Interaction with EI-AED
			Uncertain risk of VTE with limited mobility
			Inadvertent removal of patch
Progesterone only	POP		Interaction with EI-AED
			Irregular bleeding
	DMPA	Four times per year	Bone density issues
			Irregular bleeding
			Potential weight gain
	Implant	3 y	Irregular bleeding
			Insertion concerns
	LNG-IUD	5 y	May need anesthesia for insertion and removal
			Inability to check strings
			Initial irregular bleeding
Surgical	Endometrial ablation		Amenorrhea rates low
			No long-term data
			Legal and ethical issues
	Hysterectomy	Amenorrhea	Legal and ethical issues
			Permanent sterilization

COC indicates combined oral contraceptive; EI-AED, enzyme-inducing anti-epileptic drugs; LNG-IUD, levonorgestrel intrauterine device; POP, progesterone-only pills; VTE, venous thromboembolism.

are just as likely to be sexually active as their peers and have a higher incidence of sexual abuse.[15] Issues of consent and confidentiality regarding reproductive health care provided by physicians to minor adolescents are complex. Most states recognize the rights of a teenager to consent for confidential services around diagnosis and treatment of issues such as sexually transmitted infections, contraception, and pregnancy care; however, when the patient is cognitively impaired, the issue of consent is more complicated and may require discussion about legal guardianship or medical power of attorney status for the families.[16]

OVERVIEW OF MENSTRUAL MANAGEMENT

The decision for menstrual suppression is based on a discussion with the patient and parents or guardians, clinical considerations (eg, anemia), and social context (eg, hygiene, risk of abuse/pregnancy). It is important to discuss that any

menstrual suppression does not change the risk of abuse or sexually transmitted infections. The patient's cognitive disabilities may complicate the decision about menstrual intervention. Similar to the use of suppressive hormonal treatment in the nondisabled population, the decision to suppress menses in teenagers with physical disabilities is based on whether the patient believes this will help her better manage her life. In contrast, when families of adolescents with severe intellectual disabilities ask for menstrual suppression, the issues are more complicated if there is no clear medical indication, such as heavy bleeding or dysmenorrhea. When the stated reasons for suppression are an inability of caregivers to deal with menses or fear of abuse or pregnancy, further investigation into the patient's circumstances and safety is warranted. If the issue is mainly to get assistance at school, then health care providers can help families to address the student's needs with the school.

There are several important issues that need to be considered in menstrual management. No matter what method is used, it is difficult to make patients completely and reliably amenorrheic. For any teenager, having unscheduled bleeding may be worse than having scheduled controlled withdrawal bleeds but may be especially difficult for teenagers who rely on others for hygiene assistance. For teenagers in wheelchairs, even minimal weight gain can be the difference between the ability to transfer themselves or having to rely on someone else, thereby limiting independence. It is important to set outcome goals (eg, no periods, scheduled bleeding 3 times a year, no interference with activities) with the adolescent and her family and periodically reassess whether the goals have been reached or whether changes are indicated. In a large cohort of teenagers with developmental disabilities, it took an average of 1.5 hormonal methods before satisfaction was reached (range, 1–4). The most commonly selected initial method of suppression was the extended or continuous oral contraceptive pill (42.3%), followed by the patch (20%), expectant management (14.9%), depot medroxyprogesterone acetate (DMPA [11.6%]), and the levonorgestrel intrauterine device (LNG-IUD [2.8%]). There was a significant decrease in the selection of DMPA as the initial choice for menstrual suppression noted over time.[2] Gonadotropin-releasing hormone agonists are not generally recommended for long-term menstrual suppression because of adverse effects such as decreased bone density, except in cases of precocious puberty.[2]

The following overview focuses on how the use of hormonal methods for menstrual suppression may specifically affect teenagers with intellectual and/or physical disabilities (Table 2). As recommended by ACOG and AAP,[17] a pelvic examination is not necessary before 21 years of age or to start hormonal medications.[18] Extensive reviews of contraception methods have been published and will not be addressed in this report.[19]

Estrogen-Containing Methods

Combined Oral Contraceptives

Combined oral contraceptives (COCs) are often used in a continuous or extended-cycle fashion to limit the amount of bleeding. Because complete amenorrhea is difficult[20] to obtain and reported in only 62% of individuals, scheduled withdrawal bleeds every 3 to 4 months may be more helpful to patients with disabilities than unpredictable breakthrough bleeding.[21,22] For those teenagers with difficulty swallowing, there are chewable COCs that can also be put into food or crushed and given through a gastrostomy tube.[23] A Cochrane review examining efficacy and safety of continuous or extended-cycle versus monthly cycle use of combined oral contraceptives concludes that extended-cycle pills have similar contraceptive efficacy and safety profiles to monthly cycle pills. Some studies suggest that menstrual symptoms of headaches, genital irritation, tiredness, bloating, and menstrual pain may be less in extended-cycle regimens.[24]

Combined Contraceptive Patch

The combined contraceptive patch may be useful in patients who have difficulty swallowing pills. It can be used in an off-label continuous weekly fashion with similar breakthrough bleeding patterns as the continuous oral contraceptive pill.[25] Because some patients with developmental disabilities may attempt to pull off the patch, placement high on the back or buttocks is helpful.

Vaginal Ring

The monthly placement of a vaginal ring is another delivery form of combined hormones. The ring has enough hormones for 35 days, and leaving it in for 28 days at a time can provide continuous hormones in an off-label use.[22] However, the physical and privacy concerns of having another person place the ring intravaginally for teenagers without adequate dexterity or with intellectual disabilities have severely limited its use in this population. Bleeding profile for the ring when used continuously shows a rate of 8% for amenorrhea and 19% for spotting.[26]

Special Considerations: Venous Thrombotic Events and Estrogen-Containing Methods

The use of estrogen-containing hormones increases the risk of venous thrombotic events (VTEs). The risk of VTEs is higher for formulations with increasing doses of estrogen (compare 20 to 35 µg ethinyl estradiol) and likely higher with newer generations of progestins and for women using the combined contraceptive patch and the vaginal ring, although there are conflicting studies.[27–29]

The data on estrogen-containing hormones and VTEs have led to concerns about the risk of VTE for patients in wheelchairs; however, there are no data to provide guidance on this type of immobility in teenagers. Immobility is not a contraindication in the medical eligibility criteria for contraception per Centers for Disease Control and Prevention (CDC) recommendation.[30] Although the use of estrogen-containing contraceptives is not contraindicated in teenagers with mobility issues, a thorough family history can decrease the likelihood of an inherited thrombophilia. Health care providers can consider using the lowest-dose estrogen COCs that contain a first- or second-generation progestin, such as norethindrone and levonorgestrel for teenagers with limited mobility, because these progestins have been shown to be likely associated with lower rates of VTE.[19,27,28]

Progestin-Only Methods

Oral Progestins

Oral progestins can be used cyclically for teenagers with anovulation to induce menses or continuously to cause amenorrhea. Because the lowest dose daily progestin, known as the "minipill," only has a 20% rate of amenorrhea[31] and has to be taken at the same time every day, higher daily doses of oral progestins such as medroxyprogesterone (10–40 mg) or norethindrone (5–15 mg) have been attempted to achieve amenorrhea (as well as pain control in patients with endometriosis). Amenorrhea rates are not consistently reported. Although not well studied in teenagers, mood changes related to all progestins have been described.[32]

Depot Medroxyprogesterone Acetate

DMPA, the intramuscular and now subcutaneous injection, has been used for years as both a contraceptive and for menstrual suppression. The rate of amenorrhea is 50% to 60% at 1 year and 80% at 5 years.[33]

There are 2 specific areas of concern for use of DMPA in teenagers with disabilities.

1. Weight gain: the weight gain (average 13 pounds in 4 years, according to package insert) associated with the use of this medication is troubling for all teenagers, but for teenagers with mobility issues, even a small amount of weight gain may complicate transfers and could impede independence. There appears to be more weight gain in obese teenagers and in teenagers whose weight increases >5%

over baseline weight in the first 3 months of use.[34]

2. Bone health: there have been significant concerns around the effects of DMPA on bone mineral density (BMD), which led to a "black box warning" from the US Food and Drug Administration (FDA) to limit its use to 2 years. It is specifically of concern to teenagers, because girls accrue approximately 30% to 40% of their bone mass during adolescence. The rate of BMD loss decreases with longer duration of the DMPA use. The World Health Organization,[35] ACOG,[36] and Society for Adolescent Health and Medicine[37] have advised that health care providers interpret the 2-year duration limit individually and discuss with the patient and families whether DMPA is the best option for them in the context of relative risks and benefits.[35] In teenagers with disabilities and limited mobility, BMD may already be lower, but it is not clear whether this is actually associated with increased fracture risk.[38] The bone-density loss appears reversible after stopping the DMPA; however, for teenagers with limited mobility, no data are available.[39]

In summary, the use of DMPA in teenagers in wheelchairs can be considered for menstrual suppression after careful counseling and assessment of any contraindications to estrogen and considering whether the potential risk of decreased BMD is outweighed by the need for the suppression. The AAP and ACOG do not support the use of bone-density screening if long-term use of DMPA seems prudent, including in adolescents with limited mobility, unless fractures have occurred.[36,39] Calcium and vitamin D intake may be optimized per current guidelines.[40,41]

Levonorgestrel Intrauterine Device

LNG-IUDs have been used extensively in adult women and, although not approved by the FDA for adolescents younger than 18 years, more recently have been advocated for use in teenagers for birth control by national organizations because of their excellent contraceptive effect.[42] The original LNG-IUD dispenses 20 μg of levonorgestrel daily with a 50% dose reduction at 5 years. It is well tolerated with a 5-year duration and amenorrhea rates of approximately 50% at 1 year.[43] It has been used in women with disabilities and medical conditions that exclude estrogen use.

Several recent studies have addressed LNG-IUD use in teenagers with intellectual disabilities. Satisfactory outcomes by families were reported in 1 study,[44] and a 50% amenorrhea rate in 7 of 14 teenagers in another.[45] From a larger Canadian cohort, among 26 adolescents with disabilities (mean age, 15.4 years) who chose LNG-IUD insertion, 3 patients had LNG-IUD expulsions (11.2%), and another 2 had the LNG-IUD removed because of spotting and low positioning. Amenorrhea was noted at 1 year in all 21 patients who continued using the LNG-IUD.[2] As described for most patients in these series, the LNG-IUD can be inserted or removed under sedation or anesthesia, or if having another surgical procedure, could be inserted at the same time. The expulsion rate of the LNG-IUD is slightly higher in nulliparous women (approximately 3%–4%)[46] and is reported at 8% in teenagers with disabilities combining all published studies.[47] Whether ultrasonography before insertion of the LNG-IUD in this population is helpful to predict successful insertion is under discussion. A uterine length of 6 to 10 cm is recommended for 1 LNG-IUD; a newer, slightly smaller 3-year version does not have that recommendation. Although preinsertion ultrasonographic measurements were recommended in 1 report,[45] another study on 26 LNG-IUD insertions in adolescents with developmental disabilities showed that of 5 patients who had cavity length of less than 6 cm measured by ultrasonography, 4 had a successful insertion of the LNG-IUD.[47]

A sudden increase in vaginal bleeding may indicate LNG-IUD expulsion, and families are educated to look for this potential sign. If the families notice the increase in bleeding and the LNG-IUD string cannot be checked in the office because of patient intolerance of the examination, ultrasonography for device location can be performed. A newer, slightly smaller, and lower-dose device, 13.5-mg LNG-IUD (Skyla, Bayer HealthCare Pharmaceuticals, Wayne, NJ) has recently become available in the United States, is approved by the FDA for patients younger than 18 years, and is effective for 3 years. Although the decreased size may be helpful to address placement and expulsion in nulliparous women, the initial bleeding profile reported on the product insert gives significantly lower amenorrhea rates (12% after 3 years)[48] than the 5-year LNG–IUD, which may be an important factor to consider.

Progestin Implant

Use of the etonogestrel single-rod implant for menstrual suppression in teenagers with disabilities is limited because of the continued concern regarding the unpredictable bleeding patterns that are associated with the implant. Amenorrhea is approximately 13% after 1 year, with many days of spotting each month.[49] Insertion and removal requires patient cooperation, which may be an issue for some teenagers with intellectual disabilities.

Special Considerations
Seizures and Hormonal Contraception

For patients with epilepsy taking anticonvulsant medications, interactions with hormones are described. Many anticonvulsants and some other neuropsychiatric medications induce the hepatic cytochrome P450 system and, thus, interfere with contraceptive efficacy and cycle control reliability. As a result, COCs can cause irregular bleeding, and higher doses of COCs may be indicated to achieve amenorrhea. The CDC medical eligibility criteria categorize the estrogen-containing methods and the progesterone-only pill as category 3 for contraception (ie, risks outweigh the benefits) for enzyme-inducing anticonvulsant agents. In general, hormonal contraceptives do not affect the efficacy of anticonvulsant medications, with the 1 exception of lamotrigine, which can have decreased efficacy when combined with a COC. The lamotrigine dose may need to be adjusted, and discussion with the prescribing physician is recommended when starting a COC (CDC medical eligibility criteria, category 3).[50] LNG-IUDs, injectables, and implants are recommended for patients on anticonvulsant medication. For the progesterone injectables (medroxyprogesterone acetate), some experts recommend dosing on an every-10-week schedule if irregular bleeding continues.[51] Finally, cyclical or catamenial epilepsy and other cyclic menstrual symptoms may be a clinically significant problem for some patients, and suppression of hormone fluctuations can be helpful.[52]

Herbal Supplements

Because the use of complementary medicine is widespread and increasing in the population, pediatricians can advise families that the use of these compounds can interfere with the hormonal medications.[53] For example, St John's wort is known to decrease the bioavailability of oral contraceptives, which might interfere with contraceptive efficacy and may lead to spotting.[54,55] Other herbals have been implicated in increasing bleeding risk as well as in hepatotoxicity.[56]

Nonhormonal Methods

Nonsteroidal antiinflammatory drugs can be used to help with dysmenorrhea as well as with heavy bleeding. Studies show a small decrease in flow when nonsteroidal antiinflammatory drugs are used around the clock during the menses.[57]

A new oral antifibrinolytic medication, tranexamic acid, was approved by the FDA for heavy menses in 2009. It can be taken for up to 5 days of menses and results in 40% lighter bleeding.[58]

Surgical Requests and Options

Parents may ask the pediatrician about surgical interventions, especially endometrial ablation or hysterectomy, for their daughter with severe intellectual disabilities, in the hope that it will help with menstrual bleeding, behavior changes, or perceived or expressed dysmenorrhea or because of concerns about the risk of pregnancy. Surgical interventions in these cases have clear ethical and legal implications because most of patients with intellectual disabilities cannot give their own consent.

Endometrial Ablation

Endometrial ablation destroys most or all of the endometrium and was designed for women who have completed childbearing to alleviate heavy cycles. The rates of amenorrhea range from 13% to 83%, and complications include pain, cramping, and continued bleeding as well as the need for additional procedures. Ablation leads to only relative infertility, and birth control is still recommended, because pregnancy after an ablation may have complications. Because of this relative infertility, there are legal implications for use in teenagers with disabilities (see Hysterectomy). There are no studies on use of ablation in adolescents including long-term consequences and

outcomes, and therefore, endometrial ablation is not recommended for this age group.[12]

Hysterectomy

Families sometimes request hysterectomy for menstrual management in their daughter with severe intellectual disability. When hysterectomy is requested, it is critical to delineate why the family desires this intervention. It may be considered the ideal way to achieve birth control and amenorrhea. This is a complex and controversial issue and can cause conflict between health care providers and families. A hysterectomy (removal of the uterus and cervix) does not prevent behavioral hormonal concerns. Hysterectomy in the adolescent years for medical indications is extremely rare for teenagers, with or without disabilities. Laws regarding sterilization in minors with intellectual disabilities, hysterectomy, and consent issues vary from state to state. There is a network of legal experts on disability with offices in every state (http://www.ndrn.org/about/paacap-network.html). In most jurisdictions, sterilization of women with known cognitive impairments has specific legal oversight mandated.

Referral to a gynecologist with experience in this area may be considered as well as an ethics consultation and legal representation for the patient as part of the review process. The ACOG has guidelines regarding permanent sterilization.[59]

CONCLUSIONS

The pediatrician plays a pivotal role during the sometimes difficult pubertal transition for patients with physical and intellectual disabilities, when concerns about menstruation, sexuality, and fertility come to the forefront. Pediatricians should assist with anticipatory guidance for patients and families by normalizing menses as an expected part of life, helping with the management of menses, and referring to experts as needed for more complicated concerns.

COMMITTEE ON ADOLESCENCE, 2014–2015

Paula K. Braverman, MD, Chairperson
William P. Adelman, MD
Elizabeth M. Alderman, MD
Cora C. Breuner, MD, MPH
David A. Levine, MD
Arik V. Marcell, MD, MPH
Rebecca F. O'Brien, MD

LIAISONS

Lauren Zapata, MD – *Centers for Disease Control and Prevention*
Laurie L. Hornberger, MD, MPH – *Section on Adolescent Health*
Margo Lane, MD, FRCPC – *Canadian Pediatric Society*
Benjamin Shain, MD, PhD – *American Academy of Child and Adolescent Psychiatry*
Julie Strickland, MD – *American College of Obstetricians and Gynecologists*

STAFF

Karen Smith
James Baumberger, MPP

ABBREVIATIONS

AAP: American Academy of Pediatrics
ACOG: American College of Obstetricians and Gynecologists
BMD: bone mineral density
CDC: Centers for Disease Control and Prevention
COC: combined oral contraceptive
DMPA: depot medroxyprogesterone acetate
FDA: US Food and Drug Administration
LNG-IUD: levonorgestrel intrauterine device
VTE: venous thrombotic event

REFERENCES

1. Zacharin M, Savasi I, Grover S. The impact of menstruation in adolescents with disabilities related to cerebral palsy. *Arch Dis Child.* 2010;95(7):526–530

2. Kirkham YA, Allen L, Kives S, Caccia N, Spitzer RF, Ornstein MP. Trends in menstrual concerns and suppression in adolescents with developmental disabilities. *J Adolesc Health.* 2013;53(3):407–412

3. Murphy NA, Elias ER. Sexuality of children and adolescents with developmental disabilities. *Pediatrics.* 2006;118(1):398–403

4. US Census Bureau. School-Aged Children with Disabilities in U.S. Metropolitan Areas: 2010. Available at: https://www.census.gov/prod/2011pubs/acsbr10-12.pdf. Accessed May 4, 2015

5. Pratt HD, Greydanus DE. Intellectual disability (mental retardation) in children and adolescents. *Prim Care.* 2007;34(2):375–386, abstract ix

6. Siddiqi SU, Van Dyke DC, Donohoue P, McBrien DM. Premature sexual development in individuals with neurodevelopmental disabilities. *Dev Med Child Neurol.* 1999;41(6):392–395

7. Knickmeyer RC, Wheelwright S, Hoekstra R, Baron-Cohen S. Age of menarche in girls with autism spectrum conditions. *Dev Med Child Neurol.* 2006;48(12):1007–1008

8. American College of Obstetricians and Gynecologists. ACOG Committee Opinion No. 349, November 2006: Menstruation in girls and adolescents: using the menstrual cycle as a vital sign. *Obstet Gynecol.* 2006;108(5):1323–1328

9. Kinon BJ, Gilmore JA, Liu H, Halbreich UM. Hyperprolactinemia in response to antipsychotic drugs: characterization across comparative clinical trials. *Psychoneuroendocrinology.* 2003;28(suppl 2):69–82

10. Joffe H, Hayes FJ. Menstrual cycle dysfunction associated with neurologic and psychiatric disorders: their treatment in adolescents. *Ann N Y Acad Sci.* 2008;1135:219–229

11. Emans SJ, Divasta A. Amenorrhea in the adolescent. In: Emans SJ, Laufer MR, eds. *Emans, Laufer, Goldstein's Pediatric and Adolescent Gynecology,* 6th ed. Philadelphia, PA: Lippincott Williams & Wilkins; 2012:135–158

12. American College of Obstetricians and Gynecologists. Menstrual manipulation for adolescents with disabilities. ACOG Committee Opinion No. 448. *Obstet Gynecol.* 2009;114(6):1428–1431

13. Burke LM, Kalpakjian CZ, Smith YR, Quint EH. Gynecologic issues of adolescents with Down syndrome, autism, and cerebral palsy. *J Pediatr Adolesc Gynecol.* 2010;23(1):11–15

14. Hagan JF Jr, Shaw JS, Duncan PM, eds. *Bright Futures: Guidelines for Health Supervision of Infants, Children, and Adolescents,* 3rd ed. Elk Grove Village, IL: American Academy of Pediatrics; 2008

15. Cheng MM, Udry JR. Sexual behaviors of physically disabled adolescents in the United States. *J Adolesc Health.* 2002;31(1):48–58

16. McDonnell WM; American Academy of Pediatrics, Committee on Medical Liability and Risk Management. Adolescent health care. In: Donn SM, McAbee GN, eds. *Medicolegal Issues in Pediatrics.* Elk Grove Village, IL: American Academy of Pediatrics; 2012:131–140

17. Braverman PK, Breech L, and the Committee on Adolescence. Clinical Report. Gynecologic Examination for Adolescents in the Pediatric Office Setting. *Pediatrics* 2010; *126:3 583-590; published ahead of print August 30, 2010, doi:*10.1542/peds.2010-1564

18. American College of Obstetricians and Gynecologists. ACOG Committee Opinion No. 534: well-woman visit. *Obstet Gynecol.* 2012;120(2 pt 1):421–424

19. Committee on Adolescence. Contraception for adolescents. *Pediatrics.* 2014;134(4). Available at: www.pediatrics.org/cgi/content/full/134/4/e1244

20. Gold MA, Duffy K. Extended cycling or continuous use of hormonal contraceptives for female adolescents. *Curr Opin Obstet Gynecol.* 2009;21(5):407–411

21. Hee L, Kettner LO, Vejtorp M. Continuous use of oral contraceptives: an overview of effects and side-effects. *Acta Obstet Gynecol Scand.* 2013;92(2):125–136

22. Jacobson JC, Likis FE, Murphy PA. Extended and continuous combined contraceptive regimens for menstrual suppression. *J Midwifery Womens Health.* 2012;57(6):585–592

23. First chewable oral contraceptive. *FDA Consum.* 2004;38(2):4

24. Edelman A, Micks E, Gallo MF, Jensen JT, Grimes DA. Continuous or extended cycle vs. cyclic use of combined hormonal contraceptives for contraception. *Cochrane Database Syst Rev.* 2014;7(7):CD004695

25. Stewart FH, Kaunitz AM, Laguardia KD, Karvois DL, Fisher AC, Friedman AJ. Extended use of transdermal norelgestromin/ethinyl estradiol: a randomized trial. *Obstet Gynecol.* 2005;105(6):1389–1396

26. Sulak PJ, Smith V, Coffee A, Witt I, Kuehl AL, Kuehl TJ. Frequency and management of breakthrough bleeding with continuous use of the transvaginal contraceptive ring: a randomized controlled trial. *Obstet Gynecol.* 2008;112(3):563–571

27. Lidegaard Ø, Nielsen LH, Skovlund CW, Skjeldestad FE, Løkkegaard E. Risk of venous thromboembolism from use of oral contraceptives containing different progestogens and oestrogen doses: Danish cohort study, 2001-9. *BMJ.* 2011;343:d6423

28. Lidegaard Ø, Løkkegaard E, Jensen A, Skovlund CW, Keiding N. Thrombotic stroke and myocardial infarction with hormonal contraception. *N Engl J Med.* 2012;366(24):2257–2266

29. Hugon-Rodin J, Gompel A, Plu-Bureau G. Epidemiology of hormonal contraceptives-related venous thromboembolism. *Eur J Endocrinol.* 2014;171(6):R221–R230

30. United States Medical Eligibility Criteria (US MEC) for Contraceptive Use. 2010. Available at: www.cdc.gov/reproductivehealth/unintendedpregnancy/usmec.htm. Accessed May 4, 2015

31. Broome M, Fotherby K. Clinical experience with the progestogen-only pill. *Contraception.* 1990;42(5):489–495

32. Ott MA, Shew ML, Ofner S, Tu W, Fortenberry JD. The influence of hormonal contraception on mood and sexual interest among adolescents. *Arch Sex Behav.* 2008;37(4):605–613

33. Arias RD, Jain JK, Brucker C, Ross D, Ray A. Changes in bleeding patterns with depot medroxyprogesterone acetate subcutaneous injection 104 mg. *Contraception.* 2006;74(3):234–238

34. Lopez LM, Edelman A, Chen M, Otterness C, Trussell J, Helmerhorst FM. Progestin-only contraceptives: effects on weight. *Cochrane Database Syst Rev.* 2013;7(7):CD008815

35. World Health Organization. Technical Consultation on the Effects of Hormonal Contraception on Bone Health: Summary Report. Geneva, Switzerland: World Health Organization: 2005. Available at: http://whqlibdoc.who.int/hq/2007/WHO_RHR_07.08_eng.pdf. Accessed May 4, 2015

36. American College of Obstetricians and Gynecologists. Committee Opinion No. 602: depot medroxyprogesterone acetate and bone effects. *Obstet Gynecol.* 2014;123(6):1398–1402

37. Cromer BA, Scholes D, Berenson A, Cundy T, Clark MK, Kaunitz AM; Society for Adolescent Medicine. Depot medroxyprogesterone acetate and bone mineral density in adolescents--the Black Box Warning: a Position Paper of the Society for Adolescent Medicine. *J Adolesc Health.* 2006;39(2):296–301

38. Lopez LM, Chen M, Mullins S, Curtis KM, Helmerhorst FM. Steroidal contraceptives and bone fractures in women: evidence from observational studies. *Cochrane Database Syst Rev.* 2012;8:CD009849

39. Bachrach LK, Sills IN; Section on Endocrinology. Clinical report—bone densitometry in children and adolescents. *Pediatrics.* 2011;127(1):189–194

40. Zacharin M. Assessing the skeleton in children and adolescents with disabilities: avoiding pitfalls, maximising outcomes. A guide for the general paediatrician. *J Paediatr Child Health.* 2009;45(6):326–331

41. Golden NH, Abrams SA; Committee on Nutrition. Optimizing bone health in children and adolescents. *Pediatrics.* 2014;134(4). Available at: www.pediatrics.org/cgi/content/full/134/4/e1229

42. Committee on Adolescent Health Care Long-Acting Reversible Contraception Working Group, The American College of Obstetricians and Gynecologists. ACOG Committee Opinion No. 539: adolescents and long-acting reversible contraception: implants and intrauterine devices. *Obstet Gynecol.* 2012;120(4):983–988

43. Stoegerer-Hecher E, Kirchengast S, Huber JC, Hartmann B. Amenorrhea and BMI as independent determinants of patient satisfaction in LNG-IUD users: cross-sectional study in a Central European district. *Gynecol Endocrinol.* 2012;28(2):119–124

44. Hillard PJ. Menstrual suppression with the levonorgestrel intrauterine system in girls with developmental delay. *J Pediatr Adolesc Gynecol.* 2012;25(5):308–313

45. Pillai M, O'Brien K, Hill E. The levonorgestrel intrauterine system (Mirena) for the treatment of menstrual problems in adolescents with medical disorders, or physical or learning disabilities. *BJOG.* 2010;117(2):216–221

46. Alton TM, Brock GN, Yang D, Wilking DA, Hertweck SP, Loveless MB. Retrospective review of intrauterine device in adolescent and young women. *J Pediatr Adolesc Gynecol.* 2012;25(3):195–200

47. Savasi I, Jayasinghe K, Moore P, Jayasinghe Y, Grover SR. Complication rates associated with levonorgestrel intrauterine system use in adolescents with developmental disabilities. *J Pediatr Adolesc Gynecol.* 2014;27(1):25–28

48. SKYLA. (levonorgestrel-releasing intrauterine system) [package insert]. Available at: http://labeling.bayerhealthcare.com/html/products/pi/Skyla_PI.pdf. Accessed May 4, 2015

49. Hubacher D, Lopez L, Steiner MJ, Dorflinger L. Menstrual pattern

changes from levonorgestrel subdermal implants and DMPA: systematic review and evidence-based comparisons. *Contraception.* 2009;80(2):113–118

50. Wegner I, Edelbroek PM, Bulk S, Lindhout D. Lamotrigine kinetics within the menstrual cycle, after menopause, and with oral contraceptives. *Neurology.* 2009;73(17):1388–1393

51. Guillemette T, Yount SM. Contraception and antiepileptic drugs. *J Midwifery Womens Health.* 2012;57(3):290–295

52. Verrotti A, D'Egidio C, Agostinelli S, Verrotti C, Pavone P. Diagnosis and management of catamenial seizures: a review. *Int J Womens Health.* 2012;4:535–541

53. Izzo AA, Ernst E. Interactions between herbal medicines and prescribed drugs: an updated systematic review. *Drugs.* 2009;69(13):1777–1798

54. Murphy PA, Kern SE, Stanczyk FZ, Westhoff CL. Interaction of St. John's Wort with oral contraceptives: effects on the pharmacokinetics of norethindrone and ethinyl estradiol, ovarian activity and breakthrough bleeding. *Contraception.* 2005;71(6):402–408

55. Pfrunder A, Schiesser M. Gerbers, Haszhke M, Bitzer J, Drewe J. Interaction of St. John's wort with low dose oral contraceptive therapy: a randomized controlled trial. *J Clin Pharmacol.* 2003;56(6):683–690

56. Teschke R, Frenzel C, Glass X, Schulze J, Eickhoff A. Herbal hepatotoxicity: a critical review. *Br J Clin Pharmacol.* 2013;75(3):630–636

57. Lethaby A, Duckitt K, Farquhar C. Non-steroidal anti-inflammatory drugs for heavy menstrual bleeding. *Cochrane Database Syst Rev.* 2013;1(1):CD000400

58. Leminen H, Hurskainen R. Tranexamic acid for the treatment of heavy menstrual bleeding: efficacy and safety. *Int J Womens Health.* 2012;4:413–421

59. American College of Obstetricians and Gynecologists. ACOG Committee Opinion No. 371: sterilization of women, including those with mental disabilities. *Obstet Gynecol.* 2007;110(1):217–220

Mind-Body Therapies in Children and Youth

• •

- *Clinical Report*

CLINICAL REPORT   Guidance for the Clinician in Rendering Pediatric Care

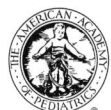

American Academy
of Pediatrics

DEDICATED TO THE HEALTH OF ALL CHILDREN™

Mind-Body Therapies in Children and Youth

SECTION ON INTEGRATIVE MEDICINE

abstract

Mind-body therapies are popular and are ranked among the top 10 complementary and integrative medicine practices reportedly used by adults and children in the 2007–2012 National Health Interview Survey. A growing body of evidence supports the effectiveness and safety of mind-body therapies in pediatrics. This clinical report outlines popular mind-body therapies for children and youth and examines the best-available evidence for a variety of mind-body therapies and practices, including biofeedback, clinical hypnosis, guided imagery, meditation, and yoga. The report is intended to help health care professionals guide their patients to nonpharmacologic approaches to improve concentration, help decrease pain, control discomfort, or ease anxiety.

DOI: 10.1542/peds.2016-1896

PEDIATRICS (ISSN Numbers: Print, 0031-4005; Online, 1098-4275).

Copyright © 2016 by the American Academy of Pediatrics

FINANCIAL DISCLOSURE: The authors have indicated they do not have a financial relationship relevant to this article to disclose.

FUNDING: No external funding.

POTENTIAL CONFLICT OF INTEREST: The authors have indicated they have no potential conflicts of interest to disclose.

To cite: AAP SECTION ON INTEGRATIVE MEDICINE. Mind-Body Therapies in Children and Youth. *Pediatrics.* 2016;138(3): e20161896

INTRODUCTION

Mind-body therapies and practices (eg, meditation and yoga) are among the top 10 complementary therapies reportedly used by adults and children in the 2007–2012 National Health Interview Survey.[1] Mind-body therapies focus on the interaction between the mind and the body, with the intent to use the mind to influence physical functions and directly affect health. Complementary therapies, such as yoga, meditation, mindfulness-based stress reduction (MBSR), hypnotherapy, guided imagery, and biofeedback, embrace this concept. Data from the 2012 National Health Interview Survey show that 3.7% of US children 4 to 17 years of age used mind-body approaches. Mind-body therapies were used slightly more in older youth aged 13 to 17 years, more than twice as often among females versus males (5.7% vs 1.7%), and less often in the South (2.4%). Children and youth were more likely to use mind-body therapies if they experienced pain-related conditions or emotional, behavioral, or mental conditions and if they received specialty or mental health care. The most common reasons for the use of mind-body approaches were to improve overall health and feel better, to reduce stress level or relax, for general wellness or disease prevention, and to feel better emotionally.[2] Children are very capable of engaging in self-care skills such as mind-body therapies,[3] and there are many mind-body skills that children and adolescents can learn and apply throughout life.[4]

A growing body of evidence supports the effectiveness and safety of mind-body therapies in pediatrics. In this clinical report, relevant evidence regarding biofeedback, clinical hypnosis, guided imagery, meditation/MBSR, and yoga is reviewed so that pediatric health care providers are better prepared to answer parent questions and provide patient-centered, evidence-based care. For each therapy reviewed, recommendations regarding indications and precautions are provided. The level of evidence based on data from published clinical trials and systematic reviews is described (Table 1). Key outcomes discussed in association with mind-body therapies and practices include focused concentration, decreased pain, and reduced anxiety.

SUMMARIES OF RELEVANT EVIDENCE BY TOPIC

Biofeedback

"Every change in the physiological state is accompanied by an appropriate change in the mental-emotional state, conscious or unconscious, and conversely every change in the mental-emotional state is accompanied by a change in the physiological state."[33]

Biofeedback is defined as the use of electronic or electromechanical equipment to measure and then feed-back information about physiologic processes to an individual. These physiologic processes can then be controlled by the individual for therapeutic purposes. Feedback can be provided in auditory, visual, kinesthetic, or multimedia formats and even now in the form of "video games for the body."[34] This makes biofeedback, in its many forms, particularly relevant as an option for today's tech-savvy youth.

Although direct clinical observation can provide clues to a patient's physiologic state and level of autonomic nervous system (ANS) arousal, it is primarily subjective and, therefore, unreliable. In addition, many patients (pediatric, adolescent, or adult) may subjectively state that they "feel relaxed," but objectively they may not be relaxed at all, at least as defined by measurable physiologic phenomena, especially those that reflect the relative balance of sympathetic and parasympathetic nervous system activity. Therefore, biofeedback can be an invaluable tool for the pediatric health care provider to help gauge what topics, thoughts, and other phenomena trigger mind/body arousal in children and adolescents. The benefits for pediatric patients include allowing them to observe the immediate, convincing, objective mind-body interactions, literally seeing that a "change in the mind (thoughts and/or feelings) can immediately lead to a change in the body's physiological response."[4,35] Interested clinicians can be certified in biofeedback by the Biofeedback Certification International Alliance.[36,37] The Biofeedback Certification International Alliance certifies individuals who meet education and training standards in biofeedback and progressively recertifies those who advance their knowledge through continuing education.

Research over the past 30 years has shown that children and adolescents are good at self-regulation[36] and capable of voluntarily modulating physiologic processes, including peripheral temperature, muscle activity, breathing, brain electrical activity, and certain aspects of immune function, such as salivary immunoglobulin A secretion.[35] The most common forms of biofeedback that reflect the balance of the ANS include the following: (1) peripheral temperature (measuring the temperature change in hands or

fingers), (2) heart rate variability (measuring the beat-to-beat variation in heart rate patterns over time), (3) electrodermal activity (measuring sweat gland activity), (4) electromyography (measuring muscle activity), (5) EEG (measuring brain wave activity), (6) capnometry (measuring exhaled carbon dioxide), and (7) pneumography (measuring the movements of the chest and stomach associated with breathing).[34]

Biofeedback technology has evolved to the point that there are now several low-cost, portable products available that allow for training at home and school, thereby supporting greater generalization of the skill into real-life settings. Enhancing an individual's context awareness in real-life settings by using biomonitoring and providing real-time feedback is an emerging e-health trend.[38] Home biofeedback systems with multimedia game formats are available for personal computers as well as for smart phones and tablet devices.

The user-friendly technologies listed in Table 2 can make practice of these self-regulation skills more enjoyable and effective as they measure a variety of physiologic functions, such as heart rate variability, skin conductance, and peripheral temperature. Like other mind-body skills, it is important that pediatric patients use these skills on a regular basis both for prevention and for acute situational relief, as they eventually learn to control and ultimately reset their ANS response patterns and master the mind-body connection.

Conclusions

Research suggests benefits of peripheral forms of biofeedback for children and adolescents, particularly for headache (tension type and migraine), asthma, enuresis, and rehabilitation applications, as well as EEG biofeedback (neurofeedback)

TABLE 1 Evidence Summary by Topic

Study, year (design)	Sample Size, N	Age, y	Study Goal	Intervention	Outcomes
Biofeedback					
Knox et al, 2011 (clinical trial)[5]	24	9–17	Examined changes in anxiety and depression	Heart rate variability biofeedback based on a session-by-session protocol	Biofeedback-assisted relaxation training can be useful in decreasing anxiety and depressive symptoms
Palermo et al, 2010 (meta-analysis)[6]	1247 (25 studies)	9–17	Quantify the effects of psychological therapies for the management of chronic pain in youth	Cognitive-behavioral therapy, relaxation therapy, and biofeedback	Omnibus cognitive-behavioral therapy, relaxation therapy, and biofeedback all produced significant and positive effects on pain reduction
Monastra et al, 2005 (review)[7]	N/A	6–19	Effects of EEG biofeedback on ADHD	EEG biofeedback	EEG biofeedback was determined to be "probably efficacious" for the treatment of ADHD
Eccleston et al, 2002 (systematic review)[8]	808	6–18	Efficacy of psychological therapy of children and adolescents with chronic pain	Variety of biofeedback modalities	Treatments examined are effective in reducing the severity and frequency of chronic pain
Clinical hypnosis					
Rutten et al, 2013 (systematic review)[9]	108	5–18	Assess efficacy of HT in pediatric patients with FAP and IBS	Gut-directed HT	Therapeutic effects of HT seem superior to standard medical care in children with FAP or IBS
Accardi and Milling, 2009 (systematic review)[10]	528	3–19	Effectiveness of hypnosis in reducing procedure-related pain	Hypnosis	Hypnosis was more effective than standard medical care or control at relieving pain in children during medical procedures
Vlieger et al, 2007 (RCT)[11]	53	8–18	Effectiveness of hypnosis for FAP and IBS	6 sessions of 50 min over a 3-mo period of gut-directed HT	Gut-directed HT is highly effective in the treatment of children with longstanding FAP or IBS
Richardson et al, 2006 (systematic review)[12]	313	3–18	Effectiveness of hypnosis for procedure-related pain and distress in pediatric patients with cancer	Hypnosis	Hypnosis has the potential to reduce procedure-related pain and distress in pediatric patients with cancer
Butler et al, 2005 (RCT)[13]	44	4–15	Examine whether hypnotic relaxation could reduce distress for children who undergo VCUG	Hypnosis	Results indicate significant benefits for the hypnosis group
Calipel et al, 2005 (RCT)[14]	50	2–11	Efficacy of hypnosis on anxiety and perioperative behavioral disorders	Hypnosis	Hypnosis alleviates preoperative anxiety
Guided imagery					
Weigensberg et al, 2014 (RCT)[15]	35	14–17	Determine the effects of the mind-body modality of IGI in obese Latino adolescents	12 weekly sessions of a lifestyle education plus IGI program	The IGI group showed significant reductions in leisure sedentary behavior and increases in moderate physical activity
van Tilburg et al, 2009 (pilot study)[16]	34	6–15	Test a home-based, guided imagery treatment protocol using audio and video recordings	2-mo guided imagery treatment	Guided imagery treatment plus medical care was superior to standard medical care only for the treatment of abdominal pain
Weydert et al, 2006 (RCT)[17]	22	5–18	Evaluated the therapeutic effect of guided imagery for children with recurrent abdominal pain	4 weekly sessions of guided imagery with progressive muscle relaxation	Significantly greater decrease in the number of days with pain
Meditation and MBSR					
Britton et al, 2014 (RCT, pilot)[18]	101	11.7 (mean)	Effects of a nonelective, classroom-based, teacher-implemented, mindfulness meditation intervention on standard clinical measures of mental health and affect	6-wk program with daily mindfulness meditation practice	Both control and intervention groups decreased significantly on clinical syndrome subscales and affect but did not differ in the extent of their improvements
Sibinga et al, 2014 (RCT)[19]	43	13–21	Explore the specific effects of MBSR for urban youth	8 weekly 2-h MBSR sessions and a 3-h retreat	MBSR did not result in statistically significant differences in self-reported survey outcomes of interest but was associated with qualitative outcomes of increased calm, conflict avoidance, self-awareness, and self-regulation for urban youth

TABLE 1 Continued

Study, year (design)	Sample Size, N	Age, y	Study Goal	Intervention	Outcomes
Sibinga et al, 2013 (RCT)[20]	41	11–14	Effects of a school-based MBSR program for young urban males	12-session programs of MBSR	Results provide cautious support that MBSR enhances self-regulatory processes for urban male youth, including improved psychological symptoms and enhanced coping
Sibinga et al, 2016[21] (RCT)	300	12 (mean)	Ameliorate the negative effects of stress and trauma among low-income, minority, middle-school public school students	12-wk program	MBSR students had significantly lower levels of somatization, depression, negative affect, negative coping, rumination, self-hostility, and posttraumatic symptom severity
Barnes et al, 2012 (RCT)[22]	62	15–17	Impact of TM on LVM in African-American youth at increased risk of development of cardiovascular disease	15-min TM sessions twice/day for 4 mo	TM decreased LVM index in prehypertensive African-American adolescents
Wright et al, 2011 (RCT)[19]	121	14–15	Impact on ABP in African-American patients at increased risk of development of essential hypertension	BAM each weekday, 10-min sessions for 3 mo	BAM participants showed significant reductions in self-reported hostility and 24-h systolic ABP
Flook et al 2010 (RCT)[23]	64	7–9	Evaluate school-based program of MAPs	30-min MAPs, twice/week for 8 wk	Stronger effect of MAPs on children with executive function difficulties
Biegel et al 2009 (RCT)[24]	102	14–18	Assess the effect of the MBSR program for adolescents with heterogeneous diagnoses in an outpatient psychiatric facility	8 weekly MBSR classes, meeting 2 h/wk	MBSR may be a beneficial adjunct to outpatient mental health treatment of adolescents
Barnes et al, 2004 (RCT)[25]	100	15–17	Determine the impact of stress reduction on blood pressure in adolescents by the TM program	15-min TM sessions, twice/day for 4 mo	Beneficial impact of the TM program in youth at risk of the development of hypertension
Barnes et al, 2003 (RCT)[26]	45	15–18	Determine the effect of stress reduction via the TM program on school rule infractions in adolescents	15-min TM sessions, twice/day for 4 mo	TM program conducted in the school setting has a beneficial effect on absenteeism, rule infractions, and suspension rates
Yoga					
Hagins et al, 2013 (RCT)[27]	30	10–11	Effects of yoga on physiologic response to behavioral stressor tasks	50 min yoga, 3 times/wk for 15 wk	No significant differences in physiologic responses to behavioral stressors between groups
Telles et al, 2013 (RCT)[28]	98	8–13	Effects of yoga on physical fitness, cognitive performance, self-esteem	45 min yoga, 5 d/wk for 3 mo	Social self-esteem higher in control versus yoga group, whereas general and parental self-esteem improved
Khalsa et al, 2012 (RCT)[29]	121	15–19	Evaluate potential mental health benefits of yoga for adolescents in secondary school	30–40 min yoga, 2–3 times/wk for 11 wk	Measures of anger, resilience and fatigue/inertia significantly improved
Nidhi et al, 2012 (RCT)[30]	72	15–18	Efficacy of yoga on glucose metabolism and blood lipid values in adolescent girls with PCOS	60 min yoga, 7 d/wk for 12 wk	Fasting insulin, fasting blood glucose, and insulin resistance were significantly improved
White, 2012 (RCT)[31]	155	8–11	Efficacy of yoga to reduce perceived stress, enhance coping abilities, self-esteem, and self-regulation	60 min yoga, 1 d/wk for 8 wk, as well as 10 min yoga homework 6 d/wk	Self-esteem and self-regulation increased in both groups, whereas the yoga group reported greater appraisal of stress and greater frequency of coping
Mendelson et al, 2010 (RCT)[32]	97	9.7 and 10.6 (mean)	Improve adjustment among chronically stressed and disadvantaged youth	45 min yoga, 4 d/wk for 12 wk	Significant improvement in the RSQ Involuntary Engagement Scale and component subscales for rumination, intrusive thoughts, and emotional arousal

ABP, ambulatory blood pressure; ADHD, attention-deficit/ hyperactivity disorder; BAM, breathing awareness meditation; HT, hypnotherapy; IGI, Interactive Guided Imagery; LVM, left ventricular mass; MAP, mindful awareness practice; N/A, not available; PCOS, polycystic ovary syndrome; RSQ, Responses to Stress Questionnaire; VCUG, voiding cystourethrography.

for attention-deficit/hyperactivity disorder. Positive evidence for other indications (eg, insomnia, chronic pain syndromes, and anxiety disorders) exists but is not conclusive. Biofeedback applications for the treatment of functional gastrointestinal tract disorders is an area of particular promise.[54] Biofeedback offers a particularly attractive form of self-regulation for today's youth, given their interest in and comfort with technology. There are no significant contraindications to the use of biofeedback, and the

TABLE 2 Demonstrated Safety and Efficacy of Biofeedback-Based Treatments in a Variety of Childhood Conditions

Biofeedback-Based Treatment Technique	Condition	Reference
sEMG and peripheral temperature	Migraine, muscle tension, headache	Andrasik and Schwartz, 2006[39]; Nestoriuc et al, 2008[40]
Variety of biofeedback modalities	Chronic pain syndromes	Eccleston et al, 2002[8]; Palermo et al, 2010[6]
sEMG pelvic floor biofeedback; anorectal EMG biofeedback; manometric feedback	Functional disorders of elimination	Culbert and Banez 2007,[41] 2008[42]; Palsson et al, 2004[43]; Weydert et al, 2003[44]
Sophisticated multichannel sEMG biofeedback	Developmental disabilities and neuromuscular challenges	Bolek, 2006[45]; Brütsch et al, 2011[46]; Wang and Reid, 2011[47];
EEG biofeedback (also termed neurofeedback)	Attention-deficit/hyperactivity disorder	Wang and Reid, 2011[47]; Monastra et al, 2005[7]; Vernon et al, 2004[48]
Heart rate variability biofeedback	Performance anxiety	Knox et al, 2011[5]
Bifrontal sEMG biofeedback	Asthma	Lehrer et al, 2002[49]
sEMG biofeedback	Various learning disorders	Carter and Russell, 1985[50]; Hoy et al 2011[51]
Specific biofeedback training targeting lowered sympathetic nervous system arousal	Sleep disorders	Barowsky et al, 1990[52]; Morin et al, 2006[53]

sEMG, surface electromyography.

only barrier may be financial in that both home and professional health care biofeedback hardware/software packages can be somewhat expensive and third-party health care insurance payers do not consistently cover biofeedback treatment. A selection of resources for pediatric health care providers is provided in Table 3.

Clinical Hypnosis

Clinical hypnosis in children and adolescents has seen a surge in both research and clinical application in the past 30 years, although its use in children dates back >200 years.[55] Hypnosis is defined variably by several professional societies.[56] Perhaps best stated, "when we are in hypnosis, we intensify our attention, decrease our peripheral awareness and become more receptive to new ideas and associations whenever we reinforce, rewire, reframe or otherwise alter the neurophysiological networks we call 'experience.' Trance is what happens when we engage in changing our minds.... Hypnosis is a skill set involving interpersonal communication designed to facilitate therapeutic change in maladaptive psycho-physiological reflexes."[56] Pediatric health care providers should understand that hypnotherapy in children is a well-established therapeutic modality, and it should not be confused with or misperceived as the

inappropriate practice of hypnosis by entertainers.

Clinical hypnosis, when provided by appropriately trained individuals, is an adjunctive therapy that can be used by pediatric health care providers to assist in managing conditions that they are already otherwise licensed to treat. For example, a pediatrician may use clinical hypnosis to help a child dealing with enuresis, irritable bowel syndrome (IBS), or anxiety. A licensed mental health practitioner may use clinical hypnosis to help children with anxiety, depression, or posttraumatic stress disorder (PTSD). However, a mental health practitioner should not use clinical hypnosis for a child with IBS without physician comanagement, and pediatricians should not use this technique for PTSD without collaborating with a mental health practitioner.

Case series and clinical trials of clinical hypnosis first appeared in the 1970s and 1980s. Since then, the literature has grown and includes clinical trials, Cochrane reviews, and neuroimaging studies.[55–59] However, high-quality randomized controlled trials (RCTs) with clear methodologies remain lacking. Clinical hypnosis involves establishing a strong rapport with patients and individualizing the therapy to the specific goals and

characteristics of the patient. This situation precludes a standardized approach, and large randomized studies of individualized approaches are difficult to conduct.

Functional Abdominal Pain

A few studies have evaluated the effectiveness of hypnosis for functional abdominal pain (FAP) and IBS. Vlieger et al[11] randomly assigned 52 children to either hypnosis with an experienced clinician or standard care, which included dietary guidance, medication as needed, and supportive counseling. Twelve sessions over 3 months led to marked improvement in pain frequency and severity in patients in the hypnosis group compared with control patients at the end of the intervention and at 1-year follow-up.[11] A later follow-up study at 5 years showed a significantly higher remission rate in the hypnosis group compared with the control group (68% vs 20%; $P = .005$).[60] A systematic review of 3 trials for FAP and IBS in children and adolescents showed superior efficacy over standard care.[9]

Pain Management

Numerous small trials have shown the efficacy of clinical hypnosis for procedural as well as for chronic pain. Butler et al[13] compared hypnosis with breathing and relaxation techniques for procedure-related pain and anxiety during

TABLE 3 Resources by Topic

Resources	Web Sites, Books, DVDs, etc
Biofeedback	
Biofeedback Certification International Alliance	www.bcia.org
Inner Balance	www.heartmath.com
Interactive games (Healing Rhythms, Journey to Wild Divine)	www.wilddivine.com
"eSense" temperature and sweat gland activity (electrodermal activity) sensors	http://www.mindfield.de/en/biofeedback/products/esense/esense-skin-response
Tinke	http://www.zensorium.com/tinke/
Hypnosis	
Video: "magic glove" technique, performed by Dr Leora Kuttner[a]	http://www.youtube.com/watch?v=cyApK8Z_SQQ
Dr Laurence Sugarman's 70-minute DVD[a]	Sugarman L. *Hypnosis in Pediatric Practice: Imaginative Medicine in Action* [DVD and booklet]. Carmarthen, United Kingdom: Crown House Publishing; 2006
National Pediatric Hypnosis Training Institute	www.nphti.org
American Society of Clinical Hypnosis	www.asch.net
Society for Clinical and Experimental Hypnosis	www.sceh.us
Guided imagery	
Health Journeys: Guided Meditation and Imagery	http://www.healthjourneys.com
Kaiser Permanente: Guided Imagery (podcasts)	https://healthy.kaiserpermanente.org/health/care/!ut/p/a0/FchBDoMgEADAt_iAzYZEYfFmhH6hhdsGiZIlGELt99seZ9DjC33hO-3cUy18_uxCLD22md9bqnCnLVZ8okd_Nd4zoysVAocj_o9bT-GM6lzVap2MBamIBCGsgEWPBohoUkKp8UErXjnTZxmGL2IKPpI!/
Shambala Kids: Guided Imagery and Relaxation Audio CDs	http://shambalakids.com/index.php?option=com_content&view=category&id=40&Itemid=419&lang=us
Stress Free Kids Indigo Dreams Audio CDs	http://www.stressfreekids.com/category/cds/children-cds
Academy for Guided Imagery	http://acadgi.com
Meditation and MBSR	
For health professionals:	
Mind-Body STREAM program	https://mind-bodyhealth.osu.edu
For parents:	
Everyday Blessings: The Inner Work of Mindful Parenting	Kabat-Zinn M, Kabat-Zinn J. *Everyday Blessings: The Inner Work of Mindful Parenting*. New York, NY: Hyperion; 1998
Growing Happiness	http://growing-happiness.com/mindfulness-training-for-parents/
Meditation for children	http://www.freemeditation.com/online-meditation/meditation-for-children/
For teens:	
Mindfulness for Teens	http://mindfulnessforteens.com
Mindfulness Retreats	http://ibme.info/
Learning to Breathe	http://learning2breathe.org/
UCSD Center for Mindfulness Professional Training	http://mbpti.org/
UCSD Center for Mindfulness blog	https://ucsdcfm.wordpress.com/tag/ron-epstein/
UMass Medical School Center for Mindfulness	http://www.umassmed.edu/cfm/training/
UCLA Mindful Awareness Research Center	http://marc.ucla.edu/
Yoga	
Global Family Yoga	http://globalfamilyyoga.com/
International Association of Yoga Therapists	http://iayt.org/
Kripalu Yoga in the Schools	http://nccam.nih.gov/health/yoga
Yoga Alliance	http://www.yogaalliance.org/
Yoga Calm	http://www.yogacalm.org/
Yoga for the Special Child	http://www.specialyoga.com/
Yoga in Schools	http://yogainschools.org
YogaKids	http://yogakids.com/

STREAM, Skills Training for Resilience, Effectiveness, and Mindfulness; UCLA, University of California, Los Angeles; UCSD, University of California, San Diego; UMass, University of Massachusetts.

[a] The technique should never be used for entertainment, should only be used by appropriately trained providers, and should only be used in clinical situations for which the provider already has competence in treating.

voiding cystourethrography. Moderate effect sizes for symptom reduction were noted by parents, medical staff, and research observers; and procedure length was reduced by 14 minutes in the hypnosis group. A trial comparing preprocedure hypnosis with midazolam for anesthesia for abdominal surgery showed reduced anxiety at the time of induction as well as improved behavior outcomes at 1 and 7 days after surgery for the hypnosis group.[14] Two systematic reviews concluded that there is promising evidence for hypnosis for acute procedure-related pain.[10,12]

Conclusions

Research suggests benefits of clinical hypnosis for children and adolescents, particularly for FAP, IBS, and pain management. Promising evidence for its application for other indications (eg, enuresis, tics/Tourette syndrome, migraine, and anxiety) exists but is not conclusive. There are few absolute contraindications to the use of hypnosis. The technique should be used only by appropriately trained providers and in clinical situations in which the provider already is competent managing without the inclusion of hypnosis. A selection of practical resources (eg, videos) for pediatric health care providers is provided in Table 3.

Guided Imagery

Guided imagery is a powerful mind-body technique that invokes all of the senses (sight, sound, taste, touch, smell, and movement). Imagery has a rich history in healing traditions throughout the world. Guided imagery and clinical hypnosis have significant overlap, and many studies combine these modalities. Strengths of guided imagery treatment include that it is not invasive and has flexibility of use in different age ranges (preschool-aged through adolescents and adults) and in various settings (outpatient, inpatient, and acute care). The use of guided imagery has been shown to produce measurable physiologic changes in stress and immune biomarkers.[61] Challenges in the use of imagery include variable training, acceptance of a novel therapy by patient and practitioner, familiarity with and access to high-quality resources, and relative lack of randomized controlled outcome studies in children. Due caution is indicated in patients with a history of physical, sexual, or emotional abuse or those with PTSD, in which case coordination of care with a qualified mental health expert is strongly advisable.

An evidence base for the use of guided imagery in adults is present, and an evidence base in children is growing. In 1 adult RCT, guided imagery in 96 patients with newly diagnosed breast cancer showed significant correlation with improved mood and quality of life.[62] For example, a second adult RCT that used guided imagery was correlated with an increase in numbers and activity of beneficial immune function (T helper cells, natural killer cells, lymphokine-activated killer cells, and favorable interleukin-1β levels) in 80 patients with breast cancer in active treatment.[63] An example of a pediatric RCT that used guided imagery involved a 12-week lifestyle intervention trial in 29 Latino adolescents with obesity, in which weekly interactive guided imagery sessions were associated with a statistically significant reduction in salivary cortisol, improved physical activity, and promotion of health behavior change in the treatment group.[15] A second RCT combined guided imagery with progressive muscle relaxation in 22 children ages 5 to 18 years with a diagnosis of recurrent abdominal pain. Guided imagery with progressive muscle relaxation in 4 weekly sessions was associated with a statistically significant reduction in days with pain throughout the 2-month follow-up period.[17] Home-based audio-recorded guided imagery also has been shown to be effective in the reduction of recurrent abdominal pain in a treatment group of 34 children ages 6 to 15 years who were randomly assigned to receive guided imagery versus standard care. Results were maintained throughout the 6-month follow-up period.[16]

In addition to these RCTs, other small studies that showed efficacy of guided imagery have been conducted for a variety of medical conditions, including asthma,[64] sickle cell disease,[65] procedural anxiety,[66] and posttraumatic stress.[67] Both imagery and hypnosis may be combined successfully with other mind-body

therapies, such as biofeedback, to enhance relaxation.[68] Regulated training for guided imagery does not exist at this time.

Conclusions

Guided imagery appears to be a promising complementary therapy for children and adolescents, with very low reports of adverse effects. Guided imagery as a therapeutic intervention has been shown to have positive effects on psychological functioning, stress reduction, and pain management. Caution is advised in patients with a history of previous emotional, sexual, or physical abuse to avoid an unintended triggering of posttraumatic stress symptoms. Consultation with a mental health practitioner is advised if questions about appropriateness of use exist in this context. More RCTs in children are needed for this noninvasive therapy in the pediatric clinical setting. A selection of guided imagery Web resources is provided in Table 3.

Meditation and MBSR

Meditation

Meditation practices for children and youth have become increasingly popular in schools and medical settings alike. Meditation is the practice of intentional attention training and consists of a number of different specific approaches. Research on meditation in children and youth consists primarily of 2 types of meditation: mindfulness meditation and concentration meditation.

Research on meditation in diverse populations of adults has accumulated sufficiently to provide convincing high-level evidence for reproducible benefits of meditation in mental health and pain management.[69-71] In addition, data suggest that greater levels of mindfulness in adulthood may mitigate some of the negative health effects of adverse childhood experiences.[72] The literature in children and youth, however, is less developed and, although suggestive of benefit, is just beginning to emerge.[73-76] To provide the highest level of available evidence regarding the specific effect(s) attributable to meditation instruction for children and youth, conclusions in this report are based on findings from RCTs with active control conditions.

Mindfulness Meditation

Mindfulness meditation is aimed at enhancing individuals' innate capacity to be purposefully aware of their present-moment emotional, cognitive, and sensory experiences. Through instruction in formal and informal meditation techniques, this capacity for purposeful, moment-by-moment, nonjudgmental awareness develops, along with the ability to shift attention. Several RCTs in youth have evaluated the MBSR program, which has established instructor training through the University of Massachusetts School of Medicine's Center for Mindfulness and has been well researched in adults.[77] Youth-adapted MBSR programs have been found to be beneficial in improving mental health symptoms, coping, and self-regulatory processes and decreasing blood pressure when used in both primary prevention[18-21,78,79] and treatment settings.[80] In children 7 to 9 years of age, an RCT of school-based mindful awareness practice instruction versus a reading program did not show differences by treatment group overall but did reveal improvements in mindful awareness practice participants in executive function among children with lower executive function skills at baseline.[24]

Concentration Meditation

Concentration meditation involves focusing attention on 1 specific thing, such as a word, phrase, or object.[23] A Cochrane review found current research inadequate to suggest meditation for attention-deficit/

hyperactivity disorder and suggested additional trials.[81] Active-controlled RCTs and active-control programs of concentration meditation in children and youth have included both transcendental meditation (TM) and the relaxation response. Compared with active-control programs, TM has been shown to lead to decreases in blood pressure and left ventricular hypertrophy among African-American adolescents with prehypertension[22,25] as well as fewer negative school behaviors, such as absenteeism.[26] Relaxation response has been associated with improvements in self-esteem.[82]

Conclusions

Research on structured meditation programs for children and youth is suggestive of benefits, particularly related to improvements in mental health, coping, and self-regulation as well as decreasing hypertension and negative school behaviors. Although there are structured training and certification programs for a number of meditation programs (including MBSR, TM, and mindfulness-based cognitive therapy), there is no formal credentialing or licensure for meditation instruction. Costs vary depending on the format of instruction and are increasingly, but not universally, covered by insurance. Although these results are encouraging, careful attention should be paid to elements of implementation and dissemination to maintain high-quality, effective meditation instruction for children and youth.

Yoga

The word yoga is derived from the Sanskrit word *yuj* meaning "union." An ancient Indian practice, yoga has been classified by the National Center for Complementary and Integrative Health as a mind-body medicine modality.[83] According to the 2007 National Health Interview Survey,[84]

yoga was the fifth most commonly used complementary therapy practice among all children ages 2 to 17 years, with ~1.5 million children practicing yoga in the previous year. In a survey of children and adolescents with chronic pain, yoga was preferred by 32% as their first choice of complementary therapy.[85] Therapeutic yoga is the practice of uniting the mind, the body, and the spirit through mindfulness of breathing and body postures to improve stress coping, lessen pain, and improve specific health conditions. Although not completely understood, yoga effects changes in the parasympathetic nervous system, positively affecting heart rate variability.[86]

Fourteen controlled studies[27-32,87-94] and 4 systematic reviews[95-98] were identified, and all uncontrolled trials and those in which yoga was not the sole treatment intervention[99] were eliminated from consideration. The conclusions of the systematic reviews can be summarized as follows: yoga appears to be a promising complementary therapy for children and adolescents, especially for those with pain and emotional, mental, and behavioral conditions, with very few reported adverse effects. However, a lack of methodologic and statistical rigor, including small sample sizes, absence of randomization, and a high degree of variability between intervention methods, limits the ability to recommend yoga as a primary intervention for any particular population. On the basis of the 14 individual controlled studies, yoga appears to be a promising complementary therapy and stress-management tool for children and adolescents, with very low reports of adverse effects. Yoga as a therapeutic intervention has positive effects on psychological functioning, especially in children coping with emotional, mental, and behavioral health problems. Specifically, research has shown that educational curricula incorporating stress-management programs improve academic performance, self-esteem, classroom behaviors, concentration, and emotional balance,[98] suggesting that schools may be an ideal setting to bring yoga to a heterogeneous, socioeconomically diverse sample of children. In addition, in 4 controlled trials, yoga was shown to positively influence metabolic and hormonal variables. Given the increasing prevalence of obesity and metabolic dysfunction in children, coupled with the relative safety and cost-effectiveness of yoga as an intervention, more research in this population is needed. Limitations of reviewed studies include small sample sizes, high attrition rates, lack of evaluator blinding, reliance on self-report measures, and heterogeneity of intervention and control designs. Well-designed controlled trials of yoga for conditions with strong stress-modulated components are warranted. Excellent candidate conditions include asthma, IBS, inflammatory bowel diseases, juvenile idiopathic arthritis, and fibromyalgia. Given the preference for yoga in studies in children with chronic pain, coupled with biological plausibility for response, limited potential for adverse effects, and promising pilot data, there is a great need for controlled studies in this population.

Conclusions

Yoga appears to be a promising complementary therapy and stress-management tool for children and adolescents, with very low reports of adverse effects. Yoga, as a therapeutic intervention, has positive effects on psychological functioning, especially in children coping with emotional, mental, and behavioral health problems. Yoga generally is not billed for and reimbursed as an insurance-covered therapy. Yoga instructors and centers establish a fee for service (per session or as a package for a set number of classes) on the basis of

community-established standards. The Yoga Alliance[100] sets guidelines for yoga teacher certification in the United States. A selection of yoga Web resources is provided in Table 3.

CONCLUSIONS AND RECOMMENDATIONS

This report examines the best-available evidence for a variety of mind-body therapies and practices in children and youth, including biofeedback, clinical hypnosis, guided imagery, meditation, and yoga. The evidence varies in terms of quantity and quality but generally is supportive of mind-body therapies and practices as safe and potentially effective in common and debilitating conditions, including pain and anxiety. Additional potential benefits for school-aged children include improved concentration and self-esteem. Pediatric health care providers are encouraged to facilitate an open dialog with their patients about their use of complementary therapies and to become familiar with mind-body therapies and practices as nonpharmacologic options to improve mood, behavior, and quality of life, which are of great interest and relevance to children, youth, and their parents/caregivers.

LEAD AUTHORS

Sunita Vohra, MD, FAAP, Past Chairperson, *AAP Section on Integrative Medicine*
Hilary McClafferty, MD, FAAP

CONTRIBUTING AUTHORS

David Becker, MD, FAAP
Christina Bethell, PhD, MBA, MPH
Timothy Culbert, MD, FAAP
Susanne King-Jones, PhD
Larry Rosen, MD, FAAP
Erica Sibinga, MD, FAAP

SECTION ON INTEGRATIVE MEDICINE EXECUTIVE COMMITTEE, 2014–2015

Hilary McClafferty, MD, FAAP, Chairperson
Erica Sibinga, MD, FAAP
Michelle Bailey, MD, FAAP
Timothy Culbert, MD, FAAP
Joy Weydert, MD, FAAP
Melanie Brown, MD, FAAP

STAFF

Teri Salus, MPA, CPC

ABBREVIATIONS

ANS: autonomic nervous system
FAP: functional abdominal pain
IBS: irritable bowel syndrome
MBSR: mindfulness-based stress reduction
PTSD: posttraumatic stress disorder
RCT: randomized controlled trial
TM: transcendental meditation

REFERENCES

1. Black LI, Clarke TC, Barnes PM, Stussman BJ, Nahin RL. Use of complementary health approaches among children aged 4-17 years in the United States: National Health Interview Survey, 2007-2012. *Natl Health Stat Rep.* 2015;(78):1–19

2. Data Resource Center for Child and Adolescent Health. The National Health Interview Survey (NHIS). Child Complementary and Alternative Medicine (CAM) supplement. Data Resource Center for Child and Adolescent Health; 2012. Available at: http://childhealthdata.org/learn/nhis. Accessed December 10, 2015

3. Sussman D, Culbert T. Pediatric self-regulation. In: Levine MD, Carey WB, Crocker AC, eds. *Developmental-Behavioral Pediatrics.* 3rd ed. Philadelphia, PA: WB Saunders; 1999:911–922

4. Kohen DP. A pediatric perspective on mind-body medicine. In: Culbert T, Olness K, eds. *Integrative Pediatrics.* New York, NY: Oxford University Press; 2009:267–301

5. Knox M, Lentini J, Cummings T, McGrady A, Whearty K, Sancrant L. Game-based biofeedback for paediatric anxiety and depression. *Ment Health Fam Med.* 2011;8(3):195–203

6. Palermo TM, Eccleston C, Lewandowski AS, Williams AC, Morley S. Randomized controlled trials of psychological therapies for management of chronic pain in children and adolescents: an updated meta-analytic review. *Pain.* 2010;148(3):387–397

7. Monastra VJ, Lynn S, Linden M, Lubar JF, Gruzelier J, LaVaque TJ. Electroencephalographic biofeedback in the treatment of attention-deficit/hyperactivity disorder. *Appl Psychophysiol Biofeedback.* 2005;30(2):95–114

8. Eccleston C, Morley S, Williams A, Yorke L, Mastroyannopoulou K. Systematic review of randomised controlled trials of psychological therapy for chronic pain in children and adolescents, with a subset meta-analysis of pain relief. *Pain.* 2002;99(1–2):157–165

9. Rutten JM, Reitsma JB, Vlieger AM, Benninga MA. Gut-directed hypnotherapy for functional abdominal pain or irritable bowel syndrome in children: a systematic review. *Arch Dis Child.* 2013;98(4):252–257

10. Accardi MC, Milling LS. The effectiveness of hypnosis for reducing procedure-related pain in children and adolescents: a comprehensive methodological review. *J Behav Med.* 2009;32(4):328–339

11. Vlieger AM, Menko-Frankenhuis C, Wolfkamp SC, Tromp E, Benninga MA. Hypnotherapy for children with functional abdominal pain or irritable bowel syndrome: a randomized controlled trial. *Gastroenterology.* 2007;133(5):1430–1436

12. Richardson J, Smith JE, McCall G, Pilkington K. Hypnosis for procedure-related pain and distress in pediatric cancer patients: a systematic review of effectiveness and methodology related to hypnosis interventions. *J Pain Symptom Manage.* 2006;31(1):70–84

13. Butler LD, Symons BK, Henderson SL, Shortliffe LD, Spiegel D. Hypnosis reduces distress and duration of an invasive medical procedure for children. *Pediatrics.* 2005;115(1). Available at: www.pediatrics.org/cgi/content/full/115/1/e77

14. Calipel S, Lucas-Polomeni MM, Wodey E, Ecoffey C. Premedication in children: hypnosis versus midazolam. *Paediatr Anaesth.* 2005;15(4):275–281

15. Weigensberg MJ, Lane CJ, Ávila Q, et al. Imagine HEALTH: results from a randomized pilot lifestyle intervention for obese Latino adolescents using Interactive Guided ImagerySM. *BMC Complement Altern Med.* 2014;14:1–13

16. van Tilburg MA, Chitkara DK, Palsson OS, et al. Audio-recorded guided imagery treatment reduces functional abdominal pain in children: a pilot study. *Pediatrics.* 2009;124(5). Available at: www.pediatrics.org/cgi/content/full/124/5/e890

17. Weydert JA, Shapiro DE, Acra SA, Monheim CJ, Chambers AS, Ball TM. Evaluation of guided imagery as treatment for recurrent abdominal pain in children: a randomized controlled trial. *BMC Pediatr.* 2006;6:1–10

18. Britton WB, Lepp NE, Niles HF, Rocha T, Fisher NE, Gold JS. A randomized controlled pilot trial of classroom-based mindfulness meditation compared to an active control condition in sixth-grade children. *J Sch Psychol.* 2014;52(3):263–278

19. Sibinga EM, Perry-Parrish C, Thorpe K, Mika M, Ellen JM. A small mixed-method RCT of mindfulness instruction for urban youth. *Explore (NY).* 2014;10(3):180–186

20. Sibinga EM, Perry-Parrish C, Chung SE, Johnson SB, Smith M, Ellen JM. School-based mindfulness instruction for urban male youth: a small randomized controlled trial. *Prev Med.* 2013;57(6):799–801

21. Sibinga EM, Webb L, Ghazarian SR, Ellen JM. School-based mindfulness instruction: an RCT. *Pediatrics.* 2016;137(1):e20152532

22. Barnes VA, Kapuku GK, Treiber FA. Impact of transcendental meditation on left ventricular mass in African American adolescents. *Evid Based Complement Alternat Med.* 2012;2012:923153

23. Sibinga EMS, Kemper KJ. Complementary, holistic, and integrative medicine: meditation practices for pediatric health. *Pediatr Rev.* 2010;31(12):e91–e103

24. Flook L, Smalley SL, Kitil MJ, et al. Effects of mindful awareness practices on executive functions in elementary school children. *J Appl Sch Psychol.* 2010;26(1):70–95

25. Barnes VA, Treiber FA, Johnson MH. Impact of transcendental meditation on ambulatory blood pressure in African-American adolescents. *Am J Hypertens.* 2004;17(4):366–369

26. Barnes VA, Bauza LB, Treiber FA. Impact of stress reduction on negative school behavior in adolescents. *Health Qual Life Outcomes.* 2003;1(10):1–7

27. Hagins M, Haden SC, Daly LA. A randomized controlled trial on the effects of yoga on stress reactivity in 6th grade students. *Evid Based Complement Alternat Med.* 2013;2013:607134

28. Telles S, Singh N, Bhardwaj AK, Kumar A, Balkrishna A. Effect of yoga or physical exercise on physical, cognitive and emotional measures in children: a randomized controlled trial. *Child Adolesc Psychiatry Ment Health.* 2013;7(1):1–16

29. Khalsa SB, Hickey-Schultz L, Cohen D, Steiner N, Cope S. Evaluation of the mental health benefits of yoga in a secondary school: a preliminary randomized controlled trial. *J Behav Health Serv Res.* 2012;39(1):80–90

30. Nidhi R, Padmalatha V, Nagarathna R, Amritanshu R. Effect of holistic yoga program on anxiety symptoms in adolescent girls with polycystic ovarian syndrome: a randomized control trial. *Int J Yoga.* 2012;5(2):112–117

31. White LS. Reducing stress in school-age girls through mindful yoga. *J Pediatr Health Care.* 2012;26(1):45–56

32. Mendelson T, Greenberg MT, Dariotis JK, Gould LF, Rhoades BL, Leaf PJ. Feasibility and preliminary outcomes of a school-based mindfulness intervention for urban youth. *J Abnorm Child Psychol.* 2010;38(7):985–994

33. Green E, Green A, Walters ED. Voluntary control of internal states: psychological and physiological. *J Transpers Psychol.* 1970;2(1):1–26

34. Culbert T. Biofeedback with children and adolescents. In: Schaefer C, ed. *Innovative Psychotherapy in Child and Adolescent Therapy.* 2nd ed. Hoboken, NJ: Wiley; 1999

35. Schwartz MS, Andrasik FE, eds. *Biofeedback: A Practitioners Guide.* 4th ed. New York, NY: Guilford Press; 2015

36. Attanasio V, Andrasik F, Burke C. Clinical issues in utilizing biofeedback with children. *Clin Biofeedback Health.* 1985;8(2):134–141

37. Biofeedback Certification International Alliance. Become board certified. Available at: www.bcia.org/i4a/pages/index.cfm?pageid=1. Accessed December 10, 2015

38. Liu C, Zhu Q, Holroyd KA, Seng EK. Status and trends of mobile-health applications for iOS devices: a developer's perspective. *J Syst Softw.* 2011;84(11):2022–2033

39. Andrasik F, Schwartz MS. Behavioral assessment and treatment of pediatric headache. *Behav Modif.* 2006;30(1):93–113

40. Nestoriuc Y, Martin A, Rief W, Andrasik F. Biofeedback treatment for headache disorders: a comprehensive efficacy review. *Appl Psychophysiol Biofeedback.* 2008;33(3):125–140

41. Culbert TP, Banez GA. Integrative approaches to childhood constipation and encopresis. *Pediatr Clin North Am.* 2007;54(6):927–947, xi

42. Culbert TP, Banez GA. Wetting the bed: integrative approaches to nocturnal enuresis. *Explore (NY).* 2008;4(3):215–220

43. Palsson OS, Heymen S, Whitehead WE. Biofeedback treatment for functional anorectal disorders: a comprehensive efficacy review. *Appl Psychophysiol Biofeedback.* 2004;29(3):153–174

44. Weydert JA, Ball TM, Davis MF. Systematic review of treatments for recurrent abdominal pain. *Pediatrics.* 2003;111(1):e1–e11

45. Bolek JE. Use of multiple-site performance-contingent SEMG reward programming in pediatric rehabilitation: a retrospective review. *Appl Psychophysiol Biofeedback.* 2006;31(3):263–272

46. Brütsch K, Koenig A, Zimmerli L, et al. Virtual reality for enhancement of robot-assisted gait training in children with central gait disorders. *J Rehabil Med.* 2011;43(6):493–499

47. Wang M, Reid D. Virtual reality in pediatric neurorehabilitation: attention deficit hyperactivity disorder, autism and cerebral palsy. *Neuroepidemiology.* 2011;36(1):2–18

48. Vernon D, Frick A, Gruzelier J. Neurofeedback as a treatment for ADHD: a methodological review with implications for future research. *J Neurother.* 2004;8(2):53–82

49. Lehrer P, Feldman J, Giardino N, Song HS, Schmaling K. Psychological aspects of asthma. *J Consult Clin Psychol.* 2002;70(3):691–711

50. Carter JL, Russell HL. Use of EMG biofeedback procedures with learning disabled children in a clinical and an educational setting. *J Learn Disabil.* 1985;18(4):213–216

51. Hoy MM, Egan MY, Feder KP. A systematic review of interventions to improve handwriting. *Can J Occup Ther.* 2011;78(1):13–25

52. Barowsky EI, Moskowitz J, Zweig JB. Biofeedback for disorders of initiating and maintaining sleep. *Ann N Y Acad Sci.* 1990;602(1):97–103

53. Morin CM, Bootzin RR, Buysse DJ, Edinger JD, Espie CA, Lichstein KL. Psychological and behavioral treatment of insomnia:update of the recent evidence (1998-2004). *Sleep.* 2006;29(11):1398–1414

54. Chiarioni G, Whitehead WE. The role of biofeedback in the treatment of gastrointestinal disorders. *Nat Clin Pract Gastroenterol Hepatol.* 2008;5(7):371–382

55. Kohen DP, Olness K. *Hypnosis and Hypnotherapy With Children.* 4th ed. New York, NY: Routledge; 2011

56. Kohen DP, Kaiser P. Clinical hypnosis with children and adolescents—What? Why? How? Origins, applications, and efficacy. *Children.* 2014;1(2):74–98

57. Kohen DP, Zajac R. Self-hypnosis training for headaches in children and adolescents. *J Pediatr.* 2007;150(6):635–639

58. Sugarman LI, Wester WC. *Therapeutic Hypnosis With Children and Adolescents.* 2nd ed. Carmarthen, United Kingdom: Crown House Publishing; 2013

59. Raz A. Does neuroimaging of suggestion elucidate hypnotic trance? *Int J Clin Exp Hypn.* 2011;59(3):363–377

60. Vlieger AM, Rutten JM, Govers AM, Frankenhuis C, Benninga MA. Long-term follow-up of gut-directed hypnotherapy vs. standard care in children with functional abdominal pain or irritable bowel syndrome. *Am J Gastroenterol.* 2012;107(4):627–631

61. Astin JA, Shapiro SL, Eisenberg DM, Forys KL. Mind-body medicine: state of the science, implications for practice. *J Am Board Fam Pract.* 2003;16(2):131–147

62. Walker LG, Walker MB, Ogston K, et al. Psychological, clinical and pathological effects of relaxation training and guided imagery during primary chemotherapy. *Br J Cancer.* 1999;80(1–2):262–268

63. Eremin O, Walker MB, Simpson E, et al. Immuno-modulatory effects of relaxation training and guided imagery in women with locally advanced breast cancer undergoing multimodality therapy: a randomised controlled trial. *Breast.* 2009;18(1):17–25

64. Kapoor VG, Bray MA, Kehle TJ. Asthma and anxiety disorders: relaxation and guided imagery as a school-based treatment. *Can J Sch Psychol.* 2007;25(4):311–327

65. Dobson CE, Byrne MW. Original research: using guided imagery to manage pain in young children with sickle cell disease. *Am J Nurs.* 2014;114(4):26–36, 37, 47

66. Forsner M, Norström F, Nordyke K, Ivarsson A, Lindh V. Relaxation and guided imagery used with 12-year-olds during venipuncture in a school-based screening study. *J Child Health Care.* 2014;18(3):241–252

67. Staples JK, Abdel Atti JA, Gordon JS. Mind-body skills groups for posttraumatic stress disorder and depression symptoms in Palestinian children and adolescents in Gaza. *Int J Stress Manag.* 2011;18(3):246–262

68. Shockey DP, Menzies V, Glick DF, Taylor AG, Boitnott A, Rovnyak V. Preprocedural distress in children with cancer: an intervention using biofeedback and relaxation. *J Pediatr Oncol Nurs.* 2013;30(3):129–138

69. Goyal M, Singh S, Sibinga EM, et al. Meditation programs for psychological stress and well-being: a systematic review and meta-analysis. *JAMA Intern Med.* 2014;174(3):357–368

70. Orme-Johnson DW, Barnes VA. Effects of the transcendental meditation technique on trait anxiety: a meta-analysis of randomized controlled trials. *J Altern Complement Med.* 2014;20(5):330–341

71. Ager K, Albrecht NJ, Cohen M. Mindfulness in Schools Research Project: exploring students' perspectives of mindfulness. *Psychology (Irvine)*. 2015;6(7):896–914

72. Whitaker RC, Dearth-Wesley T, Gooze RA, Becker BD, Gallagher KC, McEwen BS. Adverse childhood experiences, dispositional mindfulness, and adult health. *Prev Med*. 2014;67:147–153

73. Burke CA. Mindfulness-based approaches with children and adolescents: a preliminary review of current research in an emergent field. *J Child Fam Stud*. 2010;19(2):133–144

74. Zenner C, Herrnleben-Kurz S, Walach H. Mindfulness-based interventions in schools-a systematic review and meta-analysis. *Front Psychol*. 2014;5:1–20

75. Harnett PH, Dawe S. The contribution of mindfulness-based therapies for children and families and proposed conceptual integration. *Child Adolesc Ment Health*. 2012;17(4):195–208

76. Weare K. Evidence for the impact of mindfulness on children and young people. The Mindfulness in Schools Project in association with Mood Disorders Centre. 2012. Available at: http://mindfulnessinschools.org/wp-content/uploads/2013/02/MiSP-Research-Summary-2012.pdf. Accessed January 15, 2015

77. Kabat-Zinn J, Hanh TN. *Full Catastrophe Living: Using the Wisdom of Your Body and Mind to Face Stress, Pain, and Illness*. 15th ed. New York, NY: Bantham Dell; 2009

78. Wright LB, Gregoski MJ, Tingen MS, Barnes VA, Treiber FA. Impact of stress reduction interventions on hostility and ambulatory systolic blood pressure in African American adolescents. *J Black Psychol*. 2011;37(2):210–233

79. Kallapiran K, Koo S, Kirubakaran R, Hancock K. Effectiveness of mindfulness in improving mental health symptoms of children and adolescents: a meta-analysis. *Child Adolesc Ment Health*. 2015;20(4):182–194

80. Biegel GM, Brown KW, Shapiro SL, Schubert CM. Mindfulness-based stress reduction for the treatment of adolescent psychiatric outpatients: a randomized clinical trial. *J Consult Clin Psychol*. 2009;77(5):855–866

81. Krisanaprakornkit T, Ngamjarus C, Witoonchart C, Piyavhatkul N. Meditation therapies for attention-deficit/hyperactivity disorder (ADHD). *Cochrane Database Syst Rev*. 2010;6:CD006507

82. Benson H, Kornhaber A, Kornhaber C, LeChanu MN. Increases in positive psychological characteristics with a new relaxation-response curriculum in high school students. *J Res Dev Educ*. 1994;27(4):226–231

83. National Center for Complementary and Integrative Health. Yoga. Available at: https://nccih.nih.gov/health/yoga. Updated 2015. Accessed January 2015

84. Data Resource Center for Child and Adolescent Health. National profile of complementary and alternative medicine (CAM) use for children with emotional, mental or behavioral conditions or problems (2-17 years). Available at: www.childhealthdata.org/docs/drc/emb-profile_9-27-12.pdf. Updated 2012. Accessed October 2014

85. Tsao JC, Meldrum M, Kim SC, Jacob MC, Zeltzer LK. Treatment preferences for CAM in children with chronic pain. *Evid Based Complement Alternat Med*. 2007;4(3):367–374

86. Khattab K, Khattab AA, Ortak J, Richardt G, Bonnemeier H. Iyengar yoga increases cardiac parasympathetic nervous modulation among healthy yoga practitioners. *Evid Based Complement Alternat Med*. 2007;4(4):511–517

87. Berger DL, Silver EJ, Stein RE. Effects of yoga on inner-city children's well-being: a pilot study. *Altern Ther Health Med*. 2009;15(5):36–42

88. Noggle JJ, Steiner NJ, Minami T, Khalsa SB. Benefits of yoga for psychosocial well-being in a US high school curriculum: a preliminary randomized controlled trial. *J Dev Behav Pediatr*. 2012;33(3):193–201

89. Nidhi R, Padmalatha V, Nagarathna R, Amritanshu R. Effects of a holistic yoga program on endocrine parameters in adolescents with polycystic ovarian syndrome: a randomized controlled trial. *J Altern Complement Med*. 2013;19(2):153–160

90. Khalsa SB, Butzer B, Shorter SM, Reinhardt KM, Cope S. Yoga reduces performance anxiety in adolescent musicians. *Altern Ther Health Med*. 2013;19(2):34–45

91. Kuttner L, Chambers CT, Hardial J, Israel DM, Jacobson K, Evans K. A randomized trial of yoga for adolescents with irritable bowel syndrome. *Pain Res Manag*. 2006;11(4):217–224

92. Carei TR, Fyfe-Johnson AL, Breuner CC, Brown MA. Randomized controlled clinical trial of yoga in the treatment of eating disorders. *J Adolesc Health*. 2010;46(4):346–351

93. Seo DY, Lee S, Figueroa A, et al. Yoga training improves metabolic parameters in obese boys. *Korean J Physiol Pharmacol*. 2012;16(3):175–180

94. Nidhi R, Padmalatha V, Nagarathna R, Ram A. Effect of a yoga program on glucose metabolism and blood lipid levels in adolescent girls with polycystic ovary syndrome. *Int J Gynaecol Obstet*. 2012;118(1):37–41

95. Galantino ML, Galbavy R, Quinn L. Therapeutic effects of yoga for children: a systematic review of the literature. *Pediatr Phys Ther*. 2008;20(1):66–80

96. Birdee GS, Yeh GY, Wayne PM, Phillips RS, Davis RB, Gardiner P. Clinical applications of yoga for the pediatric population: a systematic review. *Acad Pediatr*. 2009;9(4):212.–220

97. Kaley-Isley LC, Peterson J, Fischer C, Peterson E. Yoga as a complementary therapy for children and adolescents: a guide for clinicians. *Psychiatry (Edgmont)*. 2010;7(8):20–32

98. Kraag G, Zeegers MP, Kok G, Hosman C, Abu-Saad HH. School programs targeting stress management in children and adolescents: a meta-analysis. *J Sch Psychol*. 2006;44(6):449–472

99. Rosen L, French A, Sullivan G; RYT-200. Complementary, holistic, and integrative medicine: yoga. *Pediatr Rev*. 2015;36(10):468–474

100. Yoga Alliance. Credentialing. Available at: https://www.yogaalliance.org/Credentialing. Accessed December 10, 2015

Out-of-Home Placement for Children and Adolescents With Disabilities—Addendum: Care Options for Children and Adolescents With Disabilities and Medical Complexity

• *Clinical Report*

CLINICAL REPORT Guidance for the Clinician in Rendering Pediatric Care

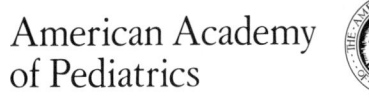

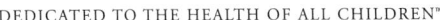

DEDICATED TO THE HEALTH OF ALL CHILDREN™

Out-of-Home Placement for Children and Adolescents With Disabilities— Addendum: Care Options for Children and Adolescents With Disabilities and Medical Complexity

Sandra L. Friedman, MD, MPH, FAAP, Kenneth W. Norwood Jr, MD, FAAP, COUNCIL ON CHILDREN WITH DISABILITIES

abstract

Children and adolescents with significant intellectual and developmental disabilities and complex medical problems require safe and comprehensive care to meet their medical and psychosocial needs. Ideally, such children and youth should be cared for by their families in their home environments. When this type of arrangement is not possible, there should be exploration of appropriate, alternative noncongregate community-based settings, especially alternative family homes. Government funding sources exist to support care in the community, although there is variability among states with regard to the availability of community programs and resources. It is important that families are supported in learning about options of care. Pediatricians can serve as advocates for their patients and their families to access community-based services and to increase the availability of resources to ensure that the option to live in a family home is available to all children with complex medical needs.

This document is copyrighted and is property of the American Academy of Pediatrics and its Board of Directors. All authors have filed conflict of interest statements with the American Academy of Pediatrics. Any conflicts have been resolved through a process approved by the Board of Directors. The American Academy of Pediatrics has neither solicited nor accepted any commercial involvement in the development of the content of this publication.

Clinical reports from the American Academy of Pediatrics benefit from expertise and resources of liaisons and internal (AAP) and external reviewers. However, clinical reports from the American Academy of Pediatrics may not reflect the views of the liaisons or the organizations or government agencies that they represent.

The guidance in this report does not indicate an exclusive course of treatment or serve as a standard of medical care. Variations, taking into account individual circumstances, may be appropriate.

All clinical reports from the American Academy of Pediatrics automatically expire 5 years after publication unless reaffirmed, revised, or retired at or before that time.

DOI: 10.1542/peds.2016-3216

PEDIATRICS (ISSN Numbers: Print, 0031-4005; Online, 1098-4275).

To cite: Friedman SL, Norwood KW, AAP COUNCIL ON CHILDREN WITH DISABILITIES. Out-of-Home Placement for Children and Adolescents With Disabilities—Addendum: Care Options for Children and Adolescents With Disabilities and Medical Complexity. Pediatrics. 2016;138(6):e20163216

INTRODUCTION

The clinical report "Out-of-Home Placement for Children and Adolescents With Disabilities,"[1] published by the American Academy of Pediatrics (AAP) Council on Children with Disabilities in October 2014, provides information about the option of pediatric congregate care settings for children with complex medical conditions and severe developmental disabilities whose families cannot or choose not to care for them in their own family home. The children and youth (referring to "adolescents") discussed in the article are those who have significant medical complexity and medical fragility, often requiring 24-hour skilled care for medical stability or survival. Although the Council on Children With

Disabilities believes that all children, including those with complex medical conditions and technology dependencies, ideally are cared for in their own homes and with their families whenever possible, for some children and their families, this may not be a safe or sustainable option. The clinical report, written in response to the expressed needs for information by AAP members, was not intended to endorse out-of-home placement for children with severe disabilities and complex medical conditions but rather describes the one option of out-of-home congregate care when children cannot live with their families. This addendum responds to reader requests for additional information about noncongregate, family-based out-of-home options, supplementing but not repeating or replacing the content of the original publication.

AAP POLICIES/CLINICAL REPORTS IN SUPPORT OF CHILDREN LIVING WITH FAMILIES

The AAP has been, and continues to be, a strong advocate for providing all children and youth with environments that foster optimal physical and psychosocial development. The psychosocial and cognitive benefits of living with a family in a nurturing home environment have long been established.[2] As such, children with disabilities, like all other children, develop better in the context of a loving and supportive environment. The AAP promotes comprehensive and coordinated supports and services for children and youth with special health care needs within the context of the medical home and medical community.[3] The basic tenets of the medical home are in line with the Developmental Disabilities Assistance and Bill of Rights Act of 2000[4] and the Americans With Disabilities Act,[5] which are laws that support all people with disabilities to live in their homes and communities

as fully integrated members of society. The AAP endorses permanent family and community environments for all children, with adequate and accessible community services to support children with all types of needs and their families.[6] The AAP values partnerships among parents, primary care providers, and the community to improve outcomes of children with disabilities.[7] The AAP provides resources for providers to support the care of children with complex heath care needs in the home, including those who are dependent on technology.[8] For example, the AAP *Guidelines for Pediatric Home Care* offers information to support children with special health care needs in the home setting, including information about respite, in-home nursing care, and medical day treatment programs for children with complex medical conditions.[9]

IMPORTANCE OF NURTURING FAMILY SETTINGS

Children with significant disabilities and complex medical conditions, like all children, need stable homes with loving families and caregivers who provide the essential physical and emotional resources to promote well-being. There is a consensus among the disability community, consistent with federal disability laws like the Americans with Disabilities Act,[5] that all children should reside with families – their own, whenever possible, or another family when that is not an option. Much has been written about the significance of an enriched, interactive environment on child development and attachment. Pediatric skilled nursing facilities are a type of congregate, institutional setting that may provide care to children and youth with severe disabilities and significant medical complexity who require 24-hour skilled nursing care. Children in skilled nursing facilities do not have the advantage of being in a

small setting with a family that provides consistent care. It has also been noted that children cared for by different providers working in shifts, such as in pediatric skilled nursing facilities, develop less strong emotional connections with caregivers compared with children being cared for in family homes.[10]

Research has documented the deleterious effects on development and attachment for children without disabilities who reside in settings that lack adequate stimuli for learning and bonding with caregivers. Findings from neurobiology have deepened our understanding of the vital role of the parent-child relationship in early development. Custodial care in large institutions has been characterized historically as "warehousing" individuals and denying opportunities for social interaction, engagement in stimulating activities, and individualized processes of care. Studies in Romanian orphanages have shown the importance of a nurturing and enriched environment on children's developmental outcomes. Although these studies were not focused specifically on children with significant disabilities and associated medical conditions,[11-14] they underscore the importance of stable and loving environments in which all children can develop a close bond with their caregiver(s).

Well-established factors that contribute to healthy development that are embedded in most families are missing in even the best congregate care setting.[15] Factors inherent in congregate care that distinguish it from a family and render it potentially harmful to children include (1) large ratio of children to caregivers; (2) absence of a primary caregiver for each child; (3) turnover of caregivers; (4) inferior cognitive, linguistic, and socioemotional stimulation; (5) regimented schedules and lack of spontaneity in child-adult interactions; and (6) limited peer-to-peer interaction.[15]

Problems with attachment can occur when young children are raised in socially deprived environments.[16] Conversely, resilience in children has been strongly associated with stable and supportive relationships with attuned and responsive adults, particularly with parents.[17,] The relationships and experiences of early childhood influence the long-term well-being of individuals.[18] Strong family functioning mediates against adverse neighborhood and environmental conditions,[19] and a strong community with reduced potential stressors also ensures better health outcomes in children.[20]

More recently, national attention has been directed to the effects of toxic stress on children residing in environments that do not provide adequate supports to promote optimal development, early literacy, and better academic outcomes. Exposure to adverse environments can have lifelong negative effects on a child's development.[2] Similarly, we know that children who are abused and neglected, whether in familial or congregate settings, are at risk for long-lasting negative effects on developmental and psychosocial well-being. There is convincing evidence about the importance of early identification and intervention of children who are abused and neglected.[21] Some children exposed to traumatic experiences in the home do require removal to a safe, nurturing environment, such as foster care. Evidence shows, however, that young children can recover after placement in a nurturing home with an attuned and responsive parent.

Some studies have found that children with disabilities, in general, are at increased risk of abuse, both in congregate settings and in their own family homes,[22–25] although in a systematic review of population-based studies, a weak association

was found between disability and abuse and neglect.[26] It is imperative that all children, including those with developmental disabilities and medical complexity, are provided with safe and secure environments that meet their physical and psychosocial needs.

FAMILY AND PARENT FACTORS FOR CHOOSING HOME VERSUS OUT-OF-HOME CARE

Most families want to care for their children in their home, have expertise about their children's needs, and make decisions that support their children's best interests.[27] In a review of technology-dependent children and their families, Wei Wang and Barnard[28] noted that it is more cost-effective to discharge children to home care, which also normalizes their care. Berry et al[29] conducted a retrospective analysis of more than 2 million acute care hospital discharges in the United States in 2012 for patients from 0 to 21 years of age, evaluating discharge to home health care and postacute care facilities. Analysis of discharge data revealed that 5.5% of these patients were discharged to home health care, and 1.1% were discharged to postacute care facilities. Children and youth who accessed these services had longer hospitalizations and greater medical complexity (eg, use of technology and multiple chronic medical problems). However, most children and youth with these complex medical issues do not use these resources and also use them significantly less than adults. Significant variability of use also was found on the basis of geographic location, race, and ethnicity.[29]

Parents who care for their children at home have been noted to do best when supported by professionals who value their input and work together with them toward common goals.[30] To support families, programs have been developed to

train them to care for their child with medical complexity in the home setting.[31] Although some families caring for a child with complex medical needs may experience less time for other activities and work loss to care for their child with special health care needs,[32,33] there is evidence that raising a child with chronic medical conditions has positive effects on family cohesion and appreciation for life.[34] However, home care is demanding and can affect the quality of life of these children and their families. Currently, the demand for in-home nursing is greater than the supply, and there are many geographic areas where it is especially difficult to find adequate nursing support. In a recent comparison of parent and child physical and mental health outcomes when children with complex conditions and technology dependencies are cared for at home, in long-term care settings, and in medical day-care settings, Caicedo found no differences in parent/guardian perception of child health outcomes, but the highest levels of parent physical health and vigor were experienced by the parents of children in long-term care settings.[35] The dynamic interplay of the function of parents and their children (in this case, with cerebral palsy) also was described by Murphy et al,[36] who found significant correlations between parent and child physical health, mental health, psychosocial function, and health-related quality of life. When considering placement options, the needs of both the child and the family warrant consideration.

Children with special health care needs who have disabilities experience more severe health conditions and unmet routine and specialty care needs compared with those without significant disabilities.[37–39] This disparity is most notable for adolescents with significant limitations, those living below or near poverty, those residing in the South and West, and those of Hispanic or non-Hispanic "other" (not white or black) ethnicity.[40] These children have greater medical complexity and technology dependence, placing increasing demands on caregivers.[41] Unmet care requirements may lead some families to explore different care options, such as in-home nursing, personal care and home health and therapies, and other care options such as host homes and medical foster care.[42–44]

Bruns[45] noted that the decision to place a child in a setting outside the family home is complex and involves multiple factors, including need for additional assistance, significant medical care needs, and financial concerns. Rosenau et al[46] evaluated reasons for placement of children with developmental disabilities (not limited to children with complex medical needs) in congregate care settings in Texas and found that this decision usually is influenced by stress-related situations that were worsened by lack of resources and/ or alternative options of care. The study found that another factor influencing parental decisions regarding placement in congregate settings was the availability or absence of a trusted, knowledgeable facilitator with the time and energy necessary to assist them to explore family-based alternatives.

CARE OPTIONS OTHER THAN THE FAMILY HOME AND CONGREGATE SETTINGS

Medical, surgical, and technological advances over the years have resulted in more children surviving with disabilities and/or complex medical conditions. Most children with disabilities or complex medical conditions are cared for in their homes, where they receive supports, services, and medical care.[47,48] The 2012–2013 National Core Indicators Survey, in collaboration with the National Association of Directors of

Developmental Disabilities Services and the Human Services Research Institute, captured data on more than 13 000 adults with intellectual and developmental disability who received services from state developmental disabilities agencies in 26 states. Those surveyed included a small subset of individuals between ages 18 and 22 years identified as having severe to profound developmental disabilities. Ticha et al[49] found that the vast majority of these youth are living with families; 69% lived with their own family, and 4.5% lived with host families. The majority of the remaining individuals lived in small community settings (21.9%, of which 2.6% were living on their own; 5.8% were living in provider-run settings of 1 to 3 people; and 9% were living in provider-run settings of 4 to 6 people). Only 1.3% lived in large provider-run settings with 7 to 15 people, and 3.8% lived in institutional settings.

When families believe they cannot care for their child in their home, other noncongregate family-based options may be possible. These may include host families, shared care arrangements, and voluntary foster care. One type of family-based alternative is placement in the home of a relative who is able to provide care. Support may be available for care by relatives through Medicaid Home and Community Based Waivers (discussed later). Although higher placement stability has been found in kinship settings for children removed because of neglect or maltreatment, problems such as higher rates of poverty and living in disadvantaged neighborhoods have been associated with kinship placements, particularly when the biological family faces those same disadvantages. Overall, kinship placements are considered to be more positive, with greater family and cultural connections,[50] although some studies indicate that more data are needed to better understand their

true benefits compared with other placements.[51,52]

Children with complex medical needs also can be placed with another family who can care for them through medical foster care or host home arrangements. Medical foster care is an option of care for children with special health care needs and disabilities to live with families who are specially trained to provide needed supports and services. This option is available in some but not all states.[53,54] Approaches have been developed to recruit, train, and support alternative families to be able to care for children with medical complexity in their homes as an alternative to congregate placement.[41–43] Many states offer family-based alternatives that include the use of host families, shared care, shared parenting, life sharing, and voluntary foster care. In these alternative care arrangements, the child's parents retain legal authority yet delegate the child's care to families who are trained and supported to care for children with special health care needs.[35] Forty-eight states report use of host family options.[55] An Internet search found that more than half of states offer out-of-home family-based alternatives to congregate care to children in their Medicaid waiver programs (discussed later). Texas, for example, offers host family homes funded by Medicaid Home and Community-Based Services waivers that parents of children living in nursing facilities can choose as a voluntary placement option, enabling family life for their child with their continued involvement or shared parenting arrangements. Availability of these host family options in Texas has contributed to the significant reduction of nursing facility use by children younger than 22 years since 2002.[56]

CURRENT STATE/POLICY IMPLICATIONS

The availability, flexibility, and capacity to develop robust plans rapidly to support children with complex medical needs in a family home vary by state and local community. The availability and type of services and supports are affected by decisions made at the state level on which services and supports to offer, how to fund programs, and eligibility for services. An additional complication is the coverage, or lack thereof, provided by private insurance companies.

Medicaid Home and Community-Based Services (HCBS, also commonly referred to as "waivers") funding exists in all states, although states vary in terms of the specific services they offer. HCBS is one of the most flexible types of funding to pay for services and can be used to access different community supports.[57] HCBS can be used to provide both in-home and out-of-home support. In-home supports can include respite, personal assistance, homemaker, and other specialist care. In some states, parents can become personal care assistants and be paid for the care they provide to their children.[58] HCBS also can be used for out-of-home supports such as respite, medical day-care programs, and living arrangements such as medical foster care and host homes.

Children with complex medical needs and developmental disabilities are often eligible for Medicaid, which must cover all necessary medical services for eligible children. For families with income levels too high for Medicaid, some states provide additional funding.[59] The Tax Equity and Fiscal Responsibility Act of 1982 State Plan Option allows states to provide Medicaid coverage to children and youth with severe disabilities who require care at a level provided in congregate care facilities but who receive care at home.[60] Most states also have a Medicaid Buy-In program, whereby

families may be eligible to pay relatively low premiums to obtain Medicaid coverage that can be used for services they otherwise would be unable to afford.[60] Despite these payment options, there continues to be a lack of adequate financial and staffing support for families of children with disabilities and medical complexity.

Families, providers, and their allies need to know the options that exist in their communities. Several resources are available in each state that can assist medical providers and families in obtaining information on care options, including Governors' Councils on Developmental Disabilities, state protection and advocacy organizations, and University Centers on Excellence in Developmental Disabilities. All states also have advocacy organizations, such as the Arc and Family Voices.

CONCLUSIONS

Family life with caring and loving caregivers should be the goal for every child with disabilities and medical complexity. Additional funding and resources are needed for community supports, and families require more care options for their children. Waitlists for services need to be shorter, with larger pools of home-based providers and more respite services for family caregivers. It should be a priority of the nation and states to improve policies and financing that promote services and supports for children and youth with disabilities and medical complexity to live in their own family homes or alternative family homes when that is not possible. Advocacy is needed to ensure that the option to live in a family home is available to all children with complex medical needs across this country. Community pediatricians should consider advocating for system changes that would lead to more comprehensive community

resources that promote home care for children and youth with severe intellectual and developmental disabilities and complex medical problems. For those children who are in more restrictive environments, there should be ongoing assessment of their needs and exploration of appropriate home-based services that may lead to discharge. Most important, all children and youth with significant disabilities and medical complexity should be cared for in safe environments that provide comprehensive supports to meet their medical and psychosocial needs.

ACKNOWLEDGMENTS

We acknowledge Alison Barkoff, JD, Director of Advocacy, Center for Public Representation, Bazelon Center for Mental Health Law; Amy Hewitt, PhD, Director Research and Training Center on Community Living, Institute on Community Integration, University of Minnesota; Andrew J. Imparato, Executive Director, Association of University Centers on Disabilities, and Nancy Rosenau, PhD, Immediate Past Executive Director, EveryChild Inc, for their contributions to this document.

LEAD AUTHORS

Sandra L. Friedman, MD, MPH, FAAP
Kenneth W. Norwood, Jr, MD, FAAP

COUNCIL ON CHILDREN WITH DISABILITIES EXECUTIVE COMMITTEE, 2015–2016

Kenneth W. Norwood, Jr, MD, FAAP, Chairperson
Richard C. Adams, MD, FAAP
Timothy J. Brei, MD, FAAP
Lynn F. Davidson, MD, FAAP
Beth Ellen Davis, MD, MPH, FAAP
Sandra L. Friedman, MD, MPH, FAAP
Amy J. Houtrow, MD, PhD, MPH, FAAP
Susan L. Hyman, MD, FAAP
Dennis Z. Kuo, MD, MHS, FAAP
Garey H. Noritz, MD, FAAP
Larry Yin, MD, MSPH, FAAP
Nancy A. Murphy, MD, FAAP, Immediate Past Chairperson
Miriam Kalichman, MD, FAAP, Immediate Past Member and 2014 Clinical Report Coauthor

LIAISONS

Peter J. Smith, MD, MA, FAAP – *Section on Developmental and Behavioral Pediatrics*

Georgina Peacock, MD, MPH, FAAP – *Centers for Disease Control and Prevention*

Marie Mann, MD, MPH, FAAP – *Maternal and Child Health Bureau*

Jennifer Bolden Pitre, MA, JD – *Family Voices*

STAFF

Stephanie Mucha, MPH

ABBREVIATIONS

AAP: American Academy of Pediatrics
HCBS: Home and Community-Based Services

REFERENCES

1. Friedman SL, Kalichman MA; Council on Children with Disabilities; Council on Children with Disabilities. Out-of-home placement for children and adolescents with disabilities. *Pediatrics.* 2014;134(4):836–846

2. Shonkoff JP, Garner AS; Committee on Psychosocial Aspects of Child and Family Health; Committee on Early Childhood, Adoption, and Dependent Care; Section on Developmental and Behavioral Pediatrics. The lifelong effects of early childhood adversity and toxic stress. *Pediatrics.* 2012;129(1). Available at: www.pediatrics.org/cgi/content/full/129/1/e232

3. Strickland B, McPherson M, Weissman G, van Dyck P, Huang ZJ, Newacheck P. Access to the medical home: results of the national survey of children with special health care needs. *Pediatrics.* 2004;113(suppl 5):1485–1492

4. The Developmental Disabilities Assistance and Bill of Rights Act. Pub L No. 106–402, 114 Stat 1677 (2000)

5. Americans With Disabilities Act. Pub L No. 101-336, 104 Stat 327 (1990)

6. Johnson CP, Kastner TA; American Academy of Pediatrics Committee/Section on Children With Disabilities. Helping families raise children with special health care needs at home. *Pediatrics.* 2005;115(2):507–511

7. Murphy NA, Carbone PS; American Academy of Pediatrics, Council on Children With Disabilities. Parent-provider-community partnerships: optimizing outcomes for children with disabilities. *Pediatrics.* 2011;128(4):795–802

8. Elias ER, Murphy NA; Council on Children with Disabilities. Home care of children and youth with complex health care needs and technology dependencies. *Pediatrics.* 2012;129(5):996–1005

9. Libby C, Imaizumi SO, eds; American Academy of Pediatrics, Section on Home Care. *Guidelines for Pediatric Home Health Care.* 2nd ed. Elk Grove Village, IL: American Academy of Pediatrics; 2009

10. The Anne E. Casey Foundation. *Every Kid Needs a Family: Giving Children in the Child Welfare System the Best Chance for Success.* May 19, 2015. Available at: www.aecf.org/resources/every-kid-needs-a-family/. Accessed June 15, 2016

11. Berens AE, Nelson CA. The science of early adversity: is there a role for large institutions in the care of vulnerable children? *Lancet.* 2015;386(9991):388–398

12. Nelson CA. A neurobiological perspective on early human deprivation. *Child Dev Perspect.* 2007;1(1):13–18

13. Nelson CA III, Zeanah CH, Fox NA, Marshall PJ, Smyke AT, Guthrie D. Cognitive recovery in socially deprived young children: the Bucharest Early Intervention Project. *Science.* 2007;318(5858):1937–1940

14. Carlson EA, Sampson MC, Sroufe LA. Implications of attachment theory and research for developmental-behavioral pediatrics. *J Dev Behav Pediatr.* 2003;24(5):364–379

15. *A. R. Ex Rel Root v Dudek,* Fla Dist Ct 31 F Supp 3d 1363 (2014)

16. Smyke AT, Dumitrescu A, Zeanah CH. Attachment disturbances in young children. I: The continuum of caretaking casualty. *J Am Acad Child Adolesc Psychiatry.* 2002;41(8):972–982

17. Center on the Developing Child at Harvard University. The science of neglect: The persistent absence of responsive care disrupts the developing brain (Working Paper 12). Available at: http://developingchild.harvard.edu/wp-content/uploads/2012/05/The-Science-of-Neglect-The-Persistent-Absence-of-Responsive-Care-Disrupts-the-Developing-Brain.pdf. Accessed June 15, 2016

18. Center on the Developing Child at Harvard University. The foundations of lifelong health are built in early childhood. Available at: http://developingchild.harvard.edu/wp-content/uploads/2010/05/Foundations-of-Lifelong-Health.pdf. Accessed June 15, 2016

19. Fan Y, Chen Q. Family functioning as a mediator between neighborhood conditions and children's health: evidence from a national survey in the United States. *Soc Sci Med.* 2012;74(12):1939–1947

20. Jutte DP, Miller JL, Erickson DJ. Neighborhood adversity, child health, and the role for community development. *Pediatrics.* 2015;135(suppl 2):S48–S57

21. Perry BD. Childhood experience and expression of genetic potential: what childhood neglect tells us about nature and nurture. *Brain Mind.* 2002;3(1):79–100

22. Jones L, Bellis MA, Wood S, et al. Prevalence and risk of violence against children with disabilities: a systematic review and meta-analysis of observational studies. *Lancet.* 2012;380(9845):899–907

23. Slayter E, Springer C. Child welfare-involved youth with intellectual disabilities: pathways into and placements in foster care. *Intellect Dev Disabil.* 2011;49(1):1–13

24. Wissink IB, van Vugt E, Moonen X, Stams GJ, Hendriks J. Sexual abuse involving children with an intellectual disability (ID): a narrative review. *Res Dev Disabil.* 2015;36:20–35

25. Euser S, Alink LR, Tharner A, van IJzendoorn MH, Bakermans-Kranenburg MJ. The prevalence of child sexual abuse in out-of-home care: increased risk for children with a mild intellectual disability. *J Appl Res Intellect Disabil.* 2016;29(1):83–92

26. Govindshenoy M, Spencer N. Abuse of the disabled child: a systematic review of population-based studies. *Child Care Health Dev.* 2007;33(5):552–558

27. Knox M, Parmenter TR, Atkinson N, Yazbeck M. Family control: the views of families who have a child with an intellectual disability. *J Appl Res Intellect Disabil.* 2000;13(1):17–28

28. Wang KW, Barnard A. Technology-dependent children and their families: a review. *J Adv Nurs.* 2004;45(1):36–46

29. Berry JG, Hall M, Dumas H, et al. Pediatric hospital discharges to home health and postacute facility care: a national study. *JAMA Pediatr.* 2016;170(4):326–333

30. Lindblad BM, Rasmussen BH, Sandman PO. Being invigorated in parenthood: parents' experiences of being supported by professionals when having a disabled child. *J Pediatr Nurs.* 2005;20(4):288–297

31. Steinhorn DM, Msall M, Keen M. A Successful Model for the Provision of Care to Medically Complex and Technology-dependent Children. February 14, 2015. Almost Home Kids. Available at: https://www.researchgate.net/publication/268048362_A_Successful_Model_for_the_Provision_of_Care_to_Medically_Complex_and_Technology-dependent_Children_Introduction_Summary. Accessed June 15, 2016

32. Helitzer DL, Cunningham-Sabo LD, VanLeit B, Crowe TK. Perceived changes in self-image and coping strategies of mothers of children with disabilities. *Occup Ther J Res.* 2002;22:25–33

33. Okumura MJ, Van Cleave J, Gnanasekaran S, Houtrow A. Understanding factors associated with work loss for families caring for CSHCN. *Pediatrics.* 2009;124(suppl 4):S392–S398

34. Case-Smith J. Parenting a child with a chronic medical condition. *Am J Occup Ther.* 2004;58(5):551–560

35. Caicedo C. Health and functioning of families of children with special health care needs cared for in home care, long-term care, and medical day care settings. *J Dev Behav Pediatr.* 2015;36(5):352–361

36. Murphy N, Caplin DA, Christian BJ, Luther BL, Holobkov R, Young PC. The function of parents and their children with cerebral palsy. *PM R.* 2011;3(2):98–104

37. Boudreau AA, Perrin JM, Goodman E, Kurowski D, Cooley WC, Kuhlthau K. Care coordination and unmet specialty care among children with special health care needs. *Pediatrics.* 2014;133(6):1046–1053

38. Mayer ML, Skinner AC, Slifkin RT; National Survey of Children With Special Health Care Needs. Unmet need for routine and specialty care: data from the national survey of children with special health care needs. *Pediatrics.* 2004;113(2). Available at: www.pediatrics.org/cgi/content/full/113/2/e109

39. Kuo DZ, Goudie A, Cohen E, et al. Inequities in health care needs for children with medical complexity. *Health Aff (Millwood).* 2014;33(12):2190–2198

40. Huang ZJ, Kogan MD, Yu SM, Strickland B. Delayed or forgone care among children with special health care needs: an analysis of the 2001 National Survey of Children With Special Health Care Needs. *Ambul Pediatr.* 2005;5(1):60–67

41. McDowell BC, Duffy C, Parkes J. Service use and family-centred care in young people with severe cerebral palsy: a population-based, cross-sectional clinical survey. *Disabil Rehabil.* 2015;37(25):2324–2329

42. Houtrow AJ, Okumura MJ, Hilton JF, Rehm RS. Profiling health and health-related services for children with special health care needs with and without disabilities. *Acad Pediatr.* 2011;11(6):508–516

43. Every Child Inc. Available at: www.everychildtexas.org. Accessed June 15, 2016

44. Rosenau N. Do we really mean families for all children? Permanency planning for children with developmental disabilities (Policy Research Brief). Minneapolis, MN: Institute on Community Integration, University of Minnesota; 2000;11(2). Available at: https://ici.umn.edu/products/prb/112/default.html. Accessed October 14, 2016

45. Bruns DA. Leaving home at an early age: parents' decisions about out-of-home placement for young children with complex medical needs. *Ment Retard.* 2000;38(1):50–60

46. Rosenau N, Sheppard L, Tucker E. Pathways to and from congregate care for children with developmental disabilities. Every Child Inc. October 27, 2010. Available at: http://everychildtexas.org/Pathwaystofrom41BD102.pdf. Accessed June 15, 2016

47. Cohen E, Kuo DZ, Agrawal R, et al. Children with medical complexity: an emerging population for clinical and research initiatives. *Pediatrics.* 2011;127(3):529–538

48. Glendinning C, Kirk S, Guiffrida A, Lawton D. Technology-dependent children in the community: definitions, numbers and costs. *Child Care Health Dev.* 2001;27(4):321–334

49. Ticha R, Anderson L, Hewitt A. *Analyses of National Core Indicators on Community Living and Support Options for Children With Intellectual and Developmental Disabilities With Significant Support Needs.* Minneapolis, MN: Research and Training Center on Community Living, University of Minnesota; 2015

50. Texas Department of Family and Protective Services. Kinship Care. Available at: https://www.dfps.state.tx.us/Adoption_and_Foster_Care/Kinship_Care/. Accessed October 21, 2016

51. Font SA. Is higher placement stability in kinship foster care by virtue or design? *Child Abuse Negl.* 2015;42:99–111

52. Winokur M, Holtan A, Batchelder KE. Kinship care for the safety, permanency, and well-being of children removed from the home for maltreatment. *Cochrane Database Syst Rev.* 2014;(1):CD006546

53. Diaz A, Edwards S, Neal WP, et al. Foster children with special needs: The Children's Aid Society experience. *Mt Sinai J Med.* 2004;71(3):166–169

54. Sharieff GQ, Hostetter S, Silva PD. Foster parents of medically fragile children can improve their BLS scores:

results of a demonstration project. *Pediatr Emerg Care.* 2001;17(2):93–95

55. Coucouvanis K, Prouty R, Charlie Lakin K. Own home and host family options growing rapidly as more than 70% of residential service recipients with ID/DD in 2004 live in settings of 6 or fewer. *Ment Retard.* 2005;43(4):307–309

56. Planning P, Report F-BA. As Required by S.B. 368, 77th Legislature, Regular Session, 2001. Texas Health and Human Services Commission. Available at: www.hhsc.state.tx.us/reports/2015/SB-368-Permanency-Planning-July-2015.pdf. Accessed June 16, 2016

57. Centers for Medicare and Medicaid Services. Fact sheet: summary of key provisions of the 1915(c) Home and Community Based Services (HCBS) waivers final rule (CMS2249 F/2296 F). Available at: https://www.cms.gov/Medicare-Medicaid-Coordination/Fraud-Prevention/Medicaid-Integrity-Education/Downloads/hcbs-tk1-gen-overview-factsheet.pdf. Accessed October 21, 2016

58. Niesz H, Martino P. States that allow family members to act as personal care assistants (OLR Research Report). February 21, 2003. Available at: www.cga.ct.gov/2003/rpt/2003-R-0040.htm. Accessed June 16, 2016

59. Catalyst Center. Your questions about the Medicaid Expansion Provision of the Affordable Care Act. Available at: http://southeastgenetics.org/aca/medicaid-expansionQA_0.pdf. Accessed October 21, 2016

60. National Disability Navigator Resource Collaborative. Fact Sheet 15: Medicaid Buy-In. Available at: www.nationaldisabilitynavigator.org/ndnrc-materials/fact-sheets/fact-sheet-15. Accessed June 16, 2016

Oxygen Targeting in Extremely Low Birth Weight Infants

• •

- *Clinical Report*

CLINICAL REPORT   Guidance for the Clinician in Rendering Pediatric Care

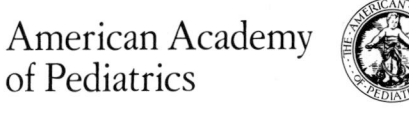

American Academy
of Pediatrics
DEDICATED TO THE HEALTH OF ALL CHILDREN™

Oxygen Targeting in Extremely Low Birth Weight Infants

James J. Cummings, MD, FAAP, Richard A. Polin, MD, FAAP, COMMITTEE ON FETUS AND NEWBORN

abstract

The use of supplemental oxygen plays a vital role in the care of the critically ill preterm infant, but the unrestricted use of oxygen can lead to unintended harms, such as chronic lung disease and retinopathy of prematurity. An overly restricted use of supplemental oxygen may have adverse effects as well. Ideally, continuous monitoring of tissue and cellular oxygen delivery would allow clinicians to better titrate the use of supplemental oxygen, but such monitoring is not currently feasible in the clinical setting. The introduction of pulse oximetry has greatly aided the clinician by providing a relatively easy and continuous estimate of arterial oxygen saturation, but pulse oximetry has several practical, technical, and physiologic limitations. Recent randomized clinical trials comparing different pulse oximetry targets have been conducted to better inform the practice of supplemental oxygen use. This clinical report discusses the benefits and limitations of pulse oximetry for assessing oxygenation, summarizes randomized clinical trials of oxygen saturation targeting, and addresses implications for practice.

Clinical reports from the American Academy of Pediatrics benefit from expertise and resources of liaisons and internal (AAP) and external reviewers. However, clinical reports from the American Academy of Pediatrics may not reflect the views of the liaisons or the organizations or government agencies that they represent.

The guidance in this report does not indicate an exclusive course of treatment or serve as a standard of medical care. Variations, taking into account individual circumstances, may be appropriate.

All clinical reports from the American Academy of Pediatrics automatically expire 5 years after publication unless reaffirmed, revised, or retired at or before that time.

DOI: 10.1542/peds.2016-1576

PEDIATRICS (ISSN Numbers: Print, 0031-4005; Online, 1098-4275).

INTRODUCTION

The discovery of oxygen is attributed to Polish scientist Michal Sędziwój in 1604, and a series of observations by John Mayow, Carl Wilhelm Scheele, and Joseph Priestley established the necessity of oxygen for life. In the early 1940s, Wilson et al[1] demonstrated that the use of 70% oxygen reduced periodic breathing in preterm infants. In 1949, investigators studying breathing irregularities in newborn infants recommended using 40% to 50% oxygen for all preterm infants immediately after birth for as long as 1 month.[2]

In 1951, two physicians, Kate Campbell in Melbourne, Australia, and Mary Crosse in Birmingham, England, suggested that unrestricted use of oxygen was associated with an increased risk of retrolental fibroplasia (now called retinopathy of prematurity [ROP]).[3,4] Several small clinical studies during the next few years confirmed this suggestion and recommended restricted use of supplemental oxygen.[5–9] In those studies, there was a trend toward increased mortality in the oxygen-restricted

To cite: Cummings JJ, Polin RA, AAP COMMITTEE ON FETUS AND NEWBORN. Oxygen Targeting in Extremely Low Birth Weight Infants. *Pediatrics.* 2016;138(2):e20161576

infants, although it did not reach statistical significance.[5-7,9] Therefore, restricted oxygen use in preterm infants gained general acceptance, despite estimates of 16 additional deaths for every case of blindness prevented.[10]

Because measurement of arterial oxygen tension was not yet feasible clinically, none of the earlier studies of oxygen supplementation and ROP were able to correlate measures of blood or tissue oxygenation with increased risk of ROP. In 1977, a large, 5-center, prospective observational study could not demonstrate a correlation between high partial pressure of oxygen in arterial blood (Pao_2) and ROP but did find a strong association of ROP with cumulative supplemental oxygen exposure.[11] In 1987, a small randomized study of transcutaneous oxygen monitoring in infants with a birth weight <1300 g found a significantly lower rate of ROP in infants who were managed with continuous oxygenation measures versus standard intermittent oxygenation assessment.[12]

In the ensuing decades, numerous observational studies have indicated that the incidence of ROP and bronchopulmonary dysplasia could be reduced by restricted use of oxygen. In 2007, the *Guidelines for Perinatal Care* recommended an oxygen saturation range of 85% to 95%.[13] Recently completed randomized trials using nearly identical trial designs have now provided additional evidence regarding the effects of varying saturation targets in the NICU. The present clinical report discusses the benefits and limitations of pulse oximetry for assessing oxygenation, summarizes randomized clinical trials of oxygen saturation targeting, and addresses implications for practice.

PULSE OXIMETRY: ITS USES AND LIMITATIONS IN MONITORING OXYGEN DELIVERY

Principles of Pulse Oximetry

Pulse oximeters measure the differential absorption of red and infrared light by oxyhemoglobin and deoxyhemoglobin. In neonates and young infants, light is transmitted through a distal extremity and sensed by a detector placed on the opposite side of the extremity. Pulsatile blood flow results in fluctuations in blood volume, thereby changing the distance the light has to travel. Detecting this variable component of light transmission allows pulse oximeters to eliminate signals attributable to nonarterial blood elements, such as venous blood, skin, connective tissue, muscle, and bone, directly measuring the relative amounts of oxyhemoglobin and deoxyhemoglobin in arterial blood and reporting saturation (Spo_2).

Limitations of Pulse Oximetry for Monitoring Tissue Oxygenation

Device Limitations

Accuracy. The accuracy of pulse oximetry is determined by comparison of Spo_2 with the measured saturation of arterial blood (Sao_2). Most manufacturers report an SD of the difference between Spo_2 and actual Sao_2 of 3 points for neonates. However, because 1 SD on each side of the mean includes approximately 68% of the measurements, nearly one-third of the measurements will fall outside that range. For example, an Spo_2 reading of 88% could reflect an actual Sao_2 between 85% and 91% in 68% of infants but may fall outside a range of 82% to 94% in up to 5% of infants.

The accuracy of pulse oximetry also depends on the range of saturations being measured. Reports of increased inaccuracy at the lower ranges of saturation values commonly encountered in the NICU are of great concern. For oximetry saturation readings in the 85% to 89% range, early studies reported that actual arterial saturations were as much as 10 points lower.[14,15] These findings have been confirmed in the most recently developed devices using signal extraction technology to reduce motion artifact; in 1 study, 39% of oximeter readings in the 85% to 89% range had arterial saturations below that range, with 25% of those readings having an actual Sao_2 <80%.[16] This finding is consistent with a previous observation that using an 85% to 89% Spo_2 range resulted in Pao_2 values much lower than expected.[17] In addition, pulse oximeters are only calibrated down to 80%; saturations below this level are extrapolated and may therefore be subject to even greater error.

Averaging Times. Pulse oximeters do not give instantaneous readings of Spo_2 because aberrant signals can make the device response erratic. Modern devices use time-averaging (typically, from 2–16 seconds) over several heartbeats to smooth out the displayed readings. In general, longer averaging times result in a more stable value with fewer false alarms; however, longer averaging times are also less sensitive to brief deviations in saturation outside the targeted range. Longer averaging times not only reduce the detection of desaturations that are either brief (<30 seconds) or marked (<70%) but also overestimate the duration of some detected events by combining 2 or more shorter events.[18,19] Shorter averaging time will detect more events but result in more false alarms. Studies have not been able to demonstrate that averaging times alter the amount of time actually spent outside targeted ranges. However, a particular concern is the potential for delayed detection of hypoxemic events.

Pulse Oximeter Algorithms. Pulse oximeters do not measure oxygen saturation directly but derive

Spo_2 from an internal reference table generated from empirical measurements of Sao_2 in healthy adult subjects. No pulse oximeter uses calibration data derived from Sao_2 measurements in critically ill patients or even in well infants. Although the effect of age on pulse oximeter accuracy has not been studied, at least 1 study has shown that in critically ill adult patients, changes in Spo_2 tend to overestimate actual changes in Sao_2, and this discrepancy worsened with decreasing hemoglobin concentrations.[20]

Relationship Between Sao_2 and Pao_2

Oxygen delivery depends on 2 factors: oxygen content of the arterial blood and blood flow. Oxygen content is determined by hemoglobin-oxygen saturation and, to a much lesser extent, by dissolved oxygen; both hemoglobin saturation and dissolved content depend on the prevailing Pao_2. Although the relationship between Sao_2 and Pao_2 is reasonably linear at Sao_2 values <80%, the slope of that relationship changes at Sao_2 levels >80%, resulting in large changes in Pao_2 with small changes in Sao_2. This relationship is even more exaggerated in the presence of hemoglobin F, which shifts the oxyhemoglobin dissociation curve to the left. Given that Spo_2 is, at best, an estimate of Sao_2, Spo_2 measurements become poor predictors of actual Pao_2 levels, particularly when the infant is receiving supplemental oxygen.

Fetal Versus Adult Hemoglobin

Absent a history of intrauterine transfusion, all extremely low birth weight neonates have high concentrations (>95%) of hemoglobin F in their blood. Hemoglobin F has a higher affinity for oxygen than does hemoglobin A and enhances tissue oxygen delivery at lower Sao_2 levels. As the amount of hemoglobin A relative to hemoglobin F increases in the blood (eg, after a red blood cell transfusion), this ability diminishes. Because the absorption spectrum for hemoglobin F is similar to hemoglobin A, there is no effect on the correlation between Spo_2 and Sao_2.

Clinical Variables Affecting Oxygen Saturation Targeting

Few studies have examined ways to best target a specific oxygen saturation range in preterm infants. Manually maintaining oxygen saturation targets in a given range depends on several factors, including: (1) technology (ie, setting Spo_2 alarm limits); (2) personnel (bedside nurses); and (3) the clinical stability of the patient. Although automated, closed-loop systems of oxygen delivery have been developed, they are not approved for clinical use in the United States.[21]

Alarm Limits

Alarm limits must be distinguished from targets. Targets represent the clinical goal, and alarm limits are used to achieve that goal. In clinical practice, alarm limits typically are set at or slightly beyond the target range. Some monitoring systems allow the use of "alerts" or "soft" alarms, which are less disruptive (being either visual, or at a lower volume or frequency) but warn that a parameter is about to reach an alarm limit. In these cases, the alerts are set within the targets, and the alarm limits may be set wider.

From a human engineering perspective, there are 2 problems with the setting of alarm limits. First, the majority of alarms do not require intervention. Most are either false (eg, a displaced probe or electrode) or are so brief that an intervention is not required. Second, the sheer number of alarms that go off in a busy NICU in a single day can total in the thousands, leading to desensitization. Both issues can lead to disregard of alarms, either deliberately or unintentionally; this condition has been termed "alarm fatigue" and is one reason why providers change alarm limits from those ordered. Clucas et al[22] observed that in infants weighing <1500 g, the lower alarm limit was set correctly 91% of the time, but the upper alarm limit was set correctly only 23% of the time. This differential compliance with low versus high alarms could be attributable to an increased tendency for the high alarm limit to be reached, the assumption that hypoxemia is more detrimental than hyperoxemia, and/or the fact that many monitors automatically reset to a high alarm limit of 100% when first turned on.[23]

A balance must be struck between setting alarm limits too narrow (increasing the number of unnecessary alarms) or too wide (decreasing the safety margin for intervention). Studies have shown that matching the alarm limits with the target range is associated with more time spent within the target range.[24,25]

Personnel

In the multicenter COT (Canadian Oxygen Trial), study participants were maintained within the intended Spo_2 range between 68% and 79% of the time. Nurses from one of the centers identified several factors as important in targeting a specific saturation range, including: (1) education; (2) prompt response times; and (3) a favorable nurse-to-patient ratio.[26] Targets in the Canadian trial were achieved significantly more often than in other randomized studies,[25,27] even though those studies also used educational interventions and process algorithms.[24,28] Even in studies in which favorable nurse-to-patient ratios were believed to exist, infants spent 33% to 38% of the time outside their target ranges.[20,25] Maintaining infants in a given target range is an extremely labor-intensive process, as evidenced by studies showing that multiple manual adjustments per hour only achieved target ranges approximately 50% of the time.[29] Using a fully automated oxygen-controlling system improved targeting by 7% over manual control.[30]

An additional concern is that manual documentation of hyperoxemic and hypoxemic episodes results in significant underreporting of such events.[31,32] Better tracking of saturation targeting can be accomplished by using third-party data extraction technology[33] or by using the histogram feature available on some monitoring equipment.[27,34]

Stability of the Saturation Signal in Clinical Settings

Preterm infants who require respiratory support are at increased risk of straying outside desired oxygen saturation targets, particularly if they are receiving supplemental oxygen. Because these infants often have desaturations during routine care (eg, repositioning, feeding, suctioning), it was once common practice to increase supplemental oxygen just before delivering such care (ie, preoxygenation). Preoxygenation also has been used commonly during intubation or other invasive procedures. Such practices may be harmful.[35] Instead, oxygen saturation values should be monitored closely, with measures to increase oxygenation used only as needed to maintain Spo_2 within the target range.

RANDOMIZED CLINICAL TRIALS OF OXYGEN TARGETING

The optimal saturation range for preterm infants in the NICU has remained elusive for more than 70 years. Although studies performed more than 50 years ago suggested an increased mortality associated with restricted oxygen administration,[36] observational trials performed in the era of continuous Spo_2

monitoring suggest that mortality is unchanged, with target Spo_2 ranges as low as 70%.[37] In addition, data from the Vermont Oxford Network indicate that the incidences of ROP and bronchopulmonary dysplasia are lower when a lower oxygen saturation range is targeted.[38] However, because these were observational studies, no cause-and-effect relationship can be inferred.

The first published randomized controlled trial (RCT) of differential targeting of oxygen saturations was the STOP-ROP (Supplemental Therapeutic Oxygen for Prethreshold Retinopathy of Prematurity) trial, published in 2000.[39] This study randomized infants to treatment when they reached "prethreshold" ROP, at an average postnatal age of 10 weeks. In this multicenter trial, 649 infants with prethreshold ROP were randomized to a saturation range of 89% to 94% (conventional arm) or 96% to 99% (supplemental arm). Progression to threshold ROP was not significantly different between groups in the total population; however, significant benefit was observed for infants in the high oxygen saturation arm who did not have "plus disease" (abnormal dilation and tortuosity of posterior pole blood vessels). On the negative side, infants in the high-oxygen saturation arm experienced an increased length of supplemental oxygen therapy and more often received diuretics at 50 weeks' postmenstrual age.

A second RCT that randomized infants to treatment at a later postnatal age was the BOOST (Benefits of Oxygen Saturation Targeting) trial (*N* = 358 infants), which hypothesized that maintaining higher oxygen saturation target ranges (95%–98% vs 93%–96%) would improve growth and neurodevelopmental outcomes.[40] The pulse oximeters in both groups were modified to read a targeted value in the range of 93% to 96%.

The study reported no benefit to the higher saturation range but did find, similar to the STOP-ROP trial, that infants in the high-saturation arm had significant increases in length of oxygen therapy, supplemental oxygen at 36 weeks' corrected gestation, and home oxygen.

In 2003, an international meeting of clinical trials experts, statisticians, neonatologists, ophthalmologists, and developmental pediatricians was convened to harmonize the planned RCTs of different target saturation ranges to be able to conduct a prospective individual patient meta-analysis of the data after completion of the follow-up phase of the individual trials (NeOProM [Neonatal Oxygenation Prospective Meta-analysis]).[41] Investigators from all 3 planned studies agreed, including SUPPORT (Surfactant Positive Airway Pressure and Pulse Oximetry Trial), sponsored by the *Eunice Kennedy Shriver* National Institute for Child Health and Human Development; the BOOST-II United Kingdom, Australia, and New Zealand study groups; and the COT trial. Although there were small differences in study design and outcome measures (Table 1), the studies were similar in terms of the population enrolled, methods, interventions tested, and outcomes collected. All studies were masked by the use of pulse oximeters that read 3% above or below the infant's actual saturation value within the 85% to 95% range. Outside the range of study saturation values ($\leq$84% and $\geq$96%), true saturation values were displayed. The primary outcome of the NeOProM study was a composite of death or disability at 18 to 24 months of corrected age. It was estimated that 5000 infants would be needed to detect a 4% difference in the rate of death or disability.[42]

The first of these 3 RCTs to be published was SUPPORT.[43] In this study, infants between 24[0/7] weeks' and 27[6/7] weeks' gestational age

TABLE 1 RCTs of Differing Pulse Oximetry Targets

Study	Primary Outcome	Primary Outcome Results	Other Findings
STOP-ROP[39]	Rate of progression to threshold ROP (89%–94% vs 96%–99%) $N = 649$	No significant differences	• Higher saturation range exhibited worsening of chronic lung disease and longer duration of hospitalization
BOOST[40]	Growth and developmental outcomes (91%–94% vs 95%–98%) $N = 358$	No significant differences	• Higher saturation range required oxygen for a longer period of time, dependence on oxygen at 36 wk postmenstrual age, and need for home oxygen
SUPPORT[43,44]	Death, severe ROP, or both (85%–89% vs 91%–95%) $N = 1316$	No significant differences	• Severe ROP significantly more common in the higher Sa_{O_2} range • Increased mortality in the lower Sa_{O_2} range at 18–22 mo of corrected age • No significant difference in the composite outcome of death or neurodevelopmental impairment at 18–22 mo
BOOST II[45–48]	Death or neurodevelopmental impairment at 18–22 mo of corrected for prematurity (85%–89% vs 91%–95%) $N = 2448$	No significant differences in a pooled analysis of all 3 trials[47] No significant difference in individual trial analyses[46,48] In a post hoc analysis combining 2 of the 3 trials, the primary outcome occurred in 492 (48.1%) of 1022 in the lower target group versus 437 (43.1%) of 1013 in the higher target group (RR, 1.11 [95% CI, 1.01–1.23]; $P = .023$)[46]	• Change in oximeter algorithm during the study • Study stopped before complete enrollment • Severe ROP significantly more common in the higher Sa_{O_2} range • Significantly increased necrotizing enterocolitis at the lower saturation range • Significantly increased mortality at hospital discharge in the lower Sa_{O_2} range with the revised oximeter algorithm
COT[49]	Death before a corrected age of 18 mo or survival with ≥1 of the following: gross motor disability, cognitive or language delay, severe hearing loss, and bilateral blindness (85%–89% vs 91%–95%) $N = 1201$	No significant differences	• Change in oximeter algorithm during the study • No difference in mortality • Targeting the lower saturation range reduced the postmenstrual age at last use of oxygen therapy

COT, Canadian Oxygen Trial; BOOST, Benefits of Oxygen Saturation Targeting; STOP, Supplemental Therapeutic Oxygen for Prethreshold Retinopathy of Prematurity; SUPPORT, Surfactant Positive Airway Pressure and Pulse Oximetry Trial.

($N = 1316$) were randomized to the 2 different oxygen saturation ranges (85%–89% or 91%–95%) and also to either CPAP or intubation and surfactant, in a factorial design. Oxygen saturation targeting was initiated within 2 hours of birth. The primary outcome was a composite of severe ROP (defined as the presence of threshold retinopathy, need for surgical intervention, or the use of bevacizumab), death before discharge from the hospital, or both. The oximeters in SUPPORT used an older software algorithm that subsequently was updated for the other RCTs.

The composite primary outcome in SUPPORT did not differ significantly between the lower and the higher oxygen saturation groups (28.3% vs 32.1%; relative risk [RR], 0.90; 95% confidence interval [CI], 0.76–1.06). However, death before discharge from the NICU was significantly different, occurring in 19.9% of infants in the lower oxygen saturation group and 16.2% of infants in the higher oxygen saturation group (RR, 1.27; 95% CI, 1.01–1.60), with a number-needed-to-harm of 27. In contrast, the rate of severe ROP among survivors was 8.6% in the lower saturation group versus 17.9% in the higher saturation group (RR, 0.52 [95% CI, 0.37–0.73]), with a number-needed-to-benefit of 11.

At 18 to 22 months of corrected age, death or neurodevelopmental impairment occurred in 30.2% of infants in the lower oxygen saturation group and 27.5% of those in the higher oxygen saturation group (RR, 1.12 [95% CI, 0.94–1.32]).[44] Mortality remained significantly higher in the lower oxygen saturation group (22.1% vs 18.2%; RR, 1.25 [95% CI, 1.00–1.25]). No significant differences were detected in neurodevelopmental impairment, cerebral palsy, or blindness.

The next RCT published was BOOST-II, from the United Kingdom, Australia, and New Zealand.[45] Oxygen saturation targeting began in the first

24 hours of life but not as early as in the SUPPORT study. During these trials, investigators in the United Kingdom found that the standard oximeters (Masimo Corporation, Irvine, California) returned an unexpectedly low number of oxygen saturation values between 87% and 90%. They discovered that there was a shift-up in the oximeter calibration curve that caused values between 87% and 90% to read 1% to 2% higher. A new software algorithm was expected to improve oxygen saturation targeting, although that was not tested. The United Kingdom and Australian investigators began using oximeters with the new software approximately halfway through the trial. However, the New Zealand trial oximeters were not modified, because enrollment had already been completed. Of 2448 infants enrolled in BOOST-II, 1187 (48.5%) were monitored with oximeters incorporating the new software.

Because of the increased mortality in the lower oxygen saturation range in SUPPORT, the BOOST-II Data Safety and Monitoring Board conducted a safety analysis in December 2010.[50] In the 1187 infants monitored with the revised algorithm, those assigned to the lower target range had a significantly increased mortality rate at 36 weeks' gestational age (23.1% vs 15.9%; RR, 1.45 [95% CI, 1.15–1.84]). However, among the entire study population (N = 2448), there was no significant difference. The rate of ROP requiring treatment was reduced in the lower saturation group (10.6% vs 13.5%; RR, 0.79 [95% CI, 0.63–1.00]), and the rate of necrotizing enterocolitis requiring surgery or causing death was increased in that group (10.4% vs 8.0%; RR, 1.32 [95% CI, 1.02–1.68]). The rate of bronchopulmonary dysplasia was unaffected. Although a recent report combining outcomes for 2 of the 3 BOOST-II sites found a significant difference in the composite outcome of death or disability by 2 years of age in a post hoc analysis,[46] a pooled analysis from all 3 BOOST-II sites, as originally planned, showed no significant difference in this outcome between the 2 arms (46.8% in the lower vs 43.4% in the higher saturation group; P = .10).[47]

Two-year outcomes for the COT were published.[49] The primary outcome measure for this study was the rate of death (before 18 months of age) or survival with 1 or more disabilities (gross motor disability, severe hearing loss, bilateral blindness, and cognitive or language delay). Infants were randomly assigned to the lower saturation group or higher saturation group in the first 24 hours of life. Similar to BOOST-II, the calibration software for the oximeter was changed at the midpoint in the study. The number of infants enrolled was 1201, of whom 538 were monitored with oximeters using the new software. There was no difference in the primary composite outcome (51.6% in the lower vs 49.7% in the higher saturation range). Mortality was 16.6% in the 85% to 89% group and 15.3% in the 91% to 95% group. Infants in the lower saturation group had a shorter duration of supplemental oxygen but no changes in any other outcomes. Use of the revised oximeter software had no effect on the primary outcome or mortality.

Saugstad and Aune[51] published a systematic review of the 5 oxygen saturation trials. In total, 4911 infants were enrolled in the studies. At the time of this meta-analysis (in 2014), the composite outcome of death or severe neurosensory disability at 18 to 24 months of age was only available for SUPPORT and COT, and there was no difference in that composite outcome between groups. The RR of mortality using the original software in the BOOST-II and COT trials was 1.04 (95% CI, 0.88–1.22). With the revised software (COT and BOOST-II United Kingdom and Australia), the RR of mortality in the lower saturation arm was 1.41 (95% CI, 1.14–1.74). For all 5 trials (SUPPORT; BOOST-II United Kingdom, Australia, and New Zealand; and COT), the risk of mortality was increased (RR, 1.18 [95% CI, 1.04–1.34]). Severe ROP was significantly reduced in the low saturation group (RR, 0.74 [95% CI, 0.59–0.92]), and the risk of necrotizing enterocolitis was increased (RR, 1.25 [95% CI, 1.05–1.49]). The rates of bronchopulmonary dysplasia, patent ductus arteriosus, and intraventricular hemorrhage grades 2 through 4 were not significantly different.

A more recent systematic review[52] of the 5 oxygen saturation trials concluded that although infants randomly assigned to the more liberal oxygen target ranges had higher survival rates (relative effect, 1.18 [95% CI, 1.03–1.36]) to discharge, the quality of evidence (assessed by using the Grading of Recommendations Assessment, Development and Evaluation approach[53]) for this estimate of effect was low for 1 or more of the following reasons: (1) the pulse oximeter algorithm was modified partway into the study; (2) the distribution of Spo_2 values did not achieve the planned degree of separation (the median Spo_2 in the 85% to 89% groups was >90%); (3) the BOOST-II trials were stopped prematurely on the basis of this outcome; and (4) the COT trial did not report on this outcome explicitly. In addition, although the investigators noted that necrotizing enterocolitis occurred less frequently in the higher saturation arms, there were no significant differences in bronchopulmonary dysplasia, ROP, hearing loss, or death or disability at 24 months of age.[52]

The mechanism(s) by which maintaining lower oxygen saturation levels might increase the risk of death is unclear, as the data from these trials suggest that tissue hypoxia was unlikely to be a factor.[23] In particular, in the SUPPORT trial, the proportion of infants with median oxygen saturations <85% was no different between the low and high saturation groups.[43] Conversely, a post hoc analysis from the SUPPORT trial found a disproportionally higher mortality rate in small-for-gestational-age infants in the lower oxygen saturation target group, suggesting a possible interaction[54]; if this observation can be confirmed in the other oxygen saturation trials, and more importantly in the individual patient analysis, it would suggest that small-for-gestational-age infants may be more vulnerable to lower oxygen saturations.

In the 5 RCTs discussed in this report, the degree to which individual infants may have been harmed or benefited by the oxygen saturation targets to which they were assigned is not clear.[55] Specifically, it would be helpful to know whether an individual infant's outcome correlated with the amount of time he or she spent within, above, or below the target oxygen saturation range. This information is particularly relevant to ROP because avoiding hypoxemic episodes may be as important as avoiding hyperoxemic episodes.[56–59] The preplanned individual patient meta-analysis of these trials (NeOProM) may shed some light on these critical questions.

CONCLUSIONS

Establishing a target range for oxygen saturation in infants of extremely low birth weight has both clinical and practical considerations, and the ideal target range remains an elusive goal. Nevertheless, data from several well-designed RCTs can inform practice. Pending additional data, including the individual patient meta-analysis (NeOProM), the following can be concluded:

1. The ideal physiologic target range for oxygen saturation for infants of extremely low birth weight is likely patient-specific and dynamic and depends on various factors, including gestational age, chronologic age, underlying disease, and transfusion status.

2. The ideal physiologic target range is a compromise among negative outcomes associated with either hyperoxemia (eg, ROP, bronchopulmonary dysplasia) or hypoxemia (eg, necrotizing enterocolitis, cerebral palsy, death). Recent RCTs suggest that a targeted oxygen saturation range of 90% to 95% may be safer than 85% to 89%, at least for some infants. However, the ideal oxygen saturation range for extremely low birth weight infants remains unknown.

3. Alarm limits are used to avoid potentially harmful extremes of hyperoxemia or hypoxemia. Given the limitations of pulse oximetry and the uncertainty that remains regarding the ideal oxygen saturation target range for infants of extremely low birth weight, these alarm limits could be fairly wide. Regardless of the chosen target, an upper alarm limit approximately 95% while the infant remains on supplemental oxygen is reasonable. A lower alarm limit will generally need to extend somewhat below the lower target, as it must take into account practical and clinical considerations, as well as the steepness of the oxygen saturation curve at lower saturations.

LEAD AUTHORS

James J. Cummings, MD, FAAP
Richard A. Polin, MD, FAAP

COMMITTEE ON FETUS AND NEWBORN, 2014–2015

Kristi L. Watterberg, MD, FAAP, Chairperson
Brenda Poindexter, MD, FAAP
James J. Cummings, MD, FAAP
William E. Benitz, MD, FAAP
Eric C. Eichenwald, MD, FAAP
Brenda B. Poindexter, MD, FAAP
Dan L. Stewart, MD, FAAP
Susan W. Aucott, MD, FAAP
Jay P. Goldsmith, MD, FAAP
Karen M. Puopolo, MD, PhD, FAAP
Kasper S. Wang, MD, FAAP

PAST COMMITTEE MEMBERS

Richard A. Polin, MD, FAAP
Waldemar A. Carlo, MD, FAAP

CONSULTANT

Waldemar A. Carlo, MD, FAAP

LIAISONS

Tonse N.K. Raju, MD, DCH, FAAP – *National Institutes of Health*
CAPT Wanda D. Barfield, MD, MPH, FAAP – *Centers for Disease Control and Prevention*
Erin L. Keels, APRN, MS, NNP-BC – *National Association of Neonatal Nurses*
Thierry Lacaze, MD – *Canadian Paediatric Society*
James Goldberg, MD – *American College of Obstetricians and Gynecologists*

STAFF

Jim R. Couto, MA

ABBREVIATIONS

CI: confidence interval
Pao_2: partial pressure of oxygen in arterial blood
ROP: retinopathy of prematurity
RR: relative risk
Sao_2: measured saturation of arterial blood
Spo_2: pulse oxygen saturation

FINANCIAL DISCLOSURE: The authors have indicated they do not have a financial relationship relevant to this article to disclose.

FUNDING: No external funding.

POTENTIAL CONFLICTS OF INTEREST: Dr Cummings is a consultant for ONY, Inc and Windtree Therapeutics (formerly Discovery Laboratories). Dr Polin is a consultant for Windtree Therapeutics and Fisher & Paykel.

REFERENCES

1. Wilson J, Long S, Howard P. Respiration of premature infants: response to variations of oxygen and to increased carbon dioxide in inspired air. *Am J Dis Child.* 1942;63(6):1080–1085

2. Howard PJ, Bauer AR. Irregularities of breathing in the newborn period. *Am J Dis Child.* 1949;77(5):592–609

3. Campbell K. Intensive oxygen therapy as a possible cause of retrolental fibroplasia; a clinical approach. *Med J Aust.* 1951;2(2):48–50

4. Crosse V. The problem of retrolental fibroplasia in the city of Birmingham. *Trans Ophthalmol Soc U K.* 1951;71:609–612

5. Lanman JT, Guy LP, Dancis J. Retrolental fibroplasia and oxygen therapy. *J Am Med Assoc.* 1954;155(3):223–226

6. Engle MA, Baker DH, Baras I, Freemond A, Laupus WE, Norton EW. Oxygen administration and retrolental fibroplasia. *AMA Am J Dis Child.* 1955;89(4):399–413

7. Kinsey VE. Retrolental fibroplasia; cooperative study of retrolental fibroplasia and the use of oxygen. *AMA Arch Opthalmol.* 1956;56(4):481–543

8. Patz A, Hoeck LE, De La Cruz E. Studies on the effect of high oxygen administration in retrolental fibroplasia. I. Nursery observations. *Am J Ophthalmol.* 1952;35(9):1248–1253

9. Weintraub DH, Tabankin A. Relationship of retrolental fibroplasia to oxygen concentration. *J Pediatr.* 1956;49(1):75–79

10. Bolton DP, Cross KW. Further observations on cost of preventing retrolental fibroplasia. *Lancet.* 1974;1(7855):445–448

11. Kinsey VE, Arnold HJ, Kalina RE, et al. PaO2 levels and retrolental fibroplasia: a report of the cooperative study. *Pediatrics.* 1977;60(5):655–668

12. Bancalari E, Flynn J, Goldberg RN, et al. Transcutaneous oxygen monitoring and retinopathy of prematurity. *Adv Exp Med Biol.* 1987;220:109–113

13. American Academy of Pediatrics and the American College of Obstetricians and Gynecologists. *Guidelines for Perinatal Care.* 6th ed. Elk Grove Village, IL: American Academy of Pediatrics; 2007

14. Brockway J, Hay WW Jr. Prediction of arterial partial pressure of oxygen with pulse oxygen saturation measurements. *J Pediatr.* 1998;133(1):63–66

15. Workie FA, Rais-Bahrami K, Short BL. Clinical use of new-generation pulse oximeters in the neonatal intensive care unit. *Am J Perinatol.* 2005;22(7):357–360

16. Rosychuk RJ, Hudson-Mason A, Eklund D, Lacaze-Masmonteil T. Discrepancies between arterial oxygen saturation and functional oxygen saturation measured with pulse oximetry in very preterm infants. *Neonatology.* 2012;101(1):14–19

17. Quine D, Stenson BJ. Arterial oxygen tension (Pao2) values in infants <29 weeks of gestation at currently targeted saturations. *Arch Dis Child Fetal Neonatal Ed.* 2009;94(1):F51–F53

18. Ahmed SJ, Rich W, Finer NN. The effect of averaging time on oximetry values in the premature infant. *Pediatrics.* 2010;125(1). Available at: www.pediatrics.org/cgi/content/full/125/1/e115

19. Vagedes J, Poets CF, Dietz K. Averaging time, desaturation level, duration and extent. *Arch Dis Child Fetal Neonatal Ed.* 2013;98(3):F265–F266

20. Perkins GD, McAuley DF, Giles S, Routledge H, Gao F. Do changes in pulse oximeter oxygen saturation predict equivalent changes in arterial oxygen saturation? *Crit Care.* 2003;7(4):R67

21. Claure N, Bancalari E. Automated closed loop control of inspired oxygen concentration. *Respir Care.* 2013;58(1):151–161

22. Clucas L, Doyle LW, Dawson J, Donath S, Davis PG. Compliance with alarm limits for pulse oximetry in very preterm infants. *Pediatrics.* 2007;119(6):1056–1060

23. Sola A, Golombek SG, Montes Bueno MT, et al. Safe oxygen saturation targeting and monitoring in preterm infants: can we avoid hypoxia and hyperoxia? *Acta Paediatr.* 2014;103(10):1009–1018

24. Clarke A, Yeomans E, Elsayed K, et al. A randomised crossover trial of clinical algorithm for oxygen saturation targeting in preterm infants with frequent desaturation episodes. *Neonatology.* 2015;107(2):130–136

25. Hagadorn JI, Furey AM, Nghiem TH, et al; AVIOx Study Group. Achieved versus intended pulse oximeter saturation in infants born less than 28 weeks' gestation: the AVIOx study. *Pediatrics.* 2006;118(4):1574–1582

26. Armbruster J, Schmidt B, Poets CF, Bassler D. Nurses' compliance with alarm limits for pulse oximetry: qualitative study. *J Perinatol.* 2010;30(8):531–534

27. Lim K, Wheeler KI, Gale TJ, et al. Oxygen saturation targeting in preterm infants receiving continuous positive airway pressure. *J Pediatr.* 2014;164(4):730–736.e1

28. Ford SP, Leick-Rude MK, Meinert KA, et al. Overcoming barriers to oxygen saturation targeting. *Pediatrics.* 2006;118(suppl 2):S177–S186

29. van der Eijk AC, Dankelman J, Schutte S, Simonsz HJ, Smit BJ. An observational study to quantify manual adjustments of the inspired oxygen fraction in extremely low birth weight infants. *Acta Paediatr.* 2012;101(3):e97–e104

30. Waitz M, Schmid MB, Fuchs H, Mendler MR, Dreyhaupt J, Hummler HD. Effects of automated adjustment of the inspired oxygen on fluctuations of arterial and regional cerebral tissue oxygenation in preterm infants with frequent desaturations. *J Pediatr.* 2015;166(2):240–244.e1

31. Brockmann PE, Wiechers C, Pantalitschka T, Diebold J, Vagedes J, Poets CF. Under-recognition of

alarms in a neonatal intensive care unit. *Arch Dis Child Fetal Neonatal Ed.* 2013;98(6):F524–F527

32. Ruiz TL, Trzaski JM, Sink DW, Hagadorn JI. Transcribed oxygen saturation vs oximeter recordings in very low birth weight infants. *J Perinatol.* 2014;34(2):130–135

33. Cirelli J, McGregor C, Graydon B, James A. Analysis of continuous oxygen saturation data for accurate representation of retinal exposure to oxygen in the preterm infant. *Stud Health Technol Inform.* 2013;183:126–131

34. Bizzarro MJ, Li FY, Katz K, Shabanova V, Ehrenkranz RA, Bhandari V. Temporal quantification of oxygen saturation ranges: an effort to reduce hyperoxia in the neonatal intensive care unit. *J Perinatol.* 2014;34(1):33–38

35. Sola A, Saldeño YP, Favareto V. Clinical practices in neonatal oxygenation: where have we failed? What can we do? *J Perinatol.* 2008;28(suppl 1):S28–S34

36. Askie LM, Henderson-Smart DJ, Ko H. Restricted versus liberal oxygen exposure for preventing morbidity and mortality in preterm or low birth weight infants. *Cochrane Database Syst Rev.* 2009;(1):CD001077

37. Tin W, Milligan DW, Pennefather P, Hey E. Pulse oximetry, severe retinopathy, and outcome at one year in babies of less than 28 weeks gestation. *Arch Dis Child Fetal Neonatal Ed.* 2001;84(2):F106–F110

38. Payne NR, LaCorte M, Karna P, et al; Breathsavers Group, Vermont Oxford Network Neonatal Intensive Care Quality Improvement Collaborative. Reduction of bronchopulmonary dysplasia after participation in the Breathsavers Group of the Vermont Oxford Network Neonatal Intensive Care Quality Improvement Collaborative. *Pediatrics.* 2006;118(suppl 2):S73–S77

39. The STOP-ROP Multicenter Study Group. Supplemental Therapeutic Oxygen for Prethreshold Retinopathy of Prematurity (STOP-ROP), a randomized, controlled trial. I: primary outcomes. *Pediatrics.* 2000;105(2):295–310

40. Askie LM, Henderson-Smart DJ, Irwig L, Simpson JM. Oxygen-saturation targets and outcomes in extremely preterm infants. *N Engl J Med.* 2003;349(10):959–967

41. Cole CH, Wright KW, Tarnow-Mordi W, Phelps DL; Pulse Oximetry Saturation Trial for Prevention of Retinopathy of Prematurity Planning Study Group. Resolving our uncertainty about oxygen therapy. *Pediatrics.* 2003;112(6 pt 1):1415–1419

42. Askie LM, Brocklehurst P, Darlow BA, Finer N, Schmidt B, Tarnow-Mordi W; NeOProM Collaborative Group. NeOProM: Neonatal Oxygenation Prospective Meta-analysis Collaboration study protocol. *BMC Pediatr.* 2011;11(6):6

43. Carlo WA, Finer NN, Walsh MC, et al; SUPPORT Study Group of the Eunice Kennedy Shriver NICHD Neonatal Research Network. Target ranges of oxygen saturation in extremely preterm infants. *N Engl J Med.* 2010;362(21):1959–1969

44. Vaucher YE, Peralta-Carcelen M, Finer NN, et al; SUPPORT Study Group of the Eunice Kennedy Shriver NICHD Neonatal Research Network. Neurodevelopmental outcomes in the early CPAP and pulse oximetry trial. *N Engl J Med.* 2012;367(26):2495–2504

45. Stenson BJ, Tarnow-Mordi WO, Darlow BA, et al; BOOST II United Kingdom Collaborative Group; BOOST II Australia Collaborative Group; BOOST II New Zealand Collaborative Group. Oxygen saturation and outcomes in preterm infants. *N Engl J Med.* 2013;368(22):2094–2104

46. Tarnow-Mordi W, Stenson B, Kirby A, et al; BOOST-II Australia and United Kingdom Collaborative Groups. Outcomes of two trials of oxygen-saturation targets in preterm infants. *N Engl J Med.* 2016;374(8):749–760

47. Cummings JJ, Lakshminrusimha S, Polin RA. The BOOST trials and the pitfalls of post hoc analyses. *N Engl J Med.* 2016, In press

48. Darlow BA, Marschner SL, Donoghoe M, et al Randomized controlled trial of oxygen saturation targets in very preterm infants: two year outcomes. *J Pediatr.* 2014;165(1):30–35.e2

49. Schmidt B, Whyte RK, Asztalos EV, et al; Canadian Oxygen Trial (COT) Group. Effects of targeting higher vs lower arterial oxygen saturations on death or disability in extremely preterm infants: a randomized clinical trial. *JAMA.* 2013;309(20):2111–2120

50. Stenson B, Brocklehurst P, Tarnow-Mordi W; UK BOOST II trial; Australian BOOST II trial; New Zealand BOOST II trial. Increased 36-week survival with high oxygen saturation target in extremely preterm infants. *N Engl J Med.* 2011;364(17):1680–1682

51. Saugstad OD, Aune D. Optimal oxygenation of extremely low birth weight infants: a meta-analysis and systematic review of the oxygen saturation target studies. *Neonatology.* 2014;105(1):55–63

52. Manja V, Lakshminrusimha S, Cook DJ. Oxygen saturation target range for extremely preterm infants: a systematic review and meta-analysis. *JAMA Pediatr.* 2015;169(4):332–340

53. Guyatt GH, Oxman AD, Schünemann HJ, Tugwell P, Knottnerus A. GRADE guidelines: a new series of articles in the Journal of Clinical Epidemiology. *J Clin Epidemiol.* 2011;64(4):380–382

54. Walsh MC, Di Fiore JM, Martin RJ, Gantz M, Carlo WA, Finer N. Association of oxygen target and growth status with increased mortality in small for gestational age infants: further analysis of the Surfactant, Positive Pressure and Pulse Oximetry Randomized Trial. *JAMA Pediatr.* 2016;170(3):292–294

55. Bateman D, Polin RA. A lower oxygen-saturation target decreases retinopathy of prematurity but increases mortality in premature infants. *J Pediatr.* 2013;163(5):1528–1529

56. Thomas WJ, Rauser M, Dovich JA, Dustin L, Flaxel CJ. Oxygen saturation in premature infants at risk for threshold retinopathy of prematurity. *Eur J Ophthalmol.* 2011;21(2):189–193

57. Di Fiore JM, Bloom JN, Orge F, et al. A higher incidence of intermittent hypoxemic episodes is associated with severe retinopathy of prematurity. *J Pediatr.* 2010;157(1):69–73

58. Kaufman DA, Zanelli SA, Gurka MJ, Davis M, Richards CP, Walsh BK. Time outside targeted oxygen saturation range and retinopathy of prematurity. *Early Hum Dev.* 2014;90(suppl 2):S35–S40

59. York JR, Landers S, Kirby RS, Arbogast PG, Penn JS. Arterial oxygen fluctuation and retinopathy of prematurity in very-low-birth-weight infants. *J Perinatol.* 2004;24(2):82–87

ERRATA

Errors occurred in the article by Cummings et al, titled "Oxygen Targeting in Extremely Low Birth Weight Infants" published in the August 2016 issue of *Pediatrics* (2016;138(2):e20161576; doi:10.1542/peds.2016-1576).

On page e6, under the section heading Randomized Clinical Trials of Oxygen Targeting, in paragraph 8, on lines 30-32, this reads: "a pooled analysis from all 3 BOOST-II sites, as originally planned, showed no significant difference in this outcome." This should have read: "a pooled analysis from all 3 BOOST-II sites showed no significant difference in this outcome."

On page e9, under References, reference # 47 reads: "Cummings JJ, Lakshminrusimha S, Polin RA. The BOOST trials and the pitfalls of post hoc analyses. *N Engl J Med* 2016, in press." This has been updated and should now read: "Cummings JJ, Lakshminrusimha S, Polin RA. Oxygen saturation targets in preterm infants [Letter to the Editor]. Reply: Tarnow-Mordi WO, Stenson B, Kirby A. *N Engl J Med* 2016;375(2):186-188."

doi:10.1542/peds.2016-2904

Parental Presence During Treatment of Ebola or Other Highly Consequential Infection

• •

- *Clinical Report*

CLINICAL REPORT   Guidance for the Clinician in Rendering Pediatric Care

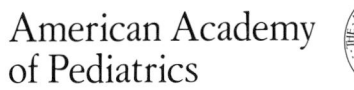
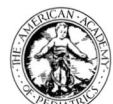

American Academy
of Pediatrics

DEDICATED TO THE HEALTH OF ALL CHILDREN™

Parental Presence During Treatment of Ebola or Other Highly Consequential Infection

H. Dele Davies, MD, MS, MHCM, FAAP, Carrie L. Byington, MD, FAAP, COMMITTEE ON INFECTIOUS DISEASES

abstract

This clinical report offers guidance to health care providers and hospitals on options to consider regarding parental presence at the bedside while caring for a child with suspected or proven Ebola virus disease (Ebola) or other highly consequential infection. Options are presented to help meet the needs of the patient and the family while also posing the least risk to providers and health care organizations. The optimal way to minimize risk is to limit contact between the person under investigation or treatment and family members/caregivers whenever possible while working to meet the emotional support needs of both patient and family. At times, caregiver presence may be deemed to be in the best interest of the patient, and in such situations, a strong effort should be made to limit potential risks of exposure to the caregiver, health care providers, and the community. The decision to allow parental/caregiver presence should be made in consultation with a team including an infectious diseases expert and state and/or local public health authorities and should involve consideration of many factors, depending on the stage of investigation and management, including (1) a careful history, physical examination, and investigations to elucidate the likelihood of the diagnosis of Ebola or other highly consequential infection; (2) ability of the facility to offer appropriate isolation for the person under investigation and family members and to manage Ebola; (3) ability to recognize and exclude people at increased risk of worse outcomes (eg, pregnant women); and (4) ability of parent/caregiver to follow instructions, including appropriate donning and doffing of personal protective equipment.

Clinical reports from the American Academy of Pediatrics benefit from expertise and resources of liaisons and internal (AAP) and external reviewers. However, clinical reports from the American Academy of Pediatrics may not reflect the views of the liaisons or the organizations or government agencies that they represent.

The guidance in this report does not indicate an exclusive course of treatment or serve as a standard of medical care. Variations, taking into account individual circumstances, may be appropriate.

All clinical reports from the American Academy of Pediatrics automatically expire 5 years after publication unless reaffirmed, revised, or retired at or before that time.

DOI: 10.1542/peds.2016-1891

PEDIATRICS (ISSN Numbers: Print, 0031-4005; Online, 1098-4275).

Copyright © 2016 by the American Academy of Pediatrics

FINANCIAL DISCLOSURE: The authors have indicated they do not have a financial relationship relevant to this article to disclose.

FUNDING: No external funding.

POTENTIAL CONFLICT OF INTEREST: The authors have indicated they have no potential conflicts of interest to disclose.

To cite: Davies HD, Byington CL, AAP COMMITTEE ON INFECTIOUS DISEASES. Parental Presence During Treatment of Ebola or Other Highly Consequential Infection. *Pediatrics.* 2016;138(3):e20161891

BACKGROUND

During the peak of the Ebola virus disease (Ebola) outbreak in West Africa, the American Academy of Pediatrics (AAP) held regular weekly conference calls with the Centers for Disease Control and Prevention

(CDC) to identify issues of concern to health care practitioners and to address them using the best available information. One of the most frequently asked questions was how to handle parental or legal guardian presence in the setting of a child with suspected or confirmed Ebola. As a result, consultations were held with infectious diseases and infection-control experts who had already handled suspected cases in the United States, and the literature was reviewed for the best possible guidance. Bioethicists and family-centered care experts also were consulted. It was clear that there was not a single approach that was uniformly viewed as creating the greatest safety for health care providers, while also fully taking into consideration the ongoing social and emotional needs of the child and his or her parents or legal guardians. Given the strong ongoing requests for such guidance, the AAP developed this clinical report to offer guidance to health care providers and hospitals regarding options to consider that could meet the needs of the patient and the family while also posing the least risk to providers and health care organizations. Although this guidance is based primarily on the opinions of experts, the principles proposed are ones that have been vetted carefully and represent consensus intended to enable health care providers and health systems and organizations that care for children to consider these important issues in their preparedness plans before the arrival of any child suspected of having Ebola or similar highly consequential infectious diseases. Because sufficient data do not yet exist to create an evidence-based policy, as data accumulate both in the United States and worldwide on the appropriate care for children with Ebola, this consensus guidance will be reevaluated.

> **Goal:** To provide guidance for health care providers and health care organizations to consider when determining the extent of legal guardian presence at the bedside of a child with suspected or confirmed Ebola virus disease (Ebola).
>
> **Intended Audience:** Pediatric health care providers, transport teams providing care to children, and hospital and ambulatory care centers providing care to children.
>
> **Definition of a caregiver for this guidance:** Parent or legal guardian; in the event a parent or legal guardian cannot be present at the bedside, an alternate adult caregiver (such as a relative) may be designated.

Advance preparedness planning can mitigate risk, reduce material and operational losses, improve financial stability, strengthen the medical home, and help promote the health of children in the community.[1] Children need psychosocial support and comfort from their caregivers in times of extreme stress.[2-5] Pediatric health care providers generally support parental or legal guardian presence during prehospital and interhospital transport by emergency medical services personnel, emergency care, inpatient care, invasive medical procedures, and resuscitation attempts. However, adaptations and limitations may apply to this approach when a child is suspected or confirmed to have Ebola or another similarly transmitted disease of high consequence.

Because of the risk to other family members,[6] it is preferable to minimize contact between the patient under investigation and family members whenever possible, while working to meet the emotional support needs of both patient and family.[7] There may be times when caregiver presence may be deemed to be in the best interest of the patient. Efforts made surrounding caregiver presence with a child that is suspected or confirmed to have Ebola or another similarly transmitted disease of high consequence must limit potential risks of exposure to the caregiver, health care providers, and the community.[8,9] Although there are limited evidence-based criteria to inform practice, factors that should be considered when determining the extent and conditions of caregiver presence are discussed in the following sections.

CAREGIVER PRESENCE DURING INITIAL EVALUATION OF A SYMPTOMATIC CHILD

(Example: initial presentation to an ambulatory care center or hospital emergency department)

During initial presentation to a health care provider, caregivers will likely accompany the child. Health care providers, in consultation with state and/or local public health authorities, will need to evaluate the child to determine whether the child is

- a "person under investigation" (PUI) (with a plan to test for Ebola)[10] or

- not a PUI (with no plan to test for Ebola).

While this initial evaluation of the child is being conducted, the following guidance should be considered:

- All people accompanying the child must be evaluated to determine whether they are at risk of Ebola (or another disease in question)[11] and symptomatic. If these people refuse evaluation, public health authorities should be contacted promptly. If they are both at risk of and symptomatic of illness, the facility should offer isolation for the adult(s) and activate their adult care protocols. If these adults refuse isolation and care, public health authorities should be notified immediately.

- Discuss with any female caregivers of child-bearing age whether they potentially could be pregnant (consider pregnancy test) because of the increased risk of severe illness and death as well as fetal loss and pregnancy-associated hemorrhage.[12,13] If a caregiver could be pregnant, consider removing her from the isolation room because of the increased risks to her and her fetus if she were to contract Ebola.

- All adult caregivers accompanying the child who are asymptomatic should be placed in appropriate personal protective equipment (PPE)[14] and roomed with the child until determination of the child's status (PUI versus not a PUI) is made.[10]

- If the child is not a PUI, then the health care facility should treat the child and caregivers according to standard procedure. If the child is a PUI, then the child may be evaluated in the hospital emergency department per protocol. At this time, family contact with the PUI should be limited to 1 parent or legal guardian wearing appropriate PPE. All other family members (beyond the 1 parent who is wearing appropriate PPE) or others accompanying the index patient should wait in a separate area pending determination by public health and/or the local infection-control expert. These experts also will determine the need for any specific infection-control actions toward the accompanying people or other contacts of the index patient.

Siblings and other children:

- If a sibling or another child who arrived with the family is determined to be at risk of Ebola or other illness in question,[15] and the child is symptomatic, that child should also be medically

evaluated. Cohorting of siblings is not permissible if there is any uncertainty that both have the same illness.

Alternate arrangements should be made for the care of all asymptomatic siblings or other children accompanying the family. Siblings or other children who cannot wear the appropriate PPE (because of size, developmental level, etc) should wait in a separate room with supervision while alternate arrangements are made. The latter scenario would be the expected one for children in most situations.

CAREGIVER PRESENCE DURING INPATIENT CARE OF A CHILD WHO IS A PUI OR CONFIRMED CASE

Making the decision to allow caregiver presence:

- Consider the ability of your hospital to care for an Ebola patient (is your hospital designated by the CDC as a frontline, assessment, or treatment center?) and follow the CDC guidelines for your level of institution[16] to determine whether the patient should be retained at your institution.

- A care team conference should be convened immediately to make the decision. Care members should include the attending physician, nursing staff designee, and hospital administrative designee. The care team might also benefit from the inclusion of a medical director of infection control or designee, an ethics committee designee, a child life designee, a designee from the local/state department of public health, and the parent or caregiver. If possible, the care team conference should be convened before arrival of the patient if there is sufficient warning and knowledge of who is accompanying him or her.

- Consider the child's age, developmental level, acuity, and ability to follow directions and cooperate with caregivers.

- Consider available hospital resources to care for both the child and the caregiver in the event the caregiver must be quarantined or isolated. Consider available hospital resources (eg, PPE supply, staffing to train and observe the caregiver in donning and doffing PPE, etc) to support caregiver presence at the bedside or to provide parental support via videoconferencing or other technology that enables the ability to monitor from outside the room. The abilities of the caregiver to don and doff PPE safely, tolerate wearing PPE, and comply with all infection-control policies are also important considerations. Institutional and local public health policies for quarantine and restrictions should also be reviewed and considered.

- Consider whether the caregiver has health considerations that may increase the risk of illness or complicate the use of PPE. A pregnant caregiver should not stay with a child who is a PUI or a confirmed case because of the very high risk of death for an Ebola-infected pregnant woman and her fetus.[13]

- Consider the impact to other children if the caregiver is the sole provider for other children in the family.

- Consider the risk to health care providers and other patients and their families/visitors.

ACTION TOWARD THE SAFETY OF THE CAREGIVER IN SUSPECTED OR PROVEN EBOLA

Options for implementation:

- Consider the following options once an assessment of age, development level, risk of transmission, and acuity of the child are determined:

  o Option 1: Caregiver remains in a separate room with videoconferencing capability with which to interact with the child and be (remotely) involved in the child's care.[7,17,18]

o Option 2: Caregiver remains at the bedside if able to show proficiency with PPE and staff is available to observe doffing and donning, as often as allowed by PPE tolerance and hospital guidelines, following the recommendations described previously.

o Option 3 (combined): Caregiver primarily spends time in a separate room with videoconferencing capability and joins the child at the bedside intermittently.

If options 2 or 3 are chosen:

• Only 1 caregiver should be designated to provide bedside support and comfort to the child for the course of the illness. The caregiver must be informed of the potential risks associated with close contact with a symptomatic child. Informed consent must be obtained and documented, in which the caregiver acknowledges the risks and consents to enter the child's room.

o Although families may find it exceedingly difficult to designate a single bedside caregiver, this recommendation is based on infection-control guidance,[19] resource and staffing considerations, and minimizing the number of individuals (caregivers and health care staff) placed at risk of illness.

o Additional caregivers may remain engaged with the child through the use of videoconferencing.[18]

• The caregiver must agree to and be willing to comply with CDC guidance for monitoring and movement of exposed individuals[20] and the recommendations of the local state/county health department.

• The caregiver must agree to comply at all times with directions from hospital personnel, including leaving the bedside

if it is determined to be in the best interest of the patient or the caregiver.

• Caregiver visits should be scheduled and controlled to allow for the following:

o Screening for Ebola or other illness (eg, fever and other symptoms) before entering or upon arrival to the hospital. The caregiver must not be experiencing symptoms compatible with the illness in question. The state and/or local public health department and responsible health care provider should be involved in determining the procedure for surveillance and monitoring of the caregiver while he or she is both inside and outside the room.

o Evaluating the risk to the health of the caregiver and his or her ability to comply fully with infection-control precautions.

o Providing instruction daily, before entry into the patient care area, on hand hygiene, limiting surfaces touched, and the use of PPE according to the current facility policy while in the patient's room.

o Compliance with policies intended to reduce potential exposure to caregivers and other hospital staff, patients and visitors, and the community.

• The caregiver must be able to and agree to follow CDC recommendations for safely donning and doffing PPE,[19] must be trained in proper procedure, and must be observed and assisted during the donning and doffing processes by hospital infection-control personnel.

• The caregiver must wear CDC-recommended PPE before entering the room and during all contact with the child. This must be, at a minimum, the same level of CDC-recommended PPE worn by

health care workers caring for the child. Higher-level PPE may be considered for the parent or caregiver if it allows for increased comfort over prolonged periods (airflow) or improves the child's ability to interact with parent (full clear face shield).

• The caregiver should limit his or her exposure to blood and body fluids while at the child's bedside. The caregiver should not change the child's diaper, assist with personal hygiene after urination or defecation, or clean up blood or body fluids.

• The caregiver must agree to follow all infection-control protocols and procedures established by the hospital.

• The caregiver's movement within the rest of the health care facility should be restricted to the patient care area and, if available, designated spaces or waiting areas for these caregivers,[18] along with any other restrictions that may be stipulated by the state and local health departments.

• The caregiver must agree to and be willing to comply with any additional guidelines provided by the hospital, health care providers, and public health authorities.

• Confidentiality must be strictly maintained at all times. Without a full understanding of the extraordinary precautions and controls built in by institutions to minimize risk to other patients and the public, there are significant potential negative consequences to a confidentiality breech in which information about the nature or circumstance of the illness of a patient with Ebola is revealed without clear explanation of what, if any, implications this may have to the public. Examples of such consequences that were noted among institutions that cared for patients with Ebola in the United States during the recent outbreak included health care workers known to work in the unit caring for the patient being publicly shunned and their children being removed from invitations to events, among others. There is also the risk that other patients, without appropriate information, have an exaggerated sense of risk and unnecessarily decide to shun the institution providing care for these patients. Parents/caregivers should be advised not to communicate with members of the press, on social media, or through other forums the nature of their own or their child's exposure or illness.[21] Doing so may subject the child and family members to unwanted scrutiny or behaviors from the public, both during hospitalization and after discharge, and this possibility should be explained to the parents/caregivers. The child should be admitted under a protocol that prohibits the announcement of his or her presence, and the hospital should avoid giving information to anyone other than the parents, even if the parents consent to disclosure, to protect the privacy interest of the minor child.

- For any of the 3 options, particularly for option 1, if videoconferencing is not available, audiotaping advice/bedtime stories also may help to support the psychosocial health of the child. In addition, family pictures may be placed in the child's room, along with family notes for older children, all of which should be appropriately discarded and destroyed upon discharge to maintain infection control.

Preparing Hospital Plans

- The hospital should engage in risk management each time the policy is implemented.

- If the caregiver should develop symptoms concerning for Ebola, the hospital should be prepared to either provide care

or transfer to a designated adult biocontainment unit treatment center for evaluation, admission, and treatment.[16]

- Vaccination should be considered in the future. Recently, a recombinant, replication-competent vesicular stomatitis virus vectored vaccine expressing a surface glycoprotein of Zaire Ebolavirus (rVSV-ZEBOV) was shown to be 100% protective in preventing disease among 4123 contacts of persons with Ebola.[22] This vaccine, also shown to be safe, holds promise for future prevention among contacts and will likely be a major mechanism of protection of health care workers and close contacts of infected people, but guidelines for use have not yet been developed, nor has its use been evaluated in children.

SPECIAL CONSIDERATIONS WHEN DEATH IS IMMINENT AND/OR AFTER A CHILD HAS DIED

Certain diseases, such as Ebola, are most infectious just before and after death[23]; the risk of exposure to these diseases may be highest at this time. For this reason, consideration of whether a caregiver or other loved ones are allowed access during this critical time with the attendant risks should involve all of the factors discussed previously in "Action Toward the Safety of the Caregiver in Suspected or Proven Ebola."

- Consider options related to memory tokens. Only materials that can be autoclaved can be used to create any memory tokens.

- Have a chaplain or other support person immediately available to family and caregivers.

- Work with pastoral care on having a service via videoconferencing, if desired by family members.

ACKNOWLEGMENTS

The AAP acknowledges the significant contributions of the CDC Children's Preparedness Unit throughout the Ebola Public Health Emergency and in the development of this clinical report. The committee specifically thanks Dr Eric Dziuban, MD, DTM, FAAP; Dr Stephanie Griese, MD, MPH, FAAP; Dr Georgina Peacock, MD, MPH, FAAP; Dr Cynthia Hinton, PhD, MS, MPH; Mr Michael Bartenfeld, MA; and Ms Wendy Ruben, MS, CHES.

COMMITTEE ON INFECTIOUS DISEASES, 2015–2016

Carrie L. Byington, MD, FAAP, Chairperson
Yvonne A. Maldonado, MD, FAAP, Vice Chairperson
Elizabeth D. Barnett MD, FAAP
H. Dele Davies, MD, MS, MHCM, FAAP
Kathryn M. Edwards, MD, FAAP
Ruth Lynfield, MD, FAAP
Flor M. Munoz, MD, FAAP
Dawn Nolt, MD, FAAP
Ann-Christine Nyquist, MD, MSPH, FAAP
Mobeen H. Rathore, MD, FAAP
Mark H. Sawyer, MD, FAAP
William J. Steinbach, MD, FAAP
Tina Q. Tan, MD, FAAP
Theoklis E. Zaoutis, MD, MSCE, FAAP

EX OFFICIO

David W. Kimberlin, MD, FAAP – *Red Book* Editor
Michael T. Brady, MD, FAAP – *Red Book* Associate Editor
Mary Anne Jackson, MD, FAAP – *Red Book* Associate Editor
Sarah S. Long, MD, FAAP – *Red Book* Associate Editor
Henry H. Bernstein, DO, MHCM, FAAP – *Red Book* Online Associate Editor
H. Cody Meissner, MD, FAAP – Visual *Red Book* Associate Editor

CONTRIBUTOR

Steven E. Krug, MD, FAAP, *Disaster Preparedness Advisory Council*

LIAISONS

Douglas Campos-Outcalt, MD, MPA – *American Academy of Family Physicians*
Karen M. Farizo, MD – *US Food and Drug Administration*
Marc Fischer, MD, FAAP – *Centers for Disease Control and Prevention*
Bruce G. Gellin, MD, MPH – *National Vaccine Program Office*
Richard L. Gorman, MD, FAAP – *National Institutes of Health*

Natasha Halasa, MD, MPH, FAAP – *Pediatric Infectious Diseases Society*

Joan L. Robinson, MD – *Canadian Pediatric Society*

Marco Aurelio Palazzi Safadi, MD – *Sociedad Latinoamericana de Infectologia Pediatrica*

Jane F. Seward, MBBS, MPH, FAAP – *Centers for Disease Control and Prevention*

Geoffrey R. Simon, MD, FAAP – *Committee on Practice Ambulatory Medicine*

Jeffrey R. Starke, MD, FAAP – *American Thoracic Society*

STAFF

Jennifer M. Frantz, MPH

ABBREVIATIONS

AAP: American Academy of Pediatrics
CDC: Centers for Disease Control and Prevention
Ebola: Ebola virus disease
PPE: personal protective equipment
PUI: person under investigation

REFERENCES

1. Disaster Preparedness Advisory Council; Committee On Pediatric Emergency Medicine. Ensuring the health of children in disasters. *Pediatrics*. 2015;136(5):e1407–e1417

2. Suzuki LK, Kato PM. Psychosocial support for patients in pediatric oncology: the influences of parents, schools, peers, and technology. *J Pediatr Oncol Nurs*. 2003;20(4):159–174

3. Woodgate RL. Social support in children with cancer: a review of the literature. *J Pediatr Oncol Nurs*. 1999;16(4):201–213

4. Schaffer HR, Callender WM. Psychologic effects of hospitalization in infancy. *Pediatrics*. 1959;24(4):528–539

5. Bush JP, Melamed BG, Sheras PL, Greenbaum PE. Mother-child patterns of coping with anticipatory medical stress. *Health Psychol*. 1986;5(2):137–157

6. Kanapathipillai R. Ebola virus disease—current knowledge. *N Engl J Med*. 2014;371(13):e18

7. Mehrotra P, Shane AL, Milstone AM. Family-centered care and high-consequence pathogens: thinking outside the room. *JAMA Pediatr*. 2015;169(11):985–986

8. Suwantarat N, Apisarnthanarak A. Risks to healthcare workers with emerging diseases: lessons from MERS-CoV, Ebola, SARS, and avian flu. *Curr Opin Infect Dis*. 2015;28(4):349–361

9. Kilmarx PH, Clarke KR, Dietz PM, et al; Centers for Disease Control and Prevention. Ebola virus disease in health care workers—Sierra Leone, 2014. *MMWR Morb Mortal Wkly Rep*. 2014;63(49):1168–1171

10. Centers for Disease Control and Prevention. Case definition for Ebola virus disease (EVD). Available at: www.cdc.gov/vhf/ebola/healthcare-us/evaluating-patients/case-definition.html. Accessed July 13, 2015

11. Centers for Disease Control and Prevention. CDC Health Advisory: Guidelines for Evaluation of US Patients Suspected of Having Ebola Virus Disease. Atlanta, GA: Centers for Disease Control and Prevention; August 1, 2014. Available at: www.cdc.gov/vhf/ebola/healthcare-us/evaluating-patients/case-definition.html. Accessed July 13, 2015

12. Mupapa K, Mukundu W, Bwaka MA, et al. Ebola hemorrhagic fever and pregnancy. *J Infect Dis*. 1999;179(suppl 1):S11–S12

13. Kitching A, Walsh A, Morgan D. Ebola in pregnancy: risk and clinical outcomes. *BJOG*. 2015;122(3):287

14. Centers for Disease Control and Prevention. Identify, isolate, inform: emergency department evaluation and management of patients under investigation for Ebola virus disease. Available at: www.cdc.gov/vhf/ebola/pdf/ed-algorithm-management-patients-possible-ebola.pdf. Accessed July 13, 2015

15. Centers for Disease Control and Prevention. Epidemiologic risk factors to consider when evaluating a person for exposure to Ebola virus. Available at: www.cdc.gov/vhf/ebola/exposure/risk-factors-when-evaluating-person-for-exposure.html. Accessed May 2, 2016

16. Centers for Disease Control and Prevention. Ebola virus disease. Hospital preparedness: a tiered approach. Available at: www.cdc.gov/vhf/ebola/healthcare-us/preparing/assessment-hospitals.html. Accessed May 2, 2016

17. Yang NH, Dharmar M, Hojman NM, et al. Videoconferencing to reduce stress among hospitalized children. *Pediatrics*. 2014;134(1). Available at: www.pediatrics.org/cgi/content/full/134/1/e169

18. DeBiasi RL, Song X, Cato K, et al; CNHS Ebola Response Task Force. Preparedness, evaluation and care of pediatric patients under investigation for Ebola virus disease: experience from a pediatric designated care facility. *J Pediatric Infect Dis Soc*. 2016;5(1):68–75

19. Centers for Disease Control and Prevention. Guidance on personal protective equipment (PPE) to be used by healthcare workers during management of patients with confirmed Ebola or persons under investigation (PUIs) for Ebola who are clinically unstable or have bleeding, vomiting, or diarrhea in U.S. hospitals, including procedures for donning and doffing PPE. Available at: www.cdc.gov/vhf/ebola/healthcare-us/ppe/guidance.html. Accessed May 2, 2016

20. Centers for Disease Control and Prevention. Notes on the interim U.S. guidance for monitoring and movement of persons with potential Ebola virus exposure. Available at: www.cdc.gov/vhf/ebola/exposure/monitoring-and-movement-of-persons-with-exposure.html. Accessed May 2, 2016

21. Shultz JM, Baingana F, Neria Y. The 2014 Ebola outbreak and mental health: current status and recommended response. *JAMA*. 2015;313(6):567–568

22. Henao-Restrepo AM, Longini IM, Egger M, et al. Efficacy and effectiveness of an rVSV-vectored vaccine expressing Ebola surface glycoprotein: interim results from the Guinea ring vaccination cluster-randomised trial. *Lancet*. 2015;386(9996):857–866

23. Dowell SF, Mukunu R, Ksiazek TG, Khan AS, Rollin PE, Peters CJ. Transmission of Ebola hemorrhagic fever: a study of risk factors in family members, Kikwit, Democratic Republic of the Congo, 1995. Commission de Lutte contre les Epidémies à Kikwit. *J Infect Dis*. 1999;179(suppl 1):S87–S91

The Pediatrician's Role in Optimizing School Readiness

• *Policy Statement*

POLICY STATEMENT   Organizational Principles to Guide and Define the Child Health
Care System and/or Improve the Health of all Children

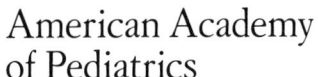
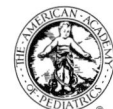

American Academy
of Pediatrics

DEDICATED TO THE HEALTH OF ALL CHILDREN™

The Pediatrician's Role in Optimizing School Readiness

COUNCIL ON EARLY CHILDHOOD, COUNCIL ON SCHOOL HEALTH

abstract

School readiness includes not only the early academic skills of children but also their physical health, language skills, social and emotional development, motivation to learn, creativity, and general knowledge. Families and communities play a critical role in ensuring children's growth in all of these areas and thus their readiness for school. Schools must be prepared to teach all children when they reach the age of school entry, regardless of their degree of readiness. Research on early brain development emphasizes the effects of early experiences, relationships, and emotions on creating and reinforcing the neural connections that are the basis for learning. Pediatricians, by the nature of their relationships with families and children, may significantly influence school readiness. Pediatricians have a primary role in ensuring children's physical health through the provision of preventive care, treatment of illness, screening for sensory deficits, and monitoring nutrition and growth. They can promote and monitor the social-emotional development of children by providing anticipatory guidance on development and behavior, by encouraging positive parenting practices, by modeling reciprocal and respectful communication with adults and children, by identifying and addressing psychosocial risk factors, and by providing community-based resources and referrals when warranted. Cognitive and language skills are fostered through timely identification of developmental problems and appropriate referrals for services, including early intervention and special education services; guidance regarding safe and stimulating early education and child care programs; and promotion of early literacy by encouraging language-rich activities such as reading together, telling stories, and playing games. Pediatricians are also well positioned to advocate not only for children's access to health care but also for high-quality early childhood education and evidence-based family supports such as home visits, which help provide a foundation for optimal learning.

DOI: 10.1542/peds.2016-2293

PEDIATRICS (ISSN Numbers: Print, 0031-4005; Online, 1098-4275).

FINANCIAL DISCLOSURE: The authors have indicated they do not have a financial relationship relevant to this article to disclose.

FUNDING: No external funding.

POTENTIAL CONFLICT OF INTEREST: The authors have indicated they have no potential conflicts of interest to disclose.

To cite: AAP COUNCIL ON EARLY CHILDHOOD and AAP COUNCIL ON SCHOOL HEALTH. The Pediatrician's Role in Optimizing School Readiness. *Pediatrics.* 2016;138(3):e20162293

COMPONENTS OF SCHOOL READINESS

Children's readiness for school, according to the National Education Goals Panel, consists of the following elements: physical health and motor development, social and emotional development, approaches to learning, language development, and cognition and general knowledge.[1] The National Education Goals Panel advocates for a broader concept of school readiness that includes not only children's readiness for school but also schools' readiness for children as well as the family and community supports and services that contribute to school success. Thus, the responsibility for school readiness of the child lies not only with the child but also with the families, communities, and schools that shape his or her development.[2] Families need to provide a safe, stable, and nurturing environment in which trust and confidence allow children to take advantage of learning experiences.[3] Parents should read aloud to their children, preferably daily, as well as expand their children's language through responsive verbal interactions, and engage them in active and stimulating play. Communities need to provide high-quality prenatal and intrapartum care, including home visits for families at significant risk; stimulating early education and child care experiences; healthy nutrition and housing for children; appropriate child protective services; and early interventions for children at risk of developmental delays.[4] Communities also have the responsibility of reducing environmental toxins, developing safe areas for play, and providing means for all families to access quality medical and dental care.[4] Schools need to meet the individual needs and abilities of children who come from a wide range of environmental and emotional experiences.[2] The technical report by the American Academy of Pediatrics (AAP) on school readiness

provides an excellent description of school readiness issues; this policy statement addresses the role of the pediatrician in promoting school readiness.[5] It is understood that, even with best intentions, not all of the physical, emotional, and social factors that can adversely affect school performance will be identifiable by a pediatrician before school entry, but to the extent that it is practical, pediatricians may significantly influence school readiness.

EARLY BRAIN DEVELOPMENT AND SCHOOL READINESS

The importance of school readiness has become increasingly apparent with recent research on early brain development, which emphasizes the effects that early experiences and relationships have on the brain's foundational architecture and subsequent function. Early learning is integrated, cumulative, and nonlinear, with critical periods of proliferation and pruning of neuronal synapses.[6] Neural connections are created and modified by the child's social and environmental interactions; repetition helps strengthen neural pathways. Learning is influenced not only by individual learning styles but by emotions and specific settings and situations.[7,8] This early plasticity can be a double-edged sword, because chronically chaotic, stressful, and otherwise adverse environments can be toxic to the development of important brain structures, such as the hippocampus and prefrontal cortex. Safe, stable, and nurturing relationships, on the other hand, mitigate this kind of "toxic stress," providing a strong foundation for future learning.[9] The literature on early brain development shows that a child's caregivers exert a tremendous influence, both positive and negative, on early learning. These findings take on special significance in view of the factors that have been identified as affecting school readiness, namely

physical health and motor skill development, social and emotional development, individual learning differences, language development, and cognitive abilities.[10] Certainly, within the context of a medical home, which provides compassionate, coordinated, family-centered, accessible, and culturally sensitive care, the pediatrician will have a foremost role in monitoring the critical elements of early experiences that foster school readiness.[11]

ROLE OF THE PEDIATRICIAN IN PROMOTING SCHOOL READINESS

Physical Well-being

The effect of physical well-being on school readiness is indisputable, and optimizing physical health has always been a primary goal of the pediatrician.[12,13] *Bright Futures* provides comprehensive health supervision guidelines within the context of the family-physician partnership and emphasizes effective communication strategies and shared goals.[14] Health supervision includes monitoring growth; identifying obesity, food insecurity, or abnormal growth patterns; and encouraging physical activity and attainment of motor skills, and emphasizing the effects of high-quality, accredited child care and early education programs such as Head Start on school readiness. Pediatricians, through their advocacy, can help ensure that existing surveillance programs, such as Early and Periodic Screening, Diagnosis, and Treatment (EPSDT), are aligned with *Bright Futures* guidelines.[15,16] The pediatrician screens children for exposure to lead and other environmental toxins, as indicated, and identifies vision and hearing deficits as early as possible. The pediatrician has a crucial role in treating chronic health problems and minimizing the effects of these problems on physical stamina and development.[17] Pediatricians can also help ensure that children with chronic illnesses have access to quality early learning experiences despite their health concerns. In addition, the pediatrician has the responsibility of reporting suspected child abuse and monitoring and supporting children in foster and kinship care. Pediatricians may also be advocates for accessible health care for all children, including home visits and food subsidy programs that help minimize the gap in health care services for the disadvantaged.[17]

Social-Emotional Well-being

The pediatrician's influence on the social-emotional well-being of the child begins with the identification of risk factors such as maternal depression, parental history of early childhood adversity, parental discord, or other family psychosocial stressors, such as poverty, that could interfere with initial parent-infant bonding. The critical influence of early attachment on later behavior and development is overwhelmingly supported by research.[3,18,19] The pediatrician also provides anticipatory guidance regarding behaviors, such as infant crying, sleeping, and feeding, as well as parental self-care. A parent's perceived success or failure with these early challenges can set the tone for how he or she approaches subsequent difficult behaviors, such as tantrums or toileting problems. Positive parenting techniques should also be discussed. Physicians can model appropriate adult-child interactions within the office and provide materials and resources to help promote healthy parent-child relationships.[20] The physician often has the opportunity to help parents recognize differences in temperament that may influence parent-child interactions.[9] Pediatricians are often asked to give advice about behavior concerns and appropriate disciplinary strategies. Emphasis should be placed on the

3 essential components of effective discipline: (1) a positive, supportive parent-child relationship with many opportunities for "times in" throughout the day; (2) the use of positive reinforcement strategies, including praise, to increase desired behaviors; and (3) the purposeful and appropriate use of strategies such as ignoring, redirection, "time out," or removal of privileges to reduce undesired behaviors.[21] The use of corporal punishment should be discouraged, because harsh disciplinary strategies often have a deleterious effect on the parent-child relationship by promoting aggressive behaviors on the part of the child.[9] Consideration of cultural differences must always be part of this process.[22] For children or families who present with significant behavioral/ emotional issues or children who have experienced significant exposure to toxic stressors, the pediatrician can offer support and guidance and referral to behavioral health professionals who can provide evidence-based interventions.[23] Integrated models of mental health care often allow families better access to services.

Cognitive and Language Development

Cognitive and language development can be promoted by sharing with families the powerful information on early brain development that emphasizes the essential role that parents play in their child's learning. Families may need guidance regarding the importance of touch, movement, and gestures in learning.[24,25] Optimal early childhood environments in and outside the home encourage exploration, mentor basic skills, celebrate developmental advances, rehearse and extend new skills, protect from inappropriate disapproval and punishment, and provide a rich and responsive language environment.[26] Exposure to television and other media is not recommended for children younger

than 2 years, and the need for limitations and restrictions on media use and attention to media quality can be raised with parents and other caregivers of children of all ages.[27] Pediatricians can promote early language development and literacy by encouraging parents to read and spend time with their children every day if possible and by participating in programs such as Reach Out and Read.[28] For parents with limited reading skills, pediatricians can model storytelling; educate parents as to the value of using books to identify words, numbers, colors, and objects; and emphasize the power of the spoken word on brain development and cognition.[29] Physicians should foster the 5 "Rs" of early childhood education: "reading" together daily; "rhyming," talking, playing together; establishing "routines" around meals, play, and sleep; "rewarding" everyday successes; and supporting nurturing reciprocal "relationships."[5]

Pediatricians have responsibility for early screening for developmental problems, such as autism, intellectual disability, and attention-deficit/ hyperactivity disorder, with subsequent referral for intervention services and diagnostic clarification as available.[30] Pediatricians may also help parents recognize a child's individual strengths and weaknesses in learning and provide resources that can help the child succeed within this framework. Guidance regarding the importance of early education and child care quality and the availability of these resources will also be helpful to families as they seek healthy and stimulating environments for their children. Pediatricians can contribute to child care and school guides to assist parents in selecting and monitoring child care programs and working with schools to enhance the academic success of their children. Pediatricians can encourage parents to take an active interest in their child's education by suggesting that parents visit the child's school and meet with the teacher before school entry, have regular communication with the teacher, and advocate for appropriate school services, especially for children with developmental concerns. Finally, pediatricians can advocate for high-quality educational services in the community, as measured by objective quality-rating systems or accreditation, including efforts such as early intervention services and Head Start.[31]

CONCLUSIONS

In summary, the concept of school readiness encompasses the entirety of a child's physical, cognitive, and social-emotional attributes, which serve as the foundation for early brain development and learning. A team effort among families, the medical home, child care/early intervention, schools, and communities provides the experiences, relationships, and interactions that shape the learning process and serve as building blocks for later success in school and in life. Pediatricians, in their role as medical home providers, have the opportunity to substantially influence school readiness. Not only do pediatricians address physical health concerns, but they also are uniquely suited to address developmental and behavioral health concerns of the child and family and to promote healthy relationships and interactions that encourage future resilience. Beyond the influence that pediatricians have on individual families, they can lend their voices as advocates for appropriate mental health, early education, and child care; basic health care services; and safe, healthy living conditions for children and families.

RECOMMENDATIONS FOR PEDIATRICIANS

1. Optimal physical well-being is critical to school readiness.

Pediatricians promote this in all of their work around health issues. Pediatricians are encouraged to use the comprehensive guidelines provided by *Bright Futures* to ensure adequate and appropriate health supervision.

2. Pediatricians should promote social-emotional well-being necessary for school readiness by establishing a partnership with the family to (1) foster safe, stable, and nurturing relationships through age-appropriate anticipatory guidance[14,32]; (2) address behavior concerns in a proactive, skills-building fashion, recognizing that temperament may play a role; (3) identify and mitigate psychosocial risks for toxic stress, such as child abuse and neglect, maternal depression, inadequate food or shelter, and domestic violence; (4) help families access community resources, including evidence-based home-visiting programs, such as Nurse Family Partnership, Family Check Up, Parent Child Home Program, and Parents as Teachers[33]; and (5) facilitate access to evidence-based mental health services when indicated.[34–37]

3. Families have a critical role in promoting cognitive and language development of their children, both of which greatly influence school readiness. Pediatricians are encouraged to share information on early brain development[9,38] and the role that families play in their child's early learning.[5,32,39] Pediatricians can discuss with families the need for providing optimal learning environments rich with reading materials (eg, www.reachoutandread.org), opportunities for exploration (eg, www.circleofsecurity.net), and praise. Pediatricians should support whenever possible opportunities for the utilization of strategies to improve school readiness, such as colocation of

parent-child specialists (http://www.rain.org/littlesteps/Healthy%20Steps%20User%20Manual.pdf) and videotaping/reviewing of parent-child interactions.[40]

4. Pediatric providers can promote the 5 Rs of early childhood education by encouraging parents to read together daily as a favorite family activity that strengthens family relationships and builds language, literacy, and social-emotional skills that last a lifetime; rhyme, play, sing, talk, and cuddle with their young children throughout the day (children develop language skills, problem-solving ability, and relationships through play); create and sustain routines for children around sleep, meals, and play (children need to know what caregivers expect from them and what they can expect from those who care for them); provide frequent rewards for everyday successes, especially for effort toward worthwhile goals such as helping (praise from those the child loves and respects is among the most powerful of rewards); and remember that relationships that are nurturing and secure provide the foundation of healthy child development.[5]

5. Pediatricians should identify children at risk of developmental problems through the use of valid screening tests, behavioral observations, and attention to parent concerns.[30] Pediatricians can make timely referrals for appropriate early intervention services and further evaluation for diagnostic clarification. Pediatricians should familiarize themselves with suitable community resources and understand their state's laws that mandate public school intervention for children identified as high risk of school or learning problems.

6. All children would benefit from access to high-quality early education programs. Pediatricians can link children from low-income or disadvantaged households to such programs (eg, Headstart) in an effort to minimize the gap in early learning experiences. Pediatricians can collaborate with professionals from other disciplines who have relevant expertise (eg, early childhood education, infant mental health, public health practitioners) and with key stakeholders (eg, early intervention agencies, Zero to Three) to minimize toxic stressors and to establish a solid foundation for positive early childhood experiences. Pediatricians can assist families in identifying the characteristics of quality child care facilities.

7. Pediatricians can advocate for services and supports that will allow children to be successful in school and in life; opportunities for advocacy occur not only within the pediatrician's office and community but also in regional, national, or international venues.

RECOMMENDATIONS FOR POLICY MAKERS

1. The AAP supports state and federal funding for quality preschool, child care, and child development programs (eg, Head Start) that promote developmentally appropriate activities in a stimulating, nurturing, and safe environment.

2. The AAP supports the incorporation of components of school readiness into pediatric residency training. Residency continuity practices can integrate the recommendations for pediatricians listed above regarding the promotion of school readiness into their competency-based curriculum.

3. The AAP supports funding for parent-child programs that help build the positive interactions and appropriate attachments that are the cornerstones of healthy social-emotional development and an essential component for school readiness.

4. The AAP supports funding for community, state, and federal programs that ensure adequate housing, health care, and nutrition for children in their formative years and that provide safe environments in which children can explore and play.

5. The AAP supports research into the ways in which school readiness can be most effectively achieved and the dissemination of this information to families and other child care providers/educators.

LEAD AUTHORS

P. Gail Williams, MD, FAAP
Jeffrey Okamoto, MD, FAAP

COUNCIL ON EARLY CHILDHOOD EXECUTIVE COMMITTEE, 2015–2016

Dina Lieser, MD, FAAP, Chairperson
Beth DelConte, MD, FAAP
Elaine Donoghue, MD, FAAP
Marian Earls, MD, FAAP
Danette Glassy, MD, FAAP
Terri McFadden, MD, FAAP
Alan Mendelsohn, MD, FAAP
Seth Scholer, MD, FAAP
Jennifer Takagishi, MD, FAAP
Douglas Vanderbilt, MD, FAAP
P. Gail Williams, MD, FAAP

LIAISONS

Abbey Alkon, RN, PNP, PhD – *National Association of Pediatric Nurse Practitioners*
Lynette Fraga, PhD – *Child Care Aware*
Barbara U. Hamilton, MA – *Maternal and Child Health Bureau*
Laurel Hoffmann, MD – *AAP Section on Pediatric Trainees*
Claire Lerner, LCSW – *Zero to Three*
David Willis, MD, FAAP – *Maternal and Child Health Bureau*

STAFF

Charlotte O. Zia, MPH, CHES

COUNCIL ON SCHOOL HEALTH EXECUTIVE COMMITTEE, 2015–2016

Breena Holmes, MD, FAAP, Chairperson
Mandy Allison, MD, MEd, MSPH, FAAP
Richard Ancona, MD, FAAP
Elliott Attisha, DO, FAAP
Nathaniel Beers, MD, MPA, FAAP
Cheryl De Pinto, MD, MPH, FAAP
Peter Gorski, MD, MPA, FAAP
Chris Kjolhede, MD, MPH, FAAP
Marc Lerner, MD, FAAP
Adrienne Weiss-Harrison, MD, FAAP
Thomas Young, MD, FAAP

FORMER EXECUTIVE COMMITTEE MEMBER

Jeffrey Okamoto, MD, FAAP, Immediate Past Chairperson

LIAISONS

Nina Fekaris, MS, BSN, RN, NCSN – *National Association of School Nurses*
Veda Johnson, MD, FAAP – *School-Based Health Alliance*
Sheryl Kataoka, MD, MSHS – *American Academy of Child and Adolescent Psychiatry*
Sandra Leonard, DNP, RN, FNP – *Centers for Disease Control and Prevention*

STAFF

Madra Guinn-Jones, MPH

ABBREVIATION

AAP: American Academy of Pediatrics

REFERENCES

1. National Education Goals Panel. National Education Goals Report: building a nation of learners, 1999. Washington, DC: National Educational Goals Panel; 1999. Available at: http://govinfo.library.unt.edu/negp/reports/99rpt.pdf. Accessed April 4, 2014

2. Rafoth MA, Buchenauer EL, Crissman KK, Halko JK. *School Readiness—Preparing Children for Kindergarten and Beyond: Information for Parents.* Bethesda, MD: National Association for School Psychologists; 2004. Available at: www.nasponline.org/resources/handouts/schoolreadiness.pdf. Accessed April 4, 2014

3. Edwards CP, Sheridan SM, Knoche LL. Parent-child relationships in early learning. Baker E, Peterson P, McGaw B, eds. *International Encyclopedia of*

Education. Oxford, United Kingdom: Elsevier; 2010:438–443

4. Halle T, Zaff J. *Background for community level work on school readiness, reviewing the literature on contributing factors on school readiness: Final report to the Knight Foundation*. Bethesda, MD: Child Trends; 2000. Accessed April 4, 2014. Available at

5. High PC; Committee on Early Childhood, Adoption and Dependent Care; Council on School Health. School readiness [technical report]. *Pediatrics*. 2008;121(4). Available at: www.pediatrics.org/cgi/content/full/121/4/e1008. Reaffirmed September 2013

6. Huttenlocher PR, Dabholkar AS. Regional differences in synaptogenesis in human cerebral cortex. *J Comp Neurol*. 1997;387(2):167–178

7. Families and Work Institute. *Rethinking the Brain: New Insights into Early Development*. Executive summary of the Conference on Brain Development in Young Children: New Frontiers for Research, Policy and Practice. Chicago, IL: University of Chicago; 1996

8. Scott LO, Lynn SJ, Ruscio J, Beyerstein BL. *50 Great Myths of Popular Psychology: Shattering Widespread Misconceptions About Human Behavior*. Hoboken, NJ: Wiley-Blackwell; 2010

9. Garner AS, Shonkoff JP; Committee on Psychosocial Aspects of Child and Family Health; Committee on Early Childhood, Adoption, and Dependent Care; Section on Developmental and Behavioral Pediatrics. Early childhood adversity, toxic stress, and the role of the pediatrician: translating developmental science into lifelong health. *Pediatrics*. 2012;129(1):e224–e231

10. Rhode Island Kids Count. Getting ready: findings from the National School Readiness Indicators Initiative. Providence, RI: Rhode Island Kids Count; 2005. Available at: www.gettingready.org/matriarch/MultiPiecePage.asp_Q_PageID_E_318_A_PageName_E_NationalSchoolReadinessIndicat. Accessed April 4, 2014

11. Medical Home Initiatives for Children With Special Needs Project Advisory Committee. The medical home [policy statement]. *Pediatrics*. 2002;110(1). Available at: www.pediatrics.org/cgi/content/full/110/1/184. Reaffirmed May 2008

12. Fransoo RR, Roos NP, Martens PJ, Heaman M, Levin B, Chateau D. How health status affects progress and performance in school: a population-based study. *Can J Public Health*. 2008;99(4):344–349

13. Currie J. Health disparities and gaps in school readiness. *Future Child*. 2005;15(1):117–138

14. Hagan JF, Shaw JS, Duncan P, eds. *Bright Futures: Guidelines for Health Supervision of Infants, Children and Adolescents*. 3rd ed, pocket guide. Elk Grove Village, IL: American Academy of Pediatrics; 2008

15. American Academy of Pediatrics. *Pediatricians' Provision of Preventive Care and Use of Health Supervision Guidelines. Periodic Survey of Fellows No. 56: Executive Summary*. Elk Grove Village, IL: American Academy of Pediatrics; 2004

16. Centers for Medicare and Medicaid Services. Early and periodic screening, diagnosis and treatment. Available at: www.medicaid.gov. Accessed April 4, 2014

17. Schor EL, Abrams M, Shea K. Medicaid: health promotion and disease prevention for school readiness. *Health Aff (Millwood)*. 2007;26(2):420–429

18. Webster-Stratton C, Reid MJ. Strengthening social and emotional competence in young children—the foundation for early school readiness and success. *Infants Young Child*. 2004;17(2):96–113

19. Belsky J, Fearon RM. Infant-mother attachment security, contextual risk, and early development: a moderational analysis. *Dev Psychopathol*. 2002;14(2):293–310

20. Mendelsohn AL, Huberman HS, Berkule SB, Brockmeyer CA, Morrow LM, Dreyer BP. Primary care strategies for promoting parent-child interactions and school readiness in at-risk families: the Bellevue Project for Early Language, Literacy, and Education Success. *Arch Pediatr Adolesc Med*. 2011;165(1):33–41

21. Committee on Psychosocial Aspects of Child and Family Health. Guidance for effective discipline. *Pediatrics*. 1998;101(4):723–728. Reaffirmed May 2012

22. Committee on Pediatric Workforce. Culturally effective pediatric care: education and training issues [policy statement]. *Pediatrics*. 2004;114(2):1677–1685. Reaffirmed February 2008

23. Foy JM, Perrin J; Task Force on Mental Health. Enhancing pediatric mental health care: strategies for preparing a community. *Pediatrics*. 2010;125(suppl 3):S75–S86

24. Maggi S, Irwin LG, Siddiqi A, Poureslami I, Hertzman E, Hertzman C. *Analytic and Strategic Review Paper: International Perspectives on Early Child Development, Human Early Learning Partnership*. Geneva, Switzerland: World Health Organization; 2005

25. Cabrera D, Cotosi L. The world at our fingertips: the connection between touch and learning. *Sci Am Mind*. 2010;21(4):36–41

26. Ramey CT, Ramey SL. Prevention of intellectual disabilities: early interventions to improve cognitive development. *Prev Med*. 1998;27(2):224–232

27. Gentile DA, Oberg C, Sherwood NE, Story M, Walsh DA, Hogan M. Well-child visits in the video age: pediatricians and the American Academy of Pediatrics' guidelines for children's media use. *Pediatrics*. 2004;114(5):1235–1241

28. High PC, LaGasse L, Becker S, Ahlgren I, Gardner A. Literacy promotion in primary care pediatrics: can we make a difference? *Pediatrics*. 2000;105(4 pt 2):927–934

29. Ferry AL, Hespos SJ, Waxsman S. Categorization in 3- and 4-month-old infants: an advantage of words over tones. *Child Dev*. 2010;81(2):472–479

30. Council on Children With Disabilities; Section on Developmental Behavioral Pediatrics; Bright Futures Steering Committee; Medical Home Initiatives for Children With Special Needs Project Advisory Committee. Identifying infants and young children with developmental disorders in the medical home: an algorithm for developmental

surveillance and screening. *Pediatrics*. 2006;118(1):405–420. Reaffirmed December 2009

31. Committee on Early Childhood, Adoption, and Dependent Care. Quality education and child care from birth to kindergarten. *Pediatrics*. 2005;115(1):187–191. Reaffirmed December 2009

32. Milteer R, Ginsburg KR; Council on Communications and Media; Committee on Psychosocial Aspects of Child and Family Health. The importance of play in promoting healthy child development and maintaining strong parent-child bond: focus on children in poverty. *Pediatrics*. 2007;129(1). Available at: www.pediatrics.org/cgi/content/full/129/1/e204

33. Council on Community Pediatrics. The role of preschool home-visiting programs in improving children's developmental and health outcomes. *Pediatrics*. 2009;123(2):598–603

34. The Incredible Years. Parents, Teachers, and Child Training Series. Available at: http://incredibleyears.com/. Accessed April 4, 2014

35. PCIT International. Parent-child interaction therapy. Available at: www.pcit.org. Accessed April 4, 2014

36. Triple P—Positive Parenting Program. Available at: www.triplep.net/glo-en/home/. Accessed April 4, 2014

37. American Academy of Pediatrics. *Addressing Mental Health Concerns in Primary Care: A Clinician's Toolkit*. Elk Grove Village, IL: American Academy of Pediatrics; 2010

38. Shonkoff JP, Garner AS; Committee on Psychosocial Aspects of Child and Family Health; Committee on Early Childhood, Adoption, and Dependent Care; Section on Developmental and Behavioral Pediatrics. The lifelong effects of early childhood adversity and toxic stress. *Pediatrics*. 2012;129(1):e232–e246

39. American Academy of Pediatrics. Literacy toolkit. Elk Grove Village, IL: American Academy of Pediatrics. Available at: www.aap.org/en-us/advocacy-and-policy/aap-health-initiatives/Literacy-Toolkit/Pages/Toolkit.aspx. Accessed April 4, 2014

40. Mendelsohn AL, Valdez PT, Flynn V, et al. Use of videotaped interactions during pediatric well-child care: impact at 33 months on parenting and on child development. *J Dev Behav Pediatr*. 2007;28(3):206–212

Poverty and Child Health in the United States

- *Policy Statement*

POLICY STATEMENT Organizational Principles to Guide and Define the Child Health
Care System and/or Improve the Health of all Children

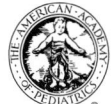

American Academy
of Pediatrics

DEDICATED TO THE HEALTH OF ALL CHILDREN™

Poverty and Child Health in the United States

COUNCIL ON COMMUNITY PEDIATRICS

abstract

Almost half of young children in the United States live in poverty or near poverty. The American Academy of Pediatrics is committed to reducing and ultimately eliminating child poverty in the United States. Poverty and related social determinants of health can lead to adverse health outcomes in childhood and across the life course, negatively affecting physical health, socioemotional development, and educational achievement. The American Academy of Pediatrics advocates for programs and policies that have been shown to improve the quality of life and health outcomes for children and families living in poverty. With an awareness and understanding of the effects of poverty on children, pediatricians and other pediatric health practitioners in a family-centered medical home can assess the financial stability of families, link families to resources, and coordinate care with community partners. Further research, advocacy, and continuing education will improve the ability of pediatricians to address the social determinants of health when caring for children who live in poverty. Accompanying this policy statement is a technical report that describes current knowledge on child poverty and the mechanisms by which poverty influences the health and well-being of children.

DOI: 10.1542/peds.2016-0339

PEDIATRICS (ISSN Numbers: Print, 0031-4005; Online, 1098-4275).

Copyright © 2016 by the American Academy of Pediatrics

To cite: AAP COUNCIL ON COMMUNITY PEDIATRICS. Poverty and Child Health in the United States. *Pediatrics.* 2016; 137(4):e20160339

STATEMENT OF THE PROBLEM

Poverty is an important social determinant of health and contributes to child health disparities. Children who experience poverty, particularly during early life or for an extended period, are at risk of a host of adverse health and developmental outcomes through their life course.[1] Poverty has a profound effect on specific circumstances, such as birth weight, infant mortality, language development, chronic illness, environmental exposure, nutrition, and injury. Child poverty also influences genomic function and brain development by exposure to toxic stress,[2] a condition characterized by "excessive or prolonged activation of the physiologic stress response systems in the absence of the buffering protection afforded by stable, responsive relationships."[3] Children living in poverty are at increased risk of difficulties with self-regulation and executive function, such as inattention, impulsivity, defiance, and poor peer relationships.[4] Poverty can make parenting difficult, especially in the context of concerns about inadequate food, energy, transportation, and housing.

Child poverty is associated with lifelong hardship. Poor developmental and psychosocial outcomes are accompanied by a significant financial burden, not just for the children and families who experience them but also for the rest of society. Children who do not complete high school, for example, are more likely to become teenage parents, to be unemployed, and to be incarcerated, all of which exact heavy social and economic costs.[5] A growing body of research shows that child poverty is associated with neuroendocrine dysregulation that may alter brain function and may contribute to the development of chronic cardiovascular, immune, and psychiatric disorders.[6] The economic cost of child poverty to society can be estimated by anticipating future lost productivity and increased social expenditure. A study compiled before 2008 projected a total cost of approximately $500 billion each year through decreased productivity and increased costs of crime and health care,[7] nearly 4% of the gross domestic product. Other studies of "opportunity youth," young people 16 to 24 years of age who are neither employed nor in school, derived similar results, generating cohort aggregate lifetime costs in the trillions.[8]

Child poverty is greater in the United States than in most countries with comparable resources. In a 2012 report from the United Nations Children's Fund,[9] the United States ranked 34th of 35 member nations of the Organization for Economic Cooperation and Development, a reflection of the rate of child

poverty during and immediately after the Great Recession of 2007–2009. A later 2014 report from the Organization for Economic Cooperation and Development[10] ranked the United States 35th of 40 nations, only above Chile, Mexico, Romania, Turkey, and Israel. This policy statement specifically addresses child poverty in the United States but reflects the 2015 United Nations' Sustainability Goal to end poverty in all its forms everywhere.[11]

According to 2014 Census data, an estimated 21.1% of all US children younger than 18 years (15.5 million) lived in households designated as "poor" (ie, in 2014, incomes below 100% of the federal poverty level [FPL] of $24 230 for a family of 4*) and 42.9% (over 31.5 million) lived in households designated as "poor, near poor, or low income" (ie, incomes up to 200% of the FPL). Nearly 9.3% (6.8 million) lived in households of deep poverty (ie, incomes below 50% of the FPL).[12] In 2014, an estimated 16 million children lived in families who received Supplemental Nutrition Assistance Program (SNAP) benefits.[13] Between 2007 and 2010, foreclosures affected 5.3 million children.[14]

Demographics have a profound influence on the likelihood that a family or community will experience poverty or low income. For example, African American, Hispanic, and

---

* The FPL is determined by comparing a family's pretax cash income to an income poverty threshold that is 3 times the cost of a minimum food diet. This measure does not take into account government benefits (eg, SNAP), income tax credits, or family expenses (eg, child care, income taxes) and has not fundamentally changed since 1969 except for annual adjustments for food price inflation. In 2010, the SPM was instituted to provide a more comprehensive measure of a family's financial circumstances. The SPM includes the value of certain federal in-kind benefits, federal tax benefits, and family expenses. For additional details on these measures, see the accompanying technical report, "Mediators and Adverse Effects of Child Poverty in the United States."

American Indian/Alaska Native children are 3 times more likely to live in poverty than are white and Asian children.[15] Infants and toddlers more commonly live in poverty than do older children.

Children may be born into poverty, remain in a poor household throughout childhood, or, most commonly, rotate in and out of poverty over time. Approximately 37% of all children live in poverty for some period during their childhood.[16] Children who are born into poverty and live persistently in poor conditions are at greatest risk of adverse outcomes. However, even short-term spells of poverty can expose children to hardships, such as food insecurity, housing insecurity/ homelessness, loss of health care, and school disruptions.

Equality of opportunity is central to the American dream and is reflected by social mobility or the potential of intergenerational economic betterment. However, social mobility is difficult to measure, because the usual method compares incomes of 30-year-old persons against the incomes of their parents. Despite the difficulties, most researchers agree that social mobility in the United States has faltered as the wealth and opportunity gaps between rich and poor have widened in the past decade. In comparison with European and other wealthy industrialized countries, social mobility in the United States ranks among the lowest.[17] A 2015 Pew Charitable Trusts report documented that the effect of parental income advantage is persistent over all levels of parental income but is especially strong for children born to wealthy families. Persistent parental economic advantage means that a son's income is strongly influenced by his father's, indicating low social mobility. The result is a dramatic decline of the possibility of economic improvement for the poor.[18] Poor children tend to remain poor and live in neighborhoods of low opportunity. Wealthy children continue to be wealthy as adults and enjoy academic and employment advantages.

The drag on social mobility resulting from income and opportunity inequality is even more striking for people of color. During the recovery of the Great Recession, income inequality in the United States accelerated, with 91% of the gains going to the top 1% of families.[19] Left out of the recovery were African American families who, during the downturn, lost an average of 35% of their accumulated wealth.[20] African American unemployment increased, home ownership decreased, and child poverty deepened to approximately 46% of children younger than 6 years.[21] Because social mobility is lowest for people in the lowest income quartile, half of African American children who are poor as young children will remain poor as adults, approximately twice as many as white adults similarly exposed to poverty as children.[22]

Although legacy residential segregation and environmental racism persist as regions of deep poverty in mostly urban areas,[23] the epidemiology of poverty has shifted over the past decade, in part because of the housing crisis and the Great Recession. Since 2008, suburbs have experienced larger and faster increases in poverty than either urban or rural areas.[24] This significant shift in the location and demographics of children and families dealing with financial stress makes necessary a reevaluation of the current engagement and service delivery systems that may not meet this emerging need.[25]

Because pediatricians work to prevent childhood diseases during health supervision visits and with anticipatory guidance, the early detection and management of poverty-related disorders is an important, emerging component of pediatric scope of practice. With

improved understanding of the root causes and distal effects of poverty, pediatricians can apply interventions in practice to help address the toxic effects of poverty on children and families. They also can advocate for programs and policies to ameliorate early childhood adverse events related to poverty. Pediatricians have the opportunity to screen for risk factors for adversity, to identify family strengths that are protective against toxic stress, and to provide referrals to community organizations that support and assist families in economic stress. This policy statement builds on previous policies related to child health equity,[26] housing insecurity,[27] and early childhood adversity.[3] The accompanying technical report from the American Academy of Pediatrics (AAP), "Mediators and Adverse Effects of Child Poverty in the United States,"[28] supports this statement by describing current knowledge on childhood poverty and the mechanisms by which poverty influences the health and well-being of children.

WHAT WORKS TO AMELIORATE THE EFFECTS OF CHILD POVERTY

Programs that help poor families and children take many forms and often involve stakeholders from multiple communities, including governmental, private nonprofit, faith-based, business, and other philanthropic organizations. The following paragraphs describe several antipoverty and safety net programs that are particularly important for child health and well-being. These programs help families by increasing access to cash, providing "near-cash" benefits, and investing in child development.

Individual program outcomes, including financial cost-benefit estimates, are documented where possible. However, the cumulative

effect of safety net programs has been demonstrably positive. Longitudinal studies from 1967 to 2012 that used the Supplemental Poverty Measure (SPM) revealed that government programs have had a significant effect on family poverty. Without these programs, the rate of child poverty would have increased to 31% in 2012, 13 percentage points more than the actual SPM child poverty rate of 18%. Therefore, the income supports and direct benefits provided by these government programs have cut family poverty almost in half, from an estimated 31% to approximately 16%.[29]

Tax Policies and Direct Financial Aid

The earned income tax credit (EITC) is a refundable federal tax credit that helps low-income families. The EITC helps reduce poverty by incentivizing employment and supplementing income for low-wage workers. In 2012, 25 states had established their own state-level credits to supplement the federal credit.[30] The Center on Budget and Policy Priorities estimates that the federal EITC lifted 3.1 million children out of poverty in 2011.[31] The EITC has been shown to increase workforce participation among single women with children and help families pay for basic essentials.[32] Additional research also has connected the EITC to improvements in infant health. An analysis of families who received the largest EITC under the 1990s expansions of the credit showed lower rates of low birth weight children, fewer preterm births, and increased prenatal care among these families.[33]

The child tax credit provides tax refunds to low-income working families who pay payroll taxes but who might not owe federal income tax. Although only partially refundable, this direct cash benefit in 2012 helped approximately 1.6 million children and their families maintain an income above the FPL.[34]

Taken together, the EITC and child tax credit represent tax policies that reduce childhood poverty and its effects.

Temporary Assistance for Needy Families (TANF) is a block grant program by which the federal government provides money for states to fund work and family support programs with specific goals and time limits. The Personal Responsibility and Work Reconciliation Act of 1996 (often referred to as welfare reform) created TANF to replace Aid to Families with Dependent Children, thereby creating block grants for state administration, work requirements for eligibility, and lifetime limits on receipt of federal support. Because of unchanging federal funding levels and limits of the amount of time individuals can access benefits, the number of families receiving TANF has decreased, despite the increased need since the Great Recession. National TANF caseloads, especially those receiving cash benefits, have declined by 50% since 1996, with state caseload reductions varying from 25% to 80% despite the steadily increasing numbers of families in poverty and deep poverty.[35] The latitude that states have to designate how the funds are used adds to the limitation of TANF as a national safety net program.

Income stagnation in recent decades and the erosion of purchasing power have contributed to the financial instability of working poor families.[36] Raising the minimum wage has been shown to help some low-income families reach 200% of the FPL and to be considered out of poverty.[37] The benefit to children of improved family income stability is both general and specific. Financial stability means that basic needs, such as housing and transportation, are more dependable and family stress may be reduced. School readiness and academic performance

of children are sensitive to family income. In a 1999 analysis by the Brookings Institute, statistically significant increases in math and reading performance were associated with only a $1000 increase in family annual income.[38] A retrospective review of population data drawn from the Panel Study of Economic Dynamics and covering the years 1968 to 2005 correlated the date of birth and family income during early childhood with eventual adult educational and economic attainment. The results suggest that an increase in annual family income of only $3000 during early childhood may result in significant improvements on both SAT scores and adult labor market success measured by an earnings increase of almost 20%. The association is strongest at the low end of the family income scale and becomes statistically nonsignificant for wealthy families.[39]

Work requirements for cash and other benefits have been advanced, especially since welfare reform in the 1990s, as a way to promote self-sufficiency and reduce welfare rolls. However, as a consequence of young mothers being required to work, infants may be placed in child care at a very early age, and mothers often require a patchwork of solutions, some of which may be substandard.[40] Quality child care and early childhood education are extremely important for the promotion of cognitive and socioemotional development of infants and toddlers.[41] Yet, child care may cost as much as housing in most areas of the United States, 25% of the budget of a family with 2 children, and infant care can cost as much as college.[42] Many working families benefit from the dependent care tax credit for the cost of child care, allowing those families to place their children in a certified or higher-quality environment.[43] However, working families who do not have sufficient income to pay taxes are

not able to realize this support for their children, because the credit is not refundable or paid to families before taxation.[44] Therefore, some of the most at-risk children who might benefit from high-quality early childhood education are not eligible for financial support.

Access to Comprehensive Health Care

Children in poverty who otherwise would not have access to health care have greatly benefited from Medicaid and the Children's Health Insurance Program (CHIP) and many provisions and protections of the Patient Protection and Affordable Care Act. From 1984 through 2013, the rate of uninsured poor children decreased by 70%, from approximately 29% to just over 8%. During the first 3 months of 2014, the uninsured rate for poor children dropped further to 6.6%.[45] As a measure of benefit from expanded coverage, children enrolled in Medicaid or CHIP are more likely to access preventive care than are uninsured children.[46,47] In addition, CHIP has resulted in a 9.8% increase in the coverage of children with chronic illness and a 6.4% decrease in uninsured children in the general population.[48] In 2009, CHIP programs expanded access to comprehensive care by covering dental, mental health, and substance abuse services in addition to medical and surgical care for all eligible near-poor children.[49]

Early Childhood Education

Early Head Start and Head Start are federally funded, community-based programs for low-income families with young children. Early Head Start serves pregnant women and families with infants and toddlers up to 3 years of age; Head Start serves families with preschool-aged children 3 to 5 years of age. In fiscal year 2011, the programs served more than 900 000 children nationally, with a budget of $7 billion. These programs provide educational, nutritional, health, and social services. In addition to child care and preschool services, Early Head Start and Head Start offer prenatal education, job-training and adult education, and assistance in accessing housing and insurance.[50] However, Early Head Start presently serves only approximately 3% of low-income families.[51] The Child Care Development Block Grants Act of 2014 and subsequent appropriations also provide child care subsidies for low-income working families and funds to improve child care quality, in addition to new and needed protections to keep children safe and healthy when they are being cared for outside the home.[52]

Early childhood interventions have been found to have a high rate of return in both human and financial terms. Early interventions in high-risk situations have the highest return, presumably through mitigating the effects of toxic stress by providing nurturance, stimulation, and nutrition. Child benefits include improved cognitive functioning, improved self-regulation, and advancement of development in all domains. Research as early as 2005 by the Rand Corporation found a range of return on investment from $1.80 to $17 for each dollar spent on early childhood interventions.[53] More recent studies of preschool (birth to age 5 years) education estimate a return on investment as high as 14% per year on the basis of improved academic and occupation outcomes, in addition to lowered costs of remedial education and juvenile justice involvement.[54]

Nutrition Support

The Supplemental Nutrition Program for Women, Infants, and Children (WIC) is a federal assistance program of the US Department of Agriculture that was first established in 1974 with the aim of improving the health of low-income women, infants, and

children. WIC provides nutrition education, growth monitoring, and breastfeeding promotion and support in addition to food for pregnant and postpartum women, infants, and children younger than 5 years with incomes less than 185% of the FPL.[55]

WIC is associated with improved outcomes in pregnancy and early childhood development. A series of reports from the US Department of Agriculture has shown that WIC participation for low-income women decreased the rates of prematurity and infant mortality and increased involvement in prenatal care.[56] The promotion of breastfeeding has resulted in significant improvements in the rate and duration of exclusive breastfeeding among WIC participants.[57] Studies of the postinfancy period also have shown that WIC increases the quality of children's diets, with increases in micronutrient intake and resulting decreases in iron-deficiency anemia. Children participating in WIC have scored higher on assessments of mental development at 2 years of age than similar children who were not participating in the program. In addition, children whose mothers participated in WIC when they were in utero have also been shown to perform better on reading assessments than similar children of mothers who did not use the program.[58]

SNAP, formerly referred to as "food stamps," uses an electronic benefits card to provide nutrition assistance to low-income individuals and families. As with other federal programs, eligibility depends on income, age, family size, and citizenship. More than 45 million Americans currently receive SNAP benefits each month, including approximately 20 million children.[59] Using the SPM, SNAP benefits reduce both the rate (decrease of 4.4% attributable to SNAP from 2000 to 2009) and, more importantly, the

depth of poverty for children in the poorest of poor families.[60]

The National School Lunch Program is a federally funded program that provides low-cost and free breakfasts, lunches, and, on a limited basis, summer food to school-aged children. The federal program supplies both public and private nonprofit schools with food and cash incentives. The meals are produced in accordance with the Dietary Guidelines for Americans. In 2012, 31.6 million children each day were served low-cost and free lunches at a total cost of $11.6 billion.[61] Students from families with an income less than 130% of the FPL are eligible to receive free meals, and those from families with an income less than 185% of the FPL are eligible for reduced-price meals. A recent analysis estimated that, using these guidelines, more than half of all US public school students are eligible to receive free or reduced-price meals.[62]

Nutrition support, such as WIC and SNAP, address undernutrition, but other forms of malnutrition, such as obesity, also may be responsive to supplemental programs. For instance, a recent study in preschool-aged children found that those who participated in Head Start had a healthier BMI at school entry than did children who did not have the benefit of food provided by federal subsidy.[63]

Home Visiting

The Maternal, Infant, and Early Child Home Visiting (MIECHV) Program was established as part of the Affordable Care Act in 2010. It provides support for federal, state, and community governments to implement established and proven home visiting programs for at-risk children. The stated goals of MIECHV are to improve maternal and newborn health; prevent child injuries, abuse, neglect, or maltreatment; reduce emergency department visits; improve school readiness and achievement; reduce crime or domestic violence; improve family economic self-sufficiency; and improve coordination and referrals for other community resources and supports.[64]

MIECHV has identified 19 evidence-based interventions that target families with pregnant mothers and children younger than 5 years.[65,66] One example of an MIECHV program with evidence of success is the Nurse-Family Partnership. First-time, low-income mothers are enrolled during the prenatal period and visited weekly by nurses trained in a validated curriculum beginning in the second trimester. The benefit-cost ratio for high-risk mothers has been calculated at 5.68 to 1.[67]

Family and Parenting Support in the Medical Home

Programs designed for the pediatric medical home provide opportunities for low-cost, population-based preventive intervention with low-income families. An awareness of the protective factors that are present in children and families can help pediatricians to build on their strengths during health promotion conversations. A commonly used instrument to assess protective factors in high-risk families is available through the FRIENDS National Resource Center.[68] The Protective Factor Survey is used to assess current status as well as change over time in family resiliency, social connectedness, quality of attachment, and knowledge of child development.

In a medical home adapted to the needs of families in poverty, parents have the opportunities and resources to promote resilience in their young children, giving them the capacity to adapt to adversity and buffering the effects of stress. Healthy Steps for Young Children, a manual-based primary care strategy, and programs such as Incredible Years and Triple P, which integrate behavioral health

into primary care, have been shown to promote responsive parenting and address common behavioral and developmental concerns.[69–73] Early literacy promotion in the medical home with programs such as Reach Out and Read advances reading readiness by approximately 6 months when compared with controls.[74] In addition, parents in Reach Out and Read practices are 4 times as likely to read to their children and more likely to spend time with their children in interactive play[75] than are families who are not in Reach Out and Read. Another program, the Video Interaction Project (VIP), combines early literacy with guided parent-child interactions that support family relationships and social development of children.[70]

The AAP has promoted the National Center for Medical-Legal Partnerships model, which provides legal aid collocated with health services, especially to families in poverty. A pilot study of medical-legal partnerships found that addressing the social determinants of health by providing legal services and helping families negotiate safety net organizations improves child health outcomes, reduces unnecessary urgent visits, and raises overall child well-being.[76]

Care coordination, a fundamental service of the medical home model, can link families with community resources and support interagency coordination to address basic concerns such as food and energy insecurity. An example of a robust case management initiative is Health Leads,[77] an enhanced primary care strategy that uses college volunteers as advocates and advanced resource management techniques, which has improved coordination of care and utilization of collocated social services by low-income families with the intent of reducing the social barriers to good health.

Early Identification of Families in Need of Services

To link families to services as early as possible, pediatricians can use screening tools that have high sensitivity and specificity. The WE CARE survey[78] is a brief set of questions that alerts the pediatrician to families experiencing stress related to poverty. In the policy statement "Promoting Food Security for All Children," the AAP recommends the use of a 2-question survey that has a high sensitivity to detect food insecurity.[79,80] A single question, "Do you have difficulty making ends meet at the end of the month?" may be enough to alert the pediatrician with 98% sensitivity to a need for linking families to community resources.[81] Inquiring whether families have moved frequently in the past year or have lived with another family for financial reasons will reveal housing insecurity.[82]

Effective early identification of families in need may facilitate prevention services, including nutritional supplements for young children, preventive health services, age-appropriate learning opportunities, and socioemotional support of parents. Program evaluation has supported this multifaceted approach in multiple countries and settings.[83] Analyses by Nobel Prize–winning economist James Heckman reveal that early prevention activities targeted toward disadvantaged children have high rates of economic returns, much higher than remediation efforts later in childhood or adult life.[84] For example, the Perry Preschool Program showed an average rate of return of $8.74 for every dollar invested in early childhood education.[85] Targeted interventions foster protective factors, including responsive, nurturing, cognitively stimulating, consistent, and stable parenting by either birth parents or other consistent adults. Early childhood experiences that promote relational health lead to secure attachment, effective self-regulation and sleep, normal development of the neuroendocrine system, healthy stress-response systems, and positive changes in the architecture of the developing brain.[86,87] Perhaps the most important protective factors are those that attenuate the toxic stress effects of childhood poverty on early brain and child development.[3,5,88]

Interventions for Adolescents and Parents of Young Children

In recent years, there has been a growing focus on "2-generation" strategies to reduce poverty and improve outcomes for low-income families. Two-generation strategies focus on helping low-income children and their parents simultaneously through high-quality interventions.[89] For example, a 2-generation program may enroll parents into job training at the same time as children are enrolled into quality child care. This type of approach aims to improve a family's earning potential as well as the child's developmental outcomes. Improved coordination of programs and services for low-income families is essential to a 2-generation strategy.

Recent research suggests that noncognitive skills, such as perseverance, empathy, and self-efficacy, remain malleable during adolescence[90] and build on the cognitive skills developed during early childhood. Interventions such as adolescent mentoring, residential training (eg, Job Corps), and workplace-based apprenticeship programs can increase academic achievement, employment success, and other nonacademic accomplishments over the life span.[90]

RECOMMENDATIONS

As the health care system increasingly focuses on efforts to improve quality and contain costs,

there may be new opportunities to restructure the health care delivery system in ways that can improve care for children in low-income families. Policy decisions in other countries, such as the United Kingdom,[91] also may inform these efforts. Incentivizing care coordination and team-based care may help more children access quality health care through patient- and family-centered medical homes (FCMHs). Medical homes also can help families address unmet social and economic needs by using partners, such as community health workers, within the health care team.[92,93] As previously noted, home visiting is supported through the MIECHV.

State reforms and integrated health delivery systems in some regions are providing incentives for population health approaches, facilitating collaboration in healthy neighborhood initiatives.[94] Collaborators with health care organizations may include education systems, social services, faith-based groups, and community development organizations. Although all children may benefit from greater collaboration between health care organizations and community resources, children in poor and low-income families may experience even greater gains.

Opportunities for Public Policy Advocacy

Public policy efforts are needed to protect the health of children affected by poverty and to help families become economically secure. The specific recommendations made in this and the following section are based on positive outcomes in peer-reviewed literature or preliminary studies that show sufficient promise that rigorous long-term evaluations are underway.

- Invest in young children. Funding quality early childhood programs can have a significant financial return on investment, but more

importantly, making healthy development of young children a national priority while addressing social determinants of health helps families and communities build a foundation for lifelong health.

- Protect and expand funding for essential benefits programs that assist low-income and poor children. Invest in children's health and development by appropriately funding evidence-based programs, including Early Head Start and Head Start, Medicaid, CHIP, WIC, home visiting, SNAP, school meal programs and other programs that increase access to healthy food, and Child Care Development Block Grant–funded programs. Streamline enrollment and renewal processes for public benefit programs.[95]

- Support 2-generation strategies that focus on helping children and parents simultaneously. Promote the coordination and alignment of adult- and child-focused programs, policies, and systems.

- Support and expand strategies that promote employment and that increase parental income. Programs that increase low-income parents' earnings have been shown to improve child outcomes. Support policies that help parents increase family income, including higher minimum wages, education and job-training programs, and the EITC, child tax credit, and child and dependent care tax credit.

- Support policy measures that improve community infrastructure, including affordable housing and public spaces. Ensure that all children have safe outdoor play areas as well as healthy, safe, and affordable housing.

- Improve access to quality health care and create incentives to improve population health with the goal of reducing health disparities. Strategies to improve quality and reduce costs should include care coordination and team-based care that help families address nonmedical health-related concerns, such as food, housing, and utilities. Pediatricians and health care systems should be encouraged to partner with other stakeholders to advance community-level strategies that improve health and reduce disparities among populations of varying income levels.

- Enhance health care financing to support comprehensive care for at-risk families. All benefit plans should include coverage for enhanced services in the medical home for families in poverty. Care coordination, team-delivered care, and coverage for mental health services provided by pediatricians are examples of these enhanced services.

- Make a national commitment to fully fund home visiting programs for all children living in low-income or poor households. The Bureau of Maternal and Child Health has identified 19 programs, including but not limited to Nurse-Family Partnership, Early Head Start, Healthy Families America, and Parents as Teachers, that target families with pregnant women or children younger than 5 years.

- Support integrated models of care in the medical home that promote effective parenting and school readiness, such as Healthy Steps, Reach Out and Read, VIP, Incredible Years, Medical Legal Partnerships, and Positive Parenting Program. Both Medicaid and education funding agencies should provide support in the medical home for parenting and literacy promotion.

- Improve national poverty definitions and measures. The FPL underestimates the extent and depth of poverty in the United States. The SPM is an improvement, but more research

is necessary to quantify the extent of poverty in the United States and its effects on children and families so that effective responses can be developed and promoted.

- Support a comprehensive research agenda to improve the understanding of the effects of poverty on children and to identify and refine interventions that improve child health outcomes. Research is needed to identify better ways to measure how poverty affects children, what works to help families in poverty, and how to translate the information gained into real solutions for the poor.

Opportunities for Community Practice

The following recommendations address how individual pediatricians can support the health and well-being of children living in poverty. Adaptations of the medical home to acknowledge the complex challenges that confront poor families require surveillance on the part of the practitioner of both risk and protective factors that characterize each family.

- Create a medical home that acknowledges and is sensitive to the needs of families living in poverty. Although every family wants to provide the best resources and care to their children, economic barriers can stand in the way. All members of the care team and practice should become familiar with some of the common challenges faced by poor families. Recognizing problems such as transportation barriers, difficult work schedules, and competing financial issues can help practices effectively communicate and partner with families. An enhanced medical home providing integrated care for families in poverty is informed by the understanding that emotional care of the family, including recognizing

maternal depression, is within the scope of practice for community pediatricians and that the effects of toxic stress on children can be ameliorated by supportive, secure relational health during early childhood.

- Screen for risk factors within social determinants of health during patient encounters. Practices can use a brief written screener or verbally ask family members questions about basic needs, such as food, housing, and heat. Screening for basic needs can help uncover not only obvious but also less apparent economic difficulties experienced by families. As patient-centered medical homes continue to develop, care coordinators will fulfill the role of community liaison for families in poverty, connecting them with needed resources.

- Consider implementing integrated medical home programs, such as Healthy Steps, Reach Out and Read, Health Leads, and VIP, in addition to primary care integration with mental health interventions such as Incredible Years and Triple P. These programs help parents develop the capacity and confidence to build resilience in their children and improve the ability of the family to cope with adversity. Bright Futures guidelines provide the most comprehensive recommendations for health supervision and are enhanced by strategies to advance behavioral health care into the pediatric medical home and to address the social determinants of health.

- Identify and build on family strengths and protective factors. Although families in poverty face many challenges, each family has strengths, capabilities, and protective factors. Pediatricians can strive to identify and build on protective factors within families, such as cohesion, humor, support networks, skills, and spiritual and cultural beliefs.[96,97] By approaching families from a strengths-based perspective, pediatricians can help build trust and identify the assets on which a family can draw to effectively address problems and care for their children.

- Collaborate with community organizations to help families address unmet basic needs and assist with family stressors. When unmet basic needs and poverty-associated risks are identified, pediatricians can refer families to appropriate community services and public programs. Key partners may include local and state public health departments, legal services, social work organizations, food pantries, faith-based organizations, and community development organizations. Some communities also may have innovative financial literacy programs that are helpful.[98] Practices may partner with local home visiting programs, community mental health services, and parent support groups that can help families address parenting challenges and other stressors.

- Engage with early intervention programs and schools to promote learning and academic achievement. Education professionals are often very involved in efforts to help children from low-income backgrounds with academic achievement and also may participate in initiatives focused on basic needs, such as feeding programs, clothing drives, and health screenings. Pediatricians can actively participate with these efforts as well as early intervention programs, after-school programs, tutoring programs, and social services provided through the school district.

- Promote the MIECHV program. Pediatricians should be familiar with local MIECHV programs and how to connect their patients with home visiting programs on the state and local levels. Pediatricians and the AAP should be aware that the MIECHV continually reviews home visiting programs for inclusion in the MIECHV and can submit programs for review that they have found successful. Opportunities for enhanced communication between the FCMH and home-visiting programs may be explored, including the possibility of collocation of visitors in the FCMH as an integrated service model.

- Support community programs that enhance the involvement of fathers in the lives of their children. Pediatricians can be an important support resource and advocate for community-based fatherhood initiatives. When possible, nonresidential fathers should be involved in all aspects of pediatric care.

- Advance strategies to address family and child mental health and development. Pediatricians are strongly encouraged to include routine screening for maternal depression at every health supervision visit during the first year of life and to be able to provide an appropriate referral for treatment when depression is suspected. Pediatricians can advocate for increased resources to address mental health and behavioral issues in poor communities, including separate payment for screening for parental depression and for care coordination activities.

- Advocate for public policies that support all children and help mitigate the effects of poverty on child health. Pediatricians can serve as important advocates for policies that help children and families in poverty. Pediatricians can add a unique voice to poverty-related advocacy by reframing poverty as an evidence-based health concern with lifelong health, social, and economic consequences.

CONCLUSIONS

Poverty and other adverse social determinants have a detrimental effect on child health and are root causes of child health inequity in the United States. Knowledge is expanding rapidly, especially regarding the neurobiological effects of poverty and related environmental stressors on the developing human brain as well as the life course of chronic illness. Understanding the causative relation between early childhood poverty and adult health status should inform and influence the decisions of policy makers, researchers, and community pediatricians. The evidence strongly suggests that the FCMH with its enhanced capabilities is an essential asset in efforts to ameliorate the adverse effects of poverty on children.

The AAP considers child poverty in the United States unacceptable and detrimental to the health and well-being of children and is committed to its elimination. The AAP calls for concerted action by its state chapters as well as governmental, private, nonprofit, faith-based, philanthropic, and other advocacy organizations to reduce child poverty by supporting and expanding existing programs that have been shown to work and to make efforts to develop, identify, and promote other potentially effective policies and programs. In 1935, the US Congress passed the Social Security Act and in 1965 enacted Medicare. Together, these 2 pieces of legislation have greatly reduced and nearly eliminated poverty in the elderly. It is time to enact similar reforms to eliminate child poverty. By embracing the policies and enacting the recommendations in this statement, the AAP joins with governmental, philanthropic, private, and other health care organizations in a concerted and dedicated effort to eliminate child poverty in the United States.

ACKNOWLEDGMENTS

We acknowledge the following University of California–Los Angeles pediatric and med-peds residents for their research contributions to this policy statement: Natalie Cerda, MD, Jeremy Lehman Fox, MD, Neil A. Gholkar, MD, Lydia Soo-Hyun Kim, MD, MPH, Rachel J. Klein, MD, Ashley E. Lewis Hunter, MD, Sarah J. Maufe, MD, Colin L. Robinson, MD, MPH, Joseph R. Rojas, MD, and Weiyi Tan, MD, MPH.

LEAD AUTHORS

James H. Duffee, MD, MPH, FAAP
Alice A. Kuo, MD, PhD, FAAP
Benjamin A. Gitterman, MD, FAAP

COUNCIL ON COMMUNITY PEDIATRICS EXECUTIVE COMMITTEE, 2015–2016

Benjamin A. Gitterman, MD, FAAP, Chairperson
Patricia J. Flanagan MD, FAAP, Vice-Chairperson
William H. Cotton, MD, FAAP
Kimberley J. Dilley, MD, MPH, FAAP
James H. Duffee, MD, MPH, FAAP
Andrea E. Green, MD, FAAP
Virginia A. Keane, MD, FAAP
Scott D. Krugman, MD, MS, FAAP
Julie M. Linton, MD, FAAP
Carla D. McKelvey, MD, MPH, FAAP
Jacqueline L. Nelson, MD, FAAP

LIAISONS

Jacqueline R. Dougé, MD, MPH, FAAP –
Chairperson, Public Health Special Interest Group
Janna Gewirtz O'Brien, MD – *Section on Medical Students, Residents, and Fellowship Trainees*

FORMER EXECUTIVE COMMITTEE MEMBERS

Lance A. Chilton, MD, FAAP
Thresia B. Gambon, MD, FAAP
Alice A. Kuo, MD, PhD, FAAP
Gonzalo J. Paz-Soldan, MD, FAAP
Barbara Zind, MD, FAAP

FORMER LIAISONS

Toluwalase Ajayi, MD – *Section on Medical Students, Residents, and Fellowship Trainees*
Ricky Y. Choi, MD, MPH, FAAP – *Chairperson, Immigrant Health Special Interest Group*
Frances J. Dunston, MD, MPH, FAAP – *Commission to End Health Care Disparities*
M. Edward Ivancic, MD, FAAP – *Chairperson, Rural Health Special Interest Group*

CONTRIBUTORS

John M. Pascoe, MD, MPH, FAAP
David Wood, MD, MPH, FAAP

CONSULTANT

Anne Brown Rodgers, Science Writer

STAFF

Camille Watson, MS

COMMITTEE ON PSYCHOSOCIAL ASPECTS OF CHILD AND FAMILY HEALTH, 2015–2016

Michael Yogman, MD, FAAP, Chairperson
Nerissa Bauer, MD, MPH, FAAP
Thresia B. Gambon, MD, FAAP
Arthur Lavin, MD, FAAP
Keith M. Lemmon, MD, FAAP
Gerri Mattson, MD, FAAP
Jason Richard Rafferty, MD, MPH, EdM
Lawrence Sagin Wissow, MD, MPH, FAAP

LIAISONS

Sharon Berry, PhD, LP – *Society of Pediatric Psychology*
Terry Carmichael, MSW – *National Association of Social Workers*
Edward Christophersen, PhD, FAAP – *Society of Pediatric Psychology*
Norah Johnson, PhD, RN, CPNP-BC – *National Association of Pediatric Nurse Practitioners*
Leonard Read Sulik, MD, FAAP – *American Academy of Child and Adolescent Psychiatry*

CONSULTANT

George J. Cohen, MD, FAAP

STAFF

Stephanie Domain, MS, CHES

ABBREVIATIONS

AAP: American Academy of Pediatrics
CHIP: Children's Health Insurance Program
EITC: earned income tax credit
FCMH: family-centered medical home
FPL: federal poverty level
MIECHV: Maternal, Infant, and Early Child Home Visiting
SNAP: Supplemental Nutrition Assistance Program
SPM: Supplemental Poverty Measure
TANF: Temporary Assistance for Needy Families
VIP: Video Interaction Project
WIC: Supplemental Nutrition Program for Women, Infants, and Children

---

REFERENCES

1. Brooks-Gunn J, Duncan GJ. The effects of poverty on children. *Future Child.* 1997;7(2):55–71

2. Blair C, Granger DA, Willoughby M, et al; FLP Investigators. Salivary cortisol mediates effects of poverty and parenting on executive functions in early childhood. *Child Dev.* 2011;82(6):1970–1984

3. Garner AS, Shonkoff JP; Committee on Psychosocial Aspects of Child and Family Health; Committee on Early Childhood, Adoption, and Dependent Care; Section on Developmental and Behavioral Pediatrics. Early childhood adversity, toxic stress, and the role of the pediatrician: translating developmental science into lifelong health. *Pediatrics.* 2012;129(1). Available at: www.pediatrics.org/cgi/content/full/129/1/e224

4. Boyle CA, Boulet S, Schieve LA, et al. Trends in the prevalence of developmental disabilities in US children, 1997-2008. *Pediatrics.* 2011;127(6):1034–1042

5. Belfield CR, Levin HM, eds. *The Price We Pay: Economic and Social Consequences of Inadequate Education.* Washington, DC: Brookings Press; 2007

6. Shonkoff JP, Garner AS; Committee on Psychosocial Aspects of Child and Family Health; Committee on Early Childhood, Adoption, and Dependent Care; Section on Developmental and Behavioral Pediatrics. The lifelong effects of early childhood adversity and toxic stress. *Pediatrics.* 2012;129(1). Available at: www.pediatrics.org/cgi/content/full/129/1/e232

7. Holzer H, Schanzenbach DW, Duncan GJ, Ludwig J. The economic costs of childhood poverty in the United States. *J Child Poverty.* 2008;14(1):41–61

8. Belfield CR, Levin HM, Rosen R. The economic value of opportunity youth. Washington, DC: Corporation for National and Community Service; 2012. Available at: www.serve.gov/new-images/council/pdf/econ_value_opportunity_youth.pdf. Accessed January 11, 2016

9. UNICEF Innocenti Research Centre. Measuring child poverty: new league

tables of child poverty in the world's rich countries. Florence, Italy: UNICEF Innocenti Research Centre; 2012. Innocenti Report Card 10. Available at: www.unicef-irc.org/publications/pdf/rc10_eng.pdf. Accessed January 11, 2016

10. Organization for Economic Cooperation and Development. Child poverty. Available at: www.oecd.org/els/soc/CO2_2_ChildPoverty_Jan2014.pdf. Accessed January 11, 2016

11. United Nations. Sustainable Development Goals. Goal 1: end poverty in all its forms everywhere. Available at: www.un.org/sustainabledevelopment/poverty/. Accessed January 11, 2016

12. DeNavas-Walt C, Proctor BD; US Census Bureau. Current population reports, P60-252, income and poverty in the United States: 2014. Washington, DC: US Government Printing Office; 2015

13. US Census Bureau. One in five children receive food stamps, Census Bureau reports. Available at: www.census.gov/newsroom/press-releases/2015/cb15-16.html. Accessed September 28, 2015

14. Kids Count Data Center. 2011 Kids Count Data Book. Available at: http://datacenter.kidscount.org. Accessed July 31, 2015

15. The Annie E. Casey Foundation. 2013 Kids Count Data Book. Available at: www.aecf.org/MajorInitiatives/KIDSCOUNT.aspx?rules=2. Accessed July 31, 2015

16. Ratcliffe C, McKernan SM. Childhood poverty persistence: facts and consequences. Urban Institute Brief. June 2010. Available at: www.urban.org/UploadedPDF/412126-child-poverty-persistence.pdf. Accessed July 31, 2015

17. Isaacs JB. International comparisons of economic mobility. In: Isaacs JB, Sawhill IV, Haskins R, eds. Getting ahead or losing ground: economic mobility in America. Washington, DC: The Brookings Institution; 2008:37–44. Available at: www.brookings.edu/~/media/Research/Files/Reports/2008/2/economic%20mobility%20sawhill/02_economic_mobility_sawhill.pdf. Accessed January 11, 2016

18. Mitnik PA, Grusky DB. Economic mobility in the United States. 2015. Philadelphia, PA: Pew Charitable Trusts, Russell Sage Foundation; 2015. Available at: www.pewtrusts.org/~/media/assets/2015/07/fsm-irs-report_artfinal.pdf. Accessed December 27, 2015

19. Saez E. Striking it richer: the evolution of top incomes in the United States. Berkeley, CA: University of California Berkeley; 2015. Available at: http://eml.berkeley.edu/~saez/saez-UStopincomes-2013.pdf. Accessed December 27, 2015

20. Stiglitz J. Inequality in America: a policy agenda for a stronger future. Ann Am Acad Pol Soc Sci. 2015;657(1):8–20

21. Economic Policy Institute. The state of working America: key numbers. African Americans. Available at: http://stateofworkingamerica.org/files/book/factsheets/african-americans.pdf. Accessed December 27, 2015

22. Wagmiller RL, Adelman RM. Childhood and intergenerational poverty. New York, NY: National Center for Children in Poverty; 2009. Available at: www.nccp.org/publications/pub_909.html. Accessed December 27, 2015

23. Bolin B, Grineski S, Collins T. The geography of despair. Hum Ecol Rev. 2005;12(2):156–168

24. Kneebone B. Confronting Suburban Poverty in America. Washington, DC: Brookings Press; 2013

25. Joint Center's Health Policy Institute. Building stronger communities for better health. 2004. Available at: www.racialequitytools.org/resourcefiles/jointcenter3.pdf. Accessed December 28, 2015

26. Council on Community Pediatrics and Committee on Native American Child Health. Policy statement—health equity and children's rights. Pediatrics. 2010;125(4):838–849

27. Council on Community Pediatrics. Providing care for children and adolescents facing homelessness and housing insecurity. Pediatrics. 2013;131(6):1206–1210

28. Pascoe JM, Wood DL, Kuo A, Duffee JH; Committee on Psychosocial Aspects of Child and Family Health; Council on Community Pediatrics. Mediators and adverse effects of child poverty in the United States. Pediatrics. 2016;137(4):e20160340

29. Fox L, Garfinkel I, Kaushal N, Waldfogel J, Wimer C. Waging War on Poverty: Historical Trends in Poverty Using the Supplemental Poverty Measure. Cambridge, MA: National Bureau of Economic Research; 2014. Working Paper 19789. Available at: www.nber.org/papers/w19789. Accessed July 31, 2015

30. Center on Budget and Policy Priorities. Policy basics: the earned income tax credit. January 2014. Available at: www.cbpp.org/files/policybasics-eitc.pdf. Accessed July 31, 2015

31. Center on Budget and Policy Priorities. Earned income tax credit promotes work, encourages children's success at school, research finds. April 2013. Available at: www.cbpp.org/files/6-26-12tax.pdf\. Accessed July 31, 2015

32. Leibman J. The impact of the earned income tax credit on incentives and income distribution. In: Poterba JM, ed. Tax Policy and the Economy. Cambridge, MA: MIT Press; 1998:83–120

33. Hoynes HW, Miller DL, Simon D. The EITC: linking income to real health outcomes [policy brief]. Davis, CA: University of California Davis Center for Poverty Research; 2013. Available at: http://poverty.ucdavis.edu/research-paper/policy-brief-linking-eitc-income-real-health-outcomes. Accessed July 31, 2015

34. Center on Budget and Policy Priorities. Policy basics: the child tax credit. January 2014. Available at: www.cbpp.org/files/policybasics-ctc.pdf. Accessed July 31, 2015

35. Center on Budget and Policy Priorities. TANF weakening as a safety-net for poor families. March 2012. Available at: www.cbpp.org/files/3-13-12tanf.pdf. Accessed July 31, 2015

36. Hernandez DJ. Declining fortunes of children in middle-class families: economic inequality and child well-being in the 21st century. New York, NY: Foundation for Child Development; 2011. Available at: http://fcd-us.org/sites/default/files/2011%20Declining%20Fortunes_0.pdf. Accessed July 31, 2015

37. Dube A. Minimum wages and the distribution of family incomes. UMass Amherst Working Paper.

2013. Available at: https://dl.dropboxusercontent.com/u/15038936/Dube_MinimumWagesFamilyIncomes.pdf. Accessed July 31, 2015

38. Issacs JB, Magnuson K. Income and education as predictors of children's school readiness. Washington, DC: Brookings Institute; 2011. Available at: www.brookings.edu/research/reports/2011/12/15-school-readiness-isaacs. Accessed July 31, 2015

39. Duncan GJ, Ziol-Guest KM, Kalil A. Early-childhood poverty and adult attainment, behavior, and health. *Child Dev.* 2010;81(1):306–325

40. Knox V, London A, Scoot E. Welfare reform, work, and child care. MDRC policy brief. 2003. Available at: www.mdrc.org/sites/default/files/policybrief_40.pdf. Accessed July 31, 2015

41. Cohen J, Ewen D. Infants and toddlers in child care [policy brief]. Washington, DC: Zero to Three; 2008. Available at: http://main.zerotothree.org/site/DocServer/Infants_and_Toddlers_in_Child_Care_Brief.pdf?docID=6561. Accessed July 31, 2015

42. Allegretto S. Basic family budgets: working families' incomes often fail to meet living expenses around the U.S. Economic Policy Institute; 2005. Available at: www.epi.org/publication/bp165/. Accessed July 31, 2015

43. MacGillvary J, Lucia L. Economic impacts of early care and education in California. Berkley, CA: UC Berkley Center for Labor Research and Education; 2011. Available at: http://laborcenter.berkeley.edu/pdf/2011/child_care_report0811.pdf. Accessed July 31, 2015

44. Tax Policy Center. Taxation and the family. How does the tax system subsidize child care expenses? 2015. Available at: www.taxpolicycenter.org/briefing-book/key-elements/family/child-care-subsidies.cfm. Accessed July 31, 2015

45. National Health Interview Survey Early Release Program. Health insurance coverage: early release of estimates from the National Health Interview Survey, January–March 2014. Available at: www.cdc.gov/nchs/data/nhis/earlyrelease/insur201409.pdf. Accessed January 11, 2016

46. Abdus S, Selden TM. Adherence with recommended well-child visits has grown, but large gaps persist among various socioeconomic groups. *Health Aff (Millwood).* 2013;32(3):508–515

47. Perry CD, Kenney GM. Preventive care for children in low-income families: how well do Medicaid and state children's health insurance programs do? *Pediatrics.* 2007;120(6). Available at: www.pediatrics.org/cgi/content/full/120/6/e1393

48. Howell EM, Kenney GM. The impact of the Medicaid/CHIP expansions on children: a synthesis of the evidence. *Med Care Res Rev.* 2012;69(4):372–396

49. Racine AD, Long TF, Helm ME, et al; Committee on Child Health Financing. Children's Health Insurance Program (CHIP): accomplishments, challenges, and policy recommendations. *Pediatrics.* 2014;133(3). Available at: www.pediatrics.org/cgi/content/full/133/3/e784

50. Head Start Program. Head Start Program facts fiscal year 2011. Available at: http://eclkc.ohs.acf.hhs.gov/hslc/mr/factsheets/2011-hs-program-factsheet.html. Accessed July 31, 2015

51. DiLaruro E. Learning, thriving and ready to succeed. Zero to Three; 2009. Available at: http://main.zerotothree.org/site/DocServer/EHSsinglesMar5.pdf?docID=7884. Accessed July 31, 2015

52. Administration for Children and Families, Office of Child Care. OCC fact sheet. Available at: www.acf.hhs.gov/programs/occ/fact-sheet-occ. Accessed January 19, 2016

53. Karoly LA, Kilburn MR, Cannon JS. Proven benefits of early childhood interventions [research brief]. Santa Monica, CA: Rand Corporation; 2005. Available at: www.rand.org/content/dam/rand/pubs/research_briefs/2005/RAND_RB9145.pdf. Accessed July 31, 2015

54. Heckman JJ. The case for investing in disadvantaged young children. In: *Big Ideas for Children: Investing in Our Nation's Future.* Washington, DC: First Focus; 2008:49–58

55. Special Supplemental Nutrition Program for Women, Infants, and Children. WIC eligibility requirements. Available at: www.fns.usda.gov/wic/howtoapply/eligibilityrequirements.htm. Accessed July 31, 2015

56. Colman S, Nichols-Barrer IP, Redline JE, Devaney BL, Ansell SV, Joyce T. Effects of the Special Supplemental Nutrition Program for Women, Infants, and Children (WIC): a review of recent research. Alexandria, VA: US Department of Agriculture, Food and Nutrition Service; 2012. Report WIC-12-WM. Available at: www.mathematica-mpr.com/~/media/publications/pdfs/nutrition/wic_research_review.pdf. Accessed January 11, 2016

57. Suchman A, Mendelson M, Patlan KL, Freeman B, Gotlieb R, Connor P. *WIC Participant and Program Characteristics 2012.* Prepared by Insight Policy Research under contract no. AG-3198-C-11-0010. Alexandria, VA: Food and Nutrition Service, US Department of Agriculture; 2013

58. Jackson MI. Early childhood WIC participation, cognitive development and academic achievement. *Soc Sci Med.* 2015;126:145–153

59. Executive Office of the President of the United States. Long-term benefits of the Supplemental Nutrition Assistance Program. December 2015. Available at: https://www.whitehouse.gov/sites/whitehouse.gov/files/documents/SNAP_report_final_nonembargo.pdf. Accessed January 11, 2016

60. US Department of Agriculture, Economic Research Service. SNAP benefits alleviate the intensity and incidence of poverty. Available at: www.ers.usda.gov/amber-waves/2012-june/snap-benefits.aspx#.VolJcBHVStV. Accessed January 11, 2016

61. US Department of Agriculture, Food and Nutrition Service. National School Lunch Program. Available at: www.fns.usda.gov/sites/default/files/NSLPFactSheet.pdf. Accessed July 31, 2015

62. Southern Education Foundation. A New Majority Research Bulletin: low income students now a majority in the nation's public schools. Atlanta, GA: Southern Education Foundation; 2015. Available at: www.southerneducation.org/Our-Strategies/Research-and-Publications/New-Majority-Diverse-Majority-Report-Series/

A-New-Majority-2015-Update-Low-Income-Students-Now. Accessed July 31, 2015

63. Lumeng JC, Kaciroti N, Sturza J, et al. Changes in body mass index associated with head start participation. *Pediatrics*. 2015;135(2). Available at: www.pediatrics.org/cgi/content/full/135/2/e449

64. US Department of Health and Human Services. Maternal, Infant, and Early Childhood Home Visiting Program. Available at: http://mchb.hrsa.gov/programs/homevisiting/index.html. Accessed July 31, 2015

65. Health Resources and Services Administration. Home visiting models. Available at: http://mchb.hrsa.gov/programs/homevisiting/models.html. Accessed July 31, 2015

66. Avellar S, Paulsell D, Sama-Miller E, Del Grosso P, Akers L, Kleinman R. Home visiting evidence of effectiveness review: executive summary. Washington, DC: Office of Planning, Research and Evaluation, Administration for Children and Families, US Department of Health and Human Services; 2015. Available at: http://homvee.acf.hhs.gov/HomVEE_Executive_Summary_2015.pdf. Accessed January 3, 2016

67. Olds D. The nurse–family partnership: an evidence-based preventive intervention. *Infant Ment Health J.* 2006;27(1):5–25

68. National Center for Community-Based Child Abuse Prevention. Protective Factors Survey. Available at: http://friendsnrc.org/protective-factors-survey. Accessed July 31, 2015

69. Zuckerman B. Promoting early literacy in pediatric practice: twenty years of reach out and read. *Pediatrics*. 2009;124(6):1660–1665

70. Mendelsohn AL, Dreyer BP, Brockmeyer CA, Berkule-Silberman SB, Morrow LM. Fostering early development and school readiness in pediatric settings. In: Dickinson D, Neuman SB, eds. *Handbook of Early Literacy Research*. Vol. 3. New York, NY: Guilford; 2011:279–294

71. Minkovitz CS, Strobino D, Mistry KB, et al. Healthy Steps for Young Children: sustained results at 5.5 years.

Pediatrics. 2007;120(3). Available at: www.pediatrics.org/cgi/content/full/120/3/e658

72. Perrin EC, Sheldrick RC, McMenamy JM, Henson BS, Carter AS. Improving parenting skills for families of young children in pediatric settings: a randomized clinical trial. *JAMA Pediatr.* 2014;168(1):16–24

73. Bauer NS, Webster-Stratton C. Prevention of behavioral disorders in primary care. *Curr Opin Pediatr.* 2006;18(6):654–660

74. Diener ML, Hobson Rohrer W, Byington CL. Kindergarten readiness and performance of Latino children participating in Reach Out and Read. *J Community Med Health Educ.* 2012;2:133

75. Mendelsohn AL, Mogilner LN, Dreyer BP, et al. The impact of a clinic-based literacy intervention on language development in inner-city preschool children. *Pediatrics*. 2001;107(1):130–134

76. Weintraub D, Rodgers MA, Botcheva L, et al. Pilot study of medical-legal partnership to address social and legal needs of patients. *J Health Care Poor Underserved*. 2010;21(2 suppl):157–168

77. Vasan A, Solomon BS. Use of colocated multidisciplinary services to address family psychosocial needs at an urban pediatric primary care clinic. *Clin Pediatr (Phila)*. 2015;54(1):25–32

78. Garg A, Butz AM, Dworkin PH, Lewis RA, Thompson RE, Serwint JR. Improving the management of family psychosocial problems at low-income children's well-child care visits: the WE CARE Project. *Pediatrics*. 2007;120(3):547–558

79. Council on Community Pediatrics; Committee on Nutrition. Promoting food security for all children. *Pediatrics*. 2015;136(5). Available at: www.pediatrics.org/cgi/content/full/136/5/e1431

80. Hager ER, Quigg AM, Black MM, et al. Development and validity of a 2-item screen to identify families at risk for food insecurity. *Pediatrics*. 2010;126(1). Available at: www.pediatrics.org/cgi/content/full/126/1/e26

81. Brcic V, Eberdt C, Kaczorowski J. Development of a tool to identify poverty in a family practice setting: a pilot study. *Int J Family Med.* 2011;2011:812182

82. Cutts DB, Meyers AF, Black MM, et al. US housing insecurity and the health of very young children. *Am J Public Health*. 2011;101(8):1508–1514

83. Shonkoff JP, Richter L, van der Gaag J, Bhutta ZA. An integrated scientific framework for child survival and early childhood development. *Pediatrics*. 2012;129(2). Available at: www.pediatrics.org/cgi/content/full/129/2/e460

84. Heckman JJ. Skill formation and the economics of investing in disadvantaged children. *Science*. 2006;312(5782):1900–1902

85. Barnett WS. Benefit-cost analysis of preschool education. 2004. Available at: http://nieer.org/resources/files/BarnettBenefits.ppt. Accessed July 31, 2015

86. Yoshikawa H, Aber JL, Beardslee WR. The effects of poverty on the mental, emotional, and behavioral health of children and youth: implications for prevention. *Am Psychol.* 2012;67(4):272–284

87. McEwen BS, Gianaros PJ. Central role of the brain in stress and adaptation: links to socioeconomic status, health, and disease. *Ann N Y Acad Sci.* 2010;1186:190–222

88. Johnson SB, Riley AW, Granger DA, Riis J. The science of early life toxic stress for pediatric practice and advocacy. *Pediatrics*. 2013;131(2):319–327

89. Woodrow Wilson School of Public and International Affairs at Princeton University; Brookings Institution. Helping parents, helping children: two-generation mechanisms. *Future Child*. 2014;24(1):1–170. Available at: www.princeton.edu/futureofchildren/publications/journals/journal_details/index.xml?journalid=81. Accessed January 11, 2016

90. Heckman JJ, Kautz T. Fostering and measuring skills: interventions that improve character and cognition. In: Heckman JJ, Humphries JE, Kautz T, eds. *The Myth of Achievement Tests: The GED and the Role of Character in*

American Life. Chicago, IL: University of Chicago Press; 2014:293–317

91. Waldfogel J. Tackling child poverty and improving child well-being: lessons from Britain. Report for First Focus and Foundation for Child Development. 2010. Available at: http://fcd-us.org/resources/tackling-child-poverty-and-improving-child-well-being-lessons-britain. Accessed July 31, 2015

92. Antonelli RC, McAllister JW, Popp J. Making care coordination a critical component of the pediatric health system: a multidisciplinary framework. The Commonwealth Fund; 2009. Available at: www.commonwealthfund.org/publications/fund-reports/2009/may/making-care-coordination-a-critical-component-of-the-pediatric-health-system. Accessed July 31, 2015

93. Rosenthal EL, Brownstein JN, Rush CH, et al. Community health workers: part of the solution. *Health Aff (Millwood)*. 2010;29(7):1338–1342

94. Nationwide Children's. Healthy neighborhoods, healthy families. Available at: www.nationwidechildrens.org/healthy-neighborhoods-healthy-families. Accessed July 31, 2015

95. The Annie E. Casey Foundation. Improving access to public benefits helping eligible individuals and families get the income supports they need. April 2010. Available at: www.aecf.org/~/media/Pubs/Topics/Economic%20Security/Family%20Economic%20Supports/ImprovingAccesstoPublicBenefitsHelpingEligibl/BenefitsAccess41410.pdf. Accessed July 31, 2015

96. US Department of Health and Human Services; Administration for Children and Families; Office of Head Start; USA.gov. Training guides for the Head Start Learning Community: abstracts. 2000. Available at: http://eclkc.ohs.acf.hhs.gov/hslc/tta-system/pd/pds/Cultivating%20a%20Learning%20Organization/TrainingGuidesf.htm. Accessed July 31, 2015

97. Center for the Study of Social Policy; American Academy of Pediatrics. Primary health partners. Promoting children's health and resiliency: a strengthening families approach. Available at: www.cssp.org/reform/strengthening-families/messaging-at-the-intersection/Messaging-at-the-Intersections_Primary-Health.pdf. Accessed July 31, 2015

98. The Neighborhood Developers. Available at: www.theneighborhooddevelopers.org/money-wise/. Accessed July 31, 2015

Preventing Obesity and Eating Disorders in Adolescents

• *Clinical Report*

CLINICAL REPORT Guidance for the Clinician in Rendering Pediatric Care

American Academy
of Pediatrics

DEDICATED TO THE HEALTH OF ALL CHILDREN™

Preventing Obesity and Eating Disorders in Adolescents

Neville H. Golden, MD, FAAP, Marcie Schneider, MD, FAAP, Christine Wood, MD, FAAP,
COMMITTEE ON NUTRITION, COMMITTEE ON ADOLESCENCE, SECTION ON OBESITY

abstract

Obesity and eating disorders (EDs) are both prevalent in adolescents. There are concerns that obesity prevention efforts may lead to the development of an ED. Most adolescents who develop an ED did not have obesity previously, but some teenagers, in an attempt to lose weight, may develop an ED. This clinical report addresses the interaction between obesity prevention and EDs in teenagers, provides the pediatrician with evidence-informed tools to identify behaviors that predispose to both obesity and EDs, and provides guidance about obesity and ED prevention messages. The focus should be on a healthy lifestyle rather than on weight. Evidence suggests that obesity prevention and treatment, if conducted correctly, do not predispose to EDs.

DOI: 10.1542/peds.2016-1649

PEDIATRICS (ISSN Numbers: Print, 0031-4005; Online, 1098-4275).

Copyright © 2016 by the American Academy of Pediatrics

FINANCIAL DISCLOSURE: The authors have indicated they do not have a financial relationship relevant to this article to disclose.

FUNDING: No external funding.

POTENTIAL CONFLICT OF INTEREST: The authors have indicated they have no potential conflicts of interest to disclose.

To cite: Golden NH, Schneider M, Wood C, AAP COMMITTEE ON NUTRITION. Preventing Obesity and Eating Disorders in Adolescents. Pediatrics. 2016;138(3):e20161649

INTRODUCTION

The prevalence of childhood obesity has increased dramatically over the past few decades in the United States and other countries, and obesity during adolescence is associated with significant medical morbidity during adulthood.[1] Eating disorders (EDs) are the third most common chronic condition in adolescents, after obesity and asthma.[2] Most adolescents who develop an ED did not have obesity previously, but some adolescents may misinterpret what "healthy eating" is and engage in unhealthy behaviors, such as skipping meals or using fad diets in an attempt to "be healthier," the result of which could be the development of an ED.[3] Messages from pediatricians addressing obesity and reviewing constructive ways to manage weight can be safely and supportively incorporated into health care visits. Avoiding certain weight-based language and using motivational interviewing (MI) techniques may improve communication and promote successful outcomes when providing weight-management counseling.[4]

This clinical report complements existing American Academy of Pediatrics (AAP) reports on EDs[5] and obesity prevention.[6] The aim is to address the interaction between obesity prevention and EDs in teenagers and to stress that obesity prevention does not promote the development of EDs in adolescents. This report provides the pediatrician with office-based, evidence-informed tools to identify behaviors that predispose to both obesity and EDs and to provide guidance about obesity and ED prevention messages.

INCREASING PREVALENCE OF ADOLESCENT OBESITY

Data from the NHANES on adolescent obesity prevalence revealed that, in 2011–2012, 20.5% of 12- to 19-year-olds were obese (BMI ≥95th percentile according to the 2000 sex-specific BMI-for-age growth charts of the Centers for Disease Control and Prevention).[7,8] Combining the definitions of overweight (BMI between the 85th and 95th percentiles) and obesity, according to the NHANES 2011–2012 data, 34.5% of 12- to 19-year-olds were overweight or obese.[7,8] Disparities exist in obesity rates among minority youth, with Hispanic, American Indian, and African-American adolescents having the highest prevalence of obesity. Over the past 30 years, the rate of childhood obesity has more than doubled, and the rate of adolescent obesity has quadrupled. However, more recent data over the past 9 years between 2003–2004 and 2011–2012 have revealed no significant changes in obesity prevalence in youth or adults. Although halting the increase in the rate of obesity is a step in the right direction, the prevalence of obesity remains high, and its health care burden and costs remain significant.[9]

RELATIONSHIP BETWEEN CHILDHOOD OBESITY AND ADULT HEALTH STATUS

Most studies have found that children and adolescents who are obese, especially those in the higher range of BMI percentiles, are more likely to be obese as adults.[10-12] The health consequences of obesity can manifest during childhood, but the longer a person is obese, the more at risk he

or she is for adult health problems. A high adolescent BMI increases adult diabetes and coronary artery disease risks by nearly threefold and fivefold, respectively.[13] Type 2 diabetes is one of the most serious complications of childhood obesity. Risks of other common comorbid conditions, such as hypertension, abnormal lipid profiles, nonalcoholic fatty liver disease, gallstones, gastroesophageal reflux, polycystic ovary syndrome, obstructive sleep apnea, asthma, and bone and joint problems, are significantly increased in both obese adolescents and adults who were obese as adolescents.[1,14-16] In addition, the psychosocial morbidities associated with childhood obesity, such as depression, poor self-esteem, and poor quality of life, are of significant concern.[17-19]

PREVALENCE OF EDS IN CHILDREN AND ADOLESCENTS AND CHANGES IN DSM-5 DIAGNOSTIC CRITERIA

The onset of EDs usually is during adolescence, with the highest prevalence in adolescent girls, but EDs increasingly are being recognized in children as young as 5 to 12 years.[20-22] Increased prevalence rates also have been noted in males and minority youth.[23] The peak age of onset for anorexia nervosa (AN) is early to mid-adolescence, and the peak age of onset for bulimia nervosa (BN) is late adolescence. Although overall incidence rates have been stable, there has been a notable increase in the incidence of AN in 15- to 19-year-old girls.[24] In the United States from 1999 to 2006, hospitalizations for EDs increased 119% for children younger than 12 years.[25] The lifetime prevalences of AN, BN, and binge eating disorder in adolescent females are 0.3%, 0.9%, and 1.6%, respectively.[26] The reported female-to-male ratio is 9:1, but increasing numbers of males with EDs are being recognized, especially among younger age groups.[20-22]

The *Diagnostic and Statistical Manual of Mental Disorders, Fifth Edition* (DSM-5) criteria for EDs are listed in Table 1.[27] The diagnostic criteria for both AN and BN in the DSM-5 are less stringent than in the *Diagnostic and Statistical Manual of Mental Disorders, Fourth Edition, Text Revision*, so the numbers of reported cases likely will increase. For AN, the 85% expected body weight threshold and the amenorrhea criterion from the *Diagnostic and Statistical Manual of Mental Disorders, Fourth Edition, Text Revision*, both have been eliminated in the DSM-5. For BN, DSM-5 modifications from the previous edition include reducing the threshold of the frequency of binge eating and inappropriate compensatory behaviors (self-induced vomiting, periods of starvation, compulsive exercising or the use of laxatives, diuretics, or diet pills) from twice a week for 3 months to once a week for 3 months. Binge eating disorder now is officially recognized in the DSM-5 as a distinct disorder characterized by recurrent episodes of bingeing at least once a week for 3 months, but without compensatory behaviors, and is associated with the development of obesity.[28] "Atypical AN" describes a subset of patients who lost a significant amount of weight and then returned to normal weight but who continue to have preoccupations with body shape and weight, comparable to patients with "classic" AN.

MEDICAL COMPLICATIONS ASSOCIATED WITH EDS

The medical complications of EDs have been well described elsewhere.[5] In general, medical complications are either the result of physiologic adaptations to the effects of malnutrition or a consequence of unhealthy weight-control behaviors. Young people who have lost large amounts of weight or lost weight too rapidly can develop hypothermia, bradycardia, hypotension, and orthostasis even if their current weight is in the normal range.[29,30] Rapid weight loss can be associated with acute pancreatitis and gallstone formation. Electrolyte disturbances can occur secondary to self-induced vomiting or the use of laxatives or diuretics or can develop when food is reintroduced after prolonged periods of dietary restriction (the so-called refeeding syndrome). Dietary restriction can lead to primary or secondary amenorrhea in adolescent girls of even normal weight as a result of the suppression of the hypothalamic-pituitary-ovarian axis, which is mediated in part by leptin.[31] Prolonged amenorrhea results in a low-estrogen state, which can contribute to osteoporosis.[23]

THE INTERACTION BETWEEN EDS AND OBESITY PREVENTION IN ADOLESCENTS

Most adolescents who develop an ED were not previously overweight. However, it is not unusual for an ED to begin with a teenager "trying to eat healthy."[32] Some adolescents and their parents misinterpret obesity prevention messages and begin eliminating foods they consider to be "bad" or "unhealthy."[32] US Food and Drug Administration–mandated nutrition facts on food labels list percent daily values based on a 2000-kcal diet. Moderately active adolescent girls require approximately 2200 kcal/day, and moderately active adolescent boys require 2800 kcal/day for normal growth and development. Teenagers who are athletes require even higher caloric intakes.[33] Strict adherence to a 2000-kcal/day diet may lead to an energy deficit and weight loss for many growing teenagers.

Adolescents who are overweight may adopt disordered eating behaviors while attempting to lose weight. In cross-sectional studies, adolescents who are overweight have been shown to engage in self-induced vomiting or laxative use more frequently than

TABLE 1 Key Features of DSM-5 Diagnostic Criteria for Feeding Disorders and EDs

AN
- Restriction of food eaten leading to lower than expected body weight
- Intense fear of weight gain or being fat
- Body image distortion
  Types: restricting or binge eating/purging
BN
- Binge eating in which
  o a larger amount of food is eaten within a 2-hour period compared with peers; and
  o there is a perceived lack of control during the time of the binge
- Repeated use of unhealthy behaviors after a binge to prevent weight gain: (vomiting; abuse of laxatives, diuretics, or other medications; food restriction; or excessive exercise)
- Behaviors occur at least once a week for 3 months
- Self-worth is overly based on body shape and weight
- Behaviors occur distinctly apart from AN
Binge-eating disorder
- Recurrent episodes of binge eating in which
  o a larger amount of food is eaten within a 2-hour period compared with peers; and
  o there is a perceived lack of control during the time of the binge
  Bingeing episodes are associated with at least 3 of the following:
  o eating faster than normal;
  o eating until overly full;
  o eating large quantities of food when not hungry;
  o eating alone because of embarrassment about the quantity of food eaten; and
  o feeling badly emotionally after eating
- Upset about bingeing
- Bingeing behavior occurs at least once a week for 3 months
- Bingeing is not followed by the use of unhealthy behaviors to purge and does not occur during AN or BN
Avoidant/restrictive food intake disorder
- A feeding problem that results in at least one of the following:
  o significant weight loss or failure to meet the expected weight or height gain in children;
  o significant nutritional deficiency;
  o dependence on nonfood nutrition, such as nasogastric feedings or oral nutritional supplements; or
  o marked interference with psychosocial functioning
- The problem is not attributable to food availability or cultural ideas
- The problem is
  o not attributable to AN, and there is no distortion in body image; and
  o not attributable to another condition, medical or mental
Other specified feeding disorder or ED
  Atypical AN: all criteria for anorexia, but weight is normal
  BN (of low frequency and/or limited duration): all criteria except for frequency
  Binge-eating disorder (of low frequency and/or limited duration): all criteria except for frequency
  Purging disorder: recurrent purging in an effort to lose weight without bingeing

Source: DSM-5.[27]

their normal-weight peers.[34,35] Some adolescents who were overweight or obese previously can go on to develop a full ED.[3,30,32] In 1 study in adolescents seeking treatment of an ED, 36.7% had a previous weight greater than the 85th percentile for age and sex.[3] Initial attempts to lose weight by eating in a healthy manner may progress to severe dietary restriction, skipping of meals, prolonged periods of starvation, or the use of self-induced vomiting, diet pills, or laxatives. Initial attempts

to increase physical activity may progress to compulsive and excessive exercise, even to the point at which the teenager awakens at night to exercise or continues excess exercise despite injury. EDs that develop in the context of previous obesity can present with challenges that delay treatment of the ED.[32] At first, weight loss is praised and reinforced by family members, friends, and health care providers, but ongoing excessive preoccupation with weight loss can lead to social isolation, irritability, difficulty concentrating, profound fear of gaining the lost weight back, and body image distortion. If the pediatrician only focuses on weight loss without identifying the associated concerning symptoms and signs, an underlying ED may be missed.

EVIDENCE-BASED MANAGEMENT STRATEGIES ASSOCIATED WITH BOTH OBESITY AND EDS IN TEENAGERS

Cross-sectional and longitudinal observational studies have identified the following certain behaviors associated with both obesity and EDs in adolescents:

1. *Dieting.* Dieting, defined as caloric restriction with the goal of weight loss, is a risk factor for both obesity and EDs. In a large prospective cohort study in 9- to 14-year-olds (N = 16 882) followed for 2 years, dieting was associated with greater weight gain and increased rates of binge eating in both boys and girls.[36] Similarly, in a prospective observational study in 2516 adolescents enrolled in Project Eating Among Teens (Project EAT) followed for 5 years, dieting behaviors were associated with a twofold increased risk of becoming overweight and a 1.5-fold increased risk of binge eating at 5-year follow-up after adjusting for weight status at baseline.[37] Stice et al[38] showed that girls without obesity who dieted in the ninth grade were 3 times more likely to be overweight in the 12th grade compared with nondieters. These findings and others[36,38,39] suggest that dieting is counterproductive to weight-management efforts. Dieting also can predispose to EDs. In a large prospective cohort study in students 14 to 15 years of age followed for 3 years, dieting was the most important predictor of a developing ED. Students who severely restricted their energy intake and skipped meals were 18 times more likely to develop an ED than those who did not diet; those who dieted at a moderate level had a fivefold increased risk.[40]

2. *Family meals.* Family meals have been associated with improved dietary intake and provide opportunities for modeling behavior by parents, even though family meals have not been shown to prevent obesity across ethnic groups.[41–43] A higher frequency of family meals is associated with improved dietary quality, as evidenced by increased consumption of fruits, vegetables, grains, and calcium-rich foods and fiber and reduced consumption of carbonated beverages.[44] Eating family meals together 7 or more times per week resulted in families consuming 1 serving more of fruits and vegetables per day compared with families who had no meals together. These improvements in dietary intake were sustained 5 years later during young adulthood.[45] Family meals also have been shown to protect girls from disordered eating behaviors.[46–48] Most recently, a prospective study in more than 13 000 preadolescents and adolescents found that eating family dinners most days or every day during the previous year was protective against purging behaviors, binge eating, and frequent dieting. The trend was similar in both females and males, although not statistically significant in males.[48] In girls, family meals perceived to be enjoyable were protective from extreme weight-control behaviors.[46] Postulates for why family meals are protective include the following: families will consume healthier foods than teenagers would choose on their own; parents can model healthy food choices; family meals provide a time for teenagers and parents to interact; and parents can monitor their child's eating and address issues earlier when they are aware of their child's eating behavior.[49]

3. *Weight talk.* Weight talk by family members refers to comments made by family members about their own weight or comments made to the child by parents to encourage weight loss. Even well-intended comments can be perceived as hurtful by the child or adolescent. Several studies have found that parental weight talk, whether it involves encouraging their children to diet or talking about their own dieting, is linked to overweight[37,50] and EDs.[51] Project EAT linked weight talk to higher rates of overweight 5 years later. Loth et al[51] interviewed patients in recovery from EDs and found that weight talk affected them negatively. Parents who had conversations about weight had adolescents who were more likely to engage in dieting, unhealthy weight-control behaviors, and binge eating. However, if the focus of the conversation was only on healthful eating behaviors, overweight adolescents were less likely to diet and to use unhealthy weight-control behaviors.[52]

4. *Weight teasing.* In overweight adolescents, weight teasing by peers or family members is experienced by 40% of early adolescent females (mean age: 12.8 ± 0.7 years), 28.2% of middle adolescent females (mean age: 15.9 ± 0.8 years), 37% of early adolescent males, and 29% of middle adolescent males.[53] Family weight teasing predicts the development of overweight status, binge eating, and extreme weight-control behaviors in girls and overweight status in boys. Adolescent girls who were teased

about their weight at baseline were at approximately twice the risk of being overweight 5 years later.[37] A 10-year longitudinal study found that the prevalence of weight teasing did not decrease as children matured into young adults, despite the fact that the relationship between bullying and obesity had received a great deal of attention in the news.[53] A group of subjects who were studied in their young teenage years were studied again in young adulthood to evaluate the role of hurtful weight-related comments and eating behaviors (n = 1902; mean age: 25 years). For both males and females, hurtful weight-related comments from family members and significant others were associated with the use of unhealthy weight-control behaviors and binge eating in both males and females.[54]

5. *Healthy body image.* Approximately half of teenage girls and one-quarter of teenage boys are dissatisfied with their bodies; these numbers are higher in overweight teenagers.[55] Body dissatisfaction is a known risk factor for both EDs and disordered eating; higher scores of body dissatisfaction are associated with more dieting and unhealthy weight-control behaviors in both boys and girls, reduced physical activity in girls, and more binge eating in boys.[56] Body dissatisfaction and disordered eating occur in minority populations and are not limited to white girls and boys.[57] Adolescents who were more satisfied with their bodies were more likely to report parental and peer attitudes that encouraged healthful eating and exercising to be fit, rather than dieting; they were less likely to report personal weight-related concerns and behaviors.[58]

MI IS USEFUL IN ADDRESSING WEIGHT-RELATED ISSUES

MI was developed by Miller and Rollnick in 1991 to treat patients with addiction. Although MI has been well studied in adults with addictions and obesity, fewer studies have evaluated the effect of MI on patients with EDs and the use of MI in children and adolescents.[59–61] Studies to date on the use of MI for patients with EDs[60,61] and for children and adolescents with obesity have been promising.[62–65] The most recent book on MI by Miller and Rollnick defines MI as "a collaborative, goal-oriented style of communication with particular attention to the language of change. It is designed to strengthen personal motivation for and commitment to a specific goal by eliciting and exploring the person's own reasons for change within an atmosphere of acceptance and compassion."[66] This counseling approach involves 4 broad processes listed in Table 2.[67]

A study conducted through the AAP Pediatric Research in Office Settings (PROS) network assessed the effect of MI delivered by pediatricians and found that pediatricians and dietitians who used MI to counsel families with overweight children were successful in reducing children's BMI percentile by 3.1 more points than a control group in which MI was not used.[68] The AAP Web and mobile app called "Change Talk: Childhood Obesity" (http://ihcw.aap.org/resources) uses an interactive virtual practice environment to train pediatricians about the basics of MI. Pediatricians can successfully facilitate their patients' lifestyle behavior changes. Concerns from pediatricians and parents that obesity counseling can lead to an ED can be addressed by understanding the effectiveness of family-centered MI to promote healthy behaviors.

TABLE 2 The Counseling Processes of MI

- Engaging
  Establishing a working relationship with the patient
- Focusing
  Identifying how change is being discussed in the conversation
- Evoking
  Encouraging the patient to explore and discuss the need to change
- Planning for change
  Planning for change with the patient once the patient demonstrates the readiness to change

WHAT TO DO IF AN ED IS SUSPECTED

The pediatrician often is the first professional consulted by a parent or the school when there is a concern about a possible ED. Height, weight, and BMI should be plotted on the 2000 growth charts available from the Centers for Disease Control and Prevention (www.cdc.gov/growthcharts), and the current data should be compared with as many previous data points as possible. A BMI below the fifth percentile is underweight and may indicate an ED. Other possible indicators of an ED include missed menstrual periods in girls, an unusually rapid decline in BMI, or engaging in disordered eating behaviors by normal-weight and overweight adolescents who are dissatisfied with their body image. Early diagnosis and intervention are associated with improved outcome.[69] EDs are best evaluated and managed by a multidisciplinary health care team, with the pediatrician as an important member of that team.[70] A thorough physical examination and review of systems can help to identify any underlying medical and psychiatric causes for weight loss. This comprehensive clinical assessment has been described in detail elsewhere.[5] High-risk eating and activity behaviors and clinical findings of concern are outlined in Table 3. The pediatrician may feel comfortable performing this evaluation or may prefer to refer the patient to a specialized ED center, if one is available in the

TABLE 3 High-Risk Eating and Activity Behaviors and Clinical Findings of Concern

High-risk eating and activity behaviors
- Severe dietary restriction (<500 kcal/d)
- Skipping of meals to lose weight
- Prolonged periods of starvation
- Self-induced vomiting
- Use of diet pills, laxatives, or diuretics
- Compulsive and excessive exercise
- Social isolation, irritability, profound fear of gaining weight, body image distortion

Clinical findings of concern
- Rapid weight loss
- Falling off percentiles for weight and BMI
- Amenorrhea in girls
- Presence of vital sign instability
  o Bradycardia (heart rate <50 beats/minute during the day)
  o Hypotension (<90/45 mm Hg)
  o Hypothermia (body temperature <96°F [<35.6°C])
  o Orthostasis (increase in pulse >20 beats/min) or decrease in blood pressure (>20 mm Hg systolic or >10 mm Hg diastolic) on standing

TABLE 4 Principles of Family-Based Treatment of EDs and Role of the Pediatrician

Principles of treatment
- Parents are not to blame
- Parents are vital to therapeutic success
- Parents are responsible for weight restoration
- Separate the child from the illness
- Nonauthoritarian approach

Three phases of treatment
- Phase 1: parents restore patient's weight
- Phase 2: control transferred back to the child or adolescent
- Phase 3: focuses on adolescent developmental issues and termination of treatment

Examples of the role the pediatrician can play
- Act as a consultant to the parents and therapist
- Explain the medical seriousness of the ED
- Monitor and manage the medical status of the adolescent
- Empower the parents in decision-making
- Communicate with the patient, family, and therapist

local community. A psychological assessment by a mental health professional can assist with the evaluation for comorbid psychiatric illnesses (eg, affective or anxiety disorders).

In children and adolescents with AN and BN, family-based therapy (FBT), in which the parents control the refeeding process, has been shown to be an effective first-line method of treatment.[71,72] With FBT, the pediatrician can assist with monitoring the patient for weight gain and vital sign stability and can communicate with the patient, family, and therapist. Becoming familiar with the general principles of FBT can assist the pediatrician in understanding his or her role in this form of treatment (Table 4).[73]

AN INTEGRATED APPROACH TO OBESITY AND ED PREVENTION FOCUSES ON HEALTHY FAMILY-BASED LIFESTYLE MODIFICATION

Obesity prevention and treatment, if conducted correctly, does not predispose to EDs. On the contrary, randomized controlled trials of obesity prevention programs have shown a reduction in the use of self-induced vomiting or diet pill use to control weight[74] and a decrease in concerns about weight in the intervention groups.[75]

Family involvement in the treatment of both adolescent obesity and EDs has been determined to be more effective than an adolescent-only focus.[73,76] An integrated approach to the prevention of obesity and EDs focuses less on weight and more

on healthy family-based lifestyle modification that can be sustained. Pediatricians can encourage parents to be healthy role models and supportively manage the food environment by creating easy accessibility to healthy foods (eg, fruits, vegetables, whole grains, beans and other legumes, and water) and by limiting the availability of sweetened beverages, including those containing artificial sweeteners, and other foods containing refined carbohydrates. Discussions between pediatricians and parents about increasing physical activity and limiting the amount of total entertainment screen time to less than 2 hours/day are important and may lead to changes in family behavior.[77] Another area of prevention is avoiding the presence of a television in the teenager's bedroom, because having a television in the room predicts significantly less physical activity as well as poorer dietary intakes compared with not having a television in the room.[78,79] Other evidence-based approaches encourage parents to include more family meals, home-prepared meals, and meals with less distractions as well as fewer discussions about weight and about dieting.[6,80] Understanding that poor body image can lead to an ED, parents should avoid comments about body weight and discourage dieting efforts that may inadvertently result in EDs and body dissatisfaction.

ROLE OF THE PEDIATRICIAN IN THE PREVENTION OF OBESITY AND EDS IN ADOLESCENTS

Observations that can be concluded from current research summarized in this report to help prevent weight-related problems including both obesity and EDs include the following:

1. Discourage dieting, skipping of meals, or the use of diet pills; instead, encourage and support the implementation of healthy

eating and physical activity behaviors that can be maintained on an ongoing basis. The focus should be on healthy living and healthy habits rather than on weight.

2. Promote a positive body image among adolescents. Do not encourage body dissatisfaction or focus on body dissatisfaction as a reason for dieting.

3. Encourage more frequent family meals.

4. Encourage families not to talk about weight but rather to talk about healthy eating and being active to stay healthy. Do more at home to facilitate healthy eating and physical activity.

5. Inquire about a history of mistreatment or bullying in overweight and obese teenagers and address this issue with patients and their families.

6. Carefully monitor weight loss in an adolescent who needs to lose weight to ensure the adolescent does not develop the medical complications of semistarvation.

Time constraints in a busy pediatric practice are significant. Weight issues can be a topic of sensitivity and therefore can be time consuming. The evidence-based suggestions in this report can be implemented in relatively brief encounters and can be an excellent first step for teenagers and families to promote a healthy lifestyle.

LEAD AUTHORS

Neville H. Golden, MD, FAAP
Marcie Schneider, MD, FAAP
Christine Wood, MD, FAAP

COMMITTEE ON NUTRITION, 2014–2015

Stephen Daniels, MD, PhD, FAAP, Chairperson
Steven Abrams, MD, FAAP
Mark Corkins, MD, FAAP
Sarah de Ferranti, MD, FAAP
Neville H. Golden, MD, FAAP
Sheela N. Magge, MD, MSCE, FAAP
Sarah Schwarzenberg, MD, FAAP

LIAISONS

Jeff Critch, MD – *Canadian Pediatric Society*
Van Hubbard, MD, PhD, FAAP – *National Institutes of Health*
Kelley Scanlon, PhD – *Centers for Disease Control and Prevention*
Valery Soto, MS, RD, LD – *US Department of Agriculture*

STAFF

Debra Burrowes, MHA
Tamar Haro

COMMITTEE ON ADOLESCENCE, 2014–2015

Paula K. Braverman, MD, FAAP, Chairperson
William Adelman, MD, FAAP
Elizabeth M. Alderman, MD, FAAP, FSAHM
Cora C. Breuner, MD, MPH, FAAP
David A. Levine, MD, FAAP
Arik V. Marcell, MD, MPH, FAAP
Rebecca O'Brien, MD, FAAP

LIAISONS

Margo Lane, MD, FAAP, FRCPC – *Canadian Pediatric Society*
Julie Strickland, MD – *American College of Obstetricians and Gynecologists*
Benjamin Shain, MD, PhD – *American Academy of Child and Adolescent Psychiatry*

STAFF

Karen Smith
James Baumberger, MPP

SECTION ON OBESITY EXECUTIVE COMMITTEE, 2014–2015

Stephen Pont, MD, MPH, FAAP, Chairperson
Christopher Bolling, MD, FAAP
Stephen Cook, MD, MPH, FAAP
Lenna Liu, MD, MPH, FAAP
Robert Schwartz, MD, FAAP
Wendelin Slusser, MD, MS, FAAP

STAFF

Mala Thapar, MPH
Jeanne Lindros, MPH

ABBREVIATIONS

AAP: American Academy of Pediatrics
AN: anorexia nervosa
BN: bulimia nervosa
DSM-5: *Diagnostic and Statistical Manual of Mental Disorders, Fifth Edition*
ED: eating disorder
FBT: family-based therapy
MI: motivational interviewing

REFERENCES

1. Inge TH, King WC, Jenkins TM, et al. The effect of obesity in adolescence on adult health status. *Pediatrics.* 2013;132(6):1098–1104

2. Fisher M, Golden NH, Katzman DK, et al. Eating disorders in adolescents: a background paper. *J Adolesc Health.* 1995;16(6):420–437

3. Lebow J, Sim LA, Kransdorf LN. Prevalence of a history of overweight and obesity in adolescents with restrictive eating disorders. *J Adolesc Health.* 2015;56(1): 19–24

4. Puhl RM, Peterson JL, Luedicke J. Parental perceptions of weight terminology that providers use with youth. *Pediatrics.* 2011;128(4). Available at: www.pediatrics.org/cgi/content/full/128/4/e786

5. Rosen DS; American Academy of Pediatrics Committee on Adolescence. Identification and management of eating disorders in children and adolescents. *Pediatrics.* 2010;126(6):1240–1253

6. Daniels SR, Hassink SG; Committee on Nutrition. The role of the pediatrician in primary prevention of obesity. *Pediatrics.* 2015;136(1). Available at: www.pediatrics.org/cgi/content/full/136/1/e275

7. Ogden CL, Carroll MD, Kit BK, Flegal KM. Prevalence of childhood and adult obesity in the United States, 2011-2012. *JAMA.* 2014;311(8):806–814

8. National Center for Health Statistics. Health, United States, 2011: with special features on socioeconomic status and health. Hyattsville, MD: US Department of Health and Human Services; 2012. Available at: www.cdc.gov/nchs/data/hus/hus11.pdf. Accessed November 10, 2015

9. Trasande L, Elbel B. The economic burden placed on healthcare systems by childhood obesity. *Expert Rev Pharmacoecon Outcomes Res.* 2012;12(1):39–45

10. The NS, Suchindran C, North KE, Popkin BM, Gordon-Larsen P. Association of adolescent obesity with risk of severe obesity in adulthood. *JAMA.* 2010;304(18):2042–2047

11. Whitaker RC, Wright JA, Pepe MS, Seidel KD, Dietz WH. Predicting obesity in young adulthood from childhood and parental obesity. *N Engl J Med.* 1997;337(13):869–873

12. Guo SS, Chumlea WC. Tracking of body mass index in children in relation to overweight in adulthood. *Am J Clin Nutr.* 1999;70(1):145S–148S

13. Tirosh A, Shai I, Afek A, et al. Adolescent BMI trajectory and risk of diabetes versus coronary disease. *N Engl J Med.* 2011;364(14):1315–1325

14. Freedman DS, Khan LK, Serdula MK, Dietz WH, Srinivasan SR, Berenson GS. The relation of childhood BMI to adult adiposity: the Bogalusa Heart Study. *Pediatrics.* 2005;115(1):22–27

15. Li C, Ford ES, Zhao G, Mokdad AH. Prevalence of pre-diabetes and its association with clustering of cardiometabolic risk factors and hyperinsulinemia among U.S. adolescents: National Health and Nutrition Examination Survey 2005-2006. *Diabetes Care.* 2009;32(2):342–347

16. Whitlock EP, Williams SB, Gold R, Smith PR, Shipman SA. Screening and interventions for childhood overweight: a summary of evidence for the US Preventive Services Task Force. *Pediatrics.* 2005;116(1). Available at: www.pediatrics.org/cgi/content/full/116/1/e125

17. French SA, Story M, Perry CL. Self-esteem and obesity in children and adolescents: a literature review. *Obes Res.* 1995;3(5):479–490

18. Strauss RS. Childhood obesity and self-esteem. *Pediatrics.* 2000;105(1). Available at: www.pediatrics.org/cgi/content/full/105/1/e15

19. Strauss RS, Pollack HA. Social marginalization of overweight children. *Arch Pediatr Adolesc Med.* 2003;157(8):746–752

20. Madden S, Morris A, Zurynski YA, Kohn M, Elliot EJ. Burden of eating disorders in 5-13-year-old children in Australia. *Med J Aust.* 2009;190(8):410–414

21. Nicholls DE, Lynn R, Viner RM. Childhood eating disorders: British national surveillance study. *Br J Psychiatry.* 2011;198(4):295–301

22. Pinhas L, Morris A, Crosby RD, Katzman DK. Incidence and age-specific presentation of restrictive eating disorders in children: a Canadian Paediatric Surveillance Program study. *Arch Pediatr Adolesc Med.* 2011;165(10):895–899

23. Golden NH, Katzman DK, Sawyer SM, et al. Update on the medical management of eating disorders in adolescents. *J Adolesc Health.* 2015;56(4):370–375

24. van Son GE, van Hoeken D, Bartelds AI, van Furth EF, Hoek HW. Time trends in the incidence of eating disorders: a primary care study in The Netherlands. *Int J Eat Disord.* 2006;39(7):565–569

25. Zhao Y, Escinosa W. *An Update on Hospitalizations for Eating Disorders, 1999 to 2009.* Rockville, MD: Agency for Health Care Policy and Research; 2011. Statistical Brief No. 120

26. Swanson SA, Crow SJ, Le Grange D, Swendsen J, Merikangas KR. Prevalence and correlates of eating disorders in adolescents. Results from the national comorbidity survey replication adolescent supplement. *Arch Gen Psychiatry.* 2011;68(7):714–723

27. American Psychiatric Association. *Diagnostic and Statistical Manual of Mental Disorders, Fifth Edition.* Washington, DC: American Psychiatric Association; 2013

28. Sonneville KR, Horton NJ, Micali N, et al. Longitudinal associations between binge eating and overeating and adverse outcomes among adolescents and young adults: does loss of control matter? *JAMA Pediatr.* 2013;167(2):149–155

29. Peebles R, Hardy KK, Wilson JL, Lock JD. Are diagnostic criteria for eating disorders markers of medical severity? *Pediatrics.* 2010;125(5). Available at: www.pediatrics.org/cgi/content/full/125/5/e1193

30. Whitelaw M, Gilbertson H, Lee KJ, Sawyer SM. Restrictive eating disorders among adolescent inpatients. *Pediatrics.* 2014;134(3). Available at: www.pediatrics.org/cgi/content/full/134/3/e758

31. Golden NH, Carlson JL. The pathophysiology of amenorrhea in the adolescent. *Ann N Y Acad Sci.* 2008;1135:163–178

32. Sim LA, Lebow J, Billings M. Eating disorders in adolescents with a history of obesity. *Pediatrics.* 2013;132(4). Available at: www.pediatrics.org/cgi/content/full/132/4/e1026

33. American Academy of Pediatrics Committee on Nutrition. *Pediatric Nutrition. 7th Edition: Adolescent Nutrition.* Elk Grove Village, IL: American Academy of Pediatrics; 2014

34. Field AE, Camargo CA Jr, Taylor CB, et al. Overweight, weight concerns, and bulimic behaviors among girls and boys. *J Am Acad Child Adolesc Psychiatry.* 1999;38(6):754–760

35. Neumark-Sztainer D, Hannan PJ. Weight-related behaviors among adolescent girls and boys: results from a national survey. *Arch Pediatr Adolesc Med.* 2000;154(6):569–577

36. Field AE, Austin SB, Taylor CB, et al. Relation between dieting and weight change among preadolescents and adolescents. *Pediatrics.* 2003;112(4):900–906

37. Neumark-Sztainer DR, Wall MM, Haines JI, Story MT, Sherwood NE, van den Berg PA. Shared risk and protective factors for overweight and disordered eating in adolescents. *Am J Prev Med.* 2007;33(5):359–369

38. Stice E, Cameron RP, Killen JD, Hayward C, Taylor CB. Naturalistic weight-reduction efforts prospectively predict growth in relative weight and onset of obesity among female adolescents. *J Consult Clin Psychol.* 1999;67(6):967–974

39. Stice E, Presnell K, Shaw H, Rohde P. Psychological and behavioral risk factors for obesity onset in adolescent girls: a prospective study. *J Consult Clin Psychol.* 2005;73(2):195–202

40. Patton GC, Selzer R, Coffey C, Carlin JB, Wolfe R. Onset of adolescent eating disorders: population based cohort study over 3 years. *BMJ.* 1999;318(7186):765–768

41. Fulkerson JA, Neumark-Sztainer D, Hannan PJ, Story M. Family meal frequency and weight status among adolescents: cross-sectional and 5-year longitudinal

associations. *Obesity (Silver Spring)*. 2008;16(11):2529–2534

42. Taveras EM, Rifas-Shiman SL, Berkey CS, et al. Family dinner and adolescent overweight. *Obes Res*. 2005;13(5):900–906

43. Sen B. Frequency of family dinner and adolescent body weight status: evidence from the national longitudinal survey of youth, 1997. *Obesity (Silver Spring)*. 2006;14(12):2266–2276

44. Neumark-Sztainer D, Hannan PJ, Story M, Croll J, Perry C. Family meal patterns: associations with sociodemographic characteristics and improved dietary intake among adolescents. *J Am Diet Assoc*. 2003;103(3):317–322

45. Larson NI, Neumark-Sztainer D, Hannan PJ, Story M. Family meals during adolescence are associated with higher diet quality and healthful meal patterns during young adulthood. *J Am Diet Assoc*. 2007;107(9):1502–1510

46. Neumark-Sztainer D, Wall M, Story M, Fulkerson JA. Are family meal patterns associated with disordered eating behaviors among adolescents? *J Adolesc Health*. 2004;35(5):350–359

47. Neumark-Sztainer D, Eisenberg ME, Fulkerson JA, Story M, Larson NI. Family meals and disordered eating in adolescents: longitudinal findings from Project EAT. *Arch Pediatr Adolesc Med*. 2008;162(1):17–22

48. Haines J, Gillman MW, Rifas-Shiman S, Field AE, Austin SB. Family dinner and disordered eating behaviors in a large cohort of adolescents. *Eat Disord*. 2010;18(1):10–24

49. Neumark-Sztainer D. Preventing obesity and eating disorders in adolescents: what can health care providers do? *J Adolesc Health*. 2009;44(3):206–213

50. Berge JM, MacLehose RF, Loth KA, Eisenberg ME, Fulkerson JA, Neumark-Sztainer D. Parent-adolescent conversations about eating, physical activity and weight: prevalence across sociodemographic characteristics and associations with adolescent weight and weight-related behaviors. *J Behav Med*. 2015;38(1):122–135

51. Loth KA, Neumark-Sztainer D, Croll JK. Informing family approaches to eating disorder prevention: perspectives of those who have been there. *Int J Eat Disord*. 2009;42(2):146–152

52. Berge JM, Maclehose R, Loth KA, Eisenberg M, Bucchianeri MM, Neumark-Sztainer D. Parent conversations about healthful eating and weight: associations with adolescent disordered eating behaviors. *JAMA Pediatr*. 2013;167(8):746–753

53. Haines J, Hannan PJ, van den Berg P, Eisenberg ME, Neumark-Sztainer D. Weight-related teasing from adolescence to young adulthood: longitudinal and secular trends between 1999 and 2010. *Obesity (Silver Spring)*. 2013;21(9):E428–E434

54. Eisenberg ME, Berge JM, Fulkerson JA, Neumark-Sztainer D. Associations between hurtful weight-related comments by family and significant other and the development of disordered eating behaviors in young adults. *J Behav Med*. 2012;35(5):500–508

55. Neumark-Sztainer D, Story M, Hannan PJ, Perry CL, Irving LM. Weight-related concerns and behaviors among overweight and nonoverweight adolescents: implications for preventing weight-related disorders. *Arch Pediatr Adolesc Med*. 2002;156(2):171–178

56. Neumark-Sztainer D, Paxton SJ, Hannan PJ, Haines J, Story M. Does body satisfaction matter? Five-year longitudinal associations between body satisfaction and health behaviors in adolescent females and males. *J Adolesc Health*. 2006;39(2):244–251

57. Neumark-Sztainer D, Croll J, Story M, Hannan PJ, French SA, Perry C. Ethnic/racial differences in weight-related concerns and behaviors among adolescent girls and boys: findings from Project EAT. *J Psychosom Res*. 2002;53(5):963–974

58. Kelly AM, Wall M, Eisenberg ME, Story M, Neumark-Sztainer D. Adolescent girls with high body satisfaction: who are they and what can they teach us? *J Adolesc Health*. 2005;37(5):391–396

59. Flattum C, Friend S, Neumark-Sztainer D, Story M. Motivational interviewing as a component of a school-based obesity prevention program for adolescent girls. *J Am Diet Assoc*. 2009;109(1):91–94

60. Sepulveda AR, Wise C, Zabala M, Todd G, Treasure J. Development and reliability of a Motivational Interviewing Scenarios Tool for Eating Disorders (MIST-ED) using a skills-based intervention among caregivers. *Eat Behav*. 2013;14(4):432–436

61. Macdonald P, Hibbs R, Corfield F, Treasure J. The use of motivational interviewing in eating disorders: a systematic review. *Psychiatry Res*. 2012;200(1):1–11

62. Carcone AI, Naar-King S, Brogan KE, et al. Provider communication behaviors that predict motivation to change in black adolescents with obesity. *J Dev Behav Pediatr*. 2013;34(8):599–608

63. Resnicow K, Davis R, Rollnick S. Motivational interviewing for pediatric obesity: conceptual issues and evidence review. *J Am Diet Assoc*. 2006;106(12):2024–2033

64. Schwartz RP, Hamre R, Dietz WH, et al. Office-based motivational interviewing to prevent childhood obesity: a feasibility study. *Arch Pediatr Adolesc Med*. 2007;161(5):495–501

65. Resnicow K, McMaster F, Bocian A, et al. Motivational interviewing and dietary counseling for obesity in primary care: an RCT. *Pediatrics*. 2015;135(4):649–657

66. Miller WR, Rollnick S. *Motivational Interviewing. Helping People Change*. 3rd ed. New York, NY: The Guilford Press; 2013

67. American Academy of Pediatrics. Motivational interviewing. Healthy Active Living for Families Implementation Guide. Available at: www.aap.org/en-us/advocacy-and-policy/aap-health-initiatives/HALF-Implementation-Guide/communicating-with-families/Pages/Motivational-Interviewing.aspx. Accessed November 10, 2015

68. Resnicow K, Harris D, Schwartz R, et al. Can brief motivational interviewing in practice reduce child body mass index? Results of a 2-year randomized controlled trial [abstr]. Presented at: *Pediatric Academic*

Societies Annual Meeting; Vancouver, British Columbia, Canada; May 4, 2014

69. Forman SF, Grodin LF, Graham DA, et al; National Eating Disorder QI Collaborative. An eleven site national quality improvement evaluation of adolescent medicine-based eating disorder programs: predictors of weight outcomes at one year and risk adjustment analyses. *J Adolesc Health.* 2011;49(6):594–600

70. Golden NH, Katzman DK, Sawyer SM, et al; Society for Adolescent Health and Medicine. Position paper of the Society for Adolescent Health and Medicine: medical management of restrictive eating disorders in adolescents and young adults. *J Adolesc Health.* 2015;56(1):121–125

71. Lock J, Le Grange D, Agras WS, Moye A, Bryson SW, Jo B. Randomized clinical trial comparing family-based treatment with adolescent-focused individual therapy for adolescents with anorexia nervosa. *Arch Gen Psychiatry.* 2010;67(10):1025–1032

72. Le Grange D, Crosby RD, Rathouz PJ, Leventhal BL. A randomized controlled comparison of family-based treatment and supportive psychotherapy for adolescent bulimia nervosa. *Arch Gen Psychiatry.* 2007;64(9):1049–1056

73. Katzman DK, Peebles R, Sawyer SM, Lock J, Le Grange D. The role of the pediatrician in family-based treatment for adolescent eating disorders: opportunities and challenges. *J Adolesc Health.* 2013;53(4):433–440

74. Austin SB, Field AE, Wiecha J, Peterson KE, Gortmaker SL. The impact of a school-based obesity prevention trial on disordered weight-control behaviors in early adolescent girls. *Arch Pediatr Adolesc Med.* 2005;159(3):225–230

75. Robinson TN, Killen JD, Kraemer HC, et al. Dance and reducing television viewing to prevent weight gain in African-American girls: the Stanford GEMS pilot study. *Ethn Dis.* 2003;13(1, suppl 1):S65–S77

76. Shrewsbury VA, Steinbeck KS, Torvaldsen S, Baur LA. The role of parents in pre-adolescent and adolescent overweight and obesity treatment: a systematic review of clinical recommendations. *Obes Rev.* 2011;12(10):759–769

77. Strasburger VC; Council on Communications and Media. Children, adolescents, obesity, and the media. *Pediatrics.* 2011;128(1):201–208

78. Barr-Anderson DJ, van den Berg P, Neumark-Sztainer D, Story M. Characteristics associated with older adolescents who have a television in their bedrooms. *Pediatrics.* 2008;121(4):718–724

79. Bauer KW, Neumark-Sztainer D, Fulkerson JA, Hannan PJ, Story M. Familial correlates of adolescent girls' physical activity, television use, dietary intake, weight, and body composition. *Int J Behav Nutr Phys Act.* 2011;8:25

80. Barlow SE; Expert Committee. Expert committee recommendations regarding the prevention, assessment, and treatment of child and adolescent overweight and obesity: summary report. *Pediatrics.* 2007;120(suppl 4):S164–S192

Prevention and Management of Procedural Pain in the Neonate: An Update

• *Policy Statement*

POLICY STATEMENT Organizational Principles to Guide and Define the Child Health
Care System and/or Improve the Health of all Children

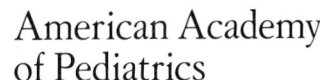
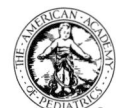

American Academy of Pediatrics

DEDICATED TO THE HEALTH OF ALL CHILDREN™

Prevention and Management of Procedural Pain in the Neonate: An Update

COMMITTEE ON FETUS AND NEWBORN and SECTION ON ANESTHESIOLOGY AND PAIN MEDICINE

abstract

The prevention of pain in neonates should be the goal of all pediatricians and health care professionals who work with neonates, not only because it is ethical but also because repeated painful exposures have the potential for deleterious consequences. Neonates at greatest risk of neurodevelopmental impairment as a result of preterm birth (ie, the smallest and sickest) are also those most likely to be exposed to the greatest number of painful stimuli in the NICU. Although there are major gaps in knowledge regarding the most effective way to prevent and relieve pain in neonates, proven and safe therapies are currently underused for routine minor, yet painful procedures. Therefore, every health care facility caring for neonates should implement (1) a pain-prevention program that includes strategies for minimizing the number of painful procedures performed and (2) a pain assessment and management plan that includes routine assessment of pain, pharmacologic and nonpharmacologic therapies for the prevention of pain associated with routine minor procedures, and measures for minimizing pain associated with surgery and other major procedures.

Previous guidance from the American Academy of Pediatrics (AAP) and the Canadian Pediatric Society addressed the need to assess neonatal pain, especially during and after diagnostic and therapeutic procedures.[1,2] These organizations also provided recommendations on preventing or minimizing pain in newborn infants and treating unavoidable pain promptly and adequately.[1,2] This statement updates previous recommendations with new evidence on the prevention, assessment, and treatment of neonatal procedural pain.

BACKGROUND

Neonates are frequently subjected to painful procedures, with the most immature infants receiving the highest number of painful events.[3–5]

Policy statements from the American Academy of Pediatrics benefit from expertise and resources of liaisons and internal (AAP) and external reviewers. However, policy statements from the American Academy of Pediatrics may not reflect the views of the liaisons or the organizations or government agencies that they represent.

The guidance in this statement does not indicate an exclusive course of treatment or serve as a standard of medical care. Variations, taking into account individual circumstances, may be appropriate.

All policy statements from the American Academy of Pediatrics automatically expire 5 years after publication unless reaffirmed, revised, or retired at or before that time.

DOI: 10.1542/peds.2015-4271

PEDIATRICS (ISSN Numbers: Print, 0031-4005; Online, 1098-4275).

To cite: AAP COMMITTEE ON FETUS AND NEWBORN and SECTION ON ANESTHESIOLOGY AND PAIN MEDICINE. Prevention and Management of Procedural Pain in the Neonate: An Update. *Pediatrics.* 2016;137(2):e20154271

Despite recommendations from the AAP and other experts, neonatal pain continues to be inconsistently assessed and inadequately managed.[2,3] A large prospective study from France in 2008 found that specific pharmacologic or nonpharmacologic analgesia was given before painful procedures in only 21% of infants, and ongoing analgesia was given in an additional 34%.[3] Thus, infants received analgesia for approximately half of the procedures performed, with wide variation among facilities.

The prevention and alleviation of pain in neonates, particularly preterm infants, is important not only because it is ethical but also because exposure to repeated painful stimuli early in life is known to have short- and long-term adverse sequelae. These sequelae include physiologic instability, altered brain development, and abnormal neurodevelopment, somatosensory, and stress response systems, which can persist into childhood.[5–15] Nociceptive pathways are active and functional as early as 25 weeks' gestation and may elicit a generalized or exaggerated response to noxious stimuli in immature newborn infants.[16]

Researchers have demonstrated that a procedure-related painful stimulus that results in increased excitability of nociceptive neurons in the dorsal horn of the spinal cord accentuates the infant's sensitivity to subsequent noxious and nonnoxious sensory stimuli (ie, sensitization).[17,18] This persistent sensory hypersensitivity can be physiologically stressful, particularly in preterm infants.[19–22] Investigators have demonstrated increased stress-related markers and elevated free radicals after even simple procedures, such as routine heel punctures or tape removal from central venous catheters,[23,24] which can adversely affect future pain perception.[8] Specific cortical pain processing occurs even in preterm

infants; however, multiple factors interact to influence the nociceptive processing and/or behavioral responses to pain.[14,16,25–27] Noxious stimuli activate these signaling pathways but also activate the central inhibitory circuits, thus altering the balance between the excitatory and inhibitory feedback mechanisms. The immaturity of the dorsal horn synaptic connectivity and descending inhibitory circuits in neonates results in poor localization and discrimination of sensory input and poor noxious inhibitory modulation, thus facilitating central nervous system sensitization to repeated noxious stimuli.[25]

ASSESSMENT OF PAIN AND STRESS IN THE NEONATE

Reliable neonatal pain assessment tools are essential for the rating and management of neonatal pain, and their use has been strongly recommended by the AAP and by international researchers, including the International Evidence-Based Group for Neonatal Pain.[1,2,28] However, the effective management of pain in the neonate remains problematic because of the inability of the infant to report his or her own pain and the challenges of assessing pain in extremely premature, ill, and neurologically compromised neonates.[29] Thus, pain assessment tools reflect surrogate measures of physiologic and behavioral responses to pain. Although numerous neonatal pain scales exist (Table 1), only 5 pain scales have been subjected to rigorous psychometric testing with the patients serving as their own controls, measuring their physiologic and behavioral responses by using the scale in question (Neonatal Facial Coding System,[30,31] Premature Infant Pain Profile [PIPP],[32–34] Neonatal Pain and Sedation Scale,[35,36] Behavioral Infant Pain Profile,[37] and Douleur Aiguë du Nouveau-né[38]). Many of the current pain assessment tools have been tested against

existing or newly developed tools and against each other to determine which is more reliable for a particular population and application, but more research is needed.[29,39]

Contextual factors such as gestational age and behavioral state may play a significant role in pain assessment and are beginning to be included in some assessment tools (eg, the PIPP-Revised).[40,41] New and emerging technologies to measure pain responses, such as near-infrared spectroscopy, amplitude-integrated electroencephalography, functional MRI, skin conductance, and heart rate variability assessment, are being investigated.[53,54] These innovations hold promise in the development of neurophysiologically based methods for assessing noxious stimuli processing at the cortical level in neonates while they are awake, sedated, or anesthetized. If the neurophysiologic measures prove to be reliable and quantifiable, these measures could be used in the future to simultaneously correlate with the physiologic and behavioral pain assessment scales to determine the most clinically useful tool(s).

Many of the tools developed to measure acute pain in neonates are multidimensional in nature and include a combination of physiologic and behavioral signs. These tools were most commonly developed to assess unventilated infants; only a few scales are validated to assess pain in infants who are ventilated through an endotracheal tube or receiving nasal continuous positive airway pressure.[42,55] Recently, investigators reported that 2 behaviorally based, one-dimensional pain assessment tools (the Behavioral Indicators of Infant Pain and the Neonatal Facial Coding System) were more sensitive in detecting behavioral cues related to pain in term neonates than the PIPP.[56]

It is unlikely that a single, comprehensive pain assessment

TABLE 1 Pain Assessment Tools for Neonates

Pain Assessment Tool	Number and GA of Infants Studied	Indicators	Intervention Studied	Validation Methodology	Intended Use
Neonatal Facial Coding System (NFCS)[30,31] (1998, 2003)	$N = 40$ 24–32 wk GA 5–56 DOL	Brow lowering Eye squeeze Nasolabial furrowing Lip opening Vertical mouth stretch Horizontal mouth stretch Taut tongue Chin quiver Lip pursing	Postoperative abdominal or thoracic surgery	Patients served as controls Interrater reliability: 0.86 Construct validity: demonstrated Feasibility: established	Acute pain Prolonged pain Postoperative pain
Premature Infant Pain Profile (PIPP)[32–34] (1996, 1999)	$N = 211, 43, 24$ Age: 28–40 wk GA	GA Behavioral state Maximum HR % Decrease in O_2 sat Brow bulge Eye squeeze Nasolabial furrow	Heel lance	Patients served as controls Internal consistency: 0.71 Construct validity: established Interrater reliability: 0.93–0.96 Intrarater reliability: 0.94–0.98	Acute pain
Neonatal Pain Agitation and Sedation Scale (NPASS)[35,36] (2010) (http://www.n-pass.com/research.html)	$N = 42$ Age: 23–40 wk GA 1–100 DOL	Crying Behavioral state Facial expressions Extremities/tone Vital signs (HR, BP, RR, O_2 sat)	Heel lance	Validated against PIPP Interrater reliability: 0.86–0.93 Internal consistency: 0.84–0.89 Construct (discriminate) validity: established Convergent validity: correlation with the PIPP scores Spearman rank correlation coefficient of 0.75 and 0.72 Test-retest reliability: 0.87	Acute pain Prolonged pain Level of sedation
Behavioral Indicators of Infant Pain (BIIP)[37] (2007)	$N = 92$ Age: 24–32 wk GA	Behavioral state Facial expressions Hand movements	Heel lance	Validated against NIPS Internal consistency: 0.82 Interrater reliability: 0.80–0.92 Construct validity: 85.9 Concurrent validity: correlations between the BIIP and NIPS = 0.64. Correlations between the BIIP and mean HR also remained moderate between GAs: earlier born = 0.33, $P < .05$; later born, $r = 0.50$, $P < .001$	Acute pain
Douleur Aiguë du Nouveau-né (DAN)[38] (1997)	$N = 42$ Age: 24–41 wk GA	Facial movements Limb movements Vocal expression	Heel lance Venipuncture	Patients served as controls Internal consistency: 0.88 Interrater reliability: 91.2 (Krippendorf)	Procedural pain
Premature Infant Pain Profile–Revised (PIPP-R)[40,41] (2014)	$N = 52, 85, 31$ Age: 25–40 wk GA	Maximum HR % Decrease in O_2 sat Brow bulge Eye squeeze Nasolabial furrow GA and behavioral state assessed if pain response detected	Retrospective comparison of PIPP and PIPP-R scores	Validated against PIPP Construct validity: established Feasibility: established	Acute pain

TABLE 1 Continued

Pain Assessment Tool	Number and GA of Infants Studied	Indicators	Intervention Studied	Validation Methodology	Intended Use
Faceless Acute Neonatal Pain Scale (FANS)[42] (2010)	N = 53 Age: 30–35 wk GA	HR change; Acute discomfort (bradycardia, desat); Limb movements; Vocal expression (must be nonintubated)	Heel lance	Validated against DAN; Interrater reliability: 0.92 (0.9–0.98); Internal consistency: Cronbach's α = 0.72; The ICC between the FANS and DAN scores was 0.88 (0.76–0.93)	Acute pain; Developed for use when the neonate's face is not completely visible related to respiratory devices
Neonatal Infant Pain Scale (NIPS)[43] (1993)	N = 38 Age: 26–47 wk GA	Facial expression; Crying; Breathing patterns; Arm movements; Leg movements; State of arousal	Needle insertion	Validated against VAS; Concurrent validity: correlations with VAS ranged from 0.53 to 0.84.; Interrater reliability: 0.92–0.97; Internal consistency: Cronbach's α's were 0.95, 0.87, and 0.88 for before, during, and after the procedures, respectively	Acute pain; Postoperative pain
Crying Requires Increased oxygen administration, Increased vital signs, Expression, Sleeplessness (CRIES)[44] (1995)	N = 24 Age: 32–60 wk GA 1382 observations	Crying; Requires O_2 to maintain sat at 95%; Increased blood pressure, HR; Expression; Sleep state	Postoperative pain	Validated against the Objective Pain Score; Interrater reliability: 0.72; Construct validity: yes; Discriminant validity: yes	Prolonged pain; Postoperative pain
COMFORTneo[45] (2009)	N = 286 Age: 24.6–42.6 wk GA 3600 assessments	Alertness; Calmness/agitation; Respiratory response in ventilated patient; Crying in spontaneously breathing patient; Body movement; Facial tension; Body muscle tone	Tertiary NICU care, including ventilation	Validated against Numeric Rating Scale; Internal consistency: Cronbach's α = 0.88 for nonventilated, 0.84 for ventilated patients; Interrater reliability: 0.79; Concurrent validity: Pearson product-moment correlation coefficient between COMFORTneo and NRS-pain = 0.54; Correlation coefficient: 0.75 (95% confidence interval: 0.70–0.79; P < .0001)	Persistent or prolonged pain; Level of sedation
COVERS Neonatal pain scale[46] (2010)	N = 21 Age: 27–40 wk GA	Crying; FiO_2 requirement; Vital signs (HR, BP, frequency of apnea/bradycardia; Facial expression; Resting state; Body movements	Heel lance	Validated different GAs against CRIES, NIPS, and PIPP; Concurrent validity: premature infants PIPP versus COVERS, r = 0.84; full-term infants NIPS versus COVERS, r = 0.95; Construct validity: baseline (P < .05); heel stick (P < .05); recovery (P < .05)	Acute pain

TABLE 1 Continued

Pain Assessment Tool	Number and GA of Infants Studied	Indicators	Intervention Studied	Validation Methodology	Intended Use
Pain Assessment in Neonates (PAIN)[47] (2002)	$N = 196$ neonates Age: 26–47 wk GA	Facial expression Cry Breathing pattern Extremity movement State of arousal FiO_2 required for sat >95% Increase in HR	Heel lance, suctioning, IV placement, circumcision, NG tube insertion, tape or IV removal	Adapted from NIPS and CRIES Inter-rater reliability: not established Correlation between the total scores on the two scales (NIPS and PAIN) was 0.93 ($P < .001$).	Acute pain
Pain Assessment Tool (PAT)[48,49] (2005)	$N = 144$ Age: 27–40 wk GA	Posture/tone Cry Sleep pattern Expression Color Respirations HR O_2 sat BP Nurse's perception	Ventilated and postoperative neonates	Validated against CRIES and VAS Interrater reliability: 0.85 Correlation between PAT and CRIES scores ($r = 0.76$) and (0.38) between the PAT score and VAS	Prolonged pain
Scale for Use in Newborns (SUN)[50] (1998)	$N = 33$ Age: 24–40 wk GA 0–214 DOL 68 procedures	CNS state Breathing Movement Tone Face HR changes Mean BP changes	Intubation PIV insertion	Validated against NIPS and COMFORT Coefficient of variation: 33 ± 8%	Acute pain
Échelle Douleur Inconfort Nouveau-Né (EDIN)[51] (2001)	$N = 76$ Age: 25–36 wk GA	Facial activity Body movements Quality of sleep Quality of contact with nurses Consolability	Acute and chronic ventilation; NEC, postoperative for PDA ligation	Patients served as controls Interrater reliability: coefficient range of 0.59–0.74 Internal consistency: Cronbach's α coefficients ranged from 0.86 to 0.94	Prolonged pain
Bernese Pain Scale for Neonates (BPSN)[52] (2004)	$N = 12$ Age: 27–41 wk GA 288 pain assessments	Alertness Duration of crying Time to calm Skin color Eyebrow bulge with eye squeeze Posture Breathing pattern	Heel lance	Validated against VAS and PIPP Concurrent and convergent validity: compared with VAS and PIPP was $r = 0.86$ and $r = 0.91$, respectively ($P < .0001$) Interrater reliability: $r = 0.86$–0.97 Intrarater reliability: $r = 0.98$–0.99	Acute pain

BP, blood pressure; CNS, central nervous system; desat, desaturation; DOL, days of life; FiO_2, fraction of inspired oxygen; GA, gestational age; HR, heart rate; ICC, intraclass correlation coefficient; IV, intravenous (catheter); NEC, necrotizing enterocolitis; NG, nasogastric; PDA, patent ductus arteriosus; PIV, peripheral intravenous (line); RR, respiratory rate; sat, saturation; VAS, visual analog scale.

tool will be satisfactory for assessing neonatal pain for all situations and in infants of all gestational ages,[39,57] although initial validation studies have been published for the PIPP-Revised in infants with a gestational age of 25 to 41 weeks.[40,41] More research needs to be performed to assess the intensity of both acute and chronic pain at the bedside, to differentiate signs and symptoms of pain from those attributable to other causes, and to understand the significance of situations when there is no perceptible response to pain.[40,41] However, even with those limitations, one can use the available evidence to choose a pain assessment tool that is appropriate for the type of pain assessed (acute, prolonged, postoperative) and advocate for the competency of the neonatal care provider team with the specific use of that tool.[58] Table 1 lists commonly used pain assessment tools and the evidence used to test them.

NONPHARMACOLOGIC TREATMENT STRATEGIES

Pediatricians and health care professionals who work with neonates have the difficult task of balancing the need for appropriate monitoring, testing, and treatment versus minimizing pain and stress to the patient. Nonpharmacologic strategies for pain management, such as swaddling combined with positioning, facilitated tucking (holding the infant in a flexed position with arms close to the trunk) with or without parental assistance, nonnutritive sucking, and massage, have all shown variable effectiveness in reducing pain and/or stress-related behaviors related to mild to moderately painful or stressful interventions.[59-63] A meta-analysis of 51 studies of nonpharmacologic interventions used during heel lance and intravenous catheter insertion found that sucking-related and swaddling/facilitated-tucking interventions were beneficial for

preterm neonates and that sucking-related and rocking/holding interventions were beneficial for term neonates, but that no benefit was evident among older infants.[64]

Skin-to-skin care (SSC), with or without sucrose or glucose administration, has been shown to decrease some measures of pain in preterm and term infants.[65] An analysis of 19 studies examining the effects of SSC on neonatal pain caused by single needle-related procedures found no statistical benefit for physiologic indicators of pain but did show benefit for composite pain score items.[65] However, some investigators have reported decreased cortisol concentrations and decreased autonomic indicators of pain in preterm infants during SSC, suggestive of a physiologic benefit.[66,67]

The effects of breastfeeding on pain response have also been investigated. A Cochrane systematic review published in 2012 found that breastfeeding during a heel lance or venipuncture was associated with significantly lower pain responses in term neonates (eg, smaller increases in heart rate and shorter crying time), compared with other nonpharmacologic interventions such as positioning, rocking, or maternal holding. Breastfeeding showed similar effectiveness to oral sucrose or glucose solutions.[68] This meta-analysis of 20 randomized controlled trials (RCTs)/quasi-RCTs also found that providing supplemental human milk via a pacifier or syringe seems to be as effective as providing sucrose or glucose for pain relief in term neonates.

Sensorial stimulation (SS), a method of gently stimulating the tactile, gustatory, auditory, and visual systems simultaneously, has shown effectiveness at decreasing pain during minor procedures such as heel lance.[69] SS is achieved by looking at and gently talking to the infant, while stroking or massaging the face

or back, and providing oral sucrose or glucose solution before a painful procedure. A systematic review of 16 studies found that SS was more effective than sucrose when all elements of SS were used,[69] and 1 study suggested that SS may play an important role in nonpharmacologic management of procedural pain for neonates.[70]

PHARMACOLOGIC TREATMENT STRATEGIES

Sucrose and Glucose

Oral sucrose is commonly used to provide analgesia to infants during mild to moderately painful procedures. It has been extensively studied for this purpose, yet many gaps in knowledge remain, including appropriate dosing, mechanism of action, soothing versus analgesic effects, and long-term consequences.[71-73] A meta-analysis of 57 studies including >4730 infants with gestational ages ranging from 25 to 44 weeks concluded that sucrose is safe and effective for reducing procedural pain from a single event.[74]

Maximum reductions in physiologic and behavioral pain indicators have been noted when sucrose was administered ~2 minutes before a painful stimulus, and the effects lasted ~4 minutes.[74-76] Procedures of longer duration, such as ophthalmologic examinations or circumcision, may require multiple doses of sucrose to provide continual analgesic effect.[76] In animal studies, the analgesic effects of sucrose appear to be a sweet-taste-mediated response of opiate, endorphin, and possibly dopamine or acetylcholine pathways; however, the mechanism of action is not well understood in human neonates.[72,77-81] An additive analgesic effect has been noted when sucrose is used in conjunction with other nonpharmacologic measures, such as nonnutritive sucking and swaddling, especially for procedures such as ophthalmologic examinations and immunizations.[74,78] Although the evidence that oral sucrose alleviates procedurally related pain and stress, as judged by clinical pain scores, appears to be strong, a small RCT found no difference in either nociceptive brain activity on electroencephalography or spinal nociceptive reflex withdrawal on electromyography between sucrose or sterile water administered to term infants before a heel lance.[73] This masked study did find, however, that clinical pain scores were decreased in the infants receiving sucrose, and several methodologic concerns limit the conclusions that can be drawn from the trial.[74]

Sucrose use is common in most nurseries; however, doses vary widely.[82] Although an optimal dose has not been determined,[74] an oral dose of 0.1 to 1 mL of 24% sucrose (or 0.2–0.5 mL/kg) 2 minutes before a painful procedure has been recommended, taking into account gestational age, severity of illness, and procedure to be performed.[71] The role and safety of long-term sucrose use for persistent, ongoing pain have not been systematically studied. One study in 107 preterm infants of <31 weeks' gestation found worse neurodevelopmental scores at 32, 36, and 40 weeks' gestational age in infants who had received >10 doses of sucrose over a 24-hour period in the first week of life, raising concerns about frequent dosing in newly born preterm infants.[83,84] In addition, 1 infant in that study developed hyperglycemia coincident with frequent sucrose dosing, which may have been related to the sucrose or to subsequently diagnosed sepsis.[83] When sucrose is used as a pain management strategy, it should be prescribed and tracked as a medication. More research is needed to better understand the effects of sucrose use for analgesia.[71,81,84]

Glucose has also been found to be effective in decreasing response to brief painful procedures. A meta-analysis of 38 RCTs that included 3785 preterm and term neonates found that the administration of 20% to 30% glucose solutions reduced pain scores and decreased crying during heel lance and venipuncture compared with water or no intervention. The authors concluded that glucose could be used as an alternative to sucrose solutions, although no recommendations about dose or timing of administration could be made.[85] As described for sucrose, however, glucose may not be effective for longer procedures. For example, an RCT found no effect of glucose on pain response during ophthalmologic examinations.[86]

Opioids, Benzodiazepines, and Other Drugs

The most common pharmacologic agents used for pain relief in newborns are opioids, with fentanyl and morphine most often used, especially for persistent pain. Analgesics and sedatives are known to be potent modulators of several G-protein–linked receptor signaling pathways in the developing brain that are implicated in the critical regulation of neural tissue proliferation, survival, and differentiation. Studies of appropriate dosing and long-term effects of these analgesics given during the neonatal period are woefully lacking and/or conflicting.[87,88] However, in their absence, it remains critical to achieve adequate pain control in newborns, both as an ethical duty and because painful experiences in the NICU can have long-term adverse effects.[7,10,19,20,89]

Studies evaluating pharmacologic prevention and treatment of mild to moderate pain have generally been limited to a specific procedure such as intubation. The AAP recommends routine pain management during procedures such as circumcision,[90] chest drain insertion and removal,[2] and nonemergency intubations.[91]

However, effective management strategies for pain and sedation during mechanical ventilation remain elusive. A recent systematic review reported limited favorable effect with selective rather than routine use of opioids for analgesia in mechanically ventilated infants.[92] Concerns have been raised for adverse short- and long-term neurodevelopmental outcomes related to the use of morphine infusions in preterm neonates.[92,93] However, a follow-up study in ninety 8- to 9-year-olds who had previously participated in 1 RCT comparing continuous morphine infusion with placebo found that low-dose morphine infusion did not affect cognition or behavior and may have had a positive effect on everyday executive functions for these children.[87]

A 2008 Cochrane systematic review found insufficient evidence to recommend the routine use of opioids in mechanically ventilated infants.[94] Although there appeared to be a reduction in pain, there were no long-term benefits favoring the treatment groups; and concerns for adverse effects, such as respiratory depression, increase in the duration of mechanical ventilation, and development of dependence and tolerance, were raised. Other short-term physiologic adverse effects of concern included hypotension, constipation, and urinary retention for morphine and bradycardia and chest wall rigidity for fentanyl.[94] Remifentanil, a shorter-acting fentanyl derivative, may be an alternative for short-term procedures and surgeries because it is not cleared by liver metabolism, but there are no studies examining its long-term effects.[95,96]

Benzodiazepines, most commonly midazolam, are frequently used in the NICU for sedation. However, because there is evidence of only minor additional analgesic effect, they may not provide much benefit. These agents can potentiate the respiratory depression and hypotension that can occur with opioids, and infants receiving them should be carefully monitored.[97] Midazolam was associated with adverse short-term effects in the NOPAIN (Neonatal Outcome and Prolonged Analgesia in Neonates) trial.[98] A systematic review in 2012 found insufficient evidence to recommend midazolam infusions for sedation in the NICU and raised safety concerns, particularly regarding neurotoxicity.[97]

Alternative medications, such as methadone,[99] ketamine, propofol, and dexmedetomidine, have been proposed for pain management in neonates; however, few, if any, studies of these agents have been performed in this population, and caution should be exercised when considering them for use because of concerns about unanticipated adverse effects and potential neurotoxic effects.[100] Although the potential benefits of using methadone for the treatment of neonatal pain include satisfactory analgesic effects and enteral bioavailability as well as prolonged duration of action related to its long half-life and lower expense compared with other opiates, safe and effective dosing regimens have yet to be developed.[101] Ketamine is a dissociative anesthetic that, in lower doses, provides good analgesia, amnesia, and sedation.[102] Although ketamine has been well studied in older populations, further research is needed to establish safety profiles for use in neonates because of concerns regarding possible neurotoxicity.[103] Propofol has been used for short procedural sedation in children because of its rapid onset and clearance. The clearance of propofol in the neonatal population is inversely related to postmenstrual age, with significant variability in its pharmacokinetics in preterm and term neonates.[104] It has also been associated with bradycardia, desaturations, and

prolonged hypotension in newborn infants.[105] Limited experience with dexmedetomidine in preterm and term infants suggests that it may provide effective sedation and analgesia. Preliminary pharmacokinetic data showed decreased clearance in preterm infants compared with term infants and a favorable safety profile over a 24-hour period.[106]

The use of oral or intravenous acetaminophen has been limited to postoperative pain control. Although intravenous acetaminophen has not been approved by the US Food and Drug Administration, preliminary data on its safety and efficacy are promising in neonates and infants and it may decrease the total amount of morphine needed to treat postoperative pain.[107–109] Nonsteroidal antiinflammatory medication use has been restricted to pharmacologic closure of patent ductus arteriosus because of concerns regarding renal insufficiency, platelet dysfunction, and the development of pulmonary hypertension.[110] An animal study suggests that cyclooxygenase-1 inhibitors are less effective in immature compared with mature animals, probably because of decreased cyclooxygenase-1 receptor expression in the spinal cord.[110] This decrease in receptor expression may explain the lack of efficacy of nonsteroidal antiinflammatory drugs in human infants.[111]

Topical Anesthetic Agents

Topical anesthesia may provide pain relief during some procedures. The most commonly studied and used topical agents in the neonatal population are tetracaine gel and Eutectic Mixture of Local Anesthetics (EMLA), a mixture of 2.5% lidocaine and 2.5% prilocaine. These agents have been found to decrease measures of pain during venipuncture, percutaneous central venous catheter insertion, and

peripheral arterial puncture.[112–114] EMLA did not decrease pain-related measures during heel lance[113] but may decrease pain measures during lumbar puncture,[115] particularly if the patient is concurrently provided with oral sucrose or glucose solution.[116] Concerns related to the use of topical anesthetics include methemaglobinemia, prolonged application times to allow absorption for optimal effectiveness, local skin irritation, and toxicity, especially in preterm infants.[117,118]

CONCLUSIONS AND RECOMMENDATIONS

In summary, there are significant research gaps regarding the assessment, management, and outcomes of neonatal pain; and there is a continuing need for studies evaluating the effects of neonatal pain and pain-prevention strategies on long-term neurodevelopmental, behavioral, and cognitive outcomes. The use of pharmacologic treatments for pain prevention and management in neonates continues to be hampered by the paucity of data on the short- and long-term safety and efficacy of these agents. At the same time, repetitive pain in the NICU has been associated with adverse neurodevelopmental, behavioral, and cognitive outcomes, calling for more research to address gaps in knowledge.[5,8,22,89,119–122] Despite incomplete data, the pediatrician and other health care professionals who care for neonates face the need to weigh both of these concerns in assessing pain and the need for pain prevention and management on a continuing basis throughout the infant's hospitalization.

Recommendations

1. Preventing or minimizing pain in neonates should be the goal of pediatricians and other health care professionals who care for neonates. To facilitate this goal, each institution should

have written guidelines, based on existing and emerging evidence, for a stepwise pain-prevention and treatment plan, which includes judicious use of procedures, routine assessment of pain, use of both pharmacologic and nonpharmacologic therapies for the prevention of pain associated with routine minor procedures, and effective medications to minimize pain associated with surgery and other major procedures.

2. Despite the significant challenges of assessing pain in this population, currently available, validated neonatal pain assessment tools should be consistently used before, during, and after painful procedures to monitor the effectiveness of pain relief interventions. In addition, the need for pain prevention and management should be assessed on a continuing basis throughout the infant's hospitalization.

3. Nonpharmacologic strategies, such as facilitated tucking, nonnutritive sucking, provision of breastfeeding or providing expressed human milk, or SS have been shown to be useful in decreasing pain scores during short-term mild to moderately painful procedures and should be consistently used.

4. Oral sucrose and/or glucose solutions can be effective in neonates undergoing mild to moderately painful procedures, either alone or in combination with other pain relief strategies. When sucrose or glucose is used as a pain management strategy, it should be prescribed and tracked as a medication; evidence-based protocols should be developed and implemented in nurseries, and more research should be conducted to better understand the effects of sucrose use for analgesia.

5. The pediatrician and other health care professionals who care for neonates must weigh potential and actual benefits and burdens when using pharmacologic treatment methods based on available evidence. Some medications can potentiate the respiratory depression and hypotension that can occur with opioids, and infants receiving them should be carefully monitored. Caution should be exercised when considering newer medications for which data in neonates are sparse or nonexistent.

6. Pediatricians, other neonatal health care providers, and family members should receive continuing education regarding the recognition, assessment, and management of pain in neonates, including new evidence as it becomes available.

7. To address the gaps in knowledge, more research should be conducted on pain assessment tools and pharmacologic and nonpharmacologic strategies to prevent or ameliorate pain. Studies on pharmacokinetics and pharmacodynamics of newer medications are needed to prevent therapeutic misadventures in the most vulnerable patients in pediatric practice.

LEAD AUTHORS

Erin Keels, APRN, MS, NNP-BC
Navil Sethna, MD, FAAP

COMMITTEE ON FETUS AND NEWBORN, 2015–2016

Kristi L. Watterberg, MD, FAAP, Chairperson
James J. Cummings, MD, FAAP
William E. Benitz, MD, FAAP
Eric C. Eichenwald, MD, FAAP
Brenda B. Poindexter, MD, FAAP
Dan L. Stewart, MD, FAAP
Susan W. Aucott, MD, FAAP
Jay P. Goldsmith, MD, FAAP
Karen M. Puopolo, MD, PhD, FAAP
Kasper S. Wang, MD, FAAP

LIAISONS

Tonse N.K. Raju, MD, DCH, FAAP — *National Institutes of Health*
Captain Wanda D. Barfield, MD, MPH, FAAP — *Centers for Disease Control and Prevention*
Erin L. Keels, APRN, MS, NNP-BC — *National Association of Neonatal Nurses*
Thierry Lacaze, MD — *Canadian Pediatric Society*
Maria Mascola, MD — *American College of Obstetricians and Gynecologists*

STAFF

Jim Couto, MA

SECTION ON ANESTHESIOLOGY AND PAIN MEDICINE EXECUTIVE COMMITTEE, 2014–2015

Joseph D. Tobias, MD, FAAP, Chairperson
Rita Agarwal, MD, FAAP, Chairperson-Elect
Corrie T.M. Anderson, MD, FAAP
Courtney A. Hardy, MD, FAAP
Anita Honkanen, MD, FAAP
Mohamed A. Rehman, MD, FAAP
Carolyn F. Bannister, MD, FAAP

LIAISONS

Randall P. Flick, MD, MPH, FAAP — *American Society of Anesthesiologists Committee on Pediatrics*
Constance S. Houck, MD, FAAP — *AAP Committee on Drugs*

STAFF

Jennifer Riefe, MEd

ABBREVIATIONS

AAP: American Academy of Pediatrics
PIPP: Premature Infant Pain Profile
RCT: randomized controlled trial
SS: sensorial stimulation
SSC: skin-to-skin care

REFERENCES

1. American Academy of Pediatrics Committee on Fetus and Newborn, Committee on Drugs, Section on Anesthesiology, Section on Surgery; Canadian Paediatric Society Fetus and Newborn Committee. Prevention and management of pain and stress in the neonate. *Pediatrics*. 2000;105(2):454–461

2. Batton DG, Barrington KJ, Wallman C; American Academy of Pediatrics

Committee on Fetus and Newborn; American Academy of Pediatrics Section on Surgery; Canadian Paediatric Society Fetus and Newborn Committee. Prevention and management of pain in the neonate: an update. *Pediatrics*. 2006;118(5):2231–2241

3. Carbajal R, Rousset A, Danan C, et al. Epidemiology and treatment of painful procedures in neonates in intensive care units. *JAMA*. 2008;300(1):60–70

4. Simons SH, van Dijk M, Anand KS, Roofthooft D, van Lingen RA, Tibboel D. Do we still hurt newborn babies? A prospective study of procedural pain and analgesia in neonates. *Arch Pediatr Adolesc Med*. 2003;157(11):1058–1064

5. Anand KJ, Aranda JV, Berde CB, et al. Summary proceedings from the neonatal pain-control group. *Pediatrics*. 2006;117(3 Suppl 1):S9–S22

6. Anand KJ. Clinical importance of pain and stress in preterm neonates. *Biol Neonate*. 1998;73(1):1–9

7. Vinall J, Grunau RE. Impact of repeated procedural pain-related stress in infants born very preterm. *Pediatr Res*. 2014;75(5):584–587

8. Doesburg SM, Chau CM, Cheung TP, et al. Neonatal pain-related stress, functional cortical activity and visual-perceptual abilities in school-age children born at extremely low gestational age. *Pain*. 2013;154(10):1946–1952

9. Hermann C, Hohmeister J, Demirakça S, Zohsel K, Flor H. Long-term alteration of pain sensitivity in school-aged children with early pain experiences. *Pain*. 2006;125(3):278–285

10. Grunau RE, Whitfield MF, Petrie-Thomas J, et al. Neonatal pain, parenting stress and interaction, in relation to cognitive and motor development at 8 and 18 months in preterm infants. *Pain*. 2009;143(1–2):138–146

11. Walker SM, Franck LS, Fitzgerald M, Myles J, Stocks J, Marlow N. Long-term impact of neonatal intensive care and surgery on somatosensory perception in children born extremely preterm. *Pain*. 2009;141(1–2):79–87

12. Beggs S, Torsney C, Drew LJ, Fitzgerald M. The postnatal reorganization of primary afferent input and dorsal horn cell receptive fields in the rat spinal cord is an activity-dependent process. *Eur J Neurosci*. 2002;16(7):1249–1258

13. Jennings E, Fitzgerald M. Postnatal changes in responses of rat dorsal horn cells to afferent stimulation: a fibre-induced sensitization. *J Physiol*. 1998;509(pt 3):859–868

14. Schmelzle-Lubiecki BM, Campbell KA, Howard RH, Franck L, Fitzgerald M. Long-term consequences of early infant injury and trauma upon somatosensory processing. *Eur J Pain*. 2007;11(7):799–809

15. Ranger M, Chau CM, Garg A, et al. Neonatal pain-related stress predicts cortical thickness at age 7 years in children born very preterm. *PLoS One*. 2013;8(10):e76702

16. Slater R, Cantarella A, Gallella S, et al. Cortical pain responses in human infants. *J Neurosci*. 2006;26(14):3662–3666

17. Ingram RA, Fitzgerald M, Baccei ML. Developmental changes in the fidelity and short-term plasticity of GABAergic synapses in the neonatal rat dorsal horn. *J Neurophysiol*. 2008;99(6):3144–3150

18. Walker SM, Meredith-Middleton J, Lickiss T, Moss A, Fitzgerald M. Primary and secondary hyperalgesia can be differentiated by postnatal age and ERK activation in the spinal dorsal horn of the rat pup. *Pain*. 2007;128(1–2):157–168

19. Holsti L, Grunau RE, Oberlander TF, Whitfield MF. Prior pain induces heightened motor responses during clustered care in preterm infants in the NICU. *Early Hum Dev*. 2005;81(3):293–302

20. Grunau RE, Holsti L, Haley DW, et al. Neonatal procedural pain exposure predicts lower cortisol and behavioral reactivity in preterm infants in the NICU. *Pain*. 2005;113(3):293–300

21. Cignacco E, Hamers J, van Lingen RA, et al. Neonatal procedural pain exposure and pain management in ventilated preterm infants during the first 14 days of life. *Swiss Med Wkly*. 2009;139(15–16):226–232

22. Bouza H. The impact of pain in the immature brain. *J Matern Fetal Neonatal Med*. 2009;22(9):722–732

23. Bellieni CV, Iantorno L, Perrone S, et al. Even routine painful procedures can be harmful for the newborn. *Pain*. 2009;147(1–3):128–131

24. Slater L, Asmerom Y, Boskovic DS, et al. Procedural pain and oxidative stress in premature neonates. *J Pain*. 2012;13(6):590–597

25. Fitzgerald M. The development of nociceptive circuits. *Nat Rev Neurosci*. 2005;6(7):507–520

26. Hohmeister J, Demirakça S, Zohsel K, Flor H, Hermann C. Responses to pain in school-aged children with experience in a neonatal intensive care unit: cognitive aspects and maternal influences. *Eur J Pain*. 2009;13(1):94–101

27. Grunau RE, Whitfield MF, Fay TB. Psychosocial and academic characteristics of extremely low birth weight (< or =800 g) adolescents who are free of major impairment compared with term-born control subjects. *Pediatrics*. 2004;114(6). Available at: www.pediatrics.org/cgi/content/full/114/6/e725

28. Anand KJ; International Evidence-Based Group for Neonatal Pain. Consensus statement for the prevention and management of pain in the newborn. *Arch Pediatr Adolesc Med*. 2001;155(2):173–180

29. Hummel P, van Dijk M. Pain assessment: current status and challenges. *Semin Fetal Neonatal Med*. 2006;11(4):237–245

30. Grunau RE, Oberlander T, Holsti L, Whitfield MF. Bedside application of the Neonatal Facial Coding System in pain assessment of premature neonates. *Pain*. 1998;76(3):277–286

31. Peters JW, Koot HM, Grunau RE, et al. Neonatal Facial Coding System for assessing postoperative pain in infants: item reduction is valid and feasible. *Clin J Pain*. 2003;19(6):353–363

32. Stevens B, Johnston C, Petryshen P, Taddio A. Premature Infant Pain Profile: development and initial validation. *Clin J Pain*. 1996;12(1):13–22

33. Ballantyne M, Stevens B, McAllister M, Dionne K, Jack A. Validation of the premature infant pain profile in the clinical setting. *Clin J Pain.* 1999;15(4):297–303

34. Jonsdottir RB, Kristjansdottir G. The sensitivity of the Premature Infant Pain Profile—PIPP to measure pain in hospitalized neonates. *J Eval Clin Pract.* 2005;11(6):598–605

35. Hummel P, Puchalski M, Creech SD, Weiss MG. Clinical reliability and validity of the N-PASS: neonatal pain, agitation and sedation scale with prolonged pain. *J Perinatol.* 2008;28(1):55–60

36. Hummel P, Lawlor-Klean P, Weiss MG. Validity and reliability of the N-PASS assessment tool with acute pain. *J Perinatol.* 2010;30(7):474–478

37. Holsti L, Grunau RE. Initial validation of the Behavioral Indicators of Infant Pain (BIIP). *Pain.* 2007;132(3):264–272

38. Carbajal R, Paupe A, Hoenn E, Lenclen R, Olivier-Martin M. [APN: evaluation behavioral scale of acute pain in newborn infants.] [Article in French]. *Arch Pediatr.* 1997;4(7):623–628

39. Cong X, McGrath JM, Cusson RM, Zhang D. Pain assessment and measurement in neonates: an updated review. *Adv Neonatal Care.* 2013;13(6):379–395

40. Stevens BJ, Gibbins S, Yamada J, et al. The premature infant pain profile-revised (PIPP-R): initial validation and feasibility. *Clin J Pain.* 2014;30(3):238–243

41. Gibbins S, Stevens BJ, Yamada J, et al. Validation of the Premature Infant Pain Profile-Revised (PIPP-R). *Early Hum Dev.* 2014;90(4):189–193

42. Milesi C, Cambonie G, Jacquot A, et al. Validation of a neonatal pain scale adapted to the new practices in caring for preterm newborns. *Arch Dis Child Fetal Neonatal Ed.* 2010;95(4):F263–F266

43. Lawrence J, Alcock D, McGrath P, Kay J, MacMurray SB, Dulberg C. The development of a tool to assess neonatal pain. *Neonatal Netw.* 1993;12(6):59–66

44. Krechel SW, Bildner J. CRIES: a new neonatal postoperative pain measurement score. Initial testing of validity and reliability. *Paediatr Anaesth.* 1995;5(1):53–61

45. van Dijk M, Roofthooft DW, Anand KJ, et al. Taking up the challenge of measuring prolonged pain in (premature) neonates: the COMFORTneo scale seems promising. *Clin J Pain.* 2009;25(7):607–616

46. Hand I, Noble L, Geiss D, Wozniak L, Hall C. COVERS Neonatal Pain Scale: development and validation. *Int J Pediatr.* 2010. Available at: www.hindawi.com/journals/ijpedi/2010/496719/. Accessed December 17, 2014

47. Hudson-Barr D, Capper-Michel B, Lambert S, Palermo TM, Morbeto K, Lombardo S. Validation of the Pain Assessment in Neonates (PAIN) scale with the Neonatal Infant Pain Scale (NIPS). *Neonatal Netw.* 2002;21(6):15–21

48. Hodgkinson K, Bear M, Thorn J, Van Blaricum S. Measuring pain in neonates: evaluating an instrument and developing a common language. *Aust J Adv Nurs.* 1994;12(1):17–22

49. Spence K, Gillies D, Harrison D, Johnston L, Nagy S. A reliable pain assessment tool for clinical assessment in the neonatal intensive care unit. *J Obstet Gynecol Neonatal Nurs.* 2005;34(1):80–86

50. Blauer T, Gerstmann D. A simultaneous comparison of three neonatal pain scales during common NICU procedures. *Clin J Pain.* 1998;14(1):39–47

51. Debillon T, Zupan V, Ravault N, Magny JF, Dehan M. Development and initial validation of the EDIN scale, a new tool for assessing prolonged pain in preterm infants. *Arch Dis Child Fetal Neonatal Ed.* 2001;85(1):F36–F41

52. Cignacco E, Mueller R, Hamers JP, Gessler P. Pain assessment in the neonate using the Bernese Pain Scale for Neonates. *Early Hum Dev.* 2004;78(2):125–131

53. Slater R, Cantarella A, Franck L, Meek J, Fitzgerald M. How well do clinical pain assessment tools reflect pain in infants? *PLoS Med.* 2008;5(6):e129

54. Smith GC, Gutovich J, Smyser C, et al. Neonatal intensive care unit stress is associated with brain development in preterm infants. *Ann Neurol.* 2011;70(4):541–549

55. Hünseler C, Merkt V, Gerloff M, Eifinger F, Kribs A, Roth B. Assessing pain in ventilated newborns and infants: validation of the Hartwig score. *Eur J Pediatr.* 2011;170(7):837–843

56. Arias MC, Guinsburg R. Differences between uni-and multidimensional scales for assessing pain in term newborn infants at the bedside. *Clinics (Sao Paulo).* 2012;67(10):1165–1170

57. Ahn Y, Jun Y. Measurement of pain-like response to various NICU stimulants for high-risk infants. *Early Hum Dev.* 2007;83(4):255–262

58. Walden M, Gibbins S. *Pain Assessment and Management: Guidelines for Practice.* 2nd ed. Glenview, IL: National Association of Neonatal Nurses; 2010

59. Morrow C, Hidinger A, Wilkinson-Faulk D. Reducing neonatal pain during routine heel lance procedures. *MCN Am J Matern Child Nurs.* 2010;35(6):346–354; quiz: 354–356

60. Axelin A, Salanterä S, Kirjavainen J, Lehtonen L. Oral glucose and parental holding preferable to opioid in pain management in preterm infants. *Clin J Pain.* 2009;25(2):138–145

61. Obeidat H, Kahalaf I, Callister LC, Froelicher ES. Use of facilitated tucking for nonpharmacological pain management in preterm infants: a systematic review. *J Perinat Neonatal Nurs.* 2009;23(4):372–377

62. Liaw JJ, Yang L, Katherine Wang KW, Chen CM, Chang YC, Yin T. Non-nutritive sucking and facilitated tucking relieve preterm infant pain during heel-stick procedures: a prospective, randomised controlled crossover trial. *Int J Nurs Stud.* 2012;49(3):300–309

63. Abdallah B, Badr LK, Hawwari M. The efficacy of massage on short and long term outcomes in preterm infants. *Infant Behav Dev.* 2013;36(4):662–669

64. Pillai Riddell RR, Racine NM, Turcotte K, et al. Non-pharmacological management of infant and young child procedural pain. *Cochrane Database Syst Rev.* 2011;20115(10):CD006275

65. Johnston C, Campbell-Yeo M, Fernandes A, Inglis D, Streiner D, Zee R. Skin-to-skin care for procedural pain

in neonates. *Cochrane Database Syst Rev.* 2014;1(1):CD008435

66. Cong X, Cusson RM, Walsh S, Hussain N, Ludington-Hoe SM, Zhang D. Effects of skin-to-skin contact on autonomic pain responses in preterm infants. *J Pain.* 2012;13(7):636–645

67. Cong X, Ludington-Hoe SM, Walsh S. Randomized crossover trial of kangaroo care to reduce biobehavioral pain responses in preterm infants: a pilot study. *Biol Res Nurs.* 2011;13(2):204–216

68. Shah PS, Herbozo C, Aliwalas LL, Shah VS. Breastfeeding or breast milk for procedural pain in neonates. *Cochrane Database Syst Rev.* 2012;12(12):CD004950

69. Bellieni CV, Tei M, Coccina F, Buonocore G. Sensorial saturation for infants' pain. *J Matern Fetal Neonatal Med.* 2012;25(suppl 1):79–81

70. Gitto E, Pellegrino S, Manfrida M, et al. Stress response and procedural pain in the preterm newborn: the role of pharmacological and non-pharmacological treatments. *Eur J Pediatr.* 2012;171(6):927–933

71. Harrison D, Beggs S, Stevens B. Sucrose for procedural pain management in infants. *Pediatrics.* 2012;130(5):918–925

72. Slater R, Cornelissen L, Fabrizi L, et al. Oral sucrose as an analgesic drug for procedural pain in newborn infants: a randomised controlled trial. *Lancet.* 2010;376(9748):1225–1232

73. Wilkinson DJ, Savulescu J, Slater R. Sugaring the pill: ethics and uncertainties in the use of sucrose for newborn infants. *Arch Pediatr Adolesc Med.* 2012;166(7):629–633

74. Stevens B, Yamada J, Lee GY, Ohlsson A. Sucrose for analgesia in newborn infants undergoing painful procedures. *Cochrane Database Syst Rev.* 2013;1(1):CD001069

75. Lefrak L, Burch K, Caravantes R, et al. Sucrose analgesia: identifying potentially better practices. *Pediatrics.* 2006;118(2 suppl 2):S197–S202

76. Johnston CC, Stremler R, Horton L, Friedman A. Effect of repeated doses of sucrose during heel stick procedure in preterm neonates. *Biol Neonate.* 1999;75(3):160–166

77. Fernandez M, Blass EM, Hernandez-Reif M, Field T, Diego M, Sanders C. Sucrose attenuates a negative electroencephalographic response to an aversive stimulus for newborns. *J Dev Behav Pediatr.* 2003;24(4):261–266

78. Blass EM, Watt LB. Suckling- and sucrose-induced analgesia in human newborns. *Pain.* 1999;83(3):611–623

79. Shide DJ, Blass EM. Opioidlike effects of intraoral infusions of corn oil and polycose on stress reactions in 10-day-old rats. *Behav Neurosci.* 1989;103(6):1168–1175

80. Anseloni VC, Ren K, Dubner R, Ennis M. A brainstem substrate for analgesia elicited by intraoral sucrose. *Neuroscience.* 2005;133(1):231–243

81. Holsti L, Grunau RE. Considerations for using sucrose to reduce procedural pain in preterm infants. *Pediatrics.* 2010;125(5):1042–1047

82. Taddio A, Yiu A, Smith RW, Katz J, McNair C, Shah V. Variability in clinical practice guidelines for sweetening agents in newborn infants undergoing painful procedures. *Clin J Pain.* 2009;25(2):153–155

83. Johnston CC, Filion F, Snider L, et al. Routine sucrose analgesia during the first week of life in neonates younger than 31 weeks' postconceptional age. *Pediatrics.* 2002;110(3):523–528

84. Johnston CC, Filion F, Snider L, et al. How much sucrose is too much sucrose [letter]? *Pediatrics.* 2007;119(1):226

85. Bueno M, Yamada J, Harrison D, et al. A systematic review and meta-analyses of nonsucrose sweet solutions for pain relief in neonates. *Pain Res Manag.* 2013;18(3):153–161

86. Costa MC, Eckert GU, Fortes BG, Fortes Filho JB, Silveira RC, Procianoy RS. Oral glucose for pain relief during examination for retinopathy of prematurity: a masked randomized clinical trial. *Clinics (Sao Paulo).* 2013;68(2):199–204

87. de Graaf J, van Lingen RA, Valkenburg AJ, et al. Does neonatal morphine use affect neuropsychological outcomes at 8 to 9 years of age? *Pain.* 2013;154(3):449–458

88. Rozé JC, Denizot S, Carbajal R, et al. Prolonged sedation and/or analgesia

and 5-year neurodevelopment outcome in very preterm infants: results from the EPIPAGE cohort. *Arch Pediatr Adolesc Med.* 2008;162(8):728–733

89. Whitfield MF, Grunau RE. Behavior, pain perception, and the extremely low-birth weight survivor. *Clin Perinatol.* 2000;27(2):363–379

90. American Academy of Pediatrics, Task Force on Circumcision. Circumcision policy statement. *Pediatrics.* 1999;103(3):686–693

91. Kumar P, Denson SE, Mancuso TJ; Committee on Fetus and Newborn, Section on Anesthesiology and Pain Medicine. Premedication for nonemergency endotracheal intubation in the neonate. *Pediatrics.* 2010;125(3):608–615

92. Bellù R, de Waal K, Zanini R. Opioids for neonates receiving mechanical ventilation: a systematic review and meta-analysis. *Arch Dis Child Fetal Neonatal Ed.* 2010;95(4):F241–F251

93. Anand KJ, Hall RW, Desai N, et al; NEOPAIN Trial Investigators Group. Effects of morphine analgesia in ventilated preterm neonates: primary outcomes from the NEOPAIN randomised trial. *Lancet.* 2004;363(9422):1673–1682

94. Bellù R, de Waal KA, Zanini R. Opioids for neonates receiving mechanical ventilation. *Cochrane Database Syst Rev.* 2008;1:CD004212

95. Choong K, AlFaleh K, Doucette J, et al. Remifentanil for endotracheal intubation in neonates: a randomised controlled trial. *Arch Dis Child Fetal Neonatal Ed.* 2010;95(2):F80–F84

96. Lago P, Tiozzo C, Boccuzzo G, Allegro A, Zacchello F. Remifentanil for percutaneous intravenous central catheter placement in preterm infant: a randomized controlled trial. *Paediatr Anaesth.* 2008;18(8):736–744

97. Ng E, Taddio A, Ohlsson A. Intravenous midazolam infusion for sedation of infants in the neonatal intensive care unit. *Cochrane Database Syst Rev.* 2012;6(6):CD002052

98. Anand KJ, Barton BA, McIntosh N, et al. Analgesia and sedation in preterm neonates who require ventilatory support: results from the NOPAIN trial. Neonatal Outcome and Prolonged

Analgesia in Neonates. *Arch Pediatr Adolesc Med.* 1999;153(4):331–338

99. Anand KJ. Pharmacological approaches to the management of pain in the neonatal intensive care unit. *J Perinatol.* 2007;27(suppl 1):S4–S11

100. Durrmeyer X, Vutskits L, Anand KJ, Rimensberger PC. Use of analgesic and sedative drugs in the NICU: integrating clinical trials and laboratory data. *Pediatr Res.* 2010;67(2):117–127

101. Chana SK, Anand KJ. Can we use methadone for analgesia in neonates? *Arch Dis Child Fetal Neonatal Ed.* 2001;85(2):F79–F81

102. Nemergut ME, Yaster M, Colby CE. Sedation and analgesia to facilitate mechanical ventilation. *Clin Perinatol.* 2013;40(3):539–558

103. Cravero JP, Havidich JE. Pediatric sedation—evolution and revolution. *Paediatr Anaesth.* 2011;21(7):800–809

104. Allegaert K, Peeters MY, Verbesselt R, et al. Inter-individual variability in propofol pharmacokinetics in preterm and term neonates. *Br J Anaesth.* 2007;99(6):864–870

105. Vanderhaegen J, Naulaers G, Van Huffel S, Vanhole C, Allegaert K. Cerebral and systemic hemodynamic effects of intravenous bolus administration of propofol in neonates. *Neonatology.* 2010;98(1):57–63

106. Chrysostomou C, Schulman SR, Herrera Castellanos M, et al. A phase II/III, multicenter, safety, efficacy, and pharmacokinetic study of dexmedetomidine in preterm and term neonates. *J Pediatr.* 2014;164(2):276–282

107. Allegaert K, van den Anker J. Pharmacokinetics and pharmacodynamics of intravenous acetaminophen in neonates. *Expert Rev Clin Pharmacol.* 2011;4(6):713–718

108. Ceelie I, de Wildt SN, van Dijk M, et al. Effect of intravenous paracetamol on postoperative morphine requirements in neonates and infants undergoing major noncardiac surgery: a randomized controlled trial. *JAMA.* 2013;309(2):149–154

109. Ohlsson A, Shah PS. Paracetamol (acetaminophen) for prevention or treatment of pain in newborns. *Cochrane Database Syst Rev.* 2015;6(6):CD011219

110. Ohlsson A, Walia R, Shah S. Ibuprofen for the treatment of patent ductus arteriosus in preterm and/or low birth weight infants. *Cochrane Database Syst Rev.* 2008;1:CD003481

111. Ririe DG, Prout HD, Barclay D, Tong C, Lin M, Eisenach JC. Developmental differences in spinal cyclooxygenase 1 expression after surgical incision. *Anesthesiology.* 2006;104(3):426–431

112. Taddio A, Ohlsson A, Einarson TR, Stevens B, Koren G. A systematic review of lidocaine-prilocaine cream (EMLA) in the treatment of acute pain in neonates. *Pediatrics.* 1998;101(2):e1

113. Kapellou O. Blood sampling in infants (reducing pain and morbidity). 2011;Apr 5: 2011. pii: 0313

114. Hall RW, Anand KJ. Pain management in newborns. *Clin Perinatol.* 2014;41(4):895–924

115. Kaur G, Gupta P, Kumar A. A randomized trial of eutectic mixture of local anesthetics during lumbar puncture in newborns. *Arch Pediatr Adolesc Med.* 2003;157(11):1065–1070

116. Biran V, Gourrier E, Cimerman P, Walter-Nicolet E, Mitanchez D, Carbajal R. Analgesic effects of EMLA cream and oral sucrose during venipuncture in preterm infants. *Pediatrics.* 2011;128(1). Available at: www. pediatrics.org/cgi/content/full/128/1/e63

117. Foster JP, Taylor C, Bredemeyer SL. Topical anaesthesia for needle-related pain in newborn infants. *Cochrane Database Syst Rev.* 2013; (1):CD010331

118. Maulidi H, McNair C, Seller N, Kirsh J, Bradley TJ, Greenway SC, Tomlinson C. Arrhythmia associated with tetracaine in an extremely low birth weight premature infant. *Pediatrics.* 2012;130(6). Available at: www. pediatrics.org/cgi/content/full/130/6/e1704

119. Harrison D, Yamada J, Stevens B. Strategies for the prevention and management of neonatal and infant pain. *Curr Pain Headache Rep.* 2010;14(2):113–123

120. Grunau R. Early pain in preterm infants: a model of long-term effects. *Clin Perinatol.* 2002;29(3):373–394, vii–viii

121. Taddio A, Shah V, Gilbert-MacLeod C, Katz J. Conditioning and hyperalgesia in newborns exposed to repeated heel lances. *JAMA.* 2002;288(7):857–861

122. Anand KJ, Johnston CC, Oberlander TF, Taddio A, Lehr VT, Walco GA. Analgesia and local anesthesia during invasive procedures in the neonate. *Clin Ther.* 2005;27(6):844–876

Prevention of Childhood Lead Toxicity

• *Policy Statement*

POLICY STATEMENT Organizational Principles to Guide and Define the Child Health
Care System and/or Improve the Health of all Children

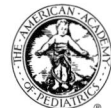

American Academy
of Pediatrics

DEDICATED TO THE HEALTH OF ALL CHILDREN™

Prevention of Childhood Lead Toxicity

COUNCIL ON ENVIRONMENTAL HEALTH

abstract

Blood lead concentrations have decreased dramatically in US children over the past 4 decades, but too many children still live in housing with deteriorated lead-based paint and are at risk for lead exposure with resulting lead-associated cognitive impairment and behavioral problems. Evidence continues to accrue that commonly encountered blood lead concentrations, even those below 5 μg/dL (50 ppb), impair cognition; there is no identified threshold or safe level of lead in blood. From 2007 to 2010, approximately 2.6% of preschool children in the United States had a blood lead concentration ≥5 μg/dL (≥50 ppb), which represents about 535 000 US children 1 to 5 years of age. Evidence-based guidance is available for managing increased lead exposure in children, and reducing sources of lead in the environment, including lead in housing, soil, water, and consumer products, has been shown to be cost-beneficial. Primary prevention should be the focus of policy on childhood lead toxicity.

DOI: 10.1542/peds.2016-1493

Accepted for publication May 5, 2016

PEDIATRICS (ISSN Numbers: Print, 0031-4005; Online, 1098-4275).

FINANCIAL DISCLOSURE: The author has indicated he does not have a financial relationship relevant to this article to disclose.

FUNDING: No external funding.

POTENTIAL CONFLICT OF INTEREST: The author has indicated he has no potential conflicts of interest to disclose.

To cite: AAP COUNCIL ON ENVIRONMENTAL HEALTH. Prevention of Childhood Lead Toxicity. *Pediatrics.* 2016;138(1):e20161493

OVERVIEW AND INTRODUCTION

Primary prevention, reducing or eliminating the myriad sources of lead in the environment of children before exposure occurs, is the most reliable and cost-effective measure to protect children from lead toxicity. Very high blood lead concentrations (eg, >100 μg/dL) can cause significant overt symptoms, such as protracted vomiting and encephalopathy, and even death. Low-level lead exposure, even at blood lead concentrations below 5 μg/dL (50 ppb), is a causal risk factor for diminished intellectual and academic abilities, higher rates of neurobehavioral disorders such as hyperactivity and attention deficits, and lower birth weight in children. No effective treatments ameliorate the permanent developmental effects of lead toxicity. Reducing lead exposure from residential lead hazards, industrial sources, contaminated foods or water, and other consumer products is an effective way to prevent or control childhood lead exposure. Lead poisoning prevention education directed at hand-washing or dust control fails to reduce children's blood lead concentrations. However, pediatricians and parents should be aware of measures to reduce the toxic effects of lead on children, including the promulgation of regulations to screen or test older housing units for lead hazards

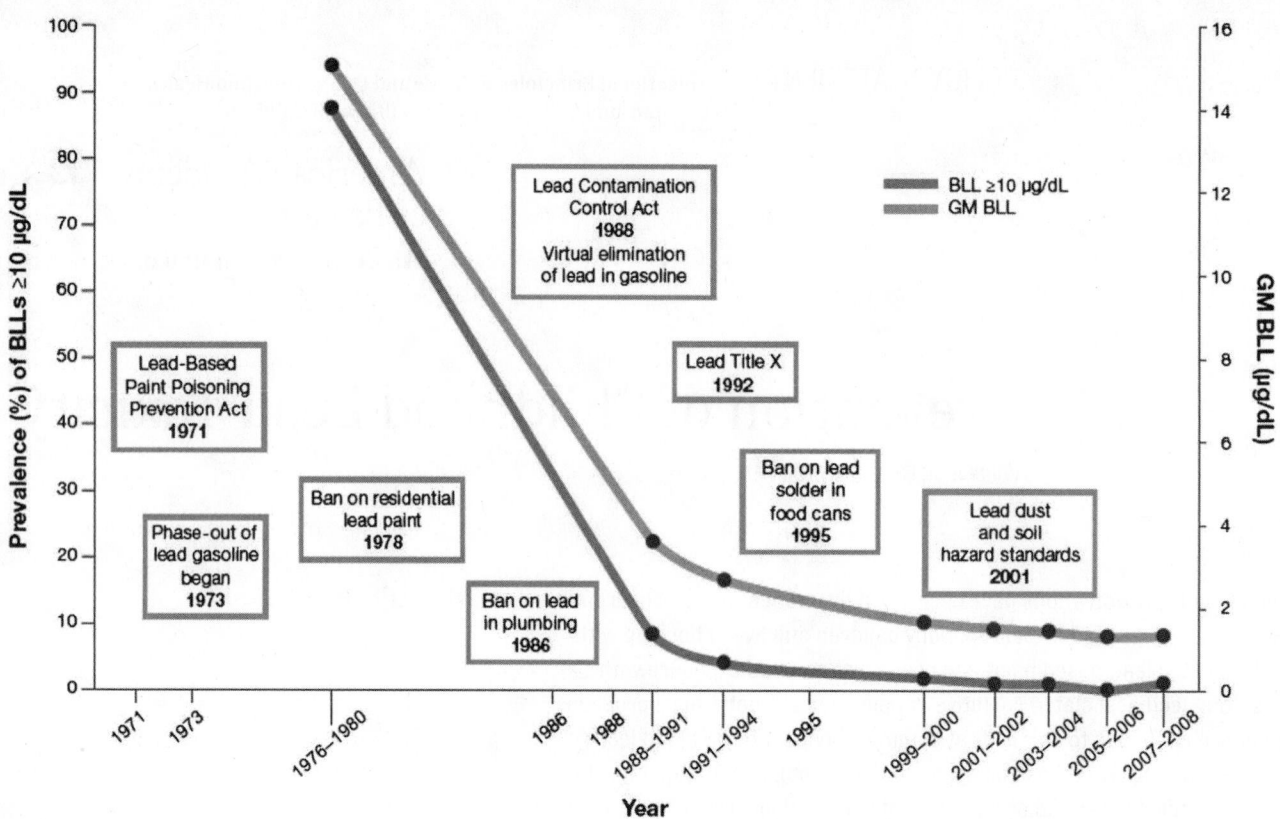

FIGURE 1
Timeline of lead poisoning prevention policies and blood lead levels in children aged 1–5 years, by year—NHANES, United States, 1971–2008. BLL, blood lead level; GM BLL, geometric mean blood lead level. Adapted from Brown et al.[1]

before occupancy and after major renovation and abatement; revision of federal standards to reduce allowable levels of lead in settled house dust, water, soil, cosmetics, and other consumer products; and enhanced protection for children who live in lead-contaminated communities or near lead-emitting industries.

SCOPE OF THE PROBLEM

Over the past 4 decades, blood lead concentrations among US children have declined dramatically since the elimination of lead from gasoline, paints, and other consumer products[1] (Fig 1, Table 1). From 1976 to 1980, blood lead concentrations among US children declined more sharply than anticipated after the phase-out of leaded gasoline.[2] In 1978, the US Consumer Product Safety Commission (CPSC) restricted

the allowable content of lead in residential paint to 0.06% (600 ppm); in 2008, it was lowered to 0.009% (90 ppm).[3,4] There have also been significant reductions in tap water lead concentrations since the US Environmental Protection Agency (EPA) promulgated the Lead and Copper Rule.[5,6] Finally, use of lead solder in canned foods and other consumer products was banned. It is difficult to accurately apportion the decline in blood lead concentrations to specific sources, but the combined effect of these regulations clearly led to the dramatic reductions in children's blood lead concentrations.[1] The key to preventing lead toxicity in children is to reduce or eliminate persistent sources of lead exposure in their environment.

Prevention of low-level lead toxicity has historically focused on anticipatory guidance, screening children's blood for lead after

exposure, and iron or calcium supplementation to reduce lead absorption.[7] Unfortunately, studies that evaluated the efficacy of parent education or provision of cleaning equipment to families failed to show significant reductions in children's blood lead concentrations.[8] Similarly, calcium and iron supplementation have not consistently been shown to be efficacious in reducing blood lead concentrations of children.[9,10] Collectively, these studies indicate that the focus of prevention should be on reducing the sources of childhood lead exposures rather than identifying children who have already been unduly exposed or attempting to ameliorate the toxic effects of lead exposure.

In 2005, the American Academy of Pediatrics (AAP) recognized that blood lead concentrations below 10 μg/dL (100 ppb) may impair cognition; no threshold for the toxic effects of lead was identified.[7] The AAP adopted a blood lead concentration >10 µg/dL (>100 ppb) as the "level of concern" recommended by the Centers for Disease Control and Prevention (CDC), which indicated the need for closer medical and public health management.[7] Extensive and compelling evidence now indicates that lead-associated cognitive deficits and behavioral problems can occur at blood lead concentrations below 5 µg/dL (50 ppb). In 2012, the US National Toxicology Program of the National Institutes of Health reported that, after other risk factors are accounted for, blood lead concentrations <5 µg/dL (<50 ppb) are strongly associated with intellectual deficits, diminished academic abilities, attention deficits, and problem behaviors (Table 2).[11] In that same year, the Advisory Committee on Childhood Lead Poisoning Prevention of the CDC concluded that there is no safe level of lead exposure and adopted the use of a reference value of ≥5 µg/dL (≥50 ppb) (based on the 97.5th percentile of blood lead concentrations from the National Health and Nutrition Examination Survey [NHANES]) to be used as a trigger to guide clinical and public health interventions.[12]

Low-level elevations in children's blood lead concentrations, even at concentrations below 5 µg/dL (50 ppb), can result in decrements in cognitive functions, as measured by IQ scores and academic performance.[13,14] For a given level of exposure, lead-associated IQ decrements are proportionately greater at the lowest blood lead concentrations. The IQ decrement associated with an increase in blood lead concentration from <1 µg/dL (<10 ppb) to 30 µg/dL (300 ppb) was 9.2 IQ points, but the decrement associated with an increase in blood lead concentration from <1 µg/dL (<10 ppb) to 10 µg/dL (100 ppb) was 6.2 IQ points.[14] The population

TABLE 1 Federal Lead Poisoning Prevention Policies

Policy or Legislation	Year	Comment
Lead Based Paint Poisoning Prevention Act	1971	First major lead-based paint legislation; addressed lead-based paint in federal housing.
Phase Out Lead in Gasoline	1973	US EPA regulated a phase-out of lead in gasoline.
Ban on Residential Paint	1978	CPSC banned lead paint in residential properties.
Safe Drinking Water Act	1986	US EPA banned use of lead pipes and lead solder in plumbing.
Housing and Community Development Act	1987	Highlighted the danger to children of lead-contaminated dust.
Lead Contamination Control Act	1988	Authorized CDC to make grants to state and local programs to screen children and to provide for education about lead poisoning.
Residential Lead-Based Paint Hazard Reduction Act, Title X	1992	Established primary prevention of lead poisoning as a national strategy.
Guidelines for the Evaluation and Control of Lead-Based Paint Hazards in Housing	1995, 2012	HUD established guidelines for evaluating and controlling residential lead-based paint hazards.
Ban Lead Solder in Food Cans	1995	FDA amended food additive regulations to ban lead solder from food cans.
Lead Safe Housing Rule	1999, 2012	Regulation issued by HUD setting forth new requirements for lead-based paint notification, evaluation, and remediation.
Hazard Standards for Lead in Paint, Dust and Soil	2001	US EPA established a definition of a lead-based paint hazard and standards for paint, dust, and soil in children's play areas.
Consumer Product Safety Improvement Act	2008	CPSC lowered the cap on lead in paint from 0.06% to 0.0009% and incorporated the Lead-Free Toy Act, setting limit on lead content in toys.
Lead Renovation, Repair and Paint Rule	2010	US EPA required contractors working on homes built before 1978 to be certified and follow lead safe guidelines.

TABLE 2 Effects of Low-Level Lead Exposure on Academic and Intellectual Abilities, Puberty, Kidney Function, Postnatal Growth, Hearing, and Other Health Endpoints

Blood Lead Concentration	Evidence Level	Health Effect
<5 µg/dL	Sufficient	Decreased academic achievement
		Lower IQ scores
		Attention-related behavior problems
		Antisocial behaviors
	Limited	Delayed puberty
		Decreased kidney function in children ≥12 y of age
<10 µg/dL	Sufficient	Delayed puberty
		Reduced postnatal growth
		Decreased hearing
	Limited	Hypersensitivity by skin prick test
	Inadequate	Asthma and eczema
		Cardiovascular effects
		Kidney function <12 y of age

From the US Department of Health and Human Services, National Institute of Environmental Health Sciences, 2012.

impact of lead on intellectual abilities is substantial. Despite the dramatic reductions in blood lead levels, lead toxicity accounts for an estimated total loss of 23 million IQ points among a 6-year cohort of contemporary US children.[15]

Focusing efforts on children who have blood lead concentrations

≥5 µg/dL (≥50 ppb) is efficient but will fail to preserve the majority of lost IQ points in US children. The *prevention paradox* refers to the concept that most disease or disability occurs in low- to moderate-risk groups. Children who have blood lead concentrations ≥5 µg/dL (≥50 ppb) will, on average, experience a lead-associated IQ deficit of 6.1 points, an IQ deficit much larger than that of children who have lower blood lead concentrations (Fig 2). Still, if the focus is only on reducing exposures for children who have a blood lead concentration ≥5 µg/dL (≥50 ppb), we will fail to preserve more than 20 million (>80% of total) of the 23 million IQ points lost among US children with lower lead exposure because there are so many more children who have low to moderate blood lead concentrations (Fig 2). No therapeutic interventions currently exist for low blood lead concentrations; therefore, prevention of exposure is paramount. For these reasons, this statement focuses heavily on how pediatricians can help *prevent* lead exposure in children.

Elevated blood lead concentrations can result in the development of behavioral problems in children, including inattention, impulsivity, aggression, and hyperactivity.[16–18] In a nationally representative study of 8- to 15-year-old US children, Froehlich et al[17] found that having a blood lead concentration >1.3 µg/dL (>13 ppb) was associated with an elevated risk for attention-deficit/hyperactivity disorder (ADHD). Children with a blood lead concentration in the lowest tertile (<0.7 µg/dL, or <7 ppb) exhibited, on average, 1 symptom of ADHD, whereas children with a blood lead concentration in the highest tertile (>1.3 µg/dL, or >13 ppb) exhibited 3 symptoms. Some critics have argued that these "subtle" shifts in behavioral symptoms are inconsequential, but this shift in the population distribution of ADHD symptoms led to an increase in the percentage of children who met criteria for ADHD from 5% to 13%. Approximately 1 in 5 cases of ADHD among US children have been attributed to lead exposure.[17]

Antisocial behaviors, including conduct disorder, delinquency, and criminal behaviors, can result from

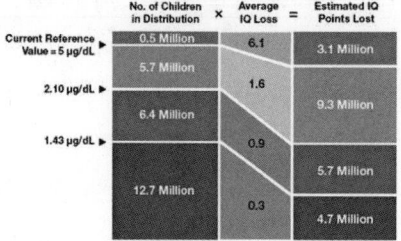

FIGURE 2
Prevention paradox. The majority of IQ points lost due to lead exposure occur in children who have low to moderate blood lead levels. Using the current reference value of 5 µg/dL, we will protect only 3.1 million IQ points (about 13% of the total). Adapted from Bellinger.[15]

a variety of risk factors, but there is substantial evidence that lead toxicity is 1 of the major risk factors for their development.[16,19–22] Needleman et al[16] found that adolescents who had higher bone lead concentrations had higher scores for delinquency and aggression. In a meta-analysis of 16 studies, Marcus et al[22] concluded that lead exposure, measured via blood lead or bone lead concentrations, was a risk factor for conduct disorder. In 2 prospective longitudinal studies, higher childhood blood lead or tooth lead concentrations resulted in higher rates of self-reported delinquent behaviors and arrests or convictions.[20,21] Reyes[23] concluded that the reduction in population mean blood lead concentrations was the major risk factor associated with the decline in severe violent behaviors over the past 3 decades.

Limited evidence implicates lead exposure in diminished kidney function in adolescents at low levels of exposure.[11] Using the NHANES, Fadrowski et al[24] found that, among 769 adolescents with a median blood lead concentration of 1.5 µg/dL (15 ppb), a doubling of the concentration led to a significant reduction in the glomerular filtration rate. It is not clear whether chronic, low-level lead exposure in childhood or adolescence is sufficient to result in chronic renal failure or whether it is the cumulative effect of a variety of risk factors that

ultimately results in the development of chronic renal failure. Still, this study is consistent with others linking lead exposure with chronic renal failure in adults.[11]

Lead can cause spontaneous abortion, low birth weight, and reduced growth in children. In a case–control study of pregnant women in Mexico City with blood lead concentrations that ranged from 1.3 µg/dL (13 ppb) to 29 (290 ppb) µg/dL, the odds for spontaneous abortion increased by 1.8 for every 5-µg/dL (50-ppb) increase in maternal blood lead concentration.[25] Early studies that examined the association of prenatal lead exposure and low birth weight or preterm birth, measured via either maternal or cord blood lead concentrations, found inconsistent results. However, in a large cohort involving more than 34 000 live births, investigators found that a 5-µg/dL (50-ppb) increase in blood lead concentrations was associated with a 61-g decrement in birth weight.[26] The National Toxicology Program concluded that maternal blood lead concentrations <5 µg/dL (<50 ppb) are associated with lower birth weight.

PREVENTING LEAD TOXICITY

Despite historical reductions in children's blood lead concentrations, preventing childhood lead toxicity remains a major public health priority in the United States. Many children who live in older, poorly maintained housing or older housing that undergoes renovation are at high risk for lead exposure. In the NHANES conducted from 2007 to 2010, approximately 2.6% of preschool children in the United States had a blood lead concentration ≥5 µg/dL (≥50 ppb), which represents about 535 000 US children 1 to 5 years of age.[12] Children who lived in older housing units experienced an increased risk for having a blood lead concentration in excess of 5 µg/dL (50 ppb); 15% of US children who lived in housing units built before 1950 had a blood lead concentration ≥5 µg/dL (≥50 ppb), whereas 4.2% of children who lived in housing built between 1950 and 1978 had a blood lead concentration ≥5 µg/dL (≥50 ppb), compared with 2.1% of children who lived in housing units built after 1978.[27] No treatments have been shown to be effective in ameliorating the permanent developmental effects of lead toxicity.[28] Finally, the economic costs of childhood lead toxicity are substantial. Despite the historical reductions in blood lead concentrations, it has been estimated that the annual cost of childhood lead exposure in the United States is $50 billion.[29] For every $1 invested to reduce lead hazards in housing units, society would benefit by an estimated $17 to $221, a cost–benefit ratio that is comparable with the cost–benefit ratio for childhood vaccines.[30]

The key to preventing lead toxicity in children is identification and elimination of the major sources of lead exposure. Primary prevention of lead exposure is now widely recognized as the optimal strategy because of the irreversible effects of low-level lead toxicity.[7,12] The primary prevention approach contrasts with practices and policies that too often have relied predominantly on detection of lead exposure only after children develop elevated blood lead concentrations.

SOURCES AND VARIABILITY OF LEAD EXPOSURE

Lead ingestion and absorption are dynamic during the first 2 years of life. Blood lead concentrations of children who live in lead-contaminated environments typically increase rapidly between 6 and 12 months of age, peak between 18 and 36 months of age, and then gradually decrease.[31] The peak in children's blood lead concentrations stems from the confluence of normal mouthing behaviors and increasing mobility.[31] Younger children also absorb lead more efficiently than older children and adults.[32] Iron deficiency can also increase the absorption of lead.[33]

A large number of housing units in the United States contain lead-based paint. In a national survey of housing conducted in 2011, it was estimated that 37 million (35%) of 106 million housing units contain lead-based paint.[34] Lead-based paint is the most common, highly concentrated source of lead exposure for children who live in older housing.[35] Paint that was used on both the interior and exterior of houses through the 1950s contained higher concentrations of lead than that of houses built in later years.[34,35] The lead concentration in paint and other media can be measured by using a hand-held instrument called the x-ray fluorescence (XRF) spectrum analyzer or by chemically analyzing paint chips.

The US Department of Housing and Urban Development (HUD) defines lead-based paint as an XRF reading ≥1 µg/cm^2 or 5000 ppm of lead in a paint chip.[36] The presence of *lead*-based *paint* is not as predictive of childhood lead exposure as a *lead paint hazard*. A lead paint hazard is defined by the EPA as "any condition that causes exposure to lead from contaminated dust, lead-contaminated soil, or lead-contaminated paint that is deteriorated, or the presence of accessible (or chewable) surfaces, friction surfaces or impact surfaces that would result in adverse human health effects."[37]

Age of the housing is a major determinant of lead paint hazards. For housing built from 1978 to 1998, 2.7% contained one or more lead paint hazards, whereas the prevalence of residential hazards increased to 11.4% of housing built from 1960 to 1977, 39% of housing built from 1940 to 1959, and 67% of housing units built before 1940.[34] Federal regulations for defining a lead paint hazard in house dust are obsolete. Federal agencies have set environmental lead standards to protect children from having a blood lead concentration ≥10 µg/dL (≥100 ppb), but it is now recognized that there is no safe level of lead exposure. Therefore, because the current standards for lead in house dust, water, and soil remain too high to protect children,[31,38] the percentage of housing that contains one or more lead paint hazards described above is an underestimate.

Lead-based paint is the major source of lead, but ingestions of lead-contaminated house dust and residential soil are the major pathways for exposure (Fig 3).[35–42] House dust, which can be contaminated by small particles of lead-based paint or track-in of lead-contaminated soil, is a major pathway of lead exposure for children who live in older, poorly maintained housing.[40] Ingestions of lead-contaminated house dust and soil are also the primary pathways of exposure for children who live in homes that were recently abated or renovated.[43–45]

Sampling house dust for lead hazards involves using a special wipe to sample a specified area, such as the floor, which is readily accessible to a child, or a window sill or window trough.[36] Windows are often more heavily contaminated than floors because exterior paints often contained higher concentrations of lead, and window troughs can act as reservoirs. Sampling house dust for lead is used to screen older housing units that may contain lead hazards at the time of purchase or rental and before occupancy; to conduct a full risk assessment that involves extensive sampling of settled dust in housing units that failed a lead hazard screen or where there is a high probability of a lead hazard;

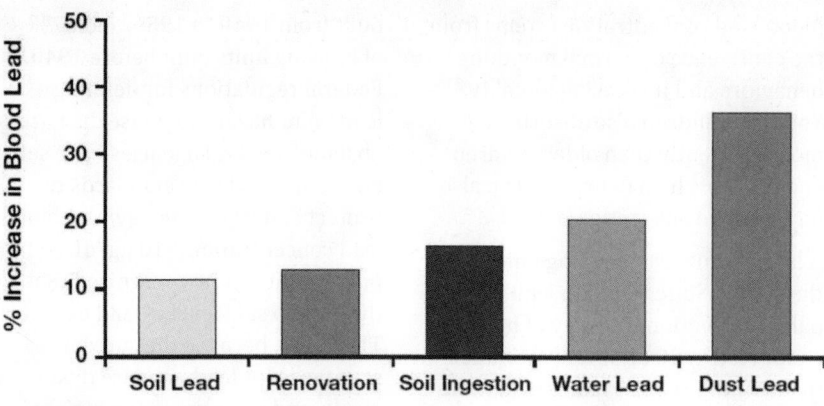

FIGURE 3
Contribution of lead exposure to children's blood lead concentrations. Adapted from Lanphear et al[31] and Spanier et al.[45]

TABLE 3 Common Sources of Lead Exposure

Source	Comment
House paint used before 1978 but especially before 1960	Deteriorated paint releases fine lead dust during home renovation.
Toys and furniture painted before 1976	
Painted toys made outside the United States	
Lead bullets, fishing sinkers, certain weights	Exposures often occur during practice in firing ranges.
Plumbing, pipes, and faucets	Lead leaches into drinking water when the pipes are connected with lead solder.
Soil contaminated by lead	Often in soil near highways and in yard of houses with exterior lead paint.
Hobbies involving soldering such as stained glass, jewelry making, pottery glazing, and miniature lead figures	Always check the labels.
Children's paint sets and art supplies	Always check the labels.
Pewter pitchers and ceramic dinner ware	
Storage batteries	
Parental occupation	Auto repair, mining, battery manufacture, pipe fitting and plumbing, welding, firing range use, ship building, painting, construction.
Folk remedies	Greta and Azarcon, Hispanic traditional medicines; Ghasard, an Indian folk medicine; and Ba-baw-saw, a Chinese herbal remedy, contain lead.
Cosmetics	Examples include Swad brand Sindoor, a cosmetic product used by traditional Hindus; Tiro, an eye cosmetic from Nigeria.
Candy from Mexico	Ingredient tamarind may contain lead.
Toy jewelry	A child died in 2006 after swallowing a metal heart charm that came with a purchase of shoes made by Reebok.

and to conduct clearance testing after repair or renovation of painted surfaces and after lead abatement, to verify that the housing unit is safe for occupancy (Table 3).[38]

Lead-contaminated soil is an important source of lead intake for children.[40,41] Lead-contaminated soil can directly contribute to children's blood lead concentrations via soil ingestion and indirectly from soil tracked indoors on shoes, which then contaminates house dust (Fig 3). Former mine and smelter communities present a particular risk to children for the ingestion of lead-contaminated soil, but lead in urban soil also is often heavily contaminated from the past use of leaded gasoline and paints. Other sources of lead in soil include weathering of lead-based exterior paint and nearby renovation or demolition activity. Soil testing is usually performed in areas where children play and the foundation perimeter. The EPA standards are 400 µg of lead per gram of soil for play areas and 1200 µg/g for the foundation perimeter.[37] Children's blood lead concentrations increase by approximately 3.8 µg/dL (38 ppb) for every 1000-ppm increase in soil lead concentration.[40]

Water is an important but often overlooked source of exposure for children, especially for infants who are formula fed.[5,46,47] Water typically contributes to approximately 20% of a child's blood lead concentrations if the water lead concentration exceeds 5 ppb (Fig 3).[31] The contribution of lead from water can be much higher for some children, especially for infants who ingest large quantities of tap water.[5,46,47] Children who reside in communities with lead service lines and inadequate anticorrosion control are also at increased risk for elevated blood lead concentrations.[48]

Phasing out leaded gasoline and creating stricter national air lead standards led to large reductions in the contribution of airborne lead to children's blood lead concentrations. Still, in some communities, such as those surrounding regional airports, airborne lead is an important source of lead exposure. Airborne lead is ingested primarily after it settles in house dust and soil where children play. Current sources of airborne lead include lead battery recycling operations, piston engine aircraft, and incinerators.[49] The contributions of airborne lead to children's blood lead concentrations are proportionately greater at the lower levels of exposure than at higher levels.[49]

Other sources of lead intake for children have been identified, such as nutritional supplements and folk medicines, ceramic dishware, and cosmetics[50–52] (Table 3).

Lead brought into the home from a worksite by a parent can also be a major source of exposure for some children.[53] Consumer products such as children's toys, lunch boxes, crayons, and lipstick that are contaminated with lead have received a great deal of attention. These products constitute a small source of lead intake for most children, but they can be the major source for an individual child. Moreover, because lead exposure is cumulative and there is no apparent threshold for the adverse effects of lead exposure, all sources of lead exposure should be eliminated. It is the responsibility of the relevant federal agencies, such as the CPSC and the Food and Drug Administration (FDA), to promulgate and enforce standards that will protect children from lead-contaminated consumer products.

RESIDENTIAL STANDARDS FOR LEAD IN PAINT, DUST, AND WATER

Lead in Paint and Dust

Under section 403 of Title X, the US Congress mandated the EPA to promulgate residential health-based lead standards that are designed to protect children from lead toxicity.[37] Standards are necessary to identify lead hazards before a child is unduly exposed and to identify the source of lead exposure for children who have blood lead concentrations ≥5 μg/dL (≥50 ppb).[31] Unless performed carefully, attempts to reduce lead exposure, such as abatement, repair, or renovation, can result in increased contamination and elevation in a child's blood lead concentration.[43–45] Dust clearance tests, which involve collecting dust from floors or windows of a home by using a lead-free material that resembles a baby wipe, should be conducted after extensive repair, renovation, or abatement of older housing units to determine whether the housing intervention was sufficient to protect

TABLE 4 Federal Standards for Lead in House Paint, House Dust, Soil, Water, Air, and Candy

Source	Standard
1. Lead-based paint (XRF)	1 μg/cm^2
2. Paint containing lead applied after August 14, 2009	90 ppm by wt
3. Testing (full risk assessment) for dust lead hazards (by wipe sampling)	
a. Floors	40 μg/ft^2
b. Interior window sills	200 μg/ft^2
4. Screening test for dust levels (by wipe sampling) to determine whether a full risk assessment is indicated	
a. Floors	25 μg/ft^2
b. Interior window sills	125 μg/ft^2
5. Dust lead clearance levels after abatement (by wipe sampling)	
a. Floors	40 μg/ft^2
b. Interior window sills	250 μg/ft^2
6. Bare residential soil	
a. Children's playground area	400 μg/g
b. Yard other than play area	1200 μg/g
7. Drinking water systems	
Exceeded if lead is above this concentration in >10% of a drinking water system's tap water samples	15 ppb (0.015 mg/L)
8. Candy likely to be consumed by small children	0.1 ppb
9. National Ambient Air Quality Standards: http://www.epa.gov/ttn/naaqs/standards/pb/s_pb_history.html	0.15 μg/m^3

Other state or local standards may vary, and the most protective standard applies. FDA has not set a standard for lead in cosmetics.
1–7, adapted from HUD.[36]
8, from FDA Guidance for Industry, November 2006.

children from lead hazards, especially in housing units built before 1960.[27,34] Property owners are required to disclose possible presence of lead-based paint in properties built before 1978 and are required to provide the blue pamphlet from the EPA, HUD, and Consumer Product Safety Commission titled "Protect Your Family From Lead in Your Home" at the time of rental or sale.

Most existing lead standards fail to protect children (Table 4). In 1978, the CPSC set the maximum paint lead concentration at 0.06% (600 ppm), because there was evidence that paint could be manufactured with this lower level of contamination.[3] Similarly, the EPA's action level of 15 ppb of lead in water, which is used to regulate water systems in the United States, is routinely (but erroneously) used as a health-based standard; it was not intended as a health-based standard, nor does it adequately protect children or pregnant women from adverse effects of lead exposure.[5,31] In 1988, the HUD established a postabatement floor dust standard of 200 μg/ft^2

because there was evidence that it was feasible to attain, not because it was demonstrated to be safe or protective. In 2001, the EPA promulgated residential lead standards of 40 μg/ft^2 for floors and 250 μg/ft^2 for window sills.[37] Unfortunately, these standards, which failed to protect children from having a blood lead concentration ≥10 μg/dL (≥100 ppb) when they were first promulgated, dictate the levels of lead contamination considered "normal" or "low," and they provide an illusion of safety.[38,40] At a floor standard of 40 μg/ft^2, the current EPA standard for floors, 50% of children were estimated to have a blood lead concentration ≥5 μg/dL (≥50 ppb); 5% of children have a blood lead concentration ≥5 μg/dL (≥50 ppb) at a median floor dust lead level of 1.5 μg/ft^2 (Fig 4).[42]

Scraping, sanding, or construction during painting, repair, renovation, or abatement of older housing can result in lead contamination of a child's environment.[41,43–45,54] In a controlled study of children with baseline blood lead concentrations

<22 μg/dL (<220 ppb), Aschengrau et al[41] reported a 6.5-μg/dL (65-ppb) *increase* in blood lead concentrations for children whose homes had undergone paint abatement. Clark et al[44] reported that 6-month-old infants were 11 times more likely to have a ≥5 μg/dL (≥50 ppb) increase in blood lead concentrations after abatement compared with older children. Spanier et al[45] reported that routine renovation of older housing was associated with a 12% higher mean blood lead concentration. These studies indicate that the levels of lead-contaminated dust generated by lead hazard control work or housing renovations can result in excessive lead exposure and absorption for children unless there is sufficient cleanup and clearance testing after the work is completed. The HUD has published technical guidelines and regulations for workers involved in lead-based paint abatement or remediation of housing.[36]

In 1992, the US Congress mandated the EPA to promulgate regulations to protect children from lead exposure resulting from housing repairs and renovation.[37] In 2011, the EPA finalized recommendations for the Lead Renovation, Repair and Painting Rule.[54] Unfortunately, the EPA failed to recommend the validated wipe-sampling method for clearance testing. Instead, it used an unvalidated cloth test, which should not be confused with the validated wipe sampling test. The white cloth test assumes that if dust is visible on a white cloth (ie, the "white glove test"), it contains a lead hazard; conversely, if there is no visible dust, it does not contain a lead hazard.[54] Although it would be valuable to have a quick test to identify the presence of a lead hazard, the white cloth test is not a validated tool and is not a reliable way to quantify the presence of a lead hazard.

Lead hazard control work can result in sizable reductions in the

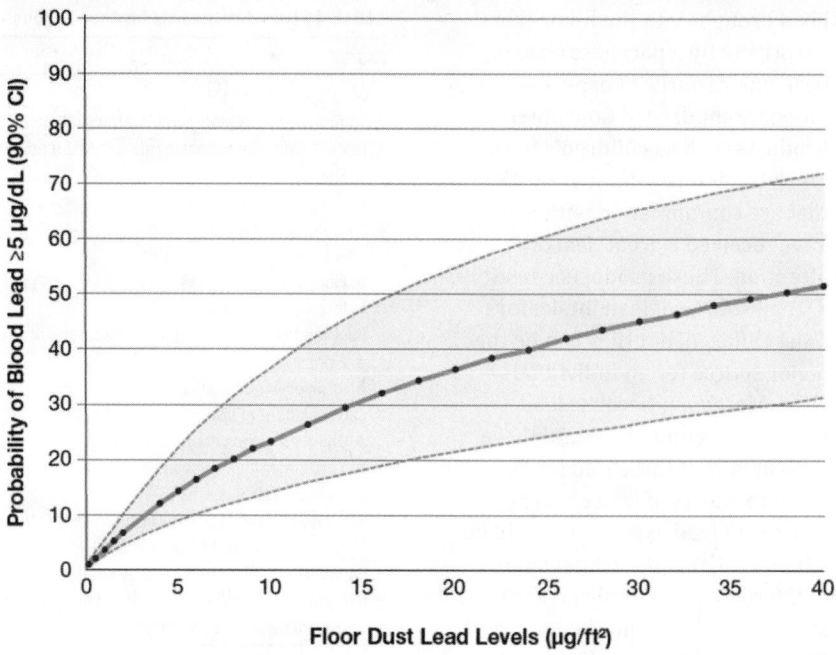

FIGURE 4
Estimated probability of blood lead concentrations ≥5 μg/dL for children living in pre-1978 housing by floor dust lead level, NHANES, 1999–2004. CI, confidence interval. Adapted from Dixon et al.[42]

magnitude of dust lead loading when proper procedures are followed and cleanup and postwork clearance testing are performed. In 1 study, dust lead levels (measured as micrograms of lead per area) immediately after professional abatement were 8.5 μg/ft², 8.0 μg/ft², and 21 μg/ft² for floors, interior window sills, and window troughs, respectively, representing reductions of more than 80% compared with preabatement levels.[55] In another study of more than 2600 housing units, postabatement dust lead levels were 12 μg/ft², 31 μg/ft², and 32 μg/ft² for floors, window sills and window troughs, respectively.[56] These levels were achieved with dust clearance testing set at 100 μg/ft² or higher, but floor dust lead levels below 5 μg/ft² can be achieved by following a specific protocol. In 1 unpublished study of more than 160 housing units built before 1978, 1 group found that it is possible to routinely meet floor lead levels below 5 μg/ft² after housing renovations costing an average of $5600

(B. Lanphear, MD, MPH, Simon Fraser University, unpublished data).

Lead in Water

The primary sources of lead in water, which can be dissolved or particulate, consist of lead service lines, lead solder, and brass fittings that contain high concentrations of lead.[5] Plumbing installed before 1986, the year a federal ban was issued on using lead pipe and lead solder and a maximum lead content of 8% by weight for brass plumbing was established, is more likely to contain higher concentrations of lead.[5] Lead services lines that are being replaced, are undergoing maintenance, or are damaged can release particles of lead that can be ingested.[57] Partial service line replacement, which is sometimes performed to minimize the cost of service line repair by water authorities, fails to reduce lead exposure.[57] Proper maintenance and ultimately full replacement of water service lines will be necessary to eliminate lead intake from water, but it must be performed with proper precautions. In the interim, water filters that are certified by the National Sanitation Foundation for lead removal can effectively reduce water lead concentrations. The EPA recommends running the cold water of residential units for up to 2 minutes to flush the lead leached from pipes out of the plumbing system, but flushing is useful only in housing units without lead service lines.[58-61] In housing units without lead service lines, and where the primary source is brass fittings or lead-soldered joints, a 1-minute flush may be sufficient, depending on the length of plumbing; for housing units with lead service lines, flushing may *increase* lead exposure, again depending on the length of the lead service lines.[58-61]

Drinking fountains in older schools can be an important source of lead exposure.[5] Unfortunately, there are no regulations for evaluating lead contamination of school drinking fountains in most states.

Implementation of the Lead and Copper Rule has significantly reduced tap water lead levels. In 1991, the US EPA set an action level for lead in water of 15 μg/L or (15 ppb).[6] Communities in which >10% of water samples taken from various taps throughout the system exceed 15 ppb are considered to be out of compliance and are required by the EPA to take action to reduce lead levels using corrosion control methods or replacement of lead service lines. The action level is used as an administrative tool to evaluate community-level exposure; it is not a health-based standard. The maximum contaminant level goal, the value the EPA deems acceptable for health, is 0.

Testing Asymptomatic Children for Elevated Blood Lead Concentrations

In the primary care office, primary prevention begins with education and counseling. Ideally, environmental assessments, such as screening older housing units, occurs before a child is born so that

parents can identify and hire trained workers to abate environmental lead exposure hazards.[12] It is especially important to conduct an environmental assessment for lead if a family resides in a housing unit built before 1960 that has undergone recent renovation, repair, or painting or if it is poorly maintained.

Screening questionnaires frequently used in the primary care setting fail to identify children who have elevated blood lead concentrations,[62] but they may be useful as a tool to identify lead hazards in children who have a blood lead concentration ≥5 μg/dL (≥50 ppb). In addition, public health agencies often use other methods of targeting children who should be screened with a blood lead test on the basis of community and residential characteristics, such as older housing. Blood lead surveillance data can be used to identify cities, communities, or housing units at higher than typical risk for lead poisoning. Technologies using geographic information system–based analyses and surveillance from electronic medical records are important tools to identify at-risk children who should have their blood lead concentration measured.

In 1991, the CDC recommended universal blood lead testing for all children.[63] In 2005, the AAP recommended that states and cities formulate their own lead screening recommendations on the basis of local data because of the wide variation in lead exposure.[7] The AAP, consistent with the CDC, recommended universal screening of children's blood for lead if they lived in communities with more than 27% of housing built before 1950 or a prevalence of blood lead concentrations ≥10 μg/dL in children 12 to 36 months old of 12% or greater.[7,12,63,64] Screening is not efficient after 36 months of age unless specific high-risk factors are identified; the likelihood of a child having a blood lead concentration >10 μg/dL after 36 months of age is low.[65] These recommendations now need to be

updated to conform to with our new understanding of lead toxicity.[11,12]

A detailed evaluation and follow-up of children who have blood lead concentrations <10 μg/dL (<100 ppb) is now indicated. Current federal regulations for clinical laboratory testing through the Clinical Laboratory Improvement Amendments of 1988[66] permit an allowable laboratory error in blood lead proficiency testing programs of ±4 μg/dL (±40 ppb) for blood lead concentrations ≤20 μg/dL (≤200 ppb). This range of error can result in children being misclassified and cause additional anxiety or false comfort when blood lead concentrations within the margin of error erroneously are interpreted as going up or down. The majority of laboratories analyzing blood lead reference materials routinely achieved laboratory error of ±2 μg/dL (±20 ppb) at blood lead concentrations ≤20 μg/dL (≤200 ppb).[67] Changing the allowable laboratory error to tighter performance requirements, such as ±2 μg/dL (±20 ppb), could decrease misclassification of children and lead to better allocation of health care resources.

Case Management of Children With a Blood Lead Concentration at or Above Reference Value

The AAP is adopting the current reference value of ≥5 μg/dL (≥50 ppb) for case management.[12] The CDC recommended that the 97.5th percentile of blood lead concentrations derived from the combination of the 2 most recent cycles of NHANES data be used to identify children who have unacceptably high exposure and to set public health goals.[12] The CDC will reconsider the reference value for children's blood lead concentrations every 4 years.[12]

After confirmatory testing, it is important to monitor children who have blood lead concentrations

TABLE 5 AAP Recommendations on Management of Childhood Lead Exposure and Poisoning

Lead Level	Recommendation
<5 µg/dL (<50 ppb)	1. Review laboratory results with family. For reference, the geometric mean blood lead concentration for US children 1–5 y old is <2 µg/dL (<20 ppb); 2.5% have a blood lead concentration ≥5 µg/dL (≥50 ppb).
	2. Repeat the blood lead concentration in 6–12 mo if the child is at high risk for lead exposure or if risk profile increases. Follow all local and state lead screening recommendations.
	3. For children initially screened before 12 mo of age, consider retesting in 3–6 mo for children at high risk; lead exposure may increase as mobility increases.
	4. Perform routine assessment of nutrition and physical and mental development and assess risk factors for iron deficiency.
	5. Provide anticipatory guidance about common sources of environmental lead exposure: paint in homes or child care facilities built before 1960, soil near roadways, take-home exposures related to adult occupations, and imported spices, cosmetics, folk remedies, and cookware.
5–14 µg/dL (50–140 ppb)	1. Perform steps as described above for blood lead concentrations <5 µg/dL (<50 ppb).
	2. Retest venous blood lead concentration within 1–3 mo to verify that the lead concentration is not rising. If it is stable or decreasing, retest the blood lead concentration in 3 mo. Refer patient to local health authorities if such resources are available. Most states require elevated blood lead concentrations be reported to the state health department. Contact the CDC at 800-CDC-INFO (800-232-4636) or www.cdc.gov/nceh/lead or the National Lead Information Center at 800-424-LEAD (5323) for resources regarding lead poisoning prevention and local childhood lead poisoning prevention programs.
	3. Take a careful environmental history to identify potential sources of exposures (see #5 above) and provide preliminary advice about reducing or eliminating exposures. Take care to consider other children who may be exposed.
	4. Provide nutritional counseling related to calcium and iron. Encourage the consumption of iron-enriched foods (eg, cereals, meats). Encourage families to sign up for the Special Supplemental Nutrition Program for Women, Infants, and Children, if eligible.
	5. Screen for iron sufficiency with adequate laboratory testing (complete blood cell count, ferritin, C-reactive protein) and provide treatment per AAP guidelines. Consider starting a multivitamin with iron.
	6. Perform structured developmental screening evaluations at child health maintenance visits, because lead's effect on development may manifest over years.
15–44 µg/dL (150–440 ppb)	1. Perform steps as described above for blood lead concentrations 5–14 µg/dL (50–140 ppb).
	2. Confirm the blood lead concentration with repeat venous sample within 1–4 wk.
	3. Abdominal radiography should be considered for children who have a history of pica for paint chips or excessive mouthing behaviors. Gut decontamination may be considered if leaded foreign bodies are visualized on radiography. Any treatment of blood lead concentrations in this range should be provided in consultation with an expert. Contact local pediatric environmental health specialty unit (www.pehsu.net or 888-347-2632) or local or regional Poison Control Center (www.aapcc.org or 800-222-1222) for guidance.
>44 µg/dL (>440 ppb)	1. Follow guidance for blood lead level 15–44 µg/dL (150–440 ppb) as listed above.
	2. Confirm the blood lead concentration with repeat venous lead level within 48 h.
	3. Consider hospitalization or chelation therapy (managed with the assistance of an experienced provider). Safety of the home or child care facility with respect to lead hazards, isolation of the lead source, family social situation, and chronicity of the exposure are factors that may influence management. Contact your regional pediatric environmental health specialty unit or Poison Control Center or the CDC for assistance.

Modified from Pediatric Environmental Health Specialty Unit. Medical Management of Childhood Lead Exposure and Poisoning (http://www.pehsu.net/_Library/facts/medical-mgmnt-childhood-lead-exposure-June-2013.pdf).

≥5 µg/dL (≥50 ppb). The pediatrician should inform the local or state health department and request an inspection of the child's house to identify and remediate any lead hazards (Table 4). Screening children for iron deficiency and insufficient dietary calcium intake is also important.[7] A detailed description of the diagnosis and treatment of significant lead toxicity (ie, ≥45 µg/dL [≥450 ppb]) is beyond the scope of this policy statement, but guidance is available in an earlier publication of the AAP[7] and through the Pediatric Environmental Health Specialty Units Web site (www.pehsu. net) (Table 5). Children who have elevated blood lead concentrations need to be monitored until environmental investigations and remediation are complete and blood lead concentrations decline.[12]

The AAP recognizes that environmental investigations will typically be conducted by local or state health or environmental departments to identify sources of lead exposure for a child who has a blood lead concentration ≥5 µg/dL (≥50 ppb). In many cases, however, the pediatrician can provide clues about possible sources of lead intake by taking a careful history.

Case management involves a thorough investigation of potential sources of lead poisoning in a child's environment, including paint, house dust, water, and soil. Case management also includes a questionnaire and visual inspection for other potential sources of lead exposure, including antique furniture, toys, ethnic folk remedies, and consumer products such as imported food, cosmetics, and ceramics.[12,50–52] It can include testing deteriorated paint on furniture, such as a crib, taking dust samples from child care settings or a family member's house, and taking soil samples from a child's play area.

SUMMARY AND RECOMMENDATIONS

Lead toxicity results in substantial, population-level effects on children's intellectual abilities, academic abilities, problem behaviors, and birth weight. Pediatricians may be well equipped to advocate for more stringent regulations to reduce sources of lead exposure and prevent childhood lead exposure. The AAP recognizes the importance of a variety of educational, enforcement, and environmental actions to reduce the number of children who are exposed to lead hazards and concur with recent detailed recommendations for prioritization of primary prevention of lead toxicity.[7,12,68–70] The AAP offers the following recommendations for government as well as pediatricians, other health care providers, and public health officials.

Recommendations for Government

1. The federal government should expand the resources currently offered by the HUD to local and state governments for lead hazard control work.

2. The federal government should provide both financial and nonfinancial resources and technical guidance through the CDC, the EPA, and the HUD to state and local public health agencies as well as environmental and housing agencies engaged in childhood lead poisoning prevention efforts.

3. The US EPA and HUD should review their protocols for identifying and mitigating residential lead hazards (eg, lead-based paint, dust, and soil) and lead-contaminated water from lead service lines or lead

solder and revise downward the allowable levels of lead in house dust, soil, paint, and water to conform with the recognition that there are no safe levels of lead.

4. The federal government should resume and expand its vital role in providing federal public health leadership in childhood lead poisoning prevention work through the CDC. Allocation of additional resources would be necessary to accomplish this goal.

5. The Centers for Medicare & Medicaid Services, which is responsible for regulating clinical laboratory testing through the Clinical Laboratory Improvement Amendments of 1988,[69] should expeditiously revise current regulations for allowable laboratory error permitted in blood lead proficiency testing programs from ± 4 µg/dL (± 40 ppb) to ± 2 µg/dL (± 20 ppb) for blood lead concentrations ≤ 20 µg/dL (≤ 200 ppb).[12] In the future, when feasible, allowable laboratory error permitted in blood lead proficiency testing programs should be reduced even more, to ± 1 µg/dL (± 10 ppb) for blood lead concentrations ≤ 20 µg/dL (≤ 200 ppb).

6. The federal government should continue to conduct the NHANES and provide national data on trends in blood lead concentrations. These newer data should be used by the CDC to periodically formulate a new reference value and guide clinical and public health interventions.

7. The federal government should continue to regularly survey children and adolescents in the NHANES for ADHD and conduct disorder by using validated diagnostic surveys from the

Diagnostic and Statistical Manual of Mental Disorders, Fifth Edition to examine the association of lower blood lead concentrations with these conditions.

8. Local or state governments, in consultation with pediatricians, should develop policies and regulations requiring the remediation of lead-contaminated housing and child care facilities, including the elimination of lead hazards during transfer of rental units or renovation or demolition of older housing.

9. State and local governments should collect, analyze, and publish blood lead test results performed in their jurisdictions and should regularly publish reports of age of housing and other risk factors for children having blood lead concentrations ≥ 5 µg/dL (≥ 50 ppb). These reports should be readily available to pediatricians, health care providers, and the public.

10. Federal, state, and local governments should provide resources for environmental evaluations and case management of children who have blood lead concentrations ≥ 5 µg/dL (≥ 50 ppb), in conjunction with the child's primary care provider.

11. State and local governments should take steps to ensure that water fountains in schools do not exceed water lead concentrations of 1 ppb.

Recommendations for Pediatricians, Health Care Providers, and Public Health Officials

1. Pediatricians are in a unique position to work with public health officials to conduct surveys of blood lead concentrations among a randomly selected,

representative sample of children in their states or communities at regular intervals to identify trends in blood lead concentrations. These periodic surveys are especially important for children who live in highly contaminated communities, such as smelter communities or regions with a historically high prevalence of lead exposure.

2. Pediatricians, heath care providers, and public health officials should routinely recommend individual environmental assessments of older housing,[12] particularly if a family resides in a housing unit built before 1960 that has undergone recent renovation, repair, or painting or that has been poorly maintained.

3. Pediatricians and public health officials should advocate for the promulgation and enforcement of strict legal standards based on empirical data that regulate allowable levels of lead in air, water, soil, house dust, and consumer products. These standards should address the major sources of lead exposure, including industrial emissions, lead paint in older housing, lead-contaminated soil, water service lines, and consumer products.

4. Pediatricians should be familiar with collection and interpretation of reports of lead hazards found in house dust, soil, paint, and water, or they should be able to refer families to a pediatrician, health care provider, or specialist who is familiar with these tools.

5. Pediatricians, women's health care providers, and public health officials should be familiar with federal, state, local, and professional recommendations or requirements for screening children and pregnant women for lead poisoning.[12,68,69]

6. Pediatricians and other primary care providers should test asymptomatic children for elevated blood lead concentrations according to federal, local, and state requirements. Immigrant, refugee, and internationally adopted children also should be tested for blood lead concentrations when they arrive in the United States because of their increased risk.[71,72] Blood lead tests do not need to be duplicated, but the pediatrician or other primary care provider should <u>attempt to verify</u> that screening was performed elsewhere and determine the result before testing is deferred during the office visit.

7. Pediatricians and other primary care health providers should conduct targeted screening of children for elevated blood lead concentrations if they are 12 to 24 months of age and live in communities or census block groups with $\geq 25\%$ of housing built before 1960 or a prevalence of children's blood lead concentrations ≥ 5 µg/dL (≥ 50 ppb) of $\geq 5\%$.

8. Pediatricians and other primary care providers should test children for elevated blood lead concentrations if they live in or visit a home or child care facility with an identified lead hazard or a home built before 1960 that is in poor repair or was renovated in the past 6 months.[7,12]

9. Pediatricians and primary care providers should work with their federal, state, and local governments to ensure that a comprehensive environmental inspection is conducted in the housing units of children who have blood lead concentrations ≥ 5 µg/dL (≥ 50 ppb) and that they receive appropriate case management.

LEAD AUTHOR

Bruce Perrin Lanphear, MD, MPH, FAAP

COUNCIL ON ENVIRONMENTAL HEALTH EXECUTIVE COMMITTEE, 2015–2016

Jennifer A. Lowry, MD, FAAP, Chairperson
Samantha Ahdoot, MD, FAAP
Carl R. Baum, MD, FACMT, FAAP
Aaron S. Bernstein, MD, MPH, FAAP
Aparna Bole, MD, FAAP
Heather Lynn Brumberg, MD, MPH, FAAP
Carla C. Campbell, MD, MS, FAAP
Bruce Perrin Lanphear, MD, MPH, FAAP
Susan E. Pacheco, MD, FAAP
Adam J. Spanier, MD, PhD, MPH, FAAP
Leonardo Trasande, MD, MPP, FAAP

FORMER EXECUTIVE COMMITTEE MEMBERS

Kevin C. Osterhoudt, MD, MSCE, FAAP
Jerome A. Paulson, MD, FAAP
Megan T. Sandel, MD, MPH, FAAP

CONTRIBUTOR

Paul Thomas Rogers, MD, FAAP

LIAISONS

John M. Balbus, MD, MPH – *National Institute of Environmental Health Sciences*
Todd A. Brubaker, DO – *Section on Medical Students, Residents, and Fellowship Trainees*
Nathaniel G. DeNicola, MD, MSc – *American College of Obstetricians and Gynecologists*
Ruth Ann Etzel, MD, PhD, FAAP – *US Environmental Protection Agency*
Mary Ellen Mortensen, MD, MS – *CDC/National Center for Environmental Health*
Mary H. Ward, PhD – *National Cancer Institute*

STAFF

Paul Spire

ABBREVIATIONS

AAP: American Academy of Pediatrics
ADHD: attention-deficit/ hyperactivity disorder
CDC: Centers for Disease Control and Prevention
CPSC: Consumer Product Safety Commission
EPA: Environmental Protection Agency
FDA: US Food and Drug Administration
HUD: Department of Housing and Urban Development
NHANES: National Health and Nutrition Examination Survey
XRF: x-ray fluorescence

REFERENCES

1. Brown MJ, Margolis S; Centers for Disease Control and Prevention. Lead in drinking water and human blood lead levels in the United States. *MMWR Suppl.* 2012;61(4 suppl 1):1–9

2. Annest JL, Pirkle JL, Makuc D, Neese JW, Bayse DD, Kovar MG. Chronological trend in blood lead levels between 1976 and 1980. *N Engl J Med.* 1983;308(23):1373–1377

3. Committee on Toxicology, Assembly of Life Sciences, National Research Council. Recommendations for the prevention of lead poisoning in children. *Nutr Rev.* 1976;34(11):321–327

4. Consumer Product Safety Commission. Final rule. Children's products containing lead; determinations regarding lead content limits on certain materials or products. *Fed Regist.* 2009;74(164):43031–43042 Available at: https://www.cpsc.gov/PageFiles/77828/leadcontent.txt. Accessed January 14, 2016

5. Triantafyllidou S, Edwards M. Lead (Pb) in tap water and in blood: implications for lead exposure in the United States. *Crit Rev Environ Sci Technol.* 2012;42(13):1297–1352

6. US Environmental Protection Agency. Drinking water regulations: maximum contaminant level goals and national primary drinking water regulations for lead and copper; Final Rule. *Fed Regist.* 1991;56(11):26460–26564

7. American Academy of Pediatrics Committee on Environmental Health. Lead exposure in children: prevention, detection, and management. *Pediatrics.* 2005;116(4):1036–1046

8. Yeoh B, Woolfenden S, Lanphear B, Ridley GF, Livingstone N. Household interventions for preventing domestic lead exposure in children. *Cochrane Database Syst Rev.* 2012;4(4):CD006047

9. Rico JA, Kordas K, López P, et al. Efficacy of iron and/or zinc supplementation on cognitive performance of lead-exposed Mexican schoolchildren: a randomized, placebo-controlled trial. *Pediatrics.* 2006;117(3). Available at: www.pediatrics.org/cgi/content/full/117/3/e518

10. Sargent JD, Dalton MA, O'Connor GT, Olmstead EM, Klein RZ. Randomized trial of calcium glycerophosphate–supplemented infant formula to prevent lead absorption. *Am J Clin Nutr.* 1999;69(6):1224–1230

11. National Toxicology Program. *Monograph on Health Effects of Low-Level Lead.* Research Triangle Park, NC: National Institute of Environmental Health Sciences; 2012:xiii, xv–148

12. Centers for Disease Control and Prevention, Advisory Committee on Childhood Lead Poisoning Prevention. *Low Level Lead Exposure Harms Children: A Renewed Call for Primary Prevention.* Atlanta, GA: Centers for Disease Control and Prevention; 2012. Available at: www.cdc.gov/nceh/lead/ACCLPP/Final_Document_030712.pdf. Accessed January 14, 2016

13. Lanphear BP, Dietrich K, Auinger P, Cox C. Cognitive deficits associated with blood lead concentrations <10 microg/dL in US children and adolescents. *Public Health Rep.* 2000;115(6):521–529

14. Lanphear BP, Hornung R, Khoury J, et al. Low-level environmental lead exposure and children's intellectual function: an international pooled analysis. *Environ Health Perspect.* 2005;113(7):894–899

15. Bellinger DC. A strategy for comparing the contributions of environmental chemicals and other risk factors to neurodevelopment of children. *Environ Health Perspect.* 2012;120(4):501–507

16. Needleman HL, Riess JA, Tobin MJ, Biesecker GE, Greenhouse JB. Bone lead levels and delinquent behavior. *JAMA.* 1996;275(5):363–369

17. Froehlich TE, Lanphear BP, Auinger P, et al. The association of tobacco and lead exposure with attention-deficit/hyperactivity disorder. *Pediatrics.* 2009;124(6). Available at: www.pediatrics.org/cgi/content/full/124/6/e1054

18. Nigg JT, Knottnerus GM, Martel MM, et al. Low blood lead levels associated with clinically diagnosed attention-deficit/hyperactivity disorder and mediated by weak cognitive control. *Biol Psychiatry.* 2008;63(3):325–331

19. Dietrich KN, Ris MD, Succop PA, Berger OG, Bornschein RL. Early exposure to lead and juvenile delinquency. *Neurotoxicol Teratol.* 2001;23(6):511–518

20. Wright JP, Dietrich KN, Ris MD, et al. Association of prenatal and childhood blood lead concentrations with criminal arrests in early adulthood. *PLoS Med.* 2008;5(5):e101

21. Fergusson DM, Boden JM, Horwood LJ. Dentine lead levels in childhood and criminal behaviour in late adolescence and early adulthood. *J Epidemiol Community Health.* 2008;62(12):1045–1050

22. Marcus DK, Fulton JJ, Clarke EJ. Lead and conduct problems: a meta-analysis. *J Clin Child Adolesc Psychol.* 2010;39(2):234–241

23. Reyes JW. Environmental policy as social policy? The impact of childhood lead exposure on crime. *BE J Econ Anal Policy.* 2007;7(1):1–41

24. Fadrowski JJ, Navas-Acien A, Tellez-Plaza M, Guallar E, Weaver VM, Furth SL. Blood lead level and kidney function in US adolescents: the Third National Health and Nutrition Examination Survey. *Arch Intern Med.* 2010;170(1):75–82

25. Borja-Aburto VH, Hertz-Picciotto I, Rojas Lopez M, Farias P, Rios C, Blanco J. Blood lead levels measured prospectively and risk of spontaneous abortion. *Am J Epidemiol.* 1999;150(6):590–597

26. Zhu M, Fitzgerald EF, Gelberg KH, Lin S, Druschel CM. Maternal low-level lead exposure and fetal growth. *Environ Health Perspect.* 2010;118(10):1471–1475

27. Jones RL, Homa DM, Meyer PA, et al. Trends in blood lead levels and blood lead testing among US children aged 1 to 5 years, 1988–2004. *Pediatrics.* 2009;123(3). Available at: www.pediatrics.org/cgi/content/full/123/3/e376

28. Dietrich KN, Ware JH, Salganik M, et al; Treatment of Lead-Exposed Children Clinical Trial Group. Effect of chelation therapy on the neuropsychological and behavioral development of lead-exposed children after school entry. *Pediatrics.* 2004;114(1):19–26

29. Trasande L, Liu Y. Reducing the staggering costs of environmental disease in children, estimated at $76.6 billion in 2008. *Health Aff (Millwood)*. 2011;30(5):863–870

30. Gould E. Childhood lead poisoning: conservative estimates of the social and economic benefits of lead hazard control. *Environ Health Perspect*. 2009;117(7):1162–1167

31. Lanphear BP, Hornung R, Ho M, Howard CR, Eberly S, Knauf K. Environmental lead exposure during early childhood [published correction appears in *J Pediatr*. 2002;140(4):490]. *J Pediatr*. 2002;140(1):40–47

32. Ziegler EE, Edwards BB, Jensen RL, Mahaffey KR, Fomon SJ. Absorption and retention of lead by infants. *Pediatr Res*. 1978;12(1):29–34

33. Wright RO, Shannon MW, Wright RJ, Hu H. Association between iron deficiency and low-level lead poisoning in an urban primary care clinic. *Am J Public Health*. 1999;89(7):1049–1053

34. US Department of Health and Human Services. *American Healthy Homes Survey. Lead and Arsenic Findings. Office of Healthy Homes and Lead Hazard Controls*. Washington, DC: US Department of Health and Human Services; 2011

35. Clark CS, Bornschein RL, Succop P, Que Hee SS, Hammond PB, Peace B. Condition and type of housing as an indicator of potential environmental lead exposure and pediatric blood lead levels. *Environ Res*. 1985;38(1):46–53

36. US Department of Housing and Urban Development. *Guidelines for the Evaluation and Control of Lead-Based Paint Hazards in Housing*. 2nd ed. Washington, DC: US Department of Housing and Urban Development; 2012

37. US Environmental Protection Agency. 40 CFR part 745. Lead; identification of dangerous levels of lead: final rule. *Fed Regist*. 2001;66(4):1206–1240

38. Lanphear BP. The paradox of lead poisoning prevention. *Science*. 1998;281(5383):1617–1618

39. Sayre JW, Charney E, Vostal J, Pless IB. House and hand dust as a potential source of childhood lead exposure. *Am J Dis Child*. 1974;127(2):167–170

40. Lanphear BP, Matte TD, Rogers J, et al. The contribution of lead-contaminated house dust and residential soil to children's blood lead levels. A pooled analysis of 12 epidemiologic studies. *Environ Res*. 1998;79(1):51–68

41. Aschengrau A, Beiser A, Bellinger D, Copenhafer D, Weitzman M. Residential lead-based-paint hazard remediation and soil lead abatement: their impact among children with mildly elevated blood lead levels. *Am J Public Health*. 1997;87(10):1698–1702

42. Dixon SL, Gaitens JM, Jacobs DE, et al. Exposure of US children to residential dust lead, 1999–2004: II. The contribution of lead-contaminated dust to children's blood lead levels. *Environ Health Perspect*. 2009;117(3):468–474

43. Amitai Y, Brown MJ, Graef JW, Cosgrove E. Residential deleading: effects on the blood lead levels of lead-poisoned children. *Pediatrics*. 1991;88(5):893–897

44. Clark S, Grote J, Wilson J, et al. Occurrence and determinants of increases in blood lead levels in children shortly after lead hazard control activities. *Environ Res*. 2004;96(2):196–205

45. Spanier AJ, Wilson S, Ho M, Hornung R, Lanphear BP. The contribution of housing renovation to children's blood lead levels: a cohort study. *Environ Health*. 2013;12:72

46. Shannon M, Graef JW. Lead intoxication from lead-contaminated water used to reconstitute infant formula. *Clin Pediatr (Phila)*. 1989;28(8):380–382

47. Edwards M, Triantafyllidou S, Best D. Elevated blood lead in young children due to lead-contaminated drinking water: Washington, DC, 2001–2004. *Environ Sci Technol*. 2009;43(5):1618–1623

48. Hanna-Attisha M, LaChance J, Sadler RC, Champney Schnepp A. Elevated blood lead levels in children associated with the Flint drinking water crisis: a spatial analysis of risk and public health response. *Am J Public Health*. 2016;106(2):283–290

49. Richmond-Bryant J, Meng Q, Davis A, et al. The influence of declining air lead levels on blood lead–air lead slope

factors in children. *Environ Health Perspect*. 2014;122(7):754–760

50. Levin R, Brown MJ, Kashtock ME, et al. Lead exposures in U.S. children, 2008: implications for prevention. *Environ Health Perspect*. 2008;116(10):1285–1293

51. Centers for Disease Control and Prevention (CDC). Lead poisoning in pregnant women who used Ayurvedic medications from India: New York City, 2011–2012. *MMWR Morb Mortal Wkly Rep*. 2012;61(33):641–646

52. Gorospe EC, Gerstenberger SL. Atypical sources of childhood lead poisoning in the United States: a systematic review from 1966–2006. *Clin Toxicol (Phila)*. 2008;46(8):728–737

53. Roscoe RJ, Gittleman JL, Deddens JA, Petersen MR, Halperin WE. Blood lead levels among children of lead-exposed workers: a meta-analysis. *Am J Ind Med*. 1999;36(4):475–481

54. US Environmental Protection Agency. 40 CFR part 745. Lead; Clearance and clearance testing requirements for the renovation, repair and painting program. *Fed Regist*. 2010;75(87):25037–25073

55. Farfel MR, Rohde C, Lees PSJ, Rooney B, Bannon DL, Derbyshire W. *Lead-Based Paint Abatement and Repair and Maintenance Study in Baltimore: Findings Based on Two Years of Follow-Up*. Washington, DC: US Environmental Protection Agency; 1998

56. Galke W, Clark S, Wilson J, et al. Evaluation of the HUD lead hazard control grant program: early overall findings. *Environ Res*. 2001;86(2):149–156

57. Del Toral MA, Porter A, Schock MR. Detection and evaluation of elevated lead release from service lines: a field study. *Environ Sci Technol*. 2013;47(16):9300–9307

58. Schock MR. Causes of temporal variability of lead in domestic plumbing systems. *Environ Monit Assess*. 1990;15(1):59–82

59. Schock MR, Lemieux FG. Challenges in addressing variability of lead in domestic plumbing. *Water Science & Technology: Water Supply*. 2010;10(5):792–798

60. Schock MR, Lytle DA. *Water Quality and Treatment: A Handbook of Community Water Supplies.* 6th ed. New York, NY: McGraw-Hill Inc; 2011

61. Schock MR, Sandvig AM, Lemieux FG, DeSantis MK. Diagnostic sampling to reveal hidden lead and copper health risks. Presented at the *15th Canadian National Conference and 6th Policy Forum on Drinking Water,* Kelowna, BC; October 21–24, 2012

62. Ossiander EM. A systematic review of screening questionnaires for childhood lead poisoning. *J Public Health Manag Pract.* 2013;19(1):E21–E29

63. Centers for Disease Control. *Preventing Lead Poisoning in Young Children: A Statement by the Centers for Disease Control and Prevention.* Atlanta, GA: US Department of Health and Human Services; 1991

64. Centers for Disease Control and Prevention. *Screening Young Children for Lead Poisoning: Guidance for State and Local Public Health Officials.* Atlanta, GA: Centers for Disease Control and Prevention; 1997

65. Karp R, Abramson J, Clark-Golden M, et al. Should we screen for lead poisoning after 36 months of age? Experience in the inner city. *Ambul Pediatr.* 2001;1(5):256–258

66. Clinical Laboratory Improvement Amendments of 1988. Pub L No. 100-578, 102 Stat 2903, 10 USC §263a (1988)

67. Parsons PJ, Geraghty C, Verostek MF. An assessment of contemporary atomic spectroscopic techniques for the determination of lead in blood and urine matrices. *Spect Act B.* 2001;56(9):1593–1604

68. Centers for Disease Control and Prevention. *Guidelines for the Identification and Management of Lead Exposure in Pregnant and Lactating Women.* Atlanta, GA: Centers for Disease Control and Prevention; 2010

69. American College of Obstetricians and Gynecologists. Committee opinion no. 533. Lead screening during pregnancy and lactation. *Obstet Gynecol.* 2012;120(2 Pt 1):416–420

70. Centers for Disease Control and Prevention. *Preventing Lead Exposure in Young Children: A Housing-Based Approach to Primary Prevention of Lead Poisoning.* Atlanta, GA: Centers for Disease Control and Prevention; 2004

71. Geltman PL, Brown MJ, Cochran J. Lead poisoning among refugee children resettled in Massachusetts, 1995 to 1999. *Pediatrics.* 2001;108(1):158–162

72. Centers for Disease Control and Prevention (CDC). Elevated blood lead levels among internationally adopted children: United States, 1998. *MMWR Morb Mortal Wkly Rep.* 2000;49(5):97–100

Recognition and Management of Medical Complexity

- *Clinical Report*

CLINICAL REPORT   Guidance for the Clinician in Rendering Pediatric Care

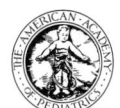

American Academy
of Pediatrics
DEDICATED TO THE HEALTH OF ALL CHILDREN™

Recognition and Management of Medical Complexity

Dennis Z. Kuo, MD, MHS, FAAP, Amy J. Houtrow, MD, PhD, MPH, FAAP, COUNCIL ON CHILDREN WITH DISABILITIES

abstract

Children with medical complexity have extensive needs for health services, experience functional limitations, and are high resource utilizers. Addressing the needs of this population to achieve high-value health care requires optimizing care within the medical home and medical neighborhood. Opportunities exist for health care providers, payers, and policy makers to develop strategies to enhance care delivery and to decrease costs. Important outcomes include decreasing unplanned hospital admissions, decreasing emergency department use, ensuring access to health services, limiting out-of-pocket expenses for families, and improving patient and family experiences, quality of life, and satisfaction with care. This report describes the population of children with medical complexity and provides strategies to optimize medical and health outcomes.

Clinical reports from the American Academy of Pediatrics benefit from expertise and resources of liaisons and internal (AAP) and external reviewers. However, clinical reports from the American Academy of Pediatrics may not reflect the views of the liaisons or the organizations or government agencies that they represent.

The guidance in this report does not indicate an exclusive course of treatment or serve as a standard of medical care. Variations, taking into account individual circumstances, may be appropriate.

All clinical reports from the American Academy of Pediatrics automatically expire 5 years after publication unless reaffirmed, revised, or retired at or before that time.

DOI: 10.1542/peds.2016-3021

PEDIATRICS (ISSN Numbers: Print, 0031-4005; Online, 1098-4275).

Copyright © 2016 by the American Academy of Pediatrics

FINANCIAL DISCLOSURE: The authors have indicated they do not have a financial relationship relevant to this article to disclose.

FUNDED: No external funding.

POTENTIAL CONFLICT OF INTEREST: The authors have indicated they have no potential conflicts of interest to disclose.

To cite: Kuo DZ, Houtrow AJ, AAP COUNCIL ON CHILDREN WITH DISABILITIES. Recognition and Management of Medical Complexity. *Pediatrics.* 2016;138(6):e20163021

INTRODUCTION

Children with medical complexity (CMC), who may also be known as "complex chronic"[1] or "medically complex,"[2] have multiple significant chronic health problems that affect multiple organ systems and result in functional limitations, high health care need or utilization, and often the need for or use of medical technology.[3,4] An example of a child with medical complexity is one with a genetic syndrome with an associated congenital heart defect, difficulty with swallowing, cerebral palsy, and a urologic condition. This child would typically require the care of a primary care physician; multiple pediatric medical subspecialists or pediatric surgical specialists, home nurses, and rehabilitative and habilitative therapists; community-based services; extensive pharmaceutical therapies; special attention to his or her nutritional needs and growth; and durable medical equipment to maintain health, maximize development, and promote function.[3]

Children and youth with special health care needs (CYSHCN), who require health and related services for a chronic physical, developmental, behavioral, or emotional condition beyond what is typically required for children,[5] have long been designated as a priority population of interest for health care policy.[6] CMC, a subset of CYSHCN because of their extensive and costly health care use, are increasingly recognized as requiring additional and specific consideration from physicians, payers, and policy makers. Approximately 1% of children, most of whom are CMC, account for up to one-third of overall health care spending for children,[7-9] an increasing percentage of pediatric hospitalizations,[10-12] and recurrent hospital admissions.[13] Evidence suggests that CMC have among the highest risk of all children for adverse medical, developmental, psychosocial, and family outcomes.[14]

The Department of Health and Human Services issued the "Strategic Framework on Multiple Chronic Conditions" in 2010,[15] emphasizing health systems change, empowering individuals, equipping clinicians with best practices, and enhancing research. In the adult health care system, selected actions include the formation of new integrated care models, clinical practice guidelines, education and training initiatives, and additional funding mechanisms for patient-centered outcomes research focusing on multiple chronic conditions.[16] Optimal care of CMC should be similarly framed, with the medical home as the foundation of an integrated care system. Most important, acknowledging and incorporating the life experiences of children, youth, and their families into the framework of understanding complexity strengthen its applicability and center the discussion on the child instead of the health care system that serves the child.

In this report, suggestions are provided for physicians, payers, and policy makers to address the growing population of CMC. The overarching goals for optimal health care for CMC are to (1) maximize health, function, development, and family functioning through coordinated patient- and family-centered care

(PFCC) and (2) provide proactive, rather than reactive, care so that critical medical and health events are averted to the extent possible. The prospective identification of CMC, proper and timely management of health care delivery, supports for self-management, and appropriate resource allocation are necessary to achieve a coordinated health care system that provides better health care, smarter use of health care dollars, higher family satisfaction, and healthier CMC.[17]

RECOGNIZING MEDICAL COMPLEXITY

Medical complexity is conceptually regarded as a combination of multiorgan system involvement from chronic health condition(s), functional limitations, ongoing use of medical technology, and high resource need/use.[3,18] However, different constructs of complexity may exist at the individual as well as the population level, which makes consistent and reliable recognition of complexity difficult. Clinicians may subjectively identify complexity on the basis of consequences of medical and/or behavioral conditions, social context, or family stressors that influence health, relevant items that may not be available in population-level data sources.[19] Because no consensus yet exists on recognizing complexity on the population level, multiple tools, such as a diagnosis classification scheme and a questionnaire, may be needed to recognize the multiple attributes of complexity.[19] Limiting the construct of complexity to high health care resource use or multiple diagnosed medical conditions that are easily identified through administrative records, without considering associated social or functional issues, may hamper the development of resources and policies needed to address complexity. In addition, such an approach does not embrace PFCC principles of incorporating

the preferences, experiences, and psychosocial needs of the family.

CMC have functional limitations, specifically, limitations in their ability to do the things typically developing children of the same age can do in their day-to-day lives. The limitations experienced may be temporary or may result in permanent disability. Functional limitations are best understood by using the framework of the World Health Organization's *International Classification of Functioning, Disability, and Health* (ICF).[20] According to the ICF framework, when a specific body system or body part's functioning is affected, the person has an impairment; when the person's total functioning is affected such that he or she has difficulty or is unable to perform tasks (eg, walking and dressing), the person has an activity limitation; and when the person is unable to fully engage in life events, he or she has a participation restriction.[20,21] For example, CMC who are unable to attend school because of their health have participation restrictions. The experience of functional limitations (or in ICF language, disability) goes beyond health status and results from the interaction of specific health conditions with environmental and personal contextual factors, such as health service use, aspects of the home and community environments, and access to resources.[21,22] Understanding the needs of CMC includes the consideration of such contextual factors.

CMC often rely on medical technology and/or ongoing supportive services for their health and well-being. This reliance on supportive care for vital functioning is why CMC, as a group, are sometimes referred to as medically fragile. The term "medically fragile" refers to continual needs for skilled services that support basic life functions necessary for survival.[23,24] When designating complexity, it is important to recognize that parents and extended family members often shoulder much of the responsibility for providing such skilled care because of the round-the-clock health care needs and limited resources from the health care financing system to support in-home services.[25] "Technology dependence" usually means that the child requires technology to compensate for the loss of a vital body function.[26] Examples of technologies include supplemental oxygen, ventilators, dialysis machines, and gastrostomy tubes. A child might also be "technology assisted" if he or she uses augmentative communication or assistive devices (eg, a wheelchair for mobility) that compensate for lost functions that are not essential for survival. "Technology assisted," as opposed to "technology dependent," is a more inclusive term and highlights the value of these technologies to help children function optimally in their day-to-day lives. The presence of either medical fragility or technology dependency/assistance alone does not constitute complexity, but both can be important components of complexity.

PFCC AS THE FOUNDATION OF THE HEALTH CARE SYSTEM

PFCC is a fundamental component of a high-performing, coordinated health care system.[27] Given the intersection of family-identified needs, child functioning, and the framework of medical complexity, PFCC should be the foundation of the health care system for CMC. With PFCC, the family is understood to be the child's primary strength and support,[28] and families are full and equal partners in shared decision-making.[29] PFCC has the potential to raise patient satisfaction and streamline care.[30] However, operationalizing PFCC in health care is frequently misinterpreted as patient education, patient engagement, or delegating excess responsibility and decision-making

to families.[29] The effective delivery of PFCC may require a shift in culture from the traditional physician-patient paradigm, leading to a collaborative partnership with shared decision-making that directly addresses family needs. In fact, such a shift has begun to take place. Ensuring that each person and family are engaged as partners in the care of CMC is 1 of 6 priorities on which the National Quality Strategy is focusing to improve health and health care quality.[27,31]

Families of CMC describe the need for effective and timely medical care, assistance with care coordination among multiple providers to improve communication between providers, decreasing duplicative services and the need for unnecessary travel and appointments, the support of multiple community-based therapists, improved access to specialized community services, and assistance with significant financial and psychological burdens. Families know how complex their circumstances are, as articulated in the care map drawn by the mother of a child with medical complexity in Fig 1. Families also report feeling abandoned by providers with the expectation that they must navigate the health care delivery system by themselves, which many families perceive to be unrealistic.[32–34] Caregivers of CMC report a median of 2 hours per week providing care coordination and >11 hours a week providing direct home care.[4] Families report having to simultaneously manage the technical aspects of care, the additional parenting responsibilities, and the challenges of navigating the maze of health care services, all while having to juggle competing family needs.[34]

The numerous and complex medical care services that CMC require lead to the highest unmet family-reported needs of all children, with nearly 50% of families reporting at least 1 unmet need.[4, 35–38] Commonly reported

unmet needs include limited access to medical subspecialty, dental, and mental health care providers and a lack of help navigating the care system.[32,39–43] More than half of families of CMC report having to stop working for pay, and 57% report having financial problems.[4] In addition, 39.4% report being very dissatisfied with medical services.[4] For CYSHCN in general, physicians already routinely underestimate the family needs for community referrals, access to care, psychological services, respite, and interpersonal communication[44–46]; the situation is likely much worse for CMC.

THE MEDICAL HOME CONCEPT AS THE FOUNDATION FOR CARE OF CMC

The medical home, whose foundation lies in community-based care for CYSHCN, serves as the standard of care for all children, including CMC.[47] In 2002, the American Academy of Pediatrics reiterated that the medical home ensures that care is accessible, family centered, continuous, comprehensive, coordinated, compassionate, and culturally effective.[48] In 2007, multiple medical societies affirmed the principles of the patient-centered medical home (PCMH). The PCMH Joint Principles state that the PCMH is "an approach to providing comprehensive primary care for children, youth and adults" and emphasize the importance of quality, safety, and appropriate payments at the practice level. The PCMH has become a cornerstone for health care payment reforms within the Affordable Care Act by establishing financial incentives for expanded primary care–based services.[49]

Effective care for CMC requires a comprehensive level of care that is seamless, accessible, and integrated for the child and family, with the medical home as the foundation. A comprehensive approach to care within a medical home may benefit

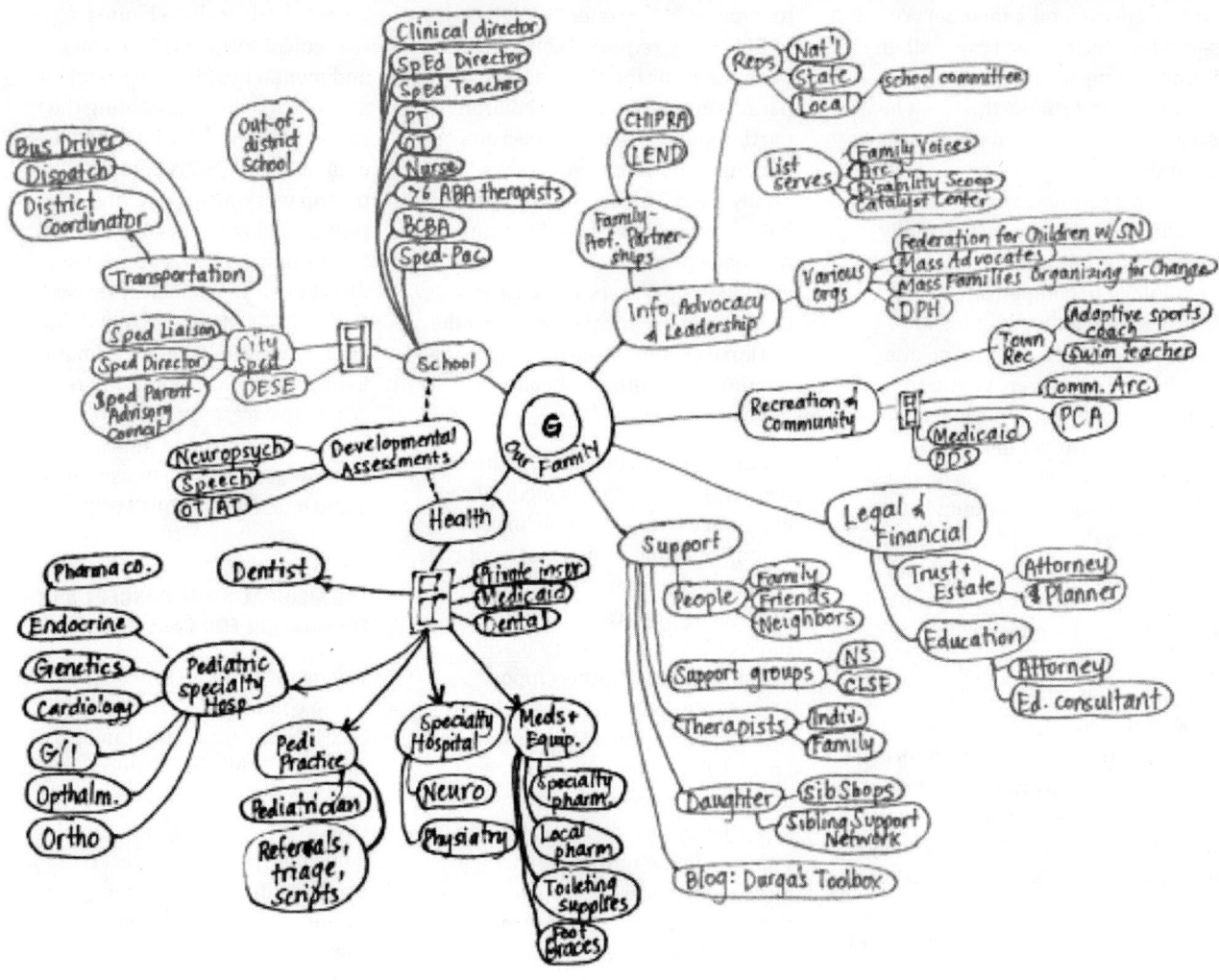

FIGURE 1
Care map created by the mother of a child with medical complexity to pictorially represent aspects of her child's life. Reprinted with permission by Cristin Lind.

CMC who have more severe needs compared with those who have less severe needs[50] but also may be harder to achieve. The medical home also is only 1 key component of care within a larger system of care for CMC.[51,52] Extensive health care needs of CMC have led to calls for a "medical neighborhood" (or "health neighborhood") with service integration, through cooperative agreements, among health care providers.[53] The medical neighborhood is built on the "collaborative care agreement," which is a comanagement agreement that delineates roles and expectations for a child's health care across disciplines. The

medical neighborhood conceptually links the primary care setting with community-based services and medical subspecialists in tertiary care settings and emphasizes appropriate transfer of information and accountability.[54,55] This arrangement between providers may be especially important as CMC transition home after an inpatient stay for surgery or illness. Some institutions have specialized transition services dedicated to this process.

Despite the surge of emphasis on the primary care–based medical home as part of health care reform, 1 recent study found that two-fifths of CMC with Medicaid insurance did not see their primary care physician in the

previous 12 months.[56] Primary care physicians have expressed limited desire to take on more children with special needs because of the time investment and limited capacity,[57,58] and in a recent study, just under half of pediatricians surveyed across the United States reported that the subspecialty setting may be best equipped to provide a medical home to CMC.[59] Barriers to community-based primary care medical homes include a lack of care coordination skills, training, payment, time, adequate staffing, and system navigation. The primary care physician may need a higher level of medical expertise and staffing support that is not readily available in many practice settings.

Primary care practices that serve as the medical home for CMC will often require practice transformation in staffing and clinical training, in addition to supportive changes at the system and payer level. Effective practice transformation requires the formation of practice-based quality-improvement teams, team-based care delivery that provides care coordination, and delivery of family-centered care with parents as improvement partners, all of which require substantial time and financial investment.[60,61] Existing research on comprehensive care in the primary care setting has generally focused on a limited number of medical conditions instead of the multiple chronic conditions found in CMC,[62] although the multiple studies of specific conditions do provide some guidance to the model of team-based care.

Ideally, the medical home concept would incorporate, in the medical neighborhood style, the extensive tertiary care services that CMC require, because CMC receive far more care in the tertiary care setting than in the primary care setting.[56] Tertiary care delivery settings range from individual specialty services, a service dedicated to a unifying condition such as cystic fibrosis, to "complex care" clinics dedicated to CMC that provide care coordinators, specific expertise to medically manage complex care, and team-based interdisciplinary services.[63] Compared with the traditional primary care setting, hospital-based complex care clinics may be better positioned to provide the care coordination and medical expertise that CMC require and, in some cases, may be the best option to be the medical home.[64,65] Some complex care clinics may not assume the responsibility of primary care, but rather coordinate and collocate the most essential specialty services

related to the underlying conditions while comanaging with primary care. Three before-and-after studies of such services, 2 of which are comanagement consultative services and the third providing primary care, suggest overall financial savings through decreased emergency department and inpatient utilization,[66–68] while acknowledging that payment models are insufficient to cover the costs of the services provided.[66] A randomized controlled trial of "enhanced" primary care, with collocation of specialty and comprehensive services, found significant reductions in serious illnesses, emergency department and inpatient admissions, and Medicaid payments.[69] Although these models are promising, they are limited to the enrolled population, and some families do not live close enough to the tertiary children's hospital setting to take full advantage of available services. In such situations, many families also express a preference to have their care closer to home.[70] This preference underscores the important role of the community-based physician as part of an integrated care model for CMC.

BUILDING THE IDEAL MODEL OF CARE DELIVERY FOR CMC

The ideal family-centered model of care for CMC builds on the foundation of the medical home concept. The medical home, in turn, fosters family-provider-community partnerships that support an integrated, community-based system of care.[71] The model of care should, first and foremost, identify and address the needs of the child and the family (including respite care, family support groups, educational support, and advocacy for resources) while simultaneously taking into account their strengths and assets. The provider should actively engage in shared decision-making with patients and families to define goals, solve problems, and plan

care.[72] Families of CMC desire that the various parts of the health care system (primary and subspecialty care, dental care, emergency care, home-nursing services, and multiple supportive components such as physical therapy, community mental health, and school-based services) work as an integrated whole. The system of care for CMC would include components of the National Consensus Framework for Systems of Care for CYSHCN, published by the Association of Maternal and Child Health Programs. In this framework, the components of a unified system of care include the following: (1) family-professional partnerships, (2) medical home, (3) insurance and financing, (4) early and continuous screening and referral, (5) easy-to-use services and supports, (6) transition to adulthood, and (7) cultural competence.[73]

Individual primary care practices should be supported, when desired, as the foundation of longitudinal, comprehensive care for CMC. Families are best supported when providers have high continuity and a thorough knowledge of the child and family, including their attitudes, beliefs, and values related to health and health care.[74] These care components are inherent to good primary care[75,76] and may be best delivered from the communities where CMC reside. Adequate financial support, dedicated resources (eg, community health workers, interpreter services), staff training, and delineation of care roles within the broader integrated care system with seamless communication between providers are required to support primary care practices in this role of medical home provider. Key care aspects include a designated staff person who acts as a care coordinator who is the identified contact for CMC and their families, as well as a personal physician who is able to perform the medical functions of the medical home. Staffing ideally accounts for adequate and appropriately trained personnel resources to support non–face-to-face care necessary in population management of CMC. Optimal care coordination requires enhancing the caregiving capabilities of families while addressing multiple domains of health care, psychosocial, and educational needs to achieve health and wellness.[77,78] Effective care coordination, in turn, is associated with favorable family-provider relations and family-child outcomes.[78,79]

The medical home is an ideal setting from which to address the educational needs of CMC who are at high risk of missed school days because of illness. Families often need the assistance of the medical home while they navigate the Individualized Education Program or 504 plans at school.[80] The medical home should provide medical information that will help the school develop programming, including physical, occupational, and speech therapy, to meet the child's needs in the least restrictive environment.[81,82] Most CMC can attend school successfully with appropriate supports, but in circumstances in which the child is unable to attend school, the medical home should be highly engaged to ensure non–school-based instruction and a return to school when medically appropriate.[83]

Pediatric medical subspecialty care is vital to the care of CMC, and many pediatric medical subspecialists are located in tertiary care centers. Regardless of where CMC receive their care, all care should be coordinated through a single provider who acts as the designated care-coordinating entity. As described previously, care coordination may be through the primary care physician, although in certain situations, a complex care service located within the hospital setting may manage or comanage the child with medical complexity

and act as the designated medical home.[65] Such an agreement may be fluid, depending on immediate need. When feasible, dedicated support, education, and communication from the pediatric medical subspecialist and tertiary care center to the community-based provider can reduce the number of visits necessary to the tertiary care center, increase adherence to the care plan, raise satisfaction for families, and decrease costs through reduced tertiary care center utilization.[50,84–87] Regardless of the setting, CMC should have periodic scheduled contact with the medical home as part of the care plan to prospectively address growth and nutrition, health maintenance and preventive care (including dental care), developmental and psychosocial needs, family functioning, medical management of underlying chronic conditions, long-term planning and palliative care (if appropriate), and early and timely intervention in the case of an adverse event. For children who receive home health services, the health maintenance visit is one of the best times to review the accuracy of home health orders, which must be signed at regular intervals.

The ideal medical home setting will have a registry of CMC to help the care team proactively identify CMC as well as support care coordination activities and functions for CMC care.[78,88] Considerations for empanelment in a registry should include a combination of diagnoses and an assessment of functional needs and supports, family-identified needs, and risk factors putting the child/youth at risk of poor outcomes. Leeway should be provided for designation in the registry, given a lack of standardized methods to identify environmental and psychosocial determinants of complexity.[19] Families should have continuous access to connect by phone, via telehealth, or through secure online

access to a knowledgeable provider to discuss health care needs of the child or be seen when an urgent situation arises. A key primary contact may be a care coordinator, in addition to the medical home provider, who is familiar with the child and family as well as the medical history and care needs. The key care team members are ideally available at all times on all days for consultations in case of emergencies and able to bridge communication between the primary care practice, specialty practice, and the emergency providers. In addition, the practice should be able to address the needs of and effectively communicate with families from diverse backgrounds. Care is negatively affected when language barriers exist[89]; therefore, as the population becomes more diverse, extra efforts should be made to enhance communication with appropriate interpreter services.

Care templates and care plans (available in the report "Achieving a Shared Plan of Care With Children and Youth With Special Health Care Needs: An Implementation Guide" from the Lucile Packard Foundation at http://www.lpfch.org/sites/ default/files/field/publications/ achieving_a_shared_plan_of_ care_implementation.pdf and the National Center for Medical Home Implementation site at https:// medicalhomeinfo.aap.org/tools-resources/Pages/For-Practices. aspx) are important adjuncts for effective comanagement.[90] The care plan should be jointly developed and maintained and implemented by the family and the provider responsible for overall coordination of care. The care plan may consist of a summary of medical needs, care providers, and goals outlined with families. A section of the care plan should address emergency care needs.[91] Care plans can also provide all parties, but particularly parents and caregivers, with a level partner relationship.[92] Electronic care plans integrated into an electronic health record have the potential to facilitate sharing between providers and families, particularly when coupled with patient/family portals. The care plan should be available in real-time and across care settings electronically as an up-to-date document.

The 2001 Institute of Medicine report "Crossing the Quality Chasm" emphasizes the ongoing challenge of achieving the full potential of health care delivery and the systemic and organizational barriers that can impede consistent delivery of effective health care.[27] Accordingly, providers and practices caring for CMC should participate in quality-improvement initiatives to improve the consistency and quality of care that is provided to CMC. Quality measures for CMC can be obtained from a combination of chart review, patient surveys, and practice surveys and may include domains from primary care, PFCC, chronic care, care coordination, and health care transition.[93] Process measures specific to a care team may include the quality of care transitions between providers, reason for referral, the ongoing relationship between the referring primary care provider and pediatric medical subspecialist, and action steps incorporated into a collaborative care plan. Considerations for outcome measures include unplanned hospitalizations, readmissions, emergency department visits, and total costs of care. Other important outcomes include perceived ease of use of health care services, family experience of care, reduction in duplicate/unnecessary testing/laboratory tests, minimization of work loss for caregivers, and child functional status and quality of life. Some measures may rely on the achievement of specific health goals, such as improving respiratory function, optimizing nutrition, or maximizing community participation

through the use of adaptive technologies and equipment.

CMC are at particular risk of adverse outcomes during the transition from pediatric to adult health care.[94] Transition planning based on the unique needs of the individual child with medical complexity should be addressed beginning by the early adolescent years so that the process is seamless and the youth does not experience a gap in health care.[95] Areas of importance include self-management, to the extent possible; optimal health and functioning; and tools necessary to navigate the health care system. A handoff between pediatric and adult providers should be arranged at the appropriate time.[95] The high prevalence of neurodevelopmental disabilities, coupled with the myriad service needs, may restrict the opportunity for independent living and raise guardianship and service issues that should be addressed proactively. A transdisciplinary model approach may be needed to fully facilitate the transition process, which often takes longer for CMC than for children without medical complexity.[96]

Pediatric residency training that focuses on caring for CMC may be helpful to prepare for the additional tasks required as the medical home provider for CMC.[97,98] Residency and postgraduate training should focus on medical care issues that are common to many CMC, including growth, nutrition and feeding, respiratory health, technology management, home health order approvals, atypical development and disability, and psychosocial assessments.[98] Not only should training focus on the attributes of care that are condition specific, but it also should emphasize the whole-child approach with attention to how conditions interact with environmental and personal modifiers, as framed by the ICF and the medical home neighborhood.

PAYMENT AND POLICY CONSIDERATIONS

New and innovative systems of payment for CMC, if properly designed, may represent an important opportunity to support the ideal model of care, improve health, and address costs for this population and, because of their outsized effect on health care costs, for the pediatric population in general. Opportunities for health care system savings may be enhanced through reducing potentially preventable, costly emergency/hospital-based care.[56] Payment reform challenges also stem from the high level of services and payments that are incurred. Hospitals may see a loss in revenue if CMC use fewer inpatient services, even while health systems see savings. However, current payment models for CMC under a fee-for-service system for many outpatient-based physicians generally have not covered the cost of providing care, especially when care involves active care coordination and other nonbillable services.[66] Psychosocial assessment and management, care plan development, communication between providers, reconciliation of home health care plans and nursing/durable equipment orders, transition between settings, and 24/7 access by specific, knowledgeable providers are key labor-intensive activities that are crucial to effective health care management of CMC. These services require appropriate compensation under any payment model.

Appropriate compensation for delivered services may entail raising fee-for-service payments, compensation for non–face-to-face activities, and upfront payments for care management by clinical and nonclinical staff. Current Procedural Technology codes have set up the infrastructure for billing for a variety of non–face-to-face services. In recent years, this area has seen an expansion of codes and services covered under those codes. Refer to coding resources from the American Academy of Pediatrics' "Coding for Medical Home Visits" and "Coding for Telehealth Services" for more details on what codes can be reported and associated values.

State Medicaid agencies are important providers of insurance coverage for many CMC. Payment initiatives, such as Health Homes from the Affordable Care Act,[99] and the rise of accountable care organizations offer the opportunity to design new care systems to meet the needs of CMC, potentially in collaboration with Medicaid agencies. CMC may be considered separately in payment models from children without medical complexity because of differing utilization patterns, such as significantly higher specialty care and mental health, and inpatient care needs.[56,100] In some cases, CMC may remain in traditional fee-for-service programs; in other cases, they are considered for managed-care models that may include bundled payments or fully capitated plans with assumption of risk. This movement has occurred because of outsized costs of care for CMC and the perceived difficulty for primary care physicians to be responsible for overall care. The assumption is that making an organization responsible for the totality of care for a given population will result in appropriate spending, reduced overall costs, and improved quality.[101,102] A national demonstration project across multiple children's hospitals is testing care planning and coordination interventions while developing a population-based payment model to support the interventions.[103] Proposed national legislation would create a national care model and accompanying payment reforms for CMC that would be centered in tertiary care children's hospitals.[104] On the state level, Texas is rolling out the STAR Kids program, a Medicaid managed-care program that enrolls children with disabilities

identified by Supplemental Security Income, with individual service assessments, plans, and accompanying benefits.[105] Challenges include the accurate identification of CMC, risk stratification, and setting appropriate payment rates that may underestimate actual need on the basis of previous outpatient claims. The longitudinal cost trajectory of CMC or the rate of return on investment remains poorly defined, along with approaches of care management that may result in improved health and cost savings for CMC as a whole or for specific subgroups of CMC.[56,106]

CONCLUSIONS AND RECOMMENDATIONS

To support the movement for additional health care reform and service delivery enhancements specifically for CMC, the following recommendations are offered.

Pediatricians and Other Pediatric Health Care Providers

- Pediatricians are encouraged to be familiar with the concepts of the medical home, particularly as they apply to CMC, including practice-based patient registries, interdisciplinary team-based care, care planning, care coordination, and care templates, and to have a familiarity with common clinical challenges such as nutrition and respiratory and technology needs.

- Pediatricians may strive to ensure that CMC have a medical home that provides team-based comprehensive care. Ideally, there would be a clearly identified provider who will be the "go to" person for comprehensive care needs who, unless otherwise stated, should be the primary care physician, as per the family's expectation.

- Pediatricians can consider assessing their practice's

willingness and capability to support care for CMC.

- Pediatricians may consider prospectively identifying CMC and including them in a practice registry for comprehensive management of health care needs. Pediatricians may use a combination of methods, such as review of billing data, resource use, family survey, or chart review. Identifying criteria may consider administrative data, survey data, and/or clinical assessments.[19]

- Pediatricians who deliver primary care in the community setting may consider augmenting their care through comanagement with providers within the tertiary care setting who may provide additional medical home/neighborhood supports. It is advised to explicitly define the locus of management and specific care roles.[65]

- Pediatricians should document and bill appropriately for complexity management and both face-to-face and non–face-to-face time for medical management and care-coordination services.

- Pediatricians are encouraged to recognize, identify, advocate for, and partner with community-based services, such as schools, therapists, and home health and family-support services, with appropriate referrals. Communication tools available may include a written or electronic care plan and the use of a dedicated care coordinator who serves as the point of contact for home nursing, school feeding, or other supportive services.

- When possible, pediatricians across the care setting, including hospitalists and pediatric medical subspecialists, can use appropriate tools to facilitate care planning, real-time communication with families and all providers, and transitions between hospital and home, community resources, and pediatric to adult settings. Such tools and mechanisms may include electronic care plans, secure messaging, electronic registries, or telehealth mechanisms, with defined electronic interoperability and communication mechanisms with the child's identified care team members.

- Pediatricians may consider the use of quality-improvement process and outcome measures and value capture tools to evaluate and improve care coordination and care management.

Payer

- Payers should provide adequate incentives for community-based providers to accept and manage CMC. Such methods may be tied to emerging quality metrics and financial incentives specific to CMC who are identified in panels of primary care providers.

- Payers should recognize the value of non–face-to-face encounters and care management that are crucial to health outcomes for CMC. For CMC in particular, payers should pay at appropriate levels for care coordination, including telephone management, telehealth, home-health and equipment documentation, population registry formation, and comanagement of CMC. In some cases, payers may consider providing the care coordination for CMC that works in partnership with the community-based medical home.

- Payers need to recognize current care management codes for CMC to allow all CMC to receive care that can be paid to all primary care physicians, without the potentially financially burdensome technology requirements.

- Payers should account for the presence and management of CMC under different payment models. Under fee-for-service models, non–face-to-face encounters

should be adequately reimbursed; under a capitated plan, appropriate care management fees should be provided with appropriate risk-adjustment strategies that account for varying levels of severity and need. Care should be taken to avoid narrow provider networks that may discriminate against patients with complex care needs.[107]

- Given the current levels of evidence, population-based payment models that support integrated care systems for CMC, incorporating a range of community-based, primary care, and hospital services, should be developed and implemented in partnership with provider and community stakeholders that continually monitor and evaluate payment levels and outcomes.

Policy

- CMC should be recognized as a distinct population of interest for policy, research, and payment reform agendas. Policy strategies applied to adults with complex conditions may not adequately service CMC who need specific attention to their unique needs.

- Residency, postgraduate, and continuing education may consider standardized learning modules and curricula specific to the management of CMC, including nutrition, development and function, care coordination, technology management, telehealth, coordinated handoffs, and PFCC. Similar considerations can be made for interprofessional training (eg, nursing, social work, community health worker, behavioral health professionals) that is essential for care coordination and integration.

- Quality measures relevant and specific to CMC should be developed and applied across systems. Such measures should be specific to children. Quality metrics

should consider child functioning, utilization (preventable emergency department and hospital encounters), and patient- and family-centered metrics (growth, parent stress, employment).

- National and state policies should require adequate health insurance and payment for medically necessary services for CMC while minimizing out-of-pocket costs, which are often barriers to needed care.

- Research agendas should drive a consensus definition of which children constitute the cohort of CMC and then address the accurate identification of CMC for population management, development and assessment of evidence-based models of care, the impact value of PFCC, the impact on health status of CMC, and the financial effect of the previous factors. Metrics should focus on health care quality, psychosocial needs, and investments in outpatient care delivery to assess the value of care delivery provided, managed, or coordinated in the medical home that may mitigate potentially preventable inpatient and emergency department use for nonurgent care.

LEAD AUTHORS

Dennis Z. Kuo, MD, MHS, FAAP
Amy J. Houtrow, MD, PhD, MPH, FAAP

COUNCIL ON CHILDREN WITH DISABILITIES EXECUTIVE COMMITTEE, 2015–2016

Kenneth W. Norwood Jr, MD, FAAP, Chairperson
Richard C. Adams, MD, FAAP
Timothy J. Brei, MD, FAAP
Lynn F. Davidson, MD, FAAP
Beth Ellen Davis, MD, MPH, FAAP
Sandra L. Friedman, MD, MPH, FAAP
Amy J. Houtrow, MD, PhD, MPH, FAAP
Susan L. Hyman, MD, FAAP
Dennis Z. Kuo, MD, MHS, FAAP
Garey H. Noritz, MD, FAAP
Larry Yin, MD, MSPH, FAAP
Nancy A. Murphy, MD, FAAP, Immediate Past Chairperson

LIAISONS

Jennifer Bolden Pitre, MA, JD – *Family Voices*
Marie Mann, MD, MPH, FAAP – *Maternal and Child Health Bureau*
Georgina Peacock, MD, MPH, FAAP – *Center for Disease Control and Prevention*
Edwin Simpser, MD, FAAP – *Section on Home Care*
Peter J. Smith, MD, MA, FAAP – *Section on Developmental and Behavioral Pediatrics*

STAFF

Stephanie Mucha, MPH

ABBREVIATIONS

CMC: children with medical complexity
CYSHCN: children and youth with special health care needs
ICF: *International Classification of Functioning, Disability, and Health*
PCMH: patient-centered medical home
PFCC: patient- and family-centered care

REFERENCES

1. Feudtner C, Christakis DA, Connell FA. Pediatric deaths attributable to complex chronic conditions: a population-based study of Washington State, 1980-1997. *Pediatrics.* 2000;106(1 pt 2):205–209

2. Srivastava R, Stone BL, Murphy NA. Hospitalist care of the medically complex child. *Pediatr Clin North Am.* 2005;52(4):1165–1187

3. Cohen E, Kuo DZ, Agrawal R, et al. Children with medical complexity: an emerging population for clinical and research initiatives. *Pediatrics.* 2011;127(3):529–538

4. Kuo DZ, Cohen E, Agrawal R, Berry JG, Casey PH. A national profile of caregiver challenges among more medically complex children with special health care needs. *Arch Pediatr Adolesc Med.* 2011;165(11):1020–1026

5. McPherson M, Arango P, Fox H, et al. A new definition of children with special health care needs. *Pediatrics.* 1998;102(1 pt 1):137–140

6. US Department of Health and Human Services. *Children with special health care needs. Campaign '87. Surgeon General's Report. Commitment to: Family-Centered, Community-Based, Coordinated Care.* Rockville, MD: US Department of Health and Human Services; 1987

7. Cohen E, Berry JG, Camacho X, Anderson G, Wodchis W, Guttmann A. Patterns and costs of health care use of children with medical complexity. *Pediatrics.* 2012;130(6). Available at: www.pediatrics.org/cgi/content/full/130/6/e1463

8. Neff JM, Sharp VL, Muldoon J, Graham J, Myers K. Profile of medical charges for children by health status group and severity level in a Washington State Health Plan. *Health Serv Res.* 2004;39(1):73–89

9. Kuo DZ, Melguizo-Castro M, Goudie A, Nick TG, Robbins JM, Casey PH. Variation in child health care utilization by medical complexity. *Matern Child Health J.* 2015;19(1):40–48

10. Burns KH, Casey PH, Lyle RE, Bird TM, Fussell JJ, Robbins JM. Increasing prevalence of medically complex children in US hospitals. *Pediatrics.* 2010;126(4):638–646

11. Simon TD, Berry J, Feudtner C, et al. Children with complex chronic conditions in inpatient hospital settings in the United States. *Pediatrics.* 2010;126(4):647–655

12. Berry JG, Hall M, Hall DE, et al. Inpatient growth and resource use in 28 children's hospitals: a longitudinal, multi-institutional study. *JAMA Pediatr.* 2013;167(2):170–177

13. Berry JG, Hall DE, Kuo DZ, et al. Hospital utilization and characteristics of patients experiencing recurrent readmissions within children's hospitals. *JAMA.* 2011;305(7):682–690

14. Bramlett MD, Read D, Bethell C, Blumberg SJ. Differentiating subgroups of children with special health care needs by health status and complexity of health care needs. *Matern Child Health J.* 2009;13(2):151–163

15. US Department of Health and Human Services. *Multiple Chronic Conditions —A Strategic Framework: Optimum Health and Quality of Life for Individuals With Multiple Chronic Conditions.* Washington, DC: Department of Health and Human Services; 2010

16. Parekh AK, Kronick R, Tavenner M. Optimizing health for persons with multiple chronic conditions. *JAMA.* 2014;312(12):1199–1200

17. Burwell SM. Setting value-based payment goals—HHS efforts to improve U.S. health care. *N Engl J Med.* 2015;372(10):897–899

18. Berry JG, Agrawal RK, Cohen E, Kuo DZ. *The Landscape of Medical Care for Children With Medical Complexity.* Overland Park, KS: Children's Hospital Association; 2013

19. Berry JG, Hall M, Cohen E, O'Neill M, Feudtner C. Ways to identify children with medical complexity and the importance of why. *J Pediatr.* 2015;167(2):229–237

20. World Health Organization. Towards a common language for functioning, disability and health. 2002. Available at: www.who.int/classifications/icf/training/icfbeginnersguide.pdf. Accessed February 8, 2016

21. Jette AM. Toward a common language for function, disability, and health. *Phys Ther.* 2006;86(5):726–734

22. Lollar DJ, Simeonsson RJ. Diagnosis to function: classification for children and youths. *J Dev Behav Pediatr.* 2005;26(4):323–330

23. Rehm RS, Bradley JF. Normalization in families raising a child who is medically fragile/technology dependent and developmentally delayed. *Qual Health Res.* 2005;15(6):807–820

24. Rehm RS, Bradley JF. The search for social safety and comfort in families raising children with complex chronic conditions. *J Fam Nurs.* 2005;11(1):59–78

25. Wells N, Krauss MW, Anderson B, et al. *What Do Families Say About Health Care for Children With Special Health Care Needs? Your Voice Counts!! The Family Partners Project report to families.* Boston, MA: Family Voices at the Federation for Children With Special Health Care Needs; 2000

26. Spratling R. Defining technology dependence in children and adolescents. *West J Nurs Res.* 2015;37(5):634–651

27. Institute of Medicine. *Crossing the Quality Chasm: A New Health System for the 21st Century.* Washington, DC: The National Academies Press; 2001

28. Committee on Hospital Care; Institute for Patient- and Family-Centered Care. Patient- and family-centered care and the pediatrician's role. *Pediatrics.* 2012;129(2):394–404

29. Kuo DZ, Houtrow AJ, Arango P, Kuhlthau KA, Simmons JM, Neff JM. Family-centered care: current applications and future directions in pediatric health care. *Matern Child Health J.* 2012;16(2):297–305

30. Kuhlthau KA, Bloom S, Van Cleave J, et al. Evidence for family-centered care for children with special health care needs: a systematic review. *Acad Pediatr.* 2011;11(2):136–143

31. Agency for Healthcare Research and Quality. About the National Quality Strategy. Available at: www.ahrq.gov/workingforquality/about.htm. Accessed February 9, 2016

32. MacKean GL, Thurston WE, Scott CM. Bridging the divide between families and health professionals' perspectives on family-centered care. *Health Expect.* 2005;8(1):74–85

33. Leiter V. Dilemmas in sharing care: maternal provision of professionally driven therapy for children with disabilities. *Soc Sci Med.* 2004;58(4):837–849

34. Ray LD. Parenting and childhood chronicity: making visible the invisible work. *J Pediatr Nurs.* 2002;17(6):424–438

35. Bitsko RH, Visser SN, Schieve LA, Ross DS, Thurman DJ, Perou R. Unmet health care needs among CSHCN with neurologic conditions. *Pediatrics.* 2009;124(suppl 4):S343–S351

36. Singh GK, Strickland BB, Ghandour RM, van Dyck PC. Geographic disparities in access to the medical home among US CSHCN. *Pediatrics.* 2009;124(suppl 4):S352–S360

37. Kane DJ, Kasehagen L, Punyko J, Carle AC, Penziner A, Thorson S. What factors are associated with state performance on provision of transition services to CSHCN? *Pediatrics.* 2009;124(suppl 4):S375–S383

38. Kenney MK. Oral health care in CSHCN: state Medicaid policy considerations. *Pediatrics.* 2009;124(suppl 4):S384–S391

39. Dusing SC, Skinner AC, Mayer ML. Unmet need for therapy services, assistive devices, and related services: data from the national survey of children with special health care needs. *Ambul Pediatr.* 2004;4(5):448–454

40. Warfield ME, Gulley S. Unmet need and problems accessing specialty medical and related services among children with special health care needs. *Matern Child Health J.* 2006;10(2):201–216

41. Mayer ML, Skinner AC, Slifkin RT; National Survey of Children With Special Health Care Needs. Unmet need for routine and specialty care: data from the National Survey of Children With Special Health Care Needs. *Pediatrics.* 2004;113(2). Available at: www.pediatrics.org/cgi/content/full/113/2/e109

42. McPherson M, Weissman G, Strickland BB, van Dyck PC, Blumberg SJ, Newacheck PW. Implementing community-based systems of services for children and youths with special health care needs: how well are we doing? *Pediatrics.* 2004;113(suppl 5):1538–1544

43. Lewis C, Robertson AS, Phelps S. Unmet dental care needs among children with special health care needs: implications for the medical home. *Pediatrics.* 2005;116(3). Available at: www.pediatrics.org/cgi/content/full/116/3/e426

44. Nolan KW, Orlando M, Liptak GS. Care coordination services for children with special health care needs: are we family-centered yet? *Fam Syst Health.* 2007;25(3):293–306

45. Liptak GS, Revell GM. Community physician's role in case management of children with chronic illnesses. *Pediatrics.* 1989;84(3):465–471

46. Houtrow AJ, Okumura MJ, Hilton JF, Rehm RS. Profiling health and health-related services for children with special health care needs with and without disabilities. *Acad Pediatr.* 2011;11(6):508–516

47. Sia C, Tonniges TF, Osterhus E, Taba S. History of the medical home concept. *Pediatrics.* 2004;113(suppl 5):1473–1478

48. American Academy of Pediatrics; Medical Home Initiatives for Children With Special Needs Project Advisory Committee. The medical home [reaffirmed May 2008]. *Pediatrics.* 2002;110(1 pt 1):184–186

49. Edwards ST, Abrams MK, Baron RJ, et al. Structuring payment to medical homes after the affordable care act. *J Gen Intern Med.* 2014;29(10):1410–1413

50. Palfrey JS, Sofis LA, Davidson EJ, Liu J, Freeman L, Ganz ML; Pediatric Alliance for Coordinated Care. The Pediatric Alliance for Coordinated Care: evaluation of a medical home model. *Pediatrics.* 2004;113(suppl 5):1507–1516

51. Bodenheimer T, Wagner EH, Grumbach K. Improving primary care for patients with chronic illness. *JAMA.* 2002;288(14):1775–1779

52. Antonelli R, Stille C, Freeman L. *Enhancing Collaboration Between Primary and Subspecialty Care Providers for Children and Youth With Special Health Care Needs.* Washington, DC: Georgetown University Center for Children and Human Development; 2005

53. Greenberg JO, Barnett ML, Spinks MA, Dudley JC, Frolkis JP. The "medical neighborhood": integrating primary and specialty care for ambulatory patients. *JAMA Intern Med.* 2014;174(3):454–457

54. Garg A, Sandel M, Dworkin PH, Kahn RS, Zuckerman B. From medical home to health neighborhood: transforming the medical home into a community-based health neighborhood. *J Pediatr.* 2012;160(4):535–536.e1

55. Meyers D, Peikes D, Genevro J, et al. *The roles of patient-centered medical homes and accountable care organizations in coordinating patient care.* Rockville, MD: Agency for Healthcare Research and Quality; 2010. AHRQ Publication No.: 11-M005-EF

56. Berry JG, Hall M, Neff J, et al. Children with medical complexity and Medicaid: spending and cost savings. *Health Aff (Millwood)*. 2014;33(12):2199–2206

57. Kuo DZ, Robbins JM, Burns KH, Casey PH. Individual and practice characteristics associated with physician provision of recommended care for children with special health care needs. *Clin Pediatr (Phila)*. 2011;50(8):704–711

58. Agrawal R, Shah P, Zebracki K, Sanabria K, Kohrman C, Kohrman AF. Barriers to care for children and youth with special health care needs: perceptions of Illinois pediatricians. *Clin Pediatr (Phila)*. 2012;51(1):39–45

59. Van Cleave J, Okumura MJ, Swigonski N, O'Connor KG, Mann M, Lail JL. Medical homes for children with special health care needs: primary care or subspecialty service [published online ahead of print October 30, 2015]? *Acad Pediatr*. doi: 10.1016/j.acap.2015.10.009

60. McAllister JW, Sherrieb K, Cooley WC. Improvement in the family-centered medical home enhances outcomes for children and youth with special healthcare needs. *J Ambul Care Manage*. 2009;32(3):188–196

61. McAllister JW, Cooley WC, Van Cleave J, Boudreau AA, Kuhlthau K. Medical home transformation in pediatric primary care—what drives change? *Ann Fam Med*. 2013;11(suppl 1):S90–S98

62. Homer CJ, Klatka K, Romm D, et al. A review of the evidence for the medical home for children with special health care needs. *Pediatrics*. 2008;122(4). Available at: www.pediatrics.org/cgi/content/full/122/4/e922

63. Berry JG, Agrawal R, Kuo DZ, et al. Characteristics of hospitalizations for patients who use a structured clinical care program for children with medical complexity. *J Pediatr*. 2011;159(2):284–290

64. Cohen E, Jovcevska V, Kuo DZ, Mahant S. Hospital-based comprehensive care programs for children with special health care needs: a systematic review. *Arch Pediatr Adolesc Med*. 2011;165(6):554–561

65. Cooley WC, Kemper AR; Medical Home Workgroup of the National Coordinating Center for the Regional Genetic and Newborn Screening Service Collaboratives. An approach to family-centered coordinated co-management for individuals with conditions identified through newborn screening. *Genet Med*. 2013;15(3):174–177

66. Gordon JB, Colby HH, Bartelt T, Jablonski D, Krauthoefer ML, Havens P. A tertiary care-primary care partnership model for medically complex and fragile children and youth with special health care needs. *Arch Pediatr Adolesc Med*. 2007;161(10):937–944

67. Casey PH, Lyle RE, Bird TM, et al. Effect of hospital-based comprehensive care clinic on health costs for Medicaid-insured medically complex children. *Arch Pediatr Adolesc Med*. 2011;165(5):392–398

68. Klitzner TS, Rabbitt LA, Chang RK. Benefits of care coordination for children with complex disease: a pilot medical home project in a resident teaching clinic. *J Pediatr*. 2010;156(6):1006–1010

69. Mosquera RA, Avritscher EB, Samuels CL, et al. Effect of an enhanced medical home on serious illness and cost of care among high-risk children with chronic illness: a randomized clinical trial. *JAMA*. 2014;312(24):2640–2648

70. Miller MR, Forrest CB, Kan JS. Parental preferences for primary and specialty care collaboration in the management of teenagers with congenital heart disease. *Pediatrics*. 2000;106(2 pt 1):264–269

71. Murphy NA, Carbone PS; American Academy of Pediatrics Council on Children With Disabilities. Parent-provider-community partnerships: optimizing outcomes for children with disabilities. *Pediatrics*. 2011;128(4):795–802

72. Godolphin W. Shared decision-making. *Healthc Q*. 2009;12 Spec:e186–e190

73. Association of Maternal and Child Health Programs. *Standards for Systems of Care for Children and Youth With Special Health Care Needs*. Washington, DC: Association of Maternal and Child Health Programs; 2014

74. Miller AR, Condin CJ, McKellin WH, Shaw N, Klassen AF, Sheps S. Continuity of care for children with complex chronic health conditions: parents' perspectives. *BMC Health Serv Res*. 2009;9:242

75. Starfield B, Simpson L. Primary care as part of US health services reform. *JAMA*. 1993;269(24):3136–3139

76. Donaldson MS, Yordy KD, Lohr KN, Vanselow NA. *Primary Care: America's Health in a New Era*. Washington, DC: Institute of Medicine; 1996

77. Antonelli RC, McAllister JW, Popp J. *Making Care Coordination a Critical Component of the Pediatric Health System: A Multidisciplinary Framework*. New York, NY: The Commonwealth Fund; 2009

78. Council on Children With Disabilities; Medical Home Implementation Project Advisory Committee. Patient- and family-centered care coordination: a framework for integrating care for children and youth across multiple systems. *Pediatrics*. 2014;133(5). Available at: www.pediatrics.org/cgi/content/full/133/5/e1451

79. Turchi RM, Berhane Z, Bethell C, Pomponio A, Antonelli R, Minkovitz CS. Care coordination for CSHCN: associations with family-provider relations and family/child outcomes. *Pediatrics*. 2009;124(suppl 4):S428–S434

80. Adams RC, Tapia C; Council on Children With Disabilities. Early intervention, IDEA Part C services, and the medical home: collaboration for best practice and best outcomes. *Pediatrics*. 2013;132(4). Available at: www.pediatrics.org/cgi/content/full/132/4/e1073

81. American Academy of Pediatrics Committee on Children with Disabilities. The pediatrician's role in development and implementation of an Individual Education Plan (IEP) and/or an Individual Family Service Plan (IFSP). *Pediatrics*. 1999;104(1 pt 1):124–127

82. Lipkin PH, Okamoto J; Council on Children with Disabilities; Council on School Health. The Individuals With Disabilities Education Act (IDEA) for children with special educational needs. *Pediatrics*. 2015;136(6).

Available at: www.pediatrics.org/cgi/content/full/136/6/e1650

83. American Academy of Pediatrics Committee on School Health. Home, hospital, and other non-school-based instruction for children and adolescents who are medically unable to attend school. *Pediatrics*. 2000;106(5):1154–1155

84. Stille CJ. Communication, comanagement, and collaborative care for children and youth with special healthcare needs. *Pediatr Ann*. 2009;38(9):498–504

85. Stiles AD, Tayloe DT Jr, Wegner SE. Comanagement of medically complex children by subspecialists, generalists, and care coordinators. *Pediatrics*. 2014;134(2):203–205

86. Cohen E, Lacombe-Duncan A, Spalding K, et al. Integrated complex care coordination for children with medical complexity: a mixed-methods evaluation of tertiary care-community collaboration. *BMC Health Serv Res*. 2012;12:366

87. Van Cleave J, Le TT, Perrin JM. Point-of-care child psychiatry expertise: the Massachusetts Child Psychiatry Access Project. *Pediatrics*. 2015;135(5):834–841

88. Wagner E. Transforming safety net clinics into patient-centered medical homes: empanelment. The Safety Net Medical Home Initiative; March 2010

89. Arthur KC, Mangione-Smith R, Meischke H, et al. Impact of English proficiency on care experiences in a pediatric emergency department. *Acad Pediatr*. 2015;15(2):218–224

90. Van Cleave J, Boudreau AA, McAllister J, Cooley WC, Maxwell A, Kuhlthau K. Care coordination over time in medical homes for children with special health care needs. *Pediatrics*. 2015;135(6):1018–1026

91. American Academy of Pediatrics Committee on Pediatric Emergency Medicine and Council on Clinical Information Technology; American

College of Emergency Physicians; Pediatric Emergency Medicine Committee. Policy statement—emergency information forms and emergency preparedness for children with special health care needs. *Pediatrics*. 2010;125(4):829–837

92. Adams S, Cohen E, Mahant S, Friedman JN, Macculloch R, Nicholas DB. Exploring the usefulness of comprehensive care plans for children with medical complexity (CMC): a qualitative study. *BMC Pediatr*. 2013;13:10

93. Chen AY, Schrager SM, Mangione-Smith R. Quality measures for primary care of complex pediatric patients. *Pediatrics*. 2012;129(3):433–445

94. Bloom SR, Kuhlthau K, Van Cleave J, Knapp AA, Newacheck P, Perrin JM. Health care transition for youth with special health care needs. *J Adolesc Health*. 2012;51(3):213–219

95. Cooley WC, Sagerman PJ; American Academy of Pediatrics; American Academy of Family Physicians; American College of Physicians; Transitions Clinical Report Authoring Group. Supporting the health care transition from adolescence to adulthood in the medical home. *Pediatrics*. 2011;128(1):182–200

96. Ciccarelli MR, Gladstone EB, Armstrong Richardson EA. Implementation of a transdisciplinary team for the transition support of medically and socially complex youth. *J Pediatr Nurs*. 2015;30(5):661–667

97. Sadof M, Gortakowski M, Stechenberg B, Carlin S. The "HEADS AT" training tool for residents: a roadmap for caring for children with medical complexity. *Clin Pediatr (Phila)*. 2015;54(12):1210–1214

98. Bogetz JF, Bogetz AL, Rassbach CE, Gabhart JM, Blankenburg RL. Caring for children with medical complexity: challenges and educational opportunities identified by pediatric residents. *Acad Pediatr*. 2015;15(6):621–625

99. Centers for Medicare and Medicaid Services. Health homes. Available at: https://www.medicaid.gov/Medicaid-CHIP-Program-Information/By-Topics/Long-Term-Services-and-Supports/Integrating-Care/Health-Homes/Health-Homes.html. Accessed February 28, 2016

100. Kuo DZ, Berry JG, Glader L, Morin MJ, Johaningsmeir S, Gordon J. Health services and health care needs fulfilled by structured clinical programs for children with medical complexity. *J Pediatr*. 2016;169:291–296.e1

101. Homer CJ, Patel KK. Accountable care organizations in pediatrics: irrelevant or a game changer for children? *JAMA Pediatr*. 2013;167(6):507–508

102. Kelleher KJ, Cooper J, Deans K, et al. Cost saving and quality of care in a pediatric accountable care organization. *Pediatrics*. 2015;135(3). Available at: www.pediatrics.org/cgi/content/full/135/3/e582

103. Children's Hospital Association. CARE award. Available at: https://www.childrenshospitals.org/Programs-and-Services/Quality-Improvement-and-Measurement/CARE-Award. Accessed January 14, 2016

104. O'Donnell R. Reforming Medicaid for medically complex children. *Pediatrics*. 2013;131(suppl 2):S160–S162

105. Texas Health and Human Services Commission. STAR Kids. Available at: www.hhsc.state.tx.us/medicaid/managed-care/mmc/star-kids.shtml. Accessed January 14, 2016

106. Coller RJ, Lerner CF, Eickhoff JC, et al. Medical complexity among children with special health care needs: a two-dimensional view [published online ahead of print November 30, 2015]. *Health Serv Res*. 2016;51(4):1644–1659

107. Summer L. *Health Plan Features: Implications of Narrow Networks and the Trade-off Between Price and Choice*. Washington, DC: Academy Health; 2014

Recommendations for Prevention and Control of Influenza in Children, 2016–2017

• *Policy Statement*

    – *PPI: AAP Partnership for Policy Implementation*
      See Appendix 2 for more information.

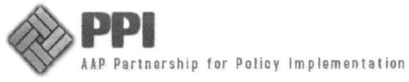

POLICY STATEMENT Organizational Principles to Guide and Define the Child Health Care System and/or Improve the Health of all Children

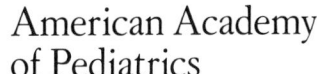

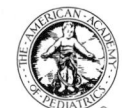

American Academy of Pediatrics

DEDICATED TO THE HEALTH OF ALL CHILDREN™

Recommendations for Prevention and Control of Influenza in Children, 2016–2017

COMMITTEE ON INFECTIOUS DISEASES

abstract

The purpose of this statement is to update recommendations for the routine use of seasonal influenza vaccine and antiviral medications for the prevention and treatment of influenza in children. The AAP recommends annual seasonal influenza immunization for *everyone* 6 months and older, including children and adolescents. Highlights for the upcoming 2016–2017 season include the following:

1. Annual universal influenza immunization is indicated with either a trivalent or quadrivalent (no preference) inactivated vaccine.

2. The 2016–2017 influenza A (H3N2) vaccine strain differs from that contained in the 2015–2016 seasonal vaccines. The 2016–2017 influenza B vaccine strain (Victoria lineage) included in the trivalent vaccine differs from that contained in the 2015–2016 seasonal trivalent vaccines (Yamagata lineage).

   a. Trivalent vaccine contains an A/California/7/2009 (H1N1)pdm09–like virus, an A/Hong Kong/4801/2014 (H3N2)–like virus, and a B/Brisbane/60/2008-like virus (B/Victoria lineage).

   b. Quadrivalent vaccine contains an additional B virus (B/Phuket/3073/2013-like virus [B/Yamagata lineage]).

3. Quadrivalent live attenuated influenza vaccine (LAIV4) should not be used in any setting during the 2016–2017 influenza season in light of the evidence for poor effectiveness of LAIV4 in recent seasons, particularly against influenza A (H1N1)pdm09 viruses.

4. All children with egg allergy can receive influenza vaccine with no additional precautions from those of routine vaccinations.

5. All HCP should receive an annual influenza vaccine, a crucial step in preventing influenza and reducing health care–associated influenza infections. Because HCP may care for or live with people at high risk of influenza-related complications, it is especially important for them to get vaccinated annually.

6. Pediatricians should attempt to promptly identify children suspected of having influenza for rapid antiviral treatment, when indicated, to reduce morbidity and mortality.

DOI: 10.1542/peds.2016-2527

PEDIATRICS (ISSN Numbers: Print, 0031-4005; Online, 1098-4275).

Copyright © 2016 by the American Academy of Pediatrics

FINANCIAL DISCLOSURE: The authors have indicated they do not have a financial relationship relevant to this article to disclose.

FUNDING: No external funding.

POTENTIAL CONFLICT OF INTEREST: The authors have indicated they have no potential conflicts of interest to disclose.

To cite: AAP COMMITTEE ON INFECTIOUS DISEASES. Recommendations for Prevention and Control of Influenza in Children, 2016–2017. *Pediatrics.* 2016;138(4):e20162527

INTRODUCTION

The American Academy of Pediatrics (AAP) recommends annual seasonal influenza vaccination for *everyone* 6 months and older, including children and adolescents, during the 2016–2017 influenza season. Special effort should be made to vaccinate people in the following groups:

- all children, including infants born preterm, aged 6 months and older (based on chronologic age) with conditions that increase the risk of complications from influenza (eg, children with chronic medical conditions, such as asthma, diabetes mellitus, hemodynamically significant cardiac disease, immunosuppression, or neurologic and neurodevelopmental disorders);

- all household contacts and out-of-home care providers of children with high-risk conditions and those younger than 5 years, especially infants younger than 6 months;

- American Indian/Alaska Native children;

- all health care personnel (HCP);

- all child care providers and staff; and

- all women who are pregnant, are considering pregnancy, are in the postpartum period, or are breastfeeding during the influenza season.

KEY POINTS RELEVANT FOR THE 2016–2017 INFLUENZA SEASON

1. **Annual seasonal influenza vaccine is recommended for everyone 6 months and older, including children and adolescents, during the 2016–2017 influenza season.** It is important that household contacts and out-of-home care providers of children younger than 5 years, especially infants

younger than 6 months, and children of any age at high risk of complications from influenza (eg, children with chronic medical conditions, such as asthma, diabetes mellitus, hemodynamically significant cardiac disease, immunosuppression, or neurologic and neurodevelopmental disorders) receive annual influenza vaccine. In the United States, more than two-thirds of children younger than 6 years and almost all children 6 years and older spend significant time in child care or school settings outside the home. Exposure to groups of children increases the risk of contracting infectious diseases. Children younger than 2 years are at increased risk of hospitalization and complications attributable to influenza. School-aged children bear a large influenza disease burden and have a significantly higher chance of seeking influenza-related medical care compared with healthy adults. Reducing influenza virus transmission (eg, by using appropriate hand hygiene and respiratory hygiene/cough etiquette) among children who attend out-of-home child care or school has been shown to decrease the burden of childhood influenza and the transmission of influenza virus to household contacts and community members of all ages.

2. The 2015–2016 influenza season was moderate overall, with lower levels of influenza activity, outpatient illness, influenza-associated hospitalization, and pediatric deaths compared with the previous season. Although the start of the season was typical in the United States, with increasing activity noted in January 2016, activity peaked in mid-March, which was later

than in the previous 3 seasons. The influenza A (H1N1)pdm09 viruses predominated overall, influenza A (H3N2) viruses were more commonly identified from October through early December, and influenza B viruses were more commonly identified from mid-April through mid-May. The majority of circulating strains matched vaccine strains well. Pediatric hospitalizations and deaths caused by influenza vary by the predominant circulating strain and from 1 season to the next (Table 1). Historically, 80% to 85% of pediatric deaths have occurred in unvaccinated children aged 6 months and older. In the past 10 seasons, the rates of hospitalization for children younger than 5 years have always exceeded the rates for children 5 through 17 years of age. As of August 20, 2016, the following data were reported by the Centers for Disease Control and Prevention (CDC) during the 2015–2016 influenza season: 85 laboratory-confirmed influenza-associated pediatric deaths occurred; 53 of these were associated with influenza A viruses, 28 of these were associated with influenza B viruses, and 3 of these were associated with an undetermined type of influenza virus. Although children with certain conditions are at higher risk of complications, 59.7% of the deaths occurred in children with no high-risk underlying medical condition. Among children hospitalized with influenza and for whom medical chart data were available, approximately 50% had no recorded underlying condition, whereas approximately 21% had underlying asthma or reactive airway disease (Fig 1).

3. In light of the evidence for poor effectiveness of quadrivalent

TABLE 1 Pediatric Deaths and Hospitalizations by Season and Predominant Strain

Influenza Season	Predominant Strain	Pediatric Deaths, n	Hospitalizations, per 100 000	
			0–4 years old	5–17 years old
2015–2016 (preliminary data)	H1N1	85	42.5	9.4
2014–2015[a]	H3N2	148	57.3	16.6
2013–2014	pH1NI	111	47.3	9.4
2012–2013	H3N2	171	67	14.6
2011–2012[a]	H3N2	37	16	4
2010–2011	H3N2	123	49.5	9.1
2009–2010	pH1NI	288	77.4	27.2
2008–2009	H1N1	137	28	5
2007–2008	H3N2	88	40.3	5.5
2006–2007	H1N1	77	34.6	2.3

Source: CDC (FluView 2015–2016 data as of August 20, 2016; available at: www.cdc.gov/flu/weekly/fluviewinteractive.htm).
[a] Vaccine strains did not change from previous influenza season.

live attenuated influenza vaccine (LAIV4) documented during the past 3 seasons, particularly against influenza A (H1N1) pdm09 viruses, LAIV4 should not be used in any setting during the 2016–2017 season. In the 2015–2016 influenza season, vaccine effectiveness of any vaccine (inactivated influenza vaccine [IIV] or live attenuated influenza vaccine [LAIV]) against influenza A and B was 47% (95% confidence interval

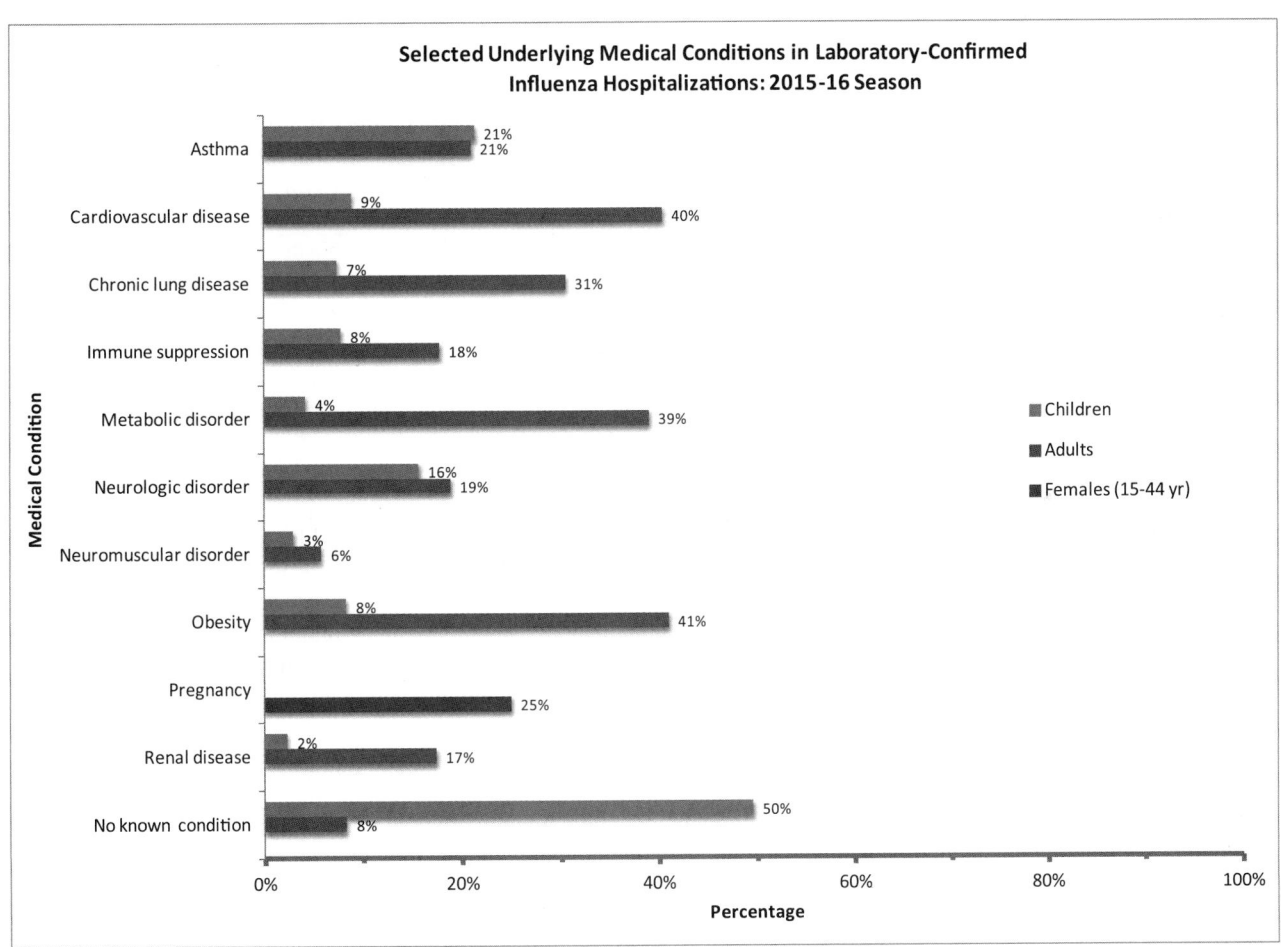

FIGURE 1

Selected underlying medical conditions in patients hospitalized with laboratory-confirmed influenza: FluSurv-NET 2015–2016. Asthma includes a medical diagnosis of asthma or reactive airway disease. Cardiovascular diseases include conditions such as coronary heart disease, cardiac valve disorders, congestive heart failure, pulmonary hypertension, and aortic stenosis (does not include hypertension disease only). Chronic lung diseases include conditions such as chronic obstructive pulmonary disease, bronchiolitis obliterans, chronic aspiration pneumonia, and interstitial lung disease. Immune suppression includes conditions such as immunoglobulin deficiency, leukemia, lymphoma, and HIV/AIDS and individuals taking immunosuppressive medications. Metabolic disorders include conditions such as diabetes mellitus and thyroid dysfunction. Neuromuscular disorders include conditions such as multiple sclerosis and muscular dystrophy. Obesity was assigned if indicated in the patient's medical chart or if BMI >30. Pregnancy percentages were calculated by using the number of female cases aged between 15 and 44 years as the denominator. Renal diseases include conditions such as acute or chronic renal failure, nephrotic syndrome, glomerulonephritis, and impaired creatinine clearance. "No known condition" indicates that the case did not have any known underlying medical condition indicated in the medical chart at the time of hospitalization. Source: CDC (FluView 2015–2016 preliminary data as of August 20, 2016; available at: gis.cdc.gov/grasp/fluview/FluHospChars.html).

[CI]: 39% to 53%) according to observational data from the US Influenza Vaccine Effectiveness Network. However, relative vaccine effectiveness against both influenza A (H1N1)pdm09 viruses (the predominant influenza strain this season) and influenza B viruses strongly favored IIV over LAIV4 among children 2 through 17 years of age. LAIV4 was not significantly effective against any influenza (all A and B viruses combined) among children 2 through 17 years of age (Table 2). In all pediatric age groups for all 3 seasons, LAIV4 did not have any statistically significant benefit in preventing influenza (all 95% CIs cross zero), whereas IIV provided statistically significant protection, albeit to differing degrees by season (Table 2). Children who received LAIV4 had more than 2.5 times higher odds of developing influenza attributable to any virus type compared with children who received IIV. For influenza A (H1N1)pdm09 viruses in particular, LAIV4 had an adjusted vaccine effectiveness of –21% (95% CI: –108% to 30%) compared with 65% for IIV (95% CI: 49% to 76%). The adjusted odds ratio was 3.67, indicating that children who received LAIV4 were almost 4 times more likely to get influenza than those who received IIV. In the 2014–2015 influenza season, data from the US Influenza Vaccine Effectiveness Network indicated that vaccine effectiveness of both IIV and LAIV4 was reduced against influenza A (H3N2) viruses for all age groups because of antigenic drift of the predominantly circulating A (H3N2) viruses. During the 2013–2014 season, observational data from the US Influenza Vaccine Effectiveness Network and 2 additional

TABLE 2 Vaccine Effectiveness Against Any Influenza in Children, by Age and Vaccine Type

Season (Predominant Strain) and Age Range	Adjusted Vaccine Effectiveness, % (95% CI)	
	LAIV4	IIV3/IIV4
2013–2014 (H1N1pdm09)		
2–17 years	2 (−53 to 37)	61 (42 to 74)
2–8 years	−39 (−156 to 25)	60 (32 to 76)
9–17 years	36 (−31 to 69)	62 (30 to 80)
2014–2015 (H3N2)		
2–17 years	9 (−18 to 29)	31 (16 to 44)
2–8 years	9 (−28 to 35)	26 (2 to 44)
9–17 years	17 (−27 to 46)	33 (9 to 51)
2015–2016 (H1N1pdm09)		
2–17 years	3 (−49 to 37)	63 (52 to 72)
2–8 years	−3 (−76 to 40)	58 (40 to 70)
9–17 years	20 (−78 to 64)	71 (52 to 82)

Source: CDC.

studies showed that LAIV4 was not effective against the predominantly circulating influenza A (H1N1)pdm09 viruses when compared with IIV in children aged 2 through 8 years. Additional research will help determine whether the interim recommendation that LAIV4 should not be used in any setting will continue for subsequent influenza seasons. Current focus should be on the administration of IIV for all children and adolescents, particularly those with underlying medical conditions associated with an elevated risk of complications from influenza.

4. **Vaccination remains the best available preventive measure against influenza.** Given the unpredictable nature of influenza each season, *any* licensed and age-appropriate IIV available should be used. The vaccine strains are predicted to be well matched to circulating strains with the intent of providing optimal protection. Vaccination is effective in reducing outpatient medical visits for illness caused by circulating influenza viruses by 50% to 75%. The universal administration of seasonal vaccine to everyone 6 months and older is still the best strategy

available for preventing illness from influenza.

5. Both trivalent and quadrivalent IIVs are available in the United States for the 2016–2017 season. To vaccinate as many people as possible for this influenza season, neither *inactivated* vaccine formulation is preferred over the other. Although manufacturers anticipate an increasing amount of quadrivalent vaccine, pediatricians should give whichever formulation is available in their communities. Both formulations contain an A/California/7/2009 (H1N1)pdm09–like virus, an A/HongKong/4801/2014 (H3N2)–like virus, and a B/Brisbane/60/2008-like virus (B/Victoria lineage). Quadrivalent influenza vaccines contain the B/Phuket/3073/2013-like virus (B/Yamagata lineage) as well. The influenza A (H3N2) virus in both formulations differs from that contained in the 2015–2016 seasonal vaccines. The influenza B virus in the trivalent formulation is the opposite lineage from that in last season's trivalent vaccine.

6. The number of seasonal influenza vaccine doses to be administered in the 2016–2017 influenza season depends on the

Number of Seasonal Influenza Doses for Children 6 Months Through 8 Years of Age

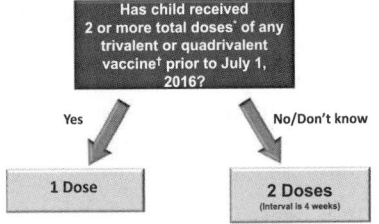

FIGURE 2

Number of 2016–2017 seasonal influenza vaccine doses for children 6 months through 8 years of age. *The 2 doses need not have been received during the same season or consecutive seasons. †Receipt of LAIV4 in the past is still expected to have primed a child's immune system, despite recent evidence for poor effectiveness. There currently are no data that suggest otherwise.

child's age at the time of the first administered dose and his or her vaccine history (Fig 2):

- Influenza vaccines are not licensed for administration to infants younger than 6 months.

- Children aged 9 years and older need only 1 dose.

- Children 6 months through 8 years of age:

  ■ Need 2 doses if they have received fewer than 2 doses of any trivalent or quadrivalent influenza vaccine (IIV or LAIV) before July 1, 2016. The interval between the 2 doses should be at least 4 weeks.

  ■ Require only 1 dose if they have previously received 2 or more total doses of any trivalent or quadrivalent influenza vaccine (IIV or LAIV) before July 1, 2016. The 2 previous doses do not need to have been received during the same influenza season or consecutive influenza seasons. Despite recent evidence for poor effectiveness of LAIV4, receipt of LAIV4 in the past is still expected to have primed a child's immune system. There currently are no data that suggest otherwise. Therefore,

children who received 2 or more doses of LAIV4 before July 1, 2016 may receive only 1 dose of IIV for the 2016–2017 season. Given the continuing circulation of H1N1pdm09 viruses as the predominant influenza A (H1N1) strain since 2009 and its inclusion in all seasonal influenza vaccines since the 2010–2011 season, this virus is no longer believed to be antigenically novel; therefore, special consideration with respect to vaccine policy is no longer necessary. Vaccination should not be delayed to obtain a specific product for either dose. Any available, age-appropriate trivalent or quadrivalent inactivated vaccine can be used. A child who receives only 1 of the 2 doses as a quadrivalent formulation is likely to be less primed against the additional B virus.

7. Pediatric offices may choose to serve as an alternate venue for providing influenza vaccination for parents and other care providers of children, if the practice is acceptable to both pediatricians and the adults who are to be vaccinated.[1] Medical liability issues and medical record documentation

requirements need to be considered before a pediatrician begins immunizing adults (see details at www.aapredbook.org/implementation). Pediatricians are reminded to document the recommendation for adult vaccination in the child's medical record. In addition, adults should still be encouraged to have a medical home and communicate their vaccination status to their primary care provider. Offering adult vaccinations in the pediatric practice setting would not be intended to undermine the adult medical home model but could serve as an additional venue for parents and other care providers of children to receive influenza vaccines. Vaccination of close contacts of children at high risk of influenza-related complications (Table 3) is intended to reduce their risk of contagion (ie, "cocooning"). The practice of cocooning also will help protect infants younger than 6 months who are too young to be immunized with influenza vaccine.

8. Pregnant women can receive influenza vaccine safely at any time during pregnancy. Pregnant women are of special concern because they are at high risk of complications from influenza. Vaccination of pregnant women

TABLE 3 People at High Risk of Influenza Complications and Therefore Recommended for Antiviral Treatment of Suspected or Confirmed Influenza

Children aged <2 years

Adults aged ≥65 years

Persons with chronic pulmonary (including asthma), cardiovascular (except hypertension alone), renal, hepatic, hematologic (including sickle cell disease), or metabolic disorders (including diabetes mellitus) or neurologic and neurodevelopment conditions (including disorders of the brain, spinal cord, peripheral nerve, and muscle such as cerebral palsy, epilepsy [seizure disorders], stroke, intellectual disability, moderate to severe developmental delay, muscular dystrophy, or spinal cord injury)

Persons with immunosuppression, including that caused by medications or by HIV infection

Women who are pregnant or postpartum (within 2 weeks after delivery)

Persons aged <19 y who are receiving long-term aspirin therapy

American Indian/Alaska Native persons

Residents of nursing homes and other chronic care facilities

Adapted from the CDC. Antiviral agents for the treatment and chemoprophylaxis of influenza: recommendations of the Advisory Committee on Immunization Practices (ACIP). *MMWR Recomm Rep.* 2011;60(RR-1):1–24.

also provides protection for their infants, potentially for as long as 6 months through the transplacental transfer of antibodies. For example, 1 recent study documented that infants born to women reporting influenza vaccination during pregnancy had risk reductions of 70% for laboratory-confirmed influenza and 81% for influenza hospitalizations in their first 6 months.

9. Once seasonal influenza vaccine is available locally, pediatricians or vaccine administrators should encourage immunization of HCP, notify parents and caregivers of vaccine availability and the importance of annual vaccination, and immunize children 6 months and older per recommendations, especially those at high risk of complications from influenza. HCP should ideally provide vaccination by the end of October, if possible. This is particularly important for children who need 2 doses of influenza vaccine to achieve optimal protection before the circulation of influenza viruses in the community. Provider endorsement plays a major role in patient acceptance and vaccine uptake. Prompt initiation of influenza vaccination and continuing to vaccinate throughout the influenza season, whether influenza is circulating (or has circulated) in the community, are important components of an effective vaccination strategy. Although there is no evidence that waning immunity from administering the vaccine early increases the risk of infection in children, recent literature raises the possibility that very early vaccination of adults, particularly the elderly, might contribute to reduced protection later in the

influenza season. Until there is definitive information that determines whether waning immunity influences vaccine effectiveness, the influenza vaccine should not be delayed until a later date, because this increases the likelihood of missing influenza vaccination altogether. Further evaluation is needed before any policy change in timing is made.

10. Providers may continue to offer vaccine until June 30th of each year, marking the end of the influenza season, because influenza is so unpredictable. Protective immune responses generally persist in children throughout the influenza season. Although peak influenza activity in the United States tends to occur in January through March, influenza activity can occur in early fall (October) or in late spring (end of May) and may have more than 1 disease peak. This approach also provides ample opportunity to administer a second dose of vaccine to children 6 months through 8 years of age when indicated, as detailed previously in key point 6. This approach also allows for optimal ability to immunize international travelers, who may be exposed to influenza year-round, depending on destination.

11. HCP, influenza campaign organizers, and public health agencies are encouraged to collaborate to develop improved strategies for planning, distribution, communication, and administration of vaccines.

- Plan to make seasonal influenza vaccine easily accessible for all children. Examples include sending alerts to families that vaccine is available (eg, e-mails, texts, letters, and patient portals); creating walk-in influenza vaccination clinics; extending hours beyond routine

times during peak vaccination periods; administering influenza vaccine during both well and sick visits; considering how to immunize parents, adult caregivers, and siblings at the same time in the same office setting as children[1]; and working with other institutions (eg, schools, child care programs, local public health departments, and religious organizations) or alternative care sites, such as emergency departments, to expand venues for administering vaccine. If a child receives an influenza vaccine outside of his or her medical home, such as at a pharmacy, retail-based clinic, or another practice, appropriate documentation of vaccination should be provided to the patient for his or her medical home and entered into the state or regional immunization registry as required by state law.

- Concerted efforts among the aforementioned groups, plus vaccine manufacturers, distributors, and payers, also are necessary to prioritize distribution appropriately to the primary care office setting and patient-centered medical home before other venues, especially when vaccine supplies are delayed or limited. Similar efforts should be made to assuage the vaccine supply discrepancy between privately insured patients and those eligible for vaccination through the Vaccines for Children program. Without an intranasal influenza vaccine recommended for this 2016–2017 season, the AAP is working closely with manufacturers to make available an adequate supply with geographically wide and timely distribution of inactivated vaccine products for pediatric-aged patients.

- Public health will benefit from pediatricians' discussions about vaccine safety, effectiveness, and indications, particularly since LAIV4 should not be used during the 2016–2017 season because of its poor effectiveness against influenza A (H1N1) pdm09 viruses during the 2013–2014 and 2015–2016 influenza seasons in the United States. Pediatricians can influence vaccine acceptance by explaining the importance of annual influenza vaccination for children, emphasizing when a second dose of vaccine is indicated, and explaining why the intranasal formulation is not available this season. The AAP and CDC are developing communication resources to convey these important messages and to help the public understand this influenza recommendation. Resources will be available on *Red Book* Online (www.aapredbook.org/flu).

- HCP should act as role models for both their patients and colleagues by receiving influenza vaccination annually and by letting others know that they have received vaccine, highlighting the safety and effectiveness of annual influenza vaccination. Influenza vaccination programs for HCP benefit the health of employees, their patients, and members of the community. Mandatory influenza immunization for all HCP is ethical, just, and necessary to improve patient safety.[2] Employees of health care institutions are obligated to act in the best interests of the health of their patients and to honor the requirement of causing no harm.

12. Antiviral medications also are important in the control of influenza but are not a substitute for influenza vaccination. The neuraminidase inhibitors (NAIs)

oral oseltamivir (Tamiflu; Roche Laboratories, Nutley, NJ) and inhaled zanamivir (Relenza; GlaxoSmithKline, Research Triangle Park, NC) are the only antiviral medications that are recommended for chemoprophylaxis or treatment of influenza in children during the 2016–2017 season. Peramivir (Rapivab; BioCryst Pharmaceuticals, Durham, NC), a third NAI, was licensed on December 19, 2014, for use in adults 18 years or older and is being studied in children. Intravenous use of peramivir is approved for adults. Intravenous zanamivir remains investigational but can be used in consultation with infectious diseases specialists, and it may also be obtained on a compassionate-use basis for seriously ill children, as currently supported by the US Food and Drug Administration (FDA) through the manufacturer, GlaxoSmithKline. This information is especially important for those who are immunocompromised or who cannot tolerate or absorb orally or enterically administered oseltamivir. Intravenous zanamivir is being studied in pediatric patients, but the manufacturer has not publicly released any information regarding any plans to file for licensure in adults or children. Recent viral surveillance and resistance data from the CDC and the World Health Organization (WHO) indicate that the majority of currently circulating influenza viruses likely to cause influenza in North America during the 2016–2017 season continue to be susceptible to oseltamivir, zanamivir, and peramivir. If a newly emergent oseltamivir- or peramivir-resistant virus is a concern, the use of intravenous zanamivir may be feasible.

Amantadine and rimantadine (adamantanes that block M2 proton channels) should not be used to treat influenza in 2016–2017, because circulating influenza A viruses continue to have extremely high levels of resistance to these drugs, which also are not effective against influenza B viruses. Because resistance characteristics can change over the duration of a treatment course, especially in severely immunocompromised people who may receive prolonged courses, pediatricians can verify susceptibility data for circulating strains at the start of the influenza season and monitor the data throughout the season. Up-to-date information can be found on the AAP Web site (www.aap.org or www.aapredbook.org/flu), through state-specific AAP chapter Web sites, or on the CDC Web site (www.cdc.gov/flu/index.htm).

SEASONAL INFLUENZA VACCINES

Before the 2013–2014 influenza season, only trivalent influenza vaccines that included a single influenza B strain were available. Since the 1980s, 2 antigenically distinct lineages (ie, Victoria or Yamagata) of influenza B viruses have circulated globally. Vaccination against 1 B viral lineage confers little cross-protection against the other B viral lineage. Thus, trivalent vaccines offer limited immunity against circulating influenza B strains of the lineage not present in the vaccine. Furthermore, in recent years, it has proven difficult to predict consistently which B lineage will predominate during a given influenza season. Therefore, a quadrivalent influenza vaccine with influenza B strains of *both* lineages would be predicted to offer additional protection, but there is no evidence

TABLE 4 Recommended Seasonal Influenza Vaccines for Different Age Groups: United States, 2016–2017 Influenza Season

Vaccine	Trade Name	Manufacturer	Presentation	Thimerosal Mercury Content, µg Hg/0.5-mL dose	Age Group
Inactivated					
IIV3	Fluzone High-Dose	Sanofi Pasteur	0.5-mL prefilled syringe	0	≥65 years
IIV3	Fluvirin	Seqirus	0.5-mL prefilled syringe	≤1.0	≥4 years
			5.0-mL multidose vial	25	≥4 years
IIV3	Afluria	Seqirus	0.5-mL prefilled syringe	0	≥9 years[a]
			5.0-mL multidose vial	24.5	≥9 years[a] via needle/syringe 18–64 years via jet injector
aIIV3	Fluad	Seqirus	0.5-mL prefilled syringe	0	≥65 years
ccIIV4	Flucelvax	Seqirus	0.5-mL prefilled syringe	0	≥4 years
IIV4	Fluzone	Sanofi Pasteur	0.25-mL prefilled syringe	0	6–35 months
			0.5-mL prefilled syringe	0	≥36 months
			0.5-mL vial	0	≥36 months
			5.0-mL multidose vial	25	≥6 months
IIV4	Fluzone Intradermal	Sanofi Pasteur	0.1-mL prefilled microinjection	0	18–64 years
IIV4	Fluarix	GlaxoSmithKline	0.5-mL prefilled syringe	0	≥3 years
IIV4	FluLaval	ID Biomedical Corporation of Quebec (distributed by GlaxoSmithKline)	0.5-mL prefilled syringe	0	≥3 years
			5.0-mL multidose vial	<25	≥3 years
Recombinant					
RIV3	Flublok	Protein Sciences	0.5-mL vial	0	≥18 years

Sources: AAP Committee on Infectious Diseases. Recommendations for prevention and control of influenza in children, 2015–2016. *Pediatrics.* 2015;136(4):792–808; Grohskopf LA, Sokolow LZ, Broder KR, et al. Prevention and control of seasonal influenza with vaccines: recommendations of the Advisory Committee on Immunization Practices (ACIP)—United States, 2016-2017 influenza season. *MMWR Recomm Rep.* 2016;65(RR-3):1-54. Implementation guidance on supply, pricing, payment, Current Procedural Terminology (CPT) coding, and liability issues can be found at www.aapredbook.org/implementation. aIIV, adjuvanted inactivated influenza vaccine.

[a] Age indication per the package insert is ≥5 years; however, the Advisory Committee on Immunization Practices recommends Afluria not be used in children 6 months through 8 years of age because of increased reports of febrile reactions noted in this age group. If no other age-appropriate, licensed inactivated seasonal influenza vaccine is available for a child 5 through 8 years of age who has a medical condition that increases the child's risk of influenza complications, Afluria can be used; however, pediatricians should discuss with the parents or caregivers the benefits and risks of influenza vaccination with Afluria before administering this vaccine.

at this time that quadrivalent vaccine is more effective.

IIVs

For the 2016–2017 season, IIVs will be available for intramuscular injection in both trivalent (IIV3) and quadrivalent (IIV4) formulations. IIVs do not contain live virus. The available intramuscular formulations and age groups for which use is approved are presented in Table 4. The intramuscular formulations can be used in children with and without chronic medical conditions. The most common adverse events after IIV3 administration are local injection site pain and tenderness. Fever occurs within 24 hours after immunization in approximately 10% to 35% of children younger than 2 years but rarely in older children and adults. Mild systemic symptoms, such as nausea, lethargy, headache, muscle aches, and chills, may occur after administration of IIV3.

Intramuscular formulations of IIV4 are available from several manufacturers. Different formulations have different age indications, but there are brands licensed for use in children as young as 6 months of age. In children, the most common injection site adverse reactions were pain, redness, and swelling. The most common systemic adverse events were drowsiness, irritability, loss of appetite, fatigue, muscle aches, headache, arthralgia, and gastrointestinal tract symptoms. These events were reported with comparable frequency among participants receiving the licensed comparator IIV3. IIV4 is an acceptable vaccine for people 6 months or older when otherwise appropriate and may offer broader protection against circulating influenza B strains than IIV3.

An intradermal formulation of IIV4 is licensed and available for use in persons 18 through 64 years of age. Intradermal vaccine administration involves a microinjection with a shorter needle than needles used for intramuscular administration. The most common adverse events are redness, induration, swelling, pain, and itching, which occur at the site of administration. There is no preference for intramuscular or intradermal immunization with IIV4 in persons 18 through 64 years of age. Therefore, pediatricians may choose to use either the intramuscular or intradermal product for their young adult patients and for any adults they are vaccinating in their office.

During the 2 influenza seasons spanning 2010–2012, there were increased reports of febrile seizures in the United States in young children who received IIV3 and the 13-valent pneumococcal conjugate vaccine (PCV [PCV13]) concomitantly. Subsequent retrospective analyses of past seasons have revealed a slight increase in the risk of febrile seizures in children 6 through 23 months of age when vaccines are given concomitantly with IIV. For example, although 1 study found that IIV3 was not independently associated with a risk of febrile seizures, an increased risk of febrile seizures was noted when IIV3 was administered on the same day as either PCV or diphtheria-tetanus-acellular pertussis (DTaP) vaccine. Data on which dose in the series for either of these vaccines were not documented. The concomitant administration of IIV3, PCV, and DTaP was associated with the greatest relative risk estimate, corresponding to a maximum additional 30 febrile seizure cases per 100 000 children vaccinated, compared with the administration of the vaccines on separate days. In contrast, data from the FDA's Postlicensure Rapid Immunization Safety Monitoring (PRISM) program, the largest vaccine safety surveillance program in the United States, revealed that there was no significant increase in febrile seizures associated with concomitant administration of these 3 vaccines in children 6 to 59 months of age during the 2010–2011 season. Although the possibility of increased risk of febrile seizures cannot be ruled out, simultaneous administration of IIV with PCV13 and/or other vaccines for the 2016–2017 influenza season continues to be recommended when these vaccines are indicated. Overall, the benefits of timely vaccination with same-day administration of IIV and PCV or DTaP outweigh the risk of febrile seizures, which rarely have any long-term sequelae, with simultaneous administration.

Two trivalent influenza vaccines manufactured with the use of newer technologies will also be available for people 18 years or older during the 2016–2017 season: trivalent recombinant hemagglutinin influenza vaccine (RIV3) and trivalent cell culture–based inactivated influenza vaccine (ccIIV3), both administered intramuscularly. RIV3 is a recombinant baculovirus-expressed hemagglutinin vaccine produced in cell culture. The most frequently reported adverse events after the administration of RIV3 and ccIIV3 are pain, headache, myalgia, and fatigue. RIV3 and ccIIV3 have been shown to be efficacious against influenza disease in randomized controlled efficacy trials. A quadrivalent cell culture–based inactivated influenza vaccine (ccIIV4), administered intramuscularly, also will be available for people 4 years and older during the 2016–2017 season. Studies showed noninferiority of ccIIV4 compared with ccIIV3; ccIIV4 elicited a robust immune response in both children and adults. ccIIV4 has a similar safety profile to ccIIV3 and other licensed trivalent influenza vaccines. In children aged 4 through 17 years, injection site tenderness and erythema were the most common (≥10%) local reactions, and the most common (≥10%) systemic reactions included sleepiness/fatigue and irritability/headache.

In November 2015, the FDA licensed a trivalent, MF-59–adjuvanted IIV for people 65 years and older. This vaccine is the first adjuvanted influenza vaccine marketed in the United States. Adjuvants elicit a more robust immune response, which could lead to a reduction in the number of doses required for children. The vaccine is currently being studied in children.

Table 4 summarizes information on the types of IIVs licensed for children and adults during the 2016–2017 season. More than 1 product may be appropriate for a given patient. Vaccination should not be delayed to obtain a specific product.

A large body of scientific evidence shows that thimerosal-containing vaccines are not associated with an increased risk of autism spectrum disorders in children. Thimerosal from vaccines has not been linked to any other medical condition. As such, the AAP extends its strongest support to the current WHO recommendations to retain the use of thimerosal as a preservative in multiuse vials in the global vaccine supply. Some people may still raise concerns about the minute amounts of thimerosal in some IIV formulations (Table 4), and in some states, including California, Delaware, Illinois, Missouri, New York, and Washington, there is legislated restriction on the use of thimerosal-containing vaccines. The benefits of protecting children against the known risks of influenza are clear. Therefore, to the extent authorized by state law, children should receive any available formulation of IIV rather than delaying vaccination while waiting for reduced-thimerosal-content or thimerosal-free vaccines. Although some formulations of IIV contain a trace amount of thimerosal, thimerosal-free IIV products can be obtained (Table 4). Vaccine manufacturers are delivering increasing amounts of thimerosal-free influenza vaccine each year.

Vaccine Effectiveness and LAIV

The AAP supports the decision by the CDC that LAIV4 not be used in any setting during the 2016–2017 influenza season. This interim recommendation follows 3 influenza seasons during which observational data from the US Influenza Vaccine

Effectiveness Network revealed that LAIV performed poorly (see Table 2). The 2015–2016 influenza season was the first season in which an updated influenza A (H1N1) pdm09 LAIV virus strain was used in response to unexpectedly low vaccine effectiveness for LAIV against influenza A (H1N1)pdm09 viruses in the 2013–2014 influenza season. Despite this virus strain adjustment, LAIV was not effective against influenza A (H1N1)pdm09 and influenza B viruses among children 2 through 17 years of age. Results of relative vaccine effectiveness favored IIV over LAIV for both influenza A (H1N1)pdm09 viruses among children in this age range.

During the 2014–2015 influenza season, the predominant circulating influenza A (H3N2) viruses were antigenically distinct from the influenza A (H3N2) vaccine viruses, resulting in reduced vaccine effectiveness against influenza A (H3N2) viruses in all ages. In contrast to what had been anticipated from previous studies, LAIV did not offer greater protection than IIV against the drifted H3N2 viruses. During the 2013–2014 season, observational data from the US Influenza Vaccine Effectiveness Network and 2 additional studies showed that LAIV was not effective against the predominantly circulating influenza A (H1N1) pdm09 viruses when compared with IIV in children 2 through 8 years of age.

INFLUENZA VACCINES AND EGG ALLERGY

Although most IIV vaccines are produced in eggs and contain measurable amounts of egg protein, recent data have shown that IIV administered in a single, age-appropriate dose is well tolerated by recipients with a history of egg allergy of any severity. Recent

literature has shown that egg allergy does not impart an increased risk of anaphylactic reaction to vaccination with IIV. A 2012 review of published data found no instances of anaphylaxis among 4172 egg-allergic patients, 513 of whom had a history of severe egg allergy, after vaccination with influenza vaccine; some did have milder reactions. According to a Vaccine Safety Datalink study, the rate of anaphylaxis after IIV3 administration is about 1 per 1 000 000 doses (10 cases in almost 7.5 million doses given alone from 2009 to 2011). This rate is not different from those of other vaccines, including ones that do not contain egg. Although a waiting period of 30 minutes after vaccination for patients with egg allergy was previously recommended, this study also found that the onset of symptoms of anaphylaxis after receiving any vaccine began more than 30 minutes later in 21 of 29 cases. In addition, ccIIV4 is anticipated to be available for people 4 years and older during the 2016–2017 season.

The Joint Task Force on Practice Parameters, representing the American Academy of Allergy, Asthma, and Immunology and the American College of Allergy, Asthma, and Immunology, states that special precautions regarding medical setting and waiting periods after the administration of IIV to egg-allergic recipients beyond those recommended for any vaccine are no longer warranted. Therefore, the algorithm used beginning in the 2011–2012 influenza season to guide vaccination precautions on the basis of the severity of the allergic reaction to eggs is not necessary. The recommended waiting period for influenza vaccine, as for any vaccine, is 15 minutes after vaccination for all vaccine recipients to decrease the risk of injury should they faint. Standard vaccination practice should

include the ability to respond to acute hypersensitivity reactions.[3]

VACCINE STORAGE AND ADMINISTRATION

The AAP Storage and Handling Tip Sheet provides resources for practices to develop comprehensive vaccine management protocols to keep the temperature for vaccine storage constant during a power failure or other disaster (https://www.aap.org/en-us/Documents/immunization_disasterplanning.pdf). Any of the influenza vaccines can be administered at the same visit with all other recommended routine vaccines.

Intramuscular Vaccine

IIVs for intramuscular injection are shipped and stored at 2° to 8°C (36°–46°F); frozen vaccines should not be used. These vaccines are administered intramuscularly into the anterolateral thigh of infants and young children and into the deltoid muscle of older children and adults. The volume of vaccine is age dependent; infants and toddlers 6 months through 35 months of age should receive a dose of 0.25 mL, and all persons 3 years (36 months) and older should receive a dose of 0.5 mL. A 0.5-mL unit dose of any IIV should not be split into 2 separate 0.25-mL doses because of safety concerns for lack of sterility, variance with the package insert, and potential compliance difficulties with vaccine excise taxes.

Intradermal Vaccine

IIVs for intradermal injection are shipped and stored at 2° to 8°C (36°–46°F). These vaccines are administered intradermally only to people 18 through 64 years of age, preferably over the deltoid muscle, and only using the device included in the vaccine package. Vaccine is supplied in a single-dose, prefilled microinjection system (0.1 mL) for adults. The package insert contains the full administration details of this product.

CURRENT RECOMMENDATIONS

Seasonal influenza vaccination with IIV is recommended for all children 6 months and older. LAIV should *not* be used. Children and adolescents with certain underlying medical conditions have an elevated risk of complications from influenza, which include the following:

- asthma or other chronic pulmonary diseases, including cystic fibrosis;

- hemodynamically significant cardiac disease;

- immunosuppressive disorders or therapy;

- HIV infection;

- sickle cell anemia and other hemoglobinopathies;

- diseases that necessitate long-term aspirin therapy, including juvenile idiopathic arthritis or Kawasaki disease;

- chronic renal dysfunction;

- chronic metabolic disease, including diabetes mellitus;

- any condition that can compromise respiratory function or handling of secretions or that can increase the risk of aspiration, such as neurodevelopmental disorders, spinal cord injuries, seizure disorders, or neuromuscular abnormalities; and

- pregnancy.

Additional vaccination efforts should be made for the following groups to prevent transmission of influenza to those at risk, unless contraindicated:

- Household contacts and out-of-home care providers of children younger than 5 years and of at-risk children of all ages

- Any woman who is pregnant or considering pregnancy, is in the postpartum period, or is breastfeeding during the influenza season. Studies have shown that infants born to immunized women have better influenza-related health outcomes compared with infants of unimmunized women. However, according to Internet-based panel surveys conducted by the CDC, only approximately 50% of pregnant women reported receiving an influenza vaccine during the 2014–2015 season, even though both pregnant women and their infants are at higher risk of complications. In addition, data from some studies suggest that influenza vaccination in pregnancy may decrease the risk of preterm birth and infants being small for gestational age. Breastfeeding also is recommended to protect against influenza viruses by activating innate antiviral mechanisms, specifically type 1 interferons. In addition, the breast milk of mothers vaccinated during the third trimester contains higher levels of influenza-specific immunoglobulin A. Greater exclusivity of breastfeeding in the first 6 months of life decreases the episodes of respiratory illness with fever in infants of vaccinated mothers. Pregnant women can receive influenza vaccine safely during any trimester.

- American Indian/Alaska Native children and adolescents

- HCP or health care volunteers. Despite the AAP recommendation for mandatory influenza immunization for all health care personnel,[2] many remain unvaccinated. With an increasing number of organizations mandating influenza vaccine, coverage among HCP increased to 77% in the 2014–2015 season. The optimal prevention of influenza in the health care setting depends on the vaccination of at least 90% of

HCP, which is consistent with the national *Healthy People 2020* target for annual influenza vaccination among HCP. However, overall vaccination rates for this group remain consistently below this goal. The AAP recently reaffirmed its support for a mandatory influenza vaccination policy for all HCP nationwide.[2] Mandating influenza vaccine for all HCP is ethical, just, and necessary to improve patient safety, especially because HCP frequently come into contact with patients at high risk of influenza illness in their clinical settings. For the prevention and control of influenza, all HCP must continue to put the health and safety of patients first.

- Close contacts of immunosuppressed people

CONTRAINDICATIONS AND PRECAUTIONS

Minor illnesses, with or without fever, are not contraindications to the use of influenza vaccines, particularly among children with mild upper respiratory infection symptoms or allergic rhinitis. Children with moderate to severe febrile illness, based on the judgment of the clinician, should not be vaccinated with IIV until resolution of the illness. Infants younger than 6 months should also not be vaccinated with IIV. A previous severe allergic reaction (ie, anaphylaxis involving cardiovascular changes, respiratory or gastrointestinal tract symptoms, or reactions that necessitate the use of epinephrine) to influenza vaccine, regardless of the component suspected of being responsible for the reaction, continues to be a contraindication to future receipt of the vaccine.

The estimated risk of Guillain-Barré syndrome (GBS) is low, especially in children. As a precaution, people who are not at high risk of severe influenza and who are known to have experienced GBS within 6 weeks of influenza vaccination generally should not be vaccinated. However, the benefits of influenza vaccination might outweigh the risks for certain people who have a history of GBS and who also are at high risk of severe complications from influenza.

SURVEILLANCE

Information about influenza surveillance is available through the CDC Voice Information System (influenza update: 888-232-3228) or at www.cdc.gov/flu/index.htm. Although current influenza season data on circulating strains do not necessarily predict which and in what proportion strains will circulate in the subsequent season, it is instructive to be aware of 2015–2016 influenza surveillance data and use them as a guide to empirical therapy until current seasonal data are available from the CDC. Information is posted weekly on the CDC Web site (www.cdc.gov/flu/weekly/fluactivitysurv.htm). The AAP offers "What's the Latest With the Flu" (http://www.aap.org/disasters/flu) messages to highlight those details most relevant for AAP members and child care providers on a monthly basis during influenza season.

VACCINE IMPLEMENTATION

These updated recommendations for the prevention and control of influenza in children may have considerable operational and fiscal effects on pediatric practice. Therefore, the AAP has developed implementation guidance on supply, payment, coding, and liability issues; these documents can be found at http://redbook.solutions.aap.org/ss/vaccine-policy-guidance.aspx.

In addition, the AAP's Partnership for Policy Implementation has developed a series of definitions with the use of accepted health information technology standards to assist in the implementation of this guideline in computer systems and quality measurement efforts. This document is available at www2.aap.org/informatics/PPI.html.

The interim recommendation that LAIV should not be used in any setting during the 2016–2017 season could have supply and financial effects on health care settings that have already preordered their influenza vaccines. The AAP is advocating with the manufacturer to appropriately address reimbursement for LAIV. In response to a decrease in overall influenza vaccine supply (ie, LAIV represented approximately 8% of an anticipated 171–176 million doses), manufacturers may adjust their production capacities of IIV.

USE OF ANTIVIRAL MEDICATIONS

Oral oseltamivir remains the antiviral drug of choice for the management of influenza infections. Inhaled zanamivir is an equally acceptable alternative for patients who do not have chronic respiratory disease. However, it is more difficult to administer. Antiviral resistance to either drug can emerge, necessitating continuous population-based assessment that is conducted by the CDC. If local or national influenza surveillance data indicate the emergence of an influenza strain with a known antiviral resistance profile, then empirical treatment can be directed toward that strain with an effective antiviral agent. During the 2015–2016 season, the great majority of influenza strains were susceptible to oseltamivir, zanamivir, and peramivir. In contrast, high levels of resistance to amantadine and rimantadine exist, so these drugs should not be used in the upcoming season unless resistance patterns change significantly.

- Current treatment guidelines for antiviral medications (Table 5) are unchanged for the 2016–2017 season and are applicable to both infants and children with suspected influenza when strains are known to be circulating in the community or when infants or children are tested and confirmed to have influenza.

- Oseltamivir is available in capsule and oral suspension formulations. The commercially manufactured liquid formulation has a concentration of 6 mg/mL. If the commercially manufactured oral suspension is not available, the capsule may be opened and the contents mixed with simple syrup or Ora-Sweet SF (sugar-free) by retail pharmacies to a final concentration of 6 mg/mL (Table 5).

- Continuous monitoring of the epidemiology, change in severity, and resistance patterns of influenza strains may lead to new guidance.

Regardless of influenza vaccination status and whether the onset of illness has been <48 hours, treatment should be *offered* as early as possible for the following individuals (Table 6):

- any hospitalized child clinically presumed to have influenza disease or with severe, complicated, or progressive illness attributable to influenza; and

- influenza infection of any severity in children at high risk of complications of influenza infection (Table 3).

Treatment should be *considered* for the following individuals (Table 6):

- any otherwise healthy child clinically presumed to have influenza disease (the greatest effect on outcome will occur if treatment can be initiated within 48 hours of illness onset but still should be considered if later in the course of illness); and

- children clinically presumed to have influenza disease and whose siblings or household contacts either are younger than 6 months or who have underlying medical conditions that predispose them to complications of influenza.

TABLE 5 Recommended Dosage and Schedule of Influenza Antiviral Medications for Treatment and Chemoprophylaxis for the 2016–2017 Influenza Season: United States

Medication	Treatment (5 Days)	Chemoprophylaxis (10 Days)
Oseltamivir[a]		
Adults	75 mg twice daily	75 mg once daily
Children aged ≥12 months		
Body weight		
≤15 kg (≤33 lb)	30 mg twice daily	30 mg once daily
>15–23 kg (33–51 lb)	45 mg twice daily	45 mg once daily
>23–40 kg (>51–88 lb)	60 mg twice daily	60 mg once daily
>40 kg (>88 lb)	75 mg twice daily	75 mg once daily
Infants aged 9–11 months[b]	3.5 mg/kg per dose twice daily	3.5 mg/kg per dose once daily
Term infants aged 0–8 months[b]	3 mg/kg per dose twice daily	3 mg/kg per dose once daily for infants 3–8 months; not recommended for infants <3 months old unless situation is judged critical, because of limited safety and efficacy data in this age group
Preterm infants	See details[c]	
Zanamivir[d]		
Adults	10 mg (two 5-mg inhalations) twice daily	10 mg (two 5-mg inhalations) once daily
Children (≥7 years for treatment, ≥5 years for chemoprophylaxis)	10 mg (two 5-mg inhalations) twice daily	10 mg (two 5-mg inhalations) once daily

Sources: CDC. Antiviral agents for the treatment and chemoprophylaxis of influenza: recommendations of the Advisory Committee on Immunization Practices (ACIP). *MMWR Recomm Rep.* 2011;60(RR-1):1–24; Kimberlin DW, Acosta EP, Prichard MN, et al; National Institute of Allergy and Infectious Diseases Collaborative Antiviral Study Group. Oseltamivir pharmacokinetics, dosing, and resistance among children aged <2 y with influenza. *J Infect Dis.* 2013;207(5):709–720.

[a] Oseltamivir is administered orally without regard to meals, although administration with meals may improve gastrointestinal tolerability. Oseltamivir is available as Tamiflu in 30-mg, 45-mg, and 75-mg capsules and as a powder for oral suspension that is reconstituted to provide a final concentration of 6 mg/mL. For the 6-mg/mL suspension, a 30-mg dose is given with 5 mL oral suspension, a 45-mg dose is given with 7.5 mL oral suspension, a 60-mg dose is given with 10 mL oral suspension, and a 75-mg dose is given with 12.5 mL oral suspension. If the commercially manufactured oral suspension is not available, a suspension can be compounded by retail pharmacies (final concentration is also 6 mg/mL), based on instructions that are present in the package label. In patients with renal insufficiency, the dose should be adjusted on the basis of creatinine clearance. For the treatment of patients with creatinine clearance of 10–30 mL/min: 75 mg, once daily, for 5 d. For chemoprophylaxis of patients with creatinine clearance of 10–30 mL/min: 30 mg, once daily, for 10 d after exposure or 75 mg, once every other day, for 10 d after exposure (5 doses). See www.cdc.gov/flu/professionals/antivirals/antiviral-drug-resistance.htm.

[b] Approved by the FDA for children as young as 2 weeks of age. Given preliminary pharmacokinetic data and limited safety data, oseltamivir can be used to treat influenza in both term and preterm infants from birth because benefits of therapy are likely to outweigh possible risks of treatment.

[c] Oseltamivir dosing for preterm infants. The weight-based dosing recommendation for preterm infants is lower than for term infants. Preterm infants may have lower clearance of oseltamivir because of immature renal function, and doses recommended for full-term infants may lead to very high drug concentrations in this age group. Limited data from the National Institute of Allergy and Infectious Diseases Collaborative Antiviral Study Group provides the basis for dosing preterm infants by using their postmenstrual age (gestational age + chronological age): 1.0 mg/kg per dose, orally, twice daily, for those <38 weeks' postmenstrual age; 1.5 mg/kg per dose, orally, twice daily, for those 38 through 40 weeks' postmenstrual age; 3.0 mg/kg per dose, orally, twice daily, for those >40 weeks' postmenstrual age. For extremely preterm infants (<28 weeks), consult a pediatric infectious diseases physician.

[d] Zanamivir is administered by inhalation with the use of a proprietary "Diskhaler" device distributed together with the medication. Zanamivir is a dry powder, not an aerosol, and should not be administered using nebulizers, ventilators, or other devices typically used for administering medications in aerosolized solutions. Zanamivir is not recommended for people with chronic respiratory diseases, such as asthma or chronic obstructive pulmonary disease, which increase the risk of bronchospasm.

Reviews of available studies by the CDC, the WHO, and independent investigators have consistently found that timely oseltamivir treatment can reduce the duration of fever and illness symptoms and the risks of complications, including those resulting in hospitalization and death. However, treatment efficacy has not yet been evaluated among hospitalized children or children with comorbid conditions in randomized trials. Although no prospective comparative data exist to date, multiple retrospective studies and meta-analyses have been conducted to determine the role of NAIs in treating severe influenza. Most experts support use of NAIs to reduce complications and hospitalizations, but less agreement exists on the use of NAIs in low-risk populations in whom the benefits are likely modest.

Importantly, treatment with oseltamivir for children with serious, complicated, or progressive disease presumptively or definitively caused by influenza, irrespective of influenza vaccination status or whether illness began greater than 48 hours before admission, continues to be recommended by the AAP, CDC, and Infectious Diseases Society of America. Earlier treatment provides better clinical responses. However, treatment after 48 hours of symptoms in adults and children with moderate to severe disease or with progressive disease has been shown to provide some benefit and should be strongly considered. In previous years, the use of double-dose oseltamivir, particularly for those hospitalized with severe illness caused by influenza A (H1N1)pdm09, was believed to provide better outcomes compared with standard dosing. However, published data from a randomized prospective trial with 75% of subjects younger than 15 years documented no benefit of double-dose therapy over standard-dose therapy.

Dosages of antiviral agents for both treatment and chemoprophylaxis in children are shown in Table 5

TABLE 6 Summary of Antiviral Treatment of Clinical Influenza During the 2016–2017 Season

Offer Treatment as Soon as Possible to Children…	Consider Treatment as Soon as Possible for…
Hospitalized with presumed influenza	Any healthy child with presumed influenza
Hospitalized for severe, complicated, or progressive illness attributable to influenza	Healthy children with presumed influenza, who live at home with a sibling or household contact that is <6 months old or has a medical condition that predisposes to complications
With presumed influenza (of any severity) and at high risk of complications	

(for all ages, including doses for preterm infants that have not been evaluated by the FDA) and on the CDC Web site (www.cdc.gov/flu/professionals/antivirals/index.htm). Children younger than 2 years are at an increased risk of hospitalization and complications attributable to influenza. The FDA has licensed oseltamivir for children as young as 2 weeks of age. Given preliminary pharmacokinetic data and limited safety data, the AAP believes that oseltamivir can be used to treat influenza in both term and preterm infants from birth because benefits of therapy are likely to outweigh the possible risks of treatment.

In adverse event data collected systematically in prospective trials, vomiting was the only adverse effect seen more often with oseltamivir compared with placebo when studied in children aged 1 through 12 years (ie, 15% of treated vs 9% receiving placebo). In addition, after reports from Japan of oseltamivir-attributable neuropsychiatric adverse effects, a review of controlled clinical trial data and ongoing surveillance failed to establish a link between this drug and neurologic or psychiatric events. Information is available at www.gene.com/download/pdf/tamiflu_prescribing.pdf and www.fda.gov/downloads/advisorycommittees/committeesmeetingmaterials/pediatricadvisorycommittee/ucm302449.pdf.

Clinical judgment (on the basis of underlying conditions, disease severity, time since symptom onset, and local influenza activity) is

an important factor in treatment decisions for pediatric patients who present with influenza-like illness. Antiviral treatment should be started as soon as possible after illness onset and should not be delayed while waiting for a definitive influenza test result, because early therapy provides the best outcomes. Influenza diagnostic tests vary by method, availability, processing time, sensitivity, and cost (Table 7), all of which should be considered in making the best clinical judgment. Testing should be performed when timely results will be available to influence clinical management or infection control measures. Although decisions on treatment and infection control can be made on the basis of positive rapid antigen test results, negative results should not be used in a similar fashion because of the suboptimal sensitivity and potential for false-negative results. Positive results of rapid influenza tests are helpful, because they may reduce additional testing to identify the cause of the child's influenza-like illness. Available FDA-approved rapid molecular assays are highly sensitive and specific diagnostic tests performed in less than 20 minutes with the use of RNA detection. These molecular assays or polymerase chain reaction (PCR) test confirmation are preferred in hospitalized patients because they are more sensitive compared with antigen detection. Presumptive antiviral treatment in high-risk and hospitalized patients should be started before receiving rapid test, molecular assay, or PCR results. Immunofluorescence assays may be an alternative to PCR testing,

although the sensitivity is lower. Early detection, prompt antiviral treatment, and infection-control interventions can lead to improved individual patient outcomes and allow for effective cohorting and disease containment.

Persons with suspected influenza who present with an uncomplicated febrile illness should be offered treatment with antiviral medications if they are at higher risk of influenza complications (Table 3). Any otherwise healthy child who has a similar uncomplicated presentation should be considered for antiviral medication, particularly if he or she is in contact with other children who either are younger than 6 months or who have underlying medical conditions that predispose them to complications of influenza. If there is a local shortage of antiviral medications, local public health authorities should provide additional guidance on testing and treatment. In past years, local shortages of oseltamivir suspension have occurred because of uneven drug distribution, although national shortages have not occurred since 2009, particularly given the availability of the capsule formulation that can be made into a suspension for young children (Table 5).

Randomized placebo-controlled studies showed that oseltamivir and zanamivir were efficacious when administered as chemoprophylaxis to household contacts after a family member had laboratory-confirmed influenza. During the 2009 pandemic, the emergence of oseltamivir resistance was noted among people

TABLE 7 Comparison of Types of Influenza Diagnostic Tests Ordered by Test Accuracy and Time to Results

Influenza Diagnostic Test	Method	Availability	Typical Processing Time	Sensitivity, %	Distinguishing Subtype Strains of Influenza A	Cost
Rapid influenza molecular assays	RNA detection	Wide	<20 minutes	86–100	No	$$$
Rapid influenza diagnostic tests	Antigen detection	Wide	<15 minutes	10–70	No	$
Nucleic Acid Amplification Tests (including reverse transcriptase–PCR)	RNA detection	Limited	1–8 hours	86–100	Yes	$$$
Direct and indirect Immunofluorescence assays	Antigen detection	Wide	1–4 hours	70–100	No	$
Rapid cell culture (shell vials and cell mixtures)	Virus isolation	Limited	1–3 days	100	Yes	$$
Viral cell culture	Virus isolation	Limited	3–10 days	100	Yes	$$

Adapted from the CDC. Guidance for clinicians on the use of rapid influenza diagnostic tests. Available at: www.cdc.gov/flu/professionals/diagnosis/clinician_guidance_ridt.htm. Accessed June 8, 2016.

receiving postexposure prophylaxis, highlighting the need to be aware of the possibility of emerging resistance in this population. Decisions on whether to administer antiviral chemoprophylaxis should take into account the exposed person's risk of influenza complications, vaccination status, the type and duration of contact, recommendations from local or public health authorities, and clinical judgment. Optimally, postexposure chemoprophylaxis should only be used when antiviral agents can be started within 48 hours of exposure; the lower dose for prophylaxis should not be used for the treatment of symptomatic children. Early, full-treatment doses provided to high-risk symptomatic patients without waiting for laboratory confirmation is an alternate strategy.

Although vaccination is the preferred approach to the prevention of infection, chemoprophylaxis during an influenza outbreak, as defined by the CDC (http://www.cdc.gov/ophss/csels/dsepd/ss1978/lesson1/section11.html), is recommended in the following situations:

- for children at high risk of complications from influenza for whom influenza vaccine is contraindicated;
- for children at high risk during the 2 weeks after influenza

vaccination, when optimal immunity is achieved;

- for family members or HCP who are unimmunized and are likely to have ongoing, close exposure to unimmunized children at high risk or unimmunized infants and toddlers who are younger than 24 months;

- for control of influenza outbreaks for unimmunized staff and children in a closed institutional setting with children at high risk (eg, extended-care facilities);

- as a supplement to vaccination among children at high risk, including children who are immunocompromised and who may not respond with sufficient protective immune responses after vaccination;

- as postexposure prophylaxis for family members and close contacts of an infected person if those persons are at high risk of complications from influenza; and

- for children at high risk and their family members and close contacts, as well as HCP, when circulating strains of influenza virus in the community are not matched with seasonal influenza vaccine strains, on the basis of current data from the CDC and local health departments.

These recommendations apply to routine circumstances, but it should be noted that guidance may change on the basis of updated recommendations from the CDC in concert with antiviral availability, local resources, clinical judgment, recommendations from local or public health authorities, risk of influenza complications, type and duration of exposure contact, and change in epidemiology or severity of influenza. Chemoprophylaxis is not recommended for infants younger than 3 months unless the situation is judged critical because of limited efficacy data in this age group.

Chemoprophylaxis should not be considered a substitute for vaccination. Influenza vaccine should always be offered before and within the influenza season when not contraindicated, even after influenza virus has been circulating in the community. Antiviral medications currently licensed are important adjuncts to influenza vaccination for the control and prevention of influenza disease. Toxicities may be associated with antiviral agents; indiscriminate use might limit availability. Pediatricians should inform recipients of antiviral chemoprophylaxis that the risk of influenza is lowered but still remains while taking the medication, and susceptibility to influenza returns when the medication is discontinued. Oseltamivir use is not a contraindication to vaccination with IIV. For recommendations on treatment and chemoprophylaxis against influenza, see Tables 5 and 6. Among some high-risk people, both vaccination and antiviral chemoprophylaxis may be considered. Updates will be available at www.aapredbook.org/flu and www.cdc.gov/flu/professionals/antivirals/index.htm.

FUTURE DIRECTIONS

For the 2016–2017 season, postmarketing safety and real-time vaccine effectiveness data will be analyzed as they become available. Continued evaluation of the safety, immunogenicity, and effectiveness of influenza vaccine, especially for children younger than 2 years, is important. The potential role of previous influenza vaccination on overall vaccine effectiveness by vaccine formulation, virus strain, and subject age in preventing outpatient medical visits, hospitalizations, and deaths continues to be evaluated. Furthermore, complete analysis of quadrivalent vaccines is needed as the number of formulations of IIV4 increase. In addition, with limited data on the use of NAIs in hospitalized children or in children with comorbid conditions, prospective randomized clinical trials in this population are warranted. In addition, to administer antiviral therapy optimally in hospitalized patients with influenza who cannot tolerate oral or inhaled antiviral agents, FDA-approved intravenous NAIs for children also are needed. A single-dose, intranasal drug, lananimivir octanoate, needs further research as a potential option for influenza prophylaxis in children.

The interim recommendation that LAIV4 not be used in children will be reevaluated for future influenza seasons, although it is recognized that analyses of LAIV effectiveness in the United States during the 2016–2017 influenza season will be limited. Data on the vaccine effectiveness of LAIV4 against a matched H3N2 virus strain are lacking. Analyses of LAIV effectiveness also differ somewhat between the CDC and other groups in the United States and abroad. This discrepancy may be attributable to varied sample sizes, dissimilar rates of vaccine exposure history in different populations, interference with the addition of the fourth vaccine antigen in the quadrivalent formulation, or other unknown factors. In addition, it recently has been documented that LAIV is well tolerated in children with a history of anaphylaxis after exposure to egg, similar to IIV. This finding could be clinically useful in the future.

Immunizing all HCP, a crucial step in efforts to reduce health care–associated influenza infections, serves as an example to patients, highlighting the safety and effectiveness of annual vaccination. Ongoing efforts should include broader implementation and evaluation of mandatory vaccination programs in both inpatient and outpatient settings. Further investigation into the extent of offering immunization of parents and adult child care providers in the pediatric office setting; the level of family contact satisfaction with this practice; how practices handle the logistic, liability, legal, and financial barriers that limit or complicate this service; and most important, how this practice will affect disease rates in children and adults is needed. There is also a need for more systematic health services research on influenza vaccine uptake and refusal as well as the identification of methods to enhance uptake.

Efforts should be made to create adequate outreach and infrastructure to facilitate the optimal distribution of vaccine so that more people are immunized. Pediatricians also might consider becoming more involved in pandemic preparedness and disaster-planning efforts. A bidirectional partner dialog between pediatricians and public health decision-makers assists efforts to address children's issues during the initial state, regional, and local plan-development stages. Additional information can be found at www.aap.org/disasters/resourcekit.

With the increased demand for vaccination during each influenza season, the AAP and the CDC recommend vaccine administration at any visit to the medical home during influenza season when it is not contraindicated, at specially arranged vaccine-only sessions, and through cooperation with community sites, schools, and child care centers to provide influenza vaccine. If alternate venues, including pharmacies and other retail-based clinics, are used for vaccination, a system of patient record transfer is beneficial in maintaining the accuracy of immunization records. Immunization information systems should be used whenever available. Two-dimensional barcodes have been used to facilitate more efficient and accurate documentation of vaccine administration, with limited experience to date. Additional information concerning current vaccines shipped with two-dimensional barcodes can be found at www.cdc.gov/vaccines/programs/iis/2d-vaccine-barcodes/. Access to care issues, lack of immunization records, and questions regarding who can provide consent may be addressed by linking children (eg, those in foster care or refugee, immigrant, or homeless children) with a medical home, by using all health care encounters as vaccination opportunities, and more consistently by using immunization registry data. Innovative strategies of capturing those who usually prefer the intranasal formulation would be valuable given the recent recommendation to not use LAIV this season.

Development efforts continue for a universal influenza vaccine that induces broader protection and eliminates the need for annual vaccination. In addition, the development of a safe, immunogenic vaccine for infants younger than 6 months is essential. Studies on the effectiveness and safety of influenza vaccines containing adjuvants that enhance immune responses to influenza vaccines are ongoing. Finally, efforts to improve the vaccine development process to allow for a shorter interval between the identification of vaccine strains and vaccine production continue. Pediatricians can remain informed during the influenza season by following the AAP *Red Book* Online Influenza Resource Page (www.aapredbook.org/flu).

ACKNOWLEDGMENTS

This AAP policy statement was prepared in parallel with CDC recommendations and reports. Much of this statement is based on literature reviews, analyses of unpublished data, and deliberations of CDC staff in collaboration with the Advisory Committee on Immunization Practices Influenza Working Group, with liaison from the AAP.

COMMITTEE ON INFECTIOUS DISEASES, 2016–2017

Carrie L. Byington, MD, FAAP, Chairperson
Yvonne A. Maldonado, MD, FAAP, Vice Chairperson
Elizabeth D. Barnett MD, FAAP
James D. Campbell, MD, FAAP
H. Dele Davies, MD, FAAP
Ruth Lynfield, MD, FAAP
Flor M. Munoz, MD, FAAP
Dawn L. Nolt, MD, MPH FAAP
Ann-Christine Nyquist, MD, MSPH, FAAP
Sean T. O'Leary, MD, MD, MPH, FAAP
Mobeen H. Rathore, MD, FAAP
Mark H. Sawyer, MD, FAAP
William J. Steinbach, MD, FAAP

Tina Q. Tan, MD, FAAP
Theoklis E. Zaoutis, MD, MSCE, FAAP

FORMER COMMITTEE MEMBERS

John S. Bradley MD, FAAP
Kathryn M. Edwards, MD, FAAP

EX OFFICIO

Henry H. Bernstein, DO, MHCM, FAAP — *Red Book* Online Associate Editor
Michael T. Brady, MD, FAAP, *Red Book* Associate Editor
Mary Anne Jackson, MD, FAAP, *Red Book* Associate Editor
David W. Kimberlin, MD, FAAP — *Red Book* Editor
Sarah S. Long, MD, FAAP — *Red Book* Associate Editor
H. Cody Meissner, MD, FAAP — Visual *Red Book* Associate Editor

CONTRIBUTORS

Stuart T. Weinberg, MD, FAAP — *Partnership for Policy Implementation*
Tiffany Wang, BA — Research Assistant, *Cohen Children's Medical Center of NY*
Meredith Kline — Research Assistant, *Cohen Children's Medical Center of NY*
Elise Seyferth, BA— Research Assistant, *Cohen Children's Medical Center of NY*
Julia Bratic, BA— Research Assistant, *Cohen Children's Medical Center of NY*
Casidhe-Nicole Bethancourt, BA — Research Assistant, *Cohen Children's Medical Center of NY*
John M. Kelso, MD, FAAP — *Division of Allergy, Asthma, and Immunology, Scripps Clinic, San Diego, CA*

LIAISONS

Douglas Campos-Outcalt, MD, MPA- *American Academy of Family Physicians*
Amanda C. Cohn, MD, FAAP — *Centers for Disease Control and Prevention*
Karen M. Farizo, MD — *US Food and Drug Administration*
Marc Fischer, MD, FAAP — *Centers for Disease Control and Prevention*
Bruce G. Gellin, MD, MPH — *National Vaccine Program Office*
Richard L. Gorman, MD, FAAP — *National Institutes of Health*
Natasha Halasa, MD, MPH, FAAP — *Pediatric Infectious Diseases Society*
Joan L. Robinson, MD — *Canadian Paediatric Society*
Jamie Deseda-Tous, MD — *Sociedad Latinoamericana de Infectologia Pediatrica*
Geoffrey R. Simon, MD, FAAP — *Committee on Practice Ambulatory Medicine*
Jeffrey R. Starke, MD, FAAP — *American Thoracic Society*

STAFF

Jennifer M. Frantz, MPH

ABBREVIATIONS

AAP: American Academy of Pediatrics
ccIIV3: trivalent cell culture-based inactivated influenza vaccine
ccIIV4: quadrivalent cell culture-based inactivated influenza vaccine
CDC: Centers for Disease Control and Prevention
CI: confidence interval
DTaP: diphtheria-tetanus-acellular pertussis
FDA: US Food and Drug Administration
GBS: Guillain-Barré syndrome
HCP: health care personnel
IIV: inactivated influenza vaccine
IIV3: trivalent inactivated influenza vaccine
IIV4: quadrivalent inactivated influenza vaccine
LAIV: live attenuated influenza vaccine
LAIV4: quadrivalent live attenuated influenza vaccine
NAI: neuraminidase inhibitor
PCR: polymerase chain reaction
PCV: pneumococcal conjugate vaccine
RIV3: trivalent recombinant influenza vaccine
WHO: World Health Organization

REFERENCES

1. Lessin HR, Edwards KM; Committee on Practice and Ambulatory Medicine; Committee on Infectious Diseases. Immunizing parents and other close family contacts in the pediatric office setting. *Pediatrics*. 2012;129(1). Available at: www.pediatrics.org/cgi/content/full/129/1/e247

2. American Academy of Pediatrics, Committee on Infectious Diseases. Policy statement: Influenza immunization for all health care personnel: keep it mandatory. *Pediatrics*. 2015;136(4):809–818

3. American Academy of Pediatrics Committee on Pediatric Emergency Medicine. Preparation for emergencies in the offices of pediatricians and pediatric primary care providers. *Pediatrics*. 2007;120(1):200–212. Reaffirmed June 2011

ADDITIONAL RESOURCES

American Academy of Pediatrics Committee on Pediatric Emergency Medicine; American Academy of Pediatrics Committee on Medical Liability; Task Force on Terrorism. The pediatrician and disaster preparedness. *Pediatrics*. 2006;117(2):560–565. Reaffirmed September 2013

American Academy of Pediatrics. Influenza. In: Kimberlin DW, Brady MT, Jackson MA, Long SS, eds. *Red Book: 2015 Report of the Committee on Infectious Diseases*. 30th ed. Elk Grove Village, IL: American Academy of Pediatrics; 2015:476–493. Available at: http://aapredbook.aappublications.org/flu

Chan-Tack KM, Kim C, Moruf A, Birnkrant DB. Clinical experience with intravenous zanamivir under an Emergency IND program in the United States (2011-2014). *Antivir Ther*. 2015;20(5):561–564

Committee on Infectious Diseases. Recommendations for prevention and control of influenza in children, 2015–2016. *Pediatrics*. 2015;136(4):792–808

Des Roches A, Paradis L, Gagnon R, et al; Public Health Agency of Canada/Canadian Institutes of Health Research Influenza Research Network. Egg-allergic patients can be safely vaccinated against influenza. *J Allergy Clin Immunol*. 2012;130(5):1213–1216.e1

Englund JA, Walter EB, Fairchok MP, Monto AS, Neuzil KM. A comparison of 2 influenza vaccine schedules in 6- to 23-month-old children. *Pediatrics*. 2005;115(4):1039–1047

Fiore AE, Fry A, Shay D, Gubareva L, Bresee JS, Uyeki TM; Centers for Disease Control and Prevention. Antiviral agents for the treatment and chemoprophylaxis of influenza—recommendations of the Advisory Committee on Immunization Practices (ACIP). *MMWR Recomm Rep*. 2011;60(1 RR-1):1–24

Frey SE, Reyes MR, Reynales H, et al. Comparison of the safety and immunogenicity of an MF59®-adjuvanted with a non-adjuvanted seasonal influenza vaccine in elderly subjects. *Vaccine*. 2014;32(39):5027–5034

Grohskopf LA, Sokolow LZ, Broder KR, et al. Prevention and control of influenza with vaccines: recommendations of the Advisory Committee on Immunization Practices, United States, 2016-17 influenza season. *MMWR Morb Mortal Wkly Rep*. 2016;65(RR-3):1–54

Haber P, Moro PL, Cano M, et al. Post-licensure surveillance of trivalent live-attenuated influenza vaccine in children aged 2–18 years, Vaccine Adverse Event Reporting System, United States, July 2005–June 2012. *J Pediatric Infect Dis Soc*. 2015;4(3):205–213

Harper SA, Bradley JS, Englund JA, et al; Expert Panel of the Infectious Diseases Society of America. Seasonal influenza in adults and children—diagnosis, treatment, chemoprophylaxis, and institutional outbreak management: clinical practice guidelines of the Infectious Diseases Society of America. *Clin Infect Dis*. 2009;48(8):1003–1032

Jefferson T, Jones MA, Doshi P, et al. Neuraminidase inhibitors for preventing and treating influenza in healthy adults and children. *Cochrane Database Syst Rev*. 2014;4:CD008965

Kelso JM, Greenhawt MJ, Li JT, et al. Adverse reactions to vaccines practice parameter 2012 update. *J Allergy Clin Immunol*. 2012;130(1):25–43

Kelso JM, Greenhawt MJ, Li JT; Joint Task Force on Practice Parameters. Update on influenza vaccination of egg allergic patients. *Ann Allergy Asthma Immunol*. 2013;111(4):301–302

Kimberlin DW, Acosta EP, Prichard MN, et al; National Institute of Allergy and Infectious Diseases Collaborative Antiviral Study Group. Oseltamivir pharmacokinetics, dosing, and resistance among children aged <2 years with influenza. *J Infect Dis*. 2013;207(5):709–720

McNeil MM, Weintraub ES, Duffy J, et al. Risk of anaphylaxis after vaccination in children and adults. *J Allergy Clin Immunol*. 2016;137(3):868–878

Pickering LK, Baker CJ, Freed GL, et al; Infectious Diseases Society of America. Immunization programs for infants, children, adolescents, and adults: clinical practice guidelines by the Infectious Diseases Society of America. *Clin Infect Dis*. 2009;49(6):817–840

Sawyer MH, Simon G, Byington C. Vaccines and febrile seizures: quantifying the risk. *Pediatrics*. 2016;138(1):e20160976

Schlaudecker EP, Steinhoff MC, Omer SB, et al. IgA and neutralizing antibodies to influenza a virus in human milk: a randomized trial of antenatal influenza immunization. *PLoS One*. 2013;8(8):e70867

Shakib JH, Korgenski K, Presson AP, et al. Influenza in infants born to women vaccinated during pregnancy. *Pediatrics*. 2016;137(6):e20152360

South East Asia Infectious Disease Clinical Research Network. Effect of double dose oseltamivir on clinical and virological outcomes in children and adults admitted to hospital with severe influenza: double blind randomised controlled trial. *BMJ*. 2013;346:f3039

Turner PJ, Southern J, Andrews NJ, Miller E, Erlewyn-Lajeunesse M; SNIFFLE Study Investigators. Safety of live attenuated influenza vaccine in atopic children with egg allergy. *J Allergy Clin Immunol*. 2015;136(2):376–381

Turner PJ, Southern J, Andrews NJ, Miller E, Erlewyn-Lajeunesse M; SNIFFLE-2 Study Investigators. Safety of live attenuated influenza vaccine in young people with egg allergy: multicentre prospective cohort study. *BMJ*. 2015;351:h6291

Recommendations for Serogroup B Meningococcal Vaccine for Persons 10 Years and Older

• *Policy Statement*

POLICY STATEMENT   Organizational Principles to Guide and Define the Child Health
Care System and/or Improve the Health of all Children

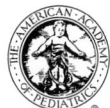

American Academy
of Pediatrics

DEDICATED TO THE HEALTH OF ALL CHILDREN™

Recommendations for Serogroup B Meningococcal Vaccine for Persons 10 Years and Older

COMMITTEE ON INFECTIOUS DISEASES

abstract

This policy statement provides recommendations for the prevention of serogroup B meningococcal disease through the use of 2 newly licensed serogroup B meningococcal vaccines: MenB-FHbp (Trumenba; Wyeth Pharmaceuticals, a subsidiary of Pfizer, Philadelphia, PA) and MenB-4C (Bexsero; Novartis Vaccines, Siena, Italy). Both vaccines are approved for use in persons 10 through 25 years of age. MenB-FHbp is licensed as a 2- or 3-dose series, and MenB-4C is licensed as a 2-dose series for all groups. Either vaccine is recommended for routine use in persons 10 years and older who are at increased risk of serogroup B meningococcal disease (category A recommendation). Persons at increased risk of meningococcal serogroup B disease include the following: (1) persons with persistent complement component diseases, including inherited or chronic deficiencies in C3, C5–C9, properdin, factor D, or factor H or persons receiving eculizumab (Soliris; Alexion Pharmaceuticals, Cheshire, CT), a monoclonal antibody that acts as a terminal complement inhibitor by binding C5 and inhibiting cleavage of C5 to C5A; (2) persons with anatomic or functional asplenia, including sickle cell disease; and (3) healthy persons at increased risk because of a serogroup B meningococcal disease outbreak. Both serogroup B meningococcal vaccines have been shown to be safe and immunogenic and are licensed by the US Food and Drug Administration for individuals between the ages of 10 and 25 years. On the basis of epidemiologic and antibody persistence data, the American Academy of Pediatrics agrees with the Advisory Committee on Immunization Practices of the Centers for Disease Control and Prevention that either vaccine may be administered to healthy adolescents and young adults 16 through 23 years of age (preferred ages are 16 through 18 years) to provide short-term protection against most strains of serogroup B meningococcal disease (category B recommendation).

DOI: 10.1542/peds.2016-1890

PEDIATRICS (ISSN Numbers: Print, 0031-4005; Online, 1098-4275).

Copyright © 2016 by the American Academy of Pediatrics

FINANCIAL DISCLOSURE: The authors have indicated they do not have a financial relationship relevant to this article to disclose.

FUNDING: No external funding.

POTENTIAL CONFLICT OF INTEREST: The authors have indicated they have no potential conflicts of interest to disclose.

To cite: AAP COMMITTEE ON INFECTIOUS DISEASES. Recommendations for Serogroup B Meningococcal Vaccine for Persons 10 Years and Older. *Pediatrics*. 2016;138(3): e20161890

INTRODUCTION

There are 12 known serogroups of *Neisseria meningitidis*, as determined by antigens of the *N meningitidis* polysaccharide capsule. Six serogroups (A, B, C, W, X, and Y) are responsible for invasive human disease. Serogroups A and X are currently rare in the United States. Before October 2014, 4 vaccines were licensed for the prevention of meningococcal disease: 2 quadrivalent meningococcal conjugate vaccines (MenACWY [Menveo; Novartis, Siena, Italy] and Menactra [Sanofi Pasteur; Swiftwater, PA]), a bivalent meningococcal conjugate vaccine (serogroups C and Y) combined with a *Haemophilus influenzae* type b conjugate vaccine (MenHibrix; GlaxoSmithKline; Brentford, United Kingdom), and a quadrivalent meningococcal polysaccharide vaccine (Menomune; Sanofi Pasteur). In October 2014, the first serogroup B meningococcal vaccine, MenB-FHbp (Trumenba; Wyeth Pharmaceuticals, a subsidiary of Pfizer, Philadelphia, PA), was licensed. The second serogroup B meningococcal vaccine, MenB-4C (Bexsero; Novartis Vaccines; Siena, Italy), was licensed in January 2015. Both vaccines are licensed for use in persons 10 through 25 years of age. MenB-FHbp is administered as a 3-dose series for those at increased risk of serogroup B meningococcal disease and as a 2-dose series for those not at increased risk (Table 1). MenB-4C is administered as a 2-dose series for all groups. On February 26, 2015, the Advisory Committee on Immunization Practices (ACIP) of the Centers for Disease Control and Prevention (CDC) recommended the routine use of MenB vaccines in persons 10 years and older at increased risk of serogroup B meningococcal disease (category A recommendation*). On June 24,

---

*Category A recommendations are made for all persons in an age- or risk factor–based group. Category B recommendations are made for individual clinical decision-making.

TABLE 1 Increased Risk Groups Recommended for the Different Meningococcal Vaccines

MenACWY	MenB
Complement deficiency[a]	Complement deficiency[a]
Anatomic/functional asplenia[b]	Anatomic/functional asplenia[b]
Outbreak[c]	Outbreak[c]
Microbiologists[d]	Microbiologists[d]
Travelers[e]	
First-year college students[f]	
Military recruits	

Sources: refs 1–4.
[a] Inherited or chronic deficiencies of C3, C5–C9, properdin, factor D, or factor H or those receiving eculizumab.
[b] Includes sickle cell disease.
[c] The CDC defines outbreaks and those at risk.[5]
[d] Only microbiologists who routinely work with *N meningitidis*.
[e] To areas with hyperendemic or epidemic meningococcal disease.
[f] Unvaccinated or inadequately vaccinated first-year college students who live in residence halls.

2015, the ACIP stated that healthy adolescents and young adults 16 through 23 years of age (preferred ages, 16 through 18 years) who are not at increased risk of serogroup B meningococcal disease may be considered for vaccination with an MenB vaccine to provide short-term protection against most strains of serogroup B meningococcal disease (category B recommendation), but routine immunization is not recommended. The age groups reflected in the recommendation were determined by epidemiologic and antibody persistence data.

Previous meningococcal vaccines have relied on the polysaccharide antigens from serogroups A, C, W, and Y. Protein conjugation of these polysaccharide antigens enhanced immunogenicity. However, the polysaccharide capsule of *N meningitidis* serogroup B is poorly immunogenic, even among those who experience serogroup B meningococcal disease.[6] The immunochemical structure of the serogroup B meningococcal polysaccharide is similar to human glycoproteins, including certain intracellular adhesion molecules.[6] The induction of antibodies to serogroup B meningococcal polysaccharide capsular antigens might result in unacceptable adverse events. For theoretical safety reasons, a serogroup B meningococcal vaccine was designed to contain

nonpolysaccharide antigens. MenB-FHbp is a bivalent vaccine consisting of 2 different recombinant lipidated factor H binding protein (FHbp) antigens, one from FHbp subfamily A and one from FHbp subfamily B. MenB-4C is a multicomponent vaccine consisting of 3 recombinant proteins from *N meningitidis* (FHbp, neisserial adhesion A [NadA], and neisserial heparin binding antigen protein [NHBA]) and an outer membrane vesicle containing Por A P.14 (New Zealand epidemic strain N298/254).

Although in 2015 meningococcal disease caused by any serogroup in the United States was rare, invasive meningococcal disease is a serious illness. Each case can be life-threatening. The United States currently is experiencing historically low levels of meningococcal disease caused by all serogroups, with an incidence of 0.18 per 100 000 population (CDC, unpublished data, 2013). The incidence of meningococcal disease caused by all serogroups has declined. Serogroup B disease incidence has declined despite the fact that serogroup B is not contained in any of the existing conjugate polysaccharide meningococcal vaccines. Approximately 50 to 60 cases of serogroup B meningococcal disease occur annually in adolescents and young adults 11 through 24 years of age in the United States.

A majority of these (80%) occur in individuals 16 through 23 years of age (CDC, unpublished data). Despite a number of recent outbreaks on college campuses, the incidence of serogroup B meningococcal disease in college students (0.09 per 100 000) is similar to or lower than the incidence in all 18- through 23-year-olds (0.14 per 100 000) and noncollege students (0.21 per 100 000) (CDC, unpublished data). A routine adolescent MenB vaccine recommendation would be estimated to prevent 15 to 29 cases and 2 to 5 deaths per year, assuming that all eligible persons were immunized. A recommendation for routine MenB vaccination of college students only is estimated to prevent 10 cases and 1 death per year (CDC, unpublished data).

Certain individuals are known to have an increased susceptibility to invasive meningococcal disease.[1] These individuals are currently recommended to be vaccinated with a quadrivalent meningococcal conjugate vaccine (MenACWY).[1] Many, but not all, of these groups are also at increased risk of invasive disease attributable to *N meningitidis* serogroup B (Table 1). Persons with persistent complement component deficiencies, including inherited or chronic deficiencies in C3, C5–C9, properdin, factor D, or factor H, have up to a 10 000-fold increased risk of meningococcal disease and can experience recurrent disease.[1,2] Individuals receiving eculizumab (Soliris; Alexion Pharmaceuticals, Cheshire, CT), a monoclonal antibody that binds to C5 and inhibits the terminal portion of the complement pathway, are at increased risk of invasive meningococcal disease, including serogroup B meningococcus.[3] Eculizumab is approved for the treatment of atypical hemolytic-uremic syndrome and paroxysmal nocturnal hemoglobinuria.[3] Five of 326 subjects (1.5%) in clinical trials of eculizumab developed invasive meningococcal disease despite previous immunization with a meningococcal vaccine.[3] The package insert does not describe the serogroups of these 5 meningococcal infections.[3] However, serogroup B meningococcal disease in eculizumab recipients has been described. Persons with functional or anatomic asplenia, including sickle cell disease, appear to be at increased risk of invasive meningococcal disease and have a higher case fatality rate (40%–70%) from meningococcal disease than healthy populations.[4] The increased risk of meningococcal infection in patients with asplenia is less than that for invasive pneumococcal disease.[1] Data describing immune responses to MenB vaccines in populations with complement deficiency and asplenia have not yet been published. Microbiologists who routinely work with *N meningitidis* have an attack rate of 13 per 100 000. This attack rate in microbiologists is several-fold higher than that in the general population.[1] Because microbiologists are not in the pediatric age range, recommendations for microbiologists will not be included in recommendations from the American Academy of Pediatrics (AAP) but are included in the ACIP recommendations.

The vast majority of all cases of meningococcal disease occurring in the United States are sporadic (97%–98%). However, outbreaks of meningococcal disease continue to occur and often receive media attention because of the severity of invasive meningococcal disease. In recent years, outbreaks of serogroup B meningococcal disease have occurred on several different college campuses. Data from 2 recent outbreaks on college campuses (spring 2013 through spring 2014) noted a 200- to 1400-fold increase in risk of meningococcal disease among students at these colleges during the outbreak period (CDC, unpublished data).

A comparison of risk groups for the quadrivalent meningococcal conjugate vaccine and the recently licensed serogroup B meningococcal vaccines is presented in Table 1. Persons at increased risk and for whom administration of the quadrivalent meningococcal vaccine (MenACWY) is recommended but for whom the serogroup B meningococcal vaccine is not recommended routinely include the following: (1) persons who travel to or reside in countries in which meningococcal disease is hyperendemic or epidemic, (2) first-year college students living in residence halls, and (3) military recruits. Serogroup B meningococcal vaccine is currently not recommended for travel to any area of the world.[1] College students have a lower risk of serogroup B meningococcal disease than the general population of a similar age (college students compared with 18- through 23-year-olds: 0.09 per 100 000 and 0.14 per 100 000, respectively).

The safety and immunogenicity of both serogroup B meningococcal vaccines (MenB-4C and MenB-FHbp) have been evaluated in numerous published clinical trials[7-16] (and in unpublished data[†]). Both vaccines appear to provide

---

[†]Unpublished data from the following sources: Safety and Immunogenicity of Novartis Meningococcal B Vaccine Formulated With OMV Manufactured at Two Sites, in Healthy Adolescents Aged 11–17 Years; T Vesikari et al. Immunogenicity, Safety, and Tolerability of Bivalent rLP2086 Meningococcal Group B Vaccine Administered Concomitantly With Tdap-IPV Vaccine to Healthy Adolescents. (Clinical Trials Registration: NCT01323270); Safety, Tolerability, and Immunogenicity of MCV4, Tdap Vaccine When Administered Concomitantly in Healthy Subjects Aged ≥10 to <13 Years; Safety and Tolerability of a Meningococcal Serogroup B Bivalent Recombinant Lipoprotein (rLP2086) Vaccine Given in Healthy Subjects Aged ≥10 to <26 Years; T Vesikari et al. Meningococcal Serogroup B Bivalent rLP2086 Vaccine Elicits Broad and Robust Serum Bactericidal Responses in Healthy Adolescents; and Open Label Safety and Immunogenicity in Meningococcal Laboratory Workers.

short-term immunogenicity in healthy populations.[7-16] Studies on vaccine efficacy are not available. Licensure was based on the ability of the vaccines to elicit detection of bactericidal antibody that is presumed to indicate protection. Studies regarding antibody persistence are limited. Immunogenicity studies in populations at increased risk of invasive meningococcal disease have not been completed. MenB-FHbp has been administered concomitantly with the following: quadrivalent human papillomavirus (HPV) vaccine (Gardasil; Merck & Co, Kenilworth, NJ)[16] but not 9-valent HPV vaccine; with MenACWY (unpublished data); with tetanus toxoid, reduced diphtheria toxoid, and acellular pertussis, adsorbed (Tdap) vaccine (Adacel; Sanofi Pasteur [unpublished data]); and with Tdap/inactivated poliovirus vaccine (Repevax; Sanofi Pasteur [this vaccine is not licensed in the United States; unpublished data]). Immune responses were noninferior for HPV-6, HPV-11, and HPV-16[16] and for MenACWY and tetanus, diphtheria, and pertussis antigens (unpublished data) when MenB-FHbp was administered concomitantly. For HPV-18, noninferiority criteria (lower bound of the 95% confidence interval of geometric mean titer [GMT] ratio >0.67) were not met for the GMT ratio at 1 month after the third quadrivalent HPV vaccination (lower bound of 95% confidence interval for GMT ratio was 0.62); however, for each HPV vaccine type, more than 99% of subjects achieved seroconversion.[16]

In clinical trials, both MenB vaccines were safe, with few serious adverse events (all resolved without sequelae).[7-16] There were no deaths considered to be related to either vaccine. Local and systemic adverse

TABLE 2 Local and Systemic Adverse Events Reported in Clinical Trials for MenB-4C and MenB-FHbp

Adverse Event	MenB-4C (Bexsero), %	MenB-FHbp (Trumenba), %
Severe pain at injection site	20–29	5–8
Fever ≥38%	1–5	2–8
Headache (severe)	4–6	1
Fatigue (severe)	4–6	1–4
Muscle pain (severe)	12–13	1–3
Joint pain (severe)	2	1
Use of antipyretic medication	NA	17–28

Sources: refs 7–16; unpublished data. NA, not applicable.

events noted in clinical trials are included in Table 2.[7-16]

Both MenB vaccines were licensed for use in the United States under an accelerated approval pathway. Both vaccine manufacturers are required to conduct postmarketing studies to confirm effectiveness against a panel of diverse meningococcal group stains. Important data, including duration of immunogenicity, the proportion of serogroup B meningococcal strains covered by each vaccine in different geographic areas, and other data needed to provide guidance for recommendations for MenB vaccines, are not yet available. Theoretical concerns exist regarding autoimmune disease after receipt of a vaccine containing FHbp antigen.[17] Additional postlicensure safety data are also needed and will be reviewed by the ACIP and the AAP as they become available.

RECOMMENDATIONS

1. Persons 10 years and older at increased risk of meningococcal disease should receive an MenB vaccine routinely (category A recommendation for all 3 of the following groups):

   (a) persons with persistent complement component deficiencies, including inherited or chronic deficiencies in C3, C5–C9, properdin, factor D, or factor H or those receiving eculizumab;

   (b) persons with anatomic or functional asplenia, including sickle cell disease; and

   (c) healthy persons identified to be at increased risk because of a serogroup B meningococcal disease outbreak (defined by local health department on the basis of CDC criteria[5]); these persons should receive an MenB vaccine series if their treating health care providers, in consultation with their local health or state departments, determine they are appropriate candidates on the basis of CDC criteria.[5]

2. An MenB vaccine series is not routinely recommended, but it may be administered to adolescents and young adults 16 through 23 years of age to provide short-term protection against diverse strains of serogroup B meningococcal disease (category B recommendation). If an MenB vaccine is administered, the preferred age for MenB vaccination is 16 through 18 years of age. This age preference is based on limited data on antibody persistence and the peak ages of invasive serogroup B meningococcal disease.

The MenB vaccines are routinely recommended for individuals at increased risk of disease (category A recommendation) but not for low-risk adolescents and young adults in the age range for which the vaccines are licensed (Table 1). Instead, a permissive or category B recommendation was made for low-risk individuals. The ACIP recommendation for MenB vaccine in low-risk adolescents

TABLE 3 Summary of Cost-effectiveness Analysis of Different Strategies for Adolescent Vaccination, United States

Strategy	Cases Prevented, n	Deaths Prevented, n	NNV to Prevent Cases	NNV to Prevent Deaths	Cost by QALY, $
Series at 11 years	15	2	203 000	1 512 000	$8 700 000
Series at 16 years	28	5	107 000	788 000	$4 100 000
Series at 18 years	29	5	102 000	638 000	$3 700 000
College students	9	1	368 000	2 297 080	$9 400 000

Sources: ref 5; unpublished data, key model assumptions presented at ACIP meeting, June 2015; and methods described in MacNeil et al.[18] NNV, number needed to vaccinate; QALY, quality-adjusted life-year.

and young adults is based on the very low incidence of serogroup B meningococcal disease in persons who are not at high risk and lack of availability of certain data that would be valuable in developing policy. For these reasons, the ACIP determined that there were insufficient data to make a routine recommendation that all adolescents be vaccinated with an MenB vaccine. The AAP also considered the difficulty of delivering multiple vaccine doses to adolescents, the cost of the vaccine series, and the unfavorable cost-effectiveness evaluation (ACIP meeting, unpublished data, June 2015; methods described in MacNeil et al[18]; Table 3) while developing these recommendations. This restrictive recommendation allows treating clinicians to determine which adolescents and young adults might receive benefit from receiving a series of one of the MenB vaccines. If the clinician and family discuss the MenB vaccine and the MenB vaccine is not administered, the discussion and decision should be documented in the patient's health record.

Specific epidemiologic data or guidelines are not available to assist treating clinicians to determine who should receive the MenB vaccine series. Estimates from the CDC indicate that fewer than 60 cases of meningococcal B disease occur each year in the United States among young persons between 11 and 21 years of age. Universal vaccination of the annual cohort of 4 million persons at 16 or 18 years of age would prevent an estimated maximum of 28 cases. Universal vaccination of all college students

is estimated to prevent, at most, 10 cases and 1 death. Except during outbreaks, the available data do not suggest an increased rate of MenB disease among college students relative to non–college students of the same age group.[19]

Pediatricians are encouraged to discuss the availability of the MenB vaccines with families. Discussion should include the low incidence of MenB disease and the unknown efficacy of the vaccines (licensure was based on the ability of the vaccines to induce a presumed concentration of protective antibodies). MenACWY vaccine administration is recommended for college freshman because of increased invasive meningococcal disease attributable to serogroups in the conjugate meningococcal vaccine in college students, particularly in college freshmen living in residence halls; however, this is not the case for serogroup B meningococcal disease. This apparent dichotomy in the incidence of the different meningococcal serogroups in college students is not understood. Colleges and universities may recommend or even require the MenB vaccine for students. The treating clinician should discuss the benefits, risks, and costs with patients and their families and then work with them to determine what is in their best interest.

When used, MenB vaccine should be administered as either a 2-dose series of MenB-4C or as a 3-dose series of MenB-FHbp. A 2-dose series of MenB-FHbp was recently licensed by the Food and Drug

Administration. The 2-dose series of MenB-FHbp should be administered at day 0, and the second dose should be administered no sooner than 6 months after the first dose. The 2-dose series of Men-FHbp should not be used for persons at increased risk of meningococcal B disease (Table 1 lists persons at increased risk) or for persons for whom immediate protection is optimal. The inclusion of the 2-dose series of MenB-FHbp in formal recommendations will be made in conjunction with the ACIP of the CDC when additional data are available, including longer-term antibody persistence after a 2-dose series. On the basis of available data and expert opinion, either MenB vaccine may be administered concomitantly with other vaccines indicated for this age, but at a different anatomic site, if feasible. The first dose of MenB-4C should be administered at day 0, and the second dose should be administered $\geq$1 month later; the 3-dose series of MenB-FHbp should be administered on a 0-, 1- to 2-, and 6-month schedule. Because there are no data on the interchangeability of the 2 MenB vaccines and each vaccine uses very different protein antigens, the same vaccine must be used for all doses to complete the full series. Providers need to communicate to patients which product was given so that the same vaccine is used for subsequent doses.

PRECAUTIONS AND CONTRAINDICATIONS

Before administering MenB vaccines, treating clinicians should consult the package insert for a full list of precautions, warnings, and contraindications. Pregnancy and breastfeeding are precautions, because neither vaccine has been evaluated in these situations. A severe allergic reaction to a previous dose of MenB vaccine or any of its components is a contradiction. Adverse events occurring after the administration of any vaccine should be reported to the Vaccine Adverse Event Reporting System (VAERS). Reports can be submitted to VAERS online, by fax, or by mail. Additional information about VAERS is available by telephone (1-800-822-7963) or online (http://vaers.gov).

COMMITTEE ON INFECTIOUS DISEASES, 2015–2016

Carrie L. Byington, MD, FAAP, Chairperson
Yvonne A. Maldonado, MD, FAAP, Vice Chairperson
Elizabeth D. Barnett, MD, FAAP
H. Dele Davies, MD, FAAP
Kathryn M. Edwards, MD, FAAP
Ruth Lynfield, MD, FAAP
Flor M. Munoz, MD, FAAP
Dawn L. Nolt, MD, FAAP
Ann-Christine Nyquist, MD, MSPH, FAAP
Mobeen H. Rathore, MD, FAAP
Mark H. Sawyer, MD, FAAP
William J. Steinbach, MD, FAAP
Tina Q. Tan, MD, FAAP
Theoklis E. Zaoutis, MD, MSCE, FAAP

EX OFFICIO

Henry H. Bernstein, DO, MHCM, FAAP – *Red Book* Online Associate Editor
Michael T. Brady, MD, FAAP – *Red Book* Associate Editor
Mary Anne Jackson, MD, FAAP – *Red Book* Associate Editor
David W. Kimberlin, MD, FAAP – *Red Book* Editor
Sarah S. Long, MD, FAAP – *Red Book* Associate Editor
H. Cody Meissner, MD, FAAP – Visual *Red Book* Associate Editor

LIAISONS

Douglas Campos-Outcalt, MD, MPA – *American Academy of Family Physicians*
Amanda C. Cohn, MD, FAAP – *Centers for Disease Control and Prevention*
Karen M. Farizo, MD – *US Food and Drug Administration*
Marc Fischer, MD, FAAP – *Centers for Disease Control and Prevention*
Bruce G. Gellin, MD, MPH – *National Vaccine Program Office*

Richard L. Gorman, MD, FAAP – *National Institutes of Health*
Natasha Halasa, MD, MPH, FAAP – *Pediatric Infectious Diseases Society*
Joan L. Robinson, MD – *Canadian Paediatric Society*
Jamie Deseda-Tous, MD – *Sociedad Latinoamericana de Infectologia Pediatrica*
Geoffrey R. Simon, MD, FAAP – *Committee on Practice Ambulatory Medicine*
Jeffrey R. Starke, MD, FAAP – *American Thoracic Society*

STAFF

Jennifer M. Frantz, MPH

ABBREVIATIONS

AAP: American Academy of Pediatrics
ACIP: Advisory Committee on Immunization Practices
CDC: Centers for Disease Control and Prevention
FHbp: factor H binding protein
GMT: geometric mean titer
HPV: human papillomavirus
Tdap: tetanus toxoid, reduced diphtheria toxoid, and acellular pertussis, adsorbed
VAERS: Vaccine Adverse Event Reporting System

REFERENCES

1. Cohn AC, MacNeil JR, Clark TA, et al; Centers for Disease Control and Prevention. Prevention and control of meningococcal disease: recommendations of the Advisory Committee on Immunization Practices (ACIP). *MMWR Recomm Rep.* 2013;62(RR-2):1–28

2. Densen P. Complement deficiencies and meningococcal disease. *Clin Exp Immunol.* 1991;86(suppl 1):57–62

3. Alexion Pharmaceuticals. Soliris [package insert]. Cheshire, CT: Alexion Pharmaceuticals, Inc; April 2014. Available at: http://soliris.net/sites/default/files/assets/soliris_pi.pdf. Accessed January 21, 2016

4. Balmer P, Falconer M, McDonald P, et al. Immune response to meningococcal serogroup C conjugate vaccine in asplenic individuals. *Infect Immun.* 2004;72(1):332–337

5. Centers for Disease Control and Prevention. Interim guidance for control of serogroup B meningococcal disease outbreaks in organizational settings. Available at: www.cdc.gov/meningococcal/downloads/interim-guidance.pdf. Accessed January 21, 2016

6. Finne J, Leinonen M, Mäkelä PH. Antigenic similarities between brain components and bacteria causing meningitis. Implications for vaccine development and pathogenesis. *Lancet.* 1983;2(8346):355–357

7. Santolaya ME, O'Ryan ML, Valenzuela MT, et al; V72P10 Meningococcal B Adolescent Vaccine Study Group. Immunogenicity and tolerability of a multicomponent meningococcal serogroup B (4CMenB) vaccine in healthy adolescents in Chile: a phase 2b/3 randomised, observer-blind, placebo-controlled study. *Lancet.* 2012;379(9816):617–624

8. Santolaya ME, O'Ryan M, Valenzuela MT, et al. Persistence of antibodies in adolescents 18-24 months after immunization with one, two, or three doses of 4CMenB meningococcal serogroup B vaccine. *Hum Vaccin Immunother.* 2013;9(11):2304–2310

9. Kimura A, Toneatto D, Kleinschmidt A, Wang H, Dull P. Immunogenicity and safety of a multicomponent meningococcal serogroup B vaccine and a quadrivalent meningococcal CRM197 conjugate vaccine against serogroups A, C, W-135, and Y in adults who are at increased risk for occupational exposure to meningococcal isolates. *Clin Vaccine Immunol.* 2011;18(3):483–486

10. Read RC, Baxter D, Chadwick DR, et al. Effect of a quadrivalent meningococcal ACWY glycoconjugate or a serogroup B meningococcal vaccine on meningococcal carriage: an observer-blind, phase 3 randomised clinical trial. *Lancet.* 2014;384(9960):2123–2131

11. Block SL, Szenborn L, Daly W, et al. Comparative evaluation of two different investigational meningococcal ABCWY vaccine formulations in adolescents and young adults. Presented at: Infectious Disease Week; October 8–12, 2014; Philadelphia, PA. Available at: https://idsa.confex.com/idsa/2014/webprogram/

Paper46007.html. Accessed January 21, 2016

12. Toneatto D, Ismaili S, Ypma E, Vienken K, Oster P, Dull P. The first use of an investigational multicomponent meningococcal serogroup B vaccine (4CMenB) in humans. *Hum Vaccin.* 2011;7(6):646–653

13. Marshall HS, Richmond PC, Nissen MD, et al. A phase 2 open-label safety and immunogenicity study of a meningococcal B bivalent rLP2086 vaccine in healthy adults. *Vaccine.* 2013;31(12):1569–1575

14. Sheldon EA, Schwartz H, Jiang Q, Giardina PC, Perez JL. A phase 1, randomized, open-label, active-controlled trial to assess the safety of a meningococcal serogroup B bivalent rLP2086 vaccine in healthy adults. *Hum Vaccin Immunother.* 2012;8(7):888–895

15. Richmond PC, Marshall HS, Nissen MD, et al; 2001 Study Investigators. Safety, immunogenicity, and tolerability of meningococcal serogroup B bivalent recombinant lipoprotein 2086 vaccine in healthy adolescents: a randomised, single-blind, placebo-controlled, phase 2 trial. *Lancet Infect Dis.* 2012;12(8):597–607

16. Senders S, Bhuyan P, Jiang Q, et al. Immunogenicity, tolerability and safety in adolescents of bivalent rLP2086, a meningococcal serogroup B vaccine, coadministered with quadrivalent human papilloma virus vaccine. *J Clin Infect Dis.* 2016;35(5):548–554

17. Costa I, Pajon R, Granoff DM. Human factor H (FH) impairs protective meningococcal anti-FHbp antibody responses and the antibodies enhance FH binding. *MBio.* 2014;5(5):e01625–e14

18. MacNeil JR, Rubin L, Folaranmi T, Ortega-Sanchez IR, Patel M, Martin SW; ABCs Team. Cost-effectiveness of conjugate meningococcal vaccination strategies in the United States. *Pediatrics.* 2005;115(5):1220–1232

19. Centers for Disease Control and Prevention. Use of serogroup B meningococcal vaccines in adolescents and young adults: recommendations of the Advisory Committee on Immunization Practices, 2015. *MMWR Morb Mortal Wkly Rep.* 2015;64(41):1171–1176

Recommended Childhood and Adolescent Immunization Schedule—United States, 2017

- *Policy Statement*

POLICY STATEMENT Organizational Principles to Guide and Define the Child Health
Care System and/or Improve the Health of all Children

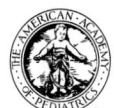

American Academy
of Pediatrics

DEDICATED TO THE HEALTH OF ALL CHILDREN™

Recommended Childhood and Adolescent Immunization Schedule—United States, 2017

COMMITTEE ON INFECTIOUS DISEASES

The 2017 recommended childhood and adolescent immunization schedules have been approved by the American Academy of Pediatrics, the Advisory Committee on Immunization Practices of the Centers for Disease Control and Prevention, the American Academy of Family Physicians, and the American College of Obstetricians and Gynecologists. The schedules are revised annually to reflect current recommendations for the use of vaccines licensed by the US Food and Drug Administration.

The 2017 format of Fig 1 is similar to the 2016 schedule consisting of a single table for persons from birth through 18 years of age. The yellow bars indicate the recommended age range for all children and contain a notation indicating the recommended dose number by age. The green bars indicate the recommended catch-up age. The purple bars designate the range for immunization for certain groups at high risk. The blue bars indicate the range of recommended doses for persons in non–high-risk groups who may receive a vaccine, subject to individual decision-making. The white boxes show the ages at which a vaccine is not recommended routinely. The columns that begin with a gray-shaded box indicate vaccine recommendations for school entry and at adolescent visits. The following specific changes have been made to the 2017 schedule:

- A column has been added for adolescents at 16 years of age. This age group has been separated from 17- to 18-year-olds to emphasize the need for a meningococcal conjugate vaccine (MenACWY) booster dose at age 16.

- Reference to live attenuated influenza vaccine (LAIV) has been removed from the influenza vaccine row.

- A blue bar has been added to the human papillomavirus (HPV) vaccine row at 9 to 10 years to indicate that, even in the absence of a high-risk condition, children may receive HPV vaccine series at this age.

DOI: 10.1542/peds.2016-4007

PEDIATRICS (ISSN Numbers: Print, 0031-4005; Online, 1098-4275).

Copyright © 2017 by the American Academy of Pediatrics

FINANCIAL DISCLOSURE: The authors have indicated they do not have a financial relationship relevant to this article to disclose.

FUNDING: No potential funding.

POTENTIAL CONFLICT OF INTEREST: The authors have indicated they have no potential conflicts of interest to disclose.

To cite: AAP COMMITTEE ON INFECTIOUS DISEASES. Recommended Childhood and Adolescent Immunization Schedule—United States, 2017. *Pediatrics.* 2017;139(3):e20164007

Figure 2 is the catch-up immunization schedule offering recommendations for children and adolescents who start late or are >1 month behind. As in previous years, the catch-up schedule is divided into sections for children ages 4 months through 6 years and children and adolescents ages 7 through 18 years. No changes have been made to the 2017 catch-up immunization figure. Tables (job aids) are available to assist in the clarification of the recommended use of *Haemophilus influenzae* type b, pneumococcal, and pertussis-containing vaccines as a function of age; the number of doses previously administered; and the time interval since the last dose.

Figure 3 is a new table that addresses which vaccines may be indicated for persons aged 0 through 18 years who have a specific medical indication. This figure indicates vaccines that may be administered during pregnancy or to children and adolescents with an immunocompromising condition; kidney, heart, or liver disease; a cochlear implant; a cerebrospinal fluid leak; asplenia; a complement deficiency; or diabetes. Figure 3 in the childhood/adolescent schedule is similar to Fig 2 in the adult immunization schedule.

Footnotes contain recommendations for routine vaccination, for catch-up vaccination, as well as for vaccination of children and adolescents with high-risk conditions or in special circumstances. Recommendations in the figures should be read with the corresponding footnotes. Changes have been made to the following footnotes:

- Hepatitis B. Updated recommendations reflect that a monovalent birth dose should be administered to all newborns within 24 hours of birth. Revised wording indicates that infants born to hepatitis B surface antigen (HBsAg)–positive mothers should be tested for HBsAg and antibody to HBsAg at 9 through 12 months (rather than 9 through 18 months).

- *Haemophilus influenzae* type b. Comvax vaccine (Merck, Whitehouse Station, NJ) has been removed because the vaccine is no longer commercially available and all available doses have expired. Hiberix (GlaxoSmithKline Biologicals, Rixensart, Belgium) has been added to the list of vaccines that may be used for a primary vaccination series.

- Pneumococcal conjugate. References to PCV7 vaccine have been removed because all children who may have received PCV7 as part of a primary series have now aged out of the recommendation for pneumococcal vaccine.

- Influenza. Wording has been added to indicate that LAIV is not recommended for the 2016–2017 influenza season.

- Meningococcal ACWY. Recommendations now include vaccination of children with HIV infection.

- Meningococcal B. Wording has been modified to note that persons aged 16 through 23 years may be vaccinated on the basis of clinical discretion. Updated recommendations regarding a 2-dose Trumenba (Wyeth Pharmaceuticals, Philadelphia, PA) schedule have been added.

- Tdap. Revised wording indicates a preference for administration of 1 dose for pregnant adolescents, and this dose should be administered as early as possible in the 27- to 36-week gestational age period. Wording is changed to indicate that for children aged 7 through 10 years who receive Tdap as part of a catch-up series, either Tdap or Td may be administered for the adolescent dose at 11 through 12 years.

- Human papillomavirus. Wording reflects that the number of recommended doses is based on age at administration of the first dose. Two doses are recommended for persons starting the series before their 15th birthday, whereas 3 doses are recommended for those who start the series on or after their 15th birthday and for persons with certain immunocompromising conditions. 2vHPV (Cervarix ; GlaxoSmithKline Biologicals, Rixensart, Belgium) has been removed from the schedule because this vaccine is no longer available and all available doses expired before January 1, 2017.

In addition to publication of the schedules in this issue of *Pediatrics*, the 2017 version of Figs 1 through 3, the catch-up schedule, the footnotes, and job aids are available at the AAP Web site (https://redbook. solutions.aap.org/selfserve/ssPage. aspx?SelfServeContentId=Immunization_ Schedules) and the Centers for Disease Control and Prevention Web site (https://www.cdc.gov/vaccines/ schedules/). A parent-friendly vaccine schedule for children and adolescents is available at http://www.cdc.gov/ vaccines/schedules/index.html. An adult immunization schedule is published in February of each year and is available at www.cdc.gov/ vaccines.

Clinically significant adverse events that follow immunization should be reported to the Vaccine Adverse Event Reporting System (VAERS). Guidance about how to obtain and complete a VAERS form can be obtained at www.vaers.hhs.gov or by calling 800-822-7967. Additional information can be found in the *Red Book* and at *Red Book* Online (http:// aapredbook.aappublications.org/). Statements from the Advisory Committee on Immunization Practices of the Centers for Disease Control and Prevention that contain detailed recommendations for individual vaccines, including recommendations for children with high-risk conditions, are available at www.cdc.gov/vaccines/pubs/ACIP-list.htm. Information on new vaccine releases, vaccine supplies, and interim recommendations resulting from vaccine shortages and statements on specific vaccines can be found at www.aapredbook.org/news/vaccstatus.shtml and www.cdc.gov/vaccines/pubs/ACIP-list.htm.

COMMITTEE ON INFECTIOUS DISEASE, 2016-2017

Carrie L. Byington, MD, FAAP, Chairperson

Yvonne A. Maldonado, MD, FAAP, Vice Chairperson

Elizabeth D. Barnett, MD, FAAP

James D. Campbell, MD, FAAP

H. Dele Davies, MD, MS, MHCM, FAAP

Ruth Lynfield, MD, FAAP

Flor M. Munoz, MD, FAAP

Dawn Nolt, MD, MPH, FAAP

Ann Christine Nyquist, MD, MSPH, FAAP

Sean O'Leary, MD, MPH, FAAP

Mobeen H. Rathore, MD, FAAP

Mark H. Sawyer, MD, FAAP

William J. Steinbach, MD, FAAP

Tina Q. Tan, MD, FAAP

Theoklis E. Zaoutis, MD, MSCE, FAAP

EX OFFICIO

David W. Kimberlin, MD, FAAP – *Red Book* Editor

Michael T. Brady, MD, FAAP – *Red Book* Associate Editor

Mary Anne Jackson, MD, FAAP – *Red Book* Associate Editor

Sarah S. Long, MD, FAAP – *Red Book* Associate Editor

Henry H. Bernstein, DO, MHCM, FAAP – *Red Book* Online Associate Editor

H. Cody Meissner, MD, FAAP – Visual *Red Book* Associate Editor

LIAISONS

Douglas Campos-Outcalt, MD, MPA – *American Academy of Family Physicians*

Amanda C. Cohn, MD, FAAP – *Centers for Disease Control and Prevention*

Karen M. Farizo, MD – *US Food and Drug Administration*

Marc Fischer, MD, FAAP – *Centers for Disease Control and Prevention*

Bruce G. Gellin, MD, MPH – *National Vaccine Program Office*

Richard L. Gorman, MD, FAAP – *National Institutes of Health*

Natasha Halasa, MD, MPH, FAAP – *Pediatric Infectious Diseases Society*

Joan L. Robinson, MD – *Canadian Paediatric Society*

Jamie Deseda-Tous, MD – *Sociedad Latinoamericana de Infectologia Pediatrica (SLIPE)*

Geoffrey R. Simon, MD, FAAP – *Committee on Practice Ambulatory Medicine*

Jeffrey R. Starke, MD, FAAP – *American Thoracic Society*

STAFF

Jennifer M. Frantz, MPH

Role of the School Nurse in Providing School Health Services

• *Policy Statement*

POLICY STATEMENT Organizational Principles to Guide and Define the Child Health
Care System and/or Improve the Health of all Children

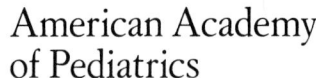
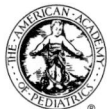

American Academy
of Pediatrics

DEDICATED TO THE HEALTH OF ALL CHILDREN™

Role of the School Nurse in Providing School Health Services

COUNCIL ON SCHOOL HEALTH

abstract

The American Academy of Pediatrics recognizes the important role school nurses play in promoting the optimal biopsychosocial health and well-being of school-aged children in the school setting. Although the concept of a school nurse has existed for more than a century, uniformity among states and school districts regarding the role of a registered professional nurse in schools and the laws governing it are lacking. By understanding the benefits, roles, and responsibilities of school nurses working as a team with the school physician, as well as their contributions to school-aged children, pediatricians can collaborate with, support, and promote school nurses in their own communities, thus improving the health, wellness, and safety of children and adolescents.

DOI: 10.1542/peds.2016-0852

PEDIATRICS (ISSN Numbers: Print, 0031-4005; Online, 1098-4275).

To cite: AAP COUNCIL ON SCHOOL HEALTH. Role of the School Nurse in Providing School Health Services. *Pediatrics.* 2016;137(6):e20160852

INTRODUCTION

Traditionally, the school nursing role was designed to support educational achievement by promoting student attendance. The first school nurse, Lina Rogers, was appointed in 1902 to tend to the health of 8671 students in 4 separate schools in New York City. Her early success in reducing absenteeism led to the hiring of 12 more nurses. Within 1 year, medical exclusions decreased by 99%.[1]

Over the past century, the role of the school nurse has expanded to include critical components, such as surveillance, chronic disease management, emergency preparedness, behavioral health assessment, ongoing health education, extensive case management, and much more. Although the position has taken on a more comprehensive approach, the core focus of keeping students healthy and in school remains unchanged. School attendance is essential for academic success.

School nurses provide both individual and population health through their daily access to large numbers of students, making them well positioned to address and coordinate the health care needs of children and adolescents. The impact of social determinants of health are felt in the school setting and well known to school nurses.[2,3] School nursing is a specialized practice of professional nursing that advances the well-being, academic success, and lifelong achievement and health of students. To that end, school nurses understand and educate about normal development; promote health and safety, including a healthy environment; intervene with actual and potential health problems; provide case-management services; and actively collaborate with physicians who work in schools, such as medical advisors and team physicians, families, community service providers, and health care providers, to build student and family capacity for adaptation, self-management, self-advocacy, and learning.[4,5]

School nurses and pediatricians, both community- and school-based, working together can be a great example of team-based care, defined as the provision of comprehensive health services to individuals, families, and/or their communities by at least 2 health professionals who work collaboratively along with patients, family caregivers, and community service providers on shared goals within and across settings to achieve care that is safe, effective, patient-centered, timely, efficient, and equitable. The principles of team-based health care are as follows: shared goals, clear roles, mutual trust, effective communication, and measurable processes and outcomes.[6,7] As a health care team member, school nurses connect students and their families to the medical home and can support coordination of care.[8–10]

As more children with special health care needs attend school, the school nurse plays a vital role in disease management, often working closely with children and their parents to reinforce the medical home's recommendations and provide treatment(s) during the school day. Feedback mechanisms regarding student response to the treatment

plan in school are critical to timely medical management in areas such as attention-deficit/hyperactivity disorder, diabetes, life-threatening allergies, asthma, and seizures as well as for the growing population of children with behavioral health concerns. School nurses play an important role in interpreting medical recommendations within the educational environment and, for example, may participate in the development of action plans for epilepsy management and safe transportation of a child with special health care needs.[11,12] School nurses may also provide insight to a student's pediatrician when attendance concerns, parental noncompliance with medical home goals, or even neglect or abuse is suspected. In addition, with increased awareness recently about such issues as head injuries, the school nurse is poised to offer on-site assessment of the student's postconcussion progress and adaptations required in the educational plan.[13]

School nurses are also participants in public health arenas, such as immunization, obesity prevention, substance abuse assessment, tobacco control, and asthma education. Their daily presence in the school setting further augments and potentiates the pediatrician's professional interventions with individual children and adolescents.[14]

Collaboration among pediatricians, families, school staff, school physicians, and school nurses is increasingly critical to optimal health care in both office and community settings. This policy statement describes the crucial aspects of the school nurse's role, its relationship to pediatric practice, and recommendations to facilitate productive working relationships benefiting all school-aged children and adolescents. An important and more detailed reference for school health, *School Health: Policy and Practice*, provides a more in-depth

description about health and schools, including a comprehensive chapter on school health services, including school nurses.[15]

BACKGROUND

During the past few decades, major legal, medical, and societal changes have critically influenced the need for registered professional nurses (hereafter referred to as school nurse) in the school setting.

Legal Changes

Social attitudes that promote inclusion, as well as state and federal laws such as the Individuals With Disabilities Act (Pub L No. 101-476 [1990]) and section 504 of the Rehabilitation Act of 1973 (Pub L No. 93-112), specify disability rights and access to education, resulting in more children requiring and receiving nursing care and other health-related services in school.[16,17]

The Privacy, Security, and Breach Notification Rules of the Health Insurance Portability and Accountability Act of 1996 (Pub L No. 104-191) and Family Educational Rights and Privacy Act (Pub L No. 93-380 [1974]) laws impose important privacy protections for a student's health information. However, myths and misunderstanding among parents, pediatricians, and school nurses about these laws can inadvertently hinder efficient, efficacious, and cost-effective case management of student health care needs. School nurses work with parents to educate, facilitate, and expedite necessary communication between schools and the medical home. School nurses facilitate parental permissions for information exchange and serve as a link between parent and pediatrician to establish essential and effective individualized health care plans for students at school.

Medical Changes

Survival rates of preterm infants have increased to more than 80% of infants born at 26 weeks' gestation and to more than 90% of infants born after 27 weeks' gestation, resulting in an increase in the number of children with moderate to severe disabilities and learning or behavioral problems.[18,19]

Chronic illnesses also are on the rise. In 2010, 215 000 people younger than 20 years in the United States had a diagnosis of either type 1 or type 2 diabetes.[20] The prevalence of food allergies among children younger than 18 years increased from 3.4% in 1997–1999 to 5.1% in 2009–2011.[21] An average of 1 in 10 school-aged children has asthma,[22] contributing to more than 13 million missed school days per year.[23] As the number of students with chronic conditions grows, the need for health care at school has increased.[24] The rise in enrollment of students with special health care needs increases the need for school nurses and school health services.[25]

Caring for children with chronic conditions in schools requires registered professional school nurses. However, the reality is that school nurse staffing patterns vary widely across the United States.[14] When a school nurse is not available at all times, the American Academy of Pediatrics, the National Association of School Nurses, and the American Nurses Association recommend that delegated, unlicensed assistive personnel be trained and supervised in the knowledge, skills, and composure to deliver specific school health services under the guidance of a registered nurse. The delegation of nursing duties must be consistent with the requirements of state nurse practice acts, state regulations, and guidelines provided by professional nursing organizations.[26] Delegation does not obviate the need for continued advocacy for full-time professional school nurses in each

building. American Academy of Pediatrics' policy has previously supported ratios of 1 school nurse to 750 students in the healthy student population and 1:225 for student populations requiring daily professional nursing services. However, the use of a ratio for workload determination in school nursing is inadequate to fill the increasingly complex health needs of students.[27,28]

Societal Changes

Families face multiple barriers to adequate health care, including accessibility, availability, and affordability. Many working parents also fear job loss if they are absent from work to attend a child's medical appointment, forcing them to leave illnesses and chronic conditions unattended.[29] The availability of school nurses to children and families helps to increase access to the medical home for comprehensive care as well as to essential public health functions, such as immunization or obesity prevention.

Schools and school nurses can partner with medical homes and public health agencies to increase access to or to deliver vaccines. The presence of registered nurses in schools is correlated with fewer immunization exemptions in schools.[30] School nurses can improve vaccine uptake among students and staff by providing accurate information about vaccines. They can also remind students, families, and staff of immunization schedules and retrieve and update immunization records for state-specific reporting requirements.

Increasing rates of obesity over the past several decades represent alarming risks for the current and future health of children and adolescents. The percentage of children 6 to 11 years of age with obesity increased from 7% in 1980 to nearly 18% in 2012, with more than

one-third of children now overweight or obese.[31]

The immediate and long-term effects on health range from cardiovascular disease and diabetes mellitus to social problems because of stigmatization.[31] The school nurse, with his or her daily presence in school and access to large populations of students, is well positioned to prevent and/or intervene on this health issue through (1) implementing BMI screenings and referrals to the medical home as needed, (2) collaborating with food service personnel and administrators to advocate for and to provide nutritional meals and snacks, (3) working with school staff to promote opportunities for physical activity, (4) educating parents about healthy lifestyles, and (5) involving the community providers and organizations in these efforts.

School-based health centers complement school nursing services by delivering a continuum of diagnostic and treatment services on-site and collaborating for prevention, early intervention, and harm-reduction services. To be most effective, school nurses and school-based health center staff need to develop close communication and referral systems, similar to school nurses and any medical home.[32]

Another societal change is the increase in students identified with mental or behavioral health issues. One in five young people between the ages of 4 and 17 years experiences symptoms of minor to severe mental/behavioral health problems. One in ten children and adolescents has a mental illness severe enough to cause some level of impairment; yet, in any given year, only about 12% of children in need of mental health services actually receive them.[33] Pediatricians, both community- and school-based, and school nurses need to collaborate to advocate for professional resources addressing this burgeoning problem that affects both their practices.[9]

Health care reform, including how health care is financed and delivered, is a significant societal change. In addition to improving quality of health care, cost containment is a major aim of health care reform. Working closely with parents, school staff, and community pediatricians, school nurses are well positioned to help contain costs. Initiatives such as chronic disease management, early detection of behavioral health issues, and obesity prevention are just a few examples of how school nurses contribute to significant cost savings for the health care system. There is growing evidence that full-time school nurse staffing results in cost savings for society. In 1 study, for each dollar spent on school nurses, $2.20 was saved in parent loss of work time, teacher time, and procedures performed in school rather than in a more costly health care setting.[34]

Healthy Students Are Better Learners

Understanding the complex factors that lead to academic underachievement, poor school attendance, student drop out, and poor health outcomes is critical for the practicing community and school pediatrician, the educational community, and lawmakers alike. Physical and emotional health problems rank high among the factors contributing to chronic absenteeism (missing 10% or more of school days for any reason), a key risk factor for failing to complete school.[35] Health-related problems contributing to academic underachievement are a primary responsibility of the medical home, the family, and the school health services team led by the school nurse in the health office on a daily basis. A growing body of research indicates that school nurses can improve attendance by reducing illness rates

through education about preventive health care, early recognition of disease processes, improving chronic disease management, and increasing return-to-class rates.[36] Of the students seen by the school nurse for illness or injury, 95% were able to return to the classroom. Without a school nurse, unlicensed personnel who are uncertain what to do medically are at risk of sending children home from school or to the emergency department needlessly.[37]

The presence of a coordinated school health program, often led by school nurses, contributes to both educational achievement and the educational system.[38] School nurses can provide key leadership in all the components of the Whole School, Whole Community, Whole Child model.[39] Direct health services provided by a school nurse are linked to positive academic achievement. With a nurse in the school, other school staff, including teachers, divert less time from their primary job responsibilities to deal with student health issues.[40]

CONCLUSIONS

School nurses, working with pediatric patient-centered medical homes, school physicians, and families, are in a critical position to identify unmet health needs of large populations of children and adolescents in the school setting. Promoting the presence of a qualified school nurse in every school and a school physician in every district fosters the close interdependent relationship between health and education. Academic achievement, improved attendance, and better graduation rates can be a direct result of a coordinated team effort among the medical, family, and educational homes all recognizing that good health and strong education cannot be separated.

RECOMMENDATIONS

1. Pediatricians can advocate for a minimum of 1 full-time professional school nurse in every school with medical oversight from a school physician in every school district as the optimal staffing to ensure the health and safety of students during the school day.

2. Pediatricians can ask school-related questions, including about health problems contributing to chronic absenteeism, at each visit and provide relevant information directly to the school. Electronic health records should include the name of the patient's school and primary contact at the school. Health Information Exchange requirements, as defined in stage 3 of Meaningful Use, should permit the direct exchange of school-related information collected in the pediatrician's office at each visit, including attendance and health problems contributing to absenteeism.

3. Pediatricians can establish a working relationship with school nurses to improve chronic condition management. Establishing an agreed-upon method of communication with the use of standardized forms and securing permission to exchange information are ways to facilitate this relationship. Communication and collaboration will also aid in the development of Individualized Health Care Plans, care coordination, and planning for transition from pediatric to adult health care.

4. Pediatricians can include school nurses as important team members in the delivery of health care for children and adolescents and in the design of integrated health systems, including school-based health centers.

LEAD AUTHORS

Breena Welch Holmes, MD
Anne Sheetz, MPH, RN

COUNCIL ON SCHOOL HEALTH EXECUTIVE COMMITTEE, 2015–2016

Breena Welch Holmes, MD, FAAP, Chairperson
Mandy Allison, MD, MEd, MSPH, FAAP
Richard Ancona, MD, FAAP
Elliott Attisha, DO, FAAP
Nathaniel Beers, MD, MPA, FAAP
Cheryl De Pinto, MD, MPH, FAAP
Peter Gorski, MD, MPA, FAAP
Chris Kjolhede, MD, MPH, FAAP
Marc Lerner, MD, FAAP
Adrienne Weiss-Harrison, MD, FAAP
Thomas Young, MD, FAAP

CONSULTANT

Anne Sheetz, MPH, RN

LIAISONS

Nina Fekaris, MS, BSN, RN, NCSN – *National Association of School Nurses*
Veda Johnson, MD, FAAP – *School-Based Health Alliance*
Sheryl Kataoka, MD, MSHS – *American Academy of Child and Adolescent Psychiatry*
Sandra Leonard, DNP, RN, FNP – *Centers for Disease Control and Prevention*

FORMER EXECUTIVE COMMITTEE MEMBERS

Cynthia DiLaura Devore, MD, FAAP, Past Chairperson
Jeffrey Okamoto, MD, FAAP, Immediate Past Chairperson
Mark Minier, MD, FAAP

FORMER LIAISONS

Carolyn Duff, RN, MS, NCSN – *National Association of School of Nurses*
Linda Grant, MD, MPH, FAAP – *American School Health Association*
Elizabeth Mattey, MSN, RN, NCSN – *National Association of School Nurses*
Mary Vernon-Smiley, MD, MPH, MDiv – *Centers for Disease Control and Prevention*

STAFF

Madra Guinn-Jones, MPH

REFERENCES

1. Zaiger D. Historical perspectives of school nursing. In: Selekman J, ed. *School Nursing: A Comprehensive Text.* 2nd ed. Philadelphia, PA: F.A. Davis; 2013:2–24

2. National Association of School Nurses. Resolution: public health as the foundation of school nursing practice. Available at: www.nasn.org/Portals/0/statements/resolutionph.pdf. Accessed April 15, 2015

3. American Academy of Pediatrics, Council on Community Pediatrics. Policy statement: community pediatrics: navigating the intersection of medicine, public health and social determinants. *Pediatrics.* 2013;131(3):623–628

4. National Association of School Nurses. Position statement: definition of school nursing. Available at: http://nasnupgrade.winxweb.com/PolicyAdvocacy/PositionPapersand Reports/NASNPositionState mentsFullView/tabid/462/ArticleId/87/Role-of-the-School-Nurse-Revised-2011. Accessed May 12, 2014

5. Devore CD, Wheeler LS; American Academy of Pediatrics, Council on School Health. Policy statement: role of the school physician. *Pediatrics.* 2013;131(1):178–182

6. Mitchell P, Wynia M, Golden R, et al *Core Principles and Values of Effective Team-Based Health Care.* Washington, DC: National Academies Press; 2012

7. Committee on Pediatric Workforce. Policy statement: scope of practice issues in the delivery of pediatric health care. *Pediatrics.* 2013;131(6):1211–1216

8. American Academy of Pediatrics, Medical Home Initiatives for Children With Special Needs Project Advisory Committee. Policy statement: the medical home. *Pediatrics.* 2002;110(1):184–186. Reaffirmed May 2008

9. Council on Children With Disabilities and Medical Home Implementation Project Advisory Committee. Policy statement: patient- and family-centered care coordination: a framework for integrating care for children and youth across multiple systems. *Pediatrics.* 2014;133(5). Available at: www.pediatrics.org/cgi/content/full/133/5/e1451

10. McAllister JW, Presler E, Cooley WC. Practice-based care coordination: a medical home essential. *Pediatrics.* 2007;120(3). Available at: www.pediatrics.org/cgi/content/full/120/3/e723

11. Hartman AL, Devore CD ; American Academy of Pediatrics, Section on Neurology, Council on School Health. Rescue medicine for epilepsy in education settings. *Pediatrics.* 2016;137(1):e2015–3876

12. American Academy of Pediatrics, Committee on Injury, Violence, and Poison Prevention. School bus transportation of children with special health care needs. *Pediatrics.* 2001;108(2):516–518. Reaffirmed May 2013

13. Halstead ME, McAvoy K, Devore CD, Carl R, Lee M, Logan K; Council on Sports Medicine and Fitness; Council on School Health. Clinical report: returning to learning following a concussion. *Pediatrics.* 2013;132(5):948–957

14. Robert Wood Johnson Foundation. Unlocking the potential of school nursing: keeping children healthy, in school, and ready to learn. *Charting Nursing's Future.* Princeton, NJ: Robert Wood Johnson Foundation; 2010;14:1–8. Available at: www.rwjf.org/content/dam/farm/reports/issue_briefs/2010/rwjf64263. Accessed May 12, 2014

15. American Academy of Pediatrics, Council on School Health. *School Health: Policy and Practice.* 6th ed. Elk Grove Village, IL: American Academy of Pediatrics; 2004

16. Gibbons L, Lehr K, Selekman J. Federal laws protecting children and youth with disabilities in the schools. In: Selekman J, ed. *School Nursing: A Comprehensive Text.* 2nd ed. Philadelphia, PA: F.A. Davis; 2013:257–283

17. Raymond JA. The integration of children dependent on medical technology into public schools. *J Sch Nurs.* 2009;25(3):186–194

18. Allen MC, Cristofalo EA, Kim C. Outcomes of preterm infants: morbidity replaces mortality. *Clin Perinatol.* 2011;38(3):441–454

19. Roberts G, Lim J, Doyle LW, Anderson PJ. High rates of school readiness difficulties at 5 years of age in very preterm infants compared with term controls. *J Dev Behav Pediatr.* 2011;32(2):117–124

20. Centers for Disease Control and Prevention. National diabetes fact sheet, 2011. Available at: www.cdc.gov/diabetes/pubs/pdf/ndfs_2011.pdf. Accessed May 12, 2014

21. Jackson KD, Howie LD, Akinbami LJ. Trends in allergic conditions among children: United States, 1997-2011, no. 121. Atlanta, GA: National Center for Health Statistics; May 2013. Available at: www.cdc.gov/nchs/data/databriefs/db121.htm#summary. Accessed May 12, 2014

22. Forum on Child and Family Statistics. America's children: key national indicators of well-being, 2013. Available at: www.childstats.gov/americaschildren/glance.asp. Accessed May 12, 2014

23. McCarthy AM, Kelly MW, Reed D. Medication administration practices of school nurses. *J Sch Health*. 2000;70(9):371–376

24. Van Cleave J, Gortmaker SL, Perrin JM. Dynamics of obesity and chronic health conditions among children and youth. *JAMA*. 2010;303(7):623–630

25. Clements KM, Barfield WD, Ayadi MF, Wilber N. Preterm birth-associated cost of early intervention services: an analysis by gestational age. *Pediatrics*. 2007;119(4). Available at: www.pediatrics.org/cgi/content/full/119/4/e866

26. American Academy of Pediatrics, Council on School Health. Policy statement: guidance for the administration of medication in school. *Pediatrics*. 2009;124(4):1244–1251. Reaffirmed February 2013

27. Magalnick H, Mazyck D; American Academy of Pediatrics, Council on School Health. Policy statement: role of the school nurse in providing school health services. *Pediatrics*. 2008;121(5):1052–1056

28. National Association of School Nurses. Position statement: school nurse workload: staffing for safe care. Available at: www.nasn.org/PolicyAdvocacy/PositionPapersandReports/NASNPositionStatementsFullView/tabid/462/ArticleId/803/School-Nurse-Workload-Staffing-for-Safe-Care-Adopted-January-2015. Accessed April 15, 2015

29. Smolensky E, Gootman JA, eds. *Working Families and Growing Kids: Caring for Children and Adolescents*. Washington, DC: National Academies Press; 2003

30. Salmon DA, Omer SB, Moulton LH, et al. Exemptions to school immunization requirements: the role of school-level requirements, policies, and procedures. *Am J Public Health*. 2005;95(3):436–440

31. Centers for Disease Control and Prevention. Childhood obesity facts. Available at: www.cdc.gov/healthyschools/obesity/facts.htm. Accessed September 30, 2015

32. Council on School Health. Policy statement: school-based health centers and pediatric practice. *Pediatrics*. 2012;129(2):387–393

33. Substance Abuse and Mental Health Services Administration. *Mental Health, United States, 2010*. Rockville, MD: Substance Abuse and Mental Health Services Administration; 2012. HHS Publication (SMA) 12-4681

34. Wang LY, Vernon-Smiley M, Gapinski MA, Desisto M, Maughan E, Sheetz A. Cost-benefit study of school nursing services. *JAMA Pediatr*. 2014;168(7):642–648

35. Moonie S, Sterling DA, Figgs LW, Castro M. The relationship between school absence, academic performance, and asthma status. *J Sch Health*. 2008;78(3):140–148

36. Basch CE. Healthier students are better learners: high-quality, strategically planned, and effectively coordinated school health programs must be a fundamental mission of schools to help close the achievement gap. *J Sch Health*. 2011;81(10):650–662

37. Pennington N, Delaney E. The number of students sent home by school nurses compared to unlicensed personnel. *J Sch Nurs*. 2008;24(5):290–297

38. Vinciullo FM, Bradley BJ. A correlational study of the relationship between a coordinated school health program and school achievement: a case for school health. *J Sch Nurs*. 2009;25(6):453–465

39. Association for Supervision and Curriculum Development. Whole school, whole community, whole child: a collaborative approach to learning and health. 2014. Available at: www.ascd.org/ASCD/pdf/siteASCD/publications/wholechild/wscc-a-collaborative-approach.pdf. Accessed September 30, 2015

40. Baisch MJ, Lundeen SP, Murphy MK. Evidence-based research on the value of school nurses in an urban school system. *J Sch Health*. 2011;81(2):74–80

Safe Sleep and Skin-to-Skin Care in the Neonatal Period for Healthy Term Newborns

- *Clinical Report*

CLINICAL REPORT   Guidance for the Clinician in Rendering Pediatric Care

American Academy
of Pediatrics

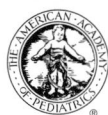

DEDICATED TO THE HEALTH OF ALL CHILDREN™

Safe Sleep and Skin-to-Skin Care in the Neonatal Period for Healthy Term Newborns

Lori Feldman-Winter, MD, MPH, FAAP, Jay P. Goldsmith, MD, FAAP, COMMITTEE ON FETUS AND NEWBORN, TASK FORCE ON SUDDEN INFANT DEATH SYNDROME

abstract

Skin-to-skin care (SSC) and rooming-in have become common practice in the newborn period for healthy newborns with the implementation of maternity care practices that support breastfeeding as delineated in the World Health Organization's "Ten Steps to Successful Breastfeeding." SSC and rooming-in are supported by evidence that indicates that the implementation of these practices increases overall and exclusive breastfeeding, safer and healthier transitions, and improved maternal-infant bonding. In some cases, however, the practice of SSC and rooming-in may pose safety concerns, particularly with regard to sleep. There have been several recent case reports and case series of severe and sudden unexpected postnatal collapse in the neonatal period among otherwise healthy newborns and near fatal or fatal events related to sleep, suffocation, and falls from adult hospital beds. Although these are largely case reports, there are potential dangers of unobserved SSC immediately after birth and throughout the postpartum hospital period as well as with unobserved rooming-in for at-risk situations. Moreover, behaviors that are modeled in the hospital after birth, such as sleep position, are likely to influence sleeping practices after discharge. Hospitals and birthing centers have found it difficult to develop policies that will allow SSC and rooming-in to continue in a safe manner. This clinical report is intended for birthing centers and delivery hospitals caring for healthy newborns to assist in the establishment of appropriate SSC and safe sleep policies.

DOI: 10.1542/peds.2016-1889

PEDIATRICS (ISSN Numbers: Print, 0031-4005; Online, 1098-4275).

Copyright © 2016 by the American Academy of Pediatrics

FINANCIAL DISCLOSURE: The authors have indicated they do not have a financial relationship relevant to this article to disclose.

FUNDING: No external funding.

POTENTIAL CONFLICT OF INTEREST: The authors have indicated they have no potential conflicts of interest to disclose.

To cite: Feldman-Winter L, Goldsmith JP, AAP COMMITTEE ON FETUS AND NEWBORN, AAP TASK FORCE ON SUDDEN INFANT DEATH SYNDROME. Safe Sleep and Skin-to-Skin Care in the Neonatal Period for Healthy Term Newborns. *Pediatrics.* 2016;138(3):e20161889

INTRODUCTION

Definition of Skin-to-Skin Care and Rooming-In

Skin-to-skin care (SSC) is defined as the practice of placing infants in direct contact with their mothers or other caregivers with the ventral skin of the infant facing and touching the ventral skin of the mother/

caregiver (chest-to-chest). The infant is typically naked or dressed only in a diaper to maximize the surface-to-surface contact between mother/caregiver and the infant, and the dyad is covered with prewarmed blankets, leaving the infant's head exposed. SSC is recommended for all mothers and newborns, regardless of feeding or delivery method, immediately after birth (as soon as the mother is medically stable, awake, and able to respond to her newborn) and to continue for at least 1 hour, as defined by the World Health Organization's (WHO's) "Ten Steps to Successful Breastfeeding."[1,2] SSC is also a term used to describe continued holding of the infant in the manner described above and beyond the immediate delivery period and lasting throughout infancy, whenever the mother/caregiver and infant have the opportunity. For mothers planning to breastfeed, SSC immediately after delivery and continued throughout the postpartum period also involves encouraging mothers to recognize when their infants are ready to breastfeed and providing help if needed.[2] Additional recommendations by the WHO, as part of the Baby-Friendly Hospital Initiative and endorsed by the American Academy of Pediatrics (AAP) in 2009, include the following specifications for the period of time immediately after delivery: routine procedures such as assessments and Apgar scores are conducted while SSC is underway, and procedures that may be painful or require separation should be delayed until after the first hour; if breastfeeding, these procedures should occur after the first breastfeeding is completed.[3] The AAP further delineates that the administration of vitamin K and ophthalmic prophylaxis can be delayed for at least 1 hour and up to 4 hours after delivery. The Baby-Friendly Hospital Initiative encourages continued SSC

throughout the hospital stay while rooming-in.[4]

Unless there is a medical reason for separation, such as resuscitation, SSC may be provided for all newborns. In the case of cesarean deliveries, SSC may also be provided when the mother is awake and able to respond to her infant. In some settings, SSC may be initiated in the operating room following cesarean deliveries, while in other settings SSC may begin in the recovery room. SSC for healthy newborns shall be distinguished from "kangaroo care" in this clinical report, because the latter applies to preterm newborns or infants cared for in the NICU.[5] This report is intended for mothers and infants who are well, are being cared for in the routine postpartum or mother-infant setting, and have not required resuscitation. Although sick or preterm newborns may benefit from SSC, this review is intended only for healthy term newborns. Late preterm infants (defined as a gestational age of 34–37 weeks) may also benefit from early SSC but are at increased risk of a number of early neonatal morbidities.[6]

Rooming-in is defined as allowing mothers and infants to remain together 24 hours per day while in the delivery hospital. This procedure is recommended for all mothers and their healthy newborns, regardless of feeding or delivery method, and in some cases applies to older late preterm (>35 weeks' gestation) or early term (37–39 weeks' gestation) newborns who are otherwise healthy and receiving routine care, who represent up to 70% of this population.[7] Mothers are expected to be more involved with routine care, such as feeding, holding, and bathing. Newborns may remain with their mothers unless there is a medical reason for separation for either the mother or the infant. Procedures that can be performed at the bedside can be performed while the infant is preferably being held skin-to-skin or

at least in the room with the mother. Being held skin-to-skin by the mother has been shown to decrease pain in newborns undergoing painful procedures such as blood draws.[8,9] Mothers may nap, shower, or leave the room with the expectation that the mother-infant staff members monitor the newborn at routine intervals. Mothers are encouraged to use call bells for assistance with their own care or that of their newborns.

Evidence for SSC and Rooming-In

SSC has been researched extensively as a method to provide improved physiologic stability for newborns and potential benefits for mothers. SSC immediately after birth stabilizes the newborn body temperature and can help prevent hypothermia.[10,11] SSC also helps stabilize blood glucose concentrations, decreases crying, and provides cardiorespiratory stability, especially in late preterm newborns.[12] SSC has been shown in numerous studies as a method to decrease pain in newborns being held by mothers[13–16] and fathers.[17] In preterm infants, SSC has been shown to result in improved autonomic and neurobehavioral maturation and gastrointestinal adaptation, more restful sleep patterns, less crying, and better growth.[18–21] Although not specifically studied in full-term infants, it is likely that these infants also benefit in similar ways.

SSC also benefits mothers. Immediately after birth, SSC decreases maternal stress and improves paternal perception of stress in their relationship.[22] A recent study suggested that SSC and breastfeeding within 30 minutes of birth reduce postpartum hemorrhage.[23] Experimental models indicate that mother-infant separation causes significant stress, and the consequences of this stress on the hypothalamic-pituitary-adrenal axis persist.[24] In a randomized trial examining the relationship between SSC and maternal depression and stress, both depression scores and salivary cortisol concentrations were lower over the first month among postpartum mothers providing SSC compared with mothers who were provided no guidance about SSC.[22] For breastfeeding mother-infant dyads, SSC enhances the opportunity for an early first breastfeeding, which, in turn, leads to more readiness to breastfeed, an organized breastfeeding suckling pattern, and more success in exclusive and overall breastfeeding,[12,25,26] even after cesarean deliveries.[27] Further evidence shows a benefit for mothers after cesarean deliveries who practice SSC as soon as the mother is alert and responsive in increased breastfeeding initiation, decreased time to the first breastfeeding, reduced formula supplementation, and increased bonding and maternal satisfaction.[28] Increasing rates of breastfeeding ultimately have short- and long-term health benefits, such as decreased risk of infections, obesity, cancer, and sudden infant death syndrome.[3]

The evidence for rooming-in also extends beyond infant feeding practices and is consistent with contemporary models of family-centered care.[29] Rooming-in and the maternity care practices aligned with keeping mothers and newborns together in a hospital setting were defined as best practice but not fully implemented in the post–World War II era, largely because of nursing culture and the presumption that newborns were safer in a sterile nursery environment.[30] Rooming-in leads to improved patient satisfaction.[31,32] Integrated mother-infant care leads to optimal outcomes for healthy mothers and infants, including those with neonatal abstinence syndrome.[33] Rooming-in also provides more security, may avoid newborn abductions or switches, leads to decreased infant abandonment,[34] and provides more

opportunity for supervised maternal-newborn interactions.[35] Hospital staff members caring for mother-infant dyads have more opportunities to empower mothers to care for their infants than when infant care is conducted without the mother and in a separate nursery. For the breastfeeding mother-infant dyad, rooming-in may help to support cue-based feeding, leading to increased frequency of breastfeeding, especially in the first few days[36]; decreased hyperbilirubinemia; and increased likelihood of continued breastfeeding up to 6 months.[37]

SSC and rooming-in are 2 of the important steps in the WHO's "Ten Steps to Successful Breastfeeding" and serve as the basic tenets for a baby-friendly–designated delivery hospital.[1,38,39] The Ten Steps include practices that also improve patient safety and outcomes by supporting a more physiologic transition immediately after delivery; maintaining close contact between the mother and her newborn, which decreases the risk of infection and sepsis; increasing the opportunity for the development of a protective immunologic environment; decreasing stress responses by the mother and her infant; and enhancing sleep patterns in the mother.[40-42]

SAFETY CONCERNS REGARDING IMMEDIATE SSC

Rarely are there contraindications to providing SSC; however, there are potential safety concerns to address. A newborn requiring positive-pressure resuscitation should be continuously monitored, and SSC should be postponed until the infant is stabilized.[43] Furthermore, certain conditions, such as low Apgar scores (less than 7 at 5 minutes) or medical complications from birth, may require careful observation and monitoring of the newborn during SSC and in some cases may prevent SSC.[11] Other

safety concerns are attributable to the lack of standardization in the approach, discontinuous observation of the mother-infant dyad (with lapses exceeding 10 to 15 minutes during the first few hours of life), lack of education and skills among staff supporting the dyad during transition while skin-to-skin, and unfamiliarity with the potential risks of unsafe positioning and methods of assessment that may avert problems.[44] The main concerns regarding immediate postnatal SSC include sudden unexpected postnatal collapse (SUPC), which includes any condition resulting in temporary or permanent cessation of breathing or cardiorespiratory failure.[45-48] Many, but not all, of these events are related to suffocation or entrapment. In addition, falls may occur during SSC, particularly if unobserved, and other situations or conditions may occur that prevent SSC from continuing safely.[44,49]

SUPC is a rare but potentially fatal event in otherwise healthy-appearing term newborns. The definition of SUPC varies slightly depending on the author and population studied. One definition offered by the British Association of Perinatal Medicine[50] includes any term or near-term (defined as >35 weeks' gestation in this review) infant who meets the following criteria: (1) is well at birth (normal 5-minute Apgar and deemed well enough for routine care), (2) collapses unexpectedly in a state of cardiorespiratory extremis such that resuscitation with intermittent positive-pressure ventilation is required, (3) collapses within the first 7 days of life, and (4) either dies, goes on to require intensive care, or develops encephalopathy. Other potential medical conditions should be excluded (eg, sepsis, cardiac disease) for SUPC to be diagnosed. The incidence of SUPC in the first hours to days of life varies widely because of different definitions, inclusion and exclusion criteria of newborns being described, and lack of standardized reporting and may be higher in certain settings. The incidence is estimated to be 2.6 to 133 cases per 100 000 newborns. In 1 case series, the authors described one-third of SUPC events occurring in the first 2 hours of life, one-third occurring between 2 and 24 hours of life, and the final third occurring between 1 and 7 days of life.[51] Other authors suggested that 73% of SUPC events occur in the first 2 hours of life.[52] In the case series by Pejovic and Herlenius,[51] 15 of the 26 cases of SUPC were found to have occurred during SSC in a prone position. Eighteen were in primiparous mothers, 13 occurred during unsupervised breastfeeding at <2 hours of age, and 3 occurred during smart cellular phone use by the mother. Five developed grade 2 hypoxic-ischemic encephalopathy (moderate encephalopathy), with 4 requiring hypothermia treatment. Twenty-five of the 26 cases had favorable neurologic outcomes in 1 series; however, in another review, mortality was as high as 50%, and among survivors, 50% had neurologic sequelae.[53] Experimental models suggest that autoresuscitation of breathing after hypoxic challenge takes longer with lower postnatal age and decreased core body temperature.[54]

SUPC, in some definitions, includes acute life-threatening episodes; however, the latter is presumed to be more benign. An apparent life-threatening episode, or what may be referred to as a brief resolved unexplained event, may be low risk and require simple interventions such as positional changes, brief stimulation, or procedures to resolve airway obstruction.[46,53]

Falls are another concern in the immediate postnatal period. Mothers who are awake and able to respond to their newborn infant immediately after birth may become suddenly and unexpectedly sleepy, ill, or unable to continue holding their infant. Fathers or other support people providing SSC may also suddenly become unable to continue to safely hold the newborn because of lightheadedness, fatigue, incoordination, or other factors. If a hospital staff member is not immediately available to take over, unsafe situations may occur, and newborns may fall to the floor or may be positioned in a manner that obstructs their airway.

SUGGESTIONS TO IMPROVE SAFETY IMMEDIATELY AFTER DELIVERY

Several authors have suggested mechanisms for standardizing the procedure of immediate postnatal SSC to prevent sentinel events; however, none of the checklists or procedures developed have been proven to reduce the risk. Frequent and repetitive assessments, including observation of newborn breathing, activity, color, tone, and position, may avert positions that obstruct breathing or events leading to sudden collapse.[41] In addition, continuous monitoring by trained staff members and the use of checklists may improve safety.[35] Some have suggested continuous pulse oximetry; however, there is no evidence that this practice would improve safety, and it may be impractical. Given the occurrence of events in the first few hours of life, it is prudent to consider staffing the delivery unit to permit continuous staff observation with frequent recording of neonatal vital signs. A procedure manual that is implemented in a standardized fashion and practiced with simulation drills may include sequential steps identified in Box 1.[55]

BOX 1: PROCEDURE FOR IMMEDIATE SKIN-TO-SKIN CARE

1. Delivery of newborn
2. Dry and stimulate for first breath/cry, and assess newborn
3. If the newborn is stable, place skin to skin with cord attached (with option to milk cord), clamp cord after 1 minute or after placenta delivered, and reassess newborn to permit physiological circulatory transition[56]
4. Continue to dry entire newborn except hands to allow the infant to suckle hands bathed in amniotic fluid (which smells and tastes similar to colostrum), which facilitates rooting and first breastfeeding[57]
5. Cover head with cap (optional) and place prewarmed blankets to cover body of newborn on mother's chest, leaving face exposed[58]
6. Assess Apgar scores at 1 and 5 minutes
7. Replace wet blankets and cap with dry warm blankets and cap
8. Assist and support to breastfeed

Risk stratification and associated monitoring and care may avert SUPC, falls, and suffocation.[59] High-risk situations may include infants who required resuscitation (ie, any positive-pressure ventilation), those with low Apgar scores, late preterm and early term (37–39 weeks' gestation) infants, difficult delivery, mother receiving codeine[60] or other medications that may affect the newborn (eg, general anesthesia or magnesium sulfate), sedated mother, and excessively sleepy mothers and/or newborns. Mothers may be assessed to determine their level of fatigue and sleep deprivation.[61] In situations such as those described, increased staff vigilance with continuous monitoring, as described previously, is important to assist with SSC throughout the immediate postpartum period.[62] Additional suggestions to improve safety include enhancements to the environment, such as stabilizing the ambient temperature,[63] use of appropriate lighting so that the infant's color and condition can be easily assessed, and facilitating an unobstructed view of the newborn (Box 2). Additional support persons, such as doulas and family members, may augment but not replace staff monitoring. Furthermore, staff education, appropriate staffing, and awareness of genetic risks may limit sentinel events such as SUPC. These suggestions, however, have not yet been tested in prospective studies to determine efficacy.

BOX 2. COMPONENTS OF SAFE POSITIONING FOR THE NEWBORN WHILE SKIN-TO-SKIN[62]:

1. Infant's face can be seen

2. Infant's head is in "sniffing" position

3. Infant's nose and mouth are not covered

4. Infant's head is turned to one side

5. Infant's neck is straight, not bent

6. Infant's shoulders and chest face mother

7. Infant's legs are flexed

8. Infant's back is covered with blankets

9. Mother-infant dyad is monitored continuously by staff in the delivery environment and regularly on the postpartum unit

10. When mother wants to sleep, infant is placed in bassinet or with another support person who is awake and alert

SSC may be continued while moving a mother from a delivery surface (either in a delivery room or operating room) to the postpartum maternal bed. Transitions of mother-infant dyads throughout this period, and from delivery settings to postpartum settings,

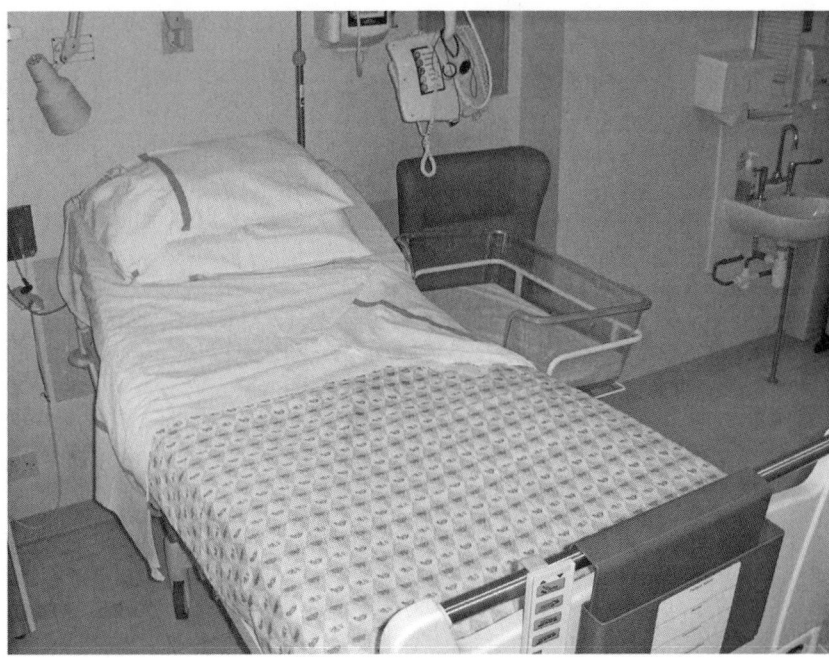

FIGURE 1
Side-car bassinet for in-hospital use. Photo courtesy of Kristin Tully, PhD.

facilitate continued bonding, thermoregulation, and increased opportunities for breastfeeding. These transitions may be accomplished safely with skilled staff members by using a standardized procedure.[64] A newborn who is not properly secured may pose a risk for falls or unsafe positioning, leading to suffocation.

SAFETY CONCERNS REGARDING ROOMING-IN

Despite all of the advantages of rooming-in, there are specific conditions that pose risks for the newborn. Many of the same concerns that occur during SSC in the immediate postnatal period continue to be of concern while rooming-in, especially if the mother and infant are sleeping together in the mother's bed on the postpartum unit.[65] In addition, breastfeeding mothers may fall asleep unintentionally while breastfeeding in bed, which can result in suffocation.[66] Infant falls may be more common in the postpartum setting because of less frequent

monitoring and increased time that a potentially fatigued mother is alone with her newborn(s).[67] The Oregon Patient Safety Review evaluated 7 hospitals that were part of 1 larger health system and identified 9 cases of newborn falls (from 22 866 births), for a rate of 3.94 falls per 10 000 births over a 2-year period from 2006 to 2007, which is higher than previous reports of 1.6 per 100 000.[68-70] It is not clear whether this higher incidence was attributable to an actual increase or better reporting. For hospitals transitioning to mother-infant dyad care (1 nurse providing care for both mother and infant) or separate mother-newborn care while rooming-in, it is important to communicate to staff that the same level of attention and care is necessary to provide optimal safety. Mothers will be naturally exhausted and potentially sleep-deprived or may sleep in short bursts.[61] They may also be unable to adjust their position or ambulate safely while carrying a newborn. The postpartum period provides unique challenges regarding falls/drops and is understudied compared with falls in the neurologically impaired or elderly patient. Checklists and scoring tools may be appropriate and have the potential to decrease these adverse events, particularly if geared to the unique needs of the postpartum period, such as short-term disability from numbness or pain, sleepiness or lethargy related to pregnancy and delivery, and effects from medication.[71]

Even though mothers and family members may be educated about the avoidance of bed-sharing, falling asleep while breastfeeding or holding the newborn during SSC is common. Staff can educate support persons and/or be immediately available to safely place newborns on a close but separate sleep surface when mothers fall asleep. Mothers may be reassured that they or their support persons can safely provide SSC and that staff will be available to assist with the transition to a safe sleep surface as needed. Mothers who have had cesarean deliveries are particularly at risk because of limited mobility and effects of anesthesia and warrant closer monitoring.[72]

Several studies examining safety while rooming-in have been conducted. Sixty-four mother-infant dyads were studied in the United Kingdom and randomly assigned to have newborns sleep in a stand-alone bassinet, a side-car bassinet (Fig 1), or the mother's bed to determine perception of safety (by video monitoring) and breastfeeding outcomes.[73] Breastfeeding was more frequent among those sharing a bed and using a side-car than a separate bassinet, but there were more hazards associated with bed-sharing than using a side-car or bassinet. Although there were no adverse events in this study, the authors concluded that the side-car provided the best opportunities for breastfeeding with the safest conditions. In a similar study

examining dyads after cesarean delivery, more hazards were associated with stand-alone bassinets than side-car bassinets. However, side-car technology for hospital beds is not yet well established in the United States, and safety data are not yet available. Given the level of disability in mothers who have had a cesarean delivery, side-car technology holds promise for improvement in the safety of the rooming-in environment.[74]

SUGGESTIONS TO IMPROVE SAFETY WHILE ROOMING-IN

Healthy mother-infant dyads are safest when kept together and cared for as a unit in a mother-infant setting. Staffing ratios are determined to meet the needs of both the mother and her newborn(s) and to ensure the best possible outcomes. The Association of Women's Health, Obstetric and Neonatal Nurses' recommendations are to have no more than 3 dyads assigned to 1 nurse to avoid situations in which nursing staff are not immediately available and able to regularly monitor the mother-infant dyads throughout the postpartum period.[75] These ratios may permit routine monitoring, rapid response to call bells, and adequate time for teaching; however, nursing staff extenders, such as health educators and nursing assistants, may augment care. Mothers and families who are informed of the risks of bed-sharing and guided to place newborns on separate sleep surfaces for sleep are more likely to follow these recommendations while in the hospital and after going home. Family members and staff can be available to assist mothers with transitioning the newborn to a safe sleep location, and regular staff supervision facilitates the recognition of sleepy family members and safer placement of the newborns in bassinets or side-cars.

SUGGESTIONS FOR ROOMING-IN

1. Use a patient safety contract with a particular focus on high-risk situations (see parent handout Newborn Safety Information for Parents[68] and sample contract[71]).

2. Monitor mothers according to their risk assessment: for example, observing every 30 minutes during nighttime and early morning hours for higher-risk dyads.[69]

3. Use fall risk assessment tools.[76]

4. Implement maternal egress testing (a modification of a tool originally designed to transfer obese patients from bed to stand, chair, or ambulation by using repetition to verify stability), especially if the mother is using medications that may affect stability in ambulating.[69]

5. Review mother-infant equipment to ensure proper function and demonstrate the appropriate use of equipment, such as bed rails and call bells, with mothers and families.

6. Publicize information about how to prevent newborn falls throughout the hospital system.

7. Use risk assessment tools to avoid hazards of SSC and rooming-in practices.[77]

TRANSITIONING TO HOME AND SAFE SLEEP BEYOND DISCHARGE

Information provided to parents at the time of hospital discharge should include anticipatory guidance about breastfeeding and sleep safety.[3,78,79] Pediatricians, hospitals, and other clinical staff should abide by AAP recommendations/guidance on breastfeeding and safe sleep, pacifier introduction, maternal smoking, use of alcohol, sleep positioning, bed-sharing, and appropriate sleep surfaces, especially when practicing SSC.[79] In addition, the AAP recommends the avoidance of practices that increase the risk of sudden and unexpected infant death, such as smoking, the use of alcohol, placing the infant in a nonsupine position for sleep, nonexclusive breastfeeding, and placing the infant to sleep (with or without another person) on sofas or chairs.[79,80] To facilitate continued exclusive breastfeeding, the coordination of postdischarge support is recommended to enable the best opportunity to meet breastfeeding goals. Mothers may be referred to peer support groups and trained lactation specialists if breastfeeding problems occur. Community support is optimized by coordination with the medical home.[81]

CONCLUSIONS

Pediatricians and other providers have important roles in the implementation of safe SSC and rooming-in practices. Safe implementation with the use of a standardized approach may prevent adverse events such as SUPC and falls.

The following suggestions support safe implementation of these practices:

1. Develop standardized methods and procedures of providing immediate and continued SSC with attention to continuous monitoring and assessment.

2. Standardize the sequence of events immediately after delivery to promote safe transition, thermoregulation, uninterrupted SSC, and direct observation of the first breastfeeding session.

3. Document maternal and newborn assessments and any changes in conditions.

4. Provide direct observation of the mother-infant dyad while in the delivery room setting.

5. Position the newborn in a manner that provides an unobstructed airway.

6. Conduct frequent assessments and monitoring of the mother-infant dyad during postpartum rooming-in settings, with particular attention to high-risk situations such as nighttime and early morning hours.

7. Assess the level of maternal fatigue periodically. If the mother is tired or sleepy, move the infant to a separate sleep surface (eg, side-car or bassinet) next to the mother's bed.

8. Avoid bed-sharing in the immediate postpartum period by assisting mothers to use a separate sleep surface for the infant.

9. Promote supine sleep for all infants. SSC may involve the prone or side position of the newborn, especially if the dyad is recumbent; therefore, it is imperative that the mother/caregiver who is providing SSC be awake and alert.

10. Train all health care personnel in standardized methods of providing immediate SSC after delivery, transitioning the mother-infant dyad, and monitoring the dyad during SSC and rooming-in throughout the delivery hospital period.

LEAD AUTHORS

Lori Feldman-Winter, MD, MPH, FAAP
Jay P. Goldsmith, MD, FAAP

TASK FORCE ON SUDDEN INFANT DEATH SYNDROME

Rachel Y. Moon, MD, FAAP, Chairperson
Robert A. Darnall, MD
Lori Feldman-Winter, MD, MPH, FAAP
Michael H. Goodstein, MD, FAAP
Fern R. Hauck, MD, MS

CONSULTANTS

Marian Willinger, PhD – *Eunice Kennedy Shriver National Institute for Child Health and Human Development*
Carrie K. Shapiro-Mendoza, PhD, MPH – *Centers for Disease Control and Prevention*

COMMITTEE ON FETUS AND NEWBORN, 2015–2016

Kristi L. Watterberg, MD, FAAP, Chairperson
James J. Cummings, MD, FAAP
William E. Benitz, MD, FAAP
Eric C. Eichenwald, MD, FAAP
Brenda B. Poindexter, MD, FAAP
Dan L. Stewart, MD, FAAP
Susan W. Aucott, MD, FAAP
Jay P. Goldsmith, MD, FAAP
Karen M. Puopolo, MD, PhD, FAAP
Kasper S. Wang, MD, FAAP

LIAISONS

Tonse N.K. Raju, MD, DCH, FAAP – *National Institutes of Health*
Wanda D. Barfield, MD, MPH, FAAP – *Centers for Disease Control and Prevention*
Erin L. Keels, APRN, MS, NNP-BC – *National Association of Neonatal Nurses*
Thierry Lacaze, MD – *Canadian Pediatric Society*
Maria Mascola, MD – *American College of Obstetricians and Gynecologists*

STAFF

Jim Couto, MA

ABBREVIATIONS

AAP: American Academy of Pediatrics
SIDS: sudden infant death syndrome
SSC: skin-to-skin care
SUPC: sudden unexpected postnatal collapse
WHO: World Health Organization

REFERENCES

1. World Health Organization. Evidence for the ten steps to successful breastfeeding. Geneva, Switzerland: World Health Organization; 1998. Available at: www.who.int/nutrition/publications/evidence_ten_step_eng.pdf. Accessed May 5, 2016

2. World Health Organization; UNICEF. Baby-Friendly Hospital Initiative: revised, updated, and expanded for integrated care. 2009. Available at: http://apps.who.int/iris/bitstream/10665/43593/1/9789241594967_eng.pdf. Accessed May 5, 2016

3. Eidelman AI, Schanler RJ; Section on Breastfeeding. Breastfeeding and the use of human milk. *Pediatrics*.

2012;129(3). Available at: www.pediatrics.org/cgi/content/full/129/3/e827

4. Baby-Friendly USA. Guidelines and evaluation criteria for facilities seeking Baby-Friendly designation. 2012. Available at: https://www.babyfriendlyusa.org/get-started/the-guidelines-evaluation-criteria. Accessed May 5, 2016

5. World Health Organization. Kangaroo mother care: a practical guide. 2003. Available at: http://apps.who.int/iris/bitstream/10665/42587/1/9241590351.pdf. Accessed May 5, 2016

6. Baley J, ; Committee on Fetus and Newborn. Skin-to-skin care for term and preterm infants in the neonatal ICU. Pediatrics. 2015;136(3):596–599

7. Horgan MJ. Management of the late preterm infant: not quite ready for prime time. Pediatr Clin North Am. 2015;62(2):439–451

8. Codipietro L, Ceccarelli M, Ponzone A. Breastfeeding or oral sucrose solution in term neonates receiving heel lance: a randomized, controlled trial. Pediatrics. 2008;122(3). Available at: www.pediatrics.org/cgi/content/full/122/3/e716

9. Gray L, Miller LW, Philipp BL, Blass EM. Breastfeeding is analgesic in healthy newborns. Pediatrics. 2002;109(4):590–593

10. Nimbalkar SM, Patel VK, Patel DV, Nimbalkar AS, Sethi A, Phatak A. Effect of early skin-to-skin contact following normal delivery on incidence of hypothermia in neonates more than 1800 g: randomized control trial. J Perinatol. 2014;34(5):364–368

11. Moore ER, Anderson GC. Randomized controlled trial of very early mother-infant skin-to-skin contact and breastfeeding status. J Midwifery Womens Health. 2007;52(2):116–125

12. Moore ER, Anderson GC, Bergman N, Dowswell T. Early skin-to-skin contact for mothers and their healthy newborn infants. Cochrane Database Syst Rev. 2012;5:CD003519

13. Johnston C, Campbell-Yeo M, Fernandes A, Inglis D, Streiner D, Zee R. Skin-to-skin care for procedural pain in neonates. Cochrane Database Syst Rev. 2014;1:CD008435

14. Kostandy R, Anderson GC, Good M. Skin-to-skin contact diminishes pain from hepatitis B vaccine injection in healthy full-term neonates. Neonatal Netw. 2013;32(4):274–280

15. Okan F, Ozdil A, Bulbul A, Yapici Z, Nuhoglu A. Analgesic effects of skin-to-skin contact and breastfeeding in procedural pain in healthy term neonates. Ann Trop Paediatr. 2010;30(2):119–128

16. Castral TC, Warnock F, Leite AM, Haas VJ, Scochi CG. The effects of skin-to-skin contact during acute pain in preterm newborns. Eur J Pain. 2008;12(4):464–471

17. Erlandsson K, Dsilna A, Fagerberg I, Christensson K. Skin-to-skin care with the father after cesarean birth and its effect on newborn crying and prefeeding behavior. Birth. 2007;34(2):105–114

18. Feldman R, Eidelman AI, Sirota L, Weller A. Comparison of skin-to-skin (kangaroo) and traditional care: parenting outcomes and preterm infant development. Pediatrics. 2002;110(1 pt 1):16–26

19. Feldman R, Weller A, Sirota L, Eidelman AI. Skin-to-skin contact (Kangaroo care) promotes self-regulation in premature infants: sleep-wake cyclicity, arousal modulation, and sustained exploration. Dev Psychol. 2002;38(2):194–207

20. Feldman R, Eidelman AI. Skin-to-skin contact (kangaroo care) accelerates autonomic and neurobehavioural maturation in preterm infants. Dev Med Child Neurol. 2003;45(4):274–281

21. Chwo M-J, Anderson GC, Good M, Dowling DA, Shiau S-HH, Chu D-M. A randomized controlled trial of early kangaroo care for preterm infants: effects on temperature, weight, behavior, and acuity. J Nurs Res. 2002;10(2):129–142

22. Mörelius E, Örtenstrand A, Theodorsson E, Frostell A. A randomised trial of continuous skin-to-skin contact after preterm birth and the effects on salivary cortisol, parental stress, depression, and breastfeeding. Early Hum Dev. 2015;91(1):63–70

23. Saxton A, Fahy K, Rolfe M, Skinner V, Hastie C. Does skin-to-skin contact and breast feeding at birth affect the rate of primary postpartum haemorrhage: results of a cohort study. Midwifery. 2015;31(11):1110–1117

24. Vetulani J. Early maternal separation: a rodent model of depression and a prevailing human condition. Pharmacol Rep. 2013;65(6):1451–1461

25. Dani C, Cecchi A, Commare A, Rapisardi G, Breschi R, Pratesi S. Behavior of the newborn during skin-to-skin. J Hum Lact. 2015;31(3):452–457

26. Dumas L, Lepage M, Bystrova K, Matthiesen A-S, Welles-Nyström B, Widström A-M. Influence of skin-to-skin contact and rooming-in on early mother-infant interaction: a randomized controlled trial. Clin Nurs Res. 2013;22(3):310–336

27. Beiranvand S, Valizadeh F, Hosseinabadi R, Pournia Y. The effects of skin-to-skin contact on temperature and breastfeeding successfulness in full-term newborns after cesarean delivery. Int J Pediatr. 2014;2014:846486

28. Stevens J, Schmied V, Burns E, Dahlen H. Immediate or early skin-to-skin contact after a Caesarean section: a review of the literature. Matern Child Nutr. 2014;10(4):456–473

29. Phillips CR. Family-Centered Maternity Care. Sudbury, MA: Jones & Bartlett Learning; 2003

30. Silberman SL. Pioneering in family-centered maternity and infant care: Edith B. Jackson and the Yale rooming-in research project. Bull Hist Med. 1990;64(2):262–287

31. Mullen K, Conrad L, Hoadley G, Iannone D. Family-centered maternity care: one hospital's quest for excellence. Nurs Womens Health. 2007;11(3):282–290

32. Martell LK. Postpartum women's perceptions of the hospital environment. J Obstet Gynecol Neonatal Nurs. 2003;32(4):478–485

33. Ordean A, Kahan M, Graves L, Abrahams R, Kim T. Obstetrical and neonatal outcomes of methadone-maintained pregnant women: a Canadian multisite cohort study. J Obstet Gynaecol Can. 2015;37(3):252–257

34. Lvoff NM, Lvoff V, Klaus MH. Effect of the baby-friendly initiative on

infant abandonment in a Russian hospital. *Arch Pediatr Adolesc Med.* 2000;154(5):474–477

35. O'Connor S, Vietze PM, Sherrod KB, Sandler HM, Altemeier WA III. Reduced incidence of parenting inadequacy following rooming-in. *Pediatrics.* 1980;66(2):176–182

36. Jaafar SH, Lee KS, Ho JJ. Separate care for new mother and infant versus rooming-in for increasing the duration of breastfeeding. *Cochrane Database Syst Rev.* 2012;9:CD006641

37. Chiou ST, Chen LC, Yeh H, Wu SR, Chien LY. Early skin-to-skin contact, rooming-in, and breastfeeding: a comparison of the 2004 and 2011 National Surveys in Taiwan. *Birth.* 2014;41(1):33–38

38. Merewood A, Patel B, Newton KN, et al Breastfeeding duration rates and factors affecting continued breastfeeding among infants born at an inner-city US Baby-Friendly hospital. *J Hum Lact.* 2007;23(2):157–164

39. Aghdas K, Talat K, Sepideh B. Effect of immediate and continuous mother-infant skin-to-skin contact on breastfeeding self-efficacy of primiparous women: a randomised control trial. *Women Birth.* 2014;27(1):37–40

40. Montgomery-Downs HE, Clawges HM, Santy EE. Infant feeding methods and maternal sleep and daytime functioning. *Pediatrics.* 2010;126(6). Available at: www.pediatrics.org/cgi/content/full/126/6/e1562

41. Takahashi Y, Tamakoshi K, Matsushima M, Kawabe T. Comparison of salivary cortisol, heart rate, and oxygen saturation between early skin-to-skin contact with different initiation and duration times in healthy, full-term infants. *Early Hum Dev.* 2011;87(3):151–157

42. Daschner FD. Nosocomial infections in maternity wards and newborn nurseries: rooming-in or not? *J Hosp Infect.* 1986;7(1):1–3

43. Swanson JR, Sinkin RA. Transition from fetus to newborn. *Pediatr Clin North Am.* 2015;62(2):329–343

44. Davanzo R, De Cunto A, Paviotti G, et al. Making the first days of life safer: preventing sudden unexpected postnatal collapse while promoting breastfeeding. *J Hum Lact.* 2015;31(1):47–52

45. Poets A, Steinfeldt R, Poets CF. Sudden deaths and severe apparent life-threatening events in term infants within 24 hours of birth. *Pediatrics.* 2011;127(4). Available at: www.pediatrics.org/cgi/content/full/127/4/e869

46. Andres V, Garcia P, Rimet Y, Nicaise C, Simeoni U. Apparent life-threatening events in presumably healthy newborns during early skin-to-skin contact. *Pediatrics.* 2011;127(4). Available at: www.pediatrics.org/cgi/content/full/127/4/e1073

47. Dageville C, Pignol J, De Smet S. Very early neonatal apparent life-threatening events and sudden unexpected deaths: incidence and risk factors. *Acta Paediatr.* 2008;97(7):866–869

48. Leow JY, Platt MP. Sudden, unexpected and unexplained early neonatal deaths in the North of England. *Arch Dis Child Fetal Neonatal Ed.* 2011;96(6):F440–F442

49. Goldsmith JP. Hospitals should balance skin-to-skin contact with safe sleep policies. *AAP News.* 2013;34(11):22

50. Nassi N, Piumelli R, Nardini V, et al. Sudden unexpected perinatal collapse and sudden unexpected early neonatal death. *Early Hum Dev.* 2013;89(suppl 4):S25–S26

51. Pejovic NJ, Herlenius E. Unexpected collapse of healthy newborn infants: risk factors, supervision and hypothermia treatment. *Acta Paediatr.* 2013;102(7):680–688

52. Becher JC, Bhushan SS, Lyon AJ. Unexpected collapse in apparently healthy newborns—a prospective national study of a missing cohort of neonatal deaths and near-death events. *Arch Dis Child Fetal Neonatal Ed.* 2012;97(1):F30–F34

53. Herlenius E, Kuhn P. Sudden unexpected postnatal collapse of newborn infants: a review of cases, definitions, risks, and preventive measures. *Transl Stroke Res.* 2013;4(2):236–247

54. Fewell JE. Protective responses of the newborn to hypoxia. *Respir Physiol Neurobiol.* 2005;149(1–3):243–255

55. Schoch DE, Lawhon G, Wicker LA, Yecco G. An interdisciplinary multidepartmental educational program toward baby friendly hospital designation. *Adv Neonatal Care.* 2014;14(1):38–43

56. Niermeyer S, Velaphi S. Promoting physiologic transition at birth: re-examining resuscitation and the timing of cord clamping. *Semin Fetal Neonatal Med.*2013;18(6):385–392

57. Widström AM, Lilja G, Aaltomaa-Michalias P, Dahllöf A, Lintula M, Nissen E. Newborn behaviour to locate the breast when skin-to-skin: a possible method for enabling early self-regulation. *Acta Paediatr.* 2011;100(1):79–85

58. Christensson K, Siles C, Moreno L, et al. Temperature, metabolic adaptation and crying in healthy full-term newborns cared for skin-to-skin or in a cot. *Acta Paediatr.* 1992;81(6–7):488–493

59. Abike F, Tiras S, Dunder I, Bahtiyar A, Akturk Uzun O, Demircan O. A new scale for evaluating the risks for in-hospital falls of newborn infants: a failure modes and effects analysis study. *Int J Pediatr.* 2010;2010:547528

60. Madadi P, Ross CJ, Hayden MR, et al. Pharmacogenetics of neonatal opioid toxicity following maternal use of codeine during breastfeeding: a case-control study. *Clin Pharmacol Ther.* 2009;85(1):31–35

61. Rychnovsky J, Hunter LP. The relationship between sleep characteristics and fatigue in healthy postpartum women. *Womens Health Issues.* 2009;19(1):38–44

62. Ludington-Hoe Sm MK, Morgan K. Infant assessment and reduction of sudden unexpected postnatal collapse risk during skin-to-skin contact. *Newborn Infant Nurs Rev.* 2014;14(1):28–33

63. Delavar M, Akbarianrad Z, Mansouri M, Yahyapour M. Neonatal hypothermia and associated risk factors at baby friendly hospital in Babol, Iran. *Ann Med Health Sci Res.* 2014;4(8, suppl 2):S99–S103

64. Elliott-Carter N, Harper J. Keeping mothers and newborns together after cesarean: how one hospital made the change. *Nurs Womens Health.* 2012;16(4):290–295

65. Thach BT. Deaths and near deaths of healthy newborn infants while bed sharing on maternity wards. *J Perinatol.* 2014;34(4):275–279

66. Feldman K, Whyte RK. Two cases of apparent suffocation of newborns during side-lying breastfeeding. *Nurs Womens Health.* 2013;17(4):337–341

67. Wallace SC; Pennsylvania Patient Safety Authority. Balancing family bonding with newborn safety. *Pennsylvania Patient Safety Advisory.* 2014;11(3). Available at: http://patientsafetyauth ority.org/ADVISORIES/AdvisoryLibrary/ 2014/Sep;11(3)/Pages/102.aspx

68. Helsley L, McDonald JV, Stewart VT. Addressing in-hospital "falls" of newborn infants. *Jt Comm J Qual Patient Saf.* 2010;36(7):327–333

69. Gaffey AD. Fall prevention in our healthiest patients: assessing risk and preventing injury for moms and babies. *J Healthc Risk Manag.* 2015;34(3):37–40

70. Monson SA, Henry E, Lambert DK, Schmutz N, Christensen RD. In-hospital falls of newborn infants: data from a multihospital health care system. *Pediatrics.* 2008;122(2). Available at: www.pediatrics.org/cgi/content/full/ 122/2/e277

71. Lockwood S, Anderson K. Postpartum safety: a patient-centered approach to fall prevention. *MCN Am J Matern Child Nurs.* 2013;38(1):15–18, quiz 19–20

72. Mahlmeister LR. Couplet care after cesarean delivery: creating a safe environment for mother and baby. *J Perinat Neonatal Nurs.* 2005;19(3):212–214

73. Ball HL, Ward-Platt MP, Heslop E, Leech SJ, Brown KA. Randomised trial of infant sleep location on the postnatal ward. *Arch Dis Child.* 2006;91(12):1005–1010

74. Tully KP, Ball HL. Postnatal unit bassinet types when rooming-in after cesarean birth: implications for breastfeeding and infant safety. *J Hum Lact.* 2012;28(4):495–505

75. Scheich B, Bingham D; AWHONN Perinatal Staffing Data Collaborative. Key findings from the AWHONN perinatal staffing data collaborative. *J Obstet Gynecol Neonatal Nurs.* 2015;44(2):317–328

76. Heafner L, Suda D, Casalenuovo N, Leach LS, Erickson V, Gawlinski A. Development of a tool to assess risk for falls in women in hospital obstetric units. *Nurs Womens Health.* 2013;17(2):98–107

77. Slogar A, Gargiulo D, Bodrock J. Tracking 'near misses' to keep newborns safe from falls. *Nurs Womens Health.* 2013;17(3):219–223

78. American Academy of Pediatrics. Education in quality improvement for pediatric practice: safe and healthy beginnings. 2012. Available at: https:// www.aap.org/en-us/professional- resources/quality-improvement/ Quality-Improvement-Innovation- Networks/Pages/Safe-and-Healthy- Beginnings-Improvement-Project.aspx. Accessed May 5, 2016

79. Moon RY; Task Force on Sudden Infant Death Syndrome. SIDS and other sleep- related infant deaths: expansion of recommendations for a safe infant sleeping environment. *Pediatrics.* 2011;128(5). Available at: www.pediatrics. org/cgi/content/full/128/5/e1341

80. Hauck FR, Thompson JM, Tanabe KO, Moon RY, Vennemann MM. Breastfeeding and reduced risk of sudden infant death syndrome: a meta-analysis. *Pediatrics.* 2011;128(1):103–110

81. Turchi RM, Antonelli RC, Norwood KW, et al; Council on Children with Disabilities and Medical Home Implementation Project Advisory Committee. Patient- and family- centered care coordination: a framework for integrating care for children and youth across multiple systems. *Pediatrics.* 2014;133(5). Available at: www.pediatrics.org/cgi/ content/full/133/5/e1451

Sexuality Education for Children and Adolescents

• *Clinical Report*

CLINICAL REPORT   Guidance for the Clinician in Rendering Pediatric Care

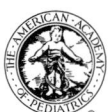

American Academy
of Pediatrics

DEDICATED TO THE HEALTH OF ALL CHILDREN™

Sexuality Education for Children and Adolescents

Cora C. Breuner, MD, MPH, Gerri Mattson, MD, MSPH, COMMITTEE ON ADOLESCENCE,
COMMITTEE ON PSYCHOSOCIAL ASPECTS OF CHILD AND FAMILY HEALTH

abstract

The purpose of this clinical report is to provide pediatricians updated research on evidence-based sexual and reproductive health education conducted since the original clinical report on the subject was published by the American Academy of Pediatrics in 2001. Sexuality education is defined as teaching about human sexuality, including intimate relationships, human sexual anatomy, sexual reproduction, sexually transmitted infections, sexual activity, sexual orientation, gender identity, abstinence, contraception, and reproductive rights and responsibilities. Developmentally appropriate and evidence-based education about human sexuality and sexual reproduction over time provided by pediatricians, schools, other professionals, and parents is important to help children and adolescents make informed, positive, and safe choices about healthy relationships, responsible sexual activity, and their reproductive health. Sexuality education has been shown to help to prevent and reduce the risks of adolescent pregnancy, HIV, and sexually transmitted infections for children and adolescents with and without chronic health conditions and disabilities in the United States.

DOI: 10.1542/peds.2016-1348

PEDIATRICS (ISSN Numbers: Print, 0031-4005; Online, 1098-4275).

Copyright © 2016 by the American Academy of Pediatrics

FINANCIAL DISCLOSURE: The authors have indicated they have no financial relationships relevant to this article to disclose.

FUNDING: No external funding.

POTENTIAL CONFLICT OF INTEREST: The authors have indicated they have no potential conflicts of interest to disclose.

To cite: Breuner CC, Mattson G, AAP COMMITTEE ON ADO-LESCENCE, AAP COMMITTEE ON PSYCHOSOCIAL ASPECTS OF CHILD AND FAMILY HEALTH. Sexuality Education for Children and Adolescents. *Pediatrics.* 2016;138(2):e20161348

INTRODUCTION

The purpose of this clinical report is to provide pediatricians with an update on the research regarding evidence-based sexual and reproductive health education that has been conducted since the original clinical report on the subject was published by the American Academy of Pediatrics (AAP) in 2001.[1] Education about sexuality that is provided by pediatricians can complement the education children obtain at school or at home,[2,3] but many pediatricians do not address it. In a review of health maintenance visits, 1 of 3 adolescent patients did not receive any information on sexuality from their pediatrician, and if they did, the conversation lasted less than 40 seconds.[4]

BACKGROUND

Children and adolescents with and without chronic health conditions and disabilities will benefit when they are provided with accurate and developmentally appropriate information about the biological, sociocultural, psychological, relational, and spiritual dimensions of sexuality. Information about sexuality can be taught and shared in schools, communities, homes, and medical offices using evidence-based interventions. Children and adolescents should be shown how to develop a safe and positive view of sexuality through age-appropriate education about their sexual health. Sexuality education can be disseminated through the 3 learning domains: cognitive (information), affective (feelings, values, and attitudes), and behavioral (communication, decision-making, and other skills).[5]

Sexuality education is more than the instruction of children and adolescents on anatomy and the physiology of biological sex and reproduction. It covers healthy sexual development, gender identity, interpersonal relationships, affection, sexual development, intimacy, and body image for all adolescents, including adolescents with disabilities, chronic health conditions, and other special needs.[6] Developing a healthy sexuality is a key developmental milestone for all children and adolescents that depends on acquiring information and forming attitudes, beliefs, and values about consent, sexual orientation, gender identity, relationships, and intimacy.[7] Healthy sexuality is influenced by ethnic, racial, cultural, personal, religious, and moral concerns. Healthy sexuality includes the capacity to promote and preserve significant interpersonal relationships; value one's body and personal health; interact with both sexes in respectful and appropriate ways; and express

affection, love, and intimacy in ways consistent with one's own values, sexual preferences, and abilities. The various dimensions of healthy sexuality comprise the anatomy, physiology, and biochemistry of the sexual response system; identity, orientation, roles, and personality; and thoughts, feelings, and relationships.[6] Ideally, children and adolescents receive accurate information on sexual health from multiple professional resources.[8,9]

All children and adolescents need to receive accurate education about sexuality to understand ultimately how to practice healthy sexual behavior. Unhealthy, exploitive, or risky sexual activity may lead to health and social problems, such as unintended pregnancy and sexually transmitted infections (STIs), including gonorrhea, *Chlamydia*, syphilis, hepatitis, herpes, human papilloma virus (HPV); HIV infection; and AIDS.[10] From a 2012 informative report by the National Campaign to Prevent Teen and Unplanned Pregnancy that surveyed 1200 high school seniors, many senior girls and boys reported having mixed feelings about the first time they had sex, with more than three-quarters responding that they would change the way their first sexual experience occurred. Interestingly, seniors in this study wanted their younger peers to know it was "fine to be a virgin" when they graduated from high school.[11]

It has been demonstrated that sexuality education interventions can prevent or reduce the risk of adolescent pregnancy HIV, and STIs for children and adolescents with and without chronic health conditions and disabilities in the United States.[12] Adolescent sexual activity and teen births and pregnancies have been decreasing since 1991, with the exception of 2005 to 2007, when there was a 5% increase in birth rates. The decrease in adolescent birth rates in the United States reflects an

increased use of contraception at first intercourse and in the use of dual methods of condoms and hormonal contraception in already sexually active teenagers.[13] Nevertheless, the United States continues to lead industrialized countries with the highest rates of adolescent pregnancy.[14] Importantly, 88% of births to adolescents 15 to 17 years of age in the United States continued to be unintended (unwanted or mistimed).[15]

Sexual health information messages are received by children and adolescents multiple times throughout the day from the media, religious organizations, schools, and family peers, parents/caregivers, and partners, although the quality of the information varies.[16,17] In an article published in 2013 on how sexually experienced adolescents in the United States receive sexual health information, parents and teachers were the source of information for 55% of girls and 43% of boys about birth control and for 59% of girls and 66% of boys about STIs/HIV.[18] Only 10% of sexually experienced adolescents reported health care providers as a source of birth control/STI/HIV information. More than 80% of adolescents 15 to 19 years of age received formal instruction about STIs, HIV, or how to say "no" to sex between 2011-2013, yet only 55% of males and 60% of females received instruction about birth control.[19] Strong support of multilevel expanded and integrative sex education is warranted now more than ever.[20]

Delivery of Sexuality Education
Pediatricians/Health Care Providers

Pediatricians are in an excellent position to provide and support longitudinal sexuality education to all children, adolescents, and young adults with and without chronic health conditions and disabilities as part of preventive health care. Over the past decade, increasing numbers of adolescents contend with sexuality in the context of their own chronic physical or mental health condition and/or developmental disability.[21,22] When sexuality is discussed routinely and openly during well-child visits for all children and adolescents in the pediatrician's office, conversations are easier to initiate, more comfortable to continue, and more effective and informative for all participants. Pediatricians and other primary care clinicians can explore the expectations of parents for their child's sexual development while providing general, factual information about sexuality and can monitor adolescent use of guidance and resources offered over time.

Pediatricians can introduce issues of physical, cognitive, and psychosexual development to parents and their children in early childhood and continue discussions at ongoing health maintenance visits throughout school age, adolescence, and young adulthood. Sharing this information can help overcome barriers to discussing the sexual development of all children and adolescents and to improve screening rates for STIs, pregnancy, and partner violence. It is also important to provide access to current accurate sexuality education and to provide access to confidential relevant information, services, and support over the course of a lifetime.[18,21] These conversations can begin with questions the family might have about the child and his or her body as well as about self-stimulation and "safe touch." With insights into the typical stages of child and adolescent sexual development, parents can better understand their own child's behaviors. For example, by recognizing that masturbation is typical toddler behavior, parents can better understand and discuss self-stimulatory behaviors of their teenager. The problem is often the inability to distinguish between behaviors that are publicly and

privately appropriate as children grow older.[23]

Often, the pediatrician can take the lead from the parent or caregiver and then ask a few gentle leading questions about how much information the family would like to receive with the child and parent together in the room. The dynamics of the sexuality education conversation can then change as the child becomes a young adolescent by asking the parent or caregiver to leave the room after the initial introductions and history taking has occurred with the parent in the room. Parents and adolescents benefit from being prepared for these changes in adolescent interactions when there will be time alone for the adolescent to engage with the pediatrician to discuss sexuality, as well as personal and mental health, drug and tobacco use, and other psychosocial issues. The importance of confidentiality and its role in adolescent health care autonomy should be discussed with both adolescents and their parents. Unlike school-based instruction, a conversation about sexuality with pediatricians can provide an opportunity for personalized information, for confidential screening of risks, and for addressing risks and enhancing existing strengths through health promotion and counseling. Children and adolescents may ask questions, discuss potentially embarrassing experiences, or reveal highly personal information to their pediatricians. Families and children may obtain education together or in a separate but coordinated manner. Prevention and counseling can be targeted to the needs of youth who are and those who are not yet sexually active and to groups at high risk of early or unsafe sexual activity, which includes children with and without chronic health conditions and disabilities.

Use of a psychosocial behavior screening tool or the Bright Futures

Previsit Questionnaire (available at https://brightfutures.aap.org/Bright%20Futures%20Documents/CoreTools11-14YearOCVisit.pdf) is a good way to address all of these topics, in addition to physical activity, nutrition, school, and relationships. The AAP policy statement on providing care for lesbian, gay, bisexual, transgender, and questioning youth, as well as other resources, offer suggestions on how to incorporate important conversations about sexual and gender identity in the health supervision visit.[24–26]

In the office setting, children and adolescents have been shown to prefer a pediatrician who is open and nonjudgmental and comfortable with discussions to address knowledge, questions, worries, or misunderstandings among children, adolescents with and without chronic health conditions and disabilities, and their parents/caregivers related to a wide range of topics. These topics include, but are not limited to, anatomy, masturbation, menstruation, erections, nocturnal emissions ("wet dreams"), sexual fantasies, sexual orientation, and orgasms. Information regarding availability and access to confidential sexual and reproductive health services and emergency contraception is important to discuss with adolescents and with parents. During these discussions, pediatricians also can address homosexual or bisexual experiences or orientation, including topics related to gender identity. It is also important to acknowledge the influence of media imagery on sexuality as it is portrayed in music and music videos, movies, pornography, and television, print, and Internet content and to address the effects of social media and sexting. According to the US Preventive Services Task Force, intensive behavioral counseling is important for all sexually active adolescents and for adults who are at increased risk of STIs.[27] Although there may not be time to address all of these topics in a brief office visit, the longitudinal relationship and annual well visit present several opportunities for discussion. In addition, more information and resources can be shared with adolescents, many of which are easily accessible and listed at the end of this report.

Most adolescents have the opportunity to explore intimacy and sexuality in a safe context, but some others experience coercion, abuse, and violence. In fact, unwanted first sexual encounters were reported in the National Survey of Family Growth among 11% of female and male subjects 18 to 24 years of age who had first intercourse before age 20 years.[28] Teenagers who report first sex at 14 years of age and younger are more likely to report that it was nonvoluntary, compared with those who were 17 to 19 years of age at sexual debut.[29] Unwanted encounters may include dating violence, stranger assaults, and intrafamilial sexual abuse/incest. Screening for sexual violence and nonconsensual sexual encounters is important when evaluating all sexually active adolescents, especially for adolescents with chronic health conditions and disabilities, because they may be more likely to be victims of sexual abuse.[5,30]

In the Schools

Formal sexuality education in schools that includes instruction about healthy sexual decision-making and STI/HIV prevention can improve the health and well-being of adolescents and young adults.[31] If comprehensive sexuality education programs are offered in the schools, positive outcomes can occur, including delay in the initiation and reduction in the frequency of sexual intercourse, a reduction in the number of sexual partners, and an

increase in condom use.[12,32] Some studies also have shown less truancy and an improvement in academic performance in those who have taken sexuality education courses.[33]

A student's experience in school with sexuality education can vary a great deal. The Sexuality Information and Education Council of the United States and the Future of Sex Education (FoSE) promote evidence-informed comprehensive school-based sexuality education appropriate to students' age, developmental abilities, and cultural background as an important part of the school curriculum at every grade.[34] A comprehensive sexuality program provides medically accurate information, recognizes the diversity of values and beliefs represented in the community, and complements and augments the sexuality education children receive from their families, religious and community groups, and health care professionals. Adolescents and most parents agree that school-based programs need to be an important source of formal education for adolescent sexual health.[35-37]

The protective influence of sexuality education is not limited to the questions about if or when to have sex, but extends to issues of partner selection, contraceptive use, and reproductive health outcomes.[38] Creating access to medically accurate comprehensive sexuality education by using an evidence-based curriculum and reducing sociodemographic disparities in its receipt remain a primary goal for improving the well-being of teenagers and young adults. Ideally, this education happens conjointly in the home and in the school.[39]

Factors that shape the content and delivery of sexuality education include state and school district policies, state education standards, funding from state and federal sources, and individual teacher comfort, knowledge, and skills. Fewer

than half of states require public schools to teach sexuality education, and even fewer states require that, if offered, sexuality education must be medically, factually, or technically accurate. State definitions of "medically accurate" vary, from requiring that the department of health review curriculum for accuracy to mandating that curriculum be based on published medical information.[40]

Two-thirds of states and the District of Columbia allow parents to remove their children from participation or opt out from sexuality education. Fewer than half of states and the District of Columbia require parents to be notified that sexuality education will be provided. Other states have specific content requirements, including "stressing abstinence" or precluding discussion of homosexuality or abortion.[41] The status of sexuality education in private schools is less well known. There is little to no information available from parochial or private scholastic institutions on the provisions of sexuality education.

Although policies exist requiring sexuality education, it may not be occurring in an unbiased and systematic manner. From the 2012 School Health Policies and Practices Survey, only 71% of US high school districts have adopted a policy specifying that human sexuality is taught. In a separate study comparing high schools, middle schools, and elementary schools, sexuality education taught in middle schools across states was more likely to be focused on "how to say no to sex" rather than other topics, with approximately 1 in 5 teenagers reporting that they first received instruction on "how to say no to sex" while in the first through fifth grade. Adolescent boys were slightly more likely than girls to be instructed on how to say no to sex or were using birth control while in middle school (52% of male teenagers, compared with 46% of female teenagers). Male teenagers were less likely than female teenagers to report first receiving instruction on methods of birth control while in high school (38% of male teenagers, compared with 47% of female teenagers).[42]

Teacher training in the United States is quite variable from district to district and school to school especially in sexuality education. The FoSE Initiative has released the National Teacher Preparation Standards for Sexuality Education to provide guidance to institutions of higher education to better prepare future teachers.[9] The FoSE teacher standards include professional disposition, diversity and equity, content knowledge, legal and professional ethics, planning, implementation, and assessment. According to these standards, teachers may benefit from receiving specialized training on human sexuality, which includes accurate and current knowledge about biological, social, and emotional stages of child and adolescent sexual development (including sexual orientation) and legal aspects of sexuality (ie, age of consent).

Professionals responsible for sexuality education may benefit from receiving training in several learning and behavior theories and how to provide age- and developmentally appropriate instruction as part of sexuality education lesson planning. Ideally, teachers would be familiar with relevant and current state and/or district laws, policies, and standards to help them choose and adapt an evidence-based and scientifically accurate curriculum that is appropriate and permissible within a school district. Ongoing professional development and participation in continuing education classes or intensive seminars is advised. Teachers can benefit from access to updated and current sexuality information, curricula, policies, laws, standards, and other

materials. The FoSE standards advise that teachers are aware of and take into account their own biases about sexuality, understand guidelines for discussion of sensitive subjects in the classroom and addressing confidentiality, and know how to address disclosure by students of sexual abuse, incest, dating violence, pregnancy, and other associated sexual health issues. The goal is for teachers to feel comfortable and committed to discussing human sexuality and to know how to conduct themselves appropriately with students as professionals both inside and outside of the classroom and school. It is important for teachers to have an appreciation for how students' diverse backgrounds and experience may affect students' personal beliefs, values, and knowledge about sexuality. In the United States, 35.5% of districts have adopted a policy stating that there is a requirement that those who teach health education must earn continuing education credits on strategies or on health-related topics. It is important for teachers to develop skills in creating a safe, respectful, and inclusive classroom.[41]

In the Home

Fundamentally, parents and caregivers can have an important role as their children's primary sexuality educators. However, a number of factors, including lack of knowledge, skills, or comfort, may impede a parent's or caregiver's successful fulfillment of that role. Health care providers, schools, faith-based institutions, the media, and professional sexuality educators are resources that guide and advise parents by providing training, resources, understanding, and encouragement. One program, "Talking Parents, Healthy Teens," aims to influence parents' skills, such as communication, monitoring, and involvement. These include intentions to talk about sex, to monitor and stay involved, and

to understand environmental barriers and facilitators that influence talking about sexuality (eg, community norms that discourage or encourage such communication).[43] By increasing parents' skills and facilitating opportunities for communication through take-home activities, the program also aims to affect the parent-adolescent relationship, further influencing adolescent behavior change (eg, the likelihood that adolescents will delay intercourse or use condoms).[44]

In one study, adolescents were asked whether they received formal instruction on 4 topics of sexuality education at home, school, church, a community center, or some other place before they were 18 years old.[42] They were specifically asked whether they spoke to their parents before the age of 18 about topics concerning sex, birth control, STIs, and HIV/AIDS prevention. Two-thirds of male and 80% of female adolescents reported having talked with a parent about at least 1 of 6 sexuality education topics ("how to say no to sex," methods of birth control, STIs, where to get birth control, how to prevent HIV/AIDS, and how to use a condom). Younger (15–17 years old) female teenagers were more likely (80%) than younger male teenagers (68%) to have talked to their parents about these topics.[42]

The medical literature supports that family and parental characteristics can dictate patterns of sexual experience among teenagers, as shown in the National Survey of Family Growth data from 2006 to 2010.[28] For example, in both male and female teenagers, a significantly smaller percentage were sexually experienced if they lived with both parents when they were 14 years of age, if their mothers had their first birth at 20 years or older, if the teenager's mother was a college graduate, or if the teenager lived with both of his or her parents.[28] Further, the approaches parents take when talking with their adolescent about sex may have a tremendous influence on the teenager.[45] Parents who dominate the conversation have teenagers who do not have as much knowledge. Conversely, parents who are engaged and comfortable talking about sexual health have teenagers who are more knowledgeable and may even be more proactive in seeking reproductive health medical services.[45]

A review of 12 studies on parental communication about sex revealed that parents who received training on this topic had better communication with their adolescents about sexuality compared with those who did not.[46] Parental conversations with their adolescents about sexuality education is correlated with a delay in sexual debut and increased use of contraception and condoms.[47] Jaccard and Levitz[45] identified multiple effective components in parent-adolescent sexual health communication, including (1) the extent of communication as measured by frequency and depth of discussions, (2) informational style, (3) the content of data that is discussed, (4) when and how the communication occurs, and (5) the overall environment where the conversation takes place.

Discussions of sexuality do not occur equally among mothers and fathers. One review found that overall, the number of discussions parents have with teenagers about sex has decreased from 1995 to 2002.[48] From a separate review covering 1980 through July 2010, mothers were the primary discussant in all interventions.[49] In reviewing the role of fathers in sexual health discussions, Kirkman et al[50] found that fathers recognized, by self-report, that they need to share the role of communication about this topic with their teenagers but that they leave the conversation to the mothers more often than not. Although mothers can also effectively teach their sons about sexuality,[51]

the relationship boys have with their fathers or other male role models plays a crucial role in their sexual health, including reducing sexual risk taking and delaying initiation of sexual intercourse, especially in those boys with a connection to their fathers, whether they live in the same home or not.[52,53]

It is clear that parents would benefit from support to improve communication with their adolescents about sex.

ABSTINENCE EDUCATION

We know that abstinence is 100% effective at preventing pregnancy and STIs; however, research has conclusively demonstrated that programs promoting abstinence-only until heterosexual marriage occurs are ineffective.[54–57] A recent systematic review examined the evidence supporting both abstinence-only programs and comprehensive sexuality education programs designed to promote abstinence from sexual intercourse. In that review, most comprehensive sexuality education programs showed efficacy in delaying initiation of intercourse in addition to promoting other protective behaviors, such as condom use. There was no evidence that abstinence-only programs effectively delayed initiation of sexual intercourse.[57] In another review of sexuality education, Cavazos-Rehg et al[35] found that the literature examining the efficacy of current school-based sexuality education programs had insufficient evidence to support the intervention of abstinence on the basis of inconsistent results across studies.

The federal government has historically provided $178 million for abstinence-only education through Title V, Section 510 of the Social Security Act in 1996, Community-Based Abstinence Education projects through the Patient Protection and Affordable Care Act, and the

Adolescent Family Life Act program. The Community-Based Abstinence Education program received the most federal funds and made direct grants to community-based organizations, including faith-based organizations. Federal guidance required all programs to adhere to an 8-point definition of abstinence-only education and prohibited programs from disseminating information on contraceptive services, sexual orientation and gender identity, and other aspects of human sexuality. Programs promoted exclusive abstinence outside of heterosexual marriage and required that contraceptive use, contraceptive methods, and specifically condoms must not be discussed except to demonstrate failure rates.[58]

The Obama administration's proposed budget for fiscal year 2014 created funding for programs that have been proven effective in reducing teen pregnancy, delaying sexual activity, or increasing contraceptive use.[32,59–61] There are still Title V–funded programs for abstinence-only programs in the schools and in other places in the community. However, most public funding now supports evidence-informed interventions that have been proven to delay onset of sexual activity, reduce numbers of partners, increase condom and contraceptive use, and decrease incidence of teen pregnancy and STIs, including HIV.[32,59–61] Private and parochial schools also have their own standards/polices and limited funding stream for sexuality education.[57]

In a 2005 study by Brückner and Bearman,[62] a review of Add Health data suggested that many teenagers who take a "virginity pledge" and intend to be abstinent before marriage fail to do so and that when these teenagers do initiate intercourse, they fail to protect themselves by using contraception. In a review of the virginity pledge movement, these researchers found that 88% of teenagers who took the pledge had initiated intercourse before marriage, compared with 99% of those who did not take the pledge. They also found that teenagers who took the pledge were less likely to use contraception after they did initiate sexual intercourse and not to seek STI screening. At 6-year follow-up, the prevalence of STIs (*Chlamydia*, gonorrhea, trichomoniasis, and HPV infection) was comparable among those who took the abstinence pledge and those who did not.[62]

The American College of Obstetricians and Gynecologists, the Society for Adolescent Health and Medicine, the AAP, the American Medical Association, the American Public Health Association, National Education Association, and the National School Boards Association oppose abstinence-only education and endorse comprehensive sexuality education that includes both abstinence promotion and accurate information about contraception, human sexuality, and STIs.[62–67]

CLINICAL GUIDANCE FOR PEDIATRICIANS

1. The pediatrician should encourage early parental discussion with children at home about sexuality, contraception, and Internet and social media use that is consistent with the child's and family's attitudes, values, beliefs, and circumstances.

2. Diverse family circumstances, such as families with same-sex parents or children who identify as lesbian, gay, bisexual, transgender, or questioning, create unique guidance needs regarding sexuality education.

3. Modeling ways to initiate talks about sexuality with children at pertinent opportunities, such as the birth of a sibling can encourage parents to answer children's questions fully and accurately.

4. Parents and adolescents are encouraged to receive information from multiple sources, including health care providers and sexuality educators, about circumstances that are associated with earlier sexual activity. Adolescents are encouraged to feel empowered through discussing strategies that allow for practicing social skills, assertiveness, control, and rejection of unwanted sexual advances and cessation of sexual activity when the partner does not consent.

5. Discussions regarding healthy relationships and intimate partner violence can be effectively included in health care visits.

6. Pediatricians are encouraged to acknowledge that sexual activity may be pleasurable but also must be engaged in responsibly.

7. Specific components of sexuality education offered in schools, religious institutions, parent organizations, and other community agencies vary based on many factors. The pediatrician can serve as a resource to each.

8. School-based comprehensive sexuality education that emphasizes prevention of unintended pregnancy and STIs should be encouraged.

9. The discussion of methods of contraception and STI and HPV cancer prevention with male and female adolescents is encouraged before the onset of sexual intercourse (see the AAP statement "Contraception and Adolescents"). It is also important to discuss consistent use of safer sex precautions with sexually active teens. Bright Futures recommendations can be used.

10. Abstinence is the most effective strategy for preventing HIV infection and other STIs, as well as for prevention of pregnancy.

11. Preparation for college entry is an excellent opportunity for pediatricians to address issues such as the effects of alcohol, marijuana, and other drug consumption on decisions about safe, consensual sexual practices.

12. Children and adolescents with special issues and disabilities may benefit from additional counseling, referrals, and sharing of online resources listed at the end of this report.

ONLINE SEXUALITY EDUCATION RESOURCES

School and Community

- United Nations Population Fund: http://www.unfpa.org/public/home/adolescents/pid/6483. *Advocates for and supports promotion of comprehensive sexuality education, provides programming guidance for both school and community settings, and advocates for wider educational opportunities for all young people and partners with civil society organizations.*

- The National Alliance to Advance Adolescent Health: http://www.thenationalalliance.org/. *Uses resources, advocacy, collaboration, and research to improve and increase access to integrated physical, behavioral, and sexual health care for adolescents.*

- The Future of Sexuality Education (FoSe): http://www.futureofsexed.org/documents/josh-fose-standards-web.pdf. *Developed the National Sexuality Education Standards for teachers to standardize and improve the quality of sexuality education provided in schools.*

- Sexuality Information and Education Council of the United States: http://www.sexedlibrary.org/index.cfm. *A resource for educators, counselors, administrators, and health professionals about human sexuality research, lesson plans, and professional development. The SexEd Library is a comprehensive online collection of lesson plans relate to sexuality education.*

- Sexual Education: Get Real: http://www.getrealeducation.org. *Get Real: Comprehensive Sex Education is a unique curriculum designed for implementation in both middle and high schools. Information provided is medically accurate and age-appropriate and can reinforce family communication and improve communication skills for healthy relationships.*

- Centers for Disease Control and Prevention Health Education Curriculum Analysis Tool: http://www.cdc.gov/healthyyouth/hecat/pdf/HECAT_Module_SH.pdf. *The Health Education Curriculum Analysis Tool can help school districts, schools, and others conduct a clear, complete, and consistent analysis of health education curricula based on the National Health Education Standards and the Centers for Disease Control and Prevention's Characteristics of an Effective Health Education Curriculum. The Health Education Curriculum Analysis Tool can help schools select or develop appropriate and effective health education curricula and can be customized to meet local community needs and conform to the curriculum requirements of the state or school district.*

Health Care Providers

- Bright Futures: http://brightfutures.aap.org/pdfs/Guidelines_PDF/9-Promoting-Healthy-Sexual-Development.pdf. *Preventive health information and recommendations about promoting healthy sexual development and sexuality to help health care providers during health supervision visits from early childhood through adolescence.*

- The Community Preventive Services Task Force: http://www.thecommunityguide.org/hiv/RRriskreduction.html. *Recommendations about interventions to promote behaviors that prevent or reduce the risk of pregnancy, HIV, and other STIs in adolescents.*

- American Congress of Obstetricians and Gynecologists: http://www.acog.org/About-ACOG/ACOG-Departments/Adolescent-Health-Care. *Information and resources about adolescent sexuality and sex education.*

Youth

- Scarleteen: http://www.scarleteen.com/. *Scarleteen is an independent, grassroots sexuality education and support organization and Web site. Founded in 1998, Scarleteen.com is visited by approximately three-quarters of a million diverse people each month worldwide, most between the ages of 15 and 25. It is the highest-ranked Web site for sex education and sexuality advice online and has held that rank through most of its tenure.*

- Sex, etc: http://sexetc.org/. Sexetc.org has comprehensive sex education information, including the following:

  o Stories written by teen staff writers and national contributors.

  o Opportunities to get involved and make a difference on sexual health issues.

  o The Sex, etc. blog, which addresses timely and relevant news.

  o Forums where teens can participate in moderated discussions with other teens.

  o "Sex in the States," which is a state-by-state guide to teens' rights to sex education, birth control, and more.

  o Videos about sexual health.

  o A sex terms glossary of almost 400 terms.

- Love is Respect: http://www.loveisrespect.org/. *Loveisrespect is a project of the National Domestic Violence Hotline and Break the Cycle. By combining our resources and capacity, we are reaching more people, building more healthy relationships, and saving more lives.*

Youth With Disabilities

- Parent Advocacy Coalition for Educational Rights: www.pacer.org. *Parent training and information center for families of children and youth with all disabilities from birth through 21 years old. Parents can find publications, workshops, and other resources about a number of topics, including sexuality and disabilities.*

- Your Child Development and Behavioral Resources: www.med.umich.edu/1libr/yourchild/disabsex.htm. *A program at the University of Michigan that houses a resource list of materials and Web sites about sexuality education for youth with disabilities for families as well as for teachers, and providers.*

- Center for Parent Information and Resources: http://www.parentcenterhub.org/repository/sexed/. *Contains information about sexuality education for students with disabilities for use with parents and teachers. The site also contains information about specific disabilities and sexuality, such as autism spectrum disorders, cerebral palsy, and spina bifida.*

Advocacy

- United Nations Population Fund: http://www.unfpa.org/public/home/adolescents/pid/6483. *Advocates for and supports promotion of comprehensive sexuality education, provides programming guidance for both school and community settings, and advocates for wider educational opportunities for all young people and partners with civil society organizations.*

- National Alliance to Advance Adolescent Health: http://www.thenationalalliance.org/. *Uses resources, advocacy, collaboration, and research to improve and increase access to integrated physical, behavioral, and sexual health care for adolescents.*

- Futures Without Violence: http://www.futureswithoutviolence.org/. *Uses advocacy, collaboration, and training with policy makers; health care, legal, and educational professionals; and others to improve responses to violence and abuse against women and children.*

- Advocates for Youth: http://www.advocatesforyouth.org/sex-education-home. *Leads efforts that help young people make informed and responsible decisions about their reproductive and sexual health and focuses its work on young people ages 14 to 25 in the United States and around the globe. There are a number of resources for multiple audiences on the Sex Education home page.*

- The National Campaign to Prevent Teen and Unplanned Pregnancy: http://thenationalcampaign.org/featured-topics/sex-education-and-effective-programs. *A series of resources that relate to sex education and a database of those sex education programs and interventions that work as well as online curricula that can be used with various audiences, including teens, college students, and others.*

LEAD AUTHORS

Cora C. Breuner, MD, MPH

Gerri Mattson, MD, MSPH

COMMITTEE ON ADOLESCENCE, 2015–2016

Cora C. Breuner, MD, MPH, FAAP, Chairperson

William P. Adelman, MD, FAAP

Elizabeth M. Alderman, MD, FSAHM, FAAP

Robert Garofalo, MD, FAAP

Arik V. Marcell, MD, MPH, FAAP

Makia E. Powers, MD MPH, FAAP

Krishna Kumari Upadhya, MD, FAAP

LIAISONS

Laurie L. Hornberger, MD, MPH, FAAP — *Section on Adolescent Health*

Margo Lane, MD, FRCPC, FAAP — *Canadian Pediatric Society*

Benjamin Shain, MD, PhD — *American Academy of Child and Adolescent Psychiatry*

Julie Strickland, MD — *American College of Obstetricians and Gynecologists*

Lauren B. Zapata, PhD, MSPH — *Centers for Disease Control and Prevention*

STAFF

Karen S. Smith

James D. Baumberger, MPP

COMMITTEE ON PSYCHOSOCIAL ASPECTS OF CHILD AND FAMILY HEALTH, 2015–2016

Michael W. Yogman, MD, FAAP, Chairperson

Nerissa S. Bauer, MD, MPH, FAAP

Thresia B. Gambon, MD, FAAP

Arthur Lavin, MD, FAAP

Keith M. Lemmon, MD, FAAP

Gerri Mattson, MD, FAAP

Jason R. Rafferty, MD, MPH, EdM

Lawrence S. Wissow, MD, MPH, FAAP

CONSULTANT

George J. Cohen, MD

LIAISONS

Sharon Berry, PhD, LP — *Society of Pediatric Psychology*

Terry Carmichael, MSW — *National Association of Social Workers*

Edward R. Christophersen, PhD, FAAP — *Society of Pediatric Psychology*

Norah L. Johnson, PhD, RN, CPNP-BC — *National Association of Pediatric Nurse Practitioners*

Leonard R. Sulik, MD — *American Academy of Child and Adolescent Psychiatry*

STAFF

Stephanie Domain, MS, CHES

Tamar M. Haro

ABBREVIATIONS

AAP: American Academy of Pediatrics

FoSE: Future of Sex Education Initiative

HPV: human papillomavirus

STI: sexually transmitted infection

REFERENCES

1. American Academy of Pediatrics, Committee on Psychosocial Aspects of Child and Family Health and Committee on Adolescence. Sexuality education for children and adolescents. *Pediatrics*. 2001;108(2):498–502

2. Gruber EL, Wang PH, Christensen JS, Grube JW, Fisher DA. Private television viewing, parental supervision, and sexual and substance use risk behaviors in adolescents [abstract]. *J Adolesc Health*. 2005;36(2):107

3. Strasburger VC; Council on Communications and Media. American Academy of Pediatrics. Policy statement—sexuality, contraception, and the media. *Pediatrics*. 2010;126(3):576–582

4. Boekeloo BO. Will you ask? Will they tell you? Are you ready to hear and respond? Barriers to physician-adolescent discussion about sexuality. *JAMA Pediatr*. 2014;168(2):111–113

5. Duncan P, Hagan JF Jr, Shaw JS. Promoting healthy sexual development and sexuality. In: *American Academy of Pediatrics. Bright Futures: Guidelines for Health Supervision of Infants, Children, and Adolescents*. Elk Grove Village, IL: American Academy of Pediatrics; 2008:169–176. Available at: https://brightfutures.aap.org/Bright%20Futures%20Documents/9-Sexuality.pdf. Accessed September 28, 2015

6. Martino SC, Elliott MN, Corona R, Kanouse DE, Schuster MA. Beyond the "big talk": the roles of breadth and repetition in parent-adolescent communication about sexual topics. *Pediatrics*. 2008;121(3). Available at: www.pediatrics.org/cgi/content/full/121/3/e612

7. Swartzendruber A, Zenilman JM. A national strategy to improve sexual health. *JAMA*. 2010;304(9):1005–1006

8. Sexuality Information and Education Council of the United States. Position Statement on Human Sexuality. Available at: www.siecus.org/index.cfm?fuseaction=page.viewPage&pageId=494&parentID=472. Accessed July 16, 2015

9. Future of Sex Education (FoSE). National Sexuality Education Standards Tools. Available at: http://www.futureofsexed.org/documents/josh-fose-standards-web.pdf. Accessed July 16, 2015

10. Jackson CA, Henderson M, Frank JW, Haw SJ. An overview of prevention of multiple risk behaviour in adolescence and young adulthood. *J Public Health (Oxf)*. 2012;34(suppl 1):i31–i40

11. Kramer A. *Girl Talk: What High School Senior Girls Have to Say About Sex, Love, and Relationships*. Washington, DC: The National Campaign to Prevent Teen and Unplanned Pregnancy; 2012

12. Chin HB, Sipe TA, Elder R, et al; Community Preventive Services Task Force. The effectiveness of group-based comprehensive risk-reduction and abstinence education interventions to prevent or reduce the risk of adolescent pregnancy, human immunodeficiency virus, and sexually transmitted infections: two systematic reviews for the Guide to Community Preventive Services. *Am J Prev Med*. 2012;42(3):272–294

13. Hamilton BE, Ventura SJ; Centers for Disease Control and Prevention, National Center for Health Statistics. Birth rates for U.S. teenagers reach historic lows for all age and ethnic groups. *NCHS Data Brief*. 2012;(89):1–8

14. United Nations. Statistics Division. Live births by age of mother and sex of child, general and age-specific fertility rates: latest available year, 2002–2011. In: *Demographic Yearbook*. New York, NY: United Nations, Statistics Division; 2012. Available at: http://unstats.un.org/unsd/demographic/products/dyb/dyb2011/Table10.pdf. Accessed July 16, 2015

15. Finer LB, Zolna MR. Unintended pregnancy in the United States: incidence and disparities, 2006. *Contraception*. 2011;84(5):478–485

16. Centers for Disease Control and Prevention. Health Education Curriculum Analysis Tool (HECAT). Available at: www.cdc.gov/HealthyYouth/HECAT/. Accessed July 16, 2015

17. Wilson SF, Strohsnitter W, Baecher-Lind L. Practices and perceptions among pediatricians regarding adolescent contraception with emphasis on intrauterine contraception. *J Pediatr Adolesc Gynecol*. 2013;26(5):281–284

18. Donaldson AA, Lindberg LD, Ellen JM, Marcell AV. Receipt of sexual health information from parents, teachers, and healthcare providers by sexually experienced U.S. adolescents. *J Adolesc Health*. 2013;53(2):235–240

19. Lindberg LD, Maddow-Zimet I, Boonstra H. Changes in adolescents' receipt of sex education, 2006-2013. *J Adolesc Health*. 2016;58(6):621–627

20. Hall KS, McDermott Sales J, Komro KA, Santelli J. The state of sex education in the United States. *J Adolesc Health*. 2016;58(6):595–597

21. Cheng MM, Udry JR. Sexual behaviors of physically disabled adolescents in the United States. *J Adolesc Health*. 2002;31(1):48–58

22. Florida Developmental Disabilities Council Inc. Developmental disabilities: an instructional manual for parents of and individuals with developmental disabilities. Available at: www.fddc.org/sites/default/files/file/publications/Sexuality%20Guide-Parents-English.pdf. Accessed July 16, 2015

23. Murphy NA, Elias ER; American Academy of Pediatrics, Council on Children With Disabilities. Sexuality of children and adolescents with developmental disabilities. *Pediatrics*. 2006;118(1):398–403

24. Committee On Adolescence. Office-based care for lesbian, gay, bisexual, transgender, and questioning youth. *Pediatrics*. 2013;132(1):198–203

25. Institute of Medicine, Committee on Lesbian, Gay, Bisexual, and Transgender Health Issues and Research Gaps and Opportunities. *The Health of Lesbian, Gay, Bisexual, and Transgender People: Building a Foundation for Better Understanding*. Washington, DC: National Academies Press; 2011

26. Spigarelli MG. Adolescent sexual orientation. *Adolesc Med State Art Rev*. 2007;18(3):508–518, vii

27. US Preventive Services Task Force. Sexually transmitted infections: behavioral counseling. Released September 2014. Available at: www.uspreventiveservicestaskforce.org/uspstf/uspsstds.htm. Accessed July 16, 2015

28. Martinez G, Copen CE, Abma JC; Centers for Disease Control and Prevention, National Center for Health Statistics. Teenagers in the United States: sexual activity, contraceptive use, and childbearing, 2006-2010 national survey of family growth. *Vital Health Stat 23*. 2011;23(31):1–35

29. Eaton DK, Kann L, Kinchen S, et al; Centers for Disease Control and Prevention (CDC). Youth risk behavior surveillance - United States, 2011. *MMWR Surveill Summ*. 2012;61(4):1–162

30. Caldas SJ, Bensy ML. The sexual maltreatment of students with disabilities in American school settings. *J Child Sex Abuse*. 2014;23(4):345–366

31. Lindberg LD, Santelli JS, Singh S. Changes in formal sex education: 1995-2002. *Perspect Sex Reprod Health*. 2006;38(4):182–189

32. Kohler PK, Manhart LE, Lafferty WE. Abstinence-only and comprehensive sex education and the initiation of sexual activity and teen pregnancy. *J Adolesc Health*. 2008;42(4):344–351

33. Advocates for Youth. *Science and Success*. 3rd ed. Programs that Work to Prevent Teen Pregnancy, HIV and STIs in the US. Washington, DC: Advocates for Youth; 2012

34. Sexuality Information and Education Council of the United States. Sexuality Education Q & A. Available at: www.siecus.org/index.cfm?fuseaction=page.viewpage&pageid=521&grandparentID=477&parentID=514. Accessed July 16, 2015

35. Cavazos-Rehg PA, Krauss MJ, Spitznagel EL, et al. Associations between sexuality education in schools and adolescent birthrates: a state-level longitudinal model. *Arch Pediatr Adolesc Med*. 2012;166(2):134–140

36. Frappier JY, Kaufman M, Baltzer F, et al. Sex and sexual health: a survey of Canadian youth and mothers. *Paediatr Child Health*. 2008;13(1):25–30

37. Merzel CR, VanDevanter NL, Middlestadt S, Bleakley A, Ledsky R, Messeri PA. Attitudinal and contextual factors associated with discussion of sexual issues during adolescent health visits. *J Adolesc Health.* 2004;35(2):108–115

38. Mueller TE, Gavin LE, Kulkarni A. The association between sex education and youth's engagement in sexual intercourse, age at first intercourse, and birth control use at first sex. *J Adolesc Health.* 2008;42(1):89–96

39. Grossman JM, Tracy AJ, Charmaraman L, Ceder I, Erkut S. Protective effects of middle school comprehensive sex education with family involvement. *J Sch Health.* 2014;84(11):739–747

40. Guttmacher Institute. State policies in brief: sex and HIV education. Available at: www.guttmacher.org/statecenter/spibs/spib_SE.pdf. Accessed July 16, 2015

41. Kann L, Telljohan S, Hunt H, Hunt P, Haller R. Health education. In: *Centers for Disease Control and Prevention. Results from the School Health Policies and Practices Study.* Atlanta, GA: Centers for Disease Control and Prevention; 2013. Available at: www.cdc.gov/healthyyouth/shpps/2012/pdf/shpps-results_2012.pdf#page=27. Accessed July 16, 2015

42. Martinez G, Abma J, Copen C. Educating teenagers about sex in the United States. *NCHS Data Brief.* 2010;(44):1–8

43. Eastman KL, Corona R, Schuster MA. Talking parents, healthy teens: a worksite-based program for parents to promote adolescent sexual health. *Prev Chronic Dis.* 2006;3(4):A126

44. Strasburger VC, Brown SS. Sex education in the 21st century. *JAMA.* 2014;312(2):125–126

45. Jaccard J, Levitz N. Counseling adolescents about contraception: towards the development of an evidence-based protocol for contraceptive counselors. *J Adolesc Health.* 2013;52(suppl 4):S6–S13

46. Wight D, Fullerton D. A review of interventions with parents to promote the sexual health of their children. *J Adolesc Health.* 2013;52(1):4–27

47. Klein JD, Sabaratnam P, Pazos B, Auerbach MM, Havens CG, Brach MJ. Evaluation of the parents as primary sexuality educators program. *J Adolesc Health.* 2005;37(suppl 3):S94–S99

48. Robert AC, Sonenstein FL. Adolescents' reports of communication with their parents about sexually transmitted diseases and birth control: 1988, 1995, and 2002. *J Adolesc Health.* 2010;46(6):532–537

49. Akers AY, Holland CL, Bost J. Interventions to improve parental communication about sex: a systematic review. *Pediatrics.* 2011;127(3):494–510

50. Kirkman M, Rosenthal DA, Feldman SS. Talking to a tiger: fathers reveal their difficulties in communicating about sexuality with adolescents. *New Dir Child Adolesc Dev.* 2002;(97):57–74

51. Jemmott LS, Outlaw FH, Jemmott JB, Brown EJ, Howard M, Hopkins B. Strengthening the bond: the Mother and Son Health Promotion Project. In: Pequegnat W, Szapocznik J, eds. *Inside Families: The Role of Families in Preventing and Adapting to HIV/AIDS.* Bethesda, MD: Sage Publications; 2000:133–151

52. King V, Sobolewski JM. Nonresident fathers' contributions to adolescent well-being. *J Marriage Fam.* 2006;68(3):537–557

53. Carlson MJ. Family structure, father involvement, and adolescent behavioral outcomes. *J Marriage Fam.* 2006;68(1):137–154

54. Ball H. Theory-based abstinence-only intervention may delay sexual initiation among black urban youth. *Perspect Sex Reprod Health.* 2010;42(2):135–136

55. Jemmott JB III, Jemmott LS, Fong GT. Efficacy of a theory-based abstinence-only intervention over 24 months: a randomized controlled trial with young adolescents. *Arch Pediatr Adolesc Med.* 2010;164(2):152–159

56. Kirby D. The impact of abstinence and comprehensive sex and STD/HIV education programs on adolescent sexual behavior. *Sexuality Research and Social Policy.* 2008;5(3):18–27

57. Trenholm C, Devaney B, Fortson K, Quay L, Wheeler J, Clark M; Mathematica Policy Research Inc. Impacts of Four Title V, Section 510 Abstinence Education Programs. Final Report. Submitted to US Department of Health and Human Services, Office of the Assistant Secretary for Planning and Evaluation. Princeton, NJ: Mathematica Policy Research Inc; 2007. Available at: www.mathematica-mpr.com/~/media/publications/PDFs/impactabstinence.pdf. Accessed July 16, 2015

58. Catalog of Federal Domestic Assistance. Community-based abstinence education. Available at: https://www.cfda.gov/index?s=program&mode=form&tab=core&id=7a526272ffcfea290497a3548fb92654. Accessed July 16, 2015

59. Ott MA, Santelli JS. Abstinence and abstinence-only education. *Curr Opin Obstet Gynecol.* 2007;19(5):446–452

60. Santelli J, Ott MA, Lyon M, Rogers J, Summers D. Abstinence-only education policies and programs: a position paper of the Society for Adolescent Medicine. *J Adolesc Health.* 2006;38(1):83–87

61. Advocates for Youth. Comprehensive sex education: research and results. Available at: www.advocatesforyouth.org/storage/advfy/documents/fscse.pdf. Accessed July 16, 2015

62. Brückner H, Bearman P. After the promise: the STD consequences of adolescent virginity pledges. *J Adolesc Health.* 2005;36(4):271–278

63. Kirby DB, Laris BA, Rolleri LA. Sex and HIV education programs: their impact on sexual behaviors of young people throughout the world. *J Adolesc Health.* 2007;40(3):206–217

64. Kirby D. *Emerging Answers: Research Findings on Programs to Reduce Teen Pregnancy.* Washington, DC: National Campaign to Prevent Teen Pregnancy; 2001

65. Manlove J, Romano-Papillo A, Ikramullah E. *Not Yet: Programs to Delay First Sex Among Teens.* Washington, DC: National Campaign to Prevent Teen Pregnancy; 2004

66. Bearman PS, Brueckner H. Promising the future: virginity pledges and first intercourse. *American Journal of Sociology.* 2001;106(4):859–912

67. Kraft JM, Kulkarni A, Hsia J, Jamieson DJ, Warner L. Sex education and adolescent sexual behavior: do community characteristics matter? *Contraception.* 2012;86(3):276–280

SIDS and Other Sleep-Related Infant Deaths: Updated 2016 Recommendations for a Safe Infant Sleeping Environment

- *Policy Statement*

POLICY STATEMENT Organizational Principles to Guide and Define the Child Health Care System and/or Improve the Health of all Children

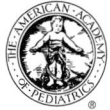

American Academy of Pediatrics

DEDICATED TO THE HEALTH OF ALL CHILDREN™

SIDS and Other Sleep-Related Infant Deaths: Updated 2016 Recommendations for a Safe Infant Sleeping Environment

TASK FORCE ON SUDDEN INFANT DEATH SYNDROME

abstract

Approximately 3500 infants die annually in the United States from sleep-related infant deaths, including sudden infant death syndrome (SIDS; International Classification of Diseases, 10th Revision [ICD-10], R95), ill-defined deaths (ICD-10 R99), and accidental suffocation and strangulation in bed (ICD-10 W75). After an initial decrease in the 1990s, the overall death rate attributable to sleep-related infant deaths has not declined in more recent years. Many of the modifiable and nonmodifiable risk factors for SIDS and other sleep-related infant deaths are strikingly similar. The American Academy of Pediatrics recommends a safe sleep environment that can reduce the risk of all sleep-related infant deaths. Recommendations for a safe sleep environment include supine positioning, the use of a firm sleep surface, room-sharing without bed-sharing, and the avoidance of soft bedding and overheating. Additional recommendations for SIDS reduction include the avoidance of exposure to smoke, alcohol, and illicit drugs; breastfeeding; routine immunization; and use of a pacifier. New evidence is presented for skin-to-skin care for newborn infants, use of bedside and in-bed sleepers, sleeping on couches/armchairs and in sitting devices, and use of soft bedding after 4 months of age. The recommendations and strength of evidence for each recommendation are included in this policy statement. The rationale for these recommendations is discussed in detail in the accompanying technical report (www.pediatrics.org/cgi/doi/10.1542/peds.2016-2940).

Policy statements from the American Academy of Pediatrics benefit from expertise and resources of liaisons and internal (AAP) and external reviewers. However, policy statements from the American Academy of Pediatrics may not reflect the views of the liaisons or the organizations or government agencies that they represent.

The guidance in this statement does not indicate an exclusive course of treatment or serve as a standard of medical care. Variations, taking into account individual circumstances, may be appropriate.

All policy statements from the American Academy of Pediatrics automatically expire 5 years after publication unless reaffirmed, revised, or retired at or before that time.

DOI: 10.1542/peds.2016-2938

PEDIATRICS (ISSN Numbers: Print, 0031-4005; Online, 1098-4275).

Copyright © 2016 by the American Academy of Pediatrics

FINANCIAL DISCLOSURE: The author has indicated she does not have a financial relationship relevant to this article to disclose.

FUNDING: No external funding.

POTENTIAL CONFLICT OF INTEREST: The author has indicated she has no potential conflicts of interest to disclose.

To cite: AAP TASK FORCE ON SUDDEN INFANT DEATH SYNDROME. SIDS and Other Sleep-Related Infant Deaths: Updated 2016 Recommendations for a Safe Infant Sleeping Environment. *Pediatrics.* 2016;138(5):e20162938

BACKGROUND

Sudden unexpected infant death (SUID), also known as sudden unexpected death in infancy, or SUDI, is a term used to describe any sudden and unexpected death, whether explained or unexplained

TABLE 1 Definitions of Terms

Bed-sharing: Parent(s) and infant sleeping together on any surface (bed, couch, chair).

Caregivers: Throughout the document, "parents" are used, but this term is meant to indicate any infant caregivers.

Cosleeping: This term is commonly used, but the task force finds it confusing, and it is not used in this document. When used, authors need to make clear whether they are referring to sleeping in close proximity (which does not necessarily entail bed-sharing) or bed-sharing.

Room-sharing: Parent(s) and infant sleeping in the same room on separate surfaces.

Sleep-related infant death: SUID that occurs during an observed or unobserved sleep period.

Sudden infant death syndrome (SIDS): Cause assigned to infant deaths that cannot be explained after a thorough case investigation, including a scene investigation, autopsy, and review of the clinical history.[1]

Sudden unexpected infant death (SUID), or sudden unexpected death in infancy (SUDI): A sudden and unexpected death, whether explained or unexplained (including SIDS), occurring during infancy.

TABLE 2 Summary of Recommendations With Strength of Recommendation

A-level recommendations

  Back to sleep for every sleep.

  Use a firm sleep surface.

  Breastfeeding is recommended.

  Room-sharing with the infant on a separate sleep surface is recommended.

  Keep soft objects and loose bedding away from the infant's sleep area.

  Consider offering a pacifier at naptime and bedtime.

  Avoid smoke exposure during pregnancy and after birth.

  Avoid alcohol and illicit drug use during pregnancy and after birth.

  Avoid overheating.

  Pregnant women should seek and obtain regular prenatal care.

  Infants should be immunized in accordance with AAP and CDC recommendations.

  Do not use home cardiorespiratory monitors as a strategy to reduce the risk of SIDS.

  Health care providers, staff in newborn nurseries and NICUs, and child care providers should endorse and model the SIDS risk-reduction recommendations from birth.

  Media and manufacturers should follow safe sleep guidelines in their messaging and advertising.

  Continue the "Safe to Sleep" campaign, focusing on ways to reduce the risk of all sleep-related infant deaths, including SIDS, suffocation, and other unintentional deaths. Pediatricians and other primary care providers should actively participate in this campaign.

B-level recommendations

  Avoid the use of commercial devices that are inconsistent with safe sleep recommendations.

  Supervised, awake tummy time is recommended to facilitate development and to minimize development of positional plagiocephaly.

C-level recommendations

  Continue research and surveillance on the risk factors, causes, and pathophysiologic mechanisms of SIDS and other sleep-related infant deaths, with the ultimate goal of eliminating these deaths entirely.

  There is no evidence to recommend swaddling as a strategy to reduce the risk of SIDS.

The following levels are based on the Strength-of-Recommendation Taxonomy (SORT) for the assignment of letter grades to each of its recommendations (A, B, or C).[2] Level A: There is good-quality patient-oriented evidence. Level B: There is inconsistent or limited-quality patient-oriented evidence. Level C: The recommendation is based on consensus, disease-oriented evidence, usual practice, expert opinion, or case series for studies of diagnosis, treatment, prevention, or screening. Note: "patient-oriented evidence" measures outcomes that matter to patients: morbidity, mortality, symptom improvement, cost reduction, and quality of life; "disease-oriented evidence" measures immediate, physiologic, or surrogate end points that may or may not reflect improvements in patient outcomes (eg, blood pressure, blood chemistry, physiologic function, pathologic findings). CDC, Centers for Disease Control and Prevention.

(including sudden infant death syndrome [SIDS] and ill-defined deaths), occurring during infancy. After case investigation, SUID can be attributed to suffocation, asphyxia, entrapment, infection, ingestions, metabolic diseases, arrhythmia-associated cardiac channelopathies, and trauma (unintentional or nonaccidental). SIDS is a subcategory of SUID and is a cause assigned to infant deaths that cannot be explained after a thorough case investigation, including a scene investigation, autopsy, and review of the clinical history.[1] (See Table 1 for definitions of terms.) The distinction between SIDS and other SUIDs, particularly those that occur during an unobserved sleep period (sleep-related infant deaths), such as unintentional suffocation, is challenging, cannot be determined by autopsy alone, and may remain unresolved after a full case investigation. Many of the modifiable and nonmodifiable risk factors for SIDS and suffocation are strikingly similar. This document focuses on the subset of SUIDs that occur during sleep.

The recommendations outlined herein were developed to reduce the risk of SIDS and sleep-related suffocation, asphyxia, and entrapment among infants in the general population. As defined by epidemiologists, risk refers to the probability that an outcome will occur given the presence of a particular factor or set of factors. Although all 19 recommendations are intended for all who care for infants, the last 4 recommendations also are directed toward health policy makers, researchers, and professionals who care for or work on behalf of infants. In addition, because certain behaviors, such as smoking, can increase risk for the infant, some recommendations are directed toward women who are pregnant or may become pregnant in the near future.

Table 2 summarizes each recommendation and provides the strength of the recommendation, which is based on the Strength-of-Recommendation Taxonomy.[2] It should be noted that there are no randomized controlled trials with regard to SIDS and other sleep-related deaths; instead, case-control studies are the standard.

The recommendations are based on epidemiologic studies that include infants up to 1 year of age. Therefore, recommendations for sleep position and the sleep environment, unless otherwise specified, are for the first year after birth. The evidence-based recommendations that follow are provided to guide health care providers in conversations with parents and others who care for infants. Health care providers are encouraged to have open and nonjudgmental conversations with families about their sleep practices. Individual medical conditions may warrant that a health care provider recommend otherwise after weighing the relative risks and benefits.

For the background literature review and data analyses on which this policy statement and recommendations are based, refer to the accompanying technical report, "SIDS and Other Sleep-Related Infant Deaths: Evidence Base for 2016 Updated Recommendations for a Safe Infant Sleeping Environment," available in the electronic pages of this issue (www.pediatrics.org/cgi/doi/10.1542/peds.2016-2940).[3]

RECOMMENDATIONS TO REDUCE THE RISK OF SIDS AND OTHER SLEEP-RELATED INFANT DEATHS

1. Back to sleep for every sleep.

To reduce the risk of SIDS, infants should be placed for sleep in a supine position (wholly on the back) for every sleep by every caregiver until the child reaches 1 year of age.[4–8] Side sleeping is not safe and is not advised.[5,7]

The supine sleep position does not increase the risk of choking and aspiration in infants, even those with gastroesophageal reflux, because infants have airway anatomy and mechanisms that protect against aspiration.[9,10] The American Academy of Pediatrics (AAP) concurs with the North American Society for Pediatric Gastroenterology and Nutrition that "the risk of SIDS outweighs the benefit of prone or lateral sleep position on GER [gastroesophageal reflux]; therefore, in most infants from birth to 12 months of age, supine positioning during sleep is recommended. ...Therefore, prone positioning is acceptable if the infant

is observed and awake, particularly in the postprandial period, but prone positioning during sleep can only be considered in infants with certain upper airway disorders in which the risk of death from GERD [gastroesophageal reflux disease] may outweigh the risk of SIDS."[11] Examples of such upper airway disorders are those in which airway-protective mechanisms are impaired, including infants with anatomic abnormalities, such as type 3 or 4 laryngeal clefts, who have not undergone antireflux surgery. There is no evidence to suggest that infants receiving nasogastric or orogastric feeds are at an increased risk of aspiration if placed in the supine position. Elevating the head of the infant's crib is ineffective in reducing gastroesophageal reflux[12] and is not recommended; in addition, elevating the head of the crib may result in the infant sliding to the foot of the crib into a position that may compromise respiration.

Preterm infants should be placed supine as soon as possible. Preterm infants are at increased risk of SIDS,[13,14] and the association between prone sleep position and SIDS among low birth weight and preterm infants is equal to, or perhaps even stronger than, the association among those born at term.[15] The task force concurs with the AAP Committee on Fetus and Newborn that "preterm infants should be placed supine for sleeping, just as term infants should, and the parents of preterm infants should be counseled about the importance of supine sleeping in preventing SIDS. Hospitalized preterm infants should be kept predominantly in the supine position, at least from the postmenstrual age of 32 weeks onward, so that they become acclimated to supine sleeping before discharge."[16] NICU personnel should endorse safe sleeping guidelines with parents of infants from the time of admission to the NICU.

As stated in the AAP clinical report, "skin-to-skin care is recommended for all mothers and newborns, regardless of feeding or delivery method, immediately following birth (as soon as the mother is medically stable, awake, and able to respond to her newborn), and to continue for at least an hour."[17] Thereafter, or when the mother needs to sleep or take care of other needs, infants should be placed supine in a bassinet. There is no evidence that placing infants on their side during the first few hours after delivery promotes clearance of amniotic fluid and decreases the risk of aspiration. Infants in the newborn nursery and infants who are rooming in with their parents should be placed in the supine position as soon as they are ready to be placed in the bassinet.

Although data to make specific recommendations as to when it is safe for infants to sleep in the prone or side position are lacking, studies establishing prone and side sleeping as risk factors for SIDS include infants up to 1 year of age. Therefore, the best evidence suggests that infants should continue to be placed supine until 1 year of age. Once an infant can roll from supine to prone and from prone to supine, the infant can be allowed to remain in the sleep position that he or she assumes. Because rolling into soft bedding is an important risk factor for SUID after 3 months of age,[18] parents and caregivers should continue to keep the infant's sleep environment clear of soft or loose bedding.

2. Use a firm sleep surface.

Infants should be placed on a firm sleep surface (eg, mattress in a safety-approved crib) covered by a fitted sheet with no other bedding or soft objects to reduce the risk of SIDS and suffocation.

A firm surface maintains its shape and will not indent or conform to the shape of the infant's head when the infant is placed on the surface.

Soft mattresses, including those made from memory foam, could create a pocket (or indentation) and increase the chance of rebreathing or suffocation if the infant is placed in or rolls over to the prone position.[19,20]

A crib, bassinet, portable crib, or play yard that conforms to the safety standards of the Consumer Product Safety Commission (CPSC), including those for slat spacing less than 2-3/8 inches, snugly fitting and firm mattresses, and no drop sides, is recommended.[21] In addition, parents and providers should check to make sure that the product has not been recalled. This is particularly important for used cribs. Cribs with missing hardware should not be used, nor should the parent or provider attempt to fix broken components of a crib, because many deaths are associated with cribs that are broken or with missing parts (including those that have presumably been fixed). Local organizations throughout the United States can help to provide low-cost or free cribs or play yards for families with financial constraints.

Bedside sleepers are attached to the side of the parental bed. The CPSC has published safety standards for these products,[22] and they may be considered by some parents as an option. However, there are no CPSC safety standards for in-bed sleepers. The task force cannot make a recommendation for or against the use of either bedside sleepers or in-bed sleepers, because there have been no studies examining the association between these products and SIDS or unintentional injury and death, including suffocation.

Only mattresses designed for the specific product should be used. Mattresses should be firm and should maintain their shape even when the fitted sheet designated for that model is used, such that there are no gaps between the mattress and the wall of the crib, bassinet, portable crib, or play yard. Pillows or cushions

should not be used as substitutes for mattresses or in addition to a mattress. Mattress toppers, designed to make the sleep surface softer, should not be used for infants younger than 1 year.

There is no evidence that special crib mattresses and sleep surfaces that claim to reduce the chance of rebreathing carbon dioxide when the infant is in the prone position reduce the risk of SIDS. However, there is no disadvantage to the use of these mattresses if they meet the safety standards as described previously.

Soft materials or objects, such as pillows, quilts, comforters, or sheepskins, even if covered by a sheet, should not be placed under a sleeping infant. If a mattress cover to protect against wetness is used, it should be tightly fitting and thin.

Infants should not be placed for sleep on beds, because of the risk of entrapment and suffocation.[23,24] In addition, portable bed rails should not be used with infants, because of the risk of entrapment and strangulation.

The infant should sleep in an area free of hazards, such as dangling cords, electric wires, and window-covering cords, because these may present a strangulation risk.

Sitting devices, such as car seats, strollers, swings, infant carriers, and infant slings, are not recommended for routine sleep in the hospital or at home, particularly for young infants.[25-30] Infants who are younger than 4 months are particularly at risk, because they may assume positions that can create a risk of suffocation or airway obstruction or may not be able to move out of a potentially asphyxiating situation. When infant slings and cloth carriers are used for carrying, it is important to ensure that the infant's head is up and above the fabric, the face is visible, and the nose and mouth are clear of obstructions.[31] After nursing, the infant should be repositioned

in the sling so that the head is up, is clear of fabric, and is not against the adult's body or the sling. If an infant falls asleep in a sitting device, he or she should be removed from the product and moved to a crib or other appropriate flat surface as soon as is safe and practical. Car seats and similar products are not stable on a crib mattress or other elevated surfaces.[32-36] Infants should not be left unattended in car seats and similar products, nor should they be placed or left in car seats and similar products with the straps unbuckled or partially buckled.[30]

3. **Breastfeeding is recommended.**

Breastfeeding is associated with a reduced risk of SIDS.[37-39] Unless contraindicated, mothers should breastfeed exclusively or feed with expressed milk (ie, not offer any formula or other nonhuman milk-based supplements) for 6 months, in alignment with recommendations of the AAP.[40]

The protective effect of breastfeeding increases with exclusivity.[39] However, any breastfeeding has been shown to be more protective against SIDS than no breastfeeding.[39]

4. **It is recommended that infants sleep in the parents' room, close to the parents' bed, but on a separate surface designed for infants, ideally for the first year of life, but at least for the first 6 months.**

There is evidence that sleeping in the parents' room but on a separate surface decreases the risk of SIDS by as much as 50%.[6,8,41,42] In addition, this arrangement is most likely to prevent suffocation, strangulation, and entrapment that may occur when the infant is sleeping in the adult bed.

The infant's crib, portable crib, play yard, or bassinet should be placed in the parents' bedroom until the child's first birthday. Although there is no specific evidence for moving an infant to his or her own room before 1 year of age, the first 6 months are particularly critical, because the rates of SIDS and other sleep-related deaths, particularly those occurring in bed-sharing situations, are highest in the first 6 months. Placing the crib close to the parents' bed so that the infant is within view and reach can facilitate feeding, comforting, and monitoring of the infant. Room-sharing reduces SIDS risk and removes the possibility of suffocation, strangulation, and entrapment that may occur when the infant is sleeping in the adult bed.

There is insufficient evidence to recommend for or against the use of devices promoted to make bed-sharing "safe." There is no evidence that these devices reduce the risk of SIDS or suffocation or are safe. Some products designed for in-bed use (in-bed sleepers) are currently under study but results are not yet available. Bedside sleepers, which attach to the side of the parental bed and for which the CPSC has published standards,[22] may be considered by some parents as an option. There are no CPSC safety standards for in-bed sleepers. The task force cannot make a recommendation for or against the use of either bedside sleepers or in-bed sleepers, because there have been no studies examining the association between these products and SIDS or unintentional injury and death, including suffocation.

Infants who are brought into the bed for feeding or comforting should be returned to their own crib or bassinet when the parent is ready to return to sleep.[7,43]

Couches and armchairs are extremely dangerous places for infants. Sleeping on couches and armchairs places infants at extraordinarily high risk of infant death, including SIDS,[4,6,7,42,43] suffocation through entrapment or wedging between seat cushions, or overlay if another person is also sharing this surface.[44] Therefore, parents and other caregivers should be especially vigilant as to their wakefulness when feeding infants or lying with infants on these surfaces.

Infants should never be placed on a couch or armchair for sleep.

The safest place for an infant to sleep is on a separate sleep surface designed for infants close to the parents' bed. However, the AAP acknowledges that parents frequently fall asleep while feeding the infant. Evidence suggests that it is less hazardous to fall asleep with the infant in the adult bed than on a sofa or armchair, should the parent fall asleep. It is important to note that a large percentage of infants who die of SIDS are found with their head covered by bedding. Therefore, no pillows, sheets, blankets, or any other items that could obstruct infant breathing or cause overheating should be in the bed. Parents should also follow safe sleep recommendations outlined elsewhere in this statement. Because there is evidence that the risk of bed-sharing is higher with longer duration, if the parent falls asleep while feeding the infant in bed, the infant should be placed back on a separate sleep surface as soon as the parent awakens.

There are specific circumstances that, in case-control studies and case series, have been shown to substantially increase the risk of SIDS or unintentional injury or death while bed-sharing, and these should be avoided at all times:

- Bed-sharing with a term normal-weight infant younger than 4 months[6,8,42,43,45,46] and infants born preterm and/or with low birth weight,[47] regardless of parental smoking status. Even for breastfed infants, there is an increased risk of SIDS when bed-sharing if younger than 4 months.[48] This appears to be a particularly vulnerable time, so if parents choose to feed their infants younger than 4 months in bed, they should be especially vigilant to not fall asleep.

- Bed-sharing with a current smoker (even if he or she does not smoke in bed) or if the mother smoked during pregnancy.[6,7,46,49,50]

- Bed-sharing with someone who is impaired in his or her alertness or ability to arouse because of fatigue or use of sedating medications (eg, certain antidepressants, pain medications) or substances (eg, alcohol, illicit drugs).[8,48,51,52]

- Bed-sharing with anyone who is not the infant's parent, including nonparental caregivers and other children.[4]

- Bed-sharing on a soft surface, such as a waterbed, old mattress, sofa, couch, or armchair.[4,6,7,42,43]

- Bed-sharing with soft bedding accessories, such as pillows or blankets.[4,53]

- The safety and benefits of cobedding for twins and higher-order multiples have not been established. It is prudent to provide separate sleep surfaces and avoid cobedding for twins and higher-order multiples in the hospital and at home.[54]

5. **Keep soft objects and loose bedding away from the infant's sleep area to reduce the risk of SIDS, suffocation, entrapment, and strangulation.**

Soft objects,[19,20,55–58] such as pillows and pillow-like toys, quilts, comforters, sheepskins, and loose bedding,[4,7,59–64] such as blankets and nonfitted sheets, can obstruct an infant's nose and mouth. An obstructed airway can pose a risk of suffocation, entrapment, or SIDS.

Infant sleep clothing, such as a wearable blanket, is preferable to blankets and other coverings to keep the infant warm while reducing the chance of head covering or entrapment that could result from blanket use.

Bumper pads or similar products that attach to crib slats or sides were originally intended to prevent injury or death attributable to head entrapment. Cribs manufactured to newer standards have a narrower distance between slats to prevent head entrapment. Because bumper pads have been implicated as a factor contributing to deaths from suffocation, entrapment, and strangulation[65,66] and because they are not necessary to prevent head entrapment with new safety standards for crib slats, they are not recommended for infants.[65,66]

6. Consider offering a pacifier at nap time and bedtime.

Although the mechanism is yet unclear, studies have reported a protective effect of pacifiers on the incidence of SIDS.[67,68] The protective effect of the pacifier is observed even if the pacifier falls out of the infant's mouth.[69,70]

The pacifier should be used when placing the infant for sleep. It does not need to be reinserted once the infant falls asleep. If the infant refuses the pacifier, he or she should not be forced to take it. In those cases, parents can try to offer the pacifier again when the infant is a little older.

Because of the risk of strangulation, pacifiers should not be hung around the infant's neck. Pacifiers that attach to infant clothing should not be used with sleeping infants.

Objects, such as stuffed toys and other items that may present a suffocation or choking risk, should not be attached to pacifiers.

For breastfed infants, pacifier introduction should be delayed until breastfeeding is firmly established.[40] Infants who are not being directly breastfed can begin pacifier use as soon as desired.

There is insufficient evidence that finger sucking is protective against SIDS.

7. Avoid smoke exposure during pregnancy and after birth.

Both maternal smoking during pregnancy and smoke in the infant's environment after birth are major risk factors for SIDS.

Mothers should not smoke during pregnancy or after the infant's birth.[71-74]

There should be no smoking near pregnant women or infants. Encourage families to set strict rules for smoke-free homes and cars and to eliminate secondhand tobacco smoke from all places in which children and other nonsmokers spend time.[75,76]

The risk of SIDS is particularly high when the infant bed-shares with an adult smoker, even when the adult does not smoke in bed.[6,7,46,49,50,77]

8. Avoid alcohol and illicit drug use during pregnancy and after birth.

There is an increased risk of SIDS with prenatal and postnatal exposure to alcohol or illicit drug use.

Mothers should avoid alcohol and illicit drugs periconceptionally and during pregnancy.[78-85]

Parental alcohol and/or illicit drug use in combination with bed-sharing places the infant at particularly high risk of SIDS.[8,51]

9. Avoid overheating and head covering in infants.

Although studies have shown an increased risk of SIDS with overheating,[86-89] the definition of overheating in these studies varies. Therefore, it is difficult to provide specific room temperature guidelines to avoid overheating.

In general, infants should be dressed appropriately for the environment, with no greater than 1 layer more than an adult would wear to be comfortable in that environment.

Parents and caregivers should evaluate the infant for signs of overheating, such as sweating or the infant's chest feeling hot to the touch.

Overbundling and covering of the face and head should be avoided.[90]

There is currently insufficient evidence to recommend the use of a fan as a SIDS risk-reduction strategy.

10. Pregnant women should obtain regular prenatal care.

There is substantial epidemiologic evidence linking a lower risk of SIDS for infants whose mothers obtain

regular prenatal care.[71-74] Pregnant women should follow guidelines for frequency of prenatal visits.[91]

11. Infants should be immunized in accordance with recommendations of the AAP and Centers for Disease Control and Prevention.

There is no evidence that there is a causal relationship between immunizations and SIDS.[92-95] Indeed, recent evidence suggests that vaccination may have a protective effect against SIDS.[96-98]

12. Avoid the use of commercial devices that are inconsistent with safe sleep recommendations.

Be particularly wary of devices that claim to reduce the risk of SIDS. Examples include, but are not limited to, wedges and positioners and other devices placed in the adult bed for the purpose of positioning or separating the infant from others in the bed. Crib mattresses also have been developed to improve the dispersion of carbon dioxide in the event that the infant ends up in the prone position during sleep. Although data do not support the claim of carbon dioxide dispersion unless there is an active dispersal component,[99] there is no harm in using these mattresses if they meet standard safety requirements. However, there is no evidence that any of these devices reduce the risk of SIDS. Importantly, the use of products claiming to increase sleep safety does not diminish the importance of following recommended safe sleep practices. Information about a specific product can be found on the CPSC Web site (www.cpsc.gov). The AAP concurs with the US Food and Drug Administration and the CPSC that manufacturers should not claim that a product or device protects against SIDS unless there is scientific evidence to that effect.

13. Do not use home cardiorespiratory monitors as a strategy to reduce the risk of SIDS.

The use of cardiorespiratory monitors has not been documented to decrease the incidence of SIDS.[100–103] These devices are sometimes prescribed for use at home to detect apnea or bradycardia and, when pulse oximetry is used, decreases in oxyhemoglobin saturation for infants at risk of these conditions. In addition, routine in-hospital cardiorespiratory monitoring before discharge from the hospital has not been shown to detect infants at risk of SIDS. There are no data that other commercial devices that are designed to monitor infant vital signs reduce the risk of SIDS.

14. **Supervised, awake tummy time is recommended to facilitate development and to minimize development of positional plagiocephaly.**

Although there are no data to make specific recommendations as to how often and how long it should be undertaken, the task force concurs with the AAP Committee on Practice and Ambulatory Medicine and Section on Neurologic Surgery that "a certain amount of prone positioning, or 'tummy time,' while the infant is awake and being observed is recommended to help prevent the development of flattening of the occiput and to facilitate development of the upper shoulder girdle strength necessary for timely attainment of certain motor milestones."[104]

Diagnosis, management, and other prevention strategies for positional plagiocephaly, such as avoidance of excessive time in car seats and changing the infant's orientation in the crib, are discussed in detail in the AAP clinical report on positional skull deformities.[104]

15. **There is no evidence to recommend swaddling as a strategy to reduce the risk of SIDS.**

Swaddling, or wrapping the infant in a light blanket, is often used as a strategy to calm the infant and encourage the use of the supine position. There is a high risk of death if a swaddled infant is

placed in or rolls to the prone position.[88,105,106] If infants are swaddled, they should always be placed on the back. Swaddling should be snug around the chest but allow for ample room at the hips and knees to avoid exacerbation of hip dysplasia. When an infant exhibits signs of attempting to roll, swaddling should no longer be used.[88,105,106] There is no evidence with regard to SIDS risk related to the arms swaddled in or out. These decisions about swaddling should be made on an individual basis, depending on the physiologic needs of the infant.

16. **Health care professionals, staff in newborn nurseries and NICUs, and child care providers should endorse and model the SIDS risk-reduction recommendations from birth.**[107–109]

Staff in NICUs should model and implement all SIDS risk-reduction recommendations as soon as the infant is medically stable and well before anticipated discharge.

Staff in newborn nurseries should model and implement these recommendations beginning at birth and well before anticipated discharge.

All physicians, nurses, and other health care providers should receive education on safe infant sleep. Health care providers should screen for and recommend safe sleep practices at each visit for infants up to 1 year old. Families who do not have a safe sleep space for their infant should be provided with information about low-cost or free cribs or play yards.

Hospitals should ensure that hospital policies are consistent with updated safe sleep recommendations and that infant sleep spaces (bassinets, cribs) meet safe sleep standards.

All state regulatory agencies should require that child care providers receive education on safe infant sleep and implement safe sleep practices. It is preferable that they have written policies.

17. **Media and manufacturers should follow safe sleep guidelines in their messaging and advertising.**

Media exposures (including movie, television, magazines, newspapers, and Web sites), manufacturer advertisements, and store displays affect individual behavior by influencing beliefs and attitudes.[107,109] Media and advertising messages contrary to safe sleep recommendations may create misinformation about safe sleep practices.[110]

18. **Continue the "Safe to Sleep" campaign, focusing on ways to reduce the risk of all sleep-related infant deaths, including SIDS, suffocation, and other unintentional deaths. Pediatricians and other primary care providers should actively participate in this campaign.**

Public education should continue for all who care for infants, including parents, child care providers, grandparents, foster parents, and babysitters, and should include strategies for overcoming barriers to behavior change.

The campaign should continue to have a special focus on the black and American Indian/Alaskan Native populations because of the higher incidence of SIDS and other sleep-related infant deaths in these groups.

The campaign should specifically include strategies to increase breastfeeding while decreasing bed-sharing, and eliminating tobacco smoke exposure. The campaign should also highlight the circumstances that substantially increase the risk of SIDS or unintentional injury or death while bed-sharing, as listed previously.

These recommendations should be introduced before pregnancy and ideally in secondary school curricula to both males and females and incorporated into courses developed to train teenaged and adult babysitters. The importance of maternal preconceptional health, infant breastfeeding, and the avoidance of substance use (including alcohol and smoking) should be included in this training.

Safe sleep messages should be reviewed, revised, and reissued at least every 5 years to address the next generation of new parents and products on the market.

19. **Continue research and surveillance on the risk factors, causes, and pathophysiologic mechanisms of SIDS and other sleep-related infant deaths, with the ultimate goal of eliminating these deaths altogether.**

Education campaigns need to be evaluated, and innovative intervention methods need to be encouraged and funded.

Continued research and improved surveillance on the etiology and pathophysiologic basis of SIDS should be funded.

Standardized protocols for death scene investigations, as per Centers for Disease Control and Prevention protocol, should continue to be implemented. Comprehensive autopsies, including full external and internal examination of all major organs and tissues including the brain; complete radiographs; metabolic testing; and toxicology screening should be performed. Training about how to conduct a comprehensive death scene investigation offered to medical examiners, coroners, death scene investigators, first responders, and law enforcement should continue; and resources to maintain training and conduct of these investigations need to be allocated. In addition, child death reviews, with involvement of pediatricians and other primary care providers, should be supported and funded.

Improved and widespread surveillance of SIDS and SUID cases should be implemented and funded.

Federal and private funding agencies should remain committed to all

aspects of the aforementioned research.

ACKNOWLEDGMENTS

We acknowledge the contributions provided by others to the collection and interpretation of data examined in preparation of this report. We are particularly grateful for the independent biostatistical report submitted by Robert W. Platt, PhD.

LEAD AUTHOR

Rachel Y. Moon, MD, FAAP

TASK FORCE ON SUDDEN INFANT DEATH SYNDROME

Rachel Y. Moon, MD, FAAP, Chairperson
Robert A. Darnall, MD
Lori Feldman-Winter, MD, MPH, FAAP
Michael H. Goodstein, MD, FAAP
Fern R. Hauck, MD, MS

CONSULTANTS

Marian Willinger, PhD – Eunice Kennedy Shriver *National Institute for Child Health and Human Development*
Carrie K. Shapiro-Mendoza, PhD, MPH – *Centers for Disease Control and Prevention*

STAFF

James Couto, MA

ABBREVIATIONS

AAP: American Academy of Pediatrics
CPSC: Consumer Product Safety Commission
SIDS: sudden infant death syndrome
SUID: sudden unexpected infant death

REFERENCES

1. Willinger M, James LS, Catz C. Defining the sudden infant death syndrome (SIDS): deliberations of an expert panel convened by the National Institute of Child Health and Human Development. *Pediatr Pathol.* 1991;11(5):677–684

2. Ebell MH, Siwek J, Weiss BD, et al. Strength of recommendation taxonomy (SORT): a patient-centered approach to grading evidence in the medical literature. *Am Fam Physician.* 2004;69(3):548–556

3. Moon RY; AAP Task Force on Sudden Infant Death Syndrome. SIDS and other sleep-related infant deaths: Evidence base for 2016 updated recommendations for a safe infant sleeping environment. *Pediatrics.* 2016;138(5):e20162940

4. Hauck FR, Herman SM, Donovan M, et al. Sleep environment and the risk of sudden infant death syndrome in an urban population: the Chicago Infant Mortality Study. *Pediatrics.* 2003; 111(5 pt 2):1207–1214

5. Li DK, Petitti DB, Willinger M, et al. Infant sleeping position and the risk of sudden infant death syndrome in California, 1997-2000. *Am J Epidemiol.* 2003;157(5):446–455

6. Blair PS, Fleming PJ, Smith IJ, et al; CESDI SUDI Research Group. Babies sleeping with parents: case-control study of factors influencing the risk of the sudden infant death syndrome. *BMJ.* 1999;319(7223):1457–1461

7. Fleming PJ, Blair PS, Bacon C, et al; Confidential Enquiry into Stillbirths and Deaths Regional Coordinators and Researchers. Environment of infants during sleep and risk of the sudden infant death syndrome: results of 1993-5 case-control study for confidential inquiry into stillbirths and deaths in infancy. *BMJ.* 1996;313(7051):191–195

8. Carpenter RG, Irgens LM, Blair PS, et al. Sudden unexplained infant death in 20 regions in Europe: case control study. *Lancet.* 2004;363(9404):185–191

9. Malloy MH. Trends in postneonatal aspiration deaths and reclassification of sudden infant death syndrome: impact of the "Back to Sleep" program. *Pediatrics.* 2002;109(4):661–665

10. Tablizo MA, Jacinto P, Parsley D, Chen ML, Ramanathan R, Keens TG. Supine sleeping position does not cause clinical aspiration in neonates in hospital newborn nurseries. *Arch Pediatr Adolesc Med.* 2007;161(5):507–510

11. Vandenplas Y, Rudolph CD, Di Lorenzo C, et al; North American Society

for Pediatric Gastroenterology Hepatology and Nutrition; European Society for Pediatric Gastroenterology Hepatology and Nutrition. Pediatric gastroesophageal reflux clinical practice guidelines: joint recommendations of the North American Society for Pediatric Gastroenterology, Hepatology, and Nutrition (NASPGHAN) and the European Society for Pediatric Gastroenterology, Hepatology, and Nutrition (ESPGHAN). *J Pediatr Gastroenterol Nutr.* 2009;49(4):498–547

12. Tobin JM, McCloud P, Cameron DJ. Posture and gastro-oesophageal reflux: a case for left lateral positioning. *Arch Dis Child.* 1997;76(3):254–258

13. Malloy MH, Hoffman HJ. Prematurity, sudden infant death syndrome, and age of death. *Pediatrics.* 1995;96(3 pt 1):464–471

14. Sowter B, Doyle LW, Morley CJ, Altmann A, Halliday J. Is sudden infant death syndrome still more common in very low birthweight infants in the 1990s? *Med J Aust.* 1999;171(8):411–413

15. Oyen N, Markestad T, Skaerven R, et al. Combined effects of sleeping position and prenatal risk factors in sudden infant death syndrome: the Nordic Epidemiological SIDS Study. *Pediatrics.* 1997;100(4):613–621

16. American Academy of Pediatrics Committee on Fetus and Newborn. Hospital discharge of the high-risk neonate. *Pediatrics.* 2008;122(5):1119–1126

17. Winter-Feldman L, Golsmith JP; American Academy of Pediatrics Committee on Fetus and Newborn. Safe sleep and skin-to-skin care in the neonatal period for healthy term newborns. *Pediatrics.* 2016;138(3):e20161889

18. Colvin JD, Collie-Akers V, Schunn C, Moon RY. Sleep environment risks for younger and older infants. *Pediatrics.* 2014;134(2):e406–e412

19. Kemp JS, Nelson VE, Thach BT. Physical properties of bedding that may increase risk of sudden infant death syndrome in prone-sleeping infants. *Pediatr Res.* 1994;36(1 pt 1): 7–11

20. Kemp JS, Livne M, White DK, Arfken CL. Softness and potential to cause rebreathing: differences in bedding used by infants at high and low risk for sudden infant death syndrome. *J Pediatr.* 1998;132(2):234–239

21. US Consumer Product Safety Commission. *Crib Safety Tips: Use Your Crib Safely*, CPSC Document 5030. Washington, DC: US Consumer Product Safety Commission; 2006

22. US Consumer Product Safety Commission. Safety standard for bedside sleepers. *Fed Reg.* 2014;79(10):2581–2589

23. Ostfeld BM, Perl H, Esposito L, et al. Sleep environment, positional, lifestyle, and demographic characteristics associated with bed sharing in sudden infant death syndrome cases: a population-based study. *Pediatrics.* 2006;118(5):2051–2059

24. Scheers NJ, Rutherford GW, Kemp JS. Where should infants sleep? A comparison of risk for suffocation of infants sleeping in cribs, adult beds, and other sleeping locations. *Pediatrics.* 2003;112(4):883–889

25. Bass JL, Bull M. Oxygen desaturation in term infants in car safety seats. *Pediatrics.* 2002;110(2 pt 1):401–402

26. Kornhauser Cerar L, Scirica CV, Stucin Gantar I, Osredkar I don'D, Neubauer D, Kinane TB. A comparison of respiratory patterns in healthy term infants placed in car safety seats and beds. *Pediatrics.* 2009;124(3). Available at: www.pediatrics.org/cgi/content/full/124/3/e396

27. Côté A, Bairam A, Deschenes M, Hatzakis G. Sudden infant deaths in sitting devices. *Arch Dis Child.* 2008;93(5):384–389

28. Merchant JR, Worwa C, Porter S, Coleman JM, deRegnier RA. Respiratory instability of term and near-term healthy newborn infants in car safety seats. *Pediatrics.* 2001;108(3):647–652

29. Willett LD, Leuschen MP, Nelson LS, Nelson RM Jr. Risk of hypoventilation in premature infants in car seats. *J Pediatr.* 1986;109(2):245–248

30. Batra EK, Midgett JD, Moon RY. Hazards associated with sitting and carrying devices for children two years and younger. *J Pediatr.* 2015;167(1):183–187

31. US Consumer Product Safety Commission. Safety Standard for Sling Carriers. *Fed Reg.* 2014;79(141):42724–42734

32. Desapriya EB, Joshi P, Subzwari S, Nolan M. Infant injuries from child restraint safety seat misuse at British Columbia Children's Hospital. *Pediatr Int.* 2008;50(5):674–678

33. Graham CJ, Kittredge D, Stuemky JH. Injuries associated with child safety seat misuse. *Pediatr Emerg Care.* 1992;8(6):351–353

34. Parikh SN, Wilson L. Hazardous use of car seats outside the car in the United States, 2003-2007. *Pediatrics.* 2010;126(2):352–357

35. Pollack-Nelson C. Fall and suffocation injuries associated with in-home use of car seats and baby carriers. *Pediatr Emerg Care.* 2000;16(2):77–79

36. Wickham T, Abrahamson E. Head injuries in infants: the risks of bouncy chairs and car seats. *Arch Dis Child.* 2002;86(3):168–169

37. Ip S, Chung M, Raman G, Trikalinos TA, Lau J. A summary of the Agency for Healthcare Research and Quality's evidence report on breastfeeding in developed countries. *Breastfeed Med.* 2009;4(suppl 1):S17–S30

38. Vennemann MM, Bajanowski T, Brinkmann B, et al; GeSID Study Group. Does breastfeeding reduce the risk of sudden infant death syndrome? *Pediatrics.* 2009;123(3). Available at: www.pediatrics.org/cgi/content/full/123/3/e406

39. Hauck FR, Thompson JM, Tanabe KO, Moon RY, Vennemann MM. Breastfeeding and reduced risk of sudden infant death syndrome: a meta-analysis. *Pediatrics.* 2011;128(1):103–110

40. Eidelman AI, Schanler RJ; Section on Breastfeeding. Breastfeeding and the use of human milk. *Pediatrics.* 2012;129(3). Available at: www.pediatrics.org/cgi/content/full/129/3/e827

41. Mitchell EA, Thompson JMD. Co-sleeping increases the risk of SIDS, but sleeping in the parents' bedroom lowers it. In: Rognum TO,

ed. *Sudden Infant Death Syndrome: New Trends in the Nineties*. Oslo, Norway: Scandinavian University Press; 1995:266–269

42. Tappin D, Ecob R, Brooke H. Bedsharing, roomsharing, and sudden infant death syndrome in Scotland: a case-control study. *J Pediatr*. 2005;147(1):32–37

43. McGarvey C, McDonnell M, Chong A, O'Regan M, Matthews T. Factors relating to the infant's last sleep environment in sudden infant death syndrome in the Republic of Ireland. *Arch Dis Child*. 2003;88(12):1058–1064

44. Rechtman LR, Colvin JD, Blair PS, Moon RY. Sofas and infant mortality. *Pediatrics*. 2014;134(5). Available at: www.pediatrics.org/cgi/content/full/134/5/e1293

45. McGarvey C, McDonnell M, Hamilton K, O'Regan M, Matthews T. An 8 year study of risk factors for SIDS: bed-sharing versus non-bed-sharing. *Arch Dis Child*. 2006;91(4):318–323

46. Vennemann MM, Hense HW, Bajanowski T, et al Bed sharing and the risk of sudden infant death syndrome: can we resolve the debate? *J Pediatr*. 2012;160(1):44–48, e42

47. Blair PS, Platt MW, Smith IJ, Fleming PJ; CESDI SUDI Research Group. Sudden infant death syndrome and sleeping position in pre-term and low birth weight infants: an opportunity for targeted intervention. *Arch Dis Child*. 2006;91(2):101–106

48. Carpenter R, McGarvey C, Mitchell EA, et al. Bed sharing when parents do not smoke: is there a risk of SIDS? An individual level analysis of five major case-control studies. *BMJ Open*. 2013;3(5):e002299

49. Arnestad M, Andersen M, Vege A, Rognum TO. Changes in the epidemiological pattern of sudden infant death syndrome in southeast Norway, 1984-1998: implications for future prevention and research. *Arch Dis Child*. 2001;85(2):108–115

50. Scragg R, Mitchell EA, Taylor BJ, et al; New Zealand Cot Death Study Group. Bed sharing, smoking, and alcohol in the sudden infant death syndrome. *BMJ*. 1993;307(6915):1312–1318

51. Blair PS, Sidebotham P, Evason-Coombe C, Edmonds M, Heckstall-Smith EM, Fleming P. Hazardous cosleeping environments and risk factors amenable to change: case-control study of SIDS in south west England. *BMJ*. 2009;339:b3666

52. Blair PS, Sidebotham P, Pease A, Fleming PJ. Bed-sharing in the absence of hazardous circumstances: is there a risk of sudden infant death syndrome? An analysis from two case-control studies conducted in the UK. *PLoS One*. 2014;9(9):e107799

53. Fu LY, Moon RY, Hauck FR. Bed sharing among black infants and sudden infant death syndrome: interactions with other known risk factors. *Acad Pediatr*. 2010;10(6):376–382

54. Tomashek KM, Wallman C; American Academy of Pediatrics Committee on Fetus and Newborn. Cobedding twins and higher-order multiples in a hospital setting. *Pediatrics*. 2007;120(6):1359–1366

55. Chiodini BA, Thach BT. Impaired ventilation in infants sleeping facedown: potential significance for sudden infant death syndrome. *J Pediatr*. 1993;123(5):686–692

56. Sakai J, Kanetake J, Takahashi S, Kanawaku Y, Funayama M. Gas dispersal potential of bedding as a cause for sudden infant death. *Forensic Sci Int*. 2008;180(2–3):93–97

57. Patel AL, Harris K, Thach BT. Inspired CO(2) and O(2) in sleeping infants rebreathing from bedding: relevance for sudden infant death syndrome. *J Appl Physiol (1985)*. 2001;91(6):2537–2545

58. Kanetake J, Aoki Y, Funayama M. Evaluation of rebreathing potential on bedding for infant use. *Pediatr Int*. 2003;45(3):284–289

59. Brooke H, Gibson A, Tappin D, Brown H. Case-control study of sudden infant death syndrome in Scotland, 1992-5. *BMJ*. 1997;314(7093):1516–1520

60. L'Hoir MP, Engelberts AC, van Well GTJ, et al. Risk and preventive factors for cot death in The Netherlands, a low-incidence country. *Eur J Pediatr*. 1998;157(8):681–688

61. Markestad T, Skadberg B, Hordvik E, Morild I, Irgens LM. Sleeping position and sudden infant death syndrome (SIDS): effect of an intervention programme to avoid prone sleeping. *Acta Paediatr*. 1995;84(4):375–378

62. Ponsonby A-L, Dwyer T, Couper D, Cochrane J. Association between use of a quilt and sudden infant death syndrome: case-control study. *BMJ*. 1998;316(7126):195–196

63. Beal SM, Byard RW. Accidental death or sudden infant death syndrome? *J Paediatr Child Health*. 1995;31(4):269–271

64. Wilson CA, Taylor BJ, Laing RM, Williams SM, Mitchell EA. Clothing and bedding and its relevance to sudden infant death syndrome: further results from the New Zealand Cot Death Study. *J Paediatr Child Health*. 1994;30(6):506–512

65. Thach BT, Rutherford GW Jr, Harris K. Deaths and injuries attributed to infant crib bumper pads. *J Pediatr*. 2007;151(3):271–274, 274.e1–274.e3

66. Scheers NJ, Woodard DW, Thach BT. Crib bumpers continue to cause infant deaths: a need for a new preventive approach. *J Pediatr*. 2016;169:93–97, e91

67. Hauck FR, Omojokun OO, Siadaty MS. Do pacifiers reduce the risk of sudden infant death syndrome? A meta-analysis. *Pediatrics*. 2005;116(5). Available at: www.pediatrics.org/cgi/content/full/116/5/e716

68. Li DK, Willinger M, Petitti DB, Odouli R, Liu L, Hoffman HJ. Use of a dummy (pacifier) during sleep and risk of sudden infant death syndrome (SIDS): population-based case-control study. *BMJ*. 2006;332(7532):18–22

69. Franco P, Scaillet S, Wermenbol V, Valente F, Groswasser J, Kahn A. The influence of a pacifier on infants' arousals from sleep. *J Pediatr*. 2000;136(6):775–779

70. Weiss PP, Kerbl R. The relatively short duration that a child retains a pacifier in the mouth during sleep: implications for sudden infant death syndrome. *Eur J Pediatr*. 2001;160(1):60–70

71. Getahun D, Amre D, Rhoads GG, Demissie K. Maternal and obstetric risk factors for sudden infant death syndrome in the United States. *Obstet Gynecol*. 2004;103(4):646–652

72. Kraus JF, Greenland S, Bulterys M. Risk factors for sudden infant death syndrome in the US Collaborative Perinatal Project. *Int J Epidemiol.* 1989;18(1):113–120

73. Paris CA, Remler R, Daling JR. Risk factors for sudden infant death syndrome: changes associated with sleep position recommendations. *J Pediatr.* 2001;139(6):771–777

74. Stewart AJ, Williams SM, Mitchell EA, Taylor BJ, Ford RP, Allen EM. Antenatal and intrapartum factors associated with sudden infant death syndrome in the New Zealand Cot Death Study. *J Paediatr Child Health.* 1995;31(5):473–478

75. Farber HJ, Walley SC, Groner JA, Nelson KE; Section on Tobacco Control. Clinical practice policy to protect children from tobacco, nicotine, and tobacco smoke [policy statement]. *Pediatrics.* 2015;136(5):1008–1017

76. Farber HJ, Groner J, Walley S, Nelson K; Section on Tobacco Control. Protecting children from tobacco, nicotine, and tobacco smoke [technical report]. *Pediatrics.* 2015;136(5). Available at: www.pediatrics.org/cgi/content/full/136/5/e1439

77. Zhang K, Wang X. Maternal smoking and increased risk of sudden infant death syndrome: a meta-analysis. *Leg Med (Tokyo).* 2013;15(3):115–121

78. Rajegowda BK, Kandall SR, Falciglia H. Sudden unexpected death in infants of narcotic-dependent mothers. *Early Hum Dev.* 1978;2(3):219–225

79. Chavez CJ, Ostrea EM Jr, Stryker JC, Smialek Z. Sudden infant death syndrome among infants of drug-dependent mothers. *J Pediatr.* 1979;95(3):407–409

80. Durand DJ, Espinoza AM, Nickerson BG. Association between prenatal cocaine exposure and sudden infant death syndrome. *J Pediatr.* 1990;117(6):909–911

81. Ward SL, Bautista D, Chan L, et al. Sudden infant death syndrome in infants of substance-abusing mothers. *J Pediatr.* 1990;117(6):876–881

82. Rosen TS, Johnson HL. Drug-addicted mothers, their infants, and SIDS. *Ann N Y Acad Sci.* 1988;533:89–95

83. Kandall SR, Gaines J, Habel L, Davidson G, Jessop D. Relationship of maternal substance abuse to subsequent sudden infant death syndrome in offspring. *J Pediatr.* 1993;123(1):120–126

84. Fares I, McCulloch KM, Raju TN. Intrauterine cocaine exposure and the risk for sudden infant death syndrome: a meta-analysis. *J Perinatol.* 1997;17(3):179–182

85. O'Leary CM, Jacoby PJ, Bartu A, D'Antoine H, Bower C. Maternal alcohol use and sudden infant death syndrome and infant mortality excluding SIDS. *Pediatrics.* 2013;131(3). Available at: www.pediatrics.org/cgi/content/full/131/3/e770

86. Fleming PJ, Gilbert R, Azaz Y, et al. Interaction between bedding and sleeping position in the sudden infant death syndrome: a population based case-control study. *BMJ.* 1990;301(6743):85–89

87. Ponsonby A-L, Dwyer T, Gibbons LE, Cochrane JA, Jones ME, McCall MJ. Thermal environment and sudden infant death syndrome: case-control study. *BMJ.* 1992;304(6822):277–282

88. Ponsonby A-L, Dwyer T, Gibbons LE, Cochrane JA, Wang Y-G. Factors potentiating the risk of sudden infant death syndrome associated with the prone position. *N Engl J Med.* 1993;329(6):377–382

89. Iyasu S, Randall LL, Welty TK, et al. Risk factors for sudden infant death syndrome among northern plains Indians. *JAMA.* 2002;288(21):2717–2723

90. Blair PS, Mitchell EA, Heckstall-Smith EM, Fleming PJ. Head covering—a major modifiable risk factor for sudden infant death syndrome: a systematic review. *Arch Dis Child.* 2008;93(9):778–783

91. American Academy of Pediatrics Committee on Fetus and Newborn; ACOG Committee on Obstetric Practice. *Guidelines for Perinatal Care.* 7th ed. Elk Grove Village, IL: American Academy of Pediatrics; 2012

92. Immunization Safety Review Committee. Stratton K, Almario DA, Wizemann TM, McCormick MC, eds. *Immunization Safety Review: Vaccinations and Sudden Unexpected Death in Infancy.* Washington, DC: National Academies Press; 2003

93. Moro PL, Arana J, Cano M, Lewis P, Shimabukuro TT. Deaths reported to the Vaccine Adverse Event Reporting System, United States, 1997-2013. *Clin Infect Dis.* 2015;61(6):980–987

94. Miller ER, Moro PL, Cano M, Shimabukuro TT. Deaths following vaccination: what does the evidence show? *Vaccine.* 2015;33(29):3288–3292

95. Moro PL, Jankosky C, Menschik D, et al. Adverse events following Haemophilus influenzae type b vaccines in the Vaccine Adverse Event Reporting System, 1990-2013. *J Pediatr.* 2015;166(4):992–997

96. Mitchell EA, Stewart AW, Clements M, Ford RPK; New Zealand Cot Death Study Group. Immunisation and the sudden infant death syndrome. *Arch Dis Child.* 1995;73(6):498–501

97. Jonville-Béra AP, Autret-Leca E, Barbeillon F, Paris-Llado J; French Reference Centers for SIDS. Sudden unexpected death in infants under 3 months of age and vaccination status—a case-control study. *Br J Clin Pharmacol.* 2001;51(3):271–276

98. Fleming PJ, Blair PS, Platt MW, Tripp J, Smith IJ, Golding J. The UK accelerated immunisation programme and sudden unexpected death in infancy: case-control study. *BMJ.* 2001;322(7290):822

99. Carolan PL, Wheeler WB, Ross JD, Kemp RJ. Potential to prevent carbon dioxide rebreathing of commercial products marketed to reduce sudden infant death syndrome risk. *Pediatrics.* 2000;105(4 pt 1):774–779

100. Hodgman JE, Hoppenbrouwers T. Home monitoring for the sudden infant death syndrome: the case against. *Ann N Y Acad Sci.* 1988;533:164–175

101. Ward SL, Keens TG, Chan LS, et al. Sudden infant death syndrome in infants evaluated by apnea programs in California. *Pediatrics.* 1986;77(4):451–458

102. Monod N, Plouin P, Sternberg B, et al. Are polygraphic and cardiopneumographic respiratory patterns useful tools for predicting the risk for sudden infant death syndrome? A 10-year study. *Biol Neonate.* 1986;50(3):147–153

103. Ramanathan R, Corwin MJ, Hunt CE, et al; Collaborative Home Infant Monitoring Evaluation (CHIME) Study Group. Cardiorespiratory events recorded on home monitors: comparison of healthy infants with those at increased risk for SIDS. *JAMA*. 2001;285(17):2199–2207

104. Laughlin J, Luerssen TG, Dias MS; Committee on Practice and Ambulatory Medicine; Section on Neurological Surgery. Prevention and management of positional skull deformities in infants. *Pediatrics*. 2011;128(6):1236–1241

105. van Sleuwen BE, Engelberts AC, Boere-Boonekamp MM, Kuis W, Schulpen TW, L'Hoir MP. Swaddling: a systematic review. *Pediatrics*. 2007;120(4). Available at: www.pediatrics.org/cgi/content/full/120/4/e1097

106. McDonnell E, Moon RY. Infant deaths and injuries associated with wearable blankets, swaddle wraps, and swaddling. *J Pediatr*. 2014;164(5):1152–1156

107. Willinger M, Ko C-W, Hoffman HJ, Kessler RC, Corwin MJ. Factors associated with caregivers' choice of infant sleep position, 1994-1998: the National Infant Sleep Position Study. *JAMA*. 2000;283(16):2135–2142

108. Brenner RA, Simons-Morton BG, Bhaskar B, et al. Prevalence and predictors of the prone sleep position among inner-city infants. *JAMA*. 1998;280(4): 341–346

109. Von Kohorn I, Corwin MJ, Rybin DV, Heeren TC, Lister G, Colson ER. Influence of prior advice and beliefs of mothers on infant sleep position. *Arch Pediatr Adolesc Med*. 2010;164(4):363–369

110. Joyner BL, Gill-Bailey C, Moon RY. Infant sleep environments depicted in magazines targeted to women of childbearing age. *Pediatrics*. 2009;124(3):e416–e422

SIDS and Other Sleep-Related Infant Deaths: Evidence Base for 2016 Updated Recommendations for a Safe Infant Sleeping Environment

• *Technical Report*

TECHNICAL REPORT

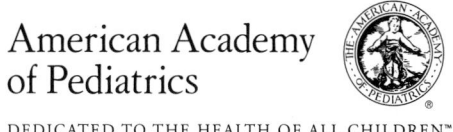

SIDS and Other Sleep-Related Infant Deaths: Evidence Base for 2016 Updated Recommendations for a Safe Infant Sleeping Environment

Rachel Y. Moon, MD, FAAP, TASK FORCE ON SUDDEN INFANT DEATH SYNDROME

abstract

Approximately 3500 infants die annually in the United States from sleep-related infant deaths, including sudden infant death syndrome (SIDS), ill-defined deaths, and accidental suffocation and strangulation in bed. After an initial decrease in the 1990s, the overall sleep-related infant death rate has not declined in more recent years. Many of the modifiable and nonmodifiable risk factors for SIDS and other sleep-related infant deaths are strikingly similar. The American Academy of Pediatrics recommends a safe sleep environment that can reduce the risk of all sleep-related infant deaths. Recommendations for a safe sleep environment include supine positioning, use of a firm sleep surface, room-sharing without bed-sharing, and avoidance of soft bedding and overheating. Additional recommendations for SIDS risk reduction include avoidance of exposure to smoke, alcohol, and illicit drugs; breastfeeding; routine immunization; and use of a pacifier. New evidence and rationale for recommendations are presented for skin-to-skin care for newborn infants, bedside and in-bed sleepers, sleeping on couches/armchairs and in sitting devices, and use of soft bedding after 4 months of age. In addition, expanded recommendations for infant sleep location are included. The recommendations and strength of evidence for each recommendation are published in the accompanying policy statement, "SIDS and Other Sleep-Related Infant Deaths: Updated 2016 Recommendations for a Safe Infant Sleeping Environment," which is included in this issue.

DOI: 10.1542/peds.2016-2940

PEDIATRICS (ISSN Numbers: Print, 0031-4005; Online, 1098-4275).

Copyright © 2016 by the American Academy of Pediatrics

FINANCIAL DISCLOSURE: The author has indicated she does not have a financial relationship relevant to this article to disclose.

FUNDING: No external funding.

POTENTIAL CONFLICT OF INTEREST: The author has indicated she has no potential conflicts of interest to disclose.

To cite: Moon RY and AAP TASK FORCE ON SUDDEN INFANT DEATH SYNDROME. SIDS and Other Sleep-Related Infant Deaths: Evidence Base for 2016 Updated Recommendations for a Safe Infant Sleeping Environment. *Pediatrics.* 2016;138(5): e20162940

SEARCH STRATEGY AND METHODOLOGY

Literature searches with the use of PubMed were conducted for each of the topics in the technical report, concentrating on articles published since 2011 (when the last technical report and policy statement were published[1,2]). All iterations of the search terms were used for each topic area. For example, the pacifier topic search combined either "SIDS,"

"SUID," "sudden death," or "cot death" with "pacifier," "dummy," "soother," and "sucking." A total of 63 new studies were judged to be of sufficiently high quality to be included in this technical report. In addition, because the data regarding bed-sharing have been conflicting, the independent opinion of a biostatistician with special expertise in perinatal epidemiology was solicited. The strength of evidence for recommendations, using the Strength-of-Recommendation Taxonomy,[3] was determined by the task force members. A draft version of the policy statement and technical report was submitted to relevant committees and sections of the American Academy of Pediatrics (AAP) for review and comment. After the appropriate revisions were made, a final version was submitted to the AAP Executive Committee for final approval.

SUDDEN UNEXPECTED INFANT DEATH AND SUDDEN INFANT DEATH SYNDROME: DEFINITIONS AND DIAGNOSTIC ISSUES

Sudden unexpected infant death (SUID), also known as sudden unexpected death in infancy (SUDI), is a term used to describe any sudden and unexpected death, whether explained or unexplained (including sudden infant death syndrome [SIDS] and ill-defined deaths), occurring during infancy. After case investigation, SUID can be attributed to causes of death such as suffocation, asphyxia, entrapment, infection, ingestions, metabolic diseases, and trauma (unintentional or nonaccidental). SIDS is a subcategory of SUID and is a cause assigned to infant deaths that cannot be explained after a thorough case investigation including autopsy, a scene investigation, and review of clinical history.[4] (See Table 1 for definitions of terms.) The distinction between SIDS and other SUIDs, particularly those that

TABLE 1 Definitions of Terms

Caregivers: Throughout the document, "parents" are used, but this term is meant to indicate any infant caregivers.

Bed-sharing: Parent(s) and infant sleeping together on any surface (bed, couch, chair).

Cosleeping: This term is commonly used, but the task force finds it confusing and it is not used in this document. When used, authors need to make clear whether they are referring to sleeping in close proximity (which does not necessarily entail bed-sharing) or bed-sharing.

Room-sharing: Parent(s) and infant sleeping in the same room on separate surfaces.

Sleep-related infant death: SUID that occurs during an observed or unobserved sleep period.

Sudden infant death syndrome (SIDS): Cause assigned to infant deaths that cannot be explained after a thorough case investigation including a scene investigation, autopsy, and review of the clinical history.[4]

Sudden unexpected infant death (SUID), or sudden unexpected death in infancy (SUDI): A sudden and unexpected death, whether explained or unexplained (including SIDS), occurring during infancy.

occur during an unobserved sleep period (ie, sleep-related infant deaths), such as unintentional suffocation, is challenging, cannot be determined by autopsy alone, and may remain unresolved after a full case investigation. A few deaths that are diagnosed as SIDS are found, with further specialized investigations, to be attributable to metabolic disorders or arrhythmia-associated cardiac channelopathies.

Although standardized guidelines for conducting thorough case investigations have been developed (http://www.cdc.gov/sids/pdf/suidi-form2-1-2010.pdf),[5] these guidelines have not been uniformly adopted across the >2000 US medical examiner and coroner jurisdictions.[6] Information from emergency responders, scene investigators, and caregiver interviews may provide additional evidence to assist death certifiers (ie, medical examiners and coroners) in accurately determining the cause of death. However, death certifiers represent a diverse group with varying levels of skill and education. In addition, there are diagnostic preferences. Recently, much attention has focused on reporting differences among death certifiers. On one extreme, some certifiers have abandoned the use of SIDS as a cause-of-death explanation.[6] At the other extreme, some certifiers will not classify a death as suffocation in the absence of a pathologic marker of asphyxia at autopsy (ie, pathologic findings

diagnostic of oronasal occlusion or chest compression[7]), even with strong evidence from the scene investigation suggesting a probable unintentional suffocation.

US Trends in SIDS, Other SUIDs, and Postneonatal Mortality

To monitor trends in SIDS and other SUIDs nationally, the United States classifies diseases and injuries according to the International Statistical Classification of Diseases (ICD) diagnostic codes. In the United States, the National Center for Health Statistics assigns a SIDS diagnostic code (International Classification of Diseases, 10th Revision [ICD-10] R95) if the death is classified with terminology such as SIDS (including presumed, probable, or consistent with SIDS), sudden infant death, sudden unexplained death in infancy, sudden unexpected infant death, SUID, or SUDI on the certified death certificate.[8,9] A death will be coded "other ill-defined and unspecified causes of mortality" (ICD-10 R99) if the cause of the death is reported as unknown or unspecified.[8] A death is coded "accidental suffocation and strangulation in bed" (ICD-10 W75) when the terms asphyxia, asphyxiated, asphyxiation, strangled, strangulated, strangulation, suffocated, or suffocation are reported, along with the terms bed or crib. This code also includes deaths while sleeping on couches and armchairs.

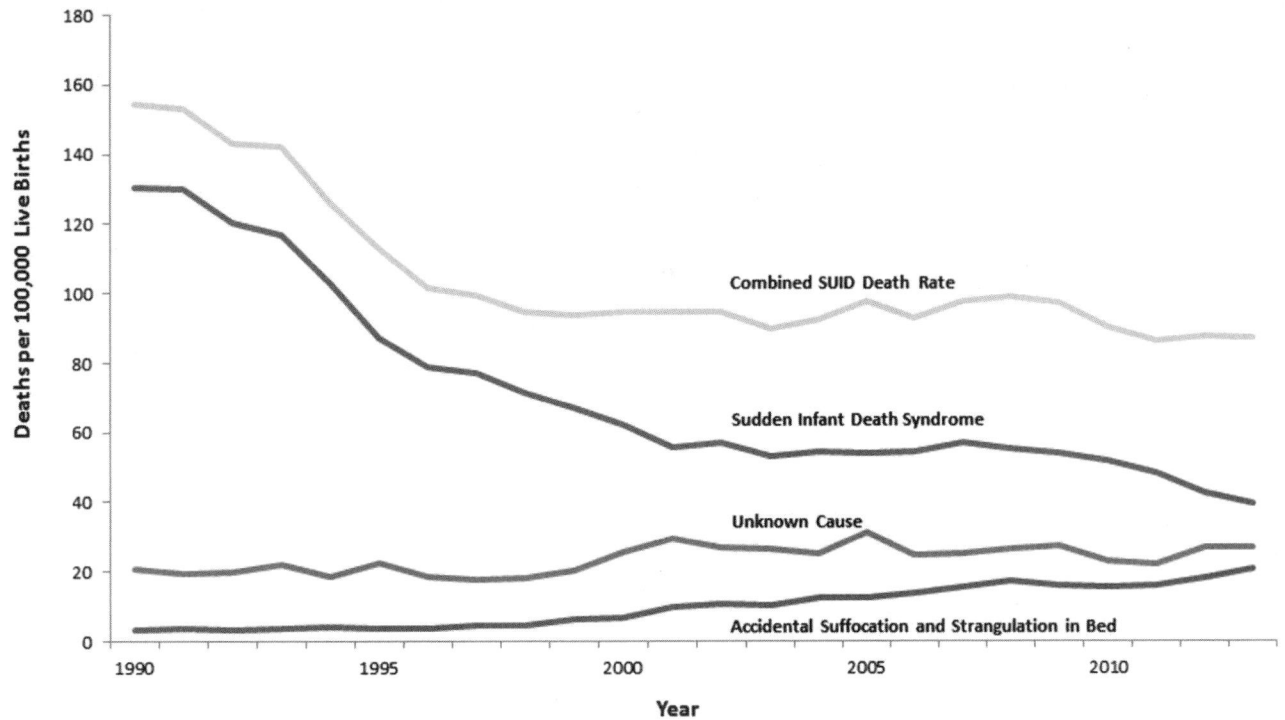

FIGURE 1

Trends in SUID by cause, 1990–2013. Source: Centers for Disease Control and Prevention/National Center for Health Statistics, National Vital Statistics System, compressed mortality file. (Figure duplicated from http://www.cdc.gov/sids/data.htm.)

Although SIDS was defined somewhat loosely until the mid-1980s, there was minimal change in the incidence of SIDS in the United States until the early 1990s. In 1992, in response to epidemiologic reports from Europe and Australia, the AAP recommended that infants be placed for sleep in a nonprone position as a strategy to reduce the risk of SIDS.[10] The "Back to Sleep" campaign (which is now known as the "Safe to Sleep" campaign[11]) was initiated in 1994 under the leadership of the National Institute of Child Health and Human Development (now the *Eunice Kennedy Shriver* National Institute of Child Health and Human Development) as a joint effort of the Maternal and Child Health Bureau of the Health Resources and Services Administration, the AAP, the SIDS Alliance (now First Candle), and the Association of SIDS and Infant Mortality Programs. Between 1992 and 2001, the SIDS rate declined,

with the most dramatic declines in the years immediately after the first nonprone sleep position recommendations, and this decline was consistent with the steady increase in the prevalence of supine sleeping (Fig 1).[12] The US SIDS rate decreased from 120 deaths per 100 000 live births in 1992 to 56 deaths per 100 000 live births in 2001, representing a reduction of 53% over 10 years. From 2001 to 2008, the rate remained constant (Fig 1) and then declined from 54 per 100 000 live births in 2009 to 40 in 2013 (the latest year that data are available). In 2013, 1561 infants died of SIDS.[13] Although SIDS rates have declined by >50% since the early 1990s, SIDS remains the leading cause of postneonatal (28 days to 1 year of age) mortality.

The all-cause postneonatal death rate follows a trend similar to the SIDS and SUID rates, with a 26% decline from 1992 to 2001 (from 314 to 231 per 100 000 live births). From 2001 until 2009, postneonatal mortality

rates also remained fairly unchanged (from 231 to 222 per 100 000 live births), and then have declined yearly since 2009 to a rate of 193 per 100 000 live births in 2013.[14] Several studies have observed that some deaths previously classified as SIDS (ICD-10 R95) are now being classified as other causes of sleep-related infant death (eg, accidental suffocation and strangulation in bed [ASSB; ICD-10 W75] or other ill-defined or unspecified causes [ICD-10 R99]),[15,16] and that at least some of the decline in SIDS rates may be explained by increasing rates of these other assigned causes of SUID.[15,17] To account for variations in death certifier classification and to more consistently track SIDS and other sleep-related infant deaths, the National Center for Health Statistics has created the special cause-of-death category SUID. The SUID category captures deaths with an underlying cause coded as ICD-10 R95, R99, and W75.[13] In 2013, SIDS accounted for 46% of the 3422

SUIDs in the United States. Similar to the SIDS rate, the SUID rate also declined in the late 2000s, from 99 per 100 000 live births in 2009 to 87 in 2013.

Racial and Ethnic Disparities

SIDS and SUID mortality rates, like other causes of infant mortality, have notable and persistent racial and ethnic disparities.[14] Despite the decline in SIDS and SUIDs in all races and ethnicities, the rate of SUIDs among non-Hispanic black (172 per 100 000 live births) and American Indian/Alaska Native (191 per 100 000 live births) infants was more than double that of non-Hispanic white infants (84 per 100 000 live births) in 2010–2013 (Fig 2). SIDS rates for Asian/Pacific Islander and Hispanic infants were much lower than the rate for non-Hispanic white infants. Furthermore, similar racial and ethnic disparities are seen with deaths attributed to both ASSB and ill-defined or unspecified deaths (Fig 2). Differences in the prevalence of supine positioning and other sleep environment conditions between racial and ethnic populations may contribute to these disparities.[18] The prevalence of supine positioning in 2010 data from the National Infant Sleep Position Study in white infants was 75%, compared with 53%, 73%, and 80% among black, Hispanic, and Asian infants, respectively (Fig 3).[19] The Pregnancy Risk Assessment Monitoring System also monitors the prevalence of infant sleep position in several states (http://www.cdc.gov/prams/pramstat/index.html). In 2011, 78% of mothers reported that they most often lay their infants on their backs for sleep (26 states reporting and most recent year available), with 80.3% of white mothers and 54% of black mothers reporting supine placement. Parent-infant bed-sharing[20–22] and the use of soft bedding are also more common among black families

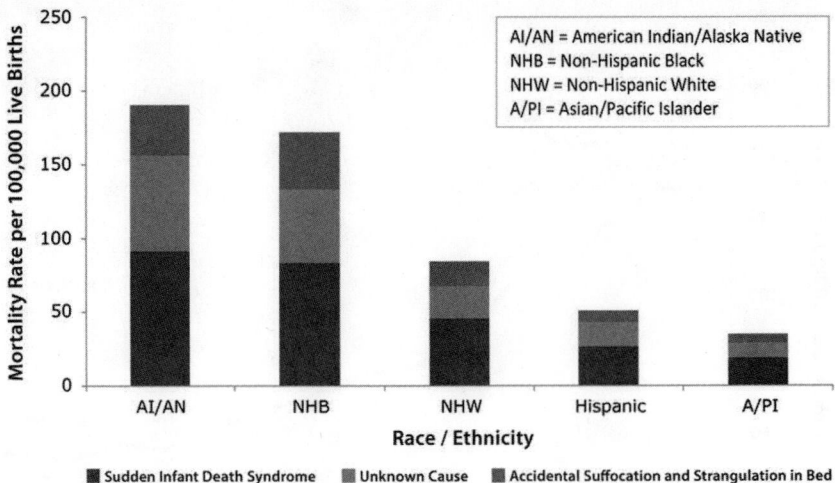

AI/AN = American Indian/Alaska Native
NHB = Non-Hispanic Black
NHW = Non-Hispanic White
A/PI = Asian/Pacific Islander

■ Sudden Infant Death Syndrome   ■ Unknown Cause   ■ Accidental Suffocation and Strangulation in Bed

FIGURE 2
SUID by race/ethnicity, 2010–2013. Source: Centers for Disease Control and Prevention/National Center for Health Statistics, National Vital Statistics System, period-linked birth/infant death data. (Figure duplicated from http://www.cdc.gov/sids/data.htm.)

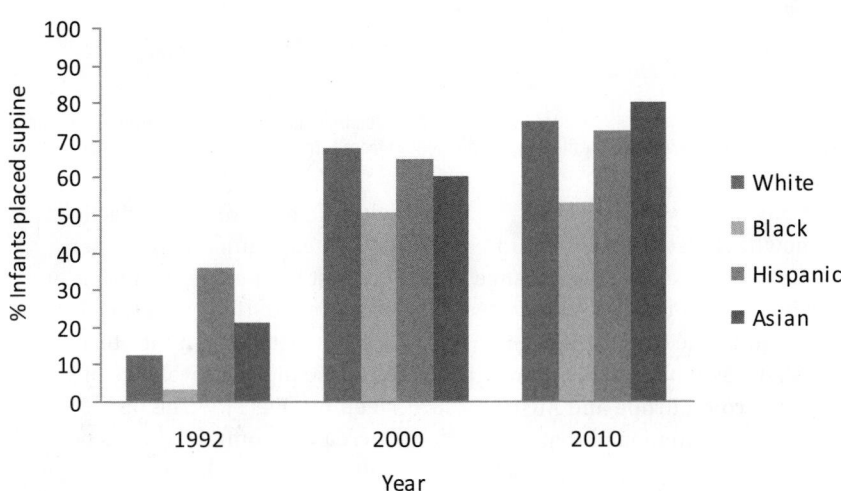

■ White
■ Black
■ Hispanic
■ Asian

FIGURE 3
Prevalence of supine sleep positioning by maternal race and ethnic origin, 1992–2010. Source: National Infant Sleep Position Study. Note that data collection for the National Infant Sleep Position Study ended in 2010.

than among other racial/ethnic groups.[23–25]

Age at Death

Ninety percent of SIDS cases occur before an infant reaches the age of 6 months.[16] SIDS peaks between 1 and 4 months of age. Although SIDS was once considered a rare event during the first month after birth, in 2004–2006 nearly 10% of cases that were coded as SIDS occurred during this period. SIDS is uncommon after 8 months of age.[16] A similar age distribution is seen for ASSB.[16]

PATHOPHYSIOLOGY AND GENETICS OF SIDS

A working model of SIDS pathogenesis includes a convergence of exogenous triggers or "stressors" (eg, prone sleep position, overbundling, airway obstruction), a critical period of development, and dysfunctional and/or immature cardiorespiratory and/or arousal systems (intrinsic vulnerability) that lead to a failure of protective responses (Fig 4).[26] The convergence of these factors may ultimately result in a combination of progressive asphyxia, bradycardia, hypotension, metabolic acidosis, and ineffectual gasping, leading to death.[27] Thus, death may occur as a result of the interaction between a vulnerable infant and a potentially asphyxiating and/or overheating sleep environment.[28]

The mechanisms responsible for intrinsic vulnerability (ie, dysfunctional cardiorespiratory and/or arousal protective responses) remain unclear but may be the result of in utero environmental conditions and/or genetically determined maldevelopment or delay in maturation. Infants who die of SIDS are more likely to have been born preterm and/or were growth restricted, which suggests a suboptimal intrauterine environment. Other adverse in utero environmental conditions include exposure to nicotine or other components of cigarette smoke and alcohol.[29]

Recent studies have explored how prenatal exposure to cigarette smoke may result in an increased risk of SIDS. In animal models, exposure to cigarette smoke or nicotine during fetal development alters the expression of the nicotinic acetylcholine receptors in areas of the brainstem important for autonomic function and alters the numbers of orexin receptors in piglets,[30,31] reduces the number of medullary serotonergic (5-hydroxytryptamine [5-HT]) neurons in the raphe obscurus in mice,[32] increases 5-HT and 5-HT turnover in Rhesus monkeys,[33] alters neuronal excitability of neurons in the nucleus tractus solitarius (a brainstem region important for sensory integration) in guinea pigs,[34] and alters fetal autonomic activity

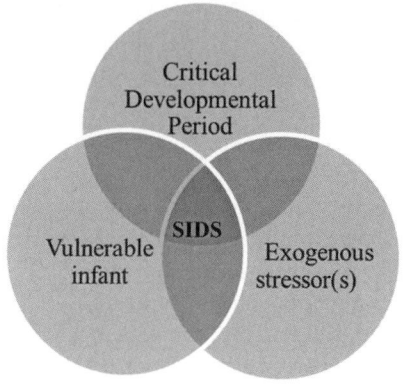

FIGURE 4
Triple risk model for SIDS. Adapted from Filiano and Kinney.[26]

and medullary neurotransmitter receptors, including nicotinic receptors, in baboons.[35–37] From a functional perspective, prenatal exposure to nicotine causes hypoventilation and increased apnea[38,39]; reduces hypercarbia and hypoxia-induced ventilator chemoreflexes in mice, rats,[38–40] and lambs[41]; and blunts arousal in response to hypoxia in rats[40] and lambs.[41]

In human infants, there are strong associations between nicotinic acetylcholine receptors and serotonergic (5-HT) receptors in the brainstem during development,[42] and there is important recent evidence of epigenetic changes in the placentas of infants with prenatal tobacco smoke exposure.[43] Prenatal exposure to tobacco smoke attenuates recovery from hypoxia in preterm infants,[44] decreases heart rate variability in preterm[45] and term[46] infants, and abolishes the normal relationship between heart rate and gestational age at birth.[45] Moreover, infants of smoking mothers exhibit impaired arousal patterns to trigeminal stimulation in proportion to urinary cotinine concentrations.[47] It is important to also note that prenatal exposure to tobacco smoke alters the normal programming of cardiovascular reflexes, such that the increase in blood pressure and heart rate in response to breathing

4% carbon dioxide or a 60° head-up tilt is greater than expected.[48] These changes in autonomic function, arousal, and cardiovascular reflexes may all increase an infant's vulnerability to SIDS.

A recent large systematic review of the neuropathologic features of unexplained SUDI, including only studies that met strict criteria, concluded that "the most consistent findings, and most likely to be pathophysiologically significant, are abnormalities of serotonergic neurotransmission in the caudal brain stem."[49] Brainstem abnormalities that involve the 5-HT system in up to 70% of infants who die of SIDS have now been confirmed in several independent data sets and laboratories.[29,50–52] These include decreased 5-hydroxytryptamine 1A (5-HT1A) receptor binding, a relative decreased binding to the 5-HT transporter, increased numbers of immature 5-HT neurons, and decreased tissue levels of 5-HT and the rate-limiting enzyme for 5-HT synthesis, tryptophan hydroxylase.[53] Moreover, there is no evidence of excessive serotonin degradation as assessed by levels of 5-hydroxyindoleacetic acid (the main metabolite of serotonin) or ratios of 5-hydroxyindoleacetic acid to serotonin.[35] This area of the brainstem plays a key role in coordinating many respiratory, arousal, and autonomic functions, and when dysfunctional, might prevent normal protective responses to stressors that commonly occur during sleep. Importantly, these findings are not confined to nuclei containing 5-HT neurons but also include relevant projection sites. Other abnormalities in brainstem projection sites have been described as well. For example, abnormalities of Phox2B immune-reactive neurons have been reported in the homologous human retrotrapezoid nucleus, a region of the brainstem that receives important 5-HT projections and is critical to carbon dioxide chemoreception and implicated in human congenital central hypoventilation syndrome.[54]

The brainstem has important reciprocal connections to the limbic system comprising both cortical and subcortical components, including the limbic cortex, hypothalamus, amygdala, and hippocampus. These areas of the brain are important in the regulation of autonomic function, particularly in response to emotional stimuli. Thus, the brainstem and limbic system constitute a key network in controlling many aspects of autonomic function. Recently, abnormalities in the dentate gyrus (a component of the hippocampus) were observed in 41% of 153 infants who died unexpectedly with no apparent cause and 43% of the subset of deaths classified as SIDS. This finding suggests that dysfunction of other brain regions interconnected with the brainstem may participate in the pathogenesis of SIDS.[55] Dentate gyrus bilamination is also found in some cases of temporal lobe epilepsy. A future potential line of investigation is a possible link in brainstem-limbic–related homeostatic instability between SIDS and sudden unexpected death in epilepsy and febrile seizures noted in some cases of sudden unexpected death in childhood.[55]

There are significant associations between brainstem 5-HT1A receptor binding abnormalities and specific SIDS risk factors, including tobacco smoking.[52] These data confirm results from earlier studies in humans[29,53] and are also consistent with studies in piglets that reveal that postnatal exposure to nicotine decreases medullary 5-HT1A receptor immunoreactivity.[56] Serotonergic neurons located in the medullary raphe and adjacent paragigantocellularis lateralis play important roles in many autonomic functions, including the control of respiration, blood pressure,

heart rate, thermoregulation, sleep and arousal, and upper airway patency. Engineered mice with decreased numbers of 5-HT neurons and rats or piglets with decreased activity secondary to 5-HT1A autoreceptor stimulation show diminished ventilator responses to carbon dioxide, dysfunctional heat production and heat loss mechanisms, and altered sleep architecture.[57] The aberrant thermoregulation in these models provides evidence for a biological substrate for the risk of SIDS associated with potentially overheating environments. In addition, mice pups with a constitutive reduction in 5-HT–producing neurons (PET1 knockout) or rat pups in which a large fraction of medullary 5-HT neurons have been destroyed with locally applied neurotoxins have a decreased ability to auto-resuscitate in response to asphyxia.[58,59] Moreover, animals with 5-HT neuron deficiency caused by direct injection of a 5-HT–selective neurotoxin had impaired arousal in response to hypoxia.[60]

Some cases of SUID have a clear genetic cause, such as medium-chain acyl-coenzyme A dehydrogenase deficiency. A recent study in California showed that the frequency of mutations for undiagnosed inborn errors of metabolism was similar in SIDS and controls and that newborn screening was effectively detecting medium-chain and very-long-chain acyl-coenzyme A dehydrogenase deficiencies that could potentially lead to SUID.[61] There is no evidence of a strong heritable contribution for SIDS; however, genetic alterations that may increase the vulnerability to SIDS have been observed. Genetic variation can take the form of common base changes (polymorphisms) that alter gene function or rare base changes (mutations) that often have highly deleterious effects. (For a comprehensive review, see Opdal

and Rognum.[62]) Several categories of physiologic functions relevant to SIDS have been examined for altered genetic makeup. Genes related to the serotonin transporter, cardiac channelopathies, and the development of the autonomic nervous system are the subject of current investigation.[63] The serotonin transporter recovers serotonin from the extracellular space and largely serves to regulate overall serotonin neuronal activity. There are reports that polymorphisms in the promoter region that enhance the efficacy of the transporter (L) allele seem to be more prevalent in infants who die of SIDS compared with polymorphisms that reduce efficacy (S)[62]; however, at least 1 study did not confirm this association.[64] It has also been reported that a polymorphism (12-repeat intron 2) of the promoter region of the serotonin transporter, which also enhances serotonin transporter efficiency, was increased in black infants who died of SIDS[63] but not in a Norwegian population.[62]

It has been estimated that 5% to 10% of infants who die of SIDS have novel mutations in the cardiac sodium or potassium channel genes, resulting in long QT syndrome, as well as in other genes that regulate channel function.[63] Some of these mutations may represent an actual cause of death, but others may contribute to causing death when combined with environmental factors, such as acidosis.[65] There is molecular and functional evidence that implicates specific SCN5A (sodium channel gene) β subunits in SIDS pathogenesis.[66] In addition, 2 rare mutations in connexin 43, a major gap junction protein, have been found in SIDS cases and not in ethnically matched controls.[67] In vitro assays of 1 mutation showed a lack of gap junction function, which could lead to ventricular arrhythmogenesis. The other mutation did not appear to have functional consequences.

A recent study also adds weight to the need to perform functional assays and morphologic studies of the altered gene products. Several of the missense variants in genes encoding cardiac channels that have been found in SIDS cases had a high prevalence in the National Heart, Lung, and Blood Institute GO Exome Sequencing Project Database.[68] A large study in a nonreferred nationwide Danish cohort estimated that up to 7.5% of SIDS cases may be explained by genetic variants in the sodium channel complex.[69] These estimates are in the range of those previously reported. However, it is important that for each channelopathy variant discovered, the biological plausibility for pathogenicity is investigated to consider it as a cause of or contributor in SIDS.

The identification of polymorphisms in genes pertinent to the embryologic origin of the autonomic nervous system in SIDS cases also lends support to the hypothesis that a genetic predisposition contributes to the etiology of SIDS. The *PACAP* (pituitary adenylate cyclase-activation polypeptide) gene and the gene of 1 of its receptors (*PAC1*) have received recent attention because of the apparent racial differences in their expression. For example, there were no associations between *PACAP* and SIDS found in white infants, but in SIDS cases in black infants a specific allele was significantly associated.[70] Although in a recent study, a strong association between variants in the *PAC1* gene and SIDS was not found, a number of potential associations between race-specific variants and SIDS were identified; these warrant further study.[71] There have also been a number of reports of polymorphisms or mutations in genes regulating inflammation,[72,73] energy production,[74–76] and hypoglycemia[77] in infants who died of SIDS, but these associations require more study to determine their importance.

RECOMMENDATIONS TO REDUCE THE RISK OF SIDS AND OTHER SLEEP-RELATED INFANT DEATHS

The recommendations outlined herein were developed to reduce the risk of SIDS and sleep-related suffocation, asphyxia, and entrapment among infants in the general population. As defined by epidemiologists, risk refers to the probability that an outcome will occur given the presence of a particular factor or set of factors. Although all recommendations are intended for all who care for infants, some recommendations are also directed toward health policy makers, researchers, and professionals who care for or work on behalf of infants. In addition, because certain behaviors, such as smoking, can increase risk for the infant, some recommendations are directed toward women who are pregnant or may become pregnant in the near future.

The recommendations, along with the strength of the recommendation, are summarized in the accompanying policy statement.[78] It should be noted that there are no randomized controlled trials with regard to SIDS and other sleep-related deaths; instead, case-control studies are the standard.

The recommendations are based on epidemiologic studies that include infants up to 1 year of age. Therefore, recommendations for sleep position and the sleep environment, unless otherwise specified, are for the first year after birth. The evidence-based recommendations that follow are provided to guide health care practitioners in conversations with parents and others who care for infants. Health care practitioners are encouraged to have open and nonjudgmental conversations with families about their sleep practices. Individual medical conditions may warrant that a health care provider make different recommendations after weighing the relative risks and benefits.

INFANT SLEEP POSITION

To reduce the risk of SIDS, infants should be placed for sleep in the supine position (wholly on the back) for every sleep period by every caregiver until 1 year of age. Side sleeping is not safe and is not advised.

The prone or side sleep position can increase the risk of rebreathing expired gases, resulting in hypercapnia and hypoxia.[79–82] The prone position also increases the risk of overheating by decreasing the rate of heat loss and increasing body temperature more than the supine position.[83,84] Evidence suggests that prone sleeping alters the autonomic control of the infant cardiovascular system during sleep, particularly at 2 to 3 months of age,[85] and may result in decreased cerebral oxygenation.[86] The prone position places infants at high risk of SIDS (odds ratio [OR]: 2.3–13.1).[87–91] In 1 US study, SIDS risk associated with the side position was similar in magnitude to that associated with the prone position (ORs: 2.0 and 2.6, respectively),[88] and a higher population-attributable risk has been reported for the side sleep position than for the prone position.[90,92] Furthermore, the risk of SIDS is exceptionally high for infants who are placed on the side and found on the stomach (OR: 8.7).[88] The side sleep position is inherently unstable, and the probability of an infant rolling to the prone position from the side sleep position is significantly greater than rolling prone from the back.[90,93] Infants who are unaccustomed to the prone position and who are placed prone for sleep are also at greater risk than those usually placed prone (adjusted OR: 8.7–45.4).[88,94,95] It is therefore critically important that every caregiver use the supine sleep position for every sleep period.

This is particularly relevant in situations in which a new caregiver is introduced: for example, when an infant is placed in foster care or an adoptive home or when an infant enters child care for the first time.

Despite these recommendations, the prevalence of supine positioning has remained stagnant for the past decade.[19] One reason often cited by parents for not using the supine sleep position is the perception that the infant is uncomfortable or does not sleep well.[96-104] However, an infant who wakes frequently is normal and should not be perceived as a poor sleeper. Physiologic studies show that infants are less likely to arouse when they are sleeping in the prone position.[105-113] The ability to arouse from sleep is an important protective physiologic response to stressors during sleep,[114-118] and the infant's ability to sleep for sustained periods may not be physiologically advantageous.

The supine sleep position does not increase the risk of choking and aspiration in infants, even in those with gastroesophageal reflux.

Parents and caregivers continue to be concerned that the infant will choke or aspirate while supine.[96-104] Parents often misconstrue coughing or gagging, which is evidence of a normal protective gag reflex, for choking or aspiration. Multiple studies in different countries have not shown an increased incidence of aspiration since the change to supine sleeping.[119-121] Parents and caregivers are often concerned about aspiration when the infant has been diagnosed with gastroesophageal reflux. The AAP concurs with the North American Society for Pediatric Gastroenterology and Nutrition that "the risk of SIDS outweighs the benefit of prone or lateral sleep position on GER [gastroesophageal reflux]; therefore, in most infants from birth to 12 months of age, supine positioning during sleep is recommended…. Therefore, prone

positioning is acceptable if the infant is observed and awake, particularly in the postprandial period, but prone positioning during sleep can only be considered in infants with certain upper airway disorders in which the risk of death from GERD [gastroesophageal reflux disease] may outweigh the risk of SIDS."[122] Examples of such upper airway disorders are those in which airway-protective mechanisms are impaired, including infants with anatomic abnormalities, such as type 3 or 4 laryngeal clefts, who have not undergone antireflux surgery. There is no evidence that infants receiving nasogastric or orogastric feedings are at increased risk of aspiration if placed in the supine position. Elevating the head of the infant's crib while the infant is supine is not effective in reducing gastroesophageal reflux[123,124]; in addition, elevating the head of the crib may result in the infant sliding to the foot of the crib into a position that may compromise respiration and therefore is not recommended.

Preterm infants should be placed supine as soon as possible.

Infants born preterm have an increased risk of SIDS,[125,126] and the association between the prone position and SIDS among low birth weight and preterm infants is equal to, or perhaps even stronger than, the association among those born at term.[94] Therefore, preterm infants should be placed supine for sleep as soon as clinical status has stabilized. The task force concurs with the AAP Committee on Fetus and Newborn that "preterm infants should be placed supine for sleeping, just as term infants should, and the parents of preterm infants should be counseled about the importance of supine sleeping in preventing SIDS. Hospitalized preterm infants should be kept predominantly in the supine position, at least from the postmenstrual age of 32 weeks onward, so that they become

acclimated to supine sleeping before discharge."[127] Furthermore, the task force believes that neonatologists, neonatal nurses, and other health care providers responsible for organizing the hospital discharge of infants from NICUs should be vigilant about endorsing the SIDS risk-reduction recommendations from birth. They should model the recommendations as soon as the infant is medically stable and significantly before the infant's anticipated discharge from the hospital. In addition, NICUs are encouraged to develop and implement policies to ensure that supine sleeping and other safe sleep practices are modeled for parents beforeo discharge from the hospital.[128,129]

As stated in the AAP clinical report, "skin-to-skin care is recommended for all mothers and newborns, regardless of feeding or delivery method, immediately following birth (as soon as the mother is medically stable, awake, and able to respond to her newborn), and to continue for at least an hour."[130] Thereafter, or when the mother needs to sleep or take care of other needs, infants should be placed supine in a bassinet.

Placing infants on the side after birth in newborn nurseries or in mother-infant rooms continues to be a concern. The practice likely occurs because of a belief among nursery staff that newborn infants need to clear their airways of amniotic fluid and may be less likely to aspirate while on the side. No evidence that such fluid will be cleared more readily while in the side position exists. Perhaps most importantly, if parents observe health care providers placing infants in the side or prone position, they are likely to infer that supine positioning is not important[131] and therefore may be more likely to copy this practice and use the side or prone position at home.[101,104,132] Infants who are rooming in with their parents or cared for in a separate newborn nursery should be placed in the supine position as soon as they are ready to be placed in the bassinet. To promote breastfeeding, placing the infant skin-to-skin with mother after delivery, with appropriate observation and/or monitoring, is the best approach. When the mother needs to sleep or take care of other needs, the infant should be placed supine in a bassinet.

Once an infant can roll from supine to prone and from prone to supine, the infant may remain in the sleep position that he or she assumes.

Parents and caregivers are frequently concerned about the appropriate strategy for infants who have learned to roll over, which generally occurs at 4 to 6 months of age. As infants mature, it is more likely that they will roll. In 1 study, 6% and 12% of 16- to 23-week-old infants placed on their backs or sides, respectively, were found in the prone position; among infants ≥24 weeks of age, 14% of those placed on their backs and 18% of those placed on their sides were found in the prone position.[133] Repositioning the sleeping infant to the supine position can be disruptive and may discourage the use of the supine position altogether. Because data to make specific recommendations as to when it is safe for infants to sleep in the prone position are lacking, the AAP recommends that all infants continue to be placed supine until 1 year of age. If the infant can roll from supine to prone and from prone to supine, the infant can then be allowed to remain in the sleep position that he or she assumes. One study analyzing sleep-related deaths reported to state child death review teams found that the predominant risk factor for sleep-related deaths in infants 4 to 12 months of age was rolling into objects in the sleep area.[134] Thus, parents and caregivers should continue to keep the infant's sleep environment

clear of soft or loose bedding and other objects. Parents may be reassured in being advised that the incidence of SIDS begins to decline after 4 months of age.[16]

SLEEP SURFACES

Infants should be placed on a firm sleep surface (eg, a mattress in a safety-approved crib) covered by a fitted sheet with no other bedding or soft objects to reduce the risk of SIDS and suffocation.

To avoid suffocation, rebreathing, and SIDS risk, infants should sleep on a firm surface (eg, safety-approved crib and mattress). The surface should be covered by a fitted sheet without any soft or loose bedding. A firm surface maintains its shape and will not indent or conform to the shape of the infant's head when the infant is placed on the surface. Soft mattresses, including those made from memory foam, could create a pocket (or indentation) and increase the chance of rebreathing or suffocation if the infant is placed in or rolls over to the prone position.[81,135]

A crib, bassinet, portable crib, or play yard that conforms to the safety standards of the Consumer Product Safety Commission (CPSC) is recommended.

Cribs should meet safety standards of the CPSC,[136] including those for slat spacing, snugly fitting and firm mattresses, and no drop sides. The AAP recommends the use of new cribs, because older cribs may no longer meet current safety standards, may have missing parts, or may be incorrectly assembled. If an older crib is to be used, care must be taken to ensure that there have been no recalls on the crib model, that all of the hardware is intact, and that the assembly instructions are available.

For some families, the use of a crib may not be possible for financial or space considerations. In addition, parents may be reluctant to place the

infant in the crib because of concerns that the crib is too large for the infant or that "crib death" (ie, SIDS) only occurs in cribs. Alternate sleep surfaces, such as portable cribs, play yards, and bassinets that meet safety standards of the CPSC,[137,138] can be used and may be more acceptable for some families because they are smaller and more portable.

Bedside sleepers are attached to the side of the parental bed. The CPSC has published safety standards for bedside sleepers,[139] and they may be considered by some parents as an option. There are no CPSC safety standards for in-bed sleepers. The task force cannot make a recommendation for or against the use of either bedside sleepers or in-bed sleepers, because there have been no studies examining the association between these products and SIDS or unintentional injury and death, including suffocation. Studies of in-bed sleepers are currently underway, but results are not yet available. Parents and caregivers should adhere to the manufacturer's guidelines regarding maximum weight of infants who use these products.[140,141] In addition, with the use of any of these products, other AAP guidelines for safe sleep outlined in this document, including supine positioning and avoidance of soft objects and loose bedding, should be followed.

Mattresses should be firm and maintain their shape even when the fitted sheet designated for that model is used, such that there are no gaps between the mattress and the wall of the bassinet, playpen, portable crib, play yard, or bedside sleeper. Only mattresses designed for the specific product should be used. Pillows or cushions should not be used as substitutes for mattresses or in addition to a mattress. Soft materials or objects, such as pillows, quilts, comforters, or sheepskins, even if covered by a sheet, should not be placed under a sleeping infant.

Mattress toppers, designed to make the sleep surface softer, should not be used for infants younger than 1 year. Any fabric on the crib walls or a canopy should be taut and firmly attached to the frame so as not to create a suffocation risk for the infant.

Infants should not be placed for sleep on adult-sized beds because of the risk of entrapment and suffocation.[142] Portable bed rails (railings installed on the side of the bed that are intended to prevent a child from falling off of the bed) should not be used with infants because of the risk of entrapment and strangulation.[143] The infant should sleep in an area free of hazards, including dangling cords, electric wires, and window-covering cords, because these may present a strangulation risk.

Recently, special crib mattresses and sleep surfaces that claim to reduce the chance of rebreathing carbon dioxide when the infant is in the prone position have been introduced. Although there are no apparent disadvantages of using these mattresses if they meet the safety standards as described previously, there are no studies that show a decreased risk of SUID/SIDS. (See section entitled "Commercial Devices" for further discussion of special mattresses.)

Sitting devices, such as car seats, strollers, swings, infant carriers, and infant slings, are not recommended for routine sleep in the hospital or at home, particularly for young infants.

Some parents choose to allow their infants to sleep in a car seat or other sitting device. Sitting devices include, but are not restricted to, car seats, strollers, swings, infant carriers, and infant slings. Parents and caregivers often use these devices, even when not traveling, because they are convenient. One study found that the average young infant spends 5.7 hours/day in a

car seat or similar sitting device.[144] However, there are multiple concerns about the use of sitting devices as a usual infant sleep location. Placing an infant in such devices can potentiate gastroesophageal reflux[145] and positional plagiocephaly. Because they still have poor head control and often experience flexion of the head while in a sitting position, infants younger than 4 months in sitting devices may be at increased risk of upper airway obstruction and oxygen desaturation.[146-150] A recent retrospective study reviewed deaths involving sitting and carrying devices (car seats, bouncers, swings, strollers, and slings) reported to the CPSC between 2004 and 2008. Of the 47 deaths analyzed, 31 occurred in car seats, 5 occurred in slings, 4 each occurred in swings and bouncers, and 3 occurred in strollers. Fifty-two percent of deaths in car seats were attributed to strangulation from straps; the others were attributed to positional asphyxia.[151] In addition, analyses of CPSC data report injuries from falls when car seats are placed on elevated surfaces,[152-156] from strangulation on unbuckled or partially buckled car seat straps,[151] and from suffocation when car seats overturn after being placed on a bed, mattress, or couch.[155] There are also reports of suffocation in infants, particularly those who are younger than 4 months, who are carried in infant sling carriers.[151,157-159] When infant slings are used for carrying, it is important to ensure that the infant's head is up and above the fabric, the face is visible, and the nose and mouth are clear of obstructions. After nursing, the infant should be repositioned in the sling so that the head is up and is clear of fabric and the airway is not obstructed by the adult's body.[151] If an infant falls asleep in a sitting device, he or she should be removed from the product and moved to a crib or other appropriate flat surface as soon as is safe and practical. Car seats and similar products are not stable on

a crib mattress or other elevated surfaces.[152-156] Infants should not be left unattended in car seats and similar products, nor should they be placed or left in car seats and similar products with the straps unbuckled or partially buckled.[151]

BREASTFEEDING

Breastfeeding is associated with a reduced risk of SIDS. The protective effect of breastfeeding increases with exclusivity. Furthermore, any breastfeeding is more protective against SIDS than no breastfeeding.

The protective role of breastfeeding on SIDS is enhanced when breastfeeding is exclusive and without formula introduction.[160-162] Studies do not distinguish between direct breastfeeding and providing expressed milk. In the Agency for Healthcare Research and Quality's "Evidence Report on Breastfeeding in Developed Countries," 6 studies were included in the SIDS-breastfeeding meta-analysis, and ever having breastfed was associated with a lower risk of SIDS (adjusted summary OR: 0.64; 95% confidence interval [CI]: 0.51–0.81).[160] The German Study of Sudden Infant Death, the largest and most recent case-control study of SIDS, found that exclusive breastfeeding at 1 month of age halved the risk of SIDS (adjusted OR: 0.48; 95% CI: 0.28–0.82).[161] Another meta-analysis of 18 case-control studies found an unadjusted summary OR for any breastfeeding of 0.40 (95% CI: 0.35–0.44) and a pooled adjusted OR of 0.55 (95% CI: 0.44–0.69) (Fig 5).[162] The protective effect of breastfeeding increased with exclusivity, with a univariable summary OR of 0.27 (95% CI: 0.24–0.31) for exclusive breastfeeding of any duration.[162]

Physiologic sleep studies showed that breastfed infants are more easily aroused from sleep than their formula-fed counterparts.[163,164] In addition, breastfeeding results in a decreased incidence of diarrhea, upper and lower respiratory infections, and other infectious diseases[165] that are associated with an increased vulnerability to SIDS and provides overall immune system benefits attributable to maternal antibodies and micronutrients in human milk.[166,167] Exclusive breastfeeding for 6 months has been found to be more protective against infectious diseases, compared with exclusive breastfeeding to 4 months of age and partial breastfeeding thereafter.[165] Furthermore, exclusive breastfeeding results in a gut microbiome that supports a normally functioning immune system and protection from infectious disease, and this commensal microbiome has been proposed as another possible mechanism or marker for protection against SIDS.[168]

INFANT SLEEP LOCATION

It is recommended that infants sleep in the parents' room, close to the parents' bed, but on a separate surface. The infant's crib, portable crib, play yard, or bassinet should be placed in the parents' bedroom, ideally for the first year of life, but at least for the first 6 months.

The terms bed-sharing and cosleeping are often used interchangeably, but they are not synonymous. Cosleeping is when parent and infant sleep in close proximity (on the same surface or different surfaces) so as to be able to see, hear, and/or touch each other.[169,170] Cosleeping arrangements can include bed-sharing or sleeping in the same room in close proximity.[170,171] Bed-sharing refers to a specific type of cosleeping when the infant is sleeping on the same surface with another person.[170] The shared surface can include a bed, sofa, or chair. Because the term cosleeping can be misconstrued and does not precisely describe sleep

Study or Subgroup	log[]	SE	Weight	IV, Fixed, 95% CI
Fleming 1996	0.058269	0.317657	12.6%	1.06 [0.57, 1.98]
Hauck 2003	-0.91629	0.319582	12.4%	0.40 [0.21, 0.75]
Klonoff-Cohen 1995	-0.89159812	0.3346305	11.4%	0.41 [0.21, 0.79]
Mitchell 1997	-0.07257	0.420337	7.2%	0.93 [0.41, 2.12]
Ponsonby 1995	-0.15082	0.401245	7.9%	0.86 [0.39, 1.89]
Vennemann 2009	-0.84397	0.239354	22.2%	0.43 [0.27, 0.69]
Wennergren 1997	-0.693147	0.21979	26.3%	0.50 [0.33, 0.77]
Total (95% CI)			100.0%	0.55 [0.44, 0.69]

Heterogeneity: Chi² = 10.08, df = 6 (P = .12); I² = 40%
Test for overall effect: Z = 5.28 (P < .00001)

FIGURE 5

Multivariable analysis of any breastfeeding versus no breastfeeding. Adapted from Hauck et al.[162] log[ ], logarithm of the OR; Weight: weighting that the study contributed to the meta-analysis (by sample size); IV, Fixed, 95% CI, fixed-effect OR with 95% CI.

arrangements, the AAP recommends the use of the terms bed-sharing and room-sharing (when the infant sleeps in the parents' room but on a separate sleep surface [crib or similar surface] close to the parents' bed) (see Table 1).

The AAP recommends room-sharing, because this arrangement decreases the risk of SIDS by as much as 50%[89, 91,172,173] and is safer than bed-sharing[89,91,172,173] or solitary sleeping (when the infant is in a separate room).[89,172] In addition, room-sharing is most likely to prevent suffocation, strangulation, and entrapment that may occur when the infant is sleeping in the adult bed. Furthermore, this arrangement allows close proximity to the infant, which will facilitate feeding, comforting, and monitoring of the infant. Most of the epidemiologic studies on which these recommendations are based include infants up to 1 year of age. Therefore, the AAP recommends that infants room-share, ideally for the first year after birth, but at least for the first 6 months. Although there is no specific evidence for moving an infant to his or her own room before 1 year of age, room-sharing during the first 6 months is especially critical because the rates of SIDS and other sleep-related deaths, particularly those occurring in bed-sharing situations, are highest during that period.

Parent-infant bed-sharing for all or part of sleep duration is common. In 1 national survey for the period

2001–2010, 46% of parents responded that they had shared a bed with their infant (8 months or younger) at some point in the preceding 2 weeks, and 13.5% reported that they usually bed-shared.[174] In another national survey, any bed-sharing was reported by 42% of mothers at 2 weeks of infant age and 27% of mothers at 12 months of infant age.[175] In a third study, almost 60% of mothers of infants from birth to 12 months of age reported bed-sharing at least once.[176] The rate of routine bed-sharing is higher among some racial/ethnic groups, including black, Hispanic, and American Indian/Alaska Native parents/infants.[20,22,174] There are often cultural and personal reasons why parents choose to bed-share, including convenience for feeding (breast or formula), comforting a fussy or sick infant, helping the infant and/or mother sleep better, bonding and attachment, and because it is a family tradition.[175,177] In addition, many parents may believe that their own vigilance is the only way that they can keep their infant safe and that the close proximity of bed-sharing allows them to maintain vigilance, even while sleeping.[178] Some parents will use bed-sharing specifically as a safety strategy if the infant sleeps in the prone position[23,178] or there is concern about environmental dangers, such as vermin or stray gunfire.[178]

Parent-infant bed-sharing continues to be highly controversial. Although electrophysiologic and behavioral studies offer a strong case for its effect in facilitating breastfeeding,[179–181] and although many parents believe that they can maintain vigilance of the infant while they are asleep and bed-sharing,[178] epidemiologic studies have shown that bed-sharing is associated with a number of conditions that are risk factors for SIDS, including soft bedding,[182–185] head covering,[186–189] and, for infants of smokers, increased exposure to tobacco smoke.[190] In addition, bed-sharing is associated with an increased risk of SIDS; a recent meta-analysis of 11 studies investigating the association of bed-sharing and SIDS showed a summary OR of 2.88 (95% CI: 1.99–4.18) with bed-sharing.[191] Furthermore, bed-sharing in an adult bed not designed for infant safety, especially when associated with other risk factors, exposes the infant to additional risks for unintentional injury and death, such as suffocation, asphyxia, entrapment, falls, and strangulation.[192,193] Infants younger than 4 months[194] and those born preterm and/or with low birth weight[195] are at the highest risk, possibly because immature motor skills and muscle strength make it difficult to escape potential threats.[191] In recent years, the concern among public health officials about bed-sharing has increased, because there have been increased reports of SUIDs occurring in high-risk sleep environments, particularly bed-sharing and/or sleeping on a couch or armchair.[196–198]

On the other hand, some breastfeeding advocacy groups encourage safer bed-sharing to promote breastfeeding,[199] and debate continues as to the safety of this sleep arrangement for low-risk, breastfed infants. In an analysis from 2 case-control studies in England (1993–1996 and 2003–2006), Blair et al[200] reported an adjusted OR of bed-sharing (excluding bed-sharing on a sofa) for infants in the absence of parental alcohol or tobacco use of 1.1 (95% CI: 0.6–2.9). For infants younger than 98 days, the OR was 1.6 (95% CI: 0.96–2.7).[200] These findings were independent of feeding method. The study lacked power to examine this association in older infants, because there was only 1 SIDS case in which bed-sharing was a factor in the absence of other risk factors. Breastfeeding was more common among bed-sharing infants, and the protective effect of breastfeeding was found only for infants who slept alone. The controls in these analyses were infants who were not bed-sharing/sofa-sharing regardless of room location; thus, they included infants who were room-sharing or sleeping in a separate room. In addition, the control infants included those whose parent(s) smoked or used alcohol. It is possible that this choice of controls overestimated their risk, leading to smaller ORs for risk among the cases (ie, biasing the results toward the null).

Carpenter et al[201] analyzed data from 19 studies across the United Kingdom, Europe, and Australasia to determine the risk of SIDS from bed-sharing when an infant is breastfed, the parents do not smoke, and the mother has not taken alcohol or drugs. When neither parent smoked, in the absence of other risk factors, the adjusted OR for bed-sharing versus room-sharing for all breastfed infants was 2.7 (95% CI: 1.4–5.3).[201] For breastfed infants younger than 3 months, in the absence of other risk factors, the adjusted OR for bed-sharing versus room-sharing was 5.1 (95% CI: 2.3–11.4). The study lacked power to examine this association in breastfed infants 3 months and older. Moreover, the large proportion of missing data for maternal alcohol and drug use is a limitation, although the authors used appropriate multiple imputation techniques for addressing these missing data.

The task force, recognizing the controversial nature of the recommendations about bed-sharing and the different methods and interpretations of these 2 sets of analyses outlined previously, requested an independent review of both articles by Dr Robert Platt, a biostatistician with expertise in perinatal epidemiology from McGill University in Canada. Dr Platt has no connection to the task force, nor does he have a vested interest in the recommendations. Dr Platt provided the following conclusion:

The fundamental difference in conclusions is that Blair et al conclude that bed-sharing in the absence of other risk factors (smoking, alcohol) does not convey an increased risk of SIDS, while Carpenter et al conclude the opposite. In both studies, the no-other-risk-factors group is limited in size, and the number of exposed cases is very small. In Blair et al, there are only 24 cases who bed-shared in the absence of these hazards. In Carpenter et al, although the total number of SIDS cases (1472) is more than 3 times the number of cases in the Blair study (400), the number of cases who bed-shared in the absence of these hazards was only 12 (personal communication, Professor Robert Carpenter, January 25, 2016). Therefore, the Carpenter results should be interpreted with some caution as well. In conclusion, both studies have strengths and weaknesses, and while on the surface the studies appear to contradict each other, I do not believe that their data support definitive differences between the 2 studies. There is some evidence of an increased risk in the no-other-risk-factor setting, in particular in the youngest age groups. However, based on concerns about sample size limitations, we are not able to say how large that increased risk is. Clearly, these data do not support a definitive conclusion that bed-sharing in the youngest age group is safe, even under less hazardous circumstances.

There is insufficient evidence to recommend for or against the use of devices promoted to make bed-sharing "safe."

There is no evidence that devices marketed to make bed-sharing "safe" reduce the risk of SIDS or suffocation or are safe. Several products designed for in-bed use are currently under study, but results are not yet available. Bedside sleepers, which attach to the side of the parental bed and for which the CPSC published standards in 2013, may be considered by some parents as an option. The task force cannot make a recommendation for or against the use of either bedside sleepers or in-bed sleepers, because there have been no studies examining the association between these products and SIDS or unintentional injury and death, including suffocation. (See section entitled "Sleep Surfaces" for further discussion of sleepers.)

Infants who are brought into the bed for feeding or comforting should be returned to their own crib or bassinet when the parent is ready to return to sleep.

Studies have found an association between bed-sharing and longer duration of breastfeeding,[202] but most of these were cross-sectional studies, which do not enable the determination of a temporal relationship: that is, whether bed-sharing promotes breastfeeding or whether breastfeeding promotes bed-sharing, and whether women who prefer one practice are also likely to prefer the other.[203] However, a more recent longitudinal study provides strong evidence that bed-sharing promotes breastfeeding duration, with the greatest effect among frequent bed-sharers.[202] Another recent study has shown that, compared with mothers who room-shared without bed-sharing, mothers who bed-shared were more likely

to report exclusive breastfeeding (adjusted OR: 2.46; 95% CI: 1.76–3.45) or partial breastfeeding (adjusted OR: 1.75; 95% CI: 1.33–2.31).[204] Although bed-sharing may facilitate breastfeeding,[175] there are other factors, such as intent, that influence successful breastfeeding.[205] Furthermore, 1 case-control study found that the risk of SIDS while bed-sharing was similar among infants in the first 4 months of life, regardless of breastfeeding status, implying that the benefits of breastfeeding do not outweigh the increased risk associated with bed-sharing for younger infants.[194] The risk of bed-sharing is higher the longer the duration of bed-sharing during the night,[91] especially when associated with other risks.[89,90,206,207] Returning the infant to the crib after bringing the infant into the bed for a short period of time is not associated with increased risk.[90,207] Therefore, after the infant is brought into the bed for feeding, comforting, and bonding, the infant should be returned to the crib when the parent is ready for sleep.

Couches and armchairs are extremely dangerous places for infants.

Sleeping on couches and armchairs places infants at an extraordinarily high risk of infant death, including SIDS,[87,89,90,173,200,207] suffocation through entrapment or wedging between seat cushions, or overlay if another person is also sharing this surface.[197] Therefore, parents and other caregivers should be especially vigilant as to their wakefulness when feeding infants or lying with infants on these surfaces. It is important to emphasize this point to mothers, because 25% of mothers in 1 study reported falling asleep during the night when breastfeeding their infant on one of these surfaces.[176] Infants should never be placed on a couch or armchair for sleep.

Guidance for parents who fall asleep while feeding their infant.

The safest place for an infant to sleep is on a separate sleep surface designed for infants close to the parent's bed. However, the AAP acknowledges that parents frequently fall asleep while feeding the infant. Evidence suggests that it is less hazardous to fall asleep with the infant in the adult bed than on a sofa or armchair, should the parent fall asleep.[87,89,90,173,200,207] It is important to note that a large percentage of infants who die of SIDS are found with their head covered by bedding.[186] Therefore, there should be no pillows, sheets, blankets, or any other items in the bed that could obstruct infant breathing[87,182] or cause overheating.[208–211] Parents should follow safe sleep recommendations outlined elsewhere in this statement. Because there is evidence that the risk of bed-sharing is higher with longer duration, if the parent falls asleep while feeding the infant in bed the infant should be placed back on a separate sleep surface as soon as the parent awakens.[89,90,206,207]

There are specific circumstances that, in case-control studies and case series, have been shown to substantially increase the risk of SIDS or unintentional injury or death while bed-sharing, and these should be avoided at all times.

The task force emphasizes that certain circumstances greatly increase the risk of bed-sharing for both breastfed and formula-fed infants. Bed-sharing is especially dangerous in the following circumstances, and these should be avoided at all times:

- when one or both parents are smokers, even if they are not smoking in bed (OR: 2.3–21.6)[89,90,191,200,201,206,212];

- when the mother smoked during pregnancy[89,90,191,206,212];

- when the infant is younger than 4 months of age, regardless of parental smoking status (OR: 4.7–10.4)[89,91,173,191,201,207,213,214];

- when the infant is born preterm and/or with low birth weight[195];

- when the infant is bed-sharing on excessively soft or small surfaces, such as waterbeds, sofas, and armchairs (OR: 5.1–66.9)[87,89,90,173,200,207];

- when soft bedding accessories such as pillows or blankets are used (OR: 2.8–4.1)[87,215];

- when there are multiple bed-sharers (OR: 5.4)[87];

- when the parent has consumed alcohol (OR: 1.66–89.7)[91,196,200,201] and/or illicit or sedating drugs[201]; and

- when the infant is bed-sharing with someone who is not a parent (OR: 5.4).[87]

A retrospective series of SIDS cases reported that mean maternal body weight was higher for bed-sharing mothers than for non–bed-sharing mothers.[216] The only case-control study to investigate the relationship between maternal body weight and bed-sharing did not find an increased risk of bed-sharing with increased maternal weight.[217]

The safety and benefits of cobedding twins and higher-order multiples have not been established. It is prudent to provide separate sleep areas and avoid cobedding (sleeping on the same sleep surface) for twins and higher-order multiples in the hospital and at home.

Cobedding of twins and other infants of multiple gestation is a frequent practice, both in the hospital setting and at home.[218] However, the benefits of cobedding twins and higher-order multiples have not been established.[219-221] Twins and higher-order multiples are often born preterm and with low birth weights, so they are at increased risk of SIDS.[125,126] Furthermore, cobedding

increases the potential for overheating and rebreathing, and size discordance between multiples may increase the risk of unintentional suffocation.[220] Most cobedded twins are placed on the side rather than supine.[218] Finally, cobedding of twins and higher-order multiples in the hospital setting may encourage parents to continue this practice at home.[220] Because the evidence for the benefits of cobedding twins and higher-order multiples is not compelling and because of the increased risk of SIDS and suffocation, the AAP believes that it is prudent to provide separate sleep areas for these infants to decrease the risk of SIDS and unintentional suffocation.

USE OF BEDDING

Keep soft objects, such as pillows, pillow-like toys, quilts, comforters, sheepskins, and loose bedding, such as blankets and nonfitted sheets, away from the infant's sleep area to reduce the risk of SIDS, suffocation, entrapment, and strangulation.

Soft objects and loose bedding can obstruct an infant's airway and increase the risk of SIDS,[87,182] suffocation, and rebreathing.[79,81,82,135,222–224] In the United States, nearly 55% of infants are placed to sleep underneath or on top of bedding such as thick blankets, quilts, and pillows.[25] The prevalence of bedding use is highest among infants whose mothers are teenagers, from minority racial groups, and among those without a college education.

Pillows, quilts, comforters, sheepskins, and other soft bedding can be hazardous when placed under the infant[87,182,210,225–229] or left loose in the infant's sleep area.[90,182,215,224,228–234] Bedding in the sleeping environment increases SIDS risk fivefold, independent of sleep position,[87,182] and this risk increases to 21-fold when the infant is placed prone.[87,182] Many infants who die of SIDS are found in the supine position but with their heads

covered by loose bedding.[90,225,226,230] In addition, infants who bed-share (share a sleep surface) have a higher SIDS risk when sleeping on a soft as opposed to a firm surface.[215]

In addition to SIDS risk, soft objects and loose bedding in the sleeping environment may also lead to unintentional suffocation.[134,224,235] A review of 66 SUID case investigations in 2011 showed that soft bedding was the most frequently reported factor among deaths classified as possible and explained unintentional suffocation deaths.[224] In addition, a CPSC report of sleep-related infant deaths in 2009–2011 found that most deaths attributed to suffocation (regardless of whether infant was sleeping in a crib, on a mattress, or in a play yard) involved extra bedding, such as pillows or blankets.[235] Soft bedding (eg, blankets and stuffed animals) may also be a stronger risk factor for sleep-related deaths among infants older than 3 months than it is for their younger counterparts, especially when infants are placed in or roll to the prone position.[134]

Parents and caregivers are likely motivated by good intentions and perceived cultural norms when they opt to use bedding for infant sleep. Qualitative studies show that parents who use bedding want to provide a comfortable and safe environment for their infant.[236] For comfort, parents may use blankets to provide warmth or to soften the sleep surface. For safety, parents may use pillows as barriers to prevent falls from adult beds or sofas or as a prop to keep their infant on the side.[236] Images of infants sleeping with blankets, pillows, and other soft objects are widespread in popular magazines targeted to families with newborn infants.[237] Parents and caregivers who see these images may perceive the use of these items as the norm, both favorable and the ideal, for infant sleep.

To avoid suffocation, rebreathing, and SIDS risk, infants should sleep on a firm surface (see section entitled "Sleep Surfaces" for a definition of a firm surface).[135] Because pillows, quilts, and comforters can obstruct the infant's airway (nose or mouth), they should never be used in the infant's sleeping environment. Infant sleep clothing, such as sleeping sacks, are designed to keep the infant warm and can be used in place of blankets to prevent the possibility of head covering or entrapment. However, care must be taken to select appropriately sized clothing and to avoid overheating. Nursing and hospital staff should model safe sleep arrangements to new parents after delivery.

Bumper pads are not recommended; they have been implicated in deaths attributable to suffocation, entrapment, and strangulation and, with new safety standards for crib slats, are not necessary for safety against head entrapment.

Bumper pads and similar products attaching to crib slats or sides are frequently used with the thought of protecting infants from injury. Initially, bumper pads were developed to prevent head entrapment between crib slats.[238] However, newer crib standards requiring crib slat spacing to be <2-3/8 inches have obviated the need for crib bumpers. In addition, infant deaths have occurred because of bumper pads. A case series by Thach et al,[239] which used 1985–2005 CPSC data, found that deaths attributed to bumper pads occurred as a result of 3 mechanisms: (1) suffocation against soft, pillow-like bumper pads; (2) entrapment between the mattress or crib and firm bumper pads; and (3) strangulation from bumper pad ties. However, a 2010 CPSC white paper that reviewed the same cases concluded that there were other confounding factors, such as the presence of pillows and/or blankets, that may have contributed to many of the deaths in this report.[240] The white paper pointed out that available

data from the scene investigations, autopsies, law enforcement records, and death certificates often lacked sufficiently detailed information to conclude how or whether bumper pads contributed to the deaths. Two more recent analyses of CPSC data also came to different conclusions. The CPSC review concluded again that there was insufficient evidence to support that bumper pads were primarily responsible for infant deaths when bumper pads were used per the manufacturer's instructions and in the absence of other unsafe sleep risk factors.[241] Scheers et al,[242] in their re-analysis, concluded that the rate of bumper pad–related deaths has increased, recognizing that changes in reporting may account for the increase, and that 67% of the deaths could have been prevented if the bumper pads had not been present. Limitations of CPSC data collection processes contribute to the difficulty in determining the risk of bumper pad use.

However, others[239,243] have concluded that the use of bumper pads only prevents minor injuries, and that the potential benefits of preventing minor injury with bumper pad use are far outweighed by the risk of serious injury, such as suffocation or strangulation. In addition, most bumper pads obscure infant and parent visibility, which may increase parental anxiety.[236,238] Other products exist that attach to crib sides or crib slats and claim to protect infants from injury; however, there are no published data that support these claims. Because of the potential for suffocation, entrapment, and strangulation and lack of evidence to support that bumper pads or similar products that attach to crib slats or sides prevent injury in young infants, the AAP does not recommend their use.

PACIFIER USE

Consider offering a pacifier at naptime and bedtime.

Multiple case-control studies[87,91,207,244–250] and 2 meta-analyses[251,252] have reported a protective effect of pacifiers on the incidence of SIDS, particularly when used at the time of the last sleep period, with decreased risk of SIDS ranging from 50% to 90%. Furthermore, 1 study found that pacifier use favorably modified the risk profile of infants who sleep in the prone/side position, bed-share, or use soft bedding.[253] The mechanism for this apparent strong protective effect is still unclear, but favorable modification of autonomic control during sleep[254] and maintaining airway patency during sleep[255] have been proposed. Physiologic studies of the effect of pacifier use on arousal are conflicting; 1 study found that pacifier use decreased arousal thresholds,[163] but others have found no effects on arousability with pacifier use.[256,257] It is common for the pacifier to fall from the mouth soon after the infant falls asleep; even so, the protective effect persists throughout that sleep period.[163,258] Two studies have shown that pacifier use is most protective when used for all sleep periods.[207,250] However, these studies also showed an increased risk of SIDS when the pacifier was usually used but not used the last time the infant was placed for sleep; the significance of these findings is yet unclear.

Although some SIDS experts and policy makers endorse pacifier use recommendations that are similar to those of the AAP,[259,260] concerns about possible deleterious effects of pacifier use have prevented others from making a recommendation for pacifier use as a risk-reduction strategy.[261] Although several observational studies[262–264] have shown a correlation between pacifiers and reduced breastfeeding duration, a recent Cochrane review comparing pacifier use and nonuse in healthy term infants who had initiated breastfeeding found that pacifier use had no effects on partial or exclusive breastfeeding rates at 3 and 4 months.[265] Furthermore, a systematic review found that the highest level of evidence (ie, from clinical trials) does not support an adverse relationship between pacifier use and breastfeeding duration or exclusivity.[266] The association between shortened duration of breastfeeding and pacifier use in observational studies likely reflects a number of complex factors, such as breastfeeding difficulties or intent to wean.[266,267] However, some have also raised the concern that studies that show no effect of pacifier introduction on breastfeeding duration or exclusivity may not account for early weaning or failure to establish breastfeeding.[268] The AAP policy statement "Breastfeeding and the Use of Human Milk" includes a recommendation that pacifiers can be used during breastfeeding but that implementation should be delayed until breastfeeding is well established.[269] Infants who are not being directly breastfed can begin pacifier use as soon as desired.

Some dental malocclusions have been found more commonly among pacifier users than nonusers, but the differences generally disappeared after pacifier cessation.[270] The American Academy of Pediatric Dentistry policy statement on oral habits states that nonnutritive sucking behaviors (ie, fingers or pacifiers) are considered normal in infants and young children and that, in general, sucking habits in children to the age of 3 years are unlikely to cause any long-term problems.[271] Pacifier use is associated with an approximate 1.2- to 2-fold increased risk of otitis media, particularly between 2 and 3 years of age.[272,273] The incidence of otitis media is generally lower in the first year after birth, especially the first 6 months, when the risk of SIDS is the highest.[274–279] However, pacifier use, once established, may persist beyond 6 months, thus increasing the risk of otitis media. Gastrointestinal tract

infections and oral colonization with *Candida* species were also found to be more common among pacifier users than nonusers.[275–277]

Because of the risk of strangulation, pacifiers should not be hung around the infant's neck. Pacifiers that attach to the infant's clothing should not be used with sleeping infants. Objects, such as stuffed toys, that may present a suffocation or choking risk, should not be attached to pacifiers.

There is insufficient evidence that finger sucking is protective against SIDS.

The literature on infant finger sucking and SIDS is extremely limited. Only 2 case-control studies have reported these results.[248,249] One study from the United States showed a protective effect of infant finger sucking (reported as "thumb sucking") against SIDS (adjusted OR: 0.43; 95% CI: 0.25–0.77), but it was less protective than pacifier use (adjusted OR: 0.07 [95% CI: 0.01–0.64] if the infant also sucked the thumb; adjusted OR: 0.08 [95% CI: 0.03–0.23] if the infant did not suck the thumb).[249] Another study from The Netherlands did not show an association between usual finger sucking (reported as "thumb sucking") and SIDS risk (OR: 1.38; 95% CI: 0.35–1.51), but the wide CI suggests that there was insufficient power to detect a significant association.[248]

PRENATAL AND POSTNATAL EXPOSURES (INCLUDING SMOKING AND ALCOHOL)

Pregnant women should obtain regular prenatal care.

There is substantial epidemiologic evidence linking a lower risk of SIDS for infants whose mothers obtain regular prenatal care.[280–283] Women should obtain prenatal care from early in the pregnancy, according to established guidelines for frequency of prenatal visits.[284]

Smoking during pregnancy, in the pregnant woman's environment, and in the infant's environment should be avoided.

Maternal smoking during pregnancy has been identified as a major risk factor in almost every epidemiologic study of SIDS.[285–288] Smoke in the infant's environment after birth has been identified as a separate major risk factor in a few studies,[286,289] although separating this variable from maternal smoking before birth is problematic. Third-hand smoke refers to residual contamination from tobacco smoke after the cigarette has been extinguished[290]; there is no research to date on the significance of third-hand smoke with regard to SIDS risk. Smoke exposure adversely affects infant arousal[291–297]; in addition, smoke exposure increases the risk of preterm birth and low birth weight, both risk factors for SIDS. The effect of tobacco smoke exposure on SIDS risk is dose-dependent. The risk of SIDS is particularly high when the infant bed-shares with an adult smoker (OR: 2.3–21.6), even when the adult does not smoke in bed.[89,90,191,200,201,206,212,298] It is estimated that one-third of SIDS deaths could be prevented if all maternal smoking during pregnancy was eliminated.[299,300] The AAP supports the elimination of all tobacco smoke exposure, both prenatally and environmentally.

Avoid alcohol and illicit drug use during pregnancy and after the infant's birth.

Several studies have specifically investigated the association of SIDS with prenatal and postnatal exposure to alcohol or illicit drug use, although substance abuse often involves more than one substance and it is often difficult to separate out these variables from each other and from smoking. However, 1 study in Northern Plains American Indian infants found that periconceptional maternal alcohol use (adjusted OR: 6.2; 95% CI: 1.6–23.3) and maternal first-trimester binge drinking (adjusted OR: 8.2; 95% CI: 1.9–35.3)[211] were associated with increased SIDS risk, independent of prenatal cigarette smoking exposure. A retrospective study from Western Australia found that a maternal alcoholism diagnosis recorded during pregnancy (adjusted hazard ratio: 6.92; 95% CI: 4.02–11.90) or within 1 year postpregnancy (adjusted hazard ratio: 8.61; 95% CI: 5.04–14.69) was associated with increased SIDS risk, and the authors estimated that at least 16.41% of SIDS deaths were attributable to maternal alcohol use disorder.[301] Another study from Denmark, based on prospective data on maternal alcohol use, has also shown a significant relationship between maternal binge drinking and postneonatal infant mortality, including SIDS.[302] Parental alcohol and/or illicit drug use in combination with bed-sharing places the infant at particularly high risk of SIDS and unintentional suffocation.[91,196]

Rat models have shown increased arousal latency to hypoxia in rat pups exposed to prenatal alcohol.[303] Furthermore, postmortem studies in Northern Plains American Indian infants showed that prenatal cigarette smoking was significantly associated with decreased serotonin receptor binding in the brainstem. In this study, the association of maternal alcohol drinking in the 3 months before or during pregnancy was of borderline significance on univariate analysis but was not significant when prenatal smoking and case versus control status was in the model.[29] However, this study had limited power for multivariate analysis because of the small sample size. One study found an association of SIDS with heavy alcohol consumption in the 2 days before the death.[304] Several studies have found a particularly strong association when alcohol consumption or illicit

drug use occurs in combination with bed-sharing.[89–91,305]

Studies investigating the relationship of illicit drug use and SIDS have focused on specific drugs or illicit drug use in general. One study found maternal cannabis use to be associated with an increased risk of SIDS (adjusted OR: 2.35; 95% CI: 1.36–4.05) at night but not during the day.[306] In utero exposure to opiates (primarily methadone and heroin) has been shown in retrospective studies to be associated with an increased risk of SIDS.[307,308] With the exception of 1 study that did not show an increased risk,[309] population-based studies have generally shown an increased risk with in utero cocaine exposure.[310–312] However, these studies did not control for confounding factors. A prospective cohort study found the SIDS rate to be significantly increased for infants exposed in utero to methadone (OR: 3.6; 95% CI: 2.5–5.1), heroin (OR: 2.3; 95% CI: 1.3–4.0), methadone and heroin (OR: 3.2; 95% CI: 1.2–8.6), and cocaine (OR: 1.6; 95% CI: 1.2–2.2), even after controlling for race/ethnicity, maternal age, parity, birth weight, year of birth, and maternal smoking.[313] In addition, a meta-analysis of studies investigating an association between in utero cocaine exposure and SIDS found an increased risk of SIDS to be associated with prenatal exposure to cocaine and illicit drugs in general.[314]

OVERHEATING, FANS, AND ROOM VENTILATION

Avoid overheating and head covering in infants.

The amount of clothing or blankets covering an infant and the room temperature are associated with an increased risk of SIDS.[208–211] Infants who sleep in the prone position have a higher risk of overheating than supine sleeping infants.[210] However,

the definition of overheating in the studies that found an increased risk of SIDS varies. It is therefore difficult to provide specific room temperature guidelines to avoid overheating.

It is unclear whether the relationship to overheating is an independent factor or merely a reflection of the increased risk of SIDS and suffocation with blankets and other potentially asphyxiating objects in the sleeping environment. Head covering during sleep is of particular concern. In 1 systematic review, the pooled mean prevalence of head covering among SIDS victims was 24.6%, compared with 3.2% among control infants.[186] It is not known whether the risk related to head covering is due to overheating, hypoxia, or rebreathing.

Some have suggested that room ventilation may be important. One study found that bedroom heating, compared with no bedroom heating, increases SIDS risk (OR: 4.5),[315] and another study showed a decreased risk of SIDS in a well-ventilated bedroom (windows and doors open; OR: 0.4).[316] In 1 study, the use of a fan appeared to reduce the risk of SIDS (adjusted OR: 0.28; 95% CI: 0.10–0.77).[317] However, because of the possibility of recall bias, the small sample size of controls who used fans (n = 36), a lack of detail about the location and types of fans used, and the weak link to a mechanism, this study should be interpreted with caution. On the basis of available data, the task force cannot make a recommendation on the use of a fan as a SIDS risk-reduction strategy.

IMMUNIZATIONS

Infants should be immunized in accordance with AAP and Centers for Disease Control and Prevention recommendations.

The incidence of SIDS peaks at a time when infants are receiving numerous immunizations. Case reports of a cluster of deaths shortly after immunization with diphtheria-tetanus toxoids-pertussis vaccine in the late 1970s created concern of a possible causal relationship between vaccinations and SIDS.[318-321] Case-control studies were performed to evaluate this temporal association. Four of the 6 studies showed no relationship between diphtheria-tetanus toxoids-pertussis vaccination and subsequent SIDS[322-325]; the other 2 suggested a temporal relationship, but only in specific subgroup analysis.[326,327] In 2003, the Institute of Medicine reviewed available data and concluded the following: "The evidence favors rejection of a causal relationship between exposure to multiple vaccinations and SIDS."[328] Several analyses of the US Vaccine Adverse Event Reporting System database have shown no relationship between vaccines and SIDS.[329-331] In addition, several large-population case-control trials consistently have found vaccines to be protective against SIDS[332-335]; however, confounding factors (social, maternal, birth, and infant medical history) may account for this protective effect.[336] It also has been theorized that the decreased SIDS rate immediately after vaccination was attributable to infants being healthier at the time of immunization, or "the healthy vaccinee effect."[337] Recent illness would both place infants at higher risk of SIDS and make them more likely to have immunizations deferred.[338]

Recent studies have attempted to control for confounding by social, maternal, birth, and infant medical history.[332,334,338] A meta-analysis of 4 studies found a multivariate summary OR for immunizations and SIDS to be 0.54 (95% CI: 0.39–0.76), indicating that the risk of SIDS is halved by immunization.[338] The evidence continues to show no causal relationship between immunizations and SIDS and suggests that vaccination may have a protective effect against SIDS.

COMMERCIAL DEVICES

Avoid the use of commercial devices that are inconsistent with safe sleep recommendations.

Risk-reduction strategies are based on the best-available evidence in large epidemiologic studies. These studies have been largely focused on the correlations between the sleep environment and SIDS. Our current understanding is that the cause of SIDS is multifactorial and that death results from the interaction between a vulnerable infant and a potentially asphyxiating sleep environment. Thus, claims that sleep devices, mattresses, or special sleep surfaces reduce the risk of SIDS must therefore be supported by epidemiologic evidence. At a minimum, any devices used should meet safety standards of the CPSC, the Juvenile Product Manufacturers Association, and ASTM International (known previously as the American Society for Testing and Materials). The AAP concurs with the US Food and Drug Administration and CPSC that manufacturers should not claim that a product or device protects against SIDS unless there is scientific evidence to that effect.

Wedges and positioning devices are often used by parents to maintain the infant in the side or supine position because of claims that these products reduce the risk of SIDS, suffocation, or gastroesophageal reflux. However, these products are frequently made with soft, compressible materials, which might increase the risk of suffocation. The CPSC has received reports of deaths attributable to suffocation and entrapment associated with wedges and positioning devices. Most of these deaths occurred when infants were placed in the prone or side position with these devices[339]; other incidents have occurred when infants have slipped out of the restraints or rolled into a prone position while using the device.[240,340] Because of

the lack of evidence that they are effective against SIDS, suffocation, or gastroesophageal reflux and because of the potential for suffocation and entrapment risk, the AAP concurs with the CPSC and the US Food and Drug Administration in warning against the use of these products. If positioning devices are used in the hospital as part of physical therapy, they should be removed from the infant sleep area well before discharge from the hospital.

Certain crib mattresses have been designed with air-permeable materials to reduce rebreathing of expired gases, in the event that an infant ends up in the prone position during sleep, and these may be preferable to those with air-impermeable materials. With the use of a head box model, Bar-Yishay et al[341] found that a permeable sleeping surface exhibited significantly better aeration properties in dispersing carbon dioxide and in preventing its accumulation. They also found the measured temperature within the head box to be substantially lower with the more permeable mattress, concluding that it was due to faster heat dissipation. This finding could be potentially protective against overheating, which has been identified as a risk factor for SIDS. Colditz et al[342] also performed studies both in vitro and in vivo, showing better diffusion and less accumulation of carbon dioxide with a mesh mattress. However, Carolan et al[343] found that even porous surfaces are associated with carbon dioxide accumulation and rebreathing thresholds unless there is an active carbon dioxide dispersal system. In addition, although rebreathing has been hypothesized to contribute to death in SIDS, particularly if the head is covered or when the infant is face down, there is no evidence that rebreathing, per se, causes SIDS and no epidemiologic evidence that these mattresses reduce the risk of SIDS. The use of "breathable" mattresses can be an acceptable alternative as long as the other manufacturing requirements are met, including being designed for a particular crib, having a firm surface, and maintaining its shape even when the fitted sheet designated for that model is used, such that there are no gaps between the mattress and the side of the crib, bassinet, portable crib, or play yard.

HOME MONITORS, SIDS, AND BRIEF RESOLVED UNEXPLAINED EVENTS (FORMERLY APPARENT LIFE-THREATENING EVENTS)

There is no evidence that apparent life-threatening events are precursors to SIDS. Furthermore, infant home cardiorespiratory monitors should not be used as a strategy to reduce the risk of SIDS.

For many years, it was believed that brief resolved unexplained events (BRUEs; formerly known as apparent life-threatening events [ALTEs]) were the predecessors of SIDS, and home apnea monitors were used as a strategy for preventing SIDS.[344] However, the use of home cardiorespiratory monitors has not been documented to decrease the incidence of SIDS.[345–348] Home cardiorespiratory monitors are sometimes prescribed for use at home to detect apnea and bradycardia and, when pulse oximetry is used, decreases in oxyhemoglobin saturation for infants at risk of these conditions.[349] Routine in-hospital cardiorespiratory monitoring before discharge from the hospital has not been shown to detect infants at risk of SIDS. There are no data that other commercial devices that are designed to monitor infant vital signs reduce the risk of SIDS.

TUMMY TIME

Supervised, awake tummy time is recommended to facilitate development and to minimize development of positional plagiocephaly.

Positional plagiocephaly, or plagiocephaly without synostosis (PWS), can be associated with a supine sleeping position (OR: 2.5).[350] It is most likely to result if the infant's head position is not varied when placed for sleep; if the infant spends little or no time in awake, supervised tummy time; and if the infant is not held in the upright position when not sleeping.[350–352] Children with developmental delay and/or neurologic injury have increased rates of PWS, although a causal relationship has not been shown.[350,353–356] In healthy normal children, the incidence of PWS decreases spontaneously from 20% at 8 months to 3% at 24 months of age.[351] Although data to make specific recommendations as to how often and how long tummy time should be undertaken are lacking, the task force concurs with the AAP Section on Neurologic Surgery that "a certain amount of prone positioning, or 'tummy time,' while the infant is awake and being observed is recommended to help prevent the development of flattening of the occiput and to facilitate development of the upper shoulder girdle strength necessary for timely attainment of certain motor milestones."[357] The AAP clinical report "Prevention and Management of Positional Skull Deformities in Infants"[357] provides additional detail on the prevention, diagnosis, and management of positional plagiocephaly.

SWADDLING

There is no evidence to recommend swaddling as a strategy to reduce the risk of SIDS. Infants who are swaddled have an increased risk of death if they are placed in or roll to the prone position. If swaddling is used, infants should always be placed on the back. When an infant exhibits signs of attempting to roll, swaddling should no longer be used.

Many cultures and newborn nurseries have traditionally used

swaddling, or wrapping the infant in a light blanket, as a strategy to soothe infants and, in some cases, to encourage sleep in the supine position. Swaddling, when done correctly, can be an effective technique to help calm infants and promote sleep.[358,359]

Some have argued that swaddling can alter certain risk factors for SIDS, thus reducing the risk of SIDS. For instance, it has been suggested that the physical restraint associated with swaddling may prevent infants placed supine from rolling to the prone position.[358] One study suggested a decrease in SIDS rate with swaddling if the infant was supine, but notably, there was an increased risk of SIDS if the infant was swaddled and placed in the prone position.[210] Although another study found a 31-fold increase in SIDS risk with swaddling, the analysis was not stratified by sleep position.[196] Although it may be more likely that parents will initially place a swaddled infant supine, this protective effect may be offset by the 12-fold increased risk of SIDS if the infant is either placed or rolls to the prone position when swaddled.[210,359] In addition, an analysis of CPSC data found that deaths associated with swaddling were most often attributed to positional asphyxia related to prone sleeping, and a large majority of sleep environments had soft bedding.[360] Thus, if swaddling is used, the infant should be placed wholly supine, and swaddling should be discontinued as soon as the infant begins to attempt to roll. Commercially available swaddle sacks are an acceptable alternative, particularly if the parent or caregiver does not know how to swaddle an infant with a conventional thin blanket. There is no evidence with regard to SIDS risk related to the arms swaddled in or out.

There is some evidence that swaddling may cause detrimental physiologic consequences. For example, it can cause an increase in respiratory rate,[361] and tight swaddling can reduce the infant's functional residual lung capacity.[358,362,363] Tight swaddling can also exacerbate hip dysplasia if the hips are kept in extension and adduction,[364–367] which is particularly important because some have advocated that the calming effects of swaddling are related to the "tightness" of the swaddling. In contrast, "loose" or incorrectly applied swaddling could result in head covering and, in some cases, strangulation if the blankets become loose in the bed. Swaddling may also possibly increase the risk of overheating in some situations, especially when the head is covered or there is infection.[368,369] However, 1 study found no increase in abdominal skin temperature when infants were swaddled in a light cotton blanket from the shoulders down.[362]

Impaired arousal has often been postulated as a mechanism contributing to SIDS, and several studies have investigated the relationship between swaddling and arousal and sleep patterns in infants. Physiologic studies have shown that, in general, swaddling decreases startling,[361] increases sleep duration, and decreases spontaneous awakenings.[370] Swaddling also decreases arousability (ie, increases cortical arousal thresholds) to a nasal pulsatile air-jet stimulus, especially in infants who are easily arousable when not swaddled.[361] One study found decreased arousability in infants at 3 months of age who were not usually swaddled and then were swaddled but no effect on arousability in routinely swaddled infants.[361] In contrast, another study has shown infants to be more easily arousable[370] and to have increased autonomic (subcortical) responses[371] to an auditory stimulus when swaddled.[371] Thus, although swaddling clearly promotes sleep and decreases the number of awakenings, the effects on arousability to an external stimulus remain unclear. Accumulating evidence suggests,

however, that routine swaddling has only minimal effects on arousal. In addition, there have been no studies investigating the effects of swaddling on arousal to more relevant stimuli such as hypoxia or hypercapnia. Finally, there is no evidence with regard to SIDS risk related to the arms swaddled in or out.

In summary, it is recognized that swaddling is one of many child care practices that can be used to calm infants, promote sleep, and encourage the use of the supine position. However, there is no evidence to recommend routine swaddling as a strategy to reduce the risk of SIDS. The risk of death is high if a swaddled infant is placed in or rolls to the prone position. If infants are swaddled, they should always be placed on the back. When an infant exhibits signs of attempting to roll, swaddling should no longer be used. Moreover, as many have advocated, swaddling must be correctly applied to avoid the possible hazards, such as hip dysplasia, head covering, and strangulation. Importantly, swaddling does not reduce the necessity to follow recommended safe sleep practices.

POTENTIAL TOXICANTS

There is no evidence substantiating a causal relationship between various toxicants to SIDS.

Many theories link various toxicants and SIDS.[372–374] Although 1 ecological study found a correlation of the maximal recorded nitrate levels of drinking water with local SIDS rates in Sweden,[375] no case-control study has shown a relationship between nitrates in drinking water and SIDS. Furthermore, an expert group in the United Kingdom analyzed data pertaining to a hypothesis that SIDS is related to toxic gases, such as antimony, phosphorus, or arsenic, being released from mattresses[376,377] and found the toxic gas hypothesis unsubstantiated.[378] Finally, 2

case-control studies found that wrapping mattresses in plastic to reduce toxic gas emission did not protect against SIDS.[230,379]

HEARING SCREENS

Current data do not support the use of newborn hearing screens as screening tests for SIDS.

One retrospective case-control study examined the use of newborn transient evoked otoacoustic emission hearing screening tests as a tool to identify infants at subsequent risk of SIDS.[380] Infants who subsequent died of SIDS did not fail their hearing tests but, compared with controls, showed a decreased signal-to-noise ratio score in the right ear only, at frequencies of 2000, 3000, and 4000 Hz. Methodologic concerns have been raised about the validity of the study methods used in this study,[381,382] and these results have not been substantiated by others. A larger, but non–peer-reviewed, report of hearing screening data in Michigan[383] and a peer-reviewed retrospective study in Hong Kong[383,384] showed no relationship between hearing screening test results and SIDS cases. Until additional data are available, hearing screening should not be considered as a valid screening tool to determine which infants may be at subsequent risk of SIDS. Furthermore, an increased risk of SIDS should not be inferred from an abnormal hearing screen result.

EDUCATIONAL INTERVENTIONS

Educational and intervention campaigns are often effective in altering practice.

Intervention campaigns for SIDS have been extremely effective, especially with regard to the avoidance of prone positioning.[385] Furthermore, primary care–based educational interventions, particularly those that address caregiver concerns and misconceptions about safe sleep recommendations, can be effective in altering practice. For instance, addressing concerns about infant comfort, choking, and aspiration while the infant is sleeping supine is helpful.[19,96,97,386] However, many families report not receiving information consistent with AAP recommendations. When a nationally representative sample of mothers of young infants were asked about information received from their pediatricians, only 54.5% had received a recommendation to place their infant supine for sleep, 19.9% had received information about appropriate sleep location, and 11.0% had received information about pacifier use.[387] Primary care providers should be encouraged to develop quality-improvement initiatives to improve adherence to safe sleep recommendations among their patients.

In addition, modeling of unsafe sleep practices by health care and child care providers may increase the prevalence of these unsafe practices.[388-390] Modeling of unsafe practices may occur because professionals are not convinced of the utility of the safe sleep recommendations or have concerns about the supine sleep position, particularly with regard to infant comfort, choking, and aspiration.[391-395] Interventions that address provider concerns are effective in improving behavior.[391,396-398]

MEDIA MESSAGES

Media and manufacturers should follow safe sleep guidelines in their messaging and advertising.

A recent study found that, in magazines targeted toward childbearing women, more than one-third of pictures of sleeping infants and two-thirds of pictures of infant sleep environments portrayed unsafe sleep positions and sleep environments.[237] Media exposures (including movie, television, magazines, newspapers, and Web

sites), manufacturer advertisements, and store displays affect individual behavior by influencing beliefs and attitudes. Frequent exposure to health-related media messages can affect individual health decisions,[399,400] and media messages have been very influential in decisions regarding sleep position.[101,104] Media and advertising messages contrary to safe sleep recommendations may create misinformation about safe sleep practices.

Media and manufacturer messaging and advertising should follow safe sleep guidelines in text, photos, and illustrations. In addition, public health departments and organizations that provide safe sleep information should review, revise, and reissue this information at least every 5 years to ensure that each generation of new parents receives appropriate information.

RECOMMENDATIONS

The recommendations for a safe infant sleeping environment to reduce the risk of both SIDS and other sleep-related infant deaths are specified in the accompanying policy statement.[78]

ACKNOWLEDGMENTS

We acknowledge the contributions provided by others to the collection and interpretation of data examined in preparation of this report. We are particularly grateful for the independent biostatistical report submitted by Robert W. Platt, PhD.

LEAD AUTHOR

Rachel Y. Moon, MD, FAAP

TASK FORCE ON SUDDEN INFANT DEATH SYNDROME

Rachel Y. Moon, MD, FAAP, Chairperson
Robert A. Darnall, MD
Lori Feldman-Winter, MD, MPH, FAAP
Michael H. Goodstein, MD, FAAP
Fern R. Hauck, MD, MS

CONSULTANTS

Marian Willinger, PhD – Eunice Kennedy Shriver National Institute for Child Health and Human Development
Carrie K. Shapiro-Mendoza, PhD, MPH – Centers for Disease Control and Prevention

STAFF

James Couto, MA

ABBREVIATIONS

AAP: American Academy of Pediatrics
ASSB: accidental suffocation or strangulation in bed
CI: confidence interval
CPSC: Consumer Product Safety Commission
ICD: International Statistical Classification of Diseases and Related Health Problems
ICD-10: International Classification of Diseases, 10th Revision
OR: odds ratio
PWS: plagiocephaly without synostosis
SIDS: sudden infant death syndrome
SUDI: sudden unexpected death in infancy
SUID: sudden unexpected infant death
5-HT: 5-hydroxytryptamine (serotonin)
5-HT1A: 5-hydroxytryptamine 1A (serotonin 1A)

REFERENCES

1. Moon RY; Task Force on Sudden Infant Death Syndrome. SIDS and other sleep-related infant deaths: expansion of recommendations for a safe infant sleeping environment. *Pediatrics.* 2011;128(5). Available at: www.pediatrics.org/cgi/content/full/128/5/e1341

2. Moon RY; Task Force on Sudden Infant Death Syndrome. SIDS and other sleep-related infant deaths: expansion of recommendations for a safe infant sleeping environment. *Pediatrics.* 2011;128(5):1030–1039

3. Ebell MH, Siwek J, Weiss BD, et al. Strength of Recommendation

Taxonomy (SORT): a patient-centered approach to grading evidence in the medical literature. *Am Fam Physician*. 2004;69(3):548–556

4. Willinger M, James LS, Catz C. Defining the sudden infant death syndrome (SIDS): deliberations of an expert panel convened by the National Institute of Child Health and Human Development. *Pediatr Pathol*. 1991;11(5):677–684

5. Centers for Disease Control and Prevention. Sudden unexplained infant death investigation reporting form (SUIDIRF). Available at: www.cdc.gov/SIDS/SUIDRF.htm. Accessed January 10, 2016

6. Camperlengo LT, Shapiro-Mendoza CK, Kim SY. Sudden infant death syndrome: diagnostic practices and investigative policies, 2004. *Am J Forensic Med Pathol*. 2012;33(3):197–201

7. Krous HF, Chadwick AE, Haas EA, Stanley C. Pulmonary intra-alveolar hemorrhage in SIDS and suffocation. *J Forensic Leg Med*. 2007;14(8):461–470

8. Kim SY, Shapiro-Mendoza CK, Chu SY, Camperlengo LT, Anderson R. Differentiating cause-of-death terminology for deaths coded as SIDS, accidental suffocation, and unknown cause: an investigation using US death certificates, 2003-2004. *Am J Forensic Sci*. 2012;57(2):364–369

9. Shapiro-Mendoza CK, Kim SY, Chu SY, Kahn E, Anderson RN. Using death certificates to characterize sudden infant death syndrome (SIDS): opportunities and limitations. *J Pediatr*. 2010;156(1):38–43

10. Kattwinkel J, Brooks J, Myerberg D; American Academy of Pediatrics Task Force on Infant Positioning and SIDS. Positioning and SIDS [published correction appears in *Pediatrics*. 1992;90(2 pt 1):264]. *Pediatrics*. 1992;89(6 pt 1):1120–1126

11. National Institute of Child Health and Human Development/National Institutes of Health. Safe to Sleep campaign. Available at: www.nichd.nih.gov/sts. Accessed September 21, 2016

12. National Infant Sleep Position Study Web site. Available at: http://sloneweb2.bu.edu/ChimeNisp/Main_Nisp.asp. Accessed January 10, 2016

13. Matthews TJ, MacDorman MF, Thoma ME. Infant mortality statistics from the 2013 period linked birth/infant death data set. *Natl Vital Stat Rep*. 2015;64(9):1–30

14. US Department of Health and Human Services. Linked birth/infant death records [CDC WONDER online database]. Available at: http://wonder.cdc.gov/lbd.html. Accessed June 1, 2016

15. Malloy MH, MacDorman M. Changes in the classification of sudden unexpected infant deaths: United States, 1992–2001. *Pediatrics*. 2005;115(5):1247–1253

16. Shapiro-Mendoza CK, Tomashek KM, Anderson RN, Wingo J. Recent national trends in sudden, unexpected infant deaths: more evidence supporting a change in classification or reporting. *Am J Epidemiol*. 2006;163(8):762–769

17. Shapiro-Mendoza CK, Kimball M, Tomashek KM, Anderson RN, Blanding S. US infant mortality trends attributable to accidental suffocation and strangulation in bed from 1984 through 2004: are rates increasing? *Pediatrics*. 2009;123(2):533–539

18. Hauck FR, Moore CM, Herman SM, et al. The contribution of prone sleeping position to the racial disparity in sudden infant death syndrome: the Chicago Infant Mortality Study. *Pediatrics*. 2002;110(4):772–780

19. Colson ER, Rybin D, Smith LA, Colton T, Lister G, Corwin MJ. Trends and factors associated with infant sleeping position: the National Infant Sleep Position Study, 1993-2007. *Arch Pediatr Adolesc Med*. 2009;163(12):1122–1128

20. Lahr MB, Rosenberg KD, Lapidus JA. Maternal-infant bedsharing: risk factors for bedsharing in a population-based survey of new mothers and implications for SIDS risk reduction. *Matern Child Health J*. 2007;11(3):277–286

21. Willinger M, Ko CW, Hoffman HJ, Kessler RC, Corwin MJ; National Infant Sleep Position Study. Trends in infant bed sharing in the United States, 1993-2000: the National Infant Sleep Position Study. *Arch Pediatr Adolesc Med*. 2003;157(1):43–49

22. Fu LY, Colson ER, Corwin MJ, Moon RY. Infant sleep location: associated maternal and infant characteristics with sudden infant death syndrome prevention recommendations. *J Pediatr*. 2008;153(4):503–508

23. Flick L, White DK, Vemulapalli C, Stulac BB, Kemp JS. Sleep position and the use of soft bedding during bed sharing among African American infants at increased risk for sudden infant death syndrome. *J Pediatr*. 2001;138(3):338–343

24. Rasinski KA, Kuby A, Bzdusek SA, Silvestri JM, Weese-Mayer DE. Effect of a sudden infant death syndrome risk reduction education program on risk factor compliance and information sources in primarily black urban communities. *Pediatrics*. 2003;111(4 pt 1). Available at: www.pediatrics.org/cgi/content/full/111/4/e347

25. Shapiro-Mendoza CK, Colson ER, Willinger M, Rybin DV, Camperlengo L, Corwin MJ. Trends in infant bedding use: National Infant Sleep Position Study, 1993–2010. *Pediatrics*. 2015;135(1):10–17

26. Filiano JJ, Kinney HC. A perspective on neuropathologic findings in victims of the sudden infant death syndrome: the triple-risk model. *Biol Neonate*. 1994;65(3-4):194–197

27. Kinney HC. Brainstem mechanisms underlying the sudden infant death syndrome: evidence from human pathologic studies. *Dev Psychobiol*. 2009;51(3):223–233

28. Goldstein RD, Trachtenberg FL, Sens MA, Harty BJ, Kinney HC. Overall postneonatal mortality and rates of SIDS. *Pediatrics*. 2016;137(1):1–10

29. Kinney HC, Randall LL, Sleeper LA, et al. Serotonergic brainstem abnormalities in Northern Plains Indians with the sudden infant death syndrome. *J Neuropathol Exp Neurol*. 2003;62(11):1178–1191

30. Browne CJ, Sharma N, Waters KA, Machaalani R. The effects of nicotine on the alpha-7 and beta-2 nicotinic acetycholine receptor subunits in the developing piglet brainstem. *Int J Dev Neurosci*. 2010;28(1):1–7

31. Hunt NJ, Waters KA, Machaalani R. Orexin receptors in the developing

piglet hypothalamus, and effects of nicotine and intermittent hypercapnic hypoxia exposures. *Brain Res.* 2013;1508:73–82

32. Cerpa VJ, Aylwin ML, Beltrán-Castillo S, et al. The alteration of neonatal raphe neurons by prenatal-perinatal nicotine: meaning for sudden infant death syndrome. *Am J Respir Cell Mol Biol.* 2015;53(4):489–499

33. Slotkin TA, Seidler FJ, Spindel ER. Prenatal nicotine exposure in rhesus monkeys compromises development of brainstem and cardiac monoamine pathways involved in perinatal adaptation and sudden infant death syndrome: amelioration by vitamin C. *Neurotoxicol Teratol.* 2011;33(3):431–434

34. Sekizawa S, Joad JP, Pinkerton KE, Bonham AC. Secondhand smoke exposure alters K+ channel function and intrinsic cell excitability in a subset of second-order airway neurons in the nucleus tractus solitarius of young guinea pigs. *Eur J Neurosci.* 2010;31(4):673–684

35. Duncan JR, Paterson DS, Hoffman JM, et al. Brainstem serotonergic deficiency in sudden infant death syndrome. *JAMA.* 2010;303(5):430–437

36. Duncan JR, Garland M, Myers MM, et al. Prenatal nicotine-exposure alters fetal autonomic activity and medullary neurotransmitter receptors: implications for sudden infant death syndrome. *J Appl Physiol (1985).* 2009;107(5):1579–1590

37. Duncan JR, Garland M, Stark RI, et al. Prenatal nicotine exposure selectively affects nicotinic receptor expression in primary and associative visual cortices of the fetal baboon. *Brain Pathol.* 2015;25(2):171–181

38. St-John WM, Leiter JC. Maternal nicotine depresses eupneic ventilation of neonatal rats. *Neurosci Lett.* 1999;267(3):206–208

39. Eugenín J, Otárola M, Bravo E, et al. Prenatal to early postnatal nicotine exposure impairs central chemoreception and modifies breathing pattern in mouse neonates: a probable link to sudden infant death syndrome. *J Neurosci.* 2008;28(51):13907–13917

40. Fewell JE, Smith FG, Ng VK. Prenatal exposure to nicotine impairs protective responses of rat pups to hypoxia in an age-dependent manner. *Respir Physiol.* 2001;127(1):61–73

41. Hafström O, Milerad J, Sundell HW. Prenatal nicotine exposure blunts the cardiorespiratory response to hypoxia in lambs. *Am J Respir Crit Care Med.* 2002;166(12 pt 1):1544–1549

42. Duncan JR, Paterson DS, Kinney HC. The development of nicotinic receptors in the human medulla oblongata: inter-relationship with the serotonergic system. *Auton Neurosci.* 2008;144(1–2):61–75

43. Wilhelm-Benartzi CS, Houseman EA, Maccani MA, et al. In utero exposures, infant growth, and DNA methylation of repetitive elements and developmentally related genes in human placenta. *Environ Health Perspect.* 2012;120(2):296–302

44. Schneider J, Mitchell I, Singhal N, Kirk V, Hasan SU. Prenatal cigarette smoke exposure attenuates recovery from hypoxemic challenge in preterm infants. *Am J Respir Crit Care Med.* 2008;178(5):520–526

45. Thiriez G, Bouhaddi M, Mourot L, et al. Heart rate variability in preterm infants and maternal smoking during pregnancy. *Clin Auton Res.* 2009;19(3):149–156

46. Fifer WP, Fingers ST, Youngman M, Gomez-Gribben E, Myers MM. Effects of alcohol and smoking during pregnancy on infant autonomic control. *Dev Psychobiol.* 2009;51(3):234–242

47. Richardson HL, Walker AM, Horne RS. Maternal smoking impairs arousal patterns in sleeping infants. *Sleep.* 2009;32(4):515–521

48. Cohen G, Vella S, Jeffery H, Lagercrantz H, Katz-Salamon M. Cardiovascular stress hyperreactivity in babies of smokers and in babies born preterm. *Circulation.* 2008;118(18):1848–1853

49. Paine SM, Jacques TS, Sebire NJ. Review: neuropathological features of unexplained sudden unexpected death in infancy: current evidence and controversies. *Neuropathol Appl Neurobiol.* 2014;40(4):364–384

50. Panigrahy A, Filiano J, Sleeper LA, et al. Decreased serotonergic receptor binding in rhombic lip-derived regions of the medulla oblongata in the sudden infant death syndrome. *J Neuropathol Exp Neurol.* 2000;59(5):377–384

51. Ozawa Y, Takashima S. Developmental neurotransmitter pathology in the brainstem of sudden infant death syndrome: a review and sleep position. *Forensic Sci Int.* 2002;130(suppl):S53–S59

52. Machaalani R, Say M, Waters KA. Serotoninergic receptor 1A in the sudden infant death syndrome brainstem medulla and associations with clinical risk factors. *Acta Neuropathol.* 2009;117(3):257–265

53. Paterson DS, Trachtenberg FL, Thompson EG, et al. Multiple serotonergic brainstem abnormalities in sudden infant death syndrome. *JAMA.* 2006;296(17):2124–2132

54. Lavezzi AM, Weese-Mayer DE, Yu MY, et al. Developmental alterations of the respiratory human retrotrapezoid nucleus in sudden unexplained fetal and infant death. *Auton Neurosci.* 2012;170(1–2):12–19

55. Kinney HC, Cryan JB, Haynes RL, et al. Dentate gyrus abnormalities in sudden unexplained death in infants: morphological marker of underlying brain vulnerability. *Acta Neuropathol.* 2015;129(1):65–80

56. Say M, Machaalani R, Waters KA. Changes in serotoninergic receptors 1A and 2A in the piglet brainstem after intermittent hypercapnic hypoxia (IHH) and nicotine. *Brain Res.* 2007;1152:17–26

57. Kinney HC, Richerson GB, Dymecki SM, Darnall RA, Nattie EE. The brainstem and serotonin in the sudden infant death syndrome. *Annu Rev Pathol.* 2009;4:517–550

58. Cummings KJ, Commons KG, Fan KC, Li A, Nattie EE. Severe spontaneous bradycardia associated with respiratory disruptions in rat pups with fewer brain stem 5-HT neurons. *Am J Physiol Regul Integr Comp Physiol.* 2009;296(6):R1783–R1796

59. Cummings KJ, Hewitt JC, Li A, Daubenspeck JA, Nattie EE. Postnatal loss of brainstem serotonin neurones compromises the ability of neonatal

rats to survive episodic severe hypoxia. *J Physiol*. 2011;589(pt 21):5247–5256

60. Darnall RA, Schneider RW, Tobia CM, Commons KG. Eliminating medullary 5-HT neurons delays arousal and decreases the respiratory response to repeated episodes of hypoxia in neonatal rat pups. *J Appl Physiol (1985)*. 2016;120(5):514–525

61. Rosenthal NA, Currier RJ, Baer RJ, Feuchtbaum L, Jelliffe-Pawlowski LL. Undiagnosed metabolic dysfunction and sudden infant death syndrome—a case-control study. *Paediatr Perinat Epidemiol*. 2015;29(2):151–155

62. Opdal SH, Rognum TO. Gene variants predisposing to SIDS: current knowledge. *Forensic Sci Med Pathol*. 2011;7(1):26–36

63. Weese-Mayer DE, Ackerman MJ, Marazita ML, Berry-Kravis EM. Sudden infant death syndrome: review of implicated genetic factors. *Am J Med Genet A*. 2007;143A(8):771–788

64. Paterson DS, Rivera KD, Broadbelt KG, et al. Lack of association of the serotonin transporter polymorphism with the sudden infant death syndrome in the San Diego Dataset. *Pediatr Res*. 2010;68(5):409–413

65. Wang DW, Desai RR, Crotti L, et al. Cardiac sodium channel dysfunction in sudden infant death syndrome. *Circulation*. 2007;115(3):368–376

66. Tan BH, Pundi KN, Van Norstrand DW, et al. Sudden infant death syndrome-associated mutations in the sodium channel beta subunits. *Heart Rhythm*. 2010;7(6):771–778

67. Van Norstrand DW, Asimaki A, Rubinos C, et al. Connexin43 mutation causes heterogeneous gap junction loss and sudden infant death. *Circulation*. 2012;125(3):474–481

68. Andreasen C, Refsgaard L, Nielsen JB, et al. Mutations in genes encoding cardiac ion channels previously associated with sudden infant death syndrome (SIDS) are present with high frequency in new exome data. *Can J Cardiol*. 2013;29(9):1104–1109

69. Winkel BG, Yuan L, Olesen MS, et al. The role of the sodium current complex in a nonreferred nationwide cohort of

sudden infant death syndrome. *Heart Rhythm*. 2015;12(6):1241–1249

70. Cummings KJ, Klotz C, Liu WQ, et al. Sudden infant death syndrome (SIDS) in African Americans: polymorphisms in the gene encoding the stress peptide pituitary adenylate cyclase-activating polypeptide (PACAP). *Acta Paediatr*. 2009;98(3):482–489

71. Barrett KT, Rodikova E, Weese-Mayer DE, et al. Analysis of PAC1 receptor gene variants in Caucasian and African American infants dying of sudden infant death syndrome. *Acta Paediatr*. 2013;102(12). Available at: www.pediatrics.org/cgi/content/full/102/12/e546

72. Ferrante L, Opdal SH, Vege A, Rognum T. Cytokine gene polymorphisms and sudden infant death syndrome. *Acta Paediatr*. 2010;99(3):384–388

73. Ferrante L, Opdal SH, Vege A, Rognum TO. IL-1 gene cluster polymorphisms and sudden infant death syndrome. *Hum Immunol*. 2010;71(4):402–406

74. Opdal SH, Rognum TO, Vege A, Stave AK, Dupuy BM, Egeland T. Increased number of substitutions in the D-loop of mitochondrial DNA in the sudden infant death syndrome. *Acta Paediatr*. 1998;87(10):1039–1044

75. Opdal SH, Rognum TO, Torgersen H, Vege A. Mitochondrial DNA point mutations detected in four cases of sudden infant death syndrome. *Acta Paediatr*. 1999;88(9):957–960

76. Santorelli FM, Schlessel JS, Slonim AE, DiMauro S. Novel mutation in the mitochondrial DNA tRNA glycine gene associated with sudden unexpected death. *Pediatr Neurol*. 1996;15(2):145–149

77. Forsyth L, Hume R, Howatson A, Busuttil A, Burchell A. Identification of novel polymorphisms in the glucokinase and glucose-6-phosphatase genes in infants who died suddenly and unexpectedly. *J Mol Med (Berl)*. 2005;83(8):610–618

78. American Academy of Pediatrics Task Force on Sudden Infant Death Syndrome. SIDS and other sleep-related infant deaths: updated 2016 recommendations for a safe infant

sleeping environment. *Pediatrics*. 2016;138(5):e20162938

79. Kanetake J, Aoki Y, Funayama M. Evaluation of rebreathing potential on bedding for infant use. *Pediatr Int*. 2003;45(3):284–289

80. Kemp JS, Thach BT. Quantifying the potential of infant bedding to limit CO2 dispersal and factors affecting rebreathing in bedding. *J Appl Physiol (1985)*. 1995;78(2):740–745

81. Kemp JS, Livne M, White DK, Arfken CL. Softness and potential to cause rebreathing: differences in bedding used by infants at high and low risk for sudden infant death syndrome. *J Pediatr*. 1998;132(2):234–239

82. Patel AL, Harris K, Thach BT. Inspired CO(2) and O(2) in sleeping infants rebreathing from bedding: relevance for sudden infant death syndrome. *J Appl Physiol (1985)*. 2001;91(6):2537–2545

83. Tuffnell CS, Petersen SA, Wailoo MP. Prone sleeping infants have a reduced ability to lose heat. *Early Hum Dev*. 1995;43(2):109–116

84. Ammari A, Schulze KF, Ohira-Kist K, et al. Effects of body position on thermal, cardiorespiratory and metabolic activity in low birth weight infants. *Early Hum Dev*. 2009;85(8):497–501

85. Yiallourou SR, Walker AM, Horne RS. Prone sleeping impairs circulatory control during sleep in healthy term infants: implications for SIDS. *Sleep*. 2008;31(8):1139–1146

86. Wong FY, Witcombe NB, Yiallourou SR, et al. Cerebral oxygenation is depressed during sleep in healthy term infants when they sleep prone. *Pediatrics*. 2011;127(3). Available at: www.pediatrics.org/cgi/content/full/127/3/e558

87. Hauck FR, Herman SM, Donovan M, et al. Sleep environment and the risk of sudden infant death syndrome in an urban population: the Chicago Infant Mortality Study. *Pediatrics*. 2003;111(5 pt 2):1207–1214

88. Li DK, Petitti DB, Willinger M, et al. Infant sleeping position and the risk of sudden infant death syndrome in California, 1997-2000. *Am J Epidemiol*. 2003;157(5):446–455

89. Blair PS, Fleming PJ, Smith IJ, et al; CESDI SUDI Research Group. Babies sleeping with parents: case-control study of factors influencing the risk of the sudden infant death syndrome. *BMJ*. 1999;319(7223):1457–1461

90. Fleming PJ, Blair PS, Bacon C, et al; Confidential Enquiry into Stillbirths and Deaths Regional Coordinators and Researchers. Environment of infants during sleep and risk of the sudden infant death syndrome: results of 1993-5 case-control study for confidential inquiry into stillbirths and deaths in infancy. *BMJ*. 1996;313(7051):191–195

91. Carpenter RG, Irgens LM, Blair PS, et al. Sudden unexplained infant death in 20 regions in Europe: case control study. *Lancet*. 2004;363(9404):185–191

92. Mitchell EA, Tuohy PG, Brunt JM, et al. Risk factors for sudden infant death syndrome following the prevention campaign in New Zealand: a prospective study. *Pediatrics*. 1997;100(5):835–840

93. Waters KA, Gonzalez A, Jean C, Morielli A, Brouillette RT. Face-straight-down and face-near-straight-down positions in healthy, prone-sleeping infants. *J Pediatr*. 1996;128(5 pt 1):616–625

94. Oyen N, Markestad T, Skaerven R, et al. Combined effects of sleeping position and prenatal risk factors in sudden infant death syndrome: the Nordic Epidemiological SIDS Study. *Pediatrics*. 1997;100(4):613–621

95. Mitchell EA, Thach BT, Thompson JMD, Williams S. Changing infants' sleep position increases risk of sudden infant death syndrome: New Zealand Cot Death Study. *Arch Pediatr Adolesc Med*. 1999;153(11):1136–1141

96. Oden RP, Joyner BL, Ajao TI, Moon RY. Factors influencing African American mothers' decisions about sleep position: a qualitative study. *J Natl Med Assoc*. 2010;102(10):870–872, 875–880

97. Colson ER, McCabe LK, Fox K, et al. Barriers to following the back-to-sleep recommendations: insights from focus groups with inner-city caregivers. *Ambul Pediatr*. 2005;5(6):349–354

98. Mosley JM, Daily Stokes S, Ulmer A. Infant sleep position: discerning

knowledge from practice. *Am J Health Behav*. 2007;31(6):573–582

99. Moon RY, Omron R. Determinants of infant sleep position in an urban population. *Clin Pediatr (Phila)*. 2002;41(8):569–573

100. Ottolini MC, Davis BE, Patel K, Sachs HC, Gershon NB, Moon RY. Prone infant sleeping despite the "Back to Sleep" campaign. *Arch Pediatr Adolesc Med*. 1999;153(5):512–517

101. Willinger M, Ko C-W, Hoffman HJ, Kessler RC, Corwin MJ. Factors associated with caregivers' choice of infant sleep position, 1994-1998: the National Infant Sleep Position Study. *JAMA*. 2000;283(16):2135–2142

102. Moon RY, Biliter WM. Infant sleep position policies in licensed child care centers after back to sleep campaign. *Pediatrics*. 2000;106(3):576–580

103. Moon RY, Weese-Mayer DE, Silvestri JM. Nighttime child care: inadequate sudden infant death syndrome risk factor knowledge, practice, and policies. *Pediatrics*. 2003;111(4 pt 1):795–799

104. Von Kohorn I, Corwin MJ, Rybin DV, Heeren TC, Lister G, Colson ER. Influence of prior advice and beliefs of mothers on infant sleep position. *Arch Pediatr Adolesc Med*. 2010;164(4):363–369

105. Kahn A, Groswasser J, Sottiaux M, Rebuffat E, Franco P, Dramaix M. Prone or supine body position and sleep characteristics in infants. *Pediatrics*. 1993;91(6):1112–1115

106. Bhat RY, Hannam S, Pressler R, Rafferty GF, Peacock JL, Greenough A. Effect of prone and supine position on sleep, apneas, and arousal in preterm infants. *Pediatrics*. 2006;118(1):101–107

107. Ariagno RL, van Liempt S, Mirmiran M. Fewer spontaneous arousals during prone sleep in preterm infants at 1 and 3 months corrected age. *J Perinatol*. 2006;26(5):306–312

108. Franco P, Groswasser J, Sottiaux M, Broadfield E, Kahn A. Decreased cardiac responses to auditory stimulation during prone sleep. *Pediatrics*. 1996;97(2): 174–178

109. Galland BC, Reeves G, Taylor BJ, Bolton DP. Sleep position, autonomic function, and arousal. *Arch Dis Child Fetal Neonatal Ed*. 1998;78(3):F189–F194

110. Galland BC, Hayman RM, Taylor BJ, Bolton DP, Sayers RM, Williams SM. Factors affecting heart rate variability and heart rate responses to tilting in infants aged 1 and 3 months. *Pediatr Res*. 2000;48(3):360–368

111. Horne RS, Ferens D, Watts AM, et al. The prone sleeping position impairs arousability in term infants. *J Pediatr*. 2001;138(6):811–816

112. Horne RS, Bandopadhayay P, Vitkovic J, Cranage SM, Adamson TM. Effects of age and sleeping position on arousal from sleep in preterm infants. *Sleep*. 2002;25(7):746–750

113. Kato I, Scaillet S, Groswasser J, et al. Spontaneous arousability in prone and supine position in healthy infants. *Sleep*. 2006;29(6):785–790

114. Phillipson EA, Sullivan CE. Arousal: the forgotten response to respiratory stimuli. *Am Rev Respir Dis*. 1978;118(5):807–809

115. Kahn A, Groswasser J, Rebuffat E, et al. Sleep and cardiorespiratory characteristics of infant victims of sudden death: a prospective case-control study. *Sleep*. 1992;15(4):287–292

116. Schechtman VL, Harper RM, Wilson AJ, Southall DP. Sleep state organization in normal infants and victims of the sudden infant death syndrome. *Pediatrics*. 1992;89(5 pt 1):865–870

117. Harper RM. State-related physiological changes and risk for the sudden infant death syndrome. *Aust Paediatr J*. 1986;22(suppl 1):55–58

118. Kato I, Franco P, Groswasser J, et al. Incomplete arousal processes in infants who were victims of sudden death. *Am J Respir Crit Care Med*. 2003;168(11):1298–1303

119. Byard RW, Beal SM. Gastric aspiration and sleeping position in infancy and early childhood. *J Paediatr Child Health*. 2000;36(4):403–405

120. Malloy MH. Trends in postneonatal aspiration deaths and reclassification of sudden infant death syndrome:

impact of the "Back to Sleep" program. *Pediatrics*. 2002;109(4):661–665

121. Tablizo MA, Jacinto P, Parsley D, Chen ML, Ramanathan R, Keens TG. Supine sleeping position does not cause clinical aspiration in neonates in hospital newborn nurseries. *Arch Pediatr Adolesc Med*. 2007;161(5):507–510

122. Vandenplas Y, Rudolph CD, Di Lorenzo C, et al; North American Society for Pediatric Gastroenterology Hepatology and Nutrition; European Society for Pediatric Gastroenterology Hepatology and Nutrition. Pediatric gastroesophageal reflux clinical practice guidelines: joint recommendations of the North American Society for Pediatric Gastroenterology, Hepatology, and Nutrition (NASPGHAN) and the European Society for Pediatric Gastroenterology, Hepatology, and Nutrition (ESPGHAN). *J Pediatr Gastroenterol Nutr*. 2009;49(4):498–547

123. Meyers WF, Herbst JJ. Effectiveness of positioning therapy for gastroesophageal reflux. *Pediatrics*. 1982;69(6):768–772

124. Tobin JM, McCloud P, Cameron DJ. Posture and gastro-oesophageal reflux: a case for left lateral positioning. *Arch Dis Child*. 1997;76(3):254–258

125. Malloy MH, Hoffman HJ. Prematurity, sudden infant death syndrome, and age of death. *Pediatrics*. 1995;96(3 pt 1):464–471

126. Sowter B, Doyle LW, Morley CJ, Altmann A, Halliday J. Is sudden infant death syndrome still more common in very low birthweight infants in the 1990s? *Med J Aust*. 1999;171(8):411–413

127. American Academy of Pediatrics Committee on Fetus and Newborn. Hospital discharge of the high-risk neonate. *Pediatrics*. 2008;122(5):1119–1126

128. Gelfer P, Cameron R, Masters K, Kennedy KA. Integrating "Back to Sleep" recommendations into neonatal ICU practice. *Pediatrics*. 2013;131(4). Available at: www.pediatrics.org/cgi/content/full/131/4e1264

129. Hwang SS, O'Sullivan A, Fitzgerald E, Melvin P, Gorman T, Fiascone JM. Implementation of safe sleep practices in the neonatal intensive care unit. *J Perinatol*. 2015;35(10):862–866

130. Feldman-Winter L, Goldsmith JP; AAP Committee on Fetus and Newborn; AAP Task Force on Sudden Infant Death Syndrome. Safe sleep and skin-to-skin care in the neonatal period for healthy term newborns. *Pediatrics*. 2016;138(3):e20161889

131. Moon RY, Oden RP, Joyner BL, Ajao TI. Qualitative analysis of beliefs and perceptions about sudden infant death syndrome (SIDS) among African-American mothers: implications for safe sleep recommendations. *J Pediatr*. 2010;157(1):92–97, e92

132. Brenner RA, Simons-Morton BG, Bhaskar B, et al. Prevalence and predictors of the prone sleep position among inner-city infants. *JAMA*. 1998;280(4):341–346

133. Willinger M, Hoffman HJ, Wu K-T, et al. Factors associated with the transition to nonprone sleep positions of infants in the United States: the National Infant Sleep Position Study. *JAMA*. 1998;280(4):329–335

134. Colvin JD, Collie-Akers V, Schunn C, Moon RY. Sleep environment risks for younger and older infants. *Pediatrics*. 2014;134(2). Available at: www.pediatrics.org/cgi/content/full/134/2/e406

135. Kemp JS, Nelson VE, Thach BT. Physical properties of bedding that may increase risk of sudden infant death syndrome in prone-sleeping infants. *Pediatr Res*. 1994;36(1 pt 1):7–11

136. US Consumer Product Safety Commission. *Crib Safety Tips: Use Your Crib Safely. CPSC Document 5030*. Washington, DC: US Consumer Product Safety Commission; 2011

137. Consumer Product Safety Commission. Safety standard for bassinets and cradles. *Fed Reg*. 2013;78(205):63019–63036

138. Consumer Product Safety Commission. Safety standard for play yards. *Fed Reg*. 2012;77(168):52220–52228

139. Consumer Product Safety Commission. Safety standards for bedside sleepers. *Fed Reg*. 2014;79(10):2581–2589

140. Jackson A, Moon RY. An analysis of deaths in portable cribs and playpens: what can be learned? *Clin Pediatr (Phila)*. 2008;47(3):261–266

141. Pike J, Moon RY. Bassinet use and sudden unexpected death in infancy. *J Pediatr*. 2008;153(4):509–512

142. Nakamura S, Wind M, Danello MA. Review of hazards associated with children placed in adult beds. *Arch Pediatr Adolesc Med*. 1999;153(10):1019–1023

143. Consumer Product Safety Commission. Safety standard for portable bed rails: final rule. *Fed Reg*. 2012;77(40):12182–12197

144. Callahan CW, Sisler C. Use of seating devices in infants too young to sit. *Arch Pediatr Adolesc Med*. 1997;151(3):233–235

145. Orenstein SR, Whitington PF, Orenstein DM. The infant seat as treatment for gastroesophageal reflux. *N Engl J Med*. 1983;309(13):760–763

146. Bass JL, Bull M. Oxygen desaturation in term infants in car safety seats. *Pediatrics*. 2002;110(2 pt 1):401–402

147. Kornhauser Cerar L, Scirica CV, Stucin Gantar I, Osredkar D, Neubauer D, Kinane TB. A comparison of respiratory patterns in healthy term infants placed in car safety seats and beds. *Pediatrics*. 2009;124(3). Available at: www.pediatrics.org/cgi/content/full/124/3/e396

148. Côté A, Bairam A, Deschenes M, Hatzakis G. Sudden infant deaths in sitting devices. *Arch Dis Child*. 2008;93(5):384–389

149. Merchant JR, Worwa C, Porter S, Coleman JM, deRegnier RA. Respiratory instability of term and near-term healthy newborn infants in car safety seats. *Pediatrics*. 2001;108(3):647–652

150. Willett LD, Leuschen MP, Nelson LS, Nelson RM Jr. Risk of hypoventilation in premature infants in car seats. *J Pediatr*. 1986;109(2):245–248

151. Batra EK, Midgett JD, Moon RY. Hazards associated with sitting and carrying devices for children two years and younger. *J Pediatr*. 2015;167(1):183–187

152. Desapriya EB, Joshi P, Subzwari S, Nolan M. Infant injuries from child restraint safety seat misuse at British

Columbia Children's Hospital. *Pediatr Int.* 2008;50(5):674–678

153. Graham CJ, Kittredge D, Stuemky JH. Injuries associated with child safety seat misuse. *Pediatr Emerg Care.* 1992;8(6):351–353

154. Parikh SN, Wilson L. Hazardous use of car seats outside the car in the United States, 2003–2007. *Pediatrics.* 2010;126(2):352–357

155. Pollack-Nelson C. Fall and suffocation injuries associated with in-home use of car seats and baby carriers. *Pediatr Emerg Care.* 2000;16(2):77–79

156. Wickham T, Abrahamson E. Head injuries in infants: the risks of bouncy chairs and car seats. *Arch Dis Child.* 2002;86(3):168–169

157. Bergounioux J, Madre C, Crucis-Armengaud A, et al. Sudden deaths in adult-worn baby carriers: 19 cases. *Eur J Pediatr.* 2015;174(12):1665–1670

158. Madre C, Rambaud C, Avran D, Michot C, Sachs P, Dauger S. Infant deaths in slings. *Eur J Pediatr.* 2014;173(12):1659–1661

159. Consumer Product Safety Commission. Safety standard for sling carriers. *Fed Reg.* 2014;79(141):42724–42734

160. Ip S, Chung M, Raman G, Trikalinos TA, Lau J. A summary of the Agency for Healthcare Research and Quality's evidence report on breastfeeding in developed countries. *Breastfeed Med.* 2009;4(suppl 1):S17–S30

161. Vennemann MM, Bajanowski T, Brinkmann B, et al; GeSID Study Group. Does breastfeeding reduce the risk of sudden infant death syndrome? *Pediatrics.* 2009;123(3). Available at: www.pediatrics.org/cgi/content/full/123/3/e406

162. Hauck FR, Thompson JM, Tanabe KO, Moon RY, Vennemann MM. Breastfeeding and reduced risk of sudden infant death syndrome: a meta-analysis. *Pediatrics.* 2011;128(1):103–110

163. Franco P, Scaillet S, Wermenbol V, Valente F, Groswasser J, Kahn A. The influence of a pacifier on infants' arousals from sleep. *J Pediatr.* 2000;136(6):775–779

164. Horne RS, Parslow PM, Ferens D, Watts AM, Adamson TM. Comparison

of evoked arousability in breast and formula fed infants. *Arch Dis Child.* 2004;89(1):22–25

165. Duijts L, Jaddoe VW, Hofman A, Moll HA. Prolonged and exclusive breastfeeding reduces the risk of infectious diseases in infancy. *Pediatrics.* 2010;126(1). Available at: www.pediatrics.org/cgi/content/full/126/1/e18

166. Heinig MJ. Host defense benefits of breastfeeding for the infant: effect of breastfeeding duration and exclusivity. *Pediatr Clin North Am.* 2001;48(1):105–123, ix

167. Kramer MS, Guo T, Platt RW, et al. Infant growth and health outcomes associated with 3 compared with 6 mo of exclusive breastfeeding. *Am J Clin Nutr.* 2003;78(2):291–295

168. Highet AR, Berry AM, Bettelheim KA, Goldwater PN. Gut microbiome in sudden infant death syndrome (SIDS) differs from that in healthy comparison babies and offers an explanation for the risk factor of prone position. *Int J Med Microbiol.* 2014;304(5–6):735–741

169. McKenna JJ, Thoman EB, Anders TF, Sadeh A, Schechtman VL, Glotzbach SF. Infant-parent co-sleeping in an evolutionary perspective: implications for understanding infant sleep development and the sudden infant death syndrome. *Sleep.* 1993;16(3):263–282

170. McKenna JJ, Ball HL, Gettler LT. Mother infant cosleeping, breastfeeding and sudden infant death syndrome: what biological anthropology has discovered about normal infant sleep and pediatric sleep medicine. *Yearb Phys Anthropol.* 2007;134(S4S):133–161

171. McKenna J. *Sleeping With Your Baby: A Parent's Guide to Cosleeping.* Washington, DC: Platypus Media, LLC; 2007

172. Mitchell EA, Thompson JMD. Co-sleeping increases the risk of SIDS, but sleeping in the parents' bedroom lowers it. In: Rognum TO, ed. *Sudden Infant Death Syndrome: New Trends in the Nineties.* Oslo, Norway: Scandinavian University Press; 1995:266–269

173. Tappin D, Ecob R, Brooke H. Bedsharing, roomsharing, and sudden

infant death syndrome in Scotland: a case-control study. *J Pediatr.* 2005;147(1):32–37

174. Colson ER, Willinger M, Rybin D, et al. Trends and factors associated with infant bed sharing, 1993-2010: the National Infant Sleep Position Study. *JAMA Pediatr.* 2013;167(11):1032–1037

175. Hauck FR, Signore C, Fein SB, Raju TN. Infant sleeping arrangements and practices during the first year of life. *Pediatrics.* 2008;122(suppl 2):S113–S120

176. Kendall-Tackett K, Cong Z, Hale TW. Mother-infant sleep locations and nighttime feeding behavior: U.S. data from the Survey of Mothers' Sleep and Fatigue. *Clin Lactation.* 2010;1(1):27–31

177. Ward TC. Reasons for mother-infant bed-sharing: a systematic narrative synthesis of the literature and implications for future research. *Matern Child Health J.* 2015;19(3):675–690

178. Joyner BL, Oden RP, Ajao TI, Moon RY. Where should my baby sleep: a qualitative study of African American infant sleep location decisions. *J Natl Med Assoc.* 2010;102(10):881–889

179. Mosko S, Richard C, McKenna J. Infant arousals during mother-infant bed sharing: implications for infant sleep and sudden infant death syndrome research. *Pediatrics.* 1997;100(5):841–849

180. McKenna JJ, Mosko SS, Richard CA. Bedsharing promotes breastfeeding. *Pediatrics.* 1997;100(2 pt 1):214–219

181. Gettler LT, McKenna JJ. Evolutionary perspectives on mother-infant sleep proximity and breastfeeding in a laboratory setting. *Am J Phys Anthropol.* 2011;144(3):454–462

182. Scheers NJ, Dayton CM, Kemp JS. Sudden infant death with external airways covered: case-comparison study of 206 deaths in the United States. *Arch Pediatr Adolesc Med.* 1998;152(6):540–547

183. Unger B, Kemp JS, Wilkins D, et al. Racial disparity and modifiable risk factors among infants dying suddenly and unexpectedly. *Pediatrics.* 2003;111(2). Available at: www.pediatrics.org/cgi/content/full/111/2/e127

184. Kemp JS, Unger B, Wilkins D, et al. Unsafe sleep practices and an analysis of bedsharing among infants dying suddenly and unexpectedly: results of a four-year, population-based, death-scene investigation study of sudden infant death syndrome and related deaths. *Pediatrics*. 2000;106(3). Available at: www.pediatrics.org/cgi/content/full/106/3/e41

185. Drago DA, Dannenberg AL. Infant mechanical suffocation deaths in the United States, 1980-1997. *Pediatrics*. 1999;103(5). Available at: www.pediatrics.org/cgi/content/full/103/5/e59

186. Blair PS, Mitchell EA, Heckstall-Smith EM, Fleming PJ. Head covering—a major modifiable risk factor for sudden infant death syndrome: a systematic review. *Arch Dis Child*. 2008;93(9):778–783

187. Baddock SA, Galland BC, Bolton DP, Williams SM, Taylor BJ. Differences in infant and parent behaviors during routine bed sharing compared with cot sleeping in the home setting. *Pediatrics*. 2006;117(5):1599–1607

188. Baddock SA, Galland BC, Taylor BJ, Bolton DP. Sleep arrangements and behavior of bed-sharing families in the home setting. *Pediatrics*. 2007;119(1). Available at: www.pediatrics.org/cgi/content/full/119/1/e200

189. Ball H. Airway covering during bed-sharing. *Child Care Health Dev*. 2009;35(5):728–737

190. Kattwinkel J, Brooks J, Keenan ME, Malloy MH; American Academy of Pediatrics. Task Force on Infant Sleep Position and Sudden Infant Death Syndrome. Changing concepts of sudden infant death syndrome: implications for infant sleeping environment and sleep position. *Pediatrics*. 2000;105(3 pt 1):650–656

191. Vennemann MM, Hense HW, Bajanowski T, et al Bed sharing and the risk of sudden infant death syndrome: can we resolve the debate? *J Pediatr*. 2012;160(1):44–48, e42

192. Ostfeld BM, Perl H, Esposito L, et al. Sleep environment, positional, lifestyle, and demographic characteristics associated with bed sharing in sudden infant death syndrome cases: a population-based study. *Pediatrics*. 2006;118(5):2051–2059

193. Scheers NJ, Rutherford GW, Kemp JS. Where should infants sleep? A comparison of risk for suffocation of infants sleeping in cribs, adult beds, and other sleeping locations. *Pediatrics*. 2003;112(4):883–889

194. Ruys JH, de Jonge GA, Brand R, Engelberts AC, Semmekrot BA. Bed-sharing in the first four months of life: a risk factor for sudden infant death. *Acta Paediatr*. 2007;96(10):1399–1403

195. Blair PS, Platt MW, Smith IJ, Fleming PJ; CESDI SUDI Research Group. Sudden infant death syndrome and sleeping position in pre-term and low birth weight infants: an opportunity for targeted intervention. *Arch Dis Child*. 2006;91(2):101–106

196. Blair PS, Sidebotham P, Evason-Coombe C, Edmonds M, Heckstall-Smith EM, Fleming P. Hazardous cosleeping environments and risk factors amenable to change: case-control study of SIDS in south west England. *BMJ*. 2009;339:b3666

197. Rechtman LR, Colvin JD, Blair PS, Moon RY. Sofas and infant mortality. *Pediatrics*. 2014;134(5). Available at: www.pediatrics.org/cgi/content/full/134/5/e1293

198. Salm Ward TC, Ngui EM. Factors associated with bed-sharing for African American and white mothers in Wisconsin. *Matern Child Health J*. 2015;19(4):720–732

199. Bartick M, Smith LJ. Speaking out on safe sleep: evidence-based infant sleep recommendations. *Breastfeed Med*. 2014;9(9):417–422

200. Blair PS, Sidebotham P, Pease A, Fleming PJ. Bed-sharing in the absence of hazardous circumstances: is there a risk of sudden infant death syndrome? An analysis from two case-control studies conducted in the UK. *PLoS One*. 2014;9(9):e107799

201. Carpenter R, McGarvey C, Mitchell EA, et al. Bed sharing when parents do not smoke: is there a risk of SIDS? An individual level analysis of five major case-control studies. *BMJ Open*. 2013;3(5):e002299

202. Huang Y, Hauck FR, Signore C, et al. Influence of bedsharing activity on breastfeeding duration among US mothers. *JAMA Pediatr*. 2013;167(11):1038–1044

203. Horsley T, Clifford T, Barrowman N, et al. Benefits and harms associated with the practice of bed sharing: a systematic review. *Arch Pediatr Adolesc Med*. 2007;161(3):237–245

204. Smith LA, Geller NL, Kellams AL, et al. Infant sleep location and breastfeeding practices in the United States, 2011-2014. *Acad Pediatr*. 2016;16(6):540–549

205. Ball HL, Howel D, Bryant A, Best E, Russell C, Ward-Platt M. Bed-sharing by breastfeeding mothers: who bed-shares and what is the relationship with breastfeeding duration? *Acta Paediatr*. 2016;105(6):628–634

206. Scragg R, Mitchell EA, Taylor BJ, et al; New Zealand Cot Death Study Group. Bed sharing, smoking, and alcohol in the sudden infant death syndrome. *BMJ*. 1993;307(6915):1312–1318

207. McGarvey C, McDonnell M, Chong A, O'Regan M, Matthews T. Factors relating to the infant's last sleep environment in sudden infant death syndrome in the Republic of Ireland. *Arch Dis Child*. 2003;88(12):1058–1064

208. Fleming PJ, Gilbert R, Azaz Y, et al. Interaction between bedding and sleeping position in the sudden infant death syndrome: a population based case-control study. *BMJ*. 1990;301(6743):85–89

209. Ponsonby A-L, Dwyer T, Gibbons LE, Cochrane JA, Jones ME, McCall MJ. Thermal environment and sudden infant death syndrome: case-control study. *BMJ*. 1992;304(6822):277–282

210. Ponsonby A-L, Dwyer T, Gibbons LE, Cochrane JA, Wang Y-G. Factors potentiating the risk of sudden infant death syndrome associated with the prone position. *N Engl J Med*. 1993;329(6):377–382

211. Iyasu S, Randall LL, Welty TK, et al. Risk factors for sudden infant death syndrome among Northern Plains Indians. *JAMA*. 2002;288(21):2717–2723

212. Arnestad M, Andersen M, Vege A, Rognum TO. Changes in the epidemiological pattern of sudden infant death syndrome in southeast

Norway, 1984-1998: implications for future prevention and research. *Arch Dis Child.* 2001;85(2):108–115

213. McGarvey C, McDonnell M, Hamilton K, O'Regan M, Matthews T. An 8 year study of risk factors for SIDS: bed-sharing versus non-bed-sharing. *Arch Dis Child.* 2006;91(4):318–323

214. Academy of Breastfeeding Medicine Protocol Committee. ABM clinical protocol #6: guideline on co-sleeping and breastfeeding. Revision, March 2008. *Breastfeed Med.* 2008;3(1):38–43

215. Fu LY, Moon RY, Hauck FR. Bed sharing among black infants and sudden infant death syndrome: interactions with other known risk factors. *Acad Pediatr.* 2010;10(6):376–382

216. Carroll-Pankhurst C, Mortimer EAJ Jr. Sudden infant death syndrome, bedsharing, parental weight, and age at death. *Pediatrics.* 2001;107(3):530–536

217. Mitchell E, Thompson J. Who cosleeps? Does high maternal body weight and duvet use increase the risk of sudden infant death syndrome when bed sharing?. *Paediatr Child Health.* 2006;11(suppl 1):14A–15A

218. Hutchison BL, Stewart AW, Mitchell EA. The prevalence of cobedding and SIDS-related child care practices in twins. *Eur J Pediatr.* 2010;169(12):1477–1485

219. Hayward K. Cobedding of twins: a natural extension of the socialization process? *MCN Am J Matern Child Nurs.* 2003;28(4):260–263

220. Tomashek KM, Wallman C; American Academy of Pediatrics Committee on Fetus and Newborn. Cobedding twins and higher-order multiples in a hospital setting. *Pediatrics.* 2007;120(6):1359–1366

221. National Association of Neonatal Nurses Board of Directors. NANN Position Statement 3045: cobedding of twins or higher-order multiples. *Adv Neonatal Care.* 2008;9(6):307–313

222. Chiodini BA, Thach BT. Impaired ventilation in infants sleeping facedown: potential significance for sudden infant death syndrome. *J Pediatr.* 1993;123(5):686–692

223. Sakai J, Kanetake J, Takahashi S, Kanawaku Y, Funayama M. Gas dispersal potential of bedding as

a cause for sudden infant death. *Forensic Sci Int.* 2008;180(2-3):93–97

224. Shapiro-Mendoza CK, Camperlengo L, Ludvigsen R, et al. Classification system for the Sudden Unexpected Infant Death Case Registry and its application. *Pediatrics.* 2014;134(1):e210–e219

225. Ponsonby A-L, Dwyer T, Couper D, Cochrane J. Association between use of a quilt and sudden infant death syndrome: case-control study. *BMJ.* 1998;316(7126):195–196

226. Mitchell EA, Scragg L, Clements M. Soft cot mattresses and the sudden infant death syndrome. *N Z Med J.* 1996;109(1023):206–207

227. Mitchell EA, Thompson JMD, Ford RPK, Taylor BJ; New Zealand Cot Death Study Group. Sheepskin bedding and the sudden infant death syndrome. *J Pediatr.* 1998;133(5):701–704

228. Kemp JS, Kowalski RM, Burch PM, Graham MA, Thach BT. Unintentional suffocation by rebreathing: a death scene and physiologic investigation of a possible cause of sudden infant death. *J Pediatr.* 1993;122(6):874–880

229. Brooke H, Gibson A, Tappin D, Brown H. Case-control study of sudden infant death syndrome in Scotland, 1992-5. *BMJ.* 1997;314(7093):1516–1520

230. Wilson CA, Taylor BJ, Laing RM, Williams SM, Mitchell EA. Clothing and bedding and its relevance to sudden infant death syndrome: further results from the New Zealand Cot Death Study. *J Paediatr Child Health.* 1994;30(6):506–512

231. Markestad T, Skadberg B, Hordvik E, Morild I, Irgens LM. Sleeping position and sudden infant death syndrome (SIDS): effect of an intervention programme to avoid prone sleeping. *Acta Paediatr.* 1995;84(4):375–378

232. L'Hoir MP, Engelberts AC, van Well GTJ, et al. Risk and preventive factors for cot death in The Netherlands, a low-incidence country. *Eur J Pediatr.* 1998;157(8):681–688

233. Beal SM, Byard RW. Accidental death or sudden infant death syndrome? *J Paediatr Child Health.* 1995;31(4):269–271

234. Schlaud M, Dreier M, Debertin AS, et al. The German case-control scene investigation study on SIDS: epidemiological approach and main results. *Int J Legal Med.* 2010;124(1):19–26

235. Chowdhury RT. *Nursery Product-Related Injuries and Deaths Among Children Under Age Five.* Washington, DC: US Consumer Product Safety Commission; 2014

236. Ajao TI, Oden RP, Joyner BL, Moon RY. Decisions of black parents about infant bedding and sleep surfaces: a qualitative study. *Pediatrics.* 2011;128(3):494–502

237. Joyner BL, Gill-Bailey C, Moon RY. Infant sleep environments depicted in magazines targeted to women of childbearing age. *Pediatrics.* 2009;124(3). Available at: www.pediatrics.org/cgi/content/full/124/3/e416

238. Moon RY. "And things that go bump in the night": nothing to fear? *J Pediatr.* 2007;151(3):237–238

239. Thach BT, Rutherford GW Jr, Harris K. Deaths and injuries attributed to infant crib bumper pads. *J Pediatr.* 2007;151(3):271–274, 274.e1–274.e3

240. Wanna-Nakamura S. White paper—unsafe sleep settings: hazards associated with the infant sleep environment and unsafe practices used by caregivers: a CPSC staff perspective. Bethesda, MD: US Consumer Product Safety Commission; July 2010

241. US Consumer Product Safety Commission. *Staff Briefing Package, Crib Bumpers Petition.* Washington, DC: US Consumer Product Safety Commission; May 15, 2013

242. Scheers NJ, Woodard DW, Thach BT. Crib bumpers continue to cause infant deaths: a need for a new preventive approach. *J Pediatr.* 2016;169:93–97.e1

243. Yeh ES, Rochette LM, McKenzie LB, Smith GA. Injuries associated with cribs, playpens, and bassinets among young children in the US, 1990-2008. *Pediatrics.* 2011;127(3):479–486

244. Tappin D, Brooke H, Ecob R, Gibson A. Used infant mattresses and sudden infant death syndrome in

Scotland: case-control study. *BMJ.* 2002;325(7371):1007–1012

245. Arnestad M, Andersen M, Rognum TO. Is the use of dummy or carry-cot of importance for sudden infant death? *Eur J Pediatr.* 1997;156(12):968–970

246. Mitchell EA, Taylor BJ, Ford RPK, et al. Dummies and the sudden infant death syndrome. *Arch Dis Child.* 1993;68(4):501–504

247. Fleming PJ, Blair PS, Pollard K, et al; CESDI SUDI Research Team. Pacifier use and sudden infant death syndrome: results from the CESDI/SUDI case control study. *Arch Dis Child.* 1999;81(2):112–116

248. L'Hoir MP, Engelberts AC, van Well GTJ, et al. Dummy use, thumb sucking, mouth breathing and cot death. *Eur J Pediatr.* 1999;158(11):896–901

249. Li DK, Willinger M, Petitti DB, Odouli R, Liu L, Hoffman HJ. Use of a dummy (pacifier) during sleep and risk of sudden infant death syndrome (SIDS): population based case-control study. *BMJ.* 2006;332(7532):18–22

250. Vennemann MM, Bajanowski T, Brinkmann B, Jorch G, Sauerland C, Mitchell EA; GeSID Study Group. Sleep environment risk factors for sudden infant death syndrome: the German Sudden Infant Death Syndrome Study. *Pediatrics.* 2009;123(4):1162–1170

251. Hauck FR, Omojokun OO, Siadaty MS. Do pacifiers reduce the risk of sudden infant death syndrome? A meta-analysis. *Pediatrics.* 2005;116(5). Available at: www.pediatrics.org/cgi/content/full/116/5/e716

252. Mitchell EA, Blair PS, L'Hoir MP. Should pacifiers be recommended to prevent sudden infant death syndrome? *Pediatrics.* 2006;117(5):1755–1758

253. Moon RY, Tanabe KO, Yang DC, Young HA, Hauck FR. Pacifier use and SIDS: evidence for a consistently reduced risk. *Matern Child Health J.* 2012;16(3):609–614

254. Franco P, Chabanski S, Scaillet S, Groswasser J, Kahn A. Pacifier use modifies infant's cardiac autonomic controls during sleep. *Early Hum Dev.* 2004;77(1-2):99–108

255. Tonkin SL, Lui D, McIntosh CG, Rowley S, Knight DB, Gunn AJ. Effect of pacifier use on mandibular position in preterm infants. *Acta Paediatr.* 2007;96(10):1433–1436

256. Hanzer M, Zotter H, Sauseng W, Pfurtscheller K, Müller W, Kerbl R. Pacifier use does not alter the frequency or duration of spontaneous arousals in sleeping infants. *Sleep Med.* 2009;10(4):464–470

257. Odoi A, Andrew S, Wong FY, Yiallourou SR, Horne RS. Pacifier use does not alter sleep and spontaneous arousal patterns in healthy term-born infants. *Acta Paediatr.* 2014;103(12):1244–1250

258. Weiss PP, Kerbl R. The relatively short duration that a child retains a pacifier in the mouth during sleep: implications for sudden infant death syndrome. *Eur J Pediatr.* 2001;160(1):60–70

259. Nederlands Centrum Jeugdgezondheit. Safe sleeping for your baby. Available at: www.wiegedood.nl/files/download_vs_engels.pdf. Accessed January 10, 2016

260. Foundation for the Study of Infant Deaths. Factfile 2. Research background to the Reduce the Risk of Cot Death advice by the Foundation for the Study of Infant Deaths. Available at: www.cotmattress.net/SIDS-Guidelines.pdf. Accessed January 10, 2016

261. Canadian Paediatric Society Community Paediatrics Committee. Recommendations for the use of pacifiers. *Paediatr Child Health.* 2003;8(8):515–528

262. Aarts C, Hörnell A, Kylberg E, Hofvander Y, Gebre-Medhin M. Breastfeeding patterns in relation to thumb sucking and pacifier use. *Pediatrics.* 1999;104(4). Available at: www.pediatrics.org/cgi/content/full/104/4/e50

263. Benis MM. Are pacifiers associated with early weaning from breastfeeding? *Adv Neonatal Care.* 2002;2(5):259–266

264. Scott JA, Binns CW, Oddy WH, Graham KI. Predictors of breastfeeding duration: evidence from a cohort study. *Pediatrics.* 2006;117(4). Available at: www.pediatrics.org/cgi/content/full/117/4/e646

265. Jaafar SH, Jahanfar S, Angolkar M, Ho JJ. Pacifier use versus no pacifier use in breastfeeding term infants for increasing duration of breastfeeding. *Cochrane Database Syst Rev.* 2011;3:CD007202

266. O'Connor NR, Tanabe KO, Siadaty MS, Hauck FR. Pacifiers and breastfeeding: a systematic review. *Arch Pediatr Adolesc Med.* 2009;163(4):378–382

267. Alm B, Wennergren G, Möllborg P, Lagercrantz H. Breastfeeding and dummy use have a protective effect on sudden infant death syndrome. *Acta Paediatr.* 2016;105(1):31–38

268. Howard CR, Howard FM, Lanphear B, et al. Randomized clinical trial of pacifier use and bottle-feeding or cupfeeding and their effect on breastfeeding. *Pediatrics.* 2003;111(3):511–518

269. Eidelman AI, Schanler RJ; Section on Breastfeeding. Breastfeeding and the use of human milk. *Pediatrics.* 2012;129(3). Available at: www.pediatrics.org/cgi/content/full/129/3/e827

270. Larsson Erik. The effect of dummy-sucking on the occlusion: a review. *Eur J Orthodont.* 1986;8(2):127–130

271. American Academy of Pediatric Dentistry, Council on Clinical Affairs. Policy statement on oral habits. Chicago, IL: American Academy of Pediatric Dentistry; 2000. Available at: www.aapd.org/media/Policies_Guidelines/P_OralHabits.pdf. Accessed January 10, 2016

272. Niemelä M, Uhari M, Möttönen M. A pacifier increases the risk of recurrent acute otitis media in children in day care centers. *Pediatrics.* 1995;96(5 pt 1):884–888

273. Niemelä M, Pihakari O, Pokka T, Uhari M. Pacifier as a risk factor for acute otitis media: a randomized, controlled trial of parental counseling. *Pediatrics.* 2000;106(3):483–488

274. Jackson JM, Mourino AP. Pacifier use and otitis media in infants twelve months of age or younger. *Pediatr Dent.* 1999;21(4):255–260

275. Daly KA, Giebink GS. Clinical epidemiology of otitis media. *Pediatr Infect Dis J.* 2000;19(5 suppl):S31–S36

276. Darwazeh AM, al-Bashir A. Oral candidal flora in healthy infants. *J Oral Pathol Med.* 1995;24(8):361–364

277. North K, Fleming P, Golding J. Pacifier use and morbidity in the first six months of life. *Pediatrics.* 1999;103(3). Available at: www.pediatrics.org/cgi/content/full/103/3/E34

278. Niemelä M, Uhari M, Hannuksela A. Pacifiers and dental structure as risk factors for otitis media. *Int J Pediatr Otorhinolaryngol.* 1994;29(2):121–127

279. Uhari M, Mäntysaari K, Niemelä M. A meta-analytic review of the risk factors for acute otitis media. *Clin Infect Dis.* 1996;22(6):1079–1083

280. Getahun D, Amre D, Rhoads GG, Demissie K. Maternal and obstetric risk factors for sudden infant death syndrome in the United States. *Obstet Gynecol.* 2004;103(4):646–652

281. Kraus JF, Greenland S, Bulterys M. Risk factors for sudden infant death syndrome in the US Collaborative Perinatal Project. *Int J Epidemiol.* 1989;18(1):113–120

282. Paris CA, Remler R, Daling JR. Risk factors for sudden infant death syndrome: changes associated with sleep position recommendations. *J Pediatr.* 2001;139(6):771–777

283. Stewart AJ, Williams SM, Mitchell EA, Taylor BJ, Ford RP, Allen EM. Antenatal and intrapartum factors associated with sudden infant death syndrome in the New Zealand Cot Death Study. *J Paediatr Child Health.* 1995;31(5):473–478

284. American Academy of Pediatrics Committee on Fetus and Newborn; ACOG Committee on Obstetric Practice. *Guidelines for Perinatal Care.* 7th ed. Elk Grove Village, IL: American Academy of Pediatrics; 2012

285. MacDorman MF, Cnattingius S, Hoffman HJ, Kramer MS, Haglund B. Sudden infant death syndrome and smoking in the United States and Sweden. *Am J Epidemiol.* 1997;146(3):249–257

286. Schoendorf KC, Kiely JL. Relationship of sudden infant death syndrome to maternal smoking during and after pregnancy. *Pediatrics.* 1992;90(6):905–908

287. Malloy MH, Kleinman JC, Land GH, Schramm WF. The association of maternal smoking with age and cause of infant death. *Am J Epidemiol.* 1988;128(1):46–55

288. Haglund B, Cnattingius S. Cigarette smoking as a risk factor for sudden infant death syndrome: a population-based study. *Am J Public Health.* 1990;80(1):29–32

289. Mitchell EA, Ford RP, Stewart AW, et al. Smoking and the sudden infant death syndrome. *Pediatrics.* 1993;91(5):893–896

290. Winickoff JP, Friebely J, Tanski SE, et al. Beliefs about the health effects of "thirdhand" smoke and home smoking bans. *Pediatrics.* 2009;123(1). Available at: www.pediatrics.org/cgi/content/full/123/1/e74

291. Tirosh E, Libon D, Bader D. The effect of maternal smoking during pregnancy on sleep respiratory and arousal patterns in neonates. *J Perinatol.* 1996;16(6):435–438

292. Franco P, Groswasser J, Hassid S, Lanquart JP, Scaillet S, Kahn A. Prenatal exposure to cigarette smoking is associated with a decrease in arousal in infants. *J Pediatr.* 1999;135(1):34–38

293. Horne RS, Ferens D, Watts AM, et al. Effects of maternal tobacco smoking, sleeping position, and sleep state on arousal in healthy term infants. *Arch Dis Child Fetal Neonatal Ed.* 2002;87(2):F100–F105

294. Sawnani H, Jackson T, Murphy T, Beckerman R, Simakajornboon N. The effect of maternal smoking on respiratory and arousal patterns in preterm infants during sleep. *Am J Respir Crit Care Med.* 2004;169(6):733–738

295. Lewis KW, Bosque EM. Deficient hypoxia awakening response in infants of smoking mothers: possible relationship to sudden infant death syndrome. *J Pediatr.* 1995;127(5):691–699

296. Chang AB, Wilson SJ, Masters IB, et al. Altered arousal response in infants exposed to cigarette smoke. *Arch Dis Child.* 2003;88(1):30–33

297. Parslow PM, Cranage SM, Adamson TM, Harding R, Horne RS. Arousal and ventilatory responses to hypoxia in sleeping infants: effects of maternal smoking [published correction appears in *Respir Physiol Neurobiol.* 2004;143(1):99]. *Respir Physiol Neurobiol.* 2004;140(1):77–87

298. Zhang K, Wang X. Maternal smoking and increased risk of sudden infant death syndrome: a meta-analysis. *Leg Med (Tokyo).* 2013;15(3):115–121

299. Mitchell EA, Milerad J. Smoking and the sudden infant death syndrome. *Rev Environ Health.* 2006;21(2):81–103

300. Dietz PM, England LJ, Shapiro-Mendoza CK, Tong VT, Farr SL, Callaghan WM. Infant morbidity and mortality attributable to prenatal smoking in the U.S. *Am J Prev Med.* 2010;39(1):45–52

301. O'Leary CM, Jacoby PJ, Bartu A, D'Antoine H, Bower C. Maternal alcohol use and sudden infant death syndrome and infant mortality excluding SIDS. *Pediatrics.* 2013;131(3). Available at: www.pediatrics.org/cgi/content/full/131/3/e770

302. Strandberg-Larsen K, Grønboek M, Andersen AM, Andersen PK, Olsen J. Alcohol drinking pattern during pregnancy and risk of infant mortality. *Epidemiology.* 2009;20(6):884–891

303. Sirieix CM, Tobia CM, Schneider RW, Darnall RA. Impaired arousal in rat pups with prenatal alcohol exposure is modulated by GABAergic mechanisms. *Physiol Rep.* 2015;3(6):e12424

304. Alm B, Wennergren G, Norvenius G, et al. Caffeine and alcohol as risk factors for sudden infant death syndrome: Nordic Epidemiological SIDS Study. *Arch Dis Child.* 1999;81(2):107–111

305. James C, Klenka H, Manning D. Sudden infant death syndrome: bed sharing with mothers who smoke. *Arch Dis Child.* 2003;88(2):112–113

306. Williams SM, Mitchell EA, Taylor BJ. Are risk factors for sudden infant death syndrome different at night? *Arch Dis Child.* 2002;87(4):274–278

307. Rajegowda BK, Kandall SR, Falciglia H. Sudden unexpected death in infants of narcotic-dependent mothers. *Early Hum Dev.* 1978;2(3):219–225

308. Chavez CJ, Ostrea EM Jr, Stryker JC, Smialek Z. Sudden infant death syndrome among infants of drug-dependent mothers. *J Pediatr.* 1979;95(3):407–409

309. Bauchner H, Zuckerman B, McClain M, Frank D, Fried LE, Kayne H. Risk of sudden infant death syndrome among infants with in utero exposure to cocaine. *J Pediatr.* 1988;113(5):831–834

310. Durand DJ, Espinoza AM, Nickerson BG. Association between prenatal cocaine exposure and sudden infant death syndrome. *J Pediatr.* 1990;117(6):909–911

311. Ward SL, Bautista D, Chan L, et al. Sudden infant death syndrome in infants of substance-abusing mothers. *J Pediatr.* 1990;117(6):876–881

312. Rosen TS, Johnson HL. Drug-addicted mothers, their infants, and SIDS. *Ann N Y Acad Sci.* 1988;533:89–95

313. Kandall SR, Gaines J, Habel L, Davidson G, Jessop D. Relationship of maternal substance abuse to subsequent sudden infant death syndrome in offspring. *J Pediatr.* 1993;123(1):120–126

314. Fares I, McCulloch KM, Raju TN. Intrauterine cocaine exposure and the risk for sudden infant death syndrome: a meta-analysis. *J Perinatol.* 1997;17(3):179–182

315. Ponsonby AL, Dwyer T, Kasl SV, Cochrane JA. The Tasmanian SIDS Case-Control Study: univariable and multivariable risk factor analysis. *Paediatr Perinat Epidemiol.* 1995;9(3):256–272

316. McGlashan ND. Sudden infant deaths in Tasmania, 1980-1986: a seven year prospective study. *Soc Sci Med.* 1989;29(8):1015–1026

317. Coleman-Phox K, Odouli R, Li DK. Use of a fan during sleep and the risk of sudden infant death syndrome. *Arch Pediatr Adolesc Med.* 2008;162(10):963–968

318. Hutcheson R. DTP vaccination and sudden infant deaths—Tennessee. *MMWR Morb Mortal Wkly Rep.* 1979;28:131–132

319. Hutcheson R. Follow-up on DTP vaccination and sudden infant deaths—Tennessee. *MMWR.* 1979;28:134–135

320. Bernier RH, Frank JA Jr, Dondero TJ Jr, Turner P. Diphtheria-tetanus toxoids-pertussis vaccination and sudden infant deaths in Tennessee. *J Pediatr.* 1982;101(3):419–421

321. Baraff LJ, Ablon WJ, Weiss RC. Possible temporal association between diphtheria-tetanus toxoid-pertussis vaccination and sudden infant death syndrome. *Pediatr Infect Dis.* 1983;2(1):7–11

322. Griffin MR, Ray WA, Livengood JR, Schaffner W. Risk of sudden infant death syndrome after immunization with the diphtheria-tetanus-pertussis vaccine. *N Engl J Med.* 1988;319(10):618–623

323. Hoffman HJ, Hunter JC, Damus K, et al. Diphtheria-tetanus-pertussis immunization and sudden infant death: results of the National Institute of Child Health and Human Development Cooperative Epidemiological Study of Sudden Infant Death Syndrome risk factors. *Pediatrics.* 1987;79(4):598–611

324. Taylor EM, Emergy JL. Immunization and cot deaths. *Lancet.* 1982;2(8300):721

325. Flahault A, Messiah A, Jougla E, Bouvet E, Perin J, Hatton F. Sudden infant death syndrome and diphtheria/tetanus toxoid/pertussis/poliomyelitis immunisation. *Lancet.* 1988;1(8585):582–583

326. Walker AM, Jick H, Perera DR, Thompson RS, Knauss TA. Diphtheria-tetanus-pertussis immunization and sudden infant death syndrome. *Am J Public Health.* 1987;77(8):945–951

327. Jonville-Bera AP, Autret E, Laugier J. Sudden infant death syndrome and diphtheria-tetanus-pertussis-poliomyelitis vaccination status. *Fundam Clin Pharmacol.* 1995;9(3):263–270

328. Immunization Safety Review Committee. Stratton K, Almario DA, Wizemann TM, McCormick MC, eds. *Immunization Safety Review: Vaccinations and Sudden Unexpected Death in Infancy.* Washington, DC: National Academies Press; 2003

329. Miller ER, Moro PL, Cano M, Shimabukuro TT. Deaths following vaccination: what does the evidence show? *Vaccine.* 2015;33(29):3288–3292

330. Moro PL, Arana J, Cano M, Lewis P, Shimabukuro TT. Deaths reported to the Vaccine Adverse Event Reporting System, United States, 1997-2013. *Clin Infect Dis.* 2015;61(6):980–987

331. Moro PL, Jankosky C, Menschik D, et al. Adverse events following Haemophilus influenzae type b vaccines in the Vaccine Adverse Event Reporting System, 1990-2013. *J Pediatr.* 2015;166(4):992–997

332. Mitchell EA, Stewart AW, Clements M; New Zealand Cot Death Study Group. Immunisation and the sudden infant death syndrome. *Arch Dis Child.* 1995;73(6):498–501

333. Jonville-Béra AP, Autret-Leca E, Barbeillon F, Paris-Llado J; French Reference Centers for SIDS. Sudden unexpected death in infants under 3 months of age and vaccination status—a case-control study. *Br J Clin Pharmacol.* 2001;51(3):271–276

334. Fleming PJ, Blair PS, Platt MW, Tripp J, Smith IJ, Golding J. The UK accelerated immunisation programme and sudden unexpected death in infancy: case-control study. *BMJ.* 2001;322(7290):822

335. Müller-Nordhorn J, Hettler-Chen CM, Keil T, Muckelbauer R. Association between sudden infant death syndrome and diphtheria-tetanus-pertussis immunisation: an ecological study. *BMC Pediatr.* 2015;15:1

336. Fine PEM, Chen RT. Confounding in studies of adverse reactions to vaccines. *Am J Epidemiol.* 1992;136(2):121–135

337. Virtanen M, Peltola H, Paunio M, Heinonen OP. Day-to-day reactogenicity and the healthy vaccinee effect of measles-mumps-rubella vaccination. *Pediatrics.* 2000;106(5). Available at: www.pediatrics.org/cgi/content/full/106/5/e62

338. Vennemann MM, Höffgen M, Bajanowski T, Hense HW, Mitchell EA. Do immunisations reduce the risk for SIDS? A meta-analysis. *Vaccine.* 2007;25(26):4875–4879

339. Centers for Disease Control and Prevention. Suffocation deaths associated with use of infant sleep positioners—United States, 1997-2011. *MMWR Morb Mortal Wkly Rep.* 2012;61(46):933–937

340. US Consumer Product Safety Commission. Deaths prompt CPSC, FDA warning on infant sleep positioners. Available at: www.cpsc.gov/en/Newsroom/News-Releases/2010/

Deaths-prompt-CPSC-FDA-warning-on-infant-sleep-position. Accessed September 21, 2016

341. Bar-Yishay E, Gaides M, Goren A, Szeinberg A. Aeration properties of a new sleeping surface for infants. *Pediatr Pulmonol.* 2011;46(2):193–198

342. Colditz PB, Joy GJ, Dunster KR. Rebreathing potential of infant mattresses and bedcovers. *J Paediatr Child Health.* 2002;38(2):192–195

343. Carolan PL, Wheeler WB, Ross JD, Kemp RJ. Potential to prevent carbon dioxide rebreathing of commercial products marketed to reduce sudden infant death syndrome risk. *Pediatrics.* 2000;105(4 Pt 1):774–779

344. Steinschneider A. Prolonged apnea and the sudden infant death syndrome: clinical and laboratory observations. *Pediatrics.* 1972;50(4):646–654

345. Hodgman JE, Hoppenbrouwers T. Home monitoring for the sudden infant death syndrome: the case against. *Ann N Y Acad Sci.* 1988;533:164–175

346. Ward SL, Keens TG, Chan LS, et al. Sudden infant death syndrome in infants evaluated by apnea programs in California. *Pediatrics.* 1986;77(4):451–458

347. Monod N, Plouin P, Sternberg B, et al. Are polygraphic and cardiopneumographic respiratory patterns useful tools for predicting the risk for sudden infant death syndrome? A 10-year study. *Biol Neonate.* 1986;50(3):147–153

348. Ramanathan R, Corwin MJ, Hunt CE, et al; Collaborative Home Infant Monitoring Evaluation (CHIME) Study Group. Cardiorespiratory events recorded on home monitors: comparison of healthy infants with those at increased risk for SIDS. *JAMA.* 2001;285(17):2199–2207

349. American Academy of Pediatrics Committee on Fetus and Newborn. Apnea, sudden infant death syndrome, and home monitoring. *Pediatrics.* 2003;111(4 pt 1):914–917

350. Hutchison BL, Thompson JM, Mitchell EA. Determinants of nonsynostotic plagiocephaly: a case-control study. *Pediatrics.* 2003;112(4). Available at: www.pediatrics.org/cgi/content/full/112/4/e316

351. Hutchison BL, Hutchison LA, Thompson JM, Mitchell EA. Plagiocephaly and brachycephaly in the first two years of life: a prospective cohort study. *Pediatrics.* 2004;114(4):970–980

352. van Vlimmeren LA, van der Graaf Y, Boere-Boonekamp MM, L'Hoir MP, Helders PJ, Engelbert RH. Risk factors for deformational plagiocephaly at birth and at 7 weeks of age: a prospective cohort study. *Pediatrics.* 2007;119(2). Available at: www.pediatrics.org/cgi/content/full/119/2/e408

353. Miller RI, Clarren SK. Long-term developmental outcomes in patients with deformational plagiocephaly. *Pediatrics.* 2000;105(2). Available at: www.pediatrics.org/cgi/content/full/105/2/E26

354. Panchal J, Amirsheybani H, Gurwitch R, et al. Neurodevelopment in children with single-suture craniosynostosis and plagiocephaly without synostosis. *Plast Reconstr Surg.* 2001;108(6):1492–1498; discussion: 1499–1500

355. Balan P, Kushnerenko E, Sahlin P, Huotilainen M, Näätänen R, Hukki J. Auditory ERPs reveal brain dysfunction in infants with plagiocephaly. *J Craniofac Surg.* 2002;13(4):520–525; discussion: 526

356. Chadduck WM, Kast J, Donahue DJ. The enigma of lambdoid positional molding. *Pediatr Neurosurg.* 1997;26(6):304–311

357. Laughlin J, Luerssen TG, Dias MS; Committee on Practice and Ambulatory Medicine; Section on Neurological Surgery. Prevention and management of positional skull deformities in infants. *Pediatrics.* 2011;128(6):1236–1241

358. Gerard CM, Harris KA, Thach BT. Physiologic studies on swaddling: an ancient child care practice, which may promote the supine position for infant sleep. *J Pediatr.* 2002;141(3):398–403

359. van Sleuwen BE, Engelberts AC, Boere-Boonekamp MM, Kuis W, Schulpen TW, L'Hoir MP. Swaddling: a systematic review. *Pediatrics.* 2007;120(4). Available at: www.pediatrics.org/cgi/content/full/120/4/e1097

360. McDonnell E, Moon RY. Infant deaths and injuries associated

with wearable blankets, swaddle wraps, and swaddling. *J Pediatr.* 2014;164(5):1152–1156

361. Richardson HL, Walker AM, Horne RS. Influence of swaddling experience on spontaneous arousal patterns and autonomic control in sleeping infants. *J Pediatr.* 2010;157(1):85–91

362. Richardson HL, Walker AM, Horne RS. Minimizing the risks of sudden infant death syndrome: to swaddle or not to swaddle? *J Pediatr.* 2009;155(4):475–481

363. Narangerel G, Pollock J, Manaseki-Holland S, Henderson J. The effects of swaddling on oxygen saturation and respiratory rate of healthy infants in Mongolia. *Acta Paediatr.* 2007;96(2):261–265

364. Kutlu A, Memik R, Mutlu M, Kutlu R, Arslan A. Congenital dislocation of the hip and its relation to swaddling used in Turkey. *J Pediatr Orthop.* 1992;12(5):598–602

365. Chaarani MW, Al Mahmeid MS, Salman AM. Developmental dysplasia of the hip before and after increasing community awareness of the harmful effects of swaddling. *Qatar Med J.* 2002;11(1):40–43

366. Yamamuro T, Ishida K. Recent advances in the prevention, early diagnosis, and treatment of congenital dislocation of the hip in Japan. *Clin Orthop Relat Res.* 1984;(184):34–40

367. Coleman SS. Congenital dysplasia of the hip in the Navajo infant. *Clin Orthop Relat Res.* 1968;56:179–193

368. Tronick EZ, Thomas RB, Daltabuit M. The Quechua manta pouch: a caretaking practice for buffering the Peruvian infant against the multiple stressors of high altitude. *Child Dev.* 1994;65(4):1005–1013

369. Manaseki S. Mongolia: a health system in transition. *BMJ.* 1993;307(6919):1609–1611

370. Franco P, Seret N, Van Hees JN, Scaillet S, Groswasser J, Kahn A. Influence of swaddling on sleep and arousal characteristics of healthy infants. *Pediatrics.* 2005;115(5):1307–1311

371. Franco P, Scaillet S, Groswasser J, Kahn A. Increased cardiac autonomic responses to auditory

challenges in swaddled infants. *Sleep*. 2004;27(8):1527–1532

372. Patriarca M, Lyon TD, Delves HT, Howatson AG, Fell GS. Determination of low concentrations of potentially toxic elements in human liver from newborns and infants. *Analyst (Lond)*. 1999;124(9):1337–1343

373. Kleemann WJ, Weller JP, Wolf M, Tröger HD, Blüthgen A, Heeschen W. Heavy metals, chlorinated pesticides and polychlorinated biphenyls in sudden infant death syndrome (SIDS). *Int J Legal Med*. 1991;104(2):71–75

374. Erickson MM, Poklis A, Gantner GE, Dickinson AW, Hillman LS. Tissue mineral levels in victims of sudden infant death syndrome I. Toxic metals—lead and cadmium. *Pediatr Res*. 1983;17(10):779–784

375. George M, Wiklund L, Aastrup M, et al. Incidence and geographical distribution of sudden infant death syndrome in relation to content of nitrate in drinking water and groundwater levels. *Eur J Clin Invest*. 2001;31(12):1083–1094

376. Richardson BA. Sudden infant death syndrome: a possible primary cause. *J Forensic Sci Soc*. 1994;34(3):199–204

377. Sprott TJ. Cot death—cause and prevention: experiences in New Zealand 1995-2004. *J Nutr Environ Med*. 2004;14(3):221–232

378. Department of Health. *Expert Group To Investigate Cot Death Theories (Chair, Lady S. Limerick)*. London, United Kingdom: HMSO; 1998

379. Blair P, Fleming P, Bensley D, Smith I, Bacon C, Taylor E. Plastic mattresses and sudden infant death syndrome. *Lancet*. 1995;345(8951):720

380. Rubens DD, Vohr BR, Tucker R, O'Neil CA, Chung W. Newborn oto-acoustic emission hearing screening tests: preliminary evidence for a marker of susceptibility to SIDS. *Early Hum Dev*. 2008;84(4):225–229

381. Hamill T, Lim G. Otoacoustic emissions does not currently have ability to detect SIDS. *Early Hum Dev*. 2008;84(6):373

382. Krous HF, Byard RW. Newborn hearing screens and SIDS. *Early Hum Dev*. 2008;84(6):371

383. Farquhar LJ, Jennings P. Newborn hearing screen results for infants that died of SIDS in Michigan 2004-2006. *Early Hum Dev*. 2008;84(10):699

384. Chan RS, McPherson B, Zhang VW. Neonatal otoacoustic emission screening and sudden infant death syndrome. *Int J Pediatr Otorhinolaryngol*. 2012;76(10):1485–1489

385. Hauck FR, Tanabe KO. Sids. *BMJ Clin Evid*. 2009;2009(315):1–13

386. Colson ER, Levenson S, Rybin D, et al. Barriers to following the supine sleep recommendation among mothers at four centers for the Women, Infants, and Children Program. *Pediatrics*. 2006;118(2). Available at: www.pediatrics.org/cgi/content/full/118/2/e243

387. Eisenberg SR, Bair-Merritt MH, Colson ER, Heeren TC, Geller NL, Corwin MJ. Maternal report of advice received for infant care. *Pediatrics*. 2015;136(2):e315–e322

388. Colson ER, Bergman DM, Shapiro E, Leventhal JH. Position for newborn sleep: associations with parents' perceptions of their nursery experience. *Birth*. 2001;28(4):249–253

389. Mason B, Ahlers-Schmidt CR, Schunn C. Improving safe sleep environments for well newborns in the hospital setting. *Clin Pediatr (Phila)*. 2013;52(10):969–975

390. McKinney CM, Holt VL, Cunningham ML, Leroux BG, Starr JR. Maternal and infant characteristics associated with prone and lateral infant sleep positioning in Washington state, 1996-2002. *J Pediatr*. 2008;153(2):194–198, e191–e193

391. Moon RY, Calabrese T, Aird L. Reducing the risk of sudden infant death syndrome in child care and changing provider practices: lessons learned from a demonstration project. *Pediatrics*. 2008;122(4):788–798

392. Moon RY, Oden RP. Back to sleep: can we influence child care providers? *Pediatrics*. 2003;112(4):878–882

393. Lerner H, McClain M, Vance JC. SIDS education in nursing and medical schools in the United States. *J Nurs Educ*. 2002;41(8):353–356

394. Price SK, Gardner P, Hillman L, Schenk K, Warren C. Changing hospital newborn nursery practice: results from a statewide "Back to Sleep" nurses training program. *Matern Child Health J*. 2008;12(3):363–371

395. Cowan S, Pease A, Bennett S. Usage and impact of an online education tool for preventing sudden unexpected death in infancy. *J Paediatr Child Health*. 2013;49(3):228–232

396. Colson ER, Joslin SC. Changing nursery practice gets inner-city infants in the supine position for sleep. *Arch Pediatr Adolesc Med*. 2002;156(7):717–720

397. Voos KC, Terreros A, Larimore P, Leick-Rude MK, Park N. Implementing safe sleep practices in a neonatal intensive care unit. *J Matern Fetal Neonatal Med*. 2015;28(14):1637–1640

398. Goodstein MH, Bell T, Krugman SD. Improving infant sleep safety through a comprehensive hospital-based program. *Clin Pediatr (Phila)*. 2015;54(3):212–221

399. Yanovitzky I, Blitz CL. Effect of media coverage and physician advice on utilization of breast cancer screening by women 40 years and older. *J Health Commun*. 2000;5(2):117–134

400. Magazine Publishers of America; Marketing Evolution. *Measuring Media Effectiveness: Comparing Media Contribution Throughout the Purchase Funnel*. New York, NY: Magazine Publishers of America; 2006

Sports Specialization and Intensive Training in Young Athletes

- *Clinical Report*

CLINICAL REPORT Guidance for the Clinician in Rendering Pediatric Care

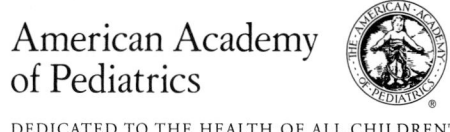

American Academy
of Pediatrics

DEDICATED TO THE HEALTH OF ALL CHILDREN™

Sports Specialization and Intensive Training in Young Athletes

Joel S. Brenner, MD, MPH, FAAP, COUNCIL ON SPORTS MEDICINE AND FITNESS

abstract

Sports specialization is becoming the norm in youth sports for a variety of reasons. When sports specialization occurs too early, detrimental effects may occur, both physically and psychologically. If the timing is correct and sports specialization is performed under the correct conditions, the athlete may be successful in reaching specific goals. Young athletes who train intensively, whether specialized or not, can also be at risk of adverse effects on the mind and body. The purpose of this clinical report is to assist pediatricians in counseling their young athlete patients and their parents regarding sports specialization and intensive training. This report supports the American Academy of Pediatrics clinical report "Overuse Injuries, Overtraining, and Burnout in Child and Adolescent Athletes."

DOI: 10.1542/peds.2016-2148

PEDIATRICS (ISSN Numbers: Print, 0031-4005; Online, 1098-4275).

Copyright © 2016 by the American Academy of Pediatrics

FINANCIAL DISCLOSURE: The authors have indicated they do not have a financial relationship relevant to this article to disclose.

FUNDING: No external funding.

POTENTIAL CONFLICT OF INTEREST: The authors have indicated they have no potential conflicts of interest to disclose.

To cite: Brenner JS and AAP COUNCIL ON SPORTS MEDICINE AND FITNESS. Sports Specialization and Intensive Training in Young Athletes. *Pediatrics.* 2016;138(3):e20162148

INTRODUCTION

Youth sports culture has changed dramatically over the past 40 years. It is less common today to see a group of young children congregate in a neighborhood to play a "pick-up" game without any adult influence. The norm has become for children and adolescents to participate in organized sports driven by coaches and parents, often with different goals for the game than its young participants. It is also less common now to have a multisport athlete in middle or high school, because the norm has become for young athletes to specialize in a single sport at younger ages. There is increased pressure to participate at a high level, to specialize in 1 sport early, and to play year-round, often on multiple teams. This increased emphasis on sports specialization has led to an increase in overuse injuries, overtraining, and burnout.

This clinical report replaces a previous American Academy of Pediatrics (AAP) policy statement entitled "Intensive Training and Sports Specialization in Young Athletes"[1] and is complementary to the AAP clinical report "Overuse Injuries, Overtraining, and Burnout in Child and Adolescent Athletes."[2] This report reviews the epidemiology of youth sports and the background of specialization, highlights specific physiologic concerns with intensive training, answers specific questions pertaining to sports specialization in athletes <18 years, and offers guidance for pediatricians to help their young athlete patients and their parents (Figure 1).

EPIDEMIOLOGY AND BACKGROUND

Participating in sports provides many benefits for youth, including developing lifelong physical activity skills, socializing with peers, building teamwork and leadership skills, improving self-esteem, and having fun. According to the 2008 National Council of Youth Sports' report on trends and participation in organized youth sports, 60 million youth aged 6 through 18 years participated in organized sports, which is an increase from 45 million in 1997.[3] The sex ratio has remained constant, with 66% of young athletes being male and 34% being female.[3] Of the 60 million young athletes reported, 27% participated in only 1 sport.[3] Participation by children aged ≤6 years increased from 6% in 1997 to 12% in 2008.[3–5] Unfortunately, 70% of children drop out of organized sports by 13 years of age.[6] According to the 2013–2014 high school athletics participation survey from the National Federation of High School Sports, 7.8 million high school students participated in sports.[7] These statistics are an underestimate of actual participation rates, because they only represent athletes who participate in the organized sports surveyed or from high schools that are members of the National Federation of High School Sports. The actual incidence of overuse and overtraining injuries is difficult to assess because of the lack of uniformity and agreement throughout the literature in the definitions used. According to some reports, overuse injuries account for 46% to 50% of all athletic injuries.[8–10] In high school athletes alone, overuse injuries represented

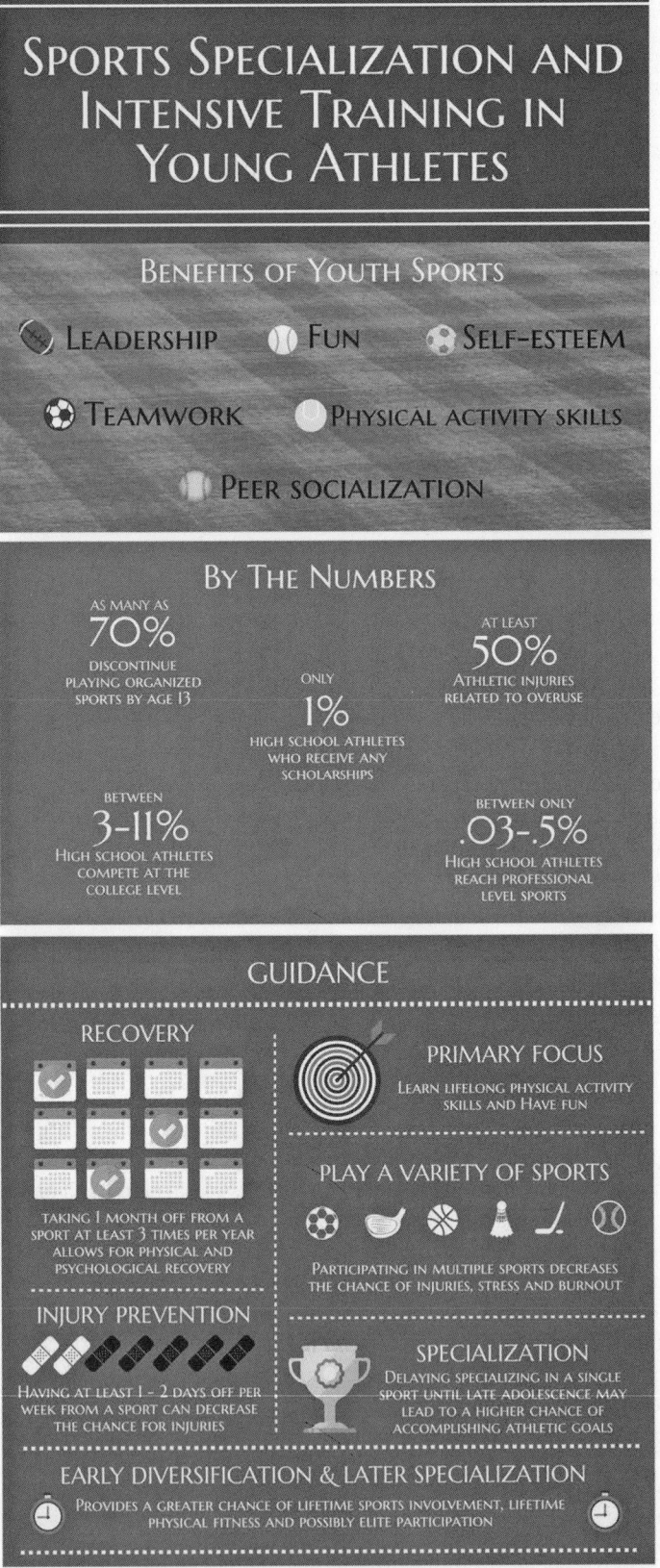

FIGURE 1
Sports Specialization and Intensive Training in Young Athletes.

7.7% of all injuries.[11] Actual injury rates vary by age, sex, and sport. Currently, no data are available on how many young athletes play year-round or on multiple teams at the same time.

Sports specialization occurs when an athlete focuses on only 1 sport, usually at the exclusion of any other and often year-round. Sports specialization appears to have increased overall, along with earlier onset, because select or travel leagues start as young as 7 years of age.[5,12,13] These leagues often are independent of school-sponsored programs and foster year-round single-sport participation.[14] Sports specialization can be divided into early specialization (ie, before puberty) and late specialization with early diversification (sampling).[4,13,15-17] The reasoning behind sports specialization is varied and includes aspirations to be one of the few who obtain a college scholarship or the even fewer who make it to the elite level of the Olympics or professional status.[4,13] Some young athletes desire to be identified as talented by coaches, the media, the sporting industry, and society as a whole.[4,13]

Year-round training in 1 sport has become more common for young athletes. Often, the motivation is for the athlete and parent to capture a piece of the very small "pie" leading to college scholarships and a professional career. Only 3.3% to 11.3% of high school athletes compete at the National Collegiate Athletic Association (NCAA) level, and only 1% receive an athletic scholarship.[4,18] In addition, only 0.03% to 0.5% of high school athletes make it to the professional level.[18] Athletes who participate in a variety of sports have fewer injuries and play sports longer than those who specialize before puberty.[1,2,4,5,19,20]

Sometimes, these are the goals of the parent and/or coaches and not necessarily the athlete. Studies have shown that parents were the strongest influence on starting a sport, and coaches influenced the decision to train intensely and specialize in a sport.[5,12,21] Even when the athlete is driven to take his or her game to the next level, evidence is mounting that specialization in a single sport before puberty may not be the best way to accomplish this goal for the majority of sports.

ATHLETE DEVELOPMENT

Long-term athlete development (LTAD) programs, which started in the 1990s in the United States, Canada, and other industrialized countries, have tried to counter the detrimental effects of early specialization and year-round sports by offering a positive framework to develop physical literacy and elite athletes.[16,22] Physical literacy has been defined as the mastering of fundamental movement skills and fundamental sports skills.[23] The ABCs (agility, balance, coordination, speed) are the basic skills required for physical literacy.[23] The shortfall of LTAD programs is that they have been based mostly on empirical evidence and are not individualized plans.[24] Many countries have also used these programs as a way to develop elite talent, thereby nurturing the rare minority instead of promoting physical activity for the great majority, as other programs promote.[25]

Five stages have been described for the late-specialization model of LTAD and include the following[16]:

1. FUNdamental
2. Training to Train
3. Training to Compete
4. Training to Win
5. Retirement/Retraining

The goal of the FUNdamental stage is to learn the fundamental movement skills and the ABCs of athleticism.[16] This stage should occur in 6- to 10-year-olds by using a positive and fun approach.[16] The Training to Train stage occurs in 10- to 14-year-olds with the goal of learning how to train and learning the basic skills of a specific sport.[16] In the Training to Train stage, there should be a ratio of 75% training to 25% competition, with the major focus on learning the basics as opposed to competition.[16] The Training to Compete stage occurs in 13- to 18-year-olds, with 50% of the time spent in developing technical and tactical skills and the other 50% on competition-specific training.[16] The Training to Win stage occurs in athletes aged ≥17 years, with the focus of training to optimize performance, with 75% of the time spent in competition (either competition-specific training activities or competitions themselves).[16] The Retirement/Retraining stage occurs when athletes stop competing permanently and possibly move into sports-related careers (ie, officiating, administration, coaching).[16] Physical and mental burnout is prevented through "prophylactic" breaks in training.[16] Athletes who decide not to continue competitive sports will still benefit from their FUNdamental stage accomplishments during their recreational activities.

The US Olympic Committee, along with National Governing Bodies, used the LTAD principles to create the American Development Model in 2014.[26] The 5 stages they created include the following:

1. Discover, Learn, and Play (ages 0–12 years)
2. Develop and Challenge (ages 10–16 years)
3. Train and Compete (ages 13–19 years)
4. Excel for High Performance or Participate and Succeed (ages ≥15 years)
5. Mentor and Thrive (for Life)[27]

Another model of sports expertise development that has been proposed is the Developmental Model of Sport Participation.[15,17,28] Two distinct pathways include either early diversification (sampling) or early specialization. The main tenants of early diversification include involvement in multiple sports and participation in deliberate play.[15,17,28] The benefits of early diversification include "experiencing different physical, cognitive, affective and psycho-social environments."[15] The foundational skills acquired are necessary to allow the athletes to successfully specialize later.[29] Diversification also allows children to experience different social interactions with peers and adults and reinforces emotional and self-regulating skills needed for the future.[15,17] "Deliberate play" has been defined as the intentional and voluntary nature of informal sport games designed to maximize inherent enjoyment.[15] Examples of deliberate play include the once common basketball in the park and backyard baseball games usually organized by children. Athletes are less likely to drop out of organized sports if they participate in informal games and sports.[29] In contrast, early specialization involves focusing on 1 sport with an emphasis on deliberate practice and very little deliberate play while focusing on performance as early as 6 years old.[15,28] "Deliberate practice" has been defined as "a highly structured activity that requires effort, generates no immediate rewards, and is motivated by the goal of improving performance rather than inherent enjoyment."[30] Early specialization assumes "talented" children can be selected early and uses a training regimen that is usually not in accordance with the child's motivation to participate in sports.[15]

Early specialization programs are designed to produce elite-level athletes, as opposed to early diversification programs, which focus on the long-term needs of children

through enjoying various activities and play.[15] Early diversification has a greater potential of minimizing dropouts while maximizing sustained participation, fostering positive peer relationships and leadership skills, and creating intrinsic motivation through participation in enjoyable activities.[15,17]

PHYSIOLOGIC AND PSYCHOLOGICAL CONCERNS WITH INTENSIVE TRAINING

Intensive training in young athletes, whether specialized or not, may potentially affect various components of their health, including cardiac, nutrition, maturation, musculoskeletal, and psychological. Musculoskeletal and psychological effects of intensive training in young athletes were covered in great detail in reports by the AAP and the American Medical Society for Sports Medicine.[2,19,20]

No studies have shown any adverse effects of intense training on the cardiovascular system of young athletes, although the number of studies is limited.[31-33] Athletes of all ages need to have a proper diet that includes an adequate amount of calories from proper sources as well as iron, calcium, and vitamin D to meet their training needs.[34] Young athletes have an additional burden because of the increased needs related to growth. The iron and calcium needs of the body are highest during the growing phases of a child and an adolescent. There is support for closely monitoring nutritional intake in all youth athletes, especially those who participate in high-intensity and endurance sports, focusing particularly on caloric intake required to meet the demands of training as well as to maintain adequate growth and development.[35]

Some female athletes experience menarche 1 to 2 years later than nonathletes but still within the normal range.[36,37] Theories proposed for this difference include lower body

fat, training, stress, undernutrition, or a sport-specific preselection bias.[37-40] Secondary amenorrhea can result from low energy availability attributable to an imbalance between energy expenditure and caloric intake. Because of the increased risk of stress fractures and lower bone density, female athletes should be monitored for amenorrhea and treated appropriately. All female athletes are at risk of developing the female athlete triad (low energy availability, menstrual dysfunction, and low bone mineral density),[35] and pediatricians should screen routinely for signs of the triad in active young females. No studies in young male athletes have shown any adverse effects on pubertal growth and maturation or adult height from intense training.[41,42]

SPORTS SPECIALIZATION

Does Specialization Lead to a Successful Performance and Career?

Most authorities agree that sports specialization, in general, leads to higher athletic "success," but the optimal timing of specialization is only now becoming clearer. Studies have shown that Division 1 NCAA athletes are more likely to have played multiple sports in high school and that their first organized sport was different from their current one.[4,43] Many examples exist of professional athletes who have learned skills that cross over to their sport by playing a variety of sports into high school and even college. There were 322 athletes invited to the 2015 National Football League Scouting Combine, 87% of whom played multiple sports in high school and 13% of whom only played football.[44] Other studies in elite athletes have shown that intense training did not start until late adolescence and that these athletes played other sports before specializing.[45,46] Reviews of studies of elite athlete specialization history by Jayanthi et al[5] and Côté et al[15] revealed that, for the majority of sports, late specialization with early diversification is most likely to lead to elite status. In addition, athletes who engaged in sport-specific training at a young age had shorter athletic careers.[15]

It has often been misquoted that to succeed, an athlete needs to have 10 000 hours of practice/competition over 10 years. The media have incorrectly extrapolated Ericsson and co-workers' studies of chess players to a formula for sports success.[30,47] Many examples exist of successful athletes who have <10 000 hours and others who have not succeeded despite having >10 000 hours of practice/competition. Other factors come into play besides sports exposure time. These may include physiologic construction (ie, a high jumper with elastic Achilles tendon) and genetic constitution.[48] For some athletes, elite status may be achieved with 10 000 hours of total deliberate play and deliberate practice time in all sports combined but only 3000 hours of sport-specific training.[28,48] Evidence is lacking that specialization before puberty is necessary to achieve elite status, and in fact, specialization before puberty is more likely to be detrimental.[5]

When Is It Appropriate and Safe to Specialize?

Current evidence suggests that delaying sport specialization for the majority of sports until after puberty (late adolescence, ~15 or 16 years of age) will minimize the risks and lead to a higher likelihood of athletic success.[4,5,13,19,20,29,49] Only 0.3% of German athletes in Olympic sports selected at the youngest level were ranked internationally, and most elite athletes specialized in their primary sport later in life.[4,46] Specialization can be divided into early versus late, with the inclusion of early diversification of multiple sports

for those who specialize later. Early diversification allows the athlete to explore a variety of sports while growing physically, cognitively, and socially in a positive environment and developing intrinsic motivation.[4,5,15,29,46,50] Young athletes can learn many important fundamental physical movement skills (ABCs) with early diversification that can then transfer over to their primary sport if they decide to specialize later.[51] By learning these skills during their developing years through deliberate play, athletes will require less deliberate practice to acquire expertise in their chosen sport.[5,15] Studies have also shown that deliberate play is crucial to normal development and attainment of elite status.[5,24] Athletes in late adolescence have the cognitive, physical, social, emotional, and motor skills needed to invest into highly specialized training.[15] They can understand the benefits and costs of intense focus on 1 sport and, just as importantly, are able to make an independent decision about investing in 1 sport.[15,29]

What Are the Risks in Specializing Too Soon or at All?

Young athletes who specialize too soon are at risk of physical, emotional, and social problems.[2,4,5,14,19,20,49] Athletes may become socially isolated from their peers and may have altered relationships with family, overdependence on others with a loss of control over their lives, arrested behavioral development, or socially maladaptive behaviors.[4,14] Specializing early with intense training can lead to overuse injuries, which can cause pain and temporary loss of playing time or may lead to early retirement from the sport.[2,4,5,19,20,29,49] The risk of injury is multifactorial, including training volume, competitive level, and pubertal maturation stage.[5,8] One study in high school athletes showed an increased risk of injury

when the training volume exceeded 16 hours per week.[52] Another study determined that sports specialization was an independent risk factor for injury and that athletes who participated in organized sports compared with free play time in a ratio of >2:1 had an increased risk of an overuse injury.[49] This same study found that young athletes who participated in more hours of organized sports per week than their age in years also had an increased risk of an overuse injury.[49] Burnout, anxiety, depression, and attrition are increased in early specializers.[2,4,5,13,19,20,53] Social isolation from peers who do not participate in the athlete's sport and lack of being exposed to a variety of sports also are concerns.[4,14] Restriction in exposure to a variety of sports can lead to the young athlete not experiencing a sport that he or she may truly enjoy, excel at playing, or want to participate in throughout his or her adult life. An additional concern is the risk of physical, emotional, and sexual abuse by the adults involved in the young athletes' lives as a result of overdependence.[4,14] Dietary and chemical manipulation are also possible.[4,14,54,55] The combination of these adverse outcomes could lead to a decrease in lifelong physical activity.[13]

Which Sports Require Early Specialization and Are Those Athletes at High Risk?

Figure skating, gymnastics, rhythmic gymnastics, and diving may require early specialization, because peak performance occurs before full physical maturation.[4,16,56] However, it is not known whether the training required for such sports poses a risk for athletes' long-term health and well-being.[29] Studies in gymnasts and figure skaters found that their training did not affect pubertal growth and maturation or adult height.[37,42] Menarche occurred later but within a normal range.[36,37] However, other studies have shown that female athletes who participate in sports requiring early sports specialization are at higher risk of overuse injuries as well as the female athlete triad.[35]

How Much Training Is Adequate to Succeed Versus Too Much?

The exact amount of training needed to succeed has not been described. The threshold to avoid injuries, burnout, and attrition has not been elucidated. The possible rule of participating in fewer hours of organized sports per week than their age in years[49] or restricting training to <16 hours per week[52] to decrease the chance of injuries needs to be validated by other long-term studies.

Do Sports-Enhancement Programs Lead to Success?

Young athletes need to learn motor development skills, social skills, and psychological skills to succeed. No studies on sports-enhancement programs in youth that only teach sport technique or "conditioning" have shown a greater chance of success despite their increased time and financial investment.

What Are the Effects of Early College Recruitment?

Talented youth are starting to be ranked nationally as early as sixth grade.[4] As colleges start to look at middle school and early high school athletes, more pressure is created for the athlete and parent to do everything possible to succeed. This situation may push athletes into playing year-round and possibly on multiple teams simultaneously to get more exposure and specializing in a single sport sooner for fear of missing their opportunity to impress a college coach. Given what is currently known about early sport specialization, this changing paradigm should be discouraged by society. The AAP, NCAA, pediatricians, parents, and other stakeholders should advocate banning national ranking of athletes

and college recruitment before the athletes' later high school years.

FUTURE DIRECTIONS

Are there genetic factors that predict success or failure of a young athlete? Success is dependent on multiple factors, with genetics playing a part.[57] It is not uncommon that an Olympic or professional athlete has an immediate relative who also played at a very high level.[48] The exact make-up of a sports gene that would guarantee athletic success has not been described, if it even exists at all.

There is a need for longitudinal data on early sport specialization and intensive training that quantify injury and burnout rates. In addition, data are needed to confirm when specialization should occur, if at all.

GUIDANCE FOR THE PEDIATRICIAN

When a pediatrician encounters athletes younger than 18 years who are considering specialization or have already specialized, the following guidance for the athlete, parents, and coaches can be helpful.

1. The primary focus of sports for young athletes should be to have fun and learn lifelong physical activity skills.

2. Participating in multiple sports, at least until puberty, decreases the chances of injuries, stress, and burnout in young athletes.

3. For most sports, specializing in a sport later (ie, late adolescence) may lead to a higher chance of the young athlete accomplishing his or her athletic goals.

4. Early diversification and later specialization provides for a greater chance of lifetime sports involvement, lifetime physical fitness, and possibly elite participation.

5. If a young athlete has decided to specialize in a single sport,

discussing his or her goals to determine whether they are appropriate and realistic is important. This discussion may involve helping the young athlete distinguish these goals from those of the parents and/or coaches.

6. It is important for parents to closely monitor the training and coaching environment of "elite" youth sports programs[14] and be aware of best practices for their children's sports.

7. Having at least a total of 3 months off throughout the year, in increments of 1 month, from their particular sport of interest will allow for athletes' physical and psychological recovery. Young athletes can still remain active in other activities to meet physical activity guidelines during the time off.

8. Young athletes having at least 1 to 2 days off per week from their particular sport of interest can decrease the chance for injuries.

9. Closely monitoring young athletes who pursue intensive training for physical and psychological growth and maturation as well as nutritional status is an important parameter for health and well-being.

RESOURCES

Epstein D. *The Sports Gene*. New York, NY: Penguin Books; 2013

Farrey T. *Game On: The All-American Race to Make Champions of Our Children*. Bristol, CT: ESPN Publishing; 2008

Hyman M. *Until It Hurts: America's Obsession With Youth Sports and How It Harms Our Kids*. Boston, MA: Beacon Press; 2010

O'Sullivan J. *Changing the Game*. New York, NY: Morgan James Publishing; 2013

O'Sullivan J. *Is It Wise to Specialize?* Seattle, WA: Amazon Digital Services, Inc; 2014

Stricker PR. *Sports Success Rx!: Your Child's Prescription for the Best Experience.* Elk Grove Village, IL: American Academy of Pediatrics; 2006

LEAD AUTHOR

Joel S. Brenner, MD, MPH, FAAP

COUNCIL ON SPORTS MEDICINE AND FITNESS EXECUTIVE COMMITTEE, 2014–2015

Joel S. Brenner, MD, MPH, FAAP, Chairperson
Cynthia R. LaBella, MD, FAAP, Chairperson-elect
Margaret A. Brooks, MD, FAAP
Alex Diamond, DO, FAAP
William Hennrikus, MD, FAAP
Amanda K. Weiss Kelly, MD, FAAP
Michele LaBotz, MD, FAAP
Kelsey Logan, MD, FAAP
Keith J. Loud, MDCM, MSc, FAAP
Kody A. Moffatt, MD, FAAP
Blaise Nemeth, MD, FAAP
Brooke Pengel, MD, FAAP

LIAISONS

Andrew J.M. Gregory, MD, FAAP – *American College of Sports Medicine*
Mark E. Halstead, MD, FAAP – *American Medical Society for Sports Medicine*
Lisa K. Kluchurosky, MEd, ATC – *National Athletic Trainers Association*

CONSULTANTS

Holly Benjamin, MD, FAAP
Neeru A. Jayanthi, MD
Tracey Zaslow, MD, FAAP

STAFF

Anjie Emanuel, MPH

ABBREVIATIONS

AAP: American Academy of Pediatrics
ABCs: agility, balance, coordination, speed
LTAD: long-term athlete development
NCAA: National Collegiate Athletic Association

REFERENCES

1. American Academy of Pediatrics, Committee on Sports Medicine and Fitness. Intensive training and sports specialization in young athletes. *Pediatrics.* 2000;106(1 pt 1):154–157. Reaffirmed October 2014

2. Brenner JS; American Academy of Pediatrics, Council on Sports Medicine and Fitness. Overuse injuries, overtraining, and burnout in child and adolescent athletes. *Pediatrics.* 2007;119(6):1242–1245. Reaffirmed June 2014

3. National Council of Youth Sports. Report on Trends and Participation in Organized Youth Sports. Available at: www.ncys.org/pdfs/2008/2008-ncys-market-research-report.pdf. Accessed December 15, 2015

4. Malina RM. Early sport specialization: roots, effectiveness, risks. *Curr Sports Med Rep.* 2010;9(6):364–371

5. Jayanthi N, Pinkham C, Dugas L, Patrick B, Labella C. Sports specialization in young athletes: evidence-based recommendations. *Sports Health.* 2013;5(3):251–257

6. O'Sullivan J. *Changing the Game.* New York, NY: Morgan James Publishing; 2013

7. National Federation of State High School Association. 2013-14 High School Athletics Participation Survey. Available at: www.nfhs.org/ParticipationStatics/PDF/2013-14_Participation_Survey_PDF.pdf. Accessed December 15, 2015

8. Luke A, Lazaro RM, Bergeron MF, et al. Sports-related injuries in youth athletes: is overscheduling a risk factor? *Clin J Sport Med.* 2011;21(4):307–314

9. Valovich McLeod TC, Decoster LC, Loud KJ, et al. National Athletic Trainers' Association position statement: prevention of pediatric overuse injuries. *J Athl Train.* 2011;46(2):206–220

10. Roos KG, Marshall SW, Kerr ZY, et al. Epidemiology of overuse injuries in collegiate and high school athletics in the United States. *Am J Sports Med.* 2015;43(7):1790–1797

11. Schroeder AN, Comstock RD, Collins CL, Everhart J, Flanigan D, Best TM. Epidemiology of overuse injuries among high-school athletes in the United States. *J Pediatr.* 2015;166(3):600–606

12. Hill GM, Simons J. A study of the sport specialization on high school athletics. *J Sport Soc Issues.* 1989;13(1):1–13

13. Mostafavifar AM, Best TM, Myer GD. Early sport specialisation, does it lead to long-term problems? *Br J Sports Med.* 2013;47(17):1060–1061

14. Malina RM. Children and adolescents in the sport culture: the overwhelming majority to the select few. *J Exerc Sci Fit.* 2009;7(2 suppl):S1–S10

15. Côté J, Lidor R, Hackfort D. ISSP position stand: to sample or to specialize? Seven postulates about youth sport activities that lead to continued participation and elite performance. *Int J Sport Exerc Psychol.* 2009;7(1):7–17

16. Balyi I. Sport system building and long-term athlete development in British Columbia. *Coaches Report.* 2001;8(1):25–28

17. Côté J, Vierimaa M. The developmental model of sport participation: 15 years after its first conceptualization. *Sci Sports.* 2014;29(suppl):S63–S69

18. National Collegiate Athletic Association. Estimated probability of competing in athletics beyond the high school interscholastic level. Available at: www.ncaa.org/sites/default/files/Probability-of-going-pro-methodology_Update2013.pdf. Accessed December 15, 2015

19. DiFiori JP, Benjamin HJ, Brenner JS, et al. Overuse injuries and burnout in youth sports: a position statement from the American Medical Society for Sports Medicine. *Br J Sports Med.* 2014;48(4):287–288

20. DiFiori JP, Benjamin HJ, Brenner J, et al. Overuse injuries and burnout in youth sports: a position statement from the American Medical Society for Sports Medicine. *Clin J Sport Med.* 2014;24(1):3–20

21. Baxter-Jones ADG, Maffulli N; TOYA Study Group. Parental influence on sport participation in elite young athletes. *J Sports Med Phys Fitness.* 2003;43(2):250–255

22. Leite N, Baker J, Sampaio J. Paths to expertise in Portuguese national

team athletes. *J Sports Sci Med.* 2009;8(4):560–566

23. Sport for Life Society. What is physical literacy? CS4L Physical Literacy. Available at: www.physicalliteracy.ca/what-is-physical-literacy. Accessed December 15, 2015

24. Ford P, De Ste Croix M, Lloyd R, et al. The long-term athlete development model: physiological evidence and application. *J Sports Sci.* 2011;29(4):389–402

25. Project Play. Playbook. Available at: http://youthreport.projectplay.us/. Accessed December 15, 2015

26. Team USA [home page]. Available at: www.teamusa.org. Accessed December 15, 2015

27. Team USA. American Development Model. Available at: www.teamusa.org/About-the-USOC/Athlete-Development/American-Development-Model. Accessed December 15, 2015

28. Côté J, Baker J, Abernethy B. Practice and play in the development of sport expertise. In: Tenenbaum G, Eklund RC, eds. *Handbook of Sport Psychology.* 3rd ed. Hoboken, NJ: John Wiley & Sons; 2007:184–202

29. Coakley J, Sheridan MP, Howard R, et al. Guidelines for participation in youth sport programs: specialization versus multiple-sport participation. Available at: http://aahperd.org/naspe2010. Accessed December 15, 2015

30. Ericsson KA, Krampe RT, Tesch-Römer C. The role of deliberate practice in the acquisition of expert performance. *Psychol Rev.* 1993;100(3):363–406

31. Rowland TW, Delaney BC, Siconolfi SF. "Athlete's heart" in prepubertal children. *Pediatrics.* 1987;79(5):800–804

32. Rowland TW, Unnithan VB, MacFarlane NG, Gibson NG, Paton JY. Clinical manifestations of the "athlete's heart" in prepubertal male runners. *Int J Sports Med.* 1994;15(8):515–519

33. Rowland T, Goff D, DeLuca P, Popowski B. Cardiac effects of a competitive road race in trained child runners. *Pediatrics.* 1997;100(3):E2

34. Sonneville KR, Gordon CM, Kocher MS, Pierce LM, Ramappa A, Field AE. Vitamin D, calcium, and dairy intakes and stress fractures among female

adolescents. *Arch Pediatr Adolesc Med.* 2012;166(7):595–600

35. De Souza MJ, Nattiv A, Joy E, et al; Expert Panel. 2014 Female Athlete Triad Coalition Consensus Statement on Treatment and Return to Play of the Female Athlete Triad: 1st International Conference held in San Francisco, California, May 2012 and 2nd International Conference held in Indianapolis, Indiana, May 2013. *Br J Sports Med.* 2014;48(4):289

36. Vadocz EA, Siegel SR, Malina RM. Age at menarche in competitive figure skaters: variation by competency and discipline. *J Sports Sci.* 2002;20(2):93–100

37. Thomis M, Claessens AL, Lefevre J, Philippaerts R, Beunen GP, Malina RM. Adolescent growth spurts in female gymnasts. *J Pediatr.* 2005;146(2):239–244

38. Malina RM. Menarche in athletes: a synthesis and hypothesis. *Ann Hum Biol.* 1983;10(1):1–24

39. Malina RM. Physical activity and training: effects on stature and the adolescent growth spurt. *Med Sci Sports Exerc.* 1994;26(6):759–766

40. Malina RM. Delayed age of menarche of athletes. *JAMA.* 1982;247(24):3312–3313

41. Malina RM. Physical growth and biological maturation of young athletes. *Exerc Sport Sci Rev.* 1994;22(1):389–433

42. Malina RM, Baxter-Jones AD, Armstrong N, et al. Role of intensive training in the growth and maturation of artistic gymnasts. *Sports Med.* 2013;43(9):783–802

43. American Medical Society for Sports Medicine. Effectiveness of early sport specialization limited in most sports, sport diversification may be better approach at young ages. Available at: www.sciencedaily.com/releases/2013/04/130423172601.htm. Accessed December 15, 2015

44. TrackingFootball.com. Available at: https://twitter.com/trckfootball. Accessed December 15, 2015

45. Vaeyens R, Güllich A, Warr CR, Philippaerts R. Talent identification and promotion programmes of Olympic athletes. *J Sports Sci.* 2009;27(13):1367–1380

46. Moesch K, Elbe A-M, Hauge M-LT, Wikman JM. Late specialization: the key to success in centimeters, grams, or seconds (cgs) sports. *Scand J Med Sci Sports.* 2011;21(6):e282–e290

47. Ericsson KA. Training history, deliberate practice and elite sports performance: an analysis in response to Tucker and Collins review—what makes champions? *Br J Sports Med.* 2013;47(9):533–535

48. Epstein D. *The Sports Gene.* New York, NY: Penguin Books; 2013

49. Jayanthi NA, LaBella CR, Fischer D, Pasulka J, Dugas LR. Sports-specialized intensive training and the risk of injury in young athletes: a clinical case-control study. *Am J Sports Med.* 2015;43(4):794–801

50. Wiersma LD. Risks and benefits of youth sport specialization: perspectives and recommendations. *Pediatr Exerc Sci.* 2000;12(1):13–22

51. Abernethy B, Baker J, Côté J. Transfer of pattern recall skills may contribute to the development of sport expertise. *Appl Cogn Psychol.* 2005;19(6):705–718

52. Rose MS, Emery CA, Meeuwisse WH. Sociodemographic predictors of sport injury in adolescents. *Med Sci Sports Exerc.* 2008;40(3):444–450

53. Capranica L, Millard-Stafford ML. Youth sport specialization: how to manage competition and training? *Int J Sports Physiol Perform.* 2011;6(4):572–579

54. Committee on Nutrition; Council on Sports Medicine and Fitness. Sports drinks and energy drinks for children and adolescents: are they appropriate? *Pediatrics.* 2011;127(6):1182–1189

55. LaBotz M, Griesemer BA; American Academy of Pediatrics, Council on Sports Medicine and Fitness. Use of performance enhancing substances. *Pediatrics.* 2016;138(1):e20161300

56. Law MP, Côté J, Ericsson KA. Characteristics of expert development in rhythmic gymnastics: a retrospective study. *Int J Sport Exerc Psychol.* 2007;5(1):82–103

57. Tucker R, Collins M. What makes champions? A review of the relative contribution of genes and training to sporting success. *Br J Sports Med.* 2012;46(8):555–561

Standard Terminology for Fetal, Infant, and Perinatal Deaths

• *Clinical Report*

CLINICAL REPORT   Guidance for the Clinician in Rendering Pediatric Care

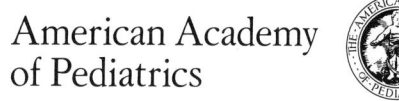

American Academy
of Pediatrics

DEDICATED TO THE HEALTH OF ALL CHILDREN™

Standard Terminology for Fetal, Infant, and Perinatal Deaths

Wanda D. Barfield, MD, MPH, COMMITTEE ON FETUS AND NEWBORN

abstract

Accurately defining and reporting perinatal deaths (ie, fetal and infant deaths) is a critical first step in understanding the magnitude and causes of these important events. In addition to obstetric health care providers, neonatologists and pediatricians should have easy access to current and updated resources that clearly provide US definitions and reporting requirements for live births, fetal deaths, and infant deaths. Correct identification of these vital events will improve local, state, and national data so that these deaths can be better addressed and prevented.

INTRODUCTION

Perinatal mortality is the combination of fetal deaths and neonatal deaths. In the United States in 2013, the fetal mortality rate for gestations of at least 20 weeks (5.96 fetal deaths per 1000 live births and fetal deaths)[1] was similar to the infant mortality rate (5.98 infant deaths per 1000 live births).[2] Depending on the definition used, fetal mortality contributes to approximately 40% to 60% of perinatal mortality. Understanding the etiologies of these events and predicting risk begins with accurately defining cases; the collection and analysis of reliable statistical data are an essential part of in-depth investigations on local, state, and national levels.

Fetal and infant deaths occur within the clinical practice of several types of health care providers. Although obstetric practitioners report fetal deaths, certain situations can occur during a delivery in which viability or possibility of survival is unclear; the pediatrician or neonatologist may attend the delivery to assess the medical condition of the fetus or infant, assess pre-viable gestational age, provide care as indicated, and report a subsequent infant death, if it occurs. Incorrectly defining and reporting fetal deaths and early infant deaths may contribute to misclassification of these important events and result in inaccurate fetal and infant mortality rates.[3] Within this context, the American Academy of Pediatrics provides definitions and reporting requirements of fetal death, live birth, and infant death to emphasize that neonatologists and pediatricians play an

This document is copyrighted and is property of the American Academy of Pediatrics and its Board of Directors. All authors have filed conflict of interest statements with the American Academy of Pediatrics. Any conflicts have been resolved through a process approved by the Board of Directors. The American Academy of Pediatrics has neither solicited nor accepted any commercial involvement in the development of the content of this publication.

The views expressed in this document are not necessarily those of the Centers for Disease Control and Prevention or the US Department of Health and Human Services.

Clinical reports from the American Academy of Pediatrics benefit from expertise and resources of liaisons and internal (AAP) and external reviewers. However, clinical reports from the American Academy of Pediatrics may not reflect the views of the liaisons or the organizations or government agencies that they represent.

The guidance in this report does not indicate an exclusive course of treatment or serve as a standard of medical care. Variations, taking into account individual circumstances, may be appropriate.

All clinical reports from the American Academy of Pediatrics automatically expire 5 years after publication unless reaffirmed, revised, or retired at or before that time.

DOI: 10.1542/peds.2016-0551

PEDIATRICS (ISSN Numbers: Print, 0031-4005; Online, 1098-4275).

To cite: Barfield WD and AAP COMMITTEE ON FETUS AND NEWBORN. Standard Terminology for Fetal, Infant, and Perinatal Deaths. Pediatrics. 2016;137(5):e20160551

important role in recording accurate and timely information surrounding these events. This role includes making the determination of the specific vital event during delivery, recording information surrounding the event on the appropriate certificate or report in compliance with state-specific requirements, and documenting information that is as complete and as accurate as possible, including the underlying cause of death, when known. Although guidance for these definitions is provided elsewhere,[4–6] it may not be readily available to pediatricians in the delivery room.

Both the collection and use of information about fetal, infant, and perinatal deaths have been hampered by lack of understanding of differences in definitions, statistical tabulations, and reporting requirements among providers and state, national, and international bodies. Distinctions can and should be made between the definition of an event and the reporting requirements for the event. The definition indicates the meaning of a term (eg, live birth, fetal death). A reporting requirement is that part of the defined event for which reporting is mandatory.

DEFINITIONS

Challenges in consistent definitions of fetal and infant death mostly stem from the perception of viability, which should not change the definition of the event. In other words, an extremely preterm infant born at 16 weeks' gestation may be defined as a live birth but is not currently viable outside of the womb. On the basis of international standards set by the World Health Organization,[7] the National Center for Health Statistics of the Centers for Disease Control and Prevention defines live birth, fetal death, infant death, and perinatal death as follows.[4]

Live Birth

A live birth is defined as the complete expulsion or extraction from the mother of a product of human conception, irrespective of the duration of pregnancy, which, after such expulsion or extraction, breathes or shows any other evidence of life, such as beating of the heart, pulsation of the umbilical cord, or definite movement of voluntary muscles, regardless of whether the umbilical cord has been cut or the placenta is attached. Heartbeats are to be distinguished from transient cardiac contractions; respirations are to be distinguished from fleeting respiratory efforts or gasps.

Fetal Death

A fetus is defined from 8 weeks after conception until term while in the uterus. Fetal death is defined as death before the complete expulsion or extraction from the mother of a product of human conception, irrespective of the duration of pregnancy that is not an induced termination of pregnancy. The death is indicated by the fact that, after such expulsion or extraction, the fetus does not breathe or show any other evidence of life such as beating of the heart, pulsation of the umbilical cord, or definite movement of voluntary muscles. Heartbeats are to be distinguished from transient cardiac contractions; respirations are to be distinguished from fleeting respiratory efforts or gasps.

For statistical purposes, fetal deaths are further subdivided as "early" (20–27 weeks' gestation) or "late" (≥28 weeks' gestation). The term "stillbirth" is also used to describe fetal deaths at 20 weeks' gestation or more. Stillbirth is not specifically divided into early and late gestations, but for international comparisons the World Health Organization defines stillbirth as at or after 28 weeks' gestation. Fetuses that die in utero before 20 weeks' gestation

are categorized specifically as miscarriages.

Infant Death

A live birth that results in death within the first year (<365 days) is defined as an infant death. Infant deaths are characterized as neonatal (<28 days) and further subdivided into early neonatal (<7 days), late neonatal (7–27 days), or postneonatal (28–364 days).

Perinatal Death

Perinatal deaths refer to a combination of fetal deaths and live births with only brief survival (days or weeks) and are grouped on the assumption that similar factors are associated with these losses. Perinatal death is not a reportable vital event, per se, but is used for statistical purposes. Three definitions of perinatal deaths are in use:

- Definition I includes infant deaths that occur at less than 7 days of age and fetal deaths with a stated or presumed period of gestation of 28 weeks or more.

- Definition II includes infant deaths that occur at less than 28 days of age and fetal deaths with a stated or presumed period of gestation of 20 weeks or more.

- Definition III includes infant deaths that occur at less than 7 days of age and fetal deaths with a stated or presumed gestation of 20 weeks or more.

From national and international perspectives, perinatal deaths have important implications for both public health and clinical interventions. However, the interpretations of these definitions vary globally on the basis of cultural perspectives, clinical definitions of viability, and availability of information. The National Center for Health Statistics currently classifies perinatal deaths according to the first 2 definitions. Definition I is used by the National Center for Health

TABLE 1 Reporting Requirements for Fetal Death According to State or Reporting Area, 2014

Criteria	State/Reporting Area
Gestational age criteria only	
All periods	Arkansas, Colorado, Georgia, Hawaii, New York,[a] Rhode Island, Virginia, Virgin Islands
≥16 weeks	Pennsylvania
≥20 weeks	Alabama, Alaska, California, Connecticut, Florida, Illinois, Indiana, Iowa, Maine, Maryland,[b] Minnesota, Nebraska, Nevada, New Jersey, North Carolina, North Dakota, Ohio, Oklahoma, Oregon, Texas, Utah, Vermont,[c] Washington, West Virginia, Wyoming
≥5 months	Puerto Rico
Both gestational age and birth weight criteria	
≥20 weeks or ≥350 g	Arizona, Idaho, Kentucky, Louisiana, Massachusetts, Mississippi, Missouri, New Hampshire, New Mexico, South Carolina, Tennessee, Wisconsin, Guam
≥20 weeks or ≥400 g	Michigan
≥20 weeks or ≥500 g	District of Columbia
Birth weight criteria only	
≥350 g	Delaware,[d] Kansas, Montana[d]
≥500 g	South Dakota

Data source: National Center for Health Statistics, National Vital Statistics Reports.
[a] Includes New York city, which has separate reporting.
[b] If gestational age is unknown, weight of ≥500 g.
[c] If gestational age is unknown, weight of ≥400 g, ≥15 ounces.
[d] If weight is unknown, ≥20 weeks' completed gestation.

Statistics and the World Health Organization to make international comparisons to account for variability in registering births and deaths between 20 and 27 weeks' gestation.[8] However, definition II is more inclusive and hence is more appropriate for monitoring perinatal deaths throughout gestation, because the majority of fetal deaths occur before 28 weeks' gestation.

REPORTING REQUIREMENTS

In the United States, states and independent reporting areas (ie, New York City; Washington, DC; and the US territories) register the certificates of live birth, death, and fetal death. These certificates/reports include clinical information. Challenges in consistent reporting of fetal death, in particular, stem from the variation in reporting requirements among states.[9] Recommended definitions and reporting requirements are issued through the Model State Vital Statistics Act and Regulations (the Model Law).[10,11] The Model Law recommends fetal death reporting for deaths that occur at 350 g birth weight or more or, if the weight is

unknown, of 20 completed weeks' gestation or more. However, states have the authority to register these vital events and might not necessarily follow the Model Law, which results in differences in birth weight and gestational age criteria for reporting fetal deaths (Table 1). States also vary in the quality of the data reported, which include missing data.[9]

All live births, regardless of gestational age, are reported as vital record events. Infant deaths involve both the reporting of a live birth event and a death event using a certificate of live birth and a certificate of death, respectively. Information from the certificate of live birth, including demographic information, selected maternal risk factors, maternal labor and delivery information, and infant weight and gestational age, is linked to information on the infant death certificate to include cause-of-death information. The fetal death certificate or report, a single document, includes maternal demographic information, selected maternal risk factors, labor and delivery information, and information about the fetus to

include weight, gestational age, and cause of death. Accurate completion of these vital records is important for generating accurate data to determine the magnitude and causes of fetal, infant, and perinatal deaths.

PRACTICAL CONSIDERATIONS

A flow diagram for the determination of appropriate reporting of perinatal deaths was developed by the National Association for Public Health Statistics and Information Systems (Fig 1). The diagram delineates the sequence of reporting and can be used in delivery rooms to appropriately report perinatal events. Induced termination of pregnancy is included in the flow diagram but is beyond the scope of this report.

In the circumstance of delivery events in which the fetus is of uncertain viability, if the infant is determined to be a live birth, the event is reported regardless of birth weight, length of gestation, survival time, or other clinical information (eg, Apgar scores). If fetal death is determined, the event is reported by the obstetric health care provider on the basis of state criteria, including

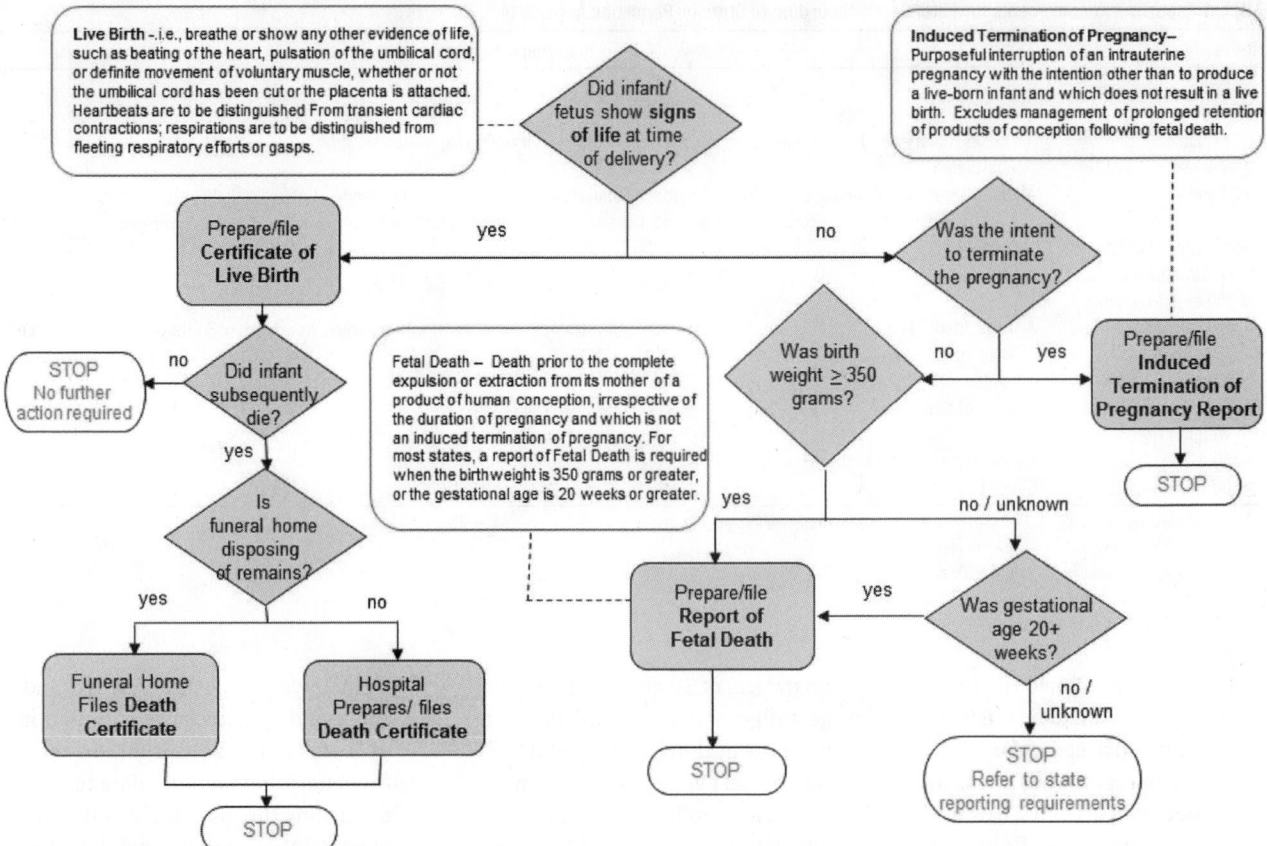

FIGURE 1
Hospital guidelines for reporting live births, infant deaths, fetal deaths, and induced terminations of pregnancy. (Adapted with permission from the National Association for Public Health Statistics and Information Systems; www.naphsis.org [available on request].)

both birth weight and gestational age. The careful use of accurate definitions is of utmost importance in medical record documentation of these events. Because there are no signs of life at delivery, fetal deaths are not assigned Apgar scores and are usually not admitted to the nursery or NICU. Postmortem examination of the fetus or infant and placenta may provide important information as to the cause of death; however, the actual evaluation and management of fetal and infant death are beyond the scope of this guidance and have been reported elsewhere.[12]

In summary, the accurate and timely reporting of live birth and fetal and infant death is the cornerstone of perinatal mortality data. Because reducing fetal and infant mortality is among the nation's health goals, accurate definitions of these events

are essential for understanding causes and researching potential solutions.

SUGGESTIONS

1. Vital events are best defined and reported as follows:

    o Live birth: The complete expulsion or extraction from the mother of a product of human conception, irrespective of the duration of pregnancy, which, after such expulsion or extraction, breathes or shows any other evidence of life such as beating of the heart, pulsation of the umbilical cord, or definite movement of voluntary muscles, regardless of whether the umbilical cord has been cut or the placenta is attached. Heartbeats are

    to be distinguished from transient cardiac contractions; respirations are to be distinguished from fleeting respiratory efforts or gasps.

    o Fetal death: Death before the complete expulsion or extraction from the mother of a product of human conception, irrespective of the duration of pregnancy that is not an induced termination of pregnancy. The death is indicated by the fact that, after such expulsion or extraction, the fetus does not breathe or show any other evidence of life such as beating of the heart, pulsation of the umbilical cord, or definite movement of voluntary muscles. Heartbeats are to be distinguished from transient cardiac contractions; respirations are to be distinguished from fleeting respiratory efforts or gasps.

- o Infant death: A live birth that results in death within the first year (<365 days).

2. Obtain accurate information on state law to file the fetal death certificate/report according to state requirements.

3. Complete reporting of live births, infant deaths, and fetal deaths (in support of obstetrician reporters) with the most accurate information possible to include pertinent demographic information, maternal medical history, and fetal or infant diagnoses.

LEAD AUTHOR

Wanda Denise Barfield, MD, MPH, FAAP
wjb5@cdc.gov

COMMITTEE ON FETUS AND NEWBORN, 2014–2015

Kristi Watterberg, MD, FAAP, Chairperson
William Benitz, MD, FAAP
James Cummings, MD, FAAP
Eric Eichenwald, MD, FAAP
Brenda Poindexter, MD, FAAP
Dan L. Stewart, MD, FAAP
Susan W. Aucott, MD, FAAP
Karen M. Puopolo, MD, FAAP
Jay P. Goldsmith, MD, FAAP

LIAISONS

Kasper S. Wang, MD, FAAP – *AAP Section on Surgery*
Thierry Lacaze, MD – *Canadian Pediatric Society*
Maria Ann Mascola, MD – *American College of Obstetricians and Gynecologists*

Tonse N.K. Raju, MD, FAAP – *National Institutes of Health*
Wanda D. Barfield, MD, MPH, FAAP – *Centers for Disease Control and Prevention*
Erin Keels, MS, APRN, NNP-BC – *National Association of Neonatal Nurses*

STAFF

Jim Couto, MA

REFERENCES

1. MacDorman MF, Gregory ECW. Fetal and perinatal mortality: United States, 2013. *Natl Vital Stat Rep.* 2015;64(8):1–8

2. Centers for Disease Control and Prevention. Deaths: final data for 2013. Available at: www.cdc.gov/nchs/data/nvsr/nvsr64/nvsr64_02.pdf. Accessed July 2015

3. MacDorman MF, Martin JA, Mathews TJ, Hoyert DL, Ventura SJ. Explaining the 2001-02 infant mortality increase: data from the linked birth/infant death data set. *Natl Vital Stat Rep.* 2005;53(12):1–22

4. Centers for Disease Control and Prevention. State definitions and reporting requirements for live births, fetal deaths, and induced terminations of pregnancy. Hyattsville, MD: National Center for Health Statistics; 1997. Available at: www.cdc.gov/nchs/data/misc/itop97.pdf. Accessed July 7, 2015

5. American Academy of Pediatrics; American College of Obstetrics and Gynecology. Appendix F: standard terminology for reporting reproductive health statistics. In: *Guidelines for Perinatal Care.* 7th ed. Elk Grove Village, IL: American Academy of Pediatrics; 2012:497–512

6. Committee on Obstetric Practice. ACOG Committee opinion: perinatal and infant mortality statistics. Number 167, December 1995. *Int J Gynaecol Obstet.* 1996;53(1):86–88

7. World Health Organization. *International Statistical Classification of Diseases and Related Health Problems,* Tenth Revision. Vol 2. Geneva, Switzerland: World Health Organization; 2006

8. World Health Organization. *Neonatal and Perinatal Mortality: Country, Regional and Global Estimates.* Geneva, Switzerland: World Health Organization; 2006

9. Martin JA, Hoyert DL. The National Fetal Death File. *Semin Perinatol.* 2002;26(1):3–11

10. Centers for Disease Control and Prevention; National Center for Health Statistics. Model State Vital Statistics Act and Regulations: 1992 revision. Hyattsville, MD: National Center for Health Statistics; 1994. Available at: www.cdc.gov/nchs/data/misc/mvsact92b.pdf. Accessed July 7, 2015

11. Centers for Disease Control and Prevention; National Center for Health Statistics. 2003 Revisions of the U.S. Standard Certificates of Live Birth and Death and the Fetal Death Report. Hyattsville, MD: National Center for Health Statistics; 2014. Available at: www.cdc.gov/nchs/nvss/vital_certificate_revisions.htm. Accessed July 7, 2015

12. American College of Obstetricians and Gynecologists. ACOG Practice Bulletin No. 102: management of stillbirth. *Obstet Gynecol.* 2009;113(3):748–761

Standardization of Inpatient Handoff Communication

- *Clinical Report*

CLINICAL REPORT   Guidance for the Clinician in Rendering Pediatric Care

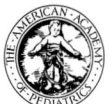

American Academy
of Pediatrics

DEDICATED TO THE HEALTH OF ALL CHILDREN™

Standardization of Inpatient Handoff Communication

Jennifer A. Jewell, MD, FAAP, COMMITTEE ON HOSPITAL CARE

abstract

Handoff communication is identified as an integral part of hospital care. Throughout medical communities, inadequate handoff communication is being highlighted as a significant risk to patients. The complexity of hospitals and the number of providers involved in the care of hospitalized patients place inpatients at high risk of communication lapses. This miscommunication and the potential resulting harm make effective handoffs more critical than ever. Although hospitalized patients are being exposed to many handoffs each day, this report is limited to describing the best handoff practices between providers at the time of shift change.

This document is copyrighted and is property of the American Academy of Pediatrics and its Board of Directors. All authors have filed conflict of interest statements with the American Academy of Pediatrics. Any conflicts have been resolved through a process approved by the Board of Directors. The American Academy of Pediatrics has neither solicited nor accepted any commercial involvement in the development of the content of this publication.

Clinical reports from the American Academy of Pediatrics benefit from expertise and resources of liaisons and internal (AAP) and external reviewers. However, clinical reports from the American Academy of Pediatrics may not reflect the views of the liaisons or the organizations or government agencies that they represent.

The guidance in this report does not indicate an exclusive course of treatment or serve as a standard of medical care. Variations, taking into account individual circumstances, may be appropriate.

All clinical reports from the American Academy of Pediatrics automatically expire 5 years after publication unless reaffirmed, revised, or retired at or before that time.

DOI: 10.1542/peds.2016-2681

PEDIATRICS (ISSN Numbers: Print, 0031-4005; Online, 1098-4275).

Copyright © 2016 by the American Academy of Pediatrics

FINANCIAL DISCLOSURE: The author has indicated she does not have a financial relationship relevant to this article to disclose.

FUNDING: No external funding.

POTENTIAL CONFLICT OF INTEREST: The author has indicated she has no potential conflicts of interest to disclose.

To cite: Jewell JA and AAP COMMITTEE ON HOSPITAL CARE. Standardization of Inpatient Handoff Communication. *Pediatrics.* 2016;138(5):e20162681

INTRODUCTION

As inpatient care becomes increasingly complex, with complicated medical problems and large volumes of information to transmit, appropriate and efficient communication among physicians is more critical than ever. According to The Joint Commission, communication breakdowns are estimated to contribute to 80% of medical errors.[1] Handoffs involve sending and receiving complete information that assists in communication of patient care responsibilities. Handoffs occur in multiple settings and among various providers, including either in-house or on-call coverage for hospitalized patients. Shift changes among physicians protect against sleep deprivation and allow for the informal review of clinical dilemmas, but they also present risks for communication failures and potential medical errors.

The medical literature indicates that handoffs can be improved[2–4] and that structured/standardized communication facilitates handoffs among group members and between shifts.[5,6] Although much of the literature focuses on trainees at academic centers, the research has widespread implications on the importance of handoffs for physicians in all fields and at all levels of training. In 1 study, the implementation of a standard handoff process among trainees decreased preventable medical errors by 30%.[7]

Many mnemonics have been developed to remind physicians about the key components of handoff communication[8,9] and these include pediatric-specific content, such as custody arrangements and social factors. In addition, maintaining a sign-out environment free of distractions and using available information technology tools can improve the efficiency and quality of information transfer.[5,10,11]

As The Joint Commission, regulators, public and private payers, physician professional organizations, and hospitals attempt to curb medical errors, there is an intense focus on handoff communication. Studies have challenged the typical belief that handoffs between physicians are efficient and effective[12] and that handoffs between experienced providers are better than between trainees.[13] Although all transitions of care benefit from appropriate handoffs, this clinical report aims to guide shift-change communication for inpatient handoffs between providers of the same service. The report also aims to improve patient care by identifying best practices for physicians who provide direct clinical care to pediatric patients in the inpatient or critical care unit. Similar principles apply to all transitions of care between units and services within a hospital (eg, PICU to pediatric ward or emergency department to pediatric ward) and at the time of discharge. However, each of these transitions has its own set of additional concerns that are not addressed in this clinical report. Throughout this report, the terms "handoff" and "sign-out" will be used interchangeably.

A new policy statement from the Committee on Pediatric Emergency Medicine of the American Academy of Pediatrics, the Pediatric Emergency Medicine Committee of the American College of Emergency Physicians, and the Pediatric Committee of the Emergency Nurses Association

entitled "Handoffs: Transitions of Care for Children in the Emergency Department" has been published simultaneously in this issue of the Journal (http://www.pediatrics.org/cgi/doi/10.1542/peds.2016-2680).

ROLE OF STANDARDIZATION

Depending on physicians' needs and responsibilities, handoff content will vary, requiring customization by individual physician groups; there is no "one size fits all" content. Once a group agrees on its customized content and processes, communication improves when the handoffs are standardized within a group. The data that are deemed important to transmit between providers during shift changes differ[14] depending on the medical discipline, role in patient care (primary service versus consulting service), setting, and medical/social complexity.[15,16] For example, the primary service needs a complete picture of the patient's overall condition, whereas the consulting service typically exchanges more focused information. Although variability between physician groups is understandable, the need for standardization within a group is undeniable.[14–16] Standardization can help the sender and receiver communicate essential data. Much attention is placed on the content of handoffs; however, equally important are standardized processes for handoffs.

Content

The content of handoffs includes information from the sender to the receiver that is needed to provide complete and seamless care. Although the complexity of patients, provider experience, and institutional factors dictate much of the oral handoff content, certain data should be conveyed in written form or be readily available (ie, in the electronic

medical record) for patients and often include the following[5,6,14,16,17]:

1. Demographic characteristics: name, medical record number, age, weight, sex, room number
2. Problem list with diagnoses and active medical issues
3. Code status
4. Medications (including oxygen, respiratory treatments, intravenous fluids, and "as needed" medications)
5. Allergies
6. Brief hospital course
7. Severity of illness
8. Pertinent history (medical, surgical, social)
9. Consulting providers
10. Tubes, lines, airways, and drains
11. Recent vital signs, including pain control
12. Diet
13. Activity, including weight-bearing status and fall risk
14. Social issues: custody arrangements, family discord
15. Action list
    ○ Pending studies (especially those requiring immediate intervention)
    ○ Tasks to be completed
16. Potential and anticipated clinical problems and contingency planning
17. Summary statement with attention to patient care/discharge goals for the hospitalization and shift, if applicable

To assist the sender with completeness and organization of the relevant information, many groups use a checklist, a structured template, and/or an acronym or mnemonic. This report does not endorse any particular acronym, but it will review technology options that may enhance handoff content. Ideally, effective and efficient handoffs combine printed materials (automatically populated by the electronic medical record, if possible) with written and verbal content. By using an automatically populated form, including much of the content details (eg, items 1–14 above), physicians may focus on the intricacies of patients' treatment and contingency plans. Individual services, hospital units, and institutions may collaborate with their quality and safety officers, residency programs, and information technology staff to determine particular approaches and optimal communication tools for specific patient populations. These tools should promote the inclusion of key factors, avoid unnecessary details, and promote a standardized handoff process.

In addition to sign-outs of individual patients, many physicians are responsible for the well-being of the units and the hospital during their shifts. Discussions between physicians about the capacity of the units and the hospital, the acuity of all patients, and any potential surge in capacity or acuity should be transmitted during handoffs.

Processes

In addition to standardized content, the processes used to transmit information may strongly influence the success of handoff communication. These processes should focus on certain human factors shown to improve performance during handoffs, regardless of discipline, and include the following[4,15-18]:

1. A consistent location and dedicated time, free of nonemergency interruptions. By ensuring that the location of sign-outs is consistent, the sender, receiver, and other members of the care team consciously and subconsciously identify that handoff communication is in process and eventually will recognize its importance. Requesting that others not interrupt the process and that nonurgent matters wait until handoffs are complete encourages the participants to remain fully engaged and focused on the task of transitioning care. Sign-outs are best conducted in a quiet environment, free from distractions. Barring extreme circumstances, operating rooms are an inappropriate location to conduct change-of-shift sign-outs; however, other types of handoffs between physicians (ie, between anesthesiologists) in the operating room are the standard of care.

2. Include other medical staff (eg, nurses and house staff) and patients/families for high-acuity or complex patients.[19] High-acuity and complex patients (eg, in the ICUs) benefit from including other team members in the handoff process. In doing so, all individuals appreciate that a new physician has assumed care of the patient, and it is an ideal time to address changes and ongoing concerns and to directly observe the patient's clinical status. Having multidisciplinary teams at the patient's bedside makes the patient and family aware that a new provider has assumed care, allows the patient and family to voice changes in care or status, and updates the patient and family with new information from the previous shift. When able and willing, patients and families may be present and encouraged to actively participate at the end of bedside handoffs.[20] Bedside sign-out is not be equated with simply introducing patients and families to oncoming physicians.

3. Make handoffs an active, real-time process. Sign-outs ideally are conducted in person (face-to-face), when possible, and include oral and written (or electronic) transmission of data. If face-to-face handoffs are not feasible, real-time communication (via phone or video-conferencing) is suggested. Written handoffs or audio messages, without the opportunity for oral communication and real-time dialog between providers, increase the potential for incomplete or unclear assessments and plans to be passed on to the next physician.[21] The optimal sign-out process offers the receiver an opportunity to ask questions. The use of read-back and verifying communication from the receiver to the sender increases the likelihood that all relevant information is transmitted and understood by the receiver. Any patient information that is transmitted by text or e-mail, including sign-outs, requires encryption to avoid violating the privacy rule of the Health Insurance Portability and Accountability Act (Pub L No. 104-191, 110 Stat. 1936 [1996]).

4. Identify the clear delineation of care responsibility from the sending to the receiving physician. The sender and receiver of handoff communication need to clearly identify when the transition of patient care is complete so that multiple physicians are not actively making clinical decisions and placing orders simultaneously. An explicit understanding of tasks assigned to the sending and receiving physicians (eg, phoning a consultant) after sign-out decreases confusion and frustration.

ROLE OF TECHNOLOGY

Technology provides a means to standardize the content for handoffs[15] and to decrease illegible writing.[10] Web-based applications have been used to decrease variability.[11] Even more complete handoffs are possible when the electronic medical record is linked automatically to handoff tools and includes demographic data, problem lists, code status, medications, allergies, consultants, historical and social information, and recent study results.[22,23] A mechanism to electronically attach contingency plans for clinical deterioration, pending studies needing review, and tasks requiring completion (without incorporating these into the permanent medical record) further enhances the handoff communication.[14,22] Some of the content standardization may be possible with existing technology, but others may require novel features developed in conjunction with electronic medical record companies, information technology leaders, and hospital administrators; for instance, an organization may construct a sign-out template in a given format for use throughout the institution. Depending on the hospital, handoff tools may be completely separate from the electronic medical record or they may be embedded within the electronic medical record. Electronic tools risk the transmission of excessive information, including outdated and inaccurate information. Cutting or copying and pasting from previous notes into a handout tool increases the likelihood of passing on irrelevant, outdated, or inaccurate information.

REVIEW PATIENT INFORMATION

Handoffs provide a mechanism to review laboratory and radiographic studies and to discuss difficult diagnoses and challenging patients. Because handoffs are conducted among colleagues, they are a routine, expected, nonthreatening, and natural way to review diagnostic and treatment plans between each shift. Collegial relationships between the sender and the receiver improve handoff communication.[18] By using

this time to "consult" with other providers, patient care is reviewed by multiple team members, errors are more likely to be recognized,[16] and unnecessary delays in diagnosis or treatment may be avoided.

FINANCIAL SUPPORT

Because most handoffs do not involve direct face-to-face patient contact and are not documented in the medical record, direct billing for these services is problematic. Other factors, including physician payment structure, will encourage or discourage appropriate handoffs.[16] For salaried physicians, schedules should include overlap time between outgoing and oncoming physician shifts to decrease the likelihood that quality handoffs are disincentivized. In addition, effective handoff communication may be identified as a performance-based quality metric for groups with quality withholds and/or incentives.

TRAINING AND MONITORING HANDOFF COMMUNICATION

Residency training programs have understood the importance of handoff communication for decades. However, the Accreditation Council on Graduate Medical Education heightened its attention to handoffs as duty hours were implemented and later revised. Currently, the Accreditation Council on Graduate Medical Education states: "Sponsoring institutions and programs must ensure and monitor effective, structured handover processes to facilitate both continuity of care and patient safety. Programs must ensure that residents are competent in communicating with team members in the handover process." Some training programs have met this requirement by mandating lectures and learning modules for house staff. Other programs monitor the sign-out process and deem residents

"competent" when they master the requisite skills. In addition, training programs provide a captive study cohort for the investigation of novel handoff strategies. Most of the literature on effective handoff communication derives from resident training and education.[4–6,17] These activities may qualify for part 4 maintenance of certification requirements of the American Board of Pediatrics if the projects are conducted under the guidance of an American Board of Pediatrics–accredited organization. Because recent pediatric research shows that a standard approach to handoffs decreases medical errors in patients,[7] internal medicine and other adult training programs are likely to reinvigorate their sign-out education efforts.

After residency training, the importance of handoff communication continues, but educational and monitoring opportunities diminish. Handoff training may occur during the onboarding process for newly hired staff.[15] Assessing providers' satisfaction with the handoff process as a quality measure and directly observing handoffs as part of ongoing quality improvement are advised.[14] Real-time feedback between senders and receivers also encourages and enhances handoff communication. To guide handoff deficiencies and to track communication failures, continuous quality-improvement methods may be used. Because research confirms that a standard approach to sign-out among trainees increases patient safety, attending physician education and training in handoff best practices may similarly enhance patient safety.

SUMMARY

1. Handoffs improve when communication is standardized by and within individual physician groups. Individual groups may

customize their sign-out process and content to meet their needs, patient needs, organizational culture, and available technology support.

2. The process of receiving and sending handoffs is optimized when sign-out is an active procedure, without interruptions, in a dedicated place, and at a dedicated time. Receiving physicians benefit from having the ability to ask questions and understand a patient's clinical course and social factors, including past and ongoing concerns. Anticipating problems and discussing interventions are recognized as a central part of effective handoff communication.

3. Computer technology can be used to improve the accuracy of handoff information. For providers who use electronic medical records, the bulk of content information is often available on computers. Providers may maximize their efficiency by conducting handoffs with the use of established technological resources and developing new, locally specific, customizable solutions. Oral and/or written sign-out is meant to complement the comprehensive patient information available in the electronic medical record, with a focus on anticipated problems and contingency planning. Exchanging too much, too little, or inaccurate data during handoffs increases patient risk.

4. Handoffs allow a time to review clinical events and studies. In addition, handoffs are an ideal time to seek advice, insight, and consultation about patients with challenging medical conditions from colleagues.

5. Time and administrative support for handoffs should be included in physicians' working hours.

6. Handoff communication is a skill requiring training and practice.

Attending physicians are likely to benefit from ongoing training and monitoring of a standard approach to handoffs.

LEAD AUTHOR

Jennifer A. Jewell, MD, FAAP

COMMITTEE ON HOSPITAL CARE, 2014–2015

Jack M. Percelay, MD, MPH, FAAP
Vanessa L. Hill, MD, FAAP
Jennifer A. Jewell, MD, FAAP
Claudia K. Preuschoff, MD, FAAP
Daniel A. Rauch, MD, FAAP
Richard A. Salerno, MD, MS, FAAP

CONSULTANTS

Charles Vinocur, MD, FAAP
Matthew Scanlon, MD, FAAP
Martin K. Wakeham, MD, FAAP

LIAISONS

Barbara Romito, MA, CCLS
Gloria Lukasiewicz, RN, BSN, MS

STAFF

Niccole Alexander, MPP

REFERENCES

1. Joint Commission Center for Transforming Healthcare releases targeted solutions tool for hand-off communications. *Jt Comm Perspect.* 2012;32(8):1, 3

2. Burton MC, Kashiwagi DT, Kirkland LL, Manning D, Varkey P. Gaining efficiency and satisfaction in the handoff process. *J Hosp Med.* 2010;5(9):547–552

3. Hinami K, Farnan JM, Meltzer DO, Arora VM. Understanding communication during hospitalist service changes: a mixed methods study. *J Hosp Med.* 2009;4(9):535–540

4. Sinha M, Shriki J, Salness R, Blackburn PA. Need for standardized sign-out in the emergency department: a survey of emergency medicine residency and pediatric emergency medicine fellowship program directors. *Acad Emerg Med.* 2007;14(2):192–196

5. Arora V, Johnson J, Lovinger D, Humphrey HJ, Meltzer DO. Communication failures in patient sign-out and suggestions for improvement: a critical incident analysis. *Qual Saf Health Care.* 2005;14(6):401–407

6. Starmer AJ, Sectish TC, Simon DW, et al. Rates of medical errors and preventable adverse events among hospitalized children following implementation of a resident handoff bundle. *JAMA.* 2013;310(21):2262–2270

7. Starmer AJ, Spector ND, Srivastava R, et al; I-PASS Study Group. Changes in medical errors after implementation of a handoff program. *N Engl J Med.* 2014;371(19):1803–1812

8. Riesenberg LA, Leitzsch J, Little BW. Systematic review of handoff mnemonics literature. *Am J Med Qual.* 2009;24(3):196–204

9. Starmer AJ, Spector ND, Srivastava R, Allen AD, Landrigan CP, Sectish TC; I-PASS Study Group. I-pass, a mnemonic to standardize verbal handoffs. *Pediatrics.* 2012;129(2):201–204

10. American College of Obstetricians and Gynecologists. ACOG Committee Opinion No. 517: communication strategies for patient handoffs. *Obstet Gynecol.* 2012;119(2 pt 1):408–411

11. Payne CE, Stein JM, Leong T, Dressler DD. Avoiding handover fumbles: a controlled trial of a structured handover tool versus traditional handover methods. *BMJ Qual Saf.* 2012;21(11):925–932

12. Chang VY, Arora VM, Lev-Ari S, D'Arcy M, Keysar B. Interns overestimate the effectiveness of their hand-off communication. *Pediatrics.* 2010;125(3):491–496

13. Horwitz LI, Rand D, Staisiunas P, et al. Development of a handoff evaluation tool for shift-to-shift physician handoffs: the Handoff CEX. *J Hosp Med.* 2013;8(4):191–200

14. Arora V, Johnson J. A model for building a standardized hand-off protocol. *Jt Comm J Qual Patient Saf.* 2006;32(11):646–655

15. Arora VM, Manjarrez E, Dressler DD, Basaviah P, Halasyamani L, Kripalani S. Hospitalist handoffs: a systematic review and task force recommendations. *J Hosp Med.* 2009;4(7):433–440

16. Cheung DS, Kelly JJ, Beach C, et al; Section of Quality Improvement

and Patient Safety, American College of Emergency Physicians. Improving handoffs in the emergency department. *Ann Emerg Med.* 2010;55(2):171–180

17. Dhingra KR, Elms A, Hobgood C. Reducing error in the emergency department: a call for standardization of the sign-out process. *Ann Emerg Med.* 2010;56(6):637–642

18. Manser T, Foster S, Gisin S, Jaeckel D, Ummenhofer W. Assessing the quality of patient handoffs at care transitions. *Qual Saf Health Care.* 2010;19(6):e44

19. Joy BF, Elliott E, Hardy C, Sullivan C, Backer CL, Kane JM. Standardized multidisciplinary protocol improves handover of cardiac surgery patients to the intensive care unit. *Pediatr Crit Care Med.* 2011;12(3):304–308

20. Gosdin CH, Vaughn L. Perceptions of physician bedside handoff with nurse and family involvement. *Hosp Pediatr.* 2012;2(1):34–38

21. Fogerty RL, Schoenfeld A, Salim Al-Damluji M, Horwitz LI. Effectiveness of written hospitalist sign-outs in answering overnight inquiries. *J Hosp Med.* 2013;8(11):609–614

22. Kim GR, Lehmann CU; Council on Clinical Information Technology. Pediatric aspects of inpatient health information technology systems [published correction appears in *Pediatrics.* 2009;123(2):604]. *Pediatrics.* 2008;122(6). Available at: www.pediatrics.org/cgi/content/full/122/6/e1287

23. Palma JP, Sharek PJ, Longhurst CA. Impact of electronic medical record integration of a handoff tool on sign-out in a newborn intensive care unit. *J Perinatol.* 2011;31(5):311–317

Substance Use Screening, Brief Intervention, and Referral to Treatment

- *Policy Statement*

POLICY STATEMENT Organizational Principles to Guide and Define the Child Health
Care System and/or Improve the Health of all Children

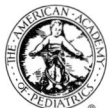

American Academy
of Pediatrics

DEDICATED TO THE HEALTH OF ALL CHILDREN™

Substance Use Screening, Brief Intervention, and Referral to Treatment

COMMITTEE ON SUBSTANCE USE AND PREVENTION

abstract

The enormous public health impact of adolescent substance use and its preventable morbidity and mortality show the need for the health care sector, including pediatricians and the medical home, to increase its capacity related to substance use prevention, detection, assessment, and intervention. The American Academy of Pediatrics published its policy statement "Substance Use Screening, Brief Intervention, and Referral to Treatment for Pediatricians" in 2011 to introduce the concepts and terminology of screening, brief intervention, and referral to treatment (SBIRT) and to offer clinical guidance about available substance use screening tools and intervention procedures. This policy statement is a revision of the 2011 SBIRT statement. An accompanying clinical report updates clinical guidance for adolescent SBIRT.

DOI: 10.1542/peds.2016-1210

PEDIATRICS (ISSN Numbers: Print, 0031-4005; Online, 1098-4275).

FINANCIAL DISCLOSURE: The authors have indicated they do not have a financial relationship relevant to this article to disclose.

FUNDING: No external funding.

POTENTIAL CONFLICT OF INTEREST: Dr Levy has indicated she has a copyright relationship with Boston Children's Hospital.

To cite: AAP COMMITTEE ON SUBSTANCE USE AND PREVENTION. Substance Use Screening, Brief Intervention, and Referral to Treatment. *Pediatrics.* 2016;138(1):e20161210

BACKGROUND

Substance use has an enormous direct and indirect public health impact on children and teenagers, ranging from prenatal exposure and complicated pregnancy outcomes to significant morbidity and mortality among adolescents and, over time, contributing to the development of many other health problems and substance use disorders. Pediatricians play a vital longitudinal role in the lives of adolescents and are uniquely positioned to effect change in adolescent patients' health knowledge, behaviors, and well-being. Guidance about substance use can be provided in many forms: preventing or delaying the onset of substance use in lower-risk patients, discouraging ongoing use and reducing harm in intermediate-risk patients, and referring patients who have developed substance use disorders for potentially life-saving treatment.

The recommendations in *Bright Futures: Guidelines for Health Supervision of Infants, Children, and Adolescents*[1] highlight the pediatrician's unique role in addressing health behavior problems throughout adolescence. Because most adolescents (83%) have contact with a physician annually, consider physicians an authoritative source of knowledge about alcohol and drugs, and are receptive to discussing substance use, medical care encounters are tremendous opportunities for addressing substance use.[2,3] The Substance Abuse and Mental Health Services Administration recommends universal screening for substance use, brief intervention, and/or referral to treatment (SBIRT) as part of routine health care.[2] Adolescents are the age group at greatest risk of experiencing substance use–related acute[3] and chronic[4] health consequences and, as such, also are most likely to derive the greatest benefit from universal SBIRT. Specific SBIRT screening tools and intervention strategies have well-documented efficacy for adult alcohol use, but fewer studies of SBIRT efficacy have been conducted in adolescents.[5–7] On the basis of a review of the limited research literature available in 2014, the US Preventive Services Task Force concluded that the evidence was insufficient to assess the efficacy of brief interventions to reduce adolescent substance use.[8,9] Despite this early conclusion, the low cost of SBIRT, minimal potential for harm, and emerging study results together support the tremendous potential for a population-level benefit from even small reductions in substance use and provide sufficient basis for the incorporation of SBIRT practices into the medical care standards for adolescents. The accompanying clinical report[10] contains clinical guidance for pediatricians and other clinicians who provide health care for adolescents.

RECOMMENDATIONS

The American Academy of Pediatrics recommends that pediatricians:

- increase their capacity in substance use detection, assessment, and intervention; and

- become familiar with adolescent SBIRT practices and their potential to be incorporated into universal screening and comprehensive care of adolescents in the medical home.

The American Academy of Pediatrics advocates for:

- the strong support of continued research to determine the most effective brief intervention strategies applicable to adolescent health care,

- health insurance providers to:

  o promote and pay for standard screening and brief intervention practices incorporated into medical home health maintenance appointments; and

  o ensure a standard mechanism for payment for confidential follow-up care of adolescents to receive continuity of care for substance use disorders; and

- parity of access and services for adolescent mental health and substance use disorder treatment compared with general adolescent care and adult health care.

LEAD AUTHORS

Sharon J.L. Levy, MD, MPH, FAAP
Janet F. Williams, MD, FAAP

COMMITTEE ON SUBSTANCE USE AND PREVENTION, 2015–2016

Sheryl A. Ryan, MD, FAAP, Chairperson
Pamela K. Gonzalez, MD, MS, FAAP
Stephen W. Patrick, MD, MPH, MS, FAAP
Joanna Quigley, MD, FAAP
Lorena Siqueira, MD, MSPH, FAAP
Leslie R. Walker, MD, FAAP

FORMER COMMITTEE MEMBERS

Sharon J.L. Levy, MD, MPH, FAAP
Janet F. Williams, MD, FAAP

LIAISONS

Vivian B. Faden, PhD – *National Institute of Alcohol Abuse and Alcoholism*
Gregory Tau, MD, PhD – *American Academy of Child and Adolescent Psychiatry*

STAFF

Renee Jarrett, MPH

ABBREVIATION

SBIRT: screening, brief intervention, and referral to treatment

REFERENCES

1. Hagan JF, Shaw JS, Duncan P, eds. *Bright Futures: Guidelines for Health Supervision of Infants, Children, and Adolescents.* 3rd ed. Elk Grove Village, IL: American Academy of Pediatrics; 2008

2. Substance Abuse and Mental Health Services Administration. Screening, brief intervention, and referral to treatment. Available at: www.samhsa.gov/sbirt. Accessed June 3, 2015

3. Centers for Disease Control and Prevention. Injury prevention and control: motor vehicles. Teen drivers: get the facts. Available at: www.cdc.gov/MotorVehicleSafety/Teen_Drivers/teendrivers_factsheet.html. Accessed June 3, 2015

4. Hingson RW, Heeren T, Winter MR. Age at drinking onset and alcohol dependence: age at onset, duration, and severity. *Arch Pediatr Adolesc Med.* 2006;160(7):739–746

5. Jonas DE, Garbutt JC, Halle RA, et al. *Behavioral Counseling After Screening for Alcohol Misuse in Primary Care: A Systematic Review and Meta-Analysis for the U.S. Preventive Services Task Force.* Rockville, MD: US Preventive Services Task Force; 2012. Available at: www.uspreventiveservicestaskforce.org/uspstf12/alcmisuse/alcomisart.htm. Accessed June 3, 2015

6. Babor TF, McRee BG, Kassebaum PA, Grimaldi PL, Ahmed K, Bray J. Screening, brief intervention, and referral to treatment (SBIRT): toward a public health approach to the management of substance abuse. *Subst Abus.* 2007;28(3):7–30

7. Madras BK, Compton WM, Avula D, Stegbauer T, Stein JB, Clark HW. Screening, brief interventions, referral to treatment (SBIRT) for illicit drug and alcohol use at multiple healthcare sites: comparison at intake and 6 months later. *Drug Alcohol Depend.* 2009;99(1–3):280–295

8. Moyer VA; US Preventive Services Task Force. Primary care behavioral interventions to reduce illicit drug

and nonmedical pharmaceutical use in children and adolescents: U.S. Preventive Services Task Force recommendation statement. *Ann Intern Med.* 2014;160(9):634–639

9. US Preventive Services Task Force. *Screening and Behavioral Counseling Interventions in Primary Care to Reduce Alcohol Misuse: Recommendation Statement.* AHRQ Publication No. 12-05171-EF-3. Rockville, MD: US Preventive Services Task Force; 2013. Available at: www.uspreventiveservicestaskforce.org/uspstf12/alcmisuse/alcmisuserfinalrs.htm. Accessed June 3, 2015

10. Levy S, Williams JF; American Academy of Pediatrics, Committee on Substance Abuse. Clinical report: substance use screening, brief intervention, and referral to treatment. *Pediatrics.* 2016

Substance Use Screening, Brief Intervention, and Referral to Treatment

- *Clinical Report*

CLINICAL REPORT Guidance for the Clinician in Rendering Pediatric Care

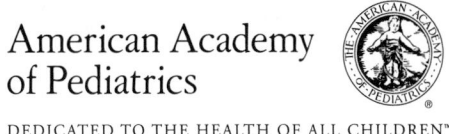

American Academy
of Pediatrics

DEDICATED TO THE HEALTH OF ALL CHILDREN™

Substance Use Screening, Brief Intervention, and Referral to Treatment

Sharon J.L. Levy, MD, MPH, FAAP, Janet F. Williams, MD, FAAP, COMMITTEE ON SUBSTANCE USE AND PREVENTION

abstract

The enormous public health impact of adolescent substance use and its preventable morbidity and mortality highlight the need for the health care sector, including pediatricians and the medical home, to increase its capacity regarding adolescent substance use screening, brief intervention, and referral to treatment (SBIRT). The American Academy of Pediatrics first published a policy statement on SBIRT and adolescents in 2011 to introduce SBIRT concepts and terminology and to offer clinical guidance about available substance use screening tools and intervention procedures. This clinical report provides a simplified adolescent SBIRT clinical approach that, in combination with the accompanying updated policy statement, guides pediatricians in implementing substance use prevention, detection, assessment, and intervention practices across the varied clinical settings in which adolescents receive health care.

DOI: 10.1542/peds.2016-1211

PEDIATRICS (ISSN Numbers: Print, 0031-4005; Online, 1098-4275).

Copyright © 2016 by the American Academy of Pediatrics

FINANCIAL DISCLOSURE: The authors have indicated they do not have a financial relationship relevant to this article to disclose.

FUNDING: No external funding.

POTENTIAL CONFLICT OF INTEREST: Dr. Levy has indicated she has a copyright relationship with Boston's Children's Hospital.

To cite: Levy SJ, Williams JF, AAP COMMITTEE ON SUBSTANCE USE AND PREVENTION. Substance Use Screening, Brief Intervention, and Referral to Treatment. Pediatrics. 2016;138(1): e20161211

INTRODUCTION

Adolescent substance use is an issue of critical importance to the American public. In 2011, a nationally representative household survey found that adults rated drug abuse as the number one health concern for adolescents.[1] These concerns are reflected in the *Healthy People 2020* objectives, which call for reducing teen substance use.[2] Alcohol, tobacco, and marijuana are the substances most often used by children and adolescents in the United States. Twenty-eight percent of students have tried alcohol by eighth grade, and 68.2% have tried alcohol by 12th grade. Twelve percent of eighth-graders and more than half of 12th-graders have been drunk at least once in their life.[3] Rates of marijuana use have increased substantially in recent years; in 2012, 45% of ninth- through 12th-graders reported ever using marijuana, and 24% reported marijuana use in the past 30 days.[4] Eight percent of teenagers reported using marijuana nearly every day, an increase of approximately 60% from 2008.[4] Decreases in tobacco use by high school students have plateaued since 2007; 41% of ninth- through 12th-graders reported having tried cigarettes and nearly one-quarter (22.4%)

reported current (past-30-day) use of tobacco in any form.[5] "Misuse" of prescription medication, especially stimulants and pain medications, continues among a substantial minority of adolescents (eg, 15% of 12th-graders[3]). Approximately half (50.4%) of 12th-graders have used any illicit drug (half of these, or 24.7%, reported the use of any illicit drug other than marijuana).[3]

Although it is common for adolescents and young adults to try psychoactive substances, it is important that this experimentation not be condoned, facilitated, or trivialized by adults. Even the first use of a psychoactive substance may result in tragic consequences, such as injury, victimization, or even fatality. Adolescence extends from approximately 12 years of age into the early 20s and is a time of intensive neurodevelopmental molding and maturation that confers greater neurodevelopmental vulnerability at a time during which risk-taking behaviors are generally more prevalent. Adolescents are particularly susceptible to risk-related injuries, including those associated with alcohol, tobacco, and other drug use.[6,7] Most alcohol and drug use consequences during adolescence are attributable not to addiction but to the fact that all substance use confers some amount of risk.[8] Substance use correlates with sexual risk-taking[9] and can complicate pregnancy outcomes. Other health complexities, such as having a chronic disease or disability, including intellectual disability, may increase an adolescent's vulnerability to both substance use and its consequences.[10,11] The neurodevelopmental changes during adolescence confer particular vulnerability to addictions.[12] The age at first substance use is inversely correlated with the lifetime incidence of developing a substance use disorder.[7,12] Adolescence is thus a most critical time period for

pediatricians, the medical home, and any other entity providing health advice to deliver clear and consistent messaging about abstaining from substance use.[13]

Bright Futures: Guidelines for Health Supervision of Infants, Children, and Adolescents[14] highlights the unique role of the pediatrician in addressing problem behaviors throughout the pediatric age range. Most adolescents (83%) have contact with a physician annually.[15] Adolescents consider physicians an authoritative source of knowledge about alcohol and drugs and are receptive to discussing substance use.[16] These findings underscore the tremendous opportunity for addressing substance use in primary care settings, the medical home, and other settings in which children and adolescents receive medical care and health advice.

The Substance Abuse and Mental Health Services Administration (SAMHSA) recommends universal substance use screening, brief intervention, and/or referral to treatment (SBIRT) as part of routine health care.[17] Capitalizing on opportunities to screen whenever and wherever adolescents receive medical care can increase the identification of risk behaviors and substance use. Because the adolescent age group is at the highest risk of experiencing substance use–related health consequences,[18] it is also the most likely to derive the most benefit from universal SBIRT. This clinical report, together with an update of the 2011 American Academy of Pediatrics (AAP) policy statement on SBIRT,[19] presents a simplified, practical clinical approach to support widespread implementation of research-informed SBIRT practices. Similar to any other patient interactions, SBIRT must be conducted with sensitivity to various patient population abilities, vulnerabilities, and needs, such as when adolescents have

chronic medical conditions or intellectual disabilities,[10,11] and with considerations to modify SBIRT techniques as needed to ensure relevance, comprehensibility, and reliability.

CONFIDENTIALITY

Confidentiality practices in the medical home are important facilitators to SBIRT practices and the care of an adolescent disclosing substance use. Protection of their confidential health care information is an essential determinant of whether adolescents will access care, answer questions honestly, and engage in and maintain a therapeutic alliance with health care professionals.[20,21] Adolescents may disclose substance use or other high-risk behaviors as a way to reveal that they want help or feel unsafe, possibly even in their own home, so a prime consideration for the pediatrician is whether maintaining confidentiality or disclosing confidential health information is in the patient's best interest.

Health care professional organizations guiding best practices in adolescent and young adult medical care, including the American Medical Association, the AAP, the American College of Obstetricians and Gynecologists, the American Academy of Family Physicians, and the Society for Adolescent Health and Medicine, have established position statements and recommendations guiding confidentiality and informed consent in this age group.[22,23] The AAP statement recommends that all children and adolescents receive comprehensive, confidential primary care, including indicated screenings, counseling, and physical and laboratory evaluations.[19] The Society for Adolescent Health and Medicine's position paper notes that participation of parents in the health care of their adolescents should usually be encouraged but not mandated.[22] The Center for Adolescent Health and the Law (CAHL.org) provides detailed information about each state's regulations that specify adolescent and parent rights, including adolescent confidentiality.

Confidentiality practices are best introduced to the patient and the parent(s) or legal guardian simultaneously before the first time the teen or "tween" (preadolescent) patient is interviewed without a parent present or when an adolescent is new to a pediatrician's practice. The "limit" to maintaining confidentiality relies on the pediatrician's clinical judgment of the need to prevent imminent harm to the patient or someone else and to protect the patient's health and safety. Adolescents often express relief that their parents will be informed of serious problems, although they may have preferences about how the information is presented. By first informing the adolescent that confidentiality can no longer be upheld and then strategizing about the disclosure, the pediatrician, with the adolescent's permission, or the patient, together with the pediatrician, can transmit the necessary information to parents while simultaneously protecting the physician-patient bond. Whether or not the adolescent's substance use poses an acute safety risk, adolescents are likely to benefit from the support and involvement of their parents in accessing recommended services and accepting the care plan. Adolescents are unlikely to follow through with referrals without the support of an adult, and even more so if they are being referred for the evaluation or treatment of something they do not believe they have, such as a severe substance use disorder (SUD), or addiction. In many cases and certainly by the time an adolescent has developed an SUD, parents are already aware or at least highly suspect that their adolescent

is engaged in substance use, although they may underestimate the extent of use or the seriousness of the situation.[24] In addition, confidentiality, intervention, and treatment are potentially influenced by a parent's substance use or active substance use disorder. Advising the substance-using parent to speak with their own physician or to seek other assistance is likely to be helpful as the pediatrician begins to work with the substance-using adolescent.

Adolescents may be less resistant to breaking confidentiality if the pediatrician and the adolescent first discuss why the disclosure is necessary, what details will be disclosed, who will disclose the details, and how disclosure will help. Teenagers may be most concerned about protecting tangential details (ie, which friends were involved, how and where they obtained substances, etc), which might be possible to keep confidential when disclosure would not substantially change the safety plan. Adolescents may be willing to include their parent(s) in a discussion of recommendations, particularly if the concerns and recommendations can be presented in a way that emphasizes positive attributes, such as the adolescent's honesty, willingness to change behavior, and/ or acceptance of further evaluation or treatment. Adolescents who agree to accept a referral without notifying their parents may be able to access services available in the school or the community. Specific laws governing the need for parental consent for SUD treatment vary by state, so legal clarification is advised. Physicians should be aware that health insurance transactions can potentially jeopardize patient confidentiality and rapport with the patient and parent: for example, when a parent's insurance policy sends the policy holder (parent) an explanation of benefits with explicit diagnostic codes about the adolescent's care.

SCREENING

Screening is a procedure applied to populations to identify individuals or groups at risk of or with a disease, condition, or symptoms. Screening is conducted so that the results can form the basis for a corresponding care plan. The best screening tools are those containing the lowest number of succinct validated questions that can elicit accurate and reliable responses. Comprehensive biopsychosocial screening, including substance use screening, is a recommended component of routine adolescent health care. The HEEADSSS mnemonic, which stands for home environment, education and employment, eating, peer-related activities, drugs, sexuality, suicide/ depression, and safety from injury and violence,[25,26] is a frequently used framework to conduct a complete psychosocial interview with adolescents, as is the SSHADESS mnemonic, a strength- and resiliency-based tool. Whether the patient responds to a written or electronic survey or provider or medical assistant questioning, the "D" in these tools triggers screening about the patient's substance use but possibly also about use by their friends or household members.

The SBIRT screening goal is to define experience with substance use along a spectrum ranging from abstinence to addiction so that this information can be used to guide the next steps of the related clinical approach, or intervention (see Table 1). Screening results broadly inform clinical care: for example, alcohol and drug use may be the source of a presenting symptom or may interfere with prescribed medications and test results. The management of inattentiveness would be different if the physician learned that the patient used marijuana (a possible cause) or a stimulant drug (a prescribing risk). Awareness about the range of possible screening results allows the pediatrician to be prepared to

TABLE 1 Substance Use Spectrum and Goals for BI

Stage	Description	BI Goals
Abstinence	The time before an individual has ever used drugs or alcohol more than a few sips.	Prevent or delay initiation of substance use through positive reinforcement and patient/parent education.
Substance use without a disorder	Limited use, generally in social situations, without related problems. Typically, use occurs at predictable times, such as on weekends.	Advise to stop. Provide counseling regarding the medical harms of substance use. Promote patient strengths.
Mild–moderate SUD	Use in high-risk situations, such as when driving or with strangers. Use associated with a problem, such as a fight, arrest, or school suspension. Use for emotional regulation, such as to relieve stress or depression. Defined as meeting 2 to 5 of the 11 criteria for an SUD in the DSM-5.	Brief assessment to explore patient-perceived problems associated with use. Give clear, brief advice to quit. Provide counseling regarding the medical harms of substance use. Negotiate a behavior change to quit or cut down. Close patient follow-up. Consider referral to SUD treatment. Consider breaking confidentiality.
Severe SUD	Loss of control or compulsive drug use associated with neurologic changes in the reward system of the brain. Defined as meeting ≥6 of the 11 criteria for an SUD in the DSM-5.	As above. Involve parents in treatment planning whenever possible. Refer to the appropriate level of care. Follow up to ensure compliance with treatment and to offer continued support.

DSM-5, *Diagnostic and Statistical Manual of Mental Disorders, Fifth Edition.*

address the range of potential patient responses.

Pediatricians' self-reported rates of routine substance use screening vary from less than 50%[27,28] to 86%,[29] although few physicians reported using a validated screening tool,[30] and most relied on clinical impressions. The most frequently cited barriers to screening were lack of time,[31] insufficient training,[32] and lack of familiarity with standardized tools.[33] Experienced pediatricians have failed to detect mild, moderate, and sometimes even severe SUDs when relying on clinical impressions alone.[34] A recent study found that when a screening tool was not used, only one-third of youth who were engaged in "excessive alcohol use" were identified.[35]

An array of validated tools is available to conduct alcohol and other substance use screening and to guide assessment for use-related problems (Table 2). The effective incorporation of screening into the pediatric practice depends on pediatricians being knowledgeable about screening options and selecting and implementing the tools most suitable for routine use in their particular care settings and patient population(s), including vulnerable patients in their care. Alcohol-only screening may be most useful with younger children, when time is very limited or when alcohol use is a particular concern. The AAP-endorsed National Institute on Alcoholism and Alcohol Abuse's "Youth Guide"[36] provides clinicians with an age-based schema to ask patients about the frequency of their drinking and their friends' drinking in the past year and to correlate the respective responses with the current and future risk of having an alcohol use disorder. The BSTAD (Brief Screener for Tobacco, Alcohol and other Drugs)[37] uses highly sensitive and specific cutoffs to identify various SUDs among adolescents 12 to 17 years of age: ≥6 days of past-year use for tobacco and >1 day of past-year use for alcohol or marijuana.[37] The Screening to Brief Intervention (S2BI) tool[38] uses a stem question and forced-response options (none, once or twice, monthly, and weekly or more)

in a sequence to reveal the frequency of past-year use of tobacco, alcohol, marijuana, and 5 other classes of substances most commonly used by adolescents (Table 3). The S2BI tool is highly sensitive and specific in discriminating among clinically relevant use-risk categories and therefore is remarkably efficient in its ability to detect severe SUDs aligned with criteria from the *Diagnostic and Statistical Manual of Mental Disorders, Fifth Edition*[39] (Table 4). Although the S2BI is not a formal diagnostic instrument, the patient's response to the question about the frequency of use in the past year correlates closely with the present likelihood of having an SUD, as follows: used "once or twice" correlates with no SUD, uses "monthly" correlates with mild or moderate SUD, and uses "weekly or more" correlates with a severe SUD (Fig 1). The CRAFFT (Car, Relax, Alone, Friends/Family, Forget, Trouble)[40] tool originally was validated to screen for substance use risk by scoring each patient's "yes" or "no" responses to 6 questions, but using the tool as an assessment to explore "yes" responses and to reveal the extent of the patient's substance use–related problems may be more effective for gathering details for use in SBIRT intervention.

Incorporating screening into the patient care visit logically assumes that the spectrum of possible screening outcomes will be addressed by using effective approaches and available resources most suitable for the particular patient population and locale. Options for pediatricians to respond to adolescent substance use screening results and to facilitate care are described by a range of "brief intervention and referral to treatment" practices.

BRIEF INTERVENTION

Brief intervention (BI) is a conversation that focuses on

encouraging healthy choices so that the risk behaviors are prevented, reduced, or stopped. In the context of SBIRT, regardless of which substance use screening tools are used, the BI strategy is identical, because it is a direct response to the reported substance use severity. BI encompasses a spectrum of potential pediatrician responses, including positive reinforcement for adolescents reporting no substance use; brief, medically based advice for those reporting use but showing no evidence of an SUD; brief motivational interventions when a mild or moderate SUD is revealed; and referral to treatment of those with a severe SUD. Using motivation-enhancing principles is compatible with all BI dialogue regarding any level of substance use and risk.

Among adolescents presenting to an ED for a substance use–related problem, BI has been shown to reduce subsequent alcohol use,[43] marijuana use,[44] and associated problems[45] and to be cost-effective compared with brief education.[46] Several BI models have been evaluated in primary care: structured intervention "5A's,"[47] "CHAT,"[48] intervention with follow-up "Healthy Choices,"[49] "MOMENT,"[50] and therapist-delivered versus computer-delivered BI.[51] All of these models have been modestly successful in showing reductions in substance use and related consequences and/or risky behaviors, although 1 trial found similar substance use reductions in both experimental and control groups.[50] Physician-implemented BI is acceptable to both teenagers[16] and clinicians.[52] Although a recent US Preventive Services Task Force[53] review found insufficient scientific basis to recommend any particular BI for addressing adolescent substance use, this clinical report reviews the current literature base to summarize expert opinion about practical BI strategies.

TABLE 2 Substance Use Screening and Assessment Tools Used With Adolescents

	Description
Brief screens	
S2BI (Screening to Brief Intervention)[38]	Single frequency-of-use question per substance
	Identifies the likelihood of a DSM-5 SUD
	Includes tobacco, alcohol, marijuana, and other/illicit drug use
	Discriminates among no use, no SUD, moderate SUD, and severe SUD
	Electronic medical record compatible
	Self- or interviewer-administered
BSTAD (Brief Screener for Tobacco, Alcohol, and Other Drugs)[37]	Identifies problematic tobacco, alcohol, and marijuana use
	Built on the NIAAA screening tool with added tobacco and "drug" questions
	Electronic medical record compatible
	Self- or interviewer-administered
NIAAA Youth Alcohol Screen (Youth Guide)[36]	Two-question alcohol screen
	Screens for friends' use and for personal use in children and adolescents aged ≥9 y
	Free resource: http://pubs.niaaa.nih.gov/publications/Practitioner/YouthGuide/YouthGuide.pdf
Brief assessment guides	
CRAFFT (Car, Relax, Alone, Friends/Family, Forget, Trouble)[40]	Quickly assesses for problems associated with substance use
	Not a diagnostic tool
GAIN (Global Appraisal of Individual Needs)[41]	Assesses for both SUDs and mental health disorders
AUDIT (Alcohol Use Disorders Identification Test)[42]	Assesses for risky drinking
	Not a diagnostic tool

Adapted with permission from American Academy of Pediatrics; Levy S, Bagley S. Substance use: initial approach in primary care. In: Adam HM, Foy JM, eds. Signs and Symptoms in Pediatrics. Elk Grove Village, IL: American Academy of Pediatrics; 2015:887–900. DSM-5, *Diagnostic and Statistical Manual of Mental Disorders, Fifth Edition*; NIAAA, National Institute on Alcohol Abuse and Alcoholism.

No Substance Use: Positive Reinforcement

It has been recommended that adolescents reporting no substance use (whether tobacco, alcohol, or other drugs) receive positive reinforcement for making this smart decision and related healthy choices.[54] Even a few positive words from a physician may delay the initiation of alcohol use by adolescents.[55] Any delay in substance use onset coincides with additional brain maturation, so abstaining may be protective against the known acute and long-term consequences of early-onset substance use. Choosing to abstain from substance use can be framed as an active decision, and the adolescent is given credit for making a healthful decision and acting on it. Although screening has never been shown to increase rates of substance use, the National Institute on Alcoholism and Alcohol Abuse recommends including a "normative

correction" statement whenever screening children or younger adolescents, such as, "I am glad to hear that you, just like most others your age, have never tried alcohol." Normative correction statements may help avoid the potential for patient misinterpretation that being screened in this case for alcohol use implies that alcohol use by the patient and at his or her age is expected and the age norm.

Substance Use Without an SUD: BI

When substance use is infrequent with a low likelihood of having an SUD, such as an S2BI screening response of using "once or twice" in the past year, the appropriate BI is to advise the patient to abstain in support of health and safety. A BI comprising clear, pointed advice to stop substance use combined with succinct mention of the negative health effects of use can lead to decreased use or abstinence in adolescent patients who use substances infrequently.[56] Brief medical advice could include statements such as, "For the sake of your health, I advise you to quit smoking marijuana. Marijuana use interferes with concentration and memory and is linked to getting lower grades at school." This BI could also recognize and leverage personal strengths and positive attributes, such as, "You are doing so well in school. I hope you will consider how your marijuana use could change all that, and whether or not that is what you really want."

Mild to Moderate SUD: Brief Motivational Intervention

Brief intervention for adolescents with mild to moderate SUD is a likely short structured conversation based on the principles of motivational interviewing,[57] through which the pediatrician respects patient autonomy while enhancing the patient's self-efficacy to institute behavior change, rather than persuading, coercing, or demanding the behavior change.[58] The core activity of BMI is to help the patient compare the benefits of continued substance use with the potential benefits of behavior change (ie, decreasing or stopping use) and ultimately take action that supports personal health and safety. The intervention is based on the premise that although adolescents who have experienced substance use–related problems can identify the potential benefits of reducing or stopping use, behavior change will not occur until the perceived benefits of giving up use outweigh the perceived "cost" and harms from continued use. For example, an adolescent may realize that marijuana use is causing tension in the relationship with his or her parents but continue to use marijuana because of perceived greater benefit from marijuana use to relieve stress or as a pleasurable activity shared with friends.

TABLE 3 S2BI Screen for Substance Use Risk Level

The following questions will ask about your use, if any, of alcohol, tobacco, and other drugs. Please answer every question by clicking on the box next to your choice.

In the past year, how many times have you used . . .
Tobacco?
-Never
-Once or twice
-Monthly
-Weekly or more
Alcohol?
-Never
-Once or twice
-Monthly
-Weekly or more
Marijuana?
-Never
-Once or twice
-Monthly
-Weekly or more
STOP if answers to all previous questions are "never." Otherwise, continue with the following questions.
In the past year, how many times have you used...
Prescription drugs that were not prescribed for you (such as pain medication or Adderall)?
-Never
-Once or twice
-Monthly
-Weekly or more
Illegal drugs (such as cocaine or Ecstasy)?
-Never
-Once or twice
-Monthly
-Weekly or more
Inhalants (such as nitrous oxide)?
-Never
-Once or twice
-Monthly
-Weekly or more
Herbs or synthetic drugs (such as salvia, "K2," or bath salts)?
-Never
-Once or twice
-Monthly
-Weekly or more

Starting an intervention with assessment questions to identify substance use frequency and associated problem severity can guide the pediatrician in deciding the next steps for patient care, namely continued conversation around behavior change managed in the medical home or referring to more specialized substance use evaluation, intervention, and/or treatment. This model optimizes the CRAFFT[40] tool as an assessment guide. For example, an adolescent patient responding "yes" to the CRAFFT question, "Have you gotten into trouble while you were using alcohol or drugs?" The pediatrician can distill these details into a fulcrum to pivot the conversation into discussing the adolescent's plans for avoiding such problems in the future. The pediatrician can assist the patient in making a specific intervention plan to record in the medical record and facilitate follow-up (Box 1).

Box 1

> The pediatrician screens a 14-year-old boy who reports monthly alcohol use. The pediatrician asks follow-up questions about patterns of use and associated problems. The patient mentions binge drinking and not always knowing how he gets home from

TABLE 4 DSM-5[39] and ICD-10 Criteria for SUD

DSM-5		ICD-10	
Criteria	Severity	Criteria	Severity
1. Use in larger amounts or for longer periods of time than intended 2. Unsuccessful efforts to cut down or quit	Severity is designated according to the number of symptoms endorsed: 0–1, no diagnosis; 2–3, mild SUD; 4–5, moderate SUD; ≥6, severe SUD	1. A strong desire or sense of compulsion to take the substance 2. Impaired capacity to control substance-taking behavior in terms of onset, termination, or level of use, as evidenced by the substance being often taken in larger amounts over a longer period than intended or any unsuccessful effort or persistent desire to cut down or control substance use	Three or more of these manifestations should have occurred together for at least 1 month or if persisting for periods of <1 month, then they have occurred together repeatedly within a 12-month period
3. Excessive time spent taking the drug		3. A psychological withdrawal state when substance use is reduced or ceased, as evidenced by the characteristic withdrawal syndrome for the substance, or use of the same (or closely related) substance with the intention of relieving or avoiding withdrawal symptoms	
4. Failure to fulfill major obligations 5. Continued use despite problems 6. Important activities given up		4. Evidence or tolerance to the effects of the substance, such that there is a need for markedly increased amounts of the substance to achieve intoxication or desired effect, or that there is a markedly diminished effect with continued use of the same amount of the substance	
7. Recurrent use in physically hazardous situations 8. Continued use despite problems		5. Preoccupation with substance use, as manifested by important alternative pleasures or interests being given up or reduced because of substance use, or a great deal of time being spent in activities necessary to obtain the substance, take the substance, or recover from its effects	
9. Tolerance 10. Withdrawal 11. Craving		6. Persisting with substance use despite clear evidence or harmful consequences, as evidenced by continued use when the person was actually aware of, or could be expected to have been aware of, the nature and extent of harm	

DSM-5, *Diagnostic and Statistical Manual of Mental Disorders, Fifth Edition*; ICD-10, International Statistical Classification of Diseases and Related Health Problems, 10th ed.

---

parties. He admits preferring not to think about it because it frightens him. The pediatrician correlates the report of 'monthly' use to a likelihood that the patient has a mild or moderate SUD, indicating the next step is intervention to reduce use. The patient is given brief advice and challenged to make a behavior change: *"As your doctor, I recommend that you stop drinking alcohol. You described having 'blackouts' from your drinking. This means that you drank enough to poison your brain cells at least temporarily, which is why at times you can't remember how you have gotten home from parties. As you*

pointed out, a teenager can get into trouble with 'blackouts,' and it sounds like you have had some frightening experiences. How do you think you can protect yourself better in the future?" The patient says that he is not going to quit drinking, but can agree to limiting himself to 2 drinks per occasion, a sharp decrease from his usual 6 to 8 drinks, because he does not want to black out again. The pediatrician gives advice about alcohol and motor vehicle-associated risks and suggests developing a safety plan. Planning is documented in the medical record and a follow-up appointment is scheduled in 3 months.

Medical home follow-up can be conducted after a few weeks of attempted behavior change to assess whether risk behaviors have diminished, remained the same, or escalated. Adolescents who are found to have met the agreed-on substance use behavior change goals can benefit from discussing the pros and cons of their decreased use and identifying any motivating factors that can be reinforced to sustain the behavior change and lead to abstinence. Adolescents who are unable to meet the behavior change goals may benefit from more extensive substance use–targeted individual counseling provided by an allied mental health professional, such

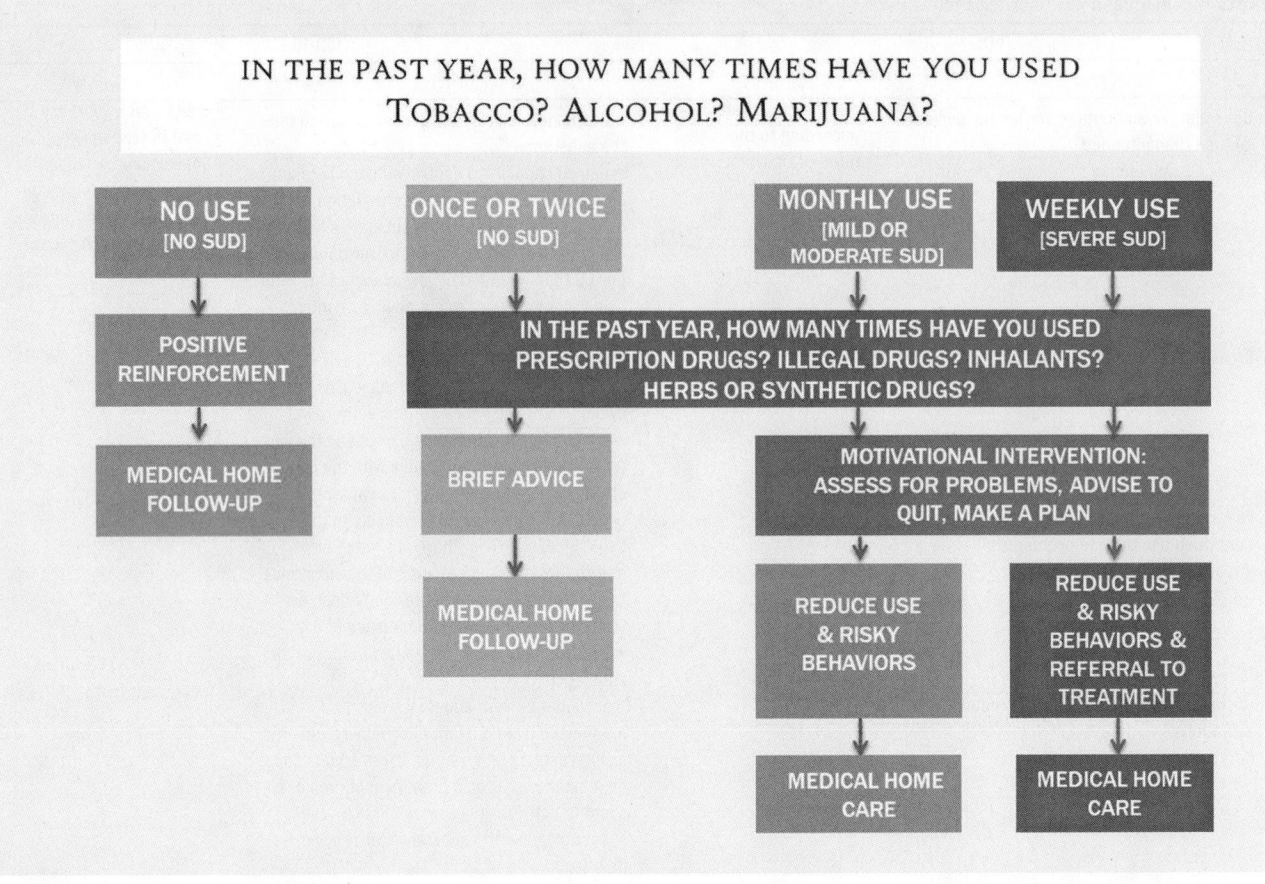

FIGURE 1
The S2BI-based approach to clinical SBIRT. S Levy, L Shrier. 2014. Boston, MA: Boston Children's Hospital. Copyright 2014, Boston Children's Hospital. Reprinted under Creative Commons Attribution-Noncommercial 4.0 International License.

as a social worker or psychologist. Referral for specific substance use evaluation and/or to psychiatric services or other available treatment options is a next step when patients have psychiatric symptomatology or cannot decrease use. When available, referral to mental health professionals within the same medical home practice setting may optimize patient compliance.

Severe SUD: Brief Intervention Focused on Referral to Treatment

Severe SUD, or addiction, is a neurologically based disorder resulting from the disruption of neurons in the reward center of the brain as the result of repeated exposure to a psychoactive substance.[59-61] The earlier an individual initiates psychoactive substance use, the more likely that

individual is to develop addiction, a nearly linear and highly significant relationship.[62-64] The S2BI tool delineates use-risk categories so that a patient reporting weekly or more frequent substance use has a high probability of a severe SUD. When addiction is likely, the next SBIRT steps are to engage the patient in a comprehensive evaluation by a substance use specialist, ensure assessment for co-occurring mental health disorders, and engage in available treatment options as soon as possible to initiate the significant behavior change that is necessary for the patient's future health and safety.

Because resistance and denial (ie, lack of insight)[65] are intrinsic SUD symptoms, the patient and/or family may be unwilling to pursue an evaluation or therapy when it is recommended. Despite this

challenge, it is important for the pediatrician to remain engaged with the patient and family and supportive during discussions and decision-making about the care options as well as throughout the entire course of care and aftercare. Motivational interviewing strategies can be helpful for encouraging an adolescent and/or the family to accept a referral (Box 2).

Box 2

In response to S2BI screening in the medical home, a 16-year-old girl reports weekly marijuana use. The pediatrician then asks questions to determine quantity, frequency, and context of use and to explore for problems. The patient says she relies on marijuana to help calm her down

TABLE 5 "911 Plan" for Adolescents at Acute Risk of Harm

Break confidentiality and notify parents of risk.

Make a verbal contract with patient not to use substances while awaiting treatment entry.

Ask parents to monitor adolescent closely while awaiting treatment entry.

If parents know adolescent is talking about self-harm, seek an emergency evaluation. Call 911, if adolescent refuses.

If parents note that the adolescent has altered mental status, seek emergency evaluation.

If the adolescent is unwilling to accept parent's rules or becomes violent or threatening, advise parents to call local police station and request emergency assistance.

when she is stressed and that she does not see the harm in it. She also states that her mother knows about her use and thinks marijuana use is bad for her, so their relationship has gotten tense over this disagreement. She was recently suspended from school when caught with marijuana. The pediatrician summarizes the situation and provides brief advice: *"It seems that you depend on marijuana to help you manage stress, and at the same time you realize marijuana use is causing tension at home and has gotten you into trouble at school. It is clear to me that you are thinking about this, and I am glad you are willing to speak with me about it. As your physician and for the sake of your health, your school work, and your relationship with your mom, I recommend that you quit your marijuana use. I would like you to speak with a colleague of mine who can help you continue thinking through the "good things" and "not so good things" about marijuana use and help you figure out what you want to do. What do you think?"* The patient agrees tentatively. The pediatrician gives her positive feedback about her willingness to discuss her marijuana use now and meet with the recommended colleague soon. The pediatrician asks the patient's permission to invite her mother into the room to discuss the plan together and mentions this would also show her that the patient is taking the concerns about her marijuana use seriously. She agrees and the patient's mother joins them for

a summary of the conversation. The counseling appointment is scheduled, and the plan is detailed in the medical record. The patient and mother are scheduled for follow-up in 1 month.

Acute Risk of Harm

Substance use screening may reveal that an adolescent patient is at risk of imminent harm and immediate attention is warranted, including screening for suicidal or homicidal ideation. Certain substance use patterns indicate acute risk, such as injection drug use, drug withdrawal symptoms, and active substance use with a past history of a drug-related emergency department visit or medically supervised withdrawal. Very high-risk behaviors include using different sedatives together, such as mixing alcohol, benzodiazepines, barbiturates, and/or opioids; frequent or excessive binge drinking, which is especially concerning for alcohol poisoning; and operating a motor vehicle coincident with alcohol or other drug use. The more recent the activity, the more immediate is the need to address the risk through mental health and/or medical intervention and to detect or confirm an SUD and other underlying or co-occurring health issues.

When an acute risk of harm is revealed, the next steps for the pediatrician are to use brief intervention techniques to facilitate a commitment from the adolescent to curtail or avoid further substance use and high-risk behaviors. Imminent risk of harm calls for the patient and pediatrician to discuss confidentiality

and disclosure, because the parent(s) nearly always should be involved in the safety plan and next steps of medical care, including how the parent(s) can support and monitor the adolescent and respond to acute concerns about safety as specialty evaluation and care services are engaged (Table 5, Box 3).

Box 3

A 17-year-old boy reports weekly use of alcohol and marijuana and monthly use of prescription medications and cocaine. The pediatrician asks follow-up questions to gauge the patient's level of acute health and safety risk. He uses marijuana to relax. He often smokes alone and sometimes drinks alone. He has frequent blackouts and explains "that's the point." He likes mixing pills with alcohol because he blacks out faster. He has thought that he may have an alcohol problem, but he does not plan to stop. He denies thoughts of hurting himself or others. The pediatrician responds: *"I am glad you spoke honestly with me today. From what you told me, I am worried about your drug use. Mixing drugs can really get you into trouble, even if you only take a couple of pills. Because I am so concerned, I want you to know that some of this information must be shared with your parents and an appointment will be made for you to speak more about your drug use with one of my colleagues. In the meantime, can you promise me that you will not use any pills or drugs at all before your next appointment? What do you think would be the best way to share the information with your parents?"*

REFERRAL TO TREATMENT

Referral to treatment describes the facilitative process through which patients identified as needing more

TABLE 6 ASAM Levels of Care for Treatment of SUDs

	Description
OUTPATIENT	
Individual counseling	Adolescents with SUDs should receive specific treatment of their substance use; general supportive counseling may be a useful adjuvant but should not be a substitute.[69] Several therapeutic modalities (motivational interviewing, cognitive behavioral therapy, contingency management, etc) have all shown promise in treating adolescents with SUDs.[70]
Group therapy	Group therapy is a mainstay of SUD treatment of adolescents with SUDs. It is a particularly attractive option because it is cost-effective and takes advantage of the developmental preference for congregating with peers. However, group therapy has not been extensively evaluated as a therapeutic modality for this age group, and existing research has produced mixed results.[69–71]
Family therapy	Family-directed therapies are the best-validated approach for treating adolescent SUDs. A number of modalities have all been shown to be effective. Family counseling typically targets domains that figure prominently in the etiology of SUDs in adolescents: family conflict, communication, parental monitoring, discipline, child abuse/neglect, and parental SUDs.[69]
Intensive outpatient program (IOP)	IOPs serve as an intermediate level of care for patients who have needs that are too complex for outpatient treatment but do not require inpatient services. These programs allow individuals to continue with their daily routine and practice newly acquired recovery skills both at home and at work. IOPs generally comprise a combination of supportive group therapy, educational groups, family therapy, individual therapy, relapse prevention and life skills, 12-step recovery, case management, and after-care planning. The programs range from 2 to 9 hours per day, 2 to 5 times per week, and last 1 to 3 months. These programs are appealing because they provide a plethora of services in a relatively short period of time.[72]
Partial hospital program	Partial hospitalization is a short-term, comprehensive outpatient program in affiliation with a hospital that is designed to provide support and treatment of patients with SUDs. The services offered at these programs are more concentrated and intensive than regular outpatient treatment because they are structured throughout the entire day and offer medical monitoring in addition to individual and group therapy. Participants typically attend sessions for 7 or 8 hours per day, at least 5 days per week, for 1–3 weeks. As with IOPs, patients return home in the evenings and have a chance to practice newly acquired recovery skills.[73]
OUTPATIENT	
Detoxification	Detoxification refers to the medical management of symptoms of withdrawal. Medically supervised detoxification is indicated for any adolescent who is at risk for withdrawing from alcohol or benzodiazepines and may also be helpful for adolescents withdrawing from opioids, cocaine, or other substances. Detoxification may be an important first step but is not considered definitive treatment. Patients who are discharged from a detoxification program should then begin either an outpatient or residential SUD treatment program.[70,71]
Acute residential treatment (ART)	ART is a short-term (days–weeks) residential placement designed to stabilize patients in crisis, often before entering a longer-term residential treatment program.[70] ART programs typically target adolescents with co-occurring mental health disorders.
Residential treatment	Residential treatment programs are highly structured live-in environments that provide therapy for those with severe SUD, mental illness, or behavioral problems that require 24-hour care. The goal of residential treatment is to promote the achievement and subsequent maintenance of long-term abstinence as well as equip each patient with both the social and coping skills necessary for a successful transition back into society. Residential treatment programs are classified by the length of the program; short-term refers to programs of ≤30 days' duration, long-term refers to programs of >30 days' duration. Residential treatment programs generally comprise individual and group therapy sessions plus medical, psychological, clinical, nutritional, and educational components. Residential facilities aim to simulate real living environments with added structure and routine to prepare individuals with the framework necessary for their lives to continue drug and alcohol free on completion of the program.[74]
Therapeutic boarding school	Therapeutic boarding schools are educational institutions that provide constant supervision for their students by professional staff. These schools offer a highly structured environment with set times for all activities, smaller, more specialized classes, and social and emotional support. In addition to the regular services offered at traditional boarding schools, therapeutic schools also provide individual and group therapy for adolescents with mental health or SUDs.[75]

extensive evaluation and treatment are able to access the appropriate services. Historically, medical encounters have been notably poor in identifying adolescents who have severe SUDs and connecting them with treatment. SAMHSA has estimated that fewer than 10% of adolescents in need of specialty substance use treatment receive it, and the majority of referrals are from the justice system.[66,67] The referral to treatment, or "RT," of SBIRT is composed of 2 distinct yet connected clinical activities: working with the adolescent and family so they accept that timely referral and treatment are necessary for the patient's health and facilitating the referral process to engage the patient and family with the appropriate professional(s) or program(s).

Deciding where to refer an adolescent in need of treatment is often complicated by limited treatment availability, insurance coverage complexities, and preferences of the adolescent and family. In most cases, pediatricians will refer adolescents with SUDs to a mental health or addiction specialist to conduct a comprehensive biopsychosocial assessment and to determine the appropriate level of care from the treatment spectrum, ranging from outpatient substance use counseling to long-term residential treatment programs. In 2001, the American Society of Addiction Medicine (ASAM) revised its comprehensive national guidelines for placement, continued stay, and discharge of patients with alcohol and other drug problems. The separate guidelines devised for adults and adolescents detail 5 broad levels of care that range from early intervention to medically managed intensive inpatient treatment and correspond to addiction severity, related problems, and potential for behavior change and recovery[68] (Table 6). Adolescents should be treated in the least-restrictive environment (ie, level of care) that supports their clinical needs. Adolescents who voluntarily accept therapeutic placement will usually engage more readily in their care, which is a key factor influencing SUD treatment success.

The Center for Substance Abuse Treatment has published evidence-based treatment and assessment protocols and manuals (available at: www.ncbi.nlm.nih.gov/books/NBK82999). To help identify treatment options throughout the country, SAMHSA maintains a comprehensive and easy-to-use Substance Abuse Treatment Facility Locator on its Web site (www.samhsa.gov/treatment/index.aspx), which also lists both a Buprenorphine Physician & Treatment Program Locator and an Opioid Treatment Program Directory. Opioid and alcohol use disorders are the primary indications for medication-assisted treatment in adult populations; medication-assisted treatment with buprenorphine or naltrexone also is an option for opioid-dependent adolescents.[76,77]

Successful addiction treatment usually involves a long recovery process during which the patient experiences more than 1 level of care. In 2013, the ASAM reconceived the notion of "patient placement" by incorporating the entire admission, treatment, and continuing care

into a single longitudinal process and encouraging the integration of addiction services with general health care, mental health, and a variety of other subjects and settings. Because clinicians and payers need to exchange information frequently and repeatedly during the treatment payment approval process, the current edition of the ASAM *National Treatment Guidelines*[68] includes a section about working effectively with managed care, particularly in the context of health care reform.

Most patients in addiction treatment consider themselves "recovering" rather than "recovered" to recognize their lifelong potential for relapse. Whether treatment begins in outpatient or inpatient care, it should continue at the level appropriate to support the patient's recovery process, which often is achieved through sequential or overlapping therapeutic levels and usually includes participation in a formal structured program, self-help groups (eg, Alcoholics Anonymous, Alateen, Narcotics Anonymous), ongoing after-care programs, and self-help recovery work.

The medical home plays a key role for all patients in recovery through many roles that include providing continuity of general medical care and rapport with the patient and family, coordinating the patient's various care specialties and services involved, and providing SUD follow-up care to detect relapse and providing support through referral and collaborative care. Relapse is not uncommon in SUDs, but anticipating it and viewing it as a learning opportunity can motivate the patient and family to re-engage in care. By collaborating with addiction medicine specialists and other mental health professionals as well as working with the family, third-party payers, and schools, among others, the pediatrician

plays an essential role in the ongoing care of children and adolescents with SUDs.

OPTIMAL STANDARDS FOR AN SUD TREATMENT PROGRAM

The following were adapted from SAMHSA and Center for Substance Abuse Treatment standards into optimal goals for inpatient or outpatient SUD treatment programs serving the pediatric population.[78] The program will:

1. View drug and alcohol use disorders as a primary disease rather than a symptom.

2. Include a comprehensive patient evaluation and a developmentally appropriate management and treatment referral plan for associated medical, emotional, and behavioral problems identified.

3. Maintain rapport with the patient's pediatrician to facilitate seamless after-care and primary care follow-up.

4. Adhere to an abstinence philosophy and consider the patient's continued use of tobacco, alcohol, or other drugs as indicating more treatment is needed rather than the program should discharge or refuse to treat.

5. Maintain a low patient-to-staff ratio.

6. Use treatment professionals who are knowledgeable in both addiction treatment and child and adolescent behavior and development.

7. Maintain separate treatment groups for individuals at varying developmental levels (adolescents, young adults, and older adults).

8. Involve the entire family in the treatment and relate to

the patients and their families with compassion and concern. Programs located as close to home as possible are preferable to facilitate family involvement, even though separation of the adolescent from the family may be indicated initially.

9. Offer patients an opportunity to continue academic and vocational education and assistance with restructuring family, school, and social life. Consider formal academic and cognitive skills assessment, because unidentified weaknesses may contribute to emotional factors contributing to the substance use.

10. Keep the family apprised of costs and financial arrangements for inpatient and outpatient care and facilitate communication with managed-care organizations.

11. Ensure that follow-up and continuing care are integral parts of the program.

Billing and payment for screening and office-based BI varies by payer. A fact sheet about coding for behavior change intervention for substance use is available on the AAP Web site (www.aap.org/en-us/professional-resources/practice-support/Coding-at-the-AAP/Pages/Private/Substance-Abuse-Coding-Fact-Sheet.aspx). Further clarification is available through the AAP coding hotline (AAPCodinghotline@aap.org).

SUMMARY

Pediatricians play a key role in preventing and curtailing adolescent substance use and associated harm, whether through direct patient care practices, multidisciplinary collaboration, or support of parenting and community efforts. Research-informed SBIRT practices can be applied across the variety of practice

settings and clinicians providing health care to adolescents. SBIRT is recognized to include the use of validated screening tools, assessing for substance use risk and problems, sharing expert health promotion and disease prevention advice, and conducting interventions that encourage substance use reduction and/or referral to treatment. (See the accompanying policy statement for further detail and recommendations.)

LEAD AUTHORS

Sharon J.L. Levy, MD, MPH, FAAP
Janet F. Williams, MD, FAAP

COMMITTEE ON SUBSTANCE USE AND PREVENTION, 2015–2016

Sheryl A. Ryan, MD, FAAP, Chairperson
Pamela K. Gonzalez, MD, MS, FAAP
Stephen W. Patrick, MD, MPH, MS, FAAP
Joanna Quigley, MD, FAAP
Lorena Siqueira, MD, MSPH, FAAP
Vincent C. Smith, MD, MPH, FAAP
Leslie R. Walker, MD, FAAP

FORMER COMMITTEE MEMBERS

Sharon J.L. Levy, MD, MPH, FAAP
Janet F. Williams, MD, FAAP

LIAISONS

Vivian B. Faden, PhD – *National Institute of Alcohol Abuse and Alcoholism*
Gregory Tau, MD, PhD – *American Academy of Child and Adolescent Psychiatry*

STAFF

Renee Jarrett, MPH

SELECTED RESOURCES FOR PEDIATRICIANS

American Academy of Child and Adolescent Psychiatry. Practice parameter for the assessment and treatment of child and adolescent substance use disorders. Available at: www.aacap.org/App_Themes/AACAP/docs/practice_parameters/substance_abuse_practice_parameter.pdf

American Academy of Pediatrics. Implementing mental health priorities in practice substance use [video]. Available at: www.aap.org/en-us/advocacy-and-policy/

aap-health-initiatives/Mental-Health/Pages/substance-use.aspx

American Academy of Pediatrics Julius B. Richmond Center of Excellence. Available at: www2.aap.org/richmondcenter

Massachusetts Department of Public Health. Adolescent SBIRT toolkit for providers. Available at: http://massclearinghouse.ehs.state.ma.us/BSASSBIRTPROG/SA1099.html

National Institute on Alcohol Abuse and Alcoholism. Alcohol screening and brief intervention for youth: a practitioner's guide. Available at: www.niaaa.nih.gov/YouthGuide

Partnership for Drug-Free Kids. The Medicine Abuse Project. Available at: http://medicineabuseproject.org/resources/health-care-providers

SELECTED RESOURCES FOR FAMILIES

American Academy of Child and Adolescent Psychiatry. Family resources. Available at: www.aacap.org/AACAP/Families_and_Youth/Family_Resources/Home.aspx

American Academy of Pediatrics. Patient/parent brochures. Available at: http://bit.ly/1LIC93Z

HealthyChildren.org. Official consumer Web site of the AAP. Available at: www.healthychildren.org/English/ages-stages/teen/substance-abuse

National Institute on Alcohol Abuse and Alcoholism. Make a difference: talk to your child about alcohol. Available at: http://pubs.niaaa.nih.gov/publications/MakeADiff_HTML/makediff.htm

National Institute on Alcohol Abuse and Alcoholism. Treatment for alcohol problems: finding and getting help. Available at: http://pubs.niaaa.nih.gov/publications/Treatment/treatment.htm

National Institute on Drug Abuse. Family checkup: positive parenting prevents drug abuse. Available at: www.drugabuse.gov/family-checkup

National Institute on Drug Abuse. NIDA for teens. Available at: http://teens.drugabuse.gov

Substance Use and Mental Health Services Administration. "Talk. They hear you". application. Available at: www.samhsa.gov/underage-drinking/mobile-application

REFERENCES

1. University of Michigan. Drug Abuse Now
    Equals Childhood Obesity as Top Health
    Concern for Kids. Vol 13. Ann Arbor,
    MI: University of Michigan, C.S. Mott
    Children's Hospital; 2011. Available at:
    http://mottnpch.org/sites/default/files/
    documents/081511toptenreport.pdf.
    Accessed July 23, 2015

2. US Department of Health and
    Human Services. Healthy People
    2020: substance abuse objectives.
    Washington, DC: US Government
    Printing Office; 2011. Available
    at: www.healthypeople.gov/2020/
    topicsobjectives2020/overview.aspx?
    topicid=40. Accessed July 23, 2015

3. Johnston LD, O'Malley PM, Bachman JG,
    Schulenberg JE, Miech RA. Monitoring
    the Future: National Survey Results
    on Drug Use, 1975–2013. Vol. I:
    Secondary School Students. Ann Arbor,
    MI: University of Michigan, Institute
    for Social Research; 2014. Available
    at www.monitoringthefuture.org/
    pubs/monographs/mtf-vol1_2013.pdf.
    Accessed July 23, 2015

4. The Partnership at DrugFree.org.
    2012 Partnership Attitude Tracking
    Study: Teens and Parents. New York,
    NY: Partnership for Drug-Free Kids;
    2013. Available at: www.drugfree.org/
    wp-content/uploads/2013/04/PATS-2012-
    FULL-REPORT2.pdf. Accessed July 23, 2015

5. Kann L, Kinchen S, Shanklin SL, et
    al; Centers for Disease Control and
    Prevention. Youth risk behavior

    surveillance—United States, 2013.
    MMWR Suppl. 2014;63(4 SS-4):1–168

6. DuRant RH, Smith JA, Kreiter SR,
    Krowchuk DP. The relationship between
    early age of onset of initial substance
    use and engaging in multiple
    health risk behaviors among young
    adolescents. *Arch Pediatr Adolesc
    Med.* 1999;153(3):286–291

7. Hingson RW, Zha W. Age of drinking
    onset, alcohol use disorders,
    frequent heavy drinking, and
    unintentionally injuring oneself and
    others after drinking. *Pediatrics.*
    2009;123(6):1477–1484

8. Weitzman ER, Nelson TF. College
    student binge drinking and the
    "prevention paradox": implications for
    prevention and harm reduction. *J Drug
    Educ.* 2004;34(3):247–265

9. Levy S, Sherritt L, Gabrielli J, Shrier
    LA, Knight JR. Screening adolescents
    for substance use-related high-risk
    sexual behaviors. *J Adolesc Health.*
    2009;45(5):473–477

10. VanDerNagel JEL, Kiewik M, Postel MG,
    et al. Capture recapture estimation
    of the prevalence of mild intellectual
    disability and substance use disorder.
    Res Dev Disabil. 2014;35(4):808–813

11. Carroll Chapman SL, Wu L-T. Substance
    abuse among individuals with
    intellectual disabilities. *Res Dev
    Disabil.* 2012;33(4):1147–1156

12. Chambers RA, Taylor JR, Potenza
    MN. Developmental neurocircuitry of
    motivation in adolescence: a critical
    period of addiction vulnerability. *Am J
    Psychiatry.* 2003;160(6):1041–1052

13. Kulig JW; American Academy of
    Pediatrics Committee on Substance
    Abuse. Tobacco, alcohol, and other
    drugs: the role of the pediatrician
    in prevention, identification, and
    management of substance abuse.
    Pediatrics. 2005;115(3):816–821

14. Hagan JF, Shaw JS, Duncan P, eds.
    *Bright Futures: Guidelines for Health
    Supervision of Infants, Children, and
    Adolescents.* 3rd ed. Elk Grove Village, IL:
    American Academy of Pediatrics; 2008

15. MacKay AP, Duran C. *Adolescent Health
    in the United States, 2007.* Atlanta, GA:
    National Center for Health Statistics,
    Centers for Disease Control and
    Prevention; 2007

16. Yoast RA, Fleming M, Balch GI.
    Reactions to a concept for physician
    intervention in adolescent alcohol use.
    J Adolesc Health. 2007;41(1):35–41

17. Substance Abuse and Mental Health
    Services Administration. About
    Screening, Brief Intervention, and
    Referral to Treatment (SBIRT).
    Available at: www.samhsa.gov/sbirt/
    about. Accessed July 23, 2015

18. Kann L, Kinchen S, Shanklin S, et al.
    Youth risk behavior surveillance—
    United States, 2013. *MMWR Surveill
    Summ.* 2014;63(4):1–172. Available at:
    www.cdc.gov/mmwr/pdf/ss/ss6304.
    pdf?utm_source=rss&utm_medium=
    rss&utm_campaign=youth-risk-
    behavior-surveillance-united-states-
    2013-pdf. Accessed July 23, 2015

19. American Academy of Pediatrics,
    Committee on Substance Abuse.
    Substance use screening, brief
    intervention, and referral to
    treatment [policy statement].
    Pediatrics. 2016

20. Ford CA, Millstein SG, Halpern-Felsher
    BL, Irwin CE Jr. Influence of
    physician confidentiality assurances
    on adolescents' willingness to
    disclose information and seek
    future health care: a randomized
    controlled trial. *JAMA.*
    1997;278(12):1029–1034

21. Ford CA, Bearman PS, Moody
    J. Foregone health care
    among adolescents. *JAMA.*
    1999;282(23):2227–2234

22. Society for Adolescent Medicine.
    Access to health care for adolescents
    and young adults. *J Adolesc Health.*
    2004;35(4):342–344

23. Coble YD, Estes EH, Head CA, et al;
    Council on Scientific Affairs, American
    Medical Association. Confidential
    health services for adolescents. *JAMA.*
    1993;269(11):1420–1424

24. Fisher SL, Bucholz KK, Reich W, et al.
    Teenagers are right—parents do not
    know much: an analysis of adolescent-
    parent agreement on reports of
    adolescent substance use, abuse,
    and dependence. *Alcohol Clin Exp Res.*
    2006;30(10):1699–1710

25. Goldenring JM, Cohen G. Getting into
    adolescent heads. *Contemp Pediatr.*
    1988;5(7):75–90

26. Goldenring JM, Rosen D. Getting into adolescent heads: an essential update. *Contemp Pediatr.* 2004;21(1):64–90

27. American Academy of Pediatrics. *Periodic Survey of Fellows #31: Practices and Attitudes Toward Adolescent Drug Screening.* Elk Grove Village, IL: American Academy of Pediatrics, Division of Child Health Research; 1997

28. Millstein SG, Marcell AV. Screening and counseling for adolescent alcohol use among primary care physicians in the United States. *Pediatrics.* 2003;111(1):114–122

29. Harris SK, Herr-Zaya K, Weinstein Z, et al. Results of a statewide survey of adolescent substance use screening rates and practices in primary care. *Subst Abus.* 2012;33(4):321–326

30. Harris SK, Csémy L, Sherritt L, et al. Computer-facilitated substance use screening and brief advice for teens in primary care: an international trial. *Pediatrics.* 2012;129(6):1072–1082

31. Barry KL, Blow FC, Willenbring ML, McCormick R, Brockmann LM, Visnic S. Use of alcohol screening and brief interventions in primary care settings: implementation and barriers. *Subst Abus.* 2004;25(1):27–36

32. O'Connor PG, Nyquist JG, McLellan AT. Integrating addiction medicine into graduate medical education in primary care: the time has come. *Ann Intern Med.* 2011;154(1):56–59

33. Van Hook S, Harris SK, Brooks T, et al; New England Partnership for Substance Abuse Research. The "Six T's": barriers to screening teens for substance abuse in primary care. *J Adolesc Health.* 2007;40(5):456–461

34. Wilson CR, Sherritt L, Gates E, Knight JR. Are clinical impressions of adolescent substance use accurate? *Pediatrics.* 2004;114(5). Available at: www.pediatrics.org/cgi/content/full/114/5/e536

35. Levy S. Brief interventions for substance use in adolescents: still promising, still unproven. *CMAJ.* 2014;186(8):565–566

36. National Institute on Alcohol Abuse and Alcoholism. Alcohol Screening and Brief Intervention for Youth: A Practitioner's Guide. Bethesda, MD: National Institute on Alcohol Abuse and Alcoholism; 2011. NIH Publication 11-7805. Available at: http://pubs.niaaa.nih.gov/publications/Practitioner/YouthGuide/YouthGuide.pdf. Accessed July 23, 2015

37. Kelly SM, Gryczynski J, Mitchell SG, Kirk A, O'Grady KE, Schwartz RP. Validity of brief screening instrument for adolescent tobacco, alcohol, and drug use. *Pediatrics.* 2014;133(5):819–826

38. Levy S, Weiss R, Sherritt L, et al. An electronic screen for triaging adolescent substance use by risk levels. *JAMA Pediatr.* 2014;168(9):822–828

39. American Psychiatric Association. *Diagnostic and Statistical Manual of Mental Disorders, Fifth Edition.* Arlington, VA: American Psychiatric Association; 2013

40. Knight JR, Shrier LA, Bravender TD, Farrell M, Vander Bilt J, Shaffer HJ. A new brief screen for adolescent substance abuse. *Arch Pediatr Adolesc Med.* 1999;153(6):591–596

41. Dennis ML, Chan YF, Funk RR. Development and validation of the GAIN Short Screener (GSS) for internalizing, externalizing and substance use disorders and crime/violence problems among adolescents and adults. *Am J Addict.* 2006;15(suppl 1):80–91

42. Saunders JB, Aasland OG, Babor TF, de la Fuente JR, Grant M. Development of the Alcohol Use Disorders Identification Test (AUDIT): WHO Collaborative Project on Early Detection of Persons with Harmful Alcohol Consumption–II. *Addiction.* 1993;88(6):791–804

43. Spirito A, Monti PM, Barnett NP, et al. A randomized clinical trial of a brief motivational intervention for alcohol-positive adolescents treated in an emergency department. *J Pediatr.* 2004;145(3):396–402

44. Bernstein E, Edwards E, Dorfman D, Heeren T, Bliss C, Bernstein J. Screening and brief intervention to reduce marijuana use among youth and young adults in a pediatric emergency department. *Acad Emerg Med.* 2009;16(11):1174–1185

45. Tait RJ, Hulse GK, Robertson SI. Effectiveness of a brief-intervention and continuity of care in enhancing attendance for treatment by adolescent substance users. *Drug Alcohol Depend.* 2004;74(3):289–296

46. Neighbors CJ, Barnett NP, Rohsenow DJ, Colby SM, Monti PM. Cost-effectiveness of a motivational intervention for alcohol-involved youth in a hospital emergency department. *J Stud Alcohol Drugs.* 2010;71(3):384–394

47. Haller DM, Meynard A, Lefebvre D, Ukoumunne OC, Narring F, Broers B. Effectiveness of training family physicians to deliver a brief intervention to address excessive substance use among young patients: a cluster randomized controlled trial. *CMAJ.* 2014;186(8):E263–E272

48. Stern SA, Meredith LS, Gholson J, Gore P, D'Amico EJ. Project CHAT: a brief motivational substance abuse intervention for teens in primary care. *J Subst Abuse Treat.* 2007;32(2):153–165

49. Murphy DA, Chen X, Naar-King S, Parsons JT; Adolescent Trials Network. Alcohol and marijuana use outcomes in the Healthy Choices motivational interviewing intervention for HIV-positive youth. *AIDS Patient Care STDS.* 2012;26(2):95–100

50. Shrier LA, Rhoads A, Burke P, Walls C, Blood EA. Real-time, contextual intervention using mobile technology to reduce marijuana use among youth: a pilot study. *Addict Behav.* 2014;39(1):173–180

51. Walton MA, Bohnert K, Resko S, et al. Computer and therapist based brief interventions among cannabis-using adolescents presenting to primary care: one year outcomes. *Drug Alcohol Depend.* 2013;132(3):646–653

52. Haller DM, Meynard A, Lefebvre D, Tylee A, Narring F, Broers B. Brief intervention addressing excessive cannabis use in young people consulting their GP: a pilot study. *Br J Gen Pract.* 2009;59(560):166–172

53. Patnode CD, O'Connor E, Rowland M, Burda BU, Perdue LA, Whitlock EP. Primary care behavioral interventions to prevent or reduce illicit drug use and nonmedical pharmaceutical use in children and adolescents: a systematic evidence review for the U.S. Preventive Services Task Force. *Ann Intern Med.* 2014;160(9):612–620

54. Ginsburg KR. Viewing our adolescent patients through a positive lens. *Contemp Pediatr.* 2007;24:65–76

55. Harris SK, Csemy L, Sherritt L, et al. Computer-facilitated screening and physician brief advice to reduce substance use among adolescent primary care patients: a multi-site international trial. *Pediatrics.* 2012;129(6):1072–1082

56. Hassan A, Harris SK, Sherritt L, et al. Primary care follow-up plans for adolescents with substance use problems. *Pediatrics.* 2009;124(1):144–150

57. Miller WR, Rollnick S. Meeting in the middle: motivational interviewing and self-determination theory. *Int J Behav Nutr Phys Act.* 2012;9:25

58. Butterworth SW. Influencing patient adherence to treatment guidelines. *J Manag Care Pharm.* 2008;14(6 suppl B):21–24

59. Nestler EJ. Molecular basis of long-term plasticity underlying addiction. *Nat Rev Neurosci.* 2001;2(2):119–128

60. Volkow ND, Li T-K. Drug addiction: the neurobiology of behaviour gone awry. *Nat Rev Neurosci.* 2004;5(12):963–970

61. Everitt BJ, Belin D, Economidou D, Pelloux Y, Dalley JW, Robbins TW. Neural mechanisms underlying the vulnerability to develop compulsive drug-seeking habits and addiction [review]. *Philos Trans R Soc Lond B Biol Sci.* 2008;363(1507):3125–3135

62. Grant BF, Dawson DA. Age of onset of drug use and its association with DSM-IV drug abuse and dependence: results from the National Longitudinal Alcohol Epidemiologic Survey. *J Subst Abuse.* 1998;10(2):163–173

63. Hingson RW, Heeren T, Winter MR. Age at drinking onset and alcohol dependence: age at onset, duration, and severity. *Arch Pediatr Adolesc Med.* 2006;160(7):739–746

64. Taioli E, Wynder EL. Effect of the age at which smoking begins on frequency of smoking in adulthood. *N Engl J Med.* 1991;325(13):968–969

65. Miller WR, Rollnick S. *Motivational Interviewing: Helping People Change.* Vol 3. New York, NY: Guilford Press; 2013

66. Substance Abuse and Mental Health Services Administration. *Results From the 2012 National Survey on Drug Use and Health: Summary of National Findings.* Rockville, MD: Substance Abuse and Mental Health Services Administration; 2013

67. Substance Abuse and Mental Health Services Administration. The TEDS Report: Substance Abuse Treatment Admissions Referred by the Criminal Justice System. Rockville, MD: Substance Abuse and Mental Health Services Administration; 2009. Available at: www.samhsa.gov/data/2k9/211/211CJadmits2k9.pdf. Accessed July 23, 2015

68. Mee-Lee D, ed. *The ASAM Criteria: Treatment Criteria for Addictive, Substance-Related, and Co-Occurring Conditions.* Carson City, NV: The Change Companies; 2013

69. Bukstein OG, Bernet W, Arnold V, et al; Work Group on Quality Issues. Practice parameter for the assessment and treatment of children and adolescents with substance use disorders. *J Am Acad Child Adolesc Psychiatry.* 2005;44(6):609–621

70. Fournier ME, Levy S. Recent trends in adolescent substance use, primary care screening, and updates in treatment options. *Curr Opin Pediatr.* 2006;18(4):352–358

71. Vaughan BL, Knight JR. Intensive drug treatment. In: Neinstein LS, Gordon C, Katzman D, Woods ER, Rosen D, eds. *Adolescent Healthcare: A Practical Guide.* 5th ed. Philadelphia, PA: Lippincott, Williams & Wilkins; 2009:671–675

72. Center for Substance Abuse Treatment. Services in intensive outpatient treatment programs. In: Substance Abuse: Clinical Issues in Intensive Outpatient Treatment. Rockville, MD: Substance Abuse and Mental Health Services Administration; 2006. Available at: www.ncbi.nlm.nih.gov/books/NBK64094. Accessed July 23, 2015

73. CIGNA. CIGNA Standards and Guidelines/Medical Necessity Criteria for Treatment of Behavioral Health and Substance Use Disorders. 2015. Available at: https://cignaforhcp.cigna.com/public/content/pdf/resourceLibrary/behavioral/medicalNecessityCriteriaDraft.pdf. Accessed October 6, 2015

74. Center for Substance Abuse Treatment. Triage and placement in treatment services. In: Substance Abuse Treatment for Adults in the Criminal Justice System. Rockville, MD: Substance Abuse and Mental Health Services Administration; 2005. Available at: www.ncbi.nlm.nih.gov/books/NBK64131. Accessed July 23, 2015

75. Center for Substance Abuse Treatment. Therapeutic communities. In: SAMHSA/CSAT Treatment Improvement Protocols. Rockville, MD: Substance Abuse and Mental Health Services Administration; 1999. Available at: www.ncbi.nlm.nih.gov/books/NBK64342. Accessed July 23, 2015

76. Gowing L, Ali R, White JM. Buprenorphine for the management of opioid withdrawal. *Cochrane Database Syst Rev.* 2009;3:CD002025

77. Woody GE, Poole SA, Subramaniam G, et al. Extended vs short-term buprenorphine-naloxone for treatment of opioid-addicted youth: a randomized trial. *JAMA.* 2008;300(17):2003–2011

78. Center for Substance Abuse Treatment. Treatment of Adolescents With Substance Abuse Disorders. Rockville, MD: US Department of Health and Human Services; 1999. Available at: http://adaiclearinghouse.org/downloads/TIP-32-Treatment-of-Adolescents-with-Substance-Use-Disorders-62.pdf. Accessed July 23, 2015

Suicide and Suicide Attempts in Adolescents

• •

• *Clinical Report*

CLINICAL REPORT   Guidance for the Clinician in Rendering Pediatric Care

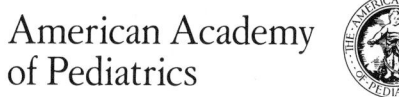

American Academy
of Pediatrics

DEDICATED TO THE HEALTH OF ALL CHILDREN™

Suicide and Suicide Attempts in Adolescents

Benjamin Shain, MD, PhD, COMMITTEE ON ADOLESCENCE

Suicide is the second leading cause of death for adolescents 15 to 19 years old. This report updates the previous statement of the American Academy of Pediatrics and is intended to assist pediatricians, in collaboration with other child and adolescent health care professionals, in the identification and management of the adolescent at risk for suicide. Suicide risk can only be reduced, not eliminated, and risk factors provide no more than guidance. Nonetheless, care for suicidal adolescents may be improved with the pediatrician's knowledge, skill, and comfort with the topic, as well as ready access to appropriate community resources and mental health professionals.

abstract

Clinical reports from the American Academy of Pediatrics benefit from expertise and resources of liaisons and internal (AAP) and external reviewers. However, clinical reports from the American Academy of Pediatrics may not reflect the views of the liaisons or the organizations or government agencies that they represent.

The guidance in this report does not indicate an exclusive course of treatment or serve as a standard of medical care. Variations, taking into account individual circumstances, may be appropriate.

All clinical reports from the American Academy of Pediatrics automatically expire 5 years after publication unless reaffirmed, revised, or retired at or before that time.

DOI: 10.1542/peds.2016-1420

PEDIATRICS (ISSN Numbers: Print, 0031-4005; Online, 1098-4275).

FINANCIAL DISCLOSURE: The author has indicated he does not have a financial relationship relevant to this article to disclose.

FUNDING: No external funding.

POTENTIAL CONFLICT OF INTEREST: The author has indicated he has no potential conflicts of interest to disclose.

To cite: Shain B and AAP COMMITTEE ON ADOLESCENCE. Suicide and Suicide Attempts in Adolescents. *Pediatrics.* 2016;138(1):e20161420

INTRODUCTION

The number of adolescent deaths that result from suicide in the United States had been increasing dramatically during recent decades until 1990, when it began to decrease modestly. From 1950 to 1990, the suicide rate for adolescents 15 to 19 years old increased by 300%,[1] but from 1990 to 2013, the rate in this age group decreased by 28%.[2] In 2013, there were 1748 suicides among people 15 to 19 years old.[2] The true number of deaths from suicide actually may be higher, because some of these deaths may have been recorded as "accidental."[3] Adolescent boys 15 to 19 years old had a completed suicide rate that was 3 times greater than that of their female counterparts,[2] whereas the rate of suicide attempts was twice as high among girls than among boys, correlating to girls tending to choose less lethal methods.[4] The ratio of attempted suicides to completed suicides among adolescents is estimated to be 50:1 to 100:1.[5]

Suicide affects young people from all races and socioeconomic groups, although some groups have higher rates than others. American Indian/ Alaska Native males have the highest suicide rate, and black females have the lowest rate of suicide. Sexual minority youth (ie, lesbian, gay, bisexual, transgender, or questioning) have more than twice the rate of suicidal ideation.[6] The 2013 Youth Risk Behavior Survey of students in grades 9 through 12 in the United States indicated that during the 12 months before the survey, 39.1% of girls and 20.8% of boys felt sad or hopeless almost every day for at least 2 weeks in a row, 16.9% of girls and 10.3% of boys had planned a suicide attempt, 10.6% of girls and 5.4% of boys had attempted suicide, and 3.6% of girls and 1.8% of boys had made a suicide attempt that required medical attention.[7]

The leading methods of suicide for the 15- to 19-year age group in 2013 were suffocation (43%), discharge of firearms (42%), poisoning (6%), and falling (3%).[2] Particular attention should be given to access to firearms, because reducing firearm access may prevent suicides. Firearms in the home, regardless of whether they are kept unloaded or stored locked, are associated with a higher risk of completed adolescent suicide.[8,9] However, in another study examining firearm security, each of the practices of securing the firearm (keeping it locked and unloaded) and securing the ammunition (keeping it locked and stored away from the firearm) were associated with reduced risk of youth shootings that resulted in unintentional or self-inflicted injury or death.[10]

Youth seem to be at much greater risk from media exposure than adults and may imitate suicidal behavior seen on television.[11] Media coverage of an adolescent's suicide may lead to cluster suicides, with the magnitude of additional deaths proportional to the amount, duration, and prominence of the media coverage.[11] A prospective study found increased suicidality with exposure to the suicide of a schoolmate.[12] Newspaper reports about suicide were associated with an increase in adolescent suicide clustering, with greater clustering associated with article front-page placement, mention of suicide or the method of suicide in the article title, and detailed description in the article text about the individual

or the suicide act.[13] More research is needed to determine the psychological mechanisms behind suicide clustering.[14,15] The National Institute of Mental Health suggests best practices for media and online reporting of deaths by suicide.[16]

ADOLESCENTS AT INCREASED RISK

Although no specific tests are capable of identifying a suicidal person, specific risk factors exist.[11,17] The health care professional should use care in interpreting risk factors, however, because risk factors are common, whereas suicide is infrequent. Of importance, the lack of most risk factors does not make an adolescent safe from suicide. Fixed risk factors include: family history of suicide or suicide attempts; history of adoption[18,19]; male gender; parental mental health problems; lesbian, gay, bisexual, or questioning sexual orientation; transgender identification; a history of physical or sexual abuse; and a previous suicide attempt. Personal mental health problems that predispose to suicide include sleep disturbances,[20] depression, bipolar disorder, substance intoxication and substance use disorders, psychosis, posttraumatic stress disorder, panic attacks, a history of aggression, impulsivity, severe anger, and pathologic Internet use (see *Internet Use* section). In particular, interview studies showed a marked higher rate of suicidal behavior with the presence of psychotic symptoms.[21] A prospective study found a 70-fold increase of acute suicidal behavior in adolescents with psychopathology that included psychosis.[22] By definition, nonsuicidal self-injury (NSSI) does not include intent to die, and risk of death is deliberately low. Nonetheless, NSSI is a risk factor for suicide attempts[23,24] and suicidal ideation.[25] More than 90% of adolescent suicide victims met criteria for a psychiatric disorder

before their death. Immediate risk factors include agitation, intoxication, and a recent stressful life event. More information is available from the American Academy of Child and Adolescent Psychiatry[26] and Gould et al.[11]

Social and environmental risk factors include bullying, impaired parent–child relationship, living outside of the home (homeless or in a corrections facility or group home), difficulties in school, neither working nor attending school, social isolation, and presence of stressful life events, such as legal or romantic difficulties or an argument with a parent. An unsupported social environment for lesbian, gay, bisexual, and transgender adolescents, for example, increases risk of suicide attempts.[27] Protective factors include religious involvement and connection between the adolescent and parents, school, and peers.[26]

Bullying

Bullying has been defined as having 3 elements: aggressive or deliberately harmful behavior (1) between peers that is (2) repeated and over time and (3) involves an imbalance of power, for example, related to physical strength or popularity, making it difficult for the victim to defend himself or herself.[28] Behavior falls into 4 categories: direct-physical (eg, assault, theft), direct-verbal (eg, threats, insults, name-calling), indirect-relational (eg, social exclusion, spreading rumors), and cyberbullying.[29] The 2013 Youth Risk Behavior Survey of students in grades 9 through 12 in the United States indicated that during the 12 months before the survey, 23.7% of girls and 15.6% of boys were bullied on school property, 21.0% of girls and 8.5% of boys were electronically bullied, and 8.7% of girls and 5.4% of boys did not go to school 1 day in the past 30 because they felt unsafe at or to or from school.[7] Studies have focused on 3 groups: those who were victims, those who were bullies, and those who were both victims and bullies (bully/victims).[30]

Reviewing 31 studies, Klomek et al[29] found a clear relationship between both bullying victimization and perpetration and suicidal ideation and behavior in children and adolescents. Females were at risk regardless of frequency, whereas males were at higher risk only with frequent bullying. A review by Arseneault et al[31] cited evidence that bullying victimization is associated with severe baseline psychopathology, as well as individual characteristics and family factors, and that the psychopathology is made significantly worse by the victimization. Being the victim of school bullying or cyberbullying is associated with substantial distress, resulting in lower school performance and school attachment.[32] Suicidal ideation and behavior were greater in those bullied with controlling for age, gender, race/ethnicity, and depressive symptomology.[33] Suicidal ideation and behavior were increased in victims and bullies and were highest in bully/victims.[34] Similar increases in suicide attempts were found comparing face-to-face bullying with cyberbullying, both for victims and bullies.[35]

Bullying predicts future mental health problems. Bullying behavior at 8 years of age was associated with later suicide attempts and completed suicides,[36] although among boys, frequent perpetration and victimization was not associated with attempts and completions after controlling for conduct and depressive symptoms. Among girls, frequent victimization was associated with later suicide attempts and completions even after controlling for conduct and depressive symptoms. High school students with the highest psychiatric impairment 4 years later were those who had been identified as at-risk for

suicide *and* experiencing frequent bullying behavior. Copeland et al[30] found that children and adolescents involved in bullying behavior had the worst outcomes when they were both bullies and victims, leading to depression, anxiety, and suicidality (suicidality only among males) as adults. Assessment for adolescents with psychopathology, other signs of emotional distress, or unusual chronic complaints should include screening for participation in bullying as victims or bullies.

Internet Use

Pathologic Internet use correlates with suicidal ideation and NSSI.[37] Self-reported daily use of video games and Internet exceeding 5 hours was strongly associated with higher levels of depression and suicidality (ideation and attempts) in adolescents.[38] A more specific problem is that adolescents with suicidal ideation may be at particular risk for searching the Internet for information about suicide-related topics.[39] Suicide-related searches were found to be associated with completed suicides among young adults.[40] Prosuicide Web sites and online suicide pacts facilitate suicidal behavior, with adolescents and young adults at particular risk.[37]

A number of factors diminish the exposure of prosuicide Web sites. Web site results from the search term, "suicide," are predominantly of institutional origin, with content largely related to research and prevention. Although there are a substantial number of sites from private senders (these sites are often antimedical, antitreatment, and pro-suicide,[41] including sites that advocate suicide or describe methods in detail[42]), suicide research and prevention sites tend to come up in searches more commonly. Clicking on links within each site keeps the reader in the site, strengthening the site's position. Methods sites and overtly prosuicide sites are

more isolated, decentralized, and unfocused; these are less prevalent among the first 100 search results, perhaps related to a recent and deliberate strategy by the internet search engines (eg, search engine optimization).[41]

Learning of another's suicide online may be another risk factor for youth.[43] Exposure to such information is through online news sites (44%), social networking sites (25%), online discussion forums (15%), and video Web sites (15%). Social networking sites have particular importance, because these may afford information on suicidal behavior of social contacts that would not otherwise be available. Fortunately, exposure to information from social networking sites does not appear related to changes in suicidal ideation, with increased exposure mitigated by greater social support. Participation in online forums, however, was associated with increases in suicidal ideation, possibly related to anonymous discussions about mental health problems. For example, suicide attempts by susceptible individuals appear to have been encouraged by such conversations.[44,45]

INTERVIEWING THE ADOLESCENT

Primary care pediatricians should be comfortable screening patients for suicide, mood disorders, and substance abuse and dependence. Ask about emotional difficulties and use of drugs and alcohol, identify lack of developmental progress, and estimate level of distress, impairment of functioning, and level of danger to self and others. Depression screening instruments shown to be valid in adolescents include the Patient Health Questionnaire (PHQ)-9 and PHQ-2.[46] If needed, a referral should be made for appropriate mental health evaluation and treatment. In areas where the resources necessary to make a timely mental health referral are lacking, pediatricians are encouraged to obtain extra training and become competent in providing a more in-depth assessment.

Suicidal ideation may be assessed by directly asking or screening via self-report. Self-administered scales can be useful for screening, because adolescents may disclose information about suicidality on self-report that they deny in person. Scales, however, tend to be oversensitive and underspecific and lack predictive value. Adolescents who endorse suicidality on a scale should be assessed clinically. Screening tools useable in a primary care setting have not been shown to have more than limited ability to detect suicide risk in adolescents,[47] consistent with the findings of an earlier review.[48] Instruments studied in adolescent groups with high prevalence of suicidal ideation and behavior showed sensitivity of 52% to 87% and specificity of 60% to 85%; the results are only generalizable to high-risk populations.[49,50] Suicide screening, at least in the school setting, does not appear to cause thoughts of suicide or other psychiatric symptoms in students.[51,52]

One approach to initiate a confidential inquiry into suicidal thoughts or concerns is to ask a general question, such as, "Have you ever thought about killing yourself or wished you were dead?" The question is best placed in the middle or toward the end of a list of questions about depressive symptoms. Regardless of the answer, the next question should be, "Have you ever done anything on purpose to hurt or kill yourself?" If the response to either question is positive, the pediatrician should obtain more detail (eg, nature of past and present thoughts and behaviors, time frame, intent, who knows and how they found out). Inquiry should include suicide plans ("If you were to kill yourself, how would you do it?"), whether there are firearms in the

home, and the response of the family. No data indicate that inquiry about suicide precipitates the behavior, even in high-risk students.[51]

The adolescent should be interviewed separately from the parent, because the patient may be more likely to withhold important information in the parent's presence. Information should also be sought from parents and others as appropriate. Although confidentiality is important in adolescent health care, for adolescents at risk to themselves or others, safety takes precedence over confidentiality; the adolescent should have this explained by the pediatrician so that he or she understands that at the onset. Pediatricians need to inform appropriate people, such as parent(s) and other providers, when they believe an adolescent is at risk for suicide and to share with the adolescent that there is a need to break confidentiality because of the risk of harm to the adolescent. As much as is possible, the sequence of events that preceded the threat should be determined, current problems and conflicts should be identified, and the degree of suicidal intent should be assessed. In addition, pediatricians should assess individual coping resources, accessible support systems, and attitudes of the adolescent and family toward intervention and follow-up.[53] Questions should also be asked to elicit known risk factors. Note that it is acceptable and, in some cases, more appropriate for the patient to be referred to a mental health specialist to access the degree of suicide intent and relevant factors such as coping mechanisms and support systems.

Care in interviewing needs to be taken, because abrupt, intrusive questions could result in a reduction of rapport and a lower likelihood of the adolescent sharing mental health concerns. This is especially true during a brief encounter for an

unrelated concern. Initial questions should be open-ended and relatively nonthreatening. Examples include "Aside from [already stated non–mental health concern], how have you been doing?" "I know that a lot of people your age have a lot going on. What kinds of things have been on your mind or stressing you lately?" "How have things been going with [school, friends, parents, sports]?" When possible, more detailed questions should then follow, particularly during routine care visits or when a mental health concern is stated or suspected.

Suicidal thoughts or comments should never be dismissed as unimportant. Statements such as, "You've come really close to killing yourself," may, if true, acknowledge the deep despair of the youth and communicate to the adolescent that the interviewer understands how serious he or she has felt about dying. Such disclosures should be met with reassurance that the patient's pleas for assistance have been heard and that help will be sought.

Serious mood disorders, such as major depressive disorder or bipolar disorder, may present in adolescents in several ways.[54] Some adolescents may come to the office with complaints similar to those of depressed adults, having symptoms, such as sad or down feelings most of the time, crying spells, guilty or worthless feelings, markedly diminished interest or pleasure in most activities, significant weight loss or weight gain or increase or decrease in appetite, insomnia or hypersomnia, fatigue or loss of energy, diminished ability to think or concentrate, and thoughts of death or suicide. The pediatrician should also look for adolescent behaviors that are characteristic of symptoms (Table 1).[54] Some adolescents may present with irritability rather than depressed mood as the main manifestation. Other adolescents present for an acute care visit with somatic symptoms, such as abdominal pain, chest pain, headache, lethargy, weight loss, dizziness and syncope, or other nonspecific symptoms[55] Others present with behavioral problems, such as truancy, deterioration in academic performance, running away from home, defiance of authorities, self-destructive behavior, vandalism, substance use disorder, sexual acting out, and delinquency.[56] Typically, symptoms of depression, mania, or a mixed state (depression and mania coexisting or rapidly alternating) can be elicited with careful questioning but may not be immediately obvious. The American Academy of Pediatrics (AAP) provides more information about adolescent bipolar disorder and the role of the pediatrician in screening, diagnosis, and management.[57]

At well-adolescent visits, adolescents who show any evidence of psychosocial or adaptive difficulties should be assessed regularly for mental health concerns and also asked about suicidal ideation, physical and sexual abuse, bullying, substance use, and sexual orientation. Depression screening is now recommended for all adolescents between the ages of 11 and 21 years of age in the third edition of *Bright Futures*.[58] The AAP developed a resource, "Addressing Mental Health Concerns in Primary Care: A Clinician's Toolkit," which is available for a fee.[59] The AAP also developed a Web site that provides resources and materials free of charge.[60] Identification and screening at acute care visits, when possible, is desirable, because mental health problems may manifest more strongly at these times.

MANAGEMENT OF THE SUICIDAL ADOLESCENT

Management depends on the degree of acute risk. Unfortunately, no one can accurately predict suicide, so

TABLE 1 Depressive Symptoms and Examples in Adolescents[54]

Signs and Symptoms of Major Depressive Disorder	Signs of Depression Frequently Seen in Youth
Depressed mood most of the day	Irritable or cranky mood; preoccupation with song lyrics that suggest life is meaningless
Decreased interest/enjoyment in once-favorite activities	Loss of interest in sports, video games, and activities with friends
Significant wt loss/gain	Failure to gain wt as normally expected; anorexia or bulimia; frequent complaints of physical illness (eg, headache, stomach ache)
Insomnia or hypersomnia	Excessive late-night TV; refusal to wake for school in the morning
Psychomotor agitation/retardation	Talk of running away from home or efforts to do so
Fatigue or loss of energy	Persistent boredom
Low self-esteem; feelings of guilt	Oppositional and/or negative behavior
Decreased ability to concentrate; indecisive	Poor performance in school; frequent absences
Recurrent thoughts of death or suicidal ideation or behavior	Recurrent suicidal ideation or behavior (threats of suicide, writing about death; giving away favorite toys or belongings)

even experts can only determine who is at higher risk. Intent is a key issue in the determination of risk. Examples of adolescents at high risk include: those with a plan or recent suicide attempt with a high probability of lethality; stated current intent to kill themselves; recent suicidal ideation or behavior accompanied by current agitation or severe hopelessness; and impulsivity and profoundly dysphoric mood associated with bipolar disorder, major depression, psychosis, or a substance use disorder. An absence of factors that indicate high risk, especially in the presence of a desire to receive help and a supportive family, suggests a lower risk but not necessarily a low risk. Low risk is difficult to determine. For example, an adolescent who has taken 8 ibuprofen tablets may have thought that it was a lethal dose and may do something more lethal the next time. Alternatively, the adolescent may have known that 8 ibuprofen tablets is not lethal and took the pills as a rehearsal for a lethal attempt. In the presence of a recent suicide attempt, the lack of current suicidal ideation may also be misleading if none of the factors that led to the attempt have changed or the reasons for the attempt are not understood. The benefit of the doubt is generally

on safety in the management of the suicidal adolescent.

The term "suicide gesture" should not be used, because it implies a low risk of suicide that may not be warranted. "Suicide attempt" is a more appropriate term for any deliberately self-harmful behavior or action that could reasonably be expected to produce self-harm and is accompanied by some degree of intent or desire for death as well as thinking by the patient at the time of the behavior that the behavior had even a small possibility of resulting in death. In a less-than-forthcoming patient, intent may be inferred by the lethality of the behavior, such as ingesting a large number of pills, or by an affirmative answer to a question such as, "At the time of your action, would you have thought it okay if you had died?"

Adolescents who initially may seem at low risk, joke about suicide, or seek treatment of repeated somatic complaints may be asking for help the only way they can. Their concerns should be assessed thoroughly. Adolescents who are judged to be at low risk of suicide should still receive close follow-up, referral for a timely mental health evaluation, or both if they should have any significant degree of dysfunction or distress from emotional or behavioral symptoms.

For adolescents who seem to be at moderate or high risk of suicide or have attempted suicide, arrangements for immediate mental health professional evaluation should be made during the office visit. Options for immediate evaluation include hospitalization, transfer to an emergency department, or a same-day appointment with a mental health professional.

Intervention should be tailored to the adolescent's needs. Adolescents with a responsive and supportive family, little likelihood of acting on suicidal impulses (eg, thought of dying with no intent or plan for suicide), and someone who can take action if there is mood or behavior deterioration may require only outpatient treatment.[17] In contrast, adolescents who have made previous attempts, exhibit a high degree of intent to commit suicide, show evidence of serious depression or other psychiatric illness, engage in substance use or have an active substance use disorder, have low impulse control, or have families who are unwilling to commit to counseling are at high risk and may require psychiatric hospitalization.

Although no controlled studies have been conducted to prove that admitting adolescents at high risk to a psychiatric unit saves lives,[17] likely the safest course of action is hospitalization, thereby placing the adolescent in a safe and protected environment. An inpatient stay will allow time for a complete medical and psychiatric evaluation with initiation of therapy in a controlled setting as well as arrangement of appropriate mental health follow-up care.

Pediatricians can enhance continuity of care and adherence to treatment recommendations by maintaining contact with suicidal adolescents even after referrals are made. Collaborative care is encouraged, because it has been shown to result in greater reduction of depressive symptoms in a primary care setting.[61] Recommendations should include that all firearms are removed from the home, because adolescents may still find access to locked guns stored in their home, and that medications, both prescription and over-the-counter, are locked up. Vigorous treatment of the underlying psychiatric disorder is important in decreasing short-term and long-term risk of suicide. Although asking the adolescent to agree to a contract against suicide has not been proven effective in preventing suicidal behavior,[17] the technique may still be helpful in assessing risk in that refusal to agree either not to harm oneself or to tell a specified person about intent to harm oneself is ominous. In addition, safety planning may help guide a patient and his or her family in what steps to take in moments of distress to ensure patient safety.

Working with a suicidal adolescent can be very difficult for those who are providing treatment. Suicide risk can only be reduced, not eliminated, and risk factors provide no more than guidance. Much of the information regarding risk factors is subjective and must be elicited from the adolescent, who may have his or her own agenda. Just as importantly, pediatricians need to be aware of their personal reactions to prevent interference in evaluation and treatment and overreaction or underreaction.

ANTIDEPRESSANT MEDICATIONS AND SUICIDE

The Food and Drug Administration (FDA) directive of October 2004 and heavy media coverage changed perceptions of antidepressant medications, and not favorably. The FDA directed pharmaceutical companies to label all antidepressant medications distributed in the United States with a "black-box warning" to alert health care providers to an increased risk of suicidality (suicidal thinking and behavior) in children and adolescents being treated with these agents. The FDA did not prohibit the use of these medications in youth but called on clinicians to balance increased risk of suicidality with clinical need and to monitor closely "for clinical worsening, suicidality, or unusual changes in behavior."[62] The warning particularly stressed the need for close monitoring during the first few months of treatment and after dose changes.

The warning by the FDA was prompted by a finding that in 24 clinical trials that involved more than 4400 child and adolescent patients and 9 different antidepressant medications, spontaneously reported suicidal ideation or behavior was present in 4% of subjects who were receiving medication and in just half that (2%) of subjects who were receiving a placebo. No completed suicides occurred during any of the studies. In the same studies, however, only a slight reduction of suicidality was found when subjects were asked directly at each visit about suicidal ideation and behavior, which was considered a contradictory finding. The method of asking directly does not rely on spontaneous reports and is considered to be more reliable than the spontaneous events report method used by the FDA to support the black-box warning.[63] In addition, a reanalysis of the data including 7 additional studies and using a more conservative model showed only a trivial 0.7% increase in the risk of suicidal ideation or behavior in those receiving antidepressant medications.[64]

Subsequent studies have addressed the validity of the black-box warning and suggest that, for appropriate youth, the risk of not prescribing antidepressant medication is significantly higher than the risk of prescribing. Gibbons et al[65] conducted a reanalysis of all sponsor-conducted randomized controlled trials of fluoxetine and venlafaxine, which included 12 adult, 4 geriatric, and 4 youth studies of fluoxetine and 21 adult trials of venlafaxine. Adult and geriatric patients treated with both medications showed decreased suicidal thoughts and behaviors, an effect mediated by the decreases of depressive symptoms with treatment. No significant treatment effect on suicidal thoughts and behaviors was found with youth treated with fluoxetine, although depressive symptoms in fluoxetine-treated patients decreased more quickly than symptoms in patients receiving placebo. There was no overall greater rate of suicidal thoughts and behaviors in the treatment groups versus the placebo groups. The finding of increased suicidal ideation and behavior in the treatment groups that formed the basis of the FDA black-box warning on antidepressant use in children and adolescents was not found in this reanalysis of the fluoxetine studies. More importantly, these reanalyses demonstrated the efficacy of fluoxetine in the treatment of depression in youth. Patients in all age and drug groups had significantly greater improvement relative to patients in placebo groups, with youth having the largest differential rate of remission over 6 weeks—46.6% of patients receiving fluoxetine versus 16.5% of those receiving placebo.[66]

Suicidal ideation and behavior are common, and suicides are vastly less common, which makes it difficult to relate a change in one to a change in the other.[63] Examining all available observational studies, Dudley et al[67] found that recent exposure to selective serotonin reuptake inhibitor medications was rare (1.6%) for young people who died by suicide, supporting the conclusion that most of the suicide victims did not have the potential benefit of antidepressants at the time of their deaths. The study suggests that whether antidepressants increase suicidal thoughts or behaviors in adolescents, few actual suicides are related to current use of the medications.

Several studies showed a negative correlation between antidepressant prescribing and completed adolescent suicide. The 28% decrease in completed suicides in the 10- to 19-year-old age group from 1990 to 2000 may have been at least partly a result of the increase in youth antidepressant prescribing over the same time period. Analyzing US data by examining prescribing and suicide in each of 588 2-digit zip code zones showed a significant ($P < .001$) 0.23-per-100 000 annual decrease in adolescent suicide with every 1% increase in antidepressant prescribing.[68] A second study analyzed county-level data during the period from1996 to1998 and found that higher selective serotonin reuptake inhibitor prescription rates significantly correlated with lower suicide rates among children and adolescents 5 to 14 years of age.[69] Using a decision analysis model, Cougnard et al[70] calculated that antidepressant treatment of children and adolescents would prevent 31.9% of suicides of depressed subjects, similar to findings in the adult (32.2%) and geriatric (32.3%) age groups.

The FDA advisory panel was aware that the black-box warning could have the unintended effect of limiting access to necessary and effective treatment[63] and reported that prescriptions of antidepressants for children and adolescents decreased by 19% in the third quarter of 2004 and 16% in the fourth quarter compared with the year before.[71] Claims data for Tennessee Medicaid showed a 33% reduction of new users of antidepressants 21 months after the black-box warning.[72] US national managed care data showed reduced diagnosing of pediatric depression and a 58% reduction of antidepressant prescribing compared with what was predicted by the preadvisory trend.[73] Decreased antidepressant prescribing was also seen with chart review.[74] Most of the reductions in diagnosing and prescribing were related to substantial reductions by primary care providers, with these reductions persisting through 2007.[75] Studies differed as to whether there was[76] or was not[73,74] a compensatory increase of psychotherapy treatment during the same time period.

Concern was expressed that the reduction of antidepressant prescribing may be related to the increase in US youth suicides from 2003 to 2004 after a decade of steady declines.[77] Gibbons et al[78] found that antidepressant prescribing for youth decreased by 22% in both the United States and the Netherlands the year after the black-box warnings in both countries and a reduction in prescribing was observed across all ages. From 2003 to 2004, the youth suicide rate in the United States increased by 14%; from 2003 to 2005, the youth suicide rate in the Netherlands increased by 49%. Across age groups, data showed a significant inverse correlation between prescribing and change in suicide rate. The authors suggested that the warnings could have had the unintended effect of increasing the rate of youth suicide.[78] Examining health insurance claims data for 1.1 million adolescents, 1.4 million young adults, and 5 million adults, the rate of psychotropic medication poisonings, a validate proxy for suicide attempts, was found to have increased significantly in adolescents (21.7%) and young adults (33.7%), but not in adults (5.2%), in the second year after the FDA black-box warning, corresponding with decreases in antidepressant prescribing (adolescents, –31.0%; young adults, –24.3%; adults, –14.5%).[79]

Regardless of whether the use of antidepressant medications changes the risk of suicide, depression is an important suicide risk factor, and careful monitoring of adolescents' mental health and behavioral status is critically important, particularly when initiating or changing treatment. Furthermore, despite the aforementioned new information, the FDA has not removed or changed the black-box warning; the warning should be discussed with parents or guardians and appropriately documented. The American Psychiatric Association and the American Academy of Child and Adolescent Psychiatry recommended a monitoring approach[63] that enlists the parents or guardians in the responsibility for monitoring and individualizing the frequency and nature of monitoring to the needs of the patient and the family. This approach potentially increases the effectiveness of monitoring and provides greater flexibility, thus reducing a barrier to prescribing. Warning signs for family members to contact the prescribing physician are listed in Table 2.[63]

SUMMARY

1. Adolescent suicide is an important public health problem.

2. Knowledge of risk factors, particularly mood disorders, psychosis, and bullying victimization and perpetration, may assist in the identification of adolescents who are at higher risk.

3. It is important to know and use appropriate techniques for interviewing potentially suicidal adolescents.

4. Mood disorders predisposing adolescents to suicide have a variety of presentations.

5. Management options depend on the degree of suicide risk.

6. Treatment with antidepressant medication is important when indicated.

TABLE 2 Treatment With Antidepressant Medication: Warning Signs for Family Members To Contact the Physician

New or more frequent thoughts of wanting to die
Self-destructive behavior
Signs of increased anxiety/panic, agitation, aggressiveness, impulsivity, insomnia, or irritability
New or more involuntary restlessness (akathesia), such as pacing or fidgeting
Extreme degree of elation or energy
Fast, driven speech
New onset of unrealistic plans or goals

ADVICE FOR PEDIATRICIANS

1. Ask questions about mood disorders, use of drugs and alcohol, suicidal thoughts, bullying, sexual orientation, and other risk factors associated with suicide in routine history taking throughout adolescence. Know the risk factors (eg, signs and symptoms of depression) associated with adolescent suicide and screen routinely for depression. Consider using a depression screening instrument, such as the PHQ-9 or PHQ-2, at health maintenance visits from 11 to 21 years of age and as needed at acute care visits.[46]

2. Educate yourself and your patients about the benefits and risks of antidepressant medications. Patients with depression should be carefully monitored, with appropriately frequent appointments and education of the family regarding warning signs for when to call you, especially after the initiation of antidepressant medication treatment and with dose changes. Recent studies suggest that, for appropriate youth, the benefits of antidepressant medications outweigh the risks.

3. Recognize the medical and psychiatric needs of the suicidal adolescent and work closely with families and health care professionals involved in the management and follow-up of youth who are at risk or have attempted suicide. Develop working relationships with emergency departments and colleagues in child and adolescent psychiatry, clinical psychology, and other mental health professions to optimally evaluate and manage the care of adolescents who are at risk for suicide. Because mental and physical health services are often provided through different systems of care, extra effort is necessary to ensure good communication, continuity, and follow-up through the medical home.

4. Because resources for adolescents and physicians vary by community, become familiar with local, state, and national resources that are concerned with treatment of psychopathology and suicide prevention in youth, including local hospitals with psychiatric units, mental health agencies, family and children's services, crisis hotlines, and crisis intervention centers. Compile the names and contact information of local mental health resources and providers and make that information available to patients/families when needed.

5. Because there is great variation among general pediatricians in training and comfort with assessing and treating patients with mental health problems, as well as in access to appropriate mental health resources, consider additional training and ongoing education in diagnosing and managing adolescent mood disorders, especially if practicing in an underserved area.

Pediatricians with fewer resources still have an important role in screening, comanaging with mental health professionals, and referring patients when necessary (as recommended in *Bright Futures, Fourth Edition*).

6. During routine evaluations and where consistent with state law, ask whether firearms are kept in the home and discuss with parents the increased risk of adolescent suicide with the presence of firearms. Specifically for adolescents at risk for suicide, advise parents to remove guns and ammunition from the house and secure supplies of prescription and over-the-counter medications.

LEAD AUTHOR

Benjamin Shain, MD, PhD

COMMITTEE ON ADOLESCENCE, 2014-2015

Paula K. Braverman, MD, Chairperson
William P. Adelman, MD
Elizabeth M. Alderman, MD, FSHAM
Cora C. Breuner, MD, MPH
David A. Levine, MD
Arik V. Marcell, MD, MPH
Rebecca F. O'Brien, MD

LIAISONS

Laurie L. Hornberger, MD, MPH – *Section on Adolescent Health*
Margo Lane, MD, FRCPC – *Canadian Pediatric Society*
Julie Strickland, MD – *American College of Obstetricians and Gynecologists*
Benjamin Shain, MD, PhD – *American Academy of Child and Adolescent Psychiatry*

STAFF

Karen Smith
James Baumberger, MPP

ABBREVIATIONS

AAP: American Academy of Pediatrics
FDA: Food and Drug Administration
NSSI: nonsuicidal self-injury
PHQ: Patient Health Questionnaire

REFERENCES

1. O'Carroll PW, Potter LB, Mercy JA. Programs for the prevention of suicide among adolescents and young adults. *MMWR Recomm Rep.* 1994;43(RR-6):1–7

2. Centers for Disease Control and Prevention. CDC Wonder [database]: mortality query. Available at: http://wonder.cdc.gov. Accessed April 24, 2015

3. American Psychiatric Association, Committee on Adolescence. *Adolescent Suicide.* Washington, DC: American Psychiatric Press; 1996

4. Grunbaum JA, Kann L, Kinchen S, et al; Centers for Disease Control and Prevention. Youth risk behavior surveillance--United States, 2003. [published corrections appear in *MMWR Morb Mortal Wkly Rep.* 2004;53(24):536 and *MMWR Morb Mortal Wkly Rep.* 2005;54(24):608] *MMWR Surveill Summ.* 2004;53(2):1–96

5. Husain SA. Current perspective on the role of psychological factors in adolescent suicide. *Psychiatr Ann.* 1990;20(3):122–127

6. Committee On Adolescence. Office-based care for lesbian, gay, bisexual, transgender, and questioning youth. *Pediatrics.* 2013;132(1):198–203

7. Kann L, Kinchen S, Shanklin SL, et al; Centers for Disease Control and Prevention (CDC). Youth risk behavior surveillance--United States, 2013. *MMWR Suppl.* 2014;63(4):1–168

8. Brent DA, Perper JA, Allman CJ, Moritz GM, Wartella ME, Zelenak JP. The presence and accessibility of firearms in the homes of adolescent suicides. A case-control study. *JAMA.* 1991;266(21):2989–2995

9. American Academy of Pediatrics, Committee on Injury and Poison Prevention. Firearm injuries affecting the pediatric population. *Pediatrics.* 1992;89(4 pt 2):788–790

10. Grossman DC, Mueller BA, Riedy C, et al. Gun storage practices and risk of youth suicide and unintentional firearm injuries. *JAMA.* 2005;293(6):707–714

11. Gould MS, Greenberg T, Velting DM, Shaffer D. Youth suicide risk and preventive interventions: a review of the past 10 years. *J Am Acad Child Adolesc Psychiatry.* 2003;42(4):386–405

12. Swanson SA, Colman I. Association between exposure to suicide and suicidality outcomes in youth. *CMAJ.* 2013;185(10):870–877

13. Gould MS, Kleinman MH, Lake AM, Forman J, Midle JB. Newspaper coverage of suicide and initiation of suicide clusters in teenagers in the USA, 1988-96: a retrospective, population-based, case-control study. *Lancet Psychiatry.* 2014;1(1):34–43

14. Haw C, Hawton K, Niedzwiedz C, Platt S. Suicide clusters: a review of risk factors and mechanisms. *Suicide Life Threat Behav.* 2013;43(1):97–108

15. Ali MM, Dwyer DS, Rizzo JA. The social contagion effect of suicidal behavior in adolescents: does it really exist? *J Ment Health Policy Econ.* 2011;14(1):3–12

16. National Institute of Mental Health. Recommendations for reporting on suicide. Available at: www.nimh.nih.gov/health/topics/suicide-prevention/recommendations-for-reporting-on-suicide.shtml. Accessed July 27, 2015

17. American Academy of Child and Adolescent Psychiatry. Practice parameter for the assessment and treatment of children and adolescents with suicidal behavior. *J Am Acad Child Adolesc Psychiatry.* 2001;40(7 Suppl):24S–51S

18. Slap G, Goodman E, Huang B. Adoption as a risk factor for attempted suicide during adolescence. *Pediatrics.* 2001;108(2). Available at: http://pediatrics.aappublications.org/content/108/2/e30

19. Keyes MA, Malone SM, Sharma A, Iacono WG, McGue M. Risk of suicide attempt in adopted and nonadopted offspring. *Pediatrics.* 2013;132(4):639–646

20. Goldstein TR, Bridge JA, Brent DA. Sleep disturbance preceding completed suicide in adolescents. *J Consult Clin Psychol.* 2008;76(1):84–91

21. Kelleher I, Lynch F, Harley M, et al. Psychotic symptoms in adolescence index risk for suicidal behavior: findings from 2 population-based

case-control clinical interview studies. *Arch Gen Psychiatry.* 2012;69(12):1277–1283

22. Kelleher I, Corcoran P, Keeley H, et al. Psychotic symptoms and population risk for suicide attempt: a prospective cohort study. *JAMA Psychiatry.* 2013;70(9):940–948

23. Asarnow JR, Porta G, Spirito A, et al. Suicide attempts and nonsuicidal self-injury in the treatment of resistant depression in adolescents: findings from the TORDIA study. *J Am Acad Child Adolesc Psychiatry.* 2011;50(8):772–781

24. Wilkinson PO. Nonsuicidal self-injury: a clear marker for suicide risk. *J Am Acad Child Adolesc Psychiatry.* 2011;50(8):741–743

25. Cox LJ, Stanley BH, Melhem NM, et al. Familial and individual correlates of nonsuicidal self-injury in the offspring of mood-disordered parents. *J Clin Psychiatry.* 2012;73(6):813–820

26. American Academy of Child and Adolescent Psychiatry Web site. Available at: www.aacap.org. Accessed July 27, 2015

27. Hatzenbuehler ML. The social environment and suicide attempts in lesbian, gay, and bisexual youth. *Pediatrics.* 2011;127(5):896–903

28. Olweus D. Bullying at school: basic facts and effects of a school based intervention program. *J Child Psychol Psychiatry.* 1994;35(7):1171–1190

29. Brunstein Klomek A, Sourander A, Gould M. The association of suicide and bullying in childhood to young adulthood: a review of cross-sectional and longitudinal research findings. *Can J Psychiatry.* 2010;55(5):282–288

30. Copeland WE, Wolke D, Angold A, Costello EJ. Adult psychiatric outcomes of bullying and being bullied by peers in childhood and adolescence. *JAMA Psychiatry.* 2013;70(4):419–426

31. Arseneault L, Bowes L, Shakoor S. Bullying victimization in youths and mental health problems: 'much ado about nothing'? *Psychol Med.* 2010;40(5):717–729

32. Schneider SK, O'Donnell L, Stueve A, Coulter RW. Cyberbullying, school bullying, and psychological distress: a regional census of high school students. *Am J Public Health.* 2012;102(1):171–177

33. Kaminski JW, Fang X. Victimization by peers and adolescent suicide in three US samples. *J Pediatr.* 2009;155(5):683–688

34. Winsper C, Lereya T, Zanarini M, Wolke D. Involvement in bullying and suicide-related behavior at 11 years: a prospective birth cohort study. *J Am Acad Child Adolesc Psychiatry.* 2012;51(3):271–282.e3

35. Hinduja S, Patchin JW. Bullying, cyberbullying, and suicide. *Arch Suicide Res.* 2010;14(3):206–221

36. Klomek AB, Sourander A, Niemelä S, et al. Childhood bullying behaviors as a risk for suicide attempts and completed suicides: a population-based birth cohort study. *J Am Acad Child Adolesc Psychiatry.* 2009;48(3):254–261

37. Durkee T, Hadlaczky G, Westerlund M, Carli V. Internet pathways in suicidality: a review of the evidence. *Int J Environ Res Public Health.* 2011;8(10):3938–3952

38. Messias E, Castro J, Saini A, Usman M, Peeples D. Sadness, suicide, and their association with video game and internet overuse among teens: results from the youth risk behavior survey 2007 and 2009. *Suicide Life Threat Behav.* 2011;41(3):307–315

39. Katsumata Y, Matsumoto T, Kitani M, Takeshima T. Electronic media use and suicidal ideation in Japanese adolescents. *Psychiatry Clin Neurosci.* 2008;62(6):744–746

40. Hagihara A, Miyazaki S, Abe T. Internet suicide searches and the incidence of suicide in young people in Japan. *Eur Arch Psychiatry Clin Neurosci.* 2012;262(1):39–46

41. Westerlund M, Hadlaczky G, Wasserman D. The representation of suicide on the Internet: implications for clinicians. *J Med Internet Res.* 2012;14(5):e122

42. Kemp CG, Collings SC. Hyperlinked suicide: assessing the prominence and accessibility of suicide websites. *Crisis.* 2011;32(3):143–151

43. Dunlop SM, More E, Romer D. Where do youth learn about suicides on the Internet, and what influence does this have on suicidal ideation? *J Child Psychol Psychiatry.* 2011;52(10):1073–1080

44. Becker K, Schmidt MH. Internet chat rooms and suicide. *J Am Acad Child Adolesc Psychiatry.* 2004;43(3):246–247

45. Becker K, Mayer M, Nagenborg M, El-Faddagh M, Schmidt MH. Parasuicide online: Can suicide websites trigger suicidal behaviour in predisposed adolescents? *Nord J Psychiatry.* 2004;58(2):111–114

46. Allgaier AK, Pietsch K, Frühe B, Sigl-Glöckner J, Schulte-Körne G. Screening for depression in adolescents: validity of the patient health questionnaire in pediatric care. *Depress Anxiety.* 2012;29(10):906–913

47. O'Connor E, Gaynes BN, Burda BU, Soh C, Whitlock EP. Screening for and treatment of suicide risk relevant to primary care: a systematic review for the U.S. Preventive Services Task Force. *Ann Intern Med.* 2013;158(10):741–754

48. Peña JB, Caine ED. Screening as an approach for adolescent suicide prevention. *Suicide Life Threat Behav.* 2006;36(6):614–637

49. Thompson EA, Eggert LL. Using the suicide risk screen to identify suicidal adolescents among potential high school dropouts. *J Am Acad Child Adolesc Psychiatry.* 1999;38(12):1506–1514

50. Holi MM, Pelkonen M, Karlsson L, et al. Detecting suicidality among adolescent outpatients: evaluation of trained clinicians' suicidality assessment against a structured diagnostic assessment made by trained raters. *BMC Psychiatry.* 2008;8:97

51. Gould MS, Marrocco FA, Kleinman M, et al. Evaluating iatrogenic risk of youth suicide screening programs: a randomized controlled trial. *JAMA.* 2005;293(13):1635–1643

52. Robinson J, Pan Yuen H, Martin C, et al. Does screening high school students for psychological distress, deliberate self-harm, or suicidal ideation cause distress--and is it acceptable? An Australian-based study. *Crisis.* 2011;32(5):254–263

53. King RA; American Academy of Child and Adolescent Psychiatry. Practice parameters for the psychiatric assessment of children and adolescents. *J Am Acad Child Adolesc Psychiatry.* 1997;36(10 Suppl):4S–20S

54. American Psychiatric Association. *Diagnostic and Statistical Manual of Mental Disorders (DS-5).* 5th ed. Washington, DC: American Psychiatric Association; 2013

55. Wolraich ML, Felice ME, Drotar D, eds. *The Classification of Child and Adolescent Mental Diagnoses in Primary Care: Diagnostic and Statistical Manual for Primary Care (DSM-PC), Child and Adolescent Version.* Elk Grove Village, IL: American Academy of Pediatrics; 1996

56. Birmaher B, Brent D, Bernet W, et al; AACAP Work Group on Quality Issues. Practice parameter for the assessment and treatment of children and adolescents with depressive disorders. *J Am Acad Child Adolesc Psychiatry.* 2007;46(11):1503–1526

57. Shain BN; COMMITTEE ON ADOLESCENCE. Collaborative role of the pediatrician in the diagnosis and management of bipolar disorder in adolescents. *Pediatrics.* 2012;130(6). Available at: http://pediatrics.aappublications.org/content/130/6/e1725

58. American Acadamy of Pediatrics. *Bright Futures: Guidelines for Health Supervision of Infants, Children, and Adolescents.* 4th ed. 2016, In press.

59. American Academy of Pediatrics, Task Force on Mental Health. *Addressing Mental Health Concerns in Primary Care: A Clinician's Toolkit.* Elk Grove Village, IL: American Academy of Pediatrics; 2010

60. American Academy of Pediatrics. Mental health initiatives. Available at: https://www.aap.org/en-us/advocacy-and-policy/aap-health-initiatives/Mental-Health/Pages/Primary-Care-Tools.aspx. Accessed July 27, 2015

61. Richardson LP, Ludman E, McCauley E, et al. Collaborative care for adolescents with depression in primary care: a randomized clinical trial. *JAMA.* 2014;312(8):809–816

62. US Food and Drug Administration. FDA public health advisory: suicidality in children and adolescents being treated with antidepressant medications. Available at: www.fda.gov/Safety/MedWatch/SafetyInformation/SafetyAlertsforHumanMedicalProducts/ucm155488.htm. Accessed July 27, 2015

63. American Psychiatric Association and American Academy of Child and Adolescent Psychiatry. The use of medication in treating childhood and adolescent depression: information for physicians. Available at: www.parentsmedguide.org/physiciansmedguide.pdf. Accessed July 27, 2015

64. Bridge JA, Iyengar S, Salary CB, et al. Clinical response and risk for reported suicidal ideation and suicide attempts in pediatric antidepressant treatment: a meta-analysis of randomized controlled trials. *JAMA.* 2007;297(15):1683–1696

65. Gibbons RD, Brown CH, Hur K, Davis J, Mann JJ. Suicidal thoughts and behavior with antidepressant treatment: reanalysis of the randomized placebo-controlled studies of fluoxetine and venlafaxine. *Arch Gen Psychiatry.* 2012;69(6):580–587

66. Gibbons RD, Hur K, Brown CH, Davis JM, Mann JJ. Benefits from antidepressants: synthesis of 6-week patient-level outcomes from double-blind placebo-controlled randomized trials of fluoxetine and venlafaxine. *Arch Gen Psychiatry.* 2012;69(6):572–579

67. Dudley M, Goldney R, Hadzi-Pavlovic D. Are adolescents dying by suicide taking SSRI antidepressants? A review of observational studies. *Australas Psychiatry.* 2010;18(3):242–245

68. Olfson M, Shaffer D, Marcus SC, Greenberg T. Relationship between antidepressant medication treatment and suicide in adolescents. *Arch Gen Psychiatry.* 2003;60(10):978–982

69. Gibbons RD, Hur K, Bhaumik DK, Mann JJ. The relationship between antidepressant prescription rates and rate of early adolescent suicide. *Am J Psychiatry.* 2006;163(11):1898–1904

70. Cougnard A, Verdoux H, Grolleau A, Moride Y, Begaud B, Tournier M. Impact of antidepressants on the risk of suicide in patients with depression in real-life conditions: a decision analysis model. *Psychol Med.* 2009;39(8):1307–1315

71. Kilgore C. Dropoff seen in prescribing of antidepressants. Clinical Psychiatry News. 2005;33(3):1–6

72. Kurian BT, Ray WA, Arbogast PG, Fuchs DC, Dudley JA, Cooper WO. Effect of regulatory warnings on antidepressant prescribing for children and adolescents. *Arch Pediatr Adolesc Med.* 2007;161(7):690–696

73. Libby AM, Brent DA, Morrato EH, Orton HD, Allen R, Valuck RJ. Decline in treatment of pediatric depression after FDA advisory on risk of suicidality with SSRIs. *Am J Psychiatry.* 2007;164(6):884–891

74. Singh T, Prakash A, Rais T, Kumari N. Decreased use of antidepressants in youth after US Food and Drug Administration black box warning. *Psychiatry (Edgmont).* 2009;6(10):30–34

75. Libby AM, Orton HD, Valuck RJ. Persisting decline in depression treatment after FDA warnings. *Arch Gen Psychiatry.* 2009;66(6):633–639

76. Valluri S, Zito JM, Safer DJ, Zuckerman IH, Mullins CD, Korelitz JJ. Impact of the 2004 Food and Drug Administration pediatric suicidality warning on antidepressant and psychotherapy treatment for new-onset depression. *Med Care.* 2010;48(11):947–954

77. Rosack J. Impact of FDA warning questioned in suicide rise. *Psychiatric News.* 2007;42(5):1–4

78. Gibbons RD, Brown CH, Hur K, et al. Early evidence on the effects of regulators' suicidality warnings on SSRI prescriptions and suicide in children and adolescents. *Am J Psychiatry.* 2007;164(9):1356–1363

79. Lu CY, Zhang F, Lakoma MD, et al. Changes in antidepressant use by young people and suicidal behavior after FDA warnings and media coverage: quasi-experimental study. *BMJ.* 2014;348:g3596

Supporting the Grieving Child and Family

- *Clinical Report*

CLINICAL REPORT   Guidance for the Clinician in Rendering Pediatric Care

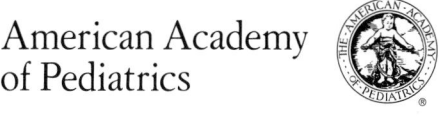

American Academy
of Pediatrics

DEDICATED TO THE HEALTH OF ALL CHILDREN™

Supporting the Grieving Child and Family

David J. Schonfeld, MD, FAAP, Thomas Demaria, PhD, COMMITTEE ON PSYCHOSOCIAL ASPECTS OF CHILD AND FAMILY HEALTH, DISASTER PREPAREDNESS ADVISORY COUNCIL

The death of someone close to a child often has a profound and lifelong effect on the child and results in a range of both short- and long-term reactions. Pediatricians, within a patient-centered medical home, are in an excellent position to provide anticipatory guidance to caregivers and to offer assistance and support to children and families who are grieving. This clinical report offers practical suggestions on how to talk with grieving children to help them better understand what has happened and its implications and to address any misinformation, misinterpretations, or misconceptions. An understanding of guilt, shame, and other common reactions, as well an appreciation of the role of secondary losses and the unique challenges facing children in communities characterized by chronic trauma and cumulative loss, will help the pediatrician to address factors that may impair grieving and children's adjustment and to identify complicated mourning and situations when professional counseling is indicated. Advice on how to support children's participation in funerals and other memorial services and to anticipate and address grief triggers and anniversary reactions is provided so that pediatricians are in a better position to advise caregivers and to offer consultation to schools, early education and child care facilities, and other child congregate care sites. Pediatricians often enter their profession out of a profound desire to minimize the suffering of children and may find it personally challenging when they find themselves in situations in which they are asked to bear witness to the distress of children who are acutely grieving. The importance of professional preparation and self-care is therefore emphasized, and resources are recommended.

abstract

This document is copyrighted and is property of the American Academy of Pediatrics and its Board of Directors. All authors have filed conflict of interest statements with the American Academy of Pediatrics. Any conflicts have been resolved through a process approved by the Board of Directors. The American Academy of Pediatrics has neither solicited nor accepted any commercial involvement in the development of the content of this publication.

Clinical reports from the American Academy of Pediatrics benefit from expertise and resources of liaisons and internal (AAP) and external reviewers. However, clinical reports from the American Academy of Pediatrics may not reflect the views of the liaisons or the organizations or government agencies that they represent.

The guidance in this report does not indicate an exclusive course of treatment or serve as a standard of medical care. Variations, taking into account individual circumstances, may be appropriate.

All clinical reports from the American Academy of Pediatrics automatically expire 5 years after publication unless reaffirmed, revised, or retired at or before that time.

DOI: 10.1542/peds.2016-2147

Accepted for publication Jun 27, 2016

PEDIATRICS (ISSN Numbers: Print, 0031-4005; Online, 1098-4275).

FINANCIAL DISCLOSURE: The authors have indicated they do not have a financial relationship relevant to this article to disclose.

FUNDING: No external funding.

POTENTIAL CONFLICT OF INTEREST: The authors have indicated they have no potential conflicts of interest to disclose.

To cite: Schonfeld DJ, Demaria T, AAP COMMITTEE ON PSYCHOSOCIAL ASPECTS OF CHILD AND FAMILY HEALTH, DISASTER PREPAREDNESS ADVISORY COUNCIL. Supporting the Grieving Child and Family. *Pediatrics.* 2016;138(3):e20162147

INTRODUCTION

At some point in their childhood, the vast majority of children will experience the death of a close family member or friend[1,2]; approximately 1 in 20 children in the United States experiences the death of a parent by the age of 16.[3] Despite the high prevalence of bereavement among children, many pediatricians are uncomfortable talking with and supporting grieving children.[4]

Bereavement is a normative experience that is universal in nature, but this does not minimize the impact of a loss. The death of someone close to a child often has a profound and lifelong effect on the child and may result in a range of both short- and long-term reactions. Pediatricians, within a patient-centered medical home, are in an excellent position to provide anticipatory guidance to caregivers before, during, and after a loss and can provide assistance and support in a number of areas, including the following:

- exploring and confirming that children understand what has occurred and what death means;

- helping to identify reactions such as guilt, fear, worry, or depressive symptoms that suggest the need for further discussion or services;

- providing reassurance to children who become concerned about their own health or those of family members;

- offering support to grieving children and their families to minimize their distress and accelerate their adjustment;

- informing families about local resources that can provide additional assistance; and

- offering advice on funeral attendance of children.

Pediatricians also can play an important role in supporting parents and other caregivers after the death of a child, even in the absence of surviving siblings.[4-6] In addition, children may experience grief in response to a range of other losses, such as separation from parents because of deployment, incarceration, or divorce, which may be helped by similar caring strategies.

This clinical report is a revision of an earlier clinical report that introduced some of the key issues that pediatricians should consider in providing support to grieving children.[7] Guidance is available elsewhere regarding how to support families faced with the impending or recent death of their child,[4,8] including practical advice on how to approach notification of parents about the death of their child in a hospital setting[8,9] or in the unique context of a disaster.[10] Because traumatic events often involve loss, complementary information on providing psychosocial support in the aftermath of a crisis can be found in a recent clinical report,[11] which may be particularly relevant to pediatricians providing care in emergency departments and intensive care settings.

IDENTIFYING CHILDREN'S LOSS EXPERIENCES

In a busy pediatric practice, it is likely that a pediatrician interacts with a child who is grieving a death virtually every week, if not every day. But many children who are grieving show few outward signs during an office visit. From an early age, children learn that questions or discussion about death make many adults uncomfortable; they learn not to talk about death in public. In the context of a recent death, children may also be reluctant to further burden grieving family members with their own concerns.

Children's questions about the impact of a personal loss can be quite poignant and/or frame the experience in concrete and direct terms that underscore the immediacy and reality of the loss to adults (eg, "If Mommy died, does that mean that she won't be here even for my birthday? How can I live the rest of my life without her?"). Adolescents who are in a better position to appreciate the secondary losses and other implications of a significant loss may raise concerns that surviving adults may not have yet appreciated (eg, "I don't know if I ever will feel comfortable having my own children when I grow up, without Mom there to help me."). When children ask such questions or make similar comments, surviving family members may become tearful and/or obviously upset. Children may misinterpret these expressions of grief triggered by their questions as evidence that the questions themselves were hurtful or inappropriate. They subsequently may remain silent and grieve alone, without support. In addition, when children lose a parent or other close family member, they are often fearful that others they count on for support may also die and leave them all alone. Children may find it particularly unsettling to observe their surviving caregivers struggling and often respond to their surviving parent(s) demonstrations of grief by offering support or assistance (eg, "Don't worry Daddy, I can help do many of the things Mommy used to do; we are going to be okay."), rather than asking for help themselves, which may convince surviving caregiver(s) that the child is coping and has no need for assistance. For this reason, it is important for pediatricians to offer to speak with children privately after a family death to identify their understanding, concerns, and reactions without children feeling that they need to protect surviving caregivers.

Caregivers who are struggling with their own personal grief may be particularly reluctant, or even unable, to recognize or accept their children's grief. The reality is that many children in this situation are grieving alone, postponing expressing their grief until a time when it feels safer, or seeking support elsewhere, such as at school or after-school programs where they can talk about their feelings and concerns with adults who have personal distance from the loss.

Young children, in particular, may not yet understand the implications the death may have for them or their family. Children and their families may wish to seek advice but view death as a normative experience that does not warrant professional assistance and may not realize that their pediatrician may be interested in helping and able to assist them. During an incidental pediatric office visit, children may be reluctant to raise the topic because they worry that they will start crying or otherwise embarrass themselves. They may be afraid to start a discussion in the pediatric office or at school because they worry that once they start to cry, they will be unable to compose themselves by the end of an office visit or a conversation at school. Children may also express their grief indirectly through their behavior or attempt to address their feelings through play. Grief is, in many ways, a private experience. Older children, especially, may elect to keep their feelings and concerns to themselves unless caring adults invite and facilitate discussion. These are among the many reasons why pediatricians may be unaware of a death involving a close family member or friend of one of their patients.

Pediatricians can increase the likelihood that children and families will bring significant losses to their attention by directly informing families, often during the initial visit and periodically thereafter, that they are interested in hearing about major changes in the lives of patients and their families, such as deaths of family members or friends, financial or marital concerns of the family, planned or recent moves, traumatic events in the local community or neighborhood, or problems or concerns at school or with peer relationships. At subsequent visits, pediatricians can ask whether any major changes or potential stressors at home, at

school, or within the community have occurred or are anticipated.[12] Practices that respond to these needs as they arise in families, by inviting conversations, expressing concern, and offering information and referral, create an atmosphere in which families are more likely to disclose their occurrence and actively seek assistance and support.

INITIATING THE CONVERSATION

Pediatricians and other caring adults often worry that asking children about the recent death of someone close to them may upset them. In the immediate aftermath of a major loss, the loss is almost always on survivors' minds. Although a question about the death may lead to an expression of sadness, it is the death itself, and not the question, that is the cause of the distress. Inviting children to express their feelings allows them to express their sadness; it does not cause it. In contrast, avoiding the subject may create more problems. Children may interpret the silence as evidence that adults are unaware of their loss, feel that their loss is trivial and unworthy of comment, are disinterested in their grief, are unwilling or unable to assist, or view the child as unable to cope even with support. Instead, the following steps can be used to initiate the conversation[13]:

- Express your concern. It is okay to be tearful or simply to let them know you feel sorry someone they care about has died.

- Be genuine; children can tell when adults are authentic. Do not tell the child you will miss her grandfather if you have never met him; instead, let the child know that you appreciate that he was important to her and you feel sorry she had to experience such a loss.

- Listen and observe; talk less. Simply being present while the child is expressing grief and

tolerating the unpleasant affect can be very helpful.

- Invite discussion using open-ended questions such as "How are you doing since your mother died?" or "How is your family coping?"

- Limit the sharing of your personal experiences. Keep the focus on the child's loss and feelings.

- Offer practical advice, such as suggestions about how to answer questions that might be posed by peers or how to talk with teachers about learning challenges.

- Offer appropriate reassurance. Do not minimize children's concerns but let them know that over time you do expect that they will become better able to cope with their distress.

- Communicate your availability to provide support over time. Do not require children or families to reach out to you for such support, but rather, make the effort to schedule follow-up appointments and reach out by phone or e-mail periodically.

Adults are often worried that they will say the wrong thing and make matters worse. In the context of talking with a patient who has recently experienced a death, caregivers may wish to consider the following suggestions[13]:

- Although well intentioned, attempts to "cheer up" individuals who are grieving are usually neither effective nor appreciated. Anything that begins with "at least" should be reconsidered (eg, "at least he isn't in pain anymore," "at least you have another brother"). Such comments may minimize professionals' discomfort in being with a child who is grieving but do not help children express and cope with their feelings.

- Do not instruct children to hide their emotions (eg, "You need to be strong; you are the man of the house now that your father has died.").

- Avoid communicating that you know how they feel (eg, "I know exactly what you are going through."). Instead, ask them to share their feelings.

- Do not tell them how they ought to feel ("You must feel angry.").

- Avoid comparisons with your own experiences. When adults share their own experiences in the context of recent loss, it shifts the focus away from the child. If your loss is perceived by the child as less important, the comparison can be insulting (eg, "I know what you are going through after the death of your father. My cat died this week."). If your experience appears worse (eg, "I understand your grandfather died. When I was your age, both my mother and father died in a car accident."), the child may feel compelled to comfort you and be reluctant to ask for help.

The use of expressive techniques, such as picture drawing or engaging children in an activity while talking with them, may be helpful in some situations in which children appear reluctant to address the topic in direct conversation. Pediatricians can also provide written information to families about how to support grieving children (eg, *After a Loved One Dies: How Children Grieve and How Parents and Other Adults Can Support Them*, which is freely available and can be accessed through the coping and adjustment Web page of the American Academy of Pediatrics at https://www.aap.org/en-us/advocacy-and-policy/aap-health-initiatives/Children-and-Disasters/Pages/Promoting-Adjustment-and-Helping-Children-Cope.aspx).[14] Books written specifically for younger children that help them develop a better understanding of death or that help children and adolescents cope and adjust with a

personal loss (eg, Guiding Your Child Through Grief is one such resource for older children[15]) can be found through recommendations of a children's librarian or at bookstores. Pediatricians can identify a few books to recommend and, ideally, may even choose to stock their offices with a couple of copies to lend to families.

CHILDREN'S DEVELOPMENTAL UNDERSTANDING OF DEATH

Before the development of object permanence, something out of view is felt to be literally "out of mind." Therefore, it is unlikely that infants in their first 6 months of life can truly grieve. But as children develop object permanence during the second half of the first year of life, they begin to acquire the ability to appreciate the possibility of true loss. It is therefore not coincidental that peek-a-boo emerges during this time period as a game played by children in all cultures, wherein the child shows heightened concern at separation and joy at reunion, as if "playing" with the idea of loss. Infants and toddlers play this game repeatedly as they try to understand and deal with the potentiality of loss. It has been suggested that peek-a-boo is one of many games that children play that might allude to loss or death. In fact, "peek-a-boo" is translated literally from Old English as "alive-or-dead." Parents who worry that it is too early to raise the topic of death with their preschool- or even school-aged children likely do not realize that they began communicating with their children about loss at an early age.

Research has shown that there are 4 concepts that children come to understand that help them make sense of, and ultimately cope with, death: irreversibility, finality (nonfunctionality), causality, and universality (inevitability).[14–19] On average, most children will develop an understanding of these concepts, outlined in Table 1, by 5

to 7 years of age. Personal loss or a terminal illness before this age has been associated with a precocious understanding of these concepts[19]; education has been shown to accelerate children's understanding as well.[20] The death of a pet in early childhood can be used as an opportunity to help young children both understand death and learn to express and cope with loss.

Understanding the concepts of death can be viewed as a necessary precondition, but not necessarily sufficient, for acceptance and adjustment. Children at a very young age can understand that death is irreversible; indeed, even toddlers come to learn "all-gone." But accepting that someone about whom you care deeply will never return is difficult even for adults. Pediatricians can counsel parents to help children understand these concepts and assess children's comprehension directly through simple questions. Parents can be encouraged to be patient with children's repetitive questions after a loss, which may occur over an extended period of time. For young children, such questions may reflect attempts to develop a more complete understanding over time as cognitive development progresses.

Misinformation or misconceptions can impair children's adjustment to loss. Literal misinterpretations are common among young children. For example, children may become resistant to attending a wake after being told that their parent's body will be placed in the casket; adults often assume this is because of a fear of dead bodies. But some children, when told that the "body" is placed in 1 location, may conclude that the head is placed elsewhere; their reluctance to attend the wake may be attributable to a fear of viewing their parent decapitated. It is best not to assume the reasons for children's worries or hesitation but instead ask what they are thinking about. Young

TABLE 1 Component Death Concepts and Implications of Incomplete Understanding for Adjustment to Loss

Irreversibility: death is a permanent phenomenon from which there is no recovery or return
• Example of incomplete understanding: the child expects the deceased to return, as if from a trip
• Implication of incomplete understanding: failure to comprehend this concept prevents the child from detaching personal ties to the deceased, a necessary first
  step in successful mourning
Finality (nonfunctionality): death is a state in which all life functions cease completely
• Example of incomplete understanding: the child worries about a buried relative being cold or in pain; the child wishes to bury food with the deceased
• Implication of incomplete understanding: may lead to preoccupation with physical suffering of the deceased and impair readjustment
Inevitability (universality): death is a natural phenomenon that no living being can escape indefinitely
• Example of incomplete understanding: the child views significant individuals (ie, self, parents) as immortal
• Implication of incomplete understanding: if the child does not view death as inevitable, he/she is likely to view death as punishment (either for actions or
  thoughts of the deceased or the child), leading to excessive guilt and shame
Causality: the child develops a realistic understanding of the causes of death
• Example of incomplete understanding: the child who relies on magical thinking is apt to assume responsibility for the death of a loved one by assuming that
  bad thoughts or unrelated actions were causative
• Implication of incomplete understanding: tends to lead to excessive guilt that is difficult for the child to resolve

Reprinted with permission from Schonfeld D. Crisis intervention for bereavement support: a model of intervention in the children's school. *Clin Pediatr (Phila)*. 1989;28(1):29.

children also may have difficulty understanding why families would choose to cremate a loved one after death. Providing developmentally appropriate explanations for parents and other caregivers to use to address common questions can be helpful and reassuring (eg, explaining to preschool-aged children that once people die, their body stops working permanently and they no longer are able to move, think, or feel pain, which is why it is okay to cremate the body, or use high temperatures to turn the body into ashes).

To minimize misinterpretations, it is best to avoid euphemisms; especially with younger children, it is important to use the word "dead" or "died." For example, a young child told that a family member is in eternal sleep may become afraid of going to sleep himself. Religious explanations can be shared with children of any age according to the wishes of their caregivers. But because religious concepts tend to be abstract and therefore more likely to be misunderstood by young children, it is important to also share with children factual information based on the physical reality. For example, a young child told only that a brother died "because he was such a good baby God wanted him back at his side" may begin to fear attending church (if this is viewed as "God's

home") and misbehave whenever brought to religious services.

Children with intellectual disabilities will generally benefit from explanations geared toward their level of cognitive functioning, followed by questions to assess the degree of comprehension and to probe for any misunderstandings. Children with neurodevelopmental disorders, such as autism spectrum disorder, may benefit from practical suggestions about communicating their feelings and needs, as well as additional support to promote coping. Children unable to communicate verbally may show their grief through nonspecific signs or behaviors, such as weight loss or head banging. To provide support after a death, parents and other caregivers can draw on the strategies and approaches that have worked with their children in the past to provide comfort when faced with other stressors and to explain challenging concepts.

ADOLESCENTS

Adolescents may have a mature conceptual understanding of death, but they still experience challenges adjusting to the death of a close family member or friend.[21] Although they are capable of rational thinking, adolescents, like adults, nonetheless benefit from additional explanation

and discussion in addition to emotional support. Although they often turn to peers for support and assistance in many situations, after the death of a close family member or friend, they can benefit from the additional physical and emotional presence of adults. Unfortunately, many adolescents receive limited explanation or support after a death. Often, surviving caregivers rely on them to take on more adult responsibilities, such as contributing to the care of younger siblings and performing more chores within the home, and may count on them to serve the role of a confidante and source of emotional support for the caregivers themselves. Pediatricians may be able to assist in such cases by encouraging adult caregivers to identify their own support, such as through faith-based organizations, community-based support groups, or professional counseling.

Juniors or seniors in high school are at a point in their development when they may be particularly vulnerable to difficulties in coping with the death of a close family member or friend. This is a time of heightened academic demands, and the common short-term negative effect on academic productivity may be compounded by the high level of academic scrutiny characteristic of applying to college. Completing high school and leaving family to pursue their own education or career is a challenging transition for adolescents and often involves stress and ambivalence. A recent death can exacerbate academic and personal challenges. Youth anticipating leaving home for school or career may feel guilty about leaving other family members who are grieving or worry that they will have difficulty coping when separated from their family, friends, and familiar supports. These young people may arrive in college to face peers who are unaware of their loss, unfamiliar with how best to provide them with support, and focused on pursuits and activities that seem incongruous with their grief. The food, people, and settings that normally provide them solace and comfort may be lacking at a time when they are most needed. Pediatricians can support these adolescents by staying connected with them during the transition and helping them and their families identify supports and resources at college and in their family's community.[13]

GUILT AND SHAME

Because of the egocentrism and magical thinking that are characteristic of young children's understanding of causality, children will often assume that there was something they did, did not do, or should have done that would have prevented the death of someone close to them and develop guilt over a death. Even older children, and indeed adults, often feel guilty when there is no logical, objective reason for them to feel responsible for a death. People may assume some responsibility because it helps them believe that, by taking actions they failed to take before, they can prevent the future deaths of others about whom they care deeply and feel more in control. For example, if a child assumes that the reason his father died was because he attended

a friend's party rather than staying home to monitor his father, he can reassure himself that his mother will be okay as long as he never leaves the home at night again. The alternative to this kind of thinking is accepting that we have limited influence over tragic events, but that reality leaves many feeling helpless. It is frightening to realize someone else we care about could die at any time, no matter what we do. But assuming fault for a death in this manner does not prevent future loss, and the resulting guilt contributes to further distress. In situations in which children's actions clearly contributed to the cause of death (eg, a child who accidentally discharges a firearm that results in the death of someone) or when children persist in feeling responsible (whether such guilt is logical), pediatricians should consider referral for counseling. In the context of ongoing support, children can be helped to either dismiss illogical guilt or come to forgive themselves for unintended actions they believe have contributed in some way to the death.

Children are also more likely to feel guilty about a death when the preexisting relationship with the deceased was ambivalent or conflicted. The relationship between adolescents and their parents often has some element of such ambivalence or conflict as the adolescent strives for independence, and conflict is more likely to be present if the deceased had a chronic mental or physical illness or problem with substance abuse or had been abusive, neglectful, or absent (eg, incarcerated or deployed). Guilt of other family members may also lead to difficulties: for example, it can distort the relationships between parents and surviving children after the death of a sibling.[22]

It is helpful for pediatricians to approach children who have lost a loved one to presume that guilt may be present, even when there is no

logical reason for it. Pediatricians can explain that they know there is nothing that the child did, failed to do, or could have done to change the outcome but wonder if the child ever believes that he or she somehow contributed to the death as many children do in similar situations. They can explain that feeling bad does not mean you did anything bad and feeling guilty does not mean you are guilty. When pediatricians help children express their guilt associated with a death, it allows children to begin to challenge their faulty assumptions about personal responsibility and promotes a refocusing on the child's feelings about the loss.

Children also may experience guilt over surviving after a sibling died or feeling relief after a death that followed a lengthy illness. In the setting of a protracted illness, family members and friends often experience anticipatory grieving. They can imagine the death and experience graduated feelings of loss, but when it becomes overwhelming they can reassure themselves that their loved one is still alive. Anticipating the death allows them to accomplish some of the "work" of grief before the death actually occurs. But this is a painful process, and at some point, many individuals in this situation will wish for the death to occur. Although they may couch this in terms of hoping for the person who is dying to be able to end his or her suffering, the death would also end some of their own emotional suffering as they anticipate the death of a loved one and free them of their responsibility to focus much of their time and efforts on the needs of the person who is critically ill. This situation can result in further guilt and complicate the grieving process.[8]

When children assume that the cause of the death was the result of the actions, inactions, or thoughts of the person who died, they may feel ashamed of the person who died and/or the death and reluctant to talk with others about their loss. Shame is also likely to complicate bereavement when the death is somehow stigmatized, such as death from suicide or resulting from criminal activity or substance abuse. This shame further isolates grieving children from the support and assistance of concerned peers and adults.

Suicide is often complicated by both guilt and shame among survivors. As a result, discussion about the cause of death is often limited, and children may struggle to understand the cause or circumstances of the death. Open communication helps prevent suicide from becoming a "family secret," which may further disrupt the grieving process. If the explanations are too simplistic, concerns may be increased. For example, if children are told only, "Your uncle killed himself because he was very, very sad," they will likely notice that extended family members and friends, who are overwhelmed with grief, may look "very, very sad" and worry that they, too, will kill themselves. A preferable explanation might aim to convey that suicide is usually the result of underlying depression or other mental health problems; it may also be related to alcohol or other substance abuse. It is important to emphasize that suicide is not generally a logical "choice" made by someone who is thinking clearly and able to consider a range of solutions to problems. In addition, children should be encouraged to communicate when they are distressed or feeling depressed, informed about where they can go for advice and assistance, and instructed not to keep in confidence when peers or others communicate to them that they are considering self-harm.[23] Sample scripts and language for discussing suicide with children at different developmental levels, prepared by the National Center for School Crisis and Bereavement,

can be used by schools to respond to a death by suicide of a student or member of the school staff (freely available at www.schoolcrisiscenter. org).

SECONDARY AND CUMULATIVE LOSSES

Although children generally show a remarkable resiliency and ability to adjust to the death of someone close to them, nonetheless, they do not "get over" a death in 6 months or a year. Rather, they spend the rest of their life accommodating the absence. In fact, many find the second year more difficult than the first. The first year after the death is filled with many anticipated challenges: the first holiday or birthday without a loved one or the first father-daughter dance after the father's death. Expectations typically are reduced (ie, the child expects to feel sad at the first special holiday without a loved one), and multiple supports are usually in place. But when these special occasions are still not joyful in the second year, children may wonder if they will ever be able to experience joy again. Unfortunately, by this point in time, the support they may have received from extended family, teachers, coaches, and others at school and in the community has probably already ended. However, the sense of loss is persistent, and without proper support it may be perceived as overwhelming. Maintaining support for children and families is important well beyond the initial period of grief.

When children experience a death of someone close to them, they lose not only the person who died (ie, the primary loss) but also everything that person had contributed or would have contributed to their life (ie, secondary losses). Common secondary losses include the following:

- change in lifestyle (eg, altered financial status of the family after the death of a parent);

- relocation resulting in a change in school and peer group;

- less interaction with friends or relatives of the person who died (eg, friends of a child's sister no longer visit after the sister dies);

- loss of shared memories;

- decreased special attention (eg, a child may no longer value participating in sports activities without his parent there to cheer for him);

- decreased availability of the surviving parent (who may need to work more hours or who becomes less available emotionally because of depression); and

- a decreased sense of safety and trust in the world.

Relationships that seemed incidental may take on new meaning after they are no longer available. For example, after the death of his sister, a younger brother may now miss the advice and guidance provided by his sister's boyfriend, who no longer visits. Other losses may not become apparent until years later. A 5-year-old girl experiencing the death of her grandmother who was her primary caregiver may not realize until many years later that she has lost her grandmother's advice and support as she faces puberty or her first date, or on the first night her newborn infant cries inconsolably. At each new milestone, the loss of someone for whom we care deeply is redefined and grief is revisited.

When children experience a death at a young age, they may also not fully understand the death or its implications. Each new developmental stage, as cognitive development advances and experience widens, may prompt a resurfacing of their grief and be accompanied by questions that permit the child to come to a more mature understanding of the death and its implications.

Subsequent losses and stressors also add to the challenge of adaptation. Children who have experienced traumatic events or significant losses in the context of sufficient support and internal capacity to cope may experience posttraumatic growth and emerge with increased resiliency and new skills to cope with future adversity. These children may shift their life goals to align more with public service; place a higher priority on family, friends, spirituality, and helping others; or become more empathic.[11,24] But in communities that are characterized by high rates of violence, poverty, and frequent deaths of peers and young family members, such supports are generally not present or are insufficient to meet the heightened need. Children in such environments do not somehow "get used to death" or become desensitized. Rather, these losses make them progressively more vulnerable to future stresses and loss. Children in these circumstances often come to appreciate that adults in their communities are unable to provide for their safety and are unwilling or unable to provide support and learn not to seek assistance from these adults because they know it is unlikely to be offered. One reason children and adolescents in these environments may instead turn to peers (and gangs) is to seek such support, which may contribute to high-risk behaviors that jeopardize their safety. They may engage in risky behaviors out of fear for their own mortality and the need to challenge these fears by engaging in the same behaviors they know to be dangerous. Only by surviving these risks can children and adolescents reassure themselves that they are safe, at least for the moment. In this context, it becomes critical that adults in our society take responsibility for ensuring that the environment is safe for children and adolescents, especially in communities characterized by violence, poverty, and frequent loss,

and that we provide them with the support and assistance they need to cope with loss and crisis.

GRIEF TRIGGERS AND ANNIVERSARY REACTIONS

Grief triggers evoke sudden reminders of the person who died that can cause powerful emotional responses in children who are grieving. Although they are most common in the first few months after the death, they may happen months or years later, although the strength of the emotions generally lessens with time. Some triggers, such as a Mother's Day activity in class or a father-daughter dance at school, are easier to identify, but grief triggers can be ubiquitous and often difficult to anticipate. A child may pass by a stranger wearing the same perfume as her aunt or hear a song that her grandfather used to sing and be reminded of the loss. Parents can work with teachers to both minimize likely triggers in school settings and create a "safety" plan wherein students know they can leave the classroom if necessary. If children know that they can leave if they need to, they are less likely to feel overwhelmed or afraid they will cry in class. As a result, they will rarely need to exit and are more able to remain within the classroom and engaged in the classwork.[13]

Anniversaries of the death, birthdays of the deceased, holidays, special events, and major transitions (eg, changing schools, graduating high school, moving homes) are also times when a loved one's absence will be acutely felt. Pediatricians can help the family find ways to meaningfully honor these events. The medical home is uniquely well suited to provide ongoing periodic bereavement support. Pediatricians should invite children and their families to reach out for assistance and advice as children adjust to the loss over time. However, many

individuals who are grieving may not anticipate the challenges posed by anniversaries or events or may feel uncomfortable imposing on the physician for advice for what they believe to be a normative and universal experience. Pediatricians can, instead, schedule follow-up appointments to coincide with such timed events (eg, just before the start of a new school year; just before the first-year anniversary of the death), when modest changes in the timing make it practical, or can call, write, or e-mail a patient/family periodically to check in and let the child and family know of their continued availability and interest. Pediatricians interested in providing significant direct bereavement support for children and families within their practice can explore coding by time for counseling and coordination of care to maximize reimbursement for these services. When the pediatrician lets the family know he or she is still concerned and available, it increases the chances that the child or family will seek advice and assistance when needed.

FUNERAL ATTENDANCE

Children, like adults, often benefit from participating in funerals, wakes, and other memorial or commemorative activities after the death of a close family member or friend. It provides them with an opportunity to grieve in the presence of family and friends while receiving their support and, as appropriate to the family, solace from their spiritual beliefs. Parents and other caregivers sometimes exclude children from funerals and wakes for fear that the experience may be upsetting or because they, themselves, are grieving and unsure whether they can provide appropriate support. Children who are excluded from memorial or funeral services often resent not being able to participate in a meaningful activity involving someone they care deeply about and may wonder what is so terrible that is being done to the loved one that it is not suitable for them to view. What they imagine is likely to be far worse than the reality.

It is best to invite children to participate in wakes, funerals, or memorial services, to the extent they wish. Begin by providing basic information in simple terms about what children can expect from the experience. For example, include information about whether there will be an open casket and anticipated cultural and religious rituals (eg, guests may be invited to place some dirt on the coffin at the gravesite), as well as how people may be expected to behave (eg, some people may be crying and very upset; humorous stories and memories may be shared). Ask children what additional information they would like and what questions they might have. Children should not be forced or coerced to participate in particular rituals or to attend the funeral or wake. If older children who had a very close relationship with the deceased (eg, teenagers whose parent has died) indicate they do not want to attend the funeral, it is helpful to explore the reason for their not wishing to attend and ask them to describe what accommodations might be made in the plans to meet their needs (eg, they prefer not to attend the wake but will attend the funeral service). But, as with all true invitations, the decision is ultimately left to the child. Families can work with children to identify alternate ways for them to recognize the death, such as a private visit to the funeral home once the casket has been closed or a visit to the gravesite after the burial. All children can be invited to make meaningful but developmentally appropriate decisions about the service of an immediate family member; they may be permitted to select a flower arrangement or a picture of the parent to be displayed at the wake.

It can be helpful to assign an adult whom the child knows well but who is not personally grieving (eg, a teacher, babysitter, or relative who is close to the child but less familiar with the deceased) to accompany and monitor the child throughout the services. If the child is fidgeting or appears distressed, the adult can suggest they go for a walk and inquire about how the child is coping with the experience. If the child prefers to stand outside of the room and hand out prayer cards, that level of participation can be accommodated without disrupting the experience for other grieving family members (ie, the child would be less able to stay outside of the room if being watched by the mother who feels it important to stand by her husband's coffin throughout the wake). Older children and adolescents may wish to invite a close friend to sit with them during the service or assist with greeting guests as they approach the room. Suggestions on how to address the needs of children related to commemoration and memorialization involving a crisis, especially in a school setting, can be found elsewhere.[11,13]

CULTURAL SENSITIVITY

Different cultures have a range of traditional practices and rituals as well as expectations around how members of their culture typically mourn the death of a family member or close friend. Although it is helpful for pediatricians to know something about these cultural differences, it is important to remember that the fundamental experience of grief is universal.

Knowledge of the common practices of a particular culture may not accurately predict how a family or individual from that culture will behave. Many families have mixed backgrounds and/or have been exposed to different cultures through their communities or schools. Parents sometimes have different beliefs or practices from their children. Families or individuals may choose to follow practices of a different culture if they seem to align better with their current preferences. Assumptions about how someone ought to mourn in a particular culture may result in a stereotype that could cloud our perceptions and make us miss opportunities to be helpful. Pediatricians should therefore ask families what they feel would be most helpful for their family or for individuals within the family.

The best approach is to be present, authentic, and honest. Approach children and their families with an open mind and heart and be guided by what you see, hear, and feel. The following are questions that may assist in this process:

- "Can you tell me how your family and your culture recognize and cope with the death of a family member?"
- "How does this fit with your own preferences at this time?"
- "Can you help me understand how I can best be of help to you and your family?"

WORKING WITH SCHOOLS

Children typically experience at least temporary academic challenges after the death of a close friend or family member. The effect the loss has on learning may first appear weeks or even months later. Some children may even respond to a death by overachieving in school. Children with learning problems that predated the loss may experience a marked worsening.

In general, it is best for the family to anticipate at least brief difficulties in learning and concentration and to establish a proactive relationship with the school to coordinate supports at school with those within the home. If schools wait for academic failure to become apparent, then school becomes a source of additional distress rather than a potential support. Instead, academic expectations should be modified as needed and supports put into place in anticipation of a possible need.

Caregivers and educators can work together to identify the level of academic work that feels appropriate and achievable at a particular point of time in the recovery process after a major loss. Some modifications that may be considered include the following:

- adapting assignments (eg, allow a student to prepare a written presentation if he feels uncomfortable with an oral presentation; substitute smaller projects for a large project that may feel overwhelming in scope);

- changing the focus or timing of a lesson (eg, excuse the student from a lesson on substance abuse if her sister recently died of a drug overdose or consider postponing it to later in the semester);

- reducing and coordinating homework and extracurricular activities so that the student is able to meet expectations for what is being required; or

- modifying or excusing the student from tests or placing more weight on grades achieved before the death.

The goal is to maintain reasonable expectations while providing the support and accommodations so that the student can achieve at that level and be prepared for successful advancement to the next grade level.[13]

Pediatricians can help provide training to schools about how best to support grieving students and provide consultation after a death has occurred involving a member of the school community.[11,13,25–27]

The Coalition to Support Grieving Students was formed to develop a set of resources broadly approved by 10 of the leading professional organizations of school professionals to guide educators and other school personnel in supporting and caring for their grieving students. The resources are available at no charge to the public at www.grievingstudents.org. The video-training modules feature expert commentary, school professionals who share their observations and advice, and bereaved children and family members who offer their own perspective on living with loss. Handouts and reference materials oriented for classroom educators, principals/administrators, and student support personnel that summarize the training videos, as well as a range of additional resources, can be downloaded from the Web site. Although developed for use by educators, the materials are applicable for the professional development of pediatric health care providers as well. Many are also appropriate for other sites where child congregate care is provided, including early learning centers, preschools, and in-home day care settings. Those caring for children younger than school age similarly benefit from the support and training that can be provided by pediatricians.

COMPLICATED MOURNING AND INDICATIONS FOR REFERRAL

In the immediate aftermath of a death, the reactions of children and adults can be quite extreme and varied. It is best to avoid the tendency to judge or try to categorize such acute reactions as either "normal" or "abnormal." If children or adults appear to be at risk of harming themselves or others, action should be immediately taken to preserve safety. Pediatricians should be aware of community resources for bereavement support. These resources may include the following:

- bereavement support groups and camps (a listing of national and regional services and resources for grieving children can be found at http://www.newyorklife.com/nyl/v/index.jsp?contentId=143564&vgnextoid=755540bf8c442310VgnVCM100000ac841cacRCRD);

- school-based programs and services;

- counselors who are interested and qualified in counseling children who are grieving; and

- other mental health professionals trained to counsel grieving children who are also experiencing depression, anxiety, or trauma symptoms.

As noted previously, adults in the family may benefit from their own support so that they do not depend unduly on their children for emotional support and so they are better able to discern and address the needs of their grieving children.

Grief from the death of a close family member or friend can dominate children's lives in the immediate aftermath of the loss, causing disinterest in engaging in previously enjoyed activities, compromising peer relationships, interfering with the ability to concentrate and learn, causing regressive or risk-taking behavior, or creating a challenge to healthy social and emotional development. But with time and adequate support, grieving children learn that their lives in the absence of the deceased, although permanently altered, nonetheless can be meaningful and increasingly characterized by moments of satisfaction and joy. Children who instead experience complicated mourning may fail to show such adjustment over time.[28] They may experience difficulty with daily functioning at school or at home that persists months after the death. They may become preoccupied with thoughts about the deceased or develop nonadaptive behaviors, such as tobacco, alcohol, or other substance use; promiscuous sexual behavior; or delinquent or other risky behaviors. Referral for counseling is particularly important in this context. More immediate or urgent referral is indicated if children show deep or sustained sadness or depression, especially if they are perceived to be at risk of suicidal behavior.

PROFESSIONAL PREPARATION AND SELF-CARE

Pediatricians often enter the profession because of a desire to help children grow, develop, and be healthy and happy. Understandably, pediatricians can find it difficult to witness children's distress as they grieve the death of someone about whom they care deeply. Many pediatricians have received limited training about how to support grieving children. It is difficult to believe you are helping people when they remain in such distress. You want to help people feel "better," but when they freely express their sorrow in the immediate aftermath of a death, it is difficult to know that you are helping them ultimately adjust and cope. Following up with children and their families over time and actively inquiring about how they are continuing to adjust will help the pediatrician support and observe the course of recovery and understand his or her role in that process. Professional preparation and education are helpful; resources are available on various professional Web sites (eg, the American Academy of Pediatrics at www. aap.org/disasters/adjustment; the Coalition to Support Grieving Students at www.grievingstudents. org; or the National Center for School Crisis and Bereavement at www. schoolcrisiscenter.org). Pediatricians can also seek out and request professional development training through professional meetings, through grand rounds, from other

continuing medical education venues, and via retreats and psychosocial rounds in hospital settings.

Children's grief may also trigger reminders of loss and other reactions in pediatricians. It may remind adults of their own losses or raise thoughts or concerns about the well-being of those they love. Children's grief is often unfiltered and pure; their questions are direct and poignant. It is difficult to witness a child's grief and not feel an effect personally. In fact, not being affected should not even be an expectation or a goal. Nonetheless, pediatricians should monitor their reactions and feelings and limit their support to what they feel ready and able to provide to any particular family at that point in time. If the family is in need of additional supportive services, the pediatrician can seek the assistance of a professional colleague in the office or through referral to someone in the community.

It is important for pediatricians to examine and understand their personal feelings about death to be effective in providing support to children who have experienced a personal loss or who are faced with their own impending death. Often, this understanding will involve an awareness of the effects of deaths of patients on pediatricians' professional and personal lives. The culture in medicine needs to acknowledge that it is understandable to feel upset when bearing witness to something that is upsetting. As professionals, pediatricians should offer support to our colleagues and seek out and accept support for ourselves.

Pediatricians who do provide support to grieving children and families often have a meaningful and lasting impact. A relatively modest effort to provide compassion and support can have a dramatic effect. It can help reduce the amount of time grieving children feel confused, isolated, and overwhelmed. Pediatricians will not

be able to take away the pain and sorrow (and should not see that as their goal), but they can significantly reduce the suffering and minimize the negative effects of loss on children's lives and developmental courses.

LEAD AUTHORS

David J. Schonfeld, MD, FAAP
Thomas Demaria, PhD

CONTRIBUTING AUTHOR

Sharon Berry, PhD, LP, ABPP

COMMITTEE ON PSYCHOSOCIAL ASPECTS OF CHILD AND FAMILY HEALTH, 2015–2016

Michael Yogman, MD, FAAP, Chairperson
Nerissa S. Bauer, MD, MPH, FAAP
Thresia Gambon, MD, FAAP
Arthur Lavin, MD, FAAP
Keith Lemmon, MD, FAAP
Gerri Mattson, MD, FAAP
Jason Rafferty, MD, MPH, EdM
Lawrence Wissow, MD, MPH, FAAP

LIAISONS

Sharon Berry, PhD, LP, ABPP – *Society of Pediatric Psychology*
Terry Carmichael, MSW – *National Association of Social Workers*
Edward R. Christopherson, PhD, FAAP (hon) – *Society of Pediatric Psychology*
Norah Johnson, PhD, RN, CPNP – *National Association of Pediatric Nurse Practitioners*
L. Read Sulik, MD – *American Academy of Child and Adolescent Psychiatry*

CONSULTANT

George Cohen, MD, FAAP

STAFF

Stephanie Domain, MS

DISASTER PREPAREDNESS ADVISORY COUNCIL

Steven E. Krug, MD, FAAP, Chairperson
Sarita Chung, MD, FAAP, Member
Daniel B. Fagbuyi, MD, FAAP, Member
Margaret C. Fisher, MD, FAAP, Member
Scott M. Needle, MD, FAAP, Member
David J. Schonfeld, MD, FAAP, Member

LIAISONS

John James Alexander, MD, FAAP – *US Food and Drug Administration*
Daniel Dodgen, PhD – *Office of the Assistant Secretary for Preparedness and Response*
Eric J. Dziuban, MD, DTM, CPH, FAAP – *Centers for Disease Control and Prevention*

Andrew L. Garrett, MD, MPH, FAAP – *Office of the Assistant Secretary for Preparedness and Response*

Ingrid Hope, RN, MSN – *Department of Homeland Security Office of Health Affairs*

Georgina Peacock, MD, MPH, FAAP – *Centers for Disease Control and Prevention*

Erica Radden, MD – *US Food and Drug Administration*

David Alan Siegel, MD, FAAP – *National Institute of Child Health and Human Development*

STAFF

Laura Aird, MS
Sean Diederich
Tamar Magarik Haro

REFERENCES

1. Ewalt P, Perkins L. The real experience of death among adolescents: an empirical study. *Soc Casework*. 1979;60(99):547–551

2. Hoven CW, Duarte CS, Lucas CP, et al. Psychopathology among New York city public school children 6 months after September 11. *Arch Gen Psychiatry*. 2005;62(5):545–552

3. Mahon MM. Children's concept of death and sibling death from trauma. *J Pediatr Nurs*. 1993;8(5):335–344

4. Wender E; Committee on Psychosocial Aspects of Child And Family Health. Supporting the family after the death of a child. *Pediatrics*. 2012;130(6):1164–1169

5. Meert KL, Eggly S, Kavanaugh K, et al. Meaning making during parent-physician bereavement meetings after a child's death. *Health Psychol*. 2015;34(4):453–461

6. Section on Hospice and Palliative Medicine; Committee on Hospital Care. Pediatric palliative care and hospice care commitments, guidelines, and recommendations. *Pediatrics*. 2013;132(5):966–972

7. American Academy of Pediatrics Committee on Psychosocial Aspects of Child and Family Health. The pediatrician and childhood bereavement. *Pediatrics*. 2000;105(2):445–447. Reaffirmed March 2013

8. Schonfeld D. Providing support for families experiencing the death of a child. In: Kreitler S, Ben-Arush MW, Martin A, eds. *Pediatric Psycho-oncology: Psychosocial Aspects and Clinical Interventions*. 2nd ed. West Sussex, United Kingdom: John Wiley & Sons Ltd; 2012:223–230

9. Leash R. *Death Notification: A Practical Guide to the Process*. Hinesburg, VT: Upper Access; 1994

10. Foltin GL, Schonfeld DJ, Shannon MW, eds. *Pediatric Terrorism and Disaster Preparedness: A Resource for Pediatricians*. Rockville, MD: Agency for Healthcare Research and Quality; 2006. AHRQ publication 06-0056-EF

11. Schonfeld D, Demaria T; Disaster Preparedness Advisory Council; Committee on Psychosocial Aspects of Child and Family Health. Providing psychosocial support to children and families in the aftermath of disaster and crisis: a guide for pediatricians. *Pediatrics*. 2015;136(4):e1120–e1130

12. Hagan JF, Shaw JS, Duncan PM, eds. *Bright Futures: Guidelines for Health Supervision of Infants, Children, and Adolescents*. 3rd ed. Elk Grove Village, IL: American Academy of Pediatrics; 2008

13. Schonfeld D, Quackenbush M. *The Grieving Student: A Teacher's Guide*. Baltimore, MD: Brookes Publishing; 2010

14. Schonfeld D, Quackenbush M. *After a Loved One Dies—How Children Grieve and How Parents and Other Adults Can Support Them*. New York, NY: New York Life Foundation; 2009

15. Emswiler M, Emswiler J. *Guiding Your Child Through Grief*. New York, NY: Bantam Books; 2000

16. Panagiotaki G, Nobes G, Ashraf A, Aubby H. British and Pakistani children's understanding of death: cultural and developmental influences. *Br J Dev Psychol*. 2015;33(1):31–44

17. Schonfeld DJ. Talking with children about death. *J Pediatr Health Care*. 1993;7(6):269–274

18. Schonfeld D. Death during childhood. In: Augustyn M, Zuckerman B, Caronna E, eds. *The Zuckerman Parker Handbook of Developmental and Behavioral Pediatrics for Primary Care*. 3rd ed. Philadelphia, PA: Lippincott Williams & Wilkins; 2011:441–445

19. Speece MW, Brent SB. Children's understanding of death: a review of three components of a death concept. *Child Dev*. 1984;55(5):1671–1686

20. Schonfeld DJ, Kappelman M. The impact of school-based education on the young child's understanding of death. *J Dev Behav Pediatr*. 1990;11(5):247–252

21. Stikkelbroek Y, Bodden DH, Reitz E, Vollebergh WA, van Baar AL. Mental health of adolescents before and after the death of a parent or sibling. *Eur Child Adolesc Psychiatry*. 2016;25(1):49–59

22. Krell R, Rabkin L. The effects of sibling death on the surviving child: a family perspective. *Fam Process*. 1979;18(4):471–477

23. Shain B; Committee on Adolescence. Suicide and suicide attempts in adolescents. *Pediatrics*. 2016;138(1):e20161420

24. Schonfeld D, Gurwitch R. Children in disasters. In: Elzouki AY, Stapleton FB, Whitley RJ, Oh W, Harfi HA, Nazer H, eds. *Textbook of Clinical Pediatrics*. 2nd ed. New York, NY: Springer; 2011:687–698

25. Schonfeld DJ. Crisis intervention for bereavement support: a model of intervention in the children's school. *Clin Pediatr (Phila)*. 1989;28(1):27–33

26. Schonfeld D, Lichtenstein R, Kline M, Speese-Linehan D. *How to Respond to and Prepare for a Crisis*. 2nd ed. Alexandria, VA: Association for Supervision and Curriculum Development; 2002

27. Schonfeld D; US Department of Education. Coping with the death of a student or staff member. *ERCMExpress*. 2007;3(2):1–12

28. Rando T. *Treatment of Complicated Mourning*. Champaign, IL: Research Press; 1993

Umbilical Cord Care in the Newborn Infant

- *Clinical Report*

CLINICAL REPORT   Guidance for the Clinician in Rendering Pediatric Care

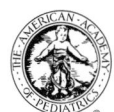

American Academy
of Pediatrics

DEDICATED TO THE HEALTH OF ALL CHILDREN™

Umbilical Cord Care in the Newborn Infant

Dan Stewart, MD, FAAP, William Benitz, MD, FAAP, COMMITTEE ON FETUS AND NEWBORN

abstract

Postpartum infections remain a leading cause of neonatal morbidity and mortality worldwide. A high percentage of these infections may stem from bacterial colonization of the umbilicus, because cord care practices vary in reflection of cultural traditions within communities and disparities in health care practices globally. After birth, the devitalized umbilical cord often proves to be an ideal substrate for bacterial growth and also provides direct access to the bloodstream of the neonate. Bacterial colonization of the cord not infrequently leads to omphalitis and associated thrombophlebitis, cellulitis, or necrotizing fasciitis. Various topical substances continue to be used for cord care around the world to mitigate the risk of serious infection. More recently, particularly in high-resource countries, the treatment paradigm has shifted toward dry umbilical cord care. This clinical report reviews the evidence underlying recommendations for care of the umbilical cord in different clinical settings.

DOI: 10.1542/peds.2016-2149

PEDIATRICS (ISSN Numbers: Print, 0031-4005; Online, 1098-4275).

Copyright © 2016 by the American Academy of Pediatrics

FINANCIAL DISCLOSURE: The authors have indicated they do not have a financial relationship relevant to this article to disclose.

FUNDING: No external funding.

POTENTIAL CONFLICT OF INTEREST: The authors have indicated they have no potential conflicts of interest to disclose.

To cite: Stewart D, Benitz W, AAP COMMITTEE ON FETUS AND NEWBORN. Umbilical Cord Care in the Newborn Infant. *Pediatrics.* 2016;138(3):e20162149

INTRODUCTION

Despite significant global progress in recent decades,[1] bacterial infections (sepsis, meningitis, and pneumonia) continue to account for approximately 700 000 neonatal deaths each year, or nearly one-quarter of the 3 million neonatal deaths that occur worldwide.[1,2] Although the magnitude of its contribution to these deaths remains uncertain, the umbilical cord may be a common portal of entry for invasive pathogenic bacteria,[3] with or without clinical signs of omphalitis. Neonatal mortality associated with bacterial contamination of the umbilical stump may therefore rank among the greatest public health opportunities of the 21st century.

Common risk factors for the development of neonatal omphalitis include unplanned home birth or septic delivery, low birth weight, prolonged rupture of membranes, umbilical catheterization, and chorioamnionitis.[4,5] In countries with limited resources, the risk of omphalitis may be 6 times greater for infants delivered at home than for hospital births.[6] Multiple studies have delineated the susceptibility of the umbilical cord to bacterial colonization. The method of caring for the umbilical cord after birth affects both bacterial colonization and time to cord separation.[7-10] The devitalized umbilical cord provides an ideal medium for bacterial growth. Sources of potentially pathogenic bacteria that colonize the umbilical cord include the mother's birth canal and various local bacterial sources at the site of delivery, most prominently the nonsterile hands of any person assisting with the delivery.[11] *Staphylococcus aureus* remains the most frequently reported organism.[5-7,12] Other common pathogens include group A and group B *Streptococci* and Gram-negative bacilli including *Escherichia coli*, *Klebsiella* species, and *Pseudomonas* species. Rarely, anaerobic and polymicrobial infections also may occur. In addition to omphalitis, tetanus in neonates can result from umbilical cord colonization, particularly in countries with limited resources. This infection results from contamination of the umbilical separation site by *Clostridium tetani* acquired from a nonsterile device used to separate the umbilical cord during the peripartum period or from application of unhygienic substances to the cord stump.

Multiple complications can occur from bacterial colonization and infection of the umbilical cord because of its direct access to the bloodstream. These complications include the development of intraabdominal abscesses, periumbilical cellulitis, thrombophlebitis in the portal and/or umbilical veins, peritonitis, and bowel ischemia.[13-16] Neonatal omphalitis may present at 4 grades of severity: (1) funisitis/umbilical discharge (an unhealthy-appearing cord with purulent, malodorous discharge), (2) omphalitis with abdominal wall cellulitis (periumbilical erythema and tenderness in addition to an unhealthy-appearing cord with

discharge), (3) omphalitis with systemic signs of infection, and (4) omphalitis with necrotizing fasciitis (umbilical necrosis with periumbilical ecchymosis, crepitus, bullae, and evidence of involvement of superficial and deep fascia; frequently associated with signs and symptoms of overwhelming sepsis and shock).[6]

The incidence of omphalitis reported in different communities varies greatly, depending on prenatal and perinatal practices, cultural variations in cord care, and delivery venue (home versus hospital). Reliable current data on rates in untreated infants are surprisingly scant. In high-resource countries, neonatal omphalitis now is rare, with an estimated incidence of approximately 1 per 1000 infants managed with dry cord care (eg, a total of 3 cases among 3518 infants described in 2 reports from Canada[17,18]). In low-income communities, omphalitis occurs in up to 8% of infants born in hospitals and in as many as 22% of infants born at home, in whom omphalitis is moderate to severe in 17% and associated with sepsis in 2%.[19] Depending on how omphalitis is defined, case-fatality rates as high as 13% have been reported.[4] The development of necrotizing fasciitis, with predictable complications from septic shock, is associated with much higher case-mortality rates.[5] These disparate observations in different settings have resulted in divergent recommendations for cord care by the World Health Organization (WHO), which advocates dry cord care for infants born in a hospital or in settings of low neonatal mortality and application of chlorhexidine solution or gel for infants born at home or in settings of high neonatal mortality.[20]

EVIDENCE-BASED PRACTICE

Best practices for antisepsis of the umbilical cord continue to remain

somewhat controversial and variable, even in high-resource countries with relatively aseptic conditions at the time of delivery. In resource-limited countries, in accordance with cultural traditions, unhygienic substances continue to be applied to the umbilicus, creating a milieu ideal for the development neonatal omphalitis. To achieve the goal of preventing omphalitis worldwide, deliveries must be clean and umbilical cord care must be hygienic. The cord should be cut with a sterile blade or scissors, preferably using sterile gloves, to prevent bacterial contamination leading to omphalitis or neonatal tetanus. As discussed later, dry cord care without the application of topical substances is preferable under most circumstances in high-resource countries and for in-hospital births elsewhere; the application of topical chlorhexidine is recommended for infants born outside the hospital setting in communities with high neonatal mortality rates.[20]

Methods of umbilical cord care have been the subject of 4 recent meta-analyses,[21-24] including 2 Cochrane reviews.[23,24] Although the scope and methodologies of these reviews differed, all 4 stratified results according to the study setting, distinguishing results reported from communities with high proportions of births at home and high neonatal mortality rates from those obtained in hospitals and settings with low neonatal mortality rates. These analyses concluded that 3 studies (including >44 000 subjects) in community settings in South Asia with a high neonatal mortality rate[3,25,26] support the effectiveness of application of 4% chlorhexidine solution or gel to the umbilical cord stump within 24 hours after birth, which results in a significant reduction in both omphalitis (relative risk [RR]: 0.48; 95% confidence interval [CI]: 0.40–0.57) and neonatal mortality

(RR: 0.81; 95% CI: 0.71–0.92) compared with dry cord care.[24] No other cord-management strategies have been evaluated systematically in such settings, but the application of traditional materials (eg, ash, herbal or other vegetal poultices, and human milk) may provide a source of contamination with pathogenic bacteria, including *C tetani*.[27] In contrast, the meta-analyses found little evidence of benefit from topical treatments for infants born in hospitals.[22-24] The meta-analyses used different criteria for inclusion of trials and compared a variety of treatments versus dry cord care or versus one another. Only a single trial[28] reported mortality data, which did not differ between topical chlorhexidine and dry care (RR: 0.11; 95% CI: 0.01–2.04). However, the low mortality rate and the small contribution made by bacterial infection[29] in these settings provide only a small opportunity for a reduction in mortality rates. In 5 such trials[30-33] analyzed by Karumbi et al,[22] no treatment was found to significantly reduce omphalitis and sepsis when compared against one another, although the sample sizes were small and the evidence was deemed of low quality.[22] The Cochrane review by Imdad et al,[23] which compared a variety of pairs of topical agents, reached similar conclusions. The most recent meta-analysis, by Sinha et al,[24] considered 2 studies[28,34] comparing chlorhexidine with dry cord care. In the first of these, 140 infants admitted to the NICU at a hospital in north India were randomly assigned to receive cord treatment with chlorhexidine solution or dry cord care.[28] Enrollment criteria included gestational age >32 weeks and birth weight >1500 g, but the provided demographic data suggest that the infants were predominantly late-preterm, and they experienced high rates of complications of prematurity (including asphyxia, respiratory distress, mechanical ventilation, and

necrotizing enterocolitis). No cases of umbilical sepsis were reported in either group, but culture-proven sepsis was more common in the dry cord care group than in the chlorhexidine group (15 of 70 vs 2 of 70; *P* = .002). These observations cannot be generalized to all healthy infants born in a hospital. The second enrolled 669 subjects, who were randomly assigned to receive treatment with chlorhexidine powder or dry cord care.[34] Cord-related adverse events (erosion, irritation, lesion, omphalitis, erythema, umbilical granuloma, purulence, bleeding, discharge, or weeping of the navel) were more common in the dry cord care group (29% vs 16%; *P* = .001), but there were no differences in serious adverse events (2.1% in both groups) or in the incidence of omphalitis (2.1% vs 0.6%; *P* = .1). Although the meta-analysis reported a significant difference in the pooled risk of omphalitis (RR: 0.48; 95% CI: 0.28–0.84), combining culture-proven sepsis cases[28] with omphalitis cases[34] is not appropriate. This analysis provides only very weak, or perhaps no, evidence for a benefit of chlorhexidine treatment.

Since 1998, the WHO has advocated the use of dry umbilical cord care in high-resource settings.[35] Dry cord care includes keeping the cord clean and leaving it exposed to air or loosely covered by a clean cloth. If it becomes soiled, the remnant of the cord is cleaned with soap and sterile water. In situations in which hygienic conditions are poor and/or infection rates are high, the WHO recommends chlorhexidine.[16]

There is some uncertainty as to the effect of chlorhexidine on mortality when applied to the umbilical cords of newborn infants in the hospital setting, but there is moderate evidence for its effects on infection prevention.[24] Although the application of chlorhexidine is regarded as safe,[35] trace levels of the compound have been detected in the

blood of infants after umbilical cord cleaning.[36,37] In addition, contact dermatitis has been reported in up to 15% of very low birth weight infants after placement of a 0.5% chlorhexidine impregnated dressing over a central venous catheter.[38] The data on the safety of chlorhexidine application are incomplete, and the amount of exposure to chlorhexidine that can be considered safe is not known.[24] In addition to the incremental increase in the cost of using chlorhexidine, the practice of reducing bacterial colonization may have the unintended consequences of selecting more virulent bacterial strains without demonstrable benefits.[24] Because the incidence of omphalitis is very low in high-resource countries and the severity is mild, the preponderance of evidence favors dry cord care.

PROMOTING NONPATHOGENIC COLONIZATION OF THE UMBILICAL CORD

Promoting colonization of the umbilical cord by nonpathogenic bacteria may prevent the development of neonatal omphalitis. By allowing neonates to "room-in" with their mothers, one can create an environment conducive for colonization from less pathogenic bacteria acquired from the mother's flora.[39] This type of colonization helps to reduce colonization and infection from potentially pathogenic organisms that are ubiquitous in the hospital environment. Over time, attempts to decrease bacterial colonization with topical antimicrobial agents may actually select for resistant and more pathogenic organisms[35] (level of evidence: III).

IMPLICATIONS FOR CLINICAL PRACTICE

1. Application of select antimicrobial agents to the umbilical cord may be beneficial for infants born at home in resource-limited

countries where the risks of omphalitis and associated sequelae are high.

2. Application of select antimicrobial agents to the umbilical cord does not provide clear benefit in the hospital setting or in high-resource countries, where reducing bacterial colonization may have the unintended consequence of selecting more virulent bacterial strains. In high-resource countries, there has been a shift away from the use of topical antimicrobial agents in umbilical cord care for this reason.

3. For deliveries outside of birthing centers or hospital settings and in resource-limited populations (eg, Native American communities), the application of prophylactic topical antimicrobial agents to the umbilical cord remains appropriate.

4. At the time of discharge, parental education regarding the signs and symptoms of omphalitis might decrease significant morbidities and even associated mortalities.

5. Of paramount importance is the need for all primary care providers to be diligent in reporting infections associated with umbilical cord care. The development of a local reporting system regarding the occurrence of omphalitis and/or its morbidities to the health care providers at the site of delivery will create more robust data, allowing for improvement in treatment paradigms in the future.

LEAD AUTHORS

Dan L. Stewart, MD, FAAP
William E. Benitz, MD, FAAP

COMMITTEE ON FETUS AND NEWBORN, 2015–2016

Kristi L. Watterberg, MD, FAAP, Chairperson
James J. Cummings, MD, FAAP
William E. Benitz, MD, FAAP
Eric C. Eichenwald, MD, FAAP
Brenda B. Poindexter, MD, FAAP

Dan L. Stewart, MD, FAAP
Susan W. Aucott, MD, FAAP
Jay P. Goldsmith, MD, FAAP
Karen M. Puopolo, MD, PhD, FAAP
Kasper S. Wang, MD, FAAP

LIAISONS

Tonse N.K. Raju, MD, DCH, FAAP – *National Institutes of Health*
Wanda D. Barfield, MD, MPH, FAAP – *Centers for Disease Control and Prevention*
Erin L. Keels, APRN, MS, NNP-BC – *National Association of Neonatal Nurses*
Thierry Lacaze, MD – *Canadian Paediatric Society*
Maria Mascola, MD – *American College of Obstetricians and Gynecologists*

STAFF

Jim R. Couto, MA

ABBREVIATIONS

CI: confidence interval
RR: relative risk
WHO: World Health Organization

REFERENCES

1. Lawn JE, Blencowe H, Oza S, et al; Lancet Every Newborn Study Group. Every Newborn: progress, priorities, and potential beyond survival. *Lancet.* 2014;384(9938):189–205

2. Liu L, Johnson HL, Cousens S, et al; Child Health Epidemiology Reference Group of WHO and UNICEF. Global, regional, and national causes of child mortality: an updated systematic analysis for 2010 with time trends since 2000. *Lancet.* 2012;379(9832):2151–2161

3. Mullany LC, Darmstadt GL, Khatry SK, et al. Topical applications of chlorhexidine to the umbilical cord for prevention of omphalitis and neonatal mortality in southern Nepal: a community-based, cluster-randomised trial. *Lancet.* 2006;367(9514):910–918

4. Güvenç H, Aygün AD, Yaşar F, Soylu F, Güvenç M, Kocabay K. Omphalitis in term and preterm appropriate for gestational age and small for gestational age infants. *J Trop Pediatr.* 1997;43(6):368–372

5. Mason WH, Andrews R, Ross LA, Wright HT Jr. Omphalitis in the newborn infant. *Pediatr Infect Dis J.* 1989;8(8):521–525

6. Sawardekar KP. Changing spectrum of neonatal omphalitis. *Pediatr Infect Dis J.* 2004;23(1):22–26

7. Verber IG, Pagan FS. What cord care—if any? *Arch Dis Child.* 1993;68(5 spec no):594–596

8. Ronchera-Oms C, Hernández C, Jimémez NV. Antiseptic cord care reduces bacterial colonization but delays cord detachment. *Arch Dis Child Fetal Neonatal Ed.* 1994;71(1):F70

9. Novack AH, Mueller B, Ochs H. Umbilical cord separation in the normal newborn. *Am J Dis Child.* 1988;142(2):220–223

10. Arad I, Eyal F, Fainmesser P. Umbilical care and cord separation. *Arch Dis Child.* 1981;56(11):887–888

11. Mullany LC, Darmstadt GL, Katz J, et al. Risk factors for umbilical cord infection among newborns of southern Nepal. *Am J Epidemiol.* 2007;165(2):203–211

12. Airede AI. Pathogens in neonatalomphalitis. *J Trop Pediatr.* 1992;38(3):129–131

13. Forshall I. Septic umbilical arteritis. *Arch Dis Child.* 1957;32(161):25–30

14. Lally KP, Atkinson JB, Woolley MM, Mahour GH. Necrotizing fasciitis: a serious sequela of omphalitis in the newborn. *Ann Surg.* 1984;199(1):101–103

15. Monu JU, Okolo AA. Neonatal necrotizing fasciitis—a complication of poor cord hygiene: report of three cases. *Ann Trop Paediatr.* 1990;10(3):299–303

16. Samuel M, Freeman NV, Vaishnav A, Sajwany MJ, Nayar MP. Necrotizing fasciitis: a serious complication of omphalitis in neonates. *J Pediatr Surg.* 1994;29(11):1414–1416

17. Dore S, Buchan D, Coulas S, et al. Alcohol versus natural drying for newborn cord care. *J Obstet Gynecol Neonatal Nurs.* 1998;27(6):621–627

18. Janssen PA, Selwood BL, Dobson SR, Peacock D, Thiessen PN. To dye or not to dye: a randomized, clinical trial of a triple dye/alcohol regime versus dry cord care. *Pediatrics.* 2003;111(1):15–20

19. Mir F, Tikmani SS, Shakoor S, et al. Incidence and etiology of omphalitis

in Pakistan: a community-based cohort study. *J Infect Dev Ctries.* 2011;5(12):828–833

20. World Health Organization. *WHO Recommendations on Postnatal Care of the Mother and Newborn.* Geneva, Switzerland: WHO Press; 2014

21. Imdad A, Mullany LC, Baqui AH, et al. The effect of umbilical cord cleansing with chlorhexidine on omphalitis and neonatal mortality in community settings in developing countries: a meta-analysis. *BMC Public Health.* 2013;13(suppl 3):S3–S15

22. Karumbi J, Mulaku M, Aluvaala J, English M, Opiyo N. Topical umbilical cord care for prevention of infection and neonatal mortality. *Pediatr Infect Dis J.* 2013;32(1):78–83

23. Imdad A, Bautista RM, Senen KA, Uy ME, Mantaring JB III, Bhutta ZA. Umbilical cord antiseptics for preventing sepsis and death among newborns. *Cochrane Database Syst Rev.* 2013;5:CD008635

24. Sinha A, Sazawal S, Pradhan A, Ramji S, Opiyo N. Chlorhexidine skin or cord care for prevention of mortality and infections in neonates. *Cochrane Database Syst Rev.* 2015;3:CD007835

25. Arifeen SE, Mullany LC, Shah R, et al. The effect of cord cleansing with chlorhexidine on neonatal mortality in rural Bangladesh: a community-based, cluster-randomised trial. *Lancet.* 2012;379(9820):1022–1028

26. Soofi S, Cousens S, Imdad A, Bhutto N, Ali N, Bhutta ZA. Topical application of chlorhexidine to neonatal umbilical cords for prevention of omphalitis and neonatal mortality in a rural district of Pakistan: a community-based,

cluster-randomised trial. *Lancet.* 2012;379(9820):1029–1036

27. Mrisho M, Schellenberg JA, Mushi AK, et al. Understanding home-based neonatal care practice in rural southern Tanzania. *Trans R Soc Trop Med Hyg.* 2008;102(7):669–678

28. Gathwala G, Sharma D, Bhakhri B. Effect of topical application of chlorhexidine for umbilical cord care in comparison with conventional dry cord care on the risk of neonatal sepsis: a randomized controlled trial. *J Trop Pediatr.* 2013;59(3):209–213

29. Centers for Disease Control and Prevention. QuickStats: leading causes of neonatal and postneonatal deaths—United States, 2002. *MMWR.* 2005;54(38):966

30. Ahmadpour-Kacho M, Zahedpasha Y, Hajian K, Javadi G, Talebian H. The effect of topical application of human milk, ethyl alcohol 96%, and silver sulfadiazine on umbilical cord separation time in newborn infants. *Arch Iran Med.* 2006;9(1):33–38

31. Erenel AS, Vural G, Efe SY, Ozkan S, Ozgen S, Erenoğlu R. Comparison of olive oil and dry-clean keeping methods in umbilical cord care as microbiological. *Matern Child Health J.* 2010;14(6):999–1004

32. Hsu WC, Yeh LC, Chuang MY, Lo WT, Cheng SN, Huang CF. Umbilical separation time delayed by alcohol application. *Ann Trop Paediatr.* 2010;30(3):219–223

33. Pezzati M, Rossi S, Tronchin M, Dani C, Filippi L, Rubaltelli FF. Umbilical cord care in premature infants: the effect of two different cord-care

regimens (salicylic sugar powder vs chlorhexidine) on cord separation time and other outcomes. *Pediatrics.* 2003;112(4):e275

34. Kapellen TM, Gebauer CM, Brosteanu O, Labitzke B, Vogtmann C, Kiess W. Higher rate of cord-related adverse events in neonates with dry umbilical cord care compared to chlorhexidine powder: results of a randomized controlled study to compare efficacy and safety of chlorhexidine powder versus dry care in umbilical cord care of the newborn. *Neonatology.* 2009;96(1):13–18

35. World Health Organization. *Care of the Umbilical Cord: A Review of the Evidence.* Geneva, Switzerland: World Health Organization; 1998

36. Aggett PJ, Cooper LV, Ellis SH, McAinsh J. Percutaneous absorption of chlorhexidine in neonatal cord care. *Arch Dis Child.* 1981;56(11):878–880

37. Johnsson J, Seeberg S, Kjellmer I. Blood concentrations of chlorhexidine in neonates undergoing routine cord care with 4% chlorhexidine gluconate solution. *Acta Paediatr Scand.* 1987;76(4):675–676

38. Garland JS, Alex CP, Mueller CD, et al. A randomized trial comparing povidone-iodine to a chlorhexidine gluconate-impregnated dressing for prevention of central venous catheter infections in neonates. *Pediatrics.* 2001;107(6):1431–1436

39. Pezzati M, Biagioli EC, Martelli E, Gambi B, Biagiotti R, Rubaltelli FF. Umbilical cord care: the effect of eight different cord-care regimens on cord separation time and other outcomes. *Biol Neonate.* 2002;81(1):38–44

Use of Performance-Enhancing Substances

- *Clinical Report*

CLINICAL REPORT   Guidance for the Clinician in Rendering Pediatric Care

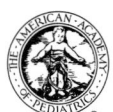

American Academy
of Pediatrics

DEDICATED TO THE HEALTH OF ALL CHILDREN™

Use of Performance-Enhancing Substances

Michele LaBotz, MD, FAAP, Bernard A. Griesemer, MD, FAAP, COUNCIL ON SPORTS MEDICINE AND FITNESS

abstract

Performance-enhancing substances (PESs) are used commonly by children and adolescents in attempts to improve athletic performance. More recent data reveal that these same substances often are used for appearance-related reasons as well. PESs include both legal over-the-counter dietary supplements and illicit pharmacologic agents. This report reviews the current epidemiology of PES use in the pediatric population, as well as information on those PESs in most common use. Concerns regarding use of legal PESs include high rates of product contamination, correlation with future use of anabolic androgenic steroids, and adverse effects on the focus and experience of youth sports participation. The physical maturation and endogenous hormone production that occur in adolescence are associated with large improvements in strength and athletic performance. For most young athletes, PES use does not produce significant gains over those seen with the onset of puberty and adherence to an appropriate nutrition and training program.

DOI: 10.1542/peds.2016-1300

PEDIATRICS (ISSN Numbers: Print, 0031-4005; Online, 1098-4275).

FINANCIAL DISCLOSURE: The authors have indicated they do not have a financial relationship relevant to this article to disclose.

FUNDING: No external funding.

POTENTIAL CONFLICT OF INTEREST: The authors have indicated they have no potential conflicts of interest to disclose.

To cite: LaBotz M, Griesemer BA, AAP COUNCIL ON SPORTS MEDICINE AND FITNESS. Use of Performance-Enhancing Substances. *Pediatrics.* 2016;138(1):e20161300

INTRODUCTION

The American Academy of Pediatrics (AAP) has published position papers, a subject review, guidelines, and textbook chapters regarding the use of performance-enhancing substances (PESs) by children and adolescents.[1-3] This clinical report updates and consolidates information on this topic. For the purposes of this report, the term "performance-enhancing substances" will be used to describe the spectrum of dietary supplements, as well as legal and illegal drugs that often are used by athletes for the purpose of improving athletic performance.

Over the last 2 decades, the availability of PESs has increased with access to Internet suppliers, proliferation, and marketing of stimulant-containing beverages, and increasing use of topically applied anabolic androgenic steroids. Although the overall use of many PESs may have declined over the past 15 years, reviews of multiple studies have prompted concern that the onset of use may be occurring increasingly in the pediatric population.[4]

EPIDEMIOLOGY OF PES USE IN THE PEDIATRIC POPULATION

Several national studies have been tracking adolescent use of PESs. Monitoring the Future (MTF) is an annual survey of 50 000 students in eighth, 10th, and 12th grade.[5] Figs 1, 2, 3, and 4 outline results and trends of PES use as noted in MTF. The Youth Risk Behavior Surveillance System (YRBSS) is a biennial survey that includes a representative cross-section of high school students in the United States. The 2013 YRBSS included surveys from more than 13 500 students and revealed prevalence rates for nonprescribed steroid use that were a bit higher than those in MTF, with 3.2% reporting lifetime use of anabolic androgenic steroids.[6] The reported number was higher in boys (4.0%) than in girls (2.2%) and indicated a significant decrease over the previous 12 years, from a high of 5.0% overall use in 2001.

The Partnership Attitude Tracking Study (PATS) is an annual survey of parents and high school students regarding behaviors and attitudes about drugs and substance abuse.[7] The 2013 PATS survey included responses from more than 3700 students. Steroid use increased slightly from 5% to 7% as compared with 2012. However, use of synthetic human growth hormone (hGH) almost doubled, from 5% to 11%, after being fairly stable from 2009–2012. The report stated that most of this increase included teenagers who reported a single episode of hGH use and that the number of teenagers who report having used hGH more often has remained consistent.

Several studies have demonstrated polypharmacy among users of PESs, with elevated rates of use of both recreational drugs and multiple PESs.[5,8,9] MTF has demonstrated a strong association between use of androstenedione, creatine, and anabolic androgenic

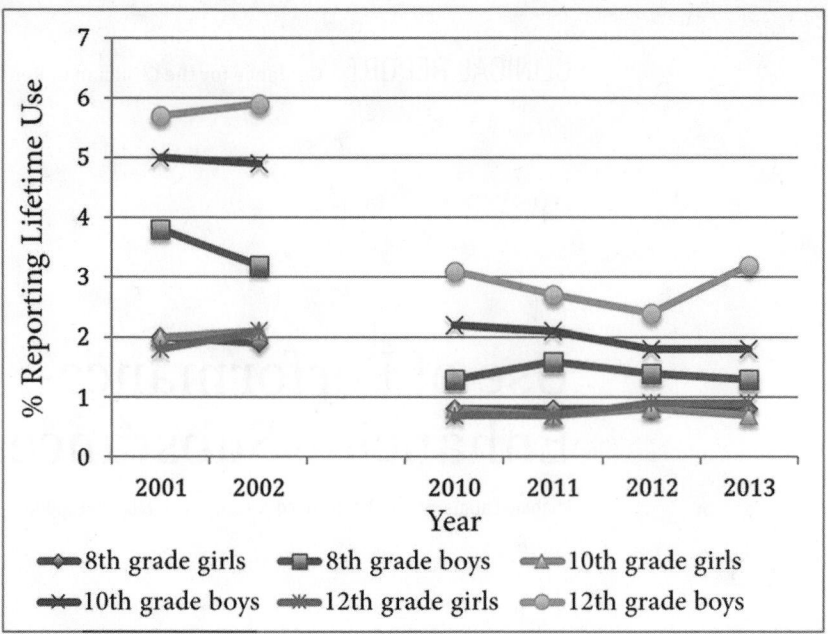

FIGURE 1
Percentage of eighth, 10th, and 12th graders reporting any lifetime use of anabolic androgenic steroids by year and sex (data from MTF, 2014).[5]

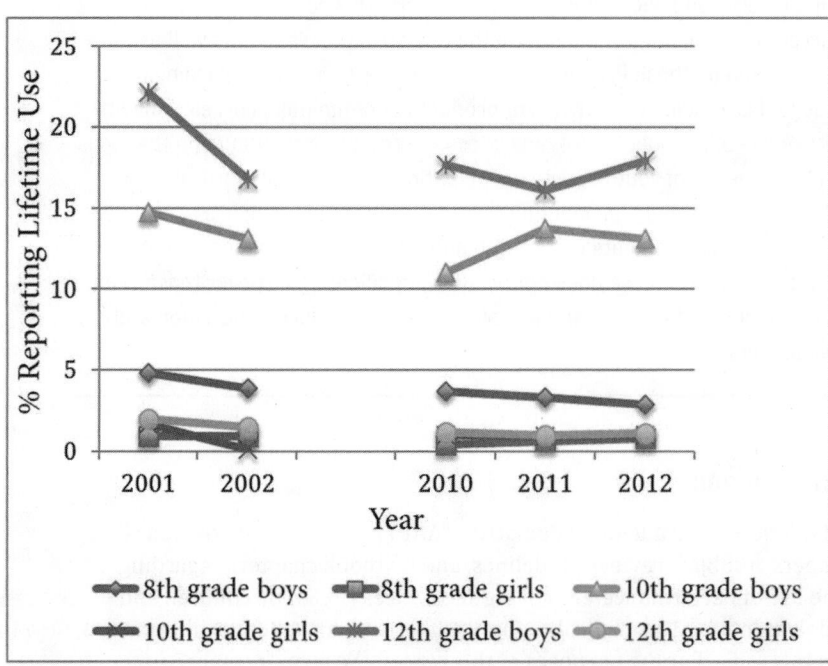

FIGURE 2
Percentage of eighth, 10th, and 12th graders reporting any lifetime use of creatine by year and sex (data from MTF, 2014).[5]

steroids. Approximately 80% of androstenedione users and more than one-third of steroid users also use creatine. Between 2010 and 2012, approximately half of androstenedione users also were

using anabolic androgenic steroids; however, this decreased to 15% in 2013. Younger creatine users are much more likely to be using multiple PESs than their older counterparts (Table 1).

TABLE 1 Polypharmacy in PES Use[5]

Grade	Creatine Users Who Also Use Androstenedione, %	Creatine users Who Also Use Anabolic Androgenic Steroids, %
8th	29	14
10th	12	8
12th	6	6

For many adolescents, use of PESs is an attempt to enhance appearance rather than performance, and many users are not actively involved in organized athletic activity. Terms such as "performance- and image-enhancing substances" and "appearance- and performance-enhancing drugs" emphasize their broader appeal.[10-13] A Minnesota study evaluating various muscle-enhancing behaviors revealed that in an urban high school population, 38.8% of boys and 18.2% of girls reported a history of protein supplement use.[11] The same study revealed rates of use in middle school for boys and girls as 29.7% and 24.7%, respectively. Although students participating in team sports were more likely to use protein supplements (24.2%), it is worth noting that use of protein supplements still was fairly high in students who were not involved in sports (18.2%).[11]

Corroborating this higher use of PESs in an athletic population, a 2012 meta-analysis revealed higher rates of steroid use in athletes than in nonathletes (odds ratio, 1.5).[14] In addition to sports participation, other correlates of PES use include body dissatisfaction,[12] higher BMI,[11] training in a commercial gym,[15] and exposure to appearance-focused media.[13] The latter was particularly true for the genre of "fitness" media, which tends to have a large focus on muscle development, as opposed to the genre of more traditional sports-reporting media. Multiple studies have revealed correlations between PES use and alcohol and drug use, as well as other risk-taking behaviors.[15-17]

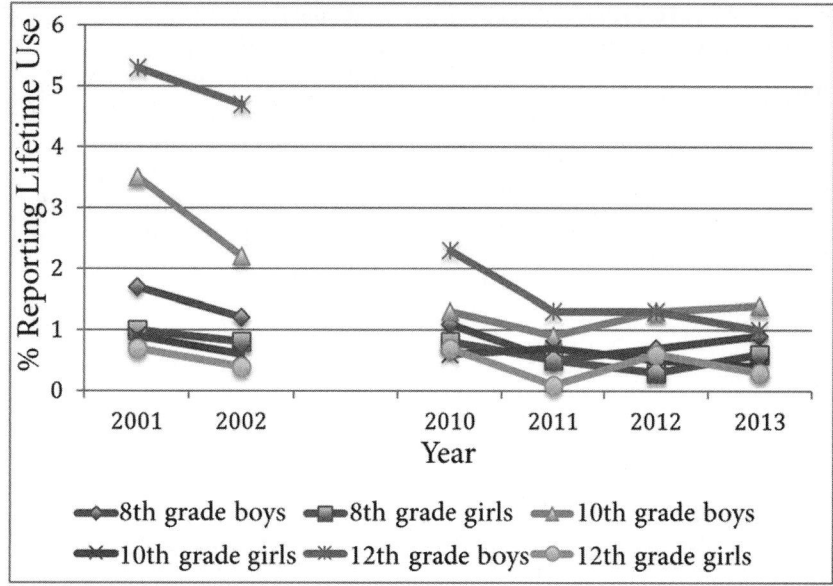

FIGURE 3
Percentage of eighth, 10th, and 12th graders reporting any lifetime use of androstenedione by year and sex (data from MTF, 2014).[5]

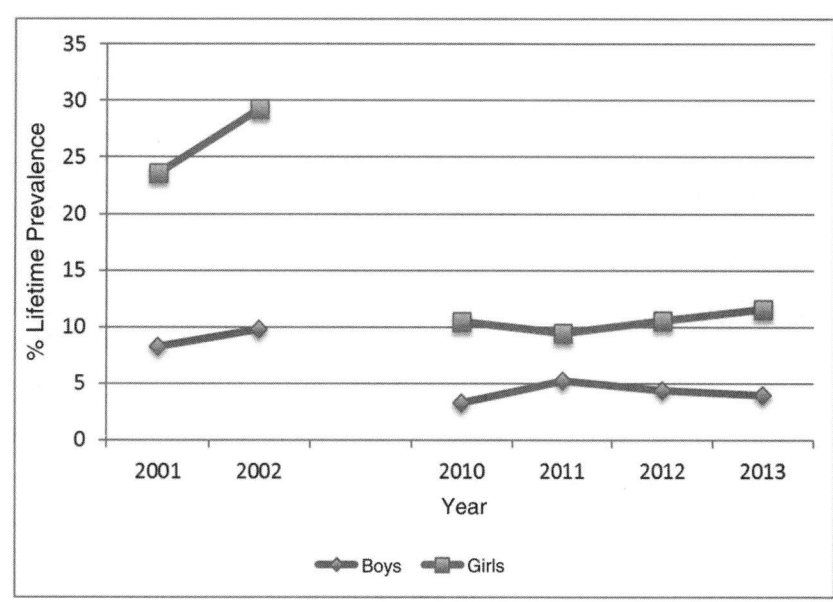

FIGURE 4
Percentage of eighth, 10th, and 12th graders reporting any lifetime use of nonprescription diet pills by sex (data from MTF, 2014).[5]

Different patterns of use have been identified between boy and girl PES users. Girls report much lower rates of using substances that are generally associated with gains in strength and muscle mass, such as creatine, androstenedione, and anabolic androgenic steroids, and these differences grow larger with age.[5] Conversely, girls report much higher rates of using nonprescription diet pills. Although this is consistent with traditional perceptions of male pursuit of muscularity and female pursuit of thinness, it is important to note that in 2013, 4% of boys reported use of diet pills in 2013, and 1% to 2% of 12th-grade girls reported use of creatine and anabolic androgenic steroids.[5,6]

It is unclear how race and ethnicity may correlate with PES use. YRBSS data revealed higher rates of steroid use in 2013 among Hispanic students (4.2%) as compared with students who identified themselves as white (2.8%) or African American (2.3%).[6] These differences were not noted for 12th graders in the 2013 MTF data, in which steroid use rates within these groups were all just under 2.0%.[5] One study revealed increased rates of steroid use among Asian students (primarily Hmong) as compared with white students, with odds ratios of 3.51 and 3.37 for boys and girls, respectively.[11] The PATS revealed that hGH use was significantly higher in African American and Hispanic teenagers as compared with white teenagers, with use rates of 15%, 13%, and 9% respectively.[7]

REGULATION OF PESs

The most commonly used PESs in the adolescent population generally are sold over the counter as dietary supplements. The Dietary Supplement Health and Education Act of 1994 (Pub L No. 103-417) created supplements as a category not subject to US Food and Drug Administration (FDA) approval for safety or efficacy before coming to market. Supplements often are intermingled with foods, beverages, and over-the-counter medications on retail shelves, and it is difficult for the consumer to differentiate products with ingredients subject to strong FDA oversight from products that are subject to the looser controls, as allowed by the Dietary Supplement Health and Education Act.

Given the lack of manufacturing oversight, consumers of these goods risk using products that are contaminated or missing ingredients. Several studies that tested protein supplements revealed that 8% to 20% of these products were

contaminated with significant amounts of heavy metals.[18] An analysis of supplements obtained from US retailers in 2007 revealed that 25% of these were contaminated with anabolic androgenic steroids, and 11% were contaminated with stimulants.[18] In 2015, the New York attorney general sent cease-and-desist letters to 4 national retailers after an investigation revealed that only 5 of 20 herbal supplement products tested consistently contained active ingredients as listed.[19]

Caffeine is unique in that it is ingested as a dietary supplement but also is contained in many foods that are common in the American diet. Although the FDA does regulate the amount of caffeine in foods (eg, soft drinks are allowed a maximum of 71 mg of caffeine/12 oz), the amount of caffeine in energy drinks and other dietary supplements is not regulated. Additional information on caffeine can be found in Fig 3, as well as the AAP clinical report "Sports Drinks and Energy Drinks for Children and Adolescents: Are They Appropriate?" which specifically states that energy drinks containing stimulants should never be consumed by children and adolescents.[20]

The Anabolic Steroid Control Acts of 1990 (Pub L No. 101-647) and 2004 (Pub L No. 108-358) classified anabolic androgenic steroids, as well as certain precursors that were previously marketed as supplements (such as androstenedione), as Schedule III drugs. The Designer Anabolic Steroid Control Act of 2014 (Pub L No. 113-260) further expanded the definition of "anabolic steroid" in part to address the expansion of synthetic prohormones that were developed after passage of the 2004 act. These prohormones are all now classified as Schedule III anabolic steroid drugs, and possession or use of any of these substances without a physician's

prescription is prohibited by state and federal laws.

SUMMARY OF PES MECHANISMS AND EFFECTS

A vast number of substances are purported to have ergogenic (ie, performance-enhancing) effects. Claims of performance enhancement with different drugs and supplements are constantly evolving. Initial claims of significant performance enhancement are often made on the Internet as well as in body-building and fitness magazines. These claims most often are unsubstantiated or based on findings from single or poorly designed studies. As these substances undergo further scrutiny, it is common for these initial claims to be debunked, and the evidence often does not support earlier assertions of performance benefit. Although it is not possible to provide a fully comprehensive list of PESs, Table 2 provides an overview of substances that are most widely known and studied in the pediatric population.

Any potential ergogenic effects of PESs can be contrasted to the great improvements in strength and athletic performance often observed in child and adolescent athletes attributable to the combined effects of training and development. Typical strength gains of approximately 30% are reported in youth resistance training programs of 8 to 20 weeks' duration.[43] Supplements or nutritional interventions that are currently available and legal cannot rival this rate of gain. The best advice for performance-related concerns in young athletes is to focus on the basics of appropriate training and nutritional practices as outlined in Table 3. PESs are not "shortcuts" to higher levels of athletic performance, and they cannot compensate for athletes who do not adhere to the basic principles of good training and nutrition.

TABLE 2 Summary Table of PES Prevalence, Effects, and Safety Concerns in Children and Adolescents

Substance	Available Prevalence Data	Usual Form of Intake	Purported Mechanism of Performance Effect	Data on Performance Effects	Potential Adverse Effects
Creatine	See Fig 1	Creatine is found in meat and fish. Approximately 3–5 g/kg uncooked meat or fish. Cooking can degrade some creatine in food. Generally ~1 g/day found in omnivore diet. Orally ingested creatine monohydrate supplement.	Delays onset of muscle fatigue during high-intensity training by adenosine triphosphate production in high intensity activities that rely upon phosphocreatine shuttle.	Performance benefit in most studies is small and primarily seen in short-duration, maximum-intensity resistance training.[21] No benefit generally shown in aerobic activities or with "on-field" athletic performance.	Short-term use at usual doses appears safe in normal adults, but has not been evaluated specifically in the pediatric population. Potential concern with impact on kidneys because of nephrotic metabolites (methylamine and formaldehyde), and specific recommendation against use for athletes at risk for kidney dysfunction.[22] May impair performance in endurance activities.
Anabolic agents	See Fig 2	Variety of testosterone derivatives. Schedule III drugs. Oral, injectable, buccal, and transdermal forms. Multiple forms often taken in "stacks" in 6- to 12-wk cycles.	Enhances net protein synthesis by increasing transcription and decreasing catabolism.	Increased strength and lean muscle mass.	Possible long-term effects on brain remodeling with adolescent AAS exposure. Premature physeal closure with decreased final adult height. Acne. Gynecomastia (irreversible). Hair loss/male pattern baldness (irreversible). Hypogonadism. Dependence. Behavior change (hypomania, irritability, aggression). Cardiomyopathy. Increased low-density lipoproteins/decreased high-density lipoproteins. Cholestatic jaundice, liver tumors.
Prohormones	See Fig 2	Variety of substances often taken in combination (stacks) and in cyclical fashion. All except for dehydroepiandrosterone (DHEA) are now scheduled drugs as a result of the Anabolic Control Act of 2005 and Designer Anabolic Steroid Act of 2014.	Purported to enhance testosterone concentrations after ingestion as well as potential direct anabolic effects.	Androstenedione and DHEA: repeated dosages do not appear to increase blood testosterone concentrations or increase muscle size or strength.[23]	Suppression of endogenous testosterone production, otherwise potentially same for testosterone as listed above.[24] Supplements contaminated with prohormones are a common cause of doping violations in organized sports.[23]
Caffeine/other stimulants	73% of children consume caffeine on any given day.[25] Median intake of those 12–19 y who ingest caffeine: 40.6 mg.[28] Nonmedical use of amphetamines in 12th grade: lifetime: 12.4%; monthly: 4.4%.[5] Overall, athletes not at greater risk for use, but boys in certain sports with higher rates: lacrosse, wrestling.[29]	Caffeine is ubiquitous in a variety of food and beverages, as well as over-the-counter diet pills and "stay awake" medication. Amphetamines often are diverted from prescription use.	Currently believed that performance benefit primarily due to central nervous system stimulation and enhanced muscle activation.	Most studies with caffeine have examined 3–6 mg/kg, but 1–3 mg/kg has been shown to have performance-enhancing effects, particularly in endurance activity.[26] This includes 4% improvements in strength of knee extensors (note: other muscle groups did not show strength improvements with caffeine); 14% in muscular endurance; and 10% to 20% improvements in time to exhaustion studies.	Tolerance. Cardiac arrhythmias (premature ventricular contractions) increased blood pressure. Headaches, irritability, sleep disruption, tremor. Gastric irritation. Increased core temperature with exertion, particularly in hot environments. Significant toxicity has been associated with ingestion of multiple energy drinks, leading to almost 1500 emergency department visits in 2011 in the 12- to 17-y age group.[27] Increased availability of pure powdered caffeine is of particular concern and is responsible for at least 2 deaths in young people (1 teaspoon of powdered caffeine is equivalent to 28 cups of coffee; FDA warning).

TABLE 2 Continued

Substance	Available Prevalence Data	Usual Form of Intake	Purported Mechanism of Performance Effect	Data on Performance Effects	Potential Adverse Effects
Protein supplements	Middle school girls: 25%. Middle school boys: 30%. High school girls: 18% High school boys: 39%.[11]	Variety of powders/bars/shakes.	Provides "building blocks" for muscle and lean tissue growth.	No performance benefit of protein supplement if diet provides adequate protein.	Contamination.
Amino acids and related compounds		Oral supplements. Individual amino acids or in combination. Diets with adequate amounts of complete proteins are replete with essential amino acids. Hydroxymethyl butyrate (HMB) is a leucine metabolite.	Arginine and citrulline produce increases in nitric oxide (see below for further discussion). β-alanine and carnosine buffer H+ accumulation (see buffer discussion below). HMB is believed to enhance repair of damaged muscle tissue.	HMB: Meta-analysis of studies on young adults reveal untrained athletes with 6.6% gains in strength, but only trivial strength impacts in trained athletes.[30] Study on elite adolescent volleyball players anaerobic power: HMB 11% improvement vs 4% with placebo.[32]	Ingestion of single amino acids may result in imbalance of others. Short-term ingestion of HMB appears safe at 6 g/day.[31]
hGH/insulinlike growth factor 1 (IGF-1)		Injectable recombinant hGH or IGF-1.	hGH acts primarily through IGF-1, resulting in increases in lean mass, decreases in fat mass.[33]	Most recent reviews do not support performance benefit.[33]	Elevated plasma glucose/insulin resistance, sodium retention and edema, myalgia/arthralgia, benign intracranial hypertension, acromegaly, cardiovascular disease, gynecomastia.[34]
Nitric oxide boosters (arginine, beetroot juice, citrulline)		Oral supplements and high nitrate-containing foods (beets most commonly studied, but also found in lettuce, spinach, radish, celery).	Nitric oxide is a potent vasodilator. Synthesized from arginine via reduction to nitrate. Citrulline is an arginine precursor.	Any potential benefit of arginine appears minimal in healthy young athletes who ingest sufficient protein.[24] Results are mixed regarding potential benefit of high nitrate-containing foods on athletic performance.[35,36] Study on junior rowers with 1.7% improvement in rowing time after repeat 500-m efforts.[37]	Supplementation with the amino acid arginine may create imbalance between other amino acids. Inorganic forms of nitrate are associated with carcinogenesis; however, current data do not support restriction of vegetable source of nitrates.[36]
Buffers		Sodium bicarbonate or sodium citrate. Carnosine and β-alanine.	Buffers the metabolic acidosis resulting from high-intensity physical activity. β-alanine is a precursor of carnosine.	Data are variable regarding endurance exercise.[38] Studies in adolescent swimmers with sodium bicarbonate reveal some swimmers with ~1-s improvement in 200-m efforts.[39] Meta-analysis β-alanine with 2.85% median improvement in exercise lasting longer than 60 s. No benefit to exercise of shorter duration.[40]	Sodium bicarbonate with significant gastric upset in ~10%. β-alanine with paresthesias at higher doses.[38]

TABLE 2 Continued

Substance	Available Prevalence Data	Usual Form of Intake	Purported Mechanism of Performance Effect	Data on Performance Effects	Potential Adverse Effects
Blood doping		Recombinant erythropoietin and synthetic analogs.	Increases oxygen delivery to exercising muscles.	Increases maximal oxygen consumption by 6%–12%.[41]	Hyperviscosity can lead to thrombogenic or embolic events. Increased cardiac afterload.[42]

CONCERNS REGARDING PES USE

The goals of the antidoping movement in sports are to protect the health of athletes and to prevent unfair competition, and use of PESs is identified in a survey of adults as the most serious issue facing sports today.[46] Potential health risks are outlined for individual substances in Table 2. In addition, the "gateway hypothesis" of adolescent substance abuse may apply with PES use. Although causation is difficult to prove, initial use of legal ergogenic supplements appears to reduce barriers to future nontherapeutic use of anabolic androgenic steroids by increasing social contacts with other users of PESs, as well as changing perceived social norms and attitudes regarding the safety and efficacy of illicit PES use.[10,47,48]

The moral implications of PES use contribute to concerns about cheating and unfair competition and may have adverse effects on the youth sports experience.[46] The top 5 issues of importance reported by children and adolescents regarding participation in sports are, in order: having fun, doing one's best, being with friends, improving skills, and being healthy. PES use shifts the focus of athletes from the pleasure and camaraderie of sports participation to that of gaining competitive advantage.

DRUG TESTING AND SCREENING

Home

Home drug tests are aggressively marketed on the Internet to parents with concerns about drug use. In a 2014 clinical report, the AAP stated it does not endorse home drug testing because of concerns about lack of efficacy, potential misinterpretation of test results, and the potential negative effect on the parent–child relationship.[49] The AAP recommends that parents' concerns about drug testing be addressed in cooperation with health care providers.

Office Based

Use of PESs often is clinically occult in the pediatric population, without reliable changes that can be detected on physical examination. *Bright Futures* contains information regarding office assessment, as well as patient and parent education and guidance when substance abuse is a concern.[50] Suggestions include screening for substance use as part of an age-appropriate comprehensive history and asking open-ended questions about substance use at home, at school, and by peers before progressing to questions about personal use.

The Preparticipation Physical Evaluation form developed by the AAP (https://www.aap.org/en-us/professional-resources/practice-support/Documents/Preparticipation-Physical-Exam-Form.pdf) contains several questions regarding use of PESs. Although sensitivity of these questions has not been studied, the questions provide an opportunity for further discussion and guidance and are as follows:

Do you drink alcohol or use other drugs?

Have you ever taken anabolic androgenic steroids or used any other performance supplement?

Have you ever taken any supplements to help you gain or lose weight or improve your performance?

The AAP does not endorse general drug use screening by pediatric health care providers but has published guidelines for drug testing in the pediatric office when there is clinical suspicion of use.[49]

High Schools

Testing in schools often is proposed not only to provide a mechanism for detecting drug use but also to serve as a deterrent. In 1995, the US Supreme Court ruled that random drug testing of student athletes does not violate the Fourth Amendment, and in 2002, the Court rendered a parallel opinion regarding students participating in other extracurricular activities.[51] Since then, schools in a number of states have initiated mandatory-random student drug testing; however, the efficacy of these programs in detecting and preventing drug use is unclear. The University Interscholastic League in Texas runs 1 of the largest high school drug testing programs in the United States. In 2013–2014, the University Interscholastic League conducted 2633 tests for anabolic androgenic steroids with 2 positive results, 7 protocol violations (ie, student did not show up for the test), and 10 inconclusive results.[52] Given the prevalence of information available on how to avoid positive anabolic-androgenic steroid (AAS) test results, it is impossible to know whether this low rate of positive results was a true reflection of reduced AAS use in this

TABLE 3 Training Principles to Enhance Athletic Performance

1. Understand that strength increases actually occur during the recovery periods after working out. Adequate recovery may require up to 48–72 h after a hard workout.
    a. Inadequate recovery will impede optimal performance gains.
    b. Low-intensity or cross-training sessions may enhance recovery in between higher-intensity workouts.
2. Training should vary in intensity, duration, and mode to enhance performance adaptations and minimize injury risk.
3. Resistance training can be an effective way to improve strength and power.
    a. The AAP policy statement on strength training in children and adolescents provides a comprehensive overview regarding safety and basic resistance training principles in the pediatric population.[44]
        i. Emphasis on appropriate supervision, technique, and equipment selection reviewed.
    b. Policy statement by the National Strength and Conditioning Association outlines more specific information on training for specific performance goals.[43]
        i. Training for strength: choose a weight that will allow completion of the following with good form and technique:
            1. Novice (<2–3 mo' experience): 10–15 repetitions for 1 set
            2. Intermediate (3–12 mo' experience): 8–12 repetitions for 1–2 sets
            3. Advanced (>12 mo' experience): 6–10 repetitions for 2–3 sets
    c. Greatest gains from a resistance training program will likely be noted after onset of peak height velocity
4. Nutrition.
    a. Adequate carbohydrates
        i. Before exercise to fuel workout and to avoid breakdown of muscle tissue
        ii. Strong evidence that carbohydrate ingestion during exercise sessions lasting longer than 1 h help athletes maintain intensity of effort; however, there is emerging evidence that small amounts of carbohydrates may be beneficial during shorter sessions as well.[45]
        iii. After exercise to build up intramuscular fuel for the next days' workouts
    b. Adequate hydration to maintain performance level throughout the workout
        i. Ensure adequate hydration before training sessions
        ii. Replenish fluid throughout period of exercise
            1. Unrestricted access to fluid during physical exertion
            2. Young athletes should be encouraged to drink to thirst
            3. Low-carbohydrate solutions (6%–8% carbohydrate) may be beneficial for training sessions longer than 30 min
                a. Sports drinks or nonacidic fruit juice diluted 1:1
            4. Assess fluid losses during exercise with pre- and postworkout weights
                a. Replenish 16–20 oz of fluid for every pound of weight lost
                b. Alter fluid replacement strategy to minimize losses in future workouts
                c. Protein after exercise and interspersed throughout the day to provide a ready pool of amino acids for muscle building throughout the recovery period
        i. Athletes consuming a balanced omnivorous diet usually with adequate protein intake
            1. Vegetarian and vegan diets often require additional planning
        ii. Protein requirements of adolescent athletes often range from 1.0 to 1.5 g protein/kg body weight/day
        iii. General rules of thumb for food protein content
            1. 8 g of protein contained in:
                a. 1 oz meat/poultry or 1/2 cup legumes or 1 cup milk/yogurt or 1 cup cooked pasta or 2 tablespoons of almond or peanut butter
                b. Examples of portion sizes:
                    i. Cooked meat or poultry: 3 oz is size of computer mouse: ~25 g protein
                    ii. 1 cup milk is about the size of a baseball: ~8 g protein
            2. Examples of food-based ways to add protein to diet:
                a. Nonfat dry milk contains 12 g protein per 1/2 cup and can be used to enrich soups/sauces/beverages
                b. Switch from traditional yogurt (7 g protein/6-oz serving) to Greek yogurt (17 g protein/6-oz serving) or cottage cheese (21 g protein/6-oz serving)
                c. Peanuts contain more protein than tree nuts with 26 g protein/100-g serving
                    i. Almonds and pistachios with 21 g protein/100-g serving
                    ii. Cashews with 18 g protein/100-g serving
                    iii. Macadamias with 8 g protein/100-g serving

population or the result of successful efforts at evading detection.

Given the association of AAS use with other risk-taking behaviors, information concerning the effects of these programs on overall rates of drug use may be pertinent. The limited number of studies evaluating school-based drug testing reveal mixed results regarding deterrent effect on use of AAS and other illicit drugs, with 1 study documenting increased rates of risk factors for future drug use.[53,54] Because of concerns regarding poor sensitivity, use of limited school resources, and potential adverse effects on student attitudes and behaviors, the AAP does not endorse widespread implementation of school-based testing.[53]

College/Elite

Athletes who are participating at collegiate, elite, or national levels are subject to specific restrictions and possible testing for a variety of ergogenic aids. Therapeutic use of certain medications by the athlete (eg, many attention-deficit/hyperactivity disorder medications, β2-agonists, diuretics) may require physician certification. Additional information for athletes and their health care providers is available as follows:

US Anti-Doping Agency (USADA) runs the antidoping program for the Olympic/Paralympic/ Pan American movements. The Web site (http://www.usada. org) includes general educational information, as well as a link to the World Anti-Doping Agency prohibited drug list.

National Collegiate Athletic Administration (NCAA) maintains Web pages providing information on its banned drug list, testing, and medical exception procedures (http://www.ncaa.org/themes/ topics/drug-testing).

National Center for Drug Free Sport administers drug-testing programs for the NCAA, as well as many professional leagues and state high school associations. The Web site (http://www.drugfreesport. com) includes additional testing information, as well as a subscription-based information center.

EDUCATION AND PREVENTION

General

Opinions of and information received from family members, school professionals, teammates, coaches, and health care providers all contribute to decision-making about PES use in the pediatric population. When adolescents are considering using PESs, the potential for benefit with PES use appears to outweigh dissuasive factors significantly.[55] Therefore, prevention efforts that are directed solely at avoidance of adverse consequences of PES use (ie, getting caught, cost) are likely to be less effective than efforts that focus on the lack of realized benefit for users of PES.

Educating athletes and families on basic training principles for pursuit of peak athletic performance may be helpful and should be emphasized as an alternative to PES use (Table 3). USADA provides a comprehensive handbook on this topic for parents, which can be accessed at http:// www.truesport.org/library/ documents/resources/nutrition_ guide/NutritionGuide.pdf.

School/Sports Team

Information contained in the AAP clinical report "The Role of Schools in Combating Illicit Substance Abuse" also is pertinent regarding PES use; however, it does not explicitly address the issue of substances that are used in pursuit of ergogenic benefit.[56] The National Institute for Drug Abuse provides teaching materials that cover use of anabolic androgenic steroids and stimulants on its Web site (http:// teens.drugabuse.gov/educators/nida-teaching-guides/mind-over-matter/ teachers-guide).

Adolescents Training and Learning to Avoid Steroids and Athletes Targeting Healthy Exercise and Nutrition Alternatives are programs designed to address PES use in adolescent boys and girls, respectively.[57] These structured, sport-centered programs are led by peers with coach facilitation and are considered by the World Anti-Doping Agency as the most rigorously studied and effective way to educate adolescents about doping.[58] Both of these programs were developed at Oregon Health and Science University, and additional information can be found at http://www.ohsu.edu/ xd/education/schools/school-of-medicine/departments/clinical-departments/medicine/divisions/ hpsm/research/index.cfm.

The Taylor Hooton Foundation provides educational resources for schools and other groups. This includes school-based presentations, as well as educational infographics and posters that can be downloaded at no cost (www.http://taylorhooton. org/education-resources/ downloads/).

Home

Many resources for parents of athletes include information on how to educate and prevent their athletes from using PESs. Publications from USADA cover a variety of issues pertinent to parents of athletes (http://www.truesport.org/library/ documents/resources/parent/ parent_handbook.pdf). Table 4 summarizes guidance for parents provided by the Partnership for Drug-Free Kids.

ADDITIONAL RESOURCES

For Health Care Professionals

Trends in PES use are subject to rapid change, with many substances having short-lived reputations as ergogenic aids. A combination of aggressive Internet marketing efforts and the lack of regulatory oversight can make it difficult to assess reliability of information sources on this topic. General information on a broad variety of specific substances is available in the *British Journal of Sports Medicine* series "A-Z of Nutritional Supplements: Dietary Supplements, Sports Nutrition Foods and Ergogenic Aids for Health and Performance (www.bjsm.bmj.com)."

For Parents and Athletes

The USADA Web site (http://www. usada.org/substances/) contains information on specific supplements and performance-enhancing drugs and information on how to assess ergogenic claims and make informed decisions regarding dietary supplement use.

SUMMARY

1. PES use is common in adolescence, and these substances are used in attempts to enhance both physical performance and appearance.

2. Throughout adolescence, use of all PESs tends to increase with age

and is higher in athletes than in nonathletes.

3. Boys are at higher risk than girls for most PES use. Other risk factors for PES use include body dissatisfaction, higher BMI, training in a commercial gym, exposure to appearance-oriented fitness media, use of alcohol or drugs, and other risk-taking behaviors.

4. PESs most commonly used by adolescents are protein supplements, creatine, and caffeine.

5. Many PESs are sold over the counter as dietary supplements. Athletes and parents often are unaware of the lack of FDA oversight of supplements and the risk of contamination with prohibited substances or absent active ingredients in these products.

6. Onset of endogenous hormone secretion during puberty, in combination with appropriate training techniques, is associated with large gains in strength and overall athletic performance. This is particularly true after the onset of peak height velocity. For most adolescent athletes, PES use will not produce significant improvements above those attained with adherence to appropriate nutrition and training fundamentals during this time.

7. It can be difficult to keep pace with the frequent reports of newly recognized PESs. Although the majority of initial reports of PES benefit are subsequently discredited after further study, it can be helpful for pediatric health care providers to steer patients and families to reputable Web-based resources for further evaluation of PES claims.

8. There is concern that initial use of over-the-counter PESs may be associated with increased risk of future anabolic steroid use and other risk-taking behaviors.

TABLE 4 Guidance for Parents With Concerns About PES Use[59]

1. Get involved
   a. Be aware of new pressures as athletes progress through different levels of participation and competition
   b. Emphasize the basics of hard work, pushing limits, teamwork, respect for competitors
   c. Give options for alternative ways to achieve peak performance
   d. Monitor any use of supplements or shakes
   e. Do not hesitate to ask directly about supplement use
   f. Provide a counterpoint for prodrug and prosupplement messages
   g. Become knowledgeable about PES
   h. Be persistent
2. Stay connected and create a strong partnership with your child's coach
   a. Get to know the team rules
   b. Keep coach informed of any pertinent issues that may be occurring in athlete's life
   c. Respect role of coach
   d. Talk to coach before or after practice, avoid sensitive discussions on game days
3. Keep lines of communication open with the athlete
   a. Emphasize the importance of good health
   b. Use the news as a starting point for discussions on PES use
   c. Emphasize that there are no shortcuts to peak performance
4. Engage health care providers if you are concerned about PES use
   a. Call provider before check-up and request that possibility of PES use addressed during examination
5. Know the warning signs of PES use
   a. Rapid changes in body shape
   b. Aggressive behavior or atypical mood swings
   c. Extreme hair growth or acne
   d. Excessive time in weight room
   e. Voice changes (especially for girls)
6. If you discover that your child is using PES
   a. Keep lines of communication open
   b. Seek outside help

Younger PES users appear to be at greater risk of polypharmacy.

LEAD AUTHORS

Michele LaBotz, MD, FAAP
Bernard A. Griesemer, MD, FAAP

COUNCIL ON SPORTS MEDICINE AND FITNESS EXECUTIVE COMMITTEE, 2014–2015

Joel S. Brenner, MD, MPH, FAAP, Chairperson
Cynthia R. LaBella, MD, FAAP, Chairperson-Elect
Margaret A. Brooks, MD, FAAP
Alex Diamond, DO, MPH, FAAP
Amanda K. Weiss Kelly, MD, FAAP
Michele LaBotz, MD, FAAP
Kelsey Logan, MD, MPH, FAAP
Keith J. Loud, MDCM, MSc, FAAP
Kody A. Moffatt, MD, FAAP
Blaise Nemeth, MD, MS, FAAP
Brooke Pengel, MD, FAAP
William Hennrikus, MD, FAAP

LIAISONS

Andrew J. M. Gregory, MD, FAAP – *American College of Sports Medicine*
Mark E. Halstead, MD, FAAP – *American Medical Society for Sports Medicine*
Lisa K. Kluchurosky, MEd, ATC – *National Athletic Trainers Association*

CONSULTANTS

Rebecca Demorest, MD, FAAP
Neeru A. Jayanthi, MD
Steven Cuff, MD, FAAP
David Smith, MD, FAAP

STAFF

Anjie Emanuel, MPH

ABBREVIATIONS

AAP: American Academy of Pediatrics
AAS: anabolic-androgenic steroid
FDA: US Food and Drug Administration
hGH: human growth hormone
MTF: Monitoring the Future
NCAA: National Collegiate Athletic Administration
PATS: Partnership Attitude Tracking Study
PES: performance-enhancing substance
USADA: US Anti-Doping Agency
YRBSS: Youth Risk Behavior Surveillance System

REFERENCES

1. Gomez J; American Academy of Pediatrics Committee on Sports Medicine and Fitness. Use of performance-enhancing substances. *Pediatrics*. 2005;115(4):1103–1106

2. American Academy of Pediatrics. Committee on Sports Medicine and Fitness. Adolescents and anabolic steroids: a subject review. *Pediatrics*. 1997;99(6):904–908

3. American Academy of Pediatrics, American Academy of Orthopaedic Surgeons. Performance enhancing substances. In: American Academy of Pediatrics, American Academy of Orthopaedic Surgeons, eds. *Care of the Young Athlete*. Elk Grove Village, IL: American Academy of Pediatrics; 2000:95–104

4. Hoffman JR, Faigenbaum AD, Ratamess NA, Ross R, Kang J, Tenenbaum G. Nutritional supplementation and anabolic steroid use in adolescents. *Med Sci Sports Exerc*. 2008;40(1):15–24

5. Johnston LD, O'Malley PM, Bachman JG, Schulenberg JE, Miech RA. Monitoring the Future: National Survey Results on Drug Use, 1975–2013, Vol. I: *Secondary School Students*. Ann Arbor, MI: Institute for Social Research, The University of Michigan; 2014

6. Kann L, Kinchen S, Shanklin SL, et al; Centers for Disease Control and Prevention (CDC). Youth risk behavior surveillance--United States, 2013. *MMWR Suppl*. 2014;63(4 SS-4):1–168

7. Partnership for Drug-Free Kids. The 2013 Partnership Attitude Tracking Study. Available at: www.drugfree.org/newsroom/pats-2013-teens-report-higher-use-of-performance-enhancing-substances. Accessed September 22, 2015

8. Hatton CK, Green GA, Ambrose PJ. Performance-enhancing drugs: understanding the risks. *Phys Med Rehabil Clin N Am*. 2014;25(4):897–913

9. Hoffman JR, Kraemer WJ, Bhasin S, et al. Position stand on androgen and human growth hormone use. *J Strength Cond Res*. 2009;23(suppl 5):S1–S59

10. Hildebrandt T, Harty S, Langenbucher JW. Fitness supplements as a gateway substance for anabolic-androgenic steroid use. *Psychol Addict Behav*. 2012;26(4):955–962

11. Eisenberg ME, Wall M, Neumark-Sztainer D. Muscle-enhancing behaviors among adolescent girls and boys. *Pediatrics*. 2012;130(6):1019–1026

12. Yager Z, O'Dea JA. Relationships between body image, nutritional supplement use, and attitudes towards doping in sport among adolescent boys: implications for prevention programs. *J Int Soc Sports Nutr*. 2014;11(1):13

13. Frison E, Vandenbosch L, Eggermont S. Exposure to media predicts use of dietary supplements and anabolic-androgenic steroids among Flemish adolescent boys. *Eur J Pediatr*. 2013;172(10):1387–1392

14. Diehl K, Thiel A, Zipfel S, Mayer J, Litaker DG, Schneider S. How healthy is the behavior of young athletes? A systematic literature review and meta-analyses. *J Sports Sci Med*. 2012;11(2):201–220

15. Dodge T, Hoagland MF. The use of anabolic androgenic steroids and polypharmacy: a review of the literature. *Drug Alcohol Depend*. 2011;114(2-3):100–109

16. Buckman JF, Farris SG, Yusko DA. A national study of substance use behaviors among NCAA male athletes who use banned performance enhancing substances. *Drug Alcohol Depend*. 2013;131(1-2):50–55

17. Buckman JF, Yusko DA, White HR, Pandina RJ. Risk profile of male college athletes who use performance-enhancing substances. *J Stud Alcohol Drugs*. 2009;70(6):919–923

18. Maughan RJ. Quality assurance issues in the use of dietary supplements, with special reference to protein supplements. *J Nutr*. 2013;143(11):1843S–1847S

19. O'Connor A. New York Attorney General targets supplements at major retailers. *New York Times*. February 3, 2015. Available at: http://well.blogs.nytimes.com/2015/02/03/new-york-attorney-general-targets-supplements-at-major-retailers/. Accessed September 23, 2015

20. Committee on Nutrition and the Council on Sports Medicine and Fitness. Sports drinks and energy drinks for children and adolescents: are they appropriate? *Pediatrics*. 2011;127(6):1182–1189

21. Hall M, Trojian TH. Creatine supplementation. *Curr Sports Med Rep*. 2013;12(4):240–244

22. Kim HJ, Kim CK, Carpentier A, Poortmans JR. Studies on the safety of creatine supplementation. *Amino Acids*. 2011;40(5):1409–1418

23. King DS, Baskerville R, Hellsten Y, et al. A-Z of nutritional supplements: dietary supplements, sports nutrition foods and ergogenic aids for health and performance: Part 34. *Br J Sports Med*. 2012;46(9):689–690

24. Castell LM, Burke LM, Stear SJ. BJSM reviews: A-Z of supplements: dietary supplements, sports nutrition foods and ergogenic aids for health and performance Part 2. *Br J Sports Med*. 2009;43(11):807–810

25. Branum AM, Rossen LM, Schoendorf KC. Trends in caffeine intake among U.S. children and adolescents. *Pediatrics*. 2014;133(3):386–393

26. Warren GL, Park ND, Maresca RD, McKibans KI, Millard-Stafford ML. Effect of caffeine ingestion on muscular strength and endurance: a meta-analysis. *Med Sci Sports Exerc*. 2010;42(7):1375–1387

27. Substance Abuse and Mental Health Services Administration, Center for Behavioral Health Statistics and Quality. *The DAWN Report: Update on Emergency Department Visits Involving Energy Drinks: A Continuing Public Health Concern*. Rockville, MD: Substance Abuse and Mental Health Services Administration; 2013

28. Ahluwalia N, Herrick K, Moshfegh A, Rybak M. Caffeine intake in children in the United States and 10-y trends: 2001-2010. *Am J Clin Nutr*. 2014;100(4):1124–1132

29. Veliz P, Boyd C, McCabe SE. Adolescent athletic participation and nonmedical Adderall use: an exploratory analysis of a performance-enhancing drug. *J Stud Alcohol Drugs*. 2013;74(5):714–719

30. Rowlands DS, Thomson JS. Effects of beta-hydroxy-beta-methylbutyrate supplementation during resistance training on strength, body composition, and muscle damage in trained and untrained young men: a meta-analysis. *J Strength Cond Res*. 2009;23(3):836–846

31. Currell K, Derave W, Everaert I, et al. A-Z of nutritional supplements: dietary

supplements, sports nutrition foods and ergogenic aids for health and performance: Part 20. *Br J Sports Med.* 2011;45(6):530–532

32. Portal S, Zadik Z, Rabinowitz J, et al. The effect of HMB supplementation on body composition, fitness, hormonal and inflammatory mediators in elite adolescent volleyball players: a prospective randomized, double-blind, placebo-controlled study. *Eur J Appl Physiol.* 2011;111(9):2261–2269

33. Liu H, Bravata DM, Olkin I, et al. Systematic review: the effects of growth hormone on athletic performance. *Ann Intern Med.* 2008;148(10):747–758

34. Baumann GP. Growth hormone doping in sports: a critical review of use and detection strategies. *Endocr Rev.* 2012;33(2):155–186

35. Sandbakk SB, Sandbakk O, Peacock O, et al Effects of acute supplementation of L-arginine and nitrate on endurance and sprint performance in elite athletes. *Nitric Oxide.* 2015;48:10–15

36. Clements WT, Lee S-R, Bloomer RJ. Nitrate ingestion: a review of the health and physical performance effects. *Nutrients.* 2014;6(11):5224–5264

37. Bond H, Morton L, Braakhuis AJ. Dietary nitrate supplementation improves rowing performance in well-trained rowers. *Int J Sport Nutr Exerc Metab.* 2012;22(4):251–256

38. Castell LM, Burke LM, Stear SJ, McNaughton LR, Harris RC. BJSM reviews: A-Z of nutritional supplements: dietary supplements, sports nutrition foods and ergogenic aids for health and performance Part 5. *Br J Sports Med.* 2010;44(1):77–78

39. Zajac A, Cholewa J, Poprzecki S, Waskiewicz Z, Langfort J. Effects of sodium bicarbonate ingestion on swim performance in youth athletes. *J Sports Sci Med.* 2009;8(1):45–50

40. Hobson RM, Saunders B, Ball G, Harris RC, Sale C. Effects of β-alanine supplementation on exercise performance: a meta-analysis. *Amino Acids.* 2012;43(1):25–37

41. Thomsen JJ, Rentsch RL, Robach P, et al. Prolonged administration of recombinant human erythropoietin increases submaximal performance more than maximal aerobic capacity. *Eur J Appl Physiol.* 2007;101(4):481–486

42. Deligiannis AP, Kouidi EI. Cardiovascular adverse effects of doping in sports. *Hellenic J Cardiol.* 2012;53(6):447–457

43. Faigenbaum AD, Kraemer WJ, Blimkie CJ, et al. Youth resistance training: updated position statement paper from the national strength and conditioning association. *J Strength Cond Res.* 2009;23(suppl 5):S60–S79

44. McCambridge TM, Stricker PR; American Academy of Pediatrics Council on Sports Medicine and Fitness. Strength training by children and adolescents. *Pediatrics.* 2008;121(4):835–840

45. Jeukendrup A. A step towards personalized sports nutrition: carbohydrate intake during exercise. *Sports Med.* 2014;44(suppl 1):S25–S33

46. US Anti-Doping Agency. *What Sport Means in America: A Study of Sport's Role in Society.* Colorado Springs, CO: US Anti-Doping Agency; 2011. Available at: www.truesport.org/library/documents/about/what_sport_means_in_america/what_sport_means_in_america.pdf. Accessed September 23, 2015

47. Dunn M, Thomas JO, Swift W, Burns L. Elite athletes' estimates of the prevalence of illicit drug use: evidence for the false consensus effect. *Drug Alcohol Rev.* 2012;31(1):27–32

48. Dunn M, Mazanov J, Sitharthan G. Predicting future anabolic-androgenic steroid use intentions with current substance use: findings from an internet-based survey. *Clin J Sport Med.* 2009;19(3):222–227

49. Levy S, Siqueira LM, Ammerman SD, et al; Committee on Substance Abuse. Testing for drugs of abuse in children and adolescents. *Pediatrics.* 2014;133(6). Available at: www.pediatrics.org/cgi/content/full/133/6/e1798

50. Hagan JF, Shaw JS, Duncan P, eds. *Bright Futures: Guidelines for Health Supervision of Infants, Children, and Adolescents.* Elk Grove Village, IL: American Academy of Pediatrics; 2008

51. *Bethel School District #43 v Fraser*, 478 U.S. 675, 106 S. Ct. 3159; 92 L. Ed. 2d 549; 1986 U.S. LEXIS 139; 54 U.S.L.W. 5054 (1986). Available at: www.uscourts.gov/ educational-resources/get-informed/supreme-court/landmark-supreme-court-cases-about-students.aspx. Accessed September 23, 2015

52. University Interscholastic League. 2013–2014 University Interscholastic League Anabolic Testing Report. Available at: https://www.uiltexas.org/health/info/2013-2014-uil-anabolic-steroid-testing-report. Accessed September 23, 2015

53. Levy S, Schizer M; Committee on Substance Abuse, American Academy of Pediatrics. Adolescent drug testing policies in schools. *Pediatrics.* 2015;135(4). Available at: www.pediatrics.org/cgi/content/full/135/4/e1107

54. Goldberg L, Elliot DL, MacKinnon DP, et al. Outcomes of a prospective trial of student-athlete drug testing: the Student Athlete Testing Using Random Notification (SATURN) study. *J Adolesc Health.* 2007;41(5):421–429

55. Goulet C, Valois P, Buist A, Côté M. Predictors of the use of performance-enhancing substances by young athletes. *Clin J Sport Med.* 2010;20(4):243–248

56. Mears CJ, Knight JR; Council on School Health, American Academy of Pediatrics; Committee on Substance Abuse, American Academy of Pediatrics. The role of schools in combating illicit substance abuse. *Pediatrics.* 2007;120(6):1379–1384

57. ATLAS and ATHENA Health Promotion and Substance Abuse Prevention. Available at: http://www.ohsu.edu/xd/education/schools/school-of-medicine/departments/clinical-departments/medicine/divisions/hpsm/research/atlas-and-athena-program.cfm. Accessed May 17, 2016

58. Kersey RD, Elliot DL, Goldberg L, et al; National Athletic Trainers' Association. National Athletic Trainers' Association position statement: anabolic-androgenic steroids. *J Athl Train.* 2012;47(5):567–588

59. Partnership for Drug-Free Kids. Parent Talk Kit: What You Need to Know Before Talking to Your Child About Performance Enhancing Substances. New York, NY: Partnership for Drug-Free Kids; 2014. Available at: http://playhealthy.drugfree.org/uploads/resources_files/Play_Healthy_Parent_Talk_Kit_2014a.pdf. Accessed September 23, 2015

The Use of Systemic and Topical Fluoroquinolones

• *Clinical Report*

CLINICAL REPORT   Guidance for the Clinician in Rendering Pediatric Care

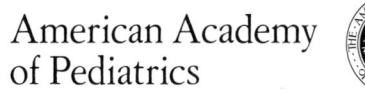 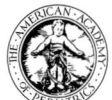

American Academy
of Pediatrics

DEDICATED TO THE HEALTH OF ALL CHILDREN™

The Use of Systemic and Topical Fluoroquinolones

Mary Anne Jackson, MD, FAAP, Gordon E. Schutze, MD, FAAP, COMMITTEE ON INFECTIOUS DISEASES

abstract

Appropriate prescribing practices for fluoroquinolones, as well as all antimicrobial agents, are essential as evolving resistance patterns are considered, additional treatment indications are identified, and the toxicity profile of fluoroquinolones in children has become better defined. Earlier recommendations for systemic therapy remain; expanded uses of fluoroquinolones for the treatment of certain infections are outlined in this report. Prescribing clinicians should be aware of specific adverse reactions associated with fluoroquinolones, and their use in children should continue to be limited to the treatment of infections for which no safe and effective alternative exists or in situations in which oral fluoroquinolone treatment represents a reasonable alternative to parenteral antimicrobial therapy.

Clinical reports from the American Academy of Pediatrics benefit from expertise and resources of liaisons and internal (AAP) and external reviewers. However, clinical reports from the American Academy of Pediatrics may not reflect the views of the liaisons or the organizations or government agencies that they represent.

The guidance in this report does not indicate an exclusive course of treatment or serve as a standard of medical care. Variations, taking into account individual circumstances, may be appropriate.

All clinical reports from the American Academy of Pediatrics automatically expire 5 years after publication unless reaffirmed, revised, or retired at or before that time.

DOI: 10.1542/peds.2016-2706

PEDIATRICS (ISSN Numbers: Print, 0031-4005; Online, 1098-4275).

Copyright © 2016 by the American Academy of Pediatrics

FINANCIAL DISCLOSURE: The authors have indicated they have no financial relationships relevant to this article to disclose.

FUNDING: No external funding.

POTENTIAL CONFLICT OF INTEREST: The authors have indicated they have no potential conflicts of interest to disclose.

To cite: Jackson MA, Schutze GE, AAP COMMITTEE ON INFECTIOUS DISEASES. The Use of Systemic and Topical Fluoroquinolones. *Pediatrics.* 2016;138(5):e20162706

OVERVIEW

Fluoroquinolones are highly active in vitro against both Gram-positive and Gram-negative pathogens, with pharmacokinetic properties that are favorable for treating a wide array of infections. The prototype quinolone antibiotic agent, nalidixic acid, was first approved by the US Food and Drug Administration (FDA) for adults in 1964 and generally is considered to be the first generation of such agents. For more than 2 decades, nalidixic acid represented the prototypic fluoroquinolone approved by the FDA and was available for children 3 months and older, but it is no longer available. Subsequent chemical modifications resulted in a series of fluoroquinolone agents with an increased antimicrobial spectrum of activity and better pharmacokinetic characteristics.

Ciprofloxacin, norfloxacin, and ofloxacin have a greater Gram-negative spectrum (with activity against *Pseudomonas aeruginosa*). In 2004, ciprofloxacin became the first fluoroquinolone agent approved for use in children 1 through 17 years of age.

Levofloxacin is often referred to as a respiratory fluoroquinolone because it has increased activity against many of the respiratory pathogens, such as *Streptococcus pneumoniae*, *Mycoplasma pneumoniae*, and *Chlamydophila pneumoniae*, while retaining activity against many of the

Gram-negative pathogens. A fourth-generation agent, moxifloxacin, displays increased activity against anaerobes while maintaining Gram-positive and Gram-negative activity and also has excellent activity against *Mycobacterium tuberculosis*; however, there are limited safety and dosing data available in children.

Animal toxicology data available with the first quinolone compounds revealed their propensity to create inflammation and subsequent destruction of weight-bearing joints in canine puppies.[1,2] This observation effectively sidelined further development or large-scale evaluation of this class of antibiotic agents in children at that time.

A policy statement summarizing the assessment of risks and benefits of fluoroquinolones in pediatric patients was published by the American Academy of Pediatrics (AAP) in 2006, and earlier recommendations remain, with updates as appropriate covered in this document.[3] The statement indicated that the parenteral fluoroquinolones were appropriate for the treatment of infections caused by multidrug-resistant pathogens for which no alternative safe and effective parenteral agent existed. However, for outpatient management, oral fluoroquinolones were only indicated when other options were intravenous (IV) treatment with other classes of antibiotic agents. In 2011, the AAP published an updated clinical report because of the increased ophthalmologic and topical use of fluoroquinolones as well as data on lack of toxicity when used in children.[4]

Quinolones that are currently approved for pediatric patients by the FDA and available in an IV and oral suspension formulation are ciprofloxacin for the indications of inhalational anthrax, plague, complicated urinary tract infections (UTIs), and pyelonephritis and levofloxacin for the indications of

inhalational anthrax and plague. A randomized, prospective, double-blind multicenter study of moxifloxacin for complicated intraabdominal infection in children, in which patients were randomly assigned to receive either moxifloxacin plus comparator drug placebo or comparator drug plus moxifloxacin placebo, was completed in July 2015, but no data are available at this time. Systemic quinolones licensed in the United States will be discussed in this report. In addition, this review will contain no discussion of the use of fluoroquinolones in infants younger than 6 months.

SAFETY

Animal Models

The original toxicology studies with quinolones documented cartilage injury in weight-bearing joints in canine puppies, with damage to the joint cartilage proportional to the degree of exposure.[1,2] Each quinolone has a different potential to cause cartilage toxicity,[5] but given a sufficiently high exposure, cartilage changes will occur in all animal models with all quinolones.

Although initial reports focused on articular cartilage, subsequent studies suggested the possibility of epiphyseal plate cartilage injury,[6] leading to fluoroquinolone clinical study designs lasting several years to assess growth potential. Data suggest that quinolone toxicity occurs as a result of concentrations present in cartilage that are sufficiently high to form chelate complexes with divalent cations, particularly magnesium, resulting in the impairment of integrin function and cartilage matrix integrity in the weight-bearing joints, which undergo chronic trauma during routine use.[7]

In studies of ciprofloxacin exposure to very young beagle puppies (one of the most sensitive animal models for quinolone toxicity), clinical evidence

of arthrotoxicity was observed during a 14-day treatment course at 90 mg/kg per day but not at 30 mg/kg per day.[8,9] Apparent joint tenderness at the higher exposure resolved 6 weeks after the last dose of ciprofloxacin. Histopathologic evidence of cartilage injury was noted in virtually all animals given 90 mg/kg per day of ciprofloxacin. At this exposure level, the observed clinical signs all occurred during and shortly after treatment but resolved by 2 months after cessation, with no recurrent signs noted during the 5-month follow-up period. Histopathologic evidence of cartilage injury was also observed at 30 mg/kg per day, the dose currently recommended for children, and inflammation occurred in fewer than half the animals at this dose but persisted for 5 months after treatment, at full skeletal maturation. The "no observed adverse event level" (NOAEL) was 10 mg/kg per day, a dose at which neither clinical nor histopathologic evidence of toxicity was present, but a dose too low for therapeutic benefit.

Similar data were developed before FDA approval of levofloxacin for adults, documenting a NOAEL at 3 mg/kg per day for IV dosing for 14 days (approximately one-quarter the current FDA-approved dose of 16 mg/kg per day for children who weigh less than 50 kg). Levofloxacin has virtually 100% bioavailability, with total drug exposure being equivalent between IV and oral formulations at the same milligram per kilogram dose.[10]

Data from a lamb model, with growth rates and activity more closely mirroring humans than juvenile beagle dogs or rats, have been reported. Gross examination of articular cartilage and microscopic examination of epiphyseal cartilage did not reveal abnormalities consistent with cartilage injury or inflammation after a 14-day drug exposure to either gatifloxacin or

TABLE 1 Rate of FDA-Defined Arthropathy 6 Weeks and 1 Year After Treatment With Ciprofloxacin or a Comparator

	Ciprofloxacin (n = 335)	Comparator (n = 349)
Arthropathy rate at 6-week follow-up,[a] n (%)	31 (9.3)	21 (6.0%)
95% CI, %		(−0.8 to 7.2)
Cumulative arthropathy rate at 1-year follow-up,[a] n (%)	46 (13.7)	33 (9.5%)
95% CI, %		(−0.6 to 9.1)
Selected musculoskeletal adverse events[b] in patients with arthropathy at 1-year follow-up	Ciprofloxacin n = 46 patients[c]	Comparator n = 33 patients[c]
Arthralgia	35 (76)	20 (61)
Abnormal joint and/or gait examination	11 (24)	8 (24)
Accidental injury	6 (13)	1 (3)
Leg pain	5 (11)	1 (3)
Back pain	4 (9)	0
Arthrosis	4 (9)	1 (3)
Bone pain	3 (7)	0
Joint disorder	2 (4)	0
Pain	2 (4)	2 (6)
Myalgia	1 (2)	4 (12)
Arm pain	0	2 (6)
Movement disorder	1 (2)	1 (3)

Data are from ref 8. CI, confidence interval.

[a] The study was designed to show that the arthropathy rate for the ciprofloxacin group did not exceed that of the comparator group by more than +6.0%. At both evaluations, the 95% CI indicated that it could not be concluded that ciprofloxacin had findings comparable to the comparator.

[b] Events occurring in 2 or more patients.

[c] A patient with arthropathy may have had more than 1 event.

ciprofloxacin that was equivalent to that achieved in children receiving therapeutic doses.[11]

Human Studies

In 2004, the FDA released data about the safety of ciprofloxacin[8] from an analysis of clinical trial 100169, which evaluated ciprofloxacin for the treatment of complicated UTI or pyelonephritis in children 1 through 17 years of age. The study was a prospective, randomized, double-blind, active-controlled, parallel-group, multinational, multicenter pediatric trial. Ciprofloxacin oral suspension was compared with oral cefixime or trimethoprim-sulfamethoxazole (TMP-SMX) in 1 stratum, and in the second stratum ciprofloxacin (IV alone or IV followed by oral suspension) was compared with a number of comparator regimens, including IV ceftazidime alone or IV ceftazidime followed by oral cefixime or TMP-SMX. Clinical end points were designed to capture any sign of cartilage or tendon

toxicity. Arthropathy rates were 9.3% for ciprofloxacin versus 6% for the comparator group (Table 1).

Adefurin et al[12] performed a systematic review of the safety data for 16 184 pediatric patients treated with ciprofloxacin by using case reports and case series and reported 1065 (6.6%) adverse events. The most frequently reported events were musculoskeletal (24%), followed by abnormal liver function tests (13%), nausea (7%), white blood cell count derangements (5.3%), vomiting (5.2%), and rash (4.7%). Arthralgia (50% of the 258 musculoskeletal adverse events) was the most common musculoskeletal adverse event reported. These data showed an estimated risk of 16 musculoskeletal adverse events per 1000 patients receiving ciprofloxacin (1.6%; 95% confidence interval: 0.9% to 2.6%), or 1 event for every 62.5 patients. All cases of arthropathy resolved or improved with medical management, which included drug withdrawal in some cases, and

none of the studies found growth inhibition.

Levofloxacin safety data were collected on a large cohort of 2523 children who participated in prospective, randomized, unblinded clinical efficacy trials. Data were collected from a community-acquired pneumonia trial in children 6 months to 16 years of age (a randomized 3:1, prospective, comparative trial in 533 levofloxacin-exposed and 179 comparator-exposed evaluable subjects) and from 2 trials assessing therapy for acute otitis media in children 6 months to 5 years of age (1 open-label noncomparative study in 204 evaluable subjects and another randomized 1:1, prospective, comparative trial in 797 levofloxacin-exposed and 810 comparator-exposed evaluable subjects).[13] In addition, after completion of the treatment trials, all subjects from both treatment arms were also offered participation in an unblinded, 12-month follow-up study for safety assessments, including musculoskeletal events.

The definitions of musculoskeletal events for tendinopathy (inflammation or rupture of a tendon as determined by physical examination and/or MRI or ultrasonography), arthritis (inflammation of a joint as evidenced by redness and/or swelling of the joint), arthralgia (pain in the joint as evidenced by complaint), and gait abnormality (limping or refusal to walk) were determined before starting the studies. The identity of study medication was known by parents, study personnel, and the subject's care providers because reports of musculoskeletal events and any other adverse events were collected during the follow-up period. An analysis of these events occurred at 1, 2, and 12 months after treatment. The analysis of disorders involving weight-bearing joints documented a statistically greater rate between the levofloxacin-treated group and comparator group at 2 months (1.9% vs 0.7%; P = .025) and at 12 months (2.9% vs 1.6%; P = .047). A history of joint pain accounted for 85% of all events, with no findings of joint abnormality when assessed by physical examination. Computed tomography or MRI was performed for 5 of the patients with musculoskeletal symptoms; no signs of structural injury were identified. No evidence of joint abnormalities was observed at 12 months in the levofloxacin group.

A long-term follow-up study (5 years) in selected subjects from this cohort was published recently.[14] The selection of the children for this long-term follow-up study was based on meeting 1 of the following criteria: (1) growth impaired or possibly growth impaired, defined as a documented height <80% of the expected height increase 12 months after treatment; (2) assessed by the investigator as having abnormal bone or joint symptoms during the original 12-month follow-up; (3) persisting musculoskeletal adverse events at the end of the original 12 months of follow-up; and (4) follow-up requested by the drug safety monitoring committee because of concerns for possible tendon/joint toxicity associated with a protocol-defined musculoskeletal disorder. Of the 2233 subjects participating in the previously described 12-month follow-up study, 124 of 1340 (9%) from the levofloxacin group and 83 of the 893 (9%) subjects in the comparator group were enrolled (207 total subjects), and 49% from each group completed the study. Although an increase in musculoskeletal events in the levofloxacin group had been noted at 12 months after treatment, the cumulative long-term outcomes of children with musculoskeletal adverse events reported during the 5-year safety study (including ongoing arthropathy, peripheral neuropathy, abnormal bone development, scoliosis, walking difficulty, myalgia, tendon disorder, hypermobility syndrome, and pain in the spine, hip, and shoulder) were slightly higher in the comparator group (0.1%) than in the levofloxacin group (0.07%). A total of 174 of 207 (84%) reviewed subjects were identified by the growth-impaired or possible growth-impaired criteria. Children from levofloxacin and comparator treatment groups had similar growth characteristics at the 5-year assessment, with equal percentages of children from each treatment group having (1) no change in height percentile, (2) an increase in percentile, or (3) a decrease in percentile. Of the 9 children that had less growth than predicted (6 of 104 [6%] from the levofloxacin group, 3 of 70 [4%] from the comparator group), none were believed by the drug monitoring safety committee to have drug-attributable growth changes. This 5-year follow-up study enrolled 48% of study participants from US sites compared with 20% from US sites enrolled in the original clinical trials.

A rare complication associated with quinolone antibiotic agents, tendon rupture, has a predilection for the Achilles tendon (and is often bilateral) and is estimated to occur at a rate of 15 to 20 per 100 000 treated patients in the adult population.[15] Advanced age, along with antecedent steroid therapy and a particular subset of underlying diseases, including hypercholesterolemia, gout, rheumatoid arthritis, end-stage renal disease/dialysis, and renal transplantation, have been identified as risk factors and prompted an FDA warning about this serious adverse event for all quinolone agents. Although rare cases of Achilles tendon rupture can follow overuse injuries in children, to date there have been no reports of Achilles tendon rupture in children in association with quinolone use. In summary, although isolated studies of fluoroquinolone antimicrobial agents have suggested possible musculoskeletal toxicity in children, there is no evidence for long-term harm at this time.

Other potential adverse reactions of fluoroquinolone-class antibiotic agents, although very uncommon in children, include central nervous system adverse effects (seizures, headaches, dizziness, lightheadedness, sleep disorders, hallucinations) and peripheral neuropathy. In data from clinical trial 100169, the rate of neurologic events described were similar between ciprofloxacin-treated and comparator-treated children.[8] Reported rates of neurologic events in the levofloxacin safety database were statistically similar between fluoroquinolone- and comparator-treated children.[16,17]

Cardiotoxicity (see Additional Risks/Conditions), disorders of glucose homeostasis (hypo- and hyperglycemia), hepatic dysfunction, renal dysfunction (interstitial nephritis and crystal nephropathy), and hypersensitivity reactions have also been reported. Practitioners should be aware that fluoroquinolone-associated photosensitivity has been described, and patients should be counseled to use appropriate sun-protection measures. Rashes were more commonly noted in association with the use of >7 days of gemifloxacin in women younger than 40 years.

RESISTANCE

Resistance has been a concern since the approval of quinolone agents, given the broad spectrum of activity and the large number of clinical indications. Multiple mechanisms of resistance have been described, including mutations leading to changes in the target enzymes DNA gyrase and DNA topoisomerase, as well as efflux pumps and alterations in membrane porins.[18] The role of plasmid-mediated quinolone resistance determinants such as *qnr* genes, continues to increase. The phenotype conferred by these genes generally shows a low-level resistance to fluoroquinolones, but it also appears to encourage additional fluoroquinolone resistance mechanisms that lead to high-level resistance.[19] Several surveillance studies have shown that after the introduction of fluoroquinolones into clinical practice, resistance rapidly develops, although less commonly in pediatric patients given the reduced use of these medications in children. In large-scale pediatric studies of levofloxacin for acute otitis media, the emergence of levofloxacin-resistant pneumococci was not shown after treatment, suggesting that the emergence of resistance during treatment is not a common event.[20] In adult patients, *Pseudomonas* resistance to both fluoroquinolones and other antimicrobial agents is problematic.[21] Data on resistance in *Escherichia coli* isolated from adults with UTIs who were seen in emergency departments in the EMERGEncy ID NET, a network of 11 geographically diverse university-affiliated institutions, suggest a low but stable rate of resistance of approximately 5%,[22] although in specific locations, rates of resistance for outpatients are closer to 10%.[23,24] Similar published data do not exist for children, although in current reports that include outpatient data, stratified by age, rates of fluoroquinolone resistance in *E coli* in children have been generally well below 3%.[24,25]

Recent data from Canadian hospitals revealed that antimicrobial resistance rates continue to be higher in older age groups as compared with children and that there is considerable variability in age-specific resistance trends for different pathogens.[26] Data available from 4 large tertiary care children's hospitals (Houston, Kansas City, San Diego, and Philadelphia) document ciprofloxacin resistance to *E coli* to range from 5% to 14% for 2014 (G.E. Schutze, MD, M.A. Jackson, MD, J. Bradley, MD, and T. Zaoutis, MD, personal communication, 2015) with rates that appear to be stable for the last 3 years. As fluoroquinolone use in pediatrics increases, it is expected that resistance will increase, as has been documented in adults. There is a clear risk of resistance in patients exposed to repeated treatment courses. Susceptibility data in patients with cystic fibrosis revealed a sharp increase in resistance to *Pseudomonas* strains when comparing rates from 2001 and 2011.[27] There is a correlation between fluoroquinolone use and the emergence of ciprofloxacin and levofloxacin resistance among Gram-negative bacilli in hospitalized children.[28] As expected, when the use of the fluoroquinolones (in particular levofloxacin) increased, the susceptibility of Gram-negative bacilli to ciprofloxacin and levofloxacin significantly decreased.[29]

ADDITIONAL RISKS/CONSIDERATIONS

The incidence of *Clostridium difficile*–associated disease in children continues to increase across the United States. The AAP Committee on Infectious Diseases emphasizes the risks related to the development of *C difficile*–associated disease, which includes exposure to antimicrobial therapy.[30] Current data suggest that clindamycin, oral cephalosporins, and fluoroquinolone-class antibiotics are associated with an increased risk of both community-acquired and hospital-acquired *C difficile*–associated disease.[31,32]

Cardiotoxicity of fluoroquinolones is well described in adults and relates to the propensity of such drugs to prolong the QT interval through blockage of the voltage-gated potassium channels, especially the rapid component of the delayed rectifier potassium current I(Kr), expressed by *HERG* (the human ether-a-go-go–related gene). Moxifloxacin has the greatest risk to prolong the QT interval and should be avoided in patients with long QT syndrome, those with hypokalemia or hypomagnesemia, those with organic heart disease including congestive heart failure, those receiving an antiarrhythmic agent from class Ia or class III (eg, quinidine and procainamide or amiodarone and sotaolo, respectively), those who are receiving a concurrent drug that prolongs the QTc interval independently, and those with hepatic insufficiency–related metabolic derangements that may promote QT prolongation. Levofloxacin also appears to prolong the QT interval, although at a lower risk than moxifloxacin. Ciprofloxacin appears to confer the lowest risk.[33] No cases of cardiotoxicity or torsades de pointes in children associated with fluoroquinolones have been reported to date.[34]

USE OF FLUOROQUINOLONES IN PEDIATRIC INFECTIONS

Conjunctivitis

Although most clinicians use a polymyxin/trimethoprim ophthalmologic solution or polymyxin/bacitracin ophthalmic ointment for the treatment of acute bacterial conjunctivitis, an increasing number of topical fluoroquinolones are approved by the FDA for this indication in adults and children older than 12 months, including levofloxacin, ofloxacin, moxifloxacin, gatifloxacin, ciprofloxacin, and besifloxacin (Table 2). Conjunctival tissue pharmacokinetic studies that use conjunctival biopsies in healthy adult volunteers with besifloxacin, gatifloxacin, and moxifloxacin have been performed. All 3 agents reached peak concentrations after 15 minutes.[35] Although drug

TABLE 2 Most Common Infections for Which Fluoroquinolones Are Effective Therapy

Infection	Primary Pathogen(s)[a]	Fluoroquinolone
Systemic antibiotic requirement[b]		
UTI	*Escherichia coli, Pseudomonas aeruginosa, Enterobacter* species, *Citrobacter* species, *Serratia* species	Ciprofloxacin[c]
Acute otitis media, sinusitis	*Streptococcus pneumoniae, Haemophilus influenzae*	Levofloxacin[d]
Pneumonia	*S pneumoniae, Mycoplasma pneumoniae* (macrolides preferred for *Mycoplasma* infections)	Levofloxacin[d]
Gastrointestinal infections	*Salmonella* species, *Shigella* species	Ciprofloxacin[c]
Topical antibiotic requirement[e]		
Conjunctivitis	*S pneumoniae, H influenza*	Besifloxacin, levofloxacin, gatifloxacin, ciprofloxacin, moxifloxacin, ofloxacin
Acute otitis externa, tympanostomy tube–associated otorrhea	*P aeruginosa, Staphylococcus aureus*, mixed Gram-positive/Gram-negative organisms	Ciprofloxacin,[f] ofloxacin

[a] Assuming that the pathogen is either documented to be susceptible or presumed to be susceptible to fluoroquinolones.

[b] If oral therapy is appropriate, use other classes of oral antibiotics if organisms are susceptible.

[c] Dose of ciprofloxacin. Oral administration: 20–40 mg/kg per day, divided every 12 hours (maximum dose: 750 mg/dose); IV administration: 20–30 mg/kg per day, divided every 8–12 hours (maximum dose: 400 mg/dose).

[d] Dose of levofloxacin. Oral or IV administration: for children 6 months to 5 years of age, 16–20 mg/kg per day divided every 12 hours; for children 5 years and older, 10 mg/kg per day once daily (maximum dose: 750 mg/dose).

[e] Systemic toxicity of fluoroquinolones is not a concern with topical therapy: the use of topical agents should be determined by suspected pathogens, efficacy for mucosal infection, tolerability, and cost. Other systemic therapy may be required for more severe infection.

[f] Available with and without corticosteroid.

concentrations are only 1 indicator of potential clinical efficacy, the utility of agents with higher concentrations is tempered by the observation of a potential increase in ocular adverse events, such as eye pain,[35] and slower corneal reepithelialization with specific agents.[36] Bacterial eradication and clinical recovery of 447 patients aged 1 through 17 years with culture-confirmed bacterial conjunctivitis were evaluated in a post hoc multicenter study investigating besifloxacin and moxifloxacin ophthalmic drops.[37] Although better clinical and microbiologic response was noted for besifloxacin compared with placebo, similar outcomes were noted when compared with moxifloxacin. Both agents were reported to be well tolerated.

External Otitis, Tympanostomy Tube–Associated Otorrhea

Recommendations for optimal care for patients with otitis externa are outlined in a review of 19 randomized controlled trials, including 2 from a primary care setting, yielding 3382 participants.[38] Topical antibiotic agents containing corticosteroids appeared to be more

effective than acetic acid solutions. Aminoglycoside-containing otic preparations were reported to cause ototoxicity if the tympanic membrane was not intact; fluoroquinolone-containing preparations represent a safer alternative to treat both otorrhea associated with tympanic membrane perforation and tympanostomy tube otorrhea. Eleven trials included aural toilet as a routine intervention, but the authors acknowledged that this treatment is not likely to be available in a typical primary care office setting.[38] The paucity of high-quality studies of antimicrobial agent–based topical therapy limited conclusions in this review. A small, prospective, randomized, open-label study in 50 patients with tympanostomy tube otorrhea or a tympanic membrane perforation showed comparable outcomes with either topical antibiotic therapy or topical plus systemic antibiotic agents.[39] For children with severe acute otitis externa, systemically administered antimicrobial agents should be considered in addition to topical therapy.[40]

Which topical antibiotic agent is best for external otitis is unclear.[41]

High-quality studies that evaluated quinolone versus nonquinolone topical solutions are limited. A systematic review of 13 meta-analyses confirmed that topical antibiotic agents were superior to placebo and noted a statistically significant advantage of quinolone agents over nonquinolone agents in the rate of microbiologic cure ($P = .035$). Safety profiles were similar between groups.[40] Similarly, Mösges et al[42] reviewed 12 relevant randomized controlled clinical studies involving 2682 patients and concluded that quinolone therapy achieved a higher cure rate ($P = .01$) and superior eradication rate ($P = .03$) than a non–fluoroquinolone-containing antibiotic-steroid combination. The clinical significance of these 2 reviews is reduced, however, when considering that bacterial persistence in the ear canal after treatment does not necessarily imply persistent acute otitis externa symptoms. A conclusion that quinolone and nonquinolone agents are similar in both microbiologic and clinical cure rates was reached in a study in more than 200 children, 90 of whom were evaluated for microbiologic response in a multicenter, randomized, parallel-group, evaluator-blinded study comparing once-daily ofloxacin drops with a 4-times-daily neomycin sulfate/polymyxin B sulfate/hydrocortisone otic suspension. Microbial eradication was documented in 95% and 94%, respectively; clinical cure was achieved in 96% and 97%, respectively.[43] Treatment with fluoroquinolone agents has been well tolerated.

Acute Otitis Media, Sinusitis, and Lower Respiratory Tract Infections

Newer fluoroquinolones show enhanced in vitro activity against S pneumoniae, compared with ciprofloxacin. The clinical need for such agents to treat respiratory tract infections has largely been driven by the emergence of multidrug-resistant strains of this pathogen, such as serotype 19A pneumococcus. Current otitis media and acute bacterial sinusitis guidelines from the AAP and Pediatric Infectious Diseases Society/Infectious Diseases Society of America guidelines on community-acquired pneumonia in children support the use of levofloxacin as an alternative therapy for those with severe penicillin allergy and for those infected with suspected multidrug-resistant pneumococcus (ie, patients in whom amoxicillin and amoxicillin-clavulanate have failed).[44-46] Pharmacokinetic data for children 6 months and older are well defined for levofloxacin, the only currently available fluoroquinolone studied for respiratory tract infections in children.[47]

Acute Bacterial Otitis Media

Clinical studies of levofloxacin and gatifloxacin have been conducted in children with recurrent or persistent otitis media but in those with not simple acute bacterial otitis media. Although studies of several fluoroquinolones have been reported, only levofloxacin is currently available in the United States. A prospective, open-label, noncomparative study of levofloxacin was performed in 205 children 6 months and older, 80% of whom were younger than 2 years. Tympanocentesis was performed at study entry and at least at 3 to 5 days into therapy for children who had treatment failure or persistent effusion. Bacterial eradication of middle-ear pathogens occurred in 88% of children, including 84% infected by pneumococci and 100% infected by Haemophilus influenzae. Levofloxacin treatment was well tolerated, with vomiting in 4% of patients documented as the most common adverse effect.[48] An evaluator-blinded, active-comparator, noninferiority multicenter study comparing levofloxacin with amoxicillin-clavulanate (1:1) involving 1305 evaluable children older than 6 months documented equivalent clinical cure rates of 75% in each treatment arm. Because tympanocentesis was not required, microbiologic cure rates could not be determined.[17]

Pneumonia

Although initially approved by the FDA for the treatment of pneumonia and acute exacerbation of chronic bronchitis in adults, ciprofloxacin therapy has not been uniformly successful in the treatment of pneumococcal pneumonia in adults at dosages initially studied 30 years ago. Failures are most likely the result of increasing pneumococcal resistance to ciprofloxacin and other fluoroquinolones documented since their first approval.[49] Ciprofloxacin is currently not considered appropriate therapy for community-acquired pneumonia in adults because of its resistance profile.

Fluoroquinolones with enhanced activity against S pneumoniae compared with ciprofloxacin (levofloxacin, moxifloxacin, gemifloxacin) have been used in adults for single-drug treatment of community-acquired pneumonia. These "respiratory tract" fluoroquinolones show in vitro activity against the most commonly isolated pathogens: S pneumoniae, H influenzae (nontypeable), and Moraxella catarrhalis as well as M pneumoniae, C pneumoniae, and Legionella pneumophila.[50-52] Although these agents are not the drugs of choice for pneumonia in previously healthy adults, they are recommended for adults with underlying comorbidities and for those who have been exposed to antibiotic agents within the previous 3 months and are, therefore, more likely to be infected with antibiotic-resistant pathogens.[53] Failures in the treatment of pneumococcal pneumonia have been reported with levofloxacin at 500 mg daily as a result of the emergence of resistance while receiving therapy or resistance from previous exposures to fluoroquinolones.[54] An increased dose of levofloxacin (750 mg daily, given for 5 days) is currently approved by the FDA for adults with pneumonia. The increase in drug exposure at the higher dose is recognized to overcome the most common mechanism for the development of fluoroquinolone resistance.[55]

Of the fluoroquinolones, only levofloxacin has been studied prospectively in children with community-acquired pneumonia, documenting efficacy in a multinational, open-label, noninferiority-design trial, compared with standard antimicrobial agents for pneumonia.[16] For children 6 months to 5 years of age, levofloxacin (oral or IV) was compared with amoxicillin-clavulanate (oral) or ceftriaxone (IV). For children 5 years and older, levofloxacin (oral) was compared with clarithromycin (oral) and levofloxacin (IV) was compared with ceftriaxone (IV) in combination with either erythromycin (IV) or clarithromycin (oral). Clinical cure rates were 94.3% in the levofloxacin-treated group and 94.0% in the comparator group, with similar rates of cure in both the younger and older age groups. Microbiologic etiologies were investigated, with *Mycoplasma* being the most frequently diagnosed pathogen, representing 32% of those receiving levofloxacin in both older and younger age groups and approximately 30% of those receiving comparator agents in both age groups. Pneumococci were infrequently documented to be the cause of pneumonia in study patients, representing only 3% to 4% of those who received levofloxacin and 3% to 5% of those receiving the comparator. Of note, the clinical response rate of 83% in children younger than 5 years, diagnosed by serologic testing with *Mycoplasma* infection and treated with amoxicillin-clavulanate, was similar to that in children treated with levofloxacin (89%), suggesting a high rate of spontaneous resolution of disease caused by *Mycoplasma* species in preschool-aged children, poor accuracy of diagnosis by serologic testing, or a clinical end-point evaluation after a treatment course that could not identify possible differences in response that may have been present in the first days of therapy.

Levofloxacin is now recognized as the preferred oral agent for children as young as 6 months of age with highly penicillin-resistant isolates (minimum inhibitory concentration of ≥ 4 μg/mL).[44] Although fluoroquinolones may represent effective therapy, they are not recommended for first-line therapy for community-acquired respiratory tract infections in children, because other better-studied and safer antimicrobial agents are available to treat the majority of the currently isolated pathogens.

Gastrointestinal Infections

Alghasham and Nahata[56] summarized the results of 12 efficacy trials by using a number of fluoroquinolone agents for infections caused by *Salmonella* and *Shigella* species, but only 2 of the 12 trials reported data on fluoroquinolones compared with nonquinolone agents. Patients were treated for typhoid fever (8 studies, including 7 for multidrug-resistant strains), invasive nontyphoid salmonellosis (1 study), and shigellosis (3 studies). Clinical and microbiologic success with fluoroquinolone therapy for these infections was similar when comparing children with adults. Recent data, however, show that fluoroquinolone resistance among isolates responsible for enteric fever in South Asia is very high (>90%), and the use of these drugs has been severely limited because of this.[57,58] Therefore, fluoroquinolones would not be an appropriate option in visitors returning from South Asia with enteric fever.

A prospective, randomized, double-blind comparative trial of acute, invasive diarrhea in febrile children in Israel was conducted by Leibovitz et al[59] comparing ciprofloxacin with intramuscular ceftriaxone in a double-dummy treatment protocol. A total of 201 children were treated and evaluated for clinical and microbiologic cure as well as for safety. Pathogens, most commonly *Shigella* and *Salmonella* species, were isolated in 121 children. Clinical and microbiologic cures were equivalent between groups.[59]

In the United States, although cases of typhoid fever and invasive salmonellosis are uncommon, there are approximately 500 000 cases of shigellosis, with 62 000 of the cases occurring in children younger than 5 years.[60] Treatment is recommended, primarily to prevent the spread of infection. Ampicillin and TMP-SMX resistance is increasing, and multidrug-resistant strains are becoming common; the National Antimicrobial Resistance Monitoring System reported that 38% of strains isolated from 1999 to 2003 were resistant to both ampicillin and TMP-SMX. A 2005 outbreak of multidrug-resistant *Shigella sonnei* infection involving 3 states was reported in the *Morbidity and Mortality Weekly Report*[61]; 89% of strains were resistant to both agents, but 100% of strains were susceptible to ciprofloxacin. Recently, however, fluoroquinolone resistance has been noted to be increasing at an alarming rate in Asia and Africa, and these resistant isolates are also starting to be seen in the United States as well.[62, 63] Treatment options for multidrug-resistant shigellosis, depending on the antimicrobial susceptibilities of the particular strain, include ciprofloxacin, azithromycin, and parenteral ceftriaxone. Nonfluoroquinolone options should be used if available.

Although ciprofloxacin has been regarded as an effective agent for traveler's diarrhea in the past, resistance rates are increasing for specific pathogens in many parts of the world. Resistance to *Campylobacter* species is particularly problematic in patients with a history of international travel. Recent data from *Campylobacter* isolates from international travel revealed fluoroquinolone resistance of approximately 61%.[64] Therefore, fluoroquinolones would not be an appropriate option in the treatment of traveler's diarrhea unless a pathogen is defined and antimicrobial susceptibilities are confirmed.

UTI

Standard empirical therapy for uncomplicated UTI in the pediatric population continues to be a cephalosporin antibiotic agent, because TMP-SMX– and amoxicillin-resistant *E coli* are increasingly common. The fluoroquinolones remain potential first-line agents only in the setting of pyelonephritis or complicated UTI when typically recommended agents are not appropriate on the basis of susceptibility data, allergy, or adverse event history. AAP policy continues to support the use of ciprofloxacin as oral therapy for UTI and pyelonephritis caused by *P aeruginosa* or other multidrug-resistant Gram-negative bacteria in children 1 through 17 years of age.[3] If ciprofloxacin is started as empirical therapy, but susceptibility data indicate a pathogen that is susceptible to other appropriate classes of antimicrobial agents, the child's therapy can be switched to a nonfluoroquinolone.

Mycobacterial Infections

The fluoroquinolones are active in vitro against mycobacteria, including *M tuberculosis* and many nontuberculous mycobacteria.[53,65] Increasing multidrug resistance in *M tuberculosis* has led to the increased use of fluoroquinolones as part of individualized, multiple-drug treatment regimens, with levofloxacin and moxifloxacin showing greater bactericidal activity than ciprofloxacin.[66] Treatment regimens that include 1 to 2 years of fluoroquinolones for multidrug-resistant and extensively drug-resistant tuberculosis have not been studied prospectively in children. Prevailing evidence supports the use of fluoroquinolones in the treatment of multidrug-resistant tuberculosis infections in children.[67,68] The extended administration of the fluoroquinolones in adults with multidrug-resistant tuberculosis has not shown serious adverse effects, and there is no evidence to date suggesting that this is different in children.[69] A recent study that focused on the use of levofloxacin for tuberculosis infection in an adult liver transplant patient population did show a risk of tenosynovitis in 18% of those treated, highlighting that the clinician needs to be aware that additional risk factors for poor

wound healing (patients older than 60 years, those taking corticosteroid drugs, and those with kidney, heart, or lung transplants [black box warning for all fluoroquinolones]) may increase the risk of musculoskeletal adverse effects.[70]

Other Uses

Ciprofloxacin and levofloxacin are among the acceptable antimicrobial agents for use in postexposure prophylaxis against *Bacillus anthracis* as well as for the treatment of many forms of anthrax (eg, cutaneous, inhalation, systemic) in children 1 month or older.[71] Ciprofloxacin is one of the antimicrobial options in postexposure prophylaxis and/or treatment of plague as well.[72,73]

Ciprofloxacin is effective in eradicating nasal carriage of *Neisseria meningitidis* (single dose, 500 mg for adults and 20 mg/kg for those older than 1 month) and preferred in nonpregnant adults. It can also be considered in younger patients as an alternative to 4 days of rifampin if ciprofloxacin-resistant isolates of *N meningitidis* have not been detected in the community.

Good penetration into the cerebrospinal fluid by certain fluoroquinolones (eg, levofloxacin) is reported, and concentrations often exceed 50% of the corresponding plasma drug concentration. In patients with tuberculosis, cerebrospinal fluid penetration, measured by the ratio of the plasma area under the concentration time curve from 0 to 24 to the cerebrospinal fluid area under the curve (0–24), was greater for levofloxacin (median: 0.74; range: 0.58–1.03) than for gatifloxacin (median: 0.48; range: 0.47–0.50) or ciprofloxacin (median: 0.26; range: 0.11–0.77).[74] In cases of multidrug-resistant, Gram-negative meningitis for which no other agents

are suitable, fluoroquinolones may represent the only treatment option.

P aeruginosa can cause skin infections (including folliculitis) after exposure to inadequately chlorinated swimming pools or hot tubs. The disease is self-limited and the majority of children will not require antimicrobial therapy, but if they do, oral fluoroquinolone agents offer a treatment option that may be preferred over parenteral nonfluoroquinolone antimicrobial therapy. In addition, fluoroquinolones may be considered as part of an antimicrobial regimen in cases of infections after penetrating skin/soft tissue injuries in the setting of water exposure when *P aeruginosa* or *Aeromonas hydrophila* may play a significant role.

A recent systematic review of empirical fluoroquinolone therapy for children with fever and neutropenia found excellent outcomes with short-term safety. It should be emphasized, however, that these data were from studies in patients with low-risk fever and neutropenia (leukemia/lymphoma), of whom only a small proportion would be expected to have a serious occult bacterial infection.[75] Ongoing investigations will help define the role for these antimicrobial agents in patients with fever and neutropenia.

SUMMARY

Fluoroquinolones are broad-spectrum agents that should be considered selectively for use in a child or adolescent for specific clinical situations, including the following: (1) infection caused by a multidrug-resistant pathogen for which there is no safe and effective alternative and (2) options for treatment include either parenteral nonfluoroquinolone therapy or oral fluoroquinolone therapy and oral therapy is preferred. In other clinical situations outlined previously, fluoroquinolones may also represent a preferred option (eg, topical fluoroquinolones in the treatment of tympanostomy tube–associated otorrhea) or an acceptable alternative to standard therapy because of concerns for antimicrobial resistance, toxicity, or characteristics of tissue penetration. If a fluoroquinolone is selected for therapy on the basis of the above considerations, practitioners should be aware that both ciprofloxacin and levofloxacin are costly.

Although adverse reactions are uncommon, because of the potential for risks of peripheral neuropathy, central nervous system effects, and cardiac, dermatologic, and hypersensitivity reactions in adults, in July 2016 the FDA added a safety announcement with updated box warnings restricting use of fluoroquinolone antibiotics in adults with acute sinusitis, acute bronchitis, and uncomplicated UTI to situations in which no other alternative treatment is available. No compelling published evidence to date supports the occurrence of sustained injury to developing bones or joints in children treated with available fluoroquinolone agents; however, FDA analysis of ciprofloxacin safety data suggests the possibility of increased musculoskeletal adverse events. Although studies were not blinded, with the potential for bias, children treated with levofloxacin both immediately after treatment and at a 12-month follow-up had an increased rate of musculoskeletal complaints but no physical evidence of joint findings. However, 5 years after treatment, no differences were seen between levofloxacin-treated and comparator-treated children. In the case of fluoroquinolones, as is appropriate with all antimicrobial agents, prescribing clinicians should verbally review common, anticipated, potential adverse events, such as rash, diarrhea, and potential musculoskeletal or neurologic events, and indicate why a fluoroquinolone is the most appropriate antibiotic agent for a child's infection.

ACKNOWLEDGMENTS

We thank Dr John S. Bradley, MD, FAAP, for his critical review and input into this manuscript.

LEAD AUTHORS

Mary Anne Jackson, MD, FAAP
Gordon E. Schutze, MD, FAAP

COMMITTEE ON INFECTIOUS DISEASES, 2016–2017

Carrie L. Byington, MD, FAAP, Chairperson
Yvonne A. Maldonado, MD, FAAP, Vice Chairperson
Elizabeth D. Barnett MD, FAAP
James D. Campbell, MD, FAAP
H. Dele Davies, MD, MS, MHCM, FAAP
Ruth Lynfield, MD, FAAP
Flor M. Munoz, MD, FAAP
Dawn Nolt, MD, FAAP
Ann-Christine Nyquist, MD, MSPH, FAAP
Sean O'Leary, MD, MPH, FAAP
Mobeen H. Rathore, MD, FAAP
Mark H. Sawyer, MD, FAAP
William J. Steinbach, MD, FAAP
Tina Q. Tan, MD, FAAP
Theoklis E. Zaoutis, MD, MSCE, FAAP

FORMER COMMITTEE MEMBERS

John S. Bradley, MD, FAAP
Kathryn M. Edwards, MD, FAAP
Gordon E. Schutze, MD, FAAP

EX OFFICIO

David W. Kimberlin, MD, FAAP – Red Book Editor
Michael T. Brady, MD, FAAP – Red Book Associate Editor
Mary Anne Jackson, MD, FAAP – Red Book Associate Editor
Sarah S. Long, MD, FAAP – Red Book Associate Editor
Henry H. Bernstein, DO, MHCM, FAAP – Red Book Online Associate Editor
H. Cody Meissner, MD, FAAP – Visual Red Book Associate Editor

LIAISONS

Douglas Campos-Outcalt, MD, MPA – American Academy of Family Physicians
Amanda C. Cohn, MD, FAAP – Centers for Disease Control and Prevention
Karen M. Farizo, MD – US Food and Drug Administration
Marc Fischer, MD, FAAP – Centers for Disease Control and Prevention
Bruce G. Gellin, MD, MPH – National Vaccine Program Office
Richard L. Gorman, MD, FAAP – National Institutes of Health
Natasha Halasa, MD, MPH, FAAP – Pediatric Infectious Diseases Society
Joan L. Robinson, MD – Canadian Paediatric Society
Jamie Deseda-Tous, MD – Sociedad Latinoamericana de Infectologia Pediatrica
Geoffrey R. Simon, MD, FAAP – Committee on Practice Ambulatory Medicine
Jeffrey R. Starke, MD, FAAP – American Thoracic Society

ABBREVIATIONS

AAP: American Academy of Pediatrics
FDA: Food and Drug Administration
IV: intravenous
TMP-SMX: trimethoprim-sulfamethoxazole
UTI: urinary tract infection

REFERENCES

1. Tatsumi H, Senda H, Yatera S, Takemoto Y, Yamayoshi M, Ohnishi K. Toxicological studies on pipemidic acid. V. Effect on diarthrodial joints of experimental animals. *J Toxicol Sci.* 1978;3(4):357–367

2. Gough A, Barsoum NJ, Mitchell L, McGuire EJ, de la Iglesia FA. Juvenile canine drug-induced arthropathy: clinicopathological studies on articular lesions caused by oxolinic and pipemidic acids. *Toxicol Appl Pharmacol.* 1979;51(1):177–187

3. Committee on Infectious Diseases. The use of systemic fluoroquinolones. *Pediatrics.* 2006;118(3):1287–1292

4. Bradley JS, Jackson MA; Committee on Infectious Diseases. The use of systemic and topical fluoroquinolones. *Pediatrics.* 2011;128(4). Available at: www.pediatrics.org/cgi/content/full/128/4/e1034

5. Patterson DR. Quinolone toxicity: methods of assessment. *Am J Med.* 1991;91(6A):35S–37S

6. Riecke K, Lozo E, ShakiBaei M, et al. Fluoroquinolone-induced lesions in the epiphyseal growth plates of immature rats. Presented at: *40th Interscience Conference on Antimicrobial Agents*

and Chemotherapy; Toronto, Canada; September 17–20, 2000

7. Sendzik J, Lode H, Stahlmann R. Quinolone-induced arthropathy: an update focusing on new mechanistic and clinical data. *Int J Antimicrob Agents.* 2009;33(3):194–200

8. US Food and Drug Administration, Division of Special Pathogen and Immunologic Drug Products. Summary of clinical review of studies submitted in a response to a pediatric written request: ciprofloxacin. Available at: www.fda.gov/downloads/drugs/ developmentapprovalprocess/ developmentresources/ucm447421.pdf. Accessed January 13, 2016

9. von Keutz E, Rühl-Fehlert C, Drommer W, Rosenbruch M. Effects of ciprofloxacin on joint cartilage in immature dogs immediately after dosing and after a 5-month treatment-free period. *Arch Toxicol.* 2004;78(7):418–424

10. US Food and Drug Administration, Division of Anti-Infective Drug Products. Review and evaluation of pharmacology and toxicology data: HFD-520. Available at: www.accessdata. fda.gov/drugsatfda_docs/nda/96/ 020634-3.pdf. Accessed June 30, 2010

11. Sansone JM, Wilsman NJ, Leiferman EM, Conway J, Hutson P, Noonan KJ. The effect of fluoroquinolone antibiotics on growing cartilage in the lamb model. *J Pediatr Orthop.* 2009;29(2):189–195

12. Adefurin A, Sammons H, Jacqz-Aigrain E, Choonara I. Ciprofloxacin safety in paediatrics: a systematic review. *Arch Dis Child.* 2011;96(9):874–880

13. Noel GJ, Bradley JS, Kauffman RE, et al. Comparative safety profile of levofloxacin in 2523 children with a focus on four specific musculoskeletal disorders. *Pediatr Infect Dis J.* 2007;26(10):879–891

14. Bradley JS, Kauffman RE, Balis DA, et al. Assessment of musculoskeletal toxicity 5 years after therapy with levofloxacin. *Pediatrics.* 2014;134(1). Available at: www.pediatrics.org/cgi/content/full/ 134/1/e146

15. Zabraniecki L, Negrier I, Vergne P, et al. Fluoroquinolone induced tendinopathy: report of 6 cases. *J Rheumatol.* 1996;23(3):516–520

16. Bradley JS, Arguedas A, Blumer JL, Sáez-Llorens X, Melkote R, Noel GJ. Comparative study of levofloxacin in the treatment of children with community-acquired pneumonia. *Pediatr Infect Dis J.* 2007;26(10):868–878

17. Noel GJ, Blumer JL, Pichichero ME, et al. A randomized comparative study of levofloxacin versus amoxicillin/ clavulanate for treatment of infants and young children with recurrent or persistent acute otitis media. *Pediatr Infect Dis J.* 2008;27(6):483–489

18. Hooper DC. Mechanisms of quinolone resistance. In: Hooper DC, Rubenstein E, eds. *Quinolone Antimicrobial Agents.* 3rd ed. Washington, DC: American Society for Microbiology Press; 2003:41–67

19. Vien TM, Minh NNQ, Thuong TC, et al. The co-selection of fluoroquinolone resistance genes in the gut flora of Vietnamese children. *PLoS One.* 2012;7(8):e42919

20. Davies TA, Leibovitz E, Noel GJ, McNeeley DF, Bush K, Dagan R. Characterization and dynamics of middle ear fluid and nasopharyngeal isolates of *Streptococcus pneumoniae* from 12 children treated with levofloxacin. *Antimicrob Agents Chemother.* 2008;52(1):378–381

21. Mesaros N, Nordmann P, Plésiat P, et al. *Pseudomonas aeruginosa*: resistance and therapeutic options at the turn of the new millennium. *Clin Microbiol Infect.* 2007;13(6):560–578

22. Talan DA, Krishnadasan A, Abrahamian FM, Stamm WE, Moran GJ; EMERGEncy ID NET Study Group. Prevalence and risk factor analysis of trimethoprim-sulfamethoxazole- and fluoroquinolone-resistant Escherichia coli infection among emergency department patients with pyelonephritis. *Clin Infect Dis.* 2008;47(9):1150–1158

23. Johnson L, Sabel A, Burman WJ, et al. Emergence of fluoroquinolone resistance in outpatient urinary *Escherichia coli* isolates. *Am J Med.* 2008;121(10):876–884

24. Boyd LB, Atmar RL, Randall GL, Hamill RJ, Steffen D, Zechiedrich L. Increased fluoroquinolone resistance with time in *Escherichia coli* from >17,000

patients at a large county hospital as a function of culture site, age, sex, and location. *BMC Infect Dis.* 2008;8:4

25. Qin X, Razia Y, Johnson JR, et al. Ciprofloxacin-resistant gram-negative bacilli in the fecal microflora of children. *Antimicrob Agents Chemother.* 2006;50(10):3325–3329

26. Adam HJ, Baxter MR, Davidson RJ, et al; Canadian Antimicrobial Resistance Alliance. Comparison of pathogens and their antimicrobial resistance patterns in paediatric, adult and elderly patients in Canadian hospitals. *J Antimicrob Chemother.* 2013;68(suppl 1):i31–i37

27. Raidt L, Idelevich EA, Dübbers A, et al. Increased prevalence and resistance of important pathogens recovered from respiratory specimens of cystic fibrosis patients during a decade. *Pediatr Infect Dis J.* 2015;34(7):700–705

28. Rose L, Coulter MM, Chan S, Hossain J, Di Pentima MC. The quest for the best metric of antibiotic use and its correlation with the emergence of fluoroquinolone resistance in children. *Pediatr Infect Dis J.* 2014;33(6):e158–e161

29. Tamma PD, Robinson GL, Gerber JS, et al. Pediatric antimicrobial susceptibility trends across the United States. *Infect Control Hosp Epidemiol.* 2013;34(12):1244–1251

30. Schutze GE, Willoughby RE; Committee on Infectious Diseases. *Clostridium difficile* infection in infants and children. *Pediatrics.* 2013;131(1):196–200

31. Deshpande A, Pasupuleti V, Thota P, et al. Community-associated Clostridium difficile infection and antibiotics: a meta-analysis. *J Antimicrob Chemother.* 2013;68(9):1951–1961

32. Slimings C, Riley TV. Antibiotics and hospital-acquired Clostridium difficile infection: update of systematic review and meta-analysis. *J Antimicrob Chemother.* 2014;69(4):881–891

33. Briasoulis A, Agarwal V, Pierce WJ. QT prolongation and torsade de pointes induced by fluoroquinolones: infrequent side effects from commonly used medications. *Cardiology.* 2011;120(2):103–110

34. Abo-Salem E, Fowler JC, Attari M, et al. Antibiotic-induced cardiac arrhythmias. *Cardiovasc Ther*. 2014;32(1):19–25

35. Torkildsen G, Proksch JW, Shapiro A, Lynch SK, Comstock TL. Concentrations of besifloxacin, gatifloxacin, and moxifloxacin in human conjunctiva after topical ocular administration. *Clin Ophthalmol*. 2010;4:331–341

36. Wagner RS, Abelson MB, Shapiro A, Torkildsen G. Evaluation of moxifloxacin, ciprofloxacin, gatifloxacin, ofloxacin, and levofloxacin concentrations in human conjunctival tissue. *Arch Ophthalmol*. 2005;123(9):1282–1283

37. Comstock TL, Paterno MR, Usner DW, Pichichero ME. Efficacy and safety of besifloxacin ophthalmic suspension 0.6% in children and adolescents with bacterial conjunctivitis: a post hoc, subgroup analysis of three randomized, double-masked, parallel-group, multicenter clinical trials. *Paediatr Drugs*. 2010;12(2):105–112

38. Kaushik V, Malik T, Saeed SR. Interventions for acute otitis externa. *Cochrane Database Syst Rev*. 2010;1:CD004740

39. Granath A, Rynnel-Dagöö B, Backheden M, Lindberg K. Tube associated otorrhea in children with recurrent acute otitis media: results of a prospective randomized study on bacteriology and topical treatment with or without systemic antibiotics. *Int J Pediatr Otorhinolaryngol*. 2008;72(8):1225–1233

40. Rosenfeld RM, Singer M, Wasserman JM, Stinnett SS. Systematic review of topical antimicrobial therapy for acute otitis externa. *Otolaryngol Head Neck Surg*. 2006;134(4 suppl):S24–S48

41. Rosenfeld RM, Schwartz SR, Cannon CR, et al. Clinical practice guideline: acute otitis externa. *Otolaryngol Head Neck Surg*. 2014;150(1 suppl):S1–S24

42. Mösges R, Nematian-Samani M, Hellmich M, Shah-Hosseini K. A meta-analysis of the efficacy of quinolone containing otics in comparison to antibiotic-steroid combination drugs in the local treatment of otitis externa. *Curr Med Res Opin*. 2011;27(10):2053–2060

43. Schwartz RH. Once-daily ofloxacin otic solution versus neomycin sulfate/polymyxin B sulfate/hydrocortisone otic suspension four times a day: a multicenter, randomized, evaluator-blinded trial to compare the efficacy, safety, and pain relief in pediatric patients with otitis externa. *Curr Med Res Opin*. 2006;22(9):1725–1736

44. Bradley JS, Byington CL, Shah SS, et al; Pediatric Infectious Diseases Society; Infectious Diseases Society of America. The management of community-acquired pneumonia in infants and children older than 3 months of age: clinical practice guidelines by the Pediatric Infectious Diseases Society and the Infectious Diseases Society of America. *Clin Infect Dis*. 2011;53(7):e25–e76

45. Lieberthal AS, Carroll AE, Chonmaitree T, et al. The diagnosis and management of acute otitis media [published correction appears in *Pediatrics*. 2014;133(2):346]. *Pediatrics*. 2013;131(3). Available at: www.pediatrics.org/cgi/content/full/131/3/e964

46. Wald ER, Applegate KE, Bordley C, et al; American Academy of Pediatrics. Clinical practice guideline for the diagnosis and management of acute bacterial sinusitis in children aged 1 to 18 years. *Pediatrics*. 2013;132(1). Available at: www.pediatrics.org/cgi/content/full/132/1/e262

47. Chien S, Wells TG, Blumer JL, et al. Levofloxacin pharmacokinetics in children. *J Clin Pharmacol*. 2005;45(2):153–160

48. Arguedas A, Dagan R, Pichichero M, et al. An open-label, double tympanocentesis study of levofloxacin therapy in children with, or at high risk for, recurrent or persistent acute otitis media. *Pediatr Infect Dis J*. 2006;25(12):1102–1109

49. Richter SS, Heilmann KP, Beekmann SE, Miller NJ, Rice CL, Doern GV. The molecular epidemiology of *Streptococcus pneumoniae* with quinolone resistance mutations. *Clin Infect Dis*. 2005;40(2):225–235

50. Factive (gemifloxacin mesylate) [package insert]. Oscient Pharmaceuticals. 2008. Available at: http://dailymed.nlm.nih.gov/dailymed/drugInfo.cfm?id=8345. Accessed July 6, 2015

51. Avelox (moxifloxacin hydrochloride) [package insert]. Schering Plough Corporation. 2015. Available at: http://dailymed.nlm.nih.gov/dailymed/drugInfo.cfm?setid=56b4f979-bf20-4908-9d7c-5536221d77f8. Accessed July 6, 2015

52. Levaquin (levofloxacin) [package insert]. Major Pharmaceuticals. 2013. Available at: http://dailymed.nlm.nih.gov/dailymed/drugInfo.cfm?setid=449ddc89-6dff-4e3e-a480-66b68389c73d. Accessed July 6, 2015

53. Mandell LA, Wunderink RG, Anzueto A, et al; Infectious Diseases Society of America; American Thoracic Society. Infectious Diseases Society of America/American Thoracic Society consensus guidelines on the management of community-acquired pneumonia in adults. *Clin Infect Dis*. 2007;44(suppl 2):S27–S72

54. Davidson R, Cavalcanti R, Brunton JL, et al. Resistance to levofloxacin and failure of treatment of pneumococcal pneumonia. *N Engl J Med*. 2002;346(10):747–750

55. Drusano GL, Louie A, Deziel M, Gumbo T. The crisis of resistance: identifying drug exposures to suppress amplification of resistant mutant subpopulations. *Clin Infect Dis*. 2006;42(4):525–532

56. Alghasham AA, Nahata MC. Clinical use of fluoroquinolones in children. *Ann Pharmacother*. 2000;34(3):347–359; quiz: 413–414

57. Qamar FN, Azmatullah A, Kazi AM, Khan E, Zaidi AK. A three-year review of antimicrobial resistance of *Salmonella enterica* serovars Typhi and Paratyphi A in Pakistan. *J Infect Dev Ctries*. 2014;8(8):981–986

58. Khanam F, Sayeed MA, Choudhury FK, et al. Typhoid fever in young children in Bangladesh: clinical findings, antibiotic susceptibility pattern and immune responses. *PLoS Negl Trop Dis*. 2015;9(4):e0003619

59. Leibovitz E, Janco J, Piglansky L, et al. Oral ciprofloxacin vs. intramuscular ceftriaxone as empiric treatment of acute invasive diarrhea in

children. *Pediatr Infect Dis J.* 2000;19(11):1060–1067

60. Scallan E, Mahon BE, Hoekstra RM, Griffin PM. Estimates of illnesses, hospitalizations and deaths caused by major bacterial enteric pathogens in young children in the United States. *Pediatr Infect Dis J.* 2013;32(3):217–221

61. Centers for Disease Control and Prevention. Outbreaks of multidrug-resistant *Shigella sonnei* gastroenteritis associated with day care centers—Kansas, Kentucky, and Missouri, 2005. *MMWR Morb Mortal Wkly Rep.* 2006;55(39):1068–1071

62. Gu B, Cao Y, Pan S, et al. Comparison of the prevalence and changing resistance to nalidixic acid and ciprofloxacin of Shigella between Europe-America and Asia-Africa from 1998 to 2009. *Int J Antimicrob Agents.* 2012;40(1):9–17

63. Bowen A, Hurd J, Hoover C, et al; Centers for Disease Control and Prevention. Importation and domestic transmission of *Shigella sonnei* resistant to ciprofloxacin—United States, May 2014-February 2015. *MMWR Morb Mortal Wkly Rep.* 2015;64(12):318–320

64. Ricotta EE, Palmer A, Wymore K, et al. Epidemiology and antimicrobial resistance of international

travel-associated *Campylobacter* infections in the United States, 2005-2011. *Am J Public Health.* 2014;104(7):e108–e114

65. American Thoracic Society; Centers for Disease Control and Prevention; Infectious Diseases Society of America. Treatment of tuberculosis. *MMWR Recomm Rep.* 2003;52(RR-11):1–77

66. Mitnick CD, Shin SS, Seung KJ, et al. Comprehensive treatment of extensively drug-resistant tuberculosis. *N Engl J Med.* 2008;359(6):563–574

67. Ettehad D, Schaaf HS, Seddon JA, Cooke GS, Ford N. Treatment outcomes for children with multidrug-resistant tuberculosis: a systematic review and meta-analysis. *Lancet Infect Dis.* 2012;12(6):449–456

68. Gegia M, Jenkins HE, Kalandadze I, Furin J. Outcomes of children treated for tuberculosis with second-line medications in Georgia, 2009-2011. *Int J Tuberc Lung Dis.* 2013;17(5):624–629

69. Thee S, Garcia-Prats AJ, Donald PR, Hesseling AC, Schaaf HS. Fluoroquinolones for the treatment of tuberculosis in children. *Tuberculosis (Edinb).* 2015;95(3):229–245

70. Torre-Cisneros J, San-Juan R, Rosso-Fernández CM, et al. Tuberculosis prophylaxis with levofloxacin in liver

transplant patients is associated with a high incidence of tenosynovitis: safety analysis of a multicenter randomized trial. *Clin Infect Dis.* 2015;60(11):1642–1649

71. Bradley JS, Peacock G, Krug SE, et al; Committee on Infectious Diseases and Disaster Preparedness Advisory Council. Pediatric anthrax clinical management. *Pediatrics.* 2014;133(5). Available at: www.pediatrics.org/cgi/content/full/133/5/e1411

72. Centers for Disease Control and Prevention. Plague. Available at: www.cdc.gov/plague/healthcare/clinicians.html. Accessed July 6, 2015

73. Inglesby TV, Dennis DT, Henderson DA, et al Plague as a biological weapon: medical and public health management. *JAMA.* 2000;283(17):2281–2290

74. Thwaites GE, Bhavnani SM, Chau TT, et al. Randomized pharmacokinetic and pharmacodynamic comparison of fluoroquinolones for tuberculous meningitis. *Antimicrob Agents Chemother.* 2011;55(7):3244–3253

75. Sung L, Manji A, Beyene J, et al. Fluoroquinolones in children with fever and neutropenia: a systematic review of prospective trials. *Pediatr Infect Dis J.* 2012;31(5):431–435

Virtual Violence

• •

• *Policy Statement*

POLICY STATEMENT   Organizational Principles to Guide and Define the Child Health
Care System and/or Improve the Health of all Children

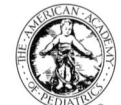

**American Academy
of Pediatrics**

DEDICATED TO THE HEALTH OF ALL CHILDREN™

Virtual Violence

COUNCIL ON COMMUNICATIONS AND MEDIA

abstract

In the United States, exposure to media violence is becoming an inescapable component of children's lives. With the rise in new technologies, such as tablets and new gaming platforms, children and adolescents increasingly are exposed to what is known as "virtual violence." This form of violence is not experienced physically; rather, it is experienced in realistic ways via new technology and ever more intense and realistic games. The American Academy of Pediatrics continues to be concerned about children's exposure to virtual violence and the effect it has on their overall health and well-being. This policy statement aims to summarize the current state of scientific knowledge regarding the effects of virtual violence on children's attitudes and behaviors and to make specific recommendations for pediatricians, parents, industry, and policy makers.

DOI: 10.1542/peds.2016-1298

PEDIATRICS (ISSN Numbers: Print, 0031-4005; Online, 1098-4275).

Copyright © 2016 by the American Academy of Pediatrics

FINANCIAL DISCLOSURE: The author has indicated he has no financial relationships relevant to this article to disclose.

FUNDING: No external funding.

POTENTIAL CONFLICT OF INTEREST: The author has indicated he has no potential conflicts of interest to disclose.

COMPANION PAPER: A companion to this article can be found online at www.pediatrics.org/cgi/doi/10.1542/peds.2016-1358.

To cite: AAP COMMITTEE ON COMMUNICATIONS AND MEDIA. Virtual Violence. *Pediatrics.* 2016;138(1):e20161298

Media violence is woven into the fabric of American children's lives. As recently as the year 2000, every G-rated movie contained violence, as did 60% of prime time television shows.[1] In 1998, the most comprehensive assessment of screen violence was completed. It estimated that the typical child will have seen 8000 murders and 100 000 other acts of violence (including rape and assault) before middle school.[2] The 1998 report was limited to television, which was appropriate at the time, because it was the primary platform exposing children to violence. Today's children experience screen violence on many different platforms, including computers, video games, and touch-screen devices, in addition to longstanding platforms, such as televisions. Increasingly, media researchers and pediatricians refer to children's "media diets" as a way of conveying the amount and type of media that is consumed. Like food diets, media diets can be healthy or unhealthy, balanced or imbalanced, or healthy in quality but unhealthy in quantity.

This policy statement uses the term "virtual violence" to discuss all forms of violence that are not experienced physically and, in particular, to encompass the extent to which children increasingly experience violence in more realistic ways than they have before. Virtual violence includes first-person shooter games and other realistic video games and applications. Furthermore, the terms "aggression" and "violence" are not used interchangeably. For the purposes of this policy statement, human *aggression* is defined as any behavior *intended* to harm another person who does not want to be harmed. The harm can be psychological or physical. *Violence* is defined as aggression that has as its goal extreme physical harm, such as injury or death. For example, a snarling dog is behaving aggressively; once it bites, it has resorted to violence. A person who verbally abuses another would not be committing an act of violence by this definition. Thus, all violent acts are aggressive, but not all aggressive acts are violent.[3] By analogy, passing a roaring monster as an avatar in a video game is experiencing virtual aggression and being shot to death in a first-person shooter game is experiencing virtual violence.

LEGISLATIVE ACTION

Although there is broad scientific consensus that virtual violence increases aggressive thoughts, feelings, and behaviors, there has been little public action to help mitigate children's exposure to it.[4] In fact, the single broadest legislative action taken by the state of California, which made it illegal to sell video games labeled for mature audiences to minors, was struck down by the US Supreme Court. It is important to note, however, that the ruling was not based on the absence of data linking media violence to aggression. Rather than rule on scientific merit, the Court invoked first-amendment protection for the games insofar as the Court construed their primary purpose to be to confer ideas and social messages.[5] Currently, there is no federal authority governing content and ratings, which are issued by the Entertainment Software Ratings Board, compliance with which is optional for industry.

EVIDENCE OF THE IMPACT OF VIRTUAL VIOLENCE

Since the first congressional hearings were held on the potential linkage between television violence and homicides in 1952, hundreds of studies exploring the effects of media violence have been conducted.[6] Notably, over the ensuing decades, media violence has evolved to become both more prevalent and more intense.[6]

Some brief mention of the types of studies performed is necessary to set the stage for the conclusions that can be, and have been, drawn. Studies have been observational and experimental as well as laboratory and field based. End points have included aggressive thoughts, angry feelings, and actual observed or reported aggression. Finally, studies have assessed short- and long-term exposure and proximate or distant aggressive actions. Accordingly, the scientific landscape is complex, because researchers have used different methods on different populations over time. Although individual research approaches may have shortcomings, when one considers the overall body of research the linkage between virtual violence and aggression has been well supported and is robust.

One research challenge has been to conclude that laboratory aggression can act as a proxy for what may happen in the real world. Consider a typical laboratory study in which subjects are randomly assigned to play a violent or nonviolent video game. They are then assessed for their willingness to administer pain in the form of unpleasant sounds (eg, mixture of fingernails scratching on blackboards, dentist drills, blow horns, and fire alarms), at a decibel of their choice within the limits of a nondamaging range, to a person who, unbeknownst to the participants, is part of the research team. Those who played a violent video game administered the sounds at a higher

level and for a longer period of time.[7] Although it is true that the situation of having a pain-inflicting auditory device at one's disposal does not occur in the real world, there is no reason to doubt the tendency or willingness to inflict pain would be less in the real world than in the laboratory, especially given study subjects' awareness that they were being observed while in the laboratory.

It is true that an experimental, real-world study that links virtual violence with real-world violence has not been conducted. Such a study will never be undertaken for several reasons, including the fact that actual violence is, fortunately, so rare that an exceedingly large sample size would be needed, and inducing and observing actual violence by manipulating subjects would never pass ethical scrutiny. But experimental linkages between virtual violence and real-world aggression have been found. For example, a recent experimental study conducted in the real world motivated parents to change their children's media diet by substituting prosocial programs in place of violent ones. This study found decreases in aggression and improvement in overall behavior.[8]

Understanding the risks of media violence can be complicated when research studies have found mixed results using varying methods. Fortunately, meta-analyses have been performed to combine the available research findings and to provide an overall estimate of the risks.[9-11] Summarizing the results of >400 studies including violent media of all types, researchers found there was a significant association between exposure to media violence and aggressive behavior (effect size: 0.19; 95% confidence interval [CI]: 0.19–0.20), aggressive thoughts (effect size: 0.18; 95% CI: 0.17–0.19), angry feelings (effect size: 0.27; 95% CI: 0.24–0.30), and physiologic arousal (effect size: 0.26; 95% CI: 0.20–0.31).[11] Another study performed a similar analysis focusing only on video games. The results, based on 140 such studies, found slightly larger negative effect sizes.[10] Some contend, rightly, that these correlations are in the small to moderate range, but they are stronger than the associations between passive smoking and lung cancer, and many municipalities have banned smoking because of that risk.[12]

PUTTING THE FINDINGS INTO PERSPECTIVE

A national discussion regarding the risks of media violence is necessary and critical for the health of our children and youth. Unfortunately, media reports frequently present "both sides" of the media violence and aggression issue by pairing a research scientist with an industry expert or spokesperson or even a contrarian academic, which creates a false equivalency and the misperception that research data and scientific consensus are lacking. A sizable majority of media researchers both in pediatrics and psychology believe that existing data show a significant link between virtual violence and aggression.[4] One might justifiably wonder why the contrarian position to media violence is so frequently presented when it is no longer presented for passive smoke exposure.

The full implications of virtual violence are best understood at a population level. Although the majority of Americans believe there is a causal relationship between screen violence and real-world aggression, most believe that they and their children are immune to these effects. The so-called third-person effect causes people to believe that other people, not themselves, but some small, susceptible fraction of people, are influenced in a way

the majority of the population is not. Stipulating that this belief is true, even if it is assumed that only 2% of the public is induced to behave more aggressively after being exposed to violent media, it can be expected that 400 000 of the 20 million viewers of the latest violent blockbuster film will exhibit increased aggression after viewing the movie, at least for a short period of time. Surely, even that figure is large enough to warrant some public attention and action.

RECOMMENDATIONS

1. Pediatricians should consider making children's "media diets" an essential part of all well-child examinations. In particular, emphasis must be placed on guiding the content of media and not only limiting quantity.[13] Impartial ratings, such as those issued by Common Sense Media, can be used to help guide selection.

2. Parents should be mindful of what shows their children watch and which games they play. When possible, they should coplay games with their children so as to have a better sense of what the games entail. Young children (under the age of 6 years) need to be protected from virtual violence. Parents should understand that young children do not always distinguish fantasy from reality. Cartoon violence can seem very real, and it can have detrimental effects. Furthermore, first-person shooter games, in which killing others is the central theme, are not appropriate for any children.

3. On state and local levels, policy makers should consider promoting legislation that provides caregivers and children better and more specific information about the content of media of all forms, especially with regard to violence, and should

enact laws that prohibit easy access to violent media for minors.

4. Pediatricians are encouraged to advocate for more child-positive media. Pediatricians should support and collaborate with the entertainment industry to create more shows and games for children of all ages that do not include violence, especially as a central theme. The American Academy of Pediatrics makes the following recommendations for the entertainment industry:

   o Avoid the glamorization of weapon carrying and the normalization of violence as an acceptable means of resolving conflict.

   o Eliminate the use of violence in a comic or sexual context or in any other situation in which violence is amusing, titillating, or trivialized.

   o Eliminate gratuitous portrayals of interpersonal violence and hateful, racist, misogynistic, or homophobic language or situations unless explicitly portraying how destructive such words and actions can be. Even so, violence does not belong in media developed for very young children.

   o If violence is used, it should be used thoughtfully as serious drama, always showing the pain and loss suffered by the victims and perpetrators.

   o Video games should not use human or other living targets or award points for killing, because this teaches children to associate pleasure and success with their ability to cause pain and suffering to others.

5. The news and information media should acknowledge the proven scientific connection between virtual violence and real-world aggression and the current consensus of credentialed experts

in this field and should avoid equating unscientific opinions and industry marketing tracts with peer-reviewed and vetted scientific research.

6. The federal government should oversee the development of a robust, valid, reliable, and "parent-centric" rating system rather than relying on industry to do so.

LEAD AUTHOR

Dimitri Christakis, MD, MPH – *Former Council on Communications and Media Executive Committee Member*

COUNCIL ON COMMUNICATIONS AND MEDIA EXECUTIVE COMMITTEE, 2014–2015

David Hill, MD, Chairperson
Nusheen Ameenuddin, MD, MPH
Yolanda (Linda) Reid Chassiakos, MD
Corinn Corss, MD
Daniel Fagbuyi, MD
Jeffrey Hutchinson, MD
Alanna Levine, MD
Claire McCarthy, MD
Robert Mendelson, MD
Megan Moreno, MD, MSEd, MPH
Wendy Sue Swanson, MD, MBE

LIAISONS

Kris Kaliebe, MD – *American Academy of Child and Adolescent Psychiatry*
Jennifer Pomeranz, JD, MPH – *American Public Health Association*
Brian Wilcox, PhD – *American Psychological Association*

STAFF

Thomas McPheron

ABBREVIATION

CI: confidence interval

REFERENCES

1. Yokota F, Thompson KM. Violence in G-rated animated films. *JAMA.* 2000;283(20):2716–2720

2. National Committee on Television Violence. *National Television Violence Study.* Vol 3. Thousand Oaks, CA: Sage Publications; 1998

3. Bushman BJ, Huesman LR. Aggression. In: Fiske ST, Gilbert DT, Linzey G, eds. *Handbook of Social Psychology.* New York, NY: John Wiley & Sons; 2010

4. Bushman BJ, Anderson CA. Understanding causality in the effects of media violence. *Am Behav Sci.* 2015;59(14):1807–1821

5. *Brown v Entertainment Merchants Association*, 131 SCt 2729 (2011)

6. H Res 278. *Investigation of radio and television programs. Hearings before a subcommittee of the Committee on Interstate and Foreign Commerce, US House of Representatives, 82nd Congress, 2nd Session.* Washington, DC: US Government Printing Office; 1952. Available at: http://babel.hathitrust.org/cgi/pt?id=uc1.b3970806;view=1up;seq=9. Accessed September 21, 2015

7. Bushman BJ, Jamieson PE, Weitz I, Romer D. Gun violence trends in movies. *Pediatrics.* 2013;132(6):1014–1018

8. Hasan Y, Begue L, Scharkow M, Bushman BJ. The more you play, the more aggressive you become: a long-term experimental study of cumulative violent video game effects on hostile expectations and aggressive behavior. *J Exp Soc Psychol.* 2013;49(2):224–227

9. Anderson CA, Bushman BJ. Effects of violent video games on aggressive behavior, aggressive cognition, aggressive affect, physiological arousal, and prosocial behavior: a meta-analytic review of the scientific literature. *Psychol Sci.* 2001;12(5):353–359

10. Anderson CA, Shibuya A, Ihori N, et al. Violent video game effects on aggression, empathy, and prosocial behavior in eastern and western countries: a meta-analytic review. *Psychol Bull.* 2010;136(2):151–173

11. Bushman BJ, Huesmann LR. Short-term and long-term effects of violent media on aggression in children and adults. *Arch Pediatr Adolesc Med.* 2006;160(4):348–352

12. Anderson CA, Bushman BJ. Media violence and the American public revisited. *Am Psychol.* 2002;57(6–7):448–450

13. Christakis DA, Garrison MM, Herrenkohl T, et al. Modifying media content for preschool children: a randomized controlled trial. *Pediatrics.* 2013;131(3):431–438

Youth Participation and Injury Risk in Martial Arts

- *Clinical Report*

CLINICAL REPORT   Guidance for the Clinician in Rendering Pediatric Care

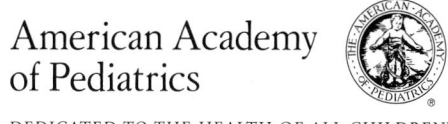

American Academy
of Pediatrics

DEDICATED TO THE HEALTH OF ALL CHILDREN™

Youth Participation and Injury Risk in Martial Arts

Rebecca A. Demorest, MD, FAAP, Chris Koutures, MD, FAAP, COUNCIL ON SPORTS MEDICINE AND FITNESS

abstract

The martial arts can provide children and adolescents with vigorous levels of physical exercise that can improve overall physical fitness. The various types of martial arts encompass noncontact basic forms and techniques that may have a lower relative risk of injury. Contact-based sparring with competitive training and bouts have a higher risk of injury. This clinical report describes important techniques and movement patterns in several types of martial arts and reviews frequently reported injuries encountered in each discipline, with focused discussions of higher risk activities. Some of these higher risk activities include blows to the head and choking or submission movements that may cause concussions or significant head injuries. The roles of rule changes, documented benefits of protective equipment, and changes in training recommendations in attempts to reduce injury are critically assessed. This information is intended to help pediatric health care providers counsel patients and families in encouraging safe participation in martial arts.

Clinical reports from the American Academy of Pediatrics benefit from expertise and resources of liaisons and internal (AAP) and external reviewers. However, clinical reports from the American Academy of Pediatrics may not reflect the views of the liaisons or the organizations or government agencies that they represent.

The guidance in this report does not indicate an exclusive course of treatment or serve as a standard of medical care. Variations, taking into account individual circumstances, may be appropriate.

All clinical reports from the American Academy of Pediatrics automatically expire 5 years after publication unless reaffirmed, revised, or retired at or before that time.

DOI: 10.1542/peds.2016-3022

PEDIATRICS (ISSN Numbers: Print, 0031-4005; Online, 1098-4275).

Copyright © 2016 by the American Academy of Pediatrics

FINANCIAL DISCLOSURE: Dr Koutures is a consultant to Neural Analytics for their clinical trials. Dr Koutures also receives royalties from SLACK Publications. Dr Demorest indicated she has no financial relationships relevant to this article to disclose.

FUNDING: No external funding.

POTENTIAL CONFLICT OF INTEREST: The authors have indicated they have no potential conflicts of interest to disclose.

INTRODUCTION

The term martial arts is derived from the "arts of Mars" (Roman god of war)[1] and presently encompasses formal combat traditions that can be practiced for self-defense, competition, physical fitness, motor development, and emotional growth. More than 6.5 million children participate in some form of martial arts in the United States.[2] Martial arts can be effective tools for building muscle strength and balance and enhancing flexibility in children and adolescents,[3,4] as well as positive interventions and activities in which to help build cognitive function, self-esteem, self-respect, and self-awareness.[5–7]

Various types of martial art disciplines can be categorized as striking (using blocks, kicks, punches, knees, and elbows to defend oneself while on one's feet[8]), grappling (taking an opponent to the ground to achieve a dominant position or use a submission hold to end a fight), weapon-based, or low-impact/meditative style with overriding philosophies that are oriented toward combat, health, or spirituality. Mixed martial arts

To cite: Demorest RA, Koutures C, AAP THE COUNCIL ON SPORTS MEDICINE AND FITNESS. Youth Participation and Injury Risk in Martial Arts. *Pediatrics.* 2016;138(6):e20163022

(MMA) involves the combination of different types of martial arts in a competitive venue.

The practice of a particular martial art or MMA involves both training and possibly competitive activities. All martial artists execute forms, which are individualized repetitive practice of movements, striking/blocking techniques, and potential use of weapons without any contact with objects or other performers. Not all martial arts practitioners progress to combat practice or competition.

For those martial arts disciplines that involve combat elements, a common training practice involves sparring. Sparring is defined as actual combat or fighting between 2 individuals that uses particular techniques of blocking, kicking, striking, and takedowns (throws from the standing position[8]), as taught by each style of martial arts and overseen by instructors. Sparring may begin at any age, as directed by the martial arts instructor, and often after learning basic movements/forms. Martial arts students are often categorized according to age and belt color, with advanced belt designations earned after proper execution of forms often combined with sparring.

Some martial arts styles require participants to use soft gear intended for head and body protection. Martial arts competitions are formal and ritualized time-measured events with referees often awarding points and supervising conduct of the performers.

EPIDEMIOLOGY OF PEDIATRIC AND ADOLESCENT MARTIAL ARTS INJURIES

Pediatric and adolescent martial arts injuries and injury risk are very difficult to quantify, stratify, and extrapolate because of:

- lack of pediatric and adolescent study populations;

- variations in injury definitions (eg, cessation of match, observed injury, reported injury, time loss injury);

- differences in study methods (competition injuries [more commonly studied] versus training injuries [less commonly studied]);

- accounting mostly for acute but not chronic injury;

- lack of consistency across studies in use of protective equipment; and

- lack of detailed, accurate, complete, or any reporting (recall bias, retrospective self-reporting, postmatch video recall).[9,10]

Most studies to date of martial arts comprise data largely from the adult population; however, when pediatric data were available, they were evaluated and are noted in this report.

In a cumulative epidemiologic study of pediatric martial arts, overall reported injury rates varied from 41 to 133 injuries per 1000 athletic exposures.[11] In a 2006 study, an estimated 128 400 children aged ≤17 years (mean age, 12.1 years; 73% male) were treated in US emergency departments for martial arts–related injuries from 1990 to 2003, with most injuries attributable to karate (79.5%).[2] Generally, martial arts injuries are not life-threatening (abrasions, contusion, sprains, and strains); however, fractures, neck injuries, dental injuries, and concussions do occur.[2,11] Overall fracture rates of 10% and higher of all documented martial arts injuries have been described in multiple articles.[2,11-13] Most reported pediatric martial arts injuries are acute.[11] Free sparring during tournaments seems to cause many overall injuries in martial arts.[14] The nature of the martial art (kicking, sparring, grappling, and takedowns) dictates the injury risk and rate. Very few catastrophic injuries are reported.[11]

Risk stratification in studies of martial arts does not show consistent results. Results are inconsistent as to whether age (younger versus older) and level (beginner versus professional/advanced) place an individual at increased or decreased risk for injury.[11,14-20] A 2005 study spanning 5 martial arts disciplines (Shotokan karate, Aikido, taekwondo, kung fu, and tai chi) found that people 18 years or older were 4 times more likely to sustain an injury compared with those younger than 18 years and that competitors with at least 3 years of experience were 2 times more likely to sustain injury compared with less experienced competitors.[14] Participants younger than 18 years doubled their risk of injury with every 2 additional hours of training per week after the first 3 hours, and those training for more than 3 hours per week had an overall increased injury risk.[14,15] One study of children and adults participating in martial arts found that those younger than 10 years had an overall lower injury rate per 1000 athletic exposures compared with all other age groups; however, when adjusting for exposure time, the 10- to 14-year-old age group had a higher injury risk per minute exposed compared with the open division.[18] To what degree skill and age may help or harm athletes continues to be researched.

Sex stratification in studies also yields inconsistent results.[2,10,11,14,15,17,21] Without significant participation of female subjects in many of these studies, more research is needed.

Injuries specific to different martial art forms are detailed in the following sections. Not all disciplines are covered, because not all disciplines have been studied in detail, especially with children and adolescents. Of note, despite kicks to the head and takedowns naturally increasing the risk of head injury, concussion rates are not well accounted for in most martial arts studies. Using mostly tournament medical reports (no postinjury data or follow-up) and retrospective information, current studies may not accurately capture concussion injury rates. Many studies do not count technical knockouts (TKOs) as concussive head injuries. More research with better epidemiologic data and methods is necessary in this field.

KARATE

Definition

Karate is a stand-up and striking martial art that started in Okinawa, Japan. The basic goal is self-defense by using punches, kicks, knees, elbows, and open hands to block an opponent's strikes and then to disable the opponent with quick strikes.[8] When takedowns are executed, they tend to be used to set up finishing strikes. Weapons are used in most styles of karate.

Injury Risk

Because much karate practiced in the United States is noncontact in nature, injury rates are lower and usually less severe than in other martial art forms. In a study of karate participants younger than 18 years, a reported injury risk over a 12-month time period of 5.6 per 100 athletes was identified.[15] One study reported a 30% rate of injury during 1 year of regular noncontact karate training. Karate focusing on technique just short of contact has been shown to have a lower injury risk compared with the contact kicks of taekwondo.[14]

The most common injuries sustained in karate include sprains/strains, contusions/abrasions, and fractures.[1,11,12,15] Karate injuries occur from being kicked (contusions), from falling (fractures), and from kicking (sprains).[2,15] Karate injuries commonly occur to the lower extremities from being kicked. Kicking injuries in less experienced individuals may occur

when landing on bony prominences as a result of punches and kicks that miss their target.[2] Free-style sparring (more common in younger athletes) accounts for fewer injuries than prearranged sparring.[15] The head and face sustain injury resulting from kicking and punching, including epistaxis.[11] Simultaneous executed punches are associated with karate injuries.

Other reported karate injuries to adolescents and adults include a blinding choroidal rupture,[22] a unilateral adrenal gland hematoma,[23] a femoral osteochondral fracture,[24] and a traumatic pseudoaneurysm of the femoral artery.[25]

TAEKWONDO

Definition

Taekwondo is a martial art and combat sport originating in Korea. The name taekwondo loosely translates into "the way of the hand and fist" and involves 80% kicks and 20% hand techniques.[8] Training involves a system of blocks, punches, and open-hand strikes and may include various takedowns or sweeps, throws, and joint locks, although it does not emphasize grappling. Sparring allows kicks to the head and requires use of soft head and body gear.

Injury Risk

Taekwondo uses contact aspects of punching and kicking, which is reflected in injury rates. Because of the various study methods, ages of study participants, and methods of reporting, as highlighted previously, reported injury rates for all ages range from 0.4 to 139.5 injures per 1000 athletic exposures, including light- and full-contact tournaments,[2,11,16] spotlighting some of the variability, validation issues, and potential unreliability of various martial arts research. In 1 study, 32% of taekwondo injuries (pediatric and adult) resulted in more than 1

week of time lost from training.[18] Another study showed a threefold increased risk of injury and a higher risk of multiple injuries in taekwondo compared with karate.[13] Of 5 martial arts disciplines (Shotokan karate, Aikido, taekwondo, kung fu, and tai chi), taekwondo had the highest number of injuries requiring time off from training (59%).[14]

Taekwondo has a high relative incidence of lower extremity injury compared with upper extremity injury because 80% of its competitive moves involve powerful, fast kicks.[13] Mechanisms for injury include being kicked, falling, and kicking.[2] Kicks to the head and face are legal and serve as point-scoring techniques in full-contact taekwondo.[10,18] Some protective equipment is used but not always hand or foot padding. Being kicked, specifically by roundhouse kicks, may cause the largest number of injuries.[2,11,18]

Common injuries sustained in taekwondo include sprains/strains, fractures, and contusions/abrasions.[2,11,18,26] Lower extremity injuries, especially of the foot, occur frequently.[2,11-13,18,27] Taekwondo participants had higher rates of bruising and soft tissue injury compared with karate athletes in 1 study.[13] Head injuries are commonly seen.[11,26] One adult study found that 82% of training injuries sustained in the preceding 12 months were mostly soft tissue injuries to the lower leg or foot; however, 1 in 20 injuries were to the head,[10] whereas another adult study supported the idea that more than 50% of adult injuries sustained in tournaments occurred to the head and neck area.[26] Although less frequent in overall number, upper extremity injuries in taekwondo may be more severe compared with lower extremity injuries.[27]

The incidence of concussion in adult taekwondo ranges from 4.6 to 50.2 per 1000 athletic exposures, potentially up to 4 times higher than that in American football.[27,28] One study of adult Olympic taekwondo kicks, measured by a simulated head target, reported that the most common kick impacts used in taekwondo had acceleration and recorded impacts equivalent to or greater than documented concussive injuries in American football.[28] Taekwondo rule changes have awarded more points for kicks aimed at the head, which may increase the risk of concussion.[27] Ineffective blocking skills may be related to risk of severe head injuries.

Other reported taekwondo injuries include bilateral radial head fractures.[29] Catastrophic taekwondo injuries have been reported, including deaths from kicks, cardiac issues, and unknown causes.[27]

JUDO

Definition

Judo originated in Japan with an emphasis on throwing or taking opponents down by using their energy against them.[8] Although striking is allowed in form work, it is not allowed in sparring. Judo starts with a standing phase and then moves after a throw or takedown to the ground phase, in which opponents are immobilized and submission holds may be used.

Injury Risk

Judo uses takedowns, throws, and flips, which use more of the upper extremities than other martial arts, such as karate and taekwondo. Strains/sprains, contusions, and fractures are the most common injury.[2,11,16] Upper extremity injuries to the shoulder, hand, wrist, and fingers are common.[2,11] Upper extremity injuries are more common in judo versus the lower extremity injuries seen more commonly in taekwondo and karate.[2] Hyperextension injury to joints may occur.[11] Youth judo athletes

sustained a higher proportion of shoulder/upper-arm injuries[2,13] and neck injuries compared with karate or taekwondo athletes.[2] Pediatric concussions were more prevalent in judo than karate.[2] Judo choking techniques can cause loss of consciousness.[30]

In judo, athletes are more likely to be injured while being thrown or flipped versus karate and taekwondo, in which most injuries are sustained by being kicked.[2,16] Improperly executed throws can injure both the attacker (if he or she drops the competitor onto himself or herself) or the defender (if he or she lands incorrectly).[2] Falling is a common pediatric mechanism for injury leading to fractures. Joint-locking techniques, in which joints are locked in full extension and thus are less able to absorb stress during falls (raising the risk of dislocations, subluxation, and fractures), can cause injury.[30] Other reported injuries sustained in judo include vertebral artery dissection,[31] embolic stroke,[32] and Paget-Schroetter syndrome (effort thrombosis of upper extremity).[33]

MUAY THAI KICKBOXING

Definition

Muay Thai kickboxing originated in Thailand and is a close combat style of martial arts that uses kicking, punching (with boxing gloves), sparring, and kick blocks.[2] Knee blows to the head or to the genital area are allowed in regular Muay Thai kickboxing, but modified competitive bouts prohibit any knee blows to the head.

Injury Risk

Muay Thai kickboxing, performed with different levels of protective equipment depending on the level, allows punches and kicks with knees and elbows specific for this discipline.[20] Limited studies exist of this discipline. Injury rates tend

to be higher in beginners compared with professionals (13.5 vs 2.79 injuries per 1000 participants).[19] However, another study reported higher injury rates in heavier weight classes (except super heavyweight).[20] Commonly reported adult injuries include soft tissue trauma, fractures (higher in more experienced athletes), and sprains and strains (higher in less experienced athletes).[19] Epistaxis (a nonprotected area) was the most frequent injury in 17- to 26-year-old competitors in 1 study.[20] Vertebral artery dissection was reported in 1 kickboxer.[34]

MIXED MARTIAL ARTS

Definition

MMA incorporates a variety of martial arts styles, from stand-up fighting, ground fighting, and throwing or takedowns, in which an opponent is forced from an upright or standing position into a grounded or more vulnerable position. Competitive bouts involve 3 to 5 rounds of fighting, each lasting 3 to 5 minutes. Contestants usually wear small gloves with exposed fingers and are barefoot. The goal of an MMA contestant is to defeat an opponent by:

- submission hold (joint lock or chokehold designed to make an opponent give up or risk injury/become unconscious);

- frank submission, in which an opponent gives up either by tapping out (tapping hand or other body part on ground to signal intent not to continue) or verbal indication (opponent unable to continue or declares stoppage of match);

- knockout or TKO (referee stops match, judging that an opponent is unable to logically or safely defend himself or herself[35,36]); or

- judge's decision at the end of the match.[36]

Injury Risk

With no reported pediatric injury studies in the literature regarding MMA, all documented injury information is from professional adult matches. Overall risk of injury has been reported as 85.1 to 228.7 per 1000 athletic exposures,[37–39] much higher than that reported in other contact sports, such as collegiate football (8.1 per 1000 athletic exposures).[40] In a 5-year review of sanctioned adult MMA fights, the injury risk over the reported 5 years was 23.6 per 100 fight participants.[38]

Lacerations, abrasions, and altered mental state are reported as the most common injuries,[21] but another study reported lacerations and upper-limb injuries (likely resulting from striking) as the most common injuries.[38] One study reported injuries, in decreasing frequency, as head injuries, lacerations, fractures, and concussion.[37]

Because of the nature of MMA, head and neck injury is a concern. Many athletes who experience TKOs receive subsequent injuries from striking the floor with their head.[36] Definitions of what constitutes a concussion vary, and studies often miss trackable injuries, making extrapolation difficult.[36]

A recent study found that head injuries accounted for 67% to 78% of total injuries in MMA.[37] In 1 study, the severe concussion rate was reported as 15.4 per 1000 athletic exposures (3% of all matches); however, only official ringside injuries documented by the ringside physician were reported, with no follow-up evaluations provided.[38] In this study, 33.7% of matches ended by TKO, despite the small number of concussions reported. Blunt force to the head resulted in the highest number of match stoppages,

suggesting a concussion rate of 48.3 per 1000 athletic exposures in 1 study.[36] Video analysis reported that the rate of match-ending head trauma was 15.9 per 100 athletic exposures (31.9% of matches).[41] All knockouts were attributable to direct head trauma, with 53.9% being strikes to the mandibular region. In the 30 seconds before match stoppage, losers sustained an average of 18.5 strikes, with 92.3% of them to the head. Cervical injury biomechanics from 4 common MMA takedown moves revealed biomechanics similar to being involved in a rear-end motor vehicle impact causing cervical spine injury.[42]

Age, weight, and fight experience did not statistically increase the injury risk in 1 study,[38] but the rate of injury was 2 times higher in amateurs than professional fighters in another study.[21] A losing fighter was 2.53 times more likely to be injured than a winning fighter.[38]

Omohyoid muscle syndrome (insidious lateral neck protrusion)[43] and vertebral artery dissection[44] have been reported in athletes participating in MMA.

OTHER MARTIAL ARTS FORMS

Kung Fu

Developed in China, kung fu is primarily a striking form of martial arts that uses low stances and powerful blocks[8] with both open and closed fists to defend against attackers. Some styles may allow throws and joint locks. Kung fu has both "hard" (meeting force with force) and "soft" (using an aggressor's strength against him or her) techniques. Kung fu is widely known for its beautiful and flowing forms.

Brazilian Jiu-Jitsu

Brazilian jiu-jitsu is a martial art based on a unique form of ground fighting in which participants are

taught to fight from the supine position. Jiu-jitsu fighters look to take their opponents to the ground and then attempt to place submission holds, often using arm bars, throws, joint locks, and takedowns.[8]

Pankration

Pankration has origins in the ancient Olympic Games, and modern versions emphasize grappling as well as limited-contact and full-contact competitions. Class C (or grappling) competition can be performed by all age groups with takedowns, ground control, and submissions allowed, but matches cannot be won by brutality or deliberate intent to cause injury. Class B (or limited-contact) competition also can be performed by all age groups and allows takedowns, ground control, submissions, and body strikes; strikes above the collarbone are not allowed. Participants wear soft gloves, helmets, and mouthguards. Head strikes are allowed in class A (full-contact) competition, which is limited to participants 18 years and older.[45]

INJURY-REDUCTION OR -PREVENTION TECHNIQUES

Headgear and Mouthguards

With many martial arts disciplines having participants deliberately target an opponent's face with strikes and kicks, protective equipment such as mouthguards, eye/face protection, and soft headgear has been used to reduce the risk of head or facial trauma. There is a paucity of studies documenting injury risk reduction in martial arts that use these protective devices.

The use of soft or other protective headgear is intended to prevent or reduce the incidence of head injuries, such as facial/scalp trauma and activity-related concussions. Although the use of padded headgear probably helps to prevent minor abrasions, lacerations, and contusions,[46] there is little evidence to support this contention. There is also a lack of data suggesting that the use of padded or other protective headgear can prevent or reduce the consequences of martial arts–related concussions. Sport-related concussions are often the result of acceleration/deceleration and rotational forces placed on the head and neck region.[47] Although unproven, there is also the potential that protective headgear in other sports may actually confer a higher risk of concussion because of a potentially perceived false sense of security for participants, parents, and instructors.

Mouthguards have been shown to reduce the incidence of dental trauma and other direct oral/facial injuries in other combat sports, such as boxing[48]; however, no solid evidence exists in the martial arts or in any other type of sport or activity that suggests a reduction in concussion incidence or severity with mouthguard use.

At the time of this writing, it cannot be recommended with any level of certainty that use of any type of protective headgear or mouthguard can reduce the risk of concussions during sparring or competitive martial arts participation. In addition, no protective device worn during MMA competitions can mitigate the potentially serious effects of chokeholds leading to near- or full suffocation, which could cause anoxic brain injury, cervical spine damage, or even vertebral artery injury, leading to cerebral vascular accidents. Additional research is needed to determine whether these theoretical concerns are encountered in young MMA participants and, if so, at what rates and levels of severity.

Many martial arts equipment companies manufacture clear plastic face guards or padded metal grilles that integrate into standard sparring headgear and do provide a significant level of eye and face protection.[46] Currently, few martial arts participants wear this type of protection, and some may regard the equipment as a nuisance or impairment to their vision or breathing. There are no published studies evaluating the use of eye protection in the martial arts.

Body Padding

Several of the combat-oriented martial arts disciplines use soft padding for arms, chest, abdominal, groin, and leg regions.[46] The padding worn by taekwondo athletes may offer some protection, but this protection may be of greatest benefit to the athlete executing the kick rather than to the recipient of the technique.[14] Although, in theory, these devices may reduce skin trauma and muscle contusions, there are no data on their efficacy in the practice of martial arts.

Rule Changes

Although some studies have identified predisposing factors for injury that include male sex, exposure to sparring and competition, and less experience, rule changes that limit sparring in the latter group may have the greatest effect on injury reduction.[49] However, other studies have found lower injury risks among less experienced youths, possibly because of less technical ability, lower body mass and strength, and an inability to generate the same level of force than older, more experienced martial artists.[14] Therefore, the exact role of rule changes limiting sparring remains uncertain.

Appropriate rule creation and enforcement have been shown to reduce injury risk. In 2000, the World Karate Federation adopted new rules regarding prohibited behavior, including excessive force used in dealing blows to permitted areas, to forbidden areas (throat, arms, legs, groin, joints, and instep), and to the face with open-hand techniques as well as dangerous or prohibited throwing techniques. Implementation of the new rules significantly lowered the relative risk of injury for competitors younger than 18 years (male and female), as well as a significant overall decrease in head injuries; however, an increase in leg injuries was also established.[17]

Training Changes

One study involving video analysis of head blows leading to concussion in competitive taekwondo participants found that close proximity between athletes and reception of a single roundhouse kick were common mechanisms of injury.[50] Another study found that young age and lack of blocking skills were risk factors for concussion in taekwondo.[51] Development of blocking skills, safety education, and rigorous enforcement of the competition rules were among the suggestions made to reduce risk of concussions in competitive taekwondo.[50,51]

Monitoring the number of martial arts training hours per week may play a role in reducing injuries. One study did not find multiple injuries or injuries requiring time away from activity in martial arts athletes younger than 18 years who trained less than 3 hours per week. Injury risk doubled with each additional 2 hours of training after the first 3 hours, although no major injuries were reported.[14]

Concussion Recognition and Safety

Although protective safety equipment may not protect against or prevent concussions, proper recognition, evaluation, management, and return to play of athletes with suspected and documented concussion injuries is important. All head injuries should be evaluated, clearly documented, and managed by a pediatrician or health care provider trained in the evaluation and management of pediatric concussions. Athletes recovering from a concussion should follow normal return-to-learn and return-to-play guidelines previously established and considered standard for concussion management.[47,52]

MEDIA INFLUENCE, PERCEPTION, AND RELATION TO YOUTH PARTICIPATION IN MMA

Professional MMA has become a sports culture sensationalized by the media. Primetime, televised showcases promote MMA as spectator events, not unlike some other American sports, with financial incentives for both participants and sponsors. MMA draws attention as entertainment venues for many. Dreams of "making it big," large paychecks, and future wealth appeal to many parents and children. In emulating what they see in the adult MMA culture, children are at risk for imitating professional MMA moves and techniques seen in mass media (eg, choking out, repetitive head blows to floor), even though these moves may not be sanctioned for their ages. Evidence also shows that exposure to media violence can increase aggressive behavior and desensitization to violence.[53] Children may try to perform risky moves learned from mass media exposure in practice or in settings with minimal or no adult supervision. As advocates of young athletes, pediatricians and pediatric health care providers can educate parents, families, coaches, teachers, and community leaders with facts on the increased susceptibility to injury if children are imitating what they see from excessive media exposure of MMA contests.

PRACTICAL CONCLUSIONS ON MARTIAL ARTS PARTICIPATION FOR THE PEDIATRIC PROVIDER

1. As a sport or activity, martial arts can provide children and adolescents with vigorous levels of physical exercise that can lead to better overall physical fitness.

2. Children and adolescents should only participate in martial arts classes or competitions supervised by instructors with appropriate training regarding proper teaching of the particular activity and understanding of a child's limitations based on age, maturity, stature, and experience. Martial arts competition and contact-based training should be delayed until children and adolescents have demonstrated adequate physical and emotional maturity during noncontact preparation and have demonstrated competency with noncontact forms, movements, and techniques.

3. In discussing selection of various disciplines and subtypes of the martial arts, the pediatric health care provider can help to discriminate between noncontact forms, which have a relatively low risk of injury, and sparring or contact forms, which confer a higher risk of injury.

4. For those martial arts disciplines that involve sparring, rigorous enforcement of rules prohibiting excessive force, dangerous movements, or blows to forbidden areas should be encouraged, with safety education promoted for all instructors, officials, and participants. Instructors and officials are encouraged to have an appropriate understanding of the rules and safety qualifications.

5. Although many martial arts disciplines require the use of soft protective headgear, there is no evidence that such devices reduce the risk of concussion. It is encouraged that participants and families also be counseled against engaging in more aggressive activities under the misconception that wearing headgear ensures increased protection against concussion.

6. Pediatric health care providers should encourage the teaching of improved defensive blocking techniques to reduce the risk of dangerous blows to the head.

7. Pediatric health care providers should support the institution of rule changes that eliminate blows to the head and conversely any points awarded for kicks or blows to the head to reduce the risk of concussions in martial arts.

8. Anticipatory guidance regarding injury risks of particular martial arts disciplines, along with proven and unproven benefits of protective equipment, are encouraged as part of a preparticipation evaluation by the pediatric health care provider.

9. Although some evidence exists that training >3 hours per week may increase injury risk, the relation of hours of training per week to particular martial arts injury risk requires more study.

10. The nature of MMA combat fighting, which includes rapid thrusts of the head to the floor and chokeholds to place an opponent into submission, confers a high risk of concussion, asphyxia, or other head and neck injury. As a result, child or adolescent participation in MMA bouts that involve these techniques should be strongly discouraged. As advocates of young athletes, pediatric health care providers can educate parents, families, coaches, teachers, and community leaders with facts on the increased susceptibility to injury if children are imitating what they see from excessive media exposure of MMA contests.

LEAD AUTHORS

Rebecca A. Demorest, MD, FAAP
Chris Koutures, MD, FAAP

ABBREVIATIONS

MMA: mixed martial arts
TKO: technical knockout

REFERENCES

1. Clements J. A short introduction to historical European martial arts. *Meibukan Magazine.* January 2006;Spec Ed 1:2–4

2. Yard EE, Knox CL, Smith GA, Comstock RD. Pediatric martial arts injuries presenting to emergency departments, United States 1990-2003. *J Sci Med Sport.* 2007;10(4):219–226

3. Padulo J, Chamari K, Chaabène H, et al. The effects of one-week training camp on motor skills in karate kids. *J Sports Med Phys Fitness.* 2014;54(6):715–724

4. Vando S, Filingeri D, Maurino L, et al. Postural adaptations in preadolescent karate athletes due to a one week karate training camp. *J Hum Kinet.* 2013;38:45–52

5. Alesi M, Bianco A, Padulo J, et al. Motor and cognitive development: the role of karate. *Muscles Ligaments Tendons J.* 2014;4(2):114–120

6. Wall RB. Tai chi and mindfulness-based stress reduction in a Boston public middle school. *J Pediatr Health Care.* 2005;19(4):230–237

7. Conant KD, Morgan AK, Muzykewicz D, Clark DC, Thiele EA. A karate program for improving self-concept and quality of life in childhood epilepsy: results of a pilot study. *Epilepsy Behav.* 2008;12(1):61–65

8. About Sports. Styles of martial arts. Available at: http://martialarts.about.com/od/styles/a/styles.htm. Accessed February 27, 2016

9. Birrer RB, Birrer CD. Unreported injuries in the martial arts. *Br J Sports Med.* 1983;17(2):131–133

10. Feehan M, Waller AE. Precompetition injury and subsequent tournament performance in full-contact taekwondo. *Br J Sports Med.* 1995;29(4):258–262

11. Pieter W. Martial arts injuries. *Med Sport Sci.* 2005;48:59–73

12. Birrer RB, Halbrook SP. Martial arts injuries. The results of a five year national survey. *Am J Sports Med.* 1988;16(4):408–410

13. Critchley GR, Mannion S, Meredith C. Injury rates in Shotokan karate. *Br J Sports Med.* 1999;33(3):174–177

14. Zetaruk MN, Violán MA, Zurakowski D, Micheli LJ. Injuries in martial arts: a comparison of five styles. *Br J Sports Med.* 2005;39(1):29–33

15. Zetaruk MN, Zurakowski D, Violan MA, Micheli LJ. Safety recommendations in Shotokan karate. *Clin J Sport Med.* 2000;10(2):117–122

16. Pocecco E, Ruedl G, Stankovic N, et al. Injuries in judo: a systematic literature review including suggestions for prevention. *Br J Sports Med.* 2013;47(18):1139–1143

17. Macan J, Bundalo-Vrbanac D, Romić G. Effects of the new karate rules on the incidence and distribution of injuries. *Br J Sports Med.* 2006;40(4):326–330, discussion 330

18. Lystad RP, Graham PL, Poulos RG. Exposure-adjusted incidence rates and severity of competition injuries in Australian amateur taekwondo athletes: a 2-year prospective study. *Br J Sports Med.* 2013;47(7):441–446

19. Gartland S, Malik MH, Lovell ME. Injury and injury rates in Muay Thai kick boxing. *Br J Sports Med.* 2001;35(5):308–313

20. Gartland S, Malik MH, Lovell M. A prospective study of injuries sustained during competitive Muay Thai kickboxing. *Clin J Sport Med.* 2005;15(1):34–36

21. McClain R, Wassermen J, Mayfield C, Berry AC, Grenier G, Suminski RR. Injury profile of mixed martial arts competitors. *Clin J Sport Med.* 2014;24(6):497–501

22. Mars JS, Pimenides D. Blinding choroidal rupture in a karateka. *Br J Sports Med.* 1995;29(4):273–274

23. Ortu M, Vaccarezza M, Trovati S, Galli M, Gervasoni C, Vella A. A martial arts injury: karate induced unilateral haematoma of the adrenal gland. *Br J Sports Med.* 2006;40(8):730–731, discussion 731

24. Mbubaegbu CE, Percy AJ. Femoral osteochondral fracture—a non-contact injury in martial arts? A case report. *Br J Sports Med.* 1994;28(3):203–205

25. Doiz E, Garrido F, Conejero R, García P, Fernández E. Acute pseudoaneurysm of the femoral artery after repeated trauma in full-contact karate practice. *Br J Sports Med.* 2008;42(12):1004–1005

26. Burke DT, Barfoot K, Bryant S, Schneider JC, Kim HJ, Levin G. Effect of implementation of safety measures in tae kwon do competition. *Br J Sports Med.* 2003;37(5):401–404

27. Pieter W, Fife GP, O'Sullivan DM. Competition injuries in taekwondo: a literature review and suggestions for prevention and surveillance. *Br J Sports Med.* 2012;46(7):485–491

28. Fife GP, O'Sullivan DM, Pieter W, Cook DP, Kaminski TW. Effects of Olympic-style taekwondo kicks on an instrumented head-form and resultant injury measures. *Br J Sports Med.* 2013;47(18):1161–1165

29. Deshmukh NV, Shah MS. Bilateral radial head fractures in a martial arts athlete. *Br J Sports Med.* 2003;37(3):270–271, discussion 271

30. STOP Sports Injuries. Preventing martial arts injuries. Available at: http://imis.sportsmed.org/AOSSMIMIS/STOP/STOP/Prevent_Injuries/Martial_Arts_Injury_Prevention.aspx. Accessed February 27, 2016

31. Lannuzel A, Moulin T, Amsallem D, Galmiche J, Rumbach L. Vertebral-artery dissection following a judo session: a case report. *Neuropediatrics.* 1994;25(2):106–108

32. McCarron MO, Patterson J, Duncan R. Stroke without dissection from a neck holding manoeuvre in martial arts. *Br J Sports Med.* 1997;31(4):346–347

33. Zigun JR, Schneider SM. "Effort" thrombosis (Paget-Schroetter's syndrome) secondary to martial arts training. *Am J Sports Med.* 1988;16(2):189–190

34. Malek AM, Halbach VV, Phatouros CC, Meyers PM, Dowd CF, Higashida RT. Endovascular treatment of a ruptured intracranial dissecting vertebral aneurysm in a kickboxer. *J Trauma.* 2000;48(1):143–145

35. Wong V. Sports lingo, activities, positions and general sports terms. In: Koutures C, Wong V, eds. *Pediatric Sports Medicine: Essentials for Office Evaluation.* Thorofare, NJ: Slack Publications; 2013:9–10

36. Reider B. Battle scars [editorial]. *Am J Sports Med.* 2014;42(6):1287–1289

37. Lystad RP, Gregory K, Wilson J. The epidemiology of injuries in mixed martial arts: a systematic review and meta-analysis. *Orthop J Sports Med.* 2014;2(1):2325967113518492

38. Ngai KM, Levy F, Hsu EB. Injury trends in sanctioned mixed martial arts competition: a 5-year review from 2002 to 2007. *Br J Sports Med.* 2008;42(8):686–689

39. Buse GJ. No holds barred sport fighting: a 10 year review of mixed martial arts competition. *Br J Sports Med.* 2006;40(2):169–172

40. National Collegiate Athletic Association. Football injuries. Available at: https://www.ncaa.org/sites/default/files/NCAA_Football_Injury_WEB.pdf. Accessed February 27, 2016

41. Hutchison MG, Lawrence DW, Cusimano MD, Schweizer TA. Head trauma in mixed martial arts. *Am J Sports Med.* 2014;42(6):1352–1358

42. Kochhar T, Back DL, Mann B, Skinner J. Risk of cervical injuries in mixed martial arts. *Br J Sports Med.* 2005;39(7):444–447

43. Lee AD, Yu A, Young SB, Battaglia PJ, Ho CJ. Omohyoid muscle syndrome in a mixed martial arts athlete: a case report. *Sports Health.* 2015;7(5):458–462

44. Slowey M, Maw G, Furyk J. Case report on vertebral artery dissection in mixed martial arts. *Emerg Med Australas.* 2012;24(2):203–206

45. United States Fight League. Pankration, grappling and mixed martial arts rules. Available at: http://fightleague.org/Rules.html. Accessed February 25, 2016

46. Woodward TW. A review of the effects of martial arts practice on health. *WMJ.* 2009;108(1):40–43

47. Halstead ME, Walter KD; Council on Sports Medicine and Fitness. American Academy of Pediatrics. Clinical report—sport-related concussion in children and adolescents. *Pediatrics.* 2010;126(3):597–615

48. Knapik JJ, Marshall SW, Lee RB, et al. Mouthguards in sport activities: history, physical properties and injury prevention effectiveness. *Sports Med.* 2007;37(2):117–144

49. Birrer RB. Trauma epidemiology in the martial arts. The results of an eighteen-year international survey. *Am J Sports Med.* 1996;24(suppl 6):S72–S79

50. Koh JO, Watkinson EJ, Yoon YJ. Video analysis of head blows leading to concussion in competition taekwondo. *Brain Inj.* 2004;18(12):1287–1296

51. Koh JO, Cassidy JD. Incidence study of head blows and concussions in competition taekwondo. *Clin J Sport Med.* 2004;14(2):72–79

52. Halstead ME, McAvoy K, Devore CD, Carl R, Lee M, Logan K; Council on Sports Medicine and Fitness; Council on School Health. Returning to learning following a concussion. *Pediatrics.* 2013;132(5):948–957

53. Council on Communications and Media. Virtual violence. *Pediatrics.* 2016;138(2). Available at: www.pediatrics.org/cgi/content/full/138/2/e20161298

Section 5

Current Policies

From the American Academy of Pediatrics
• •
(Through December 31, 2016)

- *Policy Statements*
  ORGANIZATIONAL PRINCIPLES TO GUIDE AND DEFINE THE CHILD HEALTH CARE SYSTEM
  AND TO IMPROVE THE HEALTH OF ALL CHILDREN

- *Clinical Reports*
  GUIDANCE FOR THE CLINICIAN IN RENDERING PEDIATRIC CARE

- *Technical Reports*
  BACKGROUND INFORMATION TO SUPPORT AMERICAN ACADEMY OF PEDIATRICS POLICY

AMERICAN ACADEMY OF PEDIATRICS

Policy Statements, Clinical Reports, Technical Reports

Current through January 1, 2017
The companion *Pediatric Clinical Practice Guidelines & Policies* eBook
points to the full text of all titles listed below.

2016 RECOMMENDATIONS FOR PREVENTIVE PEDIATRIC HEALTH CARE

Committee on Practice and Ambulatory Medicine and Bright Futures Periodicity Schedule Workgroup (12/15)
http://pediatrics.aappublications.org/content/137/1/e20153908

AAP PRINCIPLES CONCERNING RETAIL-BASED CLINICS

Committee on Practice and Ambulatory Medicine
ABSTRACT. The American Academy of Pediatrics views retail-based clinics (RBCs) as an inappropriate source of primary care for pediatric patients, as they fragment medical care and are detrimental to the medical home concept of longitudinal and coordinated care. This statement updates the original 2006 American Academy of Pediatrics statement on RBCs, which flatly opposed these sites as appropriate for pediatric care, discussing the shift in RBC focus and comparing attributes of RBCs with those of the pediatric medical home. (2/14)
http://pediatrics.aappublications.org/content/133/3/e794

ABUSIVE HEAD TRAUMA IN INFANTS AND CHILDREN

Cindy W. Christian, MD; Robert Block, MD; and Committee on Child Abuse and Neglect
ABSTRACT. Shaken baby syndrome is a term often used by physicians and the public to describe abusive head trauma inflicted on infants and young children. Although the term is well known and has been used for a number of decades, advances in the understanding of the mechanisms and clinical spectrum of injury associated with abusive head trauma compel us to modify our terminology to keep pace with our understanding of pathologic mechanisms. Although shaking an infant has the potential to cause neurologic injury, blunt impact or a combination of shaking and blunt impact cause injury as well. Spinal cord injury and secondary hypoxic ischemic injury can contribute to poor outcomes of victims. The use of broad medical terminology that is inclusive of all mechanisms of injury, including shaking, is required. The American Academy of Pediatrics recommends that pediatricians develop skills in the recognition of signs and symptoms of abusive head injury, including those caused by both shaking and blunt impact, consult with pediatric subspecialists when necessary, and embrace a less mechanistic term, abusive head trauma, when describing an inflicted injury to the head and its contents. (4/09, reaffirmed 3/13)
http://pediatrics.aappublications.org/content/123/5/1409

ACCESS TO OPTIMAL EMERGENCY CARE FOR CHILDREN

Committee on Pediatric Emergency Medicine
ABSTRACT. Millions of pediatric patients require some level of emergency care annually, and significant barriers limit access to appropriate services for large numbers of children. The American Academy of Pediatrics has a strong commitment to identifying barriers to access to emergency care, working to surmount these obstacles, and encouraging, through education and system changes, improved levels of emergency care available to all children. (1/07, reaffirmed 8/10, 7/14)
http://pediatrics.aappublications.org/content/119/1/161

ACCF/AHA/AAP RECOMMENDATIONS FOR TRAINING IN PEDIATRIC CARDIOLOGY

American Academy of Pediatrics Section on Cardiology and Cardiac Surgery (joint with American College of Cardiology Foundation and American Heart Association) (12/05, reaffirmed 1/09)
http://pediatrics.aappublications.org/content/116/6/1574

ACHIEVING QUALITY HEALTH SERVICES FOR ADOLESCENTS

Committee on Adolescence
ABSTRACT. This update of the 2008 statement from the American Academy of Pediatrics redirects the discussion of quality health care from the theoretical to the practical within the medical home. This statement reviews the evolution of the medical home concept and challenges the provision of quality adolescent health care within the patient-centered medical home. Areas of attention for quality adolescent health care are reviewed, including developmentally appropriate care, confidentiality, location of adolescent care, providers who offer such care, the role of research in advancing care, and the transition to adult care. (7/16)
See full text on page 521.
http://pediatrics.aappublications.org/content/138/2/e20161347

ADDRESSING EARLY CHILDHOOD EMOTIONAL AND BEHAVIORAL PROBLEMS

Council on Early Childhood, Committee on Psychosocial Aspects of Child and Family Health, and Section on Developmental and Behavioral Pediatrics
ABSTRACT. Emotional, behavioral, and relationship problems can develop in very young children, especially those living in high-risk families or communities. These early problems interfere with the normative activities of young children and their families and predict long-lasting problems across multiple domains. A growing evidence

base demonstrates the efficacy of specific family-focused therapies in reducing the symptoms of emotional, behavioral, and relationship symptoms, with effects lasting years after the therapy has ended. Pediatricians are usually the primary health care providers for children with emotional or behavioral difficulties, and awareness of emerging research about evidence-based treatments will enhance this care. In most communities, access to these interventions is insufficient. Pediatricians can improve the care of young children with emotional, behavioral, and relationship problems by calling for the following: increased access to care; increased research identifying alternative approaches, including primary care delivery of treatments; adequate payment for pediatric providers who serve these young children; and improved education for pediatric providers about the principles of evidence-based interventions. (11/16)

See full text on page 533.

http://pediatrics.aappublications.org/content/138/6/e20163023

ADDRESSING EARLY CHILDHOOD EMOTIONAL AND BEHAVIORAL PROBLEMS (TECHNICAL REPORT)

Mary Margaret Gleason, MD, FAAP; Edward Goldson, MD, FAAP; Michael W. Yogman, MD, FAAP; Council on Early Childhood; Committee on Psychosocial Aspects of Child and Family Health; and Section on Developmental and Behavioral Pediatrics

ABSTRACT. More than 10% of young children experience clinically significant mental health problems, with rates of impairment and persistence comparable to those seen in older children. For many of these clinical disorders, effective treatments supported by rigorous data are available. On the other hand, rigorous support for psychopharmacologic interventions is limited to 2 large randomized controlled trials. Access to psychotherapeutic interventions is limited. The pediatrician has a critical role as the leader of the medical home to promote well-being that includes emotional, behavioral, and relationship health. To be effective in this role, pediatricians promote the use of safe and effective treatments and recognize the limitations of psychopharmacologic interventions. This technical report reviews the data supporting treatments for young children with emotional, behavioral, and relationship problems and supports the policy statement of the same name. (11/16)

See full text on page 543.

http://pediatrics.aappublications.org/content/138/6/e20163025

ADMISSION AND DISCHARGE GUIDELINES FOR THE PEDIATRIC PATIENT REQUIRING INTERMEDIATE CARE (CLINICAL REPORT)

Committee on Hospital Care and Section on Critical Care (joint with Society of Critical Care Medicine)

ABSTRACT. During the past 3 decades, the specialty of pediatric critical care medicine has grown rapidly, leading to a number of pediatric intensive care units opening across the country. Many patients who are admitted to the hospital require a higher level of care than routine inpatient general pediatric care, yet not to the degree of intensity of pediatric critical care; therefore, an intermediate care level has been developed in institutions providing multidisciplinary subspecialty pediatric care. These patients may require frequent monitoring of vital signs and nursing interventions, but usually they do not require invasive monitoring. The admission of the pediatric intermediate care patient is guided by physiologic parameters depending on the respective organ system involved relative to an institution's resources and capacity to care for a patient in a general care environment. This report provides admission and discharge guidelines for intermediate pediatric care. Intermediate care promotes greater flexibility in patient triage and provides a cost-effective alternative to admission to a pediatric intensive care unit. This level of care may enhance the efficiency of care and make health care more affordable for patients receiving intermediate care. (5/04, reaffirmed 2/08, 1/13)

http://pediatrics.aappublications.org/content/113/5/1430

ADOLESCENT DRUG TESTING POLICIES IN SCHOOLS

Sharon Levy, MD, MPH, FAAP; Miriam Schizer, MD, MPH, FAAP; and Committee on Substance Abuse

ABSTRACT. School-based drug testing is a controversial approach to preventing substance use by students. Although school drug testing has hypothetical benefits, and studies have noted modest reductions in self-reported student drug use, the American Academy of Pediatrics opposes widespread implementation of these programs because of the lack of solid evidence for their effectiveness. (3/15)

http://pediatrics.aappublications.org/content/135/4/782

ADOLESCENT DRUG TESTING POLICIES IN SCHOOLS (TECHNICAL REPORT)

Sharon Levy, MD, MPH, FAAP; Miriam Schizer, MD, MPH, FAAP; and Committee on Substance Abuse

ABSTRACT. More than a decade after the US Supreme Court established the legality of school-based drug testing, these programs remain controversial, and the evidence evaluating efficacy and risks is inconclusive. The objective of this technical report is to review the relevant literature that explores the benefits, risks, and costs of these programs. (3/15)

http://pediatrics.aappublications.org/content/135/4/e1107

ADOLESCENT PREGNANCY: CURRENT TRENDS AND ISSUES (CLINICAL REPORT)

Jonathan D. Klein, MD, MPH, and Committee on Adolescence

ABSTRACT. The prevention of unintended adolescent pregnancy is an important goal of the American Academy of Pediatrics and our society. Although adolescent pregnancy and birth rates have been steadily decreasing, many adolescents still become pregnant. Since the last statement on adolescent pregnancy was issued by the Academy in 1998, efforts to prevent adolescent pregnancy have increased, and new observations, technologies, and prevention effectiveness data have emerged. The purpose of this clinical report is to review current trends and issues related to adolescent pregnancy, update practitioners on this topic, and review legal and policy implications of concern to pediatricians. (7/05)

http://pediatrics.aappublications.org/content/116/1/281

ADOLESCENT PREGNANCY: CURRENT TRENDS AND ISSUES—ADDENDUM
Committee on Adolescence
INTRODUCTION. The purpose of this addendum is to update pediatricians and other professionals on recent research and data regarding adolescent sexuality, contraceptive use, and childbearing since publication of the original 2005 clinical report, "Adolescent Pregnancy: Current Trends and Issues." There has been a trend of decreasing sexual activity and teen births and pregnancies since 1991, except between the years of 2005 and 2007, when there was a 5% increase in birth rates. Currently, teen birth rates in the United States are at a record low secondary to increased use of contraception at first intercourse and use of dual methods of condoms and hormonal contraception among sexually active teenagers. Despite these data, the United States continues to lead other industrialized countries in having unacceptably high rates of adolescent pregnancy, with over 700 000 pregnancies per year, the direct health consequence of unprotected intercourse. Importantly, the 2006–2010 National Survey of Family Growth (NSFG) revealed that less than one-third of 15- to 19-year-old female subjects consistently used contraceptive methods at last intercourse. (4/14)
http://pediatrics.aappublications.org/content/133/5/954

ADOLESCENTS AND HIV INFECTION: THE PEDIATRICIAN'S ROLE IN PROMOTING ROUTINE TESTING
Committee on Pediatric AIDS
ABSTRACT. Pediatricians can play a key role in preventing and controlling HIV infection by promoting risk-reduction counseling and offering routine HIV testing to adolescent and young adult patients. Most sexually active youth do not feel that they are at risk of contracting HIV and have never been tested. Obtaining a sexual history and creating an atmosphere that promotes nonjudgmental risk counseling is a key component of the adolescent visit. In light of increasing numbers of people with HIV/AIDS and missed opportunities for HIV testing, the Centers for Disease Control and Prevention recommends universal and routine HIV testing for all patients seen in health care settings who are 13 to 64 years of age. There are advances in diagnostics and treatment that help support this recommendation. This policy statement reviews the epidemiologic data and recommends that routine screening be offered to all adolescents at least once by 16 to 18 years of age in health care settings when the prevalence of HIV in the patient population is more than 0.1%. In areas of lower community HIV prevalence, routine HIV testing is encouraged for all sexually active adolescents and those with other risk factors for HIV. This statement addresses many of the real and perceived barriers that pediatricians face in promoting routine HIV testing for their patients. (10/11, reaffirmed 9/15)
http://pediatrics.aappublications.org/content/128/5/1023

ADOLESCENTS AND HUMAN IMMUNODEFICIENCY VIRUS INFECTION: THE ROLE OF THE PEDIATRICIAN IN PREVENTION AND INTERVENTION
Committee on Pediatric AIDS and Committee on Adolescence
ABSTRACT. Half of all new human immunodeficiency virus (HIV) infections in the United States occur among young people between the ages of 13 and 24. Sexual transmission accounts for most cases of HIV during adolescence. Pediatricians can play an important role in educating adolescents about HIV prevention, transmission, and testing, with an emphasis on risk reduction, and in advocating for the special needs of adolescents for access to information about HIV. (1/01, reaffirmed 10/03, 1/05)
http://pediatrics.aappublications.org/content/107/1/188

THE ADOLESCENT'S RIGHT TO CONFIDENTIAL CARE WHEN CONSIDERING ABORTION
Committee on Adolescence
ABSTRACT. In this statement, the American Academy of Pediatrics (AAP) reaffirms its position that the rights of adolescents to confidential care when considering abortion should be protected. The AAP supports the recommendations presented in the report on mandatory parental consent to abortion by the Council on Ethical and Judicial Affairs of the American Medical Association. Adolescents should be strongly encouraged to involve their parents and other trusted adults in decisions regarding pregnancy termination, and the majority of them voluntarily do so. Legislation mandating parental involvement does not achieve the intended benefit of promoting family communication, but it does increase the risk of harm to the adolescent by delaying access to appropriate medical care. The statement presents a summary of pertinent current information related to the benefits and risks of legislation requiring mandatory parental involvement in an adolescent's decision to obtain an abortion. The AAP acknowledges and respects the diversity of beliefs about abortion and affirms the value of voluntary parental involvement in decision making by adolescents. (5/96, reaffirmed 5/99, 11/02)
http://pediatrics.aappublications.org/content/97/5/746

ADVANCED PRACTICE IN NEONATAL NURSING
Committee on Fetus and Newborn
ABSTRACT. The participation of advanced practice registered nurses in neonatal care continues to be accepted and supported by the American Academy of Pediatrics. Recognized categories of advanced practice neonatal nursing are the neonatal clinical nurse specialist and the neonatal nurse practitioner. (5/09, reaffirmed 1/14)
http://pediatrics.aappublications.org/content/123/6/1606

AGE LIMITS OF PEDIATRICS
Child and Adolescent Health Action Group (5/88, reaffirmed 9/92, 1/97, 3/02, 1/06, 10/11)
http://pediatrics.aappublications.org/content/49/3/463

AGE TERMINOLOGY DURING THE PERINATAL PERIOD
Committee on Fetus and Newborn
ABSTRACT. Consistent definitions to describe the length of gestation and age in neonates are needed to compare neurodevelopmental, medical, and growth outcomes. The purposes of this policy statement are to review conventional definitions of age during the perinatal period and to recommend use of standard terminology including gestational age, postmenstrual age, chronological age, corrected age, adjusted age, and estimated date of delivery. (11/04, reaffirmed 10/07, 11/08, 1/09, 7/14)
http://pediatrics.aappublications.org/content/114/5/1362

ALCOHOL USE BY YOUTH AND ADOLESCENTS: A PEDIATRIC CONCERN

Committee on Substance Abuse

ABSTRACT. Alcohol use continues to be a major problem from preadolescence through young adulthood in the United States. Results of recent neuroscience research have substantiated the deleterious effects of alcohol on adolescent brain development and added even more evidence to support the call to prevent and reduce underaged drinking. Pediatricians should be knowledgeable about substance abuse to be able to recognize risk factors for alcohol and other substance abuse among youth, screen for use, provide appropriate brief interventions, and refer to treatment. The integration of alcohol use prevention programs in the community and our educational system from elementary school through college should be promoted by pediatricians and the health care community. Promotion of media responsibility to connect alcohol consumption with realistic consequences should be supported by pediatricians. Additional research into the prevention, screening and identification, brief intervention, and management and treatment of alcohol and other substance use by adolescents continues to be needed to improve evidence-based practices. (4/10, reaffirmed 12/14)
http://pediatrics.aappublications.org/content/125/5/1078

ALLERGY TESTING IN CHILDHOOD: USING ALLERGEN-SPECIFIC IGE TESTS (CLINICAL REPORT)

Scott H. Sicherer, MD; Robert A. Wood, MD; and Section on Allergy and Immunology

ABSTRACT. A variety of triggers can induce common pediatric allergic diseases which include asthma, allergic rhinitis, atopic dermatitis, food allergy, and anaphylaxis. Allergy testing serves to confirm an allergic trigger suspected on the basis of history. Tests for allergen-specific immunoglobulin E (IgE) are performed by in vitro assays or skin tests. The tests are excellent for identifying a sensitized state in which allergen-specific IgE is present, and may identify triggers to be eliminated and help guide immunotherapy treatment. However, a positive test result does not always equate with clinical allergy. Newer enzymatic assays based on anti-IgE antibodies have supplanted the radioallergosorbent test (RAST). This clinical report focuses on allergen-specific IgE testing, emphasizing that the medical history and knowledge of disease characteristics are crucial for rational test selection and interpretation. (12/11)
http://pediatrics.aappublications.org/content/129/1/193

ALL-TERRAIN VEHICLE INJURY PREVENTION: TWO-, THREE-, AND FOUR-WHEELED UNLICENSED MOTOR VEHICLES

Committee on Injury and Poison Prevention

ABSTRACT. Since 1987, the American Academy of Pediatrics (AAP) has had a policy about the use of motorized cycles and all-terrain vehicles (ATVs) by children. The purpose of this policy statement is to update and strengthen previous policy. This statement describes the various kinds of motorized cycles and ATVs and outlines the epidemiologic characteristics of deaths and injuries related to their use by children in light of the 1987 consent decrees entered into by the US Consumer Product Safety Commission and the manufacturers of ATVs. Recommendations are made for public, patient, and parent education by pediatricians; equipment modifications; the use of safety equipment; and the development and improvement of safer off-road trails and responsive emergency medical systems. In addition, the AAP strengthens its recommendation for passage of legislation in all states prohibiting the use of 2- and 4-wheeled off-road vehicles by children younger than 16 years, as well as a ban on the sale of new and used 3-wheeled ATVs, with a recall of all used 3-wheeled ATVs. (6/00, reaffirmed 5/04, 1/07, 5/13)
http://pediatrics.aappublications.org/content/105/6/1352

AMBIENT AIR POLLUTION: HEALTH HAZARDS TO CHILDREN

Committee on Environmental Health

ABSTRACT. Ambient (outdoor) air pollution is now recognized as an important problem, both nationally and worldwide. Our scientific understanding of the spectrum of health effects of air pollution has increased, and numerous studies are finding important health effects from air pollution at levels once considered safe. Children and infants are among the most susceptible to many of the air pollutants. In addition to associations between air pollution and respiratory symptoms, asthma exacerbations, and asthma hospitalizations, recent studies have found links between air pollution and preterm birth, infant mortality, deficits in lung growth, and possibly, development of asthma. This policy statement summarizes the recent literature linking ambient air pollution to adverse health outcomes in children and includes a perspective on the current regulatory process. The statement provides advice to pediatricians on how to integrate issues regarding air quality and health into patient education and children's environmental health advocacy and concludes with recommendations to the government on promotion of effective air-pollution policies to ensure protection of children's health. (12/04, reaffirmed 4/09)
http://pediatrics.aappublications.org/content/114/6/1699

ANTENATAL COUNSELING REGARDING RESUSCITATION AND INTENSIVE CARE BEFORE 25 WEEKS OF GESTATION (CLINICAL REPORT)

James Cummings, MD, FAAP, and Committee on Fetus and Newborn

ABSTRACT. The anticipated birth of an extremely low gestational age (<25 weeks) infant presents many difficult questions, and variations in practice continue to exist. Decisions regarding care of periviable infants should ideally be well informed, ethically sound, consistent within medical teams, and consonant with the parents' wishes. Each health care institution should consider having policies and procedures for antenatal counseling in these situations. Family counseling may be aided by the use of visual materials, which should take into consideration the intellectual, cultural, and other characteristics of the family members. Although general recommendations can guide practice, each situation is unique; thus, decision-making should be individualized. In most cases, the approach should be shared decision-making with the family, guided by considering both the likelihood of death or

morbidity and the parents' desires for their unborn child. If a decision is made not to resuscitate, providing comfort care, encouraging family bonding, and palliative care support are appropriate. (8/15)
http://pediatrics.aappublications.org/content/136/3/588

ANTERIOR CRUCIATE LIGAMENT INJURIES: DIAGNOSIS, TREATMENT, AND PREVENTION (CLINICAL REPORT)

Cynthia R. LaBella, MD, FAAP; William Hennrikus, MD, FAAP; Timothy E. Hewett, PhD, FACSM; Council on Sports Medicine and Fitness; and Section on Orthopaedics
ABSTRACT. The number of anterior cruciate ligament (ACL) injuries reported in athletes younger than 18 years has increased over the past 2 decades. Reasons for the increasing ACL injury rate include the growing number of children and adolescents participating in organized sports, intensive sports training at an earlier age, and greater rate of diagnosis because of increased awareness and greater use of advanced medical imaging. ACL injury rates are low in young children and increase sharply during puberty, especially for girls, who have higher rates of noncontact ACL injuries than boys do in similar sports. Intrinsic risk factors for ACL injury include higher BMI, subtalar joint overpronation, generalized ligamentous laxity, and decreased neuromuscular control of knee motion. ACL injuries often require surgery and/or many months of rehabilitation and substantial time lost from school and sports participation. Unfortunately, regardless of treatment, athletes with ACL injuries are up to 10 times more likely to develop degenerative arthritis of the knee. Safe and effective surgical techniques for children and adolescents continue to evolve. Neuromuscular training can reduce risk of ACL injury in adolescent girls. This report outlines the current state of knowledge on epidemiology, diagnosis, treatment, and prevention of ACL injuries in children and adolescents. (4/14)
http://pediatrics.aappublications.org/content/133/5/e1437

THE APGAR SCORE

Committee on Fetus and Newborn (joint with American College of Obstetricians and Gynecologists Committee on Obstetric Practice)
ABSTRACT. The Apgar score provides an accepted and convenient method for reporting the status of the newborn infant immediately after birth and the response to resuscitation if needed. The Apgar score alone cannot be considered as evidence of, or a consequence of, asphyxia; does not predict individual neonatal mortality or neurologic outcome; and should not be used for that purpose. An Apgar score assigned during resuscitation is not equivalent to a score assigned to a spontaneously breathing infant. The American Academy of Pediatrics and the American College of Obstetricians and Gynecologists encourage use of an expanded Apgar score reporting form that accounts for concurrent resuscitative interventions. (9/15)
http://pediatrics.aappublications.org/content/136/4/819

APNEA OF PREMATURITY (CLINICAL REPORT)

Eric C. Eichenwald, MD, FAAP, and Committee on Fetus and Newborn
ABSTRACT. Apnea of prematurity is one of the most common diagnoses in the NICU. Despite the frequency of apnea of prematurity, it is unknown whether recurrent apnea, bradycardia, and hypoxemia in preterm infants are harmful. Research into the development of respiratory control in immature animals and preterm infants has facilitated our understanding of the pathogenesis and treatment of apnea of prematurity. However, the lack of consistent definitions, monitoring practices, and consensus about clinical significance leads to significant variation in practice. The purpose of this clinical report is to review the evidence basis for the definition, epidemiology, and treatment of apnea of prematurity as well as discharge recommendations for preterm infants diagnosed with recurrent apneic events. (12/15)
http://pediatrics.aappublications.org/content/137/1/e20153757

APPLICATION OF THE RESOURCE-BASED RELATIVE VALUE SCALE SYSTEM TO PEDIATRICS

Committee on Coding and Nomenclature
ABSTRACT. The majority of public and private payers in the United States currently use the Medicare Resource-Based Relative Value Scale as the basis for physician payment. Many large group and academic practices have adopted this objective system of physician work to benchmark physician productivity, including using it, wholly or in part, to determine compensation. The Resource-Based Relative Value Scale survey instrument, used to value physician services, was designed primarily for procedural services, leading to current concerns that American Medical Association/Specialty Society Relative Value Scale Update Committee (RUC) surveys may undervalue nonprocedural evaluation and management services. The American Academy of Pediatrics is represented on the RUC, the committee charged with maintaining accurate physician work values across specialties and age groups. The Academy, working closely with other primary care and subspecialty societies, actively pursues a balanced RUC membership and a survey instrument that will ensure appropriate work relative value unit assignments, thereby allowing pediatricians to receive appropriate payment for their services relative to other services. (5/14)
http://pediatrics.aappublications.org/content/133/6/1158

ASSESSMENT AND MANAGEMENT OF INGUINAL HERNIA IN INFANTS (CLINICAL REPORT)

Kasper S. Wang, MD; Committee on Fetus and Newborn; and Section on Surgery
ABSTRACT. Inguinal hernia repair in infants is a routine surgical procedure. However, numerous issues, including timing of the repair, the need to explore the contralateral groin, use of laparoscopy, and anesthetic approach, remain unsettled. Given the lack of compelling data, consideration should be given to large, prospective, randomized controlled trials to determine best practices for the management of inguinal hernias in infants. (9/12)
http://pediatrics.aappublications.org/content/130/4/768

ATHLETIC PARTICIPATION BY CHILDREN AND ADOLESCENTS WHO HAVE SYSTEMIC HYPERTENSION

Rebecca A. Demorest, MD; Reginald L. Washington, MD; and Council on Sports Medicine and Fitness

ABSTRACT. Children and adolescents who have hypertension may be at risk for complications when exercise causes their blood pressure to rise even higher. The purpose of this statement is to update recommendations concerning the athletic participation of individuals with hypertension, including special populations such as those with spinal cord injuries or obesity, by using the guidelines from "The 36th Bethesda Conference: Eligibility Recommendations for Competitive Athletes with Cardiovascular Abnormalities"; "The Fourth Report on the Diagnosis, Evaluation, and Treatment of High Blood Pressure in Children and Adolescents"; and "The Seventh Report of the Joint National Committee on Prevention, Detection, Evaluation, and Treatment of High Blood Pressure." (5/10, reaffirmed 5/13)
http://pediatrics.aappublications.org/content/125/6/1287

ATOPIC DERMATITIS: SKIN-DIRECTED MANAGEMENT (CLINICAL REPORT)

Megha M. Tollefson, MD; Anna L. Bruckner, MD, FAAP; and Section on Dermatology

ABSTRACT. Atopic dermatitis is a common inflammatory skin condition characterized by relapsing eczematous lesions in a typical distribution. It can be frustrating for pediatric patients, parents, and health care providers alike. The pediatrician will treat the majority of children with atopic dermatitis as many patients will not have access to a pediatric medical subspecialist, such as a pediatric dermatologist or pediatric allergist. This report provides up-to-date information regarding the disease and its impact, pathogenesis, treatment options, and potential complications. The goal of this report is to assist pediatricians with accurate and useful information that will improve the care of patients with atopic dermatitis. (11/14)
http://pediatrics.aappublications.org/content/134/6/e1735

ATTENTION-DEFICIT/HYPERACTIVITY DISORDER AND SUBSTANCE ABUSE (CLINICAL REPORT)

Elizabeth Harstad, MD, MPH, FAAP; Sharon Levy, MD, MPH, FAAP; and Committee on Substance Abuse

ABSTRACT. Attention-deficit/hyperactivity disorder (ADHD) and substance use disorders are inextricably intertwined. Children with ADHD are more likely than peers to develop substance use disorders. Treatment with stimulants may reduce the risk of substance use disorders, but stimulants are a class of medication with significant abuse and diversion potential. The objectives of this clinical report were to present practical strategies for reducing the risk of substance use disorders in patients with ADHD and suggestions for safe stimulant prescribing. (6/14)
http://pediatrics.aappublications.org/content/134/1/e293

AUDITORY INTEGRATION TRAINING AND FACILITATED COMMUNICATION FOR AUTISM

Committee on Children With Disabilities

ABSTRACT. This statement reviews the basis for two new therapies for autism—auditory integration training and facilitative communication. Both therapies seek to improve communication skills. Currently available information does not support the claims of proponents that these treatments are efficacious. Their use does not appear warranted at this time, except within research protocols. (8/98, reaffirmed 5/02, 1/06, 12/09)
http://pediatrics.aappublications.org/content/102/2/431

BASEBALL AND SOFTBALL

Council on Sports Medicine and Fitness

ABSTRACT. Baseball and softball are among the most popular and safest sports in which children and adolescents participate. Nevertheless, traumatic and overuse injuries occur regularly, including occasional catastrophic injury and even death. Safety of the athlete is a constant focus of attention among those responsible for modifying rules. Understanding the stresses placed on the arm, especially while pitching, led to the institution of rules controlling the quantity of pitches thrown in youth baseball and established rest periods between pitching assignments. Similarly, field maintenance and awareness of environmental conditions as well as equipment maintenance and creative prevention strategies are critically important in minimizing the risk of injury. This statement serves as a basis for encouraging safe participation in baseball and softball. This statement has been endorsed by the Canadian Paediatric Society. (2/12, reaffirmed 7/15)
http://pediatrics.aappublications.org/content/129/3/e842

BEST PRACTICES FOR IMPROVING FLOW AND CARE OF PEDIATRIC PATIENTS IN THE EMERGENCY DEPARTMENT (TECHNICAL REPORT)

Isabel Barata, MD; Kathleen M. Brown, MD; Laura Fitzmaurice, MD; Elizabeth Stone Griffin, RN; Sally K. Snow, BSN, RN; and Committee on Pediatric Emergency Medicine (joint with American College of Emergency Physicians Pediatric Emergency Medicine Committee and Emergency Nurses Association Pediatric Committee)

ABSTRACT. This report provides a summary of best practices for improving flow, reducing waiting times, and improving the quality of care of pediatric patients in the emergency department. (12/14)
http://pediatrics.aappublications.org/content/135/1/e273

BICYCLE HELMETS

Committee on Injury and Poison Prevention

ABSTRACT. Bicycling remains one of the most popular recreational sports among children in America and is the leading cause of recreational sports injuries treated in emergency departments. An estimated 23 000 children younger than 21 years sustained head injuries (excluding the face) while bicycling in 1998. The bicycle helmet is a very effective device that can prevent the occurrence of up to 88% of serious brain injuries. Despite this, most children do not wear a helmet each time they ride a bicycle, and adolescents are particularly resistant to helmet use. Recently, a group of national experts and government agencies renewed the call for all bicyclists to wear helmets. This policy statement describes the role of the pediatrician in helping attain universal helmet use among children and teens for each bicycle ride. (10/01, reaffirmed 1/05, 2/08, 11/11)
http://pediatrics.aappublications.org/content/108/4/1030

BINGE DRINKING (CLINICAL REPORT)

Lorena Siqueira, MD, MSPH, FAAP; Vincent C. Smith, MD, MPH, FAAP; and Committee on Substance Abuse

ABSTRACT. Alcohol is the substance most frequently abused by children and adolescents in the United States, and its use is associated with the leading causes of death and serious injury at this age (ie, motor vehicle accidents, homicides, and suicides). Among youth who drink, the proportion who drink heavily is higher than among adult drinkers, increasing from approximately 50% in those 12 to 14 years of age to 72% among those 18 to 20 years of age. In this clinical report, the definition, epidemiology, and risk factors for binge drinking; the neurobiology of intoxication, blackouts, and hangovers; genetic considerations; and adverse outcomes are discussed. The report offers guidance for the pediatrician. As with any high-risk behavior, prevention plays a more important role than later intervention and has been shown to be more effective. In the pediatric office setting, it is important to ask every adolescent about alcohol use. (8/15)

http://pediatrics.aappublications.org/content/136/3/e718

BONE DENSITOMETRY IN CHILDREN AND ADOLESCENTS (CLINICAL REPORT)

Laura K. Bachrach, MD; Catherine M. Gordon, MD, MS; and Section on Endocrinology

ABSTRACT. Concerns about bone health and potential fragility in children and adolescents have led to a high interest in bone densitometry. Pediatric patients with genetic and acquired chronic diseases, immobility, and inadequate nutrition may fail to achieve expected gains in bone size, mass, and strength, leaving them vulnerable to fracture. In older adults, bone densitometry has been shown to predict fracture risk and reflect response to therapy. The role of densitometry in the management of children at risk of bone fragility is less clear. This clinical report summarizes current knowledge about bone densitometry in the pediatric population, including indications for its use, interpretation of results, and risks and costs. The report emphasizes updated consensus statements generated at the 2013 Pediatric Position Development Conference of the International Society of Clinical Densitometry by an international panel of bone experts. Some of these recommendations are evidence-based, whereas others reflect expert opinion, because data are sparse on many topics. The statements from this and other expert panels provide general guidance to the pediatrician, but decisions about ordering and interpreting bone densitometry still require clinical judgment. The interpretation of bone densitometry results in children differs from that in older adults. The terms "osteopenia" and "osteoporosis" based on bone densitometry findings alone should not be used in younger patients; instead, bone mineral content or density that falls >2 SDs below expected is labeled "low for age." Pediatric osteoporosis is defined by the Pediatric Position Development Conference by using 1 of the following criteria: ≥1 vertebral fractures occurring in the absence of local disease or high-energy trauma (without or with densitometry measurements) or low bone density for age and a significant fracture history (defined as ≥2 long bone fractures before 10 years of age or ≥3 long bone fractures before 19 years of age). Ongoing research will help define the indications and best methods for assessing bone strength in children and the clinical factors that contribute to fracture risk. The Pediatric Endocrine Society affirms the educational value of this publication. (9/16)

See full text on page 559.

http://pediatrics.aappublications.org/content/138/4/e20162398

BOXING PARTICIPATION BY CHILDREN AND ADOLESCENTS

Council on Sports Medicine and Fitness (joint with Canadian Paediatric Society Healthy Active Living and Sports Medicine Committee)

ABSTRACT. Thousands of boys and girls younger than 19 years participate in boxing in North America. Although boxing provides benefits for participants, including exercise, self-discipline, and self-confidence, the sport of boxing encourages and rewards deliberate blows to the head and face. Participants in boxing are at risk of head, face, and neck injuries, including chronic and even fatal neurologic injuries. Concussions are one of the most common injuries that occur with boxing. Because of the risk of head and facial injuries, the American Academy of Pediatrics and the Canadian Paediatric Society oppose boxing as a sport for children and adolescents. These organizations recommend that physicians vigorously oppose boxing in youth and encourage patients to participate in alternative sports in which intentional head blows are not central to the sport. (8/11, reaffirmed 2/15)

http://pediatrics.aappublications.org/content/128/3/617

BREASTFEEDING AND THE USE OF HUMAN MILK

Section on Breastfeeding

ABSTRACT. Breastfeeding and human milk are the normative standards for infant feeding and nutrition. Given the documented short- and long-term medical and neurodevelopmental advantages of breastfeeding, infant nutrition should be considered a public health issue and not only a lifestyle choice. The American Academy of Pediatrics reaffirms its recommendation of exclusive breastfeeding for about 6 months, followed by continued breastfeeding as complementary foods are introduced, with continuation of breastfeeding for 1 year or longer as mutually desired by mother and infant. Medical contraindications to breastfeeding are rare. Infant growth should be monitored with the World Health Organization (WHO) Growth Curve Standards to avoid mislabeling infants as underweight or failing to thrive. Hospital routines to encourage and support the initiation and sustaining of exclusive breastfeeding should be based on the American Academy of Pediatrics-endorsed WHO/UNICEF "Ten Steps to Successful Breastfeeding." National strategies supported by the US Surgeon General's Call to Action, the Centers for Disease Control and Prevention, and The Joint Commission are involved to facilitate breastfeeding practices in US hospitals and communities. Pediatricians play a critical role in their practices and communities as advocates of breastfeeding and thus should be knowledgeable about the health risks of not breastfeeding, the economic benefits to society of breastfeeding, and the techniques for managing and supporting the breastfeeding dyad. The "Business Case for Breastfeeding" details how mothers

can maintain lactation in the workplace and the benefits to employers who facilitate this practice. (2/12)
http://pediatrics.aappublications.org/content/129/3/e827

THE BUILT ENVIRONMENT: DESIGNING COMMUNITIES TO PROMOTE PHYSICAL ACTIVITY IN CHILDREN

Committee on Environmental Health

ABSTRACT. An estimated 32% of American children are overweight, and physical inactivity contributes to this high prevalence of overweight. This policy statement highlights how the built environment of a community affects children's opportunities for physical activity. Neighborhoods and communities can provide opportunities for recreational physical activity with parks and open spaces, and policies must support this capacity. Children can engage in physical activity as a part of their daily lives, such as on their travel to school. Factors such as school location have played a significant role in the decreased rates of walking to school, and changes in policy may help to increase the number of children who are able to walk to school. Environment modification that addresses risks associated with automobile traffic is likely to be conducive to more walking and biking among children. Actions that reduce parental perception and fear of crime may promote outdoor physical activity. Policies that promote more active lifestyles among children and adolescents will enable them to achieve the recommended 60 minutes of daily physical activity. By working with community partners, pediatricians can participate in establishing communities designed for activity and health. (5/09, reaffirmed 1/13)
http://pediatrics.aappublications.org/content/123/6/1591

CALCIUM AND VITAMIN D REQUIREMENTS OF ENTERALLY FED PRETERM INFANTS (CLINICAL REPORT)

Steven A. Abrams, MD, and Committee on Nutrition

ABSTRACT. Bone health is a critical concern in managing preterm infants. Key nutrients of importance are calcium, vitamin D, and phosphorus. Although human milk is critical for the health of preterm infants, it is low in these nutrients relative to the needs of the infants during growth. Strategies should be in place to fortify human milk for preterm infants with birth weight <1800 to 2000 g and to ensure adequate mineral intake during hospitalization and after hospital discharge. Biochemical monitoring of very low birth weight infants should be performed during their hospitalization. Vitamin D should be provided at 200 to 400 IU/day both during hospitalization and after discharge from the hospital. Infants with radiologic evidence of rickets should have efforts made to maximize calcium and phosphorus intake by using available commercial products and, if needed, direct supplementation with these minerals. (4/13)
http://pediatrics.aappublications.org/content/131/5/e1676

CARDIOVASCULAR HEALTH SUPERVISION FOR INDIVIDUALS AFFECTED BY DUCHENNE OR BECKER MUSCULAR DYSTROPHY (CLINICAL REPORT)

Section on Cardiology and Cardiac Surgery

ABSTRACT. Duchenne muscular dystrophy is the most common and severe form of the childhood muscular dystrophies. The disease is typically diagnosed between 3 and 7 years of age and follows a predictable clinical course marked by progressive skeletal muscle weakness with loss of ambulation by 12 years of age. Death occurs in early adulthood secondary to respiratory or cardiac failure. Becker muscular dystrophy is less common and has a milder clinical course but also results in respiratory and cardiac failure. The natural history of the cardiomyopathy in these diseases has not been well established. As a result, patients traditionally present for cardiac evaluation only after clinical symptoms become evident. The purpose of this policy statement is to provide recommendations for optimal cardiovascular evaluation to health care specialists caring for individuals in whom the diagnosis of Duchenne or Becker muscular dystrophy has been confirmed. (12/05, reaffirmed 1/09)
http://pediatrics.aappublications.org/content/116/6/1569

CARDIOVASCULAR MONITORING AND STIMULANT DRUGS FOR ATTENTION-DEFICIT/HYPERACTIVITY DISORDER

James M. Perrin, MD; Richard A. Friedman, MD; Timothy K. Knilans, MD; Black Box Working Group; and Section on Cardiology and Cardiac Surgery

ABSTRACT. A recent American Heart Association (AHA) statement recommended electrocardiograms (ECGs) routinely for children before they start medications to treat attention-deficit/hyperactivity disorder (ADHD). The AHA statement reflected the thoughtful work of a group committed to improving the health of children with heart disease. However, the recommendation to obtain an ECG before starting medications for treating ADHD contradicts the carefully considered and evidence-based recommendations of the American Academy of Child and Adolescent Psychiatry and the American Academy of Pediatrics (AAP). These organizations have concluded that sudden cardiac death (SCD) in persons taking medications for ADHD is a very rare event, occurring at rates no higher than those in the general population of children and adolescents. Both of these groups also noted the lack of any evidence that the routine use of ECG screening before beginning medication for ADHD treatment would prevent sudden death. The AHA statement pointed out the importance of detecting silent but clinically important cardiac conditions in children and adolescents, which is a goal that the AAP shares. The primary purpose of the AHA statement is to prevent cases of SCD that may be related to stimulant medications. The recommendations of the AAP and the rationale for these recommendations are the subject of this statement. (8/08)
http://pediatrics.aappublications.org/content/122/2/451

CARE COORDINATION IN THE MEDICAL HOME: INTEGRATING HEALTH AND RELATED SYSTEMS OF CARE FOR CHILDREN WITH SPECIAL HEALTH CARE NEEDS

Council on Children With Disabilities

ABSTRACT. Care coordination is a process that facilitates the linkage of children and their families with appropriate services and resources in a coordinated effort to achieve good health. Care coordination for children with special health care needs often is complicated because there is no single point of entry into the multiple systems of care, and complex criteria frequently determine the availability of funding and services among public and private payers. Economic and sociocultural barriers to coordination of

care exist and affect families and health care professionals. In their important role of providing a medical home for all children, primary care physicians have a vital role in the process of care coordination, in concert with the family. (11/05)
http://pediatrics.aappublications.org/content/116/5/1238

CARE OF ADOLESCENT PARENTS AND THEIR CHILDREN (CLINICAL REPORT)

Jorge L. Pinzon, MD; Veronnie F. Jones, MD; Committee on Adolescence; and Committee on Early Childhood

ABSTRACT. Teen pregnancy and parenting remain an important public health issue in the United States and the world, and many children live with their adolescent parents alone or as part of an extended family. A significant proportion of teen parents reside with their family of origin, significantly affecting the multigenerational family structure. Repeated births to teen parents are also common. This clinical report updates a previous policy statement on care of the adolescent parent and their children and addresses medical and psychosocial risks specific to this population. Challenges unique to teen parents and their children are reviewed, along with suggestions for the pediatrician on models for intervention and care. (11/12, reaffirmed 7/16)
http://pediatrics.aappublications.org/content/130/6/e1743

CARE OF THE ADOLESCENT SEXUAL ASSAULT VICTIM (CLINICAL REPORT)

Miriam Kaufman, MD, and Committee on Adolescence

ABSTRACT. Sexual assault is a broad-based term that encompasses a wide range of sexual victimizations including rape. Since the American Academy of Pediatrics published its last policy statement on sexual assault in 2001, additional information and data have emerged about sexual assault and rape in adolescents and the treatment and management of the adolescent who has been a victim of sexual assault. This report provides new information to update physicians and focuses on assessment and care of sexual assault victims in the adolescent population. (8/08)
http://pediatrics.aappublications.org/content/122/2/462

CAREGIVER-FABRICATED ILLNESS IN A CHILD: A MANIFESTATION OF CHILD MALTREATMENT (CLINICAL REPORT)

Emalee G. Flaherty, MD; Harriet L. MacMillan, MD; and Committee on Child Abuse and Neglect

ABSTRACT. Caregiver-fabricated illness in a child is a form of child maltreatment caused by a caregiver who falsifies and/or induces a child's illness, leading to unnecessary and potentially harmful medical investigations and/or treatment. This condition can result in significant morbidity and mortality. Although caregiver-fabricated illness in a child has been widely known as Munchausen syndrome by proxy, there is ongoing discussion about alternative names, including pediatric condition falsification, factitious disorder (illness) by proxy, child abuse in the medical setting, and medical child abuse. Because it is a relatively uncommon form of maltreatment, pediatricians need to have a high index of suspicion when faced with a persistent or recurrent illness that cannot be explained and that results in multiple medical procedures or when there are discrepancies between the history, physical examination, and health of a child. This report updates the previous clinical report "Beyond Munchausen Syndrome by Proxy: Identification and Treatment of Child Abuse in the Medical Setting." The authors discuss the need to agree on appropriate terminology, provide an update on published reports of new manifestations of fabricated medical conditions, and discuss approaches to assessment, diagnosis, and management, including how best to protect the child from further harm. (8/13)
http://pediatrics.aappublications.org/content/132/3/590

THE CHANGING CONCEPT OF SUDDEN INFANT DEATH SYNDROME: DIAGNOSTIC CODING SHIFTS, CONTROVERSIES REGARDING THE SLEEPING ENVIRONMENT, AND NEW VARIABLES TO CONSIDER IN REDUCING RISK

Task Force on Sudden Infant Death Syndrome

ABSTRACT. There has been a major decrease in the incidence of sudden infant death syndrome (SIDS) since the American Academy of Pediatrics (AAP) released its recommendation in 1992 that infants be placed down for sleep in a nonprone position. Although the SIDS rate continues to fall, some of the recent decrease of the last several years may be a result of coding shifts to other causes of unexpected infant deaths. Since the AAP published its last statement on SIDS in 2000, several issues have become relevant, including the significant risk of side sleeping position; the AAP no longer recognizes side sleeping as a reasonable alternative to fully supine sleeping. The AAP also stresses the need to avoid redundant soft bedding and soft objects in the infant's sleeping environment, the hazards of adults sleeping with an infant in the same bed, the SIDS risk reduction associated with having infants sleep in the same room as adults and with using pacifiers at the time of sleep, the importance of educating secondary caregivers and neonatology practitioners on the importance of "back to sleep," and strategies to reduce the incidence of positional plagiocephaly associated with supine positioning. This statement reviews the evidence associated with these and other SIDS-related issues and proposes new recommendations for further reducing SIDS risk. (11/05, reaffirmed 5/08)
http://pediatrics.aappublications.org/content/116/5/1245

CHEERLEADING INJURIES: EPIDEMIOLOGY AND RECOMMENDATIONS FOR PREVENTION

Council on Sports Medicine and Fitness

ABSTRACT. Over the last 30 years, cheerleading has increased dramatically in popularity and has evolved from leading the crowd in cheers at sporting events into a competitive, year-round sport involving complex acrobatic stunts and tumbling. Consequently, cheerleading injuries have steadily increased over the years in both number and severity. Sprains and strains to the lower extremities are the most common injuries. Although the overall injury rate remains relatively low, cheerleading has accounted for approximately 66% of all catastrophic injuries in high school girl athletes over the past 25 years. Risk factors for injuries in cheerleading include higher BMI, previous injury, cheering on harder surfaces, performing stunts, and supervision by a coach with low level of training and experience. This policy statement describes the epidemiology of cheerleading injuries and provides recommendations for injury prevention. (10/12, reaffirmed 7/15)

http://pediatrics.aappublications.org/content/130/5/966

CHEMICAL-BIOLOGICAL TERRORISM AND ITS IMPACT ON CHILDREN

Committee on Environmental Health and Committee on Infectious Diseases

ABSTRACT. Children remain potential victims of chemical or biological terrorism. In recent years, children have even been specific targets of terrorist acts. Consequently, it is necessary to address the needs that children would face after a terrorist incident. A broad range of public health initiatives have occurred since September 11, 2001. Although the needs of children have been addressed in many of them, in many cases, these initiatives have been inadequate in ensuring the protection of children. In addition, public health and health care system preparedness for terrorism has been broadened to the so-called all-hazards approach, in which response plans for terrorism are blended with plans for a public health or health care system response to unintentional disasters (eg, natural events such as earthquakes or pandemic flu or manmade catastrophes such as a hazardous-materials spill). In response to new principles and programs that have appeared over the last 5 years, this policy statement provides an update of the 2000 policy statement. The roles of both the pediatrician and public health agencies continue to be emphasized; only a coordinated effort by pediatricians and public health can ensure that the needs of children, including emergency protocols in schools or child care centers, decontamination protocols, and mental health interventions, will be successful. (9/06, reaffirmed 1/11)

http://pediatrics.aappublications.org/content/118/3/1267

CHEMICAL-MANAGEMENT POLICY: PRIORITIZING CHILDREN'S HEALTH

Council on Environmental Health

ABSTRACT. The American Academy of Pediatrics recommends that chemical-management policy in the United States be revised to protect children and pregnant women and to better protect other populations. The Toxic Substance Control Act (TSCA) was passed in 1976. It is widely recognized to have been ineffective in protecting children, pregnant women, and the general population from hazardous chemicals in the marketplace. It does not take into account the special vulnerabilities of children in attempting to protect the population from chemical hazards. Its processes are so cumbersome that in its more than 30 years of existence, the TSCA has been used to regulate only 5 chemicals or chemical classes of the tens of thousands of chemicals that are in commerce. Under the TSCA, chemical companies have no responsibility to perform premarket testing or postmarket follow-up of the products that they produce; in fact, the TSCA contains disincentives for the companies to produce such data. Voluntary programs have been inadequate in resolving problems. Therefore, chemical-management policy needs to be rewritten in the United States. Manufacturers must be responsible for developing information about chemicals before marketing. The US Environmental Protection Agency must have the authority to demand additional safety data about a chemical and to limit or stop the marketing of a chemical when there is a high degree of suspicion that the chemical might be harmful to children, pregnant women, or other populations. (4/11)

http://pediatrics.aappublications.org/content/127/5/983

CHILD ABUSE, CONFIDENTIALITY, AND THE HEALTH INSURANCE PORTABILITY AND ACCOUNTABILITY ACT

Committee on Child Abuse and Neglect

ABSTRACT. The federal Health Insurance Portability and Accountability Act (HIPAA) of 1996 has significantly affected clinical practice, particularly with regard to how patient information is shared. HIPAA addresses the security and privacy of patient health data, ensuring that information is released appropriately with patient or guardian consent and knowledge. However, when child abuse or neglect is suspected in a clinical setting, the physician may determine that release of information without consent is necessary to ensure the health and safety of the child. This policy statement provides an overview of HIPAA regulations with regard to the role of the pediatrician in releasing or reviewing patient health information when the patient is a child who is a suspected victim of abuse or neglect. This statement is based on the most current regulations provided by the US Department of Health and Human Services and is subject to future changes and clarifications as updates are provided. (12/09, reaffirmed 1/14)

http://pediatrics.aappublications.org/content/125/1/197

CHILD FATALITY REVIEW

Cindy W. Christian, MD; Robert D. Sege, MD, PhD; Committee on Child Abuse and Neglect; Committee on Injury, Violence, and Poison Prevention; and Council on Community Pediatrics

ABSTRACT. Injury remains the leading cause of pediatric mortality and requires public health approaches to reduce preventable deaths. Child fatality review teams, first established to review suspicious child deaths involving abuse or neglect, have expanded toward a public health model of prevention of child fatality through systematic review of child deaths from birth through adolescence. Approximately half of all states report reviewing child deaths from all causes, and the process of fatality review has identified effective local and state prevention strategies for reducing child deaths. This expanded approach can be a powerful tool in understanding the epidemiology and preventability of child death locally, regionally, and nationally; improving accuracy of vital statistics data; and identifying public health and legislative strategies for reducing preventable child fatalities. The American Academy of Pediatrics supports the development of federal and state legislation to enhance the child fatality review process and recommends that pediatricians become involved in local and state child death reviews. (8/10, reaffirmed 5/14)

http://pediatrics.aappublications.org/content/126/3/592

CHILD LIFE SERVICES

Committee on Hospital Care and Child Life Council

ABSTRACT. Child life programs are an important component of pediatric hospital–based care to address the psychosocial concerns that accompany hospitalization and other health care experiences. Child life specialists focus on the optimal development and well-being of infants, children, adolescents, and young adults while promoting coping skills and minimizing the adverse effects of hospitalization, health care, and/or other potentially stressful experiences. Using therapeutic play, expressive modalities, and psychological preparation as primary tools, in collaboration with the entire health care team and family, child life interventions facilitate coping and adjustment at times and under circumstances that might otherwise prove overwhelming for the child. Play and developmentally appropriate communication are used to: (1) promote optimal development; (2) educate children and families about health conditions; (3) prepare children and families for medical events or procedures; (4) plan and rehearse useful coping and pain management strategies; (5) help children work through feelings about past or impending experiences; and (6) establish therapeutic relationships with patients, siblings, and parents to support family involvement in each child's care. (4/14)

http://pediatrics.aappublications.org/content/133/5/e1471

CHILD PASSENGER SAFETY

Committee on Injury, Violence, and Poison Prevention

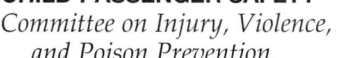

ABSTRACT. Child passenger safety has dramatically evolved over the past decade; however, motor vehicle crashes continue to be the leading cause of death of children 4 years and older. This policy statement provides 4 evidence-based recommendations for best practices in the choice of a child restraint system to optimize safety in passenger vehicles for children from birth through adolescence: (1) rear-facing car safety seats for most infants up to 2 years of age; (2) forward-facing car safety seats for most children through 4 years of age; (3) belt-positioning booster seats for most children through 8 years of age; and (4) lap-and-shoulder seat belts for all who have outgrown booster seats. In addition, a fifth evidence-based recommendation is for all children younger than 13 years to ride in the rear seats of vehicles. It is important to note that every transition is associated with some decrease in protection; therefore, parents should be encouraged to delay these transitions for as long as possible. These recommendations are presented in the form of an algorithm that is intended to facilitate implementation of the recommendations by pediatricians to their patients and families and should cover most situations that pediatricians will encounter in practice. The American Academy of Pediatrics urges all pediatricians to know and promote these recommendations as part of child passenger safety anticipatory guidance at every health-supervision visit. (3/11, reaffirmed 11/14)

http://pediatrics.aappublications.org/content/127/4/788

CHILD PASSENGER SAFETY (TECHNICAL REPORT)

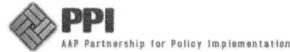

Dennis R. Durbin, MD, MSCE, and Committee on Injury, Violence, and Poison Prevention

ABSTRACT. Despite significant reductions in the number of children killed in motor vehicle crashes over the past decade, crashes continue to be the leading cause of death for children 4 years and older. Therefore, the American Academy of Pediatrics continues to recommend inclusion of child passenger safety anticipatory guidance at every health-supervision visit. This technical report provides a summary of the evidence in support of 5 recommendations for best practices to optimize safety in passenger vehicles for children from birth through adolescence that all pediatricians should know and promote in their routine practice. These recommendations are presented in the revised policy statement on child passenger safety in the form of an algorithm that is intended to facilitate their implementation by pediatricians with their patients and families. The algorithm is designed to cover the majority of situations that pediatricians will encounter in practice. In addition, a summary of evidence on a number of additional issues that affect the safety of children in motor vehicles, including the proper use and installation of child restraints, exposure to air bags, travel in pickup trucks, children left in or around vehicles, and the importance of restraint laws, is provided. Finally, this technical report provides pediatricians with a number of resources for additional information to use when providing anticipatory guidance to families. (3/11, reaffirmed 11/14)

http://pediatrics.aappublications.org/content/127/4/e1050

CHILD SEX TRAFFICKING AND COMMERCIAL SEXUAL EXPLOITATION: HEALTH CARE NEEDS OF VICTIMS (CLINICAL REPORT)

Jordan Greenbaum, MD; James E. Crawford-Jakubiak, MD, FAAP; and Committee on Child Abuse and Neglect

ABSTRACT. Child sex trafficking and commercial sexual exploitation of children (CSEC) are major public health problems in the United States and throughout the world. Despite large numbers of American and foreign youth affected and a plethora of serious physical and mental health problems associated with CSEC, there is limited information available to pediatricians regarding the nature and scope of human trafficking and how pediatricians and other health care providers may help protect children. Knowledge of risk factors, recruitment practices, possible indicators of CSEC, and common medical and behavioral health problems experienced by victims will help pediatricians recognize potential victims and respond appropriately. As health care providers, educators, and leaders in child advocacy, pediatricians play an essential role in addressing the public health issues faced by child victims of CSEC. Their roles can include working to increase recognition of CSEC, providing direct care and anticipatory guidance related to CSEC, engaging in collaborative efforts with medical and nonmedical colleagues to provide for the complex needs of youth, and educating child-serving professionals and the public. (2/15)

http://pediatrics.aappublications.org/content/135/3/566

CHILDREN, ADOLESCENTS, AND ADVERTISING
Committee on Communications

ABSTRACT. Advertising is a pervasive influence on children and adolescents. Young people view more than 40 000 ads per year on television alone and increasingly are being exposed to advertising on the Internet, in magazines, and in schools. This exposure may contribute significantly to childhood and adolescent obesity, poor nutrition, and cigarette and alcohol use. Media education has been shown to be effective in mitigating some of the negative effects of advertising on children and adolescents. (12/06, reaffirmed 3/10)
http://pediatrics.aappublications.org/content/118/6/2563

CHILDREN, ADOLESCENTS, AND TELEVISION
Committee on Public Education

ABSTRACT. This statement describes the possible negative health effects of television viewing on children and adolescents, such as violent or aggressive behavior, substance use, sexual activity, obesity, poor body image, and decreased school performance. In addition to the television ratings system and the v-chip (electronic device to block programming), media education is an effective approach to mitigating these potential problems. The American Academy of Pediatrics offers a list of recommendations on this issue for pediatricians and for parents, the federal government, and the entertainment industry. (2/01)
http://pediatrics.aappublications.org/content/107/2/423

CHILDREN, ADOLESCENTS, AND THE MEDIA
Council on Communications and Media

ABSTRACT. Media, from television to the "new media" (including cell phones, iPads, and social media), are a dominant force in children's lives. Although television is still the predominant medium for children and adolescents, new technologies are increasingly popular. The American Academy of Pediatrics continues to be concerned by evidence about the potential harmful effects of media messages and images; however, important positive and prosocial effects of media use should also be recognized. Pediatricians are encouraged to take a media history and ask 2 media questions at every well-child visit: How much recreational screen time does your child or teenager consume daily? Is there a television set or Internet-connected device in the child's bedroom? Parents are encouraged to establish a family home use plan for all media. Media influences on children and teenagers should be recognized by schools, policymakers, product advertisers, and entertainment producers. (10/13)
http://pediatrics.aappublications.org/content/132/5/958

CHILDREN, ADOLESCENTS, OBESITY, AND THE MEDIA
Council on Communications and Media

ABSTRACT. Obesity has become a worldwide public health problem. Considerable research has shown that the media contribute to the development of child and adolescent obesity, although the exact mechanism remains unclear. Screen time may displace more active pursuits, advertising of junk food and fast food increases children's requests for those particular foods and products, snacking increases while watching TV or movies, and late-night screen time may interfere with getting adequate amounts of sleep, which is a known risk factor for obesity. Sufficient evidence exists to warrant a ban on junk-food or fast-food advertising in children's TV programming. Pediatricians need to ask 2 questions about media use at every well-child or well-adolescent visit: (1) How much screen time is being spent per day? and (2) Is there a TV set or Internet connection in the child's bedroom? (7/11)
http://pediatrics.aappublications.org/content/128/1/201

CHILDREN, ADOLESCENTS, SUBSTANCE ABUSE, AND THE MEDIA
Victor C. Strasburger, MD, and Council on Communications and Media

ABSTRACT. The causes of adolescent substance use are multifactorial, but the media can play a key role. Tobacco and alcohol represent the 2 most significant drug threats to adolescents. More than $25 billion per year is spent on advertising for tobacco, alcohol, and prescription drugs, and such advertising has been shown to be effective. Digital media are increasingly being used to advertise drugs. In addition, exposure to PG-13– and R-rated movies at an early age may be a major factor in the onset of adolescent tobacco and alcohol use. The American Academy of Pediatrics recommends a ban on all tobacco advertising in all media, limitations on alcohol advertising, avoiding exposure of young children to substance-related (tobacco, alcohol, prescription drugs, illegal drugs) content on television and in PG-13– and R-rated movies, incorporating the topic of advertising and media into all substance abuse–prevention programs, and implementing media education programs in the classroom. (9/10)
http://pediatrics.aappublications.org/content/126/4/791

CHILDREN AND ADOLESCENTS AND DIGITAL MEDIA (TECHNICAL REPORT)
Yolanda (Linda) Reid Chassiakos, MD, FAAP; Jenny Radesky, MD, FAAP; Dimitri Christakis, MD, FAAP; Megan A. Moreno, MD, MSEd, MPH, FAAP; Corinn Cross, MD, FAAP; and Council on Communications and Media

ABSTRACT. Today's children and adolescents are immersed in both traditional and new forms of digital media. Research on traditional media, such as television, has identified health concerns and negative outcomes that correlate with the duration and content of viewing. Over the past decade, the use of digital media, including interactive and social media, has grown, and research evidence suggests that these newer media offer both benefits and risks to the health of children and teenagers. Evidence-based benefits identified from the use of digital and social media include early learning, exposure to new ideas and knowledge, increased opportunities for social contact and support, and new opportunities to access health promotion messages and information. Risks of such media include negative health effects on sleep, attention, and learning; a higher incidence of obesity and depression; exposure to inaccurate, inappropriate, or unsafe content and contacts; and compromised privacy and confidentiality. This technical report reviews the literature regarding these opportunities and risks, framed around clinical questions, for children from birth to adulthood. To promote health and wellness in children and adolescents, it is important to maintain adequate physical activity, healthy nutrition, good sleep hygiene, and a nurturing social environment. A healthy Family Media Use Plan (www.healthychildren.org/MediaUsePlan) that is individualized for a specific child, teenager, or family can identify an appropriate balance between screen time/online time and other activities, set boundaries for accessing content, guide displays of personal information, encourage age-appropriate critical thinking and digital literacy, and support open family communication and implementation of consistent rules about media use. (10/16)

See full text on page 569.

http://pediatrics.aappublications.org/content/138/5/e20162593

CHILDREN AS HEMATOPOIETIC STEM CELL DONORS
Committee on Bioethics

ABSTRACT. In the past half-century, hematopoietic stem cell transplantation has become standard treatment for a variety of diseases in children and adults, including selected hematologic malignancies, immunodeficiencies, hemoglobinopathies, bone marrow failure syndromes, and congenital metabolic disorders. There are 3 sources of allogeneic hematopoietic stem cells: bone marrow, peripheral blood, and umbilical cord blood; each has its own benefits and risks. Children often serve as hematopoietic stem cell donors, most commonly for their siblings. HLA-matched biological siblings are generally preferred as donors because of reduced risks of transplant-related complications as compared with unrelated donors. This statement includes a discussion of the ethical considerations regarding minors serving as stem cell donors, using the traditional benefit/burden calculation from the perspectives of both the donor and the recipient. The statement also includes an examination of the circumstances under which a minor may ethically participate as a hematopoietic stem cell donor, how the risks can be minimized, what the informed-consent process should entail, the role for a donor advocate (or some similar mechanism), and other ethical concerns. The American Academy of Pediatrics holds that minors can ethically serve as stem cell donors when specific criteria are fulfilled. (1/10)
http://pediatrics.aappublications.org/content/125/2/392

CHILDREN IN PICKUP TRUCKS
Committee on Injury and Poison Prevention

ABSTRACT. Pickup trucks have become increasingly popular in the United States. A recent study found that in crashes involving fatalities, cargo area passengers were 3 times more likely to die than were occupants in the cab. Compared with restrained cab occupants, the risk of death for those in the cargo area was 8 times higher. Furthermore, the increased use of extended-cab pickup trucks and air bag-equipped front passenger compartments creates concerns about the safe transport of children. The most effective preventive strategies are the legislative prohibition of travel in the cargo area and requirements for age-appropriate restraint use and seat selection in the cab. Parents should select vehicles that are appropriate for the safe transportation needs of the family. Physicians have an important role in counseling families and advocating public policy measures to reduce the number of deaths and injuries to occupants of pickup trucks. (10/00, reaffirmed 5/04, 1/07)
http://pediatrics.aappublications.org/content/106/4/857

CHILDREN'S HEALTH INSURANCE PROGRAM (CHIP): ACCOMPLISHMENTS, CHALLENGES, AND POLICY RECOMMENDATIONS
Committee on Child Health Financing

ABSTRACT. Sixteen years ago, the 105th Congress, responding to the needs of 10 million children in the United States who lacked health insurance, created the State Children's Health Insurance Program (SCHIP) as part of the Balanced Budget Act of 1997. Enacted as Title XXI of the Social Security Act, the Children's Health Insurance Program (CHIP; or SCHIP as it has been known at some points) provided states with federal assistance to create programs specifically designed for children from families with incomes that exceeded Medicaid thresholds but that were insufficient to enable them to afford private health insurance. Congress provided $40 billion in block grants over 10 years for states to expand their existing Medicaid programs to cover the intended populations, to erect new stand-alone SCHIP programs for these children, or to effect some combination of both options. Congress reauthorized CHIP once in 2009 under the Children's Health Insurance Program Reauthorization Act and extended its life further within provisions of the Patient Protection and Affordable Care Act of 2010. The purpose of this statement is to review the features of CHIP as it has evolved over the 16 years of its existence; to summarize what is known about the effects that the program has had on coverage, access, health status, and disparities among participants; to identify challenges that remain with respect to insuring this group of vulnerable children, including the impact that provisions of the new Affordable Care Act will have on the issue of health insurance coverage for near-poor children after 2015; and to offer recommendations on how to expand and strengthen the national commitment to provide health insurance to all children regardless of means. (2/14)
http://pediatrics.aappublications.org/content/133/3/e784

CHRONIC ABDOMINAL PAIN IN CHILDREN (CLINICAL REPORT)
Steering Committee on Quality Improvement and Management and Subcommittee on Chronic Abdominal Pain (joint with North American Society for Pediatric Gastroenterology, Hepatology, and Nutrition)

ABSTRACT. Children and adolescents with chronic abdominal pain pose unique challenges to their caregivers. Affected children and their families experience distress and anxiety that can interfere with their ability to perform regular daily activities. Although chronic abdominal pain in children is usually attributable to a functional disorder rather than organic disease, numerous misconceptions, insufficient knowledge among health care professionals, and inadequate application of knowledge may contribute to a lack of effective management. This clinical report accompanies a technical report (see page e370 in this issue) on childhood chronic abdominal pain and provides guidance for the clinician in the evaluation and

treatment of children with chronic abdominal pain. The recommendations are based on the evidence reviewed in the technical report and on consensus achieved among subcommittee members. (3/05)
http://pediatrics.aappublications.org/content/115/3/812

CHRONIC ABDOMINAL PAIN IN CHILDREN (TECHNICAL REPORT)
Steering Committee on Quality Improvement and Management and Subcommittee on Chronic Abdominal Pain (joint with North American Society for Pediatric Gastroenterology, Hepatology, and Nutrition)

ABSTRACT. Chronic abdominal pain, defined as long-lasting intermittent or constant abdominal pain, is a common pediatric problem encountered by primary care physicians, medical subspecialists, and surgical specialists. Chronic abdominal pain in children is usually functional, that is, without objective evidence of an underlying organic disorder. The Subcommittee on Chronic Abdominal Pain of the American Academy of Pediatrics and the North American Society for Pediatric Gastroenterology, Hepatology, and Nutrition has prepared this report based on a comprehensive, systematic review and rating of the medical literature. This report accompanies a clinical report based on the literature review and expert opinion.

The subcommittee examined the diagnostic and therapeutic value of a medical and psychological history, diagnostic tests, and pharmacologic and behavioral therapy. The presence of alarm symptoms or signs (such as weight loss, gastrointestinal bleeding, persistent fever, chronic severe diarrhea, and significant vomiting) is associated with a higher prevalence of organic disease. There was insufficient evidence to state that the nature of the abdominal pain or the presence of associated symptoms (such as anorexia, nausea, headache, and joint pain) can discriminate between functional and organic disorders. Although children with chronic abdominal pain and their parents are more often anxious or depressed, the presence of anxiety, depression, behavior problems, or recent negative life events does not distinguish between functional and organic abdominal pain. Most children who are brought to the primary care physician's office for chronic abdominal pain are unlikely to require diagnostic testing. Pediatric studies of therapeutic interventions were examined and found to be limited or inconclusive. (3/05)
http://pediatrics.aappublications.org/content/115/3/e370

CIRCUMCISION POLICY STATEMENT
Task Force on Circumcision

ABSTRACT. Male circumcision is a common procedure, generally performed during the newborn period in the United States. In 2007, the American Academy of Pediatrics (AAP) formed a multidisciplinary task force of AAP members and other stakeholders to evaluate the recent evidence on male circumcision and update the Academy's 1999 recommendations in this area. Evaluation of current evidence indicates that the health benefits of newborn male circumcision outweigh the risks and that the procedure's benefits justify access to this procedure for families who choose it. Specific benefits identified included prevention of urinary tract infections, penile cancer, and transmission of some sexually transmitted infections, including HIV. The American College of Obstetricians and Gynecologists has endorsed this statement. (8/12)
http://pediatrics.aappublications.org/content/130/3/585

CLASSIFYING RECOMMENDATIONS FOR CLINICAL PRACTICE GUIDELINES
Steering Committee on Quality Improvement and Management

ABSTRACT. Clinical practice guidelines are intended to improve the quality of clinical care by reducing inappropriate variations, producing optimal outcomes for patients, minimizing harm, and promoting cost-effective practices. This statement proposes an explicit classification of recommendations for clinical practice guidelines of the American Academy of Pediatrics (AAP) to promote communication among guideline developers, implementers, and other users of guideline knowledge, to improve consistency, and to facilitate user understanding. The statement describes 3 sequential activities in developing evidence-based clinical practice guidelines and related policies: (1) determination of the aggregate evidence quality in support of a proposed recommendation; (2) evaluation of the anticipated balance between benefits and harms when the recommendation is carried out; and (3) designation of recommendation strength. An individual policy can be reported as a "strong recommendation," "recommendation," "option," or "no recommendation." Use of this classification is intended to improve consistency and increase the transparency of the guideline-development process, facilitate understanding of AAP clinical practice guidelines, and enhance both the utility and credibility of AAP clinical practice guidelines. (9/04)
http://pediatrics.aappublications.org/content/114/3/874

CLIMATIC HEAT STRESS AND EXERCISING CHILDREN AND ADOLESCENTS
Council on Sports Medicine and Fitness and Council on School Health

ABSTRACT. Results of new research indicate that, contrary to previous thinking, youth do not have less effective thermoregulatory ability, insufficient cardiovascular capacity, or lower physical exertion tolerance compared with adults during exercise in the heat when adequate hydration is maintained. Accordingly, besides poor hydration status, the primary determinants of reduced performance and exertional heat-illness risk in youth during sports and other physical activities in a hot environment include undue physical exertion, insufficient recovery between repeated exercise bouts or closely scheduled same-day training sessions or rounds of sports competition, and inappropriately wearing clothing, uniforms, and protective equipment that play a role in excessive heat retention. Because these known contributing risk factors are modifiable, exertional heat illness is usually preventable. With appropriate preparation, modifications, and monitoring, most healthy children and adolescents can safely participate in outdoor sports and other physical activities through a wide range of challenging warm to hot climatic conditions. (8/11, reaffirmed 2/15)
http://pediatrics.aappublications.org/content/128/3/e741

CLINICAL GENETIC EVALUATION OF THE CHILD WITH MENTAL RETARDATION OR DEVELOPMENTAL DELAYS (CLINICAL REPORT)

John B. Moeschler, MD; Michael Shevell, MD; and Committee on Genetics

ABSTRACT. This clinical report describes the clinical genetic evaluation of the child with developmental delays or mental retardation. The purpose of this report is to describe the optimal clinical genetics diagnostic evaluation to assist pediatricians in providing a medical home for children with developmental delays or mental retardation and their families. The literature supports the benefit of expert clinical judgment by a consulting clinical geneticist in the diagnostic evaluation. However, it is recognized that local factors may preclude this particular option. No single approach to the diagnostic process is supported by the literature. This report addresses the diagnostic importance of clinical history, 3-generation family history, dysmorphologic examination, neurologic examination, chromosome analysis (≥650 bands), fragile X molecular genetic testing, fluorescence in situ hybridization studies for subtelomere chromosome rearrangements, molecular genetic testing for typical and atypical presentations of known syndromes, computed tomography and/or magnetic resonance brain imaging, and targeted studies for metabolic disorders. (6/06, reaffirmed 5/12)

http://pediatrics.aappublications.org/content/117/6/2304

CLINICAL PRACTICE POLICY TO PROTECT CHILDREN FROM TOBACCO, NICOTINE, AND TOBACCO SMOKE

Section on Tobacco Control

ABSTRACT. Tobacco dependence starts in childhood. Tobacco exposure of children is common and causes illness and premature death in children and adults, with adverse effects starting in the womb. There is no safe level of tobacco smoke exposure. Pediatricians should screen for use of tobacco and other nicotine delivery devices and provide anticipatory guidance to prevent smoking initiation and reduce tobacco smoke exposure. Pediatricians need to be aware of the different nicotine delivery systems marketed and available.

Parents and caregivers are important sources of children's tobacco smoke exposure. Because tobacco dependence is a severe addiction, to protect children's health, caregiver tobacco dependence treatment should be offered or referral for treatment should be provided (such as referral to the national smoker's quitline at 1-800-QUIT-NOW). If the source of tobacco exposure cannot be eliminated, counseling about reducing exposure to children should be provided.

Health care delivery systems should facilitate the effective prevention, identification, and treatment of tobacco dependence in children and adolescents, their parents, and other caregivers. Health care facilities should protect children from tobacco smoke exposure and tobacco promotion. Tobacco dependence prevention and treatment should be part of medical education, with knowledge assessed as part of board certification examinations. (10/15)

http://pediatrics.aappublications.org/content/136/5/1008

CLOSTRIDIUM DIFFICILE INFECTION IN INFANTS AND CHILDREN

Committee on Infectious Diseases

ABSTRACT. Infections caused by *Clostridium difficile* in hospitalized children are increasing. The recent publication of clinical practice guidelines for *C difficile* infection in adults did not address issues that are specific to children. The purpose of this policy statement is to provide the pediatrician with updated information and recommendations about *C difficile* infections affecting pediatric patients. (12/12)

http://pediatrics.aappublications.org/content/131/1/196

COCHLEAR IMPLANTS IN CHILDREN: SURGICAL SITE INFECTIONS AND PREVENTION AND TREATMENT OF ACUTE OTITIS MEDIA AND MENINGITIS

Lorry G. Rubin, MD; Blake Papsin, MD; Committee on Infectious Diseases; and Section on Otolaryngology–Head and Neck Surgery

ABSTRACT. The use of cochlear implants is increasingly common, particularly in children younger than 3 years. Bacterial meningitis, often with associated acute otitis media, is more common in children with cochlear implants than in groups of control children. Children with profound deafness who are candidates for cochlear implants should receive all age-appropriate doses of pneumococcal conjugate and Haemophilus influenzae type b conjugate vaccines and appropriate annual immunization against influenza. In addition, starting at 24 months of age, a single dose of 23-valent pneumococcal polysaccharide vaccine should be administered. Before implant surgery, primary care providers and cochlear implant teams should ensure that immunizations are up-to-date, preferably with completion of indicated vaccines at least 2 weeks before implant surgery. Imaging of the temporal bone/inner ear should be performed before cochlear implantation in all children with congenital deafness and all patients with profound hearing impairment and a history of bacterial meningitis to identify those with inner-ear malformations/cerebrospinal fluid fistulas or ossification of the cochlea. During the initial months after cochlear implantation, the risk of complications of acute otitis media may be higher than during subsequent time periods. Therefore, it is recommended that acute otitis media diagnosed during the first 2 months after implantation be initially treated with a parenteral antibiotic (eg, ceftriaxone or cefotaxime). Episodes occurring 2 months or longer after implantation can be treated with a trial of an oral antimicrobial agent (eg, amoxicillin or amoxicillin/clavulanate at a dose of approximately 90 mg/kg per day of amoxicillin component), provided the child does not appear toxic and the implant does not have a spacer/positioner, a wedge that rests in the cochlea next to the electrodes present in certain implant models available between 1999 and 2002. "Watchful waiting" without antimicrobial therapy is inappropriate for children with implants with acute otitis media. If feasible, tympanocentesis should be performed for acute otitis media, and the material should be sent for culture, but performance of this procedure should not result in an undue delay in initiating antimicrobial therapy. For patients with suspected meningitis, cerebrospinal fluid as well as middle-ear fluid, if present, should be sent for culture. Empiric antimicrobial therapy for meningitis occurring within 2 months of implantation should include an agent with broad activity against Gram-negative bacilli (eg, meropenem) plus vancomycin. For meningitis occurring 2 months or longer after implantation, standard empiric antimicrobial therapy for meningitis (eg, ceftriaxone plus vancomycin) is indicated. For patients with meningitis, urgent evaluation by an otolaryngologist is indicated for consideration of imaging and surgical exploration. (7/10)

http://pediatrics.aappublications.org/content/126/2/381

CODEINE: TIME TO SAY "NO" (CLINICAL REPORT)

Joseph D. Tobias, MD; Thomas P. Green, MD; Charles J. Coté, MD; Section on Anesthesiology and Pain Medicine; and Committee on Drugs

ABSTRACT. Codeine has been prescribed to pediatric patients for many decades as both an analgesic and an antitussive agent. Codeine is a prodrug with little inherent pharmacologic activity and must be metabolized in the liver into morphine, which is responsible for codeine's analgesic effects. However, there is substantial genetic variability in the activity of the responsible hepatic enzyme, *CYP2D6*, and, as a consequence, individual patient response to codeine varies from no effect to high sensitivity. Drug surveillance has documented the occurrence of unanticipated respiratory depression and death after receiving codeine in children, many of whom have been shown to be ultrarapid metabolizers. Patients with documented or suspected obstructive sleep apnea appear to be at particular risk because of opioid sensitivity, compounding the danger among rapid metabolizers in this group. Recently, various organizations and regulatory bodies, including the World Health Organization, the US Food and Drug Administration, and the European Medicines Agency, have promulgated stern warnings regarding the occurrence of adverse effects of codeine in children. These and other groups have or are considering a declaration of a contraindication for the use of codeine for children as either an analgesic or an antitussive. Additional clinical research must extend the understanding of the risks and benefits of both opioid and nonopioid alternatives for orally administered, effective agents for acute and chronic pain. (9/16)

See full text on page 589.

http://pediatrics.aappublications.org/content/138/4/e20162396

COLLABORATIVE ROLE OF THE PEDIATRICIAN IN THE DIAGNOSIS AND MANAGEMENT OF BIPOLAR DISORDER IN ADOLESCENTS (CLINICAL REPORT)

Benjamin N. Shain, MD, PhD, and Committee on Adolescence

ABSTRACT. Despite the complexity of diagnosis and management, pediatricians have an important collaborative role in referring and partnering in the management of adolescents with bipolar disorder. This report presents the classification of bipolar disorder as well as interviewing and diagnostic guidelines. Treatment options are described, particularly focusing on medication management and rationale for the common practice of multiple, simultaneous medications. Medication adverse effects may be problematic and better managed with

collaboration between mental health professionals and pediatricians. Case examples illustrate a number of common diagnostic and management issues. (11/12)

http://pediatrics.aappublications.org/content/130/6/e1725

COMMUNICATING WITH CHILDREN AND FAMILIES: FROM EVERYDAY INTERACTIONS TO SKILL IN CONVEYING DISTRESSING INFORMATION (TECHNICAL REPORT)

Marcia Levetown, MD, and Committee on Bioethics

ABSTRACT. Health care communication is a skill that is critical to safe and effective medical practice; it can and must be taught. Communication skill influences patient disclosure, treatment adherence and outcome, adaptation to illness, and bereavement. This article provides a review of the evidence regarding clinical communication in the pediatric setting, covering the spectrum from outpatient primary care consultation to death notification, and provides practical suggestions to improve communication with patients and families, enabling more effective, efficient, and empathic pediatric health care. (5/08, reaffirmed 5/11)

http://pediatrics.aappublications.org/content/121/5/e1441

COMMUNITY PEDIATRICS: NAVIGATING THE INTERSECTION OF MEDICINE, PUBLIC HEALTH, AND SOCIAL DETERMINANTS OF CHILDREN'S HEALTH

Council on Community Pediatrics

ABSTRACT. This policy statement provides a framework for the pediatrician's role in promoting the health and well-being of all children in the context of their families and communities. It offers pediatricians a definition of community pediatrics, emphasizes the importance of recognizing social determinants of health, and delineates the need to partner with public health to address population-based child health issues. It also recognizes the importance of pediatric involvement in child advocacy at local, state, and federal levels to ensure all children have access to a high-quality medical home and to eliminate child health disparities. This statement provides a set of specific recommendations that underscore the critical nature of this dimension of pediatric practice, teaching, and research. (2/13)

http://pediatrics.aappublications.org/content/131/3/623

COMPREHENSIVE EVALUATION OF THE CHILD WITH INTELLECTUAL DISABILITY OR GLOBAL DEVELOPMENTAL DELAYS (CLINICAL REPORT)

John B. Moeschler, MD, MS, FAAP, FACMG; Michael Shevell, MDCM, FRCP; and Committee on Genetics

ABSTRACT. Global developmental delay and intellectual disability are relatively common pediatric conditions. This report describes the recommended clinical genetics diagnostic approach. The report is based on a review of published reports, most consisting of medium to large case series of diagnostic tests used, and the proportion of those that led to a diagnosis in such patients. Chromosome microarray is designated as a first-line test and replaces the standard karyotype and fluorescent in situ hybridization subtelomere tests for the child with intellectual disability of unknown etiology. Fragile X testing remains an important first-line test. The importance of considering testing for inborn errors of metabolism in this population is supported by a recent systematic review of the literature

and several case series recently published. The role of brain MRI remains important in certain patients. There is also a discussion of the emerging literature on the use of whole-exome sequencing as a diagnostic test in this population. Finally, the importance of intentional comanagement among families, the medical home, and the clinical genetics specialty clinic is discussed. (8/14)
http://pediatrics.aappublications.org/content/134/3/e903

COMPREHENSIVE HEALTH EVALUATION OF THE NEWLY ADOPTED CHILD (CLINICAL REPORT)

Veronnie F. Jones, MD, PhD, MSPH, and Committee on Early Childhood, Adoption, and Dependent Care

ABSTRACT. Children who join families through the process of adoption often have multiple health care needs. After placement in an adoptive home, it is essential that these children have a timely comprehensive health evaluation. This evaluation should include a review of all available medical records and a complete physical examination. Evaluation should also include diagnostic testing based on the findings from the history and physical examination as well as the risks presented by the child's previous living conditions. Age-appropriate screens should be performed, including, for example, newborn screening panels, hearing, vision, dental, and formal behavioral/developmental screens. The comprehensive assessment can occur at the time of the initial visit to the physician after adoptive placement or can take place over several visits. Adopted children should be referred to other medical specialists as deemed appropriate. The Section on Adoption and Foster Care is a resource within the American Academy of Pediatrics for physicians providing care for children who are being adopted. (12/11, reaffirmed 9/15)
http://pediatrics.aappublications.org/content/129/1/e214

CONDOM USE BY ADOLESCENTS

Committee on Adolescence

ABSTRACT. Rates of sexual activity, pregnancies, and births among adolescents have continued to decline during the past decade to historic lows. Despite these positive trends, many adolescents remain at risk for unintended pregnancy and sexually transmitted infections (STIs). This policy statement has been developed to assist the pediatrician in understanding and supporting the use of condoms by their patients to prevent unintended pregnancies and STIs and address barriers to their use. When used consistently and correctly, male latex condoms reduce the risk of pregnancy and many STIs, including HIV. Since the last policy statement published 12 years ago, there is an increased evidence base supporting the protection provided by condoms against STIs. Rates of acquisition of STIs/HIV among adolescents remain unacceptably high. Interventions that increase availability or accessibility to condoms are most efficacious when combined with additional individual, small-group, or community-level activities that include messages about safer sex. Continued research is needed to inform public health interventions for adolescents that increase the consistent and correct use of condoms and promote dual protection of condoms for STI prevention with other effective methods of contraception. (10/13)
http://pediatrics.aappublications.org/content/132/5/973

CONFLICTS BETWEEN RELIGIOUS OR SPIRITUAL BELIEFS AND PEDIATRIC CARE: INFORMED REFUSAL, EXEMPTIONS, AND PUBLIC FUNDING

Committee on Bioethics

ABSTRACT. Although respect for parents' decision-making authority is an important principle, pediatricians should report suspected cases of medical neglect, and the state should, at times, intervene to require medical treatment of children. Some parents' reasons for refusing medical treatment are based on their religious or spiritual beliefs. In cases in which treatment is likely to prevent death or serious disability or relieve severe pain, children's health and future autonomy should be protected. Because religious exemptions to child abuse and neglect laws do not equally protect all children and may harm some children by causing confusion about the duty to provide medical treatment, these exemptions should be repealed. Furthermore, public health care funds should not cover alternative unproven religious or spiritual healing practices. Such payments may inappropriately legitimize these practices as appropriate medical treatment. (10/13)
http://pediatrics.aappublications.org/content/132/5/962

CONGENITAL ADRENAL HYPERPLASIA (TECHNICAL REPORT)

Section on Endocrinology and Committee on Genetics

ABSTRACT. The Section on Endocrinology and the Committee on Genetics of the American Academy of Pediatrics, in collaboration with experts from the field of pediatric endocrinology and genetics, developed this policy statement as a means of providing up-to-date information for the practicing pediatrician about current practice and controversial issues in congenital adrenal hyperplasia (CAH), including the current status of prenatal diagnosis and treatment, the benefits and problem areas of neonatal screening programs, and the management of children with nonclassic CAH. The reference list is designed to allow physicians who wish more information to research the topic more thoroughly. (12/00, reaffirmed 10/04)
http://pediatrics.aappublications.org/content/106/6/1511

CONGENITAL BRAIN AND SPINAL CORD MALFORMATIONS AND THEIR ASSOCIATED CUTANEOUS MARKERS (CLINICAL REPORT)

Mark Dias, MD, FAANS, FAAP; Michael Partington, MD, FAANS, FAAP; and Section on Neurologic Surgery

ABSTRACT. The brain, spinal cord, and skin are all derived from the embryonic ectoderm; this common derivation leads to a high association between central nervous system dysraphic malformations and abnormalities of the overlying skin. A myelomeningocele is an obvious open malformation, the identification of which is not usually difficult. However, the relationship between congenital spinal cord malformations and other cutaneous malformations, such as dimples, vascular anomalies (including infantile hemangiomata and other vascular malformations), congenital pigmented nevi or other hamartomata, or midline hairy patches may be less obvious but no less important. Pediatricians should be aware of these associations, recognize the cutaneous markers associated with congenital central nervous system malformations, and refer children with such markers to the appropriate specialist in a timely fashion for further evaluation and treatment. (9/15)

http://pediatrics.aappublications.org/content/136/4/e1105

A CONSENSUS STATEMENT ON HEALTH CARE TRANSITIONS FOR YOUNG ADULTS WITH SPECIAL HEALTH CARE NEEDS

American Academy of Pediatrics, American Academy of Family Physicians, and American College of Physicians-American Society of Internal Medicine

ABSTRACT. This policy statement represents a consensus on the critical first steps that the medical profession needs to take to realize the vision of a family-centered, continuous, comprehensive, coordinated, compassionate, and culturally competent health care system that is as developmentally appropriate as it is technically sophisticated. The goal of transition in health care for young adults with special health care needs is to maximize lifelong functioning and potential through the provision of high-quality, developmentally appropriate health care services that continue uninterrupted as the individual moves from adolescence to adulthood. This consensus document has now been approved as policy by the boards of the American Academy of Pediatrics, the American Academy of Family Physicians, and the American College of Physicians-American Society of Internal Medicine. (12/02)

http://pediatrics.aappublications.org/content/110/
Supplement_3/1304

CONSENT BY PROXY FOR NONURGENT PEDIATRIC CARE (CLINICAL REPORT)

Gary N. McAbee, DO, JD, and Committee on Medical Liability and Risk Management

ABSTRACT. Minor-aged patients are often brought to the pediatrician for nonurgent acute medical care, physical examinations, or health supervision visits by someone other than their legally authorized representative, which, in most situations, is a parent. These surrogates or proxies can be members of the child's extended family, such as a grandparent, adult sibling, or aunt/uncle; a noncustodial parent or stepparent in cases of divorce and remarriage; an adult who lives in the home but is not biologically or legally related to the child; or even a child care professional (eg, au pair, nanny). This report identifies common situations in which pediatricians may encounter "consent by proxy" for nonurgent medical care for minors, including physical examinations, and explains the potential for liability exposure associated with these circumstances. The report suggests practical steps that balance the need to minimize the physician's liability exposure with the patient's access to health care. Key issues to be considered when creating or updating office policies for obtaining and documenting consent by proxy are offered. (10/10)

http://pediatrics.aappublications.org/content/126/5/1022

CONSENT FOR EMERGENCY MEDICAL SERVICES FOR CHILDREN AND ADOLESCENTS

Committee on Pediatric Emergency Medicine and Committee on Bioethics

ABSTRACT. Parental consent generally is required for the medical evaluation and treatment of minor children. However, children and adolescents might require evaluation of and treatment for emergency medical conditions in situations in which a parent or legal guardian is not available to provide consent or conditions under which an adolescent patient might possess the legal authority to provide consent. In general, a medical screening examination and any medical care necessary and likely to prevent imminent and significant harm to the pediatric patient with an emergency medical condition should not be withheld or delayed because of problems obtaining consent. The purpose of this policy statement is to provide guidance in those situations in which parental consent is not readily available, in which parental consent is not necessary, or in which parental refusal of consent places a child at risk of significant harm. (7/11, reaffirmed 9/15)

http://pediatrics.aappublications.org/content/128/2/427

CONSUMPTION OF RAW OR UNPASTEURIZED MILK AND MILK PRODUCTS BY PREGNANT WOMEN AND CHILDREN

Committee on Infectious Diseases and Committee on Nutrition

ABSTRACT. Sales of raw or unpasteurized milk and milk products are still legal in at least 30 states in the United States. Raw milk and milk products from cows, goats, and sheep continue to be a source of bacterial infections attributable to a number of virulent pathogens, including *Listeria monocytogenes*, *Campylobacter jejuni*, *Salmonella* species, *Brucella* species, and *Escherichia coli* O157. These infections can occur in both healthy and immunocompromised individuals, including older adults, infants, young children, and pregnant women and their unborn fetuses, in whom life-threatening infections and fetal miscarriage can occur. Efforts to limit the sale of raw milk products have met with opposition from those who are proponents of the purported health benefits of consuming raw milk products, which contain natural or unprocessed factors not inactivated by pasteurization. However, the benefits of these natural factors have not been clearly demonstrated in evidence-based studies and, therefore, do not outweigh the risks of raw milk consumption. Substantial data suggest that pasteurized milk confers equivalent health benefits compared with raw milk, without the additional risk of bacterial infections. The purpose of this policy statement was to review the risks of raw milk consumption in the United States and to provide evidence of the risks of infectious complications associated with consumption of unpasteurized milk and milk products, especially among pregnant women, infants, and children. (12/13)

http://pediatrics.aappublications.org/content/133/1/175

CONTRACEPTION FOR ADOLESCENTS

Committee on Adolescence

ABSTRACT. Contraception is a pillar in reducing adolescent pregnancy rates. The American Academy of Pediatrics recommends that pediatricians develop a working knowledge of contraception to help adolescents reduce risks of and negative health consequences related to unintended pregnancy. Over the past 10 years, a number of new contraceptive methods have become available to adolescents, newer guidance has been issued on existing contraceptive methods, and the evidence base for contraception for special populations (adolescents who have disabilities, are obese, are recipients of solid organ transplants, or are HIV infected) has expanded. The Academy has addressed contraception since 1980, and this policy statement updates the 2007 statement on contraception and adolescents. It provides the pediatrician with a description and rationale for best practices in counseling and prescribing contraception for adolescents. It is supported by an accompanying technical report. (9/14)

http://pediatrics.aappublications.org/content/134/4/e1244

CONTRACEPTION FOR ADOLESCENTS (TECHNICAL REPORT)

Mary A. Ott, MD, MA, FAAP; Gina S. Sucato, MD, MPH, FAAP; and Committee on Adolescence

ABSTRACT. A working knowledge of contraception will assist the pediatrician in both sexual health promotion as well as treatment of common adolescent gynecologic problems. Best practices in adolescent anticipatory guidance and screening include a sexual health history, screening for pregnancy and sexually transmitted infections, counseling, and if indicated, providing access to contraceptives. Pediatricians' long-term relationships with adolescents and families allow them to help promote healthy sexual decision-making, including abstinence and contraceptive use. Additionally, medical indications for contraception, such as acne, dysmenorrhea, and heavy menstrual bleeding, are frequently uncovered during adolescent visits. This technical report provides an evidence base for the accompanying policy statement and addresses key aspects of adolescent contraceptive use, including the following: (1) sexual history taking, confidentiality, and counseling; (2) adolescent data on the use and side effects of newer contraceptive methods; (3) new data on older contraceptive methods; and (4) evidence supporting the use of contraceptives in adolescent patients with complex medical conditions. (9/14)

http://pediatrics.aappublications.org/content/134/4/e1257

CONTRACEPTION FOR HIV-INFECTED ADOLESCENTS (CLINICAL REPORT)

Athena P. Kourtis, MD, PhD, MPH, FAAP; Ayesha Mirza, MD, FAAP; and Committee on Pediatric AIDS

ABSTRACT. Access to high-quality reproductive health care is important for adolescents and young adults with HIV infection to prevent unintended pregnancies, sexually transmitted infections, and secondary transmission of HIV to partners and children. As perinatally HIV-infected children mature into adolescence and adulthood and new HIV infections among adolescents and young adults continue to occur in the United States, medical providers taking care of such individuals often face issues related to sexual and reproductive health. Challenges including drug interactions between several hormonal methods and antiretroviral agents make decisions regarding contraceptive options more complex for these adolescents. Dual protection, defined as the use of an effective contraceptive along with condoms, should be central to ongoing discussions with HIV-infected young women and couples wishing to avoid pregnancy. Last, reproductive health discussions need to be integrated with discussions on HIV care, because a reduction in plasma HIV viral load below the level of detection (an "undetectable viral load") is essential for the individual's health as well as for a reduction in HIV transmission to partners and children. (8/16)

See full text on page 599.

http://pediatrics.aappublications.org/content/138/3/e20161892

CONTROVERSIES CONCERNING VITAMIN K AND THE NEWBORN

Committee on Fetus and Newborn

ABSTRACT. Prevention of early vitamin K deficiency bleeding (VKDB) of the newborn, with onset at birth to 2 weeks of age (formerly known as classic hemorrhagic disease of the newborn), by oral or parenteral administration of vitamin K is accepted practice. In contrast, late VKDB, with onset from 2 to 12 weeks of age, is most effectively prevented by parenteral administration of vitamin K. Earlier concern regarding a possible causal association between parenteral vitamin K and childhood cancer has not been substantiated. This revised statement presents updated recommendations for the use of vitamin K in the prevention of early and late VKDB. (7/03, reaffirmed 5/06, 5/09, 9/14)

http://pediatrics.aappublications.org/content/112/1/191

COPARENT OR SECOND-PARENT ADOPTION BY SAME-SEX PARENTS

Committee on Psychosocial Aspects of Child and Family Health

ABSTRACT. Children who are born to or adopted by 1 member of a same-sex couple deserve the security of 2 legally recognized parents. Therefore, the American Academy of Pediatrics supports legislative and legal efforts to provide the possibility of adoption of the child by the second parent or coparent in these families. (2/02, reaffirmed 5/09)

http://pediatrics.aappublications.org/content/109/2/339

COPARENT OR SECOND-PARENT ADOPTION BY SAME-SEX PARENTS (TECHNICAL REPORT)

Committee on Psychosocial Aspects of Child and Family Health

ABSTRACT. A growing body of scientific literature demonstrates that children who grow up with 1 or 2 gay and/or lesbian parents fare as well in emotional, cognitive, social, and sexual functioning as do children whose parents are heterosexual. Children's optimal development seems to be influenced more by the nature of the relationships and interactions within the family unit than by the particular structural form it takes. (2/02, reaffirmed 5/09)

http://pediatrics.aappublications.org/content/109/2/341

CORPORAL PUNISHMENT IN SCHOOLS

Committee on School Health

ABSTRACT. The American Academy of Pediatrics recommends that corporal punishment in schools be abolished in all states by law and that alternative forms of student behavior management be used. (8/00, reaffirmed 6/03, 5/06, 2/12)

http://pediatrics.aappublications.org/content/106/2/343

COUNSELING FAMILIES WHO CHOOSE COMPLEMENTARY AND ALTERNATIVE MEDICINE FOR THEIR CHILD WITH CHRONIC ILLNESS OR DISABILITY

Committee on Children With Disabilities

ABSTRACT. The use of complementary and alternative medicine (CAM) to treat chronic illness or disability is increasing in the United States. This is especially evident among children with autism and related disorders. It may be challenging to the practicing pediatrician to distinguish among accepted biomedical treatments, unproven therapies, and alternative therapies. Moreover, there are no published guidelines regarding the use of CAM in the care of children with chronic illness or disability. To best serve the interests of children, it is important to maintain a scientific perspective, to provide balanced advice about therapeutic options, to guard against bias, and to establish and maintain a trusting relationship with families. This statement provides information and guidance for pediatricians when counseling families about CAM. (3/01, reaffirmed 1/05, 5/10)

http://pediatrics.aappublications.org/content/107/3/598

COUNSELING THE ADOLESCENT ABOUT PREGNANCY OPTIONS

Committee on Adolescence

ABSTRACT. When consulted by a pregnant adolescent, pediatricians should be able to make a timely diagnosis and to help the adolescent understand her options and act on her decision to continue or terminate her pregnancy. Pediatricians may not impose their values on the decision-making process and should be prepared to support the adolescent in her decision or refer her to a physician who can. (5/98, reaffirmed 1/01, 1/06)

http://pediatrics.aappublications.org/content/101/5/938

COUNTERING VACCINE HESITANCY (CLINICAL REPORT)

Kathryn M. Edwards, MD; Jesse M. Hackell, MD; Committee on Infectious Diseases; and Committee on Practice and Ambulatory Medicine

ABSTRACT. Immunizations have led to a significant decrease in rates of vaccine-preventable diseases and have made a significant impact on the health of children. However, some parents express concerns about vaccine safety and the necessity of vaccines. The concerns of parents range from hesitancy about some immunizations to refusal of all vaccines. This clinical report provides information about addressing parental concerns about vaccination. (8/16)

See full text on page 615.

http://pediatrics.aappublications.org/content/138/3/e20162146

CREATING HEALTHY CAMP EXPERIENCES

Council on School Health

ABSTRACT. The American Academy of Pediatrics has created recommendations for health appraisal and preparation of young people before participation in day or resident camps and to guide health and safety practices for children at camp. These recommendations are intended for parents, primary health care providers, and camp administration and health center staff. Although camps have diverse environments, there are general guidelines that apply to all situations and specific recommendations that are appropriate under special conditions. This policy statement has been reviewed and is supported by the American Camp Association. (3/11)

http://pediatrics.aappublications.org/content/127/4/794

CRITICAL ELEMENTS FOR THE PEDIATRIC PERIOPERATIVE ANESTHESIA ENVIRONMENT

Section on Anesthesiology and Pain Medicine

ABSTRACT. The American Academy of Pediatrics proposes guidance for the pediatric perioperative anesthesia environment. Essential components are identified to optimize the perioperative environment for the anesthetic care of infants and children. Such an environment promotes the safety and well-being of infants and children by reducing the risk of adverse events. (11/15)

http://pediatrics.aappublications.org/content/136/6/1200

THE CRUCIAL ROLE OF RECESS IN SCHOOL

Council on School Health

ABSTRACT. Recess is at the heart of a vigorous debate over the role of schools in promoting the optimal development of the whole child. A growing trend toward reallocating time in school to accentuate the more academic subjects has put this important facet of a child's school day at risk. Recess serves as a necessary break from the rigors of concentrated, academic challenges in the classroom. But equally important is the fact that safe and well-supervised recess offers cognitive, social, emotional, and physical benefits that may not be fully appreciated when a decision is made to diminish it. Recess is unique from, and a complement to, physical education—not a substitute for it. The American Academy of Pediatrics believes that recess is a crucial and necessary component of a child's development and, as such, it should not be withheld for punitive or academic reasons. (12/12, reaffirmed 8/16)

http://pediatrics.aappublications.org/content/131/1/183

DEALING WITH THE PARENT WHOSE JUDGMENT IS IMPAIRED BY ALCOHOL OR DRUGS: LEGAL AND ETHICAL CONSIDERATIONS (CLINICAL REPORT)

Committee on Medical Liability

ABSTRACT. An estimated 11 to 17.5 million children are being raised by a substance-abusing parent or guardian. The importance of this statistic is undeniable, particularly when a patient is brought to a pediatric office by a parent or guardian exhibiting symptoms of judgment impairment. Although the physician-patient relationship exists between the pediatrician and the minor patient, other obligations (some perceived and some real) should be considered as well. In managing encounters with impaired parents who may become disruptive or dangerous, pediatricians should be aware of their responsibilities before acting. In addition to fulfilling the duty involved with an established physician-patient relationship, the pediatrician should take reasonable care to safeguard patient confidentiality; protect the safety of the patient and other patients, visitors, and employees; and comply with reporting mandates. This clinical report identifies and discusses the legal and ethical concepts related to these circumstances. The report offers implementation suggestions when establishing anticipatory office procedures and training programs for staff on what to do (and not do) in

such situations to maximize the patient's well-being and safety and minimize the liability of the pediatrician. (9/04, reaffirmed 9/10)
http://pediatrics.aappublications.org/content/114/3/869

DEATH OF A CHILD IN THE EMERGENCY DEPARTMENT

Committee on Pediatric Emergency Medicine (joint with American College of Emergency Physicians Pediatric Emergency Medicine Committee and Emergency Nurses Association Pediatric Committee)

ABSTRACT. The American Academy of Pediatrics, American College of Emergency Physicians, and Emergency Nurses Association have collaborated to identify practices and principles to guide the care of children, families, and staff in the challenging and uncommon event of the death of a child in the emergency department in this policy statement and in an accompanying technical report. (6/14)
http://pediatrics.aappublications.org/content/134/1/198

DEATH OF A CHILD IN THE EMERGENCY DEPARTMENT (TECHNICAL REPORT)

Patricia O'Malley, MD; Isabel Barata, MD; Sally Snow, RN; and Committee on Pediatric Emergency Medicine (joint with American College of Emergency Physicians Pediatric Emergency Medicine Committee and Emergency Nurses Association Pediatric Committee)

ABSTRACT. The death of a child in the emergency department (ED) is one of the most challenging problems facing ED clinicians. This revised technical report and accompanying policy statement reaffirm principles of patient- and family-centered care. Recent literature is examined regarding family presence, termination of resuscitation, bereavement responsibilities of ED clinicians, support of child fatality review efforts, and other issues inherent in caring for the patient, family, and staff when a child dies in the ED. Appendices are provided that offer an approach to bereavement activities in the ED, carrying out forensic responsibilities while providing compassionate care, communicating the news of the death of a child in the acute setting, providing a closing ritual at the time of terminating resuscitation efforts, and managing the child with a terminal condition who presents near death in the ED. (6/14)
http://pediatrics.aappublications.org/content/134/1/e313

DEFINITION OF A PEDIATRICIAN

Committee on Pediatric Workforce

POLICY. The American Academy of Pediatrics (AAP) has developed the following definition of pediatrics and a pediatrician:

Pediatrics is the specialty of medical science concerned with the physical, mental, and social health of children from birth to young adulthood. Pediatric care encompasses a broad spectrum of health services ranging from preventive health care to the diagnosis and treatment of acute and chronic diseases.

Pediatrics is a discipline that deals with biological, social, and environmental influences on the developing child and with the impact of disease and dysfunction on development. Children differ from adults anatomically, physiologically, immunologically, psychologically, developmentally, and metabolically.

The pediatrician, a term that includes primary care pediatricians, pediatric medical subspecialists, and pediatric surgical specialists, understands this constantly changing functional status of his or her patients' incident to growth and development and the consequent changing standards of "normal" for age. A pediatrician is a physician who is concerned primarily with the health, welfare, and development of children and is uniquely qualified for these endeavors by virtue of interest and initial training. This training includes 4 years of medical school education, plus an additional year or years (usually at least 3) of intensive training devoted solely to all aspects of medical care for children, adolescents, and young adults. Maintenance of these competencies is achieved by experience, training, continuous education, self-assessment, and practice improvement.

A pediatrician is able to define accurately the child's health status and to serve as a consultant and make use of other specialists as consultants as needed, ideally in the context of, or in conjunction with, the physician-led medical home. Because the child's welfare is heavily dependent on the home and family, the pediatrician supports efforts to create a nurturing environment. Such support includes education about healthful living and anticipatory guidance for both patients and parents.

A pediatrician participates at the community level in preventing or solving problems in child health care and publicly advocates the causes of children. (3/15)
http://pediatrics.aappublications.org/content/135/4/780

DEVELOPMENTAL DYSPLASIA OF THE HIP PRACTICE GUIDELINE (TECHNICAL REPORT)

Harold P. Lehmann, MD, PhD; Richard Hinton, MD, MPH; Paola Morello, MD; Jeanne Santoli, MD; in conjunction with Steering Committee on Quality Improvement and Subcommittee on Developmental Dysplasia of the Hip

ABSTRACT. *Objective.* To create a recommendation for pediatricians and other primary care providers about their role as screeners for detecting developmental dysplasia of the hip (DDH) in children.

Patients. Theoretical cohorts of newborns.

Method. Model-based approach using decision analysis as the foundation. Components of the approach include the following:

Perspective: Primary care provider.

Outcomes: DDH, avascular necrosis of the hip (AVN).

Options: Newborn screening by pediatric examination; orthopaedic examination; ultrasonographic examination; orthopaedic or ultrasonographic examination by risk factors. Intercurrent health supervision-based screening.

Preferences: 0 for bad outcomes, 1 for best outcomes.

Model: Influence diagram assessed by the Subcommittee and by the methodology team, with critical feedback from the Subcommittee.

Evidence Sources: Medline and EMBASE search of the research literature through June 1996. Hand search of sentinel journals from June 1996 through March 1997. Ancestor search of accepted articles.

Evidence Quality: Assessed on a custom subjective scale, based primarily on the fit of the evidence to the decision model.

Results. After discussion, explicit modeling, and critique, an influence diagram of 31 nodes was created. The computer-based and the hand literature searches found 534 articles, 101 of which were reviewed by 2 or more readers. Ancestor searches of these yielded a further 17 articles for evidence abstraction. Articles came from around the globe, although primarily Europe, British Isles, Scandinavia, and their descendants. There were 5 controlled trials, each with a sample size less than 40. The remainder were case series. Evidence was available for 17 of the desired 30 probabilities. Evidence quality ranged primarily between one third and two thirds of the maximum attainable score (median: 10–21; interquartile range: 8–14). Based on the raw evidence and Bayesian hierarchical meta-analyses, our estimate for the incidence of DDH revealed by physical examination performed by pediatricians is 8.6 per 1000; for orthopaedic screening, 11.5; for ultrasonography, 25. The odds ratio for DDH, given breech delivery, is 5.5; for female sex, 4.1; for positive family history, 1.7, although this last factor is not statistically significant. Postneonatal cases of DDH were divided into mid-term (younger than 6 months of age) and late-term (older than 6 months of age). Our estimates for the mid-term rate for screening by pediatricians is 0.34/1000 children screened; for orthopaedists, 0.1; and for ultrasonography, 0.28. Our estimates for late-term DDH rates are 0.21/1000 newborns screened by pediatricians; 0.08, by orthopaedists; and 0.2 for ultrasonography. The rates of AVN for children referred before 6 months of age is estimated at 2.5/1000 infants referred. For those referred after 6 months of age, our estimate is 109/1000 referred infants. The decision model (reduced, based on available evidence) suggests that orthopaedic screening is optimal, but because orthopaedists in the published studies and in practice would differ, the supply of orthopaedists is relatively limited, and the difference between orthopaedists and pediatricians is statistically insignificant, we conclude that pediatric screening is to be recommended. The place of ultrasonography in the screening process remains to be defined because there are too few data about postneonatal diagnosis by ultrasonographic screening to permit definitive recommendations. These data could be used by others to refine the conclusions based on costs, parental preferences, or physician style. Areas for research are well defined by our model-based approach. (4/00)
http://pediatrics.aappublications.org/content/105/4/e57

DIAGNOSIS AND MANAGEMENT OF AN INITIAL UTI IN FEBRILE INFANTS AND YOUNG CHILDREN (TECHNICAL REPORT)

S. Maria E. Finnell, MD, MS; Aaron E. Carroll, MD, MS; Stephen M. Downs, MD, MS; Steering Committee on Quality Improvement and Management; and Subcommittee on Urinary Tract Infection

ABSTRACT. *Objectives.* The diagnosis and management of urinary tract infections (UTIs) in young children are clinically challenging. This report was developed to inform the revised, evidence-based, clinical guideline regarding the diagnosis and management of initial UTIs in febrile infants and young children, 2 to 24 months of age, from the American Academy of Pediatrics Subcommittee on Urinary Tract Infection.

Methods. The conceptual model presented in the 1999 technical report was updated after a comprehensive review of published literature. Studies with potentially new information or with evidence that reinforced the 1999 technical report were retained. Meta-analyses on the effectiveness of antimicrobial prophylaxis to prevent recurrent UTI were performed.

Results. Review of recent literature revealed new evidence in the following areas. Certain clinical findings and new urinalysis methods can help clinicians identify febrile children at very low risk of UTI. Oral antimicrobial therapy is as effective as parenteral therapy in treating UTI. Data from published, randomized controlled trials do not support antimicrobial prophylaxis to prevent febrile UTI when vesicoureteral reflux is found through voiding cystourethrography. Ultrasonography of the urinary tract after the first UTI has poor sensitivity. Early antimicrobial treatment may decrease the risk of renal damage from UTI.

Conclusions. Recent literature agrees with most of the evidence presented in the 1999 technical report, but meta-analyses of data from recent, randomized controlled trials do not support antimicrobial prophylaxis to prevent febrile UTI. This finding argues against voiding cystourethrography after the first UTI. (8/11)
http://pediatrics.aappublications.org/content/128/3/e749

DIAGNOSIS AND MANAGEMENT OF CHILDHOOD OBSTRUCTIVE SLEEP APNEA SYNDROME (TECHNICAL REPORT)

Carole L. Marcus, MBBCh; Lee J. Brooks, MD; Sally Davidson Ward, MD; Kari A. Draper, MD; David Gozal, MD; Ann C. Halbower, MD; Jacqueline Jones, MD; Christopher Lehmann, MD; Michael S. Schechter, MD, MPH; Stephen Sheldon, MD; Richard N. Shiffman, MD, MCIS; Karen Spruyt, PhD; Steering Committee on Quality Improvement and Management; and Subcommittee on Obstructive Sleep Apnea Syndrome

ABSTRACT. *Objective.* This technical report describes the procedures involved in developing recommendations on the management of childhood obstructive sleep apnea syndrome (OSAS).

Methods. The literature from 1999 through 2011 was evaluated.

Results and Conclusions. A total of 3166 titles were reviewed, of which 350 provided relevant data. Most articles were level II through IV. The prevalence of OSAS ranged from 0% to 5.7%, with obesity being an independent risk factor. OSAS was associated with cardiovascular, growth, and neurobehavioral abnormalities and possibly inflammation. Most diagnostic screening tests had low sensitivity and specificity. Treatment of OSAS resulted in improvements in behavior and attention and likely improvement in cognitive abilities. Primary treatment is adenotonsillectomy (AT). Data were insufficient to recommend specific surgical techniques; however, children undergoing partial tonsillectomy should be monitored for possible recurrence of OSAS. Although OSAS improved postoperatively, the proportion of patients who had residual OSAS ranged from 13% to 29% in low-risk populations to 73% when obese children were included and stricter polysomnographic criteria were used. Nevertheless, OSAS may improve after AT even in obese children, thus supporting surgery as a reasonable initial treatment. A significant number of obese patients required intubation or continuous positive airway pressure (CPAP) postoperatively, which reinforces the need for inpatient observation. CPAP was effective in the treatment of OSAS, but adherence is a major barrier. For this reason, CPAP is not recommended as first-line therapy for OSAS when AT is an option. Intranasal steroids may ameliorate mild OSAS, but follow-up is needed. Data were insufficient to recommend rapid maxillary expansion. (8/12)

http://pediatrics.aappublications.org/content/130/3/e714

DIAGNOSIS AND MANAGEMENT OF INFANTILE HEMANGIOMA (CLINICAL REPORT)

David H. Darrow, MD, DDS; Arin K. Greene, MD; Anthony J. Mancini, MD; Amy J. Nopper, MD; Section on Dermatology; Section on Otolaryngology—Head & Neck Surgery; and Section on Plastic Surgery

ABSTRACT. Infantile hemangiomas (IHs) are the most common tumors of childhood. Unlike other tumors, they have the unique ability to involute after proliferation, often leading primary care providers to assume they will resolve without intervention or consequence. Unfortunately, a subset of IHs rapidly develop complications, resulting in pain, functional impairment, or permanent disfigurement. As a result, the primary clinician has the task of determining which lesions require early consultation with a specialist. Although several recent reviews have been published, this clinical report is the first based on input from individuals representing the many specialties involved in the treatment of IH. Its purpose is to update the pediatric community regarding recent discoveries in IH pathogenesis, treatment, and clinical associations and to provide a basis for clinical decision-making in the management of IH. (9/15)

http://pediatrics.aappublications.org/content/136/4/e1060

DIAGNOSIS AND MANAGEMENT OF INFANTILE HEMANGIOMA: EXECUTIVE SUMMARY

David H. Darrow, MD, DDS; Arin K. Greene, MD; Anthony J. Mancini, MD; Amy J. Nopper, MD; Section on Dermatology; Section on Otolaryngology–Head & Neck Surgery; and Section on Plastic Surgery

ABSTRACT. Infantile hemangiomas (IHs) are the most common tumors of childhood. Unlike other tumors, they have the capacity to involute after proliferation, often leading primary care providers to assume they will resolve without intervention or consequence. However, a subset of IHs may be associated with complications, resulting in pain, functional impairment, or permanent disfigurement. As a result, the primary care provider is often called on to decide which lesions should be referred for early consultation with a specialist.

This document provides a summary of the guidance contained in the clinical report "Diagnosis and Management of Infantile Hemangioma," published concurrently in the online version of *Pediatrics* (*Pediatrics*. 2015;136[4]:e1060–e1104, available at: www.pediatrics.org/content/136/4/e1060). The report is uniquely based on input from the many specialties involved in the treatment of IH. Its purpose is to update the pediatric community about recent discoveries in IH pathogenesis, clinical associations, and treatment and to provide a knowledge base and framework for clinical decision-making in the management of IH. (9/15)

http://pediatrics.aappublications.org/content/136/4/786

DIAGNOSIS AND PREVENTION OF IRON DEFICIENCY AND IRON-DEFICIENCY ANEMIA IN INFANTS AND YOUNG CHILDREN (0–3 YEARS OF AGE) (CLINICAL REPORT)

Robert D. Baker, MD, PhD; Frank R. Greer, MD; and Committee on Nutrition

ABSTRACT. This clinical report covers diagnosis and prevention of iron deficiency and iron-deficiency anemia in infants (both breastfed and formula fed) and toddlers from birth through 3 years of age. Results of recent basic research support the concerns that iron-deficiency anemia and iron deficiency without anemia during infancy and childhood can have long-lasting detrimental effects on neurodevelopment. Therefore, pediatricians and other health care providers should strive to eliminate iron deficiency and iron-deficiency anemia. Appropriate iron intakes for infants and toddlers as well as methods for screening for iron deficiency and iron-deficiency anemia are presented. (10/10)

http://pediatrics.aappublications.org/content/126/5/1040

DIAGNOSIS OF HIV-1 INFECTION IN CHILDREN YOUNGER THAN 18 MONTHS IN THE UNITED STATES (TECHNICAL REPORT)

Jennifer S. Read, MD, MS, MPH, DTM&H, and Committee on Pediatric AIDS

ABSTRACT. The objectives of this technical report are to describe methods of diagnosis of HIV-1 infection in children younger than 18 months in the United States and to review important issues that must be considered by clinicians who care for infants and young children born to HIV-1–infected women. Appropriate HIV-1 diagnostic testing for infants and children younger than 18 months differs from that for older children, adolescents, and adults because of passively transferred maternal HIV-1 antibodies, which may be detectable in the child's bloodstream until 18 months of age. Therefore, routine serologic testing of these infants and young children is generally only informative before the age of 18 months if the test result is negative. Virologic assays, including HIV-1 DNA or RNA assays, represent the gold standard for diagnostic testing of infants and children younger than 18 months. With such testing, the diagnosis of HIV-1 infection (as well as the presumptive exclusion of HIV-1 infection) can be established within the first several weeks of life among nonbreastfed infants. Important factors that must be considered when selecting HIV-1 diagnostic assays for pediatric patients and when choosing the timing of such assays include the age of the child, potential timing of infection of the child, whether the infection status of the child's mother is known or unknown, the antiretroviral exposure history of the mother and of the child, and characteristics of the virus. If the mother's HIV-1 serostatus is unknown, rapid HIV-1 antibody testing of the newborn infant to identify HIV-1 exposure is essential so that antiretroviral prophylaxis can be initiated within the first 12 hours of life if test results are positive. For HIV-1–exposed infants (identified by positive maternal test results or positive antibody results for the infant shortly after birth), it has been recommended that diagnostic testing with HIV-1 DNA or RNA assays be performed within the first 14 days of life, at 1 to 2 months of age, and at 3 to 6 months of age. If any of these test results are positive, repeat testing is recommended to confirm the diagnosis of HIV-1 infection. A diagnosis of HIV-1 infection can be made on the basis of 2 positive HIV-1 DNA or RNA assay results. In nonbreastfeeding children younger than 18 months with no positive HIV-1 virologic test results, presumptive exclusion of HIV-1 infection can be based on 2 negative virologic test results (1 obtained at ≥2 weeks and 1 obtained at ≥4 weeks of age); 1 negative virologic test result obtained at ≥8 weeks of age; or 1 negative HIV-1 antibody test result obtained at ≥6 months of age. Alternatively, presumptive exclusion of HIV-1 infection can be based on 1 positive HIV-1 virologic test with at least 2 subsequent negative virologic test results (at least 1 of which is performed at ≥8 weeks of age) or negative HIV-1 antibody test results (at least 1 of which is performed at ≥6 months of age). Definitive exclusion of HIV-1 infection is based on 2 negative virologic test results, 1 obtained at ≥1 month of age and 1 obtained at ≥4 months of age, or 2 negative HIV-1 antibody test results from separate specimens obtained at ≥6 months of age. For both presumptive and definitive exclusion of infection, the child should have no other laboratory (eg, no positive virologic test results) or clinical (eg, no AIDS-defining conditions) evidence of HIV-1 infection. Many clinicians confirm the absence of HIV-1 infection with a negative HIV-1 antibody assay result at 12 to 18 months of age. For breastfeeding infants, a similar testing algorithm can be followed, with timing of testing starting from the date of complete cessation of breastfeeding instead of the date of birth. (12/07, reaffirmed 4/10, 2/15)

http://pediatrics.aappublications.org/content/120/6/e1547

DIAGNOSTIC IMAGING OF CHILD ABUSE

Section on Radiology

ABSTRACT. The role of imaging in cases of child abuse is to identify the extent of physical injury when abuse is present and to elucidate all imaging findings that point to alternative diagnoses. Effective diagnostic imaging of child abuse rests on high-quality technology as well as a full appreciation of the clinical and pathologic alterations occurring in abused children. This statement is a revision of the previous policy published in 2000. (4/09)

http://pediatrics.aappublications.org/content/123/5/1430

DISASTER PLANNING FOR SCHOOLS

Council on School Health

ABSTRACT. Community awareness of the school district's disaster plan will optimize a community's capacity to maintain the safety of its school-aged population in the event of a school-based or greater community crisis. This statement is intended to stimulate awareness of the disaster-preparedness process in schools as a part of a global, community-wide preparedness plan. Pediatricians, other health care professionals, first responders, public health officials, the media, school nurses, school staff, and parents all need to be unified in their efforts to support schools in the prevention of, preparedness for, response to, and recovery from a disaster. (10/08, reaffirmed 9/11)

http://pediatrics.aappublications.org/content/122/4/895

DISCLOSURE OF ADVERSE EVENTS IN PEDIATRICS

Committee on Medical Liability and Risk Management and Council on Quality Improvement and Patient Safety

ABSTRACT. Despite increasing attention to issues of patient safety, preventable adverse events (AEs) continue to occur, causing direct and consequential injuries to patients, families, and health care providers. Pediatricians generally agree that there is an ethical obligation to inform patients and families about preventable AEs and medical errors. Nonetheless, barriers, such as fear of liability, interfere with disclosure regarding preventable AEs. Changes to the legal system, improved communications skills, and carefully developed disclosure policies and programs can improve the quality and frequency of appropriate AE disclosure communications. (11/16)

See full text on page 631.

http://pediatrics.aappublications.org/content/138/6/e20163215

DISPENSING MEDICATIONS AT THE HOSPITAL UPON DISCHARGE FROM AN EMERGENCY DEPARTMENT (TECHNICAL REPORT)

Loren G. Yamamoto, MD, MPH, MBA; Shannon Manzi, PharmD; and Committee on Pediatric Emergency Medicine

ABSTRACT. Although most health care services can and should be provided by their medical home, children will be referred or require visits to the emergency department (ED) for emergent clinical conditions or injuries. Continuation of medical care after discharge from an ED is dependent on parents or caregivers' understanding of and compliance with follow-up instructions and on adherence to medication recommendations. ED visits often occur at times when the majority of pharmacies are not open and caregivers are concerned with getting their ill or injured child directly home. Approximately one-third of patients fail to obtain priority medications from a pharmacy after discharge from an ED. The option of judiciously dispensing ED discharge medications from the ED's outpatient pharmacy within the facility is a major convenience that overcomes this obstacle, improving the likelihood of medication adherence. Emergency care encounters should be routinely followed up with primary care provider medical homes to ensure complete and comprehensive care. (1/12, reaffirmed 9/15)

http://pediatrics.aappublications.org/content/129/2/e562

DISTINGUISHING SUDDEN INFANT DEATH SYNDROME FROM CHILD ABUSE FATALITIES (CLINICAL REPORT)

Kent P. Hymel, MD, and Committee on Child Abuse and Neglect (joint with National Association of Medical Examiners)

ABSTRACT. Fatal child abuse has been mistaken for sudden infant death syndrome. When a healthy infant younger than 1 year dies suddenly and unexpectedly, the cause of death may be certified as sudden infant death syndrome.

Sudden infant death syndrome is more common than infanticide. Parents of sudden infant death syndrome victims typically are anxious to provide unlimited information to professionals involved in death investigation or research. They also want and deserve to be approached in a nonaccusatory manner. This clinical report provides professionals with information and suggestions for procedures to help avoid stigmatizing families of sudden infant death syndrome victims while allowing accumulation of appropriate evidence in potential cases of infanticide. This clinical report addresses deficiencies and updates recommendations in the 2001 American Academy of Pediatrics policy statement of the same name. (7/06, reaffirmed 4/09, 3/13)

http://pediatrics.aappublications.org/content/118/1/421

DO-NOT-RESUSCITATE ORDERS FOR PEDIATRIC PATIENTS WHO REQUIRE ANESTHESIA AND SURGERY (CLINICAL REPORT)

Section on Surgery, Section on Anesthesia and Pain Medicine, and Committee on Bioethics

ABSTRACT. This clinical report addresses the topic of preexisting do-not-resuscitate (DNR) orders for children undergoing anesthesia and surgery. Pertinent issues addressed include the rights of children, surrogate decision-making, the process of informed consent, and the roles of surgeons and anesthesiologists. The reevaluation process of DNR orders called "required reconsideration" can be incorporated into the process of informed consent for surgery and anesthesia. Care should be taken to distinguish between goal-directed and procedure-directed approaches to DNR orders. By giving parents or other surrogates and clinicians the option of deciding from among full resuscitation, limitations based on procedures, or limitations based on goals, the child's needs are individualized and better served. (12/04, reaffirmed 1/09, 10/12)

http://pediatrics.aappublications.org/content/114/6/1686

DRINKING WATER FROM PRIVATE WELLS AND RISKS TO CHILDREN

Committee on Environmental Health and Committee on Infectious Diseases

ABSTRACT. Drinking water for approximately one sixth of US households is obtained from private wells. These wells can become contaminated by pollutant chemicals or pathogenic organisms and cause illness. Although the US Environmental Protection Agency and all states offer guidance for construction, maintenance, and testing of private wells, there is little regulation. With few exceptions, well owners are responsible for their own wells. Children may also drink well water at child care or when traveling. Illness resulting from children's ingestion of contaminated water can be severe. This policy statement provides recommendations for inspection, testing, and remediation for wells providing drinking water for children. (5/09, reaffirmed 1/13)

http://pediatrics.aappublications.org/content/123/6/1599

DRINKING WATER FROM PRIVATE WELLS AND RISKS TO CHILDREN (TECHNICAL REPORT)

Walter J. Rogan, MD; Michael T. Brady, MD; Committee on Environmental Health; and Committee on Infectious Diseases

ABSTRACT. Drinking water for approximately one sixth of US households is obtained from private wells. These wells can become contaminated by pollutant chemicals or pathogenic organisms, leading to significant illness. Although the US Environmental Protection Agency and all states offer guidance for construction, maintenance, and testing of private wells, there is little regulation, and with few exceptions, well owners are responsible for their own wells. Children may also drink well water at child care or when traveling. Illness resulting from children's ingestion of contaminated water can be severe. This report reviews relevant aspects of groundwater and wells; describes the common chemical and microbiologic contaminants; gives an algorithm with recommendations for inspection, testing, and remediation for wells providing drinking water for children; reviews the definitions and uses of various bottled waters; provides current estimates of costs for well testing; and provides federal, national, state, and, where appropriate, tribal contacts for more information. (5/09, reaffirmed 1/13)

http://pediatrics.aappublications.org/content/123/6/e1123

EARLY CHILDHOOD ADVERSITY, TOXIC STRESS, AND THE ROLE OF THE PEDIATRICIAN: TRANSLATING DEVELOPMENTAL SCIENCE INTO LIFELONG HEALTH

Committee on Psychosocial Aspects of Child and Family Health; Committee on Early Childhood, Adoption, and Dependent Care; and Section on Developmental and Behavioral Pediatrics

ABSTRACT. Advances in a wide range of biological, behavioral, and social sciences are expanding our understanding of how early environmental influences (the ecology) and genetic predispositions (the biologic program) affect learning capacities, adaptive behaviors, lifelong physical and mental health, and adult productivity. A supporting technical report from the American Academy of Pediatrics (AAP) presents an integrated ecobiodevelopmental framework to assist in translating these dramatic advances in developmental science into improved health across the life span. Pediatricians are now armed with new information about the adverse effects of toxic stress on brain development, as well as a deeper understanding of the early life origins of many adult diseases. As trusted authorities in child health and development, pediatric providers must now complement the early identification of developmental concerns with a greater focus on those interventions and community investments that reduce external threats to healthy brain growth. To this end, AAP endorses a developing leadership role for the entire pediatric community—one that mobilizes the scientific expertise of both basic and clinical researchers, the family-centered care of the pediatric medical home, and the public influence of AAP and its state chapters—to catalyze fundamental change in early childhood policy and services. AAP is committed to leveraging science to inform the development of innovative strategies to reduce the

precipitants of toxic stress in young children and to mitigate their negative effects on the course of development and health across the life span. (12/11, reaffirmed 7/16)
http://pediatrics.aappublications.org/content/129/1/e224

EARLY CHILDHOOD CARIES IN INDIGENOUS COMMUNITIES

Committee on Native American Child Health (joint with Canadian Paediatric Society First Nations, Inuit, and Métis Committee)

ABSTRACT. The oral health of Indigenous children of Canada (First Nations, Inuit, and Métis) and the United States (American Indian, Alaska Native) is a major child health issue: there is a high prevalence of early childhood caries (ECC) and resulting adverse health effects in this community, as well as high rates and costs of restorative and surgical treatments under general anesthesia. ECC is an infectious disease that is influenced by multiple factors, including socioeconomic determinants, and requires a combination of approaches for improvement. This statement includes recommendations for preventive oral health and clinical care for young infants and pregnant women by primary health care providers, community-based health-promotion initiatives, oral health workforce and access issues, and advocacy for community water fluoridation and fluoride-varnish program access. Further community-based research on the epidemiology, prevention, management, and microbiology of ECC in Indigenous communities would be beneficial. (5/11)
http://pediatrics.aappublications.org/content/127/6/1190

EARLY INTERVENTION, IDEA PART C SERVICES, AND THE MEDICAL HOME: COLLABORATION FOR BEST PRACTICE AND BEST OUTCOMES (CLINICAL REPORT)

Richard C. Adams, MD; Carl Tapia, MD; and Council on Children With Disabilities

ABSTRACT. The medical home and the Individuals With Disabilities Education Act Part C Early Intervention Program share many common purposes for infants and children ages 0 to 3 years, not the least of which is a family-centered focus. Professionals in pediatric medical home practices see substantial numbers of infants and toddlers with developmental delays and/or complex chronic conditions. Economic, health, and family-focused data each underscore the critical role of timely referral for relationship-based, individualized, accessible early intervention services and the need for collaborative partnerships in care. The medical home process and Individuals With Disabilities Education Act Part C policy both support nurturing relationships and family-centered care; both offer clear value in terms of economic and health outcomes. Best practice models for early intervention services incorporate learning in the natural environment and coaching models. Proactive medical homes provide strategies for effective developmental surveillance, family-centered resources, and tools to support high-risk groups, and comanagement of infants with special health care needs, including the monitoring of services provided and outcomes achieved. (9/13)
http://pediatrics.aappublications.org/content/132/4/e1073

ECHOCARDIOGRAPHY IN INFANTS AND CHILDREN

Section on Cardiology

ABSTRACT. It is the intent of this statement to inform pediatric providers on the appropriate use of echocardiography. Although on-site consultation may be impossible, methods should be established to ensure timely review of echocardiograms by a pediatric cardiologist. With advances in data transmission, echocardiography information can be exchanged, in some cases eliminating the need for a costly patient transfer. By cooperating through training, education, and referral, complete and cost-effective echocardiographic services can be provided to all children. (6/97, reaffirmed 3/03, 3/07)
http://pediatrics.aappublications.org/content/99/6/921

EFFECTS OF EARLY NUTRITIONAL INTERVENTIONS ON THE DEVELOPMENT OF ATOPIC DISEASE IN INFANTS AND CHILDREN: THE ROLE OF MATERNAL DIETARY RESTRICTION, BREASTFEEDING, TIMING OF INTRODUCTION OF COMPLEMENTARY FOODS, AND HYDROLYZED FORMULAS (CLINICAL REPORT)

Frank R. Greer, MD; Scott H. Sicherer, MD; A. Wesley Burks, MD; Committee on Nutrition; and Section on Allergy and Immunology

ABSTRACT. This clinical report reviews the nutritional options during pregnancy, lactation, and the first year of life that may affect the development of atopic disease (atopic dermatitis, asthma, food allergy) in early life. It replaces an earlier policy statement from the American Academy of Pediatrics that addressed the use of hypoallergenic infant formulas and included provisional recommendations for dietary management for the prevention of atopic disease. The documented benefits of nutritional intervention that may prevent or delay the onset of atopic disease are largely limited to infants at high risk of developing allergy (ie, infants with at least 1 first-degree relative [parent or sibling] with allergic disease). Current evidence does not support a major role for maternal dietary restrictions during pregnancy or lactation. There is evidence that breastfeeding for at least 4 months, compared with feeding formula made with intact cow milk protein, prevents or delays the occurrence of atopic dermatitis, cow milk allergy, and wheezing in early childhood. In studies of infants at high risk of atopy and who are not exclusively breastfed for 4 to 6 months, there is modest evidence that the onset of atopic disease may be delayed or prevented by the use of hydrolyzed formulas compared with formula made with intact cow milk protein, particularly for atopic dermatitis. Comparative studies of the various hydrolyzed formulas also indicate that not all formulas have the same protective benefit. There is also little evidence that delaying the timing of the introduction of complementary foods beyond 4 to 6 months of age prevents the occurrence of atopic disease. At present, there are insufficient data to document a protective effect of any dietary intervention beyond 4 to 6 months of age for the development of atopic disease. (1/08)
http://pediatrics.aappublications.org/content/121/1/183

ELECTRONIC NICOTINE DELIVERY SYSTEMS
Section on Tobacco Control
ABSTRACT. Electronic nicotine delivery systems (ENDS) are rapidly growing in popularity among youth. ENDS are handheld devices that produce an aerosolized mixture from a solution typically containing concentrated nicotine, flavoring chemicals, and propylene glycol to be inhaled by the user. ENDS are marketed under a variety of names, most commonly electronic cigarettes and e-cigarettes. In 2014, more youth reported using ENDS than any other tobacco product. ENDS pose health risks to both users and nonusers. Nicotine, the major psychoactive ingredient in ENDS solutions, is both highly addictive and toxic. In addition to nicotine, other toxicants, carcinogens, and metal particles have been detected in solutions and aerosols of ENDS. Nonusers are involuntarily exposed to the emissions of these devices with secondhand and third-hand aerosol. The concentrated and often flavored nicotine in ENDS solutions poses a poisoning risk for young children. Reports of acute nicotine toxicity from US poison control centers have been increasing, with at least 1 child death reported from unintentional exposure to a nicotine-containing ENDS solution. With flavors, design, and marketing that appeal to youth, ENDS threaten to renormalize and glamorize nicotine and tobacco product use. There is a critical need for ENDS regulation, legislative action, and counter promotion to protect youth. ENDS have the potential to addict a new generation of youth to nicotine and reverse more than 50 years of progress in tobacco control. (10/15)
http://pediatrics.aappublications.org/content/136/5/1018

ELECTRONIC PRESCRIBING IN PEDIATRICS: TOWARD SAFER AND MORE EFFECTIVE MEDICATION MANAGEMENT
Council on Clinical Information Technology
ABSTRACT. This policy statement identifies the potential value of electronic prescribing (e-prescribing) systems in improving quality and reducing harm in pediatric health care. On the basis of limited but positive pediatric data and on the basis of federal statutes that provide incentives for the use of e-prescribing systems, the American Academy of Pediatrics recommends the adoption of e-prescribing systems with pediatric functionality. The American Academy of Pediatrics also recommends a set of functions that technology vendors should provide when e-prescribing systems are used in environments in which children receive care. (3/13)
http://pediatrics.aappublications.org/content/131/4/824

ELECTRONIC PRESCRIBING IN PEDIATRICS: TOWARD SAFER AND MORE EFFECTIVE MEDICATION MANAGEMENT (TECHNICAL REPORT)
Kevin B. Johnson, MD, MS; Christoph U. Lehmann, MD; and Council on Clinical Information Technology
ABSRACT. This technical report discusses recent advances in electronic prescribing (e-prescribing) systems, including the evidence base supporting their limitations and potential benefits. Specifically, this report acknowledges that there are limited but positive pediatric data supporting the role of e-prescribing in mitigating medication errors, improving communication with dispensing pharmacists, and improving medication adherence. On the basis of these data and on the basis of federal statutes that provide incentives for the use of e-prescribing systems, the American Academy of Pediatrics recommends the adoption of e-prescribing systems with pediatric functionality. This report supports the accompanying policy statement from the American Academy of Pediatrics recommending the adoption of e-prescribing by pediatric health care providers. (3/13)
http://pediatrics.aappublications.org/content/131/4/e1350

ELECTRONIC PRESCRIBING SYSTEMS IN PEDIATRICS: THE RATIONALE AND FUNCTIONALITY REQUIREMENTS
Council on Clinical Information Technology
ABSTRACT. The use of electronic prescribing applications in pediatric practice, as recommended by the federal government and other national health care improvement organizations, should be encouraged. Legislation and policies that foster adoption of electronic prescribing systems by pediatricians should recognize both specific pediatric requirements and general economic incentives required to speed the adoption of these systems. Continued research into improving the effectiveness of these systems, recognizing the unique challenges of providing care to the pediatric population, should be promoted. (6/07)
http://pediatrics.aappublications.org/content/119/6/1229

ELECTRONIC PRESCRIBING SYSTEMS IN PEDIATRICS: THE RATIONALE AND FUNCTIONALITY REQUIREMENTS (TECHNICAL REPORT)
Robert S. Gerstle, MD; Christoph U. Lehmann, MD; and Council on Clinical Information Technology
ABSTRACT. This technical report discusses electronic prescribing systems and their limitations and potential benefits, particularly to the pediatrician in the ambulatory setting. In the report we acknowledge the benefits of integrating these systems with electronic health records and practice-management systems and recommend that the adoption of electronic prescribing systems be done in the context of ultimately moving toward an electronic health record. This technical report supports the accompanying American Academy of Pediatrics policy-statement recommendations on the adoption of electronic prescribing systems by pediatricians. (6/07)
http://pediatrics.aappublications.org/content/119/6/e1413

EMERGENCY CONTRACEPTION
Committee on Adolescence
ABSTRACT. Despite significant declines over the past 2 decades, the United States continues to have teen birth rates that are significantly higher than other industrialized nations. Use of emergency contraception can reduce the risk of pregnancy if used up to 120 hours after unprotected intercourse or contraceptive failure and is most effective if used in the first 24 hours. Indications for the use of emergency contraception include sexual assault, unprotected intercourse, condom breakage or slippage, and missed or late doses of hormonal contraceptives, including the oral contraceptive pill, contraceptive patch, contraceptive ring (ie, improper placement or loss/expulsion), and injectable contraception. Adolescents younger than 17 years must obtain a prescription from a physician to access

emergency contraception in most states. In all states, both males and females 17 years or older can obtain emergency contraception without a prescription. Adolescents are more likely to use emergency contraception if it has been prescribed in advance of need. The aim of this updated policy statement is to (1) educate pediatricians and other physicians on available emergency contraceptive methods; (2) provide current data on safety, efficacy, and use of emergency contraception in teenagers; and (3) encourage routine counseling and advance emergency-contraception prescription as 1 part of a public health strategy to reduce teen pregnancy. This policy focuses on pharmacologic methods of emergency contraception used within 120 hours of unprotected or underprotected coitus for the prevention of unintended pregnancy. Emergency contraceptive medications include products labeled and dedicated for use as emergency contraception by the US Food and Drug Administration (levonorgestrel and ulipristal) and the "off-label" use of combination oral contraceptives. (11/12, reaffirmed 7/16)
http://pediatrics.aappublications.org/content/130/6/1174

EMERGENCY CONTRACEPTION: ADDENDUM
Committee on Adolescence

This is an addendum to the American Academy of Pediatrics Policy Statement "Emergency Contraception" (*Pediatrics.* 2012;130(6):1174–1182).

In April 2013, Judge Edward Korman of the US District Court of Eastern New York directed the Food and Drug Administration (FDA) to lift the ban on over-the-counter availability of levonorgestrel-based emergency contraceptives without a prescription and without point-of-sale or age restrictions. In June 2013, the Obama administration withdrew its appeal to the Korman ruling, and the FDA allowed the 1-pill formulation Plan B One-Step (Teva Women's Health Inc, Frazer, PA) to be made available on the shelf without age restriction in the United States. The FDA granted Plan B One-Step 3 years of exclusive rights to sell the product without an age restriction. One-pill generic versions will likely be allowed to be sold on the shelf next to Plan B One-Step, but these products will require age verification and will not be sold to those younger than 17 years without a prescription. The 2-pill formulations of levonorgestrel-based emergency contraceptives will remain behind the pharmacy counter and will also not be sold to those younger than 17 years without a prescription. (2/14)
http://pediatrics.aappublications.org/content/133/3/e798

EMERGENCY INFORMATION FORMS AND EMERGENCY PREPAREDNESS FOR CHILDREN WITH SPECIAL HEALTH CARE NEEDS
Committee on Pediatric Emergency Medicine and Council on Clinical Information Technology (joint with American College of Emergency Physicians Pediatric Emergency Medicine Committee)

ABSTRACT. Children with chronic medical conditions rely on complex management plans for problems that cause them to be at increased risk for suboptimal outcomes in emergency situations. The emergency information form (EIF) is a medical summary that describes medical condition(s), medications, and special health care needs to inform health care providers of a child's special health conditions and needs so that optimal emergency medical care can be provided. This statement describes updates to EIFs, including computerization of the EIF, expanding the potential benefits of the EIF, quality-improvement programs using the EIF, the EIF as a central repository, and facilitating emergency preparedness in disaster management and drills by using the EIF. (3/10, reaffirmed 7/14, 10/14)
http://pediatrics.aappublications.org/content/125/4/829

ENDORSEMENT OF HEALTH AND HUMAN SERVICES RECOMMENDATION FOR PULSE OXIMETRY SCREENING FOR CRITICAL CONGENITAL HEART DISEASE
Section on Cardiology and Cardiac Surgery Executive Committee

ABSTRACT. Incorporation of pulse oximetry to the assessment of the newborn infant can enhance detection of critical congenital heart disease (CCHD). Recently, the Secretary of Health and Human Services (HHS) recommended that screening for CCHD be added to the uniform screening panel. The American Academy of Pediatrics (AAP) has been a strong advocate of early detection of CCHD and fully supports the decision of the Secretary of HHS.

The AAP has published strategies for the implementation of pulse oximetry screening, which addressed critical issues such as necessary equipment, personnel, and training, and also provided specific recommendations for assessment of saturation by using pulse oximetry as well as appropriate management of a positive screening result. The AAP is committed to the safe and effective implementation of pulse oximetry screening and is working with other advocacy groups and governmental agencies to promote pulse oximetry and to support widespread surveillance for CCHD.

Going forward, AAP chapters will partner with state health departments to implement the new screening strategy for CCHD and will work to ensure that there is an adequate system for referral for echocardiographic/pediatric cardiac evaluation after a positive screening result. It is imperative that AAP members engage their respective policy makers in adopting and funding the recommendations made by the Secretary of HHS. (12/11)
http://pediatrics.aappublications.org/content/129/1/190

ENHANCING PEDIATRIC WORKFORCE DIVERSITY AND PROVIDING CULTURALLY EFFECTIVE PEDIATRIC CARE: IMPLICATIONS FOR PRACTICE, EDUCATION, AND POLICY MAKING
Committee on Pediatric Workforce

ABSTRACT. This policy statement serves to combine and update 2 previously independent but overlapping statements from the American Academy of Pediatrics (AAP) on culturally effective health care (CEHC) and workforce diversity. The AAP has long recognized that with the ever-increasing diversity of the pediatric population in the United States, the health of all children depends on the ability of all pediatricians to practice culturally effective care. CEHC can be defined as the delivery of care within the context of appropriate physician knowledge, understanding, and appreciation of all cultural distinctions, leading to optimal health outcomes. The AAP believes that CEHC is a critical social value and that the knowledge and skills necessary for providing CEHC can be taught and acquired through focused curricula across the spectrum of lifelong learning.

This statement also addresses workforce diversity, health disparities, and affirmative action. The discussion of diversity is broadened to include not only race, ethnicity, and language but also cultural attributes such as gender, religious beliefs, sexual orientation, and disability, which may affect the quality of health care. The AAP believes that efforts must be supported through health policy and advocacy initiatives to promote the delivery of CEHC and to overcome educational, organizational, and other barriers to improving workforce diversity. (9/13, reaffirmed 10/15)

http://pediatrics.aappublications.org/content/132/4/e1105

ENSURING THE HEALTH OF CHILDREN IN DISASTERS

Disaster Preparedness Advisory Council and Committee on Pediatric Emergency Medicine

ABSTRACT. Infants, children, adolescents, and young adults have unique physical, mental, behavioral, developmental, communication, therapeutic, and social needs that must be addressed and met in all aspects of disaster preparedness, response, and recovery. Pediatricians, including primary care pediatricians, pediatric medical subspecialists, and pediatric surgical specialists, have key roles to play in preparing and treating families in cases of disasters. Pediatricians should attend to the continuity of practice operations to provide services in time of need and stay abreast of disaster and public health developments to be active participants in community planning efforts. Federal, state, tribal, local, and regional institutions and agencies that serve children should collaborate with pediatricians to ensure the health and well-being of children in disasters. (10/15)

http://pediatrics.aappublications.org/content/136/5/e1407

EPIDEMIOLOGY AND DIAGNOSIS OF HEALTH CARE–ASSOCIATED INFECTIONS IN THE NICU (TECHNICAL REPORT)

Committee on Fetus and Newborn and Committee on Infectious Diseases

ABSTRACT. Health care–associated infections in the NICU are a major clinical problem resulting in increased morbidity and mortality, prolonged length of hospital stays, and increased medical costs. Neonates are at high risk for health care–associated infections because of impaired host defense mechanisms, limited amounts of protective endogenous flora on skin and mucosal surfaces at time of birth, reduced barrier function of neonatal skin, the use of invasive procedures and devices, and frequent exposure to broad-spectrum antibiotics. This statement will review the epidemiology and diagnosis of health care–associated infections in newborn infants. (3/12, reaffirmed 2/16)

http://pediatrics.aappublications.org/content/129/4/e1104

EQUIPMENT FOR GROUND AMBULANCES

American Academy of Pediatrics (joint with American College of Emergency Physicians, American College of Surgeons Committee on Trauma, Emergency Medical Services for Children, Emergency Nurses Association, National Association of EMS Physicians, and National Association of State EMS Officials)

On January 1, 2014, the American Academy of Pediatrics, American College of Emergency Physicians, American College of Surgeons Committee on Trauma, Emergency Medical Services for Children, Emergency Nurses Association, National Association of EMS Physicians, and National Association of State EMS Officials coauthored a joint policy statement, "Equipment for Ground Ambulances" (*Prehosp Emerg Care.* 2014;19[1]:92–97). The full text of the joint policy statement is available at: http://informahealthcare.com/doi/full/10.3109/10903127.2013.851312. Copyright © 2014 Informa Plc. (8/14)

http://pediatrics.aappublications.org/content/134/3/e919

ERADICATING POLIO: HOW THE WORLD'S PEDIATRICIANS CAN HELP STOP THIS CRIPPLING ILLNESS FOREVER (CLINICAL REPORT)

Walter A. Orenstein, MD, FAAP, and Committee on Infectious Diseases

ABSTRACT. The American Academy of Pediatrics strongly supports the Polio Eradication and Endgame Strategic Plan of the Global Polio Eradication Initiative. This plan was endorsed in November 2012 by the Strategic Advisory Group of Experts on Immunization of the World Health Organization and published by the World Health Organization in April 2013. As a key component of the plan, it will be necessary to stop oral polio vaccine (OPV) use globally to achieve eradication, because the attenuated viruses in the vaccine rarely can cause polio. The plan includes procedures for elimination of vaccine-associated paralytic polio and circulating vaccine-derived polioviruses (cVDPVs). cVDPVs can proliferate when vaccine viruses are transmitted among susceptible people, resulting in mutations conferring both the neurovirulence and transmissibility characteristics of wild polioviruses. Although there are 3 different types of wild poliovirus strains, the polio eradication effort has already resulted in the global elimination of type 2 poliovirus for more than a decade. Type 3 poliovirus may be eliminated because the wild type 3 poliovirus was last detected in 2012. Thus, of the 3 wild types, only wild type 1 poliovirus is still known to be circulating and causing disease. OPV remains the key vaccine for eradicating wild polioviruses in polio-infected countries because it induces high levels of systemic immunity to prevent paralysis and intestinal immunity to reduce transmission. However, OPV is a rare cause of paralysis and the substantial decrease in wild-type disease has resulted in estimates that the vaccine is causing more polio-related paralysis annually in recent years than the wild virus. The new endgame strategic plan calls for stepwise removal of the type 2 poliovirus component from trivalent oral vaccines, because type 2 wild poliovirus appears to have been eradicated (since 1999) and yet is the main cause of cVDPV outbreaks and approximately 40% of vaccine-associated paralytic polio cases. The Endgame and Strategic Plan will be accomplished by shifting from trivalent OPV to bivalent OPV (containing types 1 and 3 poliovirus only). It will be necessary to introduce trivalent inactivated poliovirus vaccine (IPV) into routine immunization programs in all countries using OPV to provide population immunity to type 2 before the switch from trivalent OPV to bivalent OPV. The Global Polio Eradication Initiative hopes to achieve global eradication of polio by 2018 with this strategy, after which all OPV use will be stopped. Challenges expected for adding IPV into routine immunization schedules include higher cost of IPV compared with OPV, cold-chain capacity limits, more complex administration of vaccine because IPV requires injections as opposed to oral administration, and inferior intestinal immunity conferred by IPV. The goal of this report is to help pediatricians understand the change in strategy and outline ways that pediatricians can help global polio eradication efforts, including advocating for the resources needed to accomplish polio eradication and for incorporation of IPV into routine immunization programs in all countries. (12/14)

http://pediatrics.aappublications.org/content/135/1/196

ESSENTIAL CONTRACTUAL LANGUAGE FOR MEDICAL NECESSITY IN CHILDREN

Committee on Child Health Financing

ABSTRACT. The previous policy statement from the American Academy of Pediatrics, "Model Language for Medical Necessity in Children," was published in July 2005. Since that time, there have been new and emerging delivery and payment models. The relationship established between health care providers and health plans should promote arrangements that are beneficial to all who are affected by these contractual arrangements. Pediatricians play an important role in ensuring that the needs of children are addressed in these emerging systems. It is important to recognize that health care plans designed for adults may not meet the needs of children. Language in health care contracts should reflect the health care needs of children and families. Informed pediatricians can make a difference in the care of children and influence the role of primary care physicians in the new paradigms. This policy highlights many of the important elements pediatricians should assess as providers develop a role in emerging care models. (7/13)

http://pediatrics.aappublications.org/content/132/2/398

ESTABLISHING A STANDARD PROTOCOL FOR THE VOIDING CYSTOURETHROGRAPHY (CLINICAL REPORT)

Dominic Frimberger, MD; Maria-Gisela Mercado-Deane, MD, FAAP; Section on Urology; and Section on Radiology

ABSTRACT. The voiding cystourethrogram (VCUG) is a frequently performed test to diagnose a variety of urologic conditions, such as vesicoureteral reflux. The test results determine whether continued observation or an interventional procedure is indicated. VCUGs are ordered by many specialists and primary care providers, including pediatricians, family practitioners, nephrologists, hospitalists, emergency department physicians, and urologists. Current protocols for performing and interpreting a VCUG are based on the International Reflux Study in 1985. However, more recent information provided by many national and international institutions suggests a need to refine those recommendations. The lead author of the 1985 study, R.L. Lebowitz, agreed to and participated in the current protocol. In addition, a recent survey directed to the chairpersons of pediatric radiology of 65 children's hospitals throughout the United States and Canada showed that VCUG protocols vary substantially. Recent guidelines from the American Academy of Pediatrics (AAP) recommend a VCUG for children between 2 and 24 months of age with urinary tract infections but did not specify how this test should be performed. To improve patient safety and to standardize the data obtained when a VCUG is performed, the AAP Section on Radiology and the AAP Section on Urology initiated the current VCUG protocol to create a consensus on how to perform this test. (10/16)

See full text on page 639.

http://pediatrics.aappublications.org/content/138/5/e20162590

ETHICAL AND POLICY ISSUES IN GENETIC TESTING AND SCREENING OF CHILDREN

Committee on Bioethics and Committee on Genetics (joint with American College of Medical Genetics and Genomics)

ABSTRACT. The genetic testing and genetic screening of children are commonplace. Decisions about whether to offer genetic testing and screening should be driven by the best interest of the child. The growing literature on the psychosocial and clinical effects of such testing and screening can help inform best practices. This policy statement represents recommendations developed collaboratively by the American Academy of Pediatrics and the American College of Medical Genetics and Genomics with respect to many of the scenarios in which genetic testing and screening can occur. (2/13)

http://pediatrics.aappublications.org/content/131/3/620

ETHICAL CONSIDERATIONS IN RESEARCH WITH SOCIALLY IDENTIFIABLE POPULATIONS

Committee on Native American Child Health and Committee on Community Health Services

ABSTRACT. Community-based research raises ethical issues not normally encountered in research conducted in academic settings. In particular, conventional risk-benefits assessments frequently fail to recognize harms that can occur in socially identifiable populations as a result of research participation. Furthermore, many such communities require more stringent measures of beneficence that must be applied directly to the participating communities. In this statement, the American Academy of Pediatrics sets forth recommendations for minimizing harms that may result from community-based research by emphasizing community involvement in the research process. (1/04, reaffirmed 10/07, 1/13)

http://pediatrics.aappublications.org/content/113/1/148

ETHICAL CONTROVERSIES IN ORGAN DONATION AFTER CIRCULATORY DEATH

Committee on Bioethics

ABSTRACT. The persistent mismatch between the supply of and need for transplantable organs has led to efforts to increase the supply, including controlled donation after circulatory death (DCD). Controlled DCD involves organ

recovery after the planned withdrawal of life-sustaining treatment and the declaration of death according to the cardiorespiratory criteria. Two central ethical issues in DCD are when organ recovery can begin and how to manage conflicts of interests. The "dead donor rule" should be maintained, and donors in cases of DCD should only be declared dead after the permanent cessation of circulatory function. Permanence is generally established by a 2- to 5-minute waiting period. Given ongoing controversy over whether the cessation must also be irreversible, physicians should not be required to participate in DCD. Because the preparation for organ recovery in DCD begins before the declaration of death, there are potential conflicts between the donor's and recipient's interests. These conflicts can be managed in a variety of ways, including informed consent and separating the various participants' roles. For example, informed consent should be sought for premortem interventions to improve organ viability, and organ procurement organization personnel and members of the transplant team should not be involved in the discontinuation of life-sustaining treatment or the declaration of death. It is also important to emphasize that potential donors in cases of DCD should receive integrated interdisciplinary palliative care, including sedation and analgesia. (4/13)
http://pediatrics.aappublications.org/content/131/5/1021

ETHICAL ISSUES WITH GENETIC TESTING IN PEDIATRICS
Committee on Bioethics
ABSTRACT. Advances in genetic research promise great strides in the diagnosis and treatment of many childhood diseases. However, emerging genetic technology often enables testing and screening before the development of definitive treatment or preventive measures. In these circumstances, careful consideration must be given to testing and screening of children to ensure that use of this technology promotes the best interest of the child. This statement reviews considerations for the use of genetic technology for newborn screening, carrier testing, and testing for susceptibility to late-onset conditions. Recommendations are made promoting informed participation by parents for newborn screening and limited use of carrier testing and testing for late-onset conditions in the pediatric population. Additional research and education in this developing area of medicine are encouraged. (6/01, reaffirmed 1/05, 1/09)
http://pediatrics.aappublications.org/content/107/6/1451

ETHICS AND THE CARE OF CRITICALLY ILL INFANTS AND CHILDREN
Committee on Bioethics
ABSTRACT. The ability to provide life support to ill children who, not long ago, would have died despite medicine's best efforts challenges pediatricians and families to address profound moral questions. Our society has been divided about extending the life of some patients, especially newborns and older infants with severe disabilities. The American Academy of Pediatrics (AAP) supports individualized decision making about life-sustaining medical treatment for all children, regardless of age. These decisions should be jointly made by physicians and parents, unless good reasons require invoking established child protective services to contravene parental authority. At this time, resource allocation (rationing) decisions about which children should receive intensive care resources should be made clear and explicit in public policy, rather than be made at the bedside. (7/96, reaffirmed 10/99, 6/03)
http://pediatrics.aappublications.org/content/98/1/149

EVALUATING CHILDREN WITH FRACTURES FOR CHILD PHYSICAL ABUSE (CLINICAL REPORT)
Emalee G. Flaherty, MD; Jeannette M. Perez-Rossello, MD; Michael A. Levine, MD; William L. Hennrikus, MD; Committee on Child Abuse and Neglect; Section on Radiology; Section on Endocrinology; and Section on Orthopaedics (joint with Society for Pediatric Radiology)
Fractures are common injuries caused by child abuse. Although the consequences of failing to diagnose an abusive injury in a child can be grave, incorrectly diagnosing child abuse in a child whose fractures have another etiology can be distressing for a family. The aim of this report is to review recent advances in the understanding of fracture specificity, the mechanism of fractures, and other medical diseases that predispose to fractures in infants and children. This clinical report will aid physicians in developing an evidence-based differential diagnosis and performing the appropriate evaluation when assessing a child with fractures. (1/14)
http://pediatrics.aappublications.org/content/133/2/e477

EVALUATING FOR SUSPECTED CHILD ABUSE: CONDITIONS THAT PREDISPOSE TO BLEEDING (TECHNICAL REPORT)
Shannon L. Carpenter, MD, MS; Thomas C. Abshire, MD; James D. Anderst, MD, MS; Section on Hematology/Oncology; and Committee on Child Abuse and Neglect
ABSTRACT. Child abuse might be suspected when children present with cutaneous bruising, intracranial hemorrhage, or other manifestations of bleeding. In these cases, it is necessary to consider medical conditions that predispose to easy bleeding/bruising. When evaluating for the possibility of bleeding disorders and other conditions that predispose to hemorrhage, the pediatrician must consider the child's presenting history, medical history, and physical examination findings before initiating a laboratory investigation. Many medical conditions can predispose to easy bleeding. Before ordering laboratory tests for a disease, it is useful to understand the biochemical basis and clinical presentation of the disorder, condition prevalence, and test characteristics. This technical report reviews the major medical conditions that predispose to bruising/bleeding and should be considered when evaluating for abusive injury. (3/13, reaffirmed 7/16)
http://pediatrics.aappublications.org/content/131/4/e1357

EVALUATING INFANTS AND YOUNG CHILDREN WITH MULTIPLE FRACTURES (CLINICAL REPORT)
Carole Jenny, MD, MBA, FAAP, for Committee on Child Abuse and Neglect
ABSTRACT. Infants and toddlers with multiple unexplained fractures are often victims of inflicted injury. However, several medical conditions can also cause multiple fractures in children in this age group. In this report, the differential diagnosis of multiple fractures is

presented, and diagnostic testing available to the clinician is discussed. The hypothetical entity "temporary brittle-bone disease" is examined also. Although frequently offered in court cases as a cause of multiple infant fractures, there is no evidence that this condition actually exists. (9/06)

http://pediatrics.aappublications.org/content/118/3/1299

EVALUATION AND MANAGEMENT OF CHILDREN AND ADOLESCENTS WITH ACUTE MENTAL HEALTH OR BEHAVIORAL PROBLEMS. PART I: COMMON CLINICAL CHALLENGES OF PATIENTS WITH MENTAL HEALTH AND/OR BEHAVIORAL EMERGENCIES (CLINICAL REPORT)

Thomas H. Chun, MD, MPH, FAAP; Sharon E. Mace, MD, FAAP, FACEP; Emily R. Katz, MD, FAAP; and Committee on Pediatric Emergency Medicine (joint with American College of Emergency Physicians Pediatric Emergency Medicine Committee)

INTRODUCTION. Mental health problems are among the leading contributors to the global burden of disease. Unfortunately, pediatric populations are not spared of mental health problems. In the United States, 21% to 23% of children and adolescents have a diagnosable mental health or substance use disorder. Among patients of emergency departments (EDs), 70% screen positive for at least 1 mental health disorder, 23% meet criteria for 2 or more mental health concerns, 45% have a mental health problem resulting in impaired psychosocial functioning, and 10% of adolescents endorse significant levels of psychiatric distress at the time of their ED visit. In pediatric primary care settings, the reported prevalence of mental health and behavioral disorders is between 12% to 22% of children and adolescents.

Although the American Academy of Pediatrics (AAP) has published a policy statement on mental health competencies and a Mental Health Toolkit for pediatric primary care providers, no such guidelines or resources exist for clinicians who care for pediatric mental health emergencies. This clinical report supports the 2006 joint policy statement of the AAP and American College of Emergency Physicians (ACEP) on pediatric mental health emergencies, with the goal of addressing the knowledge gaps in this area. The report is written primarily from the perspective of ED clinicians, but it is intended for all clinicians who care for children and adolescents with acute mental health and behavioral problems.

Recent epidemiologic studies of mental health visits have revealed a rapid burgeoning of both ED and primary care visits. An especially problematic trend is the increase in "boarding" of psychiatric patients in the ED and inpatient pediatric beds (ie, extended stays lasting days or even weeks). Although investigation of boarding practices is still in its infancy, the ACEP and the American Medical Association have both expressed concern about it, because it significantly taxes the functioning and efficiency of both the ED and hospital, and mental health services may not be available in the ED.

In addition, compared with other pediatric care settings, ED patients are known to be at higher risk of mental health disorders, including depression, anxiety, posttraumatic stress disorder, and substance abuse. These mental health conditions may be unrecognized not only by treating clinicians but also by the child/adolescent and his or her parents. A similar phenomenon has been described with suicidal patients. Individuals who have committed suicide frequently visited a health care provider in the months preceding their death. Although a minority of suicidal patients present with some form of self-harm, many have vague somatic complaints (eg, headache, gastrointestinal tract distress, back pain, concern for a sexually transmitted infection) masking their underlying mental health condition.

Despite studies demonstrating moderate agreement between emergency physicians and psychiatrists in the assessment and management of patients with mental health problems, ED clinicians frequently cite lack of training and confidence in their abilities as barriers to caring for patients with mental health emergencies. Another study of emergency medicine and pediatric emergency medicine training programs found that formal training in psychiatric problems is not required nor offered by most programs. Pediatric primary care providers report similar barriers to caring for their patients with mental health problems.

Part I of this clinical report focuses on the issues relevant to patients presenting to the ED with a mental health chief complaint and covers the following topics:

• Medical clearance of pediatric psychiatric patients
• Suicidal ideation and suicide attempts
• Involuntary hospitalization
• Restraint of the agitated patient
  — Verbal restraint
  — Chemical restraint
  — Physical restraint
• Coordination with the medical home

Part II discusses challenging patients with primarily medical or indeterminate presentations, in which the contribution of an underlying mental health condition may be unclear or a complicating factor, including:

• Somatic symptom and related disorders
• Adverse effects to psychiatric medications
  — Antipsychotic adverse effects
  — Neuroleptic malignant syndrome
  — Serotonin syndrome
• Children with special needs in the ED (autism spectrum and developmental disorders)
• Mental health screening in the ED

An executive summary of this clinical report can be found at www.pediatrics.org/cgi/doi/10.1542/peds.2016-1571. (8/16)

See full text on page 647.

http://pediatrics.aappublications.org/content/138/3/e20161570

EVALUATION AND MANAGEMENT OF CHILDREN AND ADOLESCENTS WITH ACUTE MENTAL HEALTH OR BEHAVIORAL PROBLEMS. PART I: COMMON CLINICAL CHALLENGES OF PATIENTS WITH MENTAL HEALTH AND/OR BEHAVIORAL EMERGENCIES—EXECUTIVE SUMMARY (CLINICAL REPORT)

Thomas H. Chun, MD, MPH, FAAP; Sharon E. Mace, MD, FAAP, FACEP; Emily R. Katz, MD, FAAP; and Committee on Pediatric Emergency Medicine (joint with American College of Emergency Physicians Pediatric Emergency Medicine Committee)

ABSTRACT. The number of children and adolescents seen in emergency departments (EDs) and primary care settings for mental health problems has skyrocketed in recent years, with up to 23% of patients in both settings having diagnosable mental health conditions. Even when a mental health problem is not the focus of an ED or primary care visit, mental health conditions, both known and occult, may challenge the treating clinician and complicate the patient's care.

Although the American Academy of Pediatrics has published a policy statement on mental health competencies and a Mental Health Toolkit for pediatric primary care providers, no such guidelines or resources exist for clinicians who care for pediatric mental health emergencies. Many ED and primary care physicians report a paucity of training and lack of confidence in caring for pediatric psychiatry patients. The 2 clinical reports (www.pediatrics.org/cgi/doi/10.1542/peds.2016-1570 and www.pediatrics.org/cgi/doi/10.1542/peds.2016-1573) support the 2006 joint policy statement of the American Academy of Pediatrics and the American College of Emergency Physicians on pediatric mental health emergencies, with the goal of addressing the knowledge gaps in this area. Although written primarily from the perspective of ED clinicians, they are intended for all clinicians who care for children and adolescents with acute mental health and behavioral problems.

The clinical reports are organized around the common clinical challenges pediatric caregivers face, both when a child or adolescent presents with a psychiatric chief complaint or emergency (part I) and also when a mental health condition may be an unclear or complicating factor in a non–mental health clinical presentation (part II). Part II of the clinical reports (www.pediatrics.org/cgi/doi/10.1542/peds.2016-1573) includes discussions of somatic symptom and related disorders, adverse effects of psychiatric medications including neuroleptic malignant syndrome and serotonin syndrome, caring for children with special needs such as autism and developmental disorders, and mental health screening. This executive summary is an overview of part I of the clinical reports. The full text of the below topics can be accessed online at (www.pediatrics.org/cgi/doi/10.1542/peds.2016-1570). (8/16)

See full text on page 671.

http://pediatrics.aappublications.org/content/138/3/e20161571

EVALUATION AND MANAGEMENT OF CHILDREN WITH ACUTE MENTAL HEALTH OR BEHAVIORAL PROBLEMS. PART II: RECOGNITION OF CLINICALLY CHALLENGING MENTAL HEALTH RELATED CONDITIONS PRESENTING WITH MEDICAL OR UNCERTAIN SYMPTOMS (CLINICAL REPORT)

Thomas H. Chun, MD, MPH, FAAP; Sharon E. Mace, MD, FAAP, FACEP; Emily R. Katz, MD, FAAP; and Committee on Pediatric Emergency Medicine (joint with American College of Emergency Physicians Pediatric Emergency Medicine Committee)

INTRODUCTION. Part I of this clinical report (http://www.pediatrics.org/cgi/doi/10.1542/peds.2016-1570) discusses the common clinical issues that may be encountered in caring for children and adolescents presenting to the emergency department (ED) or primary care setting with a mental health condition or emergency and includes the following:

- Medical clearance of pediatric psychiatric patients
- Suicidal ideation and suicide attempts
- Involuntary hospitalization
- Restraint of the agitated patient
  — Verbal restraint
  — Chemical restraint
  — Physical restraint
- Coordination with the medical home

Part II discusses the challenges a pediatric clinician may face when evaluating patients with a mental health condition, which may be contributing to or a complicating factor for a medical or indeterminate clinical presentation. Topics covered include the following:

- Somatic symptom and related disorders
- Adverse effects of psychiatric medications
  — Antipsychotic adverse effects
  — Neuroleptic malignant syndrome
  — Serotonin syndrome
- Children with special needs (autism spectrum disorders [ASDs] and developmental disorders [DDs])
- Mental health screening

The report is written primarily from the perspective of ED clinicians, but it is intended for all clinicians who care for children and adolescents with acute mental health and behavioral problems. An executive summary of this clinical report can be found at http://www.pediatrics.org/cgi/doi/10.1542/peds.2016-1574. (8/16)

See full text on page 681.

http://pediatrics.aappublications.org/content/138/3/e20161573

EVALUATION AND MANAGEMENT OF CHILDREN WITH ACUTE MENTAL HEALTH OR BEHAVIORAL PROBLEMS. PART II: RECOGNITION OF CLINICALLY CHALLENGING MENTAL HEALTH RELATED CONDITIONS PRESENTING WITH MEDICAL OR UNCERTAIN SYMPTOMS—EXECUTIVE SUMMARY (CLINICAL REPORT)

Thomas H. Chun, MD, MPH, FAAP; Sharon E. Mace, MD, FAAP, FACEP; Emily R. Katz, MD, FAAP; and Committee on Pediatric Emergency Medicine (joint with American College of Emergency Physicians Pediatric Emergency Medicine Committee)

ABSTRACT. The number of children and adolescents seen in emergency departments (EDs) and primary care settings for mental health problems has skyrocketed in recent years, with up to 23% of patients in both settings having diagnosable mental health conditions. Even when a mental health problem is not the focus of an ED or primary care visit, mental health conditions, both known and occult, may challenge the treating clinician and complicate the patient's care.

Although the American Academy of Pediatrics (AAP) has published a policy statement on mental health competencies and a Mental Health Toolkit for pediatric primary care providers, no such guidelines or resources exist for clinicians who care for pediatric mental health emergencies. Many ED and primary care physicians report paucity of training and lack of confidence in caring for pediatric psychiatry patients. The 2 clinical reports support the 2006 joint policy statement of the AAP and the American College of Emergency Physicians on pediatric mental health emergencies, with the goal of addressing the knowledge gaps in this area. Although written primarily from the perspective of ED clinicians, it is intended for all clinicians who care for children and adolescents with acute mental health and behavioral problems. They are organized around the common clinical challenges pediatric caregivers face, both when a child or adolescent presents with a psychiatric chief complaint or emergency (part I) and when a mental health condition may be an unclear or complicating factor in a non-mental health ED presentation (part II). Part I of the clinical reports includes discussions of Medical Clearance of Pediatric Psychiatric Patients; Suicide and Suicidal Ideation; Restraint of the Agitated Patient Including Verbal, Chemical, and Physical Restraint; and Coordination of Care With the Medical Home, and it can be accessed online at www.pediatrics.org/cgi/doi/10.1542/peds.2016-1570. This executive summary is an overview of part II of the clinical reports. Full text of the following topics can be accessed online at www.pediatrics.org/cgi/doi/10.1542/peds.2016-1573. (8/16)

See full text on page 707.

http://pediatrics.aappublications.org/content/138/3/e20161574

EVALUATION AND MANAGEMENT OF THE INFANT EXPOSED TO HIV-1 IN THE UNITED STATES (CLINICAL REPORT)

Peter L. Havens, MD; Lynne M. Mofenson, MD; and Committee on Pediatric AIDS

ABSTRACT. The pediatrician plays a key role in the prevention of mother-to-child transmission of HIV-1 infection. For infants born to women with HIV-1 infection identified during pregnancy, the pediatrician ensures that antiretroviral prophylaxis is provided to the infant to decrease the risk of acquiring HIV-1 infection and promotes avoidance of postnatal HIV-1 transmission by advising HIV-1–infected women not to breastfeed. The pediatrician should perform HIV-1 antibody testing for infants born to women whose HIV-1 infection status was not determined during pregnancy or labor. For HIV-1–exposed infants, the pediatrician monitors the infant for early determination of HIV-1 infection status and for possible short- and long-term toxicity from antiretroviral exposures. Provision of chemoprophylaxis for *Pneumocystis jiroveci* pneumonia and support of families living with HIV-1 by providing counseling to parents or caregivers are also important components of care. (12/08, reaffirmed 8/15)

http://pediatrics.aappublications.org/content/123/1/175

EVALUATION AND MANAGEMENT OF THE INFANT EXPOSED TO HIV-1 IN THE UNITED STATES—ADDENDUM

Peter L. Havens, MD; Lynne M. Mofenson, MD; and Committee on Pediatric AIDS

The following paragraph is an addendum to the clinical report "Evaluation and Management of the Infant Exposed to HIV-1 in the United States" (*Pediatrics* 2009;123[1]:175–187). It pertains to the section with the heading "HIV-1 Testing of the Infant if the Mother's HIV-1 Infection Status Is Unknown":

For newborn infants whose mother's HIV-1 serostatus is unknown, the newborn infant's health care provider should perform rapid HIV-1 antibody testing on the mother or the infant as soon as possible after birth with appropriate consent as required by state and local law. These test results should be available as early as possible and certainly within 12 hours after birth and can be used to guide initiation of infant antiretroviral prophylaxis. Rapid HIV-1 antibody testing, by using either blood or saliva, is licensed for the diagnosis of HIV infection in adults. Rapid HIV-1 antibody testing of women in labor and delivery units at 16 US hospitals identified a prevalence of undiagnosed HIV infection of 7 of 1000 women and demonstrated a sensitivity of 100% and specificity of 99.9% by using several rapid test kits. Positive predictive value was 90% compared with 76% for enzyme immunoassay. However, the use of these tests in infants is neither well described nor licensed. Sherman et al evaluated 7 HIV-1 rapid tests on stored samples from 116 HIV-exposed infants and compared the findings to standard HIV enzyme immunoassay testing. In the youngest cohort tested (median age, 1.5 months; range, 3–7 weeks), sensitivity of rapid testing was greater than 99%. In a subsequent study using whole blood, sensitivities ranged between 93.3% and 99.3% in infants younger than 3 months by using 5 rapid tests. In both of these studies, rapid HIV-1 rapid tests failed to identify some HIV-infected infants. Oral fluid testing has been demonstrated to have a negative predictive value of >99% in HIV-exposed children older than 12 months. However, when used for screening infants with a median age of 1.5 months (range, birth to 6 months), oral fluid testing had a sensitivity less than 90% and failed to detect 14 of 63 HIV-infected infants (22.2%). On the basis of these

findings, only blood should be used to perform rapid HIV-1 antibody testing in newborn infants. Furthermore, rapid testing of the mother, by using either blood or saliva, is preferred over rapid testing in her infant (blood only) because of increased sensitivity in identifying HIV-1 infection. (11/12, reaffirmed 8/15)
http://pediatrics.aappublications.org/content/130/6/64

EVALUATION AND REFERRAL FOR DEVELOPMENTAL DYSPLASIA OF THE HIP IN INFANTS (CLINICAL REPORT)

Brian A. Shaw, MD, FAAOS, FAAP; Lee S. Segal, MD,
*   FAAOS, FAAP; and Section on Orthopaedics*

ABSTRACT. Developmental dysplasia of the hip (DDH) encompasses a wide spectrum of clinical severity, from mild developmental abnormalities to frank dislocation. Clinical hip instability occurs in 1% to 2% of full-term infants, and up to 15% have hip instability or hip immaturity detectable by imaging studies. Hip dysplasia is the most common cause of hip arthritis in women younger than 40 years and accounts for 5% to 10% of all total hip replacements in the United States. Newborn and periodic screening have been practiced for decades, because DDH is clinically silent during the first year of life, can be treated more effectively if detected early, and can have severe consequences if left untreated. However, screening programs and techniques are not uniform, and there is little evidence-based literature to support current practice, leading to controversy. Recent literature shows that many mild forms of DDH resolve without treatment, and there is a lack of agreement on ultrasonographic diagnostic criteria for DDH as a disease versus developmental variations. The American Academy of Pediatrics has not published any policy statements on DDH since its 2000 clinical practice guideline and accompanying technical report. Developments since then include a controversial US Preventive Services Task Force "inconclusive" determination regarding usefulness of DDH screening, several prospective studies supporting observation over treatment of minor ultrasonographic hip variations, and a recent evidence-based clinical practice guideline from the American Academy of Orthopaedic Surgeons on the detection and management of DDH in infants 0 to 6 months of age. The purpose of this clinical report was to provide literature-based updated direction for the clinician in screening and referral for DDH, with the primary goal of preventing and/or detecting a dislocated hip by 6 to 12 months of age in an otherwise healthy child, understanding that no screening program has eliminated late development or presentation of a dislocated hip and that the diagnosis and treatment of milder forms of hip dysplasia remain controversial. (11/16)
    See full text on page 717.
http://pediatrics.aappublications.org/content/138/6/e20163107

EVALUATION AND REFERRAL OF CHILDREN WITH SIGNS OF EARLY PUBERTY (CLINICAL REPORT)

Paul Kaplowitz, MD, PhD, FAAP; Clifford Bloch, MD,
*   FAAP; and Section on Endocrinology*

ABSTRACT. Concerns about possible early pubertal development are a common cause for referral to pediatric medical subspecialists. Several recent studies have suggested that onset of breast and/or pubic hair development may be occurring earlier than in the past. Although there is a chance of finding pathology in girls with signs of puberty before 8 years of age and in boys before 9 years of age, the vast majority of these children with signs of apparent puberty have variations of normal growth and physical development and do not require laboratory testing, bone age radiographs, or intervention. The most common of these signs of early puberty are premature adrenarche (early onset of pubic hair and/or body odor), premature thelarche (nonprogressive breast development, usually occurring before 2 years of age), and lipomastia, in which girls have apparent breast development which, on careful palpation, is determined to be adipose tissue. Indicators that the signs of sexual maturation may represent true, central precocious puberty include progressive breast development over a 4- to 6-month period of observation or progressive penis and testicular enlargement, especially if accompanied by rapid linear growth. Children exhibiting these true indicators of early puberty need prompt evaluation by the appropriate pediatric medical subspecialist. Therapy with a gonadotropin-releasing hormone agonist may be indicated, as discussed in this report. (12/15)
http://pediatrics.aappublications.org/content/137/1/e20153732

EVALUATION FOR BLEEDING DISORDERS IN SUSPECTED CHILD ABUSE (CLINICAL REPORT)

James D. Anderst, MD, MS; Shannon L. Carpenter, MD, MS;
*   Thomas C. Abshire, MD; Section on Hematology/Oncology;*
*   and Committee on Child Abuse and Neglect*

ABSTRACT. Bruising or bleeding in a child can raise the concern for child abuse. Assessing whether the findings are the result of trauma and/or whether the child has a bleeding disorder is critical. Many bleeding disorders are rare, and not every child with bruising/bleeding concerning for abuse requires an evaluation for bleeding disorders. In some instances, however, bleeding disorders can present in a manner similar to child abuse. The history and clinical evaluation can be used to determine the necessity of an evaluation for a possible bleeding disorder, and prevalence and known clinical presentations of individual bleeding disorders can be used to guide the extent of the laboratory testing. This clinical report provides guidance to pediatricians and other clinicians regarding the evaluation for bleeding disorders when child abuse is suspected. (3/13, reaffirmed 7/16)
http://pediatrics.aappublications.org/content/131/4/e1314

THE EVALUATION OF CHILDREN IN THE PRIMARY CARE SETTING WHEN SEXUAL ABUSE IS SUSPECTED (CLINICAL REPORT)

Carole Jenny, MD, MBA; James E. Crawford-Jakubiak, MD;
*   and Committee on Child Abuse and Neglect*

ABSTRACT. This clinical report updates a 2005 report from the American Academy of Pediatrics on the evaluation of sexual abuse in children. The medical assessment of suspected child sexual abuse should include obtaining a history, performing a physical examination, and obtaining appropriate laboratory tests. The role of the physician includes determining the need to report suspected sexual abuse; assessing the physical, emotional, and behavioral consequences of sexual abuse; providing information to parents about how to support their child;

and coordinating with other professionals to provide comprehensive treatment and follow-up of children exposed to child sexual abuse. (7/13)

http://pediatrics.aappublications.org/content/132/2/e558

THE EVALUATION OF SEXUAL BEHAVIORS IN CHILDREN (CLINICAL REPORT)

Nancy D. Kellogg, MD, and Committee on Child Abuse and Neglect

ABSTRACT. Most children will engage in sexual behaviors at some time during childhood. These behaviors may be normal but can be confusing and concerning to parents or disruptive or intrusive to others. Knowledge of age-appropriate sexual behaviors that vary with situational and environmental factors can assist the clinician in differentiating normal sexual behaviors from sexual behavior problems. Most situations that involve sexual behaviors in young children do not require child protective services intervention; for behaviors that are age-appropriate and transient, the pediatrician may provide guidance in supervision and monitoring of the behavior. If the behavior is intrusive, hurtful, and/or age-inappropriate, a more comprehensive assessment is warranted. Some children with sexual behavior problems may reside or have resided in homes characterized by inconsistent parenting, violence, abuse, or neglect and may require more immediate intervention and referrals. (8/09, reaffirmed 3/13)

http://pediatrics.aappublications.org/content/124/3/992

THE EVALUATION OF SUSPECTED CHILD PHYSICAL ABUSE (CLINICAL REPORT)

Cindy W. Christian, MD, FAAP, and Committee on Child Abuse and Neglect

ABSTRACT. Child physical abuse is an important cause of pediatric morbidity and mortality and is associated with major physical and mental health problems that can extend into adulthood. Pediatricians are in a unique position to identify and prevent child abuse, and this clinical report provides guidance to the practitioner regarding indicators and evaluation of suspected physical abuse of children. The role of the physician may include identifying abused children with suspicious injuries who present for care, reporting suspected abuse to the child protection agency for investigation, supporting families who are affected by child abuse, coordinating with other professionals and community agencies to provide immediate and long-term treatment to victimized children, providing court testimony when necessary, providing preventive care and anticipatory guidance in the office, and advocating for policies and programs that support families and protect vulnerable children. (4/15)

http://pediatrics.aappublications.org/content/135/5/e1337

EVIDENCE FOR THE DIAGNOSIS AND TREATMENT OF ACUTE UNCOMPLICATED SINUSITIS IN CHILDREN: A SYSTEMATIC REVIEW (TECHNICAL REPORT)

Michael J. Smith, MD, MSCE

In 2001, the American Academy of Pediatrics published clinical practice guidelines for the management of acute bacterial sinusitis (ABS) in children. The technical report accompanying those guidelines included 21 studies that assessed the diagnosis and management of ABS in children. This update to that report incorporates studies of pediatric ABS that have been performed since 2001. Overall, 17 randomized controlled trials of the treatment of sinusitis in children were identified and analyzed. Four randomized, double-blind, placebo-controlled trials of antimicrobial therapy have been published. The results of these studies varied, likely due to differences in inclusion and exclusion criteria. Because of this heterogeneity, formal meta-analyses were not performed. However, qualitative analysis of these studies suggests that children with greater severity of illness at presentation are more likely to benefit from antimicrobial therapy. An additional 5 trials compared different antimicrobial therapies but did not include placebo groups. Six trials assessed a variety of ancillary treatments for ABS in children, and 3 focused on subacute sinusitis. Although the number of pediatric trials has increased since 2001, there are still limited data to guide the diagnosis and management of ABS in children. Diagnostic and treatment guidelines focusing on severity of illness at the time of presentation have the potential to identify those children most likely to benefit from antimicrobial therapy and at the same time minimize unnecessary use of antibiotics. (6/13)

http://pediatrics.aappublications.org/content/132/1/e284

AN EVIDENCE-BASED REVIEW OF IMPORTANT ISSUES CONCERNING NEONATAL HYPERBILIRUBINEMIA (TECHNICAL REPORT)

Stanley Ip, MD; Mei Chung, MPH; John Kulig, MD, MPH; Rebecca O'Brien, MD; Robert Sege, MD, PhD; Stephan Glicken, MD; M. Jeffrey Maisels, MB, BCh; Joseph Lau, MD; Steering Committee on Quality and Improvement; and Subcommittee on Hyperbilirubinemia

ABSTRACT. This article is adapted from a published evidence report concerning neonatal hyperbilirubinemia with an added section on the risk of blood exchange transfusion (BET). Based on a summary of multiple case reports that spanned more than 30 years, we conclude that kernicterus, although infrequent, has at least 10% mortality and at least 70% long-term morbidity. It is evident that the preponderance of kernicterus cases occurred in infants with a bilirubin level higher than 20 mg/dL. Given the diversity of conclusions on the relationship between peak bilirubin levels and behavioral and neurodevelopmental outcomes, it is apparent that the use of a single total serum bilirubin level to predict long-term outcomes is inadequate and will lead to conflicting results. Evidence for efficacy of treatments for neonatal hyperbilirubinemia was limited. Overall, the 4 qualifying studies showed that phototherapy had an absolute risk-reduction rate of 10% to 17% for prevention of serum bilirubin levels higher than 20 mg/dL in healthy infants with jaundice. There is no evidence to suggest that phototherapy for neonatal hyperbilirubinemia has any long-term adverse neurodevelopmental effects. Transcutaneous measurements of bilirubin have a linear correlation to total serum bilirubin and may be useful as screening devices to detect clinically significant jaundice and decrease the need for serum bilirubin determinations. Based on our review of the risks associated with BETs from 15 studies consisting mainly of infants born before 1970, we conclude that the

mortality within 6 hours of BET ranged from 3 per 1000 to 4 per 1000 exchanged infants who were term and without serious hemolytic diseases. Regardless of the definitions and rates of BET-associated morbidity and the various pre-exchange clinical states of the exchanged infants, in many cases the morbidity was minor (eg, postexchange anemia). Based on the results from the most recent study to report BET morbidity, the overall risk of permanent sequelae in 25 sick infants who survived BET was from 5% to 10%. (7/04)
http://pediatrics.aappublications.org/content/114/1/e130

EXCESSIVE SLEEPINESS IN ADOLESCENTS AND YOUNG ADULTS: CAUSES, CONSEQUENCES, AND TREATMENT STRATEGIES (TECHNICAL REPORT)

Richard P. Millman; MD; Working Group on Sleepiness in Adolescents/Young Adults; and Committee on Adolescence

ABSTRACT. Adolescents and young adults are often excessively sleepy. This excessive sleepiness can have a profound negative effect on school performance, cognitive function, and mood and has been associated with other serious consequences such as increased incidence of automobile crashes. In this article we review available scientific knowledge about normal sleep changes in adolescents (13–22 years of age), the factors associated with chronic insufficient sleep, the effect of insufficient sleep on a variety of systems and functions, and the primary sleep disorders or organic dysfunctions that, if untreated, can cause excessive daytime sleepiness in this population. (6/05)
http://pediatrics.aappublications.org/content/115/6/1774

EXPERT WITNESS PARTICIPATION IN CIVIL AND CRIMINAL PROCEEDINGS

Committee on Medical Liability and Risk Management

ABSTRACT. The interests of the public and both the medical and legal professions are best served when scientifically sound and unbiased expert witness testimony is readily available in civil and criminal proceedings. As members of the medical community, patient advocates, and private citizens, pediatricians have ethical and professional obligations to assist in the administration of justice. The American Academy of Pediatrics believes that the adoption of the recommendations outlined in this statement will improve the quality of medical expert witness testimony in legal proceedings and, thereby, increase the probability of achieving outcomes that are fair, honest, and equitable. Strategies for enforcing guidance and promoting oversight of expert witnesses are proposed. (6/09)
http://pediatrics.aappublications.org/content/124/1/428

EXPOSURE TO NONTRADITIONAL PETS AT HOME AND TO ANIMALS IN PUBLIC SETTINGS: RISKS TO CHILDREN (CLINICAL REPORT)

Larry K. Pickering, MD; Nina Marano, DVM, MPH; Joseph A. Bocchini, MD; Frederick J. Angulo, DVM, PhD; and Committee on Infectious Diseases

ABSTRACT. Exposure to animals can provide many benefits during the growth and development of children. However, there are potential risks associated with animal exposures, including exposure to nontraditional pets in the home and animals in public settings. Educational materials, regulations, and guidelines have been developed to minimize these risks. Pediatricians, veterinarians, and other health care professionals can provide advice on selection of appropriate pets as well as prevention of disease transmission from nontraditional pets and when children contact animals in public settings. (10/08, reaffirmed 12/11, 6/15)
http://pediatrics.aappublications.org/content/122/4/876

EYE EXAMINATION IN INFANTS, CHILDREN, AND YOUNG ADULTS BY PEDIATRICIANS

Committee on Practice and Ambulatory Medicine and Section on Ophthalmology (joint with American Association of Certified Orthoptists, American Association for Pediatric Ophthalmology and Strabismus, and American Academy of Ophthalmology)

ABSTRACT. Early detection and prompt treatment of ocular disorders in children is important to avoid lifelong visual impairment. Examination of the eyes should be performed beginning in the newborn period and at all well-child visits. Newborns should be examined for ocular structural abnormalities, such as cataract, corneal opacity, and ptosis, which are known to result in visual problems. Vision assessment beginning at birth has been endorsed by the American Academy of Pediatrics, the American Association for Pediatric Ophthalmology and Strabismus, and the American Academy of Ophthalmology. All children who are found to have an ocular abnormality or who fail vision assessment should be referred to a pediatric ophthalmologist or an eye care specialist appropriately trained to treat pediatric patients. (4/03, reaffirmed 5/07)
http://pediatrics.aappublications.org/content/111/4/902

THE EYE EXAMINATION IN THE EVALUATION OF CHILD ABUSE (CLINICAL REPORT)

Alex V. Levin, MD, MHSc; Cindy W. Christian, MD; Committee on Child Abuse and Neglect; and Section on Ophthalmology

ABSTRACT. Retinal hemorrhage is an important indicator of possible abusive head trauma, but it is also found in a number of other conditions. Distinguishing the type, number, and pattern of retinal hemorrhages may be helpful in establishing a differential diagnosis. Identification of ocular abnormalities requires a full retinal examination by an ophthalmologist using indirect ophthalmoscopy through a pupil that has been pharmacologically dilated. At autopsy, removal of the eyes and orbital tissues may also reveal abnormalities not discovered before death. In previously well young children who experience unexpected apparent life-threatening events with no obvious cause, children with head trauma that results in significant intracranial hemorrhage and brain injury, victims of abusive head trauma, and children with unexplained death, premortem clinical eye examination and postmortem examination of the eyes and orbits may be helpful in detecting abnormalities that can help establish the underlying etiology. (7/10, reaffirmed 12/15)
http://pediatrics.aappublications.org/content/126/2/376

FACILITIES AND EQUIPMENT FOR THE CARE OF PEDIATRIC PATIENTS IN A COMMUNITY HOSPITAL (CLINICAL REPORT)

Committee on Hospital Care

ABSTRACT. Many children who require hospitalization are admitted to community hospitals that are more accessible for families and their primary care physicians but vary substantially in their pediatric resources. The intent of this clinical report is to provide basic guidelines for furnishing and equipping a pediatric area in a community hospital. (5/03, reaffirmed 5/07, 8/13)

http://pediatrics.aappublications.org/content/111/5/1120

FAILURE TO THRIVE AS A MANIFESTATION OF CHILD NEGLECT (CLINICAL REPORT)

Robert W. Block, MD; Nancy F. Krebs, MD; Committee on Child Abuse and Neglect; and Committee on Nutrition

ABSTRACT. Failure to thrive is a common problem in infancy and childhood. It is most often multifactorial in origin. Inadequate nutrition and disturbed social interactions contribute to poor weight gain, delayed development, and abnormal behavior. The syndrome develops in a significant number of children as a consequence of child neglect. This clinical report is intended to focus the pediatrician on the consideration, evaluation, and management of failure to thrive when child neglect may be present. Child protective services agencies should be notified when the evaluation leads to a suspicion of abuse or neglect. (11/05, reaffirmed 1/09)

http://pediatrics.aappublications.org/content/116/5/1234

FALLS FROM HEIGHTS: WINDOWS, ROOFS, AND BALCONIES

Committee on Injury and Poison Prevention

ABSTRACT. Falls of all kinds represent an important cause of child injury and death. In the United States, approximately 140 deaths from falls occur annually in children younger than 15 years. Three million children require emergency department care for fall-related injuries. This policy statement examines the epidemiology of falls from heights and recommends preventive strategies for pediatricians and other child health care professionals. Such strategies involve parent counseling, community programs, building code changes, legislation, and environmental modification, such as the installation of window guards and balcony railings. (5/01, reaffirmed 10/04, 5/07, 6/10)

http://pediatrics.aappublications.org/content/107/5/1188

FAMILIES AFFECTED BY PARENTAL SUBSTANCE USE (CLINICAL REPORT)

Vincent C. Smith, MD, MPH, FAAP; Celeste R. Wilson, MD, FAAP; and Committee on Substance Use and Prevention

ABSTRACT. Children whose parents or caregivers use drugs or alcohol are at increased risk of short- and long-term sequelae ranging from medical problems to psychosocial and behavioral challenges. In the course of providing health care services to children, pediatricians are likely to encounter families affected by parental substance use and are in a unique position to intervene. Therefore, pediatricians need to know how to assess a child's risk in the context of a parent's substance use. The purposes of this clinical report are to review some of the short-term effects of maternal substance use during pregnancy and long-term implications of fetal exposure; describe typical medical, psychiatric, and behavioral symptoms of children and adolescents in families affected by substance use; and suggest proficiencies for pediatricians involved in the care of children and adolescents of families affected by substance use, including screening families, mandated reporting requirements, and directing families to community, regional, and state resources that can address needs and problems. (7/16)

See full text on page 731.

http://pediatrics.aappublications.org/content/138/2/e20161575

FAMILIES AND ADOPTION: THE PEDIATRICIAN'S ROLE IN SUPPORTING COMMUNICATION (CLINICAL REPORT)

Committee on Early Childhood, Adoption, and Dependent Care

ABSTRACT. Each year, more children join families through adoption. Pediatricians have an important role in assisting adoptive families in the various challenges they may face with respect to adoption. The acceptance of the differences between families formed through birth and those formed through adoption is essential in promoting positive emotional growth within the family. It is important for pediatricians to be informed about adoption and to share this knowledge with adoptive families. Parents need ongoing advice with respect to adoption issues and need to be supported in their communication with their adopted children. (12/03)

http://pediatrics.aappublications.org/content/112/6/1437

FATHERS' ROLES IN THE CARE AND DEVELOPMENT OF THEIR CHILDREN: THE ROLE OF PEDIATRICIANS (CLINICAL REPORT)

Michael Yogman, MD, FAAP; Craig F. Garfield, MD, FAAP; and Committee on Psychosocial Aspects of Child and Family Health

ABSTRACT. Fathers' involvement in and influence on the health and development of their children have increased in a myriad of ways in the past 10 years and have been widely studied. The role of pediatricians in working with fathers has correspondingly increased in importance. This report reviews new studies of the epidemiology of father involvement, including nonresidential as well as residential fathers. The effects of father involvement on child outcomes are discussed within each phase of a child's development. Particular emphasis is placed on (1) fathers' involvement across childhood ages and (2) the influence of fathers' physical and mental health on their children. Implications and advice for all child health providers to encourage and support father involvement are outlined. (6/16)

See full text on page 747.

http://pediatrics.aappublications.org/content/138/1/e20161128

THE FEMALE ATHLETE TRIAD (CLINICAL REPORT)

Amanda K. Weiss Kelly, MD, FAAP; Suzanne Hecht, MD, FACSM; and Council on Sports Medicine and Fitness

ABSTRACT. The number of girls participating in sports has increased significantly since the introduction of Title XI in 1972. As a result, more girls have been able to experience the social, educational, and health-related benefits of sports participation. However, there are risks associated with sports participation, including the female athlete triad. The triad was originally recognized as the interrelationship of amenorrhea, osteoporosis, and disordered eating, but our understanding has evolved to recognize that each of the components of the triad exists on a spectrum from optimal health to disease. The triad occurs when energy intake does not adequately compensate for exercise-related energy expenditure, leading to adverse effects on reproductive, bone, and cardiovascular health. Athletes can present with a single component or any combination of the components. The triad can have a more significant effect on the health of adolescent athletes than on adults because adolescence is a critical time for bone mass accumulation. This report outlines the current state of knowledge on the epidemiology, diagnosis, and treatment of the triad conditions. (7/16)

See full text on page 765.

http://pediatrics.aappublications.org/content/138/2/e20160922

FETAL ALCOHOL SPECTRUM DISORDERS (CLINICAL REPORT)

Janet F. Williams, MD, FAAP; Vincent C. Smith, MD, MPH, FAAP; and Committee on Substance Abuse

ABSTRACT. Prenatal exposure to alcohol can damage the developing fetus and is the leading preventable cause of birth defects and intellectual and neurodevelopmental disabilities. In 1973, fetal alcohol syndrome was first described as a specific cluster of birth defects resulting from alcohol exposure in utero. Subsequently, research unequivocally revealed that prenatal alcohol exposure causes a broad range of adverse developmental effects. Fetal alcohol spectrum disorder (FASD) is the general term that encompasses the range of adverse effects associated with prenatal alcohol exposure. The diagnostic criteria for fetal alcohol syndrome are specific, and comprehensive efforts are ongoing to establish definitive criteria for diagnosing the other FASDs. A large and growing body of research has led to evidence-based FASD education of professionals and the public, broader prevention initiatives, and recommended treatment approaches based on the following premises:

- Alcohol-related birth defects and developmental disabilities are completely preventable when pregnant women abstain from alcohol use.

- Neurocognitive and behavioral problems resulting from prenatal alcohol exposure are lifelong.

- Early recognition, diagnosis, and therapy for any condition along the FASD continuum can result in improved outcomes.

- During pregnancy:
  - no amount of alcohol intake should be considered safe;
  - there is no safe trimester to drink alcohol;
  - all forms of alcohol, such as beer, wine, and liquor, pose similar risk; and
  - binge drinking poses dose-related risk to the developing fetus. (10/15)

http://pediatrics.aappublications.org/content/136/5/e1395

FEVER AND ANTIPYRETIC USE IN CHILDREN (CLINICAL REPORT)

Janice E. Sullivan, MD; Henry C. Farrar, MD; Section on Clinical Pharmacology and Therapeutics; and Committee on Drugs

ABSTRACT. Fever in a child is one of the most common clinical symptoms managed by pediatricians and other health care providers and a frequent cause of parental concern. Many parents administer antipyretics even when there is minimal or no fever, because they are concerned that the child must maintain a "normal" temperature. Fever, however, is not the primary illness but is a physiologic mechanism that has beneficial effects in fighting infection. There is no evidence that fever itself worsens the course of an illness or that it causes long-term neurologic complications. Thus, the primary goal of treating the febrile child should be to improve the child's overall comfort rather than focus on the normalization of body temperature. When counseling the parents or caregivers of a febrile child, the general well-being of the child, the importance of monitoring activity, observing for signs of serious illness, encouraging appropriate fluid intake, and the safe storage of antipyretics should be emphasized. Current evidence suggests that there is no substantial difference in the safety and effectiveness of acetaminophen and ibuprofen in the care of a generally healthy child with fever. There is evidence that combining these 2 products is more effective than the use of a single agent alone; however, there are concerns that combined treatment may be more complicated and contribute to the unsafe use of these drugs. Pediatricians should also promote patient safety by advocating for simplified formulations, dosing instructions, and dosing devices. (2/11, reaffirmed 7/16)

http://pediatrics.aappublications.org/content/127/3/580

FINANCING GRADUATE MEDICAL EDUCATION TO MEET THE NEEDS OF CHILDREN AND THE FUTURE PEDIATRICIAN WORKFORCE

Committee on Pediatric Workforce

ABSTRACT. The American Academy of Pediatrics (AAP) believes that an appropriately financed graduate medical education (GME) system is critical to ensuring that sufficient numbers of trained pediatricians are available to provide optimal health care to all children. A shortage of pediatric medical subspecialists and pediatric surgical specialists currently exists in the United States, and this shortage is likely to intensify because of the growing numbers of children with chronic health problems and special health care needs. It is equally important to maintain the supply of primary care pediatricians. The AAP, therefore, recommends that children's hospital GME positions funded by the Health Resources and Services Administration be increased to address this escalating demand for pediatric health services. The AAP also recommends that GME funding for pediatric physician training provide full financial support for all years of training necessary to meet program requirements. In addition, all other entities that gain from GME training should participate in its funding in a manner that does not influence curriculum, requirements, or outcomes. Furthermore, the AAP supports funding for training innovations that improve the health of children. Finally, the AAP recommends that all institutional recipients of GME funding allocate these funds directly to the settings where training occurs in a transparent manner. (3/16)

See full text on page 777.

http://pediatrics.aappublications.org/content/137/4/e20160211

FINANCING OF PEDIATRIC HOME HEALTH CARE

Committee on Child Health Financing and Section on
Home Care

ABSTRACT. In certain situations, home health care has been shown to be a cost-effective alternative to inpatient hospital care. National health expenditures reveal that pediatric home health costs totaled $5.3 billion in 2000. Medicaid is the major payer for pediatric home health care (77%), followed by other public sources (22%). Private health insurance and families each paid less than 1% of pediatric home health expenses. The most important factors affecting access to home health care are the inadequate supply of clinicians and ancillary personnel, shortages of home health nurses with pediatric expertise, inadequate payment, and restrictive insurance and managed care policies. Many children must stay in the NICU, PICU, and other pediatric wards and intermediate care areas at a much higher cost because of inadequate pediatric home health care services. The main financing problem pertaining to Medicaid is low payment to home health agencies at rates that are insufficient to provide beneficiaries access to home health services. Although home care services may be a covered benefit under private health plans, most do not cover private-duty nursing (83%), home health aides (45%), or home physical, occupational, or speech therapy (33%) and/or impose visit or monetary limits or caps. To advocate for improvements in financing of pediatric home health care, the American Academy of Pediatrics has developed several recommendations for public policy makers, federal and state Medicaid offices, private insurers, managed care plans, Title V officials, and home health care professionals. These recommendations will improve licensing, payment, coverage, and research related to pediatric home health services. (8/06)

http://pediatrics.aappublications.org/content/118/2/834

FIREARM-RELATED INJURIES AFFECTING THE PEDIATRIC POPULATION

Council on Injury, Violence, and Poison Prevention
Executive Committee

ABSTRACT. The absence of guns from children's homes and communities is the most reliable and effective measure to prevent firearm-related injuries in children and adolescents. Adolescent suicide risk is strongly associated with firearm availability. Safe gun storage (guns unloaded and locked, ammunition locked separately) reduces children's risk of injury. Physician counseling of parents about firearm safety appears to be effective, but firearm safety education programs directed at children are ineffective. The American Academy of Pediatrics continues to support a number of specific measures to reduce the destructive effects of guns in the lives of children and adolescents, including the regulation of the manufacture, sale, purchase, ownership, and use of firearms; a ban on semiautomatic assault weapons; and the strongest possible regulations of handguns for civilian use. (10/12)

http://pediatrics.aappublications.org/content/130/5/e1416

FIREWORKS-RELATED INJURIES TO CHILDREN

Committee on Injury and Poison Prevention

ABSTRACT. An estimated 8500 individuals, approximately 45% of them children younger than 15 years, were treated in US hospital emergency departments during 1999 for fireworks-related injuries. The hands (40%), eyes (20%), and head and face (20%) are the body areas most often involved. Approximately one third of eye injuries from fireworks result in permanent blindness. During 1999, 16 people died as a result of injuries associated with fireworks. Every type of legally available consumer (so-called "safe and sane") firework has been associated with serious injury or death. In 1997, 20 100 fires were caused by fireworks, resulting in $22.7 million in direct property damage. Fireworks typically cause more fires in the United States on the Fourth of July than all other causes of fire combined on that day. Pediatricians should educate parents, children, community leaders, and others about the dangers of fireworks. Fireworks for individual private use should be banned. Children and their families should be encouraged to enjoy fireworks at public fireworks displays conducted by professionals rather than purchase fireworks for home or private use. (7/01, reaffirmed 1/05, 2/08, 10/11, 11/14)

http://pediatrics.aappublications.org/content/108/1/190

FLUORIDE USE IN CARIES PREVENTION IN THE PRIMARY CARE SETTING (CLINICAL REPORT)

Melinda B. Clark, MD, FAAP; Rebecca L. Slayton, DDS,
PhD; and Section on Oral Health

ABSTRACT. Dental caries remains the most common chronic disease of childhood in the United States. Caries is a largely preventable condition, and fluoride has proven effectiveness in the prevention of caries. The goals of this clinical report are to clarify the use of available fluoride modalities for caries prevention in the primary care setting and to assist pediatricians in using fluoride to achieve maximum protection against dental caries while minimizing the likelihood of enamel fluorosis. (8/14)

http://pediatrics.aappublications.org/content/134/3/626

FOLIC ACID FOR THE PREVENTION OF NEURAL TUBE DEFECTS

Committee on Genetics

ABSTRACT. The American Academy of Pediatrics endorses the US Public Health Service (USPHS) recommendation that all women capable of becoming pregnant consume 400 µg of folic acid daily to prevent neural tube defects (NTDs). Studies have demonstrated that periconceptional folic acid supplementation can prevent 50% or more of NTDs such as spina bifida and anencephaly. For women who have previously had an NTD-affected pregnancy, the Centers for Disease Control and Prevention (CDC) recommends increasing the intake of folic acid to 4000 µg per day beginning at least 1 month before conception and continuing through the first trimester. Implementation of these recommendations is essential

for the primary prevention of these serious and disabling birth defects. Because fewer than 1 in 3 women consume the amount of folic acid recommended by the USPHS, the Academy notes that the prevention of NTDs depends on an urgent and effective campaign to close this prevention gap. (8/99, reaffirmed 11/02, 1/07, 5/12)
http://pediatrics.aappublications.org/content/104/2/325

FOLLOW-UP MANAGEMENT OF CHILDREN WITH TYMPANOSTOMY TUBES
Section on Otolaryngology and Bronchoesophagology
ABSTRACT. The follow-up care of children in whom tympanostomy tubes have been placed is shared by the pediatrician and the otolaryngologist. Guidelines are provided for routine follow-up evaluation, perioperative hearing assessment, and the identification of specific conditions and complications that warrant urgent otolaryngologic consultation. These guidelines have been developed by a consensus of expert opinions. (2/02)
http://pediatrics.aappublications.org/content/109/2/328

FORGOING LIFE-SUSTAINING MEDICAL TREATMENT IN ABUSED CHILDREN
Committee on Child Abuse and Neglect and Committee on Bioethics
ABSTRACT. A decision to forgo life-sustaining medical treatment (LSMT) for a critically ill child injured as the result of abuse should be made using the same criteria as those used for any critically ill child. The parent or guardian of an abused child may have a conflict of interest when a decision to forgo LSMT risks changing the legal charge faced by a parent, guardian, relative, or acquaintance from assault to manslaughter or homicide. If a physician suspects that a parent or guardian is not acting in a child's best interest, further review and consultation should be sought in hopes of resolving the conflict. A guardian ad litem who will represent the child's interests regarding LSMT should be appointed in all cases in which a parent or guardian may have a conflict of interest. (11/00, reaffirmed 6/03, 10/06, 4/09)
http://pediatrics.aappublications.org/content/106/5/1151

FORGOING MEDICALLY PROVIDED NUTRITION AND HYDRATION IN CHILDREN (CLINICAL REPORT)
Douglas S. Diekema, MD, MPH; Jeffrey R. Botkin, MD, MPH; and Committee on Bioethics
ABSTRACT. There is broad consensus that withholding or withdrawing medical interventions is morally permissible when requested by competent patients or, in the case of patients without decision-making capacity, when the interventions no longer confer a benefit to the patient or when the burdens associated with the interventions outweigh the benefits received. The withdrawal or withholding of measures such as attempted resuscitation, ventilators, and critical care medications is common in the terminal care of adults and children. In the case of adults, a consensus has emerged in law and ethics that the medical administration of fluid and nutrition is not fundamentally different from other medical interventions such as use of ventilators; therefore, it can be forgone or withdrawn when a competent adult or legally authorized surrogate requests withdrawal or when the intervention no longer provides a net benefit to the patient. In pediatrics, forgoing or withdrawing medically administered fluids and nutrition has been more controversial because of the inability of children to make autonomous decisions and the emotional power of feeding as a basic element of the care of children. This statement reviews the medical, ethical, and legal issues relevant to the withholding or withdrawing of medically provided fluids and nutrition in children. The American Academy of Pediatrics concludes that the withdrawal of medically administered fluids and nutrition for pediatric patients is ethically acceptable in limited circumstances. Ethics consultation is strongly recommended when particularly difficult or controversial decisions are being considered. (7/09, reaffirmed 1/14)
http://pediatrics.aappublications.org/content/124/2/813

THE FUTURE OF PEDIATRICS: MENTAL HEALTH COMPETENCIES FOR PEDIATRIC PRIMARY CARE
Committee on Psychosocial Aspects of Child and Family Health and Task Force on Mental Health
ABSTRACT. Pediatric primary care clinicians have unique opportunities and a growing sense of responsibility to prevent and address mental health and substance abuse problems in the medical home. In this report, the American Academy of Pediatrics proposes competencies requisite for providing mental health and substance abuse services in pediatric primary care settings and recommends steps toward achieving them. Achievement of the competencies proposed in this statement is a goal, not a current expectation. It will require innovations in residency training and continuing medical education, as well as a commitment by the individual clinician to pursue, over time, educational strategies suited to his or her learning style and skill level. System enhancements, such as collaborative relationships with mental health specialists and changes in the financing of mental health care, must precede enhancements in clinical practice. For this reason, the proposed competencies begin with knowledge and skills for systems-based practice. The proposed competencies overlap those of mental health specialists in some areas; for example, they include the knowledge and skills to care for children with attention-deficit/hyperactivity disorder, anxiety, depression, and substance abuse and to recognize psychiatric and social emergencies. In other areas, the competencies reflect the uniqueness of the primary care clinician's role: building resilience in all children; promoting healthy lifestyles; preventing or mitigating mental health and substance abuse problems; identifying risk factors and emerging mental health problems in children and their families; and partnering with families, schools, agencies, and mental health specialists to plan assessment and care. Proposed interpersonal and communication skills reflect the primary care clinician's critical role in overcoming barriers (perceived and/or experienced by children and families) to seeking help for mental health and substance abuse concerns. (6/09, reaffirmed 8/13)
http://pediatrics.aappublications.org/content/124/1/410

GASTROESOPHAGEAL REFLUX: MANAGEMENT GUIDANCE FOR THE PEDIATRICIAN (CLINICAL REPORT)

Jenifer R. Lightdale, MD, MPH; David A. Gremse, MD; and Section on Gastroenterology, Hepatology, and Nutrition

ABSTRACT. Recent comprehensive guidelines developed by the North American Society for Pediatric Gastroenterology, Hepatology, and Nutrition define the common entities of gastroesophageal reflux (GER) as the physiologic passage of gastric contents into the esophagus and gastroesophageal reflux disease (GERD) as reflux associated with troublesome symptoms or complications. The ability to distinguish between GER and GERD is increasingly important to implement best practices in the management of acid reflux in patients across all pediatric age groups, as children with GERD may benefit from further evaluation and treatment, whereas conservative recommendations are the only indicated therapy in those with uncomplicated physiologic reflux. This clinical report endorses the rigorously developed, well-referenced North American Society for Pediatric Gastroenterology, Hepatology, and Nutrition guidelines and likewise emphasizes important concepts for the general pediatrician. A key issue is distinguishing between clinical manifestations of GER and GERD in term infants, children, and adolescents to identify patients who can be managed with conservative treatment by the pediatrician and to refer patients who require consultation with the gastroenterologist. Accordingly, the evidence basis presented by the guidelines for diagnostic approaches as well as treatments is discussed. Lifestyle changes are emphasized as first-line therapy in both GER and GERD, whereas medications are explicitly indicated only for patients with GERD. Surgical therapies are reserved for children with intractable symptoms or who are at risk for life-threatening complications of GERD. Recent black box warnings from the US Food and Drug Administration are discussed, and caution is underlined when using promoters of gastric emptying and motility. Finally, attention is paid to increasing evidence of inappropriate prescriptions for proton pump inhibitors in the pediatric population. (4/13)

http://pediatrics.aappublications.org/content/131/5/e1684

GENERIC PRESCRIBING, GENERIC SUBSTITUTION, AND THERAPEUTIC SUBSTITUTION

Committee on Drugs (5/87, reaffirmed 6/93, 5/96, 6/99, 5/01, 5/05, 10/08, 10/12)

http://pediatrics.aappublications.org/content/79/5/835

GLOBAL CLIMATE CHANGE AND CHILDREN'S HEALTH

Council on Environmental Health

ABSTRACT. Rising global temperatures are causing major physical, chemical, and ecological changes in the planet. There is wide consensus among scientific organizations and climatologists that these broad effects, known as "climate change," are the result of contemporary human activity. Climate change poses threats to human health, safety, and security, and children are uniquely vulnerable to these threats. The effects of climate change on child health include: physical and psychological sequelae of weather disasters; increased heat stress; decreased air quality; altered disease patterns of some climate-sensitive infections; and food, water, and nutrient insecurity in vulnerable regions. The social foundations of children's mental and physical health are threatened by the specter of far-reaching effects of unchecked climate change, including community and global instability, mass migrations, and increased conflict. Given this knowledge, failure to take prompt, substantive action would be an act of injustice to all children. A paradigm shift in production and consumption of energy is both a necessity and an opportunity for major innovation, job creation, and significant, immediate associated health benefits. Pediatricians have a uniquely valuable role to play in the societal response to this global challenge. (10/15)

http://pediatrics.aappublications.org/content/136/5/992

GLOBAL CLIMATE CHANGE AND CHILDREN'S HEALTH (TECHNICAL REPORT)

Samantha Ahdoot, MD, FAAP; Susan E. Pacheco, MD, FAAP; and Council on Environmental Health

ABSTRACT. Rising global temperature is causing major physical, chemical, and ecological changes across the planet. There is wide consensus among scientific organizations and climatologists that these broad effects, known as climate change, are the result of contemporary human activity. Climate change poses threats to human health, safety, and security. Children are uniquely vulnerable to these threats. The effects of climate change on child health include physical and psychological sequelae of weather disasters, increased heat stress, decreased air quality, altered disease patterns of some climate-sensitive infections, and food, water, and nutrient insecurity in vulnerable regions. Prompt implementation of mitigation and adaptation strategies will protect children against worsening of the problem and its associated health effects. This technical report reviews the nature of climate change and its associated child health effects and supports the recommendations in the accompanying policy statement on climate change and children's health. (10/15)

http://pediatrics.aappublications.org/content/136/5/e1468

GRADUATE MEDICAL EDUCATION AND PEDIATRIC WORKFORCE ISSUES AND PRINCIPLES

Task Force on Graduate Medical Education Reform (6/94)

http://pediatrics.aappublications.org/content/93/6/1018

GUIDANCE FOR EFFECTIVE DISCIPLINE

Committee on Psychosocial Aspects of Child and Family Health

ABSTRACT. When advising families about discipline strategies, pediatricians should use a comprehensive approach that includes consideration of the parent-child relationship, reinforcement of desired behaviors, and consequences for negative behaviors. Corporal punishment is of limited effectiveness and has potentially deleterious side effects. The American Academy of Pediatrics recommends that parents be encouraged and assisted in the development of methods other than spanking for managing undesired behavior. (4/98, reaffirmed 3/01, 1/05, 5/12, 4/14)

http://pediatrics.aappublications.org/content/101/4/723

GUIDANCE FOR THE ADMINISTRATION OF MEDICATION IN SCHOOL

Council on School Health

ABSTRACT. Many children who take medications require them during the school day. This policy statement is designed to guide prescribing health care professionals, school physicians, and school health councils on the administration of medications to children at school. All districts and schools need to have policies and plans in place for safe, effective, and efficient administration of medications at school. Having full-time licensed registered nurses administering all routine and emergency medications in schools is the best situation. When a licensed registered nurse is not available, a licensed practical nurse may administer medications. When a nurse cannot administer medication in school, the American Academy of Pediatrics supports appropriate delegation of nursing services in the school setting. Delegation is a tool that may be used by the licensed registered school nurse to allow unlicensed assistive personnel to provide standardized, routine health services under the supervision of the nurse and on the basis of physician guidance and school nursing assessment of the unique needs of the individual child and the suitability of delegation of specific nursing tasks. Any delegation of nursing duties must be consistent with the requirements of state nurse practice acts, state regulations, and guidelines provided by professional nursing organizations. Long-term, emergency, and short-term medications; over-the-counter medications; alternative medications; and experimental drugs that are administered as part of a clinical trial are discussed in this statement. This statement has been endorsed by the American School Health Association. (9/09, reaffirmed 2/13)

http://pediatrics.aappublications.org/content/124/4/1244

GUIDANCE ON MANAGEMENT OF ASYMPTOMATIC NEONATES BORN TO WOMEN WITH ACTIVE GENITAL HERPES LESIONS (CLINICAL REPORT)

Committee on Infectious Diseases and Committee on Fetus and Newborn

ABSTRACT. Herpes simplex virus (HSV) infection of the neonate is uncommon, but genital herpes infections in adults are very common. Thus, although treating an infant with neonatal herpes is a relatively rare occurrence, managing infants potentially exposed to HSV at the time of delivery occurs more frequently. The risk of transmitting HSV to an infant during delivery is determined in part by the mother's previous immunity to HSV. Women with primary genital HSV infections who are shedding HSV at delivery are 10 to 30 times more likely to transmit the virus to their newborn infants than are women with recurrent HSV infection who are shedding virus at delivery. With the availability of commercial serological tests that reliably can distinguish type-specific HSV antibodies, it is now possible to determine the type of maternal infection and, thus, further refine management of infants delivered to women who have active genital HSV lesions. The management algorithm presented herein uses both serological and virological studies to determine the risk of HSV transmission to the neonate who is delivered to a mother with active herpetic genital lesions and tailors management accordingly. The algorithm does not address the approach to asymptomatic neonates delivered to women with a history of genital herpes but no active lesions at delivery. (1/13)

http://pediatrics.aappublications.org/content/131/2/e635

GUIDELINES FOR CARE OF CHILDREN IN THE EMERGENCY DEPARTMENT

Committee on Pediatric Emergency Medicine (joint with American College of Emergency Physicians Pediatric Committee and Emergency Nurses Association Pediatric Committee)

ABSTRACT. Children who require emergency care have unique needs, especially when emergencies are serious or life-threatening. The majority of ill and injured children are brought to community hospital emergency departments (EDs) by virtue of their geography within communities. Similarly, emergency medical services (EMS) agencies provide the bulk of out-of-hospital emergency care to children. It is imperative, therefore, that all hospital EDs have the appropriate resources (medications, equipment, policies, and education) and staff to provide effective emergency care for children. This statement outlines resources necessary to ensure that hospital EDs stand ready to care for children of all ages, from neonates to adolescents. These guidelines are consistent with the recommendations of the Institute of Medicine's report on the future of emergency care in the United States health system. Although resources within emergency and trauma care systems vary locally, regionally, and nationally, it is essential that hospital ED staff and administrators and EMS systems' administrators and medical directors seek to meet or exceed these guidelines in efforts to optimize the emergency care of children they serve. This statement has been endorsed by the Academic Pediatric Association, American Academy of Family Physicians, American Academy of Physician Assistants, American College of Osteopathic Emergency Physicians, American College of Surgeons, American Heart Association, American Medical Association, American Pediatric Surgical Association, Brain Injury Association of America, Child Health Corporation of America, Children's National Medical Center, Family Voices, National Association of Children's Hospitals and Related Institutions, National Association of EMS Physicians, National Association of Emergency Medical Technicians, National Association of State EMS Officials, National Committee for Quality Assurance, National PTA, Safe Kids USA, Society of Trauma Nurses, Society for Academic Emergency Medicine, and The Joint Commission. (9/09, reaffirmed 4/13, 2/16)

http://pediatrics.aappublications.org/content/124/4/1233

GUIDELINES FOR DEVELOPING ADMISSION AND DISCHARGE POLICIES FOR THE PEDIATRIC INTENSIVE CARE UNIT (CLINICAL REPORT)

Committee on Hospital Care and Section on Critical Care (joint with Society of Critical Care Medicine Pediatric Section Admission Criteria Task Force)

ABSTRACT. These guidelines were developed to provide a reference for preparing policies on admission to and discharge from pediatric intensive care units. They represent a consensus opinion of physicians, nurses, and allied health care professionals. By using this document as a framework for developing multidisciplinary admission and discharge policies, use of pediatric intensive care units can be optimized and patients can receive the level of care appropriate for their condition. (4/99, reaffirmed 5/05, 2/08, 1/13)

http://pediatrics.aappublications.org/content/103/4/840

GUIDELINES FOR HOME CARE OF INFANTS, CHILDREN, AND ADOLESCENTS WITH CHRONIC DISEASE

Committee on Children With Disabilities (7/95, reaffirmed 4/00, 1/06)

http://pediatrics.aappublications.org/content/96/1/161

GUIDELINES FOR MONITORING AND MANAGEMENT OF PEDIATRIC PATIENTS BEFORE, DURING, AND AFTER SEDATION FOR DIAGNOSTIC AND THERAPEUTIC PROCEDURES: UPDATE 2016 (CLINICAL REPORT)

Charles J. Coté, MD, FAAP; Stephen Wilson, DMD, MA, PhD; and American Academy of Pediatrics (joint with American Academy of Pediatric Dentistry)

ABSTRACT. The safe sedation of children for procedures requires a systematic approach that includes the following: no administration of sedating medication without the safety net of medical/dental supervision, careful presedation evaluation for underlying medical or surgical conditions that would place the child at increased risk from sedating medications, appropriate fasting for elective procedures and a balance between the depth of sedation and risk for those who are unable to fast because of the urgent nature of the procedure, a focused airway examination for large (kissing) tonsils or anatomic airway abnormalities that might increase the potential for airway obstruction, a clear understanding of the medication's pharmacokinetic and pharmacodynamic effects and drug interactions, appropriate training and skills in airway management to allow rescue of the patient, age- and size-appropriate equipment for airway management and venous access, appropriate medications and reversal agents, sufficient numbers of staff to both carry out the procedure and monitor the patient, appropriate physiologic monitoring during and after the procedure, a properly equipped and staffed recovery area, recovery to the presedation level of consciousness before discharge from medical/dental supervision, and appropriate discharge instructions. This report was developed through a collaborative effort of the American Academy of Pediatrics and the American Academy of Pediatric Dentistry to offer pediatric providers updated information and guidance in delivering safe sedation to children. (6/16)

See full text on page 787.

http://pediatrics.aappublications.org/content/138/1/e20161212

GUIDELINES FOR PEDIATRIC CANCER CENTERS

Section on Hematology/Oncology

ABSTRACT. Since the American Academy of Pediatrics published guidelines for pediatric cancer centers in 1986 and 1997, significant changes in the delivery of health care have prompted a review of the role of tertiary medical centers in the care of pediatric patients. The potential effect of these changes on the treatment and survival rates of children with cancer led to this revision. The intent of this statement is to delineate personnel and facilities that are essential to provide state-of-the-art care for children and adolescents with cancer. This statement emphasizes the importance of board-certified pediatric hematologists/oncologists, pediatric subspecialty consultants, and appropriately qualified pediatric medical subspecialists and pediatric surgical specialists overseeing the care of all pediatric and adolescent cancer patients and the need for facilities available only at a tertiary center as essential for the initial management and much of the follow-up for pediatric and adolescent cancer patients. (6/04, reaffirmed 10/08)

http://pediatrics.aappublications.org/content/113/6/1833

GUIDELINES FOR PEDIATRIC CARDIOVASCULAR CENTERS

Section on Cardiology and Cardiac Surgery

ABSTRACT. Pediatric cardiovascular centers should aim to provide high-quality therapeutic outcomes for infants and children with congenital and acquired heart diseases. This policy statement describes critical elements and organizational features of centers in which high-quality outcomes have the greatest likelihood of occurring. Center elements include noninvasive diagnostic modalities, cardiac catheterization, cardiovascular surgery, and cardiovascular intensive care. These elements should be organizationally united in centers in which pediatric cardiac physician specialists and specialized pediatric staff work together to achieve and surpass existing quality-of-care benchmarks. (3/02, reaffirmed 10/07)

http://pediatrics.aappublications.org/content/109/3/544

GUIDELINES FOR THE DETERMINATION OF BRAIN DEATH IN INFANTS AND CHILDREN: AN UPDATE OF THE 1987 TASK FORCE RECOMMENDATIONS (CLINICAL REPORT)

Thomas A. Nakagawa, MD; Stephen Ashwal, MD; Mudit Mathur, MD; Mohan Mysore, MD; Section on Critical Care; and Section on Neurology (joint with Society of Critical Care Medicine and Child Neurology Society)

ABSTRACT. *Objective.* To review and revise the 1987 pediatric brain death guidelines.

Methods. Relevant literature was reviewed. Recommendations were developed using the GRADE system.

Conclusions and Recommendations.

1. Determination of brain death in term newborns, infants and children is a clinical diagnosis based on the absence of neurologic function with a known irreversible cause of coma. Because of insufficient data in the literature, recommendations for preterm infants less than 37 weeks' gestational age are not included in this guideline.

2. Hypotension, hypothermia, and metabolic disturbances should be treated and corrected and medications that can interfere with the neurologic examination and apnea testing should be discontinued allowing for adequate clearance before proceeding with these evaluations.

3. Two examinations including apnea testing with each examination separated by an observation period are required. Examinations should be performed by different attending physicians. Apnea testing may be performed by the same physician. An observation period

of 24 hours for term newborns (37 weeks' gestational age) to 30 days of age, and 12 hours for infants and children (> 30 days to 18 years) is recommended. The first examination determines the child has met the accepted neurologic examination criteria for brain death. The second examination confirms brain death based on an unchanged and irreversible condition. Assessment of neurologic function following cardiopulmonary resuscitation or other severe acute brain injuries should be deferred for 24 hours or longer if there are concerns or inconsistencies in the examination.

4. Apnea testing to support the diagnosis of brain death must be performed safely and requires documentation of an arterial $Paco_2$ 20 mm Hg above the baseline and ≥ 60 mm Hg with no respiratory effort during the testing period. If the apnea test cannot be safely completed, an ancillary study should be performed.

5. Ancillary studies (electroencephalogram and radionuclide cerebral blood flow) are not required to establish brain death and are not a substitute for the neurologic examination. Ancillary studies may be us d to assist the clinician in making the diagnosis of brain death (1) when components of the examination or apnea testing cannot be completed safely due to the underlying medical condition of the patient; (2) if there is uncertainty about the results of the neurologic examination; (3) if a medication effect may be present; or (4) to reduce the inter-examination observation period. When ancillary studies are used, a second clinical examination and apnea test should be performed and components that can be completed must remain consistent with brain death. In this instance the observation interval may be shortened and the second neurologic examination and apnea test (or all components that are able to be completed safely) can be performed at any time thereafter.

6. Death is declared when the above criteria are fulfilled. (8/11, reaffirmed 1/15)

http://pediatrics.aappublications.org/content/128/3/e720

GUIDELINES FOR THE ETHICAL CONDUCT OF STUDIES TO EVALUATE DRUGS IN PEDIATRIC POPULATIONS (CLINICAL REPORT)

Robert E. Shaddy, MD; Scott C. Denne, MD; Committee on Drugs; and Committee on Pediatric Research

ABSTRACT. The proper ethical conduct of studies to evaluate drugs in children is of paramount importance to all those involved in these types of studies. This report is an updated revision to the previously published guidelines from the American Academy of Pediatrics in 1995. Since the previous publication, there have been great strides made in the science and ethics of studying drugs in children. There have also been numerous legislative and regulatory advancements that have promoted the study of drugs in children while simultaneously allowing for the protection of this particularly vulnerable group. This report summarizes these changes and advances and provides a framework from which to guide and monitor the ethical conduct of studies to evaluate drugs in children. (3/10, reaffirmed 1/14)

http://pediatrics.aappublications.org/content/125/4/850

GUIDELINES ON FORGOING LIFE-SUSTAINING MEDICAL TREATMENT

Committee on Bioethics (3/94, reaffirmed 11/97, 10/00, 1/04, 1/09, 10/12)

http://pediatrics.aappublications.org/content/93/3/532

GUIDING PRINCIPLES FOR MANAGED CARE ARRANGEMENTS FOR THE HEALTH CARE OF NEWBORNS, INFANTS, CHILDREN, ADOLESCENTS, AND YOUNG ADULTS

Committee on Child Health Financing

ABSTRACT. By including the precepts of primary care and the medical home in the delivery of services, managed care can be effective in increasing access to a full range of health care services and clinicians. A carefully designed and administered managed care plan can minimize patient under- and overutilization of services, as well as enhance quality of care. Therefore, the American Academy of Pediatrics urges the use of the key principles outlined in this statement in designing and implementing managed care programs for newborns, infants, children, adolescents, and young adults to maximize the positive potential of managed care for pediatrics. (10/13)

http://pediatrics.aappublications.org/content/132/5/e1452

GUIDING PRINCIPLES FOR PEDIATRIC HOSPITAL MEDICINE PROGRAMS

Section on Hospital Medicine

ABSTRACT. Pediatric hospital medicine programs have an established place in pediatric medicine. This statement speaks to the expanded roles and responsibilities of pediatric hospitalists and their integrated role among the community of pediatricians who care for children within and outside of the hospital setting. (9/13)

http://pediatrics.aappublications.org/content/132/4/782

GYNECOLOGIC EXAMINATION FOR ADOLESCENTS IN THE PEDIATRIC OFFICE SETTING (CLINICAL REPORT)

Paula K. Braverman, MD; Lesley Breech, MD; and Committee on Adolescence

ABSTRACT. The American Academy of Pediatrics promotes the inclusion of the gynecologic examination in the primary care setting within the medical home. Gynecologic issues are commonly seen by clinicians who provide primary care to adolescents. Some of the most common concerns include questions related to pubertal development; menstrual disorders such as dysmenorrhea, amenorrhea, oligomenorrhea, and abnormal uterine bleeding; contraception; and sexually transmitted and non–sexually transmitted infections. The gynecologic examination is a key element in assessing pubertal status and documenting physical findings. Most adolescents do not need an internal examination involving a speculum or bimanual examination. However, for cases in which more extensive examination is needed, the primary care office with the primary care clinician who has established rapport and trust with the patient is often the best setting for pelvic examination. This report reviews the gynecologic examination, including indications for the pelvic examination in adolescents and the approach to this examination in the office setting. Indications for referral to a gynecologist are included. The pelvic examination may be successfully completed when conducted without pressure and

approached as a normal part of routine young women's health care. (8/10, reaffirmed 5/13)
http://pediatrics.aappublications.org/content/126/3/583

HANDOFFS: TRANSITIONS OF CARE FOR CHILDREN IN THE EMERGENCY DEPARTMENT

Committee on Pediatric Emergency Medicine (joint with American College of Emergency Physicians Pediatric Emergency Medicine Committee and Emergency Nurses Association Pediatric Committee)

ABSTRACT. Transitions of care (ToCs), also referred to as handoffs or sign-outs, occur when the responsibility for a patient's care transfers from 1 health care provider to another. Transitions are common in the acute care setting and have been noted to be vulnerable events with opportunities for error. Health care is taking ideas from other high-risk industries, such as aerospace and nuclear power, to create models of structured transition processes. Although little literature currently exists to establish 1 model as superior, multiorganizational consensus groups agree that standardization is warranted and that additional work is needed to establish characteristics of ToCs that are associated with clinical or practice outcomes. The rationale for structuring ToCs, specifically those related to the care of children in the emergency setting, and a description of identified strategies are presented, along with resources for educating health care providers on ToCs. Recommendations for development, education, and implementation of transition models are included. (10/16)
See full text on page 821.
http://pediatrics.aappublications.org/content/138/5/e20162680

HEAD LICE (CLINICAL REPORT)

Cynthia D. Devore, MD, FAAP; Gordon E. Schutze, MD, FAAP; Council on School Health; and Committee on Infectious Diseases

ABSTRACT. Head lice infestation is associated with limited morbidity but causes a high level of anxiety among parents of school-aged children. Since the 2010 clinical report on head lice was published by the American Academy of Pediatrics, newer medications have been approved for the treatment of head lice. This revised clinical report clarifies current diagnosis and treatment protocols and provides guidance for the management of children with head lice in the school setting. (4/15)
http://pediatrics.aappublications.org/content/135/5/e1355

HEALTH AND MENTAL HEALTH NEEDS OF CHILDREN IN US MILITARY FAMILIES (CLINICAL REPORT)

Benjamin S. Siegel, MD; Beth Ellen Davis, MD, MPH; Committee on Psychosocial Aspects of Child and Family Health; and Section on Uniformed Services

ABSTRACT. The wars in Afghanistan and Iraq have been challenging for US uniformed service families and their children. Almost 60% of US service members have family responsibilities. Approximately 2.3 million active duty, National Guard, and Reserve service members have been deployed since the beginning of the wars in Afghanistan and Iraq (2001 and 2003, respectively), and almost half have deployed more than once, some for up to 18 months' duration. Up to 2 million US children have been exposed to a wartime deployment of a loved one in the past 10 years. Many service members have returned from combat deployments with symptoms of posttraumatic stress disorder, depression, anxiety, substance abuse, and traumatic brain injury. The mental health and well-being of spouses, significant others, children (and their friends), and extended family members of deployed service members continues to be significantly challenged by the experiences of wartime deployment as well as by combat mortality and morbidity. The medical system of the Department of Defense provides health and mental health services for active duty service members and their families as well as activated National Guard and Reserve service members and their families. In addition to military pediatricians and civilian pediatricians employed by military treatment facilities, nonmilitary general pediatricians care for >50% of children and family members before, during, and after wartime deployments. This clinical report is for all pediatricians, both active duty and civilian, to aid in caring for children whose loved ones have been, are, or will be deployed. (5/13)
http://pediatrics.aappublications.org/content/131/6/e2002

HEALTH CARE FOR YOUTH IN THE JUVENILE JUSTICE SYSTEM

Committee on Adolescence

ABSTRACT. Youth in the juvenile correctional system are a high-risk population who, in many cases, have unmet physical, developmental, and mental health needs. Multiple studies have found that some of these health issues occur at higher rates than in the general adolescent population. Although some youth in the juvenile justice system have interfaced with health care providers in their community on a regular basis, others have had inconsistent or nonexistent care. The health needs of these youth are commonly identified when they are admitted to a juvenile custodial facility. Pediatricians and other health care providers play an important role in the care of these youth, and continuity between the community and the correctional facility is crucial. This policy statement provides an overview of the health needs of youth in the juvenile correctional system, including existing resources and standards for care, financing of health care within correctional facilities, and evidence-based interventions. Recommendations are provided for the provision of health care services to youth in the juvenile correctional system as well as specific areas for advocacy efforts. (11/11)
http://pediatrics.aappublications.org/content/128/6/1219

HEALTH CARE ISSUES FOR CHILDREN AND ADOLESCENTS IN FOSTER CARE AND KINSHIP CARE

Council on Foster Care, Adoption, and Kinship Care; Committee on Adolescence; and Council on Early Childhood

ABSTRACT. Children and adolescents who enter foster care often do so with complicated and serious medical, mental health, developmental, oral health, and psychosocial problems rooted in their history of childhood trauma. Ideally, health care for this population is provided in a pediatric medical home by physicians who are familiar with the sequelae of childhood trauma and adversity. As youth with special health care needs, children and adolescents in foster care require more frequent monitoring of their health status, and pediatricians have a critical role in ensuring the well-being of children in out-of-home care through the provision of high-quality pediatric health services, health care coordination, and advocacy on their behalves. (9/15)

http://pediatrics.aappublications.org/content/136/4/e1131

HEALTH CARE ISSUES FOR CHILDREN AND ADOLESCENTS IN FOSTER CARE AND KINSHIP CARE (TECHNICAL REPORT)

Moira A. Szilagyi, MD, PhD; David S. Rosen, MD, MPH; David Rubin, MD, MSCE; Sarah Zlotnik, MSW, MSPH; Council on Foster Care, Adoption, and Kinship Care; Committee on Adolescence; and Council on Early Childhood

ABSTRACT. Children and adolescents involved with child welfare, especially those who are removed from their family of origin and placed in out-of-home care, often present with complex and serious physical, mental health, developmental, and psychosocial problems rooted in childhood adversity and trauma. As such, they are designated as children with special health care needs. There are many barriers to providing high-quality comprehensive health care services to children and adolescents whose lives are characterized by transience and uncertainty. Pediatricians have a critical role in ensuring the well-being of children in out-of-home care through the provision of high-quality pediatric health services in the context of a medical home, and health care coordination and advocacy on their behalf. This technical report supports the policy statement of the same title. (9/15)

http://pediatrics.aappublications.org/content/136/4/e1142

HEALTH CARE OF YOUTH AGING OUT OF FOSTER CARE

Council on Foster Care, Adoption, and Kinship Care and Committee on Early Childhood

ABSTRACT. Youth transitioning out of foster care face significant medical and mental health care needs. Unfortunately, these youth rarely receive the services they need because of lack of health insurance. Through many policies and programs, the federal government has taken steps to support older youth in foster care and those aging out. The Fostering Connections to Success and Increasing Adoptions Act of 2008 (Pub L No. 110-354) requires states to work with youth to develop a transition plan that addresses issues such as health insurance. In addition, beginning in 2014, the Patient Protection and Affordable Care Act of 2010 (Pub L No. 111-148) makes youth aging out of foster care eligible for Medicaid coverage until age 26 years, regardless of income. Pediatricians can support youth aging out of foster care by working collaboratively with the child welfare agency in their state to ensure that the ongoing health needs of transitioning youth are met. (11/12)

http://pediatrics.aappublications.org/content/130/6/1170

HEALTH CARE SUPERVISION FOR CHILDREN WITH WILLIAMS SYNDROME

Committee on Genetics

ABSTRACT. This set of guidelines is designed to assist the pediatrician to care for children with Williams syndrome diagnosed by clinical features and with regional chromosomal microdeletion confirmed by fluorescence in situ hybridization. (5/01, reaffirmed 5/05, 1/09)

http://pediatrics.aappublications.org/content/107/5/1192

HEALTH EQUITY AND CHILDREN'S RIGHTS

Council on Community Pediatrics and Committee on Native American Child Health

ABSTRACT. Many children in the United States fail to reach their full health and developmental potential. Disparities in their health and well-being result from the complex interplay of multiple social and environmental determinants that are not adequately addressed by current standards of pediatric practice or public policy. Integrating the principles and practice of child health equity—children's rights, social justice, human capital investment, and health equity ethics—into pediatrics will address the root causes of child health disparities.

Promoting the principles and practice of equity-based clinical care, child advocacy, and child- and family-centered public policy will help to ensure that social and environmental determinants contribute positively to the health and well-being of children. The American Academy of Pediatrics and pediatricians can move the national focus from documenting child health disparities to advancing the principles and practice of child health equity and, in so doing, influence the worldwide practice of pediatrics and child health. All pediatricians, including primary care practitioners and medical and surgical subspecialists, can incorporate these principles into their practice of pediatrics and child health. Integration of these principles into competency-based training and board certification will secure their assimilation into all levels of pediatric practice. (3/10, reaffirmed 10/13)

http://pediatrics.aappublications.org/content/125/4/838

HEALTH INFORMATION TECHNOLOGY AND THE MEDICAL HOME

Council on Clinical Information Technology

ABSTRACT. The American Academy of Pediatrics (AAP) supports development and universal implementation of a comprehensive electronic infrastructure to support pediatric information functions of the medical home. These functions include (1) timely and continuous management and tracking of health data and services over a patient's lifetime for all providers, patients, families, and guardians, (2) comprehensive organization and secure transfer of health data during patient-care transitions between providers, institutions, and practices, (3) establishment and maintenance of central coordination of a patient's health information among multiple repositories (including personal health records and information exchanges), (4) translation of evidence into actionable clinical decision support, and (5) reuse of archived clinical data for continuous quality improvement. The AAP supports universal, secure, and vendor-neutral portability of health information for all patients contained within the medical home across all care settings (ambulatory practices, inpatient settings, emergency departments, pharmacies, consultants, support service providers, and therapists) for multiple purposes including direct care, personal health records, public health, and registries. The AAP also supports financial incentives that promote the development of information tools that meet the needs of pediatric workflows and that appropriately recognize the added value of medical homes to pediatric care. (4/11, reaffirmed 7/15)

http://pediatrics.aappublications.org/content/127/5/978

HEALTH SUPERVISION FOR CHILDREN WITH ACHONDROPLASIA (CLINICAL REPORT)

Tracy L. Trotter, MD; Judith G. Hall, OC, MD; and Committee on Genetics

ABSTRACT. Achondroplasia is the most common condition associated with disproportionate short stature. Substantial information is available concerning the natural history and anticipatory health supervision needs in children with this dwarfing disorder. Most children with achondroplasia have delayed motor milestones, problems with persistent or recurrent middle-ear dysfunction, and bowing of the lower legs. Less often, infants and children may have serious health consequences related to hydrocephalus, craniocervical junction compression, upper-airway obstruction, or thoracolumbar kyphosis. Anticipatory care should be directed at identifying children who are at high risk and intervening to prevent serious sequelae. This report is designed to help the pediatrician care for children with achondroplasia and their families. (9/05, reaffirmed 5/12)

http://pediatrics.aappublications.org/content/116/3/771

HEALTH SUPERVISION FOR CHILDREN WITH DOWN SYNDROME (CLINICAL REPORT)

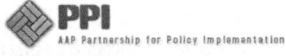

Marilyn J. Bull, MD, and Committee on Genetics

ABSTRACT. These guidelines are designed to assist the pediatrician in caring for the child in whom a diagnosis of Down syndrome has been confirmed by chromosome analysis. Although a pediatrician's initial contact with the child is usually during infancy, occasionally the pregnant woman who has been given a prenatal diagnosis of Down syndrome will be referred for review of the condition and the genetic counseling provided. Therefore, this report offers guidance for this situation as well. (7/11)

http://pediatrics.aappublications.org/content/128/2/393

HEALTH SUPERVISION FOR CHILDREN WITH FRAGILE X SYNDROME (CLINICAL REPORT)

Joseph H. Hersh, MD; Robert A. Saul, MD; and Committee on Genetics

ABSTRACT. Fragile X syndrome (an *FMR1*–related disorder) is the most commonly inherited form of mental retardation. Early physical recognition is difficult, so boys with developmental delay should be strongly considered for molecular testing. The characteristic adult phenotype usually does not develop until the second decade of life. Girls can also be affected with developmental delay. Because multiple family members can be affected with mental retardation and other conditions (premature ovarian failure and tremor/ataxia), family history information is of critical importance for the diagnosis and management of affected patients and their families. This report summarizes issues for fragile X syndrome regarding clinical diagnosis, laboratory diagnosis, genetic counseling, related health problems, behavior management, and age-related health supervision guidelines. The diagnosis of fragile X syndrome not only involves the affected children but also potentially has significant health consequences for multiple generations in each family. (4/11)

http://pediatrics.aappublications.org/content/127/5/994

HEALTH SUPERVISION FOR CHILDREN WITH MARFAN SYNDROME (CLINICAL REPORT)

Brad T. Tinkle, MD, PhD; Howard M. Saal, MD; and Committee on Genetics

ABSTRACT. Marfan syndrome is a systemic, heritable connective tissue disorder that affects many different organ systems and is best managed by using a multidisciplinary approach. The guidance in this report is designed to assist the pediatrician in recognizing the features of Marfan syndrome as well as caring for the individual with this disorder. (9/13)

http://pediatrics.aappublications.org/content/132/4/e1059

HEALTH SUPERVISION FOR CHILDREN WITH NEUROFIBROMATOSIS (CLINICAL REPORT)

Joseph H. Hersh, MD, and Committee on Genetics

ABSTRACT. Neurofibromatosis 1 is a multisystem disorder that primarily involves the skin and nervous system. Its population prevalence is 1 in 3500. The condition usually is recognized in early childhood, when cutaneous manifestations are apparent. Although neurofibromatosis 1 is associated with marked clinical variability, most affected children do well from the standpoint of their growth and development. Some features of neurofibromatosis 1 are present at birth, and others are age-related abnormalities of tissue proliferation, which necessitate periodic monitoring to address ongoing health and developmental needs and to minimize the risk of serious medical complications. This clinical report provides a review of the clinical criteria needed to establish a diagnosis, the inheritance pattern of neurofibromatosis 1, its major clinical and developmental manifestations, and guidelines for monitoring and providing intervention to maximize the growth, development, and health of an affected child. (3/08)

http://pediatrics.aappublications.org/content/121/3/633

HEALTH SUPERVISION FOR CHILDREN WITH PRADER-WILLI SYNDROME (CLINICAL REPORT)

Shawn E. McCandless, MD, and Committee on Genetics

ABSTRACT. This set of guidelines was designed to assist the pediatrician in caring for children with Prader-Willi syndrome diagnosed by clinical features and confirmed by molecular testing. Prader-Willi syndrome provides an excellent example of how early diagnosis and management can improve the long-term outcome for some genetic disorders. (12/10)

http://pediatrics.aappublications.org/content/127/1/195

HEALTH SUPERVISION FOR CHILDREN WITH SICKLE CELL DISEASE

Section on Hematology/Oncology and Committee on Genetics

ABSTRACT. Sickle cell disease (SCD) is a group of complex genetic disorders with multisystem manifestations. This statement provides pediatricians in primary care and subspecialty practice with an overview of the genetics, diagnosis, clinical manifestations, and treatment of SCD. Specialized comprehensive medical care decreases morbidity and mortality during childhood. The provision of comprehensive care is a time-intensive endeavor that includes ongoing patient and family education,

periodic comprehensive evaluations and other disease-specific health maintenance services, psychosocial care, and genetic counseling. Timely and appropriate treatment of acute illness is critical, because life-threatening complications develop rapidly. It is essential that every child with SCD receive comprehensive care that is coordinated through a medical home with appropriate expertise. (3/02, reaffirmed 1/06, 1/11, 2/16)
http://pediatrics.aappublications.org/content/109/3/526

HEARING ASSESSMENT IN INFANTS AND CHILDREN: RECOMMENDATIONS BEYOND NEONATAL SCREENING (CLINICAL REPORT)

PPI
AAP Partnership for Policy Implementation

Allen D. "Buz" Harlor Jr, MD; Charles Bower, MD;
Committee on Practice and Ambulatory Medicine; and
Section on Otolaryngology–Head and Neck Surgery

ABSTRACT. Congenital or acquired hearing loss in infants and children has been linked with lifelong deficits in speech and language acquisition, poor academic performance, personal-social maladjustments, and emotional difficulties. Identification of hearing loss through neonatal hearing screening, regular surveillance of developmental milestones, auditory skills, parental concerns, and middle-ear status and objective hearing screening of all infants and children at critical developmental stages can prevent or reduce many of these adverse consequences. This report promotes a proactive, consistent, and explicit process for the early identification of children with hearing loss in the medical home. An algorithm of the recommended approach has been developed to assist in the detection and documentation of, and intervention for, hearing loss. (9/09)
http://pediatrics.aappublications.org/content/124/4/1252

HELPING CHILDREN AND FAMILIES DEAL WITH DIVORCE AND SEPARATION (CLINICAL REPORT)

George J. Cohen, MD, FAAP; Carol C. Weitzman, MD,
FAAP; Committee on Psychosocial Aspects of Child
and Family Health; and Section on Developmental and
Behavioral Pediatrics

ABSTRACT. For the past several years in the United States, there have been more than 800 000 divorces and parent separations annually, with over 1 million children affected. Children and their parents can experience emotional trauma before, during, and after a separation or divorce. Pediatricians can be aware of their patients' behavior and parental attitudes and behaviors that may indicate family dysfunction and that can indicate need for intervention. Age-appropriate explanation and counseling for the child and advice and guidance for the parents, as well as recommendation of reading material, may help reduce the potential negative effects of divorce. Often, referral to professionals with expertise in the social, emotional, and legal aspects of the separation and its aftermath may be helpful for these families. (11/16)
See full text on page 835.
http://pediatrics.aappublications.org/content/138/6/e20163020

HIGH-DEDUCTIBLE HEALTH PLANS

Committee on Child Health Financing

ABSTRACT. High-deductible health plans (HDHPs) are insurance policies with higher deductibles than conventional plans. The Medicare Prescription Drug Improvement and Modernization Act of 2003 linked many HDHPs with tax-advantaged spending accounts. The 2010 Patient Protection and Affordable Care Act continues to provide for HDHPs in its lower-level plans on the health insurance marketplace and provides for them in employer-offered plans. HDHPs decrease the premium cost of insurance policies for purchasers and shift the risk of further payments to the individual subscriber. HDHPs reduce utilization and total medical costs, at least in the short term. Because HDHPs require out-of-pocket payment in the initial stages of care, primary care and other outpatient services as well as elective procedures are the services most affected, whereas higher-cost services in the health care system, incurred after the deductible is met, are unaffected. HDHPs promote adverse selection because healthier and wealthier patients tend to opt out of conventional plans in favor of HDHPs. Because the ill pay more than the healthy under HDHPs, families with children with special health care needs bear an increased cost burden in this model. HDHPs discourage use of nonpreventive primary care and thus are at odds with most recommendations for improving the organization of health care, which focus on strengthening primary care.

This policy statement provides background information on HDHPs, discusses the implications for families and pediatric care providers, and suggests courses of action. (4/14)
http://pediatrics.aappublications.org/content/133/5/e1461

HIGH-DEDUCTIBLE HEALTH PLANS AND THE NEW RISKS OF CONSUMER-DRIVEN HEALTH INSURANCE PRODUCTS

Committee on Child Health Financing

ABSTRACT. Consumer-driven health care is the most noteworthy development in health insurance since the widespread adoption of health maintenance organizations and preferred provider organizations in the 1980s. The most common consumer-driven health plan is the high-deductible health plan, which is essentially a catastrophic health insurance plan, often linked with tax-advantaged spending accounts, with very high deductibles, fewer benefits, and higher cost-sharing than conventional health maintenance organization or preferred provider organization plans. The financial risks are significant under high-deductible health plans, especially for low- to moderate-income families and for families whose children have special health care needs. Of concern for pediatricians are the potential quality risks that are predictable in high-deductible health plans, in which families are likely to delay or avoid seeking care, especially preventive care (if it is not exempted from the deductible), when they are faced with paying for care before the deductible is met. This policy statement provides background information on the most common consumer-driven health plan model, discusses the implications for pediatricians and families, and offers recommendations pertaining to health plan product design, education, practice administration, and research. (3/07)
http://pediatrics.aappublications.org/content/119/3/622

HIV TESTING AND PROPHYLAXIS TO PREVENT MOTHER-TO-CHILD TRANSMISSION IN THE UNITED STATES

Committee on Pediatric AIDS

ABSTRACT. Universal HIV testing of pregnant women in the United States is the key to prevention of mother-to-child transmission of HIV. Repeat testing in the third trimester and rapid HIV testing at labor and delivery are additional strategies to further reduce the rate of perinatal HIV transmission. Prevention of mother-to-child transmission of HIV is most effective when antiretroviral drugs are received by the mother during her pregnancy and continued through delivery and then administered to the infant after birth. Antiretroviral drugs are effective in reducing the risk of mother-to-child transmission of HIV even when prophylaxis is started for the infant soon after birth. New rapid testing methods allow identification of HIV-infected women or HIV-exposed infants in 20 to 60 minutes. The American Academy of Pediatrics recommends documented, routine HIV testing for all pregnant women in the United States after notifying the patient that testing will be performed, unless the patient declines HIV testing ("opt-out" consent or "right of refusal"). For women in labor with undocumented HIV-infection status during the current pregnancy, immediate maternal HIV testing with opt-out consent, using a rapid HIV antibody test, is recommended. Positive HIV antibody screening test results should be confirmed with immunofluorescent antibody or Western blot assay. For women with a positive rapid HIV antibody test result, antiretroviral prophylaxis should be administered promptly to the mother and newborn infant on the basis of the positive result of the rapid antibody test without waiting for results of confirmatory HIV testing. If the confirmatory test result is negative, then prophylaxis should be discontinued. For a newborn infant whose mother's HIV serostatus is unknown, the health care professional should perform rapid HIV antibody testing on the mother or on the newborn infant, with results reported to the health care professional no later than 12 hours after the infant's birth. If the rapid HIV antibody test result is positive, antiretroviral prophylaxis should be instituted as soon as possible after birth but certainly by 12 hours after delivery, pending completion of confirmatory HIV testing. The mother should be counseled not to breastfeed the infant. Assistance with immediate initiation of hand and pump expression to stimulate milk production should be offered to the mother, given the possibility that the confirmatory test result may be negative. If the confirmatory test result is negative, then prophylaxis should be stopped and breastfeeding may be initiated. If the confirmatory test result is positive, infants should receive antiretroviral prophylaxis for 6 weeks after birth, and the mother should not breastfeed the infant. (11/08, reaffirmed 6/11, 11/14)

http://pediatrics.aappublications.org/content/122/5/1127

HOME, HOSPITAL, AND OTHER NON–SCHOOL-BASED INSTRUCTION FOR CHILDREN AND ADOLESCENTS WHO ARE MEDICALLY UNABLE TO ATTEND SCHOOL

Committee on School Health

ABSTRACT. The American Academy of Pediatrics recommends that school-aged children and adolescents obtain their education in school in the least restrictive setting, that is, the setting most conducive to learning for the particular student. However, at times, acute illness or injury and chronic medical conditions preclude school attendance. This statement is meant to assist evaluation and planning for children to receive non–school-based instruction and to return to school at the earliest possible date. (11/00, reaffirmed 6/03, 5/06)

http://pediatrics.aappublications.org/content/106/5/1154

HOME CARE OF CHILDREN AND YOUTH WITH COMPLEX HEALTH CARE NEEDS AND TECHNOLOGY DEPENDENCIES (CLINICAL REPORT)

Ellen Roy Elias, MD; Nancy A. Murphy, MD; and Council on Children With Disabilities

ABSTRACT. Children and youth with complex medical issues, especially those with technology dependencies, experience frequent and often lengthy hospitalizations. Hospital discharges for these children can be a complicated process that requires a deliberate, multistep approach. In addition to successful discharges to home, it is essential that pediatric providers develop and implement an interdisciplinary and coordinated plan of care that addresses the child's ongoing health care needs. The goal is to ensure that each child remains healthy, thrives, and obtains optimal medical home and developmental supports that promote ongoing care at home and minimize recurrent hospitalizations. This clinical report presents an approach to discharging the child with complex medical needs with technology dependencies from hospital to home and then continually addressing the needs of the child and family in the home environment. (4/12)

http://pediatrics.aappublications.org/content/129/5/996

HONORING DO-NOT-ATTEMPT-RESUSCITATION REQUESTS IN SCHOOLS

Council on School Health and Committee on Bioethics

ABSTRACT. Increasingly, children and adolescents with complex chronic conditions are living in the community. Federal legislation and regulations facilitate their participation in school. Some of these children and adolescents and their families may wish to forego life-sustaining medical treatment, including cardiopulmonary resuscitation, because they would be ineffective or because the risks outweigh the benefits. Honoring these requests in the school environment is complex because of the limited availability of school nurses and the frequent lack of supporting state legislation and regulations. Understanding and collaboration on the part of all parties is essential. Pediatricians have an important role in helping school nurses incorporate a specific action plan into the student's individualized health care plan. The action plan should include both communication and comfort-care plans. Pediatricians who work directly with schools can also help implement policies, and professional organizations can advocate for regulations and legislation that enable students and their families to effectuate their preferences. (4/10, reaffirmed 7/13, 8/16)

http://pediatrics.aappublications.org/content/125/5/1073

HOSPITAL DISCHARGE OF THE HIGH-RISK NEONATE

Committee on Fetus and Newborn

ABSTRACT. This policy statement updates the guidelines on discharge of the high-risk neonate first published by the American Academy of Pediatrics in 1998. As with the earlier document, this statement is based, insofar as possible, on published, scientifically derived information. This updated statement incorporates new knowledge about risks and medical care of the high-risk neonate, the timing of discharge, and planning for care after discharge. It also refers to other American Academy of Pediatrics publications that are relevant to these issues. This statement draws on the previous classification of high-risk infants into 4 categories: (1) the preterm infant; (2) the infant with special health care needs or dependence on technology; (3) the infant at risk because of family issues; and (4) the infant with anticipated early death. The issues of deciding when discharge is appropriate, defining the specific needs for follow-up care, and the process of detailed discharge planning are addressed as they apply in general to all 4 categories; in addition, special attention is directed to the particular issues presented by the 4 individual categories. Recommendations are given to aid in deciding when discharge is appropriate and to ensure that all necessary care will be available and well coordinated after discharge. The need for individualized planning and physician judgment is emphasized. (11/08, reaffirmed 5/11)

http://pediatrics.aappublications.org/content/122/5/1119

THE HOSPITAL RECORD OF THE INJURED CHILD AND THE NEED FOR EXTERNAL CAUSE-OF-INJURY CODES

Committee on Injury and Poison Prevention

ABSTRACT. Proper record-keeping of emergency department visits and hospitalizations of injured children is vital for appropriate patient management. Determination and documentation of the circumstances surrounding the injury event are essential. This information not only is the basis for preventive counseling, but also provides clues about how similar injuries in other youth can be avoided. The hospital records have an important secondary purpose; namely, if sufficient information about the cause and mechanism of injury is documented, it can be subsequently coded, electronically compiled, and retrieved later to provide an epidemiologic profile of the injury, the first step in prevention at the population level. To be of greatest use, hospital records should indicate the "who, what, when, where, why, and how" of the injury occurrence and whether protective equipment (eg, a seat belt) was used. The pediatrician has two important roles in this area: to document fully the injury event and to advocate the use of standardized external cause-of-injury codes, which allow such data to be compiled and analyzed. (2/99, reaffirmed 5/02, 5/05, 10/08, 10/13)

http://pediatrics.aappublications.org/content/103/2/524

HOSPITAL STAY FOR HEALTHY TERM NEWBORN INFANTS

William E. Benitz, MD, FAAP, and Committee on Fetus and Newborn

ABSTRACT. The hospital stay of the mother and her healthy term newborn infant should be long enough to allow identification of problems and to ensure that the mother is sufficiently recovered and prepared to care for herself and her newborn at home. The length of stay should be based on the unique characteristics of each mother-infant dyad, including the health of the mother, the health and stability of the newborn, the ability and confidence of the mother to care for herself and her

newborn, the adequacy of support systems at home, and access to appropriate follow-up care in a medical home. Input from the mother and her obstetrical care provider should be considered before a decision to discharge a newborn is made, and all efforts should be made to keep a mother and her newborn together to ensure simultaneous discharge. (4/15)

http://pediatrics.aappublications.org/content/135/5/948

HUMAN EMBRYONIC STEM CELL (HESC) AND HUMAN EMBRYO RESEARCH

Committee on Pediatric Research and Committee on Bioethics

ABSTRACT. Human embryonic stem cell research has emerged as an important platform for the understanding and treatment of pediatric diseases. From its inception, however, it has raised ethical concerns based not on the use of stem cells themselves but on objections to the source of the cells—specifically, the destruction of preimplantation human embryos. Despite differences in public opinion on this issue, a large majority of the public supports continued research using embryonic stem cells. Given the possible substantial benefit of stem cell research on child health and development, the American Academy of Pediatrics believes that funding and oversight for human embryo and embryonic stem cell research should continue. (10/12)

http://pediatrics.aappublications.org/content/130/5/972

HUMAN IMMUNODEFICIENCY VIRUS AND OTHER BLOOD-BORNE VIRAL PATHOGENS IN THE ATHLETIC SETTING

Committee on Sports Medicine and Fitness

ABSTRACT. Because athletes and the staff of athletic programs can be exposed to blood during athletic activity, they have a very small risk of becoming infected with human immunodeficiency virus, hepatitis B virus, or hepatitis C virus. This statement, which updates a previous position statement of the American Academy of Pediatrics, discusses sports participation for athletes infected with these pathogens and the precautions needed to reduce the risk of infection to others in the athletic setting. Each of the recommendations in this statement is dependent upon and intended to be considered with reference to the other recommendations in this statement and not in isolation. (12/99, reaffirmed 1/05, 1/09, 11/11, 2/15)

http://pediatrics.aappublications.org/content/104/6/1400

HUMAN MILK, BREASTFEEDING, AND TRANSMISSION OF HUMAN IMMUNODEFICIENCY VIRUS IN THE UNITED STATES

Committee on Pediatric AIDS (11/95, reaffirmed 11/99, 11/03, 2/08)

http://pediatrics.aappublications.org/content/96/5/977

HUMAN MILK, BREASTFEEDING, AND TRANSMISSION OF HUMAN IMMUNODEFICIENCY VIRUS TYPE 1 IN THE UNITED STATES (TECHNICAL REPORT)

Committee on Pediatric AIDS

ABSTRACT. Transmission of human immunodeficiency virus type 1 (HIV-1) through breastfeeding has been conclusively demonstrated. The risk of such transmission has been quantified, the timing has been clarified, and certain risk factors for breastfeeding transmission

have been identified. In areas where infant formula is accessible, affordable, safe, and sustainable, avoidance of breastfeeding has represented one of the main components of mother-to-child HIV-1 transmission prevention efforts for many years. In areas where affordable and safe alternatives to breastfeeding may not be available, interventions to prevent breastfeeding transmission are being investigated. Complete avoidance of breastfeeding by HIV-1-infected women has been recommended by the American Academy of Pediatrics and the Centers for Disease Control and Prevention and remains the only means by which prevention of breastfeeding transmission of HIV-1 can be absolutely ensured. This technical report summarizes the information available regarding breastfeeding transmission of HIV-1. (11/03, reaffirmed 1/07)
http://pediatrics.aappublications.org/content/112/5/1196

HYPOTHERMIA AND NEONATAL ENCEPHALOPATHY (CLINICAL REPORT)

Committee on Fetus and Newborn

ABSTRACT. Data from large randomized clinical trials indicate that therapeutic hypothermia, using either selective head cooling or systemic cooling, is an effective therapy for neonatal encephalopathy. Infants selected for cooling must meet the criteria outlined in published clinical trials. The implementation of cooling needs to be performed at centers that have the capability to manage medically complex infants. Because the majority of infants who have neonatal encephalopathy are born at community hospitals, centers that perform cooling should work with their referring hospitals to implement education programs focused on increasing the awareness and identification of infants at risk for encephalopathy, and the initial clinical management of affected infants. (5/14)
http://pediatrics.aappublications.org/content/133/6/1146

IDENTIFICATION AND CARE OF HIV-EXPOSED AND HIV-INFECTED INFANTS, CHILDREN, AND ADOLESCENTS IN FOSTER CARE

Committee on Pediatric AIDS

ABSTRACT. As a consequence of the expanding human immunodeficiency virus (HIV) epidemic and major advances in medical management of HIV-exposed and HIV-infected persons, revised recommendations are provided for HIV testing of infants, children, and adolescents in foster care. Updated recommendations also are provided for the care of HIV-exposed and HIV-infected persons who are in foster care. (7/00, reaffirmed 3/03, 2/08, 6/11)
http://pediatrics.aappublications.org/content/106/1/149

IDENTIFICATION AND EVALUATION OF CHILDREN WITH AUTISM SPECTRUM DISORDERS (CLINICAL REPORT)

PPI
AAP Partnership for Policy Implementation

Chris Plauché Johnson, MD, MEd; Scott M. Myers, MD; and Council on Children With Disabilities

ABSTRACT. Autism spectrum disorders are not rare; many primary care pediatricians care for several children with autism spectrum disorders. Pediatricians play an important role in early recognition of autism spectrum disorders, because they usually are the first point of contact for parents. Parents are now much more aware of the early signs of autism spectrum disorders because of frequent coverage in the media; if their child demonstrates any of the published signs, they will most likely raise their concerns to their child's pediatrician. It is important that pediatricians be able to recognize the signs and symptoms of autism spectrum disorders and have a strategy for assessing them systematically. Pediatricians also must be aware of local resources that can assist in making a definitive diagnosis of, and in managing, autism spectrum disorders. The pediatrician must be familiar with developmental, educational, and community resources as well as medical subspecialty clinics. This clinical report is 1 of 2 documents that replace the original American Academy of Pediatrics policy statement and technical report published in 2001. This report addresses background information, including definition, history, epidemiology, diagnostic criteria, early signs, neuropathologic aspects, and etiologic possibilities in autism spectrum disorders. In addition, this report provides an algorithm to help the pediatrician develop a strategy for early identification of children with autism spectrum disorders. The accompanying clinical report addresses the management of children with autism spectrum disorders and follows this report on page 1162 [available at www.pediatrics.org/cgi/content/full/120/5/1162]. Both clinical reports are complemented by the toolkit titled *"Autism: Caring for Children With Autism Spectrum Disorders: A Resource Toolkit for Clinicians,"* which contains screening and surveillance tools, practical forms, tables, and parent handouts to assist the pediatrician in the identification, evaluation, and management of autism spectrum disorders in children. (11/07, reaffirmed 9/10, 8/14)
http://pediatrics.aappublications.org/content/120/5/1183

IDENTIFICATION AND MANAGEMENT OF EATING DISORDERS IN CHILDREN AND ADOLESCENTS (CLINICAL REPORT)

David S. Rosen, MD, MPH, and Committee on Adolescence

ABSTRACT. The incidence and prevalence of eating disorders in children and adolescents has increased significantly in recent decades, making it essential for pediatricians to consider these disorders in appropriate clinical settings, to evaluate patients suspected of having these disorders, and to manage (or refer) patients in whom eating disorders are diagnosed. This clinical report includes a discussion of diagnostic criteria and outlines the initial evaluation of the patient with disordered eating. Medical complications of eating disorders may affect any organ system, and careful monitoring for these complications is required. The range of treatment options, including pharmacotherapy, is described in this report. Pediatricians are encouraged to advocate for legislation and policies that ensure appropriate services for patients with eating disorders, including medical care, nutritional intervention, mental health treatment, and care coordination. (11/10)
http://pediatrics.aappublications.org/content/126/6/1240

IDENTIFYING INFANTS AND YOUNG CHILDREN WITH DEVELOPMENTAL DISORDERS IN THE MEDICAL HOME: AN ALGORITHM FOR DEVELOPMENTAL SURVEILLANCE AND SCREENING

PPI
AAP Partnership for Policy Implementation

Council on Children With Disabilities, Section on Developmental and Behavioral Pediatrics, Bright Futures Steering Committee, and Medical Home Initiatives for Children With Special Needs Project Advisory Committee

ABSTRACT. Early identification of developmental disorders is critical to the well-being of children and their families. It is an integral function of the primary care medical home and an appropriate responsibility of all pediatric health care professionals. This statement provides an algorithm as a strategy to support health care professionals in developing a pattern and practice for addressing developmental concerns in children from birth through 3 years of age. The authors recommend that developmental surveillance be incorporated at every well-child preventive care visit. Any concerns raised during surveillance should be promptly addressed with standardized developmental screening tests. In addition, screening tests should be administered regularly at the 9-, 18-, and 30-month visits. (Because the 30-month visit is not yet a part of the preventive care system and is often not reimbursable by third-party payers at this time, developmental screening can be performed at 24 months of age. In addition, because the frequency of regular pediatric visits decreases after 24 months of age, a pediatrician who expects that his or her patients will have difficulty attending a 30-month visit should conduct screening during the 24-month visit.) The early identification of developmental problems should lead to further developmental and medical evaluation, diagnosis, and treatment, including early developmental intervention. Children diagnosed with developmental disorders should be identified as children with special health care needs, and chronic-condition management should be initiated. Identification of a developmental disorder and its underlying etiology may also drive a range of treatment planning, from medical treatment of the child to family planning for his or her parents. (7/06, reaffirmed 12/09, 8/14)

http://pediatrics.aappublications.org/content/118/1/405

IMMERSION IN WATER DURING LABOR AND DELIVERY (CLINICAL REPORT)

Committee on Fetus and Newborn (joint with American College of Obstetricians and Gynecologists Committee on Obstetric Practice)

ABSTRACT. Immersion in water has been suggested as a beneficial alternative for labor, delivery, or both and over the past decades has gained popularity in many parts of the world. Immersion in water during the first stage of labor may be associated with decreased pain or use of anesthesia and decreased duration of labor. However, there is no evidence that immersion in water during the first stage of labor otherwise improves perinatal outcomes, and it should not prevent or inhibit other elements of care. The safety and efficacy of immersion in water during the second stage of labor have not been established, and immersion in water during the second stage of labor has not been associated with maternal or fetal benefit. Given these facts and case reports of rare but serious adverse effects in the newborn, the practice of immersion in the second stage of labor (underwater delivery) should be considered an experimental procedure that only should be performed within the context of an appropriately designed clinical trial with informed consent. Facilities that plan to offer immersion in the first stage of labor need to establish rigorous protocols for candidate selection, maintenance and cleaning of tubs and immersion pools, infection control procedures, monitoring of mothers and fetuses at appropriate intervals while immersed, and immediately and safely moving women out of the tubs if maternal or fetal concerns develop. (3/14)

http://pediatrics.aappublications.org/content/133/4/758

IMMUNIZATION FOR *STREPTOCOCCUS PNEUMONIAE* INFECTIONS IN HIGH-RISK CHILDREN

Committee on Infectious Diseases

ABSTACT. Routine use of the pneumococcal conjugate vaccines (PCV7 and PCV13), beginning in 2000, has resulted in a dramatic reduction in the incidence of invasive pneumococcal disease (IPD) attributable to serotypes of *Streptococcus pneumoniae* contained in the vaccines. The Advisory Committee on Immunization Practices of the Centers for Disease Control and Prevention and the American Academy of Pediatrics recommend the expanded use of PCV13 in children 6 through 18 years of age with certain conditions that place them at elevated risk of IPD. This statement provides recommendations for the use of PCV13 in children 6 through 18 years. A single dose of PCV13 should be administered to certain children in this age group who are at elevated risk of IPD. Recommendations for the use of PCV13 in healthy children and for pneumococcal polysaccharide vaccine (PPSV23) remain unchanged. (11/14)

http://pediatrics.aappublications.org/content/134/6/1230

IMMUNIZATION INFORMATION SYSTEMS

Committee on Practice and Ambulatory Medicine

ABSTRACT. The American Academy of Pediatrics continues to support the development and implementation of immunization information systems, previously referred to as immunization registries, and other systems for the benefit of children, pediatricians, and their communities. Pediatricians and others must be aware of the value that immunization information systems have for society, the potential fiscal influences on their practice, the costs and benefits, and areas for future improvement. (9/06, reaffirmed 10/11)

http://pediatrics.aappublications.org/content/118/3/1293

IMMUNIZING PARENTS AND OTHER CLOSE FAMILY CONTACTS IN THE PEDIATRIC OFFICE SETTING (TECHNICAL REPORT)

Herschel R. Lessin, MD; Kathryn M. Edwards, MD; Committee on Practice and Ambulatory Medicine; and Committee on Infectious Diseases

ABSTRACT. Additional strategies are needed to protect children from vaccine-preventable diseases. In particular, very young infants, as well as children who are immunocompromised, are at especially high risk for developing the serious consequences of vaccine-preventable diseases and cannot be immunized completely. There is some evidence that children who become infected with these diseases are exposed to pathogens through household contacts, particularly from parents or other close family contacts. Such infections likely are attributable to adults who are not fully protected from these diseases, either because their immunity to vaccine-preventable diseases has waned over time or because they have not received a vaccine. There are many challenges that have added to low adult immunization rates in the United States. One option to increase immunization coverage for parents and close family contacts of infants and vulnerable children is to provide alternative locations for these adults to be immunized, such as the pediatric office setting. Ideally, adults should receive immunizations in their medical homes; however, to provide greater protection to these adults and reduce the exposure of children to pathogens, immunizing parents or other adult family contacts in the pediatric office setting could increase immunization coverage for this population to protect themselves as well as children to whom they provide care. (12/11)

http://pediatrics.aappublications.org/content/129/1/e247

THE IMPACT OF MARIJUANA POLICIES ON YOUTH: CLINICAL, RESEARCH, AND LEGAL UPDATE

Committee on Substance Abuse and Committee on Adolescence

ABSTRACT. This policy statement is an update of the American Academy of Pediatrics policy statement "Legalization of Marijuana: Potential Impact on Youth," published in 2004. Pediatricians have special expertise in the care of children and adolescents and may be called on to advise legislators about the potential impact of changes in the legal status of marijuana on adolescents. Parents also may look to pediatricians for advice as they consider whether to support state-level initiatives that propose to legalize the use of marijuana for medical and nonmedical purposes or to decriminalize the possession of small amounts of marijuana. This policy statement provides the position of the American Academy of Pediatrics on the issue of marijuana legalization. The accompanying technical report reviews what is currently known about the relationships of marijuana use with health and the developing brain and the legal status of marijuana and adolescents' use of marijuana to better understand how change in legal status might influence the degree of marijuana use by adolescents in the future. (2/15)

http://pediatrics.aappublications.org/content/135/3/584

THE IMPACT OF MARIJUANA POLICIES ON YOUTH: CLINICAL, RESEARCH, AND LEGAL UPDATE (TECHNICAL REPORT)

Seth Ammerman, MD, FAAP; Sheryl Ryan, MD, FAAP; William P. Adelman, MD, FAAP; Committee on Substance Abuse; and Committee on Adolescence

ABSTRACT. This technical report updates the 2004 American Academy of Pediatrics technical report on the legalization of marijuana. Current epidemiology of marijuana use is presented, as are definitions and biology of marijuana compounds, side effects of marijuana use, and effects of use on adolescent brain development. Issues concerning medical marijuana specifically are also addressed. Concerning legalization of marijuana, 4 different approaches in the United States are discussed: legalization of marijuana solely for medical purposes, decriminalization of recreational use of marijuana, legalization of recreational use of marijuana, and criminal prosecution of recreational (and medical) use of marijuana. These approaches are compared, and the latest available data are presented to aid in forming public policy. The effects on youth of criminal penalties for marijuana use and possession are also addressed, as are the effects or potential effects of the other 3 policy approaches on adolescent marijuana use. Recommendations are included in the accompanying policy statement. (2/15)

http://pediatrics.aappublications.org/content/135/3/e769

IMPACT OF MUSIC, MUSIC LYRICS, AND MUSIC VIDEOS ON CHILDREN AND YOUTH

Council on Communications and Media

ABSTRACT. Music plays an important role in the socialization of children and adolescents. Popular music is present almost everywhere, and it is easily available through the radio, various recordings, the Internet, and new technologies, allowing adolescents to hear it in diverse settings and situations, alone or shared with friends. Parents often are unaware of the lyrics to which their children are listening because of the increasing use of downloaded music and headphones. Research on popular music has explored its effects on schoolwork, social interactions, mood and affect, and particularly behavior. The effect that popular music has on children's and adolescents' behavior and emotions is of paramount concern. Lyrics have become more explicit in their references to drugs, sex, and violence over the years, particularly in certain genres. A teenager's preference for certain types of music could be correlated or associated with certain behaviors. As with popular music, the perception and the effect of music-video messages are important, because research has reported that exposure to violence, sexual messages, sexual stereotypes, and use of substances of abuse in music videos might produce significant changes in behaviors and attitudes of young viewers. Pediatricians and parents should be aware of this information. Furthermore, with the evidence portrayed in these studies, it is essential for pediatricians and parents to take a stand regarding music lyrics. (10/09)

http://pediatrics.aappublications.org/content/124/5/1488

THE IMPACT OF SOCIAL MEDIA ON CHILDREN, ADOLESCENTS, AND FAMILIES (CLINICAL REPORT)

Gwenn Schurgin O'Keeffe, MD; Kathleen Clarke-Pearson, MD; and Council on Communications and Media

ABSTRACT. Using social media Web sites is among the most common activity of today's children and adolescents. Any Web site that allows social interaction is considered a social media site, including social networking sites such as Facebook, MySpace, and Twitter; gaming sites and virtual worlds such as Club Penguin, Second Life, and the Sims; video sites such as YouTube; and blogs. Such sites offer today's youth a portal for entertainment and communication and have grown exponentially in recent years. For this reason, it is important that parents become aware of the nature of social media sites, given that not all of them are healthy environments for children and adolescents. Pediatricians are in a unique position to help families understand these sites and to encourage healthy use and urge parents to monitor for potential problems with cyberbullying, "Facebook depression," sexting, and exposure to inappropriate content. (3/11)
http://pediatrics.aappublications.org/content/127/4/800

THE IMPORTANCE OF PLAY IN PROMOTING HEALTHY CHILD DEVELOPMENT AND MAINTAINING STRONG PARENT-CHILD BOND: FOCUS ON CHILDREN IN POVERTY (CLINICAL REPORT)

Regina M. Milteer, MD; Kenneth R. Ginsburg, MD, MSEd; Council on Communications and Media; and Committee on Psychosocial Aspects of Child and Family Health

ABSTRACT. Play is essential to the social, emotional, cognitive, and physical well-being of children beginning in early childhood. It is a natural tool for children to develop resiliency as they learn to cooperate, overcome challenges, and negotiate with others. Play also allows children to be creative. It provides time for parents to be fully engaged with their children, to bond with their children, and to see the world from the perspective of their child. However, children who live in poverty often face socioeconomic obstacles that impede their rights to have playtime, thus affecting their healthy social-emotional development. For children who are underresourced to reach their highest potential, it is essential that parents, educators, and pediatricians recognize the importance of lifelong benefits that children gain from play. (12/11, reaffirmed 9/15)
http://pediatrics.aappublications.org/content/129/1/e204

THE IMPORTANCE OF PLAY IN PROMOTING HEALTHY CHILD DEVELOPMENT AND MAINTAINING STRONG PARENT-CHILD BONDS (CLINICAL REPORT)

Kenneth R. Ginsburg, MD, MSEd; Committee on Communications; and Committee on Psychosocial Aspects of Child and Family Health

ABSTRACT. Play is essential to development because it contributes to the cognitive, physical, social, and emotional well-being of children and youth. Play also offers an ideal opportunity for parents to engage fully with their children. Despite the benefits derived from play for both children and parents, time for free play has been markedly reduced for some children. This report addresses a variety of factors that have reduced play, including a hurried lifestyle, changes in family structure, and increased attention to academics and enrichment activities at the expense of recess or free child-centered play. This report offers guidelines on how pediatricians can advocate for children by helping families, school systems, and communities consider how best to ensure that play is protected as they seek the balance in children's lives to create the optimal developmental milieu. (1/07)
http://pediatrics.aappublications.org/content/119/1/182

IMPROVING SUBSTANCE ABUSE PREVENTION, ASSESSMENT, AND TREATMENT FINANCING FOR CHILDREN AND ADOLESCENTS

Committee on Child Health Financing and Committee on Substance Abuse

ABSTRACT. The numbers of children, adolescents, and families affected by substance abuse have sharply increased since the early 1990s. The American Academy of Pediatrics recognizes the scope and urgency of this problem and has developed this policy statement for consideration by Congress, federal and state agencies, employers, national organizations, health care professionals, health insurers, managed care organizations, advocacy groups, and families. (10/01)
http://pediatrics.aappublications.org/content/108/4/1025

THE INAPPROPRIATE USE OF SCHOOL "READINESS" TESTS

Committee on Early Childhood, Adoption, and Dependent Care and Committee on School Health (3/95, reaffirmed 4/98, 1/04, 4/10)

http://pediatrics.aappublications.org/content/95/3/437

INCIDENTAL FINDINGS ON BRAIN AND SPINE IMAGING IN CHILDREN (CLINICAL REPORT)

Cormac O. Maher, MD, FAAP; Joseph H. Piatt Jr, MD, FAAP; and Section on Neurologic Surgery

ABSTRACT. In recent years, the utilization of diagnostic imaging of the brain and spine in children has increased dramatically, leading to a corresponding increase in the detection of incidental findings of the central nervous system. Patients with unexpected findings on imaging are often referred for subspecialty evaluation. Even with rational use of diagnostic imaging and subspecialty consultation, the diagnostic process will always generate unexpected findings that must be explained and managed. Familiarity with the most common findings that are discovered incidentally on diagnostic imaging of the brain and spine will assist the pediatrician in providing counseling to families and in making recommendations in conjunction with a neurosurgeon, when needed, regarding additional treatments and prognosis. (3/15)
http://pediatrics.aappublications.org/content/135/4/e1084

INCORPORATING RECOGNITION AND MANAGEMENT OF PERINATAL AND POSTPARTUM DEPRESSION INTO PEDIATRIC PRACTICE (CLINICAL REPORT)

Marian F. Earls, MD, and Committee on Psychosocial Aspects of Child and Family Health

ABSTRACT. Every year, more than 400 000 infants are born to mothers who are depressed, which makes perinatal depression the most underdiagnosed obstetric complication in America. Postpartum depression leads to increased costs of medical care, inappropriate medical care, child abuse and neglect, discontinuation of breastfeeding, and family dysfunction and adversely affects early brain development. Pediatric practices, as medical homes, can establish a system to implement postpartum depression screening and to identify and use community resources for the treatment and referral of the depressed mother and support for the mother-child (dyad) relationship. This system would have a positive effect on the health and well-being of the infant and family. State chapters of the American Academy of Pediatrics, working with state Early Periodic Screening, Diagnosis, and Treatment (EPSDT) and maternal and child health programs, can increase awareness of the need for perinatal depression screening in the obstetric and pediatric periodicity of care schedules and ensure payment. Pediatricians must advocate for workforce development for professionals who care for very young children and for promotion of evidence-based interventions focused on healthy attachment and parent-child relationships. (10/10, reaffirmed 12/14)

http://pediatrics.aappublications.org/content/126/5/1032

INCREASING ANTIRETROVIRAL DRUG ACCESS FOR CHILDREN WITH HIV INFECTION

Committee on Pediatric AIDS and Section on International Child Health

ABSTRACT. Although there have been great gains in the prevention of pediatric HIV infection and provision of antiretroviral therapy for children with HIV infection in resource-rich countries, many barriers remain to scaling up HIV prevention and treatment for children in resource-limited areas of the world. Appropriate testing technologies need to be made more widely available to identify HIV infection in infants. Training of practitioners in the skills required to care for children with HIV infection is required to increase the number of children receiving antiretroviral therapy. Lack of availability of appropriate antiretroviral drug formulations that are easily usable and inexpensive is a major impediment to optimal care for children with HIV. The time and energy spent trying to develop liquid antiretroviral formulations might be better used in the manufacture of smaller pill sizes or crushable tablets, which are easier to dispense, transport, store, and administer to children. (4/07, reaffirmed 4/10, 4/16)

http://pediatrics.aappublications.org/content/119/4/838

INCREASING IMMUNIZATION COVERAGE

Committee on Practice and Ambulatory Medicine and Council on Community Pediatrics

ABSTRACT. In 1977, the American Academy of Pediatrics issued a statement calling for universal immunization of all children for whom vaccines are not contraindicated. In 1995, the policy statement "Implementation of the Immunization Policy" was published by the American Academy of Pediatrics, followed in 2003 with publication of the first version of this statement, "Increasing Immunization Coverage." Since 2003, there have continued to be improvements in immunization coverage, with progress toward meeting the goals set forth in *Healthy People 2010*. Data from the 2007 National Immunization Survey showed that 90% of children 19 to 35 months of age have received recommended doses of each of the following vaccines: inactivated poliovirus (IPV), measles-mumps-rubella (MMR), varicella-zoster virus (VZB), hepatitis B virus (HBV), and *Haemophilus influenzae* type b (Hib). For diphtheria and tetanus and acellular pertussis (DTaP) vaccine, 84.5% have received the recommended 4 doses by 35 months of age. Nevertheless, the *Healthy People 2010* goal of at least 80% coverage for the full series (at least 4 doses of DTaP, 3 doses of IPV, 1 dose of MMR, 3 doses of Hib, 3 doses of HBV, and 1 dose of varicella-zoster virus vaccine) has not yet been met, and immunization coverage of adolescents continues to lag behind the goals set forth in *Healthy People 2010*. Despite these encouraging data, a vast number of new challenges that threaten continued success toward the goal of universal immunization coverage have emerged. These challenges include an increase in new vaccines and new vaccine combinations as well as a significant number of vaccines currently under development; a dramatic increase in the acquisition cost of vaccines, coupled with a lack of adequate payment to practitioners to buy and administer vaccines; unanticipated manufacturing and delivery problems that have caused significant shortages of various vaccine products; and the rise of a public antivaccination movement that uses the Internet as well as standard media outlets to advance a position, wholly unsupported by any scientific evidence, linking vaccines with various childhood conditions, particularly autism. Much remains to be accomplished by physician organizations; vaccine manufacturers; third-party payers; the media; and local, state, and federal governments to ensure dependable vaccine supply and payments that are sufficient to continue to provide immunizations in public and private settings and to promote effective strategies to combat unjustified misstatements by the antivaccination movement.

Pediatricians should work individually and collectively at the local, state, and national levels to ensure that all children without a valid contraindication receive all childhood immunizations on time. Pediatricians and pediatric organizations, in conjunction with government agencies such as the Centers for Disease Control and Prevention, must communicate effectively with parents to maximize their understanding of the overall safety and efficacy of vaccines. Most parents and children have not experienced many of the vaccine-preventable diseases, and the general public is not well informed about the risks and sequelae of these conditions. A number of recommendations are included for pediatricians, individually and collectively, to support further progress toward the goal of universal immunization coverage of all children for whom vaccines are not contraindicated. (5/10)

http://pediatrics.aappublications.org/content/125/6/1295

INDICATIONS FOR MANAGEMENT AND REFERRAL OF PATIENTS INVOLVED IN SUBSTANCE ABUSE

Committee on Substance Abuse

ABSTRACT. This statement addresses the challenge of evaluating and managing the various stages of substance use by children and adolescents in the context of pediatric practice. Approaches are suggested that would assist the pediatrician in differentiating highly prevalent experimental and occasional use from more severe use with adverse consequences that affect emotional, behavioral, educational, or physical health. Comorbid psychiatric conditions are common and should be evaluated and treated simultaneously by child and adolescent mental health specialists. Guidelines for referral based on severity of involvement using established patient treatment-matching criteria are outlined. Pediatricians need to become familiar with treatment professionals and facilities in their communities and to ensure that treatment for adolescent patients is appropriate based on their developmental, psychosocial, medical, and mental health needs. The family should be encouraged to participate actively in the treatment process. (7/00)

http://pediatrics.aappublications.org/content/106/1/143

THE INDIVIDUALS WITH DISABILITIES EDUCATION ACT (IDEA) FOR CHILDREN WITH SPECIAL EDUCATIONAL NEEDS (CLINICAL REPORT)

Paul H. Lipkin, MD, FAAP; Jeffrey Okamoto, MD, FAAP; Council on Children With Disabilities; and Council on School Health

ABSTRACT. The pediatric health care provider has a critical role in supporting the health and well-being of children and adolescents in all settings, including early intervention (EI), preschool, and school environments. It is estimated that 15% of children in the United States have a disability. The Individuals with Disabilities Education Act entitles every affected child in the United States from infancy to young adulthood to a free appropriate public education through EI and special education services. These services bolster development and learning of children with various disabilities. This clinical report provides the pediatric health care provider with a summary of key components of the most recent version of this law. Guidance is also provided to ensure that every child in need receives the EI and special education services to which he or she is entitled. (11/15)

http://pediatrics.aappublications.org/content/136/6/e1650

INDOOR ENVIRONMENTAL CONTROL PRACTICES AND ASTHMA MANAGEMENT (CLINICAL REPORT)

Elizabeth C. Matsui, MD, MHS, FAAP; Stuart L. Abramson, MD, PhD, AE-C, FAAP; Megan T. Sandel, MD, MPH, FAAP; Section on Allergy and Immunology; and Council on Environmental Health

ABSTRACT. Indoor environmental exposures, particularly allergens and pollutants, are major contributors to asthma morbidity in children; environmental control practices aimed at reducing these exposures are an integral component of asthma management. Some individually tailored environmental control practices that have been shown to reduce asthma symptoms and exacerbations are similar in efficacy and cost to controller medications. As a part of developing tailored strategies regarding environmental control measures, an environmental history can be obtained to evaluate the key indoor environmental exposures that are known to trigger asthma symptoms and exacerbations, including both indoor pollutants and allergens. An environmental history includes questions regarding the presence of pets or pests or evidence of pests in the home, as well as knowledge regarding whether the climatic characteristics in the community favor dust mites. In addition, the history focuses on sources of indoor air pollution, including the presence of smokers who live in the home or care for children and the use of gas stoves and appliances in the home. Serum allergen-specific immunoglobulin E antibody tests can be performed or the patient can be referred for allergy skin testing to identify indoor allergens that are most likely to be clinically relevant. Environmental control strategies are tailored to each potentially relevant indoor exposure and are based on knowledge of the sources and underlying characteristics of the exposure. Strategies include source removal, source control, and mitigation strategies, such as high-efficiency particulate air purifiers and allergen-proof mattress and pillow encasements, as well as education, which can be delivered by primary care pediatricians, allergists, pediatric pulmonologists, other health care workers, or community health workers trained in asthma environmental control and asthma education. (10/16)

See full text on page 847.

http://pediatrics.aappublications.org/content/138/5/e20162589

INFANT FEEDING AND TRANSMISSION OF HUMAN IMMUNODEFICIENCY VIRUS IN THE UNITED STATES

Committee on Pediatric AIDS

ABSTRACT. Physicians caring for infants born to women infected with HIV are likely to be involved in providing guidance to HIV-infected mothers on appropriate infant feeding practices. It is critical that physicians are aware of the HIV transmission risk from human milk and the current recommendations for feeding HIV-exposed infants in the United States. Because the only intervention to completely prevent HIV transmission via human milk is not to breastfeed, in the United States, where clean water and affordable replacement feeding are available, the American Academy of Pediatrics recommends that HIV-infected mothers not breastfeed their infants, regardless of maternal viral load and antiretroviral therapy. (1/13, reaffirmed 4/16)

http://pediatrics.aappublications.org/content/131/2/391

INFANT METHEMOGLOBINEMIA: THE ROLE OF DIETARY NITRATE IN FOOD AND WATER (CLINICAL REPORT)

Frank R. Greer, MD; Michael Shannon, MD; Committee on Nutrition; and Committee on Environmental Health

ABSTRACT. Infants for whom formula may be prepared with well water remain a high-risk group for nitrate poisoning. This clinical report reinforces the need for testing of well water for nitrate content. There seems to be little or no risk of nitrate poisoning from commercially prepared infant foods in the United States. However, reports of nitrate poisoning from home-prepared vegetable foods for infants continue to occur. Breastfeeding infants are not

at risk of methemoglobinemia even when mothers ingest water with very high concentrations of nitrate nitrogen (100 ppm). (9/05, reaffirmed 4/09)
http://pediatrics.aappublications.org/content/116/3/784

INFECTION PREVENTION AND CONTROL IN PEDIATRIC AMBULATORY SETTINGS
Committee on Infectious Diseases
ABSTRACT. Since the American Academy of Pediatrics published a statement titled "Infection Control in Physicians' Offices" (*Pediatrics.* 2000;105[6]:1361–1369), there have been significant changes that prompted this updated statement. Infection prevention and control is an integral part of pediatric practice in ambulatory medical settings as well as in hospitals. Infection prevention and control practices should begin at the time the ambulatory visit is scheduled. All health care personnel should be educated regarding the routes of transmission and techniques used to prevent transmission of infectious agents. Policies for infection prevention and control should be written, readily available, updated annually, and enforced. The standard precautions for hospitalized patients from the Centers for Disease Control and Prevention, with a modification from the American Academy of Pediatrics exempting the use of gloves for routine diaper changes and wiping a well child's nose or tears, are appropriate for most patient encounters. As employers, pediatricians are required by the Occupational Safety and Health Administration to take precautions to identify and protect employees who are likely to be exposed to blood or other potentially infectious materials while on the job. Key principles of standard precautions include hand hygiene (ie, use of alcohol-based hand rub or hand-washing with soap [plain or antimicrobial] and water) before and after every patient contact; implementation of respiratory hygiene and cough-etiquette strategies for patients with suspected influenza or infection with another respiratory tract pathogen to the extent feasible; separation of infected, contagious children from uninfected children when feasible; safe handling and disposal of needles and other sharp medical devices and evaluation and implementation of needle-safety devices; appropriate use of personal protective equipment such as gloves, gowns, masks, and eye protection; and appropriate sterilization, disinfection, and antisepsis. (9/07, reaffirmed 8/10, 1/15)
http://pediatrics.aappublications.org/content/120/3/650

INFECTIOUS COMPLICATIONS WITH THE USE OF BIOLOGIC RESPONSE MODIFIERS IN INFANTS AND CHILDREN (CLINICAL REPORT)
H. Dele Davies, MD, FAAP, and Committee on Infectious Diseases
ABSTRACT. Biologic response modifiers (BRMs) are substances that interact with and modify the host immune system. BRMs that dampen the immune system are used to treat conditions such as juvenile idiopathic arthritis, psoriatic arthritis, or inflammatory bowel disease and often in combination with other immunosuppressive agents, such as methotrexate and corticosteroids. Cytokines that are targeted include tumor necrosis factor α; interleukins (ILs) 6, 12, and 23; and the receptors for IL-1α (IL-1A) and IL-1β (IL-1B) as well as other molecules. Although the risk varies with the class of BRM, patients receiving immune-dampening BRMs generally are at increased risk of infection or reactivation with mycobacterial infections (*Mycobacterium tuberculosis* and nontuberculous mycobacteria), some viral (herpes simplex virus, varicella-zoster virus, Epstein-Barr virus, hepatitis B) and fungal (histoplasmosis, coccidioidomycosis) infections, as well as other opportunistic infections. The use of BRMs warrants careful determination of infectious risk on the basis of history (including exposure, residence, and travel and immunization history) and selected baseline screening test results. Routine immunizations should be given at least 2 weeks (inactivated or subunit vaccines) or 4 weeks (live vaccines) before initiation of BRMs whenever feasible, and inactivated influenza vaccine should be given annually. Inactivated and subunit vaccines should be given when needed while taking BRMs, but live vaccines should be avoided unless under special circumstances in consultation with an infectious diseases specialist. If the patient develops a febrile or serious respiratory illness during BRM therapy, consideration should be given to stopping the BRM while actively searching for and treating possible infectious causes. (7/16)
See full text on page 861.
http://pediatrics.aappublications.org/content/138/2/e20161209

INFLUENZA IMMUNIZATION FOR ALL HEALTH CARE PERSONNEL: KEEP IT MANDATORY
Committee on Infectious Diseases
ABSTRACT. The purpose of this statement is to reaffirm the American Academy of Pediatrics' support for a mandatory influenza immunization policy for all health care personnel. With an increasing number of organizations requiring influenza vaccination, coverage among health care personnel has risen to 75% in the 2013 to 2014 influenza season but still remains below the Healthy People 2020 objective of 90%. Mandatory influenza immunization for all health care personnel is ethical, just, and necessary to improve patient safety. It is a crucial step in efforts to reduce health care–associated influenza infections. (9/15)
http://pediatrics.aappublications.org/content/136/4/809

INFORMED CONSENT IN DECISION-MAKING IN PEDIATRIC PRACTICE
Committee on Bioethics
ABSTRACT. Informed consent should be seen as an essential part of health care practice; parental permission and childhood assent is an active process that engages patients, both adults and children, in health care. Pediatric practice is unique in that developmental maturation allows, over time, for increasing inclusion of the child's and adolescent's opinion in medical decision-making in clinical practice and research. (7/16)
See full text on page 885.
http://pediatrics.aappublications.org/content/138/2/e20161484

INFORMED CONSENT IN DECISION-MAKING IN PEDIATRIC PRACTICE (TECHNICAL REPORT)

Aviva L. Katz, MD, FAAP; Sally A. Webb, MD, FAAP; and Committee on Bioethics

ABSTRACT. Informed consent should be seen as an essential part of health care practice; parental permission and childhood assent is an active process that engages patients, both adults and children, in their health care. Pediatric practice is unique in that developmental maturation allows, over time, for increasing inclusion of the child's and adolescent's opinion in medical decision-making in clinical practice and research. This technical report, which accompanies the policy statement "Informed Consent in Decision-Making in Pediatric Practice," was written to provide a broader background on the nature of informed consent, surrogate decision-making in pediatric practice, information on child and adolescent decision-making, and special issues in adolescent informed consent, assent, and refusal. It is anticipated that this information will help provide support for the recommendations included in the policy statement. (7/16)

See full text on page 895.

http://pediatrics.aappublications.org/content/138/2/e20161485

INHALANT ABUSE (CLINICAL REPORT)

Janet F. Williams, MD; Michael Storck, MD; Committee on Substance Abuse; and Committee on Native American Child Health

ABSTRACT. Inhalant abuse is the intentional inhalation of a volatile substance for the purpose of achieving an altered mental state. As an important, yet-underrecognized form of substance abuse, inhalant abuse crosses all demographic, ethnic, and socioeconomic boundaries, causing significant morbidity and mortality in school-aged and older children. This clinical report reviews key aspects of inhalant abuse, emphasizes the need for greater awareness, and offers advice regarding the pediatrician's role in the prevention and management of this substance abuse problem. (5/07)

http://pediatrics.aappublications.org/content/119/5/1009

INJURIES ASSOCIATED WITH INFANT WALKERS

Committee on Injury and Poison Prevention

ABSTRACT. In 1999, an estimated 8800 children younger than 15 months were treated in hospital emergency departments in the United States for injuries associated with infant walkers. Thirty-four infant walker-related deaths were reported from 1973 through 1998. The vast majority of injuries occur from falls down stairs, and head injuries are common. Walkers do not help a child learn to walk; indeed, they can delay normal motor and mental development. The use of warning labels, public education, adult supervision during walker use, and stair gates have all been demonstrated to be insufficient strategies to prevent injuries associated with infant walkers. To comply with the revised voluntary standard (ASTM F977-96), walkers manufactured after June 30, 1997, must be wider than a 36-in doorway or must have a braking mechanism designed to stop the walker if 1 or more wheels drop off the riding surface, such as at the top of a stairway. Because data indicate a considerable risk of major and minor injury and even death from the use of infant walkers, and because there is no clear benefit from their use, the American Academy of Pediatrics recommends a ban on the manufacture and sale of mobile infant walkers. If a parent insists on using a mobile infant walker, it is vital that they choose a walker that meets the performance standards of ASTM F977-96 to prevent falls down stairs. Stationary activity centers should be promoted as a safer alternative to mobile infant walkers. (9/01, reaffirmed 1/05, 2/08, 10/11, 11/14)

http://pediatrics.aappublications.org/content/108/3/790

INJURIES IN YOUTH SOCCER (CLINICAL REPORT)

Chris G. Koutures, MD; Andrew J. M. Gregory, MD; and Council on Sports Medicine and Fitness

ABSTRACT. Injury rates in youth soccer, known as football outside the United States, are higher than in many other contact/collision sports and have greater relative numbers in younger, preadolescent players. With regard to musculoskeletal injuries, young females tend to suffer more knee injuries, and young males suffer more ankle injuries. Concussions are fairly prevalent in soccer as a result of contact/collision rather than purposeful attempts at heading the ball. Appropriate rule enforcement and emphasis on safe play can reduce the risk of soccer-related injuries. This report serves as a basis for encouraging safe participation in soccer for children and adolescents. (1/10, reaffirmed 5/13)

http://pediatrics.aappublications.org/content/125/2/410

INJURY RISK OF NONPOWDER GUNS (TECHNICAL REPORT)

Committee on Injury, Violence, and Poison Prevention

ABSTRACT. Nonpowder guns (ball-bearing [BB] guns, pellet guns, air rifles, paintball guns) continue to cause serious injuries to children and adolescents. The muzzle velocity of these guns can range from approximately 150 ft/second to 1200 ft/second (the muzzle velocities of traditional firearm pistols are 750 ft/second to 1450 ft/second). Both low- and high-velocity nonpowder guns are associated with serious injuries, and fatalities can result from high-velocity guns. A persisting problem is the lack of medical recognition of the severity of injuries that can result from these guns, including penetration of the eye, skin, internal organs, and bone. Nationally, in 2000, there were an estimated 21840 (coefficient of variation: 0.0821) injuries related to nonpowder guns, with approximately 4% resulting in hospitalization. Between 1990 and 2000, the US Consumer Product Safety Commission reported 39 nonpowder gun–related deaths, of which 32 were children younger than 15 years. The introduction of high-powered air rifles in the 1970s has been associated with approximately 4 deaths per year. The advent of war games and the use of paintball guns have resulted in a number of reports of injuries, especially to the eye. Injuries associated with nonpowder guns should receive prompt medical management similar to the management of firearm-related injuries, and nonpowder guns should never be characterized as toys. (11/04, reaffirmed 2/08, 10/11)

http://pediatrics.aappublications.org/content/114/5/1357

IN-LINE SKATING INJURIES IN CHILDREN AND ADOLESCENTS

Committee on Injury and Poison Prevention and Committee on Sports Medicine and Fitness

ABSTRACT. In-line skating has become one of the fastest-growing recreational sports in the United States. Recent studies emphasize the value of protective gear in reducing the incidence of injuries. Recommendations are provided for parents and pediatricians, with special emphasis on the novice or inexperienced skater. (4/98, reaffirmed 1/02, 1/06, 1/09, 11/11)

http://pediatrics.aappublications.org/content/101/4/720

INSTITUTIONAL ETHICS COMMITTEES

Committee on Bioethics

ABSTRACT. In hospitals throughout the United States, institutional ethics committees (IECs) have become a standard vehicle for the education of health professionals about biomedical ethics, for the drafting and review of hospital policy, and for clinical ethics case consultation. In addition, there is increasing interest in a role for the IEC in organizational ethics. Recommendations are made about the membership and structure of an IEC, and guidelines are provided for those serving on an ethics committee. (1/01, reaffirmed 1/04, 1/09, 10/12, 7/14)

http://pediatrics.aappublications.org/content/107/1/205

INSTRUMENT-BASED PEDIATRIC VISION SCREENING POLICY STATEMENT

Section on Ophthalmology and Committee on Practice and Ambulatory Medicine (joint with American Academy of Ophthalmology, American Association for Pediatric Ophthalmology and Strabismus, and American Association of Certified Orthoptists)

ABSTRACT. A policy statement describing the use of automated vision screening technology (instrument-based vision screening) is presented. Screening for amblyogenic refractive error with instrument-based screening is not dependent on behavioral responses of children, as when visual acuity is measured. Instrument-based screening is quick, requires minimal cooperation of the child, and is especially useful in the preverbal, preliterate, or developmentally delayed child. Children younger than 4 years can benefit from instrument-based screening, and visual acuity testing can be used reliably in older children. Adoption of this new technology is highly dependent on third-party payment policies, which could present a significant barrier to adoption. (10/12)

http://pediatrics.aappublications.org/content/130/5/983

INSUFFICIENT SLEEP IN ADOLESCENTS AND YOUNG ADULTS: AN UPDATE ON CAUSES AND CONSEQUENCES (TECHNICAL REPORT)

Judith Owens, MD, MPH, FAAP; Adolescent Sleep Working Group; and Committee on Adolescence

ABSTRACT. Chronic sleep loss and associated sleepiness and daytime impairments in adolescence are a serious threat to the academic success, health, and safety of our nation's youth and an important public health issue. Understanding the extent and potential short- and long-term repercussions of sleep restriction, as well as the unhealthy sleep practices and environmental factors that contribute to sleep loss in adolescents, is key in setting public policies to mitigate these effects and in counseling patients and families in the clinical setting. This report reviews the current literature on sleep patterns in adolescents, factors contributing to chronic sleep loss (ie, electronic media use, caffeine consumption), and health-related consequences, such as depression, increased obesity risk, and higher rates of drowsy driving accidents. The report also discusses the potential role of later school start times as a means of reducing adolescent sleepiness. (8/14)

http://pediatrics.aappublications.org/content/134/3/e921

INSURANCE COVERAGE OF MENTAL HEALTH AND SUBSTANCE ABUSE SERVICES FOR CHILDREN AND ADOLESCENTS: A CONSENSUS STATEMENT

American Academy of Pediatrics and Others (10/00)

http://pediatrics.aappublications.org/content/106/4/860

INTENSIVE TRAINING AND SPORTS SPECIALIZATION IN YOUNG ATHLETES

Committee on Sports Medicine and Fitness

ABSTRACT. Children involved in sports should be encouraged to participate in a variety of different activities and develop a wide range of skills. Young athletes who specialize in just one sport may be denied the benefits of varied activity while facing additional physical, physiologic, and psychologic demands from intense training and competition.

This statement reviews the potential risks of high-intensity training and sports specialization in young athletes. Pediatricians who recognize these risks can have a key role in monitoring the health of these young athletes and helping reduce risks associated with high-level sports participation. (7/00, reaffirmed 11/04, 1/06, 5/09, 10/14)

http://pediatrics.aappublications.org/content/106/1/154

INTERFERON-γ RELEASE ASSAYS FOR DIAGNOSIS OF TUBERCULOSIS INFECTION AND DISEASE IN CHILDREN (TECHNICAL REPORT)

Jeffrey R. Starke, MD, FAAP, and Committee on Infectious Diseases

ABSTRACT. Tuberculosis (TB) remains an important problem among children in the United States and throughout the world. Although diagnosis and treatment of infection with *Mycobacterium tuberculosis* (also referred to as latent tuberculosis infection [LTBI] or TB infection) remain the lynchpins of TB prevention, there is no diagnostic reference standard for LTBI. The tuberculin skin test (TST) has many limitations, including difficulty in administration and interpretation, the need for a return visit by the patient, and false-positive results caused by significant cross-reaction with *Mycobacterium bovis*–bacille Calmette-Guérin (BCG) vaccines and many nontuberculous mycobacteria. Interferon-γ release assays (IGRAs) are blood tests that measure ex vivo T-lymphocyte release of interferon-γ after stimulation by antigens specific for *M tuberculosis*. Because these antigens are not found on *M bovis*–BCG or most nontuberculous mycobacteria, IGRAs are more specific tests than the TST, yielding fewer false-positive results. However, IGRAs have little advantage over the TST in sensitivity, and both methods have

reduced sensitivity in immunocompromised children, including children with severe TB disease. Both methods have a higher positive predictive value when applied to children with risk factors for LTBI. Unfortunately, neither method distinguishes between TB infection and TB disease. The objective of this technical report is to review what IGRAs are most useful for: (1) increasing test specificity in children who have received a BCG vaccine and may have a false-positive TST result; (2) using with the TST to increase sensitivity for finding LTBI in patients at high risk of developing progression from LTBI to disease; and (3) helping to diagnose TB disease. (11/14)
http://pediatrics.aappublications.org/content/134/6/e1763

INTIMATE PARTNER VIOLENCE: THE ROLE OF THE PEDIATRICIAN (CLINICAL REPORT)
Jonathan D. Thackeray, MD; Roberta Hibbard, MD; M. Denise Dowd, MD, MPH; Committee on Child Abuse and Neglect; and Committee on Injury, Violence, and Poison Prevention
ABSTRACT. The American Academy of Pediatrics and its members recognize the importance of improving the physician's ability to recognize intimate partner violence (IPV) and understand its effects on child health and development and its role in the continuum of family violence. Pediatricians are in a unique position to identify abused caregivers in pediatric settings and to evaluate and treat children raised in homes in which IPV may occur. Children exposed to IPV are at increased risk of being abused and neglected and are more likely to develop adverse health, behavioral, psychological, and social disorders later in life. Identifying IPV, therefore, may be one of the most effective means of preventing child abuse and identifying caregivers and children who may be in need of treatment and/or therapy. Pediatricians should be aware of the profound effects of exposure to IPV on children. (4/10, reaffirmed 1/14)
http://pediatrics.aappublications.org/content/125/5/1094

IODINE DEFICIENCY, POLLUTANT CHEMICALS, AND THE THYROID: NEW INFORMATION ON AN OLD PROBLEM
Council on Environmental Health
ABSTRACT. Many women of reproductive age in the United States are marginally iodine deficient, perhaps because the salt in processed foods is not iodized. Iodine deficiency, per se, can interfere with normal brain development in their offspring; in addition, it increases vulnerability to the effects of certain environmental pollutants, such as nitrate, thiocyanate, and perchlorate. Although pregnant and lactating women should take a supplement containing adequate iodide, only about 15% do so. Such supplements, however, may not contain enough iodide and may not be labeled accurately. The American Thyroid Association recommends that pregnant and lactating women take a supplement with adequate iodide. The American Academy of Pediatrics recommends that pregnant and lactating women also avoid exposure to excess nitrate, which would usually occur from contaminated well water, and thiocyanate, which is in cigarette smoke. Perchlorate is currently a candidate for regulation as a

water pollutant. The Environmental Protection Agency should proceed with appropriate regulation, and the Food and Drug Administration should address the mislabeling of the iodine content of prenatal/lactation supplements. (5/14)
http://pediatrics.aappublications.org/content/133/6/1163

LACTOSE INTOLERANCE IN INFANTS, CHILDREN, AND ADOLESCENTS (CLINICAL REPORT)
Melvin B. Heyman, MD, MPH, for Committee on Nutrition
ABSTRACT. The American Academy of Pediatrics Committee on Nutrition presents an updated review of lactose intolerance in infants, children, and adolescents. Differences between primary, secondary, congenital, and developmental lactase deficiency that may result in lactose intolerance are discussed. Children with suspected lactose intolerance can be assessed clinically by dietary lactose elimination or by tests including noninvasive hydrogen breath testing or invasive intestinal biopsy determination of lactase (and other disaccharidase) concentrations. Treatment consists of use of lactase-treated dairy products or oral lactase supplementation, limitation of lactose-containing foods, or dairy elimination. The American Academy of Pediatrics supports use of dairy foods as an important source of calcium for bone mineral health and of other nutrients that facilitate growth in children and adolescents. If dairy products are eliminated, other dietary sources of calcium or calcium supplements need to be provided. (9/06, reaffirmed 8/12)
http://pediatrics.aappublications.org/content/118/3/1279

"LATE-PRETERM" INFANTS: A POPULATION AT RISK (CLINICAL REPORT)
William A. Engle, MD; Kay M. Tomashek, MD; Carol Wallman, MSN; and Committee on Fetus and Newborn
ABSTRACT. Late-preterm infants, defined by birth at 34 through 36 weeks' gestation, are less physiologically and metabolically mature than term infants. Thus, they are at higher risk of morbidity and mortality than term infants. The purpose of this report is to define "late preterm," recommend a change in terminology from "near term" to "late preterm," present the characteristics of late-preterm infants that predispose them to a higher risk of morbidity and mortality than term infants, and propose guidelines for the evaluation and management of these infants after birth. (12/07, reaffirmed 5/10)
http://pediatrics.aappublications.org/content/120/6/1390

LAWN MOWER-RELATED INJURIES TO CHILDREN
Committee on Injury and Poison Prevention
ABSTRACT. Lawn mower-related injuries to children are relatively common and can result in severe injury or death. Many amputations during childhood are caused by power mowers. Pediatricians have an important role as advocates and educators to promote the prevention of these injuries. (6/01, reaffirmed 10/04, 5/07, 6/10)
http://pediatrics.aappublications.org/content/107/6/1480

LAWN MOWER-RELATED INJURIES TO CHILDREN (TECHNICAL REPORT)

Committee on Injury and Poison Prevention

ABSTRACT. In the United States, approximately 9400 children younger than 18 years receive emergency treatment annually for lawn mower-related injuries. More than 7% of these children require hospitalization, and power mowers cause a large proportion of the amputations during childhood. Prevention of lawn mower-related injuries can be achieved by design changes of lawn mowers, guidelines for mower operation, and education of parents, child caregivers, and children. Pediatricians have an important role as advocates and educators to promote the prevention of these injuries. (6/01, reaffirmed 10/04, 5/07, 6/10)
http://pediatrics.aappublications.org/content/107/6/e106

LEARNING DISABILITIES, DYSLEXIA, AND VISION

Section on Ophthalmology and Council on Children With Disabilities (joint with American Academy of Ophthalmology, American Association for Pediatric Ophthalmology and Strabismus, and American Association of Certified Orthoptists)

ABSTRACT. Learning disabilities, including reading disabilities, are commonly diagnosed in children. Their etiologies are multifactorial, reflecting genetic influences and dysfunction of brain systems. Learning disabilities are complex problems that require complex solutions. Early recognition and referral to qualified educational professionals for evidence-based evaluations and treatments seem necessary to achieve the best possible outcome. Most experts believe that dyslexia is a language-based disorder. Vision problems can interfere with the process of learning; however, vision problems are not the cause of primary dyslexia or learning disabilities. Scientific evidence does not support the efficacy of eye exercises, behavioral vision therapy, or special tinted filters or lenses for improving the long-term educational performance in these complex pediatric neurocognitive conditions. Diagnostic and treatment approaches that lack scientific evidence of efficacy, including eye exercises, behavioral vision therapy, or special tinted filters or lenses, are not endorsed and should not be recommended. (7/09, reaffirmed 7/14)
http://pediatrics.aappublications.org/content/127/3/e818

LEARNING DISABILITIES, DYSLEXIA, AND VISION (TECHNICAL REPORT)

Sheryl M. Handler, MD; Walter M. Fierson, MD; and Section on Ophthalmology and Council on Children With Disabilities (joint with American Academy of Ophthalmology, American Association for Pediatric Ophthalmology and Strabismus, and American Association of Certified Orthoptists)

ABSTRACT. Learning disabilities constitute a diverse group of disorders in which children who generally possess at least average intelligence have problems processing information or generating output. Their etiologies are multifactorial and reflect genetic influences and dysfunction of brain systems. Reading disability, or dyslexia, is the most common learning disability. It is a receptive language-based learning disability that is characterized by difficulties with decoding, fluent word recognition, rapid automatic naming, and/or reading-comprehension skills. These difficulties typically result from a deficit in the phonologic component of language that makes it difficult to use the alphabetic code to decode the written word. Early recognition and referral to qualified professionals for evidence-based evaluations and treatments are necessary to achieve the best possible outcome. Because dyslexia is a language-based disorder, treatment should be directed at this etiology. Remedial programs should include specific instruction in decoding, fluency training, vocabulary, and comprehension. Most programs include daily intensive individualized instruction that explicitly teaches phonemic awareness and the application of phonics. Vision problems can interfere with the process of reading, but children with dyslexia or related learning disabilities have the same visual function and ocular health as children without such conditions. Currently, there is inadequate scientific evidence to support the view that subtle eye or visual problems cause or increase the severity of learning disabilities. Because they are difficult for the public to understand and for educators to treat, learning disabilities have spawned a wide variety of scientifically unsupported vision-based diagnostic and treatment procedures. Scientific evidence does not support the claims that visual training, muscle exercises, ocular pursuit-and-tracking exercises, behavioral/perceptual vision therapy, "training" glasses, prisms, and colored lenses and filters are effective direct or indirect treatments for learning disabilities. There is no valid evidence that children who participate in vision therapy are more responsive to educational instruction than children who do not participate. (3/11)
http://pediatrics.aappublications.org/content/127/3/e818

LEGALIZATION OF MARIJUANA: POTENTIAL IMPACT ON YOUTH

Committee on Substance Abuse and Committee on Adolescence

ABSTRACT. As experts in the health care of children and adolescents, pediatricians may be called on to advise legislators concerning the potential impact of changes in the legal status of marijuana on adolescents. Parents, too, may look to pediatricians for advice as they consider whether to support state-level initiatives that propose to legalize the use of marijuana for medical purposes or to decriminalize possession of small amounts of marijuana. This policy statement provides the position of the American Academy of Pediatrics on the issue of marijuana legalization, and the accompanying technical report (available online) reviews what is currently known about the relationship between adolescents' use of marijuana and its legal status to better understand how change might influence the degree of marijuana use by adolescents in the future. (6/04)
http://pediatrics.aappublications.org/content/113/6/1825

LEGALIZATION OF MARIJUANA: POTENTIAL IMPACT ON YOUTH (TECHNICAL REPORT)

Committee on Substance Abuse and Committee on Adolescence

ABSTRACT. This technical report provides historical perspectives and comparisons of various approaches to the legal status of marijuana to aid in forming public policy. Information on the impact that decriminalization and legalization of marijuana could have on adolescents, in addition to concerns surrounding medicinal

use of marijuana, are also addressed in this report. Recommendations are included in the accompanying policy statement. (6/04)
http://pediatrics.aappublications.org/content/113/6/e632

LEVELS OF NEONATAL CARE
Committee on Fetus and Newborn
ABSTRACT. Provision of risk-appropriate care for newborn infants and mothers was first proposed in 1976. This updated policy statement provides a review of data supporting evidence for a tiered provision of care and reaffirms the need for uniform, nationally applicable definitions and consistent standards of service for public health to improve neonatal outcomes. Facilities that provide hospital care for newborn infants should be classified on the basis of functional capabilities, and these facilities should be organized within a regionalized system of perinatal care. (8/12, reaffirmed 9/15)
http://pediatrics.aappublications.org/content/130/3/587

THE LIFELONG EFFECTS OF EARLY CHILDHOOD ADVERSITY AND TOXIC STRESS (TECHNICAL REPORT)
Jack P. Shonkoff, MD; Andrew S. Garner, MD, PhD; Committee on Psychosocial Aspects of Child and Family Health; Committee on Early Childhood, Adoption, and Dependent Care; and Section on Developmental and Behavioral Pediatrics
ABSTRACT. Advances in fields of inquiry as diverse as neuroscience, molecular biology, genomics, developmental psychology, epidemiology, sociology, and economics are catalyzing an important paradigm shift in our understanding of health and disease across the lifespan. This converging, multidisciplinary science of human development has profound implications for our ability to enhance the life prospects of children and to strengthen the social and economic fabric of society. Drawing on these multiple streams of investigation, this report presents an ecobiodevelopmental framework that illustrates how early experiences and environmental influences can leave a lasting signature on the genetic predispositions that affect emerging brain architecture and long-term health. The report also examines extensive evidence of the disruptive impacts of toxic stress, offering intriguing insights into causal mechanisms that link early adversity to later impairments in learning, behavior, and both physical and mental well-being. The implications of this framework for the practice of medicine, in general, and pediatrics, specifically, are potentially transformational. They suggest that many adult diseases should be viewed as developmental disorders that begin early in life and that persistent health disparities associated with poverty, discrimination, or maltreatment could be reduced by the alleviation of toxic stress in childhood. An ecobiodevelopmental framework also underscores the need for new thinking about the focus and boundaries of pediatric practice. It calls for pediatricians to serve as both front-line guardians of healthy child development and strategically positioned, community leaders to inform new science-based strategies that build strong foundations for educational achievement, economic productivity, responsible citizenship, and lifelong health. (12/11, reaffirmed 7/16)
http://pediatrics.aappublications.org/content/129/1/e232

LITERACY PROMOTION: AN ESSENTIAL COMPONENT OF PRIMARY CARE PEDIATRIC PRACTICE
Council on Early Childhood
ABSTRACT. Reading regularly with young children stimulates optimal patterns of brain development and strengthens parent-child relationships at a critical time in child development, which, in turn, builds language, literacy, and social-emotional skills that last a lifetime. Pediatric providers have a unique opportunity to encourage parents to engage in this important and enjoyable activity with their children beginning in infancy. Research has revealed that parents listen and children learn as a result of literacy promotion by pediatricians, which provides a practical and evidence-based opportunity to support early brain development in primary care practice. The American Academy of Pediatrics (AAP) recommends that pediatric providers promote early literacy development for children beginning in infancy and continuing at least until the age of kindergarten entry by (1) advising all parents that reading aloud with young children can enhance parent-child relationships and prepare young minds to learn language and early literacy skills; (2) counseling all parents about developmentally appropriate shared-reading activities that are enjoyable for children and their parents and offer language-rich exposure to books, pictures, and the written word; (3) providing developmentally appropriate books given at health supervision visits for all high-risk, low-income young children; (4) using a robust spectrum of options to support and promote these efforts; and (5) partnering with other child advocates to influence national messaging and policies that support and promote these key early shared-reading experiences. The AAP supports federal and state funding for children's books to be provided at pediatric health supervision visits to children at high risk living at or near the poverty threshold and the integration of literacy promotion, an essential component of pediatric primary care, into pediatric resident education. This policy statement is supported by the AAP technical report "School Readiness" and supports the AAP policy statement "Early Childhood Adversity, Toxic Stress, and the Role of the Pediatrician: Translating Developmental Science Into Lifelong Health." (7/14)
http://pediatrics.aappublications.org/content/134/2/404

LONG-TERM FOLLOW-UP CARE FOR PEDIATRIC CANCER SURVIVORS (CLINICAL REPORT)
Section on Hematology/Oncology (joint with Children's Oncology Group)
ABSTRACT. Progress in therapy has made survival into adulthood a reality for most children, adolescents, and young adults diagnosed with cancer today. Notably, this growing population remains vulnerable to a variety of long-term therapy-related sequelae. Systematic ongoing follow-up of these patients, therefore, is important for providing for early detection of and intervention for potentially serious late-onset complications. In addition, health counseling and promotion of healthy lifestyles are important aspects of long-term follow-up care to promote risk reduction for health problems that commonly present during adulthood. Both general and subspecialty pediatric health care providers are playing an increasingly

important role in the ongoing care of childhood cancer survivors, beyond the routine preventive care, health supervision, and anticipatory guidance provided to all patients. This report is based on the guidelines that have been developed by the Children's Oncology Group to facilitate comprehensive long-term follow-up of childhood cancer survivors (www.survivorshipguidelines.org). (3/09, reaffirmed 4/13)
http://pediatrics.aappublications.org/content/123/3/906

MAINTAINING AND IMPROVING THE ORAL HEALTH OF YOUNG CHILDREN
Section on Oral Health
ABSTRACT. Oral health is an integral part of the overall health of children. Dental caries is a common and chronic disease process with significant short- and long-term consequences. The prevalence of dental caries for the youngest of children has not decreased over the past decade, despite improvements for older children. As health care professionals responsible for the overall health of children, pediatricians frequently confront morbidity associated with dental caries. Because the youngest children visit the pediatrician more often than they visit the dentist, it is important that pediatricians be knowledgeable about the disease process of dental caries, prevention of the disease, and interventions available to the pediatrician and the family to maintain and restore health. (11/14, reaffirmed 12/14)
http://pediatrics.aappublications.org/content/134/6/1224

MALE ADOLESCENT SEXUAL AND REPRODUCTIVE HEALTH CARE (CLINICAL REPORT)
Arik V. Marcell, MD, MPH; Charles Wibbelsman, MD; Warren M. Seigel, MD; and Committee on Adolescence
ABSTRACT. Male adolescents' sexual and reproductive health needs often go unmet in the primary care setting. This report discusses specific issues related to male adolescents' sexual and reproductive health care in the context of primary care, including pubertal and sexual development, sexual behavior, consequences of sexual behavior, and methods of preventing sexually transmitted infections (including HIV) and pregnancy. Pediatricians are encouraged to address male adolescent sexual and reproductive health on a regular basis, including taking a sexual history, performing an appropriate examination, providing patient-centered and age-appropriate anticipatory guidance, and delivering appropriate vaccinations. Pediatricians should provide these services to male adolescent patients in a confidential and culturally appropriate manner, promote healthy sexual relationships and responsibility, and involve parents in age-appropriate discussions about sexual health with their sons. (11/11)
http://pediatrics.aappublications.org/content/128/6/e1658

MALE CIRCUMCISION (TECHNICAL REPORT)
Task Force on Circumcision
ABSTRACT. Male circumcision consists of the surgical removal of some, or all, of the foreskin (or prepuce) from the penis. It is one of the most common procedures in the world. In the United States, the procedure is commonly performed during the newborn period. In 2007,

the American Academy of Pediatrics (AAP) convened a multidisciplinary workgroup of AAP members and other stakeholders to evaluate the evidence regarding male circumcision and update the AAP's 1999 recommendations in this area. The Task Force included AAP representatives from specialty areas as well as members of the AAP Board of Directors and liaisons representing the American Academy of Family Physicians, the American College of Obstetricians and Gynecologists, and the Centers for Disease Control and Prevention. The Task Force members identified selected topics relevant to male circumcision and conducted a critical review of peer-reviewed literature by using the American Heart Association's template for evidence evaluation.

Evaluation of current evidence indicates that the health benefits of newborn male circumcision outweigh the risks; furthermore, the benefits of newborn male circumcision justify access to this procedure for families who choose it. Specific benefits from male circumcision were identified for the prevention of urinary tract infections, acquisition of HIV, transmission of some sexually transmitted infections, and penile cancer. Male circumcision does not appear to adversely affect penile sexual function/sensitivity or sexual satisfaction. It is imperative that those providing circumcision are adequately trained and that both sterile techniques and effective pain management are used. Significant acute complications are rare. In general, untrained providers who perform circumcisions have more complications than well-trained providers who perform the procedure, regardless of whether the former are physicians, nurses, or traditional religious providers.

Parents are entitled to factually correct, nonbiased information about circumcision and should receive this information from clinicians before conception or early in pregnancy, which is when parents typically make circumcision decisions. Parents should determine what is in the best interest of their child. Physicians who counsel families about this decision should provide assistance by explaining the potential benefits and risks and ensuring that parents understand that circumcision is an elective procedure. The Task Force strongly recommends the creation, revision, and enhancement of educational materials to assist parents of male infants with the care of circumcised and uncircumcised penises. The Task Force also strongly recommends the development of educational materials for providers to enhance practitioners' competency in discussing circumcision's benefits and risks with parents.

The Task Force made the following recommendations:

- Evaluation of current evidence indicates that the health benefits of newborn male circumcision outweigh the risks, and the benefits of newborn male circumcision justify access to this procedure for those families who choose it.

- Parents are entitled to factually correct, nonbiased information about circumcision that should be provided before conception and early in pregnancy, when parents are most likely to be weighing the option of circumcision of a male child.

- Physicians counseling families about elective male circumcision should assist parents by explaining, in a nonbiased manner, the potential benefits and risks and by ensuring that they understand the elective nature of the procedure.

- Parents should weigh the health benefits and risks in light of their own religious, cultural, and personal preferences, as the medical benefits alone may not outweigh these other considerations for individual families.

- Parents of newborn boys should be instructed in the care of the penis, regardless of whether the newborn has been circumcised or not.

- Elective circumcision should be performed only if the infant's condition is stable and healthy.

- Male circumcision should be performed by trained and competent practitioners, by using sterile techniques and effective pain management.

- Analgesia is safe and effective in reducing the procedural pain associated with newborn circumcision; thus, adequate analgesia should be provided whenever newborn circumcision is performed.

  — Nonpharmacologic techniques (eg, positioning, sucrose pacifiers) alone are insufficient to prevent procedural and postprocedural pain and are not recommended as the sole method of analgesia. They should be used only as analgesic adjuncts to improve infant comfort during circumcision.

  — If used, topical creams may cause a higher incidence of skin irritation in low birth weight infants, compared with infants of normal weight; penile nerve block techniques should therefore be chosen for this group of newborns.

- Key professional organizations (AAP, the American Academy of Family Physicians, the American College of Obstetricians and Gynecologists, the American Society of Anesthesiologists, the American College of Nurse Midwives, and other midlevel clinicians such as nurse practitioners) should work collaboratively to:

  — Develop standards of trainee proficiency in the performance of anesthetic and procedure techniques, including suturing;

  — Teach the procedure and analgesic techniques during postgraduate training programs;

  — Develop educational materials for clinicians to enhance their own competency in discussing the benefits and risks of circumcision with parents;

  — Offer educational materials to assist parents of male infants with the care of both circumcised and uncircumcised penises.

- The preventive and public health benefits associated with newborn male circumcision warrant third-party reimbursement of the procedure.

The American College of Obstetricians and Gynecologists has endorsed this technical report. (8/12)
http://pediatrics.aappublications.org/content/130/3/e756

MALTREATMENT OF CHILDREN WITH DISABILITIES (CLINICAL REPORT)

Roberta A. Hibbard, MD; Larry W. Desch, MD; Committee on Child Abuse and Neglect; and Council on Children With Disabilities

ABSTRACT. Widespread efforts are being made to increase awareness and provide education to pediatricians regarding risk factors of child abuse and neglect. The purpose of this clinical report is to ensure that children with disabilities are recognized as a population that is also at risk of maltreatment. Some conditions related to a disability can be confused with maltreatment. The need for early recognition and intervention of child abuse and neglect in this population, as well as the ways that a medical home can facilitate the prevention and early detection of child maltreatment, are the subject of this report. (5/07, reaffirmed 1/11, 4/16)
http://pediatrics.aappublications.org/content/119/5/1018

MANAGEMENT OF CHILDREN WITH AUTISM SPECTRUM DISORDERS (CLINICAL REPORT)

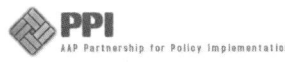

Scott M. Myers, MD; Chris Plauché Johnson, MD, MEd; and Council on Children With Disabilities

ABSTRACT. Pediatricians have an important role not only in early recognition and evaluation of autism spectrum disorders but also in chronic management of these disorders. The primary goals of treatment are to maximize the child's ultimate functional independence and quality of life by minimizing the core autism spectrum disorder features, facilitating development and learning, promoting socialization, reducing maladaptive behaviors, and educating and supporting families. To assist pediatricians in educating families and guiding them toward empirically supported interventions for their children, this report reviews the educational strategies and associated therapies that are the primary treatments for children with autism spectrum disorders. Optimization of health care is likely to have a positive effect on habilitative progress, functional outcome, and quality of life; therefore, important issues, such as management of associated medical problems, pharmacologic and nonpharmacologic intervention for challenging behaviors or coexisting mental health conditions, and use of complementary and alternative medical treatments, are also addressed. (11/07, reaffirmed 9/10, 8/14)
http://pediatrics.aappublications.org/content/120/5/1162

MANAGEMENT OF DENTAL TRAUMA IN A PRIMARY CARE SETTING (CLINICAL REPORT)

Martha Ann Keels, DDS, PhD, and Section on Oral Health

ABSTRACT. The American Academy of Pediatrics and its Section on Oral Health have developed this clinical report for pediatricians and primary care physicians regarding the diagnosis, evaluation, and management of dental trauma in children aged 1 to 21 years. This report was developed through a comprehensive search and analysis of the medical and dental literature and expert consensus. Guidelines published and updated by the International Association of Dental Traumatology (www.dentaltraumaguide.com) are an excellent resource for both dental and nondental health care providers. (1/14)
http://pediatrics.aappublications.org/content/133/2/e466

MANAGEMENT OF FOOD ALLERGY IN THE SCHOOL SETTING (CLINICAL REPORT)

Scott H. Sicherer, MD; Todd Mahr, MD; and Section on Allergy and Immunology

ABSTRACT. Food allergy is estimated to affect approximately 1 in 25 school-aged children and is the most common trigger of anaphylaxis in this age group. School food-allergy management requires strategies to reduce the risk of ingestion of the allergen as well as procedures to recognize and treat allergic reactions and anaphylaxis. The role of the pediatrician or pediatric health care provider may include diagnosing and documenting a potentially life-threatening food allergy, prescribing self-injectable epinephrine, helping the child learn how to store and use the medication in a responsible manner, educating the parents of their responsibility to implement prevention strategies within and outside the home environment, and working with families, schools, and students in developing written plans to reduce the risk of anaphylaxis and to implement emergency treatment in the event of a reaction. This clinical report highlights the role of the pediatrician and pediatric health care provider in managing students with food allergies. (11/10)

http://pediatrics.aappublications.org/content/126/6/1232

MANAGEMENT OF NEONATES WITH SUSPECTED OR PROVEN EARLY-ONSET BACTERIAL SEPSIS (CLINICAL REPORT)

Richard A. Polin, MD, and Committee on Fetus and Newborn

ABSTRACT. With improved obstetrical management and evidence-based use of intrapartum antimicrobial therapy, early-onset neonatal sepsis is becoming less frequent. However, early-onset sepsis remains one of the most common causes of neonatal morbidity and mortality in the preterm population. The identification of neonates at risk for early-onset sepsis is frequently based on a constellation of perinatal risk factors that are neither sensitive nor specific. Furthermore, diagnostic tests for neonatal sepsis have a poor positive predictive accuracy. As a result, clinicians often treat well-appearing infants for extended periods of time, even when bacterial cultures are negative. The optimal treatment of infants with suspected early-onset sepsis is broad-spectrum antimicrobial agents (ampicillin and an aminoglycoside). Once a pathogen is identified, antimicrobial therapy should be narrowed (unless synergism is needed). Recent data suggest an association between prolonged empirical treatment of preterm infants (≥5 days) with broad-spectrum antibiotics and higher risks of late onset sepsis, necrotizing enterocolitis, and mortality. To reduce these risks, antimicrobial therapy should be discontinued at 48 hours in clinical situations in which the probability of sepsis is low. The purpose of this clinical report is to provide a practical and, when possible, evidence-based approach to the management of infants with suspected or proven early-onset sepsis. (4/12, reaffirmed 2/16)

http://pediatrics.aappublications.org/content/129/5/1006

MANAGEMENT OF PEDIATRIC TRAUMA

Committee on Pediatric Emergency Medicine; Council on Injury, Violence, and Poison Prevention; Section on Critical Care; Section on Orthopaedics; Section on Surgery; and Section on Transport Medicine (joint with Pediatric Trauma Society and Society of Trauma Nurses Pediatric Committee)

ABSTRACT. Injury is still the number 1 killer of children ages 1 to 18 years in the United States (http://www.cdc.gov/nchs/fastats/children.htm). Children who sustain injuries with resulting disabilities incur significant costs not only for their health care but also for productivity lost to the economy. The families of children who survive childhood injury with disability face years of emotional and financial hardship, along with a significant societal burden. The entire process of managing childhood injury is enormously complex and varies by region. Only the comprehensive cooperation of a broadly diverse trauma team will have a significant effect on improving the care of injured children. (7/16)

See full text on page 913.

http://pediatrics.aappublications.org/content/138/2/e20161569

MANAGEMENT OF TYPE 2 DIABETES MELLITUS IN CHILDREN AND ADOLESCENTS (TECHNICAL REPORT)

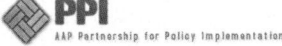

Shelley C. Springer, MD, MBA, MSc, JD; Janet Silverstein, MD; Kenneth Copeland, MD; Kelly R. Moore, MD; Greg E. Prazar, MD; Terry Raymer, MD, CDE; Richard N. Shiffman, MD; Vidhu V. Thaker, MD; Meaghan Anderson, MS, RD, LD, CDE; Stephen J. Spann, MD, MBA; and Susan K. Flinn, MA

ABSTRACT. *Objective.* Over the last 3 decades, the prevalence of childhood obesity has increased dramatically in North America, ushering in a variety of health problems, including type 2 diabetes mellitus (T2DM), which previously was not typically seen until much later in life. This technical report describes, in detail, the procedures undertaken to develop the recommendations given in the accompanying clinical practice guideline, "Management of Type 2 Diabetes Mellitus in Children and Adolescents," and provides in-depth information about the rationale for the recommendations and the studies used to make the clinical practice guideline's recommendations.

Methods. A primary literature search was conducted relating to the treatment of T2DM in children and adolescents, and a secondary literature search was conducted relating to the screening and treatment of T2DM's comorbidities in children and adolescents. Inclusion criteria were prospectively and unanimously agreed on by members of the committee. An article was eligible for inclusion if it addressed treatment (primary search) or 1 of 4 comorbidities (secondary search) of T2DM, was published in 1990 or later, was written in English, and included an abstract. Only primary research inquiries were considered; review articles were considered if they included primary data or opinion. The research population had to constitute children and/or adolescents with an existing diagnosis of T2DM; studies of adult patients were considered if at least

10% of the study population was younger than 35 years. All retrieved titles, abstracts, and articles were reviewed by the consulting epidemiologist.

Results. Thousands of articles were retrieved and considered in both searches on the basis of the aforementioned criteria. From those, in the primary search, 199 abstracts were identified for possible inclusion, 58 of which were retained for systematic review. Five of these studies were classified as grade A studies, 1 as grade B, 20 as grade C, and 32 as grade D. Articles regarding treatment of T2DM selected for inclusion were divided into 4 major subcategories on the basis of type of treatment being discussed: (1) medical treatments (32 studies); (2) nonmedical treatments (9 studies); (3) provider behaviors (8 studies); and (4) social issues (9 studies). From the secondary search, an additional 336 abstracts relating to comorbidities were identified for possible inclusion, of which 26 were retained for systematic review. These articles included the following: 1 systematic review of literature regarding comorbidities of T2DM in adolescents; 5 expert opinions presenting global recommendations not based on evidence; 5 cohort studies reporting natural history of disease and comorbidities; 3 with specific attention to comorbidity patterns in specific ethnic groups (case-control, cohort, and clinical report using adult literature); 3 reporting an association between microalbuminuria and retinopathy (2 case-control, 1 cohort); 3 reporting the prevalence of nephropathy (cohort); 1 reporting peripheral vascular disease (case series); 2 discussing retinopathy (1 case-control, 1 position statement); and 3 addressing hyperlipidemia (American Heart Association position statement on cardiovascular risks; American Diabetes Association consensus statement; case series). A breakdown of grade of recommendation shows no grade A studies, 10 grade B studies, 6 grade C studies, and 10 grade D studies. With regard to screening and treatment recommendations for comorbidities, data in children are scarce, and the available literature is conflicting. Therapeutic recommendations for hypertension, dyslipidemia, retinopathy, microalbuminuria, and depression were summarized from expert guideline documents and are presented in detail in the guideline. The references are provided, but the committee did not independently assess the supporting evidence. Screening tools are provided in the Supplemental Information. (1/13)
http://pediatrics.aappublications.org/content/131/2/e648

MARIJUANA: A CONTINUING CONCERN FOR PEDIATRICIANS

Committee on Substance Abuse
ABSTRACT. Marijuana, the common name for products derived from the plant *Cannabis sativa,* is the most common illicit drug used by children and adolescents in the United States. Despite growing concerns by the medical profession about the physical and psychological effects of its active ingredient, Δ-9-tetrahydrocannabinol, survey data continue to show that increasing numbers of young people are using the drug as they become less concerned about its dangers. (10/99, reaffirmed 4/03)
http://pediatrics.aappublications.org/content/104/4/982

MATERNAL PHENYLKETONURIA

Committee on Genetics
ABSTRACT. Elevated maternal phenylalanine concentrations during pregnancy are teratogenic and may result in growth retardation, microcephaly, significant developmental delays, and birth defects in the offspring of women with poorly controlled phenylketonuria during pregnancy. Women of childbearing age with all forms of phenylketonuria, including mild variants such as mild hyperphenylalaninemia, should receive counseling concerning their risks for adverse fetal effects, optimally before conceiving. The best outcomes occur when strict control of maternal phenylalanine concentration is achieved before conception and continued throughout pregnancy. Included are brief descriptions of novel treatments for phenylketonuria. (8/08, reaffirmed 1/13)
http://pediatrics.aappublications.org/content/122/2/445

MATERNAL-FETAL INTERVENTION AND FETAL CARE CENTERS (CLINICAL REPORT)

Committee on Bioethics (joint with American College of Obstetricians and Gynecologists Committee on Ethics)
ABSTRACT. The past 2 decades have yielded profound advances in the fields of prenatal diagnosis and fetal intervention. Although fetal interventions are driven by a beneficence-based motivation to improve fetal and neonatal outcomes, advancement in fetal therapies raises ethical issues surrounding maternal autonomy and decision-making, concepts of innovation versus research, and organizational aspects within institutions in the development of fetal care centers. To safeguard the interests of both the pregnant woman and the fetus, the American College of Obstetricians and Gynecologists and the American Academy of Pediatrics make recommendations regarding informed consent, the role of research subject advocates and other independent advocates, the availability of support services, the multidisciplinary nature of fetal intervention teams, the oversight of centers, and the need to accumulate maternal and fetal outcome data. (7/11)
http://pediatrics.aappublications.org/content/128/2/e473

MEDIA AND YOUNG MINDS

Council on Communications and Media
ABSTRACT. Infants, toddlers, and preschoolers are now growing up in environments saturated with a variety of traditional and new technologies, which they are adopting at increasing rates. Although there has been much hope for the educational potential of interactive media for young children, accompanied by fears about their overuse during this crucial period of rapid brain development, research in this area still remains limited. This policy statement reviews the existing literature on television, videos, and mobile/interactive technologies; their potential for educational benefit; and related health concerns for young children (0 to 5 years of age). The statement also highlights areas in which pediatric providers can offer specific guidance to families in managing their young children's media use, not only in terms of content or time limits, but also emphasizing the importance of parent-child shared media use and allowing the child time to take part in other developmentally healthy activities. (10/16)
See full text on page 925.
http://pediatrics.aappublications.org/content/138/5/e20162591

MEDIA EDUCATION

Committee on Communications and Media

ABSTRACT. The American Academy of Pediatrics recognizes that exposure to mass media (eg, television, movies, video and computer games, the Internet, music lyrics and videos, newspapers, magazines, books, advertising) presents health risks for children and adolescents but can provide benefits as well. Media education has the potential to reduce the harmful effects of media and accentuate the positive effects. By understanding and supporting media education, pediatricians can play an important role in reducing harmful effects of media on children and adolescents. (9/10)

http://pediatrics.aappublications.org/content/126/5/1012

MEDIA USE BY CHILDREN YOUNGER THAN 2 YEARS

Council on Communications and Media

ABSTRACT. In 1999, the American Academy of Pediatrics (AAP) issued a policy statement addressing media use in children. The purpose of that statement was to educate parents about the effects that media—both the amount and the content—may have on children. In one part of that statement, the AAP recommended that "pediatricians should urge parents to avoid television viewing for children under the age of two years." The wording of the policy specifically *discouraged* media use in this age group, although it is frequently misquoted by media outlets as no media exposure in this age group. The AAP believed that there were significantly more potential negative effects of media than positive ones for this age group and, thus, advised families to thoughtfully consider media use for infants. This policy statement reaffirms the 1999 statement with respect to media use in infants and children younger than 2 years and provides updated research findings to support it. This statement addresses (1) the lack of evidence supporting educational or developmental benefits for media use by children younger than 2 years, (2) the potential adverse health and developmental effects of media use by children younger than 2 years, and (3) adverse effects of parental media use (background media) on children younger than 2 years. (10/11)

http://pediatrics.aappublications.org/content/128/5/1040

MEDIA USE IN SCHOOL-AGED CHILDREN AND ADOLESCENTS

Council on Communications and Media

ABSTRACT. This policy statement focuses on children and adolescents 5 through 18 years of age. Research suggests both benefits and risks of media use for the health of children and teenagers. Benefits include exposure to new ideas and knowledge acquisition, increased opportunities for social contact and support, and new opportunities to access health-promotion messages and information. Risks include negative health effects on weight and sleep; exposure to inaccurate, inappropriate, or unsafe content and contacts; and compromised privacy and confidentiality. Parents face challenges in monitoring their children's and their own media use and in serving as positive role models. In this new era, evidence regarding healthy media use does not support a one-size-fits-all approach. Parents and pediatricians can work together to develop a Family Media Use Plan (www. healthychildren.org/MediaUsePlan) that considers their children's developmental stages to individualize an appropriate balance for media time and consistent rules about media use, to mentor their children, to set boundaries for accessing content and displaying personal information, and to implement open family communication about media. (10/16)

See full text on page 933.

http://pediatrics.aappublications.org/content/138/5/e20162592

MEDIA VIOLENCE

Council on Communications and Media

ABSTRACT. Exposure to violence in media, including television, movies, music, and video games, represents a significant risk to the health of children and adolescents. Extensive research evidence indicates that media violence can contribute to aggressive behavior, desensitization to violence, nightmares, and fear of being harmed. Pediatricians should assess their patients' level of media exposure and intervene on media-related health risks. Pediatricians and other child health care providers can advocate for a safer media environment for children by encouraging media literacy, more thoughtful and proactive use of media by children and their parents, more responsible portrayal of violence by media producers, and more useful and effective media ratings. Office counseling has been shown to be effective. (10/09)

http://pediatrics.aappublications.org/content/124/5/1495

MEDIATORS AND ADVERSE EFFECTS OF CHILD POVERTY IN THE UNITED STATES (TECHNICAL REPORT)

John M. Pascoe, MD, MPH, FAAP; David L. Wood, MD, MPH, FAAP; James H. Duffee, MD, MPH, FAAP; Alice Kuo, MD, PhD, MEd, FAAP; Committee on Psychosocial Aspects of Child and Family Health; and Council on Community Pediatrics

ABSTRACT. The link between poverty and children's health is well recognized. Even temporary poverty may have an adverse effect on children's health, and data consistently support the observation that poverty in childhood continues to have a negative effect on health into adulthood. In addition to childhood morbidity being related to child poverty, epidemiologic studies have documented a mortality gradient for children aged 1 to 15 years (and adults), with poor children experiencing a higher mortality rate than children from higher-income families. The global great recession is only now very slowly abating for millions of America's children and their families. At this difficult time in the history of our nation's families and immediately after the 50th anniversary year of President Lyndon Johnson's War on Poverty, it is particularly germane for the American Academy of Pediatrics, which is "dedicated to the health of all children," to publish a research-supported technical report that examines the mediators associated with the long-recognized adverse effects of child poverty on children and their families. This technical report draws on research from a number of disciplines, including physiology, sociology, psychology, economics, and epidemiology, to describe the present state of knowledge regarding poverty's negative impact on children's health and development. Children inherit not only their parents' genes but also the family ecology and its social milieu. Thus, parenting skills, housing, neighborhood, schools, and other factors (eg, medical care) all have complex relations to each other and influence how each child's genetic canvas is expressed. Accompanying this technical report is a policy statement that describes specific actions that pediatricians and other child advocates can take to attenuate the negative effects of the mediators identified in this technical report and improve the well-being of our nation's children and their families. (3/16)

See full text on page 941.

http://pediatrics.aappublications.org/content/137/4/e20160340

MEDICAID POLICY STATEMENT

Committee on Child Health Financing

ABSTRACT. Medicaid insures 39% of the children in the United States. This revision of the 2005 Medicaid Policy Statement of the American Academy of Pediatrics reflects opportunities for changes in state Medicaid programs resulting from the 2010 Patient Protection and Affordable Care Act as upheld in 2012 by the Supreme Court. Policy recommendations focus on the areas of benefit coverage, financing and payment, eligibility, outreach and enrollment, managed care, and quality improvement. (4/13)

http://pediatrics.aappublications.org/content/131/5/e1697

MEDICAL CONCERNS IN THE FEMALE ATHLETE

Committee on Sports Medicine and Fitness

ABSTRACT. Female children and adolescents who participate regularly in sports may develop certain medical conditions, including disordered eating, menstrual dysfunction, and decreased bone mineral density. The pediatrician can play an important role in monitoring the health of young female athletes. This revised policy statement provides updated and expanded information for pediatricians on these health concerns as well as recommendations for evaluation, treatment, and ongoing assessments of female athletes. (9/00, reaffirmed 5/05, 5/08)

http://pediatrics.aappublications.org/content/106/3/610

MEDICAL CONDITIONS AFFECTING SPORTS PARTICIPATION (CLINICAL REPORT)

Stephen G. Rice, MD, PhD, MPH, and Council on Sports Medicine and Fitness

ABSTRACT. Children and adolescents with medical conditions present special issues with respect to participation in athletic activities. The pediatrician can play an important role in determining whether a child with a health condition should participate in certain sports by assessing the child's health status, suggesting appropriate equipment or modifications of sports to decrease the risk of injury, and educating the athlete, parent(s) or guardian, and coach regarding the risks of injury as they relate to the child's condition. This report updates a previous policy statement and provides information for pediatricians on sports participation for children and adolescents with medical conditions. (4/08, reaffirmed 5/11, 6/14)

http://pediatrics.aappublications.org/content/121/4/841

MEDICAL COUNTERMEASURES FOR CHILDREN IN PUBLIC HEALTH EMERGENCIES, DISASTERS, OR TERRORISM

Disaster Preparedness Advisory Council

ABSTRACT. Significant strides have been made over the past 10 to 15 years to develop medical countermeasures (MCMs) to address potential disaster hazards, including chemical, biological, radiologic, and nuclear threats. Significant and effective collaboration between the pediatric health community, including the American Academy of Pediatrics, and federal partners, such as the Office of the Assistant Secretary for Preparedness and Response, Centers for Disease Control and Prevention, Federal Emergency Management Agency, National Institutes of Health, Food and Drug Administration, and other federal agencies, over the past 5 years has resulted in substantial gains in addressing the needs of children related to disaster preparedness in general and MCMs in particular. Yet, major gaps still remain related to MCMs for children, a population highly vulnerable to the effects of exposure to such threats, because many vaccines and pharmaceuticals approved for use by adults as MCMs do not yet have pediatric formulations, dosing information, or safety information. As a result, the nation's stockpiles and other caches (designated supply of MCMs) where pharmacotherapeutic and other MCMs are stored are less prepared to address the needs of children compared with those of adults in the event of a disaster. This policy statement provides recommendations to close the remaining gaps for the development and use of MCMs in children during public health emergencies or disasters. The progress made by federal agencies to date to address the needs of children and the shared commitment of collaboration that characterizes the current relationship between the pediatric health community and the federal agencies responsible for MCMs should encourage all child advocates to invest the necessary energy and resources now to complete the process of remedying the remaining significant gaps in preparedness. (1/16)

See full text on page 961.

http://pediatrics.aappublications.org/content/137/2/e20154273

MEDICAL EMERGENCIES OCCURRING AT SCHOOL

Council on School Health

ABSTRACT. Children and adults might experience medical emergency situations because of injuries, complications of chronic health conditions, or unexpected major illnesses that occur in schools. In February 2001, the American Academy of Pediatrics issued a policy statement titled "Guidelines for Emergency Medical Care in Schools" (available at: http://aappolicy.aappublications. org/cgi/content/full/pediatrics;107/2/435). Since the release of that statement, the spectrum of potential individual student emergencies has changed significantly. The increase in the number of children with special health care needs and chronic medical conditions attending schools and the challenges associated with ensuring that schools have access to on-site licensed health care professionals on an ongoing basis have added to increasing the risks of medical emergencies in schools. The goal of this statement is to increase pediatricians' awareness of schools' roles in preparing for individual student emergencies and to provide recommendations for primary care and school

physicians on how to assist and support school personnel. (10/08, reaffirmed 9/11)
http://pediatrics.aappublications.org/content/122/4/887

THE MEDICAL HOME

Medical Home Initiatives for Children With Special Needs Project Advisory Committee (7/02, reaffirmed 5/08)
http://pediatrics.aappublications.org/content/110/1/184

MEDICAL STAFF APPOINTMENT AND DELINEATION OF PEDIATRIC PRIVILEGES IN HOSPITALS (CLINICAL REPORT)

Daniel A. Rauch, MD; Committee on Hospital Care; and Section on Hospital Medicine

ABSTRACT. The review and verification of credentials and the granting of clinical privileges are required of every hospital to ensure that members of the medical staff are competent and qualified to provide specified levels of patient care. The credentialing process involves the following: (1) assessment of the professional and personal background of each practitioner seeking privileges; (2) assignment of privileges appropriate for the clinician's training and experience; (3) ongoing monitoring of the professional activities of each staff member; and (4) periodic reappointment to the medical staff on the basis of objectively measured performance. We examine the essential elements of a credentials review for initial and renewed medical staff appointments along with suggested criteria for the delineation of clinical privileges. Sample forms for the delineation of privileges can be found on the American Academy of Pediatrics Committee on Hospital Care Web site (http://www.aap.org/visit/cmte19.htm). Because of differences among individual hospitals, no 1 method for credentialing is universally applicable. The medical staff of each hospital must, therefore, establish its own process based on the general principles reviewed in this report. The issues of medical staff membership and credentialing have become very complex, and institutions and medical staffs are vulnerable to legal action. Consequently, it is advisable for hospitals and medical staffs to obtain expert legal advice when medical staff bylaws are constructed or revised. (3/12, reaffirmed 2/16)
http://pediatrics.aappublications.org/content/129/4/797

MEDICAL VERSUS NONMEDICAL IMMUNIZATION EXEMPTIONS FOR CHILD CARE AND SCHOOL ATTENDANCE

Committee on Practice and Ambulatory Medicine, Committee on Infectious Diseases, Committee on State Government Affairs, Council on School Health, and Section on Administration and Practice Management

ABSTRACT. Routine childhood immunizations against infectious diseases are an integral part of our public health infrastructure. They provide direct protection to the immunized individual and indirect protection to children and adults unable to be immunized via the effect of community immunity. All 50 states, the District of Columbia, and Puerto Rico have regulations requiring proof of immunization for child care and school attendance as a public health strategy to protect children in these settings and to secondarily serve as a mechanism to promote timely immunization of children by their caregivers. Although all states and the District of Columbia have mechanisms to exempt school attendees from specific immunization requirements for medical reasons, the majority also have a heterogeneous collection of regulations and laws that allow nonmedical exemptions from childhood immunizations otherwise required for child care and school attendance. The American Academy of Pediatrics (AAP) supports regulations and laws requiring certification of immunization to attend child care and school as a sound means of providing a safe environment for attendees and employees of these settings. The AAP also supports medically indicated exemptions to specific immunizations as determined for each individual child. The AAP views nonmedical exemptions to school-required immunizations as inappropriate for individual, public health, and ethical reasons and advocates for their elimination. (8/16)
See full text on page 973.
http://pediatrics.aappublications.org/content/138/3/e20162145

MEDICATION-ASSISTED TREATMENT OF ADOLESCENTS WITH OPIOID USE DISORDERS

Committee on Substance Use and Prevention

ABSTRACT. Opioid use disorder is a leading cause of morbidity and mortality among US youth. Effective treatments, both medications and substance use disorder counseling, are available but underused, and access to developmentally appropriate treatment is severely restricted for adolescents and young adults. Resources to disseminate available therapies and to develop new treatments specifically for this age group are needed to save and improve lives of youth with opioid addiction. (8/16)
See full text on page 981.
http://pediatrics.aappublications.org/content/138/3/e20161893

MENSTRUAL MANAGEMENT FOR ADOLESCENTS WITH DISABILITIES (CLINICAL REPORT)

Elisabeth H. Quint, MD; Rebecca F. O'Brien, MD; and Committee on Adolescence (joint with the North American Society for Pediatric and Adolescent Gynecology)

ABSTRACT. The onset of menses for adolescents with physical or intellectual disabilities can affect their independence and add additional concerns for families at home, in schools, and in other settings. The pediatrician is the primary health care provider to explore and assist with the pubertal transition and menstrual management. Menstrual management of both normal and abnormal cycles may be requested to minimize hygiene issues, premenstrual symptoms, dysmenorrhea, heavy or irregular bleeding, contraception, and conditions exacerbated by the menstrual cycle. Several options are available for menstrual management, depending on the outcome that is desired, ranging from cycle regulation to complete amenorrhea. The use of medications or the request for surgeries to help with the menstrual cycles in teenagers with disabilities has medical, social, legal, and ethical implications. This clinical report is designed to help guide pediatricians in assisting adolescent females with intellectual and/or physical disabilities and their families in making decisions related to successfully navigating menarche and subsequent menstrual cycles. (6/16)
See full text on page 987.
http://pediatrics.aappublications.org/content/138/1/e20160295

METRIC UNITS AND THE PREFERRED DOSING OF ORALLY ADMINISTERED LIQUID MEDICATIONS

Committee on Drugs

ABSTRACT. Medication overdoses are a common, but preventable, problem among children. Volumetric dosing errors and the use of incorrect dosing delivery devices are 2 common sources of these preventable errors for orally administered liquid medications. To reduce errors and increase precision of drug administration, milliliter-based dosing should be used exclusively when prescribing and administering liquid medications. Teaspoon- and tablespoon-based dosing should not be used. Devices that allow for precise dose administration (preferably syringes with metric markings) should be used instead of household spoons and should be distributed with the medication. (3/15)

http://pediatrics.aappublications.org/content/135/4/784

MIND-BODY THERAPIES IN CHILDREN AND YOUTH (CLINICAL REPORT)

Section on Integrative Medicine

ABSTRACT. Mind-body therapies are popular and are ranked among the top 10 complementary and integrative medicine practices reportedly used by adults and children in the 2007–2012 National Health Interview Survey. A growing body of evidence supports the effectiveness and safety of mind-body therapies in pediatrics. This clinical report outlines popular mind-body therapies for children and youth and examines the best-available evidence for a variety of mind-body therapies and practices, including biofeedback, clinical hypnosis, guided imagery, meditation, and yoga. The report is intended to help health care professionals guide their patients to nonpharmacologic approaches to improve concentration, help decrease pain, control discomfort, or ease anxiety. (8/16)

See full text on page 999.

http://pediatrics.aappublications.org/content/138/3/e20161896

MINORS AS LIVING SOLID-ORGAN DONORS (CLINICAL REPORT)

Lainie Friedman Ross, MD, PhD; J. Richard Thistlethwaite Jr, MD, PhD; and Committee on Bioethics

ABSTRACT. In the past half-century, solid-organ transplantation has become standard treatment for a variety of diseases in children and adults. The major limitation for all transplantation is the availability of donors, and the gap between demand and supply continues to grow despite the increase in living donors. Although rare, children do serve as living donors, and these donations raise serious ethical issues. This clinical report includes a discussion of the ethical considerations regarding minors serving as living donors, using the traditional benefit/burden calculus from the perspectives of both the donor and the recipient. The report also includes an examination of the circumstances under which a minor may morally participate as a living donor, how to minimize risks, and what the informed-consent process should entail. The American Academy of Pediatrics holds that minors can morally serve as living organ donors but only in exceptional circumstances when specific criteria are fulfilled. (8/08, reaffirmed 5/11)

http://pediatrics.aappublications.org/content/122/2/454

MODEL CONTRACTUAL LANGUAGE FOR MEDICAL NECESSITY FOR CHILDREN

Committee on Child Health Financing

ABSTRACT. The term "medical necessity" is used by Medicare and Medicaid and in insurance contracts to refer to medical services that are generally recognized as appropriate for the diagnosis, prevention, or treatment of disease and injury. There is no consensus on how to define and apply the term and the accompanying rules and regulations, and as a result there has been substantial variation in medical-necessity definitions and interpretations. With this policy statement, the American Academy of Pediatrics hopes to encourage insurers to adopt more consistent medical-necessity definitions that take into account the needs of children. (7/05, reaffirmed 10/11)

http://pediatrics.aappublications.org/content/116/1/261

MOLECULAR GENETIC TESTING IN PEDIATRIC PRACTICE: A SUBJECT REVIEW (CLINICAL REPORT)

Committee on Genetics

ABSTRACT. Although many types of diagnostic and carrier testing for genetic disorders have been available for decades, the use of molecular methods is a relatively recent phenomenon. Such testing has expanded the range of disorders that can be diagnosed and has enhanced the ability of clinicians to provide accurate prognostic information and institute appropriate health supervision measures. However, the proper application of these tests may be difficult because of their scientific complexity and the potential for negative, sometimes unexpected, consequences for many patients. The purposes of this subject review are to provide background information on molecular genetic tests, to describe specific testing modalities, and to discuss some of the benefits and risks specific to the pediatric population. It is likely that pediatricians will use these testing methods increasingly for their patients and will need to evaluate critically their diagnostic and prognostic implications. (12/00, reaffirmed 5/07)

http://pediatrics.aappublications.org/content/106/6/1494

MOTOR DELAYS: EARLY IDENTIFICATION AND EVALUATION (CLINICAL REPORT)

Garey H. Noritz, MD; Nancy A. Murphy, MD; and Neuromotor Screening Expert Panel

ABSTRACT. Pediatricians often encounter children with delays of motor development in their clinical practices. Earlier identification of motor delays allows for timely referral for developmental interventions as well as diagnostic evaluations and treatment planning. A multidisciplinary expert panel developed an algorithm for the surveillance and screening of children for motor delays within the medical home, offering guidance for the initial workup and referral of the child with possible delays in motor development. Highlights of this clinical report include suggestions for formal developmental screening at the 9-, 18-, 30-, and 48-month well-child visits; approaches to the neurologic examination, with emphasis on the assessment of muscle tone; and initial diagnostic approaches for medical home providers. Use of diagnostic tests to evaluate children with motor delays are described, including brain MRI for children with high muscle tone, and measuring serum creatine kinase concentration of

those with decreased muscle tone. The importance of pursuing diagnostic tests while concurrently referring patients to early intervention programs is emphasized. (5/13)
http://pediatrics.aappublications.org/content/131/6/e2016

NEONATAL DRUG WITHDRAWAL (CLINICAL REPORT)

Mark L. Hudak, MD; Rosemarie C. Tan, MD, PhD; Committee on Drugs; and Committee on Fetus and Newborn

ABSTRACT. Maternal use of certain drugs during pregnancy can result in transient neonatal signs consistent with withdrawal or acute toxicity or cause sustained signs consistent with a lasting drug effect. In addition, hospitalized infants who are treated with opioids or benzodiazepines to provide analgesia or sedation may be at risk for manifesting signs of withdrawal. This statement updates information about the clinical presentation of infants exposed to intrauterine drugs and the therapeutic options for treatment of withdrawal and is expanded to include evidence-based approaches to the management of the hospitalized infant who requires weaning from analgesics or sedatives. (1/12, reaffirmed 2/16)
http://pediatrics.aappublications.org/content/129/2/e540

THE NEW MORBIDITY REVISITED: A RENEWED COMMITMENT TO THE PSYCHOSOCIAL ASPECTS OF PEDIATRIC CARE

Committee on Psychosocial Aspects of Child and Family Health

ABSTRACT. In 1993, the American Academy of Pediatrics adopted the policy statement "The Pediatrician and the 'New Morbidity.'" Since then, social difficulties, behavioral problems, and developmental difficulties have become a main part of the scope of pediatric practice, and recognition of the importance of these areas has increased. This statement reaffirms the Academy's commitment to prevention, early detection, and management of behavioral, developmental, and social problems as a focus in pediatric practice. (11/01)
http://pediatrics.aappublications.org/content/108/5/1227

NEWBORN SCREENING EXPANDS: RECOMMENDATIONS FOR PEDIATRICIANS AND MEDICAL HOMES—IMPLICATIONS FOR THE SYSTEM (CLINICAL REPORT)

PPI
AAP Partnership for Policy Implementation

Newborn Screening Authoring Committee

ABSTRACT. Advances in newborn screening technology, coupled with recent advances in the diagnosis and treatment of rare but serious congenital conditions that affect newborn infants, provide increased opportunities for positively affecting the lives of children and their families. These advantages also pose new challenges to primary care pediatricians, both educationally and in response to the management of affected infants. Primary care pediatricians require immediate access to clinical and diagnostic information and guidance and have a proactive role to play in supporting the performance of the newborn screening system. Primary care pediatricians must develop office policies and procedures to ensure that newborn screening is conducted and that results are transmitted to them in a timely fashion; they must also develop strategies to use

should these systems fail. In addition, collaboration with local, state, and national partners is essential for promoting actions and policies that will optimize the function of the newborn screening systems and ensure that families receive the full benefit of them. (1/08)
http://pediatrics.aappublications.org/content/121/1/192

NEWBORN SCREENING FOR BILIARY ATRESIA (TECHNICAL REPORT)

Kasper S. Wang, MD, FAAP, FACS; Section on Surgery; and Committee on Fetus and Newborn (joint with Childhood Liver Disease Research Network)

ABSTRACT. Biliary atresia is the most common cause of pediatric end-stage liver disease and the leading indication for pediatric liver transplantation. Affected infants exhibit evidence of biliary obstruction within the first few weeks after birth. Early diagnosis and successful surgical drainage of bile are associated with greater survival with the child's native liver. Unfortunately, because noncholestatic jaundice is extremely common in early infancy, it is difficult to identify the rare infant with cholestatic jaundice who has biliary atresia. Hence, the need for timely diagnosis of this disease warrants a discussion of the feasibility of screening for biliary atresia to improve outcomes. Herein, newborn screening for biliary atresia in the United States is assessed by using criteria established by the Discretionary Advisory Committee on Heritable Disorders in Newborns and Children. Published analyses indicate that newborn screening for biliary atresia by using serum bilirubin concentrations or stool color cards is potentially life-saving and cost-effective. Further studies are necessary to evaluate the feasibility, effectiveness, and costs of potential screening strategies for early identification of biliary atresia in the United States. (11/15)
http://pediatrics.aappublications.org/content/136/6/e1663

NONDISCRIMINATION IN PEDIATRIC HEALTH CARE

Committee on Pediatric Workforce

ABSTRACT. This policy statement is a revision of a 2001 statement and articulates the positions of the American Academy of Pediatrics on nondiscrimination in pediatric health care. It addresses both pediatricians who provide health care and the infants, children, adolescents, and young adults whom they serve. (10/07, reaffirmed 6/11, 1/15)
http://pediatrics.aappublications.org/content/120/4/922

NONINITIATION OR WITHDRAWAL OF INTENSIVE CARE FOR HIGH-RISK NEWBORNS

Committee on Fetus and Newborn

ABSTRACT. Advances in medical technology have led to dilemmas in initiation and withdrawal of intensive care of newborn infants with a very poor prognosis. Physicians and parents together must make difficult decisions guided by their understanding of the child's best interest. The foundation for these decisions consists of several key elements: (1) direct and open communication between the health care team and the parents of the child with regard to the medical status, prognosis, and treatment options; (2) inclusion of the parents as active participants in the decision process; (3) continuation of comfort care even when intensive care is not being provided; and

(4) treatment decisions that are guided primarily by the best interest of the child. (2/07, reaffirmed 5/10, 6/15)
http://pediatrics.aappublications.org/content/119/2/401

NONINVASIVE RESPIRATORY SUPPORT (CLINICAL REPORT)

James J. Cummings, MD, FAAP; Richard A. Polin, MD, FAAP; and Committee on Fetus and Newborn

ABSTRACT. Mechanical ventilation is associated with increased survival of preterm infants but is also associated with an increased incidence of chronic lung disease (bronchopulmonary dysplasia) in survivors. Nasal continuous positive airway pressure (nCPAP) is a form of noninvasive ventilation that reduces the need for mechanical ventilation and decreases the combined outcome of death or bronchopulmonary dysplasia. Other modes of noninvasive ventilation, including nasal intermittent positive pressure ventilation, biphasic positive airway pressure, and high-flow nasal cannula, have recently been introduced into the NICU setting as potential alternatives to mechanical ventilation or nCPAP. Randomized controlled trials suggest that these newer modalities may be effective alternatives to nCPAP and may offer some advantages over nCPAP, but efficacy and safety data are limited. (12/15)
http://pediatrics.aappublications.org/content/137/1/e20153758

NONORAL FEEDING FOR CHILDREN AND YOUTH WITH DEVELOPMENTAL OR ACQUIRED DISABILITIES (CLINICAL REPORT)

Richard C. Adams, MD, FAAP; Ellen Roy Elias, MD, FAAP; and Council on Children With Disabilities

ABSTRACT. The decision to initiate enteral feedings is multifaceted, involving medical, financial, cultural, and emotional considerations. Children who have developmental or acquired disabilities are at risk for having primary and secondary conditions that affect growth and nutritional well-being. This clinical report provides (1) an overview of clinical issues in children who have developmental or acquired disabilities that may prompt a need to consider nonoral feedings, (2) a systematic way to support the child and family in clinical decisions related to initiating nonoral feeding, (3) information on surgical options that the family may need to consider in that decision-making process, and (4) pediatric guidance for ongoing care after initiation of nonoral feeding intervention, including care of the gastrostomy tube and skin site. Ongoing medical and psychosocial support is needed after initiation of nonoral feedings and is best provided through the collaborative efforts of the family and a team of professionals that may include the pediatrician, dietitian, social worker, and/or therapists. (11/14)
http://pediatrics.aappublications.org/content/134/6/e1745

NONTHERAPEUTIC USE OF ANTIMICROBIAL AGENTS IN ANIMAL AGRICULTURE: IMPLICATIONS FOR PEDIATRICS (TECHNICAL REPORT)

Jerome A. Paulson, MD, FAAP; Theoklis E. Zaoutis, MD, MSCE, FAAP; Council on Environmental Health; and Committee on Infectious Diseases

ABSTRACT. Antimicrobial resistance is one of the most serious threats to public health globally and threatens our ability to treat infectious diseases. Antimicrobial-resistant infections are associated with increased morbidity, mortality, and health care costs. Infants and children are affected by transmission of susceptible and resistant food zoonotic pathogens through the food supply, direct contact with animals, and environmental pathways. The overuse and misuse of antimicrobial agents in veterinary and human medicine is, in large part, responsible for the emergence of antibiotic resistance. Approximately 80% of the overall tonnage of antimicrobial agents sold in the United States in 2012 was for animal use, and approximately 60% of those agents are considered important for human medicine. Most of the use involves the addition of low doses of antimicrobial agents to the feed of healthy animals over prolonged periods to promote growth and increase feed efficiency or at a range of doses to prevent disease. These nontherapeutic uses contribute to resistance and create new health dangers for humans. This report describes how antimicrobial agents are used in animal agriculture, reviews the mechanisms of how such use contributes to development of resistance, and discusses US and global initiatives to curb the use of antimicrobial agents in agriculture. (11/15)
http://pediatrics.aappublications.org/content/136/6/e1670

OFFICE-BASED CARE FOR LESBIAN, GAY, BISEXUAL, TRANSGENDER, AND QUESTIONING YOUTH

Committee on Adolescence

ABSTRACT. The American Academy of Pediatrics issued its last statement on homosexuality and adolescents in 2004. Although most lesbian, gay, bisexual, transgender, and questioning (LGBTQ) youth are quite resilient and emerge from adolescence as healthy adults, the effects of homophobia and heterosexism can contribute to health disparities in mental health with higher rates of depression and suicidal ideation, higher rates of substance abuse, and more sexually transmitted and HIV infections. Pediatricians should have offices that are teen-friendly and welcoming to sexual minority youth. Obtaining a comprehensive, confidential, developmentally appropriate adolescent psychosocial history allows for the discovery of strengths and assets as well as risks. Referrals for mental health or substance abuse may be warranted. Sexually active LGBTQ youth should have sexually transmitted infection/HIV testing according to recommendations of the Sexually Transmitted Diseases Treatment Guidelines of the Centers for Disease Control and Prevention based on sexual behaviors. With appropriate assistance and care, sexual minority youth should live healthy, productive lives while transitioning through adolescence and young adulthood. (6/13)
http://pediatrics.aappublications.org/content/132/1/198

OFFICE-BASED CARE FOR LESBIAN, GAY, BISEXUAL, TRANSGENDER, AND QUESTIONING YOUTH (TECHNICAL REPORT)

David A. Levine, MD, and Committee on Adolescence

ABSTRACT. The American Academy of Pediatrics issued its last statement on homosexuality and adolescents in 2004. This technical report reflects the rapidly expanding medical and psychosocial literature about sexual minority youth. Pediatricians should be aware that some youth in their care may have concerns or questions about their

sexual orientation or that of siblings, friends, parents, relatives, or others and should provide factual, current, nonjudgmental information in a confidential manner. Although most lesbian, gay, bisexual, transgender, and questioning (LGBTQ) youth are quite resilient and emerge from adolescence as healthy adults, the effects of homophobia and heterosexism can contribute to increased mental health issues for sexual minority youth. LGBTQ and MSM/WSW (men having sex with men and women having sex with women) adolescents, in comparison with heterosexual adolescents, have higher rates of depression and suicidal ideation, higher rates of substance abuse, and more risky sexual behaviors. Obtaining a comprehensive, confidential, developmentally appropriate adolescent psychosocial history allows for the discovery of strengths and assets as well as risks. Pediatricians should have offices that are teen-friendly and welcoming to sexual minority youth. This includes having supportive, engaging office staff members who ensure that there are no barriers to care. For transgender youth, pediatricians should provide the opportunity to acknowledge and affirm their feelings of gender dysphoria and desires to transition to the opposite gender. Referral of transgender youth to a qualified mental health professional is critical to assist with the dysphoria, to educate them, and to assess their readiness for transition. With appropriate assistance and care, sexual minority youth should live healthy, productive lives while transitioning through adolescence and young adulthood. (6/13)
http://pediatrics.aappublications.org/content/132/1/e297

OFFICE-BASED COUNSELING FOR UNINTENTIONAL INJURY PREVENTION (CLINICAL REPORT)

H. Garry Gardner, MD, and Committee on Injury, Violence, and Poison Prevention

ABSTRACT. Unintentional injuries are the leading cause of death for children older than 1 year. Pediatricians should include unintentional injury prevention as a major component of anticipatory guidance for infants, children, and adolescents. The content of injury-prevention counseling varies for infants, preschool-aged children, school-aged children, and adolescents. This report provides guidance on the content of unintentional injury-prevention counseling for each of those age groups. (1/07)
http://pediatrics.aappublications.org/content/119/1/202

OFF-LABEL USE OF DRUGS IN CHILDREN

Committee on Drugs

ABSTRACT. The passage of the Best Pharmaceuticals for Children Act and the Pediatric Research Equity Act has collectively resulted in an improvement in rational prescribing for children, including more than 500 labeling changes. However, off-label drug use remains an important public health issue for infants, children, and adolescents, because an overwhelming number of drugs still have no information in the labeling for use in pediatrics. The purpose of off-label use is to benefit the individual patient. Practitioners use their professional judgment to determine these uses. As such, the term "off-label" does not imply an improper, illegal, contraindicated, or investigational use. Therapeutic decision-making must always

rely on the best available evidence and the importance of the benefit for the individual patient. (2/14)
http://pediatrics.aappublications.org/content/133/3/563

OPHTHALMOLOGIC EXAMINATIONS IN CHILDREN WITH JUVENILE RHEUMATOID ARTHRITIS (CLINICAL REPORT)

James Cassidy, MD; Jane Kivlin, MD; Carol Lindsley, MD; James Nocton, MD; Section on Rheumatology; and Section on Ophthalmology

ABSTRACT. Unlike the joints, ocular involvement with juvenile rheumatoid arthritis is most often asymptomatic; yet, the inflammation can cause serious morbidity with loss of vision. Scheduled slit-lamp examinations by an ophthalmologist at specific intervals can detect ocular disease early, and prompt treatment can prevent vision loss. (5/06)
http://pediatrics.aappublications.org/content/117/5/1843

OPTIMIZING BONE HEALTH IN CHILDREN AND ADOLESCENTS (CLINICAL REPORT)

Neville H. Golden, MD; Steven A. Abrams, MD; and Committee on Nutrition

ABSTRACT. The pediatrician plays a major role in helping optimize bone health in children and adolescents. This clinical report reviews normal bone acquisition in infants, children, and adolescents and discusses factors affecting bone health in this age group. Previous recommended daily allowances for calcium and vitamin D are updated, and clinical guidance is provided regarding weight-bearing activities and recommendations for calcium and vitamin D intake and supplementation. Routine calcium supplementation is not recommended for healthy children and adolescents, but increased dietary intake to meet daily requirements is encouraged. The American Academy of Pediatrics endorses the higher recommended dietary allowances for vitamin D advised by the Institute of Medicine and supports testing for vitamin D deficiency in children and adolescents with conditions associated with increased bone fragility. Universal screening for vitamin D deficiency is not routinely recommended in healthy children or in children with dark skin or obesity because there is insufficient evidence of the cost–benefit of such a practice in reducing fracture risk. The preferred test to assess bone health is dual-energy x-ray absorptiometry, but caution is advised when interpreting results in children and adolescents who may not yet have achieved peak bone mass. For analyses, z scores should be used instead of T scores, and corrections should be made for size. Office-based strategies for the pediatrician to optimize bone health are provided. This clinical report has been endorsed by American Bone Health. (9/14)
http://pediatrics.aappublications.org/content/134/4/e1229

ORAL AND DENTAL ASPECTS OF CHILD ABUSE AND NEGLECT (CLINICAL REPORT)

Nancy Kellogg, MD, and Committee on Child Abuse and Neglect (joint with American Academy of Pediatric Dentistry)

ABSTRACT. In all 50 states, physicians and dentists are required to report suspected cases of abuse and neglect to social service or law enforcement agencies. The purpose of this report is to review the oral and dental aspects of

physical and sexual abuse and dental neglect and the role of physicians and dentists in evaluating such conditions. This report addresses the evaluation of bite marks as well as perioral and intraoral injuries, infections, and diseases that may cause suspicion for child abuse or neglect. Physicians receive minimal training in oral health and dental injury and disease and, thus, may not detect dental aspects of abuse or neglect as readily as they do child abuse and neglect involving other areas of the body. Therefore, physicians and dentists are encouraged to collaborate to increase the prevention, detection, and treatment of these conditions. (12/05, reaffirmed 1/09, 1/14)
http://pediatrics.aappublications.org/content/116/6/1565

ORAL HEALTH CARE FOR CHILDREN WITH DEVELOPMENTAL DISABILITIES (CLINICAL REPORT)

Kenneth W. Norwood Jr, MD; Rebecca L. Slayton, DDS, PhD; Council on Children With Disabilities; and Section on Oral Health
ABSTRACT. Children with developmental disabilities often have unmet complex health care needs as well as significant physical and cognitive limitations. Children with more severe conditions and from low-income families are particularly at risk with high dental needs and poor access to care. In addition, children with developmental disabilities are living longer, requiring continued oral health care. This clinical report describes the effect that poor oral health has on children with developmental disabilities as well as the importance of partnerships between the pediatric medical and dental homes. Basic knowledge of the oral health risk factors affecting children with developmental disabilities is provided. Pediatricians may use the report to guide their incorporation of oral health assessments and education into their well-child examinations for children with developmental disabilities. This report has medical, legal, educational, and operational implications for practicing pediatricians. (2/13)
http://pediatrics.aappublications.org/content/131/3/614

ORGANIC FOODS: HEALTH AND ENVIRONMENTAL ADVANTAGES AND DISADVANTAGES (CLINICAL REPORT)

Joel Forman, MD; Janet Silverstein, MD; Committee on Nutrition; and Council on Environmental Health
ABSTRACT. The US market for organic foods has grown from $3.5 billion in 1996 to $28.6 billion in 2010, according to the Organic Trade Association. Organic products are now sold in specialty stores and conventional supermarkets. Organic products contain numerous marketing claims and terms, only some of which are standardized and regulated.

In terms of health advantages, organic diets have been convincingly demonstrated to expose consumers to fewer pesticides associated with human disease. Organic farming has been demonstrated to have less environmental impact than conventional approaches. However, current evidence does not support any meaningful nutritional benefits or deficits from eating organic compared with conventionally grown foods, and there are no well-powered human studies that directly demonstrate health benefits or disease protection as a result of consuming an organic diet. Studies also have not demonstrated any detrimental or disease-promoting effects from an organic diet. Although organic foods regularly command a significant price premium, well-designed farming studies demonstrate that costs can be competitive and yields comparable to those of conventional farming techniques. Pediatricians should incorporate this evidence when discussing the health and environmental impact of organic foods and organic farming while continuing to encourage all patients and their families to attain optimal nutrition and dietary variety consistent with the US Department of Agriculture's MyPlate recommendations.

This clinical report reviews the health and environmental issues related to organic food production and consumption. It defines the term "organic," reviews organic food-labeling standards, describes organic and conventional farming practices, and explores the cost and environmental implications of organic production techniques. It examines the evidence available on nutritional quality and production contaminants in conventionally produced and organic foods. Finally, this report provides guidance for pediatricians to assist them in advising their patients regarding organic and conventionally produced food choices. (10/12)
http://pediatrics.aappublications.org/content/130/5/e1406

ORGANIZED SPORTS FOR CHILDREN AND PREADOLESCENTS

Committee on Sports Medicine and Fitness and Committee on School Health
ABSTRACT. Participation in organized sports provides an opportunity for young people to increase their physical activity and develop physical and social skills. However, when the demands and expectations of organized sports exceed the maturation and readiness of the participant, the positive aspects of participation can be negated. The nature of parental or adult involvement can also influence the degree to which participation in organized sports is a positive experience for preadolescents. This updates a previous policy statement on athletics for preadolescents and incorporates guidelines for sports participation for preschool children. Recommendations are offered on how pediatricians can help determine a child's readiness to participate, how risks can be minimized, and how child-oriented goals can be maximized. (6/01, reaffirmed 1/05, 6/11)
http://pediatrics.aappublications.org/content/107/6/1459

OUT-OF-HOME PLACEMENT FOR CHILDREN AND ADOLESCENTS WITH DISABILITIES (CLINICAL REPORT)

Sandra L. Friedman, MD, MPH; Miriam A. Kalichman, MD; and Council on Children With Disabilities
ABSTRACT. The vast majority of children and youth with chronic and complex health conditions who also have intellectual and developmental disabilities are cared for in their homes. Social, legal, policy, and medical changes through the years have allowed for an increase in needed support within the community. However, there continues to be a relatively small group of children who live in various types of congregate care settings. This clinical report describes these settings and the care and services that are provided in them. The report also discusses reasons families choose out-of-home placement for their children, barriers to placement, and potential effects of this decision

on family members. We examine the pediatrician's role in caring for children with severe intellectual and developmental disabilities and complex medical problems in the context of responding to parental inquiries about out-of-home placement and understanding factors affecting these types of decisions. Common medical problems and care issues for children residing outside the family home are reviewed. Variations in state and federal regulations, challenges in understanding local systems, and access to services are also discussed. (9/14)

http://pediatrics.aappublications.org/content/134/4/836

OUT-OF-HOME PLACEMENT FOR CHILDREN AND ADOLESCENTS WITH DISABILITIES—ADDENDUM: CARE OPTIONS FOR CHILDREN AND ADOLESCENTS WITH DISABILITIES AND MEDICAL COMPLEXITY (CLINICAL REPORT)

Sandra L. Friedman, MD, MPH, FAAP; Kenneth W. Norwood Jr, MD, FAAP; and Council on Children With Disabilities

ABSTRACT. Children and adolescents with significant intellectual and developmental disabilities and complex medical problems require safe and comprehensive care to meet their medical and psychosocial needs. Ideally, such children and youth should be cared for by their families in their home environments. When this type of arrangement is not possible, there should be exploration of appropriate, alternative noncongregate community-based settings, especially alternative family homes. Government funding sources exist to support care in the community, although there is variability among states with regard to the availability of community programs and resources. It is important that families are supported in learning about options of care. Pediatricians can serve as advocates for their patients and their families to access community-based services and to increase the availability of resources to ensure that the option to live in a family home is available to all children with complex medical needs. (11/16)

See full text on page 1013.

http://pediatrics.aappublications.org/content/138/6/e20163216

OUT-OF-SCHOOL SUSPENSION AND EXPULSION

Council on School Health

ABSTRACT. The primary mission of any school system is to educate students. To achieve this goal, the school district must maintain a culture and environment where all students feel safe, nurtured, and valued and where order and civility are expected standards of behavior. Schools cannot allow unacceptable behavior to interfere with the school district's primary mission. To this end, school districts adopt codes of conduct for expected behaviors and policies to address unacceptable behavior. In developing these policies, school boards must weigh the severity of the offense and the consequences of the punishment and the balance between individual and institutional rights and responsibilities. Out-of-school suspension and expulsion are the most severe consequences that a school district can impose for unacceptable behavior. Traditionally, these consequences have been reserved for offenses deemed especially severe or dangerous and/ or for recalcitrant offenders. However, the implications and consequences of out-of-school suspension and expulsion and "zero-tolerance" are of such severity that their application and appropriateness for a developing child require periodic review. The indications and effectiveness of exclusionary discipline policies that demand automatic or rigorous application are increasingly questionable. The impact of these policies on offenders, other children, school districts, and communities is broad. Periodic scrutiny of policies should be placed not only on the need for a better understanding of the educational, emotional, and social impact of out-of-school suspension and expulsion on the individual student but also on the greater societal costs of such rigid policies. Pediatricians should be prepared to assist students and families affected by out-of-school suspension and expulsion and should be willing to guide school districts in their communities to find more effective and appropriate alternatives to exclusionary discipline policies for the developing child. A discussion of preventive strategies and alternatives to out-of-school suspension and expulsion, as well as recommendations for the role of the physician in matters of out-of-school suspension and expulsion are included. School-wide positive behavior support/positive behavior intervention and support is discussed as an effective alternative. (2/13)

http://pediatrics.aappublications.org/content/131/3/e1000

OVERCROWDING CRISIS IN OUR NATION'S EMERGENCY DEPARTMENTS: IS OUR SAFETY NET UNRAVELING?

Committee on Pediatric Emergency Medicine

ABSTRACT. Emergency departments (EDs) are a vital component in our health care safety net, available 24 hours a day, 7 days a week, for all who require care. There has been a steady increase in the volume and acuity of patient visits to EDs, now with well over 100 million Americans (30 million children) receiving emergency care annually. This rise in ED utilization has effectively saturated the capacity of EDs and emergency medical services in many communities. The resulting phenomenon, commonly referred to as ED overcrowding, now threatens access to emergency services for those who need them the most. As managers of the pediatric medical home and advocates for children and optimal pediatric health care, there is a very important role for pediatricians and the American Academy of Pediatrics in guiding health policy decision-makers toward effective solutions that promote the medical home and timely access to emergency care. (9/04, reaffirmed 5/07, 6/11, 7/16)

http://pediatrics.aappublications.org/content/114/3/878

OVERUSE INJURIES, OVERTRAINING, AND BURNOUT IN CHILD AND ADOLESCENT ATHLETES (CLINICAL REPORT)

Joel S. Brenner, MD, MPH, and Council on Sports Medicine and Fitness

ABSTRACT. Overuse is one of the most common etiologic factors that lead to injuries in the pediatric and adolescent athlete. As more children are becoming involved in organized and recreational athletics, the incidence of overuse injuries is increasing. Many children are participating in sports year-round and sometimes on multiple teams simultaneously. This overtraining can lead to burnout, which may have a detrimental effect on the child participating in sports as a lifelong healthy activity. One contributing factor to overtraining may be parental pressure to compete and succeed. The purpose of this clinical report is to assist pediatricians in identifying and counseling at-risk children and their families. This report supports the American Academy of Pediatrics policy statement on intensive training and sport specialization. (6/07, reaffirmed 3/11, 6/14)

http://pediatrics.aappublications.org/content/119/6/1242

OXYGEN TARGETING IN EXTREMELY LOW BIRTH WEIGHT INFANTS (CLINICAL REPORT)

James J. Cummings, MD, FAAP; Richard A. Polin, MD, FAAP; and Committee on Fetus and Newborn

ABSTRACT. The use of supplemental oxygen plays a vital role in the care of the critically ill preterm infant, but the unrestricted use of oxygen can lead to unintended harms, such as chronic lung disease and retinopathy of prematurity. An overly restricted use of supplemental oxygen may have adverse effects as well. Ideally, continuous monitoring of tissue and cellular oxygen delivery would allow clinicians to better titrate the use of supplemental oxygen, but such monitoring is not currently feasible in the clinical setting. The introduction of pulse oximetry has greatly aided the clinician by providing a relatively easy and continuous estimate of arterial oxygen saturation, but pulse oximetry has several practical, technical, and physiologic limitations. Recent randomized clinical trials comparing different pulse oximetry targets have been conducted to better inform the practice of supplemental oxygen use. This clinical report discusses the benefits and limitations of pulse oximetry for assessing oxygenation, summarizes randomized clinical trials of oxygen saturation targeting, and addresses implications for practice. (7/16)

See full text on page 1023.

http://pediatrics.aappublications.org/content/138/2/e20161576

PALLIATIVE CARE FOR CHILDREN

Committee on Bioethics and Committee on Hospital Care

ABSTRACT. This statement presents an integrated model for providing palliative care for children living with a life-threatening or terminal condition. Advice on the development of a palliative care plan and on working with parents and children is also provided. Barriers to the provision of effective pediatric palliative care and potential solutions are identified. The American Academy of Pediatrics recommends the development and broad availability of pediatric palliative care services based on child-specific guidelines and standards. Such services will require widely distributed and effective palliative care education of pediatric health care professionals. The Academy offers guidance on responding to requests for hastening death, but does not support the practice of physician-assisted suicide or euthanasia for children. (8/00, reaffirmed 6/03, 10/06, 2/12)

http://pediatrics.aappublications.org/content/106/2/351

PARENT-PROVIDER-COMMUNITY PARTNERSHIPS: OPTIMIZING OUTCOMES FOR CHILDREN WITH DISABILITIES (CLINICAL REPORT)

Nancy A. Murphy, MD; Paul S. Carbone, MD; and Council on Children With Disabilities

ABSTRACT. Children with disabilities and their families have multifaceted medical, developmental, educational, and habilitative needs that are best addressed through strong partnerships among parents, providers, and communities. However, traditional health care systems are designed to address acute rather than chronic conditions. Children with disabilities require high-quality medical homes that provide care coordination and transitional care, and their families require social and financial supports. Integrated community systems of care that promote participation of all children are needed. The purpose of this clinical report is to explore the challenges of developing effective community-based systems of care and to offer suggestions to pediatricians and policy-makers regarding the development of partnerships among children with disabilities, their families, and health care and other providers to maximize health and well-being of these children and their families. (9/11)

http://pediatrics.aappublications.org/content/128/4/795

PARENTAL LEAVE FOR RESIDENTS AND PEDIATRIC TRAINING PROGRAMS

Section on Medical Students, Residents, and Fellowship Trainees and Committee on Early Childhood

ABSTRACT. The American Academy of Pediatrics (AAP) is committed to the development of rational, equitable, and effective parental leave policies that are sensitive to the needs of pediatric residents, families, and developing infants and that enable parents to spend adequate and good-quality time with their young children. It is important for each residency program to have a policy for parental leave that is written, that is accessible to residents, and that clearly delineates program practices regarding parental leave. At a minimum, a parental leave policy for residents and fellows should conform legally with the Family Medical Leave Act as well as with respective state laws and should meet institutional requirements of the Accreditation Council for Graduate Medical Education for accredited programs. Policies should be well formulated and communicated in a culturally sensitive manner. The AAP advocates for extension of benefits consistent with the Family Medical Leave Act to all residents and interns beginning at the time that pediatric residency training begins. The AAP recommends that regardless of gender, residents who become parents should be guaranteed 6 to 8 weeks, at a minimum, of parental leave with pay after the infant's birth. In addition, in conformance with federal law, the resident should be allowed to extend the leave time when necessary by using paid vacation time or leave without pay. Coparenting, adopting, or fostering of a child should entitle the resident, regardless of gender, to the same amount of paid leave (6–8 weeks) as a person who takes maternity/paternity leave. Flexibility, creativity, and advanced planning are necessary to arrange schedules that optimize resident education and experience, cultivate equity in sharing workloads, and protect

pregnant residents from overly strenuous work experiences at critical times of their pregnancies. (1/13)
http://pediatrics.aappublications.org/content/131/2/387

PARENTAL PRESENCE DURING TREATMENT OF EBOLA OR OTHER HIGHLY CONSEQUENTIAL INFECTION (CLINICAL REPORT)

H. Dele Davies, MD, MS, MHCM, FAAP; Carrie L. Byington, MD, FAAP; and Committee on Infectious Diseases

ABSTRACT. This clinical report offers guidance to health care providers and hospitals on options to consider regarding parental presence at the bedside while caring for a child with suspected or proven Ebola virus disease (Ebola) or other highly consequential infection. Options are presented to help meet the needs of the patient and the family while also posing the least risk to providers and health care organizations. The optimal way to minimize risk is to limit contact between the person under investigation or treatment and family members/caregivers whenever possible while working to meet the emotional support needs of both patient and family. At times, caregiver presence may be deemed to be in the best interest of the patient, and in such situations, a strong effort should be made to limit potential risks of exposure to the caregiver, health care providers, and the community. The decision to allow parental/caregiver presence should be made in consultation with a team including an infectious diseases expert and state and/or local public health authorities and should involve consideration of many factors, depending on the stage of investigation and management, including (1) a careful history, physical examination, and investigations to elucidate the likelihood of the diagnosis of Ebola or other highly consequential infection; (2) ability of the facility to offer appropriate isolation for the person under investigation and family members and to manage Ebola; (3) ability to recognize and exclude people at increased risk of worse outcomes (eg, pregnant women); and (4) ability of parent/caregiver to follow instructions, including appropriate donning and doffing of personal protective equipment. (8/16)
See full text on page 1035.
http://pediatrics.aappublications.org/content/138/3/e20161891

PATENT DUCTUS ARTERIOSUS IN PRETERM INFANTS

William E. Benitz, MD, FAAP, and Committee on Fetus and Newborn

ABSTRACT. Despite a large body of basic science and clinical research and clinical experience with thousands of infants over nearly 6 decades, there is still uncertainty and controversy about the significance, evaluation, and management of patent ductus arteriosus in preterm infants, resulting in substantial heterogeneity in clinical practice. The purpose of this clinical report is to summarize the evidence available to guide evaluation and treatment of preterm infants with prolonged ductal patency in the first few weeks after birth. (12/15)
http://pediatrics.aappublications.org/content/137/1/e20153730

PATIENT- AND FAMILY-CENTERED CARE AND THE PEDIATRICIAN'S ROLE

Committee on Hospital Care and Institute for Patient- and Family-Centered Care

ABSTRACT. Drawing on several decades of work with families, pediatricians, other health care professionals, and policy makers, the American Academy of Pediatrics provides a definition of patient- and family-centered care. In pediatrics, patient- and family-centered care is based on the understanding that the family is the child's primary source of strength and support. Further, this approach to care recognizes that the perspectives and information provided by families, children, and young adults are essential components of high-quality clinical decision-making, and that patients and family are integral partners with the health care team. This policy statement outlines the core principles of patient- and family-centered care, summarizes some of the recent literature linking patient- and family-centered care to improved health outcomes, and lists various other benefits to be expected when engaging in patient- and family-centered pediatric practice. The statement concludes with specific recommendations for how pediatricians can integrate patient- and family-centered care in hospitals, clinics, and community settings, and in broader systems of care, as well. (1/12)
http://pediatrics.aappublications.org/content/129/2/394

PATIENT- AND FAMILY-CENTERED CARE AND THE ROLE OF THE EMERGENCY PHYSICIAN PROVIDING CARE TO A CHILD IN THE EMERGENCY DEPARTMENT

Committee on Pediatric Emergency Medicine (joint with American College of Emergency Physicians)

ABSTRACT. Patient- and family-centered care is an approach to health care that recognizes the role of the family in providing medical care; encourages collaboration between the patient, family, and health care professionals; and honors individual and family strengths, cultures, traditions, and expertise. Although there are many opportunities for providing patient- and family-centered care in the emergency department, there are also challenges to doing so. The American Academy of Pediatrics and the American College of Emergency Physicians support promoting patient dignity, comfort, and autonomy; recognizing the patient and family as key decision-makers in the patient's medical care; recognizing the patient's experience and perspective in a culturally sensitive manner; acknowledging the interdependence of child and parent as well as the pediatric patient's evolving independence; encouraging family-member presence; providing information to the family during interventions; encouraging collaboration with other health care professionals; acknowledging the importance of the patient's medical home; and encouraging institutional policies for patient- and family-centered care. (11/06, reaffirmed 6/09, 10/11, 9/15)
http://pediatrics.aappublications.org/content/118/5/2242

PATIENT- AND FAMILY-CENTERED CARE COORDINATION: A FRAMEWORK FOR INTEGRATING CARE FOR CHILDREN AND YOUTH ACROSS MULTIPLE SYSTEMS

Council on Children With Disabilities and Medical Home Implementation Project Advisory Committee

ABSTRACT. Understanding a care coordination framework, its functions, and its effects on children and families is critical for patients and families themselves, as well as for pediatricians, pediatric medical subspecialists/surgical specialists, and anyone providing services to children and families. Care coordination is an essential element of a transformed American health care delivery system that emphasizes optimal quality and cost outcomes, addresses family-centered care, and calls for partnership across various settings and communities. High-quality, cost-effective health care requires that the delivery system include elements for the provision of services supporting the coordination of care across settings and professionals. This requirement of supporting coordination of care is generally true for health systems providing care for all children and youth but especially for those with special health care needs. At the foundation of an efficient and effective system of care delivery is the patient-/family-centered medical home. From its inception, the medical home has had care coordination as a core element. In general, optimal outcomes for children and youth, especially those with special health care needs, require interfacing among multiple care systems and individuals, including the following: medical, social, and behavioral professionals; the educational system; payers; medical equipment providers; home care agencies; advocacy groups; needed supportive therapies/services; and families. Coordination of care across settings permits an integration of services that is centered on the comprehensive needs of the patient and family, leading to decreased health care costs, reduction in fragmented care, and improvement in the patient/family experience of care. (4/14)
http://pediatrics.aappublications.org/content/133/5/e1451

PATIENT- AND FAMILY-CENTERED CARE OF CHILDREN IN THE EMERGENCY DEPARTMENT (TECHNICAL REPORT)

Nanette Dudley, MD; Alice Ackerman, MD, MBA; Kathleen M. Brown, MD; Sally K. Snow, BSN, RN; and Committee on Pediatric Emergency Medicine (joint with American College of Emergency Physicians Pediatric Emergency Medicine Committee and Emergency Nurses Association Pediatric Committee)

ABSTRACT. Patient- and family-centered care is an approach to the planning, delivery, and evaluation of health care that is grounded in a mutually beneficial partnership among patients, families, and health care professionals. Providing patient- and family-centered care to children in the emergency department setting presents many opportunities and challenges. This revised technical report draws on previously published policy statements and reports, reviews the current literature, and describes the present state of practice and research regarding patient- and family-centered care for children in the emergency department setting as well as some of the complexities of providing such care. (12/14)
http://pediatrics.aappublications.org/content/135/1/e255

PATIENT SAFETY IN THE PEDIATRIC EMERGENCY CARE SETTING

Committee on Pediatric Emergency Medicine

ABSTRACT. Patient safety is a priority for all health care professionals, including those who work in emergency care. Unique aspects of pediatric care may increase the risk of medical error and harm to patients, especially in the emergency care setting. Although errors can happen despite the best human efforts, given the right set of circumstances, health care professionals must work proactively to improve safety in the pediatric emergency care system. Specific recommendations to improve pediatric patient safety in the emergency department are provided in this policy statement. (12/07, reaffirmed 6/11, 7/14)
http://pediatrics.aappublications.org/content/120/6/1367

PAYMENT FOR TELEPHONE CARE

Section on Telephone Care and Committee on Child Health Financing

ABSTRACT. Telephone care in pediatrics requires medical judgment, is associated with practice expense and medical liability risk, and can often substitute for more costly face-to-face care. Despite this, physicians are infrequently paid by patients or third-party payors for medical services provided by telephone. As the costs of maintaining a practice continue to increase, pediatricians are increasingly seeking payment for the time and work involved in telephone care. This statement reviews the role of telephone care in pediatric practice, the current state of payment for telephone care, and the practical issues associated with charging for telephone care services, a service traditionally provided gratis to patients and families. Specific recommendations are presented for appropriate documenting, reporting, and billing for telephone care services. (10/06)
http://pediatrics.aappublications.org/content/118/4/1768

PEDESTRIAN SAFETY

Committee on Injury, Violence, and Poison Prevention

ABSTRACT. Each year, approximately 900 pediatric pedestrians younger than 19 years are killed. In addition, 51000 children are injured as pedestrians, and 5300 of them are hospitalized because of their injuries. Parents should be warned that young children often do not have the cognitive, perceptual, and behavioral abilities to negotiate traffic independently. Parents should also be informed about the danger of vehicle back-over injuries to toddlers playing in driveways. Because posttraumatic stress syndrome commonly follows even minor pedestrian injury, pediatricians should screen and refer for this condition as necessary. The American Academy of Pediatrics supports community- and school-based strategies that minimize a child's exposure to traffic, especially to high-speed, high-volume traffic. Furthermore, the American Academy of Pediatrics supports governmental and industry action that would lead to improvements in vehicle design, driver manuals, driver education, and data collection for the purpose of reducing pediatric pedestrian injury. (7/09, reaffirmed 8/13)
http://pediatrics.aappublications.org/content/124/2/802

PEDIATRIC AND ADOLESCENT MENTAL HEALTH EMERGENCIES IN THE EMERGENCY MEDICAL SERVICES SYSTEM (TECHNICAL REPORT)

Margaret A. Dolan, MD; Joel A. Fein, MD, MPH; and Committee on Pediatric Emergency Medicine

ABSTRACT. Emergency department (ED) health care professionals often care for patients with previously diagnosed psychiatric illnesses who are ill, injured, or having a behavioral crisis. In addition, ED personnel encounter children with psychiatric illnesses who may not present to the ED with overt mental health symptoms. Staff education and training regarding identification and management of pediatric mental health illness can help EDs overcome the perceived limitations of the setting that influence timely and comprehensive evaluation. In addition, ED physicians can inform and advocate for policy changes at local, state, and national levels that are needed to ensure comprehensive care of children with mental health illnesses. This report addresses the roles that the ED and ED health care professionals play in emergency mental health care of children and adolescents in the United States, which includes the stabilization and management of patients in mental health crisis, the discovery of mental illnesses and suicidal ideation in ED patients, and approaches to advocating for improved recognition and treatment of mental illnesses in children. The report also addresses special issues related to mental illness in the ED, such as minority populations, children with special health care needs, and children's mental health during and after disasters and trauma. (4/11, reaffirmed 7/14)
http://pediatrics.aappublications.org/content/127/5/e1356

PEDIATRIC ANTHRAX CLINICAL MANAGEMENT (CLINICAL REPORT)

John S. Bradley, MD, FAAP, FIDSA, FPIDS; Georgina Peacock, MD, MPH, FAAP; Steven E. Krug, MD, FAAP; William A. Bower, MD, FIDSA; Amanda C. Cohn, MD; Dana Meaney-Delman, MD, MPH, FACOG; Andrew T. Pavia, MD, FAAP, FIDSA; Committee on Infectious Diseases; and Disaster Preparedness Advisory Council

ABSTRACT. Anthrax is a zoonotic disease caused by *Bacillus anthracis*, which has multiple routes of infection in humans, manifesting in different initial presentations of disease. Because *B anthracis* has the potential to be used as a biological weapon and can rapidly progress to systemic anthrax with high mortality in those who are exposed and untreated, clinical guidance that can be quickly implemented must be in place before any intentional release of the agent. This document provides clinical guidance for the prophylaxis and treatment of neonates, infants, children, adolescents, and young adults up to the age of 21 (referred to as "children") in the event of a deliberate *B anthracis* release and offers guidance in areas where the unique characteristics of children dictate a different clinical recommendation from adults. (4/14)
http://pediatrics.aappublications.org/content/133/5/e1411

PEDIATRIC ANTHRAX CLINICAL MANAGEMENT: EXECUTIVE SUMMARY

John S. Bradley, MD, FAAP, FIDSA, FPIDS; Georgina Peacock, MD, MPH, FAAP; Steven E. Krug, MD, FAAP; William A. Bower, MD, FIDSA; Amanda C. Cohn, MD; Dana Meaney-Delman, MD, MPH, FACOG; Andrew T. Pavia, MD, FAAP, FIDSA; Committee on Infectious Diseases; and Disaster Preparedness Advisory Council

The use of *Bacillus anthracis* as a biological weapon is considered a potential national security threat by the US government. *B anthracis* has the ability to be used as a biological weapon and to cause anthrax, which can rapidly progress to systemic disease with high mortality in those who are untreated. Therefore, clear plans for managing children after a *B anthracis* bioterror exposure event must be in place before any intentional release of the agent. This document provides a summary of the guidance contained in the clinical report (appendices cited in this executive summary refer to those in the clinical report) for diagnosis and management of anthrax, including antimicrobial treatment and postexposure prophylaxis (PEP), use of antitoxin, and recommendations for use of anthrax vaccine in neonates, infants, children, adolescents, and young adults up to the age of 21 years (referred to as "children"). (4/14)
http://pediatrics.aappublications.org/content/133/5/940

PEDIATRIC ASPECTS OF INPATIENT HEALTH INFORMATION TECHNOLOGY SYSTEMS (TECHNICAL REPORT)

Christoph U. Lehmann, MD, FAAP, FACMI, and Council on Clinical Information Technology

ABSTRACT. In the past 3 years, the Health Information Technology for Economic and Clinical Health Act accelerated the adoption of electronic health records (EHRs) with providers and hospitals, who can claim incentive monies related to meaningful use. Despite the increase in adoption of commercial EHRs in pediatric settings, there has been little support for EHR tools and functionalities that promote pediatric quality improvement and patient safety, and children remain at higher risk than adults for medical errors in inpatient environments. Health information technology (HIT) tailored to the needs of pediatric health care providers can improve care by reducing the likelihood of errors through information assurance and minimizing the harm that results from errors. This technical report outlines pediatric-specific concepts, child health needs and their data elements, and required functionalities in inpatient clinical information systems that may be missing in adult-oriented HIT systems with negative consequences for pediatric inpatient care. It is imperative that inpatient (and outpatient) HIT systems be adapted to improve their ability to properly support safe health care delivery for children. (2/15)
http://pediatrics.aappublications.org/content/135/3/e756

PEDIATRIC CARE RECOMMENDATIONS FOR FREESTANDING URGENT CARE FACILITIES

Committee on Pediatric Emergency Medicine

ABSTRACT. Treatment of children at freestanding urgent care facilities has become common in pediatric health care. Well-managed freestanding urgent care facilities can improve the health of the children in their communities, integrate into the medical community, and provide a safe, effective adjunct to, but not a replacement for, the medical home or emergency department. Recommendations are provided for optimizing freestanding urgent care facilities' quality, communication, and collaboration in caring for children. (4/14)
http://pediatrics.aappublications.org/content/133/5/950

PEDIATRIC FELLOWSHIP TRAINING

Federation of Pediatric Organizations (7/04)
http://pediatrics.aappublications.org/content/114/1/295

PEDIATRIC MENTAL HEALTH EMERGENCIES IN THE EMERGENCY MEDICAL SERVICES SYSTEM

Committee on Pediatric Emergency Medicine (joint with American College of Emergency Physicians)

ABSTRACT. Emergency departments are vital in the management of pediatric patients with mental health emergencies. Pediatric mental health emergencies are an increasing part of emergency medical practice because emergency departments have become the safety net for a fragmented mental health infrastructure that is experiencing critical shortages in services in all sectors. Emergency departments must safely, humanely, and in a culturally and developmentally appropriate manner manage pediatric patients with undiagnosed and known mental illnesses, including those with mental retardation, autistic spectrum disorders, and attention-deficit/hyperactivity disorder and those experiencing a behavioral crisis. Emergency departments also manage patients with suicidal ideation, depression, escalating aggression, substance abuse, posttraumatic stress disorder, and maltreatment and those exposed to violence and unexpected deaths. Emergency departments must address not only the physical but also the mental health needs of patients during and after mass-casualty incidents and disasters. The American Academy of Pediatrics and the American College of Emergency Physicians support advocacy for increased mental health resources, including improved pediatric mental health tools for the emergency department, increased mental health insurance coverage, and adequate reimbursement at all levels; acknowledgment of the importance of the child's medical home; and promotion of education and research for mental health emergencies. (10/06, reaffirmed 6/09, 4/13)
http://pediatrics.aappublications.org/content/118/4/1764

PEDIATRIC OBSERVATION UNITS (CLINICAL REPORT)

Gregory P. Conners, MD, MPH, MBA; Sanford M. Melzer, MD, MBA; Committee on Hospital Care; and Committee on Pediatric Emergency Medicine

ABSTRACT. Pediatric observation units (OUs) are hospital areas used to provide medical evaluation and/or management for health-related conditions in children, typically for a well-defined, brief period. Pediatric OUs represent an emerging alternative site of care for selected groups of children who historically may have received their treatment in an ambulatory setting, emergency department, or hospital-based inpatient unit. This clinical report provides an overview of pediatric OUs, including the definitions and operating characteristics of different types of OUs, quality considerations and coding for observation services, and the effect of OUs on inpatient hospital utilization. (6/12, reaffirmed 9/15)
http://pediatrics.aappublications.org/content/130/1/172

PEDIATRIC ORGAN DONATION AND TRANSPLANTATION

Committee on Hospital Care, Section on Surgery, and Section on Critical Care

ABSTRACT. Pediatric organ donation and organ transplantation can have a significant life-extending benefit to the young recipients of these organs and a high emotional impact on donor and recipient families. Pediatricians, pediatric medical specialists, and pediatric transplant surgeons need to be better acquainted with evolving national strategies that involve organ procurement and organ transplantation to help acquaint families with the benefits and risks of organ donation and transplantation. Efforts of pediatric professionals are needed to shape public policies to provide a system in which procurement, distribution, and cost are fair and equitable to children and adults. Major issues of concern are availability of and access to donor organs; oversight and control of the process; pediatric medical and surgical consultation and continued care throughout the organ-donation and transplantation process; ethical, social, financial, and follow-up issues; insurance-coverage issues; and public awareness of the need for organ donors of all ages. (3/10, reaffirmed 3/14)
http://pediatrics.aappublications.org/content/125/4/822

PEDIATRIC PALLIATIVE CARE AND HOSPICE CARE COMMITMENTS, GUIDELINES, AND RECOMMENDATIONS

Section on Hospice and Palliative Medicine and Committee on Hospital Care

ABSTRACT. Pediatric palliative care and pediatric hospice care (PPC-PHC) are often essential aspects of medical care for patients who have life-threatening conditions or need end-of-life care. PPC-PHC aims to relieve suffering, improve quality of life, facilitate informed decision-making, and assist in care coordination between clinicians and across sites of care. Core commitments of PPC-PHC include being patient centered and family engaged; respecting and partnering with patients and families; pursuing care that is high quality, readily accessible, and equitable; providing care across the age spectrum and life span, integrated into the continuum of care; ensuring that all clinicians can provide basic palliative care and consult PPC-PHC specialists in a timely manner; and improving care through research and quality improvement efforts. PPC-PHC guidelines and recommendations include ensuring that all large health care organizations serving children with life-threatening conditions have dedicated interdisciplinary PPC-PHC teams, which should develop collaborative relationships between hospital- and community-based teams; that PPC-PHC be provided as integrated multimodal care and practiced as a cornerstone of patient safety and quality for patients with life-threatening conditions; that PPC-PHC teams should facilitate clear, compassionate, and forthright discussions about medical issues and the goals of care and support families, siblings, and health care staff; that PPC-PHC be part of all pediatric education and training curricula, be an active area of research and quality improvement, and exemplify the highest ethical standards; and that PPC-PHC services be supported by financial and regulatory arrangements to ensure access to high-quality PPC-PHC by all patients with life-threatening and life-shortening diseases. (10/13)

http://pediatrics.aappublications.org/content/132/5/966

PEDIATRIC PRIMARY HEALTH CARE

Committee on Pediatric Workforce
ABSTRACT. Primary health care is described as accessible and affordable, first contact, continuous and comprehensive, and coordinated to meet the health needs of the individual and the family being served.

Pediatric primary health care encompasses health supervision and anticipatory guidance; monitoring physical and psychosocial growth and development; age-appropriate screening; diagnosis and treatment of acute and chronic disorders; management of serious and life-threatening illness and, when appropriate, referral of more complex conditions; and provision of first contact care as well as coordinated management of health problems requiring multiple professional services.

Pediatric primary health care for children and adolescents is family centered and incorporates community resources and strengths, needs and risk factors, and sociocultural sensitivities into strategies for care delivery and clinical practice. Pediatric primary health care is best delivered within the context of a "medical home," where comprehensive, continuously accessible and affordable care is available and delivered or supervised by qualified child health specialists.

The pediatrician, because of training (which includes 4 years of medical school education, plus an additional 3 or more years of intensive training devoted solely to all aspects of medical care for children and adolescents), coupled with the demonstrated interest in and total professional commitment to the health care of infants, children, adolescents, and young adults, is the most appropriate provider of pediatric primary health care. (1/11, reaffirmed 10/13)

http://pediatrics.aappublications.org/content/127/2/397

PEDIATRIC SUDDEN CARDIAC ARREST

Section on Cardiology and Cardiac Surgery
ABSTRACT. Pediatric sudden cardiac arrest (SCA), which can cause sudden cardiac death if not treated within minutes, has a profound effect on everyone: children, parents, family members, communities, and health care providers. Preventing the tragedy of pediatric SCA, defined as the abrupt and unexpected loss of heart function, remains a concern to all. The goal of this statement is to increase the knowledge of pediatricians (including primary care providers and specialists) of the incidence of pediatric SCA, the spectrum of causes of pediatric SCA, disease-specific presentations, the role of patient and family screening, the

rapidly evolving role of genetic testing, and finally, important aspects of secondary SCA prevention. This statement is not intended to address sudden infant death syndrome or sudden unexplained death syndrome, nor will specific treatment of individual cardiac conditions be discussed. This statement has been endorsed by the American College of Cardiology, the American Heart Association, and the Heart Rhythm Society. (3/12)

http://pediatrics.aappublications.org/content/129/4/e1094

THE PEDIATRICIAN AND CHILDHOOD BEREAVEMENT

*Committee on Psychosocial Aspects of Child and
    Family Health*
ABSTRACT. Pediatricians should understand and evaluate children's reactions to the death of a person important to them by using age-appropriate and culturally sensitive guidance while being alert for normal and complicated grief responses. Pediatricians also should advise and assist families in responding to the child's needs. Sharing, family support, and communication have been associated with positive long-term bereavement adjustment. (2/00, reaffirmed 1/04, 3/13)

http://pediatrics.aappublications.org/content/105/2/445

THE PEDIATRICIAN AND DISASTER PREPAREDNESS

*Committee on Pediatric Emergency Medicine, Committee on
    Medical Liability, and Task Force on Terrorism*
ABSTRACT. Recent natural disasters and events of terrorism and war have heightened society's recognition of the need for emergency preparedness. In addition to the unique pediatric issues involved in general emergency preparedness, several additional issues related to terrorism preparedness must be considered, including the unique vulnerabilities of children to various agents as well as the limited availability of age- and weight-appropriate antidotes and treatments. Although children may respond more rapidly to therapeutic intervention, they are at the same time more susceptible to various agents and conditions and more likely to deteriorate if not monitored carefully.

The challenge of dealing with the threat of terrorism, natural disasters, and public health emergencies in the United States is daunting not only for disaster planners but also for our medical system and health professionals of all types, including pediatricians. As part of the network of health responders, pediatricians need to be able to answer concerns of patients and families, recognize signs of possible exposure to a weapon of terror, understand first-line response to such attacks, and sufficiently participate in disaster planning to ensure that the unique needs of children are addressed satisfactorily in the overall process. Pediatricians play a central role in disaster and terrorism preparedness with families, children, and their communities. This applies not only to the general pediatrician but also to the pediatric medical subspecialist and pediatric surgical specialist. Families view pediatricians as their expert resource, and most of them expect the pediatrician to be knowledgeable in areas of concern. Providing expert guidance entails educating families in anticipation of events and responding to questions during and after actual events. It is essential that pediatricians educate themselves regarding these issues of emergency preparedness.

For pediatricians, some information is currently available on virtually all of these issues in recently produced printed materials, at special conferences, in broadcasts of various types, and on the Internet. However, selecting appropriate, accurate sources of information and determining how much information is sufficient remain difficult challenges. Similarly, guidance is needed with respect to developing relevant curricula for medical students and postdoctoral clinical trainees. (2/06, reaffirmed 6/09, 9/13)

http://pediatrics.aappublications.org/content/117/2/560

THE PEDIATRICIAN WORKFORCE: CURRENT STATUS AND FUTURE PROSPECTS (TECHNICAL REPORT)

David C. Goodman, MD, MS, and Committee on
*   Pediatric Workforce*

ABSTRACT. The effective and efficient delivery of children's health care depends on the pediatrician workforce. The number, composition, and distribution of pediatricians necessary to deliver this care have been the subject of long-standing policy and professional debate. This technical report reviews current characteristics and recent trends in the pediatric workforce and couples the workforce to a conceptual model of improvement in children's health and well-being. Important recent changes in the workforce include (1) the growth in the number of pediatricians in relation to the child population, (2) increased numbers of female pediatricians and their attainment of majority gender status in the specialty, (3) the persistence of a large number of international medical graduates entering training programs, (4) a lack of ethnic and racial diversity in pediatricians compared with children, and (5) the persistence of marked regional variation in pediatrician supply. Supply models projecting the pediatric workforce are reviewed and generally indicate that the number of pediatricians per child will increase by 50% over the next 20 years. The differing methods of assessing workforce requirements are presented and critiqued. The report finds that the pediatric workforce is undergoing fundamental changes that will have important effects on the professional lives of pediatricians and children's health care delivery. (7/05)

http://pediatrics.aappublications.org/content/116/1/e156

PEDIATRICIAN WORKFORCE POLICY STATEMENT

Committee on Pediatric Workforce

ABSTRACT. This policy statement reviews important trends and other factors that affect the pediatrician workforce and the provision of pediatric health care, including changes in the pediatric patient population, pediatrician workforce, and nature of pediatric practice. The effect of these changes on pediatricians and the demand for pediatric care are discussed. The American Academy of Pediatrics (AAP) concludes that there is currently a shortage of pediatric medical subspecialists in many fields, as well as a shortage of pediatric surgical specialists. In addition, the AAP believes that the current distribution of primary care pediatricians is inadequate to meet the needs of children living in rural and other underserved areas, and more primary care pediatricians will be needed in the future because of the increasing number of children who have significant chronic health problems, changes in physician work hours, and implementation of current health reform efforts that seek to improve access to comprehensive patient- and family-centered care for all children in a medical home. The AAP is committed to being an active participant in physician workforce policy development with both professional organizations and governmental bodies to ensure a pediatric perspective on health care workforce issues. The overall purpose of this statement is to summarize policy recommendations and serve as a resource for the AAP and other stakeholders as they address pediatrician workforce issues that ultimately influence the quality of pediatric health care provided to children in the United States. (7/13)

http://pediatrics.aappublications.org/content/132/2/390

PEDIATRICIAN-FAMILY-PATIENT RELATIONSHIPS: MANAGING THE BOUNDARIES

Committee on Bioethics

ABSTRACT. All professionals are concerned about maintaining the appropriate limits in their relationships with those they serve. Pediatricians should be aware that, under normal circumstances, caring for one's own children presents significant ethical issues. Pediatricians also must strive to maintain appropriate professional boundaries in their relationships with the family members of their patients. Pediatricians should avoid behavior that patients and parents might misunderstand as having sexual or inappropriate social meaning. Romantic and sexual involvement between physicians and patients is unacceptable. The acceptance of gifts or nonmonetary compensation for medical services has the potential to affect the professional relationship adversely. (11/09, reaffirmed 1/14)

http://pediatrics.aappublications.org/content/124/6/1685

THE PEDIATRICIAN'S ROLE IN CHILD MALTREATMENT PREVENTION (CLINICAL REPORT)

Emalee G. Flaherty, MD; John Stirling Jr, MD; and
*   Committee on Child Abuse and Neglect*

ABSTRACT. It is the pediatrician's role to promote the child's well-being and to help parents raise healthy, well-adjusted children. Pediatricians, therefore, can play an important role in the prevention of child maltreatment. Previous clinical reports and policy statements from the American Academy of Pediatrics have focused on improving the identification and management of child maltreatment. This clinical report outlines how the pediatrician can help to strengthen families and promote safe, stable, nurturing relationships with the aim of preventing maltreatment. After describing some of the triggers and factors that place children at risk for maltreatment, the report describes how pediatricians can identify family strengths, recognize risk factors, provide helpful guidance, and refer families to programs and other resources with the goal of strengthening families, preventing child maltreatment, and enhancing child development. (9/10, reaffirmed 1/14)

http://pediatrics.aappublications.org/content/126/4/833

THE PEDIATRICIAN'S ROLE IN COMMUNITY PEDIATRICS
Committee on Community Health Services

ABSTRACT. This policy statement reaffirms the pediatrician's role in community pediatrics. It offers pediatricians a definition of community pediatrics and provides a set of specific recommendations that underscore the critical nature of this important dimension of the profession. (4/05, reaffirmed 1/10)
http://pediatrics.aappublications.org/content/115/4/1092

THE PEDIATRICIAN'S ROLE IN DEVELOPMENT AND IMPLEMENTATION OF AN INDIVIDUAL EDUCATION PLAN (IEP) AND/OR AN INDIVIDUAL FAMILY SERVICE PLAN (IFSP)
Committee on Children With Disabilities

ABSTRACT. The Individual Education Plan and Individual Family Service Plan are legally mandated documents developed by a multidisciplinary team assessment that specifies goals and services for each child eligible for special educational services or early intervention services. Pediatricians need to be knowledgeable of federal, state, and local requirements; establish linkages with early intervention, educational professionals, and parent support groups; and collaborate with the team working with individual children. (7/99, reaffirmed 11/02, 1/06)
http://pediatrics.aappublications.org/content/104/1/124

THE PEDIATRICIAN'S ROLE IN FAMILY SUPPORT AND FAMILY SUPPORT PROGRAMS
Committee on Early Childhood, Adoption, and Dependent Care

ABSTRACT. Children's social, emotional, and physical health; their developmental trajectory; and the neuro-circuits that are being created and reinforced in their developing brains are all directly influenced by their relationships during early childhood. The stresses associated with contemporary American life can challenge families' abilities to promote successful developmental outcomes and emotional health for their children. Pediatricians are positioned to serve as partners with families and other community providers in supporting the well-being of children and their families. The structure and support of families involve forces that are often outside the agenda of the usual pediatric health supervision visits. Pediatricians must ensure that their medical home efforts promote a holistically healthy family environment for all children. This statement recommends opportunities for pediatricians to develop their expertise in assessing the strengths and stresses in families, in counseling families about strategies and resources, and in collaborating with others in their communities to support family relationships. (11/11)
http://pediatrics.aappublications.org/content/128/6/e1680

THE PEDIATRICIAN'S ROLE IN OPTIMIZING SCHOOL READINESS
Council on Early Childhood and Council on School Health

ABSTRACT. School readiness includes not only the early academic skills of children but also their physical health, language skills, social and emotional development, motivation to learn, creativity, and general knowledge. Families and communities play a critical role in ensuring children's growth in all of these areas and thus their readiness for school. Schools must be prepared to teach all children when they reach the age of school entry, regardless of their degree of readiness. Research on early brain development emphasizes the effects of early experiences, relationships, and emotions on creating and reinforcing the neural connections that are the basis for learning. Pediatricians, by the nature of their relationships with families and children, may significantly influence school readiness. Pediatricians have a primary role in ensuring children's physical health through the provision of preventive care, treatment of illness, screening for sensory deficits, and monitoring nutrition and growth. They can promote and monitor the social-emotional development of children by providing anticipatory guidance on development and behavior, by encouraging positive parenting practices, by modeling reciprocal and respectful communication with adults and children, by identifying and addressing psychosocial risk factors, and by providing community-based resources and referrals when warranted. Cognitive and language skills are fostered through timely identification of developmental problems and appropriate referrals for services, including early intervention and special education services; guidance regarding safe and stimulating early education and child care programs; and promotion of early literacy by encouraging language-rich activities such as reading together, telling stories, and playing games. Pediatricians are also well positioned to advocate not only for children's access to health care but also for high-quality early childhood education and evidence-based family supports such as home visits, which help provide a foundation for optimal learning. (8/16)
See full text on page 1043.
http://pediatrics.aappublications.org/content/138/3/e20162293

THE PEDIATRICIAN'S ROLE IN SUPPORTING ADOPTIVE FAMILIES (CLINICAL REPORT)
Veronnie F. Jones, MD, PhD; Elaine E. Schulte, MD, MPH; Committee on Early Childhood; and Council on Foster Care, Adoption, and Kinship Care

ABSTRACT. Each year, more children join families through adoption. Pediatricians have an important role in assisting adoptive families in the various challenges they may face with respect to adoption. The acceptance of the differences between families formed through birth and those formed through adoption is essential in promoting positive emotional growth within the family. It is important for pediatricians to be aware of the adoptive parents' need to be supported in their communication with their adopted children. (9/12)
http://pediatrics.aappublications.org/content/130/4/e1040

THE PEDIATRICIAN'S ROLE IN THE EVALUATION AND PREPARATION OF PEDIATRIC PATIENTS UNDERGOING ANESTHESIA
Section on Anesthesiology and Pain Medicine

ABSTRACT. Pediatricians play a key role in helping prepare patients and families for anesthesia and surgery. The questions to be answered by the pediatrician fall into 2 categories. The first involves preparation: is the patient in optimal medical condition for surgery, and are the patient and family emotionally and cognitively ready for surgery? The second category concerns logistics: what communication and organizational needs are necessary

to enable safe passage through the perioperative process? This revised statement updates the recommendations for the pediatrician's role in the preoperative preparation of patients. (8/14)
http://pediatrics.aappublications.org/content/134/3/634

THE PEDIATRICIAN'S ROLE IN THE PREVENTION OF MISSING CHILDREN (CLINICAL REPORT)
Committee on Psychosocial Aspects of Child and Family Health
ABSTRACT. In 2002, the *Second National Incidence Studies of Missing, Abducted, Runaway, and Thrownaway Children* report was released by the US Department of Justice, providing new data on a problem that our nation continues to face. This clinical report describes the categories of missing children, the prevalence of each, and prevention strategies that primary care pediatricians can share with parents to increase awareness and education about the safety of their children. (10/04, reaffirmed 1/15)
http://pediatrics.aappublications.org/content/114/4/1100

PERSONAL WATERCRAFT USE BY CHILDREN AND ADOLESCENTS
Committee on Injury and Poison Prevention
ABSTRACT. The use of personal watercraft (PWC) has increased dramatically during the past decade as have the speed and mobility of the watercraft. A similar dramatic increase in PWC-related injury and death has occurred simultaneously. No one younger than 16 years should operate a PWC. The operator and all passengers must wear US Coast Guard-approved personal flotation devices. Other safety recommendations are suggested for parents and pediatricians. (2/00, reaffirmed 5/04, 1/07, 6/10)
http://pediatrics.aappublications.org/content/105/2/452

PESTICIDE EXPOSURE IN CHILDREN
Council on Environmental Health
ABSTRACT. This statement presents the position of the American Academy of Pediatrics on pesticides. Pesticides are a collective term for chemicals intended to kill unwanted insects, plants, molds, and rodents. Children encounter pesticides daily and have unique susceptibilities to their potential toxicity. Acute poisoning risks are clear, and understanding of chronic health implications from both acute and chronic exposure are emerging. Epidemiologic evidence demonstrates associations between early life exposure to pesticides and pediatric cancers, decreased cognitive function, and behavioral problems. Related animal toxicology studies provide supportive biological plausibility for these findings. Recognizing and reducing problematic exposures will require attention to current inadequacies in medical training, public health tracking, and regulatory action on pesticides. Ongoing research describing toxicologic vulnerabilities and exposure factors across the life span are needed to inform regulatory needs and appropriate interventions. Policies that promote integrated pest management, comprehensive pesticide labeling, and marketing practices that incorporate child health considerations will enhance safe use. (11/12)
http://pediatrics.aappublications.org/content/130/6/e1757

PESTICIDE EXPOSURE IN CHILDREN (TECHNICAL REPORT)
James R. Roberts, MD, MPH; Catherine J. Karr, MD, PhD; and Council on Environmental Health
ABSTRACT. Pesticides are a collective term for a wide array of chemicals intended to kill unwanted insects, plants, molds, and rodents. Food, water, and treatment in the home, yard, and school are all potential sources of children's exposure. Exposures to pesticides may be overt or subacute, and effects range from acute to chronic toxicity. In 2008, pesticides were the ninth most common substance reported to poison control centers, and approximately 45% of all reports of pesticide poisoning were for children. Organophosphate and carbamate poisoning are perhaps the most widely known acute poisoning syndromes, can be diagnosed by depressed red blood cell cholinesterase levels, and have available antidotal therapy. However, numerous other pesticides that may cause acute toxicity, such as pyrethroid and neonicotinoid insecticides, herbicides, fungicides, and rodenticides, also have specific toxic effects; recognition of these effects may help identify acute exposures. Evidence is increasingly emerging about chronic health implications from both acute and chronic exposure. A growing body of epidemiological evidence demonstrates associations between parental use of pesticides, particularly insecticides, with acute lymphocytic leukemia and brain tumors. Prenatal, household, and occupational exposures (maternal and paternal) appear to be the largest risks. Prospective cohort studies link early-life exposure to organophosphates and organochlorine pesticides (primarily DDT) with adverse effects on neurodevelopment and behavior. Among the findings associated with increased pesticide levels are poorer mental development by using the Bayley index and increased scores on measures assessing pervasive developmental disorder, inattention, and attention-deficit/hyperactivity disorder. Related animal toxicology studies provide supportive biological plausibility for these findings. Additional data suggest that there may also be an association between parental pesticide use and adverse birth outcomes including physical birth defects, low birth weight, and fetal death, although the data are less robust than for cancer and neurodevelopmental effects. Children's exposures to pesticides should be limited as much as possible. (11/12)
http://pediatrics.aappublications.org/content/130/6/e1765

PHOTOTHERAPY TO PREVENT SEVERE NEONATAL HYPERBILIRUBINEMIA IN THE NEWBORN INFANT 35 OR MORE WEEKS OF GESTATION (TECHNICAL REPORT)
Vinod K. Bhutani, MD, and Committee on Fetus and Newborn
ABSTRACT. *Objective.* To standardize the use of phototherapy consistent with the American Academy of Pediatrics clinical practice guideline for the management of hyperbilirubinemia in the newborn infant 35 or more weeks of gestation.
Methods. Relevant literature was reviewed. Phototherapy devices currently marketed in the United States that incorporate fluorescent, halogen, fiber-optic, or blue light-emitting diode light sources were assessed in the laboratory.

Results. The efficacy of phototherapy units varies widely because of differences in light source and configuration. The following characteristics of a device contribute to its effectiveness: (1) emission of light in the blue-to-green range that overlaps the in vivo plasma bilirubin absorption spectrum (~460–490 nm); (2) irradiance of at least 30 µW·cm–2·nm–1 (confirmed with an appropriate irradiance meter calibrated over the appropriate wavelength range); (3) illumination of maximal body surface; and (4) demonstration of a decrease in total bilirubin concentrations during the first 4 to 6 hours of exposure.

Recommendations. The intensity and spectral output of phototherapy devices is useful in predicting potential effectiveness in treating hyperbilirubinemia (group B recommendation). Clinical effectiveness should be evaluated before and monitored during use (group B recommendation). Blocking the light source or reducing exposed body surface should be avoided (group B recommendation). Standardization of irradiance meters, improvements in device design, and lower-upper limits of light intensity for phototherapy units merit further study. Comparing the in vivo performance of devices is not practical, in general, and alternative procedures need to be explored. (9/11, reaffirmed 7/14)
http://pediatrics.aappublications.org/content/128/4/e1046

PHYSICIAN HEALTH AND WELLNESS (CLINICAL REPORT)

Hilary McClafferty, MD, FAAP; Oscar W. Brown, MD, FAAP; Section on Integrative Medicine; and Committee on Practice and Ambulatory Medicine

ABSTRACT. Physician health and wellness is a critical issue gaining national attention because of the high prevalence of physician burnout. Pediatricians and pediatric trainees experience burnout at levels equivalent to other medical specialties, highlighting a need for more effective efforts to promote health and well-being in the pediatric community. This report will provide an overview of physician burnout, an update on work in the field of preventive physician health and wellness, and a discussion of emerging initiatives that have potential to promote health at all levels of pediatric training.

Pediatricians are uniquely positioned to lead this movement nationally, in part because of the emphasis placed on wellness in the Pediatric Milestone Project, a joint collaboration between the Accreditation Council for Graduate Medical Education and the American Board of Pediatrics. Updated core competencies calling for a balanced approach to health, including focus on nutrition, exercise, mindfulness, and effective stress management, signal a paradigm shift and send the message that it is time for pediatricians to cultivate a culture of wellness better aligned with their responsibilities as role models and congruent with advances in pediatric training.

Rather than reviewing programs in place to address substance abuse and other serious conditions in distressed physicians, this article focuses on forward progress in the field, with an emphasis on the need for prevention and anticipation of predictable stressors related to burnout in medical training and practice. Examples of positive progress and several programs designed to promote physician

health and wellness are reviewed. Areas where more research is needed are highlighted. (9/14)
http://pediatrics.aappublications.org/content/134/4/830

PHYSICIAN REFUSAL TO PROVIDE INFORMATION OR TREATMENT ON THE BASIS OF CLAIMS OF CONSCIENCE

Committee on Bioethics

ABSTRACT. Health care professionals may have moral objections to particular medical interventions. They may refuse to provide or cooperate in the provision of these interventions. Such objections are referred to as conscientious objections. Although it may be difficult to characterize or validate claims of conscience, respecting the individual physician's moral integrity is important. Conflicts arise when claims of conscience impede a patient's access to medical information or care. A physician's conscientious objection to certain interventions or treatments may be constrained in some situations. Physicians have a duty to disclose to prospective patients treatments they refuse to perform. As part of informed consent, physicians also have a duty to inform their patients of all relevant and legally available treatment options, including options to which they object. They have a moral obligation to refer patients to other health care professionals who are willing to provide those services when failing to do so would cause harm to the patient, and they have a duty to treat patients in emergencies when referral would significantly increase the probability of mortality or serious morbidity. Conversely, the health care system should make reasonable accommodations for physicians with conscientious objections. (11/09, reaffirmed 1/14)
http://pediatrics.aappublications.org/content/124/6/1689

PHYSICIANS' ROLES IN COORDINATING CARE OF HOSPITALIZED CHILDREN (CLINICAL REPORT)

Patricia S. Lye, MD; Committee on Hospital Care; and Section on Hospital Medicine

ABSTRACT. The care of hospitalized children and adolescents has become increasingly complex and often involves multiple physicians beyond the traditional primary care pediatrician. Hospitalists, medical subspecialists, surgical specialists, and hospital attending physicians may all participate in the care of hospitalized children and youth. This report summarizes the responsibilities of the pediatrician and other involved physicians in ensuring that children receive coordinated and comprehensive medical care delivered within the context of their medical homes as inpatients, and that care is appropriately continued on an outpatient basis. (9/10)
http://pediatrics.aappublications.org/content/126/4/829

PLANNED HOME BIRTH

Committee on Fetus and Newborn

ABSTRACT. The American Academy of Pediatrics concurs with the recent statement of the American College of Obstetricians and Gynecologists affirming that hospitals and birthing centers are the safest settings for birth in the United States while respecting the right of women to make a medically informed decision about delivery. This statement is intended to help pediatricians provide supportive, informed counsel to women considering home birth while retaining their role as child advocates and to summarize the standards of care for newborn infants born at home, which are consistent with standards for infants born in a medical care facility. Regardless of the circumstances of his or her birth, including location, every newborn infant deserves health care that adheres to the standards highlighted in this statement, more completely described in other publications from the American Academy of Pediatrics, including *Guidelines for Perinatal Care.* The goal of providing high-quality care to all newborn infants can best be achieved through continuing efforts by all participating health care providers and institutions to develop and sustain communications and understanding on the basis of professional interaction and mutual respect throughout the health care system. (4/13)

http://pediatrics.aappublications.org/content/131/5/1016

POINT-OF-CARE ULTRASONOGRAPHY BY PEDIATRIC EMERGENCY MEDICINE PHYSICIANS

Committee on Pediatric Emergency Medicine (joint with Society for Academic Emergency Medicine Academy of Emergency Ultrasound, American College of Emergency Physicians Pediatric Emergency Medicine Committee, and World Interactive Network Focused on Critical Ultrasound)

ABSTRACT. Point-of-care ultrasonography is increasingly being used to facilitate accurate and timely diagnoses and to guide procedures. It is important for pediatric emergency medicine (PEM) physicians caring for patients in the emergency department to receive adequate and continued point-of-care ultrasonography training for those indications used in their practice setting. Emergency departments should have credentialing and quality assurance programs. PEM fellowships should provide appropriate training to physician trainees. Hospitals should provide privileges to physicians who demonstrate competency in point-of-care ultrasonography. Ongoing research will provide the necessary measures to define the optimal training and competency assessment standards. Requirements for credentialing and hospital privileges will vary and will be specific to individual departments and hospitals. As more physicians are trained and more research is completed, there should be one national standard for credentialing and privileging in point-of-care ultrasonography for PEM physicians. (3/15)

http://pediatrics.aappublications.org/content/135/4/e1097

POINT-OF-CARE ULTRASONOGRAPHY BY PEDIATRIC EMERGENCY MEDICINE PHYSICIANS (TECHNICAL REPORT)

Jennifer R. Marin, MD, MSc; Resa E. Lewiss, MD; and Committee on Pediatric Emergency Medicine (joint with Society for Academic Emergency Medicine Academy of Emergency Ultrasound, American College of Emergency Physicians Pediatric Emergency Medicine Committee, and World Interactive Network Focused on Critical Ultrasound)

ABSTRACT. Emergency physicians have used point-of-care ultrasonography since the 1990s. Pediatric emergency medicine physicians have more recently adopted this technology. Point-of-care ultrasonography is used for various scenarios, particularly the evaluation of soft tissue infections or blunt abdominal trauma and procedural

guidance. To date, there are no published statements from national organizations specifically for pediatric emergency physicians describing the incorporation of point-of-care ultrasonography into their practice. This document outlines how pediatric emergency departments may establish a formal point-of-care ultrasonography program. This task includes appointing leaders with expertise in point-of-care ultrasonography, effectively training and credentialing physicians in the department, and providing ongoing quality assurance reviews.

Point-of-care ultrasonography (US) is a bedside technology that enables clinicians to integrate clinical examination findings with real-time sonographic imaging. General emergency physicians and other specialists have used point-of-care US for many years, and more recently, pediatric emergency medicine (PEM) physicians have adopted point-of-care US as a diagnostic and procedural adjunct. This technical report and accompanying policy statement provide a framework for point-of-care US training and point-of-care US integration into pediatric care by PEM physicians. (3/15)

http://pediatrics.aappublications.org/content/135/4/e1113

POSTDISCHARGE FOLLOW-UP OF INFANTS WITH CONGENITAL DIAPHRAGMATIC HERNIA (CLINICAL REPORT)

Section on Surgery and Committee on Fetus and Newborn

ABSTRACT. Infants with congenital diaphragmatic hernia often require intensive treatment after birth, have prolonged hospitalizations, and have other congenital anomalies. After discharge from the hospital, they may have long-term sequelae such as respiratory insufficiency, gastroesophageal reflux, poor growth, neurodevelopmental delay, behavior problems, hearing loss, hernia recurrence, and orthopedic deformities. Structured follow-up for these patients facilitates early recognition and treatment of these complications. In this report, follow-up of infants with congenital diaphragmatic hernia is outlined. (3/08, reaffirmed 5/11)

http://pediatrics.aappublications.org/content/121/3/627

POSTEXPOSURE PROPHYLAXIS IN CHILDREN AND ADOLESCENTS FOR NONOCCUPATIONAL EXPOSURE TO HUMAN IMMUNODEFICIENCY VIRUS (CLINICAL REPORT)

Committee on Pediatric AIDS

ABSTRACT. Exposure to human immunodeficiency virus (HIV) can occur in a number of situations unique to, or more common among, children and adolescents. Guidelines for postexposure prophylaxis (PEP) for occupational and nonoccupational (eg, sexual, needle-sharing) exposures to HIV have been published by the US Public Health Service, but they do not directly address nonoccupational HIV exposures unique to children (such as accidental exposure to human milk from a woman infected with HIV or a puncture wound from a discarded needle on a playground), and they do not provide antiretroviral drug information relevant to PEP in children.

This clinical report reviews issues of potential exposure of children and adolescents to HIV and gives recommendations for PEP in those situations. The risk of HIV transmission from nonoccupational, nonperinatal

exposure is generally low. Transmission risk is modified by factors related to the source and extent of exposure. Determination of the HIV infection status of the exposure source may not be possible, and data on transmission risk by exposure type may not exist. Except in the setting of perinatal transmission, no studies have demonstrated the safety and efficacy of postexposure use of antiretroviral drugs for the prevention of HIV transmission in nonoccupational settings. Antiretroviral therapy used for PEP is associated with significant toxicity. The decision to initiate prophylaxis needs to be made in consultation with the patient, the family, and a clinician with experience in treatment of persons with HIV infection. If instituted, therapy should be started as soon as possible after an exposure—no later than 72 hours—and continued for 28 days. Many clinicians would use 3 drugs for PEP regimens, although 2 drugs may be considered in certain circumstances. Instruction for avoiding secondary transmission should be given. Careful follow-up is needed for psychologic support, encouragement of medication adherence, toxicity monitoring, and serial HIV antibody testing. (6/03, reaffirmed 1/07, 10/08)
http://pediatrics.aappublications.org/content/111/6/1475

POSTNATAL CORTICOSTEROIDS TO PREVENT OR TREAT BRONCHOPULMONARY DYSPLASIA

Kristi L. Watterberg, MD, and Committee on Fetus and Newborn
ABSTRACT. The purpose of this revised statement is to review current information on the use of postnatal glucocorticoids to prevent or treat bronchopulmonary dysplasia in the preterm infant and to make updated recommendations regarding their use. High-dose dexamethasone (0.5 mg/kg per day) does not seem to confer additional therapeutic benefit over lower doses and is not recommended. Evidence is insufficient to make a recommendation regarding other glucocorticoid doses and preparations. The clinician must use clinical judgment when attempting to balance the potential adverse effects of glucocorticoid treatment with those of bronchopulmonary dysplasia. (9/10, reaffirmed 1/14)
http://pediatrics.aappublications.org/content/126/4/800

POSTNATAL GLUCOSE HOMEOSTASIS IN LATE-PRETERM AND TERM INFANTS (CLINICAL REPORT)

David H. Adamkin, MD, and Committee on Fetus and Newborn
ABSTRACT. This report provides a practical guide and algorithm for the screening and subsequent management of neonatal hypoglycemia. Current evidence does not support a specific concentration of glucose that can discriminate normal from abnormal or can potentially result in acute or chronic irreversible neurologic damage. Early identification of the at-risk infant and institution of prophylactic measures to prevent neonatal hypoglycemia are recommended as a pragmatic approach despite the absence of a consistent definition of hypoglycemia in the literature. (3/11, reaffirmed 6/15)
http://pediatrics.aappublications.org/content/127/3/575

POVERTY AND CHILD HEALTH IN THE UNITED STATES

Council on Community Pediatrics
ABSTRACT. Almost half of young children in the United States live in poverty or near poverty. The American Academy of Pediatrics is committed to reducing and ultimately eliminating child poverty in the United States. Poverty and related social determinants of health can lead to adverse health outcomes in childhood and across the life course, negatively affecting physical health, socioemotional development, and educational achievement. The American Academy of Pediatrics advocates for programs and policies that have been shown to improve the quality of life and health outcomes for children and families living in poverty. With an awareness and understanding of the effects of poverty on children, pediatricians and other pediatric health practitioners in a family-centered medical home can assess the financial stability of families, link families to resources, and coordinate care with community partners. Further research, advocacy, and continuing education will improve the ability of pediatricians to address the social determinants of health when caring for children who live in poverty. Accompanying this policy statement is a technical report that describes current knowledge on child poverty and the mechanisms by which poverty influences the health and well-being of children. (3/16)
See full text on page 1053.
http://pediatrics.aappublications.org/content/137/4/e20160339

PRECERTIFICATION PROCESS

Committee on Hospital Care
ABSTRACT. Precertification is a process still used by health insurance companies to control health care costs. Although we believe precertification is unnecessary and not cost-effective, in those instances where precertification is still being utilized, we suggest that the following procedures be adopted. This statement suggests guidelines that should help achieve this goal while allowing optimal access to care for children. (8/00, reaffirmed 5/05, 11/08)
http://pediatrics.aappublications.org/content/106/2/350

PREMEDICATION FOR NONEMERGENCY ENDOTRACHEAL INTUBATION IN THE NEONATE (CLINICAL REPORT)

Praveen Kumar, MD; Susan E. Denson, MD; Thomas J. Mancuso, MD; Committee on Fetus and Newborn; and Section on Anesthesiology and Pain Medicine
ABSTRACT. Endotracheal intubation is a common procedure in newborn care. The purpose of this clinical report is to review currently available evidence on use of premedication for intubation, identify gaps in knowledge, and provide guidance for making decisions about the use of premedication. (2/10, reaffirmed 8/13)
http://pediatrics.aappublications.org/content/125/3/608

PRENATAL SUBSTANCE ABUSE: SHORT- AND LONG-TERM EFFECTS ON THE EXPOSED FETUS (TECHNICAL REPORT)

Marylou Behnke, MD; Vincent C. Smith, MD; Committee on Substance Abuse; and Committee on Fetus and Newborn
ABSTRACT. Prenatal substance abuse continues to be a significant problem in this country and poses important health risks for the developing fetus. The primary care

pediatrician's role in addressing prenatal substance exposure includes prevention, identification of exposure, recognition of medical issues for the exposed newborn infant, protection of the infant, and follow-up of the exposed infant. This report will provide information for the most common drugs involved in prenatal exposure: nicotine, alcohol, marijuana, opiates, cocaine, and methamphetamine. (2/13)
http://pediatrics.aappublications.org/content/131/3/e1009

THE PRENATAL VISIT (CLINICAL REPORT)

George J. Cohen, MD, and Committee on Psychosocial Aspects of Child and Family Health
ABSTRACT. As advocates for children and their families, pediatricians can support and guide expectant parents in the prenatal period. Prenatal visits allow the pediatrician to gather basic information from expectant parents, offer them information and advice, and identify high-risk conditions that may require special care. In addition, a prenatal visit is the first step in establishing a relationship between the family and the pediatrician (the infant's medical home) and in helping the parents develop parenting skills and confidence. There are several possible formats for this first visit. The one used depends on the experience and preference of the parents, the style of the pediatrician's practice, and pragmatic issues of reimbursement. (9/09, reaffirmed 5/14)
http://pediatrics.aappublications.org/content/124/4/1227

PREPARATION FOR EMERGENCIES IN THE OFFICES OF PEDIATRICIANS AND PEDIATRIC PRIMARY CARE PROVIDERS

Committee on Pediatric Emergency Medicine
ABSTRACT. High-quality pediatric emergency care can be provided only through the collaborative efforts of many health care professionals and child advocates working together throughout a continuum of care that extends from prevention and the medical home to prehospital care, to emergency department stabilization, to critical care and rehabilitation, and finally to a return to care in the medical home. At times, the office of the pediatric primary care provider will serve as the entry site into the emergency care system, which comprises out-of-hospital emergency medical services personnel, emergency department nurses and physicians, and other emergency and critical care providers. Recognizing the important role of pediatric primary care providers in the emergency care system for children and understanding the capabilities and limitations of that system are essential if pediatric primary care providers are to offer the best chance at intact survival for every child who is brought to the office with an emergency. Optimizing pediatric primary care provider office readiness for emergencies requires consideration of the unique aspects of each office practice, the types of patients and emergencies that might be seen, the resources on site, and the resources of the larger emergency care system of which the pediatric primary care provider's office is a part. Parent education regarding prevention, recognition, and response to emergencies, patient triage, early recognition and stabilization of pediatric emergencies in the office, and timely transfer to an appropriate facility for definitive care are important responsibilities of every pediatric primary care provider. In addition, pediatric primary care providers can collaborate with out-of-hospital and hospital-based providers and advocate for the best-quality emergency care for their patients. (7/07, reaffirmed 6/11)
http://pediatrics.aappublications.org/content/120/1/200

PREPARING FOR PEDIATRIC EMERGENCIES: DRUGS TO CONSIDER (CLINICAL REPORT)

Mary A. Hegenbarth, MD, and Committee on Drugs
ABSTRACT. This clinical report provides current recommendations regarding the selection and use of drugs in preparation for pediatric emergencies. It is not intended to be a comprehensive list of all medications that may be used in all emergencies. When possible, dosage recommendations are consistent with those used in current emergency references such as the *Advanced Pediatric Life Support and Pediatric Advanced Life Support* textbooks and the recently revised American Heart Association resuscitation guidelines. (2/08, reaffirmed 10/11, 2/16)
http://pediatrics.aappublications.org/content/121/2/433

PRESCRIBING ASSISTIVE-TECHNOLOGY SYSTEMS: FOCUS ON CHILDREN WITH IMPAIRED COMMUNICATION (CLINICAL REPORT)

Larry W. Desch, MD; Deborah Gaebler-Spira, MD; and Council on Children With Disabilities
ABSTRACT. This clinical report defines common terms of use and provides information on current practice, research, and limitations of assistive technology that can be used in systems for communication. The assessment process to determine the best devices for use with a particular child (ie, the best fit of a device) is also reviewed. The primary care pediatrician, as part of the medical home, plays an important role in the interdisciplinary effort to provide appropriate assistive technology and may be asked to make a referral for assessment or prescribe a particular device. This report provides resources to assist pediatricians in this role and reviews the interdisciplinary team functional evaluation using standardized assessments; the multiple funding opportunities available for obtaining devices and ways in which pediatricians can assist families with obtaining them; the training necessary to use these systems once the devices are procured; the follow-up evaluation to ensure that the systems are meeting their goals; and the leadership skills needed to advocate for this technology. The American Academy of Pediatrics acknowledges the need for key resources to be identified in the community and recognizes that these resources are a shared medical, educational, therapeutic, and family responsibility. Although this report primarily deals with assistive technology specific for communication impairments, many of the details in this report also can aid in the acquisition and use of other types of assistive technology. (6/08, reaffirmed 1/12)
http://pediatrics.aappublications.org/content/121/6/1271

PRESCRIBING THERAPY SERVICES FOR CHILDREN WITH MOTOR DISABILITIES (CLINICAL REPORT)

Committee on Children With Disabilities

ABSTRACT. Pediatricians often are called on to prescribe physical, occupational, and speech-language therapy services for children with motor disabilities. This report defines the context in which rehabilitation therapies should be prescribed, emphasizing the evaluation and enhancement of the child's function and abilities and participation in age-appropriate life roles. The report encourages pediatricians to work with teams including the parents, child, teachers, therapists, and other physicians to ensure that their patients receive appropriate therapy services. (6/04, reaffirmed 5/07, 5/11)

http://pediatrics.aappublications.org/content/113/6/1836

PRESERVATION OF FERTILITY IN PEDIATRIC AND ADOLESCENT PATIENTS WITH CANCER (TECHNICAL REPORT)

Mary E. Fallat, MD; John Hutter, MD; Committee on Bioethics; Section on Hematology/Oncology; and Section on Surgery

ABSTRACT. Many cancers that present in children and adolescents are curable with surgery, chemotherapy, and/or radiation therapy. Potential adverse consequences of treatment include sterility, infertility, or subfertility as a result of either gonad removal or damage to germ cells from adjuvant therapy. In recent years, treatment of solid tumors and hematologic malignancies has been modified in an attempt to reduce damage to the gonads. Simultaneously, advances in assisted reproductive techniques have led to new possibilities for the prevention and treatment of infertility. This technical report reviews the topic of fertility preservation in pediatric and adolescent patients with cancer, including ethical considerations. (5/08, reaffirmed 2/12)

http://pediatrics.aappublications.org/content/121/5/e1461

PREVENTING AND TREATING HOMESICKNESS (CLINICAL REPORT)

Christopher A. Thurber, PhD; Edward Walton, MD; and Council on School Health

ABSTRACT. Homesickness is the distress and functional impairment caused by an actual or anticipated separation from home and attachment objects such as parents. It is characterized by acute longing and preoccupying thoughts of home. Almost all children, adolescents, and adults experience some degree of homesickness when they are apart from familiar people and environments. Pediatricians and other health care professionals are in a unique position to assist families in understanding the etiology, prevention, and treatment of homesickness. In the case of planned separations, such as summer camp, techniques are provided that may aid in prevention. In the case of unanticipated or traumatic separations, such as hospitalization, effective treatment strategies are available. (1/07, reaffirmed 5/12)

http://pediatrics.aappublications.org/content/119/1/192

PREVENTING OBESITY AND EATING DISORDERS IN ADOLESCENTS (CLINICAL REPORT)

Neville H. Golden, MD, FAAP; Marcie Schneider, MD, FAAP; Christine Wood, MD, FAAP; Committee on Nutrition; Committee on Adolescence; and Section on Obesity

ABSTRACT. Obesity and eating disorders (EDs) are both prevalent in adolescents. There are concerns that obesity prevention efforts may lead to the development of an ED. Most adolescents who develop an ED did not have obesity previously, but some teenagers, in an attempt to lose weight, may develop an ED. This clinical report addresses the interaction between obesity prevention and EDs in teenagers, provides the pediatrician with evidence-informed tools to identify behaviors that predispose to both obesity and EDs, and provides guidance about obesity and ED prevention messages. The focus should be on a healthy lifestyle rather than on weight. Evidence suggests that obesity prevention and treatment, if conducted correctly, do not predispose to EDs. (8/16)

See full text on page 1069.

http://pediatrics.aappublications.org/content/138/3/e20161649

PREVENTION AND MANAGEMENT OF POSITIONAL SKULL DEFORMITIES IN INFANTS (CLINICAL REPORT)

James Laughlin, MD; Thomas G. Luerssen, MD; Mark S. Dias, MD; Committee on Practice and Ambulatory Medicine; and Section on Neurological Surgery

ABSTRACT. Positional skull deformities may be present at birth or may develop during the first few months of life. Since the early 1990s, US pediatricians have seen an increase in the number of children with cranial asymmetry, particularly unilateral flattening of the occiput, likely attributable to parents following the American Academy of Pediatrics "Back to Sleep" positioning recommendations aimed at decreasing the risk of sudden infant death syndrome. Positional skull deformities are generally benign, reversible head-shape anomalies that do not require surgical intervention, as opposed to craniosynostosis, which can result in neurologic damage and progressive craniofacial distortion. Although associated with some risk of positional skull deformity, healthy young infants should be placed down for sleep on their backs. The practice of putting infants to sleep on their backs has been associated with a drastic decrease in the incidence of sudden infant death syndrome. Pediatricians need to be able to properly differentiate infants with benign skull deformities from those with craniosynostosis, educate parents on methods of proactively decreasing the likelihood of the development of occipital flattening, initiate appropriate management, and make referrals when necessary. This report provides guidance for the prevention, diagnosis, and management of positional skull deformity in an otherwise normal infant without evidence of associated anomalies, syndromes, or spinal disease. (11/11)

http://pediatrics.aappublications.org/content/128/6/1236

PREVENTION AND MANAGEMENT OF PROCEDURAL PAIN IN THE NEONATE: AN UPDATE

Committee on Fetus and Newborn and Section on Anesthesiology and Pain Medicine

ABSTRACT. The prevention of pain in neonates should be the goal of all pediatricians and health care professionals who work with neonates, not only because it is ethical but also because repeated painful exposures have the potential for deleterious consequences. Neonates at greatest risk of neurodevelopmental impairment as a result of preterm birth (ie, the smallest and sickest) are also those most likely to be exposed to the greatest number of painful stimuli in the NICU. Although there are major gaps in knowledge regarding the most effective way to prevent and relieve pain in neonates, proven and safe therapies are currently underused for routine minor, yet painful procedures. Therefore, every health care facility caring for neonates should implement (1) a pain-prevention program that includes strategies for minimizing the number of painful procedures performed and (2) a pain assessment and management plan that includes routine assessment of pain, pharmacologic and nonpharmacologic therapies for the prevention of pain associated with routine minor procedures, and measures for minimizing pain associated with surgery and other major procedures. (1/16)

See full text on page 1081.

http://pediatrics.aappublications.org/content/137/2/e20154271

PREVENTION AND TREATMENT OF TYPE 2 DIABETES MELLITUS IN CHILDREN, WITH SPECIAL EMPHASIS ON AMERICAN INDIAN AND ALASKA NATIVE CHILDREN (CLINICAL REPORT)

Committee on Native American Child Health and Section on Endocrinology

ABSTRACT. The emergence of type 2 diabetes mellitus in the American Indian/Alaska Native pediatric population presents a new challenge for pediatricians and other health care professionals. This chronic disease requires preventive efforts, early diagnosis, and collaborative care of the patient and family within the context of a medical home. (10/03, reaffirmed 10/08)

http://pediatrics.aappublications.org/content/112/4/e328

PREVENTION OF AGRICULTURAL INJURIES AMONG CHILDREN AND ADOLESCENTS

Committee on Injury and Poison Prevention and Committee on Community Health Services

ABSTRACT. Although the annual number of farm deaths to children and adolescents has decreased since publication of the 1988 American Academy of Pediatrics statement, "Rural Injuries," the rate of nonfatal farm injuries has increased. Approximately 100 unintentional injury deaths occur annually to children and adolescents on US farms, and an additional 22 000 injuries to children younger than 20 years occur on farms. Relatively few adolescents are employed on farms compared with other types of industry, yet the proportion of fatalities in agriculture is higher than that for any other type of adolescent employment. The high mortality and severe morbidity associated with farm injuries require continuing and improved injury-control strategies. This statement provides recommendations for pediatricians regarding patient and community education as well as public advocacy related to agricultural injury prevention in childhood and adolescence. (10/01, reaffirmed 1/07, 11/11)

http://pediatrics.aappublications.org/content/108/4/1016

PREVENTION OF CHILDHOOD LEAD TOXICITY

Council on Environmental Health

ABSTRACT. Blood lead concentrations have decreased dramatically in US children over the past 4 decades, but too many children still live in housing with deteriorated lead-based paint and are at risk for lead exposure with resulting lead-associated cognitive impairment and behavioral problems. Evidence continues to accrue that commonly encountered blood lead concentrations, even those below 5 µg/dL (50 ppb), impair cognition; there is no identified threshold or safe level of lead in blood. From 2007 to 2010, approximately 2.6% of preschool children in the United States had a blood lead concentration ≥5 µg/dL (≥50 ppb), which represents about 535 000 US children 1 to 5 years of age. Evidence-based guidance is available for managing increased lead exposure in children, and reducing sources of lead in the environment, including lead in housing, soil, water, and consumer products, has been shown to be cost-beneficial. Primary prevention should be the focus of policy on childhood lead toxicity. (6/16)

See full text on page 1097.

http://pediatrics.aappublications.org/content/138/1/e20161493

PREVENTION OF CHOKING AMONG CHILDREN

Committee on Injury, Violence, and Poison Prevention

ABSTRACT. Choking is a leading cause of morbidity and mortality among children, especially those aged 3 years or younger. Food, coins, and toys are the primary causes of choking-related injury and death. Certain characteristics, including shape, size, and consistency, of certain toys and foods increase their potential to cause choking among children. Childhood choking hazards should be addressed through comprehensive and coordinated prevention activities. The US Consumer Product Safety Commission (CPSC) should increase efforts to ensure that toys that are sold in retail store bins, vending machines, or on the Internet have appropriate choking-hazard warnings; work with manufacturers to improve the effectiveness of recalls of products that pose a choking risk to children; and increase efforts to prevent the resale of these recalled products via online auction sites. Current gaps in choking-prevention standards for children's toys should be reevaluated and addressed, as appropriate, via revisions to the standards established under the Child Safety Protection Act, the Consumer Product Safety Improvement Act, or regulation by the CPSC. Prevention of food-related choking among children in the United States has been inadequately addressed at the federal level. The US Food and Drug Administration should establish a systematic, institutionalized process for examining and addressing the hazards of food-related choking. This process should include the establishment of the necessary surveillance, hazard evaluation, enforcement, and public education activities to prevent food-related choking among children.

While maintaining its highly cooperative arrangements with the CPSC and the US Department of Agriculture, the Food and Drug Administration should have the authority to address choking-related risks of all food products, including meat products that fall under the jurisdiction of the US Department of Agriculture. The existing National Electronic Injury Surveillance System–All Injury Program of the CPSC should be modified to conduct more-detailed surveillance of choking on food among children. Food manufacturers should design new foods and redesign existing foods to avoid shapes, sizes, textures, and other characteristics that increase choking risk to children, to the extent possible. Pediatricians, dentists, and other infant and child health care providers should provide choking-prevention counseling to parents as an integral part of anticipatory guidance activities. (2/10)
http://pediatrics.aappublications.org/content/125/3/601

PREVENTION OF DROWNING
Committee on Injury, Violence, and Poison Prevention
ABSTRACT. Drowning is a leading cause of injury-related death in children. In 2006, fatal drowning claimed the lives of approximately 1100 US children younger than 20 years. A number of strategies are available to prevent these tragedies. As educators and advocates, pediatricians can play an important role in the prevention of drowning. (5/10)
http://pediatrics.aappublications.org/content/126/1/178

PREVENTION OF DROWNING (TECHNICAL REPORT)
Jeffrey Weiss, MD, and Committee on Injury, Violence, and Poison Prevention
ABSTRACT. Drowning is a leading cause of injury-related death in children. In 2006, approximately 1100 US children younger than 20 years died from drowning. A number of strategies are available to prevent these tragedies. As educators and advocates, pediatricians can play an important role in the prevention of drowning. (5/10)
http://pediatrics.aappublications.org/content/126/1/e253

PREVENTION OF PEDIATRIC OVERWEIGHT AND OBESITY
Committee on Nutrition
ABSTRACT. The dramatic increase in the prevalence of childhood overweight and its resultant comorbidities are associated with significant health and financial burdens, warranting strong and comprehensive prevention efforts. This statement proposes strategies for early identification of excessive weight gain by using body mass index, for dietary and physical activity interventions during health supervision encounters, and for advocacy and research. (8/03, reaffirmed 10/06)
http://pediatrics.aappublications.org/content/112/2/424

PREVENTION OF ROTAVIRUS DISEASE: UPDATED GUIDELINES FOR USE OF ROTAVIRUS VACCINE
Committee on Infectious Diseases
ABSTRACT. This statement updates and replaces the 2007 American Academy of Pediatrics statement for prevention of rotavirus gastroenteritis. In February 2006, a live oral human-bovine reassortant rotavirus vaccine (RV5 [RotaTeq]) was licensed as a 3-dose series for use in infants

in the United States. The American Academy of Pediatrics recommended routine use of RV5 in infants in the United States. In April 2008, a live, oral, human attenuated rotavirus vaccine (RV1 [Rotarix]) was licensed as a 2-dose series for use in infants in the United States. The American Academy of Pediatrics recommends routine immunization of infants in the United States with rotavirus vaccine. The American Academy of Pediatrics does not express a preference for either RV5 or RV1. RV5 is to be administered orally in a 3-dose series with doses administered at 2, 4, and 6 months of age; RV1 is to be administered orally in a 2-dose series with doses administered at 2 and 4 months of age. The first dose of rotavirus vaccine should be administered from 6 weeks through 14 weeks, 6 days of age. The minimum interval between doses of rotavirus vaccine is 4 weeks. All doses should be administered by 8 months, 0 days of age. Recommendations in this statement also address the maximum ages for doses, contraindications, precautions, and special situations for administration of rotavirus vaccine. (3/09)
http://pediatrics.aappublications.org/content/123/5/1412

PREVENTION OF SEXUAL HARASSMENT IN THE WORKPLACE AND EDUCATIONAL SETTINGS
Committee on Pediatric Workforce
ABSTRACT. The American Academy of Pediatrics is committed to working to ensure that workplaces and educational settings in which pediatricians spend time are free of sexual harassment. The purpose of this statement is to heighten awareness and sensitivity to this important issue, recognizing that institutions, clinics, and office-based practices may have existing policies. (10/06, reaffirmed 5/09, 1/12, 10/14)
http://pediatrics.aappublications.org/content/118/4/1752

THE PREVENTION OF UNINTENTIONAL INJURY AMONG AMERICAN INDIAN AND ALASKA NATIVE CHILDREN: A SUBJECT REVIEW (CLINICAL REPORT)
Committee on Native American Child Health and Committee on Injury and Poison Prevention
ABSTRACT. Among ethnic groups in the United States, American Indian and Alaska Native (AI/AN) children experience the highest rates of injury mortality and morbidity. Injury mortality rates for AI/AN children have decreased during the past quarter century, but remain almost double the rate for all children in the United States. The Indian Health Service (IHS), the federal agency with the primary responsibility for the health care of AI/AN people, has sponsored an internationally recognized injury prevention program designed to reduce the risk of injury death by addressing community-specific risk factors. Model programs developed by the IHS and tribal governments have led to successful outcomes in motor vehicle occupant safety, drowning prevention, and fire safety. Injury prevention programs in tribal communities require special attention to the sovereignty of tribal governments and the unique cultural aspects of health care and communication. Pediatricians working with AI/AN children on reservations or in urban environments are strongly urged to collaborate with tribes and the IHS to create community-based coalitions and develop programs

to address highly preventable injury-related mortality and morbidity. Strong advocacy also is needed to promote childhood injury prevention as an important priority for federal agencies and tribes. (12/99, reaffirmed 12/02 COIVPP, 5/03 CONACH, 1/06, 1/09)
http://pediatrics.aappublications.org/content/104/6/1397

PREVENTIVE ORAL HEALTH INTERVENTION FOR PEDIATRICIANS

Section on Pediatric Dentistry and Oral Health
ABSTRACT. This policy is a compilation of current concepts and scientific evidence required to understand and implement practice-based preventive oral health programs designed to improve oral health outcomes for all children and especially children at significant risk of dental decay. In addition, it reviews cariology and caries risk assessment and defines, through available evidence, appropriate recommendations for preventive oral health intervention by primary care pediatric practitioners. (12/08)
http://pediatrics.aappublications.org/content/122/6/1387

PRINCIPLES FOR THE DEVELOPMENT AND USE OF QUALITY MEASURES

Steering Committee on Quality Improvement and Management and Committee on Practice and Ambulatory Medicine
ABSTRACT. The American Academy of Pediatrics and its members are committed to improving the health care system to provide the highest-quality and safest health care for infants, children, adolescents, and young adults. This statement is intended as a guide for pediatricians and pediatric leadership on the appropriate uses of quality measures and the criteria on which they should be based. The statement summarizes the current national efforts on quality measurement and provides a set of principles for the development, use, and evaluation of quality measures for improving children's health and health care. The American Academy of Pediatrics recommends that these measures address important issues for children; be appropriate for children's health and health care, scientifically valid, and feasible; and focus on what can be improved. In addition, the American Academy of Pediatrics supports reasonable principles for the oversight and implementation of pay-for-performance programs. (2/08)
http://pediatrics.aappublications.org/content/121/2/411

PRINCIPLES OF HEALTH CARE FINANCING

Committee on Child Health Financing
ABSTRACT. The American Academy of Pediatrics advocates that all children must have health insurance coverage that ensures them access to affordable and comprehensive quality care. Access to care depends on the design and implementation of payment systems that ensure the economic viability of the medical home; support and grow the professional pediatric workforce; promote the adoption and implementation of health information technology; enhance medical education, training, and research; and encourage and reward quality-improvement programs that advance and strengthen the medical home. Health insurance plans must be portable from state to state, with

administrative procedures to eliminate breaks and gaps in coverage to ensure continuous coverage from year to year. Plans should ensure free choice of clinicians and foster coordination with public and private community-based programs for infants, children, and adolescents through the age of 26. The scope of services provided by all health plans must include preventive, acute and chronic illness, behavioral, inpatient, emergency, and home health care. These plans must be affordable and have cost-sharing policies that protect patients and families from financial strain and are without risk of loss of benefits because of plan design, current illness, or preexisting condition. (10/10, reaffirmed 4/13)
http://pediatrics.aappublications.org/content/126/5/1018

PRINCIPLES OF JUDICIOUS ANTIBIOTIC PRESCRIBING FOR UPPER RESPIRATORY TRACT INFECTIONS IN PEDIATRICS (CLINICAL REPORT)

Committee on Infectious Diseases
ABSTRACT. Most upper respiratory tract infections are caused by viruses and require no antibiotics. This clinical report focuses on antibiotic prescribing strategies for bacterial upper respiratory tract infections, including acute otitis media, acute bacterial sinusitis, and streptococcal pharyngitis. The principles for judicious antibiotic prescribing that are outlined focus on applying stringent diagnostic criteria, weighing the benefits and harms of antibiotic therapy, and understanding situations when antibiotics may not be indicated. The principles can be used to amplify messages from recent clinical guidelines for local guideline development and for patient communication; they are broadly applicable to antibiotic prescribing in general. (11/13)
http://pediatrics.aappublications.org/content/132/6/1146

PRINCIPLES OF PEDIATRIC PATIENT SAFETY: REDUCING HARM DUE TO MEDICAL CARE

Steering Committee on Quality Improvement and Management and Committee on Hospital Care
ABSTRACT. Pediatricians are rendering care in an environment that is increasingly complex, which results in multiple opportunities to cause unintended harm. National awareness of patient safety risks has grown in the 10 years since the Institute of Medicine published its report *To Err Is Human,* and patients and society as a whole continue to challenge health care providers to examine their practices and implement safety solutions. The depth and breadth of harm incurred by the practice of medicine is still being defined as reports continue to uncover a variety of avoidable errors, from those that involve specific high-risk medications to those that are more generalizable, such as patient misidentification. Pediatricians in all venues must have a working knowledge of patient-safety language, advocate for best practices that attend to risks that are unique to children, identify and support a culture of safety, and lead efforts to eliminate avoidable harm in any setting in which medical care is rendered to children. (5/11)
http://pediatrics.aappublications.org/content/127/6/1199

PROBIOTICS AND PREBIOTICS IN PEDIATRICS (CLINICAL REPORT)

Dan W. Thomas, MD; Frank R. Greer, MD; Committee on Nutrition; and Section on Gastroenterology, Hepatology, and Nutrition

ABSTRACT. This clinical report reviews the currently known health benefits of probiotic and prebiotic products, including those added to commercially available infant formula and other food products for use in children. Probiotics are supplements or foods that contain viable microorganisms that cause alterations of the microflora of the host. Use of probiotics has been shown to be modestly effective in randomized clinical trials (RCTs) in (1) treating acute viral gastroenteritis in healthy children; and (2) preventing antibiotic-associated diarrhea in healthy children. There is some evidence that probiotics prevent necrotizing enterocolitis in very low birth weight infants (birth weight between 1000 and 1500 g), but more studies are needed. The results of RCTs in which probiotics were used to treat childhood *Helicobacter pylori* gastritis, irritable bowel syndrome, chronic ulcerative colitis, and infantile colic, as well as in preventing childhood atopy, although encouraging, are preliminary and require further confirmation. Probiotics have not been proven to be beneficial in treating or preventing human cancers or in treating children with Crohn disease. There are also safety concerns with the use of probiotics in infants and children who are immunocompromised, chronically debilitated, or seriously ill with indwelling medical devices.

Prebiotics are supplements or foods that contain a non-digestible food ingredient that selectively stimulates the favorable growth and/or activity of indigenous probiotic bacteria. Human milk contains substantial quantities of prebiotics. There is a paucity of RCTs examining prebiotics in children, although there may be some long-term benefit of prebiotics for the prevention of atopic eczema and common infections in healthy infants. Confirmatory well-designed clinical research studies are necessary. (11/10)

http://pediatrics.aappublications.org/content/126/6/1217

PROCEDURES FOR THE EVALUATION OF THE VISUAL SYSTEM BY PEDIATRICIANS (CLINICAL REPORT)

Sean P. Donahue, MD, PhD, FAAP; Cynthia N. Baker, MD, FAAP; Committee on Practice and Ambulatory Medicine; and Section on Ophthalmology (joint with American Association of Certified Orthoptists, American Association for Pediatric Ophthalmology and Strabismus, and American Academy of Ophthalmology)

ABSTRACT. Vision screening is crucial for the detection of visual and systemic disorders. It should begin in the newborn nursery and continue throughout childhood. This clinical report provides details regarding methods for pediatricians to use for screening. (12/15)

http://pediatrics.aappublications.org/content/137/1/e20153597

PROFESSIONAL LIABILITY INSURANCE AND MEDICOLEGAL EDUCATION FOR PEDIATRIC RESIDENTS AND FELLOWS

Committee on Medical Liability and Risk Management

ABSTRACT. The American Academy of Pediatrics believes that pediatric residents and fellows should be fully informed of the scope and limitations of their professional liability insurance coverage while in training. The academy states that residents and fellows should be educated by their training institutions on matters relating to medical liability and the importance of maintaining adequate and continuous professional liability insurance coverage throughout their careers in medicine. (8/11)

http://pediatrics.aappublications.org/content/128/3/624

PROFESSIONALISM IN PEDIATRICS (TECHNICAL REPORT)

Mary E. Fallat, MD; Jacqueline Glover, PhD; and Committee on Bioethics

ABSTRACT. The purpose of this report is to provide a concrete overview of the ideal standards of behavior and professional practice to which pediatricians should aspire and by which students and residents can be evaluated. Recognizing that the ideal is not always achievable in the practical sense, this document details the key components of professionalism in pediatric practice with an emphasis on core professional values for which pediatricians should strive and that will serve as a moral compass needed to provide quality care for children and their families. (10/07, reaffirmed 5/11)

http://pediatrics.aappublications.org/content/120/4/e1123

PROFESSIONALISM IN PEDIATRICS: STATEMENT OF PRINCIPLES

Committee on Bioethics

ABSTRACT. The purpose of this statement is to delineate the concept of professionalism within the context of pediatrics and to provide a brief statement of principles to guide the behavior and professional practice of pediatricians. (10/07, reaffirmed 5/11)

http://pediatrics.aappublications.org/content/120/4/895

PROMOTING EDUCATION, MENTORSHIP, AND SUPPORT FOR PEDIATRIC RESEARCH

Committee on Pediatric Research

ABSTRACT. Pediatricians play a key role in advancing child health research to best attain and improve the physical, mental, and social health and well-being of all infants, children, adolescents, and young adults. Child health presents unique issues that require investigators who specialize in pediatric research. In addition, the scope of the pediatric research enterprise is transdisciplinary and includes the full spectrum of basic science, translational, community-based, health services, and child health policy research. Although most pediatricians do not directly engage in research, knowledge of research methodologies and approaches promotes critical evaluation of scientific literature, the practice of evidence-based medicine, and advocacy for evidence-based child health policy. This statement includes specific recommendations to promote further research education and support at all levels of pediatric training, from premedical to continuing medi-

cal education, as well as recommendations to increase support and mentorship for research activities. Pediatric research is crucial to the American Academy of Pediatrics' goal of improving the health of all children. The American Academy of Pediatrics continues to promote and encourage efforts to facilitate the creation of new knowledge and ways to reduce barriers experienced by trainees, practitioners, and academic faculty pursuing research. (4/14)
http://pediatrics.aappublications.org/content/133/5/943

PROMOTING FOOD SECURITY FOR ALL CHILDREN
Council on Community Pediatrics and Committee on Nutrition
ABSTRACT. Sixteen million US children (21%) live in households without consistent access to adequate food. After multiple risk factors are considered, children who live in households that are food insecure, even at the lowest levels, are likely to be sick more often, recover from illness more slowly, and be hospitalized more frequently. Lack of adequate healthy food can impair a child's ability to concentrate and perform well in school and is linked to higher levels of behavioral and emotional problems from preschool through adolescence. Food insecurity can affect children in any community, not only traditionally underserved ones. Pediatricians can play a central role in screening and identifying children at risk for food insecurity and in connecting families with needed community resources. Pediatricians should also advocate for federal and local policies that support access to adequate healthy food for an active and healthy life for all children and their families. (10/15)
http://pediatrics.aappublications.org/content/136/5/e1431

PROMOTING OPTIMAL DEVELOPMENT: SCREENING FOR BEHAVIORAL AND EMOTIONAL PROBLEMS (CLINICAL REPORT)
Carol Weitzman, MD, FAAP; Lynn Wegner, MD, FAAP; Section on Developmental and Behavioral Pediatrics; Committee on Psychosocial Aspects of Child and Family Health; and Council on Early Childhood (joint with Society for Developmental and Behavioral Pediatrics)
ABSTRACT. By current estimates, at any given time, approximately 11% to 20% of children in the United States have a behavioral or emotional disorder, as defined in the *Diagnostic and Statistical Manual of Mental Disorders, Fifth Edition*. Between 37% and 39% of children will have a behavioral or emotional disorder diagnosed by 16 years of age, regardless of geographic location in the United States. Behavioral and emotional problems and concerns in children and adolescents are not being reliably identified or treated in the US health system. This clinical report focuses on the need to increase behavioral screening and offers potential changes in practice and the health system, as well as the research needed to accomplish this. This report also (1) reviews the prevalence of behavioral and emotional disorders, (2) describes factors affecting the emergence of behavioral and emotional problems, (3) articulates the current state of detection of these problems in pediatric primary care, (4) describes barriers to screening and means to overcome those barriers, and (5) discusses potential changes at a practice and systems level that are needed to facilitate successful behavioral and emotional screening. Highlighted and discussed are the many factors at the level of the pediatric practice, health system, and society contributing to these behavioral and emotional problems. (1/15)
http://pediatrics.aappublications.org/content/135/2/384

PROMOTING THE PARTICIPATION OF CHILDREN WITH DISABILITIES IN SPORTS, RECREATION, AND PHYSICAL ACTIVITIES (CLINICAL REPORT)
Nancy A. Murphy, MD; Paul S. Carbone, MD; and Council on Children With Disabilities
ABSTRACT. The benefits of physical activity are universal for all children, including those with disabilities. The participation of children with disabilities in sports and recreational activities promotes inclusion, minimizes deconditioning, optimizes physical functioning, and enhances overall well-being. Despite these benefits, children with disabilities are more restricted in their participation, have lower levels of fitness, and have higher levels of obesity than their peers without disabilities. Pediatricians and parents may overestimate the risks or overlook the benefits of physical activity in children with disabilities. Well-informed decisions regarding each child's participation must consider overall health status, individual activity preferences, safety precautions, and availability of appropriate programs and equipment. Health supervision visits afford pediatricians, children with disabilities, and parents opportunities to collaboratively generate goal-directed activity "prescriptions." Child, family, financial, and societal barriers to participation need to be directly identified and addressed in the context of local, state, and federal laws. The goal is inclusion for all children with disabilities in appropriate activities. This clinical report discusses the importance of physical activity, recreation, and sports participation for children with disabilities and offers practical suggestions to pediatric health care professionals for the promotion of participation. (5/08, reaffirmed 1/12)
http://pediatrics.aappublications.org/content/121/5/1057

PROMOTING THE WELL-BEING OF CHILDREN WHOSE PARENTS ARE GAY OR LESBIAN
Committee on Psychosocial Aspects of Child and Family Health
ABSTRACT. To promote optimal health and well-being of all children, the American Academy of Pediatrics (AAP) supports access for all children to (1) civil marriage rights for their parents and (2) willing and capable foster and adoptive parents, regardless of the parents' sexual orientation. The AAP has always been an advocate for, and has developed policies to support, the optimal physical, mental, and social health and well-being of all infants, children, adolescents, and young adults. In so doing, the AAP has supported families in all their diversity, because the family has always been the basic social unit in which children develop the supporting and nurturing relationships with adults that they need to thrive. Children may be born to, adopted by, or cared for temporarily by married couples, nonmarried couples, single parents, grandparents, or legal guardians, and any of these may be heterosexual, gay or

lesbian, or of another orientation. Children need secure and enduring relationships with committed and nurturing adults to enhance their life experiences for optimal social-emotional and cognitive development. Scientific evidence affirms that children have similar developmental and emotional needs and receive similar parenting whether they are raised by parents of the same or different genders. If a child has 2 living and capable parents who choose to create a permanent bond by way of civil marriage, it is in the best interests of their child(ren) that legal and social institutions allow and support them to do so, irrespective of their sexual orientation. If 2 parents are not available to the child, adoption or foster parenting remain acceptable options to provide a loving home for a child and should be available without regard to the sexual orientation of the parent(s). (3/13)
http://pediatrics.aappublications.org/content/131/4/827

PROMOTING THE WELL-BEING OF CHILDREN WHOSE PARENTS ARE GAY OR LESBIAN (TECHNICAL REPORT)
Ellen C. Perrin, MD, MA; Benjamin S. Siegel, MD; and Committee on Psychosocial Aspects of Child and Family Health

ABSTRACT. Extensive data available from more than 30 years of research reveal that children raised by gay and lesbian parents have demonstrated resilience with regard to social, psychological, and sexual health despite economic and legal disparities and social stigma. Many studies have demonstrated that children's well-being is affected much more by their relationships with their parents, their parents' sense of competence and security, and the presence of social and economic support for the family than by the gender or the sexual orientation of their parents. Lack of opportunity for same-gender couples to marry adds to families' stress, which affects the health and welfare of all household members. Because marriage strengthens families and, in so doing, benefits children's development, children should not be deprived of the opportunity for their parents to be married. Paths to parenthood that include assisted reproductive techniques, adoption, and foster parenting should focus on competency of the parents rather than their sexual orientation. (3/13)
http://pediatrics.aappublications.org/content/131/4/e1374

PROMOTION OF HEALTHY WEIGHT-CONTROL PRACTICES IN YOUNG ATHLETES
Committee on Sports Medicine and Fitness

ABSTRACT. Children and adolescents are often involved in sports in which weight loss or weight gain is perceived as an advantage. This policy statement describes unhealthy weight-control practices that may be harmful to the health and/or performance of athletes. Healthy methods of weight loss and weight gain are discussed, and physicians are given resources and recommendations that can be used to counsel athletes, parents, coaches, and school administrators in discouraging inappropriate weight-control behaviors and encouraging healthy methods of weight gain or loss, when needed. (12/05)
http://pediatrics.aappublications.org/content/116/6/1557

PROTECTING CHILDREN FROM SEXUAL ABUSE BY HEALTH CARE PROVIDERS
Committee on Child Abuse and Neglect

ABSTRACT. Sexual abuse or exploitation of children is never acceptable. Such behavior by health care providers is particularly concerning because of the trust that children and their families place on adults in the health care profession. The American Academy of Pediatrics strongly endorses the social and moral prohibition against sexual abuse or exploitation of children by health care providers. The academy opposes any such sexual abuse or exploitation by providers, particularly by the academy's members. Health care providers should be trained to recognize and abide by appropriate provider-patient boundaries. Medical institutions should screen staff members for a history of child abuse issues, train them to respect and maintain appropriate boundaries, and establish policies and procedures to receive and investigate concerns about patient abuse. Each person has a responsibility to ensure the safety of children in health care settings and to scrupulously follow appropriate legal and ethical reporting and investigation procedures. (6/11, reaffirmed 10/14)
http://pediatrics.aappublications.org/content/128/2/407

PROTECTING CHILDREN FROM TOBACCO, NICOTINE, AND TOBACCO SMOKE (TECHNICAL REPORT)
Harold J. Farber, MD, MSPH, FAAP; Judith Groner, MD, FAAP; Susan Walley, MD, FAAP; Kevin Nelson, MD, PhD, FAAP; and Section on Tobacco Control

ABSTRACT. This technical report serves to provide the evidence base for the American Academy of Pediatrics' policy statements "Clinical Practice Policy to Protect Children From Tobacco, Nicotine, and Tobacco Smoke" and "Public Policy to Protect Children From Tobacco, Nicotine, and Tobacco Smoke." Tobacco use and involuntary exposure are major preventable causes of morbidity and premature mortality in adults and children. Tobacco dependence almost always starts in childhood or adolescence. Electronic nicotine delivery systems are rapidly gaining popularity among youth, and their significant harms are being documented. In utero tobacco smoke exposure, in addition to increasing the risk of preterm birth, low birth weight, stillbirth, placental abruption, and sudden infant death, has been found to increase the risk of obesity and neurodevelopmental disorders. Actions by pediatricians can help to reduce children's risk of developing tobacco dependence and reduce children's involuntary tobacco smoke exposure. Public policy actions to protect children from tobacco are essential to reduce the toll that the tobacco epidemic takes on our children. (10/15)
http://pediatrics.aappublications.org/content/136/5/e1439

PROTECTIVE EYEWEAR FOR YOUNG ATHLETES
Committee on Sports Medicine and Fitness (joint with American Academy of Ophthalmology)

ABSTRACT. The American Academy of Pediatrics and American Academy of Ophthalmology strongly recommend protective eyewear for all participants in sports in which there is risk of eye injury. Protective eyewear should be mandatory for athletes who are functionally 1-eyed and for athletes whose ophthalmologists recom-

mend eye protection after eye surgery or trauma. (3/04, reaffirmed 2/08, 6/11, 2/15)
http://pediatrics.aappublications.org/content/113/3/619

PROVIDING A PRIMARY CARE MEDICAL HOME FOR CHILDREN AND YOUTH WITH CEREBRAL PALSY (CLINICAL REPORT)

Gregory S. Liptak, MD, MPH; Nancy A. Murphy, MD; and Council on Children With Disabilities

ABSTRACT. All primary care providers will care for children with cerebral palsy in their practice. In addition to well-child and acute illness care, the role of the medical home in the management of these children includes diagnosis, planning for interventions, authorizing treatments, and follow-up. Optimizing health and well-being for children with cerebral palsy and their families entails family-centered care provided in the medical home; comanagement is the most common model. This report reviews the aspects of care specific to cerebral palsy that a medical home should provide beyond the routine health care needed by all children. (10/11, reaffirmed 11/14)
http://pediatrics.aappublications.org/content/128/5/e1321

PROVIDING A PRIMARY CARE MEDICAL HOME FOR CHILDREN AND YOUTH WITH SPINA BIFIDA (CLINICAL REPORT)

Robert Burke, MD, MPH; Gregory S. Liptak, MD, MPH; and Council on Children With Disabilities

ABSTRACT. The pediatric primary care provider in the medical home has a central and unique role in the care of children with spina bifida. The primary care provider addresses not only the typical issues of preventive and acute health care but also the needs specific to these children. Optimal care requires communication and comanagement with pediatric medical and developmental subspecialists, surgical specialists, therapists, and community providers. The medical home provider is essential in supporting the family and advocating for the child from the time of entry into the practice through adolescence, which includes transition and transfer to adult health care. This report reviews aspects of care specific to the infant with spina bifida (particularly myelomeningocele) that will facilitate optimal medical, functional, and developmental outcomes. (11/11, reaffirmed 2/15)
http://pediatrics.aappublications.org/content/128/6/e1645

PROVIDING CARE FOR CHILDREN AND ADOLESCENTS FACING HOMELESSNESS AND HOUSING INSECURITY

Council on Community Pediatrics

ABSTRACT. Child health and housing security are closely intertwined, and children without homes are more likely to suffer from chronic disease, hunger, and malnutrition than are children with homes. Homeless children and youth often have significant psychosocial development issues, and their education is frequently interrupted. Given the overall effects that homelessness can have on a child's health and potential, it is important for pediatricians to recognize the factors that lead to homelessness, understand the ways that homelessness and its causes can lead to poor health outcomes, and when possible, help children and families mitigate some of the effects of homelessness. Through practice change, partnership with community resources, awareness, and advocacy, pediatricians can help optimize the health and well-being of children affected by homelessness. (5/13)
http://pediatrics.aappublications.org/content/131/6/1206

PROVIDING CARE FOR IMMIGRANT, MIGRANT, AND BORDER CHILDREN

Council on Community Pediatrics

ABSTRACT. This policy statement, which recognizes the large changes in immigrant status since publication of the 2005 statement "Providing Care for Immigrant, Homeless, and Migrant Children," focuses on strategies to support the health of immigrant children, infants, adolescents, and young adults. Homeless children will be addressed in a forthcoming separate statement ("Providing Care for Children and Adolescents Facing Homelessness and Housing Insecurity"). While recognizing the diversity across and within immigrant, migrant, and border populations, this statement provides a basic framework for serving and advocating for all immigrant children, with a particular focus on low-income and vulnerable populations. Recommendations include actions needed within and outside the health care system, including expansion of access to high-quality medical homes with culturally and linguistically effective care as well as education and literacy programs. The statement recognizes the unique and special role that pediatricians can play in the lives of immigrant children and families. Recommendations for policies that support immigrant child health are included. (5/13)
http://pediatrics.aappublications.org/content/131/6/e2028

PROVIDING PSYCHOSOCIAL SUPPORT TO CHILDREN AND FAMILIES IN THE AFTERMATH OF DISASTERS AND CRISES (CLINICAL REPORT)

David J. Schonfeld, MD, FAAP; Thomas Demaria, PhD; Disaster Preparedness Advisory Council; and Committee on Psychosocial Aspects of Child and Family Health

ABSTRACT. Disasters have the potential to cause short- and long-term effects on the psychological functioning, emotional adjustment, health, and developmental trajectory of children. This clinical report provides practical suggestions on how to identify common adjustment difficulties in children in the aftermath of a disaster and to promote effective coping strategies to mitigate the impact of the disaster as well as any associated bereavement and secondary stressors. This information can serve as a guide to pediatricians as they offer anticipatory guidance to families or consultation to schools, child care centers, and other child congregate care sites. Knowledge of risk factors for adjustment difficulties can serve as the basis for mental health triage. The importance of basic supportive services, psychological first aid, and professional self-care are discussed. Stress is intrinsic to many major life events that children and families face, including the experience of significant illness and its treatment. The information provided in this clinical report may, therefore, be relevant for a broad range of patient encounters, even outside the context of a disaster. Most pediatricians enter the profession because of a heartfelt desire to help children and families most in need. If adequately prepared and supported, pediatricians who are able to draw on their skills to assist children, families, and communities to recover after a disaster will find the work to be particularly rewarding. (9/15) http://pediatrics.aappublications.org/content/136/4/e1120

PROVISION OF EDUCATIONALLY RELATED SERVICES FOR CHILDREN AND ADOLESCENTS WITH CHRONIC DISEASES AND DISABLING CONDITIONS

Council on Children With Disabilities

ABSTRACT. Children and adolescents with chronic diseases and disabling conditions often need educationally related services. As medical home providers, physicians and other health care professionals can assist children, adolescents, and their families with the complex federal, state, and local laws, regulations, and systems associated with these services. Expanded roles for physicians and other health care professionals in individualized family service plan, individualized education plan, and Section 504 plan development and implementation are recommended. Recent updates to the Individuals With Disabilities Education Act will also affect these services. Funding for these services by private and nonprivate sources also continue to affect the availability of these educationally related services.

The complex range of federal, state, and local laws, regulations, and systems for special education and related services for children and adolescents in public schools is beyond the scope of this statement. Readers are referred to the American Academy of Pediatrics policy statement "The Pediatrician's Role in Development and Implementation of an Individual Education Plan (IEP) and/or an Individual Family Service Plan (IFSP)" for additional background materials. The focus of this statement is the role that health care professionals have in determining and managing educationally related services in the school setting.

This policy statement is a revision of a previous statement, "Provision of Educationally Related Services for Children and Adolescents With Chronic Diseases and Disabling Conditions," published in February 2000 by the Committee on Children With Disabilities (http://aappolicy.aappublications.org/cgi/content/full/pediatrics;105/2/448). (6/07, reaffirmed 11/14) http://pediatrics.aappublications.org/content/119/6/1218

PSYCHOLOGICAL MALTREATMENT (CLINICAL REPORT)

Roberta Hibbard, MD; Jane Barlow, DPhil; Harriet MacMillan, MD; Committee on Child Abuse and Neglect (joint with American Academy of Child and Adolescent Psychiatry Child Maltreatment and Violence Committee)

ABSTRACT. Psychological or emotional maltreatment of children may be the most challenging and prevalent form of child abuse and neglect. Caregiver behaviors include acts of omission (ignoring need for social interactions) or commission (spurning, terrorizing); may be verbal or nonverbal, active or passive, and with or without intent to harm; and negatively affect the child's cognitive, social, emotional, and/or physical development. Psychological maltreatment has been linked with disorders of attachment, developmental and educational problems, socialization problems, disruptive behavior, and later psychopathology. Although no evidence-based interventions that can prevent psychological maltreatment have been identified to date, it is possible that interventions shown to be effective in reducing overall types of child maltreatment, such as the Nurse Family Partnership, may have a role to play. Furthermore, prevention before occurrence will require both the use of universal interventions aimed at promoting the type of parenting that is now recognized to be necessary for optimal child development, alongside the use of targeted interventions directed at improving parental sensitivity to a child's cues during infancy and later parent-child interactions. Intervention should, first and foremost, focus on a thorough assessment and ensuring the child's safety. Potentially effective treatments include cognitive behavioral parenting programs and other psychotherapeutic interventions. The high prevalence of psychological abuse in advanced Western societies, along with the serious consequences, point to the importance of effective management. Pediatricians should be alert to the occurrence of psychological maltreatment and identify ways to support families who have risk indicators for, or evidence of, this problem. (7/12, reaffirmed 4/16) http://pediatrics.aappublications.org/content/130/2/372

PSYCHOSOCIAL IMPLICATIONS OF DISASTER OR TERRORISM ON CHILDREN: A GUIDE FOR THE PEDIATRICIAN (CLINICAL REPORT)

Joseph F. Hagan Jr, MD; Committee on Psychosocial Aspects of Child and Family Health; and Task Force on Terrorism

ABSTRACT. During and after disasters, pediatricians can assist parents and community leaders not only by accommodating the unique needs of children but also by being cognizant of the psychological responses of children to reduce the possibility of long-term psychological morbidity. The effects of disaster on children are mediated by many factors including personal experience, parental reaction, developmental competency, gender, and the stage of disaster response. Pediatricians can be effective advocates for the child and family and at the community level and can affect national policy in support of families. In this report, specific children's responses are delineated, risk factors for adverse reactions are discussed, and advice is given for pediatricians to ameliorate the effects of disaster on children. (9/05, reaffirmed 11/14) http://pediatrics.aappublications.org/content/116/3/787

PSYCHOSOCIAL RISKS OF CHRONIC HEALTH CONDITIONS IN CHILDHOOD AND ADOLESCENCE

Committee on Children With Disabilities and Committee on Psychosocial Aspects of Child and Family Health (12/93, reaffirmed 10/96)

http://pediatrics.aappublications.org/content/92/6/876

PSYCHOSOCIAL SUPPORT FOR YOUTH LIVING WITH HIV (CLINICAL REPORT)

Jaime Martinez, MD, FAAP; Rana Chakraborty, MD, FAAP; and Committee on Pediatric AIDS

ABSTRACT. This clinical report provides guidance for the pediatrician in addressing the psychosocial needs of adolescents and young adults living with HIV, which can improve linkage to care and adherence to life-saving antiretroviral (ARV) therapy. Recent national case surveillance data for youth (defined here as adolescents

and young adults 13 to 24 years of age) revealed that the burden of HIV/AIDS fell most heavily and disproportionately on African American youth, particularly males having sex with males. To effectively increase linkage to care and sustain adherence to therapy, interventions should address the immediate drivers of ARV compliance and also address factors that provide broader social and structural support for HIV-infected adolescents and young adults. Interventions should address psychosocial development, including lack of future orientation, inadequate educational attainment and limited health literacy, failure to focus on the long-term consequences of near-term risk behaviors, and coping ability. Associated challenges are closely linked to the structural environment. Individual case management is essential to linkage to and retention in care, ARV adherence, and management of associated comorbidities. Integrating these skills into pediatric and adolescent HIV practice in a medical home setting is critical, given the alarming increase in new HIV infections in youth in the United States. (2/14)
http://pediatrics.aappublications.org/content/133/3/558

PUBLIC POLICY TO PROTECT CHILDREN FROM TOBACCO, NICOTINE, AND TOBACCO SMOKE

Section on Tobacco Control

ABSTRACT. Tobacco use and tobacco smoke exposure are among the most important health threats to children, adolescents, and adults. There is no safe level of tobacco smoke exposure. The developing brains of children and adolescents are particularly vulnerable to the development of tobacco and nicotine dependence. Tobacco is unique among consumer products in that it causes disease and death when used exactly as intended. Tobacco continues to be heavily promoted to children and young adults. Flavored and alternative tobacco products, including little cigars, chewing tobacco, and electronic nicotine delivery systems, are gaining popularity among youth. This statement describes important evidence-based public policy actions that, when implemented, will reduce tobacco product use and tobacco smoke exposure among youth and, by doing so, improve the health of children and young adults. (10/15)
http://pediatrics.aappublications.org/content/136/5/998

QUALITY EARLY EDUCATION AND CHILD CARE FROM BIRTH TO KINDERGARTEN

Committee on Early Childhood, Adoption, and Dependent Care

ABSTRACT. High-quality early education and child care for young children improves their health and promotes their development and learning. Early education includes all of a child's experiences at home, in child care, and in other preschool settings. Pediatricians have a role in promoting access to quality early education and child care beginning at birth for all children. The American Academy of Pediatrics affords pediatricians the opportunity to promote the educational and socioemotional needs of young children with other advocacy groups. (1/05, reaffirmed 12/09)
http://pediatrics.aappublications.org/content/115/1/187

RACE, ETHNICITY, AND SOCIOECONOMIC STATUS IN RESEARCH ON CHILD HEALTH

Tina L. Cheng, MD, MPH, FAAP; Elizabeth Goodman, MD, FAAP; and Committee on Pediatric Research

ABSTRACT. An extensive literature documents the existence of pervasive and persistent child health, development, and health care disparities by race, ethnicity, and socioeconomic status (SES). Disparities experienced during childhood can result in a wide variety of health and health care outcomes, including adult morbidity and mortality, indicating that it is crucial to examine the influence of disparities across the life course. Studies often collect data on the race, ethnicity, and SES of research participants to be used as covariates or explanatory factors. In the past, these variables have often been assumed to exert their effects through individual or genetically determined biologic mechanisms. However, it is now widely accepted that these variables have important social dimensions that influence health. SES, a multidimensional construct, interacts with and confounds analyses of race and ethnicity. Because SES, race, and ethnicity are often difficult to measure accurately, leading to the potential for misattribution of causality, thoughtful consideration should be given to appropriate measurement, analysis, and interpretation of such factors. Scientists who study child and adolescent health and development should understand the multiple measures used to assess race, ethnicity, and SES, including their validity and shortcomings and potential confounding of race and ethnicity with SES. The American Academy of Pediatrics (AAP) recommends that research on eliminating health and health care disparities related to race, ethnicity, and SES be a priority. Data on race, ethnicity, and SES should be collected in research on child health to improve their definitions and increase understanding of how these factors and their complex interrelationships affect child health. Furthermore, the AAP believes that researchers should consider both biological and social mechanisms of action of race, ethnicity, and SES as they relate to the aims and hypothesis of the specific area of investigation. It is important to measure these variables, but it is not sufficient to use these variables alone as explanatory for differences in disease, morbidity, and outcomes without attention to the social and biologic influences they have on health throughout the life course. The AAP recommends more research, both in the United States and internationally, on measures of race, ethnicity, and SES and how these complex constructs affect health care and health outcomes throughout the life course. (12/14)
http://pediatrics.aappublications.org/content/135/1/e225

RACIAL AND ETHNIC DISPARITIES IN THE HEALTH AND HEALTH CARE OF CHILDREN (TECHNICAL REPORT)

Glenn Flores, MD, and Committee on Pediatric Research

ABSTRACT. *Objective.* This technical report reviews and synthesizes the published literature on racial/ethnic disparities in children's health and health care.

Methods. A systematic review of the literature was conducted for articles published between 1950 and March 2007. Inclusion criteria were peer-reviewed, original research articles in English on racial/ethnic disparities in the health and health care of US children. Search terms used included "child," "disparities," and the Index Medicus terms for each racial/ethnic minority group.

Results. Of 781 articles initially reviewed, 111 met inclusion criteria and constituted the final database. Review of the literature revealed that racial/ethnic disparities in children's health and health care are quite extensive, pervasive, and persistent. Disparities were noted across the spectrum of health and health care, including in mortality rates, access to care and use of services, prevention and population health, health status, adolescent health, chronic diseases, special health care needs, quality of care, and organ transplantation. Mortality-rate disparities were noted for children in all 4 major US racial/ethnic minority groups, including substantially greater risks than white children of all-cause mortality; death from drowning, from acute lymphoblastic leukemia, and after congenital heart defect surgery; and an earlier median age at death for those with Down syndrome and congenital heart defects. Certain methodologic flaws were commonly observed among excluded studies, including failure to evaluate children separately from adults (22%), combining all nonwhite children into 1 group (9%), and failure to provide a white comparison group (8%). Among studies in the final database, 22% did not perform multivariable or stratified analyses to ensure that disparities persisted after adjustment for potential confounders.

Conclusions. Racial/ethnic disparities in children's health and health care are extensive, pervasive, and persistent, and occur across the spectrum of health and health care. Methodologic flaws were identified in how such disparities are sometimes documented and analyzed. Optimal health and health care for all children will require recognition of disparities as pervasive problems, methodologically sound disparities studies, and rigorous evaluation of disparities interventions. (3/10, reaffirmed 5/13)
http://pediatrics.aappublications.org/content/125/4/e979

RADIATION DISASTERS AND CHILDREN
Committee on Environmental Health
ABSTRACT. The special medical needs of children make it essential that pediatricians be prepared for radiation disasters, including (1) the detonation of a nuclear weapon; (2) a nuclear power plant event that unleashes a radioactive cloud; and (3) the dispersal of radionuclides by conventional explosive or the crash of a transport vehicle. Any of these events could occur unintentionally or as an act of terrorism. Nuclear facilities (eg, power plants, fuel processing centers, and food irradiation facilities) are often located in highly populated areas, and as they age, the risk of mechanical failure increases. The short- and long-term consequences of a radiation disaster are significantly greater in children for several reasons. First, children have a disproportionately higher minute ventilation, leading to greater internal exposure to radioactive gases. Children have a significantly greater risk of developing cancer even when they are exposed to radiation in utero. Finally, children and the parents of young children are more likely than are adults to develop enduring psychologic injury after a radiation disaster. The pediatrician has a critical role in planning for radiation disasters. For example, potassium iodide is of proven value for thyroid

protection but must be given before or soon after exposure to radioiodines, requiring its placement in homes, schools, and child care centers. Pediatricians should work with public health authorities to ensure that children receive full consideration in local planning for a radiation disaster. (6/03, reaffirmed 1/07)
http://pediatrics.aappublications.org/content/111/6/1455

RADIATION RISK TO CHILDREN FROM COMPUTED TOMOGRAPHY (CLINICAL REPORT)
Alan S. Brody, MD; Donald P. Frush, MD; Walter Huda, PhD; Robert L. Brent, MD, PhD; and Section on Radiology
ABSTRACT. Imaging studies that use ionizing radiation are an essential tool for the evaluation of many disorders of childhood. Ionizing radiation is used in radiography, fluoroscopy, angiography, and computed tomography scanning. Computed tomography is of particular interest because of its relatively high radiation dose and wide use. Consensus statements on radiation risk suggest that it is reasonable to act on the assumption that low-level radiation may have a small risk of causing cancer. The medical community should seek ways to decrease radiation exposure by using radiation doses as low as reasonably achievable and by performing these studies only when necessary. There is wide agreement that the benefits of an indicated computed tomography scan far outweigh the risks. Pediatric health care professionals' roles in the use of computed tomography on children include deciding when a computed tomography scan is necessary and discussing the risk with patients and families. Radiologists should be a source of consultation when forming imaging strategies and should create specific protocols with scanning techniques optimized for pediatric patients. Families and patients should be encouraged to ask questions about the risks and benefits of computed tomography scanning. The information in this report is provided to aid in decision-making and discussions with the health care team, patients, and families. (9/07)
http://pediatrics.aappublications.org/content/120/3/677

RECOGNITION AND MANAGEMENT OF IATROGENICALLY INDUCED OPIOID DEPENDENCE AND WITHDRAWAL IN CHILDREN (CLINICAL REPORT)
Jeffrey Galinkin, MD, FAAP; Jeffrey Lee Koh, MD, FAAP; Committee on Drugs; and Section on Anesthesiology and Pain Medicine
ABSTRACT. Opioids are often prescribed to children for pain relief related to procedures, acute injuries, and chronic conditions. Round-the-clock dosing of opioids can produce opioid dependence within 5 days. According to a 2001 consensus paper from the American Academy of Pain Medicine, American Pain Society, and American Society of Addiction Medicine, dependence is defined as "a state of adaptation that is manifested by a drug class specific withdrawal syndrome that can be produced by abrupt cessation, rapid dose reduction, decreasing blood level of the drug, and/or administration of an antagonist." Although the experience of many children undergoing iatrogenically induced withdrawal may be mild or goes unreported, there is currently no guidance for recognition or management of withdrawal for this population. Guidance on this subject is available only for adults and

primarily for adults with substance use disorders. The guideline will summarize existing literature and provide readers with information currently not available in any single source specific for this vulnerable pediatric population. (12/13)

http://pediatrics.aappublications.org/content/133/1/152

RECOGNITION AND MANAGEMENT OF MEDICAL COMPLEXITY (CLINICAL REPORT)

Dennis Z. Kuo, MD, MHS, FAAP; Amy J. Houtrow, MD, PhD, MPH, FAAP; and Council on Children With Disabilities

ABSTRACT. Children with medical complexity have extensive needs for health services, experience functional limitations, and are high resource utilizers. Addressing the needs of this population to achieve high-value health care requires optimizing care within the medical home and medical neighborhood. Opportunities exist for health care providers, payers, and policy makers to develop strategies to enhance care delivery and to decrease costs. Important outcomes include decreasing unplanned hospital admissions, decreasing emergency department use, ensuring access to health services, limiting out-of-pocket expenses for families, and improving patient and family experiences, quality of life, and satisfaction with care. This report describes the population of children with medical complexity and provides strategies to optimize medical and health outcomes. (11/16)

See full text on page 1115.

http://pediatrics.aappublications.org/content/138/6/e20163021

RECOGNIZING AND RESPONDING TO MEDICAL NEGLECT (CLINICAL REPORT)

Carole Jenny, MD, MBA, and Committee on Child Abuse and Neglect

ABSTRACT. A caregiver may fail to recognize or respond to a child's medical needs for a variety of reasons. An effective response by a health care professional to medical neglect requires a comprehensive assessment of the child's needs, the parents' resources, the parents' efforts to provide for the needs of the child, and options for ensuring optimal health for the child. Such an assessment requires clear, 2-way communication between the family and the health care professional. Physicians should consider the least intrusive options for managing cases of medical neglect that ensure the health and safety of the child. (12/07, reaffirmed 1/11, 2/16)

http://pediatrics.aappublications.org/content/120/6/1385

RECOMMENDATIONS FOR PREVENTION AND CONTROL OF INFLUENZA IN CHILDREN, 2016–2017

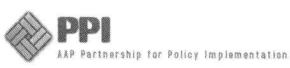

Committee on Infectious Diseases

ABSTRACT. The purpose of this statement is to update recommendations for the routine use of seasonal influenza vaccine and antiviral medications for the prevention and treatment of influenza in children. The AAP recommends annual seasonal influenza immunization for *everyone* 6 months and older, including children and adolescents. Highlights for the upcoming 2016–2017 season include the following:

1. Annual universal influenza immunization is indicated with either a trivalent or quadrivalent (no preference) inactivated vaccine.

2. The 2016–2017 influenza A (H3N2) vaccine strain differs from that contained in the 2015–2016 seasonal vaccines. The 2016–2017 influenza B vaccine strain (Victoria lineage) included in the trivalent vaccine differs from that contained in the 2015–2016 seasonal trivalent vaccines (Yamagata lineage).

   a. Trivalent vaccine contains an A/California/7/2009 (H1N1)pdm09–like virus, an A/Hong Kong/4801/2014 (H3N2)–like virus, and a B/Brisbane/60/2008-like virus (B/Victoria lineage).

   b. Quadrivalent vaccine contains an additional B virus (B/Phuket/3073/2013-like virus [B/Yamagata lineage]).

3. Quadrivalent live attenuated influenza vaccine (LAIV4) should not be used in any setting during the 2016–2017 influenza season in light of the evidence for poor effectiveness of LAIV4 in recent seasons, particularly against influenza A (H1N1)pdm09 viruses.

4. All children with egg allergy can receive influenza vaccine with no additional precautions from those of routine vaccinations.

5. All HCP should receive an annual influenza vaccine, a crucial step in preventing influenza and reducing health care–associated influenza infections. Because HCP may care for or live with people at high risk of influenza-related complications, it is especially important for them to get vaccinated annually.

6. Pediatricians should attempt to promptly identify children suspected of having influenza for rapid antiviral treatment, when indicated, to reduce morbidity and mortality. (9/16)

See full text on page 1131.

http://pediatrics.aappublications.org/content/138/4/e20162527

RECOMMENDATIONS FOR SEROGROUP B MENINGOCOCCAL VACCINE FOR PERSONS 10 YEARS AND OLDER

Committee on Infectious Diseases

ABSTRACT. This policy statement provides recommendations for the prevention of serogroup B meningococcal disease through the use of 2 newly licensed serogroup B meningococcal vaccines: MenB-FHbp (Trumenba; Wyeth Pharmaceuticals, a subsidiary of Pfizer, Philadelphia, PA) and MenB-4C (Bexsero; Novartis Vaccines, Siena, Italy). Both vaccines are approved for use in persons 10 through 25 years of age. MenB-FHbp is licensed as a 2- or 3-dose series, and MenB-4C is licensed as a 2-dose series for all groups. Either vaccine is recommended for routine use in persons 10 years and older who are at increased risk of serogroup B meningococcal disease (category A recommendation). Persons at increased risk of meningococcal serogroup B disease include the following: (1) persons with persistent complement component diseases, including inherited or chronic deficiencies in C3, C5–C9, properdin, factor D, or factor H, or persons receiving eculizumab (Soliris; Alexion Pharmaceuticals, Cheshire, CT), a monoclonal antibody that acts as a terminal complement inhibitor by binding C5 and inhibiting cleavage of C5 to C5A; (2) persons with anatomic or functional asplenia, including sickle cell disease; and (3) healthy persons at increased risk because of a serogroup B meningococcal disease outbreak. Both serogroup B meningococcal vaccines have been shown to be safe and immunogenic and are licensed by the US Food and Drug Administration for individuals between the ages of 10 and 25 years. On the basis of epidemiologic and antibody persistence data, the American Academy of Pediatrics agrees with the Advisory Committee on Immunization Practices of the Centers for Disease Control and Prevention that either vaccine may be administered to healthy adolescents and young adults 16 through 23 years of age (preferred ages are 16 through 18 years) to provide short-term protection against most strains of serogroup B meningococcal disease (category B recommendation). (8/16)

See full text on page 1151.

http://pediatrics.aappublications.org/content/138/3/e20161890

RECOMMENDATIONS FOR THE PREVENTION OF *STREPTOCOCCUS PNEUMONIAE* INFECTIONS IN INFANTS AND CHILDREN: USE OF 13-VALENT PNEUMOCOCCAL CONJUGATE VACCINE (PCV13) AND PNEUMOCOCCAL POLYSACCHARIDE VACCINE (PPSV23)

Committee on Infectious Diseases

ABSTRACT. Routine use of the 7-valent pneumococcal conjugate vaccine (PCV7), available since 2000, has resulted in a dramatic reduction in the incidence of invasive pneumococcal disease (IPD) attributable to serotypes of *Streptococcus pneumoniae* contained in the vaccine. However, IPD caused by nonvaccine pneumococcal serotypes has increased, and nonvaccine serotypes are now responsible for the majority of the remaining cases of IPD occurring in children. A 13-valent pneumococcal conjugate vaccine has been licensed by the US Food and Drug Administration, which, in addition to the 7 serotypes included in the original PCV7, contains the 6 pneumococcal serotypes responsible for 63% of IPD cases now occurring in children younger than 5 years. Because of the expanded coverage provided by PCV13, it will replace PCV7. This statement provides recommendations for (1) the transition from PCV7 to PCV13; (2) the routine use of PCV13 for healthy children and children with an underlying medical condition that increases the risk of IPD; (3) a supplemental dose of PCV13 for (*a*) healthy children 14 through 59 months of age who have completed the PCV7 series and (*b*) children 14 through 71 months of age with an underlying medical condition that increases the risk of IPD who have completed the PCV7 series; (4) "catch-up" immunization for children behind schedule; and (5) PCV13 for certain children at high risk from 6 through 18 years of age. In addition, recommendations for the use of pneumococcal polysaccharide vaccine for children at high risk of IPD are also updated. (5/10)

http://pediatrics.aappublications.org/content/126/1/186

RECOMMENDED CHILDHOOD AND ADOLESCENT IMMUNIZATION SCHEDULE—UNITED STATES, 2017

Committee on Infectious Diseases (1/17)

See full text on page 1161.

http://pediatrics.aappublications.org/content/early/2017/02/02/peds.2016-4007

RED REFLEX EXAMINATION IN NEONATES, INFANTS, AND CHILDREN

Section on Ophthalmology (joint with American Association for Pediatric Ophthalmology and Strabismus, American Academy of Ophthalmology, and American Association of Certified Orthoptists)

ABSTRACT. Red reflex testing is an essential component of the neonatal, infant, and child physical examination. This statement, which is a revision of the previous policy statement published in 2002, describes the rationale for testing, the technique used to perform this examination, and the indications for referral to an ophthalmologist experienced in the examination of children. (12/08)

http://pediatrics.aappublications.org/content/122/6/1401

REDUCING INJURY RISK FROM BODY CHECKING IN BOYS' YOUTH ICE HOCKEY

Council on Sports Medicine and Fitness

ABSTRACT. Ice hockey is an increasingly popular sport that allows intentional collision in the form of body checking for males but not for females. There is a two- to threefold increased risk of all injury, severe injury, and concussion related to body checking at all levels of boys' youth ice hockey. The American Academy of Pediatrics reinforces the importance of stringent enforcement of rules to protect player safety as well as educational interventions to decrease unsafe tactics. To promote ice hockey as a lifelong recreational pursuit for boys, the American Academy of Pediatrics recommends the expansion of non-checking programs and the restriction of body checking to elite levels of boys' youth ice hockey, starting no earlier than 15 years of age. (5/14)

http://pediatrics.aappublications.org/content/133/6/1151

REDUCING THE NUMBER OF DEATHS AND INJURIES FROM RESIDENTIAL FIRES

Committee on Injury and Poison Prevention

ABSTRACT. Smoke inhalation, severe burns, and death from residential fires are devastating events, most of which are preventable. In 1998, approximately 381 500 residential structure fires resulted in 3250 non-firefighter deaths, 17 175 injuries, and approximately $4.4 billion in property loss. This statement reviews important prevention messages and intervention strategies related to residential fires. It also includes recommendations for pediatricians regarding office anticipatory guidance, work in the community, and support of regulation and legislation that could result in a decrease in the number of fire-related injuries and deaths to children. (6/00)

http://pediatrics.aappublications.org/content/105/6/1355

REFERRAL TO PEDIATRIC SURGICAL SPECIALISTS

Surgical Advisory Panel

ABSTRACT. The American Academy of Pediatrics, with the collaboration of the Surgical Sections of the American Academy of Pediatrics, has created referral recommendations intended to serve as voluntary practice parameters to assist general pediatricians in determining when and to whom to refer their patients for pediatric surgical specialty care. It is recognized that these recommendations may be difficult to implement, because communi-

ties vary in terms of access to major pediatric medical centers. Limited access does not negate the value of the recommendations, however, because the child who needs specialized surgical and anesthetic care is best served by the skills of the appropriate pediatric surgical team. Major congenital anomalies, malignancies, major trauma, and chronic illnesses (including those associated with preterm birth) in infants and children should be managed by pediatric medical subspecialists and pediatric surgical specialists at pediatric referral centers that can provide expertise in many areas, including the pediatric medical subspecialties and surgical specialties of pediatric radiology, pediatric anesthesiology, pediatric pathology, and pediatric intensive care. The optimal management of the child with complex problems, chronic illness, or disabilities requires coordination, communication, and cooperation of the pediatric surgical specialist with the child's primary care pediatrician or physician. (1/14)
http://pediatrics.aappublications.org/content/133/2/350

REIMBURSEMENT FOR FOODS FOR SPECIAL DIETARY USE
Committee on Nutrition
ABSTRACT. Foods for special dietary use are recommended by physicians for chronic diseases or conditions of childhood, including inherited metabolic diseases. Although many states have created legislation requiring reimbursement for foods for special dietary use, legislation is now needed to mandate consistent coverage and reimbursement for foods for special dietary use and related support services with accepted medical benefit for children with designated medical conditions. (5/03, reaffirmed 1/06)
http://pediatrics.aappublications.org/content/111/5/1117

RELIEF OF PAIN AND ANXIETY IN PEDIATRIC PATIENTS IN EMERGENCY MEDICAL SYSTEMS (CLINICAL REPORT)
Joel A. Fein, MD, MPH; William T. Zempsky, MD, MPH; Joseph P. Cravero, MD; Committee on Pediatric Emergency Medicine; and Section on Anesthesiology and Pain Medicine
ABSTRACT. Control of pain and stress for children is a vital component of emergency medical care. Timely administration of analgesia affects the entire emergency medical experience and can have a lasting effect on a child's and family's reaction to current and future medical care. A systematic approach to pain management and anxiolysis, including staff education and protocol development, can provide comfort to children in the emergency setting and improve staff and family satisfaction. (10/12, reaffirmed 9/15)
http://pediatrics.aappublications.org/content/130/5/e1391

RELIGIOUS OBJECTIONS TO MEDICAL CARE
Committee on Bioethics
ABSTRACT. Parents sometimes deny their children the benefits of medical care because of religious beliefs. In some jurisdictions, exemptions to child abuse and neglect laws restrict government action to protect children or seek legal redress when the alleged abuse or neglect has

occurred in the name of religion. The American Academy of Pediatrics (AAP) believes that all children deserve effective medical treatment that is likely to prevent substantial harm or suffering or death. In addition, the AAP advocates that all legal interventions apply equally whenever children are endangered or harmed, without exemptions based on parental religious beliefs. To these ends, the AAP calls for the repeal of religious exemption laws and supports additional efforts to educate the public about the medical needs of children. (2/97, reaffirmed 10/00, 6/03, 10/06, 5/09)
http://pediatrics.aappublications.org/content/99/2/279

RESCUE MEDICINE FOR EPILEPSY IN EDUCATION SETTINGS (CLINICAL REPORT)
Adam L. Hartman, MD, FAAP; Cynthia Di Laura Devore, MD; Section on Neurology; and Council on School Health
ABSTRACT. Children and adolescents with epilepsy may experience prolonged seizures in school-associated settings (eg, during transportation, in the classroom, or during sports activities). Prolonged seizures may evolve into status epilepticus. Administering a seizure rescue medication can abort the seizure and may obviate the need for emergency medical services and subsequent care in an emergency department. In turn, this may save patients from the morbidity of more invasive interventions and the cost of escalated care. There are significant variations in prescribing practices for seizure rescue medications, partly because of inconsistencies between jurisdictions in legislation and professional practice guidelines among potential first responders (including school staff). There also are potential liability issues for prescribers, school districts, and unlicensed assistive personnel who might administer the seizure rescue medications. This clinical report highlights issues that providers may consider when prescribing seizure rescue medications and creating school medical orders and/or action plans for students with epilepsy. Collaboration among prescribing providers, families, and schools may be useful in developing plans for the use of seizure rescue medications. (12/15)
http://pediatrics.aappublications.org/content/137/1/e20153876

RESPIRATORY SUPPORT IN PRETERM INFANTS AT BIRTH
Committee on Fetus and Newborn
ABSTRACT. Current practice guidelines recommend administration of surfactant at or soon after birth in preterm infants with respiratory distress syndrome. However, recent multicenter randomized controlled trials indicate that early use of continuous positive airway pressure with subsequent selective surfactant administration in extremely preterm infants results in lower rates of bronchopulmonary dysplasia/death when compared with treatment with prophylactic or early surfactant therapy. Continuous positive airway pressure started at or soon after birth with subsequent selective surfactant administration may be considered as an alternative to routine intubation with prophylactic or early surfactant administration in preterm infants. (12/13)
http://pediatrics.aappublications.org/content/133/1/171

RESPONDING TO PARENTAL REFUSALS OF IMMUNIZATION OF CHILDREN (CLINICAL REPORT)

Douglas S. Diekema, MD, MPH, and Committee on Bioethics

ABSTRACT. The American Academy of Pediatrics strongly endorses universal immunization. However, for childhood immunization programs to be successful, parents must comply with immunization recommendations. The problem of parental refusal of immunization for children is an important one for pediatricians. The goal of this report is to assist pediatricians in understanding the reasons parents may have for refusing to immunize their children, review the limited circumstances under which parental refusals should be referred to child protective services agencies or public health authorities, and provide practical guidance to assist the pediatrician faced with a parent who is reluctant to allow immunization of his or her child. (5/05, reaffirmed 1/09, 11/12)
http://pediatrics.aappublications.org/content/115/5/1428

RESTRAINT USE ON AIRCRAFT

Committee on Injury and Poison Prevention

ABSTRACT. Occupant protection policies for children younger than 2 years on aircraft are inconsistent with all other national policies on safe transportation. Children younger than 2 years are not required to be restrained or secured on aircraft during takeoff, landing, and conditions of turbulence. They are permitted to be held on the lap of an adult. Preventable injuries and deaths have occurred in children younger than 2 years who were unrestrained in aircraft during survivable crashes and conditions of turbulence. The American Academy of Pediatrics recommends a mandatory federal requirement for restraint use for children on aircraft. The Academy further recommends that parents ensure that a seat is available for all children during aircraft transport and follow current recommendations for restraint use for all children. Physicians play a significant role in counseling families, advocating for public policy mandates, and encouraging technologic research that will improve protection of children in aircraft. (11/01, reaffirmed 5/05, 10/08)
http://pediatrics.aappublications.org/content/108/5/1218

RETURNING TO LEARNING FOLLOWING A CONCUSSION (CLINICAL REPORT)

Mark E. Halstead, MD, FAAP; Karen McAvoy, PsyD; Cynthia D. Devore, MD, FAAP; Rebecca Carl, MD, FAAP; Michael Lee, MD, FAAP; Kelsey Logan, MD, FAAP; Council on Sports Medicine and Fitness; and Council on School Health

ABSTRACT. Following a concussion, it is common for children and adolescents to experience difficulties in the school setting. Cognitive difficulties, such as learning new tasks or remembering previously learned material, may pose challenges in the classroom. The school environment may also increase symptoms with exposure to bright lights and screens or noisy cafeterias and hallways. Unfortunately, because most children and adolescents look physically normal after a concussion, school officials often fail to recognize the need for academic or environmental adjustments. Appropriate guidance and recommendations from the pediatrician may ease the transition back to the school environment and facilitate the recovery of the child or adolescent. This report serves to provide a better understanding of possible factors that may contribute to difficulties in a school environment after a concussion and serves as a framework for the medical home, the educational home, and the family home to guide the student to a successful and safe return to learning. (10/13)
http://pediatrics.aappublications.org/content/132/5/948

RITUAL GENITAL CUTTING OF FEMALE MINORS

Board of Directors (6/10)

http://pediatrics.aappublications.org/content/126/1/191

ROLE OF PEDIATRICIANS IN ADVOCATING LIFE SUPPORT TRAINING COURSES FOR PARENTS AND THE PUBLIC

Committee on Pediatric Emergency Medicine

ABSTRACT. Available literature suggests a need for both initial cardiopulmonary resuscitation basic life support training and refresher courses for parents and the public as well as health care professionals. The promotion of basic life support training courses that establish a pediatric chain of survival spanning from prevention of cardiac arrest and trauma to rehabilitative and follow-up care for victims of cardiopulmonary arrest is advocated in this policy statement and is the focus of an accompanying technical report. Immediate bystander cardiopulmonary resuscitation for victims of cardiac arrest improves survival for out-of-hospital cardiac arrest. Pediatricians will improve the chance of survival of children and adults who experience cardiac arrest by advocating for cardiopulmonary resuscitation training and participating in basic life support training courses as participants and instructors. (12/04, reaffirmed 5/07, 8/10, 8/13, 7/16)
http://pediatrics.aappublications.org/content/114/6/1676

ROLE OF PEDIATRICIANS IN ADVOCATING LIFE SUPPORT TRAINING COURSES FOR PARENTS AND THE PUBLIC (TECHNICAL REPORT)

Lee A. Pyles, MD; Jane Knapp, MD; and Committee on Pediatric Emergency Medicine

ABSTRACT. Available literature suggests a need for both initial cardiopulmonary resuscitation training and refresher courses. The establishment of a pediatric chain of survival for victims of cardiopulmonary arrest is the focus of this technical report and is advocated in the accompanying policy statement. Immediate bystander cardiopulmonary resuscitation for victims of cardiac arrest improves survival for out-of-hospital cardiac arrest. Pediatricians will improve the chance of survival of children and adults who experience cardiac arrest by advocating for basic life support training and participating in basic life support courses as participants and teachers. (12/04, reaffirmed 5/07, 8/10, 1/14)
http://pediatrics.aappublications.org/content/114/6/e761

THE ROLE OF PRESCHOOL HOME-VISITING PROGRAMS IN IMPROVING CHILDREN'S DEVELOPMENTAL AND HEALTH OUTCOMES

Council on Community Pediatrics

ABSTRACT. Child health and developmental outcomes depend to a large extent on the capabilities of families to provide a nurturing, safe environment for their infants and young children. Unfortunately, many families have insufficient knowledge about parenting skills and an

inadequate support system of friends, extended family, or professionals to help with or advise them regarding child rearing. Home-visiting programs offer a mechanism for ensuring that at-risk families have social support, linkage with public and private community services, and ongoing health, developmental, and safety education. When these services are part of a system of high-quality well-child care linked or integrated with the pediatric medical home, they have the potential to mitigate health and developmental outcome disparities. This statement reviews the history of home visiting in the United States and reaffirms the support of the American Academy of Pediatrics for home-based parenting education and support. (1/09)
http://pediatrics.aappublications.org/content/123/2/598

ROLE OF PULSE OXIMETRY IN EXAMINING NEWBORNS FOR CONGENITAL HEART DISEASE: A SCIENTIFIC STATEMENT FROM THE AHA AND AAP

William T. Mahle, MD; Jane W. Newburger, MD, MPH; G. Paul Matherne, MD; Frank C. Smith, MD; Tracey R. Hoke, MD; Robert Koppel, MD; Samuel S. Gidding, MD; Robert H. Beekman III, MD; Scott D. Grosse, PhD; on behalf of Section on Cardiology and Cardiac Surgery and Committee of Fetus and Newborn (joint with American Heart Association Congenital Heart Defects Committee of the Council on Cardiovascular Disease in the Young, Council on Cardiovascular Nursing, and Interdisciplinary Council on Quality of Care and Outcomes Research)

ABSTRACT. *Background.* The purpose of this statement is to address the state of evidence on the routine use of pulse oximetry in newborns to detect critical congenital heart disease (CCHD).

Methods and Results. A writing group appointed by the American Heart Association and the American Academy of Pediatrics reviewed the available literature addressing current detection methods for CCHD, burden of missed and/or delayed diagnosis of CCHD, rationale of oximetry screening, and clinical studies of oximetry in otherwise asymptomatic newborns. MEDLINE database searches from 1966 to 2008 were done for English-language papers using the following search terms: congenital heart disease, pulse oximetry, physical examination, murmur, echocardiography, fetal echocardiography, and newborn screening. The reference lists of identified papers were also searched. Published abstracts from major pediatric scientific meetings in 2006 to 2008 were also reviewed. The American Heart Association classification of recommendations and levels of evidence for practice guidelines were used. In an analysis of pooled studies of oximetry assessment performed after 24 hours of life, the estimated sensitivity for detecting CCHD was 69.6%, and the positive predictive value was 47.0%; however, sensitivity varied dramatically among studies from 0% to 100%. False-positive screens that required further evaluation occurred in only 0.035% of infants screened after 24 hours.

Conclusions. Currently, CCHD is not detected in some newborns until after their hospital discharge, which results in significant morbidity and occasional mortality. Furthermore, routine pulse oximetry performed on asymptomatic newborns after 24 hours of life, but before hospital discharge, may detect CCHD. Routine pulse oximetry performed after 24 hours in hospitals that have on-site pediatric cardiovascular services incurs very low cost and risk of harm. Future studies in larger populations and across a broad range of newborn delivery systems are needed to determine whether this practice should become standard of care in the routine assessment of the neonate. (8/09)
http://pediatrics.aappublications.org/content/124/2/823

THE ROLE OF SCHOOLS IN COMBATING ILLICIT SUBSTANCE ABUSE

Council on School Health and Committee on Substance Abuse

ABSTRACT. Disturbingly high levels of illicit drug use remain a problem among American teenagers. As the physical, social, and psychological "home away from home" for most youth, schools naturally assume a primary role in substance abuse education, prevention, and early identification. However, the use of random drug testing on students as a component of drug prevention programs requires additional, more rigorous scientific evaluation. Widespread implementation should await the result of ongoing studies to address the effectiveness of testing and evaluate possible inadvertent harm. If drug testing on students is conducted, it should never be implemented in isolation. A comprehensive assessment and therapeutic management program for the student who tests positive should be in place before any testing is performed. Schools have the opportunity to work with parents, health care professionals, and community officials to use programs with proven effectiveness, to identify students who show behavioral risks for drug-related problems, and to make referrals to a student's medical home. When use of an illicit substance is detected, schools can foster relationships with established health care experts to assist them. A student undergoing individualized intervention for using illicit substances merits privacy. This requires that awareness of the student's situation be limited to parents, the student's physician, and only those designated school health officials with a need to know. For the purposes of this statement, alcohol, tobacco, and inhalants are not addressed. (12/07)
http://pediatrics.aappublications.org/content/120/6/1379

ROLE OF THE MEDICAL HOME IN FAMILY-CENTERED EARLY INTERVENTION SERVICES

Council on Children With Disabilities

ABSTRACT. There is growing evidence that early intervention services have a positive influence on the developmental outcome of children with established disabilities as well as those who are considered to be "at risk" of disabilities. Various federal and state laws now mandate the establishment of community-based, coordinated, multidisciplinary, family-centered programs that are accessible to children and families. The medical home, in close collaboration with the family and the early intervention team, can play a critical role in ensuring that at-risk children receive appropriate clinical and developmental early intervention services. The purpose of this statement is to assist the pediatric health care professional in assuming a proactive role with the interdisciplinary team that provides early intervention services. (11/07)
http://pediatrics.aappublications.org/content/120/5/1153

THE ROLE OF THE PEDIATRICIAN IN PRIMARY PREVENTION OF OBESITY (CLINICAL REPORT)

Stephen R. Daniels, MD, PhD, FAAP; Sandra G. Hassink, MD, FAAP; and Committee on Nutrition

ABSTRACT. The adoption of healthful lifestyles by individuals and families can result in a reduction in many chronic diseases and conditions of which obesity is the most prevalent. Obesity prevention, in addition to treatment, is an important public health priority. This clinical report describes the rationale for pediatricians to be an integral part of the obesity-prevention effort. In addition, the 2012 Institute of Medicine report "Accelerating Progress in Obesity Prevention" includes health care providers as a crucial component of successful weight control. Research on obesity prevention in the pediatric care setting as well as evidence-informed practical approaches and targets for prevention are reviewed. Pediatricians should use a longitudinal, developmentally appropriate life-course approach to help identify children early on the path to obesity and base prevention efforts on family dynamics and reduction in high-risk dietary and activity behaviors. They should promote a diet free of sugar-sweetened beverages, of fewer foods with high caloric density, and of increased intake of fruits and vegetables. It is also important to promote a lifestyle with reduced sedentary behavior and with 60 minutes of daily moderate to vigorous physical activity. This report also identifies important gaps in evidence that need to be filled by future research. (6/15)

http://pediatrics.aappublications.org/content/136/1/e275

THE ROLE OF THE PEDIATRICIAN IN RURAL EMERGENCY MEDICAL SERVICES FOR CHILDREN

Committee on Pediatric Emergency Medicine

ABSTRACT. In rural America, pediatricians can play a key role in the development, implementation, and ongoing supervision of emergency medical services for children (EMSC). Pediatricians may represent the only source of pediatric expertise for a large region and are a vital resource for rural physicians (eg, general and family practice, emergency medicine) and other rural health care professionals (physician assistants, nurse practitioners, and emergency medical technicians), providing education about management and prevention of pediatric illness and injury; appropriate equipment for the acutely ill or injured child; and acute, chronic, and rehabilitative care. In addition to providing clinical expertise, the pediatrician may be involved in quality assurance, clinical protocol development, and advocacy, and may serve as a liaison between emergency medical services and other entities working with children (eg, school nurses, child care centers, athletic programs, and programs for children with special health care needs). (10/12, reaffirmed 9/15)

http://pediatrics.aappublications.org/content/130/5/978

ROLE OF THE PEDIATRICIAN IN YOUTH VIOLENCE PREVENTION

Committee on Injury, Violence, and Poison Prevention

ABSTRACT. Youth violence continues to be a serious threat to the health of children and adolescents in the United States. It is crucial that pediatricians clearly define their role and develop the appropriate skills to address this threat effectively. From a clinical perspective, pediatricians should become familiar with *Connected Kids: Safe, Strong, Secure,* the American Academy of Pediatrics' primary care violence prevention protocol. Using this material, practices can incorporate preventive education, screening for risk, and linkages to community-based counseling and treatment resources. As advocates, pediatricians may bring newly developed information regarding key risk factors such as exposure to firearms, teen dating violence, and bullying to the attention of local and national policy makers. This policy statement refines the developing role of pediatricians in youth violence prevention and emphasizes the importance of this issue in the strategic agenda of the American Academy of Pediatrics. (6/09)

http://pediatrics.aappublications.org/content/124/1/393

ROLE OF THE SCHOOL NURSE IN PROVIDING SCHOOL HEALTH SERVICES

Council on School Health

ABSTRACT. The American Academy of Pediatrics recognizes the important role school nurses play in promoting the optimal biopsychosocial health and well-being of school-aged children in the school setting. Although the concept of a school nurse has existed for more than a century, uniformity among states and school districts regarding the role of a registered professional nurse in schools and the laws governing it are lacking. By understanding the benefits, roles, and responsibilities of school nurses working as a team with the school physician, as well as their contributions to school-aged children, pediatricians can collaborate with, support, and promote school nurses in their own communities, thus improving the health, wellness, and safety of children and adolescents. (5/16)

See full text on page 1167.

http://pediatrics.aappublications.org/content/137/6/e20160852

ROLE OF THE SCHOOL PHYSICIAN

Council on School Health

ABSTRACT. The American Academy of Pediatrics recognizes the important role physicians play in promoting the optimal biopsychosocial well-being of children in the school setting. Although the concept of a school physician has existed for more than a century, uniformity among states and school districts regarding physicians in schools and the laws governing it are lacking. By understanding the roles and contributions physicians can make to schools, pediatricians can support and promote school physicians in their communities and improve health and safety for children. (12/12)

http://pediatrics.aappublications.org/content/131/1/178

SAFE SLEEP AND SKIN-TO-SKIN CARE IN THE NEONATAL PERIOD FOR HEALTHY TERM NEWBORNS (CLINICAL REPORT)

Lori Feldman-Winter, MD, MPH, FAAP; Jay P. Goldsmith, MD, FAAP; Committee on Fetus and Newborn; and Task Force on Sudden Infant Death Syndrome

ABSTRACT. Skin-to-skin care (SSC) and rooming-in have become common practice in the newborn period for healthy newborns with the implementation of maternity care practices that support breastfeeding as delineated in the World Health Organization's "Ten Steps to Successful Breastfeeding." SSC and rooming-in are supported by evidence that indicates that the implementation of these practices increases overall and exclusive breastfeeding, safer and healthier transitions, and improved maternal-infant bonding. In some cases, however, the practice of SSC and rooming-in may pose safety concerns, particularly with regard to sleep. There have been several recent case reports and case series of severe and sudden unexpected postnatal collapse in the neonatal period among otherwise healthy newborns and near fatal or fatal events related to sleep, suffocation, and falls from adult hospital beds. Although these are largely case reports, there are potential dangers of unobserved SSC immediately after birth and throughout the postpartum hospital period as well as with unobserved rooming-in for at-risk situations. Moreover, behaviors that are modeled in the hospital after birth, such as sleep position, are likely to influence sleeping practices after discharge. Hospitals and birthing centers have found it difficult to develop policies that will allow SSC and rooming-in to continue in a safe manner. This clinical report is intended for birthing centers and delivery hospitals caring for healthy newborns to assist in the establishment of appropriate SSC and safe sleep policies. (8/16)

See full text on page 1175.

http://pediatrics.aappublications.org/content/138/3/e20161889

SAFE TRANSPORTATION OF NEWBORNS AT HOSPITAL DISCHARGE

Committee on Injury and Poison Prevention
ABSTRACT. All hospitals should set policies that require the discharge of every newborn in a car safety seat that is appropriate for the infant's maturity and medical condition. Discharge policies for newborns should include a parent education component, regular review of educational materials, and periodic in-service education for responsible staff. Appropriate child restraint systems should become a benefit of coverage by Medicaid, managed care organizations, and other third-party insurers. (10/99, reaffirmed 1/03, 1/06, 10/08)
http://pediatrics.aappublications.org/content/104/4/986

SAFE TRANSPORTATION OF PRETERM AND LOW BIRTH WEIGHT INFANTS AT HOSPITAL DISCHARGE (CLINICAL REPORT)

Marilyn J. Bull, MD; William A. Engle, MD; Committee on Injury, Violence, and Poison Prevention; and Committee on Fetus and Newborn
ABSTRACT. Safe transportation of preterm and low birth weight infants requires special considerations. Both physiologic immaturity and low birth weight must be taken into account to properly position such infants. This clinical report provides guidelines for pediatricians and other caregivers who counsel parents of preterm and low birth weight infants about car safety seats. (4/09, reaffirmed 8/13)
http://pediatrics.aappublications.org/content/123/5/1424

SCHOOL BUS TRANSPORTATION OF CHILDREN WITH SPECIAL HEALTH CARE NEEDS

Committee on Injury and Poison Prevention (8/01, reaffirmed 1/05, 2/08, 5/13)
http://pediatrics.aappublications.org/content/108/2/516

SCHOOL HEALTH ASSESSMENTS

Committee on School Health
ABSTRACT. Comprehensive health assessments often are performed in school-based clinics or public health clinics by health professionals other than pediatricians. Pediatricians or other physicians skilled in child health care should participate in such evaluations. This statement provides guidance on the scope of in-school health assessments and the roles of the pediatrician, school nurse, school, and community. (4/00, reaffirmed 6/03, 5/06, 10/11)
http://pediatrics.aappublications.org/content/105/4/875

SCHOOL HEALTH CENTERS AND OTHER INTEGRATED SCHOOL HEALTH SERVICES

Committee on School Health
ABSTRACT. This statement offers guidelines on the integration of expanded school health services, including school-based and school-linked health centers, into community-based health care systems. Expanded school health services should be integrated so that they enhance accessibility, provide high-quality health care, link children to a medical home, are financially sustainable, and address both long- and short-term needs of children and adolescents. (1/01)
http://pediatrics.aappublications.org/content/107/1/198

SCHOOL READINESS (TECHNICAL REPORT)

Pamela C. High, MD; Committee on Early Childhood, Adoption, and Dependent Care; and Council on School Health
ABSTRACT. School readiness includes the readiness of the individual child, the school's readiness for children, and the ability of the family and community to support optimal early child development. It is the responsibility of schools to be ready for all children at all levels of readiness. Children's readiness for kindergarten should become an outcome measure for community-based programs, rather than an exclusion criterion at the beginning of the formal educational experience. Our new knowledge of early brain and child development has revealed that modifiable factors in a child's early experience can greatly affect that child's learning trajectory. Many US children enter kindergarten with limitations in their social, emotional, cognitive, and physical development that might have been significantly diminished or eliminated through early identification of and attention to child and family needs. Pediatricians have a role in promoting school readiness for all children, beginning at birth, through their practices and advocacy. The American Academy of Pediatrics affords pediatricians many opportunities to promote the physical, social-emotional, and educational health of young children, with other advocacy groups. This technical report supports American Academy of Pediatrics policy statements "Quality Early Education

and Child Care From Birth to Kindergarten" and "The Inappropriate Use of School 'Readiness' Tests." (4/08, reaffirmed 9/13)
http://pediatrics.aappublications.org/content/121/4/e1008

SCHOOL START TIMES FOR ADOLESCENTS
Adolescent Sleep Working Group, Committee on Adolescence, and Council on School Health
ABSTRACT. The American Academy of Pediatrics recognizes insufficient sleep in adolescents as an important public health issue that significantly affects the health and safety, as well as the academic success, of our nation's middle and high school students. Although a number of factors, including biological changes in sleep associated with puberty, lifestyle choices, and academic demands, negatively affect middle and high school students' ability to obtain sufficient sleep, the evidence strongly implicates earlier school start times (ie, before 8:30 AM) as a key modifiable contributor to insufficient sleep, as well as circadian rhythm disruption, in this population. Furthermore, a substantial body of research has now demonstrated that delaying school start times is an effective countermeasure to chronic sleep loss and has a wide range of potential benefits to students with regard to physical and mental health, safety, and academic achievement. The American Academy of Pediatrics strongly supports the efforts of school districts to optimize sleep in students and urges high schools and middle schools to aim for start times that allow students the opportunity to achieve optimal levels of sleep (8.5–9.5 hours) and to improve physical (eg, reduced obesity risk) and mental (eg, lower rates of depression) health, safety (eg, drowsy driving crashes), academic performance, and quality of life. (8/14)
http://pediatrics.aappublications.org/content/134/3/642

SCHOOL TRANSPORTATION SAFETY
Committee on Injury, Violence, and Poison Prevention and Council on School Health
ABSTRACT. This policy statement replaces the previous version published in 1996. It provides new information, studies, regulations, and recommendations related to the safe transportation of children to and from school and school-related activities. Pediatricians can play an important role at the patient/family, community, state, and national levels as child advocates and consultants to schools and early education programs about transportation safety. (7/07, reaffirmed 10/11)
http://pediatrics.aappublications.org/content/120/1/213

SCHOOL-BASED HEALTH CENTERS AND PEDIATRIC PRACTICE
Council on School Health
ABSTRACT. School-based health centers (SBHCs) have become an important method of health care delivery for the youth of our nation. Although they only represent 1 aspect of a coordinated school health program approach, SBHCs have provided access to health care services for youth confronted with age, financial, cultural, and geographic barriers. A fundamental principle of SBHCs is to create an environment of service coordination and collaboration that addresses the health needs and well-being of youth with health disparities or poor access to health care services. Some pediatricians have concerns that these centers are in conflict with the primary care provider's medical home. This policy provides an overview of SBHCs and some of their documented benefits, addresses the issue of potential conflict with the medical home, and provides recommendations that support the integration and coordination of SBHCs and the pediatric medical home practice. (1/12)
http://pediatrics.aappublications.org/content/129/2/387

SCHOOL-BASED MENTAL HEALTH SERVICES
Committee on School Health
ABSTRACT. More than 20% of children and adolescents have mental health problems. Health care professionals for children and adolescents must educate key stakeholders about the extent of these problems and work together with them to increase access to mental health resources. School-based programs offer the promise of improving access to diagnosis of and treatment for the mental health problems of children and adolescents. Pediatric health care professionals, educators, and mental health specialists should work in collaboration to develop and implement effective school-based mental health services. (6/04, reaffirmed 5/09)
http://pediatrics.aappublications.org/content/113/6/1839

SCOPE OF HEALTH CARE BENEFITS FOR CHILDREN FROM BIRTH THROUGH AGE 26
Committee on Child Health Financing
ABSTRACT. The optimal health of all children is best achieved with access to appropriate and comprehensive health care benefits. This policy statement outlines and defines the recommended set of health insurance benefits for children through age 26. The American Academy of Pediatrics developed a set of recommendations concerning preventive care services for children, adolescents, and young adults. These recommendations are compiled in the publication *Bright Futures: Guidelines for Health Supervision of Infants, Children, and Adolescents,* third edition. The Bright Futures recommendations were referenced as a standard for access and design of age-appropriate health insurance benefits for infants, children, adolescents, and young adults in the Patient Protection and Affordable Care Act of 2010 (Pub L No. 114–148). (11/11)
http://pediatrics.aappublications.org/content/129/1/185

SCOPE OF PRACTICE ISSUES IN THE DELIVERY OF PEDIATRIC HEALTH CARE
Committee on Pediatric Workforce
ABSTRACT. The American Academy of Pediatrics (AAP) believes that optimal pediatric health care depends on a team-based approach with supervision by a physician leader, preferably a pediatrician. The pediatrician, here defined to include not only pediatric generalists but all pediatric medical subspecialists, all surgical specialists, and internal medicine/pediatric physicians, is uniquely qualified to manage, coordinate, and supervise the entire spectrum of pediatric care, from diagnosis through all stages of treatment, in all practice settings. The AAP recognizes the valuable contributions of nonphysician

clinicians, including nurse practitioners and physician assistants, in delivering optimal pediatric care. However, the expansion of the scope of practice of nonphysician pediatric clinicians raises critical public policy and child health advocacy concerns. Pediatricians should serve as advocates for optimal pediatric care in state legislatures, public policy forums, and the media and should pursue opportunities to resolve scope of practice conflicts outside state legislatures. The AAP affirms the importance of appropriate documentation and standards in pediatric education, training, skills, clinical competencies, examination, regulation, and patient care to ensure safety and quality health care for all infants, children, adolescents, and young adults. (5/13, reaffirmed 10/15)

http://pediatrics.aappublications.org/content/131/6/1211

SCREENING EXAMINATION OF PREMATURE INFANTS FOR RETINOPATHY OF PREMATURITY

Section on Ophthalmology (joint with American Academy of Ophthalmology, American Association for Pediatric Ophthalmology and Strabismus, and American Association of Certified Orthoptists)

ABSTRACT. This statement revises a previous statement on screening of preterm infants for retinopathy of prematurity (ROP) that was published in 2006. ROP is a pathologic process that occurs only in immature retinal tissue and can progress to a tractional retinal detachment, which can result in functional or complete blindness. Use of peripheral retinal ablative therapy by using laser photocoagulation for nearly 2 decades has resulted in a high probability of markedly decreasing the incidence of this poor visual outcome, but the sequential nature of ROP creates a requirement that at-risk preterm infants be examined at proper times and intervals to detect the changes of ROP before they become permanently destructive. This statement presents the attributes on which an effective program for detecting and treating ROP could be based, including the timing of initial examination and subsequent reexamination intervals. (12/12, reaffirmed 2/16)

http://pediatrics.aappublications.org/content/131/1/189

SCREENING FOR NONVIRAL SEXUALLY TRANSMITTED INFECTIONS IN ADOLESCENTS AND YOUNG ADULTS

Committee on Adolescence (joint with Society for Adolescent Health and Medicine)

ABSTRACT. Prevalence rates of many sexually transmitted infections (STIs) are highest among adolescents. If nonviral STIs are detected early, they can be treated, transmission to others can be eliminated, and sequelae can be averted. The US Preventive Services Task Force and the Centers for Disease Control and Prevention have published chlamydia, gonorrhea, and syphilis screening guidelines that recommend screening those at risk on the basis of epidemiologic and clinical outcomes data. This policy statement specifically focuses on these curable, nonviral STIs and reviews the evidence for nonviral STI screening in adolescents, communicates the value of screening, and outlines recommendations for routine nonviral STI screening of adolescents. (6/14)

http://pediatrics.aappublications.org/content/134/1/e302

SCREENING FOR RETINOPATHY IN THE PEDIATRIC PATIENT WITH TYPE 1 DIABETES MELLITUS (CLINICAL REPORT)

Gregg T. Lueder, MD; Janet Silverstein, MD; Section on Ophthalmology; and Section on Endocrinology (joint with American Association for Pediatric Ophthalmology and Strabismus)

ABSTRACT. Diabetic retinopathy (DR) is the leading cause of blindness in young adults in the United States. Early identification and treatment of DR can decrease the risk of vision loss in affected patients. This clinical report reviews the risk factors for the development of DR and screening guidance for pediatric patients with type 1 diabetes mellitus. (7/05, reaffirmed 1/09, 7/14)

http://pediatrics.aappublications.org/content/116/1/270

SECONDHAND AND PRENATAL TOBACCO SMOKE EXPOSURE (TECHNICAL REPORT)

Dana Best, MD, MPH; Committee on Environmental Health; Committee on Native American Child Health; and Committee on Adolescence

ABSTRACT. Secondhand tobacco smoke (SHS) exposure of children and their families causes significant morbidity and mortality. In their personal and professional roles, pediatricians have many opportunities to advocate for elimination of SHS exposure of children, to counsel tobacco users to quit, and to counsel children never to start. This report discusses the harms of tobacco use and SHS exposure, the extent and costs of tobacco use and SHS exposure, and the evidence that supports counseling and other clinical interventions in the cycle of tobacco use. Recommendations for future research, policy, and clinical practice change are discussed. To improve understanding and provide support for these activities, the harms of SHS exposure are discussed, effective ways to eliminate or reduce SHS exposure are presented, and policies that support a smoke-free environment are outlined. (10/09, reaffirmed 5/14)

http://pediatrics.aappublications.org/content/124/5/e1017

SELECTING APPROPRIATE TOYS FOR YOUNG CHILDREN: THE PEDIATRICIAN'S ROLE (CLINICAL REPORT)

Committee on Early Childhood, Adoption, and Dependent Care

ABSTRACT. Play is essential for learning in children. Toys are the tools of play. Which play materials are provided and how they are used are equally important. Adults caring for children can be reminded that toys facilitate but do not substitute for the most important aspect of nurture—warm, loving, dependable relationships. Toys should be safe, affordable, and developmentally appropriate. Children do not need expensive toys. Toys should be appealing to engage the child over a period of time. Information and resources are provided in this report so pediatricians can give parents advice about selecting toys. (4/03, reaffirmed 10/06, 5/11)

http://pediatrics.aappublications.org/content/111/4/911

SELF-INJECTABLE EPINEPHRINE FOR FIRST-AID MANAGEMENT OF ANAPHYLAXIS (CLINICAL REPORT)

Scott H. Sicherer, MD; F. Estelle R. Simons, MD; and Section on Allergy and Immunology

ABSTRACT. Anaphylaxis is a severe, potentially fatal systemic allergic reaction that is rapid in onset and may cause death. Epinephrine is the primary medical therapy, and it must be administered promptly. This clinical report focuses on practical issues concerning the administration of self-injectable epinephrine for first-aid treatment of anaphylaxis in the community. The recommended epinephrine dose for anaphylaxis in children, based primarily on anecdotal evidence, is 0.01 mg/kg, up to 0.30 mg. Intramuscular injection of epinephrine into the lateral thigh (vastus lateralis) is the preferred route for therapy in first-aid treatment. Epinephrine autoinjectors are currently available in only 2 fixed doses: 0.15 and 0.30 mg. On the basis of current, albeit limited, data, it seems reasonable to recommend autoinjectors with 0.15 mg of epinephrine for otherwise healthy young children who weigh 10 to 25 kg (22–55 lb) and autoinjectors with 0.30 mg of epinephrine for those who weigh approximately 25 kg (55 lb) or more; however, specific clinical circumstances must be considered in these decisions. This report also describes several quandaries in regard to management, including the selection of dose, indications for prescribing an autoinjector, and decisions regarding when to inject epinephrine. Effective care for individuals at risk of anaphylaxis requires a comprehensive management approach involving families, allergic children, schools, camps, and other youth organizations. Risk reduction entails confirmation of the trigger, discussion of avoidance of the relevant allergen, a written individualized emergency anaphylaxis action plan, and education of supervising adults with regard to recognition and treatment of anaphylaxis. (3/07)
http://pediatrics.aappublications.org/content/119/3/638

SENSORY INTEGRATION THERAPIES FOR CHILDREN WITH DEVELOPMENTAL AND BEHAVIORAL DISORDERS

Section on Complementary and Integrative Medicine and Council on Children With Disabilities

ABSTRACT. Sensory-based therapies are increasingly used by occupational therapists and sometimes by other types of therapists in treatment of children with developmental and behavioral disorders. Sensory-based therapies involve activities that are believed to organize the sensory system by providing vestibular, proprioceptive, auditory, and tactile inputs. Brushes, swings, balls, and other specially designed therapeutic or recreational equipment are used to provide these inputs. However, it is unclear whether children who present with sensory-based problems have an actual "disorder" of the sensory pathways of the brain or whether these deficits are characteristics associated with other developmental and behavioral disorders. Because there is no universally accepted framework for diagnosis, sensory processing disorder generally should not be diagnosed. Other developmental and behavioral disorders must always be considered, and a thorough evaluation should be completed. Difficulty tolerating or processing sensory information is a characteristic that may be seen in many developmental behavioral disorders, including autism spectrum disorders, attention-deficit/hyperactivity disorder, developmental coordination disorders, and childhood anxiety disorders.

Occupational therapy with the use of sensory-based therapies may be acceptable as one of the components of a comprehensive treatment plan. However, parents should be informed that the amount of research regarding the effectiveness of sensory integration therapy is limited and inconclusive. Important roles for pediatricians and other clinicians may include discussing these limitations with parents, talking with families about a trial period of sensory integration therapy, and teaching families how to evaluate the effectiveness of a therapy. (5/12)
http://pediatrics.aappublications.org/content/129/6/1186

SEXUAL ORIENTATION AND ADOLESCENTS (CLINICAL REPORT)

Committee on Adolescence

ABSTRACT. The American Academy of Pediatrics issued its first statement on homosexuality and adolescents in 1983, with a revision in 1993. This report reflects the growing understanding of youth of differing sexual orientations. Young people are recognizing their sexual orientation earlier than in the past, making this a topic of importance to pediatricians. Pediatricians should be aware that some youths in their care may have concerns about their sexual orientation or that of siblings, friends, parents, relatives, or others. Health care professionals should provide factual, current, nonjudgmental information in a confidential manner. All youths, including those who know or wonder whether they are not heterosexual, may seek information from physicians about sexual orientation, sexually transmitted diseases, substance abuse, or various psychosocial difficulties. The pediatrician should be attentive to various potential psychosocial difficulties, offer counseling or refer for counseling when necessary and ensure that every sexually active youth receives a thorough medical history, physical examination, immunizations, appropriate laboratory tests, and counseling about sexually transmitted diseases (including human immunodeficiency virus infection) and appropriate treatment if necessary.

Not all pediatricians may feel able to provide the type of care described in this report. Any pediatrician who is unable to care for and counsel nonheterosexual youth should refer these patients to an appropriate colleague. (6/04)
http://pediatrics.aappublications.org/content/113/6/1827

SEXUALITY, CONTRACEPTION, AND THE MEDIA

Victor C. Strasburger, MD, and Council on Communications and Media

ABSTRACT. From a health viewpoint, early sexual activity among US adolescents is a potential problem because of the risk of pregnancy and sexually transmitted infections. New evidence points to the media adolescents use frequently (television, music, movies, magazines, and the Internet) as important factors in the initiation of sexual intercourse. There is a major disconnect between what mainstream media portray—casual sex and sexuality with no consequences—and what children and teenagers need—straightforward information about human sexuality and the need for contraception when having sex. Television, film, music, and the Internet are all becoming increasingly sexually explicit, yet information on abstinence, sexual responsibility, and birth control remains rare. It is unwise to promote "abstinence-only" sex education when it has been shown to be ineffective and when the media have become such an important source of information about "nonabstinence." Recommendations are presented to help pediatricians address this important issue. (8/10)

http://pediatrics.aappublications.org/content/126/3/576

SEXUALITY EDUCATION FOR CHILDREN AND ADOLESCENTS (CLINICAL REPORT)

Cora C. Breuner, MD, MPH; Gerri Mattson, MD, MSPH;
Committee on Adolescence; and Committee on Psychosocial
Aspects of Child and Family Health

ABSTRACT. The purpose of this clinical report is to provide pediatricians updated research on evidence-based sexual and reproductive health education conducted since the original clinical report on the subject was published by the American Academy of Pediatrics in 2001. Sexuality education is defined as teaching about human sexuality, including intimate relationships, human sexual anatomy, sexual reproduction, sexually transmitted infections, sexual activity, sexual orientation, gender identity, abstinence, contraception, and reproductive rights and responsibilities. Developmentally appropriate and evidence-based education about human sexuality and sexual reproduction over time provided by pediatricians, schools, other professionals, and parents is important to help children and adolescents make informed, positive, and safe choices about healthy relationships, responsible sexual activity, and their reproductive health. Sexuality education has been shown to help to prevent and reduce the risks of adolescent pregnancy, HIV, and sexually transmitted infections for children and adolescents with and without chronic health conditions and disabilities in the United States. (7/16)

See full text on page 1187.

http://pediatrics.aappublications.org/content/138/2/e20161348

SEXUALITY OF CHILDREN AND ADOLESCENTS WITH DEVELOPMENTAL DISABILITIES (CLINICAL REPORT)

Nancy A. Murphy, MD; Ellen Roy Elias, MD; for Council on
Children With Disabilities

ABSTRACT. Children and adolescents with developmental disabilities, like all children, are sexual persons. However, attention to their complex medical and functional issues often consumes time that might otherwise be invested in addressing the anatomic, physiologic, emotional, and social aspects of their developing sexuality. This report discusses issues of puberty, contraception, psychosexual development, sexual abuse, and sexuality education specific to children and adolescents with disabilities and their families. Pediatricians, in the context of the medical home, are encouraged to discuss issues of sexuality on a regular basis, ensure the privacy of each child and adolescent, promote self-care and social independence among persons with disabilities, advocate for appropriate sexuality education, and provide ongoing education for children and adolescents with developmental disabilities and their families. (7/06, reaffirmed 12/09, 7/13)

http://pediatrics.aappublications.org/content/118/1/398

SHOPPING CART–RELATED INJURIES TO CHILDREN

Committee on Injury, Violence, and Poison Prevention

ABSTRACT. Shopping cart–related injuries to children are common and can result in severe injury or even death. Most injuries result from falls from carts or cart tip-overs, and injuries to the head and neck represent three fourths of cases. The current US standard for shopping carts should be revised to include clear and effective performance criteria to prevent falls from carts and cart tip-overs. Pediatricians have an important role as educators, researchers, and advocates to promote the prevention of these injuries. (8/06, reaffirmed 4/09, 8/13)

http://pediatrics.aappublications.org/content/118/2/825

SHOPPING CART–RELATED INJURIES TO CHILDREN (TECHNICAL REPORT)

Gary A. Smith, MD, DrPH, for Committee on Injury,
Violence, and Poison Prevention

ABSTRACT. An estimated 24 200 children younger than 15 years, 20 700 (85%) of whom were younger than 5 years, were treated in US hospital emergency departments in 2005 for shopping cart–related injuries. Approximately 4% of shopping cart–related injuries to children younger than 15 years require admission to the hospital. Injuries to the head and neck represent three fourths of all injuries. Fractures account for 45% of all hospitalizations. Deaths have occurred from falls from shopping carts and cart tip-overs. Falls are the most common mechanism of injury and account for more than half of injuries associated with shopping carts. Cart tip-overs are the second most common mechanism, responsible for up to one fourth of injuries and almost 40% of shopping cart–related injuries among children younger than 2 years. Public-awareness initiatives, education programs, and parental supervision, although important, are not enough to prevent these injuries effectively. European Standard EN 1929-1:1998 and joint Australian/New Zealand Standard AS/NZS 3847.1:1999 specify requirements for the construction, performance, testing, and safety of shopping carts and have been implemented as national standards in 21 countries. A US performance standard for shopping carts (ASTM [American Society for Testing and Materials] F2372-04) was established in July 2004; however, it does not adequately address falls and cart tip-overs, which are the leading mechanisms of shopping cart–related injuries to children. The current US standard for shopping carts should be revised to include clear and effective performance criteria for shopping cart child-restraint systems and cart stability to prevent falls from carts and cart tip-overs. This is imperative to decrease the number and severity of shopping cart–related injuries to children. Recommendations from the American Academy of Pediatrics regarding prevention of shopping cart–related injuries are included in the accompanying policy statement. (8/06, reaffirmed 4/09, 8/13)

http://pediatrics.aappublications.org/content/118/2/e540

SIDS AND OTHER SLEEP-RELATED INFANT DEATHS: UPDATED 2016 RECOMMENDATIONS FOR A SAFE INFANT SLEEPING ENVIRONMENT

Task Force on Sudden Infant Death Syndrome

ABSTRACT. Approximately 3500 infants die annually in the United States from sleep-related infant deaths, including sudden infant death syndrome (SIDS; International Classification of Diseases, 10th Revision [ICD-10], R95), ill-defined deaths (ICD-10 R99), and accidental suffocation and strangulation in bed (ICD-10 W75). After an initial decrease in the 1990s, the overall death rate attributable to sleep-related infant deaths has not declined in more recent years. Many of the modifiable and nonmodifiable risk factors for SIDS and other sleep-related infant deaths are strikingly similar. The American Academy of Pediatrics recommends a safe sleep environment that can reduce the risk of all sleep-related infant deaths. Recommendations for a safe sleep environment include supine positioning, the use of a firm sleep surface, room-sharing without bed-sharing, and the avoidance of soft bedding and overheating. Additional recommendations for SIDS reduction include the avoidance of exposure to smoke, alcohol, and illicit drugs; breastfeeding; routine immunization; and use of a pacifier. New evidence is presented for skin-to-skin care for newborn infants, use of bedside and in-bed sleepers, sleeping on couches/armchairs and in sitting devices, and use of soft bedding after 4 months of age. The recommendations and strength of evidence for each recommendation are included in this policy statement. The rationale for these recommendations is discussed in detail in the accompanying technical report (www.pediatrics.org/cgi/doi/10.1542/peds.2016-2940). (10/16)

See full text on page 1201.

http://pediatrics.aappublications.org/content/138/5/e20162938

SIDS AND OTHER SLEEP-RELATED INFANT DEATHS: EVIDENCE BASE FOR 2016 UPDATED RECOMMENDATIONS FOR A SAFE INFANT SLEEPING ENVIRONMENT (TECHNICAL REPORT)

Rachel Y. Moon, MD, FAAP, and Task Force on Sudden
*   *Infant Death Syndrome*

ABSTRACT. Approximately 3500 infants die annually in the United States from sleep-related infant deaths, including sudden infant death syndrome (SIDS), ill-defined deaths, and accidental suffocation and strangulation in bed. After an initial decrease in the 1990s, the overall sleep-related infant death rate has not declined in more recent years. Many of the modifiable and nonmodifiable risk factors for SIDS and other sleep-related infant deaths are strikingly similar. The American Academy of Pediatrics recommends a safe sleep environment that can reduce the risk of all sleep-related infant deaths. Recommendations for a safe sleep environment include supine positioning, use of a firm sleep surface, room-sharing without bed-sharing, and avoidance of soft bedding and overheating. Additional recommendations for SIDS risk reduction include avoidance of exposure to smoke, alcohol, and illicit drugs; breastfeeding; routine immunization; and use of a pacifier. New evidence and rationale for recommendations are presented for skin-to-skin care for newborn infants, bedside and in-bed sleepers, sleeping

on couches/armchairs and in sitting devices, and use of soft bedding after 4 months of age. In addition, expanded recommendations for infant sleep location are included. The recommendations and strength of evidence for each recommendation are published in the accompanying policy statement, "SIDS and Other Sleep-Related Infant Deaths: Updated 2016 Recommendations for a Safe Infant Sleeping Environment," which is included in this issue. (10/16)

See full text on page 1215.

http://pediatrics.aappublications.org/content/138/5/e20162940

SKATEBOARD AND SCOOTER INJURIES

Committee on Injury, Violence, and Poison Prevention

ABSTRACT. Skateboard-related injuries account for an estimated 50 000 emergency department visits and 1500 hospitalizations among children and adolescents in the United States each year. Nonpowered scooter-related injuries accounted for an estimated 9400 emergency department visits between January and August 2000, and 90% of these patients were children younger than 15 years. Many such injuries can be avoided if children and youth do not ride in traffic, if proper protective gear is worn, and if, in the absence of close adult supervision, skateboards and scooters are not used by children younger than 10 and 8 years, respectively. (3/02, reaffirmed 5/05, 10/08, 10/13)

http://pediatrics.aappublications.org/content/109/3/542

SKIN-TO-SKIN CARE FOR TERM AND PRETERM INFANTS IN THE NEONATAL ICU (CLINICAL REPORT)

Jill Baley, MD, and Committee on Fetus and Newborn

ABSTRACT. "Kangaroo mother care" was first described as an alternative method of caring for low birth weight infants in resource-limited countries, where neonatal mortality and infection rates are high because of overcrowded nurseries, inadequate staffing, and lack of equipment. Intermittent skin-to-skin care (SSC), a modified version of kangaroo mother care, is now being offered in resource-rich countries to infants needing neonatal intensive care, including those who require ventilator support or are extremely premature. SSC significantly improves milk production by the mother and is associated with a longer duration of breastfeeding. Increased parent satisfaction, better sleep organization, a longer duration of quiet sleep, and decreased pain perception during procedures have also been reported in association with SSC. Despite apparent physiologic stability during SSC, it is prudent that infants in the NICU have continuous cardiovascular monitoring and that care be taken to verify correct head positioning for airway patency as well as the stability of the endotracheal tube, arterial and venous access devices, and other life support equipment. (8/15)

http://pediatrics.aappublications.org/content/136/3/596

SNACKS, SWEETENED BEVERAGES, ADDED SUGARS, AND SCHOOLS

Council on School Health and Committee on Nutrition

ABSTRACT. Concern over childhood obesity has generated a decade-long reformation of school nutrition policies. Food is available in school in 3 venues: federally sponsored school meal programs; items sold in

competition to school meals, such as a la carte, vending machines, and school stores; and foods available in myriad informal settings, including packed meals and snacks, bake sales, fundraisers, sports booster sales, in-class parties, or other school celebrations. High-energy, low-nutrient beverages, in particular, contribute substantial calories, but little nutrient content, to a student's diet. In 2004, the American Academy of Pediatrics recommended that sweetened drinks be replaced in school by water, white and flavored milks, or 100% fruit and vegetable beverages. Since then, school nutrition has undergone a significant transformation. Federal, state, and local regulations and policies, along with alternative products developed by industry, have helped decrease the availability of nutrient-poor foods and beverages in school. However, regular access to foods of high energy and low quality remains a school issue, much of it attributable to students, parents, and staff. Pediatricians, aligning with experts on child nutrition, are in a position to offer a perspective promoting nutrient-rich foods within calorie guidelines to improve those foods brought into or sold in schools. A positive emphasis on nutritional value, variety, appropriate portion, and encouragement for a steady improvement in quality will be a more effective approach for improving nutrition and health than simply advocating for the elimination of added sugars. (2/15)
http://pediatrics.aappublications.org/content/135/3/575

SNOWMOBILING HAZARDS
Committee on Injury and Poison Prevention
ABSTRACT. Snowmobiles continue to pose a significant risk to children younger than 15 years and adolescents and young adults 15 through 24 years of age. Head injuries remain the leading cause of mortality and serious morbidity, arising largely from snowmobilers colliding, falling, or overturning during operation. Children also were injured while being towed in a variety of conveyances by snowmobiles. No uniform code of state laws governs the use of snowmobiles by children and youth. Because evidence is lacking to support the effectiveness of operator safety certification and because many children and adolescents do not have the required strength and skills to operate a snowmobile safely, the recreational operation of snowmobiles by persons younger than 16 years is not recommended. Snowmobiles should not be used to tow persons on a tube, tire, sled, or saucer. Furthermore, a graduated licensing program is advised for snowmobilers 16 years and older. Both active and passive snowmobile injury prevention strategies are suggested, as well as recommendations for manufacturers to make safer equipment for snowmobilers of all ages. (11/00, reaffirmed 5/04, 1/07, 6/10)
http://pediatrics.aappublications.org/content/106/5/1142

SOFT DRINKS IN SCHOOLS
Committee on School Health
ABSTRACT. This statement is intended to inform pediatricians and other health care professionals, parents, superintendents, and school board members about nutritional concerns regarding soft drink consumption in schools.

Potential health problems associated with high intake of sweetened drinks are (1) overweight or obesity attributable to additional calories in the diet; (2) displacement of milk consumption, resulting in calcium deficiency with an attendant risk of osteoporosis and fractures; and (3) dental caries and potential enamel erosion. Contracts with school districts for exclusive soft drink rights encourage consumption directly and indirectly. School officials and parents need to become well informed about the health implications of vended drinks in school before making a decision about student access to them. A clearly defined, district-wide policy that restricts the sale of soft drinks will safeguard against health problems as a result of over-consumption. (1/04, reaffirmed 1/09)
http://pediatrics.aappublications.org/content/113/1/152

SPECIAL REQUIREMENTS OF ELECTRONIC HEALTH RECORD SYSTEMS IN PEDIATRICS (CLINICAL REPORT)
S. Andrew Spooner, MD, MS, and Council on Clinical Information Technology
ABSTRACT. Some functions of an electronic health record system are much more important in providing pediatric care than in adult care. Pediatricians commonly complain about the absence of these "pediatric functions" when they are not available in electronic health record systems. To stimulate electronic health record system vendors to recognize and incorporate pediatric functionality into pediatric electronic health record systems, this clinical report reviews the major functions of importance to child health care providers. Also reviewed are important but less critical functions, any of which might be of major importance in a particular clinical context. The major areas described here are immunization management, growth tracking, medication dosing, data norms, and privacy in special pediatric populations. The American Academy of Pediatrics believes that if the functions described in this document are supported in all electronic health record systems, these systems will be more useful for patients of all ages. (3/07, reaffirmed 5/12, 5/16)
http://pediatrics.aappublications.org/content/119/3/631

SPECTRUM OF NONINFECTIOUS HEALTH EFFECTS FROM MOLDS
Committee on Environmental Health
ABSTRACT. Molds are eukaryotic (possessing a true nucleus) nonphotosynthetic organisms that flourish both indoors and outdoors. For humans, the link between mold exposure and asthma exacerbations, allergic rhinitis, infections, and toxicities from ingestion of mycotoxin-contaminated foods are well known. However, the cause-and-effect relationship between inhalational exposure to mold and other untoward health effects (eg, acute idiopathic pulmonary hemorrhage in infants and other illnesses and health complaints) requires additional investigation. Pediatricians play an important role in the education of families about mold, its adverse health effects, exposure prevention, and remediation procedures. (12/06, reaffirmed 1/11)
http://pediatrics.aappublications.org/content/118/6/2582

SPECTRUM OF NONINFECTIOUS HEALTH EFFECTS FROM MOLDS (TECHNICAL REPORT)

Lynnette J. Mazur, MD, MPH; Janice Kim, MD, PhD, MPH; and Committee on Environmental Health

ABSTRACT. Molds are multicellular fungi that are ubiquitous in outdoor and indoor environments. For humans, they are both beneficial (for the production of antimicrobial agents, chemotherapeutic agents, and vitamins) and detrimental. Exposure to mold can occur through inhalation, ingestion, and touching moldy surfaces. Adverse health effects may occur through allergic, infectious, irritant, or toxic processes. The cause-and-effect relationship between mold exposure and allergic and infectious illnesses is well known. Exposures to toxins via the gastrointestinal tract also are well described. However, the cause-and-effect relationship between inhalational exposure to mold toxins and other untoward health effects (eg, acute idiopathic pulmonary hemorrhage in infants and other illnesses and health complaints) is controversial and requires additional investigation. In this report we examine evidence of fungal-related illnesses and the unique aspects of mold exposure to children. Mold-remediation procedures are also discussed. (12/06, reaffirmed 1/11)
http://pediatrics.aappublications.org/content/118/6/e1909

SPORT-RELATED CONCUSSION IN CHILDREN AND ADOLESCENTS (CLINICAL REPORT)

Mark E. Halstead, MD; Kevin D. Walter, MD; and Council on Sports Medicine and Fitness

ABSTRACT. Sport-related concussion is a "hot topic" in the media and in medicine. It is a common injury that is likely underreported by pediatric and adolescent athletes. Football has the highest incidence of concussion, but girls have higher concussion rates than boys do in similar sports. A clear understanding of the definition, signs, and symptoms of concussion is necessary to recognize it and rule out more severe intracranial injury. Concussion can cause symptoms that interfere with school, social and family relationships, and participation in sports. Recognition and education are paramount, because although proper equipment, sport technique, and adherence to rules of the sport may decrease the incidence or severity of concussions, nothing has been shown to prevent them. Appropriate management is essential for reducing the risk of long-term symptoms and complications. Cognitive and physical rest is the mainstay of management after diagnosis, and neuropsychological testing is a helpful tool in the management of concussion. Return to sport should be accomplished by using a progressive exercise program while evaluating for any return of signs or symptoms. This report serves as a basis for understanding the diagnosis and management of concussion in children and adolescent athletes. (8/10, reaffirmed 8/14)
http://pediatrics.aappublications.org/content/126/3/597

SPORTS DRINKS AND ENERGY DRINKS FOR CHILDREN AND ADOLESCENTS: ARE THEY APPROPRIATE? (CLINICAL REPORT)

Committee on Nutrition and Council on Sports Medicine and Fitness

ABSTRACT. Sports and energy drinks are being marketed to children and adolescents for a wide variety of inappropriate uses. Sports drinks and energy drinks are significantly different products, and the terms should not be used interchangeably. The primary objectives of this clinical report are to define the ingredients of sports and energy drinks, categorize the similarities and differences between the products, and discuss misuses and abuses. Secondary objectives are to encourage screening during annual physical examinations for sports and energy drink use, to understand the reasons why youth consumption is widespread, and to improve education aimed at decreasing or eliminating the inappropriate use of these beverages by children and adolescents. Rigorous review and analysis of the literature reveal that caffeine and other stimulant substances contained in energy drinks have no place in the diet of children and adolescents. Furthermore, frequent or excessive intake of caloric sports drinks can substantially increase the risk for overweight or obesity in children and adolescents. Discussion regarding the appropriate use of sports drinks in the youth athlete who participates regularly in endurance or high-intensity sports and vigorous physical activity is beyond the scope of this report. (5/11)
http://pediatrics.aappublications.org/content/127/6/1182

SPORTS SPECIALIZATION AND INTENSIVE TRAINING IN YOUNG ATHLETES (CLINICAL REPORT)

Joel S. Brenner, MD, MPH, FAAP, and Council on Sports Medicine and Fitness

ABSTRACT. Sports specialization is becoming the norm in youth sports for a variety of reasons. When sports specialization occurs too early, detrimental effects may occur, both physically and psychologically. If the timing is correct and sports specialization is performed under the correct conditions, the athlete may be successful in reaching specific goals. Young athletes who train intensively, whether specialized or not, can also be at risk of adverse effects on the mind and body. The purpose of this clinical report is to assist pediatricians in counseling their young athlete patients and their parents regarding sports specialization and intensive training. This report supports the American Academy of Pediatrics clinical report "Overuse Injuries, Overtraining, and Burnout in Child and Adolescent Athletes." (8/16)
See full text on page 1251.
http://pediatrics.aappublications.org/content/138/3/e20162148

STANDARD TERMINOLOGY FOR FETAL, INFANT, AND PERINATAL DEATHS (CLINICAL REPORT)

Wanda D. Barfield, MD, MPH, and Committee on Fetus and Newborn

ABSTRACT. Accurately defining and reporting perinatal deaths (ie, fetal and infant deaths) is a critical first step in understanding the magnitude and causes of these important events. In addition to obstetric health care providers, neonatologists and pediatricians should have easy access to current and updated resources that clearly provide US definitions and reporting requirements for live births, fetal deaths, and infant deaths. Correct identification of these vital events will improve local, state, and national data so that these deaths can be better addressed and prevented. (4/16)

See full text on page 1261.

http://pediatrics.aappublications.org/content/137/5/e20160551

STANDARDIZATION OF INPATIENT HANDOFF COMMUNICATION (CLINICAL REPORT)

Jennifer A. Jewell, MD, FAAP, and Committee on Hospital Care
ABSTRACT. Handoff communication is identified as an integral part of hospital care. Throughout medical communities, inadequate handoff communication is being highlighted as a significant risk to patients. The complexity of hospitals and the number of providers involved in the care of hospitalized patients place inpatients at high risk of communication lapses. This miscommunication and the potential resulting harm make effective handoffs more critical than ever. Although hospitalized patients are being exposed to many handoffs each day, this report is limited to describing the best handoff practices between providers at the time of shift change. (10/16)

See full text on page 1269.

http://pediatrics.aappublications.org/content/138/5/e20162681

STANDARDS FOR HEALTH INFORMATION TECHNOLOGY TO ENSURE ADOLESCENT PRIVACY

Committee on Adolescence and Council on Clinical Information Technology
ABSTRACT. Privacy and security of health information is a basic expectation of patients. Despite the existence of federal and state laws safeguarding the privacy of health information, health information systems currently lack the capability to allow for protection of this information for minors. This policy statement reviews the challenges to privacy for adolescents posed by commercial health information technology systems and recommends basic principles for ideal electronic health record systems. This policy statement has been endorsed by the Society for Adolescent Health and Medicine. (10/12)

http://pediatrics.aappublications.org/content/130/5/987

STANDARDS FOR PEDIATRIC CANCER CENTERS

Section on Hematology/Oncology
ABSTRACT. Since the American Academy of Pediatrics–published guidelines for pediatric cancer centers in 1986, 1997, and 2004, significant changes in the delivery of health care have prompted a review of the role of medical centers in the care of pediatric patients. The potential effect of these changes on the treatment and survival rates of children with cancer led to this revision. The intent of this statement is to delineate personnel, capabilities, and facilities that are essential to provide state-of-the-art care for children, adolescents, and young adults with cancer. This statement emphasizes the importance of board-certified pediatric hematologists/oncologists and appropriately qualified pediatric medical subspecialists and pediatric surgical specialists overseeing patient care and the need for specialized facilities as essential for the initial management and much of the follow-up for pediatric, adolescent, and young adult patients with cancer. For patients without practical access to a pediatric cancer center, care may be provided locally by a primary care physician or adult oncologist but at the direction of a pediatric oncologist. (7/14)

http://pediatrics.aappublications.org/content/134/2/410

STATE CHILDREN'S HEALTH INSURANCE PROGRAM ACHIEVEMENTS, CHALLENGES, AND POLICY RECOMMENDATIONS

Committee on Child Health Financing
ABSTRACT. This policy statement reviews the impressive progress of the State Children's Health Insurance Program since its enactment in 1997 and identifies outstanding challenges and state and federal policy recommendations. The American Academy of Pediatrics urges Congress to reauthorize SCHIP to strengthen its historic gains. The following set of recommended strategies for reauthorization pertain to funding, eligibility and enrollment, coverage, cost sharing, payment and provider-network capacity, and quality performance. (6/07)

http://pediatrics.aappublications.org/content/119/6/1224

STRATEGIES FOR PREVENTION OF HEALTH CARE–ASSOCIATED INFECTIONS IN THE NICU (CLINICAL REPORT)

Richard A. Polin, MD; Susan Denson, MD; Michael T. Brady, MD; Committee on Fetus and Newborn; and Committee on Infectious Diseases
ABSTRACT. Health care–associated infections in the NICU result in increased morbidity and mortality, prolonged lengths of stay, and increased medical costs. Neonates are at high risk of acquiring health care–associated infections because of impaired host-defense mechanisms, limited amounts of protective endogenous flora on skin and mucosal surfaces at time of birth, reduced barrier function of their skin, use of invasive procedures and devices, and frequent exposure to broad-spectrum antibiotic agents. This clinical report reviews management and prevention of health care–associated infections in newborn infants. (3/12, reaffirmed 2/16)

http://pediatrics.aappublications.org/content/129/4/e1085

STRENGTH TRAINING BY CHILDREN AND ADOLESCENTS

Council on Sports Medicine and Fitness
ABSTRACT. Pediatricians are often asked to give advice on the safety and efficacy of strength-training programs for children and adolescents. This statement, which is a revision of a previous American Academy of Pediatrics policy statement, defines relevant terminology and provides current information on risks and benefits of strength training for children and adolescents. (4/08, reaffirmed 6/11)

http://pediatrics.aappublications.org/content/121/4/835

SUBSTANCE USE SCREENING, BRIEF INTERVENTION, AND REFERRAL TO TREATMENT

Committee on Substance Use and Prevention

ABSTRACT. The enormous public health impact of adolescent substance use and its preventable morbidity and mortality show the need for the health care sector, including pediatricians and the medical home, to increase its capacity related to substance use prevention, detection, assessment, and intervention. The American Academy of Pediatrics published its policy statement "Substance Use Screening, Brief Intervention, and Referral to Treatment for Pediatricians" in 2011 to introduce the concepts and terminology of screening, brief intervention, and referral to treatment (SBIRT) and to offer clinical guidance about available substance use screening tools and intervention procedures. This policy statement is a revision of the 2011 SBIRT statement. An accompanying clinical report updates clinical guidance for adolescent SBIRT. (6/16)

See full text on page 1277.

http://pediatrics.aappublications.org/content/138/1/e20161210

SUBSTANCE USE SCREENING, BRIEF INTERVENTION, AND REFERRAL TO TREATMENT (CLINICAL REPORT)

Sharon J. L. Levy, MD, MPH, FAAP; Janet F. Williams, MD, FAAP; and Committee on Substance Use and Prevention

ABSTRACT. The enormous public health impact of adolescent substance use and its preventable morbidity and mortality highlight the need for the health care sector, including pediatricians and the medical home, to increase its capacity regarding adolescent substance use screening, brief intervention, and referral to treatment (SBIRT). The American Academy of Pediatrics first published a policy statement on SBIRT and adolescents in 2011 to introduce SBIRT concepts and terminology and to offer clinical guidance about available substance use screening tools and intervention procedures. This clinical report provides a simplified adolescent SBIRT clinical approach that, in combination with the accompanying updated policy statement, guides pediatricians in implementing substance use prevention, detection, assessment, and intervention practices across the varied clinical settings in which adolescents receive health care. (6/16)

See full text on page 1283.

http://pediatrics.aappublications.org/content/138/1/e20161211

SUICIDE AND SUICIDE ATTEMPTS IN ADOLESCENTS (CLINICAL REPORT)

Benjamin Shain, MD, PhD, and Committee on Adolescence

ABSTRACT. Suicide is the second leading cause of death for adolescents 15 to 19 years old. This report updates the previous statement of the American Academy of Pediatrics and is intended to assist pediatricians, in collaboration with other child and adolescent health care professionals, in the identification and management of the adolescent at risk for suicide. Suicide risk can only be reduced, not eliminated, and risk factors provide no more than guidance. Nonetheless, care for suicidal adolescents may be improved with the pediatrician's knowledge, skill, and comfort with the topic, as well as ready access to appropriate community resources and mental health professionals. (6/16)

See full text on page 1301.

http://pediatrics.aappublications.org/content/138/1/e20161420

SUPPLEMENTAL SECURITY INCOME (SSI) FOR CHILDREN AND YOUTH WITH DISABILITIES

Council on Children With Disabilities

ABSTRACT. The Supplemental Security Income (SSI) program remains an important source of financial support for low-income families of children with special health care needs and disabling conditions. In most states, SSI eligibility also qualifies children for the state Medicaid program, providing access to health care services. The Social Security Administration (SSA), which administers the SSI program, considers a child disabled under SSI if there is a medically determinable physical or mental impairment or combination of impairments that results in marked and severe functional limitations. The impairment(s) must be expected to result in death or have lasted or be expected to last for a continuous period of at least 12 months. The income and assets of families of children with disabilities are also considered when determining financial eligibility. When an individual with a disability becomes an adult at 18 years of age, the SSA considers only the individual's income and assets. The SSA considers an adult to be disabled if there is a medically determinable impairment (or combination of impairments) that prevents substantial gainful activity for at least 12 continuous months. SSI benefits are important for youth with chronic conditions who are transitioning to adulthood. The purpose of this statement is to provide updated information about the SSI medical and financial eligibility criteria and the disability-determination process. This statement also discusses how pediatricians can help children and youth when they apply for SSI benefits. (11/09, reaffirmed 2/15)

http://pediatrics.aappublications.org/content/124/6/1702

SUPPORTING THE FAMILY AFTER THE DEATH OF A CHILD (CLINICAL REPORT)

Esther Wender, MD, and Committee on Psychosocial Aspects of Child and Family Health

ABSTRACT. The death of a child can have a devastating effect on the family. The pediatrician has an important role to play in supporting the parents and any siblings still in his or her practice after such a death. Pediatricians may be poorly prepared to provide this support. Also, because of the pain of confronting the grief of family members, they may be reluctant to become involved. This statement gives guidelines to help the pediatrician provide such support. It describes the grief reactions that can be expected in family members after the death of a child. Ways of supporting family members are suggested, and other helpful resources in the community are described. The goal of this guidance is to prevent outcomes that may impair the health and development of affected parents and children. (11/12)

http://pediatrics.aappublications.org/content/130/6/1164

SUPPORTING THE GRIEVING CHILD AND FAMILY (CLINICAL REPORT)

David J. Schonfeld, MD, FAAP; Thomas Demaria, PhD; Committee on Psychosocial Aspects of Child and Family Health; and Disaster Preparedness Advisory Council

ABSTRACT. The death of someone close to a child often has a profound and lifelong effect on the child and results in a range of both short- and long-term reactions.

Pediatricians, within a patient-centered medical home, are in an excellent position to provide anticipatory guidance to caregivers and to offer assistance and support to children and families who are grieving. This clinical report offers practical suggestions on how to talk with grieving children to help them better understand what has happened and its implications and to address any misinformation, misinterpretations, or misconceptions. An understanding of guilt, shame, and other common reactions, as well an appreciation of the role of secondary losses and the unique challenges facing children in communities characterized by chronic trauma and cumulative loss, will help the pediatrician to address factors that may impair grieving and children's adjustment and to identify complicated mourning and situations when professional counseling is indicated. Advice on how to support children's participation in funerals and other memorial services and to anticipate and address grief triggers and anniversary reactions is provided so that pediatricians are in a better position to advise caregivers and to offer consultation to schools, early education and child care facilities, and other child congregate care sites. Pediatricians often enter their profession out of a profound desire to minimize the suffering of children and may find it personally challenging when they find themselves in situations in which they are asked to bear witness to the distress of children who are acutely grieving. The importance of professional preparation and self-care is therefore emphasized, and resources are recommended. (8/16)

See full text on page 1315.

http://pediatrics.aappublications.org/content/138/3/e20162147

SUPPORTING THE HEALTH CARE TRANSITION FROM ADOLESCENCE TO ADULTHOOD IN THE MEDICAL HOME (CLINICAL REPORT)

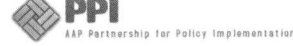

American Academy of Pediatrics, American Academy of Family Physicians, and American College of Physicians Transitions Clinical Report Authoring Group

ABSTRACT. Optimal health care is achieved when each person, at every age, receives medically and developmentally appropriate care. The goal of a planned health care transition is to maximize lifelong functioning and well-being for all youth, including those who have special health care needs and those who do not. This process includes ensuring that high-quality, developmentally appropriate health care services are available in an uninterrupted manner as the person moves from adolescence to adulthood. A well-timed transition from child- to adult-oriented health care is specific to each person and ideally occurs between the ages of 18 and 21 years. Coordination of patient, family, and provider responsibilities enables youth to optimize their ability to assume adult roles and activities. This clinical report represents expert opinion and consensus on the practice-based implementation of transition for all youth beginning in early adolescence. It provides a structure for training and continuing education to further understanding of the nature of adolescent transition and how best to support it. Primary care physicians, nurse practitioners, and physician assistants, as well as medical subspecialists, are encouraged to adopt these

materials and make this process specific to their settings and populations. (7/11, reaffirmed 8/15)

http://pediatrics.aappublications.org/content/128/1/182

SURFACTANT REPLACEMENT THERAPY FOR PRETERM AND TERM NEONATES WITH RESPIRATORY DISTRESS (CLINICAL REPORT)

Richard A. Polin, MD, FAAP; Waldemar A. Carlo, MD, FAAP; and Committee on Fetus and Newborn

ABSTRACT. Respiratory failure secondary to surfactant deficiency is a major cause of morbidity and mortality in preterm infants. Surfactant therapy substantially reduces mortality and respiratory morbidity for this population. Secondary surfactant deficiency also contributes to acute respiratory morbidity in late-preterm and term neonates with meconium aspiration syndrome, pneumonia/sepsis, and perhaps pulmonary hemorrhage; surfactant replacement may be beneficial for these infants. This statement summarizes the evidence regarding indications, administration, formulations, and outcomes for surfactant-replacement therapy. The clinical strategy of intubation, surfactant administration, and extubation to continuous positive airway pressure and the effect of continuous positive airway pressure on outcomes and surfactant use in preterm infants are also reviewed. (12/13)

http://pediatrics.aappublications.org/content/133/1/156

SWIMMING PROGRAMS FOR INFANTS AND TODDLERS

Committee on Sports Medicine and Fitness and Committee on Injury and Poison Prevention

Infant and toddler aquatic programs provide an opportunity to introduce young children to the joy and risks of being in or around water. Generally, children are not developmentally ready for swimming lessons until after their fourth birthday. Aquatic programs for infants and toddlers have not been shown to decrease the risk of drowning, and parents should not feel secure that their child is safe in water or safe from drowning after participating in such programs. Young children should receive constant, close supervision by an adult while in and around water. (4/00, reaffirmed 5/04)

http://pediatrics.aappublications.org/content/105/4/868

TACKLING IN YOUTH FOOTBALL

Council on Sports Medicine and Fitness

ABSTRACT. American football remains one of the most popular sports for young athletes. The injuries sustained during football, especially those to the head and neck, have been a topic of intense interest recently in both the public media and medical literature. The recognition of these injuries and the potential for long-term sequelae have led some physicians to call for a reduction in the number of contact practices, a postponement of tackling until a certain age, and even a ban on high school football. This statement reviews the literature regarding injuries in football, particularly those of the head and neck, the relationship between tackling and football-related injuries, and the potential effects of limiting or delaying tackling on injury risk. (10/15)

http://pediatrics.aappublications.org/content/136/5/e1419

THE TEEN DRIVER

Committee on Injury, Violence, and Poison Prevention and Committee on Adolescence

ABSTRACT. Motor vehicle–related injuries to adolescents continue to be of paramount importance to society. Since the original policy statement on the teenaged driver was published in 1996, there have been substantial changes in many state laws and much new research on this topic. There is a need to provide pediatricians with up-to-date information and materials to facilitate appropriate counseling and anticipatory guidance. This statement describes why teenagers are at greater risk of motor vehicle–related injuries, suggests topics suitable for office-based counseling, describes innovative programs, and proposes preventive interventions for pediatricians, parents, legislators, educators, and other child advocates. (12/06, reaffirmed 6/10, 7/16)

http://pediatrics.aappublications.org/content/118/6/2570

TELEMEDICINE FOR EVALUATION OF RETINOPATHY OF PREMATURITY (TECHNICAL REPORT)

Walter M. Fierson, MD, FAAP; Antonio Capone Jr, MD; and Section on Ophthalmology (joint with American Academy of Ophthalmology and American Association of Certified Orthoptists)

ABSTRACT. Retinopathy of prematurity (ROP) remains a significant threat to vision for extremely premature infants despite the availability of therapeutic modalities capable, in most cases, of managing this disorder. It has been shown in many controlled trials that application of therapies at the appropriate time is essential to successful outcomes in premature infants affected by ROP. Bedside binocular indirect ophthalmoscopy has been the standard technique for diagnosis and monitoring of ROP in these patients. However, implementation of routine use of this screening method for at-risk premature infants has presented challenges within our existing care systems, including relative local scarcity of qualified ophthalmologist examiners in some locations and the remote location of some NICUs. Modern technology, including the development of wide-angle ocular digital fundus photography, coupled with the ability to send digital images electronically to remote locations, has led to the development of telemedicine-based remote digital fundus imaging (RDFI-TM) evaluation techniques. These techniques have the potential to allow the diagnosis and monitoring of ROP to occur in lieu of the necessity for some repeated on-site examinations in NICUs. This report reviews the currently available literature on RDFI-TM evaluations for ROP and outlines pertinent practical and risk management considerations that should be used when including RDFI-TM in any new or existing ROP care structure. (12/14)

http://pediatrics.aappublications.org/content/135/1/e238

TELEMEDICINE: PEDIATRIC APPLICATIONS (TECHNICAL REPORT)

Bryan L. Burke Jr, MD, FAAP; R. W. Hall, MD, FAAP; and Section on Telehealth Care

ABSTRACT. Telemedicine is a technological tool that is improving the health of children around the world. This report chronicles the use of telemedicine by pediatricians and pediatric medical and surgical specialists to deliver inpatient and outpatient care, educate physicians and patients, and conduct medical research. It also describes the importance of telemedicine in responding to emergencies and disasters and providing access to pediatric care to remote and underserved populations. Barriers to telemedicine expansion are explained, such as legal issues, inadequate payment for services, technology costs and sustainability, and the lack of technology infrastructure on a national scale. Although certain challenges have constrained more widespread implementation, telemedicine's current use bears testimony to its effectiveness and potential. Telemedicine's widespread adoption will be influenced by the implementation of key provisions of the Patient Protection and Affordable Care Act, technological advances, and growing patient demand for virtual visits. (6/15)

http://pediatrics.aappublications.org/content/136/1/e293

TESTING FOR DRUGS OF ABUSE IN CHILDREN AND ADOLESCENTS (CLINICAL REPORT)

Sharon Levy, MD, MPH, FAAP; Lorena M. Siqueira, MD, MSPH, FAAP; and Committee on Substance Abuse

ABSTRACT. Drug testing is often used as part of an assessment for substance use in children and adolescents. However, the indications for drug testing and guidance on how to use this procedure effectively are not clear. The complexity and invasiveness of the procedure and limitations to the information derived from drug testing all affect its utility. The objective of this clinical report is to provide guidance to pediatricians and other clinicians on the efficacy and efficient use of drug testing on the basis of a review of the nascent scientific literature, policy guidelines, and published clinical recommendations. (5/14)

http://pediatrics.aappublications.org/content/133/6/e1798

TOBACCO, ALCOHOL, AND OTHER DRUGS: THE ROLE OF THE PEDIATRICIAN IN PREVENTION, IDENTIFICATION, AND MANAGEMENT OF SUBSTANCE ABUSE (CLINICAL REPORT)

John W. Kulig, MD, MPH, and Committee on Substance Abuse

ABSTRACT. Substance abuse remains a major public health concern, and pediatricians are uniquely positioned to assist their patients and families with its prevention, detection, and treatment. The American Academy of Pediatrics has highlighted the importance of such issues in a variety of ways, including its guidelines for preventive services. The harmful consequences of tobacco, alcohol, and other drug use are a concern of medical professionals who care for infants, children, adolescents, and young adults. Thus, pediatricians should include discussion of substance abuse as a part of routine health care, starting with the prenatal visit, and as part of ongoing anticipatory guidance. Knowledge of the nature and extent of the consequences of tobacco, alcohol, and other drug use as well as the physical, psychological, and social consequences is essential for pediatricians. Pediatricians should incorporate substance-abuse prevention into daily practice, acquire the skills necessary to identify young people at risk of substance abuse, and provide or facilitate assessment, intervention, and treatment as necessary. (3/05, reaffirmed 3/13)

http://pediatrics.aappublications.org/content/115/3/816

TOBACCO AS A SUBSTANCE OF ABUSE (TECHNICAL REPORT)

Tammy H. Sims, MD, MS, and Committee on Substance Abuse

ABSTRACT. Tobacco use is the leading preventable cause of morbidity and death in the United States. Because 80% to 90% of adult smokers began during adolescence, and two thirds became regular, daily smokers before they reached 19 years of age, tobacco use may be viewed as a pediatric disease. Every year in the United States, approximately 1.4 million children younger than 18 years start smoking, and many of them will die prematurely from a smoking-related disease. Moreover, there is recent evidence that adolescents report symptoms of tobacco dependence early in the smoking process, even before becoming daily smokers. The prevalence of tobacco use is higher among teenagers and young adults than among older adult populations. The critical role of pediatricians in helping to reduce tobacco use and addiction and secondhand tobacco-smoke exposure in the pediatric population includes education and prevention, screening and detection, and treatment and referral. (10/09, reaffirmed 12/14)
http://pediatrics.aappublications.org/content/124/5/e1045

TOBACCO USE: A PEDIATRIC DISEASE

Committee on Environmental Health, Committee on Substance Abuse, Committee on Adolescence, and Committee on Native American Child Health

ABSTRACT. Tobacco use and secondhand tobacco-smoke (SHS) exposure are major national and international health concerns. Pediatricians and other clinicians who care for children are uniquely positioned to assist patients and families with tobacco-use prevention and treatment. Understanding the nature and extent of tobacco use and SHS exposure is an essential first step toward the goal of eliminating tobacco use and its consequences in the pediatric population. The next steps include counseling patients and family members to avoid SHS exposures or cease tobacco use; advocacy for policies that protect children from SHS exposure; and elimination of tobacco use in the media, public places, and homes. Three overarching principles of this policy can be identified: (1) there is no safe way to use tobacco; (2) there is no safe level or duration of exposure to SHS; and (3) the financial and political power of individuals, organizations, and government should be used to support tobacco control. Pediatricians are advised not to smoke or use tobacco; to make their homes, cars, and workplaces tobacco free; to consider tobacco control when making personal and professional decisions; to support and advocate for comprehensive tobacco control; and to advise parents and patients not to start using tobacco or to quit if they are already using tobacco. Prohibiting both tobacco advertising and the use of tobacco products in the media is recommended. Recommendations for eliminating SHS exposure and reducing tobacco use include attaining universal (1) smoke-free home, car, school, work, and play environments, both inside and outside, (2) treatment of tobacco use and dependence through employer, insurance, state, and federal supports, (3) implementation and enforcement of evidence-based tobacco-control measures in local, state, national, and international jurisdictions, and (4) financial and systems support for training in and research of effective ways to prevent and treat tobacco use and SHS exposure. Pediatricians, their staff and colleagues, and the American Academy of Pediatrics have key responsibilities in tobacco control to promote the health of children, adolescents, and young adults. (10/09, reaffirmed 5/13)
http://pediatrics.aappublications.org/content/124/5/1474

TOWARD TRANSPARENT CLINICAL POLICIES

Steering Committee on Quality Improvement and Management

ABSTRACT. Clinical policies of professional societies such as the American Academy of Pediatrics are valued highly, not only by clinicians who provide direct health care to children but also by many others who rely on the professional expertise of these organizations, including parents, employers, insurers, and legislators. The utility of a policy depends, in large part, on the degree to which its purpose and basis are clear to policy users, an attribute known as the policy's transparency. This statement describes the critical importance and special value of transparency in clinical policies, guidelines, and recommendations; helps identify obstacles to achieving transparency; and suggests several approaches to overcome these obstacles. (3/08, reaffirmed 2/14)
http://pediatrics.aappublications.org/content/121/3/643

TRAMPOLINE SAFETY IN CHILDHOOD AND ADOLESCENCE

Council on Sports Medicine and Fitness

ABSTRACT. Despite previous recommendations from the American Academy of Pediatrics discouraging home use of trampolines, recreational use of trampolines in the home setting continues to be a popular activity among children and adolescents. This policy statement is an update to previous statements, reflecting the current literature on prevalence, patterns, and mechanisms of trampoline-related injuries. Most trampoline injuries occur with multiple simultaneous users on the mat. Cervical spine injuries often occur with falls off the trampoline or with attempts at somersaults or flips. Studies on the efficacy of trampoline safety measures are reviewed, and although there is a paucity of data, current implementation of safety measures have not appeared to mitigate risk substantially. Therefore, the home use of trampolines is strongly discouraged. The role of trampoline as a competitive sport and in structured training settings is reviewed, and recommendations for enhancing safety in these environments are made. (9/12, reaffirmed 7/15)
http://pediatrics.aappublications.org/content/130/4/774

THE TRANSFER OF DRUGS AND THERAPEUTICS INTO HUMAN BREAST MILK: AN UPDATE ON SELECTED TOPICS (CLINICAL REPORT)

Hari Cheryl Sachs, MD, FAAP, and Committee on Drugs

ABSTRACT. Many mothers are inappropriately advised to discontinue breastfeeding or avoid taking essential medications because of fears of adverse effects on their infants. This cautious approach may be unnecessary in many cases, because only a small proportion of medications are contraindicated in breastfeeding mothers or associated with adverse effects on their infants. Information to inform physicians about the extent of excretion for a particular drug into human milk is needed but may not

be available. Previous statements on this topic from the American Academy of Pediatrics provided physicians with data concerning the known excretion of specific medications into breast milk. More current and comprehensive information is now available on the Internet, as well as an application for mobile devices, at LactMed (http://toxnet.nlm.nih.gov). Therefore, with the exception of radioactive compounds requiring temporary cessation of breastfeeding, the reader will be referred to LactMed to obtain the most current data on an individual medication. This report discusses several topics of interest surrounding lactation, such as the use of psychotropic therapies, drugs to treat substance abuse, narcotics, galactagogues, and herbal products, as well as immunization of breastfeeding women. A discussion regarding the global implications of maternal medications and lactation in the developing world is beyond the scope of this report. The World Health Organization offers several programs and resources that address the importance of breastfeeding (see http://www.who.int/topics/breastfeeding/en/). (8/13)
http://pediatrics.aappublications.org/content/132/3/e796

TRANSITIONING HIV-INFECTED YOUTH INTO ADULT HEALTH CARE
Committee on Pediatric AIDS
ABSTRACT. With advances in antiretroviral therapy, most HIV-infected children survive into adulthood. Optimal health care for these youth includes a formal plan for the transition of care from primary and/or subspecialty pediatric/adolescent/family medicine health care providers (medical home) to adult health care provider(s). Successful transition involves the early engagement and participation of the youth and his or her family with the pediatric medical home and adult health care teams in developing a formal plan. Referring providers should have a written policy for the transfer of HIV-infected youth to adult care, which will guide in the development of an individualized plan for each youth. The plan should be introduced to the youth in early adolescence and modified as the youth approaches transition. Assessment of developmental milestones is important to define the readiness of the youth in assuming responsibility for his or her own care before initiating the transfer. Communication among all providers is essential and should include both personal contact and a written medical summary. Progress toward the transition should be tracked and, once completed, should be documented and assessed. (6/13, reaffirmed 4/16)
http://pediatrics.aappublications.org/content/132/1/192

TRANSPORTING CHILDREN WITH SPECIAL HEALTH CARE NEEDS
Committee on Injury and Poison Prevention
ABSTRACT. Children with special health care needs should have access to proper resources for safe transportation. This statement reviews important considerations for transporting children with special health care needs and provides current guidelines for the protection of children with specific health care needs, including those with a tracheostomy, a spica cast, challenging behaviors, or muscle

tone abnormalities as well as those transported in wheelchairs. (10/99, reaffirmed 1/03, 1/06, 3/13)
http://pediatrics.aappublications.org/content/104/4/988

THE TREATMENT OF NEUROLOGICALLY IMPAIRED CHILDREN USING PATTERNING
Committee on Children With Disabilities
ABSTRACT. This statement reviews patterning as a treatment for children with neurologic impairments. This treatment is based on an outmoded and oversimplified theory of brain development. Current information does not support the claims of proponents that this treatment is efficacious, and its use continues to be unwarranted. (11/99, reaffirmed 11/02, 1/06, 8/10, 4/14)
http://pediatrics.aappublications.org/content/104/5/1149

ULTRAVIOLET RADIATION: A HAZARD TO CHILDREN AND ADOLESCENTS
Council on Environmental Health and Section on Dermatology
ABSTRACT. Ultraviolet radiation (UVR) causes the 3 major forms of skin cancer: basal cell carcinoma; squamous cell carcinoma; and cutaneous malignant melanoma. Public awareness of the risk is not optimal, overall compliance with sun protection is inconsistent, and melanoma rates continue to rise. The risk of skin cancer increases when people overexpose themselves to sun and intentionally expose themselves to artificial sources of UVR. Yet, people continue to sunburn, and teenagers and adults alike remain frequent visitors to tanning parlors. Pediatricians should provide advice about UVR exposure during health-supervision visits and at other relevant times. Advice includes avoiding sunburning, wearing clothing and hats, timing activities (when possible) before or after periods of peak sun exposure, wearing protective sunglasses, and applying and reapplying sunscreen. Advice should be framed in the context of promoting outdoor physical activity. Adolescents should be strongly discouraged from visiting tanning parlors. Sun exposure and vitamin D status are intertwined. Cutaneous vitamin D production requires sunlight exposure, and many factors, such as skin pigmentation, season, and time of day, complicate efficiency of cutaneous vitamin D production that results from sun exposure. Adequate vitamin D is needed for bone health. Accumulating information suggests a beneficial influence of vitamin D on many health conditions. Although vitamin D is available through the diet, supplements, and incidental sun exposure, many children have low vitamin D concentrations. Ensuring vitamin D adequacy while promoting sun-protection strategies will require renewed attention to children's use of dietary and supplemental vitamin D. (2/11)
http://pediatrics.aappublications.org/content/127/3/588

ULTRAVIOLET RADIATION: A HAZARD TO CHILDREN AND ADOLESCENTS (TECHNICAL REPORT)
Sophie J. Balk, MD; Council on Environmental Health; and Section on Dermatology
ABSTRACT. Sunlight sustains life on earth. Sunlight is essential for vitamin D synthesis in the skin. The sun's ultraviolet rays can be hazardous, however, because excessive exposure causes skin cancer and other adverse

health effects. Skin cancer is a major public health problem; more than 2 million new cases are diagnosed in the United States each year. Ultraviolet radiation (UVR) causes the 3 major forms of skin cancer: basal cell carcinoma; squamous cell carcinoma; and cutaneous malignant melanoma. Exposure to UVR from sunlight and artificial sources early in life elevates the risk of developing skin cancer. Approximately 25% of sun exposure occurs before 18 years of age. The risk of skin cancer is increased when people overexpose themselves to sun and intentionally expose themselves to artificial sources of UVR. Public awareness of the risk is not optimal, compliance with sun protection is inconsistent, and skin-cancer rates continue to rise in all age groups including the younger population. People continue to sunburn, and teenagers and adults are frequent visitors to tanning parlors. Sun exposure and vitamin D status are intertwined. Adequate vitamin D is needed for bone health in children and adults. In addition, there is accumulating information suggesting a beneficial influence of vitamin D on various health conditions. Cutaneous vitamin D production requires sunlight, and many factors complicate the efficiency of vitamin D production that results from sunlight exposure. Ensuring vitamin D adequacy while promoting sun-protection strategies, therefore, requires renewed attention to evaluating the adequacy of dietary and supplemental vitamin D. Daily intake of 400 IU of vitamin D will prevent vitamin D deficiency rickets in infants. The vitamin D supplementation amounts necessary to support optimal health in older children and adolescents are less clear. This report updates information on the relationship of sun exposure to skin cancer and other adverse health effects, the relationship of exposure to artificial sources of UVR and skin cancer, sun-protection methods, vitamin D, community skin-cancer–prevention efforts, and the pediatrician's role in preventing skin cancer. In addition to pediatricians' efforts, a sustained public health effort is needed to change attitudes and behaviors regarding UVR exposure. (3/11)
http://pediatrics.aappublications.org/content/127/3/e791

UMBILICAL CORD CARE IN THE NEWBORN INFANT (CLINICAL REPORT)

Dan Stewart, MD, FAAP; William Benitz, MD, FAAP; and Committee on Fetus and Newborn

ABSTRACT. Postpartum infections remain a leading cause of neonatal morbidity and mortality worldwide. A high percentage of these infections may stem from bacterial colonization of the umbilicus, because cord care practices vary in reflection of cultural traditions within communities and disparities in health care practices globally. After birth, the devitalized umbilical cord often proves to be an ideal substrate for bacterial growth and also provides direct access to the bloodstream of the neonate. Bacterial colonization of the cord not infrequently leads to omphalitis and associated thrombophlebitis, cellulitis, or necrotizing fasciitis. Various topical substances continue to be used for cord care around the world to mitigate the risk of serious infection. More recently, particularly in high-resource countries, the treatment paradigm has shifted toward dry umbilical cord care. This clinical report reviews the evidence underlying recommendations for care of the umbilical cord in different clinical settings. (8/16)

See full text on page 1329.
http://pediatrics.aappublications.org/content/138/3/e20162149

UNDERINSURANCE OF ADOLESCENTS: RECOMMENDATIONS FOR IMPROVED COVERAGE OF PREVENTIVE, REPRODUCTIVE, AND BEHAVIORAL HEALTH CARE SERVICES

Committee on Adolescence and Committee on Child Health Financing

ABSTRACT. The purpose of this policy statement is to address the serious underinsurance (ie, insurance that exists but is inadequate) problems affecting insured adolescents' access to needed preventive, reproductive, and behavioral health care. In addition, the statement addresses provider payment problems that disproportionately affect clinicians who care for adolescents.

Among adolescents with insurance, particularly private health insurance, coverage of needed services is often inadequate. Benefits are typically limited in scope and amount; certain diagnoses are often excluded; and cost-sharing requirements are often too high. As a result, underinsurance represents a substantial problem among adolescents and adversely affects their health and well-being.

In addition to underinsurance problems, payment problems in the form of inadequate payment, uncompensated care for confidential reproductive services, and the failure of insurers to recognize and pay for certain billing and diagnostic codes are widespread among both private and public insurers. Payment problems negatively affect clinicians' ability to offer needed services to adolescents, especially publicly insured adolescents. (12/08, reaffirmed 8/12, 5/15)
http://pediatrics.aappublications.org/content/123/1/191

UNDERSTANDING THE BEHAVIORAL AND EMOTIONAL CONSEQUENCES OF CHILD ABUSE (CLINICAL REPORT)

John Stirling Jr, MD; Committee on Child Abuse and Neglect; and Section on Adoption and Foster Care (joint with Lisa Amaya-Jackson, MD, MPH; American Academy of Child and Adolescent Psychiatry; and National Center for Child Traumatic Stress)

ABSTRACT. Children who have suffered early abuse or neglect may later present with significant behavior problems including emotional instability, depression, and a tendency to be aggressive or violent with others. Troublesome behaviors may persist long after the abusive or neglectful environment has changed or the child has been in foster care placement. Neurobiological research has shown that early abuse results in an altered physiological response to stressful stimuli, a response that deleteriously affects the child's subsequent socialization. Pediatricians can assist caregivers by helping them recognize the abused or neglected child's altered responses, formulate more effective coping strategies, and mobilize available community resources. (9/08, reaffirmed 8/12)
http://pediatrics.aappublications.org/content/122/3/667

UPDATE OF NEWBORN SCREENING AND THERAPY FOR CONGENITAL HYPOTHYROIDISM (CLINICAL REPORT)

Susan R. Rose, MD; Section on Endocrinology; and Committee on Genetics (joint with Rosalind S. Brown, MD; American Thyroid Association; and Lawson Wilkins Pediatric Endocrine Society)

ABSTRACT. Unrecognized congenital hypothyroidism leads to mental retardation. Newborn screening and thyroid therapy started within 2 weeks of age can normalize cognitive development. The primary thyroid-stimulating hormone screening has become standard in many parts of the world. However, newborn thyroid screening is not yet universal in some countries. Initial dosage of 10 to 15 µg/kg levothyroxine is recommended. The goals of thyroid hormone therapy should be to maintain frequent evaluations of total thyroxine or free thyroxine in the upper half of the reference range during the first 3 years of life and to normalize the serum thyroid-stimulating hormone concentration to ensure optimal thyroid hormone dosage and compliance.

Improvements in screening and therapy have led to improved developmental outcomes in adults with congenital hypothyroidism who are now in their 20s and 30s. Thyroid hormone regimens used today are more aggressive in targeting early correction of thyroid-stimulating hormone than were those used 20 or even 10 years ago. Thus, newborn infants with congenital hypothyroidism today may have an even better intellectual and neurologic prognosis. Efforts are ongoing to establish the optimal therapy that leads to maximum potential for normal development for infants with congenital hypothyroidism.

Remaining controversy centers on infants whose abnormality in neonatal thyroid function is transient or mild and on optimal care of very low birth weight or preterm infants. Of note, thyroid-stimulating hormone is not elevated in central hypothyroidism. An algorithm is proposed for diagnosis and management.

Physicians must not relinquish their clinical judgment and experience in the face of normal newborn thyroid test results. Hypothyroidism can be acquired after the newborn screening. When clinical symptoms and signs suggest hypothyroidism, regardless of newborn screening results, serum free thyroxine and thyroid-stimulating hormone determinations should be performed. (6/06, reaffirmed 12/11)

http://pediatrics.aappublications.org/content/117/6/2290

UPDATED GUIDANCE FOR PALIVIZUMAB PROPHYLAXIS AMONG INFANTS AND YOUNG CHILDREN AT INCREASED RISK OF HOSPITALIZATION FOR RESPIRATORY SYNCYTIAL VIRUS INFECTION

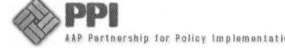

Committee on Infectious Diseases and Bronchiolitis Guidelines Committee

ABSTRACT. Palivizumab was licensed in June 1998 by the Food and Drug Administration for the reduction of serious lower respiratory tract infection caused by respiratory syncytial virus (RSV) in children at increased risk of severe disease. Since that time, the American Academy of Pediatrics has updated its guidance for the use of palivizumab 4 times as additional data became available to provide a better understanding of infants and young children

at greatest risk of hospitalization attributable to RSV infection. The updated recommendations in this policy statement reflect new information regarding the seasonality of RSV circulation, palivizumab pharmacokinetics, the changing incidence of bronchiolitis hospitalizations, the effect of gestational age and other risk factors on RSV hospitalization rates, the mortality of children hospitalized with RSV infection, the effect of prophylaxis on wheezing, and palivizumab-resistant RSV isolates. This policy statement updates and replaces the recommendations found in the 2012 *Red Book.* (7/14)

http://pediatrics.aappublications.org/content/134/2/415

UPDATED GUIDANCE FOR PALIVIZUMAB PROPHYLAXIS AMONG INFANTS AND YOUNG CHILDREN AT INCREASED RISK OF HOSPITALIZATION FOR RESPIRATORY SYNCYTIAL VIRUS INFECTION (TECHNICAL REPORT)

Committee on Infectious Diseases and Bronchiolitis Guidelines Committee

ABSTRACT. Guidance from the American Academy of Pediatrics (AAP) for the use of palivizumab prophylaxis against respiratory syncytial virus (RSV) was first published in a policy statement in 1998. Guidance initially was based on the result from a single randomized, placebo-controlled clinical trial conducted in 1996–1997 describing an overall reduction in RSV hospitalization rate from 10.6% among placebo recipients to 4.8% among children who received prophylaxis. The results of a second randomized, placebo-controlled trial of children with hemodynamically significant heart disease were published in 2003 and revealed a reduction in RSV hospitalization rate from 9.7% in control subjects to 5.3% among prophylaxis recipients. Because no additional controlled trials regarding efficacy were published, AAP guidance has been updated periodically to reflect the most recent literature regarding children at greatest risk of severe disease. Since the last update in 2012, new data have become available regarding the seasonality of RSV circulation, palivizumab pharmacokinetics, the changing incidence of bronchiolitis hospitalizations, the effects of gestational age and other risk factors on RSV hospitalization rates, the mortality of children hospitalized with RSV infection, and the effect of prophylaxis on wheezing and palivizumab-resistant RSV isolates. These data enable further refinement of AAP guidance to most clearly focus on those children at greatest risk. (7/14)

http://pediatrics.aappublications.org/content/134/2/e620

UPDATED RECOMMENDATIONS ON THE USE OF MENINGOCOCCAL VACCINES

Committee on Infectious Diseases

ABSTRACT. Since the last policy statement from the American Academy of Pediatrics (AAP) concerning meningococcal vaccine was published in 2011, 2 meningococcal conjugate vaccines have been licensed for use in infants (Hib-MenCY-TT and MenACWY-CRM). The Centers for Disease Control and Prevention (CDC) has published new recommendations, "Prevention and Control of Meningococcal Disease: Recommendations of the Advisory Committee on Immunization Practices,"

which have been endorsed by the AAP. However, the CDC recommendations were published before licensure of MenACWY-CRM for infant use. This policy statement updates the AAP recommendations for use of meningococcal vaccines in children and adolescents. A more comprehensive review of background and technical information can be found in the CDC publication. (7/14)
http://pediatrics.aappublications.org/content/134/2/400

THE USE AND MISUSE OF FRUIT JUICE IN PEDIATRICS
Committee on Nutrition
ABSTRACT. Historically, fruit juice was recommended by pediatricians as a source of vitamin C and an extra source of water for healthy infants and young children as their diets expanded to include solid foods with higher renal solute. Fruit juice is marketed as a healthy, natural source of vitamins and, in some instances, calcium. Because juice tastes good, children readily accept it. Although juice consumption has some benefits, it also has potential detrimental effects. Pediatricians need to be knowledgeable about juice to inform parents and patients on its appropriate uses. (5/01, reaffirmed 10/06, 8/13)
http://pediatrics.aappublications.org/content/107/5/1210

USE OF CHAPERONES DURING THE PHYSICAL EXAMINATION OF THE PEDIATRIC PATIENT
Committee on Practice and Ambulatory Medicine
ABSTRACT. Physicians should always communicate the scope and nature of the physical examination to be performed to the pediatric patient and his or her parent. This statement addresses the use of chaperones and issues of patient comfort, confidentiality, and privacy. The use of a chaperone should be a shared decision between the patient and physician. In some states, the use of a chaperone is mandated by state regulations. (4/11)
http://pediatrics.aappublications.org/content/127/5/991

USE OF CODEINE- AND DEXTROMETHORPHAN-CONTAINING COUGH REMEDIES IN CHILDREN
Committee on Drugs
ABSTRACT. Numerous prescription and nonprescription medications are currently available for suppression of cough, a common symptom in children. Because adverse effects and overdosage associated with the administration of cough and cold preparations in children have been reported, education of patients and parents about the lack of proven antitussive effects and the potential risks of these products is needed. (6/97, reaffirmed 5/00, 6/03, 10/06)
http://pediatrics.aappublications.org/content/99/6/918

THE USE OF COMPLEMENTARY AND ALTERNATIVE MEDICINE IN PEDIATRICS (CLINICAL REPORT)
Kathi J. Kemper, MD, MPH; Sunita Vohra, MD; Richard Walls, MD, PhD; Task Force on Complementary and Alternative Medicine; and Provisional Section on Complementary, Holistic, and Integrative Medicine
ABSTRACT. The American Academy of Pediatrics is dedicated to optimizing the well-being of children and advancing family-centered health care. Related to these goals, the American Academy of Pediatrics recognizes the increasing use of complementary and alternative

medicine in children and, as a result, the need to provide information and support for pediatricians. From 2000 to 2002, the American Academy of Pediatrics convened and charged the Task Force on Complementary and Alternative Medicine to address issues related to the use of complementary and alternative medicine in children and to develop resources to educate physicians, patients, and families. One of these resources is this report describing complementary and alternative medicine services, current levels of utilization and financial expenditures, and associated legal and ethical considerations. The subject of complementary and alternative medicine is large and diverse, and consequently, an in-depth discussion of each method of complementary and alternative medicine is beyond the scope of this report. Instead, this report will define terms; describe epidemiology; outline common types of complementary and alternative medicine therapies; review medicolegal, ethical, and research implications; review education and training for complementary and alternative medicine providers; provide resources for learning more about complementary and alternative medicine; and suggest communication strategies to use when discussing complementary and alternative medicine with patients and families. (12/08, reaffirmed 10/12, 1/13)
http://pediatrics.aappublications.org/content/122/6/1374

USE OF INHALED NITRIC OXIDE
Committee on Fetus and Newborn
ABSTRACT. Approval of inhaled nitric oxide by the US Food and Drug Administration for hypoxic respiratory failure of the term and near-term newborn provides an important new therapy for this serious condition. This statement addresses the conditions under which inhaled nitric oxide should be administered to the neonate with hypoxic respiratory failure. (8/00, reaffirmed 4/03, 12/09)
http://pediatrics.aappublications.org/content/106/2/344

USE OF INHALED NITRIC OXIDE IN PRETERM INFANTS (CLINICAL REPORT)
Praveen Kumar, MD, FAAP, and Committee on Fetus and Newborn
ABSTRACT. Nitric oxide, an important signaling molecule with multiple regulatory effects throughout the body, is an important tool for the treatment of full-term and late-preterm infants with persistent pulmonary hypertension of the newborn and hypoxemic respiratory failure. Several randomized controlled trials have evaluated its role in the management of preterm infants ≤34 weeks' gestational age with varying results. The purpose of this clinical report is to summarize the existing evidence for the use of inhaled nitric oxide in preterm infants and provide guidance regarding its use in this population. (12/13)
http://pediatrics.aappublications.org/content/133/1/164

USE OF PERFORMANCE-ENHANCING SUBSTANCES (CLINICAL REPORT)
Michele LaBotz, MD, FAAP; Bernard A. Griesemer, MD, FAAP; and Council on Sports Medicine and Fitness
ABSTRACT. Performance-enhancing substances (PESs) are used commonly by children and adolescents in attempts to improve athletic performance. More recent data reveal that these same substances often are used for

appearance-related reasons as well. PESs include both legal over-the-counter dietary supplements and illicit pharmacologic agents. This report reviews the current epidemiology of PES use in the pediatric population, as well as information on those PESs in most common use. Concerns regarding use of legal PESs include high rates of product contamination, correlation with future use of anabolic androgenic steroids, and adverse effects on the focus and experience of youth sports participation. The physical maturation and endogenous hormone production that occur in adolescence are associated with large improvements in strength and athletic performance. For most young athletes, PES use does not produce significant gains over those seen with the onset of puberty and adherence to an appropriate nutrition and training program. (6/16)

See full text on page 1337.

http://pediatrics.aappublications.org/content/138/1/e20161300

USE OF SOY PROTEIN-BASED FORMULAS IN INFANT FEEDING (CLINICAL REPORT)

Jatinder Bhatia, MD; Frank Greer, MD; and Committee on Nutrition

ABSTRACT. Soy protein-based formulas have been available for almost 100 years. Since the first use of soy formula as a milk substitute for an infant unable to tolerate a cow milk protein-based formula, the formulation has changed to the current soy protein isolate. Despite very limited indications for its use, soy protein-based formulas in the United States may account for nearly 25% of the formula market. This report reviews the limited indications and contraindications of soy formulas. It will also review the potential harmful effects of soy protein-based formulas and the phytoestrogens contained in these formulas. (5/08)

http://pediatrics.aappublications.org/content/121/5/1062

THE USE OF SYSTEMIC AND TOPICAL FLUOROQUINOLONES (CLINICAL REPORT)

Mary Anne Jackson, MD, FAAP; Gordon E. Schutze, MD, FAAP; and Committee on Infectious Diseases

ABSTRACT. Appropriate prescribing practices for fluoroquinolones, as well as all antimicrobial agents, are essential as evolving resistance patterns are considered, additional treatment indications are identified, and the toxicity profile of fluoroquinolones in children has become better defined. Earlier recommendations for systemic therapy remain; expanded uses of fluoroquinolones for the treatment of certain infections are outlined in this report. Prescribing clinicians should be aware of specific adverse reactions associated with fluoroquinolones, and their use in children should continue to be limited to the treatment of infections for which no safe and effective alternative exists or in situations in which oral fluoroquinolone treatment represents a reasonable alternative to parenteral antimicrobial therapy. (10/16)

See full text on page 1351.

http://pediatrics.aappublications.org/content/138/5/e20162706

THE USE OF TELEMEDICINE TO ADDRESS ACCESS AND PHYSICIAN WORKFORCE SHORTAGES

Committee on Pediatric Workforce

ABSTRACT. The use of telemedicine technologies by primary care pediatricians, pediatric medical subspecialists, and pediatric surgical specialists (henceforth referred to as "pediatric physicians") has the potential to transform the practice of pediatrics. The purpose of this policy statement is to describe the expected and potential impact that telemedicine will have on pediatric physicians' efforts to improve access and physician workforce shortages. The policy statement also describes how the American Academy of Pediatrics can advocate for its members and their patients to best use telemedicine technologies to improve access to care, provide more patient- and family-centered care, increase efficiencies in practice, enhance the quality of care, and address projected shortages in the clinical workforce. As the use of telemedicine increases, it is likely to impact health care access, quality, and education and costs of care. Telemedicine technologies, applied to the medical home and its collaborating providers, have the potential to improve current models of care by increasing communication among clinicians, resulting in more efficient, higher quality, and less expensive care. Such a model can serve as a platform for providing more continuous care, linking primary and specialty care to support management of the needs of complex patients. In addition, telemedicine technologies can be used to efficiently provide pediatric physicians working in remote locations with ongoing medical education, increasing their ability to care for more complex patients in their community, reducing the burdens of travel on patients and families, and supporting the medical home. On the other hand, telemedicine technologies used for episodic care by nonmedical home providers have the potential to disrupt continuity of care and to create redundancy and imprudent use of health care resources. Fragmentation should be avoided, and telemedicine, like all primary and specialty services, should be coordinated through the medical home. (6/15)

http://pediatrics.aappublications.org/content/136/1/202

USES OF DRUGS NOT DESCRIBED IN THE PACKAGE INSERT (OFF-LABEL USES)

Committee on Drugs

ABSTRACT. New regulatory initiatives have been designed to ensure that new drugs and biologicals include adequate pediatric labeling for the claimed indications at the time of, or soon after, approval. However, because such labeling may not immediately be available, off-label use (or use that is not included in the approved label) of therapeutic agents is likely to remain common in the practice of pediatrics. This policy statement was written to address questions practitioners have regarding off-label use. The purpose of off-label use is to benefit the individual patient. Practitioners may use their professional judgment to determine these uses. Practitioners should understand that the Food and Drug Administration does not regulate off-label use. (7/02, reaffirmed 10/05)

http://pediatrics.aappublications.org/content/110/1/181

VENTRICULAR FIBRILLATION AND THE USE OF AUTOMATED EXTERNAL DEFIBRILLATORS ON CHILDREN

Committee on Pediatric Emergency Medicine and Section on Cardiology and Cardiac Surgery

ABSTRACT. The use of automated external defibrillators (AEDs) has been advocated in recent years as one part of the chain of survival to improve outcomes for adult cardiac arrest victims. When AEDs first entered the market, they had not been tested for pediatric usage and rhythm interpretation. In addition, the presumption was that children do not experience ventricular fibrillation, so they would not benefit from the use of AEDs. Recent literature has shown that children do experience ventricular fibrillation, which has a better outcome than do other cardiac arrest rhythms. At the same time, the arrhythmia software on AEDs has become more extensive and validated for children, and attenuation devices have become available to downregulate the energy delivered by AEDs to allow their use on children. Pediatricians are now being asked whether AED programs should be implemented, and where they are being implemented, pediatricians are being asked to provide guidance on the use of them on children. As AED programs expand, pediatricians must advocate on behalf of children so that their needs are accounted for. For pediatricians to be able to provide guidance and ensure that children are included in AED programs, it is important for pediatricians to know how AEDs work, be up-to-date on the literature regarding pediatric fibrillation and energy delivery, and understand the role of AEDs as life-saving interventions for children. (11/07, reaffirmed 6/11, 7/14)

http://pediatrics.aappublications.org/content/120/5/1159

VIRTUAL VIOLENCE

Council on Communications and Media

ABSTRACT. In the United States, exposure to media violence is becoming an inescapable component of children's lives. With the rise in new technologies, such as tablets and new gaming platforms, children and adolescents increasingly are exposed to what is known as "virtual violence." This form of violence is not experienced physically; rather, it is experienced in realistic ways via new technology and ever more intense and realistic games. The American Academy of Pediatrics continues to be concerned about children's exposure to virtual violence and the effect it has on their overall health and well-being. This policy statement aims to summarize the current state of scientific knowledge regarding the effects of virtual violence on children's attitudes and behaviors and to make specific recommendations for pediatricians, parents, industry, and policy makers. (7/16)

See full text on page 1367.

http://pediatrics.aappublications.org/content/138/2/e20161298

VISUAL SYSTEM ASSESSMENT IN INFANTS, CHILDREN, AND YOUNG ADULTS BY PEDIATRICIANS

Committee on Practice and Ambulatory Medicine and Section on Ophthalmology (joint with American Association of Certified Orthoptists, American Association for Pediatric Ophthalmology and Strabismus, and American Academy of Ophthalmology)

ABSTRACT. Appropriate visual assessments help identify children who may benefit from early interventions to correct or improve vision. Examination of the eyes and visual system should begin in the nursery and continue throughout both childhood and adolescence during routine well-child visits in the medical home. Newborn infants should be examined using inspection and red reflex testing to detect structural ocular abnormalities, such as cataract, corneal opacity, and ptosis. Instrument-based screening, if available, should be first attempted between 12 months and 3 years of age and at annual well-child visits until acuity can be tested directly. Direct testing of visual acuity can often begin by 4 years of age, using age-appropriate symbols (optotypes). Children found to have an ocular abnormality or who fail a vision assessment should be referred to a pediatric ophthalmologist or an eye care specialist appropriately trained to treat pediatric patients. (12/15)

http://pediatrics.aappublications.org/content/137/1/e20153596

WHEN IS LACK OF SUPERVISION NEGLECT? (CLINICAL REPORT)

Kent P. Hymel, MD, and Committee on Child Abuse and Neglect

ABSTRACT. Occasionally, pediatricians become aware of children who are inadequately supervised. More frequently, pediatricians treat children for traumatic injuries or ingestions that they suspect could have been prevented with better supervision. This clinical report contains guidance for pediatricians considering a referral to a child protective services agency on the basis of suspicion of supervisory neglect. (9/06)

http://pediatrics.aappublications.org/content/118/3/1296

WIC PROGRAM

Provisional Section on Breastfeeding

ABSTRACT. This policy statement highlights the important collaboration between pediatricians and local Special Supplemental Nutrition Program for Women, Infants, and Children (WIC) programs to ensure that infants and children receive high-quality, cost-effective health care and nutrition services. Specific recommendations are provided for pediatricians and WIC personnel to help children and their families receive optimum services through a medical home. (11/01)

http://pediatrics.aappublications.org/content/108/5/1216

WITHHOLDING OR TERMINATION OF RESUSCITATION IN PEDIATRIC OUT-OF-HOSPITAL TRAUMATIC CARDIOPULMONARY ARREST

Committee on Pediatric Emergency Medicine (joint with American College of Surgeons Committee on Trauma and National Association of EMS Physicians)

ABSTRACT. This multiorganizational literature review was undertaken to provide an evidence base for determining whether recommendations for out-of-hospital termination of resuscitation could be made for children who are victims of traumatic cardiopulmonary arrest. Although there is increasing acceptance of out-of-hospital termination of resuscitation for adult traumatic cardiopulmonary arrest when there is no expectation of a good outcome, children are routinely excluded from state termination-of-resuscitation protocols. The decision to withhold resuscitative efforts in a child under specific circumstances (decapitation or dependent lividity, rigor mortis, etc) is reasonable. If there is any doubt as to the circumstances or timing of the traumatic cardiopulmonary arrest, under the current status of limiting termination of resuscitation in the field to persons older than 18 years in most states, resuscitation should be initiated and continued until arrival to the appropriate facility. If the patient has arrested, resuscitation has already exceeded 30 minutes, and the nearest facility is more than 30 minutes away, involvement of parents and family of these children in the decision-making process with assistance and guidance from medical professionals should be considered as part of an emphasis on family-centered care because the evidence suggests that either death or a poor outcome is inevitable. (3/14)
http://pediatrics.aappublications.org/content/133/4/e1104

YEAR 2007 POSITION STATEMENT: PRINCIPLES AND GUIDELINES FOR EARLY HEARING DETECTION AND INTERVENTION PROGRAMS

Joint Committee on Infant Hearing

ABSTRACT. The Joint Committee on Infant Hearing (JCIH) endorses early detection of and intervention for infants with hearing loss. The goal of early hearing detection and intervention (EHDI) is to maximize linguistic competence and literacy development for children who are deaf or hard of hearing. Without appropriate opportunities to learn language, these children will fall behind their hearing peers in communication, cognition, reading, and social-emotional development. Such delays may result in lower educational and employment levels in adulthood. To maximize the outcome for infants who are deaf or hard of hearing, the hearing of all infants should be screened at no later than 1 month of age. Those who do not pass screening should have a comprehensive audiological evaluation at no later than 3 months of age. Infants with confirmed hearing loss should receive appropriate intervention at no later than 6 months of age from health care and education professionals with expertise in hearing loss and deafness in infants and young children. Regardless of previous hearing-screening outcomes, all infants with or without risk factors should receive ongoing surveillance of communicative development beginning at 2 months of age during well-child visits in the medical home. EHDI systems should guarantee seamless transitions for infants and their families through this process. (10/07)
http://pediatrics.aappublications.org/content/120/4/898

YOUTH PARTICIPATION AND INJURY RISK IN MARTIAL ARTS (CLINICAL REPORT)

Rebecca A. Demorest, MD, FAAP; Chris Koutures, MD, FAAP; and Council on Sports Medicine and Fitness

ABSTRACT. The martial arts can provide children and adolescents with vigorous levels of physical exercise that can improve overall physical fitness. The various types of martial arts encompass noncontact basic forms and techniques that may have a lower relative risk of injury. Contact-based sparring with competitive training and bouts have a higher risk of injury. This clinical report describes important techniques and movement patterns in several types of martial arts and reviews frequently reported injuries encountered in each discipline, with focused discussions of higher risk activities. Some of these higher risk activities include blows to the head and choking or submission movements that may cause concussions or significant head injuries. The roles of rule changes, documented benefits of protective equipment, and changes in training recommendations in attempts to reduce injury are critically assessed. This information is intended to help pediatric health care providers counsel patients and families in encouraging safe participation in martial arts. (11/16)

See full text on page 1373.
http://pediatrics.aappublications.org/content/138/6/e20163022

SECTION 6

Endorsed Policies

. . . .

The American Academy of Pediatrics endorses
and accepts as its policy the following
documents from other organizations.

AMERICAN ACADEMY OF PEDIATRICS

Endorsed Policies

2015 SPCTPD/ACC/AAP/AHA TRAINING GUIDELINES FOR PEDIATRIC CARDIOLOGY FELLOWSHIP PROGRAMS (REVISION OF THE 2005 TRAINING GUIDELINES FOR PEDIATRIC CARDIOLOGY FELLOWSHIP PROGRAMS)
Robert D. Ross, MD, FAAP, FACC; Michael Brook, MD; Jeffrey A. Feinstein, MD; et al (8/15)

INTRODUCTION
Robert D. Ross, MD, FAAP, FACC; Michael Brook, MD; Peter Koenig, MD, FACC, FASE; et al (8/15)

TASK FORCE 1: GENERAL CARDIOLOGY
Alan B. Lewis, MD, FAAP, FACC; Gerard R. Martin, MD, FAAP, FACC, FAHA; Peter J. Bartz, MD, FASE; et al (8/15)

TASK FORCE 2: NONINVASIVE CARDIAC IMAGING
Shubhika Srivastava, MBBS, FAAP, FACC, FASE; Beth F. Printz, MD, PhD, FAAP, FASE; Tal Geva, MD, FACC; et al (8/15)

TASK FORCE 3: CARDIAC CATHETERIZATION
Laurie B. Armsby, MD, FAAP, FSCAI; Robert N. Vincent, MD, CM, FACC, FSCAI; Susan R. Foerster, MD, FSCAI; et al (8/15)

TASK FORCE 4: ELECTROPHYSIOLOGY
Anne M. Dubin, MD, FHRS; Edward P. Walsh, MD, FHRS; Wayne Franklin, MD, FAAP, FACC, FAHA; et al (8/15)

TASK FORCE 5: CRITICAL CARE CARDIOLOGY
Timothy F. Feltes, MD, FAAP, FACC, FAHA; Stephen J. Roth, MD, MPH, FAAP; Melvin C. Almodovar, MD; et al (8/15)

TASK FORCE 6: ADULT CONGENITAL HEART DISEASE
Karen Stout, MD, FACC; Anne Marie Valente, MD, FACC; Peter J. Bartz, MD, FASE; et al (8/15)

TASK FORCE 7: PULMONARY HYPERTENSION, ADVANCED HEART FAILURE, AND TRANSPLANTATION
Steven A. Webber, MB, ChB; Daphne T. Hsu, MD, FAAP, FACC, FAHA; D. Dunbar Ivy, MD, FAAP, FACC; et al (8/15)

TASK FORCE 8: RESEARCH AND SCHOLARLY ACTIVITY
William T. Mahle, MD, FAAP, FACC, FAHA; Anne M. Murphy, MD, FACC, FAHA; Jennifer S. Li, MD; et al (8/15)

ADVANCED PRACTICE REGISTERED NURSE: ROLE, PREPARATION, AND SCOPE OF PRACTICE
National Association of Neonatal Nurses
In recent years, the National Association of Neonatal Nurses (NANN) and the National Association of Neonatal Nurse Practitioners (NANNP) have developed several policy statements on neonatal advanced practice registered nurse (APRN) workforce, education, competency, fatigue, safety, and scope of practice. This position paper is a synthesis of previous efforts and discusses the role, preparation, and scope of practice of the neonatal APRN. (1/14)

APPROPRIATE MEDICAL CARE FOR THE SECONDARY SCHOOL-AGE ATHLETE COMMUNICATION
National Athletic Trainers' Association (2004)

APPROPRIATE USE CRITERIA FOR INITIAL TRANSTHORACIC ECHOCARDIOGRAPHY IN OUTPATIENT PEDIATRIC CARDIOLOGY
American College of Cardiology Appropriate Use Task Force
ABSTRACT. The American College of Cardiology (ACC) participated in a joint project with the American Society of Echocardiography, the Society of Pediatric Echocardiography, and several other subspecialty societies and organizations to establish and evaluate Appropriate Use Criteria (AUC) for the initial use of outpatient pediatric echocardiography. Assumptions for the AUC were identified, including the fact that all indications assumed a first-time transthoracic echocardiographic study in an outpatient setting for patients without previously known heart disease. The definitions for frequently used terminology in outpatient pediatric cardiology were established using published guidelines and standards and expert opinion. These AUC serve as a guide to help clinicians in the care of children with possible heart disease, specifically in terms of when a transthoracic echocardiogram is warranted as an initial diagnostic modality in the outpatient setting. They are also a useful tool for education and provide the infrastructure for future quality improvement initiatives as well as research in healthcare delivery, outcomes, and resource utilization.

To complete the AUC process, the writing group identified 113 indications based on common clinical scenarios and/or published clinical practice guidelines, and each indication was classified into 1 of 9 categories of common clinical presentations, including palpitations, syncope, chest pain, and murmur. A separate, independent rating panel evaluated each indication using a scoring scale of 1 to 9, thereby designating each indication as "Appropriate" (median score 7 to 9), "May Be Appropriate" (median score 4 to 6), or "Rarely Appropriate" (median score 1 to 3). Fifty-three indications were identified as Appropriate, 28 as May Be Appropriate, and 32 as Rarely Appropriate. (11/14)

BEST PRACTICE FOR INFANT SURGERY: A POSITION STATEMENT FROM THE AMERICAN PEDIATRIC SURGICAL ASSOCIATION
American Pediatric Surgical Association (9/08)

CARDIOVASCULAR RISK REDUCTION IN HIGH-RISK PEDIATRIC POPULATIONS
American Heart Association

ABSTRACT. Although for most children the process of atherosclerosis is subclinical, dramatically accelerated atherosclerosis occurs in some pediatric disease states, with clinical coronary events occurring in childhood and very early adult life. As with most scientific statements about children and the future risk for cardiovascular disease, there are no randomized trials documenting the effects of risk reduction on hard clinical outcomes. A growing body of literature, however, identifies the importance of premature cardiovascular disease in the course of certain pediatric diagnoses and addresses the response to risk factor reduction. For this scientific statement, a panel of experts reviewed what is known about very premature cardiovascular disease in 8 high-risk pediatric diagnoses and, from the science base, developed practical recommendations for management of cardiovascular risk. (*Circulation.* 2006;114:000–000.) (12/06)

CHILDREN'S SURGERY VERIFICATION PILOT DRAFT DOCUMENTS

OPTIMAL RESOURCES FOR CHILDREN'S SURGICAL CARE—DRAFT
American College of Surgeons

EXECUTIVE SUMMARY. The Task Force for Children's Surgical Care, an ad hoc multidisciplinary group of invited leaders in relevant disciplines, assembled in Rosemont, IL, initially April 30—May 1, 2012, and subsequently in 2013 and 2014 to consider approaches to optimize the delivery of children's surgical care in today's competitive national healthcare environment. Specifically, a mismatch between individual patient needs and available clinical resources for some infants and children receiving surgical care is recognized as a problem in the U.S. and elsewhere. While this phenomenon is apparent to most practitioners involved with children's surgical care, comprehensive data are not available and relevant data are imperfect. The scope of this problem is unknown at present. However, it does periodically, and possibly systematically result in suboptimal patient outcomes. The composition of the Task Force is detailed above. Support was provided by the Children's Hospital Association (CHA) and the American College of Surgeons (ACS). The group represented key disciplines and perspectives. Published literature and data were utilized when available and expert opinion when not, as the basis for these recommendations. The objective was to develop consensus recommendations that would be of use to relevant policy makers and to providers. Principles regarding resource standards, quality improvement and safety processes, data collection and a verification process were initially published in March 2014 [*J Am Coll Surg* 2014;218(3):479-487]. This document details those principles in a specific manner designed to inform and direct a verification process to be conducted by the American College of Surgeons and the ACS Committee on Children's Surgery. (11/14)

HOSPITAL PREREVIEW QUESTIONNAIRE (PRQ)—DRAFT
American College of Surgeons (11/14)

COLLABORATION IN PRACTICE: IMPLEMENTING TEAM-BASED CARE
American College of Obstetricians and Gynecologists Task Force on Collaborative Practice

INTRODUCTION. Quality, efficiency, and value are necessary characteristics of our evolving health care system. Team-based care will work toward the Triple Aim of 1) improving the experience of care of individuals and families; 2) improving the health of populations; and 3) lowering per capita costs. It also should respond to emerging demands and reduce undue burdens on health care providers. Team-based care has the ability to more effectively meet the core expectations of the health care system proposed by the Institute of Medicine. These expectations require that care be safe, effective, patient centered, timely, efficient, and equitable. This report outlines a mechanism that all specialties and practices can use to achieve these expectations.

The report was written by the interprofessional Task Force on Collaborative Practice and is intended to appeal to multiple specialties (eg, internal medicine, pediatrics, family medicine, and women's health) and professions (eg, nurse practitioners, certified nurse–midwives/certified midwives, physician assistants, physicians, clinical pharmacists, and advanced practice registered nurses). This document provides a framework for organizations or practices across all specialties to develop team-based care. In doing so, it offers a map to help practices navigate the increasingly complex and continuously evolving health care system. The guidance presented is a result of the task force's work and is based on current evidence and expert consensus. The task force challenges and welcomes all medical specialties to gather additional data on how and what types of team-based care best accomplish the Triple Aim and the Institute of Medicine's expectations of health care. (3/16)

A COMPREHENSIVE IMMUNIZATION STRATEGY TO ELIMINATE TRANSMISSION OF HEPATITIS B VIRUS INFECTION IN THE UNITED STATES
Advisory Committee on Immunization Practices and Centers for Disease Control and Prevention

SUMMARY. This report is the first of a two-part statement from the Advisory Committee on Immunization Practices (ACIP) that updates the strategy to eliminate hepatitis B virus (HBV) transmission in the United States. The report provides updated recommendations to improve prevention of perinatal and early childhood HBV transmission, including implementation of universal infant vaccination beginning at birth, and to increase vaccine coverage among previously unvaccinated children and adolescents. Strategies to enhance implementation of the recommendations include (1) establishing standing orders for administration of hepatitis B vaccination beginning at birth; (2) instituting delivery hospital policies and procedures and case management programs to improve identification of and administration of immunoprophylaxis to infants born to mothers who are hepatitis B surface antigen (HBsAg) positive and to mothers with unknown HBsAg status at the time of delivery; and (3) implementing vaccination record reviews for all children aged 11–12 years and children and adolescents aged <19 years who were born in countries with intermediate and high levels of HBV endemicity, adopting hepatitis B vaccine requirements for school entry, and integrating hepatitis B vaccination services into settings that serve adolescents. The second part of the ACIP statement, which will include updated recommendations and strategies to increase hepatitis B vaccination of adults, will be published separately. (7/06)

CONFIDENTIALITY PROTECTIONS FOR ADOLESCENTS AND YOUNG ADULTS IN THE HEALTH CARE BILLING AND INSURANCE CLAIMS PROCESS

Society for Adolescent Health and Medicine

ABSTRACT. The importance of protecting confidential health care for adolescents and young adults is well documented. State and federal confidentiality protections exist for both minors and young adults, although the laws vary among states, particularly for minors. However, such confidentiality is potentially violated by billing practices and in the processing of health insurance claims. To address this problem, policies and procedures should be established so that health care billing and insurance claims processes do not impede the ability of providers to deliver essential health care services on a confidential basis to adolescents and young adults covered as dependents on a family's health insurance plan. (3/16)

CONSENSUS COMMUNICATION ON EARLY PEANUT INTRODUCTION AND THE PREVENTION OF PEANUT ALLERGY IN HIGH-RISK INFANTS

Primary Contributors: David M. Fleischer, MD; Scott Sicherer, MD; Matthew Greenhawt, MD; Dianne Campbell, MB BS, FRACP, PhD; Edmond Chan, MD; Antonella Muraro, MD, PhD; Susanne Halken, MD; Yitzhak Katz, MD; Motohiro Ebisawa, MD, PhD; Lawrence Eichenfield, MD; Hugh Sampson, MD; Gideon Lack, MB, BCh; and George Du Toit, MB, BCh

INTRODUCTION AND RATIONALE. Peanut allergy is an increasingly troubling global health problem affecting between 1% and 3% of children in many westernized countries. Although multiple methods of measurement have been used and specific estimates differ, there appears to have been a sudden increase in the number of cases in the past 10- to 15-year period, suggesting that the prevalence might have tripled in some countries, such as the United States. Extrapolating the currently estimated prevalence, this translates to nearly 100 000 new cases annually (in the United States and United Kingdom), affecting some 1 in 50 primary school-aged children in the United States, Canada, the United Kingdom, and Australia. A similar increase in incidence is now being noted in developing countries, such as Ghana.

The purpose of this brief communication is to highlight emerging evidence for existing allergy prevention guidelines regarding potential benefits of supporting early rather than delayed peanut introduction during the period of complementary food introduction in infants. A recent study entitled "Randomized trial of peanut consumption in infants at risk for peanut allergy" demonstrated a successful 11% to 25% absolute reduction in the risk of peanut allergy in high-risk infants (and a relative risk reduction of up to 80%) if peanut was introduced between 4 and 11 months of age. In light of the significance of these findings, this document serves to better inform the decision-making process for health care providers regarding such potential benefits of early peanut introduction. More formal guidelines regarding early-life, complementary feeding practices and the risk of allergy development will follow in the next year from the National Institute of Allergy and Infectious Diseases (NIAID)–sponsored Working Group and the European Academy of Allergy and Clinical Immunology (EAACI), and thus this document should be considered interim guidance. (8/15)

CONSENSUS STATEMENT: DEFINITIONS FOR CONSISTENT EMERGENCY DEPARTMENT METRICS

American Academy of Emergency Medicine, American Association of Critical Care Nurses, American College of Emergency Physicians, Association of periOperative Registered Nurses, Emergency Department Practice Management Association, Emergency Nurses Association, and National Association of EMS Physicians (2/10)

CONSENSUS STATEMENT ON MANAGEMENT OF INTERSEX DISORDERS

International Consensus Conference on Intersex (Lawson Wilkins Pediatric Endocrine Society and European Society for Paediatric Endocrinology)

INTRODUCTION. The birth of an intersex child prompts a long-term management strategy that involves myriad professionals working with the family. There has been progress in diagnosis, surgical techniques, understanding psychosocial issues, and recognizing and accepting the place of patient advocacy. The Lawson Wilkins Pediatric Endocrine Society and the European Society for Paediatric Endocrinology considered it timely to review the management of intersex disorders from a broad perspective, review data on longer-term outcome, and formulate proposals for future studies. The methodology comprised establishing a number of working groups, the membership of which was drawn from 50 international experts in the field. The groups prepared previous written responses to a defined set of questions resulting from evidence-based review of the literature. At a subsequent gathering of participants, a framework for a consensus document was agreed. This article constitutes its final form. (8/06)

DEFINING PEDIATRIC MALNUTRITION: A PARADIGM SHIFT TOWARD ETIOLOGY-RELATED DEFINITIONS

American Society for Parenteral and Enteral Nutrition

ABSTRACT. Lack of a uniform definition is responsible for underrecognition of the prevalence of malnutrition and its impact on outcomes in children. A pediatric malnutrition definitions workgroup reviewed existing pediatric age group English-language literature from 1955 to 2011, for relevant references related to 5 domains of the definition of *malnutrition* that were *a priori* identified: anthropometric parameters, growth, chronicity of malnutrition, etiology and pathogenesis, and developmental/functional outcomes. Based on available evidence and an iterative process to arrive at multidisciplinary consensus in the group, these domains were included in the overall construct of a new definition. Pediatric malnutrition (undernutrition) is defined as an imbalance between nutrient requirements and intake that results in cumulative deficits of energy, protein, or micronutrients that may negatively affect growth, development, and other relevant outcomes. A summary of the literature is presented and a new classification scheme is proposed that incorporates chronicity, etiology, mechanisms of nutrient imbalance, severity of malnutrition, and its impact on outcomes. Based on its etiology, malnutrition is either *illness related* (secondary to 1 or more diseases/injury) or *non–illness related*, (caused by environmental/behavioral factors), or both. Future research must focus on the relationship between inflammation and illness-related malnutrition. We anticipate that the definition of malnutrition will continue to evolve with improved understanding of the processes that lead to and complicate the treatment of this condition. A uniform definition should permit future research to focus on the impact of pediatric malnutrition on functional outcomes and help solidify the scientific basis for evidence-based nutrition practices. (3/13)

DIABETES CARE FOR EMERGING ADULTS: RECOMMENDATIONS FOR TRANSITION FROM PEDIATRIC TO ADULT DIABETES CARE SYSTEMS
American Diabetes Association (11/11)

DIAGNOSIS, TREATMENT, AND LONG-TERM MANAGEMENT OF KAWASAKI DISEASE: A STATEMENT FOR HEALTH PROFESSIONALS
American Heart Association (12/04)

DIETARY RECOMMENDATIONS FOR CHILDREN AND ADOLESCENTS: A GUIDE FOR PRACTITIONERS
American Heart Association (9/05)

DIETARY REFERENCE INTAKES FOR CALCIUM AND VITAMIN D
Institute of Medicine (2011)

EMERGENCY EQUIPMENT AND SUPPLIES IN THE SCHOOL SETTING
National Association of School Nurses (1/12)

ENHANCING THE WORK OF THE HHS NATIONAL VACCINE PROGRAM IN GLOBAL IMMUNIZATIONS
National Vaccine Advisory Committee (9/13)

ETHICAL CONSIDERATION FOR INCLUDING WOMEN AS RESEARCH PARTICIPANTS
American College of Obstetricians and Gynecologists
ABSTRACT. Inclusion of women in research studies is necessary for valid inferences about health and disease in women. The generalization of results from trials conducted in men may yield erroneous conclusions that fail to account for the biologic differences between men and women. Although significant changes in research design and practice have led to an increase in the proportion of women included in research trials, knowledge gaps remain because of a continued lack of inclusion of women, especially those who are pregnant, in premarketing research trials. This document provides a historical overview of issues surrounding women as participants in research trials, followed by an ethical framework and discussion of the issues of informed consent, contraception requirements, intimate partner consent, and the appropriate inclusion of pregnant women in research studies. (11/15)

EVIDENCE REPORT: GENETIC AND METABOLIC TESTING ON CHILDREN WITH GLOBAL DEVELOPMENTAL DELAY
American Academy of Neurology and Child Neurology Society
ABSTRACT. *Objective.* To systematically review the evidence concerning the diagnostic yield of genetic and metabolic evaluation of children with global developmental delay or intellectual disability (GDD/ID).

Methods. Relevant literature was reviewed, abstracted, and classified according to the 4-tiered American Academy of Neurology classification of evidence scheme.

Results and Conclusions. In patients with GDD/ID, microarray testing is diagnostic on average in 7.8% (Class III), G-banded karyotyping is abnormal in at least 4% (Class II and III), and subtelomeric fluorescence in situ hybridization is positive in 3.5% (Class I, II, and III). Testing for X-linked ID genes has a yield of up to 42% in males with an appropriate family history (Class III). *FMR*1 testing shows full expansion in at least 2% of patients with mild to moderate GDD/ID (Class II and III), and *MeCP*2 testing is diagnostic in 1.5% of females with moderate to severe GDD/ID (Class III). Tests for metabolic disorders have a yield of up to 5%, and tests for congenital disorders of glycosylation and cerebral creatine disorders have yields of up to 2.8% (Class III). Several genetic and metabolic screening tests have been shown to have a better than 1% diagnostic yield in selected populations of children with GDD/ID. These values should be among the many factors considered in planning the laboratory evaluation of such children. (9/11)

EVIDENCE-BASED GUIDELINE UPDATE: MEDICAL TREATMENT OF INFANTILE SPASMS
American Academy of Neurology and Child Neurology Society
ABSTRACT. *Objective.* To update the 2004 American Academy of Neurology/Child Neurology Society practice parameter on treatment of infantile spasms in children.

Methods. MEDLINE and EMBASE were searched from 2002 to 2011 and searches of reference lists of retrieved articles were performed. Sixty-eight articles were selected for detailed review; 26 were included in the analysis. Recommendations were based on a 4-tiered classification scheme combining pre-2002 evidence and more recent evidence.

Results. There is insufficient evidence to determine whether other forms of corticosteroids are as effective as adrenocorticotropic hormone (ACTH) for short-term treatment of infantile spasms. However, low-dose ACTH is probably as effective as high-dose ACTH. ACTH is more effective than vigabatrin (VGB) for short-term treatment of children with infantile spasms (excluding those with tuberous sclerosis complex). There is insufficient evidence to show 'that other agents and combination therapy are effective for short-term treatment of infantile spasms. Short lag time to treatment leads to better long-term developmental outcome. Successful short-term treatment of cryptogenic infantile spasms with ACTH or prednisolone leads to better long-term developmental outcome than treatment with VGB.

Recommendations. Low-dose ACTH should be considered for treatment of infantile spasms. ACTH or VGB may be useful for short-term treatment of infantile spasms, with ACTH considered preferentially over VGB. Hormonal therapy (ACTH or prednisolone) may be considered for use in preference to VGB in infants with cryptogenic infantile spasms, to possibly improve developmental outcome. A shorter lag time to treatment of infantile spasms with either hormonal therapy or VGB possibly improves long-term developmental outcomes. (6/12)

EVIDENCE-BASED MANAGEMENT OF SICKLE CELL DISEASE: EXPERT PANEL REPORT, 2014
National Heart, Lung, and Blood Institute (2014)

EXECUTING JUVENILE OFFENDERS: A FUNDAMENTAL FAILURE OF SOCIETY
Society for Adolescent Medicine (10/04)

EXPEDITED PARTNER THERAPY FOR ADOLESCENTS DIAGNOSED WITH CHLAMYDIA OR GONORRHEA: A POSITION PAPER OF THE SOCIETY FOR ADOLESCENT MEDICINE
Society for Adolescent Medicine

ABSTRACT. Chlamydia and gonorrhea, the most frequently reported sexually transmitted infections (STIs), present substantial public health challenges among adolescents. Although these infections are easily treated with antibiotics, many adolescents are reinfected within 3–6 months, usually because their partners remain untreated. The standard approaches to notifying and treating a partner of an STI-infected patient are patient referral, whereby the patient notifies his/her partners to seek care, and provider referral, whereby the provider or public health disease intervention specialist notifies the partner and directs him/her toward treatment. These methods rely on the accuracy of the disclosed partner information as well as other limitations, such as compliance and staffing resources. Another approach to partner notification is expedited partner therapy (EPT), treating sex partners without requiring a prior clinical evaluation. In randomized trials, EPT has reduced the rates of persistent or recurrent gonorrhea and chlamydia infection; however, its routine use is limited by concerns related to liability, cost, compliance, and missed opportunities for prevention counseling. The Society for Adolescent Medicine (SAM) recommends that providers who care for adolescents should do the following: use EPT as an option for STI care among chlamydia- or gonorrhea-infected heterosexual males and females who are unlikely or unable to otherwise receive treatment; through SAM and AAP chapters, collaborate with policy makers to remove EPT legal barriers and facilitate reimbursement; and collaborate with health departments for implementation assistance. (9/09)

EXPERT PANEL ON INTEGRATED GUIDELINES FOR CARDIOVASCULAR HEALTH AND RISK REDUCTION IN CHILDREN AND ADOLESCENTS: SUMMARY REPORT
National Heart, Lung and Blood Institute
INTRODUCTION (EXCERPT). Atherosclerotic cardiovascular disease (CVD) remains the leading cause of death in North Americans, but manifest disease in childhood and adolescence is rare. By contrast, risk factors and risk behaviors that accelerate the development of atherosclerosis begin in childhood, and there is increasing evidence that risk reduction delays progression toward clinical disease. In response, the former director of the National Heart, Lung, and Blood Institute (NHLBI), Dr Elizabeth Nabel, initiated development of cardiovascular health guidelines for pediatric care providers based on a formal evidence review of the science with an integrated format addressing all the major cardiovascular risk factors simultaneously. An expert panel was appointed to develop the guidelines in the fall of 2006. (3/12)

FACULTY COMPETENCIES FOR GLOBAL HEALTH
Academic Pediatric Association Global Health Task Force
International partnerships among medical professionals from different countries are an increasingly common form of clinical and academic collaboration. Global health partnerships can include a variety of activities and serve multiple purposes in the areas of research, medical education and training, health system improvement, and clinical care. Competency domains, introduced by the Accreditation Council for Graduate Medical Education and the American Board of Medical Specialties in 1999, are now widely accepted to provide an organized, structured set of interrelated competencies, mostly for medical trainees. Although there are now competency domains and specific competencies recommended for pediatric trainees pursuing further professional training in global child health, none of these addresses competencies for faculty in global health.

In 2010 the Academic Pediatric Association established a Global Health Task Force to provide a forum for communication and collaboration for diverse pediatric academic societies and groups to advance global child health. Given the burgeoning demand for global health training, and particularly in light of a new global perspective on health education, as outlined in a Lancet Commission Report: *Health Professionals for a New Century: Transforming Education to Strengthen Health Systems in an Interdependent World,* in 2012 the Global Health Task Force noted the lack of defined faculty competencies and decided to develop a set of global health competencies for pediatric faculty engaged in the teaching and practice of global health. Using some of the principles suggested by Milner, et al. to define a competency framework, four domains were chosen, adapted from existing collaborative practice competencies. A fifth domain was added to address some of the unique challenges of global health practice encountered when working outside of one's own culture and health system. The domains are described below and specific competencies are provided for faculty working in global health research, education, administration, and clinical practice. (6/14)

FOSTER CARE MENTAL HEALTH VALUES
American Academy of Child and Adolescent Psychiatry and Child Welfare League of America (2002)

GENERAL RECOMMENDATIONS ON IMMUNIZATION: RECOMMENDATIONS OF THE ADVISORY COMMITTEE ON IMMUNIZATION PRACTICES (ACIP)

Advisory Committee on Immunization Practices

SUMMARY. This report is a revision of General Recommendations on Immunization and updates the 2002 statement by the Advisory Committee on Immunization Practices (ACIP) (CDC. General recommendations on immunization: recommendations of the Advisory Committee on Immunization Practices and the American Academy of Family Physicians. *MMWR* 2002;51[No. RR-2]). This report is intended to serve as a general reference on vaccines and immunization. The principal changes include (1) expansion of the discussion of vaccination spacing and timing; (2) an increased emphasis on the importance of injection technique/age/body mass in determining appropriate needle length; (3) expansion of the discussion of storage and handling of vaccines, with a table defining the appropriate storage temperature range for inactivated and live vaccines; (4) expansion of the discussion of altered immunocompetence, including new recommendations about use of live-attenuated vaccines with therapeutic monoclonal antibodies; and (5) minor changes to the recommendations about vaccination during pregnancy and vaccination of internationally adopted children, in accordance with new ACIP vaccine-specific recommendations for use of inactivated influenza vaccine and hepatitis B vaccine. The most recent ACIP recommendations for each specific vaccine should be consulted for comprehensive discussion. This report, ACIP recommendations for each vaccine, and other information about vaccination can be accessed at CDC's National Center for Immunization and Respiratory Diseases (proposed) (formerly known as the National Immunization Program) website at http//:www.cdc.gov/nip. (12/06)

GENETIC BASIS FOR CONGENITAL HEART DEFECTS: CURRENT KNOWLEDGE

American Heart Association

ABSTRACT. The intent of this review is to provide the clinician with a summary of what is currently known about the contribution of genetics to the origin of congenital heart disease. Techniques are discussed to evaluate children with heart disease for genetic alterations. Many of these techniques are now available on a clinical basis. Information on the genetic and clinical evaluation of children with cardiac disease is presented, and several tables have been constructed to aid the clinician in the assessment of children with different types of heart disease. Genetic algorithms for cardiac defects have been constructed and are available in an appendix. It is anticipated that this summary will update a wide range of medical personnel, including pediatric cardiologists and pediatricians, adult cardiologists, internists, obstetricians, nurses, and thoracic surgeons, about the genetic aspects of congenital heart disease and will encourage an interdisciplinary approach to the child and adult with congenital heart disease. (*Circulation.* 2007;115:3015-3038.) (6/07)

GIFTS TO PHYSICIANS FROM INDUSTRY

American Medical Association (8/01)

GUIDELINES FOR FIELD TRIAGE OF INJURED PATIENTS

Centers for Disease Control and Prevention (1/12)

GUIDELINES FOR REFERRAL OF CHILDREN AND ADOLESCENTS TO PEDIATRIC RHEUMATOLOGISTS

American College of Rheumatology (6/02, reaffirmed 5/07)

HELPING THE STUDENT WITH DIABETES SUCCEED: A GUIDE FOR SCHOOL PERSONNEL

National Diabetes Education Program (6/03)

IDENTIFYING AND RESPONDING TO DOMESTIC VIOLENCE: CONSENSUS RECOMMENDATIONS FOR CHILD AND ADOLESCENT HEALTH

Family Violence Prevention Fund (9/02)

IMPORTANCE AND IMPLEMENTATION OF TRAINING IN CARDIOPULMONARY RESUSCITATION AND AUTOMATED EXTERNAL DEFIBRILLATION IN SCHOOLS

*American Heart Association Emergency Cardiovascular Care
    Committee; Council on Cardiopulmonary, Critical Care,
    Perioperative and Resuscitation; Council on Cardiovascular
    Diseases in the Young; Council on Cardiovascular
    Nursing; Council on Clinical Cardiology; and Advocacy
    Coordinating Committee*

ABSTRACT. In 2003, the International Liaison Committee on Resuscitation published a consensus document on education in resuscitation that strongly recommended that "…instruction in CPR [cardiopulmonary resuscitation] be incorporated as a standard part of the school curriculum." The next year the American Heart Association (AHA) recommended that schools "…establish a goal to train every teacher in CPR and first aid and train all students in CPR" as part of their preparation for a response to medical emergencies on campus.

Since that time, there has been an increased interest in legislation that would mandate that school curricula include training in CPR or CPR and automated external defibrillation. Laws or curriculum content standards in 36 states (as of the 2009–2010 school year) now encourage the inclusion of CPR training programs in school curricula. The language in those laws and standards varies greatly, ranging from a suggestion that students "recognize" the steps of CPR to a requirement for certification in CPR. Not surprisingly, then, implementation is not uniform among states, even those whose laws or standards encourage CPR training in schools in the strongest language. This statement recommends that training in CPR and familiarization with automated external defibrillators (AEDs) should be required elements of secondary school curricula and provides the rationale for implementation of CPR training, as well as guidance in overcoming barriers to implementation. (2/11)

INTER-ASSOCIATION CONSENSUS STATEMENT ON BEST PRACTICES FOR SPORTS MEDICINE MANAGEMENT FOR SECONDARY SCHOOLS AND COLLEGES

National Athletic Trainers Association, National Interscholastic Athletic Administrators Association, College Athletic Trainers' Society, National Federation of State High School Associations, American College Health Association, American Orthopaedic Society for Sports Medicine, National Collegiate Athletic Association, American Medical Society for Sports Medicine, National Association of Collegiate Directors of Athletics, and National Association of Intercollegiate Athletics (7/13)

LIGHTNING SAFETY FOR ATHLETICS AND RECREATION

National Athletic Trainers' Association

ABSTRACT. *Objective.* To educate athletic trainers and others about the dangers of lightning, provide lightning-safety guidelines, define safe structures and locations, and advocate prehospital care for lightning-strike victims.

Background. Lightning may be the most frequently encountered severe-storm hazard endangering physically active people each year. Millions of lightning flashes strike the ground annually in the United States, causing nearly 100 deaths and 400 injuries. Three quarters of all lightning casualties occur between May and September, and nearly four fifths occur between 10:00 AM and 7:00 PM, which coincides with the hours for most athletic or recreational activities. Additionally, lightning casualties from sports and recreational activities have risen alarmingly in recent decades.

Recommendations. The National Athletic Trainers' Association recommends a proactive approach to lightning safety, including the implementation of a lightning-safety policy that identifies safe locations for shelter from the lightning hazard. Further components of this policy are monitoring local weather forecasts, designating a weather watcher, and establishing a chain of command. Additionally, a flash-to-bang count of 30 seconds or more should be used as a minimal determinant of when to suspend activities. Waiting 30 minutes or longer after the last flash of lightning or sound of thunder is recommended before athletic or recreational activities are resumed. Lightning safety strategies include avoiding shelter under trees, avoiding open fields and spaces, and suspending the use of land-line telephones during thunderstorms. Also outlined in this document are the prehospital care guidelines for triaging and treating lightning-strike victims. It is important to evaluate victims quickly for apnea, asystole, hypothermia, shock, fractures, and burns. Cardiopulmonary resuscitation is effective in resuscitating pulseless victims of lightning strike. Maintenance of cardiopulmonary resuscitation and first-aid certification should be required of all persons involved in sports and recreational activities. (12/00)

LONG-TERM CARDIOVASCULAR TOXICITY IN CHILDREN, ADOLESCENTS, AND YOUNG ADULTS WHO RECEIVE CANCER THERAPY: PATHOPHYSIOLOGY, COURSE, MONITORING, MANAGEMENT, PREVENTION, AND RESEARCH DIRECTIONS: A SCIENTIFIC STATEMENT FROM THE AMERICAN HEART ASSOCIATION

American Heart Association (5/13)

THE MANAGEMENT OF HYPOTENSION IN THE VERY-LOW-BIRTH-WEIGHT INFANT: GUIDELINE FOR PRACTICE

National Association of Neonatal Nurses

ABSTRACT. This guideline, released in 2011, focuses on the clinical management of systemic hypotension in the very-low-birth-weight (VLBW) infant during the first 3 days of postnatal life. (2011)

MEETING OF THE STRATEGIC ADVISORY GROUP OF EXPERTS ON IMMUNIZATION, APRIL 2012–CONCLUSIONS AND RECOMMENDATIONS

World Health Organization (5/12) (The AAP endorses the recommendation pertaining to the use of thimerosal in vaccines.)

MENSTRUATION IN GIRLS AND ADOLESCENTS: USING THE MENSTRUAL CYCLE AS A VITAL SIGN

American College of Obstetricians and Gynecologists Committee on Adolescent Health Care

ABSTRACT. Despite variations worldwide and within the U.S. population, median age at menarche has remained relatively stable—between 12 years and 13 years—across well-nourished populations in developed countries. Environmental factors, including socioeconomic conditions, nutrition, and access to preventive health care, may influence the timing and progression of puberty. A number of medical conditions can cause abnormal uterine bleeding, characterized by unpredictable timing and variable amount of flow. Clinicians should educate girls and their caretakers (eg, parents or guardians) about what to expect of a first menstrual period and the range for normal cycle length of subsequent menses. Identification of abnormal menstrual patterns in adolescence may improve early identification of potential health concerns for adulthood. It is important for clinicians to have an understanding of the menstrual patterns of adolescent girls, the ability to differentiate between normal and abnormal menstruation, and the skill to know how to evaluate the adolescent girl patient. By including an evaluation of the menstrual cycle as an additional vital sign, clinicians reinforce its importance in assessing overall health status for patients and caretakers. (12/15)

MENTAL HEALTH AND SUBSTANCE USE SCREENING AND ASSESSMENT OF CHILDREN IN FOSTER CARE

American Academy of Child and Adolescent Psychiatry and Child Welfare League of America (2003)

MULTILINGUAL CHILDREN: BEYOND MYTHS AND TOWARD BEST PRACTICES

Society for Research in Child Development

ABSTRACT. Multilingualism is an international fact of life and increasing in the United States. Multilingual families are exceedingly diverse, and policies relevant to them should take this into account. The quantity and quality of a child's exposure to responsive conversation spoken by fluent adults predicts both monolingual and multilingual language and literacy achievement. Contexts supporting optimal multilingualism involve early exposure to high quality conversation in each language, along with continued support for speaking both languages. Parents who are not fluent in English should not be told to speak

English instead of their native language to their children; children require fluent input, and fluent input in another language will transfer to learning a second or third language. Messages regarding optimal multilingual practices should be made available to families using any and all available methods for delivering such information, including home visitation programs, healthcare settings, center-based early childhood programs, and mass media. (2013)

NATIONAL ADOPTION CENTER: OPEN RECORDS
National Adoption Center
The National Adoption Center believes that it is an inalienable right of all citizens, including adopted adults, to have unencumbered access to their original birth certificates. In keeping with this position, we believe that copies of both the original and the amended birth certificate should be given to the adoptive family at the time of finalization unless specifically denied by the birthparents. In any case, the National Adoption Center advocates that the adoptee, at age 18, be granted access to his/her original birth certificate. (6/00)

NEONATAL ENCEPHALOPATHY AND NEUROLOGIC OUTCOME, SECOND EDITION
American College of Obstetricians and Gynecologists Task Force on Neonatal Encephalopathy
In the first edition of this report, the Task Force on Neonatal Encephalopathy and Cerebral Palsy outlined criteria deemed essential to establish a causal link between intrapartum hypoxic events and cerebral palsy. It is now known that there are multiple potential causal pathways that lead to cerebral palsy in term infants, and the signs and symptoms of neonatal encephalopathy may range from mild to severe, depending on the nature and timing of the brain injury. Thus, for the current edition, the Task Force on Neonatal Encephalopathy determined that a broader perspective may be more fruitful. This conclusion reflects the sober recognition that knowledge gaps still preclude a definitive test or set of markers that accurately identifies, with high sensitivity and specificity, an infant in whom neonatal encephalopathy is attributable to an acute intrapartum event. The information necessary for assessment of likelihood can be derived from a comprehensive evaluation of all potential contributing factors in cases of neonatal encephalopathy. This is the broader perspective championed in the current report. If a comprehensive etiologic evaluation is not possible, the term hypoxic–ischemic encephalopathy should best be replaced by neonatal encephalopathy because neither hypoxia nor ischemia can be assumed to have been the unique initiating causal mechanism. The title of this report has been changed from *Neonatal Encephalopathy and Cerebral Palsy: Defining the Pathogenesis and Pathophysiology* to *Neonatal Encephalopathy and Neurologic Outcome* to indicate that an array of developmental outcomes may arise after neonatal encephalopathy in addition to cerebral palsy. (4/14)

NEURODEVELOPMENTAL OUTCOMES IN CHILDREN WITH CONGENITAL HEART DISEASE: EVALUATION AND MANAGEMENT: A SCIENTIFIC STATEMENT FROM THE AMERICAN HEART ASSOCIATION
American Heart Association (7/12)

THE NEUROLOGIST'S ROLE IN SUPPORTING TRANSITION TO ADULT HEALTH CARE
Lawrence W. Brown, MD; Peter Camfield, MD, FRCPC; Melissa Capers, MA; Greg Cascino, MD; Mary Ciccarelli, MD; Claudio M. de Gusmao, MD; Stephen M. Downs, MD; Annette Majnemer, PhD, FCAHS; Amy Brin Miller, MSN; Christina SanInocencio, MS; Rebecca Schultz, PhD; Anne Tilton, MD; Annick Winokur, BS; and Mary Zupanc, MD
ABSTRACT. The child neurologist has a critical role in planning and coordinating the successful transition from the pediatric to adult health care system for youth with neurologic conditions. Leadership in appropriately planning a youth's transition and in care coordination among health care, educational, vocational, and community services providers may assist in preventing gaps in care, delayed entry into the adult care system, and/or health crises for their adolescent patients. Youth whose neurologic conditions result in cognitive or physical disability and their families may need additional support during this transition, given the legal and financial considerations that may be required. Eight common principles that define the child neurologist's role in a successful transition process have been outlined by a multidisciplinary panel convened by the Child Neurology Foundation are introduced and described. The authors of this consensus statement recognize the current paucity of evidence for successful transition models and outline areas for future consideration. *Neurology*® 2016;87:1–6. (7/16)

NONINHERITED RISK FACTORS AND CONGENITAL CARDIOVASCULAR DEFECTS: CURRENT KNOWLEDGE
American Heart Association
ABSTRACT. Prevention of congenital cardiovascular defects has been hampered by a lack of information about modifiable risk factors for abnormalities in cardiac development. Over the past decade, there have been major breakthroughs in the understanding of inherited causes of congenital heart disease, including the identification of specific genetic abnormalities for some types of malformations. Although relatively less information has been available on noninherited modifiable factors that may have an adverse effect on the fetal heart, there is a growing body of epidemiological literature on this topic. This statement summarizes the currently available literature on potential fetal exposures that might alter risk for cardiovascular defects. Information is summarized for periconceptional multivitamin or folic acid intake, which may reduce the risk of cardiac disease in the fetus, and for additional types of potential exposures that may increase the risk, including maternal illnesses, maternal therapeutic and nontherapeutic drug exposures, environmental exposures, and paternal exposures. Information is highlighted regarding definitive risk factors such as maternal rubella; phenylketonuria; pregestational diabetes; exposure to thalidomide, vitamin A cogeners, or retinoids; and indomethacin tocolysis. Caveats regarding interpretation of possible exposure-outcome relationships from case-control studies are given because this type of study has provided most of the available information. Guidelines for prospective parents that could reduce the

likelihood that their child will have a major cardiac malformation are given. Issues related to pregnancy monitoring are discussed. Knowledge gaps and future sources of new information on risk factors are described. (*Circulation.* 2007;115:2995–3014.) (6/07)

ORTHOPTISTS AS PHYSICIAN EXTENDERS
American Association for Pediatric Ophthalmology and Strabismus (5/15)

PEDIATRIC CARE IN THE EMERGENCY DEPARTMENT
Society for Academic Emergency Medicine
ABSTRACT. Physicians who have successfully completed an accredited Emergency Medicine residency and are certified in emergency medicine by the American Board of Emergency Medicine (ABEM) or the American Osteopathic Board of Emergency Medicine (AOBEM) ABEM/AOBEM or those who are certified in pediatric emergency medicine by ABEM or the American Board of Pediatrics (ABP) possess the knowledge and skills required to provide quality emergency medical care to children of all ages for a wide variety of illnesses, injuries or poisonings. To provide quality care, the emergency physician must have all necessary and age-appropriate medical equipment readily available. The emergency physician must also have access via consultation, admission, or transfer, to appropriate specialty and sub-specialty physicians, to who will provide any needed patient care after emergency department treatment. Physically separated care areas for children are not mandatory in order to provide high-quality care to patients of all ages. Although physically separate care areas for children are ideal, they are not mandatory to provide high-quality care. (11/03)

PREVENTION AND CONTROL OF MENINGOCOCCAL DISEASE: RECOMMENDATIONS OF THE ADVISORY COMMITTEE ON IMMUNIZATION PRACTICES (ACIP)
Centers for Disease Control and Prevention
SUMMARY. Meningococcal disease describes the spectrum of infections caused by *Neisseria meningitidis,* including meningitidis, bacteremia, and bacteremic pneumonia. Two quadrivalent meningococcal polysaccharide-protein conjugate vaccines that provide protection against meningococcal serogroups A, C, W, and Y (MenACWY-D [Menactra, manufactured by Sanofi Pasteur, Inc., Swiftwater, Pennsylvania] and MenACWY-CRM [Menveo, manufactured by Novartis Vaccines, Cambridge, Massachusetts]) are licensed in the United States for use among persons aged 2 through 55 years. MenACWY-D also is licensed for use among infants and toddlers aged 9 through 23 months. Quadrivalent meningococcal polysaccharide vaccine (MPSV4 [Menommune, manufactured by Sanofi Pasteur, Inc., Swiftwater, Pennsylvania]) is the only vaccine licensed for use among persons aged ≥56 years. A bivalent meningococcal polysaccharide protein conjugate vaccine that provides protection against meningococcal serogroups C and Y along with *Haemophilus influenzae* type b (Hib) (Hib-MenCY-TT [MenHibrix, manufactured by GlaxoSmithKline Biologicals, Rixensart, Belgium]) is licensed for use in children aged 6 weeks through 18 months.

This report compiles and summarizes all recommendations from CDC's Advisory Committee on Immunization Practices (ACIP) regarding prevention and control of meningococcal disease in the United States, specifically the changes in the recommendations published since 2005 (CDC. Prevention and control of meningococcal disease: recommendations of the Advisory Committee on Immunization Practices [ACIP]. *MMWR* 2005;54 Adobe PDF file [No. RR-7]). As a comprehensive summary of previously published recommendations, this report does not contain any new recommendations; it is intended for use by clinicians as a resource. ACIP recommends routine vaccination with a quadrivalent meningococcal conjugate vaccine (MenACWY) for adolescents aged 11 or 12 years, with a booster dose at age 16 years. ACIP also recommends routine vaccination for persons at increased risk for meningococcal disease (i.e., persons who have persistent complement component deficiencies, persons who have anatomic or functional asplenia, microbiologists who routinely are exposed to isolates of *N. meningitidis,* military recruits, and persons who travel to or reside in areas in which meningococcal disease is hyperendemic or epidemic). Guidelines for antimicrobial chemoprophylaxis and for evaluation and management of suspected outbreaks of meningococcal disease also are provided. (3/13)

PREVENTION OF RHEUMATIC FEVER AND DIAGNOSIS AND TREATMENT OF ACUTE STREPTOCOCCAL PHARYNGITIS
American Heart Association Rheumatic Fever, Endocarditis, and Kawasaki Disease Committee of the Council on Cardiovascular Disease in the Young; Interdisciplinary Council on Functional Genomics and Translational Biology; and Interdisciplinary Council on Quality of Care and Outcomes Research
ABSTRACT. Primary prevention of acute rheumatic fever is accomplished by proper identification and adequate antibiotic treatment of group A β-hemolytic streptococcal (GAS) tonsillopharyngitis. Diagnosis of GAS pharyngitis is best accomplished by combining clinical judgment with diagnostic test results, the criterion standard of which is the throat culture. Penicillin (either oral penicillin V or injectable benzathine penicillin) is the treatment of choice, because it is cost-effective, has a narrow spectrum of activity, and has long-standing proven efficacy, and GAS resistant to penicillin have not been documented. For penicillin-allergic individuals, acceptable alternatives include a narrow-spectrum oral cephalosporin, oral clindamycin, or various oral macrolides or azalides. The individual who has had an attack of rheumatic fever is at very high risk of developing recurrences after subsequent GAS pharyngitis and needs continuous antimicrobial prophylaxis to prevent such recurrences (secondary prevention). The recommended duration of prophylaxis depends on the number of previous attacks, the time elapsed since the last attack, the risk of exposure to GAS infections, the age of the patient, and the presence or absence of cardiac involvement. Penicillin is again the agent of choice for secondary prophylaxis, but sulfadiazine or a macrolide or azalide are acceptable alternatives in penicillin-allergic individuals. This report updates the 1995 statement by the American Heart Association Rheumatic

Fever, Endocarditis, and Kawasaki Disease Committee. It includes new recommendations for the diagnosis and treatment of GAS pharyngitis, as well as for the secondary prevention of rheumatic fever, and classifies the strength of the recommendations and level of evidence supporting them. (2/09)

PROTECTING ADOLESCENTS: ENSURING ACCESS TO CARE AND REPORTING SEXUAL ACTIVITY AND ABUSE
Society for Adolescent Medicine (11/04)

RECOMMENDED AMOUNT OF SLEEP FOR PEDIATRIC POPULATIONS: A CONSENSUS STATEMENT OF THE AMERICAN ACADEMY OF SLEEP MEDICINE
Shalini Paruthi, MD; Lee J. Brooks, MD; Carolyn D'Ambrosio, MD; Wendy A. Hall, PhD, RN; Suresh Kotagal, MD; Robin M. Lloyd, MD; Beth A. Malow, MD, MS; Kiran Maski, MD; Cynthia Nichols, PhD; Stuart F. Quan, MD; Carol L. Rosen, MD; Matthew M. Troester, DO; and Merrill S. Wise, MD

Background and Methology. Healthy sleep requires adequate duration, appropriate timing, good quality, regularity, and the absence of sleep disturbances or disorders. Sleep duration is a frequently investigated sleep measure in relation to health. A panel of 13 experts in sleep medicine and research used a modified RAND Appropriateness Method to develop recommendations regarding the sleep duration range that promotes optimal health in children aged 0–18 years. The expert panel reviewed published scientific evidence addressing the relationship between sleep duration and health using a broad set of National Library of Medicine Medical Subject Headings (MeSH) terms and no date restrictions, which resulted in a total of 864 scientific articles. The process was further guided by the Oxford grading system. The panel focused on seven health categories with the best available evidence in relation to sleep duration: general health, cardiovascular health, metabolic health, mental health, immunologic function, developmental health, and human performance. Consistent with the RAND Appropriateness Method, multiple rounds of evidence review, discussion, and voting were conducted to arrive at the final recommendations. The process to develop these recommendations was conducted over a 10-month period and concluded with a meeting held February 19–21, 2016, in Chicago, Illinois. (6/16)

REPORT OF THE NATIONAL CONSENSUS CONFERENCE ON FAMILY PRESENCE DURING PEDIATRIC CARDIO-PULMONARY RESUSCITATION AND PROCEDURES
Ambulatory Pediatric Association
INTRODUCTION. The National Consensus Conference on Family Presence during Pediatric Cardiopulmonary Resuscitation and Procedures was held in Washington, DC, on September 7–8, 2003. The concept, funding, planning and organization for the conference were the Ambulatory Pediatric Association (APA) Presidential Project of James Seidel, M.D., Ph.D. Dr. Seidel was in the final stages of preparation for chairing the conference when he died on July 25, 2003. In Dr. Seidel's absence, the conference was chaired by Deborah Parkman Henderson R.N., PhD, his co-investigator, and Jane F. Knapp, M.D., a colleague.

The National Consensus Conference on Family Presence during Pediatric Procedures and Cardiopulmonary Resuscitation was funded by a grant to the APA from the Maternal Child Health Bureau (MCHB) Partnership for Children. This meeting brought together a panel of over 20 appointed representatives from a multidisciplinary, diverse group of national organizations interested in the emergency care of children. The conference was part of a multiphase process designed with the goal of publishing consensus guidelines useful for defining policy regarding family presence (FP) during pediatric procedures and CPR in the Emergency Department (ED). It is also possible that the consensus panel recommendations could be applied to other settings.

Panel members completed a review of the literature prior to attending the conference. This review, along with results of a pre-conference questionnaire, formed the basis of the discussion during the conference. During the two day conference the participants completed the outline of the guidelines presented here. We believe these recommendations are a powerful testimony to Dr. Seidel's vision for promoting FP through multidisciplinary consensus building. Beyond that vision, however, we hope that the guidelines will make a difference in improving the quality of children's health care. (9/03)

RESPONSE TO CARDIAC ARREST AND SELECTED LIFE-THREATENING MEDICAL EMERGENCIES: THE MEDICAL EMERGENCY RESPONSE PLAN FOR SCHOOLS. A STATEMENT FOR HEALTHCARE PROVIDERS, POLICYMAKERS, SCHOOL ADMINISTRATORS, AND COMMUNITY LEADERS
American Heart Association (1/04)

SAFE AT SCHOOL CAMPAIGN STATEMENT OF PRINCIPLES
American Diabetes Association (endorsed 2/06)

SCREENING FOR IDIOPATHIC SCOLIOSIS IN ADOLESCENTS—POSITION STATEMENT
American Academy of Orthopedic Surgeons, Scoliosis Research Society, and Pediatric Orthopedic Society of North America
ABSTRACT. The Scoliosis Research Society (SRS), American Academy of Orthopedic Surgeons (AAOS), Pediatric Orthopedic Society of North America (POSNA), and American Academy of Pediatrics (AAP) believe that there has been additional useful research in the early detection and management of adolescent idiopathic scoliosis (AIS) since the review performed by the United States Preventive Services Task Force (USPSTF) in 2004. This information should be available for use by patients, treating health care providers, and policy makers in assessing the relative risks and benefits of the early identification and management of AIS.

The AAOS, SRS, POSNA, and AAP believe that there are documented benefits of earlier detection and non-surgical management of AIS, earlier identification of severe deformities that are surgically treated, and of incorporating screening of children for AIS by knowledgeable health care providers as a part of their care. (9/15)

SELECTED ISSUES FOR THE ADOLESCENT ATHLETE AND THE TEAM PHYSICIAN: A CONSENSUS STATEMENT

American Academy of Family Physicians, American Academy of Orthopaedic Surgeons, American College of Sports Medicine, American Medical Society for Sports Medicine, American Orthopaedic Society for Sports Medicine, and American Osteopathic Academy of Sports Medicine

GOAL. The goal of this document is to help the team physician improve the care of the adolescent athlete by understanding the medical, musculoskeletal and psychological factors common in this age group. To accomplish this goal, the team physician should have knowledge of and be involved with:

- Musculoskeletal injuries of the adolescent athlete, specifically those to the shoulder, knee, elbow and spine

- Medical conditions of the adolescent athlete, especially those pertaining to infectious diseases, concussion, and nutrition and supplementation

- Psychological issues related to sports specialization and overtraining. (11/08)

SKIING AND SNOWBOARDING INJURY PREVENTION

Canadian Paediatric Society

ABSTRACT. Skiing and snowboarding are popular recreational and competitive sport activities for children and youth. Injuries associated with both activities are frequent and can be serious. There is new evidence documenting the benefit of wearing helmets while skiing and snowboarding, as well as data refuting suggestions that helmet use may increase the risk of neck injury. There is also evidence to support using wrist guards while snowboarding. There is poor uptake of effective preventive measures such as protective equipment use and related policy. Physicians should have the information required to counsel children, youth and families regarding safer snow sport participation, including helmet use, wearing wrist guards for snowboarding, training and supervision, the importance of proper equipment fitting and binding adjustment, sun safety and avoiding substance use while on the slopes. (1/12)

SUPPLEMENT TO THE JCIH 2007 POSITION STATEMENT: PRINCIPLES AND GUIDELINES FOR EARLY INTERVENTION AFTER CONFIRMATION THAT A CHILD IS DEAF OR HARD OF HEARING

Joint Committee on Infant Hearing

PREFACE. This document is a supplement to the recommendations in the year 2007 position statement of the Joint Committee on Infant Hearing (JCIH) and provides comprehensive guidelines for early hearing detection and intervention (EHDI) programs on establishing strong early intervention (EI) systems with appropriate expertise to meet the needs of children who are deaf or hard of hearing (D/HH).

EI services represent the purpose and goal of the entire EHDI process. Screening and confirmation that a child is D/HH are largely meaningless without appropriate, individualized, targeted and high-quality intervention. For the infant or young child who is D/HH to reach his or her full potential, carefully designed individualized intervention must be implemented promptly, utilizing service providers with optimal knowledge and skill levels and providing services on the basis of research, best practices, and proven models.

The delivery of EI services is complex and requires individualization to meet the identified needs of the child and family. Because of the diverse needs of the population of children who are D/HH and their families, well-controlled intervention studies are challenging. At this time, few comparative effectiveness studies have been conducted. Randomized controlled trials are particularly difficult for ethical reasons, making it challenging to establish causal links between interventions and outcomes. EI systems must partner with colleagues in research to document what works for children and families and to strengthen the evidence base supporting practices.

Despite limitations and gaps in the evidence, the literature does contain research studies in which all children who were D/HH had access to the same well-defined EI service. These studies indicate that positive outcomes are possible, and they provide guidance about key program components that appear to promote these outcomes. This EI services document, drafted by teams of professionals with extensive expertise in EI programs for children who are D/HH and their families, relied on literature searches, existing systematic reviews, and recent professional consensus statements in developing this set of guidelines.

Terminology presented a challenge throughout document development. The committee noted that many of the frequently occurring terms necessary within the supplement may not reflect the most contemporary understanding and/or could convey inaccurate meaning. Rather than add to the lack of clarity or consensus and to avoid introducing new terminology to stakeholders, the committee opted to use currently recognized terms consistently herein and will monitor the emergence and/or development of new descriptors before the next JCIH consensus statement.

For purposes of this supplement:

- *Language* refers to all spoken and signed languages.

- *Early intervention* (EI), according to part C of the Individuals with Disabilities Education Improvement Act (IDEA) of 2004, is the process of providing services, education, and support to young children who are deemed to have an established condition, those who are evaluated and deemed to have a diagnosed physical or mental condition (with a high probability of resulting in a developmental delay), those who have an existing delay, or those who are at risk of developing a delay or special need that may affect their development or impede their education.

- *Communication* is used in lieu of terms such as communication options, methods, opportunities, approaches, etc.

- *Deaf or hard of hearing* (D/HH) is intended to be inclusive of all children with congenital and acquired hearing loss, unilateral and bilateral hearing loss, all degrees of hearing loss from minimal to profound, and all types of hearing loss (sensorineural, auditory neuropathy spectrum disorder, permanent conductive, and mixed).

- *Core knowledge and skills* is used to describe the expertise needed to provide appropriate EI that will optimize the development and well-being of infants/children and their families. Core knowledge and skills will differ according to the roles of individuals within the EI system (eg, service coordinator or EI provider).

This supplement to JCIH 2007 focuses on the practices of EI providers outside of the primary medical care and specialty medical care realms, rather than including the full spectrum of necessary medical, audiologic, and educational interventions. For more information about the recommendations for medical follow-up, primary care surveillance for related medical conditions, and specialty medical care and monitoring, the reader is encouraged to reference the year 2007 position statement of the JCIH as well as any subsequent revision. When an infant is confirmed to be D/HH, the importance of ongoing medical and audiologic management and surveillance both in the medical home and with the hearing health professionals, the otolaryngologist and the audiologist, cannot be overstated. A comprehensive discussion of those services is beyond the scope of this document. (3/13)

SYSTEMATIC REVIEW AND EVIDENCE-BASED GUIDELINES FOR THE MANAGEMENT OF PATIENTS WITH POSITIONAL PLAGIOCEPHALY

Congress of Neurologic Surgeons
ABSTRACT. *Background.* Positional plagiocephaly is a common problem seen by pediatricians, pediatric neurologists, and pediatric neurosurgeons. Currently, there are no evidence-based guidelines on the management of positional plagiocephaly. The topics addressed in subsequent chapters of this guideline include: diagnosis, repositioning, physical therapy, and orthotic devices.

Objective. To evaluate topics relevant to the diagnosis and management of patients with positional plagiocephaly. The rigorous systematic process in which this guideline was created is presented in this chapter.

Methods. This guideline was prepared by the Plagiocephaly Guideline Task Force, a multidisciplinary team comprised of physician volunteers (clinical experts), medical librarians, and clinical guidelines specialists. The task force conducted a series of systematic literature searches of the National Library of Medicine and the Cochrane Library, according to standard protocols described below, for each topic addressed in subsequent chapters of this guideline.

Results. The systematic literature searches returned 396 abstracts relative to the 4 main topics addressed in this guideline. The results were analyzed and are described in detail in each subsequent chapter included in this guideline.

Conclusion. Evidence-based guidelines for the management of infants with positional plagiocephaly will help practitioners manage this common disorder. (11/16)

TARGETED TUBERCULIN TESTING AND TREATMENT OF LATENT TUBERCULOSIS INFECTION

American Thoracic Society and Centers for Disease Control and Prevention (4/00) (The AAP endorses and accepts as its policy the sections of this statement as they relate to infants and children.)

TIMING OF UMBILICAL CORD CLAMPING AFTER BIRTH

American College of Obstetricians and Gynecologists Committee on Obstetric Practice (12/12)

UPDATE ON JAPANESE ENCEPHALITIS VACCINE FOR CHILDREN—UNITED STATES, MAY 2011

Centers for Disease Control and Prevention
Inactivated mouse brain-derived Japanese encephalitis (JE) vaccine (JE-MB [manufactured as JE-Vax]), the only JE vaccine that is licensed for use in children in the United States, is no longer available. This notice provides updated information regarding options for obtaining JE vaccine for U.S. children. (8/11)

WEIGHING PEDIATRIC PATIENTS IN KILOGRAMS

Emergency Nurses Association (3/12)

Appendix 1

Policies by Committee

· ·

AMERICAN ACADEMY OF PEDIATRICS
Policies by Committee

ADOLESCENT SLEEP WORKING GROUP

Insufficient Sleep in Adolescents and Young Adults: An Update on Causes and Consequences (Technical Report) (joint with Committee on Adolescence), 8/14

School Start Times for Adolescents (joint with Committee on Adolescence and Council on School Health), 8/14

BLACK BOX WORKING GROUP

Cardiovascular Monitoring and Stimulant Drugs for Attention-Deficit/Hyperactivity Disorder (joint with Section on Cardiology and Cardiac Surgery), 8/08

BOARD OF DIRECTORS

Ritual Genital Cutting of Female Minors, 6/10

BRIGHT FUTURES PERIODICITY SCHEDULE WORKGROUP

2016 Recommendations for Preventive Pediatric Health Care (joint with Committee on Practice and Ambulatory Medicine), 12/15

BRIGHT FUTURES STEERING COMMITTEE

Identifying Infants and Young Children With Developmental Disorders in the Medical Home: An Algorithm for Developmental Surveillance and Screening (joint with Council on Children With Disabilities, Section on Developmental and Behavioral Pediatrics, and Medical Home Initiatives for Children With Special Needs Project Advisory Committee), 7/06, reaffirmed 12/09, 8/14

BRONCHIOLITIS GUIDELINES COMMITTEE

Updated Guidance for Palivizumab Prophylaxis Among Infants and Young Children at Increased Risk of Hospitalization for Respiratory Syncytial Virus Infection (joint with Committee on Infectious Diseases), 7/14

Updated Guidance for Palivizumab Prophylaxis Among Infants and Young Children at Increased Risk of Hospitalization for Respiratory Syncytial Virus Infection (Technical Report) (joint with Committee on Infectious Diseases), 7/14

CARDIAC SURGERY EXECUTIVE COMMITTEE

Endorsement of Health and Human Services Recommendation for Pulse Oximetry Screening for Critical Congenital Heart Disease (joint with Section on Cardiology), 12/11

CHILD AND ADOLESCENT HEALTH ACTION GROUP (FORMERLY COUNCIL ON CHILD AND ADOLESCENT HEALTH)

Age Limits of Pediatrics, 5/88, reaffirmed 9/92, 1/97, 3/02, 1/06, 10/11

COMMITTEE ON ADOLESCENCE

Achieving Quality Health Services for Adolescents, 7/16

Adolescent Pregnancy: Current Trends and Issues (Clinical Report), 7/05

Adolescent Pregnancy: Current Trends and Issues—Addendum, 4/14

Adolescents and Human Immunodeficiency Virus Infection: The Role of the Pediatrician in Prevention and Intervention (joint with Committee on Pediatric AIDS), 1/01, reaffirmed 10/03, 1/05

The Adolescent's Right to Confidential Care When Considering Abortion, 5/96, reaffirmed 5/99, 11/02

Care of Adolescent Parents and Their Children (Clinical Report) (joint with Committee on Early Childhood), 11/12, reaffirmed 7/16

Care of the Adolescent Sexual Assault Victim (Clinical Report), 8/08

Collaborative Role of the Pediatrician in the Diagnosis and Management of Bipolar Disorder in Adolescents (Clinical Report), 11/12

Condom Use by Adolescents, 10/13

Contraception for Adolescents, 9/14

Contraception for Adolescents (Technical Report), 9/14

Counseling the Adolescent About Pregnancy Options, 5/98, reaffirmed 1/01, 1/06

Emergency Contraception, 11/12, reaffirmed 7/16

Emergency Contraception: Addendum, 2/14

Excessive Sleepiness in Adolescents and Young Adults: Causes, Consequences, and Treatment Strategies (Technical Report) (joint with Working Group on Sleepiness in Adolescents/Young Adults), 6/05

Gynecologic Examination for Adolescents in the Pediatric Office Setting (Clinical Report), 8/10, reaffirmed 5/13

Health Care for Youth in the Juvenile Justice System, 11/11

Health Care Issues for Children and Adolescents in Foster Care and Kinship Care (joint with Council on Foster Care, Adoption, and Kinship Care and Council on Early Childhood), 9/15

Health Care Issues for Children and Adolescents in Foster Care and Kinship Care (Technical Report) (joint with Council on Foster Care, Adoption, and Kinship Care and Council on Early Childhood), 9/15

Identification and Management of Eating Disorders in Children and Adolescents (Clinical Report), 11/10

The Impact of Marijuana Policies on Youth: Clinical, Research, and Legal Update (joint with Committee on Substance Abuse), 2/15

The Impact of Marijuana Policies on Youth: Clinical, Research, and Legal Update (Technical Report) (joint with Committee on Substance Abuse), 2/15

Insufficient Sleep in Adolescents and Young Adults: An Update on Causes and Consequences (Technical Report) (joint with Adolescent Sleep Working Group), 8/14

Legalization of Marijuana: Potential Impact on Youth (joint with Committee on Substance Abuse), 6/04

Legalization of Marijuana: Potential Impact on Youth (Technical Report) (joint with Committee on Substance Abuse), 6/04

Male Adolescent Sexual and Reproductive Health Care (Clinical Report), 11/11

Menstrual Management for Adolescents With Disabilities (Clinical Report) (joint with the North American Society for Pediatric and Adolescent Gynecology), 6/16

Office-Based Care for Lesbian, Gay, Bisexual, Transgender, and Questioning Youth, 6/13

Office-Based Care for Lesbian, Gay, Bisexual, Transgender, and Questioning Youth (Technical Report), 6/13

Preventing Obesity and Eating Disorders in Adolescents (Clinical Report) (joint with Committee on Nutrition and Section on Obesity), 8/16

School Start Times for Adolescents (joint with Adolescence Sleep Working Group and Council on School Health), 8/14

Screening for Nonviral Sexually Transmitted Infections in Adolescents and Young Adults (joint with Society for Adolescent Health and Medicine), 6/14

Secondhand and Prenatal Tobacco Smoke Exposure (Technical Report) (joint with Committee on Environmental Health and Committee on Native American Child Health), 10/09, reaffirmed 5/14

Sexual Orientation and Adolescents (Clinical Report), 6/04

Sexuality Education for Children and Adolescents (Clinical Report) (joint with Committee on Psychosocial Aspects of Child and Family Health), 7/16

Standards for Health Information Technology to Ensure Adolescent Privacy (joint with Council on Clinical Information Technology), 10/12

Suicide and Suicide Attempts in Adolescents (Clinical Report), 6/16

The Teen Driver (joint with Committee on Injury, Violence, and Poison Prevention), 12/06, reaffirmed 6/10, 7/16

Tobacco Use: A Pediatric Disease (joint with Committee on Environmental Health, Committee on Substance Abuse, and Committee on Native American Child Health), 10/09, reaffirmed 5/13

Underinsurance of Adolescents: Recommendations for Improved Coverage of Preventive, Reproductive, and Behavioral Health Care Services (joint with Committee on Child Health Financing), 12/08, reaffirmed 8/12, 5/15

COMMITTEE ON BIOETHICS

Children as Hematopoietic Stem Cell Donors, 1/10

Communicating With Children and Families: From Everyday Interactions to Skill in Conveying Distressing Information (Technical Report), 5/08, reaffirmed 5/11

Conflicts Between Religious or Spiritual Beliefs and Pediatric Care: Informed Refusal, Exemptions, and Public Funding, 10/13

Consent for Emergency Medical Services for Children and Adolescents (joint with Committee on Pediatric Emergency Medicine), 7/11, reaffirmed 9/15

Do-Not-Resuscitate Orders for Pediatric Patients Who Require Anesthesia and Surgery (Clinical Report) (joint with Section on Surgery and Section on Anesthesia and Pain Medicine), 12/04, reaffirmed 1/09, 10/12

Ethical and Policy Issues in Genetic Testing and Screening of Children (joint with Committee on Genetics and American College of Medical Genetics and Genomics), 2/13

Ethical Controversies in Organ Donation After Circulatory Death, 4/13

Ethical Issues With Genetic Testing in Pediatrics, 6/01, reaffirmed 1/05, 1/09

Ethics and the Care of Critically Ill Infants and Children, 7/96, reaffirmed 10/99, 6/03

Forgoing Life-Sustaining Medical Treatment in Abused Children (joint with Committee on Child Abuse and Neglect), 11/00, reaffirmed 6/03, 10/06, 4/09

Forgoing Medically Provided Nutrition and Hydration in Children (Clinical Report), 7/09, reaffirmed 1/14

Guidelines on Forgoing Life-Sustaining Medical Treatment, 3/94, reaffirmed 11/97, 10/00, 1/04, 1/09, 10/12

Honoring Do-Not-Attempt-Resuscitation Requests in Schools (joint with Council on School Health), 4/10, reaffirmed 7/13, 8/16

Human Embryonic Stem Cell (hESC) and Human Embryo Research (joint with Committee on Pediatric Research), 10/12

Informed Consent in Decision-Making in Pediatric Practice, 7/16

Informed Consent in Decision-Making in Pediatric Practice (Technical Report), 7/16

Institutional Ethics Committees, 1/01, reaffirmed 1/04, 1/09, 10/12, 7/14

Maternal-Fetal Intervention and Fetal Care Centers (Clinical Report) (joint with American College of Obstetricians and Gynecologists), 7/11

Minors as Living Solid-Organ Donors (Clinical Report), 8/08, reaffirmed 5/11

Palliative Care for Children (joint with Committee on Hospital Care), 8/00, reaffirmed 6/03, 10/06, 2/12

Pediatrician-Family-Patient Relationships: Managing the Boundaries, 11/09, reaffirmed 1/14

Physician Refusal to Provide Information or Treatment on the Basis of Claims of Conscience, 11/09, reaffirmed 1/14

Preservation of Fertility in Pediatric and Adolescent Patients With Cancer (Technical Report) (joint with Section on Hematology/Oncology and Section on Surgery), 5/08, reaffirmed 2/12

Professionalism in Pediatrics (Technical Report), 10/07, reaffirmed 5/11

Professionalism in Pediatrics: Statement of Principles, 10/07, reaffirmed 5/11

Religious Objections to Medical Care, 2/97, reaffirmed 10/00, 6/03, 10/06, 5/09

Responding to Parental Refusals of Immunization of Children (Clinical Report), 5/05, reaffirmed 1/09, 11/12

COMMITTEE ON CHILD ABUSE AND NEGLECT

Abusive Head Trauma in Infants and Children, 4/09, reaffirmed 3/13

Caregiver-Fabricated Illness in a Child: A Manifestation of Child Maltreatment (Clinical Report), 8/13

Child Abuse, Confidentiality, and the Health Insurance Portability and Accountability Act, 12/09, reaffirmed 1/14

Child Fatality Review (joint with Committee on Injury, Violence, and Poison Prevention and Council on Community Pediatrics), 8/10, reaffirmed 5/14

Child Sex Trafficking and Commercial Sexual Exploitation: Health Care Needs of Victims (Clinical Report), 2/15

Distinguishing Sudden Infant Death Syndrome From Child Abuse Fatalities (Clinical Report) (joint with National Association of Medical Examiners), 7/06, reaffirmed 4/09, 3/13

Evaluating Children With Fractures for Child Physical Abuse (Clinical Report), (joint with Section on Radiology, Section on Endocrinology, Section on Orthopaedics, and Society for Pediatric Radiology), 1/14

Evaluating for Suspected Child Abuse: Conditions That Predispose to Bleeding (Technical Report) (joint with Section on Hematology/Oncology), 3/13, reaffirmed 7/16

Evaluating Infants and Young Children With Multiple Fractures (Clinical Report), 9/06

Evaluation for Bleeding Disorders in Suspected Child Abuse (Clinical Report) (joint with Section on Hematology/Oncology), 3/13, reaffirmed 7/16

The Evaluation of Children in the Primary Care Setting When Sexual Abuse Is Suspected (Clinical Report), 7/13

The Evaluation of Sexual Behaviors in Children (Clinical Report), 8/09, reaffirmed 3/13

The Evaluation of Suspected Child Physical Abuse (Clinical Report), 4/15

The Eye Examination in the Evaluation of Child Abuse (Clinical Report) (joint with Section on Ophthalmology), 7/10, reaffirmed 12/15

Failure to Thrive as a Manifestation of Child Neglect (Clinical Report) (joint with Committee on Nutrition), 11/05, reaffirmed 1/09

Forgoing Life-Sustaining Medical Treatment in Abused Children (joint with Committee on Bioethics), 11/00, reaffirmed 6/03, 10/06, 4/09

Intimate Partner Violence: The Role of the Pediatrician (Clinical Report) (joint with Committee on Injury, Violence, and Poison Prevention), 4/10, reaffirmed 1/14

Maltreatment of Children With Disabilities (Clinical Report) (joint with Council on Children With Disabilities), 5/07, reaffirmed 1/11, 4/16

Oral and Dental Aspects of Child Abuse and Neglect (Clinical Report) (joint with American Academy of Pediatric Dentistry), 12/05, reaffirmed 1/09, 1/14

The Pediatrician's Role in Child Maltreatment Prevention (Clinical Report), 9/10, 1/14

Protecting Children From Sexual Abuse by Health Care Providers, 6/11, reaffirmed 10/14

Psychological Maltreatment (Clinical Report) (joint with American Academy of Child and Adolescent Psychiatry), 7/12, reaffirmed 4/16

Recognizing and Responding to Medical Neglect (Clinical Report), 12/07, reaffirmed 1/11, 2/16

Understanding the Behavioral and Emotional Consequences of Child Abuse (Clinical Report) (joint with Section on Adoption and Foster Care, American Academy of Child and Adolescent Psychiatry, and National Center for Child Traumatic Stress), 9/08, reaffirmed 8/12

When Is Lack of Supervision Neglect? (Clinical Report), 9/06

COMMITTEE ON CHILD HEALTH FINANCING

Children's Health Insurance Program (CHIP): Accomplishments, Challenges, and Policy Recommendations, 2/14

Essential Contractual Language for Medical Necessity in Children, 7/13

Financing of Pediatric Home Health Care (joint with Section on Home Care), 8/06

Guiding Principles for Managed Care Arrangements for the Health Care of Newborns, Infants, Children, Adolescents, and Young Adults, 10/13

High-Deductible Health Plans, 4/14

High-Deductible Health Plans and the New Risks of Consumer-Driven Health Insurance Products, 3/07

Improving Substance Abuse Prevention, Assessment, and Treatment Financing for Children and Adolescents (joint with Committee on Substance Abuse), 10/01

Medicaid Policy Statement, 4/13

Model Contractual Language for Medical Necessity for Children, 7/05, reaffirmed 10/11

Payment for Telephone Care (joint with Section on Telephone Care), 10/06

Principles of Health Care Financing, 10/10, reaffirmed 4/13

Scope of Health Care Benefits for Children From Birth Through Age 26, 11/11

State Children's Health Insurance Program Achievements, Challenges, and Policy Recommendations, 6/07

Underinsurance of Adolescents: Recommendations for Improved Coverage of Preventive, Reproductive, and Behavioral Health Care Services (joint with Committee on Adolescence), 12/08, 8/12, 5/15

COMMITTEE ON CODING AND NOMENCLATURE

Application of the Resource-Based Relative Value Scale System to Pediatrics, 5/14

COMMITTEE ON DRUGS

Codeine: Time to Say "No" (Clinical Report) (joint with Section on Anesthesiology and Pain Medicine), 9/16

Fever and Antipyretic Use in Children (Clinical Report) (joint with Section on Clinical Pharmacology and Therapeutics), 2/11, reaffirmed 7/16

Generic Prescribing, Generic Substitution, and Therapeutic Substitution, 5/87, reaffirmed 6/93, 5/96, 6/99, 5/01, 5/05, 10/08, 10/12

Guidelines for the Ethical Conduct of Studies to Evaluate Drugs in Pediatric Populations (Clinical Report) (joint with Committee on Pediatric Research), 3/10, reaffirmed 1/14

Metric Units and the Preferred Dosing of Orally Administered Liquid Medications, 3/15

Neonatal Drug Withdrawal (Clinical Report) (joint with Committee on Fetus and Newborn), 1/12, reaffirmed 2/16

Off-Label Use of Drugs in Children, 2/14

Preparing for Pediatric Emergencies: Drugs to Consider (Clinical Report), 2/08, reaffirmed 10/11, 2/16

Recognition and Management of Iatrogenically Induced Opioid Dependence and Withdrawal in Children (Clinical Report) (joint with Section on Anesthesiology and Pain Medicine), 12/13

The Transfer of Drugs and Therapeutics Into Human Breast Milk: An Update on Selected Topics (Clinical Report), 8/13

Use of Codeine- and Dextromethorphan-Containing Cough Remedies in Children, 6/97, reaffirmed 5/00, 6/03, 10/06

Uses of Drugs Not Described in the Package Insert (Off-Label Uses), 7/02, reaffirmed 10/05

COMMITTEE ON FETUS AND NEWBORN

Advanced Practice in Neonatal Nursing, 5/09, reaffirmed 1/14

Age Terminology During the Perinatal Period, 11/04, reaffirmed 10/07, 11/08, 1/09, 7/14

Antenatal Counseling Regarding Resuscitation and Intensive Care Before 25 Weeks of Gestation (Clinical Report), 8/15

The Apgar Score (joint with American College of Obstetricians and Gynecologists Committee on Obstetric Practice), 9/15

Apnea of Prematurity (Clinical Report), 12/15

Assessment and Management of Inguinal Hernia in Infants (Clinical Report) (joint with Section on Surgery), 9/12

Controversies Concerning Vitamin K and the Newborn, 7/03, reaffirmed 5/06, 5/09, 9/14

Epidemiology and Diagnosis of Health Care–Associated Infections in the NICU (Technical Report) (joint with Committee on Infectious Diseases), 3/12, reaffirmed 2/16

Guidance on Management of Asymptomatic Neonates Born to Women With Active Genital Herpes Lesions (Clinical Report) (joint with Committee on Infectious Diseases), 1/13

Hospital Discharge of the High-Risk Neonate, 11/08, reaffirmed 5/11

Hospital Stay for Healthy Term Newborn Infants, 4/15

Hypothermia and Neonatal Encephalopathy (Clinical Report), 5/14

Immersion in Water During Labor and Delivery (Clinical Report), (joint with American College of Obstetricians and Gynecologists), 3/14

"Late-Preterm" Infants: A Population at Risk (Clinical Report), 12/07, reaffirmed 5/10

Levels of Neonatal Care, 8/12, reaffirmed 9/15

Management of Neonates With Suspected or Proven Early-Onset Bacterial Sepsis (Clinical Report), 4/12, reaffirmed 2/16

Neonatal Drug Withdrawal (Clinical Report) (joint with Committee on Drugs), 1/12, reaffirmed 2/16

Newborn Screening for Biliary Atresia (Technical Report) (joint with Section on Surgery and Childhood Liver Disease Research Network), 11/15

Noninitiation or Withdrawal of Intensive Care for High-Risk Newborns, 2/07, reaffirmed 5/10, 6/15

Noninvasive Respiratory Support (Clinical Report), 12/15

Oxygen Targeting in Extremely Low Birth Weight Infants (Clinical Report), 7/16

Patent Ductus Arteriosus in Preterm Infants (Clinical Report), 12/15

Phototherapy to Prevent Severe Neonatal Hyperbilirubinemia in the Newborn Infant 35 or More Weeks of Gestation (Technical Report), 9/11, reaffirmed 7/14

Planned Home Birth, 4/13

Postdischarge Follow-up of Infants With Congenital Diaphragmatic Hernia (Clinical Report) (joint with Section on Surgery), 3/08, reaffirmed 5/11

Postnatal Corticosteroids to Prevent or Treat Bronchopulmonary Dysplasia, 9/10, reaffirmed 1/14

Postnatal Glucose Homeostasis in Late-Preterm and Term Infants (Clinical Report), 3/11, reaffirmed 6/15

Premedication for Nonemergency Endotracheal Intubation in the Neonate (Clinical Report) (joint with Section on Anesthesiology and Pain Medicine), 2/10, reaffirmed 8/13

Prenatal Substance Abuse: Short- and Long-term Effects on the Exposed Fetus (Technical Report) (joint with Committee on Substance Abuse), 2/13

Prevention and Management of Procedural Pain in the Neonate: An Update (joint with Section on Anesthesiology and Pain Medicine), 1/16

Respiratory Support in Preterm Infants at Birth, 12/13

Role of Pulse Oximetry in Examining Newborns for Congenital Heart Disease: A Scientific Statement from the AHA and AAP (joint with Section on Cardiology and Cardiac Surgery and American Heart Association Congenital Heart Defects Committee of the Council on Cardiovascular Disease in the Young, Council on Cardiovascular Nursing, and Interdisciplinary Council on Quality of Care and Outcomes Research), 8/09

Safe Sleep and Skin-to-Skin Care in the Neonatal Period for Healthy Term Newborns (Clinical Report) (joint with Task Force on Sudden Infant Death Syndrome), 8/16

Safe Transportation of Preterm and Low Birth Weight Infants at Hospital Discharge (Clinical Report) (joint with Committee on Injury, Violence, and Poison Prevention), 4/09, reaffirmed 8/13

Skin-to-Skin Care for Term and Preterm Infants in the Neonatal ICU (Clinical Report), 8/15

Standard Terminology for Fetal, Infant, and Perinatal Deaths (Clinical Report), 4/16

Strategies for Prevention of Health Care–Associated Infections in the NICU (Clinical Report) (joint with Committee on Infectious Diseases), 3/12, reaffirmed 2/16

Surfactant Replacement Therapy for Preterm and Term Neonates With Respiratory Distress (Clinical Report), 12/13

Umbilical Cord Care in the Newborn Infant (Clinical Report), 8/16

Use of Inhaled Nitric Oxide, 8/00, reaffirmed 4/03, 12/09

Use of Inhaled Nitric Oxide in Preterm Infants (Clinical Report), 12/13

COMMITTEE ON GENETICS

Clinical Genetic Evaluation of the Child With Mental Retardation or Developmental Delays (Clinical Report), 6/06, reaffirmed 5/12

Comprehensive Evaluation of the Child With Intellectual Disability or Global Developmental Delays (Clinical Report), 8/14

Congenital Adrenal Hyperplasia (Technical Report) (joint with Section on Endocrinology), 12/00, reaffirmed 10/04

Ethical and Policy Issues in Genetic Testing and Screening of Children (joint with Committee on Bioethics and American College of Medical Genetics and Genomics), 2/13

Folic Acid for the Prevention of Neural Tube Defects, 8/99, reaffirmed 11/02, 1/07, 5/12

Health Care Supervision for Children With Williams Syndrome, 5/01, reaffirmed 5/05, 1/09

Health Supervision for Children With Achondroplasia (Clinical Report), 9/05, reaffirmed 5/12

Health Supervision for Children With Down Syndrome (Clinical Report), 7/11

Health Supervision for Children With Fragile X Syndrome (Clinical Report), 4/11

Health Supervision for Children With Marfan Syndrome (Clinical Report), 9/13

Health Supervision for Children With Neurofibromatosis (Clinical Report), 3/08

Health Supervision for Children With Prader-Willi Syndrome (Clinical Report), 12/10

Health Supervision for Children With Sickle Cell Disease (joint with Section on Hematology/Oncology), 3/02, reaffirmed 1/06, 1/11, 2/16

Maternal Phenylketonuria, 8/08, reaffirmed 1/13

Molecular Genetic Testing in Pediatric Practice: A Subject Review (Clinical Report), 12/00, reaffirmed 5/07

Update of Newborn Screening and Therapy for Congenital Hypothyroidism (Clinical Report) (joint with Section on Endocrinology, American Thyroid Association, and Lawson Wilkins Pediatric Endocrine Society), 6/06, reaffirmed 12/11

COMMITTEE ON HOSPITAL CARE

Admission and Discharge Guidelines for the Pediatric Patient Requiring Intermediate Care (Clinical Report) (joint with Section on Critical Care and Society of Critical Care Medicine), 5/04, reaffirmed 2/08, 1/13

Child Life Services (joint with Child Life Council), 4/14

Facilities and Equipment for the Care of Pediatric Patients in a Community Hospital (Clinical Report), 5/03, reaffirmed 5/07, 8/13

Guidelines for Developing Admission and Discharge Policies for the Pediatric Intensive Care Unit (Clinical Report) (joint with Section on Critical Care and Society of Critical Care Medicine), 4/99, reaffirmed 5/05, 2/08, 1/13

Medical Staff Appointment and Delineation of Pediatric Privileges in Hospitals (Clinical Report) (joint with Section on Hospital Medicine), 3/12, reaffirmed 2/16

Palliative Care for Children (joint with Committee on Bioethics), 8/00, reaffirmed 6/03, 10/06, 2/12

Patient- and Family-Centered Care and the Pediatrician's Role (joint with Institute for Patient- and Family-Centered Care), 1/12

Pediatric Observation Units (Clinical Report) (joint with Committee on Pediatric Emergency Medicine), 6/12, reaffirmed 9/15

Pediatric Organ Donation and Transplantation (joint with Section on Surgery and Section on Critical Care), 3/10, reaffirmed 3/14

Pediatric Palliative Care and Hospice Care Commitments, Guidelines, and Recommendations (joint with Section on Hospice and Palliative Medicine), 10/13

Physicians' Roles in Coordinating Care of Hospitalized Children (Clinical Report) (joint with Section on Hospital Medicine), 9/10

Precertification Process, 8/00, reaffirmed 5/05, 11/08

Principles of Pediatric Patient Safety: Reducing Harm Due to Medical Care (joint with Steering Committee on Quality Improvement and Management), 5/11

Standardization of Inpatient Handoff Communication (Clinical Report), 10/16

COMMITTEE ON INFECTIOUS DISEASES

Chemical-Biological Terrorism and Its Impact on Children (joint with Committee on Environmental Health), 9/06, reaffirmed 1/11

Clostridium difficile Infection in Infants and Children, 12/12

Cochlear Implants in Children: Surgical Site Infections and Prevention and Treatment of Acute Otitis Media and Meningitis (joint with Section on Otolaryngology–Head and Neck Surgery), 7/10

Consumption of Raw or Unpasteurized Milk and Milk Products by Pregnant Women and Children (joint with Committee on Nutrition), 12/13

Countering Vaccine Hesitancy (Clinical Report) (joint with Committee on Practice and Ambulatory Medicine), 8/16

Drinking Water From Private Wells and Risks to Children (joint with Committee on Environmental Health), 5/09, reaffirmed 1/13

Drinking Water From Private Wells and Risks to Children (Technical Report) (joint with Committee on Environmental Health), 5/09, reaffirmed 1/13

Epidemiology and Diagnosis of Health Care–Associated Infections in the NICU (Technical Report) (joint with Committee on Fetus and Newborn), 3/12, reaffirmed 2/16

Eradicating Polio: How the World's Pediatricians Can Help Stop This Crippling Illness Forever (Clinical Report), 12/14

Exposure to Nontraditional Pets at Home and to Animals in Public Settings: Risks to Children (Clinical Report), 10/08, reaffirmed 12/11, 6/15

Guidance on Management of Asymptomatic Neonates Born to Women With Active Genital Herpes Lesions (Clinical Report) (joint with Committee on Fetus and Newborn), 1/13

Head Lice (Clinical Report) (joint with Council on School Health), 4/15

Immunization for *Streptococcus pneumoniae* Infections in High-Risk Children, 11/14

Immunizing Parents and Other Close Family Contacts in the Pediatric Office Setting (Technical Report) (joint with Committee on Practice and Ambulatory Medicine), 12/11

Infection Prevention and Control in Pediatric Ambulatory Settings, 9/07, reaffirmed 8/10, 1/15

Infectious Complications With the Use of Biologic Response Modifiers in Infants and Children (Clinical Report), 7/16

Influenza Immunization for All Health Care Personnel: Keep It Mandatory, 9/15

Interferon-γ Release Assays for Diagnosis of Tuberculosis Infection and Disease in Children (Technical Report), 11/14

Medical Versus Nonmedical Immunization Exemptions for Child Care and School Attendance (joint with Committee on Practice and Ambulatory Medicine, Committee on State Government Affairs, Council on School Health, and Section on Administration and Practice Management), 8/16

Nontherapeutic Use of Antimicrobial Agents in Animal Agriculture: Implications for Pediatrics (Technical Report) (joint with Council on Environmental Health), 11/15

Parental Presence During Treatment of Ebola or Other Highly Consequential Infection (Clinical Report), 8/16

Pediatric Anthrax Clinical Management (Clinical Report) (joint with Disaster Preparedness Advisory Council), 4/14

Pediatric Anthrax Clinical Management: Executive Summary (joint with Disaster Preparedness Advisory Council), 4/14

Prevention of Rotavirus Disease: Updated Guidelines for Use of Rotavirus Vaccine, 3/09

Principles of Judicious Antibiotic Prescribing for Upper Respiratory Tract Infections in Pediatrics (Clinical Report), 11/13

Probiotics and Prebiotics in Pediatrics (Clinical Report) (joint with Section on Gastroenterology, Hepatology, and Nutrition), 11/10

Promoting Food Security for All Children (joint with Council on Community Pediatrics), 10/15

Reimbursement for Foods for Special Dietary Use, 5/03, reaffirmed 1/06

The Role of the Pediatrician in Primary Prevention of Obesity (Clinical Report), 6/15

Snacks, Sweetened Beverages, Added Sugars, and Schools (joint with Council on School Health), 2/15

Sports Drinks and Energy Drinks for Children and Adolescents: Are They Appropriate? (Clinical Report) (joint with Council on Sports Medicine and Fitness), 5/11

The Use and Misuse of Fruit Juice in Pediatrics, 5/01, reaffirmed 10/06, 8/13

Use of Soy Protein-Based Formulas in Infant Feeding (Clinical Report), 5/08

COMMITTEE ON PEDIATRIC AIDS

Adolescents and HIV Infection: The Pediatrician's Role in Promoting Routine Testing, 10/11, reaffirmed 9/15

Adolescents and Human Immunodeficiency Virus Infection: The Role of the Pediatrician in Prevention and Intervention (joint with Committee on Adolescence), 1/01, reaffirmed 10/03, 1/05

Contraception for HIV-Infected Adolescents (Clinical Report), 8/16

Diagnosis of HIV-1 Infection in Children Younger Than 18 Months in the United States (Technical Report), 12/07, reaffirmed 4/10, 2/15

Evaluation and Management of the Infant Exposed to HIV-1 in the United States (Clinical Report), 12/08, reaffirmed 8/15

Evaluation and Management of the Infant Exposed to HIV-1 in the United States—Addendum, 11/12, reaffirmed 8/15

HIV Testing and Prophylaxis to Prevent Mother-to-Child Transmission in the United States, 11/08, reaffirmed 6/11, 11/14

Human Milk, Breastfeeding, and Transmission of Human Immunodeficiency Virus in the United States, 11/95, reaffirmed 11/99, 11/03, 2/08

Human Milk, Breastfeeding, and Transmission of Human Immunodeficiency Virus Type 1 in the United States (Technical Report), 11/03, reaffirmed 1/07

Identification and Care of HIV-Exposed and HIV-Infected Infants, Children, and Adolescents in Foster Care, 7/00, reaffirmed 3/03, 2/08, 6/11

Increasing Antiretroviral Drug Access for Children With HIV Infection (joint with Section on International Child Health), 4/07, reaffirmed 4/10, 4/16

Infant Feeding and Transmission of Human Immunodeficiency Virus in the United States, 1/13, reaffirmed 4/16

Postexposure Prophylaxis in Children and Adolescents for Nonoccupational Exposure to Human Immunodeficiency Virus (Clinical Report), 6/03, reaffirmed 1/07, 10/08

Psychosocial Support for Youth Living With HIV (Clinical Report), 2/14

Transitioning HIV-Infected Youth Into Adult Health Care, 6/13, reaffirmed 4/16

COMMITTEE ON PEDIATRIC EMERGENCY MEDICINE

Access to Optimal Emergency Care for Children, 1/07, reaffirmed 8/10, 7/14

Best Practices for Improving Flow and Care of Pediatric Patients in the Emergency Department (Technical Report) (joint with American College of Emergency Physicians Pediatric Emergency Medicine Committee and Emergency Nurses Association Pediatric Committee), 12/14

Consent for Emergency Medical Services for Children and Adolescents (joint with Committee on Bioethics), 7/11, reaffirmed 9/15

Death of a Child in the Emergency Department (joint with American College of Emergency Physicians and Emergency Nurses Association), 6/14

Death of a Child in the Emergency Department (Technical Report) (joint with American College of Emergency Physicians and Emergency Nurses Association), 6/14

Dispensing Medications at the Hospital Upon Discharge From an Emergency Department (Technical Report), 1/12, reaffirmed 9/15

Emergency Information Forms and Emergency Preparedness for Children With Special Health Care Needs (joint with Council on Clinical Information Technology and American College of Emergency Physicians Pediatric Emergency Medicine Committee), 3/10, reaffirmed 7/14, 10/14

Ensuring the Health of Children in Disasters (joint with Disaster Preparedness Advisory Council), 10/15

Evaluation and Management of Children and Adolescents With Acute Mental Health or Behavioral Problems. Part I: Common Clinical Challenges of Patients With Mental Health and/or Behavioral Emergencies (Clinical Report) (joint with American College of Emergency Physicians Pediatric Emergency Medicine Committee), 8/16

Evaluation and Management of Children and Adolescents With Acute Mental Health or Behavioral Problems. Part I: Common Clinical Challenges of Patients With Mental Health and/or Behavioral Emergencies—Executive Summary (Clinical Report) (joint with American College of Emergency Physicians Pediatric Emergency Medicine Committee), 8/16

Evaluation and Management of Children With Acute Mental Health or Behavioral Problems. Part II: Recognition of Clinically Challenging Mental Health Related Conditions Presenting With Medical or Uncertain Symptoms (Clinical Report) (joint with American College of Emergency Physicians Pediatric Emergency Medicine Committee), 8/16

Evaluation and Management of Children With Acute Mental Health or Behavioral Problems. Part II: Recognition of Clinically Challenging Mental Health Related Conditions Presenting With Medical or Uncertain Symptoms—Executive Summary (Clinical Report) (joint with American College of Emergency Physicians Pediatric Emergency Medicine Committee), 8/16

Guidelines for Care of Children in the Emergency Department (joint with American College of Emergency Physicians and Emergency Nurses Association), 9/09, reaffirmed 4/13, 2/16

Handoffs: Transitions of Care for Children in the Emergency Department (joint with American College of Emergency Physicians Pediatric Emergency Medicine Committee and Emergency Nurses Association Pediatric Committee), 10/16

Management of Pediatric Trauma (joint with Council on Injury, Violence, and Poison Prevention; Section on Critical Care; Section on Orthopaedics; Section on Surgery; Section on Transport Medicine; Pediatric Trauma Society; and Society of Trauma Nurses Pediatric Committee), 7/16

Overcrowding Crisis in Our Nation's Emergency Departments: Is Our Safety Net Unraveling?, 9/04, reaffirmed 5/07, 6/11, 7/16

Patient- and Family-Centered Care and the Role of the Emergency Physician Providing Care to a Child in the Emergency Department (joint with American College of Emergency Physicians), 11/06, reaffirmed 6/09, 10/11, 9/15

Patient- and Family-Centered Care of Children in the Emergency Department (Technical Report) (joint with American College of Emergency Physicians Pediatric Emergency Medicine Committee and Emergency Nurses Association Pediatric Committee), 12/14

Patient Safety in the Pediatric Emergency Care Setting, 12/07, reaffirmed 6/11, 7/14

Pediatric and Adolescent Mental Health Emergencies in the Emergency Medical Services System (Technical Report), 4/11, 7/14

Pediatric Care Recommendations for Freestanding Urgent Care Facilities, 4/14

Pediatric Mental Health Emergencies in the Emergency Medical Services System (joint with American College of Emergency Physicians), 10/06, reaffirmed 6/09, 4/13

Pediatric Observation Units (Clinical Report) (joint with Committee on Hospital Care), 6/12, reaffirmed 9/15

The Pediatrician and Disaster Preparedness (joint with Committee on Medical Liability and Task Force on Terrorism), 2/06, reaffirmed 6/09, 9/13

Point-of-Care Ultrasonography by Pediatric Emergency Medicine Physicians (joint with Society for Academic Emergency Medicine Academy of Emergency Ultrasound, American College of Emergency Physicians Pediatric Emergency Medicine Committee, and World Interactive Network Focused on Critical Ultrasound), 3/15

Point-of-Care Ultrasonography by Pediatric Emergency Medicine Physicians (Technical Report) (joint with Society for Academic Emergency Medicine Academy of Emergency Ultrasound, American College of Emergency Physicians Pediatric Emergency Medicine Committee, and World Interactive Network Focused on Critical Ultrasound), 3/15

Preparation for Emergencies in the Offices of Pediatricians and Pediatric Primary Care Providers, 7/07, reaffirmed 6/11

Relief of Pain and Anxiety in Pediatric Patients in Emergency Medical Systems (Clinical Report) (joint with Section on Anesthesiology and Pain Medicine), 10/12, reaffirmed 9/15

Role of Pediatricians in Advocating Life Support Training Courses for Parents and the Public, 12/04, reaffirmed 5/07, 8/10, 8/13, 7/16

Role of Pediatricians in Advocating Life Support Training Courses for Parents and the Public (Technical Report), 12/04, reaffirmed 5/07, 8/10, 1/14

The Role of the Pediatrician in Rural Emergency Medical Services for Children, 10/12, reaffirmed 9/15

Ventricular Fibrillation and the Use of Automated External Defibrillators on Children (joint with Section on Cardiology and Cardiac Surgery), 11/07, reaffirmed 6/11, 7/14

Withholding or Termination of Resuscitation in Pediatric Out-of-Hospital Traumatic Cardiopulmonary Arrest (joint with American College of Surgeons and National Association of EMS Physicians), 3/14

COMMITTEE ON PEDIATRIC RESEARCH

Guidelines for the Ethical Conduct of Studies to Evaluate Drugs in Pediatric Populations (Clinical Report) (joint with Committee on Drugs), 3/10, reaffirmed 1/14

Human Embryonic Stem Cell (hESC) and Human Embryo Research (joint with Committee on Bioethics), 10/12

Promoting Education, Mentorship, and Support for Pediatric Research, 4/14

Race, Ethnicity, and Socioeconomic Status in Research on Child Health, 12/14

Racial and Ethnic Disparities in the Health and Health Care of Children (Technical Report), 3/10, reaffirmed 5/13

COMMITTEE ON PEDIATRIC WORKFORCE

Definition of a Pediatrician, 3/15

Enhancing Pediatric Workforce Diversity and Providing Culturally Effective Pediatric Care: Implications for Practice, Education, and Policy Making, 9/13, reaffirmed 10/15

Financing Graduate Medical Education to Meet the Needs of Children and the Future Pediatrician Workforce, 3/16

Nondiscrimination in Pediatric Health Care, 10/07, reaffirmed 6/11, 1/15

Pediatric Primary Health Care, 1/11, reaffirmed 10/13

The Pediatrician Workforce: Current Status and Future Prospects (Technical Report), 7/05

Pediatrician Workforce Policy Statement, 7/13

Prevention of Sexual Harassment in the Workplace and Educational Settings, 10/06, reaffirmed 5/09, 1/12, 10/14

Scope of Practice Issues in the Delivery of Pediatric Health Care, 5/13, reaffirmed 10/15

The Use of Telemedicine to Address Access and Physician Workforce Shortages, 6/15

COMMITTEE ON PRACTICE AND AMBULATORY MEDICINE

2016 Recommendations for Preventive Pediatric Health Care (joint with Bright Futures Periodicity Schedule Workgroup), 12/15

AAP Principles Concerning Retail-Based Clinics, 2/14

Countering Vaccine Hesitancy (Clinical Report) (joint with Committee on Infectious Diseases), 8/16

Eye Examination in Infants, Children, and Young Adults by Pediatricians (joint with Section on Ophthalmology, American Association of Certified Orthoptists, American Association for Pediatric Ophthalmology and Strabismus, and American Academy of Ophthalmology), 4/03, reaffirmed 5/07

Hearing Assessment in Infants and Children: Recommendations Beyond Neonatal Screening (Clinical Report) (joint with Section on Otolaryngology–Head and Neck Surgery), 9/09

Immunization Information Systems, 9/06, reaffirmed 10/11

Immunizing Parents and Other Close Family Contacts in the Pediatric Office Setting (Technical Report) (joint with Committee on Infectious Diseases), 12/11

Increasing Immunization Coverage (joint with Council on Community Pediatrics), 5/10

Instrument-Based Pediatric Vision Screening Policy Statement (joint with Section on Ophthalmology, American Academy of Ophthalmology, American Association for Pediatric Ophthalmology and Strabismus, and American Association of Certified Orthoptists), 10/12

Medical Versus Nonmedical Immunization Exemptions for Child Care and School Attendance (joint with Committee on Infectious Diseases, Committee on State Government Affairs, Council on School Health, and Section on Administration and Practice Management), 8/16

Physician Health and Wellness (Clinical Report) (joint with Section on Integrative Medicine), 9/14

Prevention and Management of Positional Skull Deformities in Infants (Clinical Report) (joint with Section on Neurological Surgery), 11/11

Principles for the Development and Use of Quality Measures (joint with Steering Committee on Quality Improvement and Management), 2/08

Procedures for the Evaluation of the Visual System by Pediatricians (Clinical Report) (joint with Section on Ophthalmology, American Association of Certified Orthoptists, American Association for Pediatric Ophthalmology and Strabismus, and American Academy of Ophthalmology), 12/15

Use of Chaperones During the Physical Examination of the Pediatric Patient, 4/11

Visual System Assessment in Infants, Children, and Young Adults by Pediatricians (joint with Section on Ophthalmology, American Association of Certified Orthoptists, American Association for Pediatric Ophthalmology and Strabismus, and American Academy of Ophthalmology), 12/15

COMMITTEE ON PSYCHOSOCIAL ASPECTS OF CHILD AND FAMILY HEALTH

Addressing Early Childhood Emotional and Behavioral Problems (joint with Council on Early Childhood and Section on Developmental and Behavioral Pediatrics), 11/16

Addressing Early Childhood Emotional and Behavioral Problems (Technical Report) (joint with Council on Early Childhood and Section on Developmental and Behavioral Pediatrics), 11/16

Coparent or Second-Parent Adoption by Same-Sex Parents, 2/02, reaffirmed 5/09

Coparent or Second-Parent Adoption by Same-Sex Parents (Technical Report), 2/02, reaffirmed 5/09

Early Childhood Adversity, Toxic Stress, and the Role of the Pediatrician: Translating Developmental Science Into Lifelong Health (joint with Committee on Early Childhood, Adoption, and Dependent Care and Section on Developmental and Behavioral Pediatrics), 12/11, reaffirmed 7/16

Fathers' Roles in the Care and Development of Their Children: The Role of Pediatricians (Clinical Report), 6/16

The Future of Pediatrics: Mental Health Competencies for Pediatric Primary Care (joint with Task Force on Mental Health), 6/09, reaffirmed 8/13

Guidance for Effective Discipline, 4/98, reaffirmed 3/01, 1/05, 5/12, 4/14

Health and Mental Health Needs of Children in US Military Families (Clinical Report) (joint with Section on Uniformed Services), 5/13

Helping Children and Families Deal With Divorce and Separation (Clinical Report) (joint with Section on Developmental and Behavioral Pediatrics), 11/16

The Importance of Play in Promoting Healthy Child Development and Maintaining Strong Parent-Child Bond: Focus on Children in Poverty (Clinical Report) (joint with Council on Communications and Media), 12/11, reaffirmed 9/15

The Importance of Play in Promoting Healthy Child Development and Maintaining Strong Parent-Child Bonds (Clinical Report) (joint with Committee on Communications), 1/07

Incorporating Recognition and Management of Perinatal and Postpartum Depression Into Pediatric Practice (Clinical Report), 10/10, reaffirmed 12/14

The Lifelong Effects of Early Childhood Adversity and Toxic Stress (Technical Report) (joint with Committee on Early Childhood, Adoption, and Dependent Care and Section on Developmental and Behavioral Pediatrics), 12/11, reaffirmed 7/16

Mediators and Adverse Effects of Child Poverty in the United States (Technical Report) (joint with Council on Community Pediatrics), 3/16

The New Morbidity Revisited: A Renewed Commitment to the Psychosocial Aspects of Pediatric Care, 11/01

The Pediatrician and Childhood Bereavement, 2/00, reaffirmed 1/04, 3/13

The Pediatrician's Role in the Prevention of Missing Children (Clinical Report), 10/04, reaffirmed 1/15

The Prenatal Visit (Clinical Report), 9/09, reaffirmed 5/14

Promoting Optimal Development: Screening for Behavioral and Emotional Problems (Clinical Report) (joint with Section on Developmental and Behavioral Pediatrics, Council on Early Childhood, and Society for Developmental and Behavioral Pediatrics), 1/15

Promoting the Well-Being of Children Whose Parents Are Gay or Lesbian, 3/13

Promoting the Well-Being of Children Whose Parents Are Gay or Lesbian (Technical Report), 3/13

Providing Psychosocial Support to Children and Families in the Aftermath of Disasters and Crises (Clinical Report) (joint with Disaster Preparedness Advisory Council), 9/15

Psychosocial Implications of Disaster or Terrorism on Children: A Guide for the Pediatrician (Clinical Report) (joint with Task Force on Terrorism), 9/05, reaffirmed 11/14

Psychosocial Risks of Chronic Health Conditions in Childhood and Adolescence (joint with Committee on Children With Disabilities), 12/93, reaffirmed 10/96

Sexuality Education for Children and Adolescents (Clinical Report) (joint with Committee on Adolescence), 7/16

Supporting the Family After the Death of a Child (Clinical Report), 11/12

Supporting the Grieving Child and Family (Clinical Report) (joint with Disaster Preparedness Advisory Council), 8/16

COMMITTEE ON STATE GOVERNMENT AFFAIRS

Medical Versus Nonmedical Immunization Exemptions for Child Care and School Attendance (joint with Committee on Practice and Ambulatory Medicine, Committee on Infectious Diseases, Council on School Health, and Section on Administration and Practice Management), 8/16

COMMITTEE ON SUBSTANCE USE AND PREVENTION (FORMERLY COMMITTEE ON SUBSTANCE ABUSE)

Adolescent Drug Testing Policies in Schools, 3/15

Adolescent Drug Testing Policies in Schools (Technical Report), 3/15

Alcohol Use by Youth and Adolescents: A Pediatric Concern, 4/10, reaffirmed 12/14

Attention-Deficit/Hyperactivity Disorder and Substance Abuse (Clinical Report), 6/14

Binge Drinking (Clinical Report), 8/15

Families Affected by Parental Substance Use (Clinical Report), 7/16

Fetal Alcohol Spectrum Disorders (Clinical Report), 10/15

The Impact of Marijuana Policies on Youth: Clinical, Research, and Legal Update (joint with Committee on Adolescence), 1/15

The Impact of Marijuana Policies on Youth: Clinical, Research, and Legal Update (Technical Report) (joint with Committee on Adolescence), 1/15

Improving Substance Abuse Prevention, Assessment, and Treatment Financing for Children and Adolescents (joint with Committee on Child Health Financing), 10/01

Indications for Management and Referral of Patients Involved in Substance Abuse, 7/00

Inhalant Abuse (Clinical Report) (joint with Committee on Native American Child Health), 5/07

Legalization of Marijuana: Potential Impact on Youth (joint with Committee on Adolescence), 6/04

Legalization of Marijuana: Potential Impact on Youth (Technical Report) (joint with Committee on Adolescence), 6/04

Marijuana: A Continuing Concern for Pediatricians, 10/99, reaffirmed 4/03

Medication-Assisted Treatment of Adolescents With Opioid Use Disorders, 8/16

Prenatal Substance Abuse: Short- and Long-term Effects on the Exposed Fetus (Technical Report) (joint with Committee on Fetus and Newborn), 2/13

The Role of Schools in Combating Illicit Substance Abuse (joint with Council on School Health), 12/07

Substance Use Screening, Brief Intervention, and Referral to Treatment, 6/16

Substance Use Screening, Brief Intervention, and Referral to Treatment (Clinical Report), 6/16

Testing for Drugs of Abuse in Children and Adolescents (Clinical Report), 5/14

Tobacco, Alcohol, and Other Drugs: The Role of the Pediatrician in Prevention, Identification, and Management of Substance Abuse (Clinical Report), 3/05, reaffirmed 3/13

Tobacco as a Substance of Abuse (Technical Report), 10/09, reaffirmed 12/14

Tobacco Use: A Pediatric Disease (joint with Committee on Environmental Health, Committee on Adolescence, and Committee on Native American Child Health), 10/09, reaffirmed 5/13

COUNCIL ON CHILDREN WITH DISABILITIES (FORMERLY COMMITTEE ON CHILDREN WITH DISABILITIES AND SECTION ON CHILDREN WITH DISABILITIES)

Auditory Integration Training and Facilitated Communication for Autism, 8/98, reaffirmed 5/02, 1/06, 12/09

Care Coordination in the Medical Home: Integrating Health and Related Systems of Care for Children With Special Health Care Needs, 11/05

Counseling Families Who Choose Complementary and Alternative Medicine for Their Child With Chronic Illness or Disability, 3/01, reaffirmed 1/05, 5/10

Early Intervention, IDEA Part C Services, and the Medical Home: Collaboration for Best Practice and Best Outcomes (Clinical Report), 9/13

Guidelines for Home Care of Infants, Children, and Adolescents With Chronic Disease, 7/95, reaffirmed 4/00, 1/06

Home Care of Children and Youth With Complex Health Care Needs and Technology Dependencies (Clinical Report), 4/12

Identification and Evaluation of Children With Autism Spectrum Disorders (Clinical Report), 11/07, reaffirmed 9/10, 8/14

Identifying Infants and Young Children With Developmental Disorders in the Medical Home: An Algorithm for Developmental Surveillance and Screening (joint with Section on Developmental and Behavioral Pediatrics, Bright Futures Steering Committee, and Medical Home Initiatives for Children With Special Needs Project Advisory Committee), 7/06, reaffirmed 12/09, 8/14

The Individuals With Disabilities Education Act (IDEA) for Children With Special Educational Needs (Clinical Report) (joint with Council on School Health), 11/15

Learning Disabilities, Dyslexia, and Vision (joint with Section on Ophthalmology, American Academy of Ophthalmology, American Association for Pediatric Ophthalmology and Strabismus, and American Association of Certified Orthoptists), 7/09, reaffirmed 7/14

Learning Disabilities, Dyslexia, and Vision (Technical Report) (joint with Section on Ophthalmology, American Academy of Ophthalmology, American Association for Pediatric Ophthalmology and Strabismus, and American Association of Certified Orthoptists), 3/11

Maltreatment of Children With Disabilities (Clinical Report) (joint with Committee on Child Abuse and Neglect), 5/07, reaffirmed 1/11, 4/16

Management of Children With Autism Spectrum Disorders (Clinical Report), 11/07, reaffirmed 9/10, 8/14

Nonoral Feeding for Children and Youth With Developmental or Acquired Disabilities (Clinical Report), 11/14

Oral Health Care for Children With Developmental Disabilities (Clinical Report) (joint with Section on Oral Health), 2/13

Out-of-Home Placement for Children and Adolescents With Disabilities (Clinical Report), 9/14

Out-of-Home Placement for Children and Adolescents With Disabilities—Addendum: Care Options for Children and Adolescents With Disabilities and Medical Complexity (Clinical Report), 11/16

Parent-Provider-Community Partnerships: Optimizing Outcomes for Children With Disabilities (Clinical Report), 9/11

Patient- and Family-Centered Care Coordination: A Framework for Integrating Care for Children and Youth Across Multiple Systems (joint with Medical Home Implementation Project Advisory Committee), 4/14

The Pediatrician's Role in Development and Implementation of an Individual Education Plan (IEP) and/or an Individual Family Service Plan (IFSP), 7/99, reaffirmed 11/02, 1/06

Prescribing Assistive-Technology Systems: Focus on Children With Impaired Communication (Clinical Report), 6/08, reaffirmed 1/12

Prescribing Therapy Services for Children With Motor Disabilities (Clinical Report), 6/04, reaffirmed 5/07, 5/11

Promoting the Participation of Children With Disabilities in Sports, Recreation, and Physical Activities (Clinical Report), 5/08, reaffirmed 1/12

Providing a Primary Care Medical Home for Children and Youth With Cerebral Palsy (Clinical Report), 10/11, reaffirmed 11/14

Providing a Primary Care Medical Home for Children and Youth With Spina Bifida (Clinical Report), 11/11, reaffirmed 2/15

Provision of Educationally Related Services for Children and Adolescents With Chronic Diseases and Disabling Conditions, 6/07, reaffirmed 11/14

Psychosocial Risks of Chronic Health Conditions in Childhood and Adolescence (joint with Committee on Psychosocial Aspects of Child and Family Health), 12/93, reaffirmed 10/96

Recognition and Management of Medical Complexity (Clinical Report), 11/16

Role of the Medical Home in Family-Centered Early Intervention Services, 11/07

Sensory Integration Therapies for Children With Developmental and Behavioral Disorders (joint with Section on Complementary and Integrative Medicine), 5/12

Sexuality of Children and Adolescents With Developmental Disabilities (Clinical Report), 7/06, reaffirmed 12/09, 7/13

Supplemental Security Income (SSI) for Children and Youth With Disabilities, 11/09, reaffirmed 2/15

The Treatment of Neurologically Impaired Children Using Patterning, 11/99, reaffirmed 11/02, 1/06, 8/10, 4/14

COUNCIL ON CLINICAL INFORMATION TECHNOLOGY (FORMERLY STEERING COMMITTEE ON CLINICAL INFORMATION TECHNOLOGY, SECTION ON COMPUTERS AND OTHER TECHNOLOGIES, AND TASK FORCE ON MEDICAL INFORMATICS)

Electronic Prescribing in Pediatrics: Toward Safer and More Effective Medication Management, 3/13

Electronic Prescribing in Pediatrics: Toward Safer and More Effective Medication Management (Technical Report), 3/13

Electronic Prescribing Systems in Pediatrics: The Rationale and Functionality Requirements, 6/07

Electronic Prescribing Systems in Pediatrics: The Rationale and Functionality Requirements (Technical Report), 6/07

Emergency Information Forms and Emergency Preparedness for Children With Special Health Care Needs (joint with Committee on Pediatric Emergency Medicine and American College of Emergency Physicians Pediatric Emergency Medicine Committee), 3/10, reaffirmed 7/14, 10/14

Health Information Technology and the Medical Home, 4/11, reaffirmed 7/15

Pediatric Aspects of Inpatient Health Information Technology Systems (Technical Report), 2/15

Special Requirements of Electronic Health Record Systems in Pediatrics (Clinical Report), 3/07, reaffirmed 5/12, 5/16

Standards for Health Information Technology to Ensure Adolescent Privacy (joint with Committee on Adolescence), 10/12

COUNCIL ON COMMUNICATIONS AND MEDIA (FORMERLY COMMITTEE ON COMMUNICATIONS AND COMMITTEE ON PUBLIC EDUCATION)

Children, Adolescents, and Advertising, 12/06, reaffirmed 3/10

Children, Adolescents, and Television, 2/01

Children, Adolescents, and the Media, 10/13

Children, Adolescents, Obesity, and the Media, 7/11

Children, Adolescents, Substance Abuse, and the Media, 9/10

Children and Adolescents and Digital Media (Technical Report), 10/16

Impact of Music, Music Lyrics, and Music Videos on Children and Youth, 10/09

The Impact of Social Media on Children, Adolescents, and Families (Clinical Report), 3/11

The Importance of Play in Promoting Healthy Child Development and Maintaining Strong Parent-Child Bond: Focus on Children in Poverty (Clinical Report) (joint with Committee on Psychosocial Aspects of Child and Family Health), 12/11, reaffirmed 9/15

The Importance of Play in Promoting Healthy Child Development and Maintaining Strong Parent-Child Bonds (Clinical Report) (joint with Committee on Psychosocial Aspects of Child and Family Health), 1/07

Media and Young Minds, 10/16

Media Education, 9/10

Media Use by Children Younger Than 2 Years, 10/11

Media Use in School-Aged Children and Adolescents, 10/16

Media Violence, 10/09

Sexuality, Contraception, and the Media, 8/10

Virtual Violence, 7/16

COUNCIL ON COMMUNITY PEDIATRICS (FORMERLY COMMITTEE ON COMMUNITY HEALTH SERVICES)

Child Fatality Review (joint with Committee on Child Abuse and Neglect and Committee on Injury, Violence, and Poison Prevention), 8/10, reaffirmed 5/14

Community Pediatrics: Navigating the Intersection of Medicine, Public Health, and Social Determinants of Children's Health, 2/13

Ethical Considerations in Research With Socially Identifiable Populations (joint with Committee on Native American Child Health), 1/04, reaffirmed 10/07, 1/13

Health Equity and Children's Rights (joint with Committee on Native American Child Health), 3/10, reaffirmed 10/13

Increasing Immunization Coverage (joint with Committee on Practice and Ambulatory Medicine), 5/10

Mediators and Adverse Effects of Child Poverty in the United States (Technical Report) (joint with Committee on Psychosocial Aspects of Child and Family Health), 3/16

The Pediatrician's Role in Community Pediatrics, 4/05, reaffirmed 1/10

Poverty and Child Health in the United States, 3/16

Prevention of Agricultural Injuries Among Children and Adolescents (joint with Committee on Injury and Poison Prevention), 10/01, reaffirmed 1/07, 11/11

Promoting Food Security for All Children (joint with Committee on Nutrition), 10/15

Providing Care for Children and Adolescents Facing Homelessness and Housing Insecurity, 5/13

Providing Care for Immigrant, Migrant, and Border Children, 5/13

The Role of Preschool Home-Visiting Programs in Improving Children's Developmental and Health Outcomes, 1/09

COUNCIL ON EARLY CHILDHOOD (FORMERLY COMMITTEE ON EARLY CHILDHOOD, ADOPTION, AND DEPENDENT CARE AND COMMITTEE ON EARLY CHILDHOOD)

Addressing Early Childhood Emotional and Behavioral Problems (joint with Committee on Psychosocial Aspects of Child and Family Health and Section on Developmental and Behavioral Pediatrics), 11/16

Addressing Early Childhood Emotional and Behavioral Problems (Technical Report) (joint with Committee on Psychosocial Aspects of Child and Family Health and Section on Developmental and Behavioral Pediatrics), 11/16

Care of Adolescent Parents and Their Children (Clinical Report) (joint with Committee on Adolescence), 11/12, reaffirmed 7/16

Comprehensive Health Evaluation of the Newly Adopted Child (Clinical Report), 12/11, reaffirmed 9/15

Early Childhood Adversity, Toxic Stress, and the Role of the Pediatrician: Translating Developmental Science Into Lifelong Health (joint with Committee on Psychosocial Aspects of Child and Family Health and Section on Developmental and Behavioral Pediatrics), 12/11, reaffirmed 7/16

Families and Adoption: The Pediatrician's Role in Supporting Communication (Clinical Report), 12/03

Health Care Issues for Children and Adolescents in Foster Care and Kinship Care (joint with Council on Foster Care, Adoption, and Kinship Care and Committee on Adolescence), 9/15

Health Care Issues for Children and Adolescents in Foster Care and Kinship Care (Technical Report) (joint with Council on Foster Care, Adoption, and Kinship Care and Committee on Adolescence), 9/15

Health Care of Youth Aging Out of Foster Care (joint with Council on Foster Care, Adoption, and Kinship Care), 11/12

The Inappropriate Use of School "Readiness" Tests (joint with Committee on School Health), 3/95, reaffirmed 4/98, 1/04, 4/10

The Lifelong Effects of Early Childhood Adversity and Toxic Stress (Technical Report) (joint with Committee on Psychosocial Aspects of Child and Family Health and Section on Developmental and Behavioral Pediatrics), 12/11, reaffirmed 7/16

Literacy Promotion: An Essential Component of Primary Care Pediatric Practice, 7/14

Parental Leave for Residents and Pediatric Training Programs (joint with Section on Medical Students, Residents, and Fellowship Trainees), 1/13

The Pediatrician's Role in Family Support and Family Support Programs, 11/11

The Pediatrician's Role in Optimizing School Readiness (joint with Council on School Health), 8/16

The Pediatrician's Role in Supporting Adoptive Families (Clinical Report) (joint with Council on Foster Care, Adoption, and Kinship Care), 9/12

Promoting Optimal Development: Screening for Behavioral and Emotional Problems (Clinical Report) (joint with Section on Developmental and Behavioral Pediatrics, Committee on Psychosocial Aspects of Child and Family Health, and Society for Developmental and Behavioral Pediatrics), 1/15

Quality Early Education and Child Care From Birth to Kindergarten, 1/05, reaffirmed 12/09

School Readiness (Technical Report) (joint with Council on School Health), 4/08, reaffirmed 9/13

Selecting Appropriate Toys for Young Children: The Pediatrician's Role (Clinical Report), 4/03, reaffirmed 10/06, 5/11

COUNCIL ON ENVIRONMENTAL HEALTH (FORMERLY COMMITTEE ON ENVIRONMENTAL HEALTH)

Ambient Air Pollution: Health Hazards to Children, 12/04, reaffirmed 4/09

The Built Environment: Designing Communities to Promote Physical Activity in Children, 5/09, reaffirmed 1/13

Chemical-Biological Terrorism and Its Impact on Children (joint with Committee on Infectious Diseases), 9/06, reaffirmed 1/11

Chemical-Management Policy: Prioritizing Children's Health, 4/11

Drinking Water From Private Wells and Risks to Children (joint with Committee on Infectious Diseases), 5/09, reaffirmed 1/13

Drinking Water From Private Wells and Risks to Children (Technical Report) (joint with Committee on Infectious Diseases), 5/09, reaffirmed 1/13

Global Climate Change and Children's Health, 10/15

Global Climate Change and Children's Health (Technical Report), 10/15

Indoor Environmental Control Practices and Asthma Management (Clinical Report) (joint with Section on Allergy and Immunology), 10/16

Infant Methemoglobinemia: The Role of Dietary Nitrate in Food and Water (Clinical Report) (joint with Committee on Nutrition), 9/05, reaffirmed 4/09

Iodine Deficiency, Pollutant Chemicals, and the Thyroid: New Information on an Old Problem, 5/14

Nontherapeutic Use of Antimicrobial Agents in Animal Agriculture: Implications for Pediatrics (Technical Report) (joint with Committee on Infectious Diseases), 11/15

Organic Foods: Health and Environmental Advantages and Disadvantages (Clinical Report) (joint with Committee on Nutrition), 10/12

Pesticide Exposure in Children, 11/12

Pesticide Exposure in Children (Technical Report), 11/12

Prevention of Childhood Lead Toxicity, 6/16

Radiation Disasters and Children, 6/03, reaffirmed 1/07

Secondhand and Prenatal Tobacco Smoke Exposure (Technical Report) (joint with Committee on Native American Child Health and Committee on Adolescence), 10/09, reaffirmed 5/14

Spectrum of Noninfectious Health Effects From Molds, 12/06, reaffirmed 1/11

Spectrum of Noninfectious Health Effects From Molds (Technical Report), 12/06, reaffirmed 1/11

Tobacco Use: A Pediatric Disease (joint with Committee on Substance Abuse, Committee on Adolescence, and Committee on Native American Child Health), 10/09, reaffirmed 5/13

Ultraviolet Radiation: A Hazard to Children and Adolescents (joint with Section on Dermatology), 2/11

Ultraviolet Radiation: A Hazard to Children and Adolescents (Technical Report) (joint with Section on Dermatology), 3/11

COUNCIL ON FOSTER CARE, ADOPTION, AND KINSHIP CARE (FORMERLY SECTION ON ADOPTION AND FOSTER CARE, TASK FORCE ON FOSTER CARE, AND COMMITTEE ON EARLY CHILDHOOD, ADOPTION, AND DEPENDENT CARE)

Health Care Issues for Children and Adolescents in Foster Care and Kinship Care (joint with Committee on Adolescence and Council on Early Childhood), 9/15

Health Care Issues for Children and Adolescents in Foster Care and Kinship Care (Technical Report) (joint with Committee on Adolescence and Council on Early Childhood), 9/15

Health Care of Youth Aging Out of Foster Care (joint with Committee on Early Childhood), 11/12

The Pediatrician's Role in Supporting Adoptive Families (Clinical Report) (joint with Committee on Early Childhood), 9/12

Understanding the Behavioral and Emotional Consequences of Child Abuse (Clinical Report) (joint with Committee on Child Abuse and Neglect, American Academy of Child and Adolescent Psychiatry, and National Center for Child Traumatic Stress), 9/08, reaffirmed 8/12

COUNCIL ON INJURY, VIOLENCE, AND POISON PREVENTION (FORMERLY COMMITTEE ON INJURY, VIOLENCE, AND POISON PREVENTION)

All-Terrain Vehicle Injury Prevention: Two-, Three-, and Four-Wheeled Unlicensed Motor Vehicles, 6/00, reaffirmed 5/04, 1/07, 5/13

Bicycle Helmets, 10/01, reaffirmed 1/05, 2/08, 11/11

Child Fatality Review (joint with Committee on Child Abuse and Neglect and Council on Community Pediatrics), 8/10, reaffirmed 5/14

Child Passenger Safety, 3/11, reaffirmed 11/14

Child Passenger Safety (Technical Report), 3/11, reaffirmed 11/14

Children in Pickup Trucks, 10/00, reaffirmed 5/04, 1/07

Falls From Heights: Windows, Roofs, and Balconies, 5/01, reaffirmed 10/04, 5/07, 6/10

Firearm-Related Injuries Affecting the Pediatric Population, 10/12

Fireworks-Related Injuries to Children, 7/01, reaffirmed 1/05, 2/08, 10/11, 11/14

The Hospital Record of the Injured Child and the Need for External Cause-of-Injury Codes, 2/99, reaffirmed 5/02, 5/05, 10/08, 10/13

Injuries Associated With Infant Walkers, 9/01, reaffirmed 1/05, 2/08, 10/11, 11/14

Injury Risk of Nonpowder Guns (Technical Report), 11/04, reaffirmed 2/08, 10/11

In-line Skating Injuries in Children and Adolescents (joint with Committee on Sports Medicine and Fitness), 4/98, reaffirmed 1/02, 1/06, 1/09, 11/11

Intimate Partner Violence: The Role of the Pediatrician (Clinical Report) (joint with Committee on Child Abuse and Neglect), 4/10, reaffirmed 1/14

Lawn Mower-Related Injuries to Children, 6/01, reaffirmed 10/04, 5/07, 6/10

Lawn Mower-Related Injuries to Children (Technical Report), 6/01, reaffirmed 10/04, 5/07, 6/10

Management of Pediatric Trauma (joint with Committee on Pediatric Emergency Medicine, Section on Critical Care, Section on Orthopaedics, Section on Surgery, Section on Transport Medicine, Pediatric Trauma Society, and Society of Trauma Nurses Pediatric Committee), 7/16

Office-Based Counseling for Unintentional Injury Prevention (Clinical Report), 1/07

Pedestrian Safety, 7/09, reaffirmed 8/13

Personal Watercraft Use by Children and Adolescents, 2/00, reaffirmed 5/04, 1/07, 6/10

Prevention of Agricultural Injuries Among Children and Adolescents (joint with Committee on Community Health Services), 10/01, reaffirmed 1/07, 11/11

Prevention of Choking Among Children, 2/10

Prevention of Drowning, 5/10

Prevention of Drowning (Technical Report), 5/10

The Prevention of Unintentional Injury Among American Indian and Alaska Native Children: A Subject Review (Clinical Report) (joint with Committee on Native American Child Health), 12/99, reaffirmed 12/02, 1/06, 1/09

Reducing the Number of Deaths and Injuries From Residential Fires, 6/00

Restraint Use on Aircraft, 11/01, reaffirmed 5/05, 10/08

Role of the Pediatrician in Youth Violence Prevention, 6/09

Safe Transportation of Newborns at Hospital Discharge, 10/99, reaffirmed 1/03, 1/06, 10/08

Safe Transportation of Preterm and Low Birth Weight Infants at Hospital Discharge (Clinical Report) (joint with Committee on Fetus and Newborn), 4/09, reaffirmed 8/13

School Bus Transportation of Children With Special Health Care Needs, 8/01, reaffirmed 1/05, 2/08, 5/13

School Transportation Safety (joint with Council on School Health), 7/07, reaffirmed 10/11

Shopping Cart–Related Injuries to Children, 8/06, reaffirmed 4/09, 8/13

Shopping Cart–Related Injuries to Children (Technical Report), 8/06, reaffirmed 4/09, 8/13

Skateboard and Scooter Injuries, 3/02, reaffirmed 5/05, 10/08, 10/13

Snowmobiling Hazards, 11/00, reaffirmed 5/04, 1/07, 6/10

Swimming Programs for Infants and Toddlers (joint with Committee on Sports Medicine and Fitness), 4/00, reaffirmed 5/04

The Teen Driver (joint with Committee on Adolescence), 12/06, reaffirmed 6/10, 7/16

Transporting Children With Special Health Care Needs, 10/99, reaffirmed 1/03, 1/06, 3/13

COUNCIL ON QUALITY IMPROVEMENT AND PATIENT SAFETY

Disclosure of Adverse Events in Pediatrics (joint with Committee on Medical Liability and Risk Management), 11/16

COUNCIL ON SCHOOL HEALTH (FORMERLY COMMITTEE ON SCHOOL HEALTH AND SECTION ON SCHOOL HEALTH)

Climatic Heat Stress and Exercising Children and Adolescents (joint with Council on Sports Medicine and Fitness), 8/11, reaffirmed 2/15

Corporal Punishment in Schools, 8/00, reaffirmed 6/03, 5/06, 2/12

Creating Healthy Camp Experiences, 3/11

The Crucial Role of Recess in School, 12/12, reaffirmed 8/16

Disaster Planning for Schools, 10/08, reaffirmed 9/11

Guidance for the Administration of Medication in School, 9/09, reaffirmed 2/13

Head Lice (Clinical Report) (joint with Committee on Infectious Diseases), 4/15

Home, Hospital, and Other Non–School-based Instruction for Children and Adolescents Who Are Medically Unable to Attend School, 11/00, reaffirmed 6/03, 5/06

Honoring Do-Not-Attempt-Resuscitation Requests in Schools (joint with Committee on Bioethics), 4/10, reaffirmed 7/13, 8/16

The Inappropriate Use of School "Readiness" Tests (joint with Committee on Early Childhood, Adoption, and Dependent Care), 3/95, reaffirmed 4/98, 1/04, 4/10

The Individuals With Disabilities Education Act (IDEA) for Children With Special Educational Needs (Clinical Report) (joint with Council on Children With Disabilities), 11/15

Medical Emergencies Occurring at School, 10/08, reaffirmed 9/11

Medical Versus Nonmedical Immunization Exemptions for Child Care and School Attendance (joint with Committee on Practice and Ambulatory Medicine, Committee on Infectious Diseases, Committee on State Government Affairs, and Section on Administration and Practice Management), 8/16

Organized Sports for Children and Preadolescents (joint with Committee on Sports Medicine and Fitness), 6/01, reaffirmed 1/05, 6/11

Out-of-School Suspension and Expulsion, 2/13

The Pediatrician's Role in Optimizing School Readiness (joint with Council on Early Childhood), 8/16

Preventing and Treating Homesickness (Clinical Report), 1/07, reaffirmed 5/12

Rescue Medicine for Epilepsy in Education Settings (Clinical Report) (joint with Section on Neurology), 12/15

Returning to Learning Following a Concussion (Clinical Report) (joint with Council on Sports Medicine and Fitness), 10/13

The Role of Schools in Combating Illicit Substance Abuse (joint with Committee on Substance Abuse), 12/07

Role of the School Nurse in Providing School Health Services, 5/16

Role of the School Physician, 12/12

School Health Assessments, 4/00, reaffirmed 6/03, 5/06, 10/11

School Health Centers and Other Integrated School Health Services, 1/01

School Readiness (Technical Report) (joint with Committee on Early Childhood, Adoption, and Dependent Care), 4/08, reaffirmed 9/13

School Start Times for Adolescents (joint with Adolescent Sleep Working Group and Committee on Adolescence), 8/14

School Transportation Safety (joint with Committee on Injury, Violence, and Poison Prevention), 7/07, reaffirmed 10/11

MEDICAL HOME INITIATIVES FOR CHILDREN WITH SPECIAL NEEDS PROJECT ADVISORY COMMITTEE

Identifying Infants and Young Children With Developmental Disorders in the Medical Home: An Algorithm for Developmental Surveillance and Screening (joint with Council on Children With Disabilities, Section on Developmental and Behavioral Pediatrics, and Bright Futures Steering Committee), 7/06, reaffirmed 12/09, 8/14

The Medical Home, 7/02, reaffirmed 5/08

NEUROMOTOR SCREENING EXPERT PANEL

Motor Delays: Early Identification and Evaluation (Clinical Report), 5/13

NEWBORN SCREENING AUTHORING COMMITTEE

Newborn Screening Expands: Recommendations for Pediatricians and Medical Homes—Implications for the System (Clinical Report), 1/08

RETAIL-BASED CLINIC POLICY WORK GROUP

AAP Principles Concerning Retail-Based Clinics, 12/06, reaffirmed 1/11

SECTION ON ADMINISTRATION AND PRACTICE MANAGEMENT

Medical Versus Nonmedical Immunization Exemptions for Child Care and School Attendance (joint with Committee on Practice and Ambulatory Medicine, Committee on Infectious Diseases, Committee on State Government Affairs, Council on School Health, and Section on Administration and Practice Management), 8/16

SECTION ON ALLERGY AND IMMUNOLOGY

Allergy Testing in Childhood: Using Allergen-Specific IgE Tests (Clinical Report), 12/11

Effects of Early Nutritional Interventions on the Development of Atopic Disease in Infants and Children: The Role of Maternal Dietary Restriction, Breastfeeding, Timing of Introduction of Complementary Foods, and Hydrolyzed Formulas (Clinical Report) (joint with Committee on Nutrition), 1/08

Indoor Environmental Control Practices and Asthma Management (Clinical Report) (joint with Council on Environmental Health), 10/16

Management of Food Allergy in the School Setting (Clinical Report), 11/10

Self-injectable Epinephrine for First-Aid Management of Anaphylaxis (Clinical Report), 3/07

SECTION ON ANESTHESIOLOGY AND PAIN MEDICINE

Codeine: Time to Say "No" (Clinical Report) (joint with Committee on Drugs), 9/16

Critical Elements for the Pediatric Perioperative Anesthesia Environment, 11/15

Do-Not-Resuscitate Orders for Pediatric Patients Who Require Anesthesia and Surgery (Clinical Report) (joint with Section on Surgery and Committee on Bioethics), 12/04, reaffirmed 1/09, 10/12

The Pediatrician's Role in the Evaluation and Preparation of Pediatric Patients Undergoing Anesthesia, 8/14

Premedication for Nonemergency Endotracheal Intubation in the Neonate (Clinical Report) (joint with Committee on Fetus and Newborn), 2/10, reaffirmed 8/13

Prevention and Management of Procedural Pain in the Neonate: An Update (joint with Committee on Fetus and Newborn), 1/16

Recognition and Management of Iatrogenically Induced Opioid Dependence and Withdrawal in Children (Clinical Report) (joint with Committee on Drugs), 12/13

Relief of Pain and Anxiety in Pediatric Patients in Emergency Medical Systems (Clinical Report) (joint with Committee on Pediatric Emergency Medicine), 10/12, reaffirmed 9/15

SECTION ON BREASTFEEDING

Breastfeeding and the Use of Human Milk, 2/12

WIC Program, 11/01

SECTION ON CARDIOLOGY AND CARDIAC SURGERY

ACCF/AHA/AAP Recommendations for Training in Pediatric Cardiology (joint with American College of Cardiology Foundation and American Heart Association), 12/05, reaffirmed 1/09

Cardiovascular Health Supervision for Individuals Affected by Duchenne or Becker Muscular Dystrophy (Clinical Report), 12/05, reaffirmed 1/09

Cardiovascular Monitoring and Stimulant Drugs for Attention-Deficit/Hyperactivity Disorder (joint with Black Box Working Group), 8/08

Echocardiography in Infants and Children, 6/97, reaffirmed 3/03, 3/07

Endorsement of Health and Human Services Recommendation for Pulse Oximetry Screening for Critical Congenital Heart Disease, 12/11

Guidelines for Pediatric Cardiovascular Centers, 3/02, reaffirmed 10/07

Pediatric Sudden Cardiac Arrest, 3/12

Role of Pulse Oximetry in Examining Newborns for Congenital Heart Disease: A Scientific Statement from the AHA and AAP (joint with Committee on Fetus and Newborn and American Heart Association Congenital Heart Defects Committee of the Council on Cardiovascular Disease in the Young, Council on Cardiovascular Nursing, and Interdisciplinary Council on Quality of Care and Outcomes Research), 8/09

Ventricular Fibrillation and the Use of Automated External Defibrillators on Children (joint with Committee on Pediatric Emergency Medicine), 11/07, reaffirmed 6/11, 7/14

SECTION ON CLINICAL PHARMACOLOGY AND THERAPEUTICS

Fever and Antipyretic Use in Children (Clinical Report) (joint with Committee on Drugs), 2/11, reaffirmed 7/16

SECTION ON COMPLEMENTARY AND INTEGRATIVE MEDICINE (FORMERLY PROVISIONAL SECTION ON COMPLEMENTARY, HOLISTIC, AND INTEGRATIVE MEDICINE)

Sensory Integration Therapies for Children With Developmental and Behavioral Disorders (joint with Council on Children With Disabilities), 5/12

The Use of Complementary and Alternative Medicine in Pediatrics (Clinical Report) (joint with Task Force on Complementary and Alternative Medicine), 12/08, reaffirmed 10/12, 1/13

SECTION ON CRITICAL CARE

Admission and Discharge Guidelines for the Pediatric Patient Requiring Intermediate Care (Clinical Report) (joint with Committee on Hospital Care and Society of Critical Care Medicine), 5/04, reaffirmed 2/08, 1/13

Guidelines for Developing Admission and Discharge Policies for the Pediatric Intensive Care Unit (joint with Committee on Hospital Care and Society of Critical Care Medicine), 4/99, reaffirmed 5/05, 2/08, 1/13

Guidelines for the Determination of Brain Death in Infants and Children: An Update of the 1987 Task Force Recommendations (Clinical Report) (joint with Section on Neurology, Society of Critical Care Medicine, and Child Neurology Society), 8/11, reaffirmed 1/15

Management of Pediatric Trauma (joint with Committee on Pediatric Emergency Medicine; Council on Injury, Violence, and Poison Prevention; Section on Orthopaedics; Section on Surgery; Section on Transport Medicine; Pediatric Trauma Society; and Society of Trauma Nurses Pediatric Committee), 7/16

Pediatric Organ Donation and Transplantation (joint with Committee on Hospital Care and Section on Surgery), 3/10, reaffirmed 3/14

SECTION ON DERMATOLOGY

Atopic Dermatitis: Skin-Directed Management (Clinical Report), 11/14

Diagnosis and Management of Infantile Hemangioma (Clinical Report) (joint with Section on Otolaryngology—Head & Neck Surgery and Section on Plastic Surgery), 9/15

Diagnosis and Management of Infantile Hemangioma: Executive Summary (joint with Section on Otolaryngology—Head & Neck Surgery and Section on Plastic Surgery), 9/15

Ultraviolet Radiation: A Hazard to Children and Adolescents (joint with Council on Environmental Health), 2/11

Ultraviolet Radiation: A Hazard to Children and Adolescents (Technical Report) (joint with Council on Environmental Health), 3/11

SECTION ON DEVELOPMENTAL AND BEHAVIORAL PEDIATRICS

Addressing Early Childhood Emotional and Behavioral Problems (joint with Council on Early Childhood and Committee on Psychosocial Aspects of Child and Family Health), 11/16

Addressing Early Childhood Emotional and Behavioral Problems (Technical Report) (joint with Council on Early Childhood and Committee on Psychosocial Aspects of Child and Family Health), 11/16

Early Childhood Adversity, Toxic Stress, and the Role of the Pediatrician: Translating Developmental Science Into Lifelong Health (joint with Committee on Psychosocial Aspects of Child and Family Health and Committee on Early Childhood, Adoption, and Dependent Care), 12/11, reaffirmed 7/16

Helping Children and Families Deal With Divorce and Separation (Clinical Report) (joint with Committee on Psychosocial Aspects of Child and Family Health), 11/16

Identifying Infants and Young Children With Developmental Disorders in the Medical Home: An Algorithm for Developmental Surveillance and Screening (joint with Council on Children With Disabilities, Bright Futures Steering Committee, and Medical Home Initiatives for Children With Special Needs Project Advisory Committee), 7/06, reaffirmed 12/09, 8/14

The Lifelong Effects of Early Childhood Adversity and Toxic Stress (Technical Report) (joint with Committee on Psychosocial Aspects of Child and Family Health and Committee on Early Childhood, Adoption, and Dependent Care), 12/11, reaffirmed 7/16

Promoting Optimal Development: Screening for Behavioral and Emotional Problems (Clinical Report) (joint with Committee on Psychosocial Aspects of Child and Family Health, Council on Early Childhood, and Society for Developmental and Behavioral Pediatrics), 1/15

SECTION ON ENDOCRINOLOGY

Bone Densitometry in Children and Adolescents (Clinical Report), 9/16

Congenital Adrenal Hyperplasia (Technical Report) (joint with Committee on Genetics), 12/00, reaffirmed 10/04

SECTION ON OPHTHALMOLOGY

Eye Examination in Infants, Children, and Young Adults by Pediatricians (joint with Committee on Practice and Ambulatory Medicine, American Association of Certified Orthoptists, American Association for Pediatric Ophthalmology and Strabismus, and American Academy of Ophthalmology), 4/03, reaffirmed 5/07

The Eye Examination in the Evaluation of Child Abuse (Clinical Report) (joint with Committee on Child Abuse and Neglect), 7/10, reaffirmed 12/15

Instrument-Based Pediatric Vision Screening Policy Statement (joint with Committee on Practice and Ambulatory Medicine, American Academy of Ophthalmology, American Association for Pediatric Ophthalmology and Strabismus, and American Association of Certified Orthoptists), 10/12

Learning Disabilities, Dyslexia, and Vision (joint with Council on Children With Disabilities, American Academy of Ophthalmology, American Association for Pediatric Ophthalmology and Strabismus, and American Association of Certified Orthoptists), 7/09, reaffirmed 7/14

Learning Disabilities, Dyslexia, and Vision (Technical Report) (joint with Council on Children With Disabilities, American Academy of Ophthalmology, American Association for Pediatric Ophthalmology and Strabismus, and American Association of Certified Orthoptists), 3/11

Ophthalmologic Examinations in Children With Juvenile Rheumatoid Arthritis (Clinical Report) (joint with Section on Rheumatology), 5/06, reaffirmed 10/12

Procedures for the Evaluation of the Visual System by Pediatricians (Clinical Report) (joint with Committee on Practice and Ambulatory Medicine, American Association of Certified Orthoptists, American Association for Pediatric Ophthalmology and Strabismus, and American Academy of Ophthalmology), 12/15

Red Reflex Examination in Neonates, Infants, and Children (joint with American Association for Pediatric Ophthalmology and Strabismus, American Academy of Ophthalmology, and American Association of Certified Orthoptists), 12/08

Screening Examination of Premature Infants for Retinopathy of Prematurity (joint with American Academy of Ophthalmology, American Association for Pediatric Ophthalmology and Strabismus, and American Association of Certified Orthoptists), 12/12, reaffirmed 2/16

Screening for Retinopathy in the Pediatric Patient With Type 1 Diabetes Mellitus (Clinical Report) (joint with Section on Endocrinology and American Association for Pediatric Ophthalmology and Strabismus), 7/05, reaffirmed 1/09, 7/14

Telemedicine for Evaluation of Retinopathy of Prematurity (Technical Report) (joint with American Academy of Ophthalmology and American Association of Certified Orthoptists), 12/14

Visual System Assessment in Infants, Children, and Young Adults by Pediatricians (joint with Committee on Practice and Ambulatory Medicine, American Association of Certified Orthoptists, American Association for Pediatric Ophthalmology and Strabismus, and American Academy of Ophthalmology), 12/15

SECTION ON ORAL HEALTH (FORMERLY SECTION ON PEDIATRIC DENTISTRY AND SECTION ON PEDIATRIC DENTISTRY AND ORAL HEALTH)

Fluoride Use in Caries Prevention in the Primary Care Setting, 8/14

Maintaining and Improving the Oral Health of Young Children, 11/14, reaffirmed 12/14

Management of Dental Trauma in a Primary Care Setting (Clinical Report), 1/14

Oral Health Care for Children With Developmental Disabilities (Clinical Report) (joint with Council on Children With Disabilities), 2/13

Preventive Oral Health Intervention for Pediatricians, 12/08

SECTION ON ORTHOPAEDICS

Anterior Cruciate Ligament Injuries: Diagnosis, Treatment, and Prevention (Clinical Report) (joint with Council on Sports Medicine), 4/14

Evaluating Children With Fractures for Child Physical Abuse (Clinical Report), (joint with Committee on Child Abuse and Neglect, Section on Radiology, Section on Endocrinology, and Society for Pediatric Radiology), 1/14

Evaluation and Referral for Developmental Dysplasia of the Hip in Infants (Clinical Report), 11/16

Management of Pediatric Trauma (joint with Committee on Pediatric Emergency Medicine; Council on Injury, Violence, and Poison Prevention; Section on Critical Care; Section on Surgery; Section on Transport Medicine; Pediatric Trauma Society; and Society of Trauma Nurses Pediatric Committee), 7/16

SECTION ON OTOLARYNGOLOGY—HEAD AND NECK SURGERY

Cochlear Implants in Children: Surgical Site Infections and Prevention and Treatment of Acute Otitis Media and Meningitis (joint with Committee on Infectious Diseases), 7/10

Diagnosis and Management of Infantile Hemangioma (Clinical Report) (joint with Section on Dermatology and Section on Plastic Surgery), 9/15

Diagnosis and Management of Infantile Hemangioma: Executive Summary (joint with Section on Dermatology and Section on Plastic Surgery), 9/15

Follow-up Management of Children With Tympanostomy Tubes, 2/02

Hearing Assessment in Infants and Children: Recommendations Beyond Neonatal Screening (Clinical Report) (joint with Committee on Practice and Ambulatory Medicine), 9/09

SECTION ON PLASTIC SURGERY

Diagnosis and Management of Infantile Hemangioma (Clinical Report) (joint with Section on Dermatology and Section on Otolaryngology—Head & Neck Surgery), 9/15

Diagnosis and Management of Infantile Hemangioma: Executive Summary (joint with Section on Dermatology and Section on Otolaryngology—Head & Neck Surgery), 9/15

SECTION ON RADIOLOGY

Diagnostic Imaging of Child Abuse, 4/09

Establishing a Standard Protocol for the Voiding Cystourethrography (Clinical Report) (joint with Section on Urology), 10/16

Evaluating Children With Fractures for Child Physical Abuse (Clinical Report), (joint with Committee on Child Abuse and Neglect, Section on Endocrinology, Section on Orthopaedics, and Society for Pediatric Radiology), 1/14

Radiation Risk to Children From Computed Tomography (Clinical Report), 9/07

SECTION ON RHEUMATOLOGY

Ophthalmologic Examinations in Children With Juvenile Rheumatoid Arthritis (Clinical Report) (joint with Section on Ophthalmology), 5/06, reaffirmed 10/12

SECTION ON SURGERY

Assessment and Management of Inguinal Hernia in Infants (Clinical Report) (joint with Committee on Fetus and Newborn), 9/12

Do-Not-Resuscitate Orders for Pediatric Patients Who Require Anesthesia and Surgery (Clinical Report) (joint with Section on Anesthesia and Pain Medicine and Committee on Bioethics), 12/04, reaffirmed 1/09, 10/12

Management of Pediatric Trauma (joint with Committee on Pediatric Emergency Medicine; Council on Injury, Violence, and Poison Prevention; Section on Critical Care; Section on Orthopaedics; Section on Transport Medicine; Pediatric Trauma Society; and Society of Trauma Nurses Pediatric Committee), 7/16

Newborn Screening for Biliary Atresia (Technical Report) (joint with Committee on Fetus and Newborn and Childhood Liver Disease Research Network), 11/15

Pediatric Organ Donation and Transplantation (joint with Committee on Hospital Care and Section on Critical Care), 3/10, reaffirmed 3/14

Postdischarge Follow-up of Infants With Congenital Diaphragmatic Hernia (Clinical Report) (joint with Committee on Fetus and Newborn), 3/08, reaffirmed 5/11

Preservation of Fertility in Pediatric and Adolescent Patients With Cancer (Technical Report) (joint with Committee on Bioethics and Section on Hematology/Oncology), 5/08, reaffirmed 2/12

SECTION ON TELEHEALTH CARE (FORMERLY SECTION ON TELEPHONE CARE)

Payment for Telephone Care (joint with Committee on Child Health Financing), 10/06

Telemedicine: Pediatric Applications (Technical Report), 6/15

SECTION ON TOBACCO CONTROL

Clinical Practice Policy to Protect Children From Tobacco, Nicotine, and Tobacco Smoke, 10/15

Electronic Nicotine Delivery Systems, 10/15

Protecting Children From Tobacco, Nicotine, and Tobacco Smoke (Technical Report), 10/15

Public Policy to Protect Children From Tobacco, Nicotine, and Tobacco Smoke, 10/15

SECTION ON TRANSPORT MEDICINE

Management of Pediatric Trauma (joint with Committee on Pediatric Emergency Medicine; Council on Injury, Violence, and Poison Prevention; Section on Critical Care; Section on Orthopaedics; Section on Surgery; Pediatric Trauma Society; and Society of Trauma Nurses Pediatric Committee), 7/16

SECTION ON UNIFORMED SERVICES

Health and Mental Health Needs of Children in US Military Families (Clinical Report) (joint with Committee on Psychosocial Aspects of Child and Family Health), 5/13

SECTION ON UROLOGY

Establishing a Standard Protocol for the Voiding Cystourethrography (Clinical Report) (joint with Section on Radiology), 10/16

STEERING COMMITTEE ON QUALITY IMPROVEMENT AND MANAGEMENT

ADHD: Clinical Practice Guideline for the Diagnosis, Evaluation, and Treatment of Attention-Deficit/Hyperactivity Disorder in Children and Adolescents (Clinical Practice Guideline) (joint with Subcommittee on Attention-Deficit/Hyperactivity Disorder), 10/11

Chronic Abdominal Pain in Children (Clinical Report) (joint with Subcommittee on Chronic Abdominal Pain and North American Society for Pediatric Gastroenterology, Hepatology, and Nutrition), 3/05

Chronic Abdominal Pain in Children (Technical Report) (joint with Subcommittee on Chronic Abdominal Pain and North American Society for Pediatric Gastroenterology, Hepatology, and Nutrition), 3/05

Classifying Recommendations for Clinical Practice Guidelines, 9/04

Developmental Dysplasia of the Hip Practice Guideline (Technical Report), 4/00

Diagnosis and Management of Acute Otitis Media (Clinical Practice Guideline) (joint with American Academy of Family Physicians), 5/04

Diagnosis and Management of an Initial UTI in Febrile Infants and Young Children (Technical Report) (joint with Subcommittee on Urinary Tract Infection), 8/11

Diagnosis and Management of Childhood Obstructive Sleep Apnea Syndrome (Clinical Practice Guideline) (joint with Subcommittee on Obstructive Sleep Apnea Syndrome), 8/12

Diagnosis and Management of Childhood Obstructive Sleep Apnea Syndrome (Technical Report) (joint with Subcommittee on Obstructive Sleep Apnea Syndrome), 8/12

Early Detection of Developmental Dysplasia of the Hip (Clinical Practice Guideline), 4/00

An Evidence-Based Review of Important Issues Concerning Neonatal Hyperbilirubinemia (Technical Report) (joint with Subcommittee on Hyperbilirubinemia), 7/04

Febrile Seizures: Clinical Practice Guideline for the Long-term Management of the Child With Simple Febrile Seizures (Clinical Practice Guideline) (joint with Subcommittee on Febrile Seizures), 6/08

Management of Hyperbilirubinemia in the Newborn Infant 35 or More Weeks of Gestation (Clinical Practice Guideline) (joint with Subcommittee on Hyperbilirubinemia), 7/04

Management of Sinusitis (Clinical Practice Guideline), 9/01

Otitis Media With Effusion (Clinical Practice Guideline) (joint with Subcommittee on Otitis Media With Effusion), 5/04

Principles for the Development and Use of Quality Measures (joint with Committee on Practice and Ambulatory Medicine), 2/08

Principles of Pediatric Patient Safety: Reducing Harm Due to Medical Care (joint with Committee on Hospital Care), 5/11

Toward Transparent Clinical Policies, 3/08, reaffirmed 2/14

Urinary Tract Infection: Clinical Practice Guideline for the Diagnosis and Management of the Initial UTI in Febrile Infants and Children 2 to 24 Months (Clinical Practice Guideline) (joint with Subcommittee on Urinary Tract Infection), 8/11

SUBCOMMITTEE ON APPARENT LIFE THREATENING EVENTS

Brief Resolved Unexplained Events (Formerly Apparent Life-Threatening Events) and Evaluation of Lower-Risk Infants (Clinical Practice Guideline), 4/16

Brief Resolved Unexplained Events (Formerly Apparent Life-Threatening Events) and Evaluation of Lower-Risk Infants: Executive Summary (Clinical Practice Guideline), 4/16

SUBCOMMITTEE ON ATTENTION-DEFICIT/HYPERACTIVITY DISORDER

ADHD: Clinical Practice Guideline for the Diagnosis, Evaluation, and Treatment of Attention-Deficit/Hyperactivity Disorder in Children and Adolescents (Clinical Practice Guideline) (joint with Steering Committee on Quality Improvement and Management), 10/11

SUBCOMMITTEE ON CHRONIC ABDOMINAL PAIN

Chronic Abdominal Pain in Children (Clinical Report) (joint with Steering Committee on Quality Improvement and Management and North American Society for Pediatric Gastroenterology, Hepatology, and Nutrition), 3/05

Chronic Abdominal Pain in Children (Technical Report) (joint with Steering Committee on Quality Improvement and Management and North American Society for Pediatric Gastroenterology, Hepatology, and Nutrition), 3/05

SUBCOMMITTEE ON FEBRILE SEIZURES

Febrile Seizures: Clinical Practice Guideline for the Long-term Management of the Child With Simple Febrile Seizures (Clinical Practice Guideline) (joint with Steering Committee on Quality Improvement and Management), 6/08

Febrile Seizures: Guideline for the Neurodiagnostic Evaluation of the Child With a Simple Febrile Seizure (Clinical Practice Guideline), 2/11

SUBCOMMITTEE ON HYPERBILIRUBINEMIA

An Evidence-Based Review of Important Issues Concerning Neonatal Hyperbilirubinemia (Technical Report) (joint with Steering Committee on Quality Improvement and Management), 7/04

Management of Hyperbilirubinemia in the Newborn Infant 35 or More Weeks of Gestation (Clinical Practice Guideline) (joint with Steering Committee on Quality Improvement and Management), 7/04

SUBCOMMITTEE ON OBSTRUCTIVE SLEEP APNEA SYNDROME

Diagnosis and Management of Childhood Obstructive Sleep Apnea Syndrome (Clinical Practice Guideline) (joint with Steering Committee on Quality Improvement and Management), 8/12

Diagnosis and Management of Childhood Obstructive Sleep Apnea Syndrome (Technical Report) (joint with Steering Committee on Quality Improvement and Management), 8/12

SUBCOMMITTEE ON OTITIS MEDIA WITH EFFUSION

Otitis Media With Effusion (Clinical Practice Guideline) (joint with Steering Committee on Quality Improvement and Management), 5/04

SUBCOMMITTEE ON URINARY TRACT INFECTION

Diagnosis and Management of an Initial UTI in Febrile Infants and Young Children (Technical Report) (joint with Steering Committee on Quality Improvement and Management), 8/11

Reaffirmation of AAP Clinical Practice Guideline: The Diagnosis and Management of the Initial Urinary Tract Infection in Febrile Infants and Young Children 2–24 Months of Age (Clinical Practice Guideline), 11/16

Urinary Tract Infection: Clinical Practice Guideline for the Diagnosis and Management of the Initial UTI in Febrile Infants and Children 2 to 24 Months (Clinical Practice Guideline) (joint with Steering Committee on Quality Improvement and Management), 8/11

SURGICAL ADVISORY PANEL

Referral to Pediatric Surgical Specialists, 1/14

TASK FORCE ON CIRCUMCISION

Circumcision Policy Statement, 8/12

Male Circumcision (Technical Report), 8/12

TASK FORCE ON COMPLEMENTARY AND ALTERNATIVE MEDICINE

The Use of Complementary and Alternative Medicine in Pediatrics (Clinical Report) (joint with Provisional Section on Complementary, Holistic, and Integrative Medicine), 12/08, reaffirmed 10/12, 1/13

TASK FORCE ON GRADUATE MEDICAL EDUCATION REFORM

Graduate Medical Education and Pediatric Workforce Issues and Principles, 6/94

TASK FORCE ON MENTAL HEALTH

The Future of Pediatrics: Mental Health Competencies for Pediatric Primary Care (joint with Committee on Psychosocial Aspects of Child and Family Health), 6/09, reaffirmed 8/13

TASK FORCE ON SUDDEN INFANT DEATH SYNDROME

The Changing Concept of Sudden Infant Death Syndrome: Diagnostic Coding Shifts, Controversies Regarding the Sleeping Environment, and New Variables to Consider in Reducing Risk, 11/05, reaffirmed 5/08

Safe Sleep and Skin-to-Skin Care in the Neonatal Period for Healthy Term Newborns (Clinical Report) (joint with Committee on Fetus and Newborn), 8/16

SIDS and Other Sleep-Related Infant Deaths: Updated 2016 Recommendations for a Safe Infant Sleeping Environment, 10/16

SIDS and Other Sleep-Related Infant Deaths: Evidence Base for 2016 Updated Recommendations for a Safe Infant Sleeping Environment (Technical Report), 10/16

TASK FORCE ON TERRORISM

The Pediatrician and Disaster Preparedness (joint with Committee on Pediatric Emergency Medicine and Committee on Medical Liability), 2/06, reaffirmed 6/09, 9/13

Psychosocial Implications of Disaster or Terrorism on Children: A Guide for the Pediatrician (Clinical Report) (joint with Committee on Psychosocial Aspects of Child and Family Health), 9/05, reaffirmed 11/14

WORKING GROUP ON SLEEPINESS IN ADOLESCENTS/YOUNG ADULTS

Excessive Sleepiness in Adolescents and Young Adults: Causes, Consequences, and Treatment Strategies (Technical Report) (joint with Committee on Adolescence), 6/05

JOINT STATEMENTS

Joint Statement of the American Academy of Pediatrics, the American Academy of Child and Adolescent Psychiatry, and the National Center for Child Traumatic Stress

Behavioral and Emotional Consequences of Child Abuse (Clinical Report), 9/08, reaffirmed 8/12

Joint Statement of the American Academy of Pediatrics, the American Academy of Family Physicians, and the American College of Physicians

Supporting the Health Care Transition From Adolescence to Adulthood in the Medical Home (Clinical Report), 7/11, reaffirmed 8/15

Joint Statement of the American Academy of Pediatrics, the American Academy of Family Physicians, and the American College of Physicians-American Society of Internal Medicine

A Consensus Statement on Health Care Transitions for Young Adults With Special Health Care Needs, 12/02

Joint Statement of the American Academy of Pediatrics, the American Academy of Ophthalmology, and the American Association of Certified Orthoptists

Telemedicine for Evaluation of Retinopathy of Prematurity (Technical Report), 12/14

Joint Statement of the American Academy of Pediatrics, the American Academy of Ophthalmology, the American Association for Pediatric Ophthalmology and Strabismus, and the American Association of Certified Orthoptists

Instrument-Based Pediatric Vision Screening Policy Statement, 10/12

Screening Examination of Premature Infants for Retinopathy of Prematurity, 12/12, reaffirmed 2/16

Joint Statement of the American Academy of Pediatrics, the American Association of Certified Orthoptists, the American Association for Pediatric Ophthalmology and Strabismus, and the American Academy of Ophthalmology

Eye Examination in Infants, Children, and Young Adults by Pediatricians, 4/03, reaffirmed 5/07

Learning Disabilities, Dyslexia, and Vision, 7/09, reaffirmed 7/14

Learning Disabilities, Dyslexia, and Vision (Technical Report), 3/11

Procedures for the Evaluation of the Visual System by Pediatricians (Clinical Report), 12/15

Red Reflex Examination in Neonates, Infants, and Children, 12/08

Visual System Assessment in Infants, Children, and Young Adults by Pediatricians, 12/15

Joint Statement of the American Academy of Pediatrics, the American College of Cardiology Foundation, and the American Heart Association

ACCF/AHA/AAP Recommendations for Training in Pediatric Cardiology, 12/05, reaffirmed 1/09

Joint Statement of the American Academy of Pediatrics, the American College of Emergency Physicians, and the Emergency Nurses Association

Death of a Child in the Emergency Department, 6/14

Death of a Child in the Emergency Department (Technical Report), 6/14

Guidelines for Care of Children in the Emergency Department, 9/09, reaffirmed 4/13, 2/16

Joint Statement of the American Academy of Pediatrics, the American College of Emergency Physicians, the American College of Surgeons Committee on Trauma, Emergency Medical Services for Children, the Emergency Nurses Association, the National Association of EMS Physicians, and the National Association of State EMS Officials

Equipment for Ground Ambulances, 8/14

Joint Statement of the American Academy of Pediatrics, the American College of Emergency Physicians Pediatric Emergency Medicine Committee, and the Emergency Nurses Association Pediatric Committee

Best Practices for Improving Flow and Care of Pediatric Patients in the Emergency Department (Technical Report), 12/14

Handoffs: Transitions of Care for Children in the Emergency Department, 10/16

Patient- and Family-Centered Care of Children in the Emergency Department (Technical Report), 12/14

Joint Statement of the American Academy of Pediatrics, the American College of Surgeons Committee on Trauma, and the National Association of EMS Physicians

Withholding or Termination of Resuscitation in Pediatric Out-of-Hospital Traumatic Cardiopulmonary Arrest, 3/14

Joint Statement of the American Academy of Pediatrics, the American Thyroid Association, and the Lawson Wilkins Pediatric Endocrine Society

Update of Newborn Screening and Therapy for Congenital Hypothyroidism (Clinical Report), 6/06, reaffirmed 12/11

Joint Statement of the American Academy of Pediatrics, the Pediatric Trauma Society, and the Society of Trauma Nurses Pediatric Committee

Management of Pediatric Trauma, 7/16

Joint Statement of the American Academy of Pediatrics, the Society for Academic Emergency Medicine Academy of Emergency Ultrasound, the American College of Emergency Physicians Pediatric Emergency Medicine Committee, and the World Interactive Network Focused on Critical Ultrasound

Point-of-Care Ultrasonography by Pediatric Emergency Medicine Physicians, 3/15

Point-of-Care Ultrasonography by Pediatric Emergency Medicine Physicians (Technical Report), 3/15

Joint Statement of the American Academy of Pediatrics, the Society of Critical Care Medicine, and the Child Neurology Society

Guidelines for the Determination of Brain Death in Infants and Children: An Update of the 1987 Task Force Recommendations (Clinical Report), 8/11, reaffirmed 1/15

Joint Statement of the American Academy of Pediatrics and Others

Insurance Coverage of Mental Health and Substance Abuse Services for Children and Adolescents: A Consensus Statement, 10/00

Joint Statement of the American Academy of Pediatrics and the American Academy of Child and Adolescent Psychiatry

Psychological Maltreatment (Clinical Report), 7/12, reaffirmed 4/16

Joint Statement of the American Academy of Pediatrics and the American Academy of Family Physicians

Diagnosis and Management of Acute Otitis Media (Clinical Practice Guideline), 5/04

Joint Statement of the American Academy of Pediatrics and the American Academy of Ophthalmology

Protective Eyewear for Young Athletes, 3/04, reaffirmed 2/08, 6/11, 2/15

Joint Statement of the American Academy of Pediatrics and the American Academy of Pediatric Dentistry

Guidelines for Monitoring and Management of Pediatric Patients Before, During, and After Sedation for Diagnostic and Therapeutic Procedures: Update 2016 (Clinical Report), 6/16

Oral and Dental Aspects of Child Abuse and Neglect (Clinical Report), 12/05, reaffirmed 1/09, 1/14

Joint Statement of the American Academy of Pediatrics and the American Association for Pediatric Ophthalmology and Strabismus

Screening for Retinopathy in the Pediatric Patient With Type 1 Diabetes Mellitus (Clinical Report), 7/05, reaffirmed 1/09, 7/14

Joint Statement of the American Academy of Pediatrics and the American College of Emergency Physicians

Emergency Information Forms and Emergency Preparedness for Children With Special Health Care Needs, 3/10, reaffirmed 7/14, 10/14

Patient- and Family-Centered Care and the Role of the Emergency Physician Providing Care to a Child in the Emergency Department, 11/06, reaffirmed 6/09, 10/11, 9/15

Pediatric Mental Health Emergencies in the Emergency Medical Services System, 10/06, reaffirmed 6/09, 4/13

Joint Statement of the American Academy of Pediatrics and the American College of Emergency Physicians Pediatric Emergency Medicine Committee

Evaluation and Management of Children and Adolescents With Acute Mental Health or Behavioral Problems. Part I: Common Clinical Challenges of Patients With Mental Health and/or Behavioral Emergencies (Clinical Report), 8/16

Evaluation and Management of Children and Adolescents With Acute Mental Health or Behavioral Problems. Part I: Common Clinical Challenges of Patients With Mental Health and/or Behavioral Emergencies—Executive Summary (Clinical Report), 8/16

Evaluation and Management of Children With Acute Mental Health or Behavioral Problems. Part II: Recognition of Clinically Challenging Mental Health Related Conditions Presenting With Medical or Uncertain Symptoms (Clinical Report), 8/16

Evaluation and Management of Children With Acute Mental Health or Behavioral Problems. Part II: Recognition of Clinically Challenging Mental Health Related Conditions Presenting With Medical or Uncertain Symptoms—Executive Summary (Clinical Report), 8/16

Joint Statement of the American Academy of Pediatrics and the American College of Medical Genetics and Genomics

Ethical and Policy Issues in Genetic Testing and Screening of Children, 2/13

Joint Statement of the American Academy of Pediatrics and the American College of Obstetricians and Gynecologists

The Apgar Score, 9/15

Immersion in Water During Labor and Delivery (Clinical Report), 3/14

Maternal-Fetal Intervention and Fetal Care Centers (Clinical Report), 7/11

Joint Statement of the American Academy of Pediatrics and the American Heart Association

Role of Pulse Oximetry in Examining Newborns for Congenital Heart Disease: A Scientific Statement from the AHA and AAP, 8/09

Joint Statement of the American Academy of Pediatrics and the Canadian Paediatric Society

Boxing Participation by Children and Adolescents, 8/11, reaffirmed 2/15

Early Childhood Caries in Indigenous Communities, 5/11

Joint Statement of the American Academy of Pediatrics and the Child Life Council

Child Life Services, 4/14

Joint Statement of the American Academy of Pediatrics and the Childhood Liver Disease Research Network

Newborn Screening for Biliary Atresia (Technical Report), 11/15

Joint Statement of the American Academy of Pediatrics and the Children's Oncology Group

Long-term Follow-up Care for Pediatric Cancer Survivors (Clinical Report), 3/09, reaffirmed 4/13

Joint Statement of the American Academy of Pediatrics and the Institute for Patient- and Family-Centered Care

Patient- and Family-Centered Care and the Pediatrician's Role, 1/12

Joint Statement of the American Academy of Pediatrics and the National Association of Medical Examiners

Distinguishing Sudden Infant Death Syndrome From Child Abuse Fatalities (Clinical Report), 7/06, reaffirmed 4/09, 3/13

Joint Statement of the American Academy of Pediatrics and the North American Society for Pediatric and Adolescent Gynecology

Menstrual Management for Adolescents With Disabilities (Clinical Report), 6/16

Joint Statement of the American Academy of Pediatrics and the North American Society for Pediatric Gastroenterology, Hepatology, and Nutrition

Chronic Abdominal Pain in Children (Clinical Report), 3/05

Chronic Abdominal Pain in Children (Technical Report), 3/05

Joint Statement of the American Academy of Pediatrics and the Society for Adolescent Health Care

Screening for Nonviral Sexually Transmitted Infections in Adolescents and Young Adults, 6/14

Joint Statement of the American Academy of Pediatrics and the Society for Developmental and Behavioral Pediatrics

Promoting Optimal Development: Screening for Behavioral and Emotional Problems (Clinical Report), 1/15

Joint Statement of the American Academy of Pediatrics and the Society for Pediatric Radiology

Evaluating Children With Fractures for Child Physical Abuse (Clinical Report), 1/14

Joint Statement of the American Academy of Pediatrics and the Society of Critical Care Medicine

Admission and Discharge Guidelines for the Pediatric Patient Requiring Intermediate Care (Clinical Report), 5/04, reaffirmed 2/08, 1/13

Guidelines for Developing Admission and Discharge Policies for the Pediatric Intensive Care Unit (Clinical Report), 4/99, reaffirmed 5/05, 2/08, 1/13

Joint Statement of the Federation of Pediatric Organizations

Pediatric Fellowship Training, 7/04

ENDORSED CLINICAL PRACTICE GUIDELINES AND POLICIES

(The AAP endorses and accepts as its policy the following clinical practice guidelines and policies that have been published by other organizations.)

Academic Pediatric Association

Faculty Competencies for Global Health, 6/14

American College of Rheumatology
Guidelines for Referral of Children and Adolescents to
Pediatric Rheumatologists, 6/02, reaffirmed 5/07

American College of Surgeons
Children's Surgery Verification Pilot Draft Documents,
11/14

American College of Surgeons Committee on Trauma
An Evidence-based Prehospital Guideline for External
Hemorrhage Control (Clinical Practice Guideline),
3/14

American Diabetes Association
Diabetes Care for Emerging Adults: Recommendations
for Transition From Pediatric to Adult Diabetes Care
Systems, 11/11
Safe at School Campaign Statement of Principles,
endorsed 2/06

American Heart Association
Cardiovascular Risk Reduction in High-Risk Pediatric
Populations, 12/06
Diagnosis, Treatment, and Long-Term Management
of Kawasaki Disease: A Statement for Health
Professionals, 12/04
Dietary Recommendations for Children and Adolescents:
A Guide for Practitioners, 9/05
Genetic Basis for Congenital Heart Defects: Current
Knowledge, 6/07
Importance and Implementation of Training in
Cardiopulmonary Resuscitation and Automated
External Defibrillation in Schools, 2/11
Long-term Cardiovascular Toxicity in Children,
Adolescents, and Young Adults Who Receive Cancer
Therapy: Pathophysiology, Course, Monitoring,
Management, Prevention, and Research Directions:
A Scientific Statement From the American Heart
Association, 5/13
Neurodevelopmental Outcomes in Children With
Congenital Heart Disease: Evaluation and
Management: A Scientific Statement From the
American Heart Association, 7/12
Noninherited Risk Factors and Congenital
Cardiovascular Defects: Current Knowledge, 6/07
Prevention of Infective Endocarditis: Guidelines From
the American Heart Association (Clinical Practice
Guideline), 5/07
Prevention of Rheumatic Fever and Diagnosis and
Treatment of Acute Streptococcal Pharyngitis, 2/09
Response to Cardiac Arrest and Selected Life-
Threatening Medical Emergencies: The Medical
Emergency Response Plan for Schools. A Statement
for Healthcare Providers, Policymakers, School
Administrators, and Community Leaders, 1/04

American Medical Association
Gifts to Physicians From Industry, 8/01

American Pediatric Surgical Association
Best Practice for Infant Surgery: A Position Statement
From the American Pediatric Surgical Association,
9/08

American Society for Parenteral and Enteral Nutrition
Defining Pediatric Malnutrition: A Paradigm Shift
Toward Etiology-Related Definitions, 3/13

**American Thoracic Society and Centers for Disease
Control and Prevention**
*(The AAP endorses and accepts as its policy the sections of this
statement as they relate to infants and children.)*
Targeted Tuberculin Testing and Treatment of Latent
Tuberculosis Infection, 4/00

American Urological Association
Report on the Management of Primary Vesicoureteral
Reflux in Children (Clinical Practice Guideline), 5/97

Canadian Paediatric Society
Skiing and Snowboarding Injury Prevention, 1/12

Centers for Disease Control and Prevention
Guidelines for Field Triage of Injured Patients, 1/12
Managing Acute Gastroenteritis Among Children: Oral
Rehydration, Maintenance, and Nutritional Therapy
(Clinical Practice Guideline), 11/03
Prevention and Control of Meningococcal Disease:
Recommendations of the Advisory Committee on
Immunization Practices (ACIP), 3/13
Prevention of Perinatal Group B Streptococcal Disease:
Revised Guidelines from CDC, 2010 (Clinical Practice
Guideline), 11/10
Recommendations for Using Fluoride to Prevent and
Control Dental Caries in the United States (Clinical
Practice Guideline), 8/01
Update on Japanese Encephalitis Vaccine for Children—
United States, May 2011, 8/11

**Centers for Disease Control and Prevention, Infectious
Diseases Society of America, and American Society
of Blood and Marrow Transplantation**
Guidelines for Preventing Opportunistic Infections
Among Hematopoietic Stem Cell Transplant
Recipients (Clinical Practice Guideline), 10/00

Congress of Neurologic Surgeons
Systematic Review and Evidence-Based Guidelines
for the Management of Patients With Positional
Plagiocephaly, 11/16

Emergency Nurses Association
Weighing Pediatric Patients in Kilograms, 3/12

The Endocrine Society
Congenital Adrenal Hyperplasia Due to Steroid
21-hydroxylase Deficiency: An Endocrine Society
Clinical Practice Guideline (Clinical Practice
Guideline), 9/10

Family Violence Prevention Fund
Identifying and Responding to Domestic Violence:
Consensus Recommendations for Child and
Adolescent Health, 9/02

**Guidelines for Adolescent Depression in Primary Care
Steering Group**
Guidelines for Adolescent Depression in Primary Care
(GLAD-PC): I. Identification, Assessment, and Initial
Management (Clinical Practice Guideline), 11/07
Guidelines for Adolescent Depression in Primary Care
(GLAD-PC): II. Treatment and Ongoing Management
(Clinical Practice Guideline), 11/07

Infectious Diseases Society of America

2013 Infectious Diseases Society of America Clinical Practice Guidelines for the Immunization of the Immunocompromised Host, (Clinical Practice Guideline) 12/13

Clinical Practice Guidelines by the Infectious Diseases Society of America for the Treatment of Methicillin-Resistant *Staphylococcus aureus* Infections in Adults and Children (Clinical Practice Guideline), 2/11

Seasonal Influenza in Adults and Children—Diagnosis, Treatment, Chemoprophylaxis, and Institutional Outbreak Management: Clinical Practice Guidelines of the Infectious Diseases Society of America (Clinical Practice Guideline), 4/09

Institute of Medicine

Dietary Reference Intakes for Calcium and Vitamin D, 2011

International Consensus Conference on Intersex (Lawson Wilkins Pediatric Endocrine Society and the European Society for Paediatric Endocrinology)

Consensus Statement on Management of Intersex Disorders, 8/06

Joint Committee on Infant Hearing

Supplement to the JCIH 2007 Position Statement: Principles and Guidelines for Early Intervention After Confirmation That a Child Is Deaf or Hard of Hearing, 3/13

National Adoption Center

National Adoption Center: Open Records, 6/00

National Association of Neonatal Nurses

Advanced Practice Registered Nurse: Role, Preparation, and Scope of Practice, 1/14

The Management of Hypotension in the Very-Low-Birth-Weight Infant: Guideline for Practice, 2011

National Association of School Nurses

Emergency Equipment and Supplies in the School Setting, 1/12

National Association of State EMS Officials

National Model EMS Clinical Guidelines (Clinical Practice Guideline), 10/14

National Athletic Trainers' Association

Appropriate Medical Care for the Secondary School-Age Athlete Communication, 2004

Lightning Safety for Athletics and Recreation, 12/00

National Athletic Trainers' Association, National Interscholastic Athletic Administrators Association, College Athletic Trainers' Society, National Federation of State High School Associations, American College Health Association, American Orthopaedic Society for Sports Medicine, National Collegiate Athletic Association, American Medical Society for Sports Medicine, National Association of Collegiate Directors of Athletics, and National Association of Intercollegiate Athletics

Inter-Association Consensus Statement on Best Practices for Sports Medicine Management for Secondary Schools and Colleges, 7/13

National Consensus Project for Quality Palliative Care

Clinical Practice Guidelines for Quality Palliative Care, Third Edition, 2013

National Diabetes Education Program

Helping the Student with Diabetes Succeed: A Guide for School Personnel, 6/03

National Heart, Lung and Blood Institute

Evidence-Based Management of Sickle Cell Disease: Expert Panel Report, 2014

Expert Panel on Integrated Guidelines for Cardiovascular Health and Risk Reduction in Children and Adolescents: Summary Report, 3/12

National Institute of Allergy and Infectious Diseases

Guidelines for the Diagnosis and Management of Food Allergy in the United States: Report of the NIAID-Sponsored Expert Panel (Clinical Practice Guideline), 12/10

National Vaccine Advisory Committee

Enhancing the Work of the HHS National Vaccine Program in Global Immunizations, 9/13

North American Society for Pediatric Gastroenterology, Hepatology, and Nutrition

Guideline for the Evaluation of Cholestatic Jaundice in Infants (Clinical Practice Guideline), 8/04

Guidelines for Evaluation and Treatment of Gastroesophageal Reflux in Infants and Children (Clinical Practice Guideline), 2001

Helicobacter pylori Infection in Children: Recommendations for Diagnosis and Treatment (Clinical Practice Guideline), 11/00

Pediatric Infectious Diseases Society and Infectious Diseases Society of America

The Management of Community-Acquired Pneumonia (CAP) in Infants and Children Older Than 3 Months of Age (Clinical Practice Guideline), 10/11

Renal Physicians Association

Shared Decision-Making in the Appropriate Initiation of and Withdrawal from Dialysis, 2nd Edition (Clinical Practice Guideline), 10/10

Society for Academic Emergency Medicine

Pediatric Care in the Emergency Department, 11/03

Society for Adolescent Health and Medicine

Confidentiality Protections for Adolescents and Young Adults in the Health Care Billing and Insurance Claims Process, 3/16

Society for Adolescent Medicine

Executing Juvenile Offenders: A Fundamental Failure of Society, 10/04

Expedited Partner Therapy for Adolescents Diagnosed With Chlamydia or Gonorrhea: A Position Paper of the Society for Adolescent Medicine, 9/09

Protecting Adolescents: Ensuring Access to Care and Reporting Sexual Activity and Abuse, 11/04

Society for Research in Child Development

Multilingual Children: Beyond Myths and Toward Best Practices, 2013

Society of Critical Care Medicine, Infectious Diseases Society of America, Society for Healthcare Epidemiology of America, Surgical Infection Society, American College of Chest Physicians, American Thoracic Society, American Society of Critical Care Anesthesiologists, Association for Professionals in Infection Control and Epidemiology, Infusion Nurses Society, Oncology Nursing Society, Society of Cardiovascular and Interventional Radiology, American Academy of Pediatrics, and Healthcare Infection Control Practices Advisory Committee of the Centers for Disease Control and Prevention

Guidelines for the Prevention of Intravascular Catheter-Related Infections (Clinical Practice Guideline), 11/02

US Department of Health and Human Services

Guidelines for the Prevention and Treatment of Opportunistic Infections in HIV-Exposed and HIV-Infected Children (Clinical Practice Guideline), 11/13

Treating Tobacco Use and Dependence: 2008 Update (Clinical Practice Guideline), 5/08

World Health Organization

(The AAP endorses the recommendation pertaining to the use of thimerosal in vaccines.)

Meeting of the Strategic Advisory Group of Experts on Immunizations, April 2012–Conclusions and Recommendations, 5/12

AFFIRMATION OF VALUE CLINICAL PRACTICE GUIDELINES AND POLICIES

(These guidelines are not endorsed as policy of the American Academy of Pediatrics [AAP]. Documents that lack a clear description of the process for identifying, assessing, and incorporating research evidence are not eligible for AAP endorsement as practice guidelines. However, such documents may be of educational value to members of the AAP.)

American Society of Anesthesiologists

Practice Guidelines for the Perioperative Management of Patients with Obstructive Sleep Apnea (Clinical Practice Guideline), 5/06

National Environmental Education Foundation

Environmental Management of Pediatric Asthma: Guidelines for Health Care Providers (Clinical Practice Guideline), 8/05

National Hospice and Palliative Care Organization

Standards of Practice for Pediatric Palliative Care and Hospice (Clinical Practice Guideline), 2/09

Turner Syndrome Consensus Study Group

Care of Girls and Women With Turner Syndrome: A Guideline of the Turner Syndrome Study Group (Clinical Practice Guideline), 1/07

APPENDIX 2

PPI: AAP Partnership for Policy Implementation
· ·

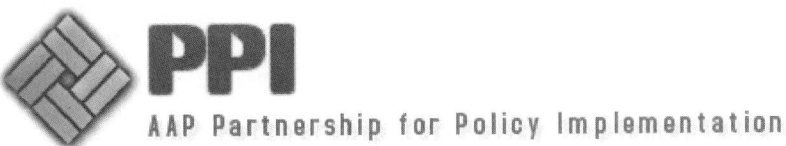

AAP Partnership for Policy Implementation

BACKGROUND

The American Academy of Pediatrics (AAP) develops policies that promote attainment of optimal physical, mental, and social health and well-being for all infants, children, adolescents, and young adults. These documents are valued highly not only by clinicians who provide direct health care to children but by members of other organizations who share similar goals and by parents, payers, and legislators. To increase clarity and action of AAP clinical guidance and recommendations for physicians at the point of care, the AAP formed the Partnership for Policy Implementation (PPI). The PPI is a group of pediatric medical informaticians who partner with authors of AAP clinical practice guidelines and clinical reports to help assure that clinical recommendations are stated with the precision needed to implement them in an electronic health record (EHR) system. Partnership for Policy Implementation volunteers focus on helping content experts develop clinical guidance that specifies exactly who is to do what, for whom, and under what circumstances.

VISION

The vision of the PPI is that all AAP clinical recommendations include clear guidance on how pediatricians can implement those recommendations into their patient care and that AAP clinical guidance can be easily incorporated within electronic health record decision-support systems.

MISSION

The mission of the PPI is to facilitate implementation of AAP recommendations at the point of care by ensuring that AAP documents are written in a practical, action-oriented fashion with unambiguous recommendations.

WHAT IS THE PPI?

The PPI is a network of pediatric informaticians who work with AAP authors and clinical practice guideline sub-committees throughout the writing process.

Contributions of the PPI to the AAP writing process include disambiguation and specification; development of clear definitions; clearly defined logic; implementation techniques; action-oriented recommendations, including clinical algorithms; transparency of evidence basis for recommendations; and health information technology (HIT) standard development.

WHAT HAS THE PPI ACCOMPLISHED?

Since inception of the PPI, more than 20 statements have been published using the PPI process, covering a wide variety of child health topics, including influenza prevention and control (*Pediatrics.* 2016;138[4]:e20162527), brief resolved unexplained events (commonly known as BRUE) (*Pediatrics.* 2016;137[5]:e20160590), respiratory syncytial virus (*Pediatrics.* 2014;134[2]:415–420), type 2 diabetes (*Pediatrics.* 2013;131[2]:364–382), and bronchiolitis (*Pediatrics.* 2014;134[5]:e1474–e1502).

One example of how a statement developed using PPI process has gained broader acceptance is the AAP annual influenza statement. Since 2007, the Centers for Disease Control and Prevention has adopted components of the PPI statement (specifically, the clinical algorithm) within its own statement on the same topic.

WHAT IS THE PPI DOING NOW?

In addition to creating practical, action-oriented guidance that pediatricians can use at the point of care, the PPI works to make it easier for these recommendations to be incorporated into electronic systems. To date, the PPI has focused its involvement on the statement development process. Involvement of the PPI during the writing process helps to produce a clear, more concise document. As these standards of care become well documented, the PPI can begin to focus on building or mapping pediatric vocabulary; once solidified, this vocabulary can be built into EHR systems. The standards of care can also be matched to various logical and functional HIT standards that already exist today. Through this work, the PPI improves AAP policy documents by providing specific guidance to pediatricians at the point of care, helping ensure that EHRs are designed to assist pediatricians in providing optimal care for children. The PPI recently developed a short video that provides an overview of its mission and process. The video is available on the PPI Web site (link below) as well as AAP YouTube channel at www.youtube.com/watch?v=woTfeoNcxn4.

For more information about the PPI, please visit its Web site (http://www2.aap.org/informatics/PPI.html) or contact Lisa Krams (lkrams@aap.org or 847/434-7663).

APPENDIX 3

American Academy
of Pediatrics Acronyms
· ·

AMERICAN ACADEMY OF PEDIATRICS

Acronyms

AACAP	American Academy of Child and Adolescent Psychiatry
AAFP	American Academy of Family Physicians
AAMC	Association of American Medical Colleges
AAOS	American Academy of Orthopaedic Surgeons
AAP	American Academy of Pediatrics
AAPD	American Academy of Pediatric Dentistry
ABM	Academy of Breastfeeding Medicine
ABMS	American Board of Medical Specialties
ABP	American Board of Pediatrics
ACBOCCSA	Advisory Committee to the Board on Community, Chapter, and State Affairs
ACBOCHW	Advisory Committee to the Board on Child Health and Wellness
ACBODIT	Advisory Committee to the Board on Development and Information Technology
ACBOE	Advisory Committee to the Board on Education
ACBOF	Advisory Committee to the Board on Finance
ACBOFA	Advisory Committee to the Board on Federal Affairs
ACBOGCH	Advisory Committee to the Board on Global Child Health
ACBOM	Advisory Committee to the Board on Membership
ACBOMS	Advisory Committee to the Board on Marketing and Sales
ACBOP	Advisory Committee to the Board on Practice
ACBOPub	Advisory Committee to the Board on Publishing
ACBOQ	Advisory Committee to the Board on Quality
ACBOR	Advisory Committee to the Board on Research
ACBOSP	Advisory Committee to the Board on Strategic Planning
ACBOSPe	Advisory Committee to the Board on Specialty Pediatrics
ACCME	Accreditation Council for Continuing Medical Education
ACEP	American College of Emergency Physicians
ACGME	Accreditation Council for Graduate Medical Education
ACIP	Advisory Committee on Immunization Practices
ACMG	American College of Medical Genetics
ACO	Accountable Care Organization
ACOG	American Congress of Obstetricians and Gynecologists
ACOP	American College of Osteopathic Pediatricians
ACP	American College of Physicians
ADAMHA	Alcohol, Drug Abuse, and Mental Health Administration
AG-M	Action Group—Multidisciplinary (Section Forum)
AG-M1	Action Group—Medical 1 (Section Forum)
AG-M2	Action Group—Medical 2 (Section Forum)
AG-S	Action Group—Surgical (Section Forum)
AHA	American Heart Association
AHA	American Hospital Association
AHRQ	Agency for Healthcare Research and Quality
ALF	Annual Leadership Forum
AMA	American Medical Association
AMCHP	Association of Maternal and Child Health Programs
AMSA	American Medical Student Association
AMSPDC	Association of Medical School Pediatric Department Chairs
AMWA	American Medical Women's Association
APA	Academic Pediatric Association
APHA	American Public Health Association
APLS	Advanced Pediatric Life Support
APPD	Association of Pediatric Program Directors
APQ	Alliance for Pediatric Quality
APS	American Pediatric Society
AQA	Ambulatory Care Quality Alliance
ASHG	American Society of Human Genetics
ASTM	American Society of Testing and Materials
BHP	Bureau of Health Professions
BIA	Bureau of Indian Affairs
BLAST	Babysitter Lessons and Safety Training
BOD	Board of Directors
BPC	Breastfeeding Promotion Consortium
CAG	Corporate Advisory Group
CAMLWG	Children, Adolescents, and Media Leadership Workgroup
CAP	College of American Pathologists
CAQI	Chapter Alliance for Quality Improvement
CATCH	Community Access to Child Health
CDC	Centers for Disease Control and Prevention

CESP	Confederation of European Specialty Pediatrics
CFMC	Chapter Forum Management Committee
CFT	Cross Functional Team
CHA	Children's Hospital Association
CHIC	Child Health Informatics Center
CHIP	Children Health Insurance Program
CMC	Council Management Committee
CME	Continuing Medical Education
CMS	Centers for Medicare & Medicaid Services
CMSS	Council of Medical Specialty Societies
CnF	Council Forum
COA	Committee on Adolescence
COB	Committee on Bioethics
COCAN	Committee on Child Abuse and Neglect
COCHF	Committee on Child Health Financing
COCIT	Council on Clinical Information Technology
COCM	Council on Communications and Media
COCME	Committee on Continuing Medical Education
COCN	Committee on Coding and Nomenclature
COCP	Council on Community Pediatrics
COCWD	Council on Children With Disabilities
COD	Committee on Drugs
CODe	Committee on Development
COEC	Council on Early Childhood
COEH	Council on Environmental Health
CoF	Committee Forum
COFCAKC	Council on Foster Care, Adoption, and Kinship Care
COFGA	Committee on Federal Government Affairs
CoFMC	Committee Forum Management Committee
COFN	Committee on Fetus and Newborn
COG	Committee on Genetics
COGME	Council on Graduate Medical Education (DHHS/HRSA)
COHC	Committee on Hospital Care
COID	Committee on Infectious Diseases
COIVPP	Committee on Injury, Violence, and Poison Prevention
COM	Committee on Membership
COMLRM	Committee on Medical Liability and Risk Management
COMSEP	Council on Medical Student Education in Pediatrics (AMSPDC)
CON	Committee on Nutrition
CONACH	Committee on Native American Child Health
COPA	Committee on Pediatric AIDS
COPACFH	Committee on Psychosocial Aspects of Child and Family Health
COPAM	Committee on Practice and Ambulatory Medicine
COPE	Committee on Pediatric Education
COPEM	Committee on Pediatric Emergency Medicine
COPR	Committee on Pediatric Research
COPW	Committee on Pediatric Workforce

COQIPS	Council on Quality Improvement and Patient Safety
CORS	Committee on Residency Scholarships
COSGA	Committee on State Government Affairs
COSH	Council on School Health
COSMF	Council on Sports Medicine and Fitness
COSUP	Committee on Substance Use and Prevention
CPS	Canadian Paediatric Society
CPTI	Community Pediatrics Training Initiative
CQN	Chapter Quality Network
CSHCN	Children With Special Health Care Needs
DHHS	Department of Health and Human Services
DOD	Department of Defense
DVC	District Vice Chairperson
EBCDLWG	Early Brain and Child Development Leadership Workgroup
EC	Executive Committee
ELWG	Epigenetics Leadership Workgroup
EMSC	Emergency Medical Services for Children
EPA	Environmental Protection Agency
EQIPP	Education in Quality Improvement for Pediatric Practice
eTACC	Electronic Translation of Academy Clinical Content
FCF	Friends of Children Fund
FDA	Food and Drug Administration
FERPA	Family Educational Rights and Privacy Act
FOPE II	Future of Pediatric Education II Project
FOPO	Federation of Pediatric Organizations
FTC	Federal Trade Commission
GME	Graduate Medical Education
HAAC	Historical Archives Advisory Committee
HBB	Helping Babies Breathe
HCCA	Healthy Child Care America
HEDIS	Health Plan Employer Data and Information Set
HHS	Health and Human Services
HIPAA	Health Insurance Portability and Accountability Act of 1996
HMO	Health Maintenance Organization
HOF	Headquarters of the Future
HQA	Hospital Quality Alliance
HRSA	Health Resources and Services Administration
HTC	Help the Children
HTPCP	Healthy Tomorrows Partnership for Children Program
IHS	Indian Health Service
IMG	International Medical Graduate
IPA	International Pediatric Association
IPC	International Pediatric Congress
IRB	Institutional Review Board
LLLI	La Leche League International
LWG	Leadership Workgroup
MCAN	Merck Childhood Asthma Network
MCH	Maternal and Child Health
MCHB	Maternal and Child Health Bureau
MCN	Migrant Clinicians Network

MHICSN-PAC	Medical Home Initiatives for Children With Special Needs Project Advisory Committee
MHLWG	Mental Health Leadership Work Group
MRT	Media Resource Team
NACHC	National Association of Community Health Centers
NAEMSP	National Association of Emergency Medical Physicians
NAEPP	National Asthma Education and Prevention Program
NAM	National Academy of Medicine
NAPNAP	National Association of Pediatric Nurse Practitioners
NASPGHAN	North American Society for Pediatric Gastroenterology, Hepatology, and Nutrition
NAWD	National Association of WIC Directors
NBME	National Board of Medical Examiners
NcBDDD	National Center on Birth Defects and Developmental Disabilities
NCE	National Conference & Exhibition
NCEPG	National Conference & Exhibition Planning Group
NCQA	National Committee for Quality Assurance
NHLBI	National Heart, Lung, and Blood Institute
NHMA	National Hispanic Medical Association
NHTSA	National Highway Traffic Safety Administration
NIAAA	National Institute on Alcohol Abuse and Alcoholism
NICHD	National Institute of Child Health and Human Development
NICHQ	National Initiative for Children's Health Quality
NIDA	National Institute on Drug Abuse
NIH	National Institutes of Health
NIMH	National Institute of Mental Health
NMA	National Medical Association
NNC	National Nominating Committee
NQF	National Quality Forum
NRHA	National Rural Health Association
NRMP	National Resident Matching Program
NRP	Neonatal Resuscitation Program
NSC	National Safety Council
NVAC	National Vaccine Advisory Committee
ODPHP	Office of Disease Prevention and Health Promotion
OED	Office of the Executive Director
OHISC	Oral Health Initiative Steering Committee
OLWG	Obesity Leadership Workgroup
P4P	Pay for Performance
PAC	Project Advisory Committee
PAHO	Pan American Health Organization
PALS	Pediatric Advanced Life Support
PAS	Pediatric Academic Societies
PCO	*Pediatric Care Online*™
PCOC	Primary Care Organizations Consortium
PCPCC	Patient-Centered Primary Care Collaborative
PCPI	Physician Consortium on Performance Improvement
PEAC	Practice Expense Advisory Committee
PECOS	Pediatric Education in Community and Office Settings
PECS	Pediatric Education in Community Settings
PEPP	Pediatric Education for Prehospital Professionals
PIR	*Pediatrics in Review*
PLA	Pediatric Leadership Alliance
PPAAC	Private Payer Advocacy Advisory Committee (COCHF Subcommittee)
PPAC	Past President's Advisory Committee
PPC-PCMH	Physician Practice Connections—Patient-Centered Medical Home (NCQA)
PPI	Partnership for Policy Implementation
PREP	Pediatric Review and Education Program
PROS	Pediatric Research in Office Settings
PSOIMG	Provisional Section on International Medical Graduates
PSOLGBTHW	Provisional Section on Lesbian, Gay, Bisexual, and Transgender Health and Wellness
PSOSILM	Provisional Section on Simulation and Innovative Learning Methods
PUPVS	Project Universal Preschool Vision Screening
QA	Quality Assurance
QI	Quality Improvement
QuIIN	Quality Improvement Innovation Network
RBPE	Resource-Based Practice Expense
RBRVS	Resource-Based Relative Value Scale
RCE	Richmond Center of Excellence
RRC	Residency Review Committee (ACGME)
RUC	AMA/Specialty Society Relative Value Scale Update Committee
RVU	Relative Value Unit
SAM	Society for Adolescent Medicine
SAMHSA	Substance Abuse and Mental Health Services Administration
SCHIP	State Children's Health Insurance Program
SDBP	Society for Developmental and Behavioral Pediatrics
SF	Section Forum
SFMC	Section Forum Management Committee
SOA	Section on Anesthesiology and Pain Medicine
SOAC	Subcommittee on Access to Care
SOAH	Section on Adolescent Health
SOAI	Section on Allergy and Immunology
SOAPM	Section on Administration and Practice Management
SOATT	Section on Advances in Therapeutics and Technology
SOB	Section on Bioethics
SOBr	Section on Breastfeeding
SOCAN	Section on Child Abuse and Neglect

SOCC	Section on Critical Care
SOCCS	Section on Cardiology and Cardiac Surgery
SOCPT	Section on Clinical Pharmacology and Therapeutics
SOD	Section on Dermatology
SODBP	Section on Developmental and Behavioral Pediatrics
SOECP	Section on Early Career Physicians
SOEM	Section on Emergency Medicine
SOEn	Section on Endocrinology
SOEp	Section on Epidemiology
SOGBD	Section on Genetics and Birth Defects
SOGHN	Section on Gastroenterology, Hepatology, and Nutrition
SOHC	Section on Home Care
SOHM	Section on Hospital Medicine
SOHO	Section on Hematology/Oncology
SOHPM	Section on Hospice and Palliative Medicine
SOICH	Section on International Child Health
SOID	Section on Infectious Diseases
SOIM	Section on Integrative Medicine
SOIMP	Section on Internal Medicine/Pediatrics
SOMP	Section on Medicine-Pediatrics
SONp	Section on Nephrology
SONPM	Section on Neonatal-Perinatal Medicine
SONS	Section on Neurological Surgery
SONu	Section on Neurology
SOOb	Section on Obesity
SOOH	Section on Oral Health
SOOHNS	Section on Otolaryngology—Head and Neck Surgery
SOOp	Section on Ophthalmology
SOOPe	Section on Osteopathic Pediatricians
SOOr	Section on Orthopaedics
SOPPSM	Section on Pediatric Pulmonology and Sleep Medicine
SOPS	Section on Plastic Surgery
SOPT	Section on Pediatric Trainees
SORa	Section on Radiology
SORh	Section on Rheumatology
SOSM	Section on Senior Members
SOSu	Section on Surgery
SOTC	Section on Telehealth Care
SOTCo	Section on Tobacco Control
SOTM	Section on Transport Medicine
SOU	Section on Urology
SOUS	Section on Uniformed Services
SPR	Society for Pediatric Research
SPWG	Strategic Planning Work Group
TA	Technical Assistance
TA	Technology Assessment
TFOA	Task Force on Access (also known as Task Force on Health Insurance Coverage and Access to Care)
TFOC	Task Force on Circumcision
TIPP	The Injury Prevention Program
TJC	The Joint Commission
UNICEF	United Nations Children's Fund
UNOS	United Network for Organ Sharing
USDA	US Department of Agriculture
WHO	World Health Organization
WIC	Special Supplemental Nutrition Program for Women, Infants, and Children

Subject Index

A

Trauma
    centers, 913–914
    dental trauma, management of, 1447
    disasters preparedness and surge, 915
    injury prevention, 914
    management of, 909–919
    medical home, rehabilitation and the, 914
    performance improvement in managing, 914
    prehospital care, 912–913
    recommendations, 915–916
    systems, 911–912
Trauma centers, 913–914
Trauma systems, 911–912
Tuberculin testing, treatment of latent tuberculosis infection and, 1522
Tuberculosis and the use of BRMs, 864–865, 869–870
Turner syndrome, 511
Tympanic membrane (TM), examination of, 285–286
Tympanometry, 280, 341
    in confirming diagnosis of otitis media with effusion, 317–318, 334
    for testing middle ear fluid, 341
Tympanostomy tubes, 325
    follow-up management of children with, 1423
    otorrhea associated with, fluoroquinolones for, 1354–1355
Type 1 diabetes mellitus (T1DM), 151
    defined, 129
Type 2 diabetes mellitus (T2DM), 125–168. *See also* Diabetes mellitus
    areas for future research, 141–142
    coding quick reference for, 165
    comorbidities of, 152, 155–160
    complementary and alternative medicine for, 160–161
    defined, 129
    depression and, 159–160
    dyslipidemia of, 157
    finger-stick BG concentrations, 137–138
    HbA1c concentrations in, 136–137
    importance of family-centered diabetes care for, 130
    insulin therapy for, 133
    key action statements on, 128, 133–141, 165
    lifestyle modification program for, 133–136
        metformin as first-line therapy, 134–136
        nutrition and physical activity, 136, 139–141
    management of, in children and adolescents, 147–163, 1448–1449
    management of newly diagnosed, 127–143
    microalbuminuria and, 158–159
    moderate-to-vigorous exercise for, 140–141
    nonalcoholic fatty liver disease and, 160
    obstructive sleep apnea and, 160
    orthopedic problems and, 160
    prevention and treatment of, 1473
    reducing screen time, 141
    retinopathy and, 157–158
    tips for healthy living, 167–168

U

UA. *See* Urinalysis (UA)
Ultrasonography, 474
    for developmental dysplasia of the hip in infants, 719
    point-of-care ultrasonography, by pediatric emergency medicine physicians, 1469
    prenatal, 475
Ultraviolet radiation, hazard to children from, 1502–1503
Umbilical cord
    care, 1325–1331, 1503
    clamping after birth, 1522
Uncomplicated acute otitis media (AOM), 279
Underinsurance of adolescents, 1503
Unintentional injury, prevention of, among American Indian and Alaska Native children, 1474–1475

United States
    childhood and adolescent immunization schedules, 1157–1161
    evaluation and management of infant exposed to HIV-1 in, 1416–1417
    health and mental health needs of children in military families, 1428
    HIV-infected adolescents in, 598
    human milk, breastfeeding, and transmission of human immunodeficiency virus in, 1433–1434
    postneonatal mortality trends in, 1214–1216
    poverty and child health in, 1049–1064, 1470
    recommended childhood and adolescent immunization schedules in, 1484
    sleep-related infant deaths in, 1214–1216
    substance use disorder/use in, 730–731
Upper respiratory tract infections, judicious antibiotic prescribing for, 1475
Urgent care facilities. *See* Freestanding urgent care facilities, pediatric care recommendations for
Urinalysis (UA)
    automated, 454
    in diagnosing urinary tract infection, 453–454
Urinary tract infections (UTIs), 441–494
    action statements on, 443–446, 451–460, 491
    algorithm for, 464
    areas for research, 460–461
    clinical practice guideline algorithm, 464
    coding quick reference for, 492
    culture in, 454–455
    diagnosis of, 443–445, 449, 451–455, 493
        automatic urinalysis, 454
        in febrile infants and young children, 443–464, 1404
        following of children after, 489
        nitrite test in, 454
        tests for, 471
        urinalysis in, 453–454
        urine testing in, 487–488
    evaluation and management of abnormalities, 472–475
    in febrile infants and young children, diagnosis and management of, 443–464, 1404
    fluoroquinolones for, 1356–1357
    follow-up, 494
    imaging after, 488–489
    literature search and, 467–482
    management of, 449–450, 455–460
        in febrile infants and young children, 443–464, 1404
    prevalence and risk factors for, 469–470
    short-term treatment of, 471–472
    symptoms of, 493
    treating, 488, 493
    ultrasonography and, 474
Urine
    collection of, 493
    obtaining samples, 471, 488
    urinary tract infections and testing, 487–488
UTIs. *See* Urinary tract infections (UTIs)

V

Vaccine(s). *See also specific vaccine*
    acceptance of, 616–617
    Advisory Committee on Immunization Practices (ACIP) recommendations, 1516
    BRMs, before, during, and after the administration of, 868–869
    to eliminate transmission of hepatitis B virus infection, 1512–1513
    exemptions, 615–616
        for child care, 969–975, 1452
        for school attendance, 969–975, 1452
    global, HHS program, 1514
    hesitancy, 614
        countering, 611–626, 1402
    historical opposition to, 615